MW01148675

# Atlas of Pelvic Anatomy and Gynecologic Surgery

## THIRD EDITION

## Michael S. Baggish, MD

Department of Obstetrics and Gynecology
St. Helena Hospital
St. Helena, California

Formerly: Chairman, Department of Obstetrics and Gynecology
Good Samaritan Hospital
Cincinnati, Ohio
Clinical Professor of Obstetrics and Gynecology
University of Cincinnati School of Medicine
Cincinnati, Ohio
Clinical Professor of Obstetrics and Gynecology
Wright State University Boonshoft School of Medicine
Dayton, Ohio

## Mickey M. Karram, MD

Director of Urogynecology
The Christ Hospital
Clinical Professor of Obstetrics and Gynecology and Urology
University of Cincinnati
Cincinnati, Ohio

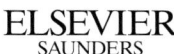

ELSEVIER
SAUNDERS

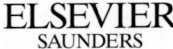

3251 Riverport Lane
St. Louis, Missouri 63043

ATLAS OF PELVIC ANATOMY AND GYNECOLOGIC SURGERY,      ISBN: 978-1-4160-5909-7
THIRD EDITION

---

### Notices

Knowledge and best practice in this field are constantly changing. As new research and experience broaden our understanding, changes in research methods, professional practices, or medical treatment may become necessary.

Practitioners and researchers must always rely on their own experience and knowledge in evaluating and using any information, methods, compounds, or experiments described herein. In using such information or methods they should be mindful of their own safety and the safety of others, including parties for whom they have a professional responsibility.

With respect to any drug or pharmaceutical products identified, readers are advised to check the most current information provided (i) on procedures featured or (ii) by the manufacturer of each product to be administered, to verify the recommended dose or formula, the method and duration of administration, and contraindications. It is the responsibility of practitioners, relying on their own experience and knowledge of their patients, to make diagnoses, to determine dosages and the best treatment for each individual patient, and to take all appropriate safety precautions.

To the fullest extent of the law, neither the Publisher nor the authors, contributors, or editors, assume any liability for any injury and/or damage to persons or property as a matter of products liability, negligence or otherwise, or from any use or operation of any methods, products, instructions, or ideas contained in the material herein.

---

**Library of Congress Cataloging-in-Publication Data**
Baggish, Michael S.
  Atlas of pelvic anatomy and gynecologic surgery / Michael S. Baggish, Mickey M. Karram.—
3rd ed.
    p. ; cm.
  Includes index.
  ISBN 978-1-4160-5909-7 (hardcover : alk. paper)  1. Pelvis—Surgery—Atlases.  2.
Generative organs, Female—Surgery—Atlases.  I. Karram, Mickey M.  II. Title.
  [DNLM:  1. Pelvis—surgery—Atlases.  2. Gynecologic Surgical Procedures—methods—Atlases.
3. Pelvis—anatomy & histology—Atlases.  WP 17 B144a 2011]
  RG104.B155 2011
  618.1'059—dc22

                                                          2010024802

*Acquisitions Editor:* Stefanie Jewell-Thomas
*Developmental Editor:* Stacey Fisher
*Publishing Services Manager:* Patricia Tannian
*Project Manager:* Claire Kramer
*Designer:* Louis Forgione

Printed in China

Last digit is the print number:  9  8  7  6  5  4  3  2  1

This book is dedicated to my wife, Leslie Ann Baggish; to my children, Jeffrey Steven Baggish, Mindy Ann Baggish, Cindy Beth Baggish, Stuart Harrison Baggish, Julia Susan Baggish; to my daughters-in-law, Doneene and Pamela Baggish; and to my grandchildren, Owen Baggish and Reagan Baggish.

*Michael S. Baggish, MD*

This Atlas is dedicated to my patients. It has been my privilege to care for each and every one of you.

*Mickey M. Karram, MD*

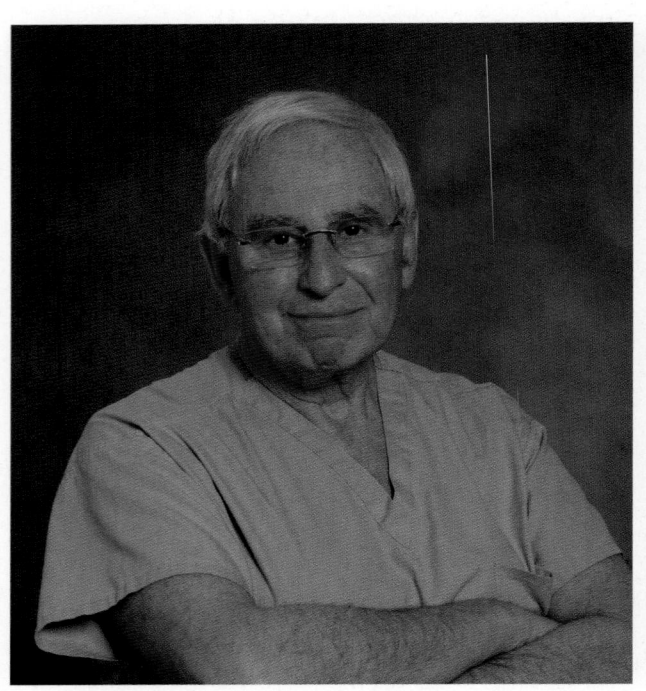

Michael S. Baggish, MD

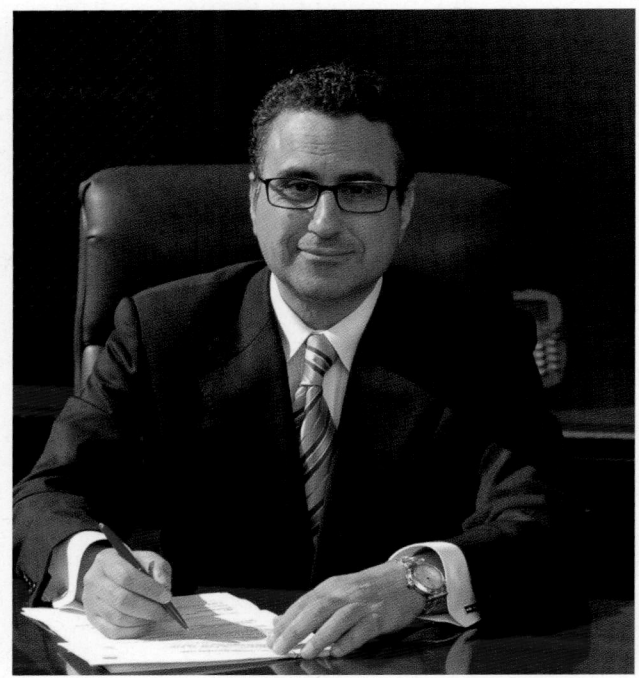

Mickey M. Karram, MD

# CONTRIBUTORS

**Brian J. Albers, MD, FACS**
Margaret Mary Community Hospital
Batesville, Indiana

**Michael S. Baggish, MD**
Department of Obstetrics and Gynecology
St. Helena Hospital
St. Helena, California

Formerly: Chairman, Department of Obstetrics and
  Gynecology
Good Samaritan Hospital
Cincinnati, Ohio
Clinical Professor of Obstetrics and Gynecology
University of Cincinnati School of Medicine
Cincinnati, Ohio
Clinical Professor of Obstetrics and Gynecology
Wright State University Boonshoft School of Medicine
Dayton, Ohio

**Jack Basil, MD, FACOG, FACS**
Tristate Gynecologic Oncology
Director, Gynecologic Oncology
Good Samaritan Hospital
Cincinnati, Ohio

**Alfred E. Bent, MD**
Professor and Head, Division of Gynecology
IWK Health Center, Dalhousie University
Halifax, Nova Scotia, Canada

**Lesley L. Breech, MD**
Associate Professor, Department of Pediatrics
Division of Adolescent Medicine
Associate Professor, Department of Obstetrics
  and Gynecology
University of Cincinnati College of Medicine
Cincinnati Children's Hospital Medical Center
Cincinnati, Ohio

**Karen S. Columbus, MD**
Cincinnati Breast Surgeons, Inc.
Cincinnati, Ohio

**Patrick Culligan, MD**
Director of Urogynecology and Reconstructive Pelvic Surgery
Atlantic Health
Morristown, New Jersey
Professor of Obstetrics, Gynecology and Reproductive Science
Mount Sinai School of Medicine
New York, New York

**Geoffrey W. Cundiff, MD, FACOG, FACS, FRCSC**
Professor of Obstetrics & Gynaecology
University of British Columbia
Vancouver, British Columbia, Canada

**Bradley R. Davis, MD, FACS, FASCRS**
Assistant Professor of Surgery
Division of Colon and Rectal Surgery
University of Cincinnati
Cincinnati, Ohio

**Roger Dmochowski, MD, FACS**
Professor of Urology
Director, Pelvic Medicine and Reconstruction Fellowship
Executive Physician for Safety
Vanderbilt University Medical Center
Nashville, Tennessee

**Tommaso Falcone, MD**
Professor and Chairman
Department of Obstetrics and Gynecology
Cleveland Clinic Foundation
Cleveland, Ohio

**John B. Gebhart, MD, MS**
Associate Professor
Department of Obstetrics and Gynecology
Fellowship Director–Urogynecology/Reconstructive
  Pelvic Surgery
Mayo Clinic
Rochester, Minnesota

**Bradley S. Hurst, MD**
Director of Assisted Reproduction
Carolinas Medical Center
Charlotte, North Carolina

**Mickey M. Karram, MD**
Director of Urogynecology
The Christ Hospital
Clinical Professor of Obstetrics and Gynecology and Urology
University of Cincinnati
Cincinnati, Ohio

**David J. Lamon, MD, FACS**
Naples Surgical Associates
Naples, Florida

**Vincent Lucente, MD, MBA**
Chief of Gynecology, St. Luke's Hospital
Medical Director, The Institute of Female Pelvic Medicine
  and Reconstructive Surgery
Clinical Professor of Obstetrics and Gynecology, Temple
  University College of Medicine
Allentown, Pennsylvania

**Michael Maggio, MD, FACS**
Good Samaritan Hospital
Cincinnati, Ohio
Dearborn County Hospital
Lawrenceburg, Indiana

**Apurva B. Pancholy, MD, FACOG**
Assistant Professor of Obstetrics and Gynecology
Division of Urogynecology
Baylor School of Medicine
Houston, Texas

**James Pavelka, MD**
Tristate Gynecologic Oncology
Director of Minimally Invasive Surgery
Department of Obstetrics and Gynecology
Good Samaritan Hospital
Cincinnati, Ohio

**W. Stuart Reynolds, MD**
Instructor in Urology
Vanderbilt University Medical Center
Nashville, Tennessee

**John A. Rock, MD**
Founding Dean & Senior Vice President for Medical Affairs
Herbert Wertheim College of Medicine
Florida International University
Miami, Florida

**Helmut F. Schellhas, MD**
Senior Gynecologic Oncologist
Good Samaritan Hospital
Cincinnati, Ohio
Adjunct Professor
Department of Obstetrics and Gynecology
University of Cincinnati Medical Center
Cincinnati, Ohio

**Donna L. Stahl, MD**
Breast Surgeon
Private Practice
Cincinnati, Ohio

**Emanuel C. Trabuco, MD, MS**
Assistant Professor of Obstetrics and Gynecology
Department of Obstetrics and Gynecology
Mayo Clinic
Rochester, Minnesota

**Christine Vaccaro, DO, FACOG**
Urogynecology Fellow
Good Samaritan Hospital
Division of Female Pelvic Medicine and Reconstructive
  Surgery
Cincinnati, Ohio

**Mark D. Walters, MD**
Professor and Vice Chair of Gynecology
Center of Urogynecology and Pelvic Floor Disorders
Obstetrics, Gynecology, and Women's Health Institute
Cleveland Clinic
Cleveland, Ohio

# PREFACE

The third edition of this continuously evolving Atlas incorporates areas of significant revision, as well as the addition of several new chapters. The table of contents has been revised to provide a more logical structure. In like fashion to previous editions, this book is logically divided into major units that are in turn subdivided into sections and finally portioned into individual chapters. This edition comprises 5 units and 123 chapters. The third edition follows our original premise, which emphasizes visual communication with photographs and drawings. In fact, we have colorized more pictures for this edition. All fixed cadaver photographs have been electronically colored to facilitate interpretation. Our artist, Joe Chovan, accomplished this work on his Apple computer using the graphics package. In this third edition we have introduced a new illustrative technique that is nicely exemplified in Chapter 31.

The Introduction to Pelvic Anatomy has been subdivided into two chapters. Chapter 2 represents all new data and new color drawings. This new material includes details of the neurological control of the pelvic viscera. Permission was obtained from Elsevier to include four Frank Netter drawings of the autonomic nervous system. Original new drawings of pelvic plexuses, the colon, the bladder, and pelvic supports complete this new chapter. Other new chapters have been added on the topics of energy devices; positioning and nerve injury; sutures, suturing techniques, and knot tying; lymph node sampling for endometrial carcinoma; radical vulvectomy with tunnel groin dissection; surgery for labial hypertrophy; minimally invasive non-hysteroscopic endometrial ablation; complications of laparoscopic surgery; robotic surgery; surgery for Meckel's diverticulum; vaginal repair of vault prolapse; obliterative procedures for prolapse; mesh kits for prolapse correction; simple vestibulectomy; repair of urethral prolapse; surgical treatment of detrusor compliance abnormalities; vulvovaginal cosmetic gynecology; and transperineal repair of rectal prolapse. In all, 20 new chapters have been added to this edition. Revisions were undertaken in many chapters and include major additions to chapters dealing with hysterectomy, vestibulectomy, avoiding ureteral injury, and surgery on the lower urinary tract.

This edition adds more than 200 pages of material to the content of the book. Our goal is to continuously add new material on the basis of surgical procedures and continuing anatomical dissections. Thus we have included new drawings depicting details of recent anatomical cadaver dissections investigating the supporting tissues of the urethra, bladder, and vagina. Interest continues to focus on whether a "perineal body" or "central tendon" actually exists. We have supplemented our drawings and still pictures with approximately 1 hour of color video material, which provides a dynamic aspect to pelvic anatomy.

We are pleased that Spanish, Italian, Polish, and Russian editions of the second edition have been published. We are especially proud that the *Atlas of Pelvic Anatomy and Gynecologic Surgery* has kindled a large degree of interest for resident gynecologists, recent graduate gynecologists, and practicing gynecologists.

Textbooks come and go. We hope this Atlas will endure the test of time. Accurate drawings and photographs are clearly desirable for the necessary sustenance of future editions. We pledge to continuously improve this book by updating material and adding new illustrations.

# ACKNOWLEDGMENTS

We wish to acknowledge Joe Chovan, our artist, who continues to exceed our expectations. The amazing skill and precision of his art work contribute in no small way to the foundations of this Atlas.

We wish to thank Shane Gamble, Jeff Feld, and Steve Potter of the Good Samaritan Hospital Audiovisual Department for their help with still and video photography. Additionally, these men spent many hours editing the authors' videos.

Dr. Baggish wishes to thank his secretaries, Anne Ulmer and Anita Zompero, for typing, editing, and creating digital disks for this book.

Dr. Karram wishes to thank his secretary, Stephanie Ramsey, for her help in preparing manuscripts for this book.

# CONTENTS

CONTENTS

# Video Table of Contents

# Principles of Pelvic Anatomy and Gynecologic Surgery

# SECTION A

## Pelvic Anatomy

UNIT 1 ■ SECTION A

# CHAPTER 1

# Introduction to Pelvic Anatomy 1

## *Michael S. Baggish, MD*

The anatomy taught in this book is based on actual cadaveric dissection. This section consists entirely of color drawings constructed from anatomic models (cadavers). This section was added to help the reader orient the dissection photographs to the overall geography of abdomen, pelvis, breasts, and extremities. In several pictures, our artist has used actual photographs of body parts (pelvic bone) into which muscles and ligaments were sketched via computer.

The following terms are used in this section to provide directive relationships: (1) *cranial* = toward the head; (2) *caudal* = toward the foot; (3) *superior* = above; (4) *inferior* = below; (5) *deep* = to the interior; (6) *superficial* = to the surface; (7) *medial* = toward the midline; (8) *lateral* = toward the side; (9) *beneath* = under; (10) *anterior* = to the belly; and (11) *posterior* = to the back.

The surgeon needs to be familiar with certain bony landmarks. The pelvic bones consist of the sacrum and coccyx, the ilium, the pubic bone, and the ischium (Fig. 1–1). The first anterior projection of the sacral vertebra is the **sacral promontory,** and the exaggerated transverse processes form the **sacral ala** (Fig. 1–2). On both anterior and posterior surfaces are the holes, or **foramina,** from which nerve roots exit. Articulating with the last sacral vertebra is the **coccyx** (Fig. 1–3). When the pelvis is observed from above (see Fig. 1–2), the iliac fossa, iliac crest, and anterior superior iliac spine are prominent. The articulations at the sacroiliac joint and the symphysis pubis mark major posterior and anterior joints, respectively. Between the two are the iliopectineal lines and the linea terminalis. Facing the pelvis, the **anterior superior iliac spine** and the **pubic tubercle** mark the boundaries of the **inguinal ligament.** The two **pubic bones** form an **arch** beneath the symphysis pubis. The rhomboid space between ischial and pubic bones is the **obturator foramen** (see Fig. 1-1). The lowest portion of the ischium forms a broad, rounded accumulation of bone referred to as the **ischial tuberosity.** Above that structure is a hemispherical socket **(acetabulum),** where the head of the femur articulates (see Fig. 1–1).

When one faces the back of the pelvis, the **sacrum** and the **sacral canal** are visible. The **ischial tuberosity, ischial spines,** and **greater** and **lesser sacral sciatic notches** are identified (Fig. 1–4). From the side, the iliac crest, ischial tuberosity, ischial spine, greater sciatic notch, and lesser sciatic notch are seen, as is the obturator foramen (Fig. 1–5).

The following ligamentous structures can be observed: Cooper's ligaments, the sacroiliac ligaments, the symphysis fibrocartilage, the sacrospinous and sacrotuberous ligaments, the inguinal ligament, the lacunar ligament, and the obturator membrane (Figs. 1–6 through 1–8). The sacrospinous and

Cooper's ligaments are utilized in pelvic reconstructive surgery, as are the pubic symphysis and the anterior longitudinal ligament (overlying the anterior sacral surface, not sketched). Large vessels and nerves cross from the abdomen to the thigh beneath the inguinal ligament and through the obturator foramen. The lacunar ligament forms the medial abutment of the femoral canal and sometimes is referred to as the pectineal portion, or extension, of the inguinal ligament.

The muscles of the pelvis that have practical and special importance for our discussion are the **obturator internus muscle,** which constitutes the "pelvic side wall" or "ovarian fossa," the **coccygeus,** the **piriformis,** and the **levator ani muscles** (Fig. 1–9).

The **obturator fascia** is a well-defined, tough structure. A particularly thickened portion of the obturator fascia is named the **arcus tendineus,** or **white line** (Fig. 1–10). The line stretches from the inner aspect of the ischial spine across the belly of the obturator internus muscle and terminates at the lower margin of the posterior pubic bone (Fig. 1–11).

The levator ani muscle takes its origin from the inferior margin of the pubic bone and the entire arcus (obturator fascia). Several anatomy texts have divided the levator into anterior and posterior portions; however, these subdivisions are artificial and have little practical value (Fig. 1–12). Functionally, the gynecologist can feel this muscle contract by performing a rectovaginal examination and requesting the patient to tighten her muscles as if holding in a bowel movement. At a point 2 cm up (cranial) from the vaginal introitus, the U-shaped muscle is felt along the side and posterior vaginal walls. A similar contraction can be felt posterior to the rectum when the anal sphincter is contracted. Insofar as the rectum is concerned, the levator component can be palpated across the posterior rectal wall. The levator ani in concert with the external sphincter ani squeezes the rectum to narrow the bowel lumen while elevating the anorectum.

The muscles and ligaments divide notches into windows (foramina). The coccygeus is overlain (deep) by the sacrospinous ligament. The piriformis muscle exits the pelvis via the **greater sciatic foramen** and is partially overlain (deep) by the sacrotuberous ligament (see Figs. 1–7 through 1–9). Internally, the hollow iliac fossa is covered by the **iliacus muscle.** At the medial margin and slightly superficial to the iliacus muscles are the **psoas major muscles.** Together with the iliacus (**iliopsoas**), the psoas major muscles pass into the thigh beneath the inguinal ligament to insert on the femur (lesser trochanter). Occasionally, the **psoas minor tendon** may be seen on the anterior surface of the psoas major muscle (Fig. 1–13).

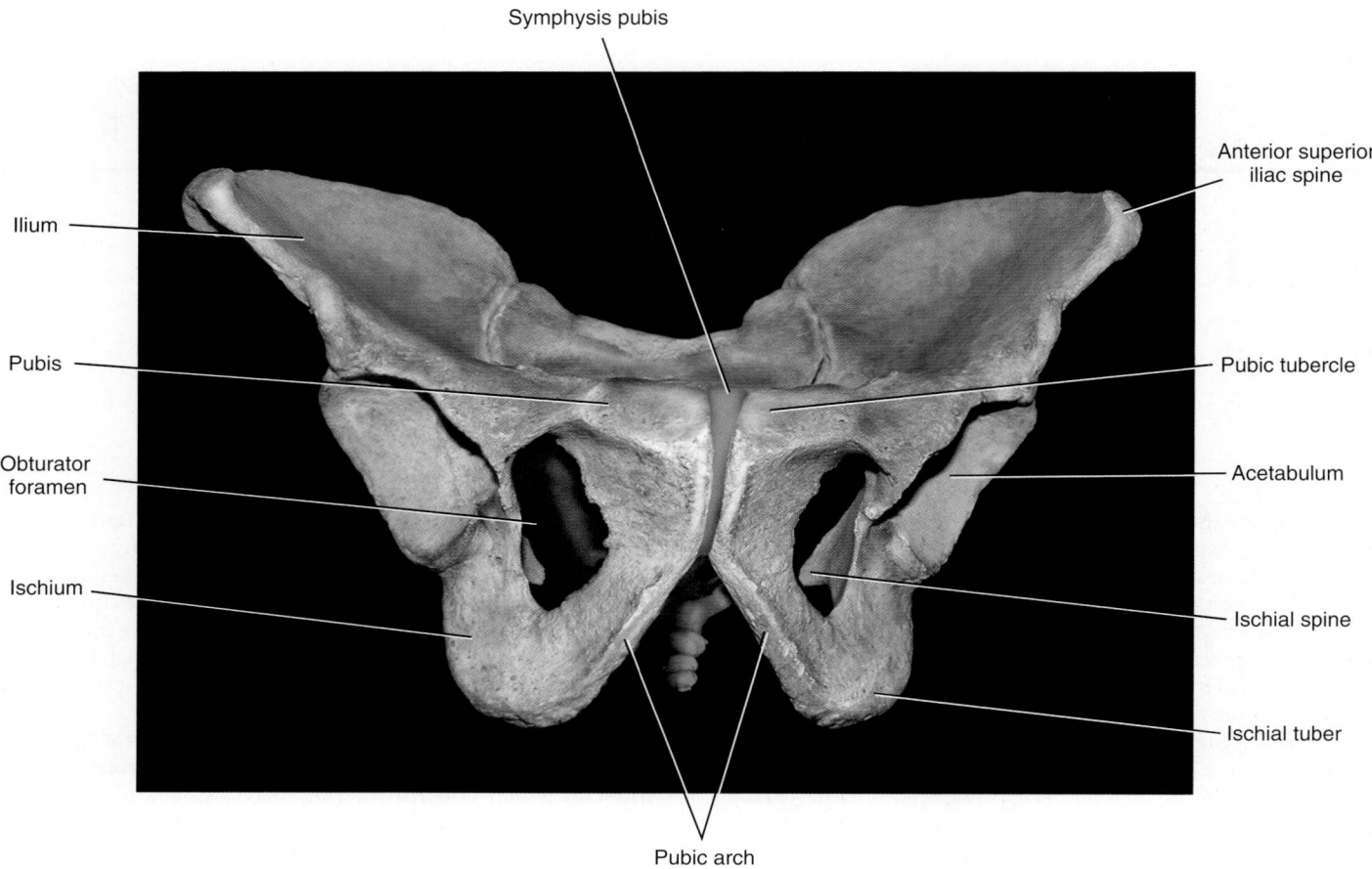

**FIGURE 1–1** The pelvic bone consists of the ilium, ischium, and pubis. The ilium is bound to the sacrum at the sacroiliac joints. This anterior aspect of the pelvis shows the pubic arch, symphysis, and obturator foramen via a head-on view.

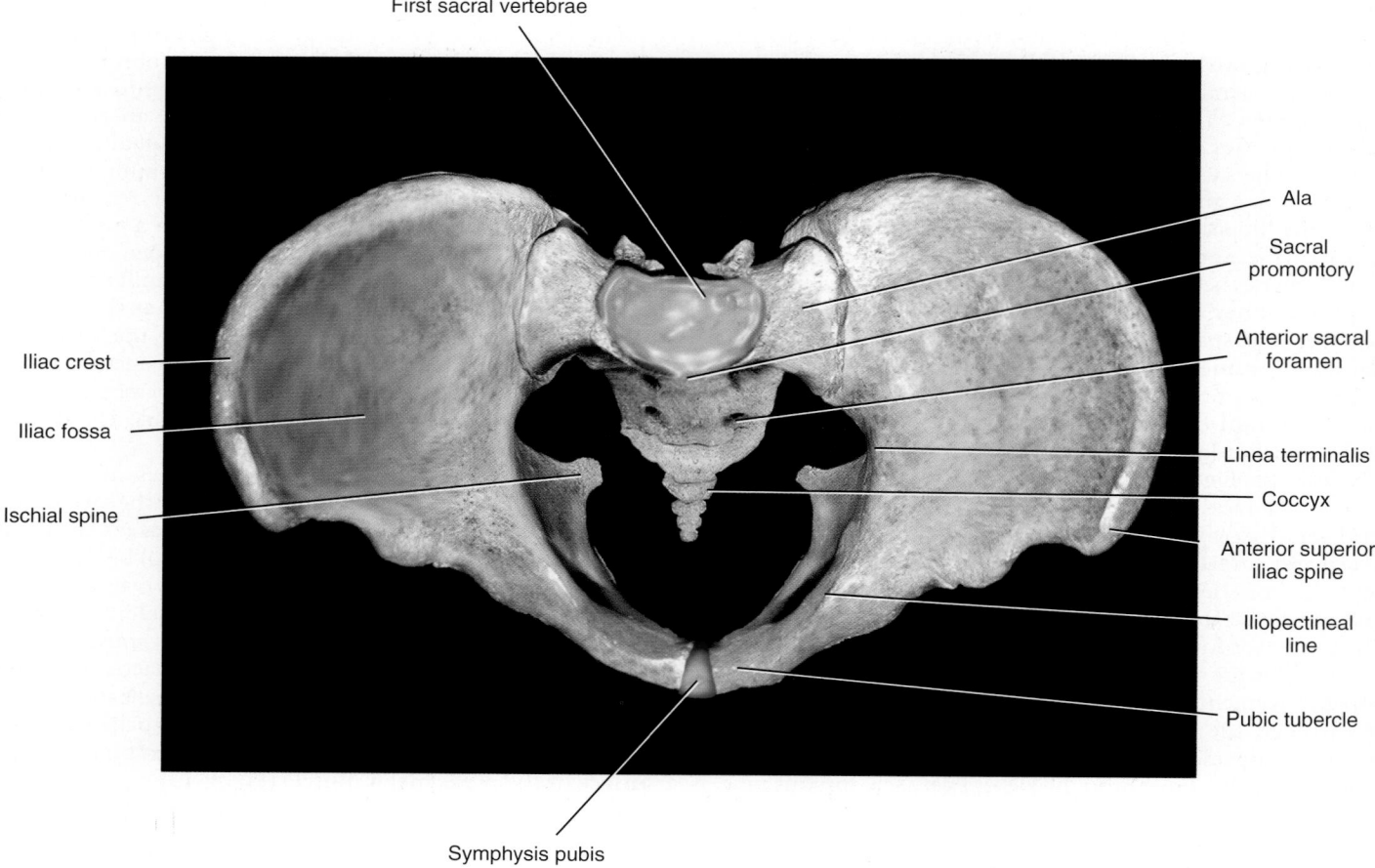

**FIGURE 1–2** This overhead view details the pelvic inlet, which is bounded anteriorly by the pubic symphysis and the pubic tubercle; laterally by the iliopectineal line and the linea terminalis; and posteriorly by the sacral alae and the first sacral vertebra. This view also nicely shows the ischial spines.

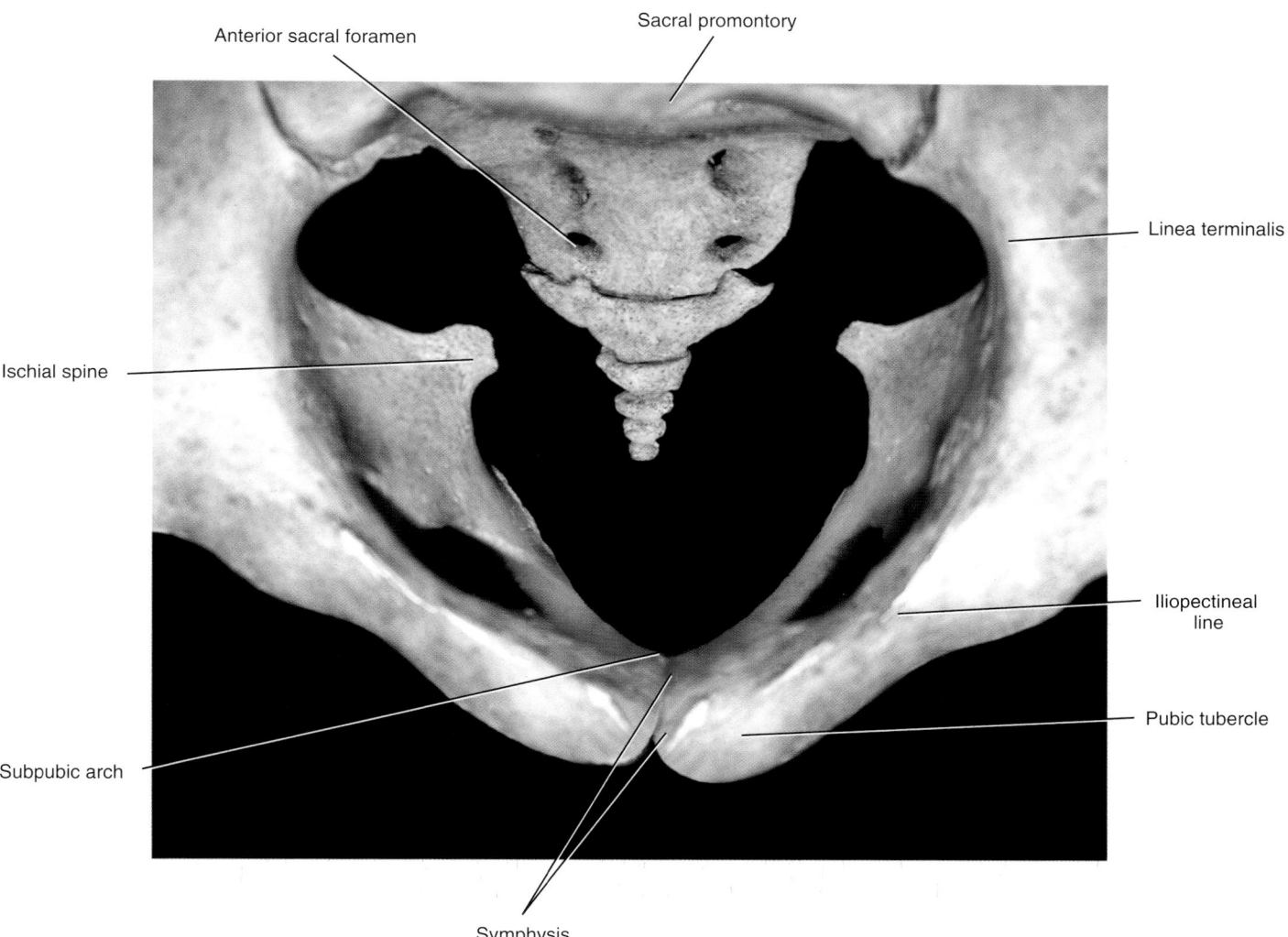

Anterior sacral foramen

Sacral promontory

Linea terminalis

Ischial spine

Iliopectineal line

Pubic tubercle

Subpubic arch

Symphysis

**FIGURE 1–3** High-power detail viewed through the pelvic inlet shows the sacrum and coccyx. The anterior sacral foramina are distinct, as are the ischial spines and the subpubic arch.

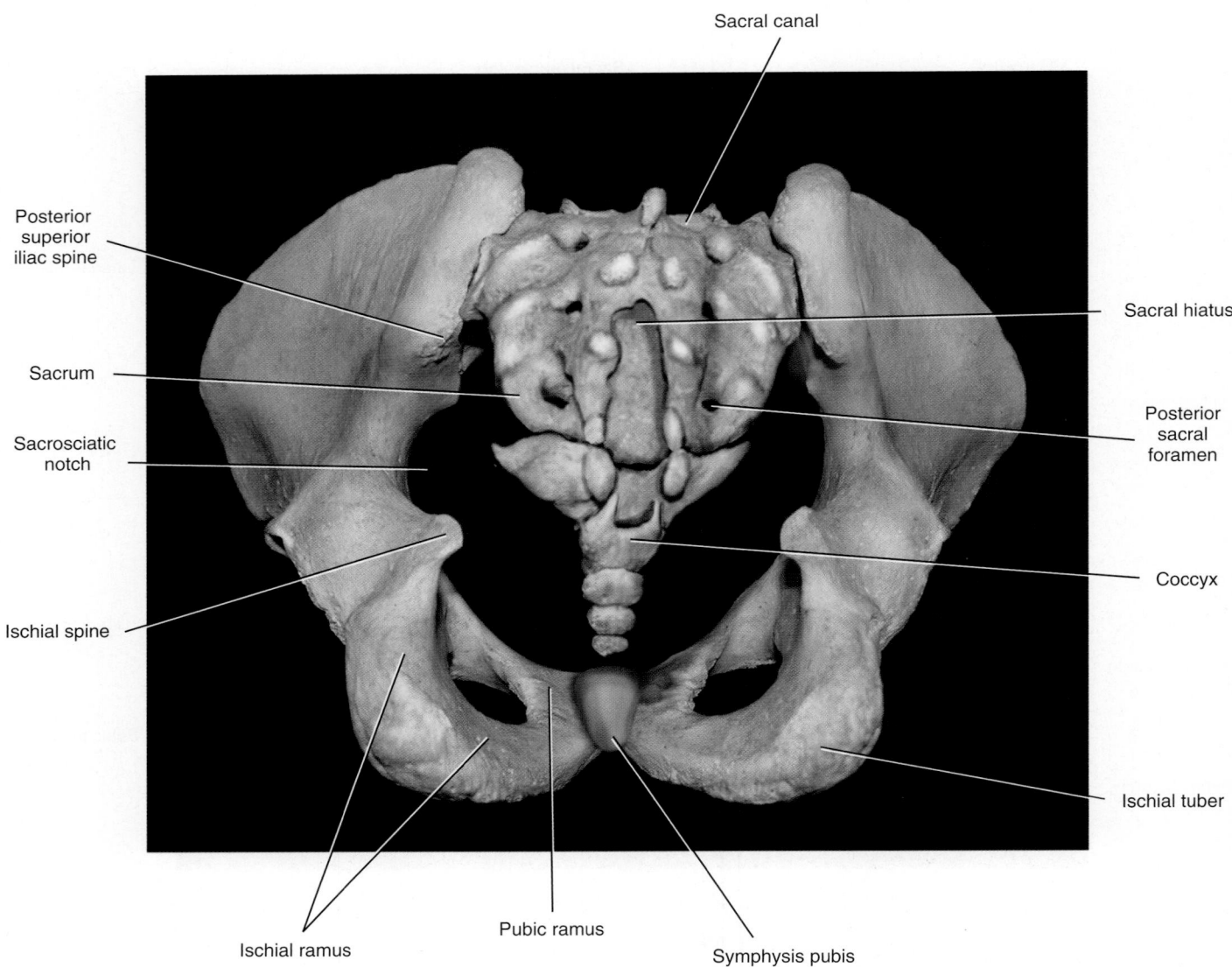

Sacral canal

Posterior
superior
iliac spine

Sacral hiatus

Sacrum

Posterior
sacral
foramen

Sacrosciatic
notch

Coccyx

Ischial spine

Ischial tuber

Ischial ramus

Pubic ramus

Symphysis pubis

**FIGURE 1–4** The posterior view of the pelvis is combined with an outlet "looking-in" perspective. The ischial tuberosity, ischial spine, and greater and lesser sacrosciatic notches are best seen from this vantage point. Posterior sacrum highlights include the sacral hiatus, sacral canal, and posterior sacral foramina.

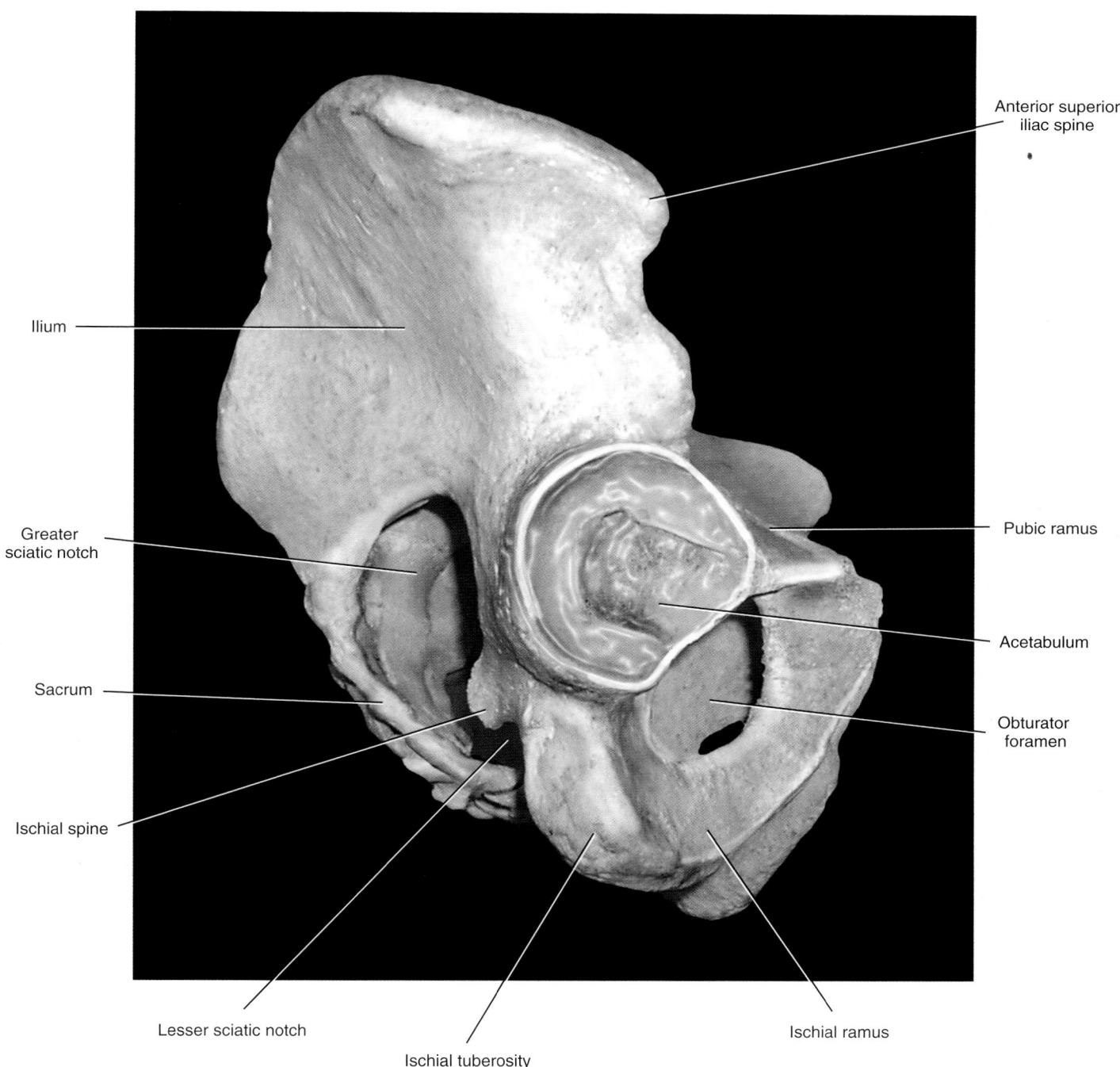

Anterior superior
iliac spine

Ilium

Greater
sciatic notch

Sacrum

Ischial spine

Pubic ramus

Acetabulum

Obturator
foramen

Lesser sciatic notch

Ischial tuberosity

Ischial ramus

**FIGURE 1–5** This right lateral view depicts the acetabulum, sacrosciatic notches, anterior superior iliac spine, and ischium.

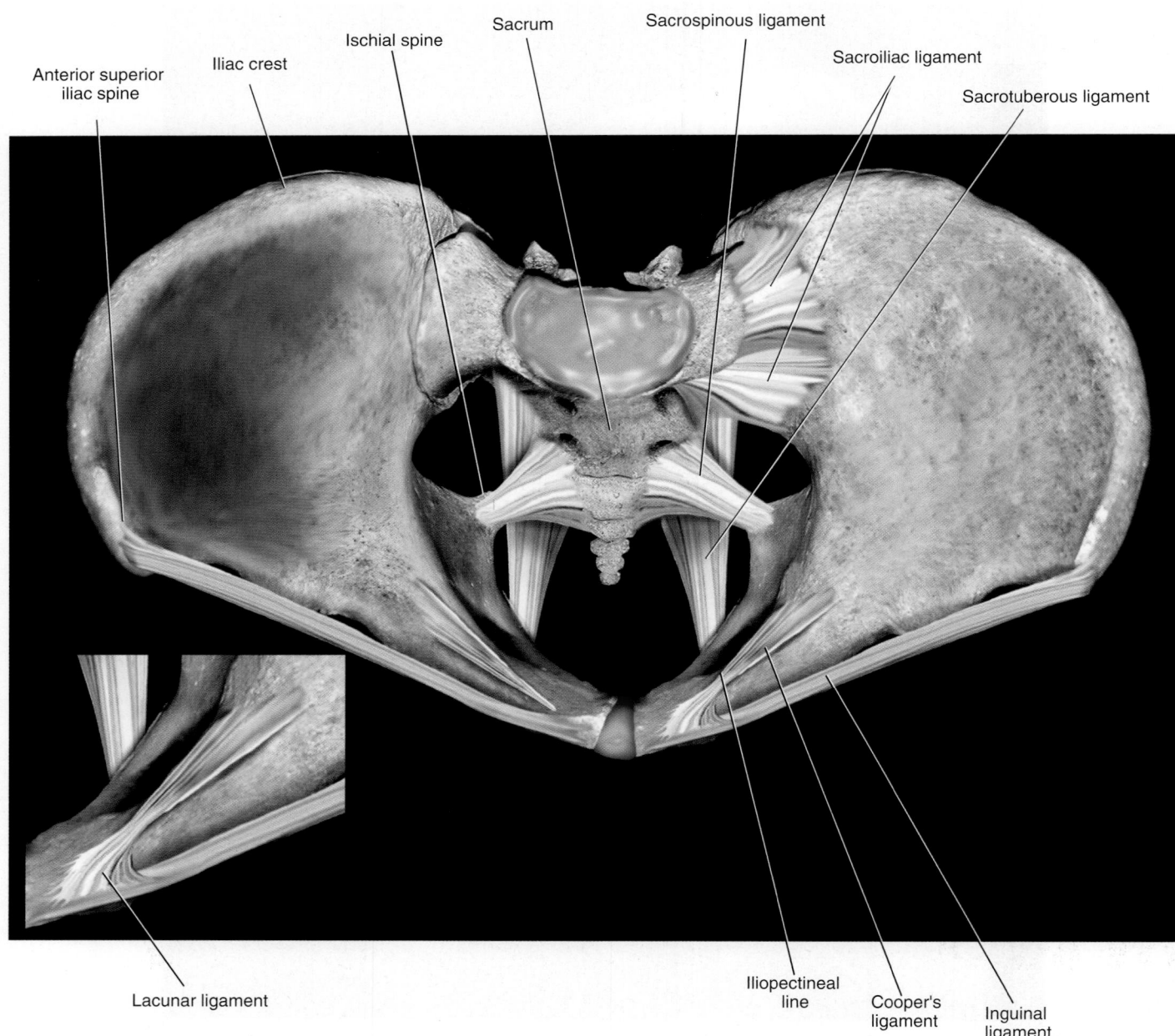

**FIGURE 1–6** The inguinal ligament stretches between the anterior superior iliac spine and the pubic tubercle. From the latter is reflected the lacunar ligament, which forms the medial boundary of the femoral canal. Cooper's ligament is a stout structure that clings to the iliopectineal line (see **inset**). Between the ischial spines and the lateral aspect of the sacrum is the sacrospinous ligament. This ligament also creates the greater and lesser sacrosciatic foramina.

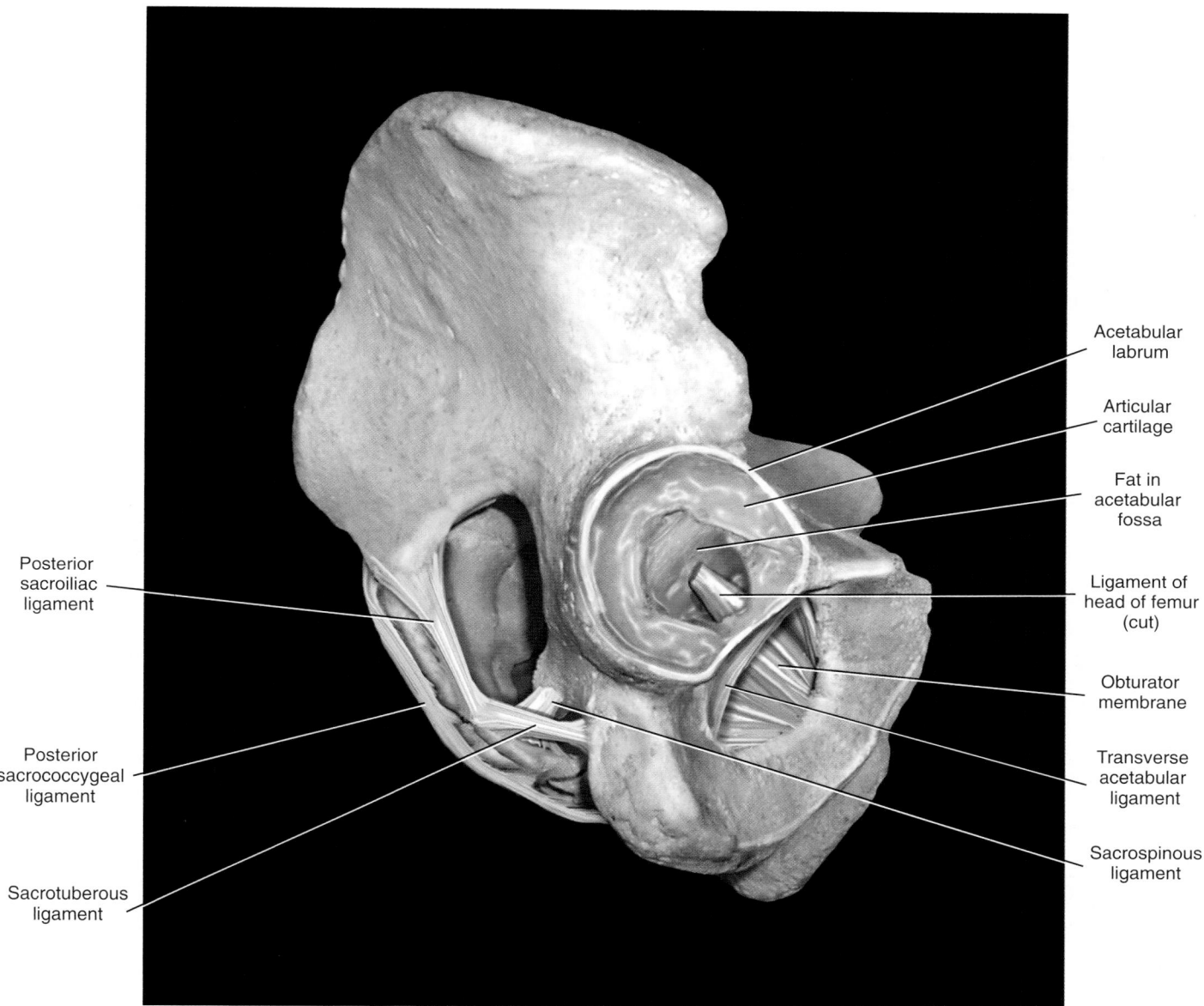

Acetabular labrum

Articular cartilage

Fat in acetabular fossa

Ligament of head of femur (cut)

Obturator membrane

Transverse acetabular ligament

Sacrospinous ligament

Posterior sacroiliac ligament

Posterior sacrococcygeal ligament

Sacrotuberous ligament

**FIGURE 1–7** This side view displays the obturator membrane, as well as the sacrotuberous ligament. The latter begins on the ischial tuberosity and terminates on the lateral margin of the sacrum.

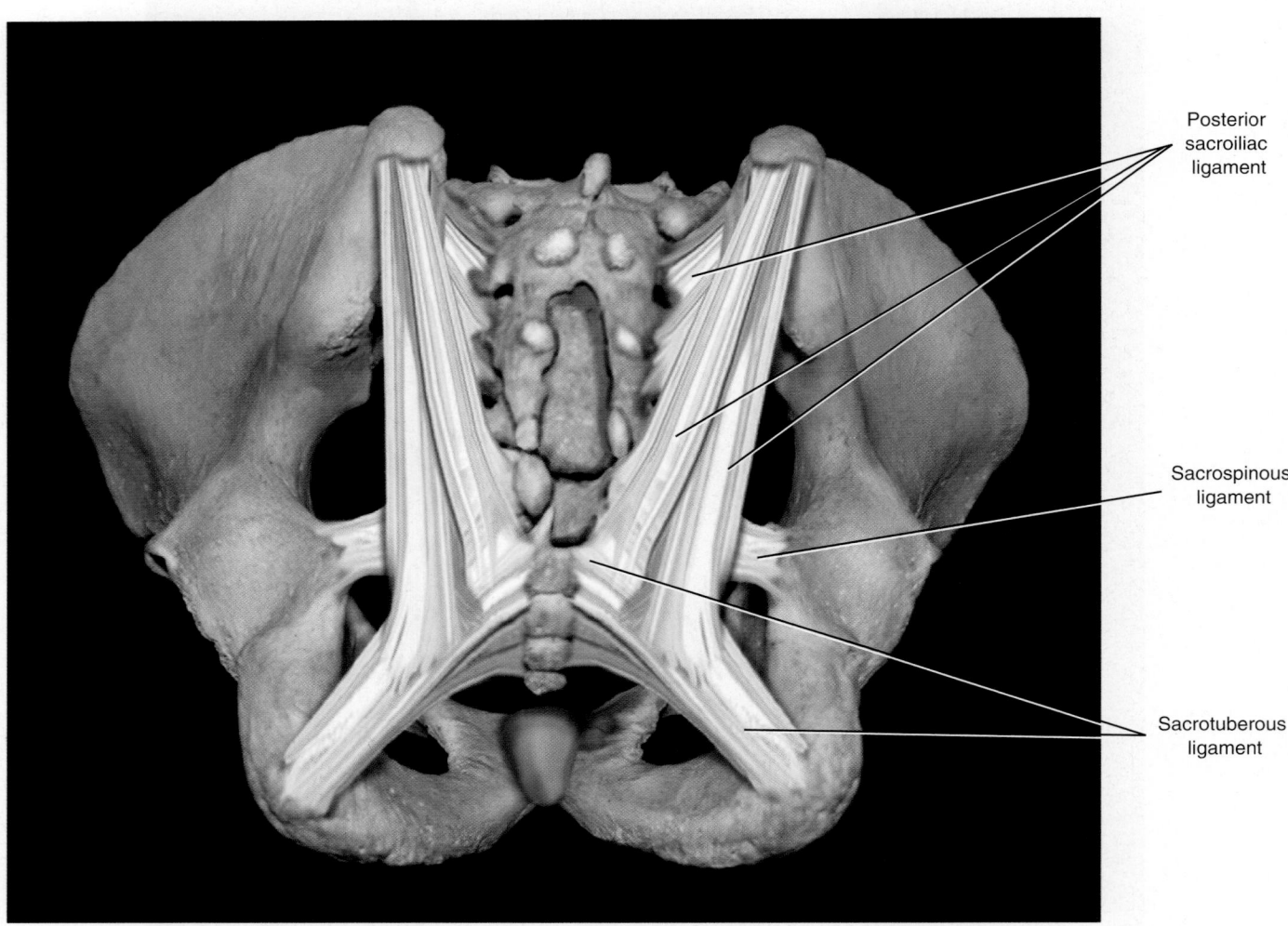

Posterior
sacroiliac
ligament

Sacrospinous
ligament

Sacrotuberous
ligament

**FIGURE 1–8** Posterior view combined with outlet view. The sacrotuberous ligament and the sacrospinous ligament cross.

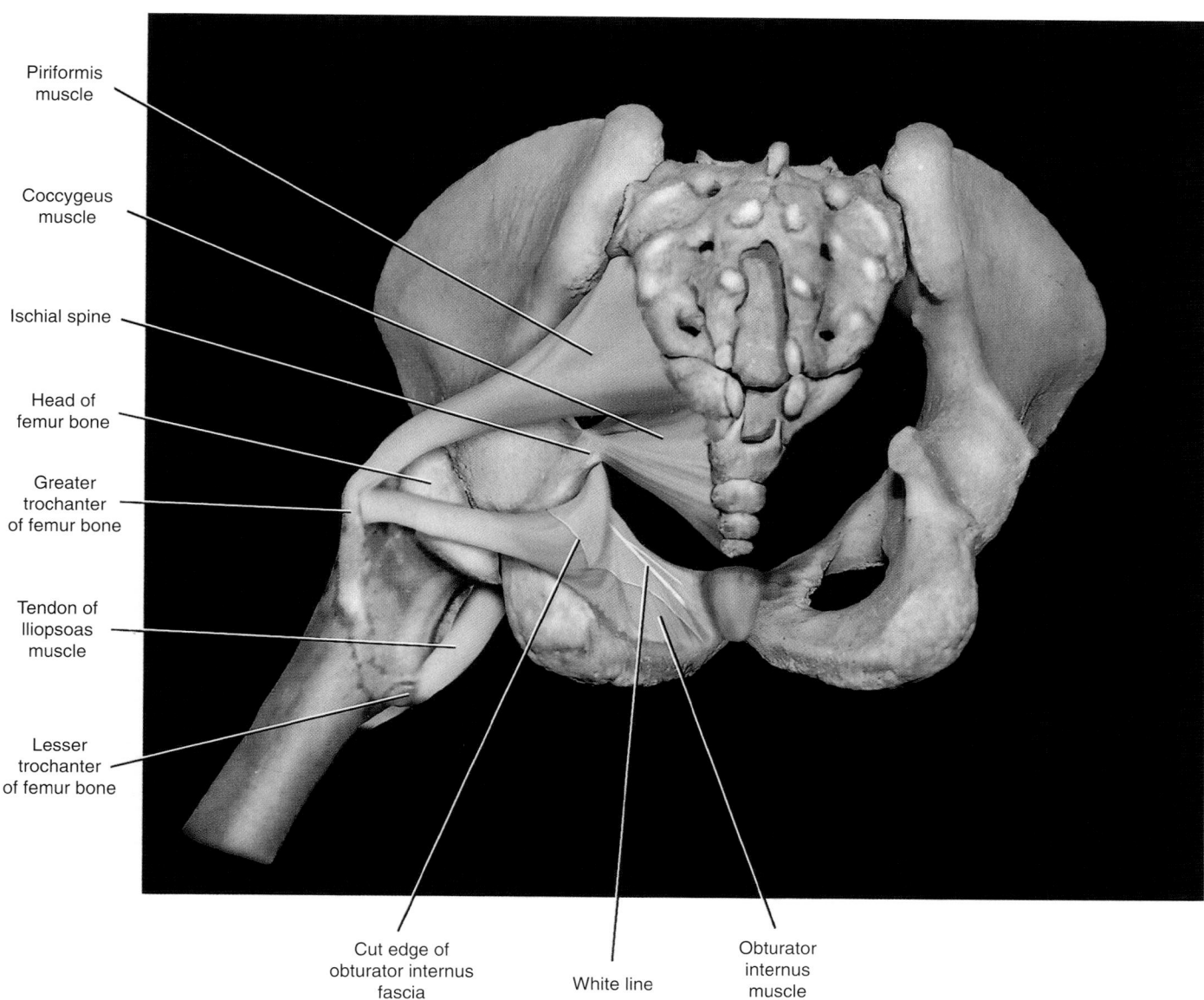

Piriformis muscle

Coccygeus muscle

Ischial spine

Head of femur bone

Greater trochanter of femur bone

Tendon of Iliopsoas muscle

Lesser trochanter of femur bone

Cut edge of obturator internus fascia

White line

Obturator internus muscle

**FIGURE 1–9** The ligaments have been eliminated. Views are through the pelvic outlet. The obturator internus, piriformis, and coccygeus are seen in sharp detail.

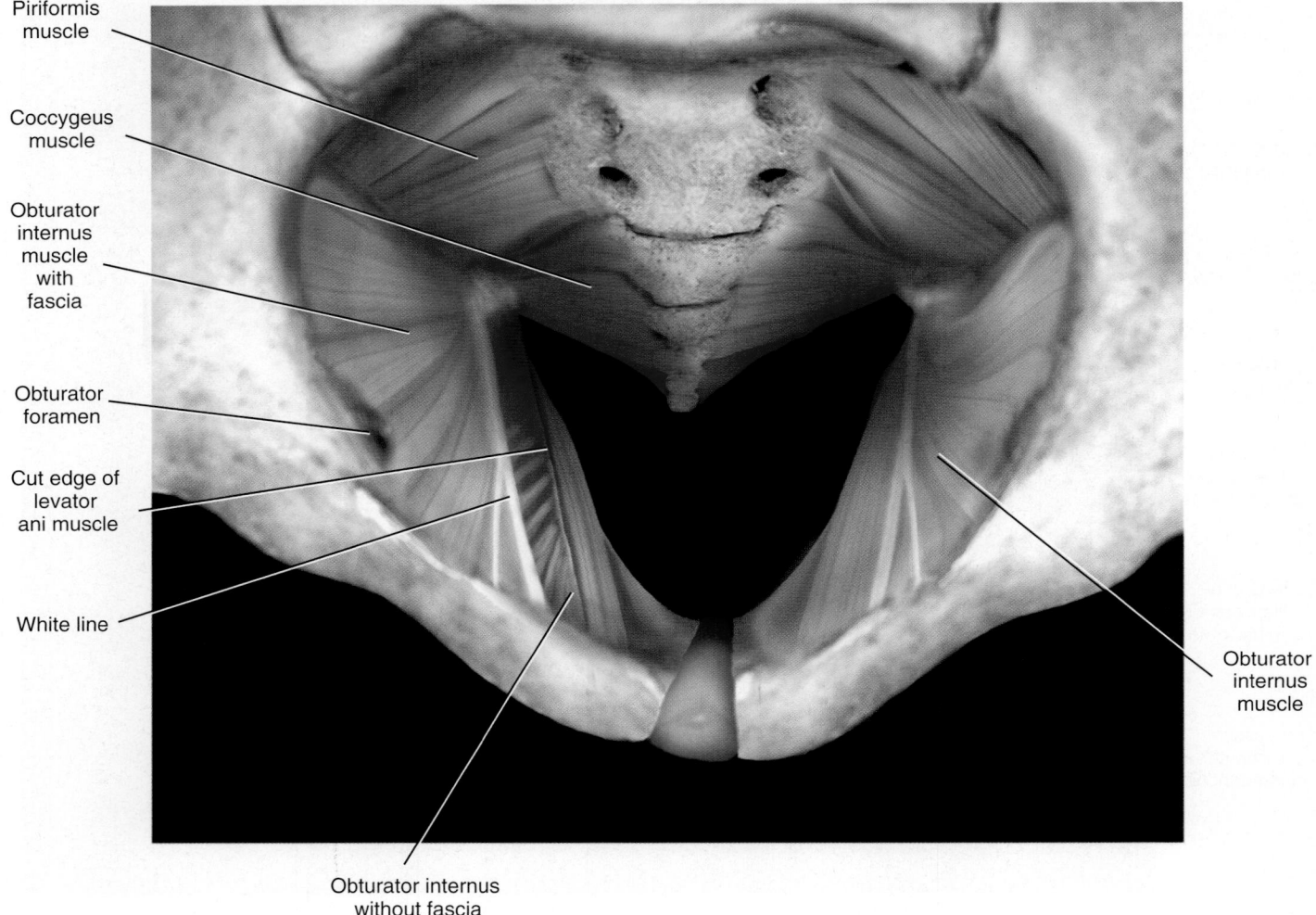

Piriformis
muscle

Coccygeus
muscle

Obturator
internus
muscle
with
fascia

Obturator
foramen

Cut edge of
levator
ani muscle

White line

Obturator
internus
muscle

Obturator internus
without fascia

**FIGURE 1–10** The large obturator internus muscle covered with tough obturator fascia forms the pelvic sidewall. The arcus tendineus, or white line, is produced by a thickened area of obturator fascia. The levator ani muscle arises from the arcus. The cut edge of the levator is shown on the patient's right side (viewer's left side). The left levator has been removed. The enclosure of the pelvis is completed by the piriformis and coccygeus muscles.

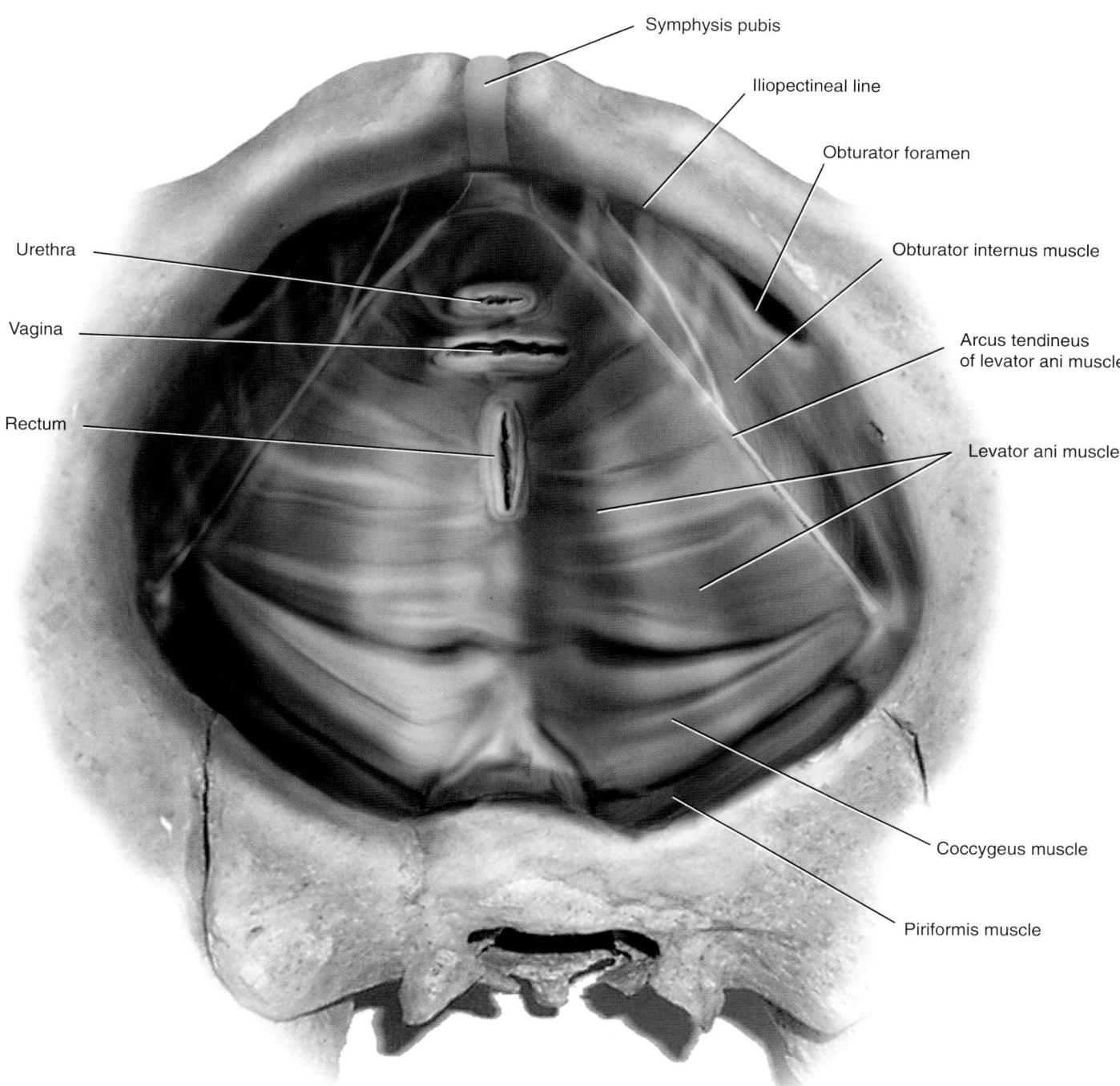

Symphysis pubis

Iliopectineal line

Obturator foramen

Obturator internus muscle

Urethra

Arcus tendineus of levator ani muscle

Vagina

Rectum

Levator ani muscle

Coccygeus muscle

Piriformis muscle

**FIGURE 1–11** This view shows the intact levator ani muscle arising along the length of the arcus tendineus. Note the exposed retropubic space, together with the cut edges of the urethra and vagina.

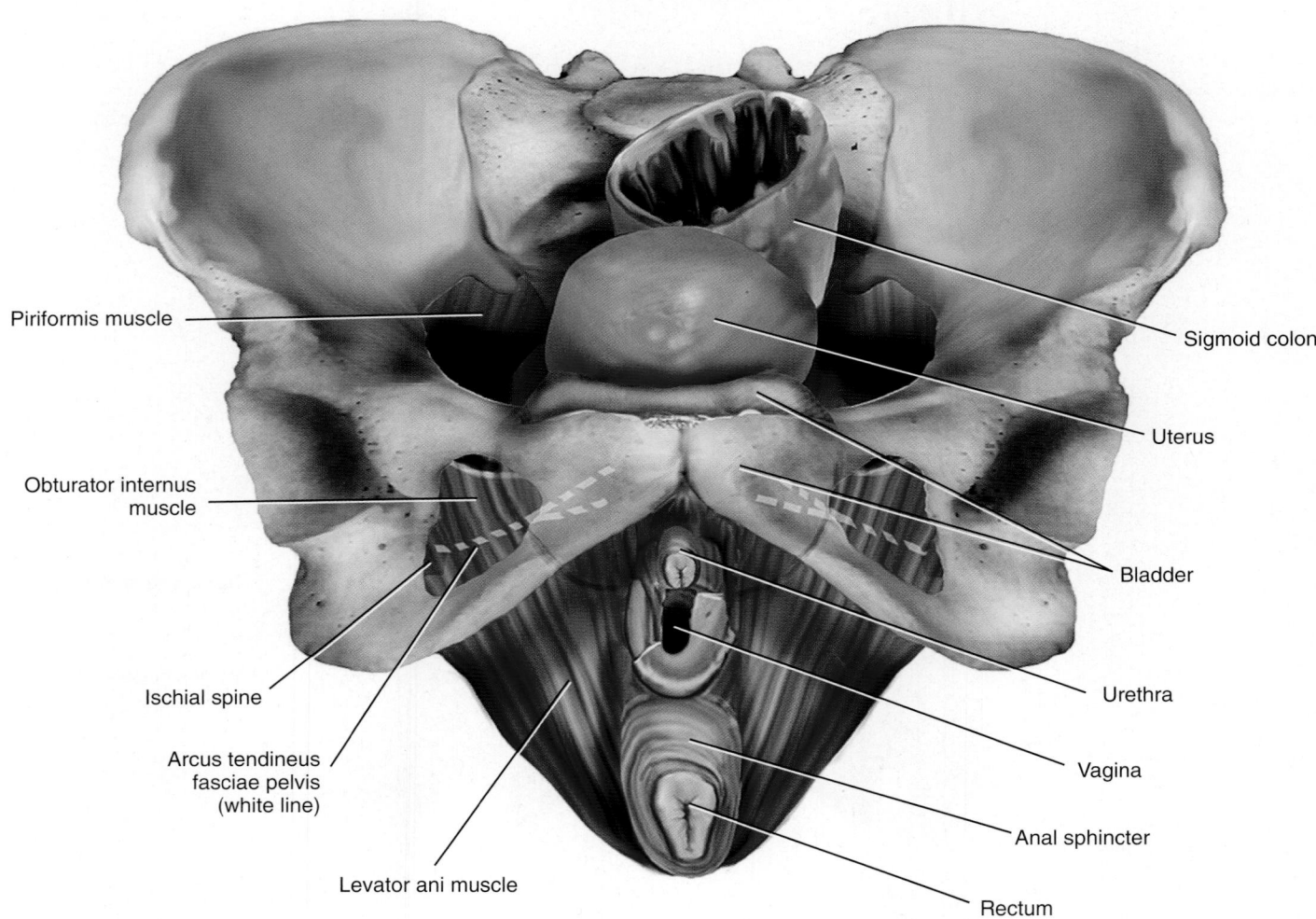

Piriformis muscle

Obturator internus
muscle

Ischial spine

Arcus tendineus
fasciae pelvis
(white line)

Levator ani muscle

Sigmoid colon

Uterus

Bladder

Urethra

Vagina

Anal sphincter

Rectum

**FIGURE 1–12** Frontal view of the funnel-like levator ani and its relationship to the vulva and superficial muscles of the perineum. The levator arises in part from the inferior margins of the pubic bone. The artist has superimposed the arcus tendineus (*dashed white line*) onto the obturator internus and pubic bone.

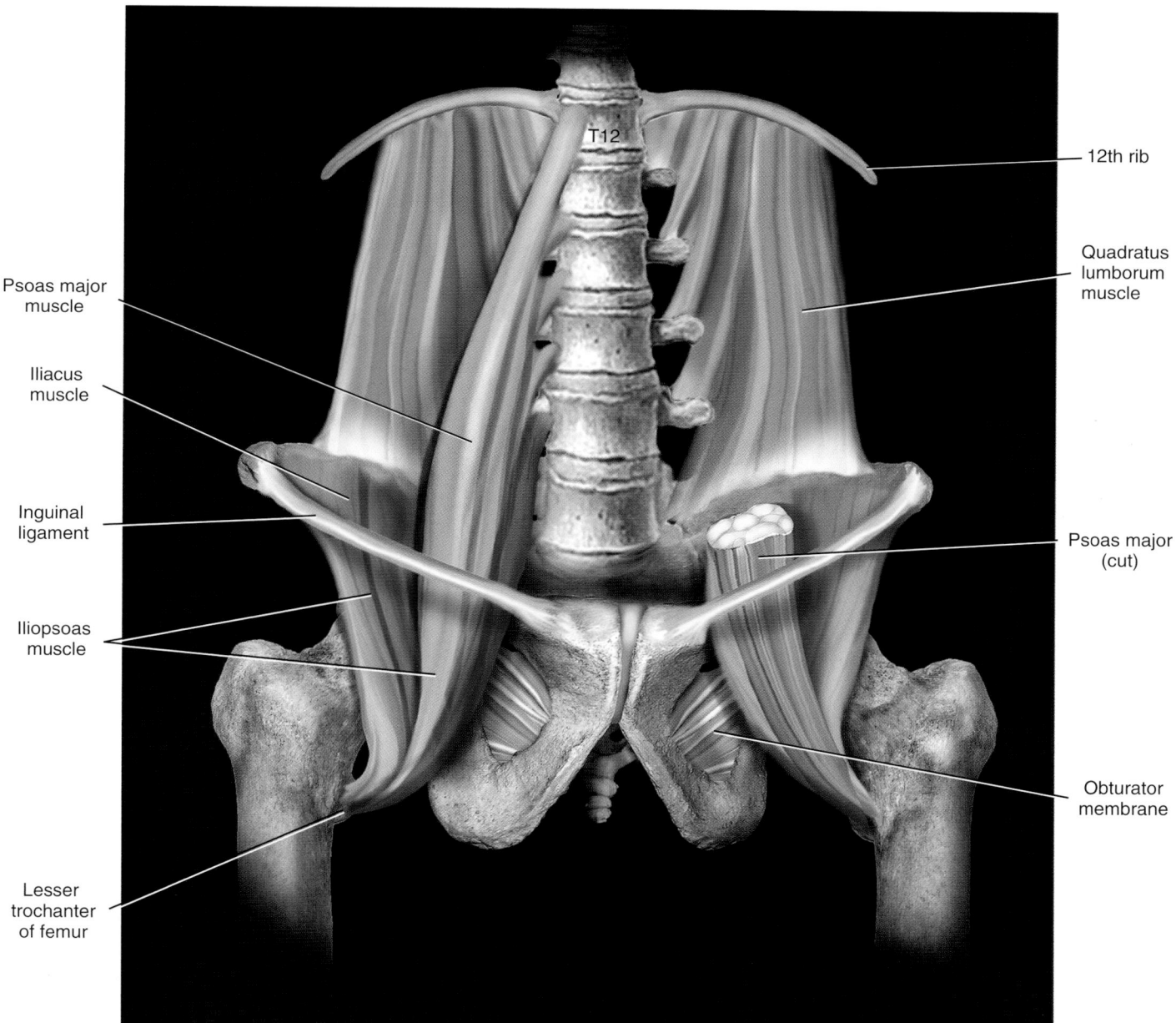

Psoas major
muscle

Iliacus
muscle

Inguinal
ligament

Iliopsoas
muscle

Lesser
trochanter
of femur

T12

12th rib

Quadratus
lumborum
muscle

Psoas major
(cut)

Obturator
membrane

**FIGURE 1–13** The large muscles of the retroperitoneum include the psoas major muscle, iliacus muscle, and quadratus lumborum muscle. The psoas and iliacus (iliopsoas) depart the abdomen and enter the thigh beneath the inguinal ligament.

The muscles of the thigh are in many cases relevant to pelvic anatomy. For example, the iliopsoas muscles leave the pelvis beneath the inguinal ligament with accompanying nerves to enter the thigh. The **sartorius muscle** is detached from the anterior superior iliac spine in radical vulvectomy surgery and transposed to cover the exposed femoral vessels. The **gracilis muscle** is utilized for pelvic reconstructive surgery as a myocutaneous graft. In addition to the muscles mentioned earlier, the gynecologist should be familiar with the **fascia lata, tensor fascia lata muscle, rectus femoris, vastus lateralis, vastus medialis, pectineus,** and **adductor longus muscles** (Figs. 1–14 and 1–15A and B).

The muscles and fascia of the abdominal wall are discussed in detail in Chapter 7.

However, the schema of the **external oblique, internal oblique, rectus abdominis,** and **transversus abdominis muscles,** and inguinal ligament are convenient to view in a single picture (Fig. 1–16).

The **inferior epigastric vessels** are identified crossing the transversus abdominis fascia from their origin in the external iliac vessels. In this drawing, the left rectus abdominis muscle has been divided and the lower muscle belly has been reflected downward (caudal) to show the details of the inferior epigastric vessels, which lie on the post sheath of the rectus abdominis muscle and the transversus fascia. The triangle formed by the inferior epigastric vessels, the inguinal ligament, and the lateral border of the rectus is **Hesselbach's triangle** (Fig. 1–17). Indirect inguinal hernias most commonly develop here (Hesselbach's triangle).

When the lower abdomen is opened, the peritoneal cavity is seen to be filled with intestines. A fat pad, the **greater omentum,** which is attached cranially to the greater curvature of the **stomach** and the **transverse colon,** hangs like an apron over the small and large intestines. Lifting the omentum reveals the **large intestine** on the periphery surrounding coils of small bowel. The large bowel is anchored normally to the parietal peritoneum along the right and left gutters (Fig. 1–18). The pelvic colon, or **sigmoid colon,** is a mobile intraperitoneal structure that is suspended by a mesocolon. The pelvic colon ranges from 5 to 35 inches in length and usually lies under the ileum. The **rectum** is 5 to 6 inches in length. It begins at the third sacral vertebra and hugs the curve of the sacrum, terminating just beyond the end of the coccyx. The rectum is covered only partially with peritoneum, with its upper third having peritoneal covering on the front and sides and the lower two thirds lying largely retroperitoneal (middle third has peritoneum in front only). The large bowel consists of **cecum, ascending colon, transverse colon, descending colon, sigmoid colon, rectum,** and **anus.**

The blood supply to the large intestine emanates from the **superior mesenteric artery** (right colon and transverse colon) and the **inferior mesenteric artery** (left flexure, left colon sigmoid colon, upper two thirds of rectum), as well as the **internal pudendal artery** (anus and lower rectum). The venous drainage is to the **hypogastric veins** to a smaller extent and to the **splenic,** or **portal, vein** to a greater extent (Fig. 1–19).

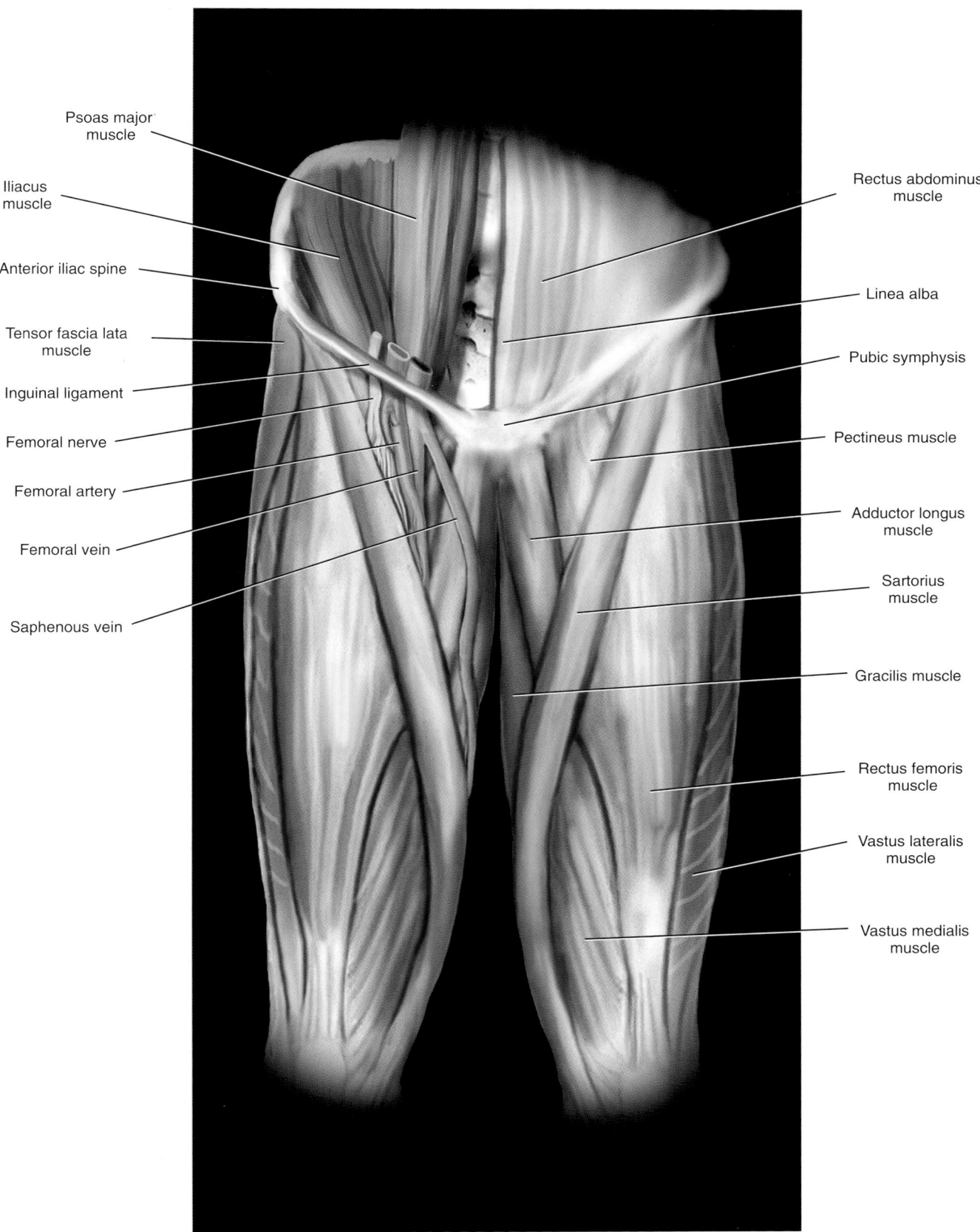

**FIGURE 1–14** Muscles of the thigh are shown, together with their relationships to the saphenous vein, femoral vessels, and femoral nerve. Note that the saphenous vein lies in the fat (dissected away) overlying the adductor longus muscle. The femoral vein is directly superficial to the pectineus muscle. The femoral artery and nerve lie on the iliopsoas muscle(s).

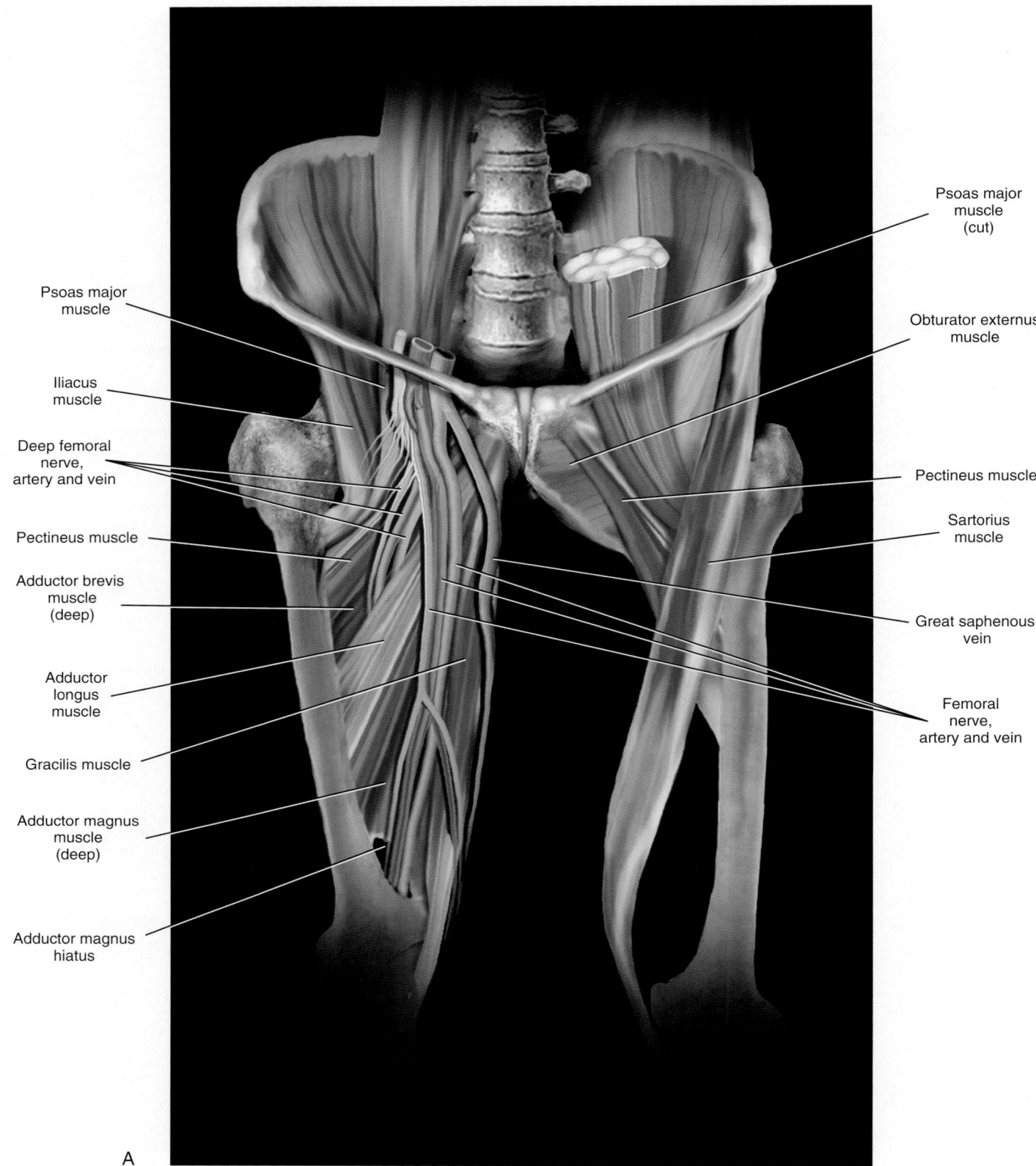

Psoas major muscle

Iliacus muscle

Deep femoral nerve, artery and vein

Pectineus muscle

Adductor brevis muscle (deep)

Adductor longus muscle

Gracilis muscle

Adductor magnus muscle (deep)

Adductor magnus hiatus

Psoas major muscle (cut)

Obturator externus muscle

Pectineus muscle

Sartorius muscle

Great saphenous vein

Femoral nerve, artery and vein

A

**FIGURE 1–15  A.** On the cadaver's right side, the sartorius muscle has been removed, as have the rectus femoris and the vasti. Similarly, the tensor fasciae latae muscle, together with the fascia lata, has been removed to expose the course of the nerves and vessels, as well as the deeper muscles.

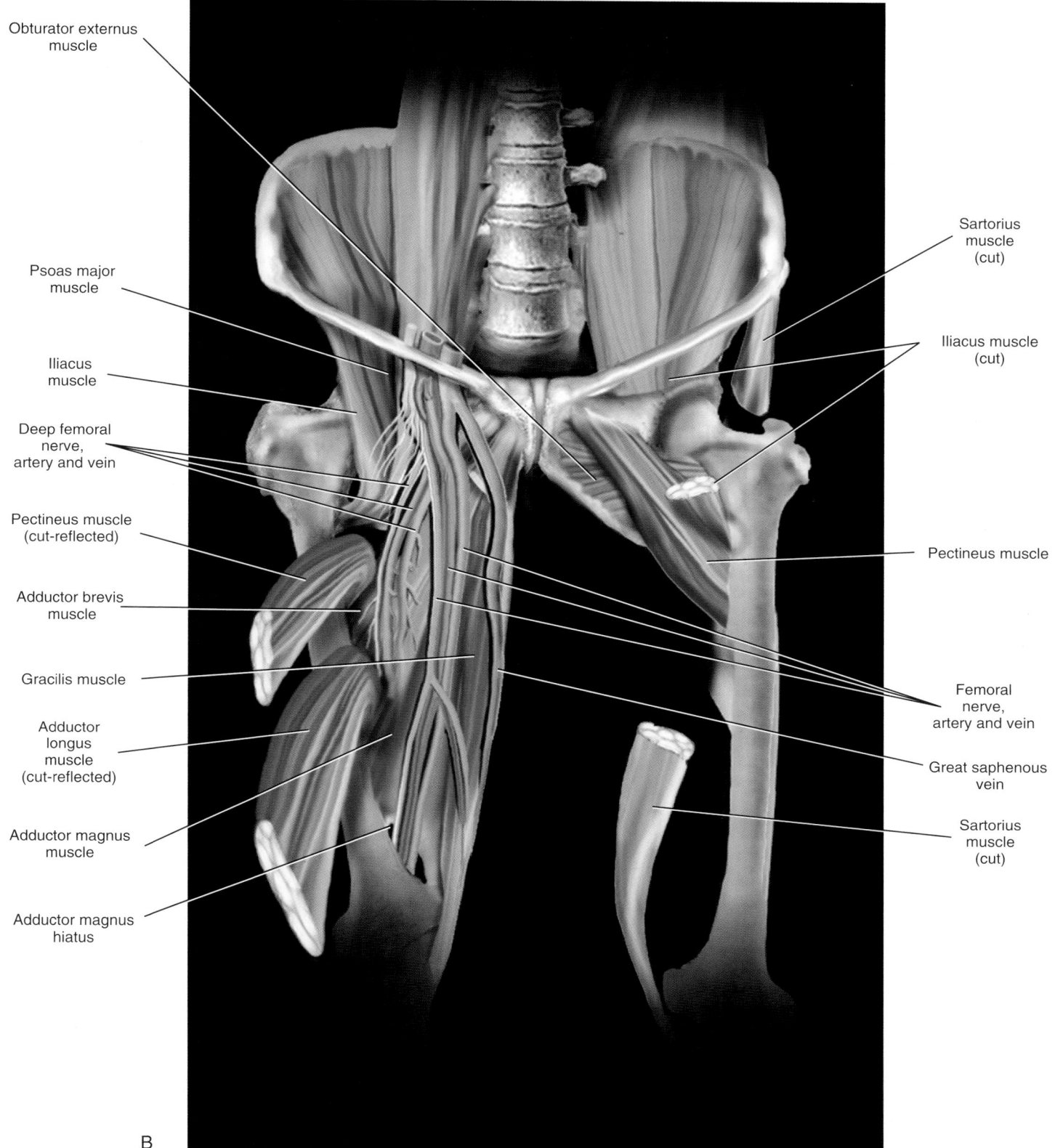

Obturator externus muscle

Psoas major muscle

Iliacus muscle

Deep femoral nerve, artery and vein

Pectineus muscle (cut-reflected)

Adductor brevis muscle

Gracilis muscle

Adductor longus muscle (cut-reflected)

Adductor magnus muscle

Adductor magnus hiatus

Sartorius muscle (cut)

Iliacus muscle (cut)

Pectineus muscle

Femoral nerve, artery and vein

Great saphenous vein

Sartorius muscle (cut)

B

**FIGURE 1–15, cont'd  B.** On the cadaver's left side, the obturator externus muscle, which covers the obturator membrane and foramen, is visible. Note the relationship of the latter to the pectineus muscle and the femoral vessels. Note that the adductor longus has been removed. On the right side, the adductor longus and pectineus muscles have been divided.

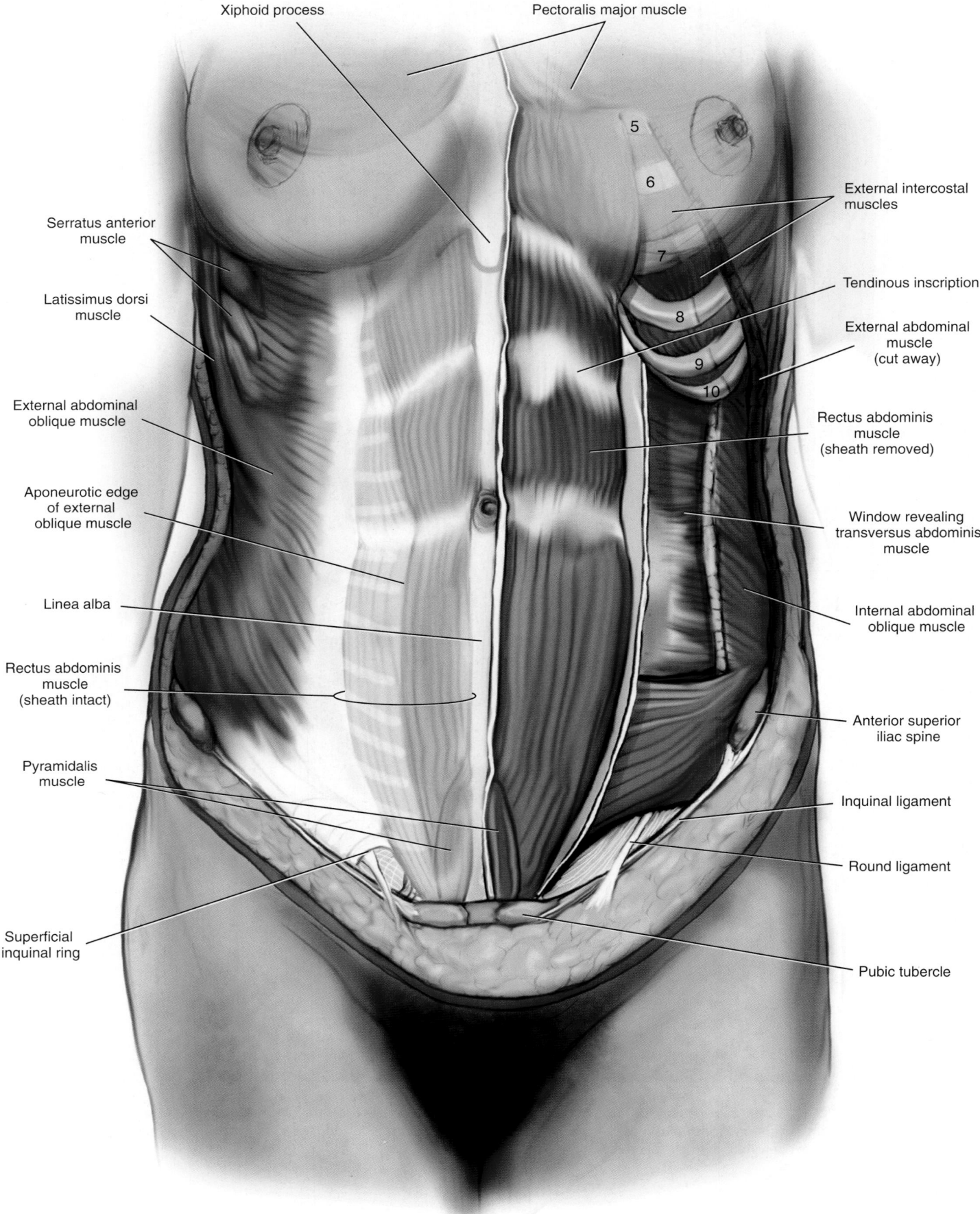

Xiphoid process

Pectoralis major muscle

Serratus anterior muscle

Latissimus dorsi muscle

External abdominal oblique muscle

Aponeurotic edge of external oblique muscle

Linea alba

Rectus abdominis muscle (sheath intact)

Pyramidalis muscle

Superficial inguinal ring

External intercostal muscles

Tendinous inscription

External abdominal muscle (cut away)

Rectus abdominis muscle (sheath removed)

Window revealing transversus abdominis muscle

Internal abdominal oblique muscle

Anterior superior iliac spine

Inquinal ligament

Round ligament

Pubic tubercle

5

6

7

8

9

10

**FIGURE 1–16** The anterior abdominal wall has been dissected deeply on the patient's left (*viewer's right*) and more superficially on the right. The anterior rectus sheath and the aponeurosis of the external oblique muscle are prominent on the right. On the left, the external oblique has been cut and largely removed. The internal oblique and transversus abdominis muscles are exposed. Note the direction of the external and internal oblique, and of the transversus fibers. The anterior rectus sheath has been opened on the left side, allowing the entire left rectus abdominis muscle to be viewed. The anterior sheath of the rectus is derived only from the fascia of the external and internal obliques below the umbilicus. At this location, the posterior sheath is derived solely from the transversus abdominis muscle.

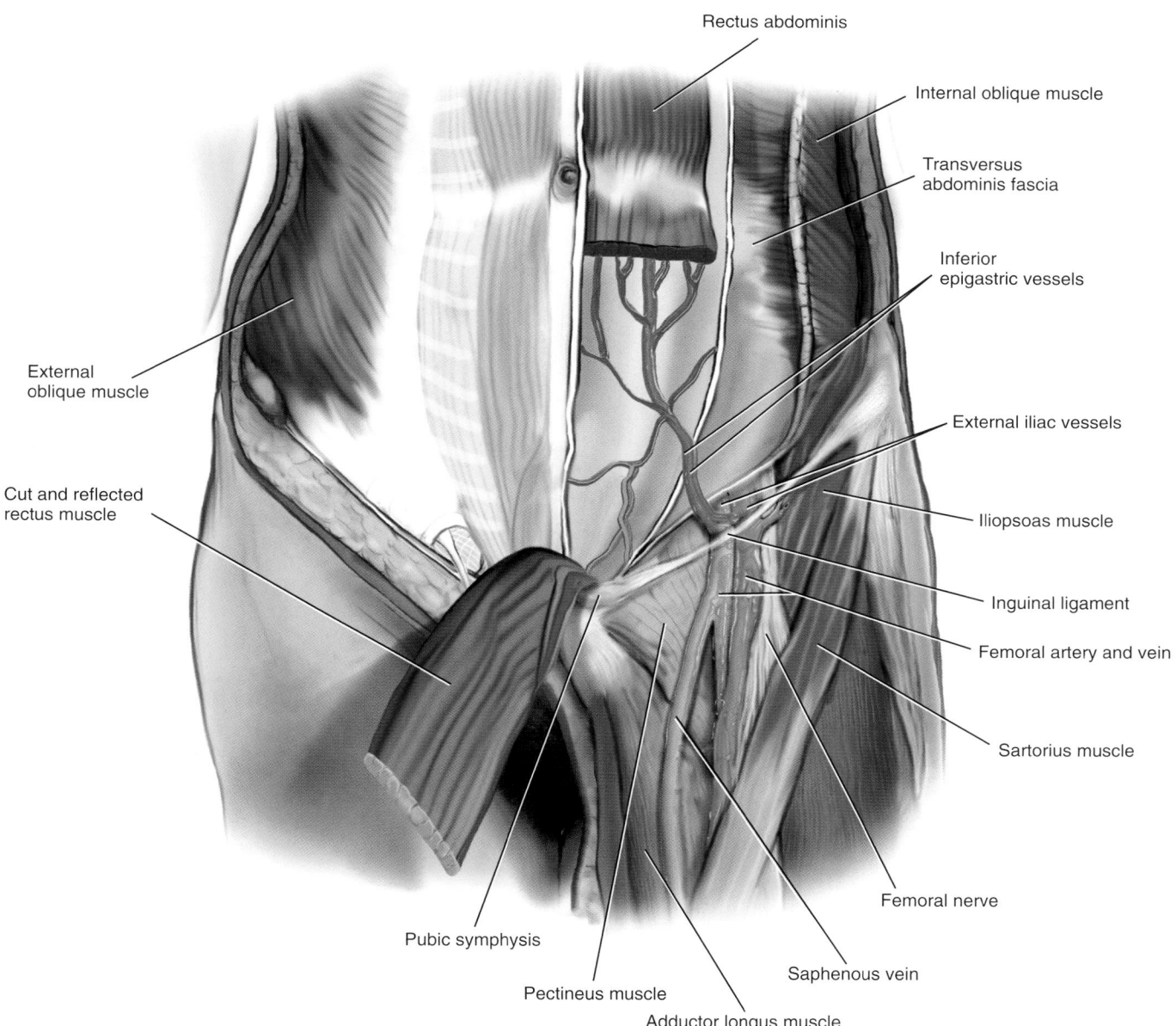

Rectus abdominis

Internal oblique muscle

Transversus abdominis fascia

Inferior epigastric vessels

External oblique muscle

External iliac vessels

Cut and reflected rectus muscle

Iliopsoas muscle

Inguinal ligament

Femoral artery and vein

Sartorius muscle

Femoral nerve

Pubic symphysis

Saphenous vein

Pectineus muscle

Adductor longus muscle

**FIGURE 1–17** The inferior epigastric vessels are important landmarks on the anterior abdominal wall, particularly because of their risk for injury during laparoscopic trocar entry. The artery arises from the lower medial aspect of the external iliac artery. The vein flows into the external iliac vein just cranial to the inguinal ligament. The femoral nerve emerges from within the substance of the psoas major muscle to be exposed directly under the tough inguinal ligament. This view shows the upper portion of the adductor longus, as well as the pectineus muscle. The latter overlies the obturator foramen (canal) and the obturator externus muscle, through which penetrate the obturator nerve plus the obturator vessels (*not shown*). Note also that the saphenous and femoral veins cross above the pectineus muscle.

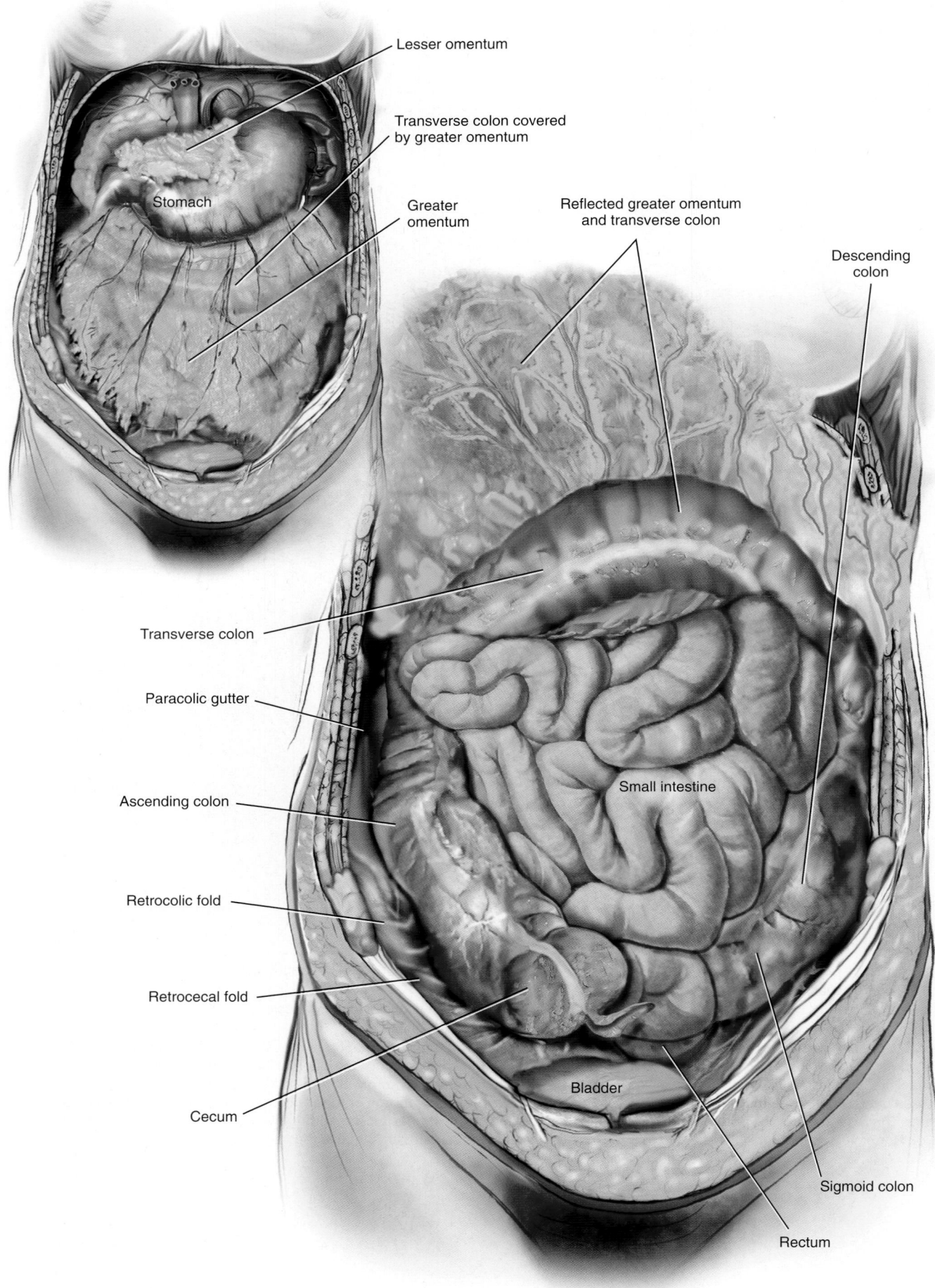

Lesser omentum

Transverse colon covered
by greater omentum

Stomach

Greater
omentum

Reflected greater omentum
and transverse colon

Descending
colon

Transverse colon

Paracolic gutter

Ascending colon

Small intestine

Retrocolic fold

Retrocecal fold

Bladder

Sigmoid colon

Cecum

Rectum

**FIGURE 1–18** The transversus fascia, which is bound to the anterior parietal peritoneum, is cut and retracted, exposing the greater omentum (**inset**). When the greater omentum itself is retracted cranially, the underlying large and small intestines dominate the abdominal cavity.

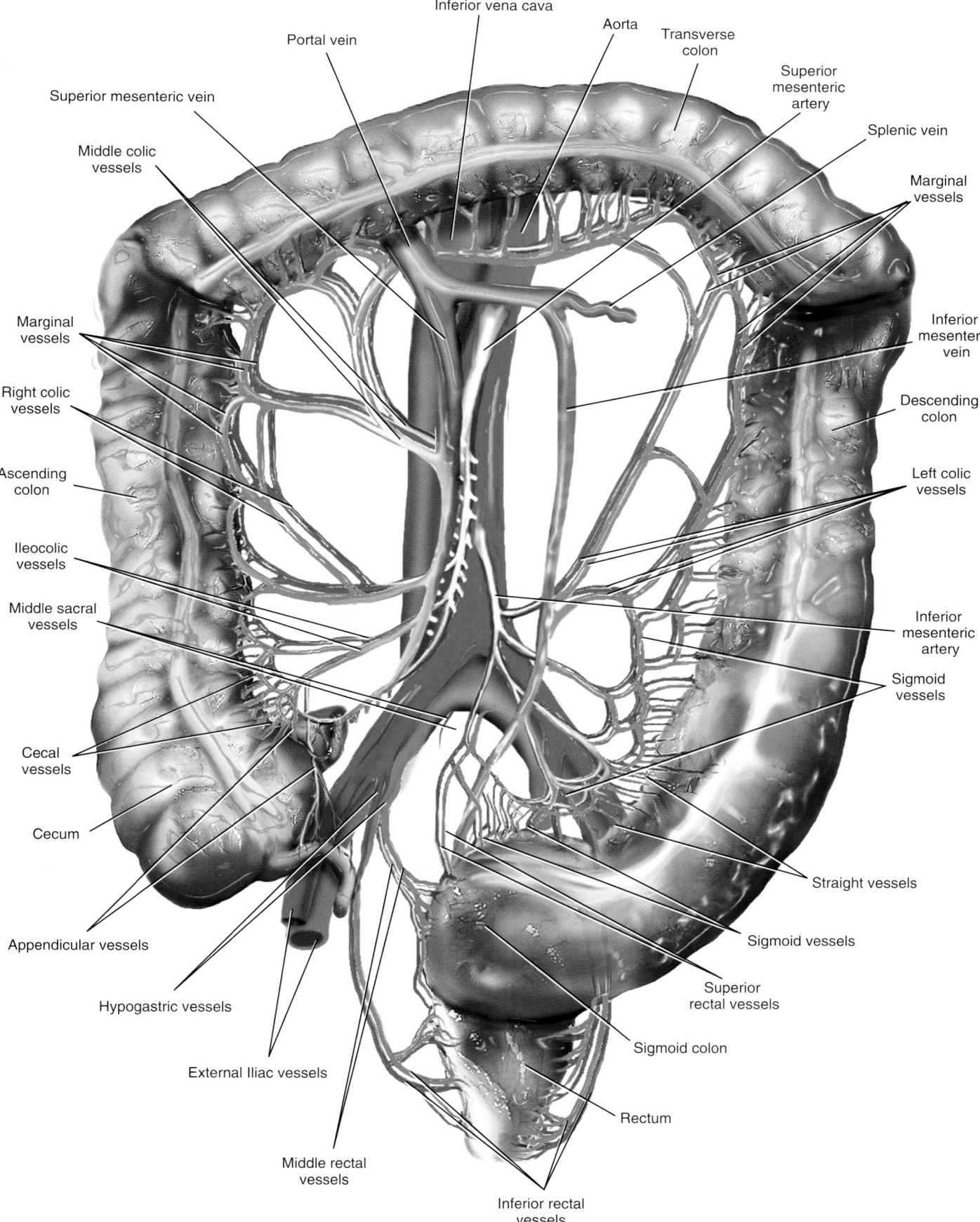

**FIGURE 1–19** The blood supply to the right colon emanates from the superior mesenteric vessels. The inferior mesenteric vessels supply the left colon and sigmoid colon. The rectum receives blood from the inferior mesenteric vessels, as well as from branches of the hypogastric vessels. The inferior rectal vessels are branches and tributaries of the internal pudendal vessels. The transverse colon receives dual supply and drainage from superior and inferior mesenteric arteries and veins.

The **small intestine** measures approximately 20 feet in length. The shortest portion of the small bowel is the **duodenum** (10 inches), which is closely related to the **stomach** at its first part and to the jejunum in its fourth part. The major portion of the small intestine consists of **jejunum** and **ileum.** The jejunum and ileum are totally surrounded by visceral peritoneum and are anchored to the posterior abdominal wall by a **mesentery.** The root of the mesentery is 6 to 8 inches in length and extends obliquely from the duodenojenunal flexure to the right colon. The small intestine itself extends from the **ligament of Treitz** to the **ileocecal valve** (Fig. 1–20). The **superior mesenteric artery** supplies the small intestine by a series of arcades. Venous drainage occurs via the **superior mesenteric vein** to the **portal vein** (Fig. 1–21). The ileum should be carefully examined 2 to 3 feet before the ileocolic junction for the presence of a finger-like projection called **Meckel's diverticulum.** This is located on the antimesenteric border. When the small and large bowels are retracted, the **uterus, adnexa,** and **urinary bladder** are brought into view (Fig. 1–22). The posterior and lateral parietal peritonei are clearly and similarly viewed but cover the underlying retroperitoneal structures. The peritoneum is incised over the **psoas major muscle.** The muscle (which may include the **psoas minor**) is exposed, and the **genitofemoral nerve** is identified. At the medial margin of the pelvic portion of the psoas muscle is the **external iliac artery.** Beneath the artery is the larger **external iliac vein.** The external iliac artery is dissected retrograde and cephalad for identification of the **common iliac artery** and **vein.** The latter are marked by the crossover of **ovarian vessels** coupled with the **ureter** (Figs. 1–22 and 1–23). The common iliac bifurcation should be identified. The **common iliac vein** is seen to lie in the crotch formed by the bifurcation of the internal and external iliac arteries. Continuing in a cephalad direction, the common iliac arteries are dissected to their origin at the bifurcation of the **abdominal aorta** at the L4–L5 interface. Just beneath (caudal to) the aortic bifurcation, the large, blue **left common iliac vein** crosses the L5 vertebral body. It next tracts beneath the right common iliac artery and joins the right common iliac vein to form the **inferior vena cava.** The **middle sacral artery** and **vein** can likewise be seen on L5–S1 vertebral bodies before descending into the sacral hollow on the sacral vertebrae.

Lateral to the psoas major muscle is the **iliacus muscle,** over which courses the **lateral femoral cutaneous nerve.** The ureter begins at the renal pelvis. It then courses on the psoas major muscle in company with the ovarian artery and veins. The ureter enters the pelvis by crossing over the common iliac vessels and then assumes a medial position relative to the hypogastric artery (see Fig. 1–23).

If the pelvic viscera are removed, details of the relationship between the **uterine artery** and the **ureter** can be easily appreciated. Similarly, the relationships of the **obturator vessels** and **nerve** to the **obturator internus muscle** and **foramen** are clear. The **external iliac artery** and **vein** cross into the thigh between the inguinal ligament and the iliopectineal line (of the pubic bone). The **femoral nerve** lies within and is protected by the substance of the **psoas major muscle** but emerges from this protection as it leaves the abdomen and enters the thigh beneath the inguinal ligament. It is therefore not surprising that compression injuries can happen when women are placed in the lithotomy position with the thigh hyperflexed or severely abducted (Figs. 1–23 and 1–24).

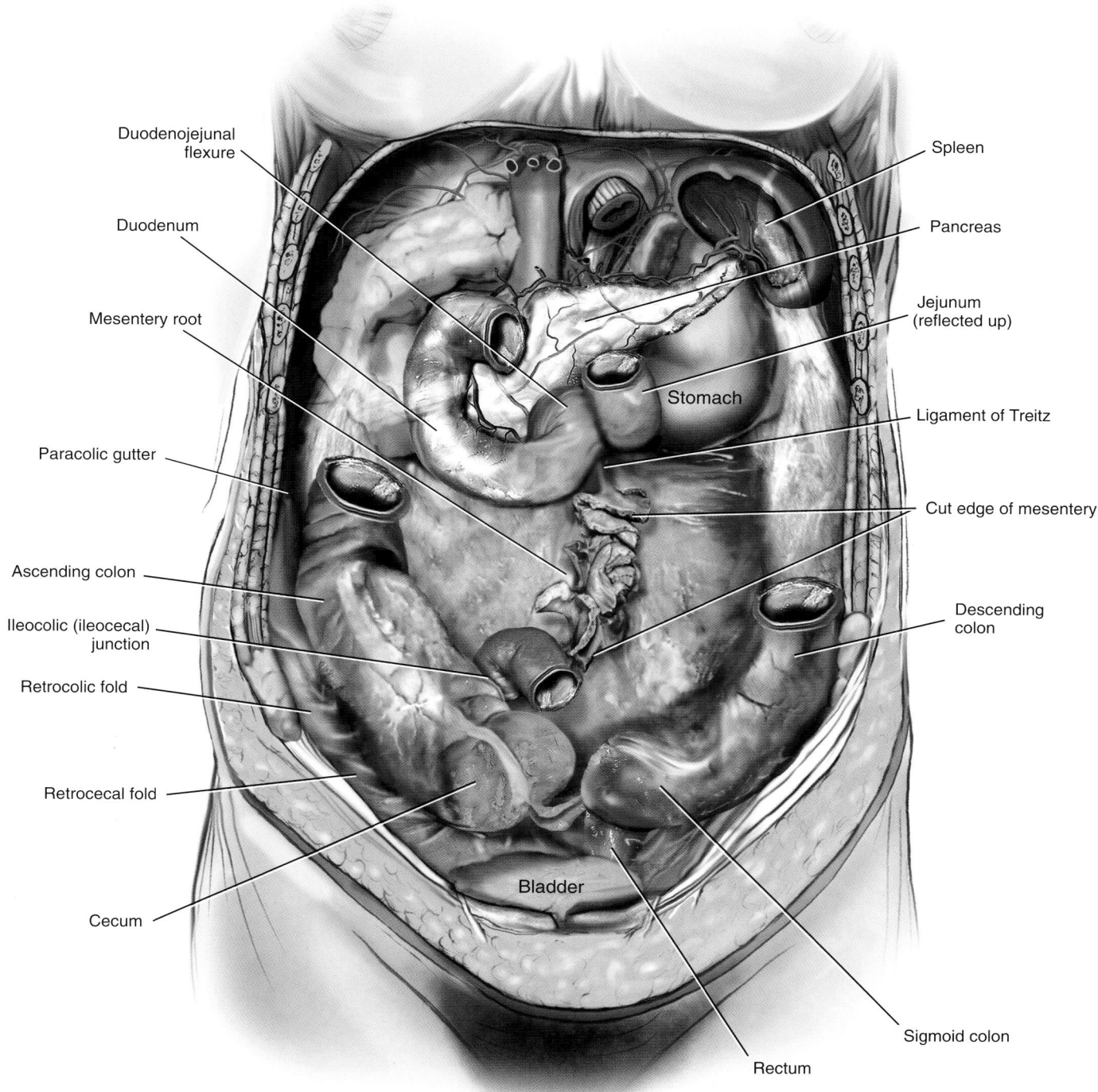

**FIGURE 1–20** The normal mesenteric attachments of the intestines are shown in this picture. The small bowel mesentery runs obliquely from left to right. The mesentery starts at the duodenojejunal flexure and ends at the cecum. The right and left sides of the colon are attached by peritoneum to the posterolateral abdominal gutters (*left* and *right*). During surgery, inspection of the small intestine should be performed systematically. The entire small bowel should be examined, beginning at the ligament of Treitz and ending at the ileocecal junction.

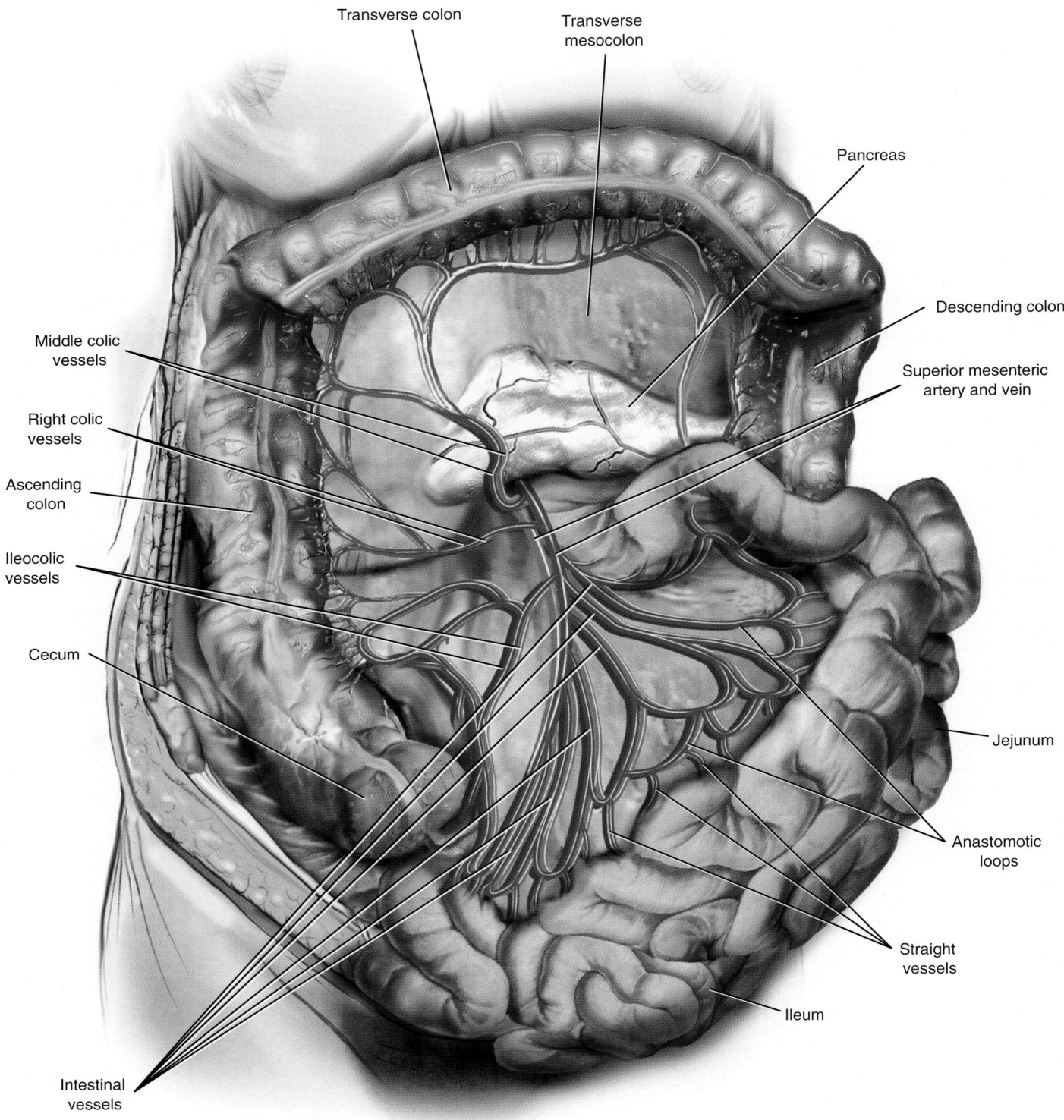

Transverse colon

Transverse mesocolon

Pancreas

Descending colon

Superior mesenteric artery and vein

Middle colic vessels

Right colic vessels

Ascending colon

Ileocolic vessels

Cecum

Jejunum

Anastomotic loops

Straight vessels

Ileum

Intestinal vessels

**FIGURE 1–21** The blood supply to the small intestine emanates from the superior mesenteric vessels. The branches of the superior mesenteric vessels are located within the fat of the small bowel mesentery and form a series of arcades as they divide distally. These arcades provide excellent overlapping circulation to the intestine. The collateral circulation is protective in cases of vascular compromise within one of the feeding branches.

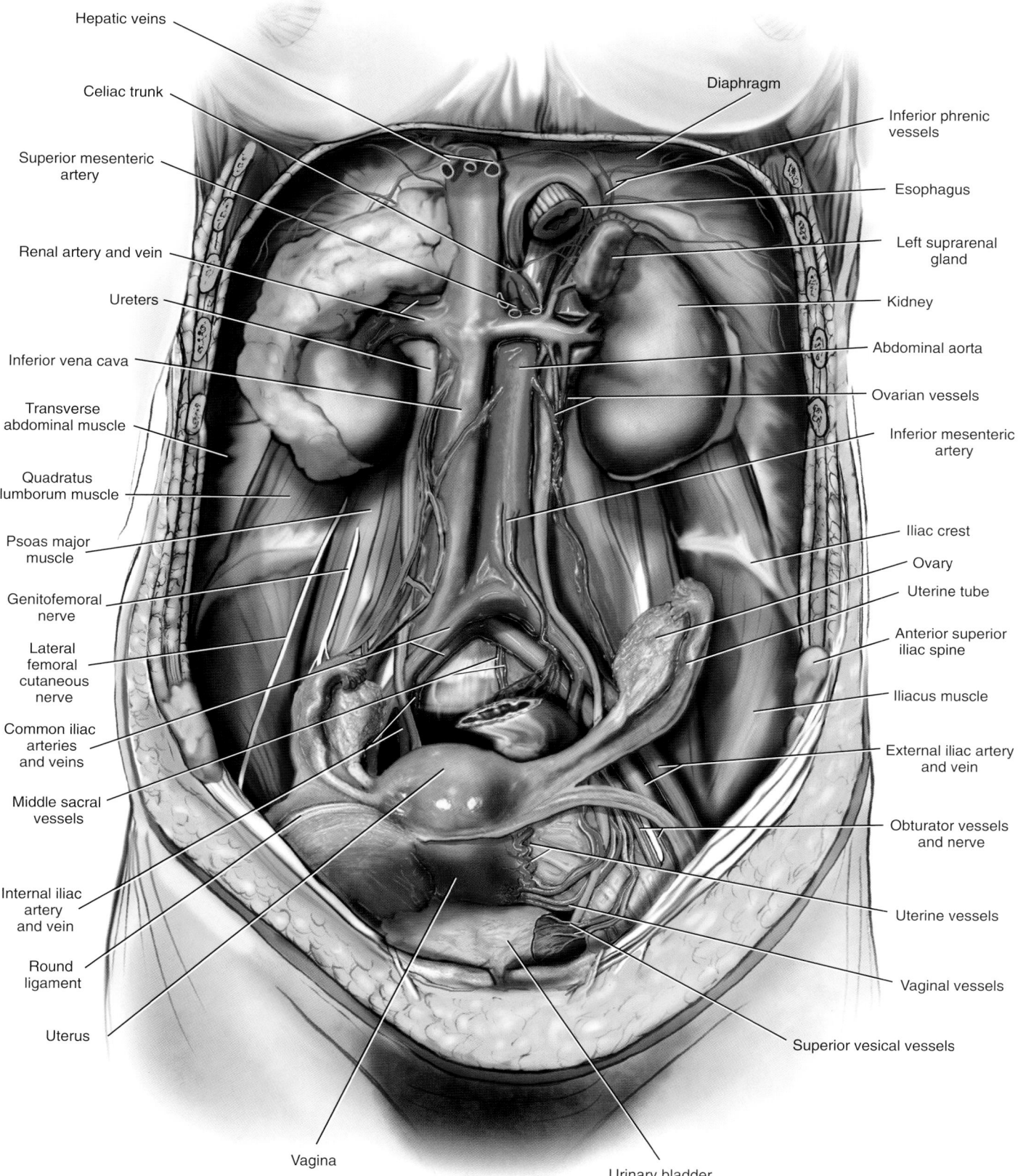

Hepatic veins

Celiac trunk

Superior mesenteric artery

Renal artery and vein

Ureters

Inferior vena cava

Transverse abdominal muscle

Quadratus lumborum muscle

Psoas major muscle

Genitofemoral nerve

Lateral femoral cutaneous nerve

Common iliac arteries and veins

Middle sacral vessels

Internal iliac artery and vein

Round ligament

Uterus

Vagina

Diaphragm

Inferior phrenic vessels

Esophagus

Left suprarenal gland

Kidney

Abdominal aorta

Ovarian vessels

Inferior mesenteric artery

Iliac crest

Ovary

Uterine tube

Anterior superior iliac spine

Iliacus muscle

External iliac artery and vein

Obturator vessels and nerve

Uterine vessels

Vaginal vessels

Superior vesical vessels

Urinary bladder

**FIGURE 1–22** The intestines have been removed. The uterus, adnexa, urinary bladder, ureters, kidneys, and rectum remain. The great vessels, as well as their branches, are exposed. Note that a deeper dissection has been performed vis-à-vis the broad ligament on the left side. The anterior leaf of the left broad ligament has been removed, exposing the course of the uterine and vaginal vessels, as well as the pelvic ureter.

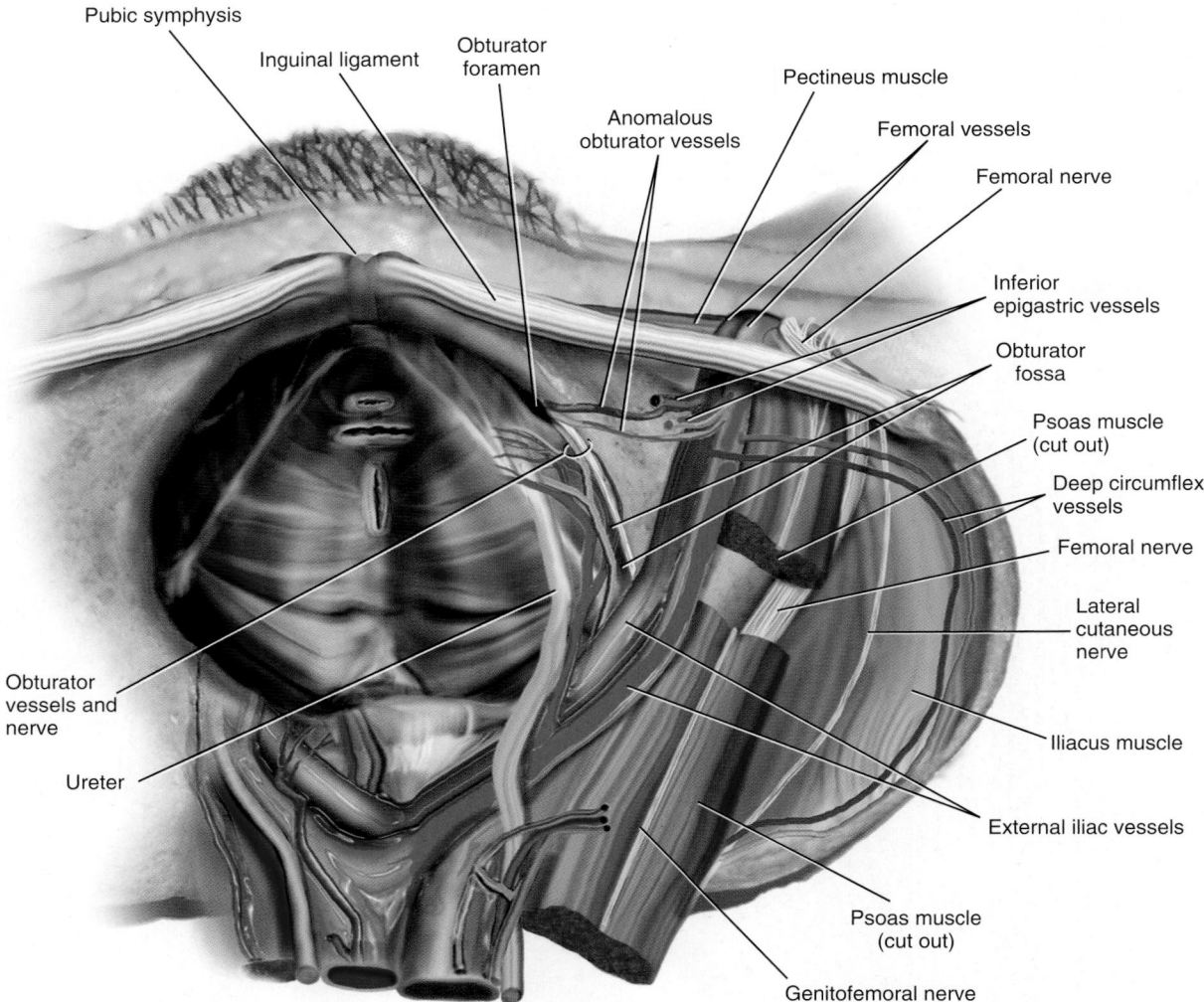

**FIGURE 1–23** The ureter descends into the pelvic cavity lying on the psoas major muscle. It is lateral to the inferior vena cava. The ureter crosses over the common iliac vessels just cranial to the iliac bifurcation. It is medial to the hypogastric artery, the obturator neurovascular bundle. At the level of the cardinal ligament, the uterine vessels cross over the ureter. This drawing illustrates the relationships of structures crossing from the abdomen beneath the inguinal ligament into the thigh. The genitofemoral nerve lies on the psoas major muscle. The lateral femoral cutaneous nerve lies on the iliacus muscle. The femoral nerve (*see cutaway*) is buried within the substance of the psoas major and emerges from the muscle just above where it crosses under the inguinal ligament.

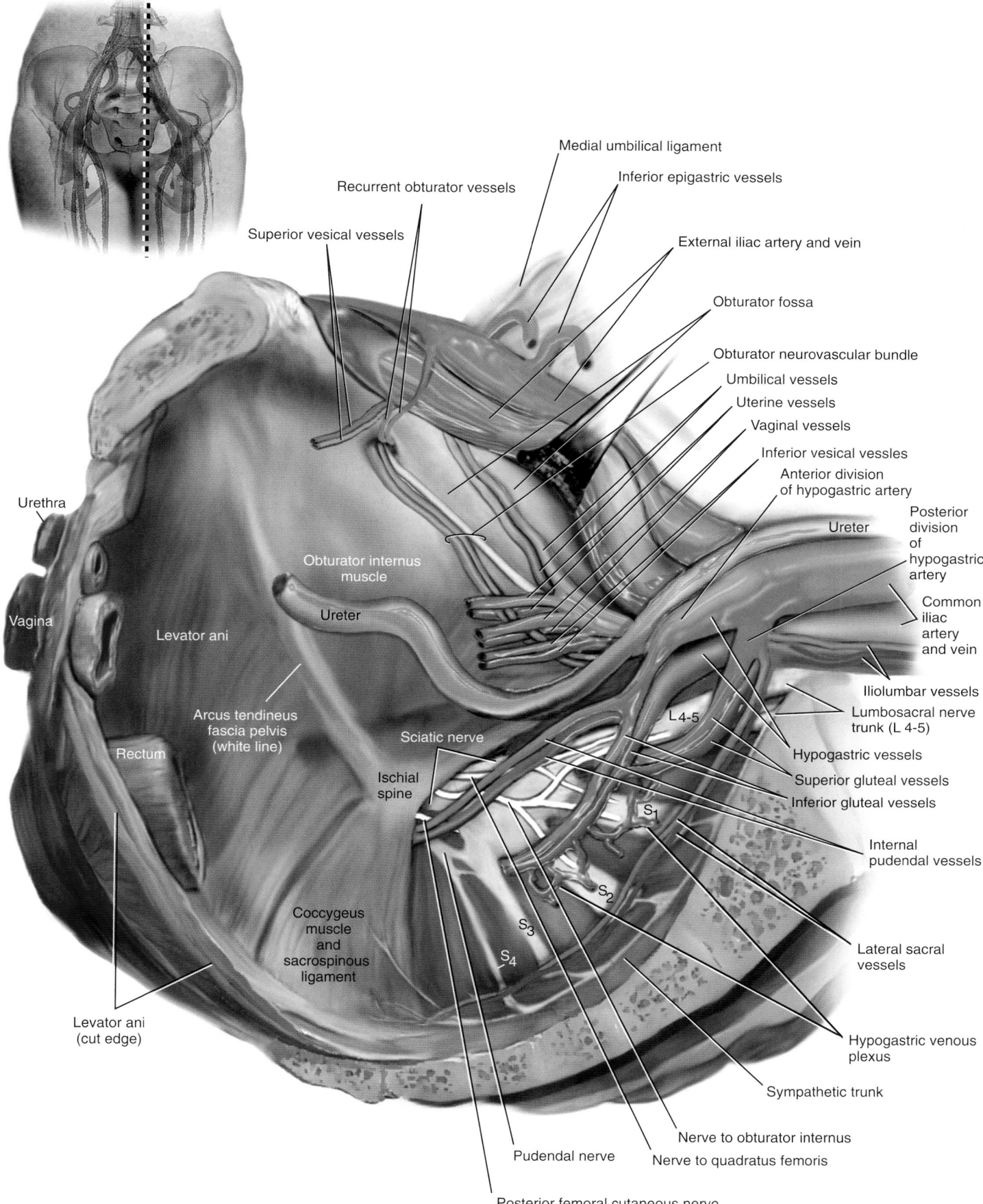

Medial umbilical ligament
Recurrent obturator vessels
Inferior epigastric vessels
Superior vesical vessels
External iliac artery and vein
Obturator fossa
Obturator neurovascular bundle
Umbilical vessels
Uterine vessels
Vaginal vessels
Inferior vesical vessels
Anterior division of hypogastric artery
Ureter
Posterior division of hypogastric artery
Common iliac artery and vein
Iliolumbar vessels
Lumbosacral nerve trunk (L 4-5)
Hypogastric vessels
Superior gluteal vessels
Inferior gluteal vessels
Internal pudendal vessels
Lateral sacral vessels
Hypogastric venous plexus
Sympathetic trunk
Nerve to obturator internus
Nerve to quadratus femoris
Pudendal nerve
Posterior femoral cutaneous nerve

Urethra
Vagina
Levator ani
Obturator internus muscle
Ureter
Arcus tendineus fascia pelvis (white line)
Rectum
Sciatic nerve
Ischial spine
Coccygeus muscle and sacrospinous ligament
Levator ani (cut edge)

L 4-5
S₁
S₂
S₃
S₄

**FIGURE 1–24** Sagittal section through the pelvis (see **inset**). The muscles enclosing the pelvis include the sidewall muscles, that is, the obturator internus, coccygeus, and piriformis. The white line, or arcus tendineus, stretches between the ischial spine and the lower margin of the pubic bone. The levator ani takes its origin from the thickened obturator internus fascia (the arcus tendineus), as well as from the lower margin of the pubic ramus. The bifurcation of the common iliac vessels is seen. The internal iliac, or hypogastric, vessels supply the pelvic viscera via several branches and tributaries. The hypogastric artery divides into a superior posterior division and an inferior anterior division. From the posterior division, the following emanate: superior gluteal vessels, lateral sacral vessels, and iliolumbar vessels. Anterior division branches include lateral umbilical, superior and inferior vesical, obturator, uterine, and vaginal. Terminal branches of the anterior division include the inferior gluteal and internal pudendal vessels. The posterior division of the hypogastric artery will lead the dissector to the sacral nerve roots and the sciatic nerve. The obturator neurovascular bundle is best exposed by retraction of the external iliac vein. The lateral umbilical vessels ascend the anterior abdominal wall supported superficial to the external iliac vessels on either side of the urachus (*not shown here*).

The sagittal cut shows details of the bony pelvis and musculature but mainly the pelvic blood supply (Figs. 1–24 and 1–25). After bifurcating from the **common iliac artery,** the **hypogastric artery** (internal iliac artery) itself immediately splits into **anterior** and **posterior divisions.** The anterior division supplies most of the pelvic viscera. The posterior division branches to form the **superior gluteal, lateral sacral,** and **iliolumbar** vessels. Following the posterior division down into the depths of the pelvis will lead to the **sacral nerve roots,** which together constitute the huge **sciatic nerve.** A vein retractor is placed carefully under the external iliac vein; an upward pull will expose the **obturator fossa** (see Fig. 1–23). When the fat is cleared from this space, the lateral margins of the fossa are seen and consist of the pubic bone and the obturator internus muscle. Several branches of the anterior division of the hypogastric artery can also be identified. These include the **lateral umbilical vessels,** the **superior vesical vessels,** and the **obturator vessels.** Variations in these vessels are common, for example, **anomalous obturator vessels** (see Fig. 1–23). The terminal branches of the anterior division are the **internal pudendal** and **inferior gluteal vessels.** The **uterine** and **vaginal vessels** may come off via a common trunk or separately (see Fig. 1–25).

The **internal pudendal artery** actually leaves the pelvis via the **greater sciatic foramen** then reenters by crossing behind and under the sacrospinous ligament to reenter the pelvis via the **lesser sciatic foramen.** The neurovascular bundle transverses the lowest portion of the obturator internus muscle and fascia (**Alcock's canal**), just medial to the ischial tuberosity (see Fig. 1–25).

The relationship of the sacrospinous and sacrotuberous ligaments to major pelvic vessels and nerves is of important clinical value in that surgery performed in this area must be precise to avoid injury to those vital structures. As can be readily observed, inaccurate placement of stitches could damage the **superior** or **inferior gluteal vessels** (or both), as well as the **sciatic nerve** (see Fig. 1–25).

Because some urethral tape-suspensory surgeries utilize the obturator foramen, the precise location of the **obturator vessels** and **nerves** is required to avoid injury to these structures. For operations involving the presacral space, knowledge of the location of the **middle sacral vessels** and emerging **sacral nerve roots** is essential (see Fig. 1–25).

Exposure of the **pelvic ureter** is a required skill for anatomists as well as for gynecologic surgeons. Any technique to accomplish the goal of ureteral identification should be easily performed with a low risk for bleeding or ureteral injury.

On the right side, the surgeon or anatomist should grasp the **cecum,** elevate it, and place light traction toward the left. The peritoneum along the **right gutter** is incised (*dashed line,* Fig. 1–26), which in turn produces great mobility. As the cecum is freed, the psoas major muscle comes into view, as do the **right ureter** and common iliac vessels. Next, the medial edge of the peritoneum, to which the ureter is closely attached, is grasped with fine forceps and placed on traction (see Fig. 1–26). The ureter can be easily separated from the peritoneal edge with a dissecting scissors, using a closed-push, open-spread technique. Thus, the ureter can be freed from the pelvic brim to the point where the **uterine arteries** cross over the ureter (Fig. 1–27). The surgeon should be aware that the **ovarian artery** and **veins** are in the same peritoneal fold as the ureter at the crossover of the common iliac artery (see Fig. 1–22). The ovarian pedicle and the ureter should be separated from one another by sharp dissection. Only after both structures are separately identified should the ovarian vessels be clamped, cut, and ligated. If short-cuts are taken in accurately identifying and securing the anatomic landmarks, ureteral injury will be inevitable.

The **left ureter** is identified by similar measures to those described for the right side of the pelvis. However, on the left, the **sigmoid colon** is grasped and pulled to the right, thereby placing tension on the left peritoneal attachment. Retroperitoneal entry and exposure are produced by incising the peritoneum along the **left paracolic gutter** (*dashed line,* Fig. 1–28). Once this is done and the loose areolar tissue dissected, the psoas major muscle comes directly into view. The muscle crosses the incision line in a perfect perpendicular direction. The left iliac vessels are identified, and medial to these is the left ureter. The left ureter proceeds deep into the pelvis to the left and in the bed of the sigmoid colon.

As the right and left ureters descend inferiorly and caudally into the depths of the pelvis, they also vector medially. At the point where the ureters encounter the uterus, they are less than a centimeter from the **uterosacral ligaments.** The ureters enter the substance of the **cardinal ligaments** at the point where the uterine vessels cross above and the vaginal vessels cross below (Fig. 1–29). To expose the lower ureter, the cardinal ligament must be dissected, that is, the ureter will be unroofed. This dissection is sharply performed and requires knowledge of the sense of direction that the ureter is taking through the cardinal ligament. A tonsil clamp creates an oblique tunnel over (superiorly and anteriorly) the ureter. The clamp is spread, thereby enlarging the space; then the cardinal ligament on each side is clamped and cut, thereby exposing the ureter as it enters the bladder, as well as securing the uterine vessels as they cross above the ureter (Figs. 1–30 through 1–33).

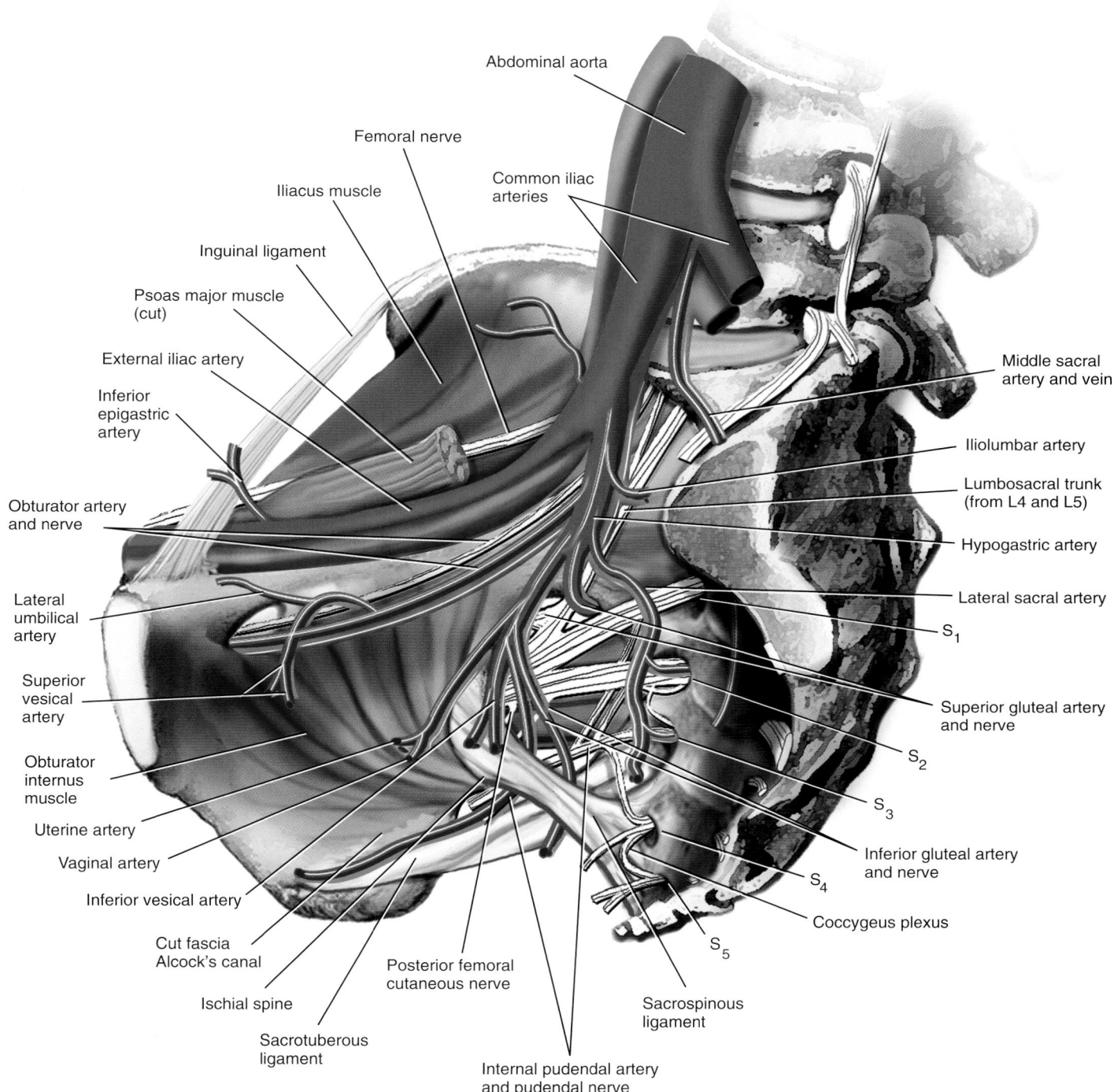

Abdominal aorta

Femoral nerve

Iliacus muscle

Common iliac arteries

Inguinal ligament

Psoas major muscle (cut)

External iliac artery

Inferior epigastric artery

Obturator artery and nerve

Lateral umbilical artery

Superior vesical artery

Obturator internus muscle

Uterine artery

Vaginal artery

Inferior vesical artery

Cut fascia Alcock's canal

Ischial spine

Sacrotuberous ligament

Posterior femoral cutaneous nerve

Internal pudendal artery and pudendal nerve

Sacrospinous ligament

Coccygeus plexus

$S_5$

$S_4$

Inferior gluteal artery and nerve

$S_3$

$S_2$

Superior gluteal artery and nerve

$S_1$

Lateral sacral artery

Hypogastric artery

Lumbosacral trunk (from L4 and L5)

Iliolumbar artery

Middle sacral artery and vein

**FIGURE 1–25** Sagittal section with several pelvic muscles removed to show the inguinal, sacrospinous, and sacrotuberous ligaments. Note the internal pudendal artery and the pudendal nerve leaving the pelvis via the superior sacrosciatic foramen and reentering via the inferior sacrosciatic foramen. At the reentry point, the pudendal neurovascular bundle enters a fascial canal created within the lowest portion of the obturator internus muscle—Alcock's canal. Note that the femoral nerve (within the substance of the psoas major muscle) emerges from within the psoas major muscle as it passes exposed beneath the inguinal ligament. The huge sciatic nerve (L4, L5, S1, S2, S3) leaves the pelvis over the piriformis muscle via the greater sacrosciatic foramen. Note that the sacrospinous and sacrotuberous ligaments form the sciatic foramina from the sacrosciatic notches.

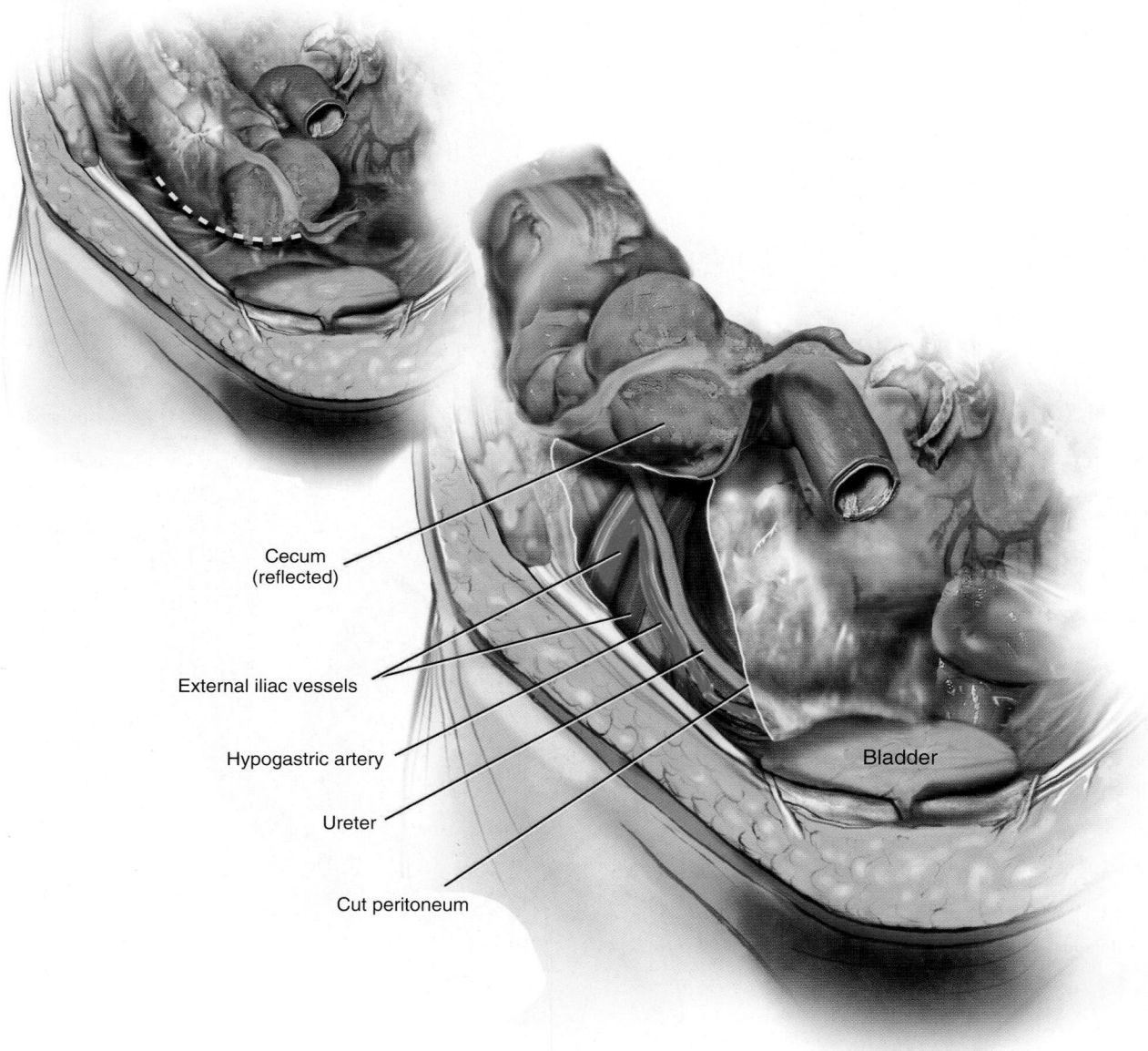

Cecum
(reflected)

External iliac vessels

Hypogastric artery

Ureter

Bladder

Cut peritoneum

**FIGURE 1–26** A quick, safe, and relatively easy technique for entering the retroperitoneal space is illustrated in this drawing. The cecum is grasped, elevated, and pulled to the left. The peritoneum (parietal) supporting the cecum to the right abdominal gutter is cut (*dashed line*). The cecum is mobilized upward. The underlying psoas major muscle, common iliac vessels, and ureter are brought into clear view. Note that the ovarian vessels have been removed in the drawing. This view is oriented from below in a cranial direction. The ovarian vessels have been removed.

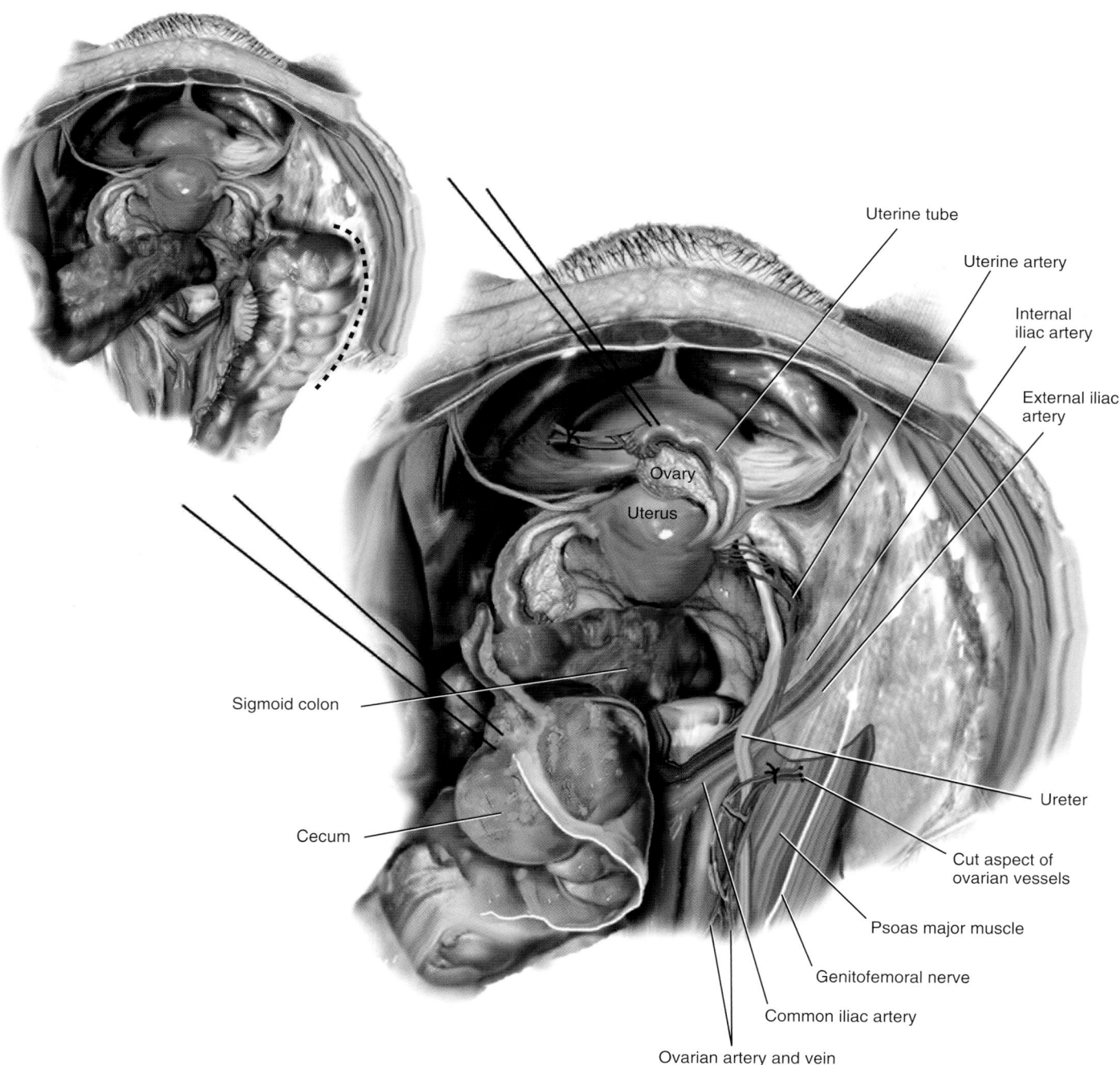

Uterine tube

Uterine artery

Internal iliac artery

External iliac artery

Ovary

Uterus

Sigmoid colon

Cecum

Ureter

Cut aspect of ovarian vessels

Psoas major muscle

Genitofemoral nerve

Common iliac artery

Ovarian artery and vein

**FIGURE 1–27** Exposure of the retroperitoneal space on the right by incising the lateral peritoneal supports, the cecum, and ascending colon (*dashed line*) allows the large bowel to be mobilized toward the left. The right common iliac vessels, the vena cava, and the ureter are brought into view. The genitofemoral nerve is seen on the surface of the psoas major muscle. The uterine vessels are shown crossing the ureter at the level of the cardinal ligament. Note the right ovarian vessels cut and ligated but overlying the ureter on the right side. This view is oriented to allow observation of the field from above, looking caudally.

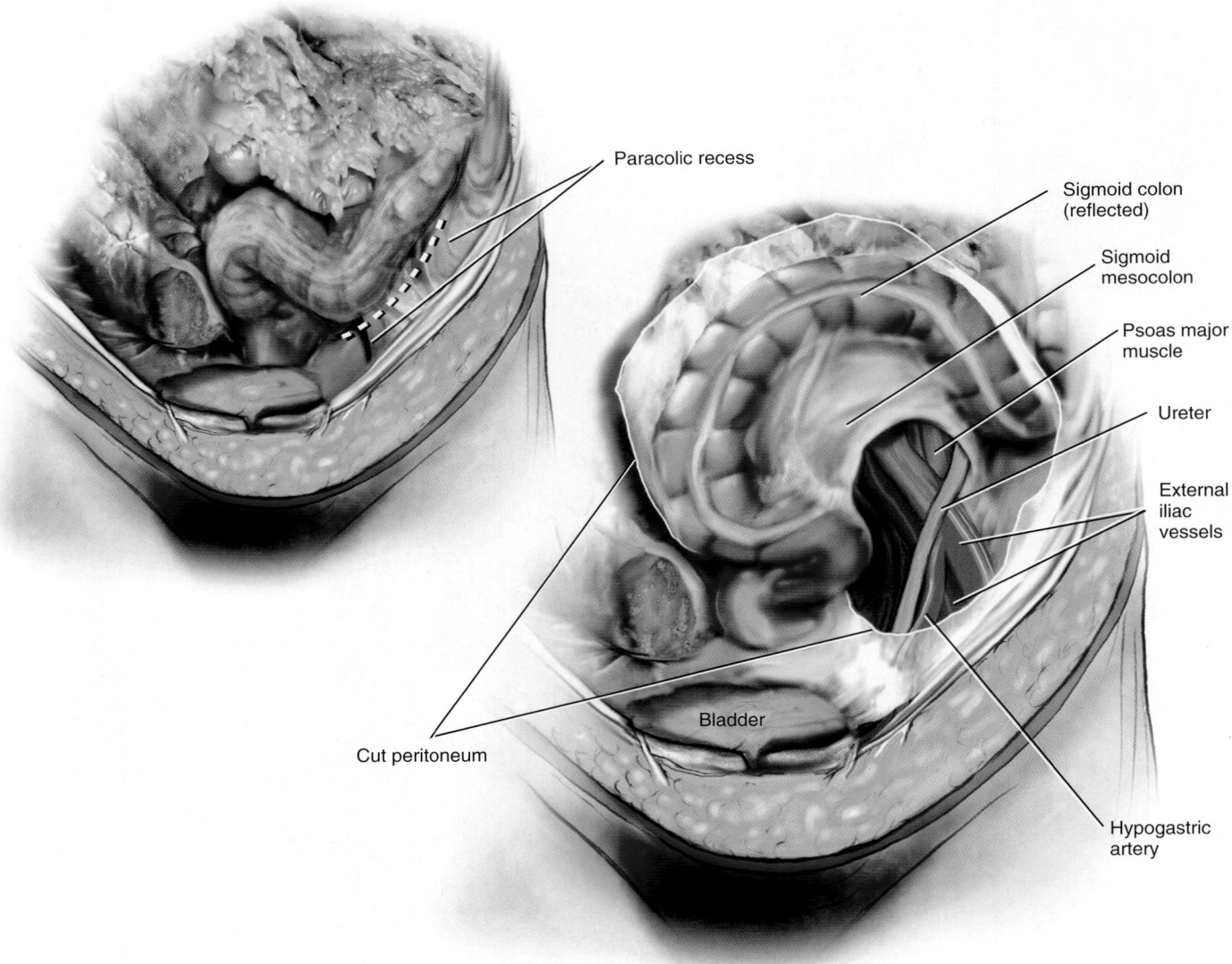

Paracolic recess

Sigmoid colon (reflected)

Sigmoid mesocolon

Psoas major muscle

Ureter

External iliac vessels

Bladder

Cut peritoneum

Hypogastric artery

**FIGURE 1–28** The technique for exposure of the retroperitoneal space on the left side is shown. The sigmoid colon is grasped, elevated, and pulled to the right. The lateral peritoneal attachments of the sigmoid and descending colon are cut along the left gutter (*dashed line* in **inset**), permitting free mobilization of the large bowel. The left psoas major crosses the sigmoid colon at a perfect 90° angle. The left common iliac vessels and the left ureter are brought into view. The left ovarian vessels, which overlie the ureter, have been removed in this drawing. The ovarian vessels (infundibulopelvic ligament) are not shown in this drawing (i.e., they have been removed).

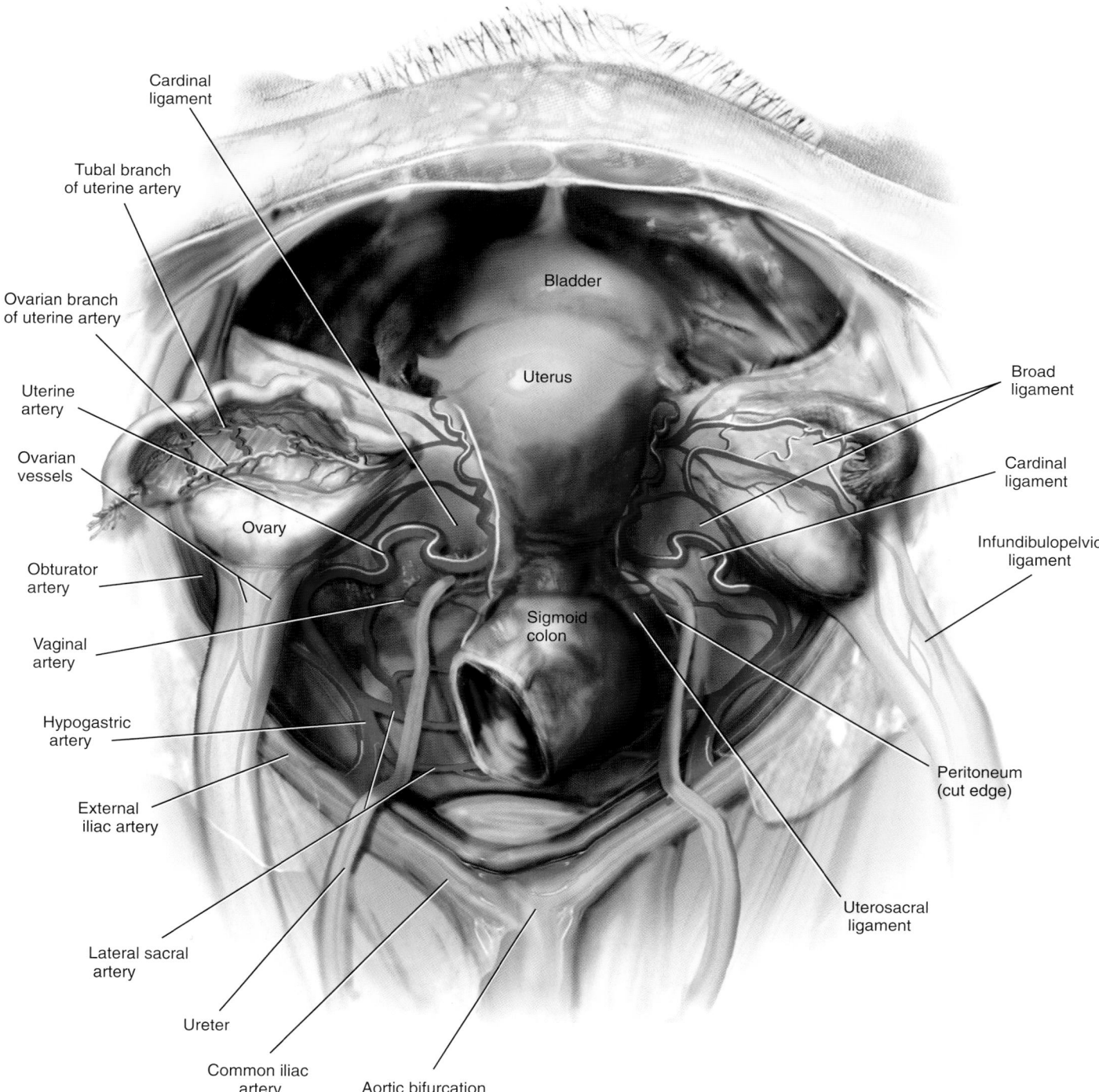

Cardinal ligament

Tubal branch of uterine artery

Ovarian branch of uterine artery

Uterine artery

Ovarian vessels

Ovary

Obturator artery

Vaginal artery

Hypogastric artery

External iliac artery

Lateral sacral artery

Ureter

Common iliac artery

Aortic bifurcation

Bladder

Uterus

Sigmoid colon

Broad ligament

Cardinal ligament

Infundibulopelvic ligament

Peritoneum (cut edge)

Uterosacral ligament

**FIGURE 1–29** This view from the back shows the course of the ureters as they descend deeply into the pelvis. Note that the ureters are closely approximated to the medial-lying hypogastric arteries. The ovarian vessels have been pulled laterally to separate them from the ureters and to better expose the ureters. The cardinal ligaments have been exposed by incising the posterior leaf of the broad ligament. Note the uterine vessels above and the vaginal vessels below as the ureters curve inward during their short journey through the cardinal ligaments. The infundibulopelvic ligament (ovarian vessels) has been retracted laterally and away from the ureters in this picture. In actual dissection, the ovarian vessels and the ureters cross over the common iliac vessels very close to one another.

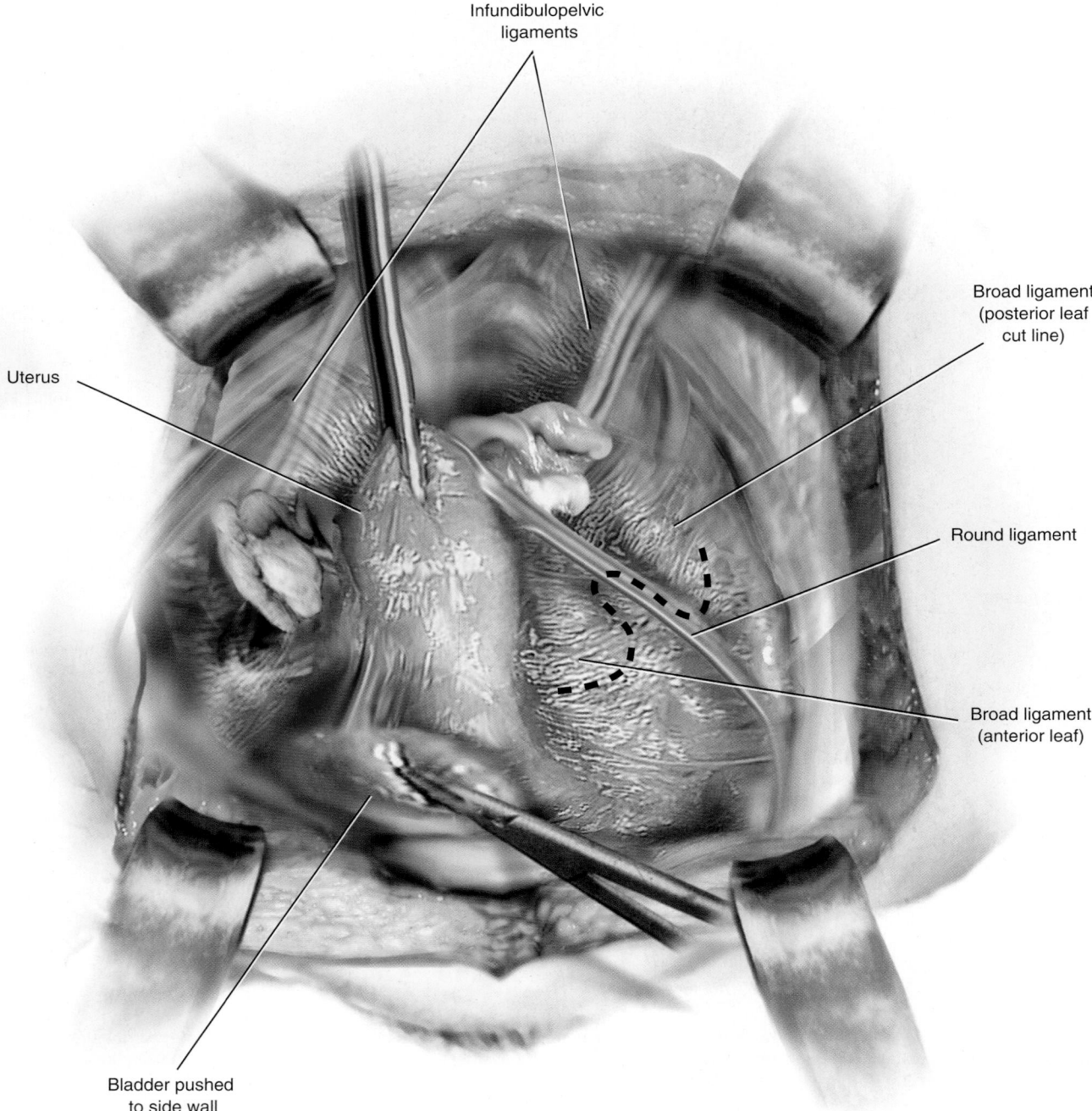

Infundibulopelvic
ligaments

Broad ligament
(posterior leaf
cut line)

Uterus

Round ligament

Broad ligament
(anterior leaf)

Bladder pushed
to side wall

**FIGURE 1–30** The uterus is pulled upward by means of a fundal clamp. This technique places the broad ligament on tension and makes it easier to see. The dashed line shows how an incision will be made through the top of the ligament and extended to open the anterior and posterior leaves.

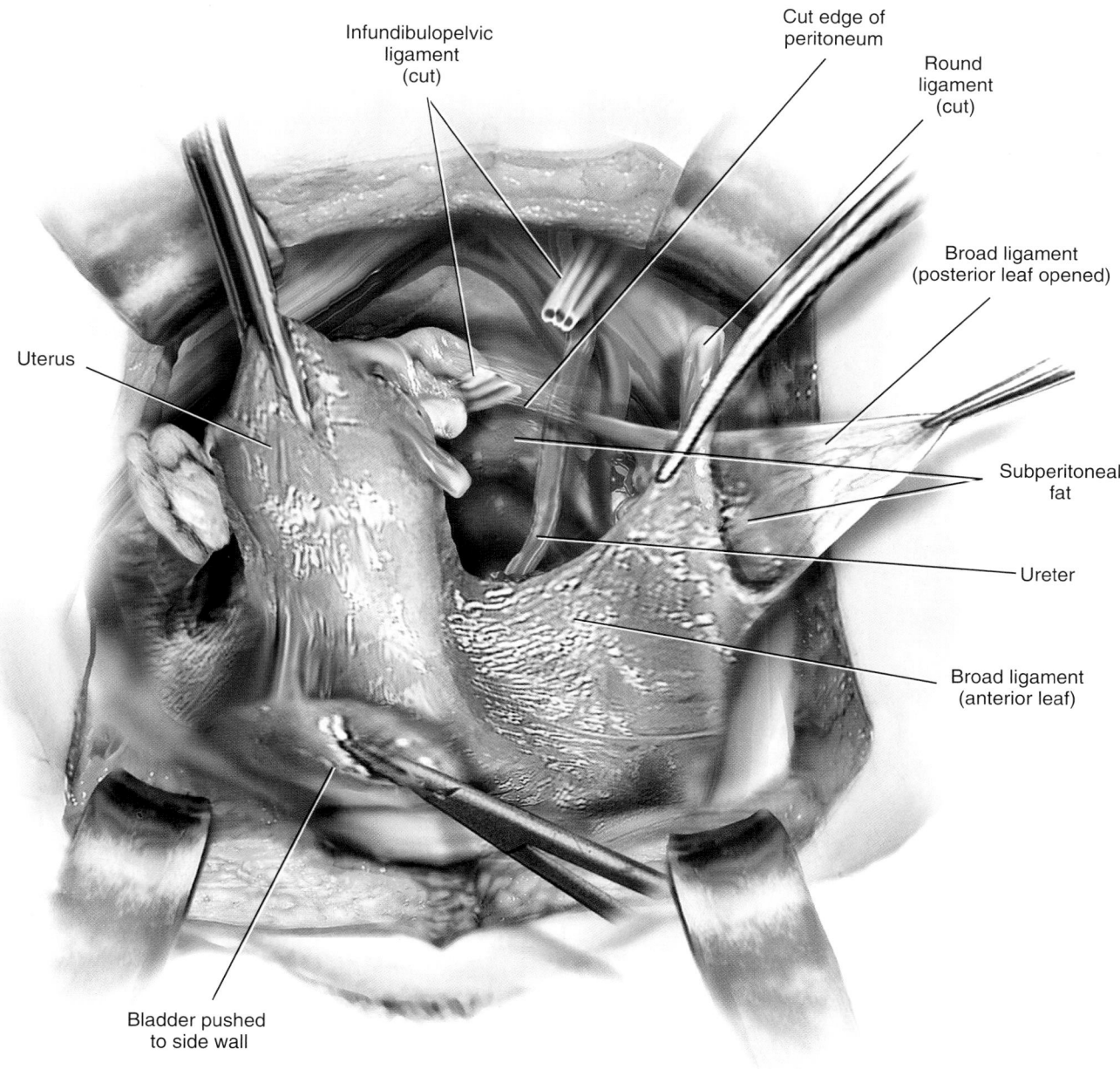

Infundibulopelvic
ligament
(cut)

Cut edge of
peritoneum

Round
ligament
(cut)

Broad ligament
(posterior leaf opened)

Uterus

Subperitoneal
fat

Ureter

Broad ligament
(anterior leaf)

Bladder pushed
to side wall

**FIGURE 1–31** The left broad ligament has been opened. The loose areolar tissues between the leaves have been dissected to expose the deeply situated left ureter.

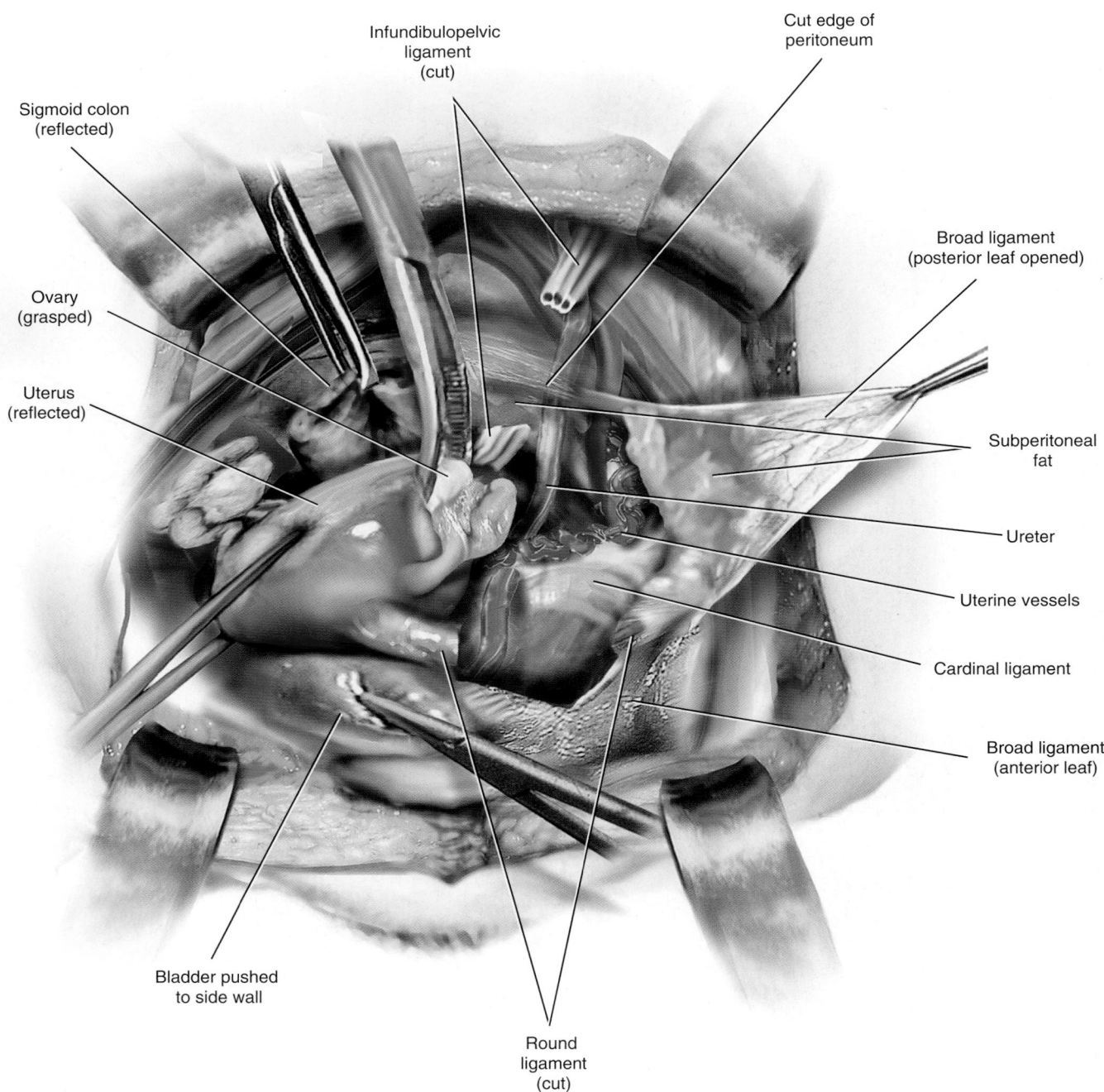

Infundibulopelvic
ligament
(cut)

Cut edge of
peritoneum

Sigmoid colon
(reflected)

Broad ligament
(posterior leaf opened)

Ovary
(grasped)

Subperitoneal
fat

Uterus
(reflected)

Ureter

Uterine vessels

Cardinal ligament

Broad ligament
(anterior leaf)

Bladder pushed
to side wall

Round
ligament
(cut)

**FIGURE 1–32** The ureter is further dissected to expose the uterine arteries crossing over the ureter.

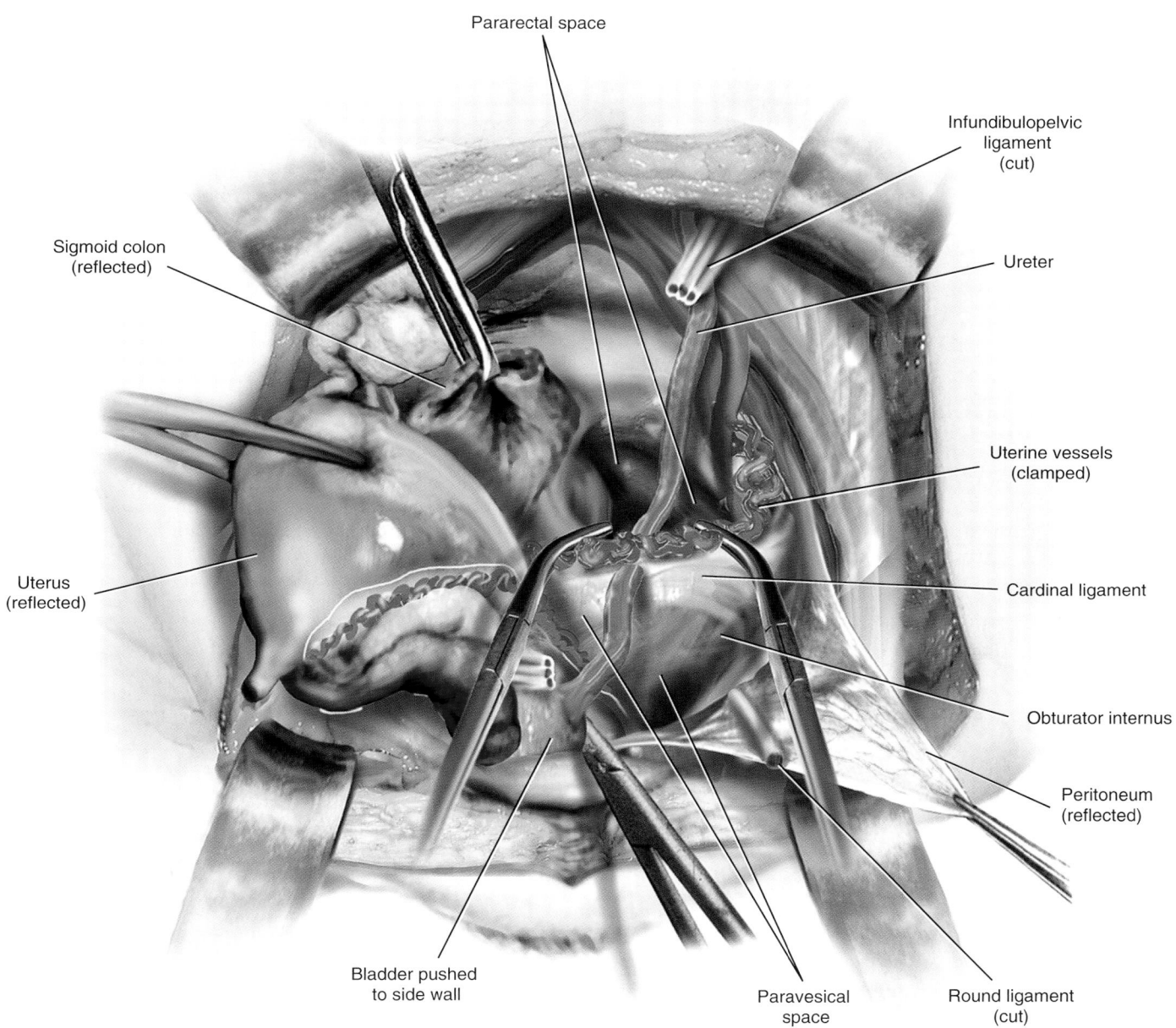

Pararectal space

Infundibulopelvic ligament (cut)

Sigmoid colon (reflected)

Ureter

Uterine vessels (clamped)

Uterus (reflected)

Cardinal ligament

Obturator internus

Peritoneum (reflected)

Bladder pushed to side wall

Paravesical space

Round ligament (cut)

**FIGURE 1–33** The uterus is rotated to stretch the ureter and uterine vessels. Tonsil clamps are placed on the uterine artery to divide it above the point where the ureter crosses under it. The entire course of the ureter is visible.

The blood supply to the uterus is generous. The **uterine artery** is a major branch of the **anterior division of the hypogastric artery.** The uterine artery in the vicinity of the junction of the cervix and uterine body splits into **ascending** and **descending branches.** The former is a coiled vessel that makes its way up the side of the uterus beneath the round ligament to the area between the junction of the tube, utero-ovarian ligament, and upper uterine corpus. At that point, the **uterine** and **ovarian arteries** anastomose (Figs. 1–34 and 1–35).

Just before the uterine artery bifurcation, the **vaginal artery** may come off a common trunk, with the uterine artery. Alternatively, the vaginal artery may arise directly as a branch of the main hypogastric artery. Several sources of collateral circulation may be observed relative to the pelvic viscera. Although the hypogastric artery may be bilaterally ligated, blood flow to the pelvic organs continues via these collaterals. The **inferior mesenteric** and **ovarian vessels** are examples of collaterals via **middle** and **inferior hemorrhoidal** connections, as well as between ovarian and uterine branches of **tubo-ovarian vessels** (see Figs. 1–34 and 1–35).

The **vagina** is a musculoepithelial tube extending from the level of the external genitals to the cervical portion of the uterus. It is a reproductive conduit in all respects, connecting the external environment to the internal genitalia. Anatomically, the vagina is anchored caudally and directly at the **introitus** by the **levator ani muscles** and **bulbocavernosus muscles.** Indirectly, other structures may contribute to the caudal vaginal support; these include the **external sphincter ani, superficial transverse perineal muscles,** and the **perineal membrane.** The anterior and posterior vaginal walls share fascial support in a manner analogous to that in unibody automobile construction with the **bladder/urethra** and **rectum/anus.** The vagina is intimately close to the **bulb of the vestibule** and **clitoral apparatus.** At the upper (cranial) end, the vagina shares support with the same structures that support the uterus. Specifically, these are the **cardinal** and **uterosacral ligaments** (Fig. 1–36).

Between the two terminals, the vagina is relatively flexible and may be easily freed from surrounding fatty tissue and loose fascia. Anteriorly and posteriorly, the potential spaces are the vesicovaginal and rectovaginal, respectively. Laterally, on either side, the free space may be identified by cutting medially to the bulbocavernosus and levator ani muscles and developing the space along the outer wall of the vagina.

The relationship of the **lower ureters** to the **uterosacral ligaments** and **anterolateral vagina** is important in that injuries to the ureters are most likely to occur in areas where there is close proximity of structures such as these. Similarly, the **cervix uteri** and **anterior fornix** of the vagina are intimately close to the bladder base (**trigone** and **interureteric ridge**). Because multiple operations (e.g., hysterectomy [vaginal and abdominal], cervical suture, colposuspension, transvaginal urethral suspensions, culdoplasty) are performed in the area,

knowledge of the anatomy of the vagina, ureters, and bladder is vital for avoiding unintended iatrogenic injury (Figs. 1–37 and 1–38).

The **hypogastric plexus** is anterior to the lower aorta and enters the presacral space from above over the retroperitoneal fat anterior to the left common iliac vein and middle sacral vessels and to the right of the inferior mesenteric vessels. As the plexus descends into the hollow of the sacrum, it typically splits into right and left divisions. The **inferior hypogastric plexuses** join other nerves to form the **pelvic plexuses,** which in turn are named for the organ with which they are associated. The hypogastric plexus is a conduit for autonomic nerves, as well as visceral pain fibers. The pelvic plexuses contain visceral and parasympathetic fibers from sacral roots 2, 3, and 4 and sympathetic fibers via the sympathetic trunks and hypogastric plexus (Figs. 1–39 and 1–40).

Several of the large nerves of the pelvis and inferior extremity originate deep in the retroperitoneum of the lower abdomen and pelvis. The plexuses include **lumbar, sacral,** and **coccygeal** (Fig. 1–41). The lumbar plexus is buried deeply beneath the substance of the psoas major muscle. The subcostal nerve sends a branch to the first lumbar nerve and should be considered part of the plexus. The following nerves emanate from the **lumbar plexus** (see Fig. 1–41):

1. Iliohypogastric
2. Ilioinguinal
3. Genitofemoral
4. Lateral femoral cutaneous
5. Obturator
6. Femoral

The **lumbosacral trunk** consists of the anterior ramus of the fifth lumbar nerve joined to the descending branch of the fourth lumbar nerve. The lumbosacral trunk and the anterior rami of sacral nerves 1, 2, and 3, as well as the upper fourth sacral anterior root, form the **sacral plexus.** The **sciatic nerve** consists of fibers from the lumbosacral trunk, as well as sacral roots 1, 2, and 3. The **pudendal nerve** springs from the second, third, and fourth sacral nerves and leaves the pelvis between the piriformis and coccygeus muscles (see Fig. 1–41).

The following additional nerves have their origin in the sacral plexus:

1. Superior gluteal
2. Inferior gluteal
3. Posterior cutaneous nerve
4. Nerve to quadratus femoris
5. Nerve to obturator internus
6. Perforating cutaneous nerve
7. Perineal branch of fourth sacral nerve

The lymph channels of the pelvis generally follow the course of the major blood vessels. The **pelvic lymph nodes** are located at various vascular and nonvascular sites (Fig. 1–42).

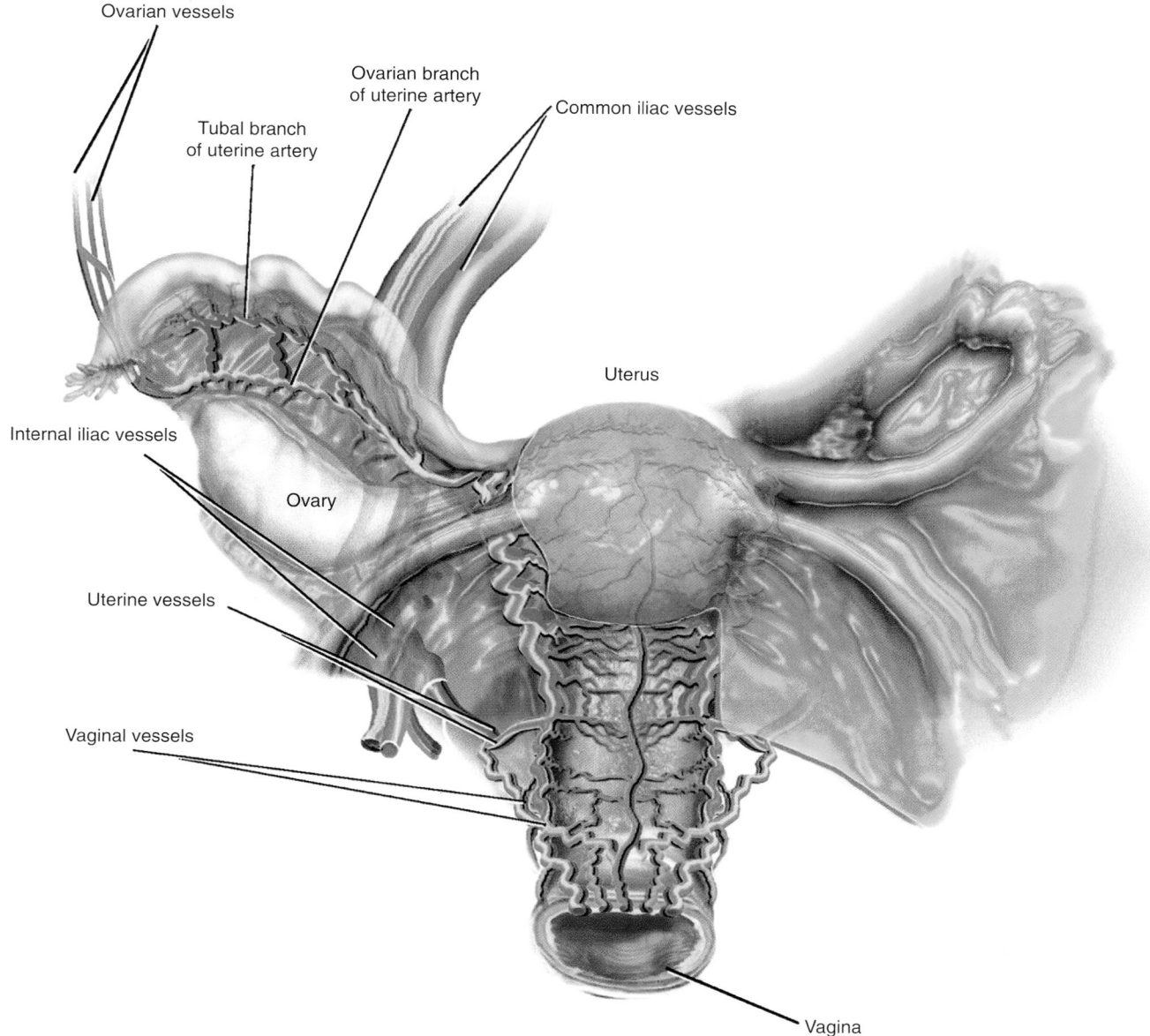

Ovarian vessels

Ovarian branch
of uterine artery

Tubal branch
of uterine artery

Common iliac vessels

Uterus

Internal iliac vessels

Ovary

Uterine vessels

Vaginal vessels

Vagina

**FIGURE 1–34** This illustration details the blood supply to the uterus and upper half of the vagina. The anterior division of the internal iliac, or hypogastric, artery branches to give off the uterine and vaginal arteries. Not uncommonly, these vessels emanate from a common arterial trunk (as illustrated here). The uterine artery passes obliquely through the lower portion of the broad ligament to reach the upper portion of the uterine cervix at a point where cervix and corpus fuse. The uterine artery divides to form an ascending branch, which heads up the side of the uterus to the level of the fundus, and a descending or cervical branch, which heads downward toward the cervix and its ultimate anastomosis with the vaginal artery. Plentiful cross-uterine anastomoses occur where the ascending branch of the uterine artery reaches the point at which the oviduct joins the fundus of the uterus. It anastomoses with the ovarian and tubal branches of the ovarian artery.

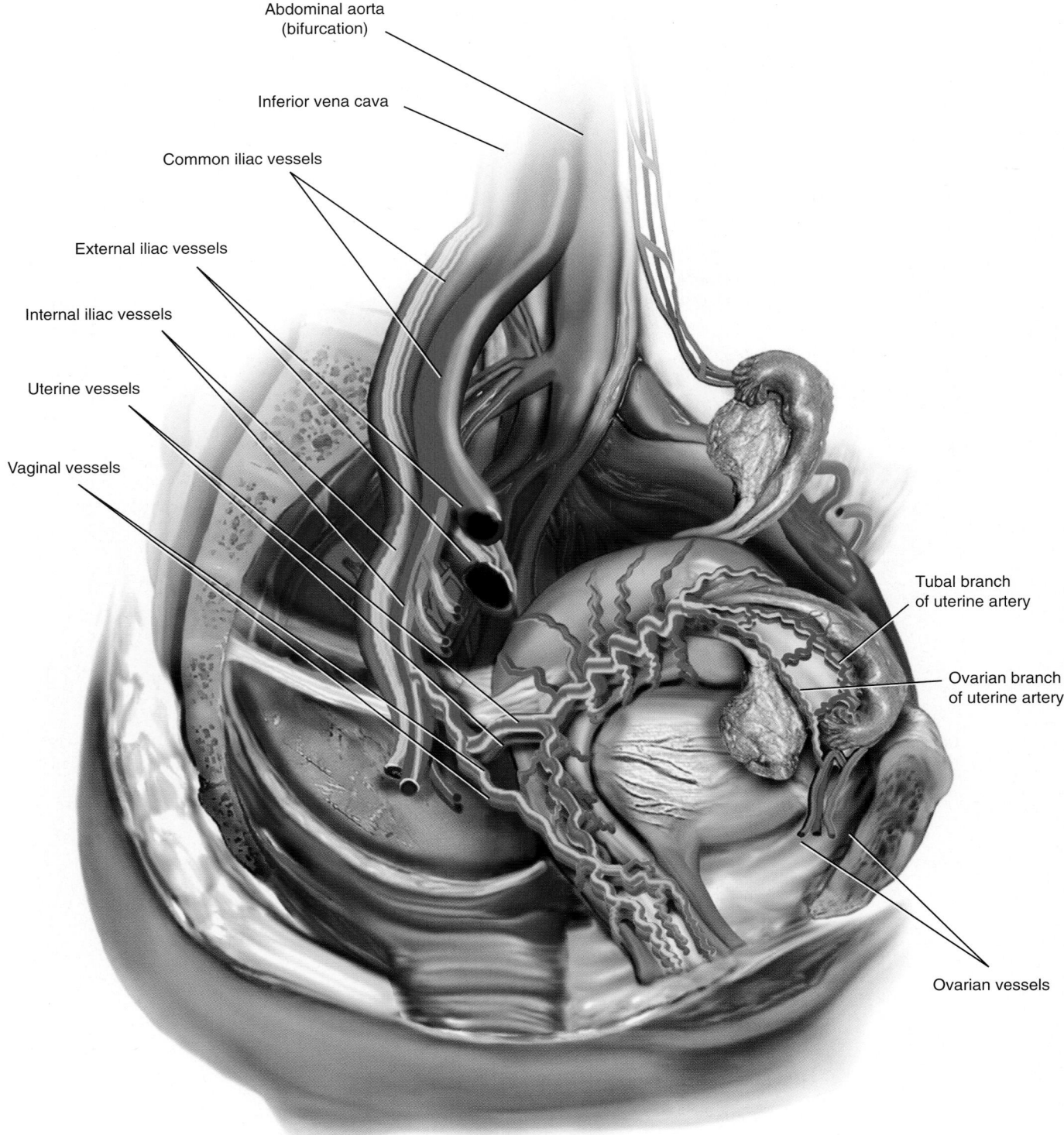

Abdominal aorta
(bifurcation)

Inferior vena cava

Common iliac vessels

External iliac vessels

Internal iliac vessels

Uterine vessels

Vaginal vessels

Tubal branch
of uterine artery

Ovarian branch
of uterine artery

Ovarian vessels

**FIGURE 1–35** Sagittal view of the uterine artery and vein. Note the close relationship of the bifurcation of the uterine vessels and the uterosacral ligaments. The main trunk of the artery is just lateral to the point where the uterosacral ligament attaches to the uterus. The anastomosis between the descending branch of the uterine artery and the vaginal artery is clearly seen. The ureter has been excluded from the drawing on the right side.

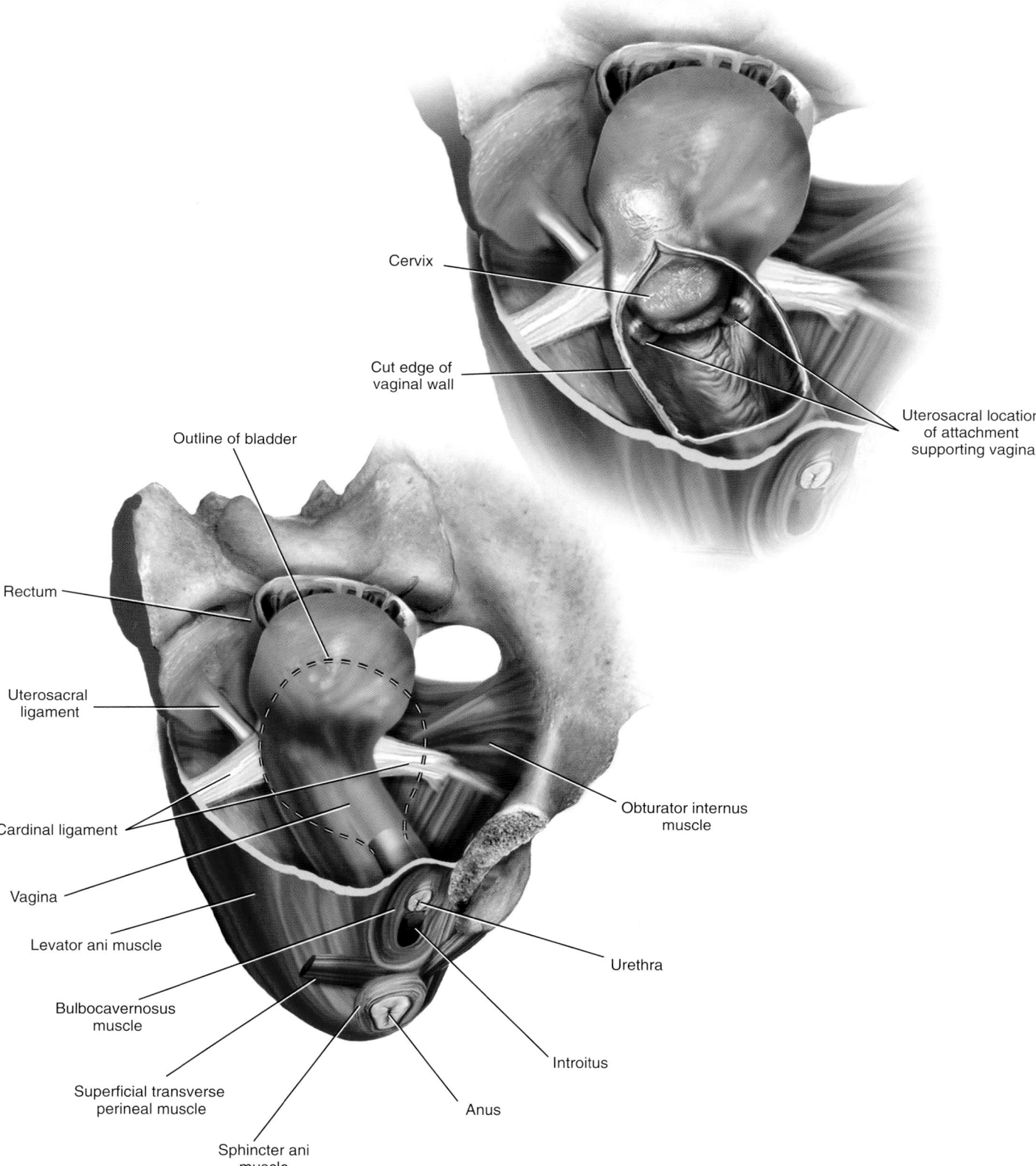

Cervix

Cut edge of
vaginal wall

Uterosacral location
of attachment
supporting vagina

Outline of bladder

Rectum

Uterosacral
ligament

Cardinal ligament

Vagina

Levator ani muscle

Bulbocavernosus
muscle

Superficial transverse
perineal muscle

Sphincter ani
muscle

Anus

Introitus

Urethra

Obturator internus
muscle

**FIGURE 1–36** This three-dimensional drawing shows the relationships of the vagina to other structures in the pelvis. The lower figure also shows the superimposed outline of the urinary bladder relative to the vagina. The upper vagina shares support with the uterus and bladder. Principally, this consists of the deep cardinal ligament and, to a lesser extent, the uterosacral ligaments. Note in the upper illustration the schematically drawn location of the portion of the uterosacral ligaments that attach to the vagina.

The lower vagina is clearly supported by the levator ani muscle, the anal sphincter, and the deep vascular structures located beneath the bulbocavernosus muscle, as well as by the commonly shared connective tissue, smooth muscle, and vessels found in the tissues between the rectum and vagina, and, likewise, between the bladder and vagina. Between these anchors, the lateral vaginal wall is not attached and opens into fat-filled paravaginal space. If the lateral wall is cut and the fat being dissected is removed, the anatomist will be looking into a retropubic (extraperitoneal) space filled with fat. If the fat is cleaned away, the obturator internus muscle is visible.

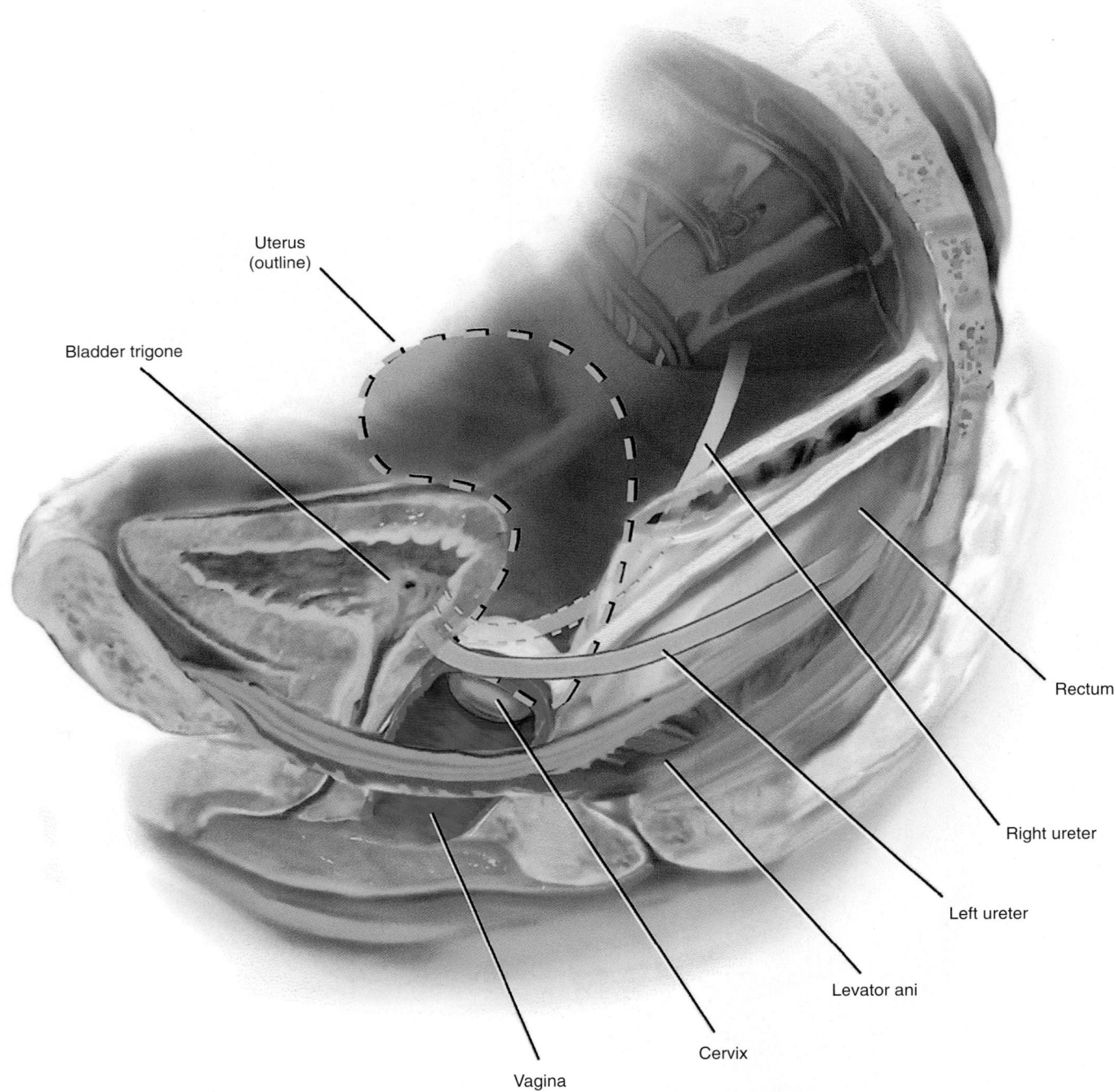

Uterus
(outline)

Bladder trigone

Rectum

Right ureter

Left ureter

Levator ani

Cervix

Vagina

**FIGURE 1–37** Sagittal view of the ureters and urinary bladder shown in relation to the vagina (*green*) and the uterus (*dark pink*). Note that the bladder base and trigone are closely applied to the anterior vaginal fornix and to the cervix, as well as to the cervicocorpal junction. The ureters cross the anterolateral aspects of the vaginal fornices just before entering the bladder wall. Sutures placed too high into the vagina during a colposuspension operation could conceivably injure the ureter(s).

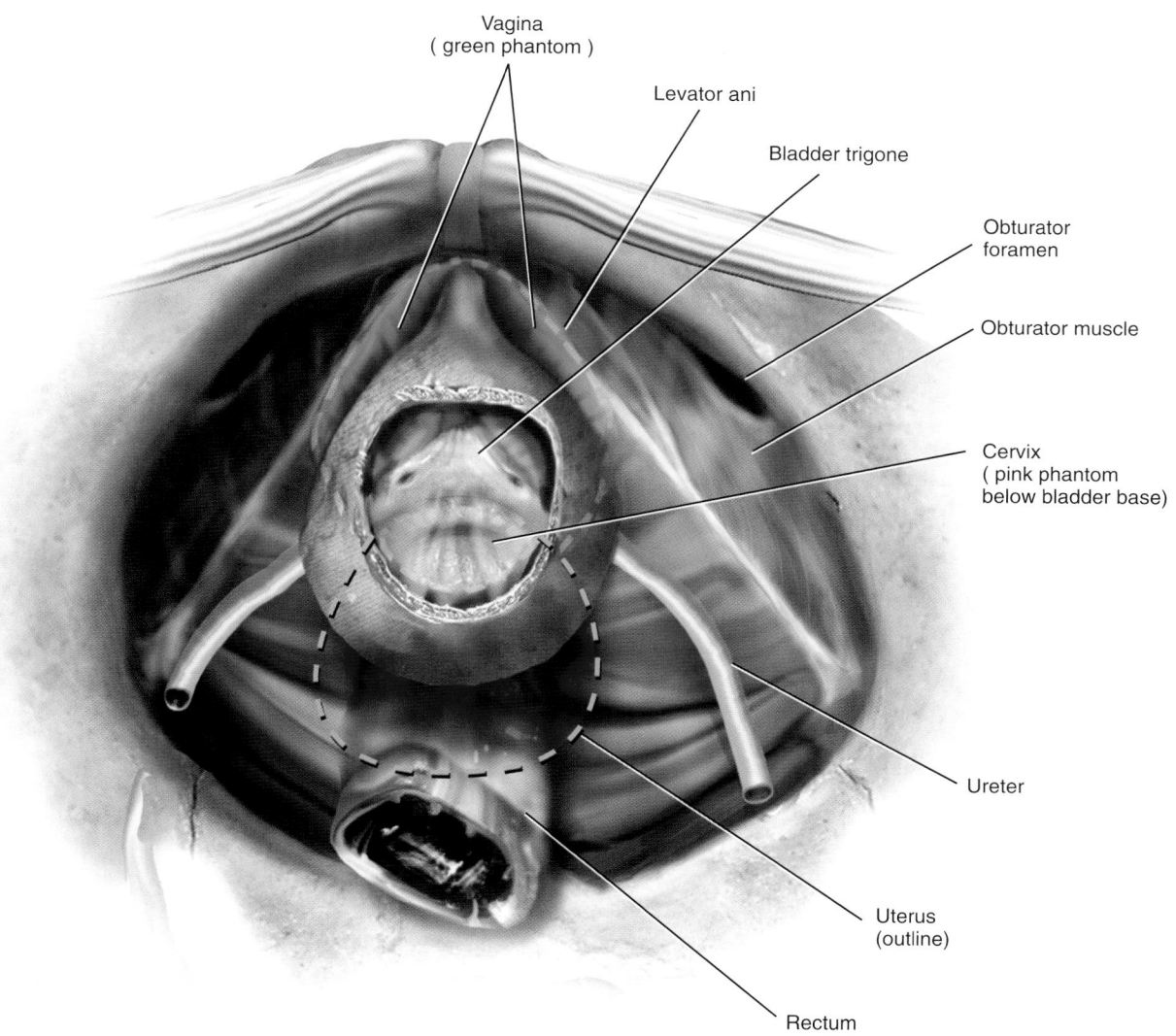

**FIGURE 1–38** This full frontal view of the bladder with an anterior window of tissue excised shows the trigone and interureteric ridge. Beneath the bladder posteriorly lies the (phantom) uterus and cervix, which are *pink*. Note that the bladder base overlies the cervix and vagina (*green*). The phantom vagina is seen because this stylized drawing has presumed to make the posterior wall of the bladder selectively transparent. Again, note that a misplaced and high suture placed in the vagina during a colposuspension could injure the terminal ureter. The ureters must traverse the tissue above the anterolateral vaginal fornices to reach the bladder.

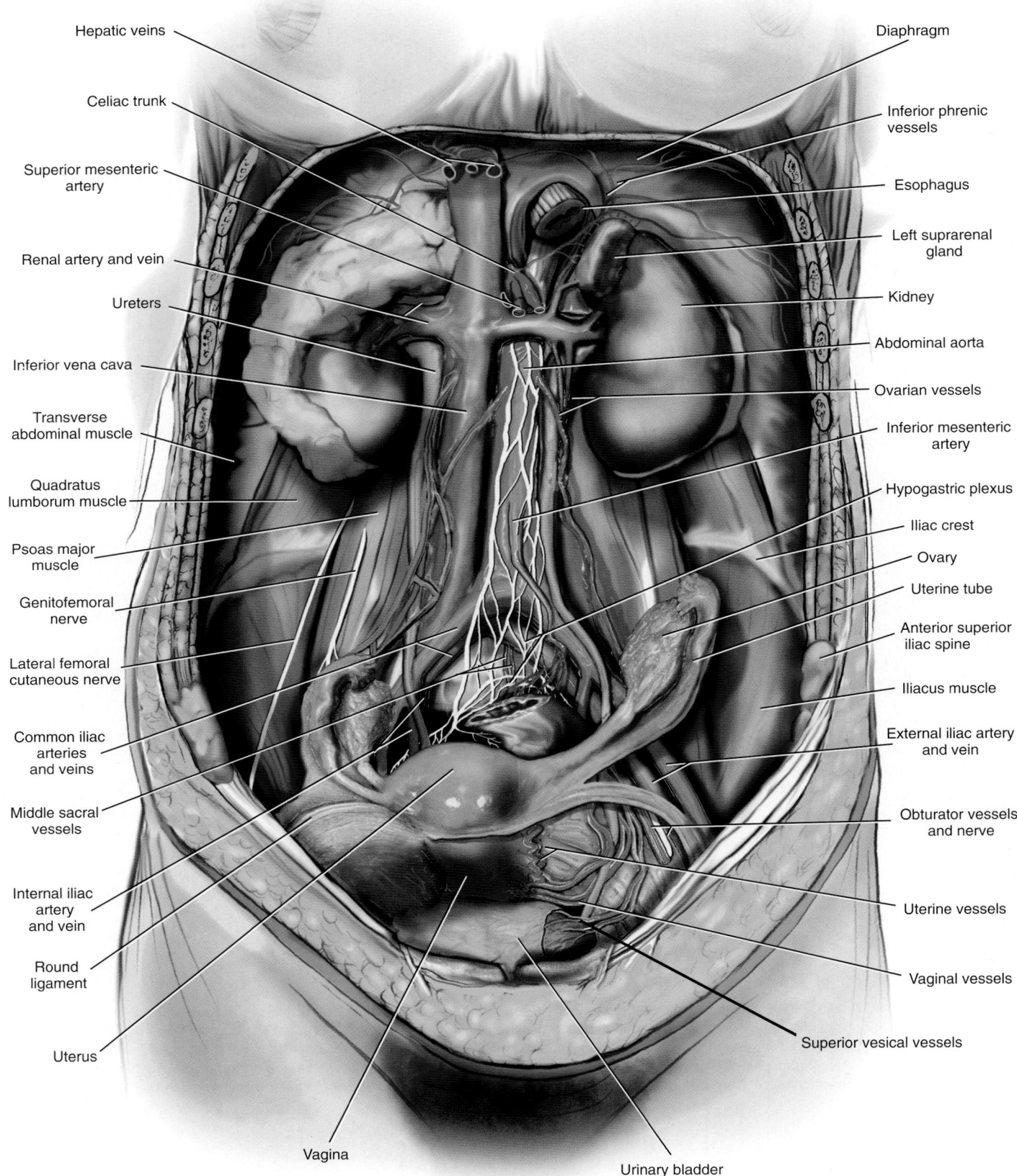

Hepatic veins

Celiac trunk

Superior mesenteric artery

Renal artery and vein

Ureters

Inferior vena cava

Transverse abdominal muscle

Quadratus lumborum muscle

Psoas major muscle

Genitofemoral nerve

Lateral femoral cutaneous nerve

Common iliac arteries and veins

Middle sacral vessels

Internal iliac artery and vein

Round ligament

Uterus

Vagina

Diaphragm

Inferior phrenic vessels

Esophagus

Left suprarenal gland

Kidney

Abdominal aorta

Ovarian vessels

Inferior mesenteric artery

Hypogastric plexus

Iliac crest

Ovary

Uterine tube

Anterior superior iliac spine

Iliacus muscle

External iliac artery and vein

Obturator vessels and nerve

Uterine vessels

Vaginal vessels

Superior vesical vessels

Urinary bladder

**FIGURE 1–39** Full view of the abdomen showing the hypogastric nerve plexus descending into the pelvis superficial to the aorta and the left common iliac vein. Below the bifurcation, the hypogastric nerve is embedded within the fat of the presacral space. The hypogastric nerve plexus is sometimes referred to as "the presacral" nerve.

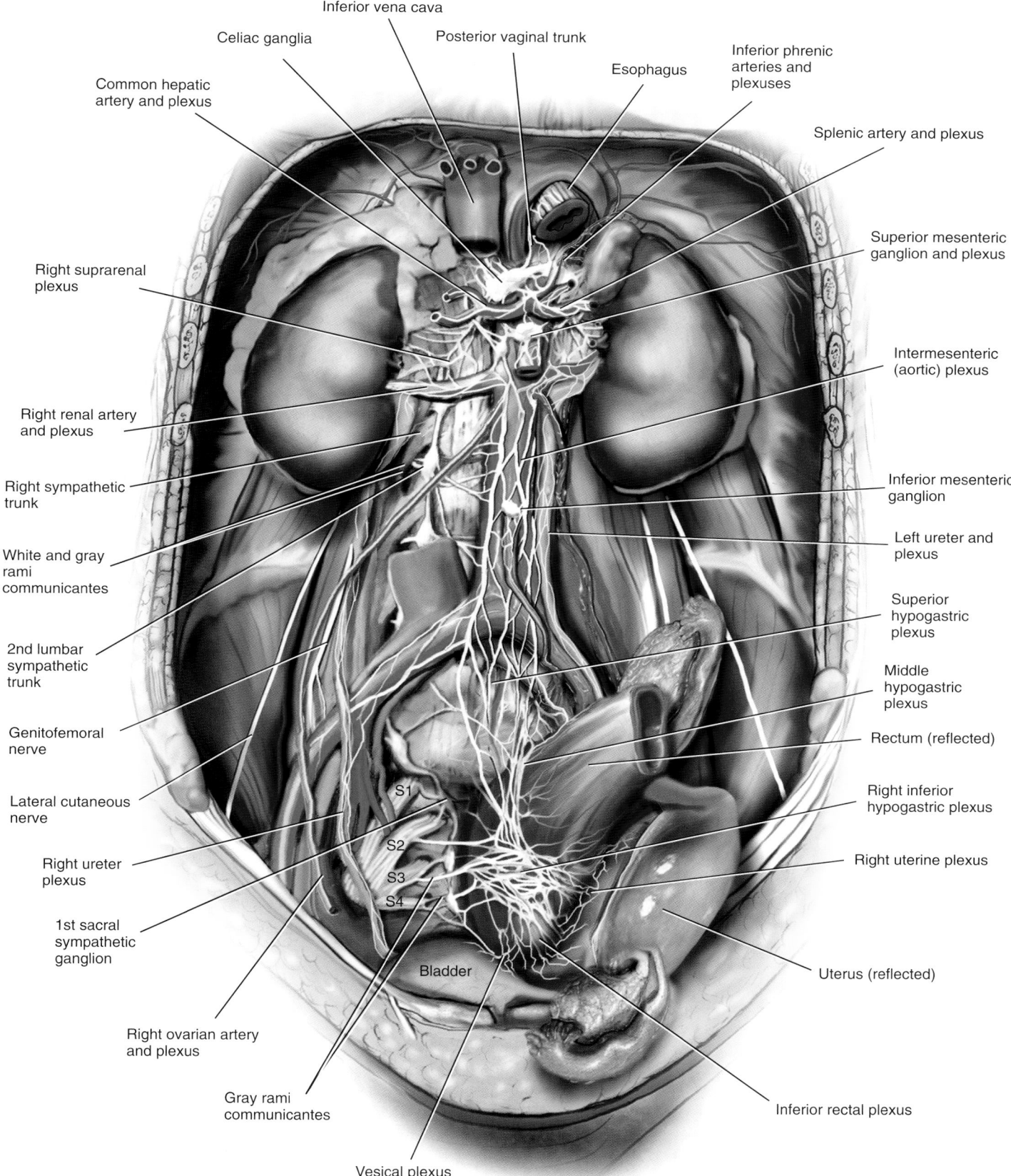

**FIGURE 1–40** The pelvic viscera are innervated via the autonomic nervous system, which can be seen as a somewhat amorphous concentration of nerve fibers and ganglia. These collections are named on that basis of the organ(s) they supply, for example, vesical, uterine. The sympathetic fibers originate in the thoracic and lumbar segments of the spinal cord and reach the pelvic organs via the hypogastric plexus. In this illustration, the superior, middle, and inferior hypogastric plexuses are shown. The parasympathetic contribution joins the inferior hypogastric plexus via the pelvic nerves (sacral nerve roots 2, 3, and 4). The picture shows the pelvic nerves and the inferior hypogastric plexus joining in the right uterine plexus.

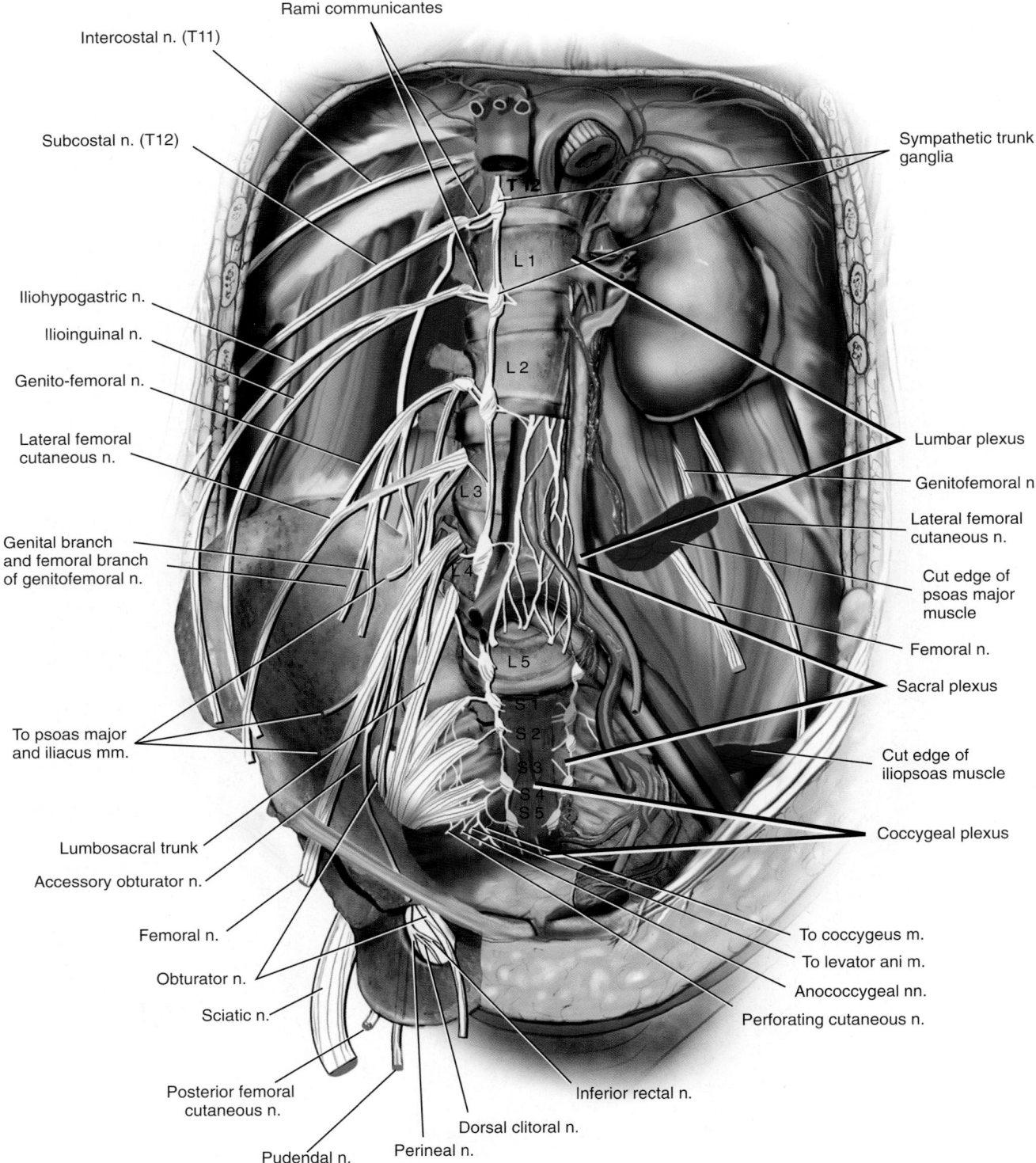

Rami communicantes

Intercostal n. (T11)

Subcostal n. (T12)

Iliohypogastric n.

Ilioinguinal n.

Genito-femoral n.

Lateral femoral
cutaneous n.

Genital branch
and femoral branch
of genitofemoral n.

To psoas major
and iliacus mm.

Lumbosacral trunk

Accessory obturator n.

Femoral n.

Obturator n.

Sciatic n.

Posterior femoral
cutaneous n.

Pudendal n.

Perineal n.

Dorsal clitoral n.

Inferior rectal n.

Perforating cutaneous n.

Anococcygeal nn.

To levator ani m.

To coccygeus m.

Coccygeal plexus

Cut edge of
iliopsoas muscle

Sacral plexus

Femoral n.

Cut edge of
psoas major
muscle

Lateral femoral
cutaneous n.

Genitofemoral n.

Lumbar plexus

Sympathetic trunk
ganglia

T 12

L 1

L 2

L 3

L 4

L 5

S 1

S 2

S 3

S 4

S 5

**FIGURE 1–41** The lumbar and sacral plexuses shown here contribute efferent and afferent fibers to the major somatic nerves of the pelvis and inferior extremity. The lumbosacral trunk and the first four sacral nerves form the sacral plexus.

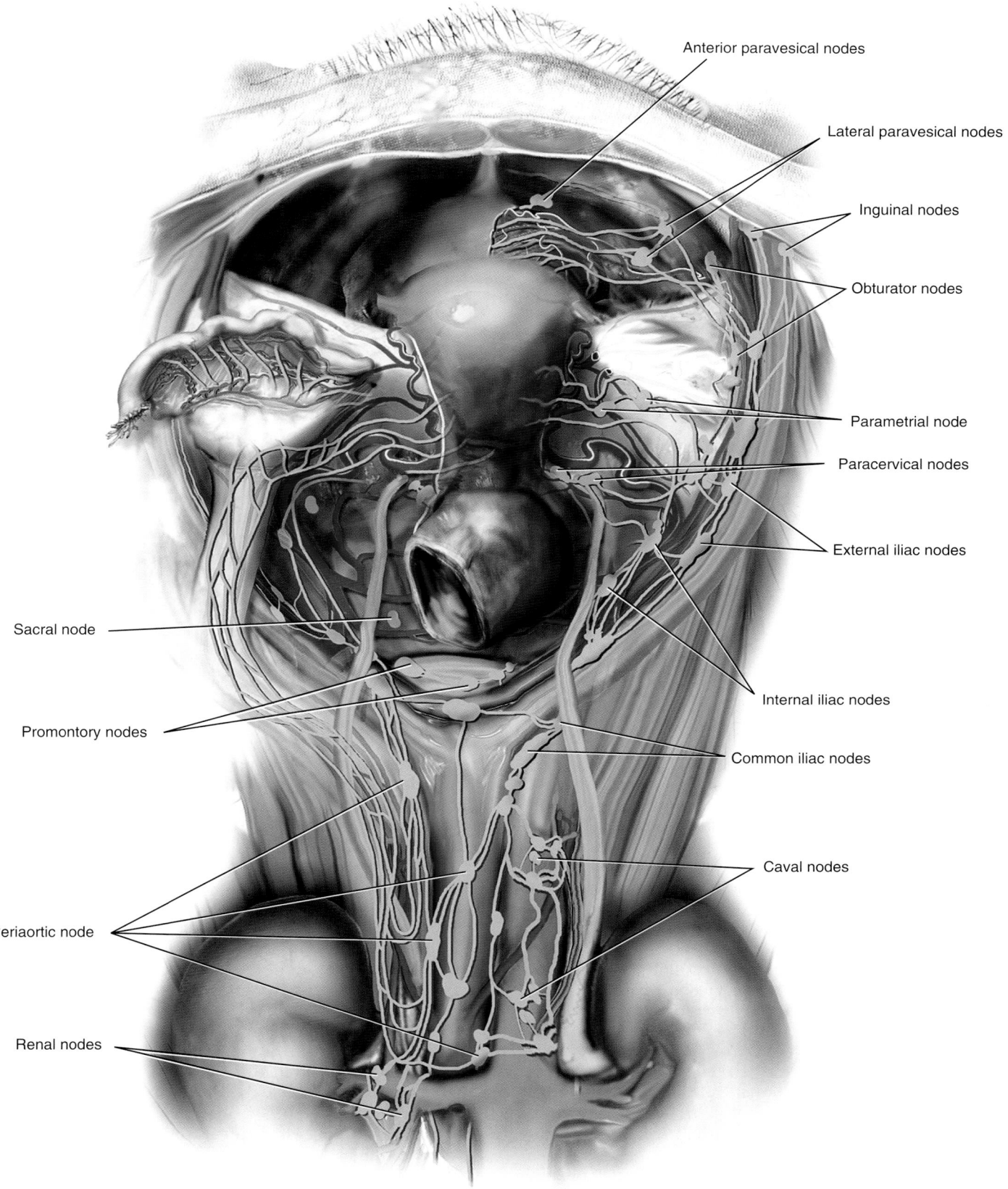

Anterior paravesical nodes

Lateral paravesical nodes

Inguinal nodes

Obturator nodes

Parametrial node

Paracervical nodes

External iliac nodes

Internal iliac nodes

Common iliac nodes

Caval nodes

Sacral node

Promontory nodes

Periaortic node

Renal nodes

**FIGURE 1–42** The lymphatic vessels and nodes of the pelvic viscera are shown. Note the relationship of the primary cervical drainage to the paracervical lymph nodes located at the point where the uterine vessels cross above the ureter. The parametrial lymph vessels draining the corpus and fundus drain into nodes located in the obturator fossa and the internal iliac nodes. The ovarian lymph vessels drain along a course following the ovarian veins to periaortic, caval, and renal lymph nodes. Lymphatics along the round ligament drain into groin lymph nodes.

From the cervix, channels drain into a series of **primary nodes:**

1. **Parametrial nodes** at the junction of the corpus and cervix located within the fat of the broad ligament.
2. **Paracervical nodes** located at the point where the uterine artery crosses over the ureter.
3. **Obturator nodes** located within the fat of the obturator fossa surrounding the obturator nerve and blood vessels.
4. **Internal iliac nodes** located along the hypogastric vein and in the crotch between the divisions of the common iliac artery.
5. **External iliac nodes** located between the artery and the vein.
6. **Sacral nodes** located along the middle sacral vessels and the sacral promontory and the lateral margins of the sacrum.

Secondary lymph nodes consist of the following:

A. The **common iliac lymph nodes,** which lie on both lateral and medial surfaces of the iliac arteries and veins.
B. The **periaortic nodes,** which lie on the anterior and lateral surfaces of the aorta from the bifurcation to the diaphragm.
C. The **inguinal lymph nodes,** above and around the femoral vein and artery and the great saphenous vein.

If one were to draw a transverse line through the middle of the cervix at the vaginal attachment, it would divide the lymphatic drainage into **superior and inferior segments,** with the former draining the **upper cervix** and **lower uterus** into the **hypogastric nodes,** and the latter draining the **lower cervix** and **upper vagina** into the **lateral sacral nodes** (Fig. 1-43).

**Interiliac nodes** are located at the bifurcation of the common iliac arteries and along the external and hypogastric vessels. Uterine fundal lymphatics may drain along the round and inguinal ligaments to the superficial and deep inguinal nodes. Similarly, the lymph vessels that drain the ovaries follow the ovarian arteries and veins, hence to the **pericaval, periaortic,** and right and left **renal nodes.**

The **vulva** consists of the labia majora, labia minora, vestibule, clitoral and periclitoral tissues, and perineum (Fig. 1-44). The **greater vulva** would include the mons veneris, crural tissues, and anal and perianal skin and structures. The **vestibule** contains many mucus-secreting glands and their ducts. The urethra and vagina also open into the vestibule. Beneath the vulvar skin is fatty subcutaneous tissue. The general contour of the vulva is largely created by fat and the deeper, Colles' fascia. The round ligaments and the vestigial canal of Nuck insert into the deep layers of fat within the labium majus.

The **pudendal vessels** and **nerves** are found within the deep fat. The neurovascular bundle emerges just medial to the ischial tuberosity on either side. Branches are given off to the anus and lower rectum, perianal skin, vulvar skin, and superficial and deep vulvar structures (Fig. 1-45). When Colles' fascia is peeled away, the **muscular structures** of the vulva are exposed. These consist of the **external** (and internal) **sphincter ani,** the **superficial transverse perineal muscle,** the **ischiocavernosus muscle,** and the **bulbocavernosus muscle.** Bridging the space between the latter three muscles stretches a tough fascial sheet, the **perineal membrane.** When the perineal membrane is opened, the underlying **levator ani** muscle is exposed. The dissector should note the topographic relationships by locating

the ischial tubers and the pubic arch, and by inserting a finger into the rectum and vagina (Fig. 1-46).

By careful dissection, the perineal muscles are separated from the underlying structures. The deep perineal cavernous apparatus is brought into view (Fig. 1-47). This consists of the **bulb of the vestibule, corpora cavernosa clitoris, clitoris body,** and **glans clitoris.** Lying on the underbelly of the **bulbocavernosus muscle** and attached to the vestibular bulb is the **Bartholin gland.** Deep to the space located between the perineal muscles is the levator ani muscle. It is curious that, in both fixed and fresh cadaver dissections, the "perineal body" cannot be found. The muscle directly beneath the perineal skin and fat is the external sphincter ani.

The **femoral triangle,** although part of the thigh, is closely linked to the anatomy of the vulva directly and to gynecologic reconstructive surgery indirectly. The muscles of the thigh were discussed and illustrated earlier (see Figs. 1-14 and 1-15). The **great saphenous vein** lies within the fat on the medial aspect of the thigh. Dissection of that large vein cranially will lead the anatomist to an oval depression filled with mesh-like connective tissue (**cribriform fascia**) and the **fossa ovalis** (Fig. 1-48). The saphenous vein empties into the large **femoral vein,** which is itself encased in a very tough **fascial compartment.** Immediately lateral to the femoral vein, likewise within its own fascial compartment, is the **femoral artery,** and lateral to it, the **femoral nerve.** Three small vessels emanating from the femoral vein (or saphenous) and femoral artery may be identified by careful dissection. These are the **superficial external pudendal,** the **superficial epigastric,** and the **superficial circumflex iliac vessels.** Medial to the femoral vein is the femoral canal, whose medial boundary lies against the lacunar ligament.

The **round ligament** encased in transversalis fascia and accompanied by the **genital branch** of the **genital femoral nerve,** as well as the **ilioinguinal nerve,** spills over the pubic bone superficial to Colles' fascia. It inserts deeply within the fat of the labium majus (see Fig. 1-48).

The **lymphatics** of the vulva drain to the thigh (groin) via lymph vessels first to the **superficial inguinal** and secondarily to the **deep inguinal lymph nodes** (femoral nodes). The former (superficial) are associated with the three superficial vessels described earlier, as well as the saphenous vein, and lie within the fat of the thigh (Fig. 1-49).

The deep inguinal (femoral) lymph nodes lie along the femoral vein and femoral canal. They drain into the external iliac nodes. The lowest of the external iliac nodes lies in the femoral canal and is known as **Cloquet's node.**

The vulvar lymphatics cross over from right to left and vice versa within the fat of the mons veneris; therefore, contralateral as well as ipsilateral lesions may drain to the groin nodes on any given side.

The relationships of the major vessels, nerves, lacunar, inguinal ligament, iliopsoas, and pectineus muscles, as well as the pubic bone, are illustrated in Figure 1-50.

In summation, the surgeon must have a precise and thorough knowledge of pelvic anatomy and specifically of the relationship of one structure to neighboring structures at every location within the pelvis. This knowledge is particularly vital when distortion is encountered because of adhesion formation. The basic anatomy is preserved within the underlying retroperitoneum.

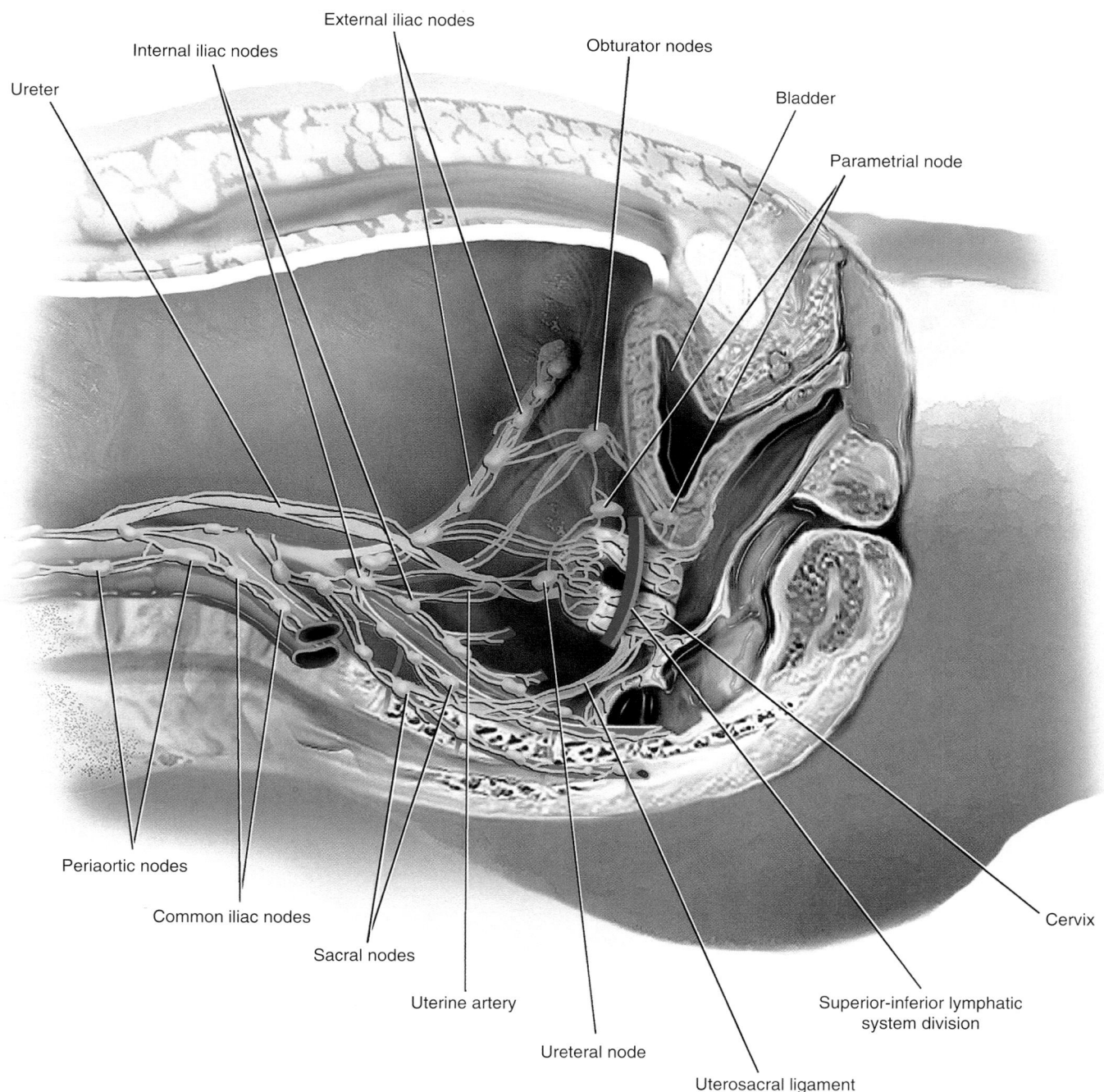

**FIGURE 1–43** This sagittal view illustrates the drainage of the upper cervix (*above the blue divisional line*) into the hypogastric nodes, as well as the lower cervix draining into the lateral sacral nodes. (After Meig's Surgical Treatment of Cancer of the Cervix, 1954, Grune and Stratton, p. 91, with permission.)

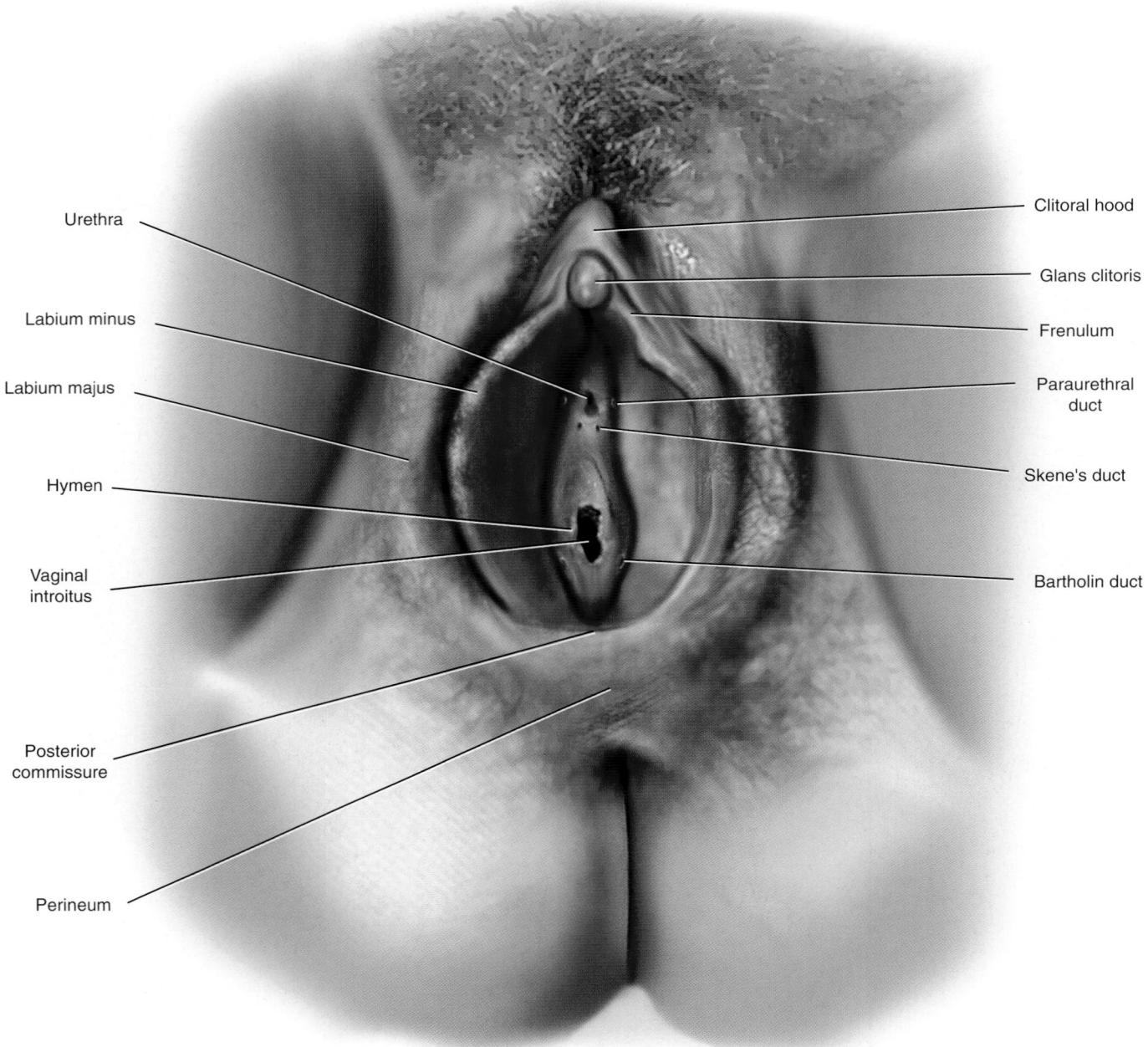

Urethra

Labium minus

Labium majus

Hymen

Vaginal introitus

Posterior commissure

Perineum

Clitoral hood

Glans clitoris

Frenulum

Paraurethral duct

Skene's duct

Bartholin duct

**FIGURE 1–44** The greater vulva consists of the external genitalia, the mons, the crura, the perineum, and the perianal skin. Mucous glands derived from endoderm are located around the vaginal introitus and the external urethral meatus and consist of the Bartholin glands/ducts and the paraurethral glands/ducts. The area of the posterior fourchette and fossa navicularis is studded with minor vestibular (mucous) glands.

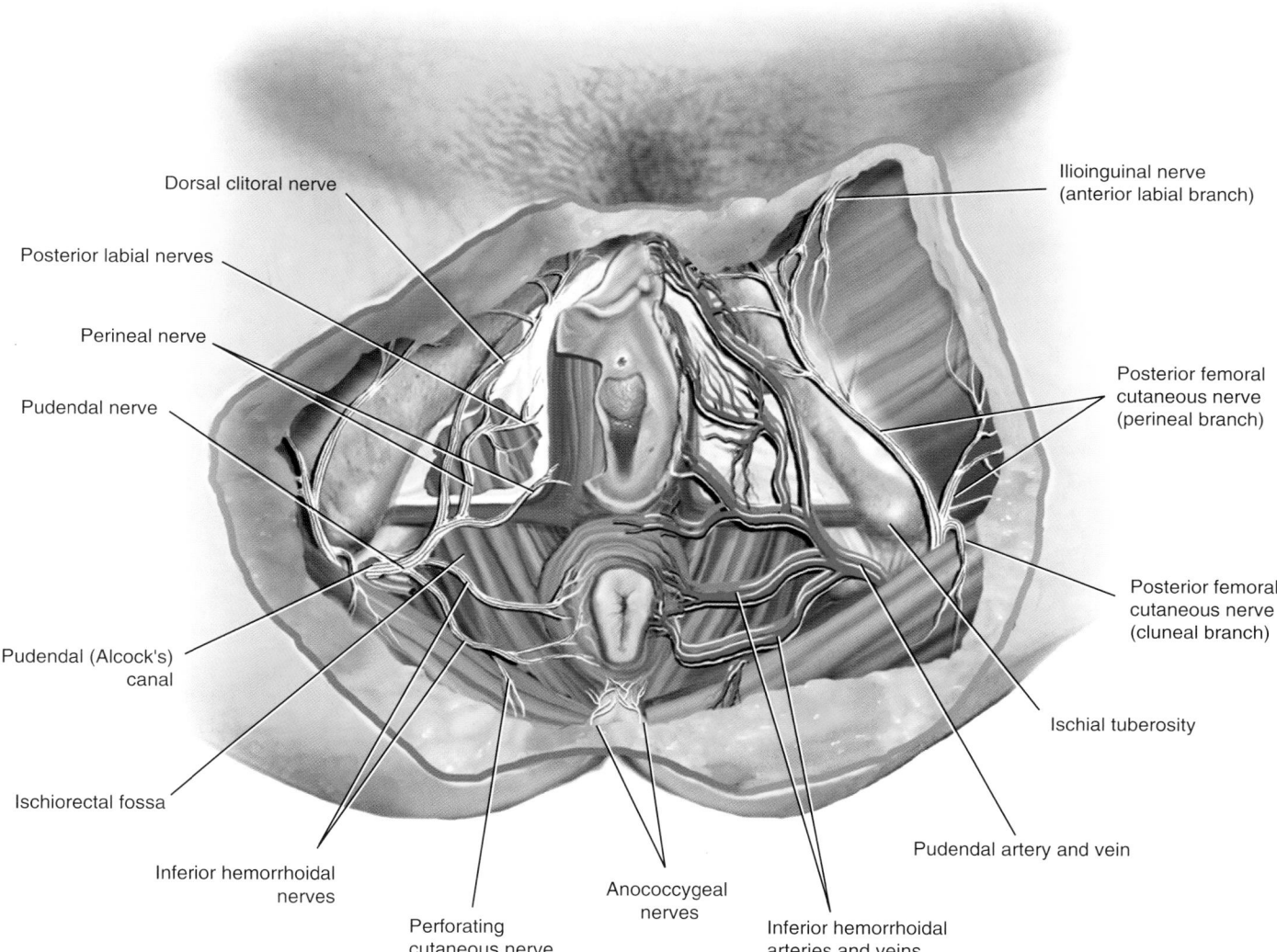

Dorsal clitoral nerve

Posterior labial nerves

Perineal nerve

Pudendal nerve

Pudendal (Alcock's) canal

Ischiorectal fossa

Inferior hemorrhoidal nerves

Perforating cutaneous nerve

Anococcygeal nerves

Inferior hemorrhoidal arteries and veins

Pudendal artery and vein

Ischial tuberosity

Posterior femoral cutaneous nerve (cluneal branch)

Posterior femoral cutaneous nerve (perineal branch)

Ilioinguinal nerve (anterior labial branch)

**FIGURE 1–45** Pudendal nerves and internal pudendal vessels emerge from Alcock's canal just medial to the ischial tuberosity. Branches pierce the fascia covering the muscles and can be found with the perineal fat. Colles' fascia has largely been stripped away in this drawing.

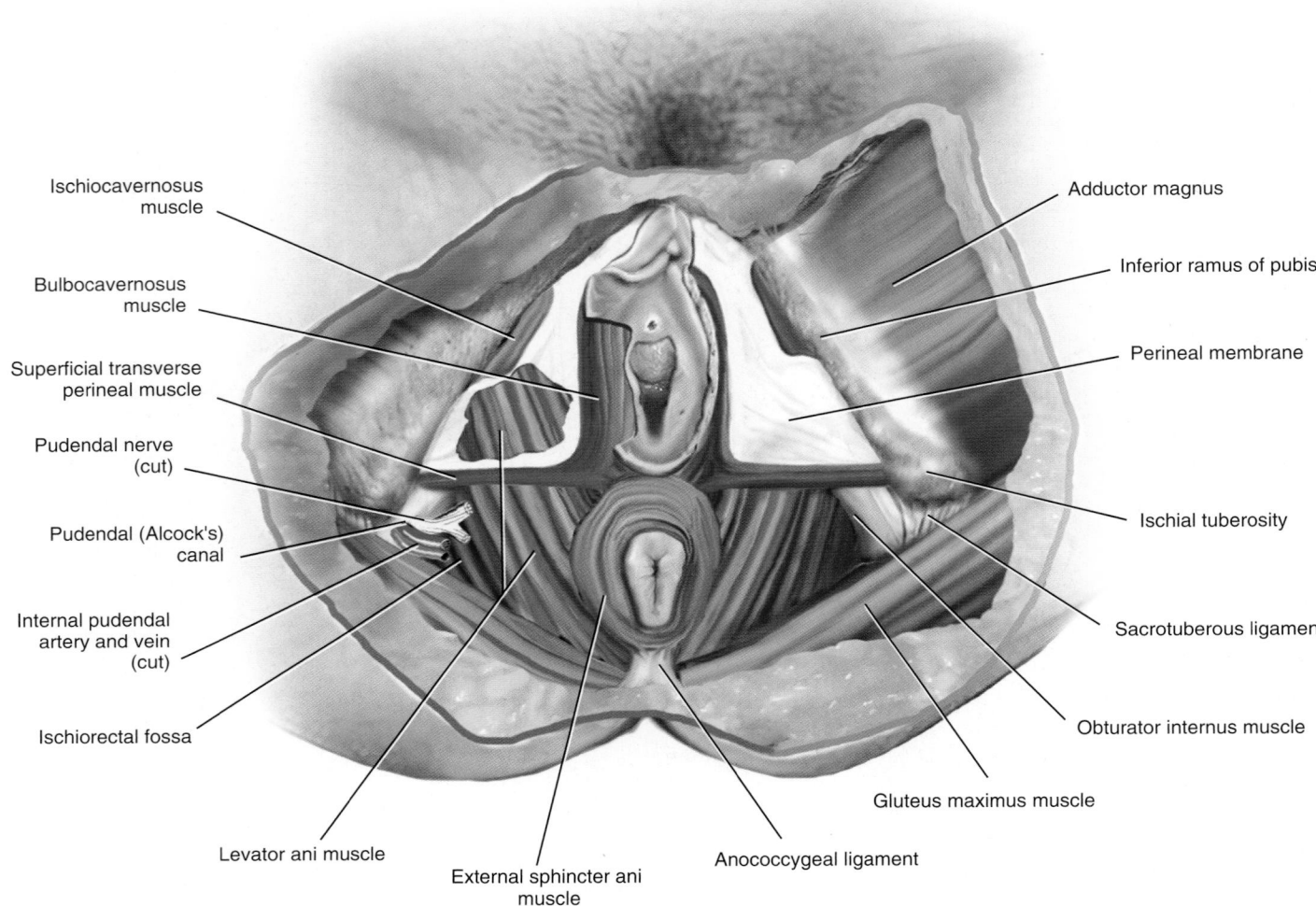

Ischiocavernosus
muscle

Bulbocavernosus
muscle

Superficial transverse
perineal muscle

Pudendal nerve
(cut)

Pudendal (Alcock's)
canal

Internal pudendal
artery and vein
(cut)

Ischiorectal fossa

Adductor magnus

Inferior ramus of pubis

Perineal membrane

Ischial tuberosity

Sacrotuberous ligament

Obturator internus muscle

Gluteus maximus muscle

Levator ani muscle

External sphincter ani
muscle

Anococcygeal ligament

**FIGURE 1–46** The muscles forming the pelvic floor are shown here. The crural area is prominently seen and felt by the adductor longus muscle. The bulbocavernosus muscle is immediately lateral to the outer wall of the vagina. The ischiocavernosus lies along the margin of the pubic ramus. Between these muscles is a tough connective tissue structure called the perineal membrane. Blending into and deep to the bulbocavernosus muscle and external sphincter ani muscle is the levator ani muscle. Between the levator ani and the ramus of the ischium is the obturator internus muscle.

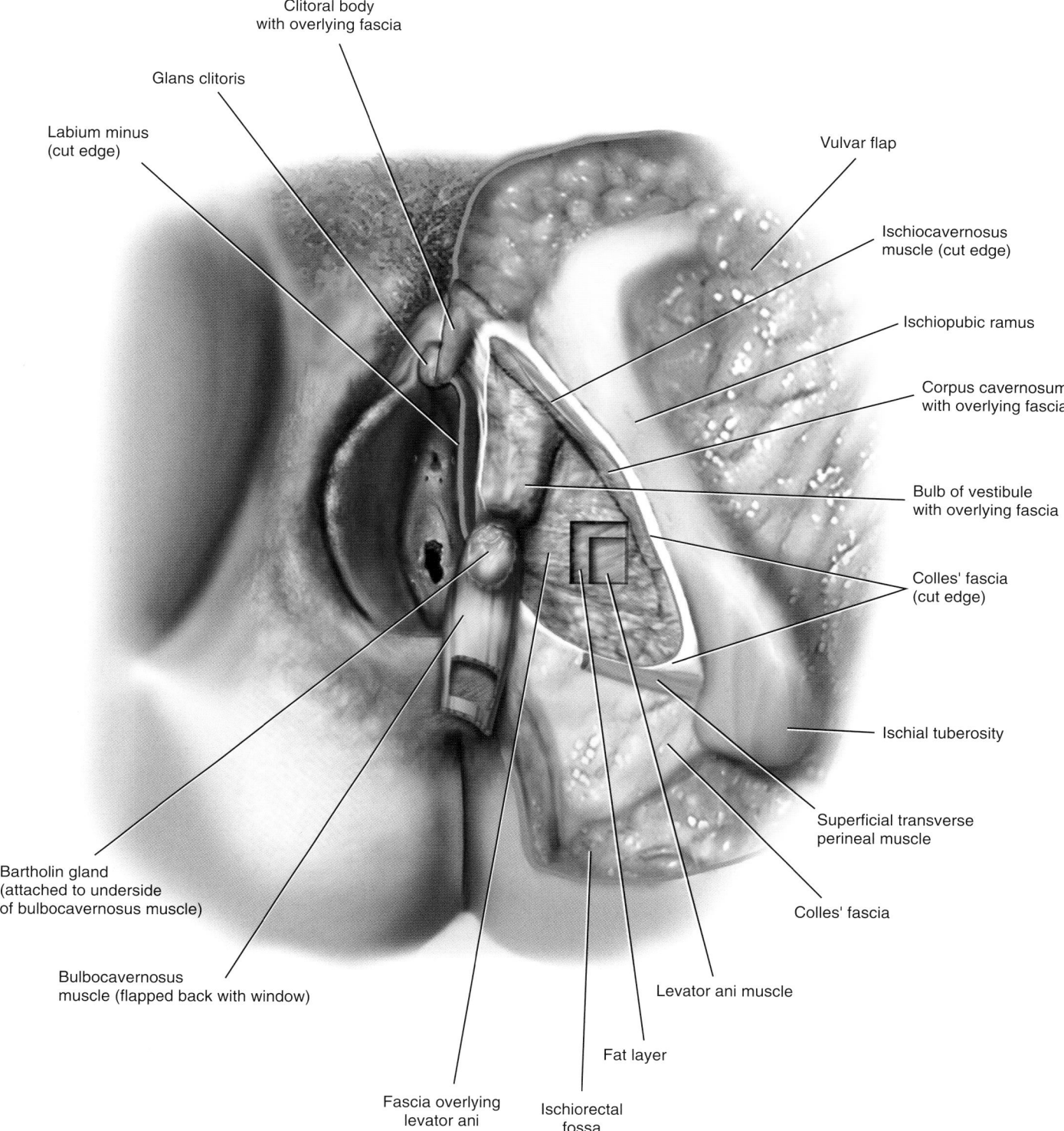

Clitoral body
with overlying fascia

Glans clitoris

Labium minus
(cut edge)

Vulvar flap

Ischiocavernosus
muscle (cut edge)

Ischiopubic ramus

Corpus cavernosum
with overlying fascia

Bulb of vestibule
with overlying fascia

Colles' fascia
(cut edge)

Ischial tuberosity

Superficial transverse
perineal muscle

Colles' fascia

Bartholin gland
(attached to underside
of bulbocavernosus muscle)

Bulbocavernosus
muscle (flapped back with window)

Levator ani muscle

Fat layer

Fascia overlying
levator ani

Ischiorectal
fossa

**FIGURE 1–47** This picture shows the bulbocavernosus muscle turned down. Clinging to its inferior margin is the Bartholin gland. The bulb of the vestibule is exposed beneath the upper portion of the muscle. Beneath the ischiocavernosus muscle is the corpus cavernosa clitoris. The two corpora (right and left) unite at the lowest margin of the symphysis pubis to form the body of the clitoris. Essentially, these cavernous structures form a virtual blood lake.

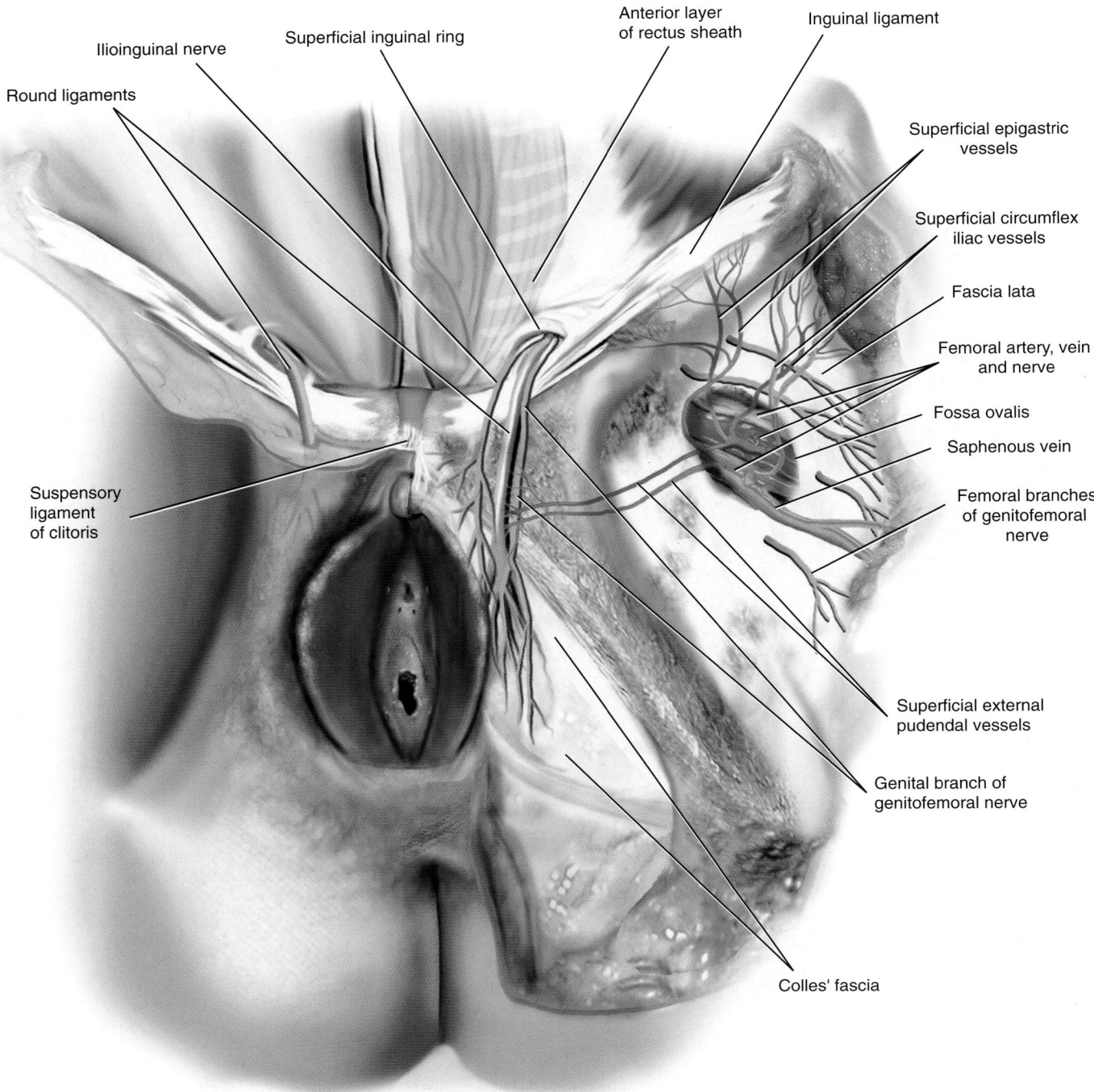

**FIGURE 1–48** The round ligament exits through the superficial inguinal ring accompanied by the ilioinguinal nerve and the genital branch of the genitofemoral nerve. These structures are buried in the fat of the mons and upper labium majus.

The fossa ovalis lies within the deeper layer of fat within the thigh. Three small blood vessels branch from the femoral artery and flow into the femoral vein. They include (1) the superficial external pudendal vessels, (2) the superficial epigastric vessels, and (3) the superficial circumflex iliac vessels. Lateral to the femoral artery is the femoral nerve. The large vein winding upward in the medial thigh fat is the saphenous vein.

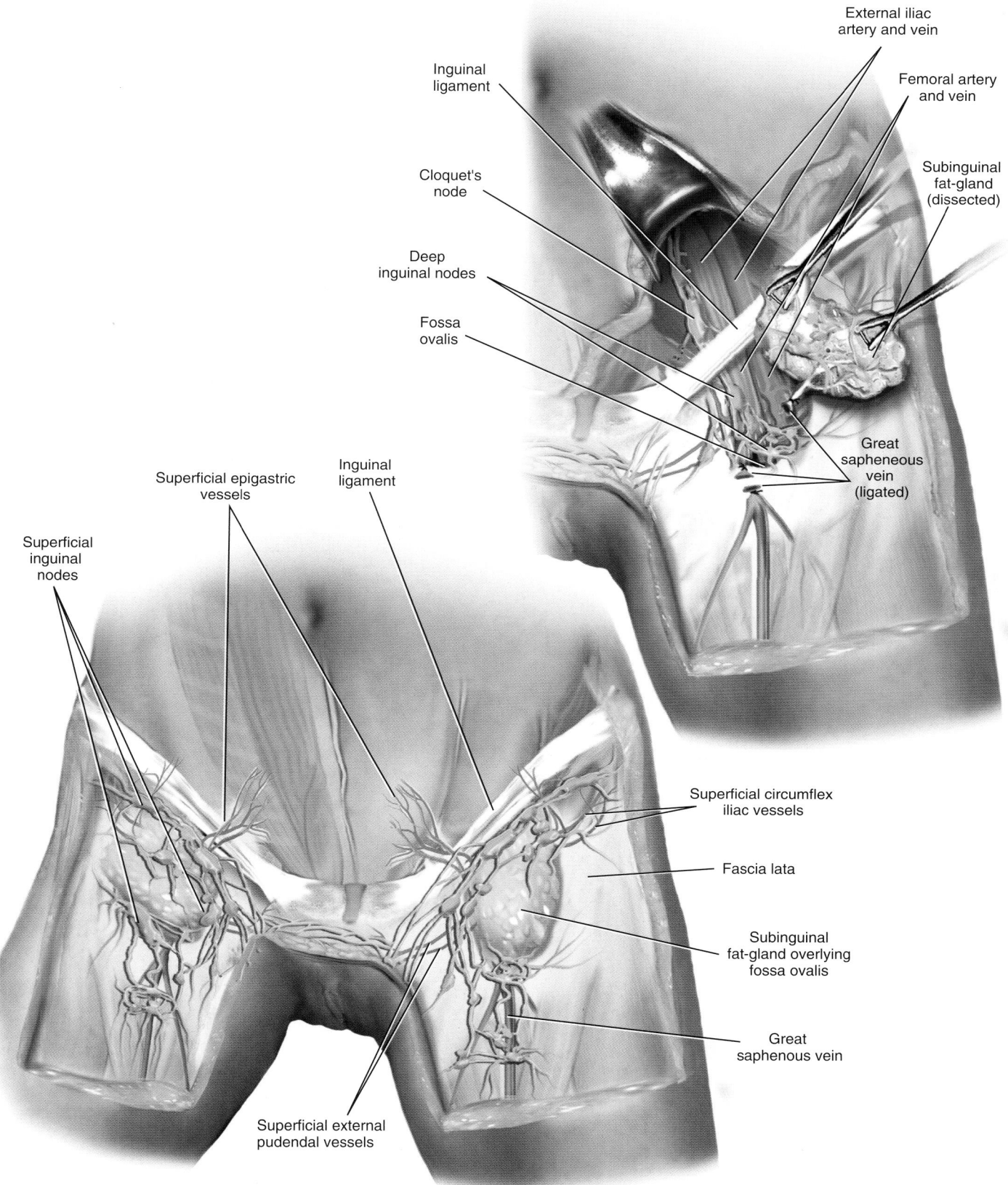

**FIGURE 1–49** The vulvar lymphatics drain first to the superficial groin (i.e., inguinal lymph nodes that are arranged in the cribriform fascia overlying the fossa ovalis and along the three superficial vessels noted in Fig. 1–48). Additional lymph nodes are located along the great saphenous vein, as are accessory saphenous tributaries.

The secondary inguinal lymph nodes consist of the femoral (deep inguinal) nodes, which are located mainly around the femoral vein and in the femoral canal. These in turn drain into the external iliac chain. The lowest of the external iliac (deep pelvic) lymph nodes lies at the top of the femoral canal and is known as Cloquet's node.

The lymphatic channels of the vulva drain ipsilaterally and contralaterally with the crossover channels located in the fat of the mons venous.

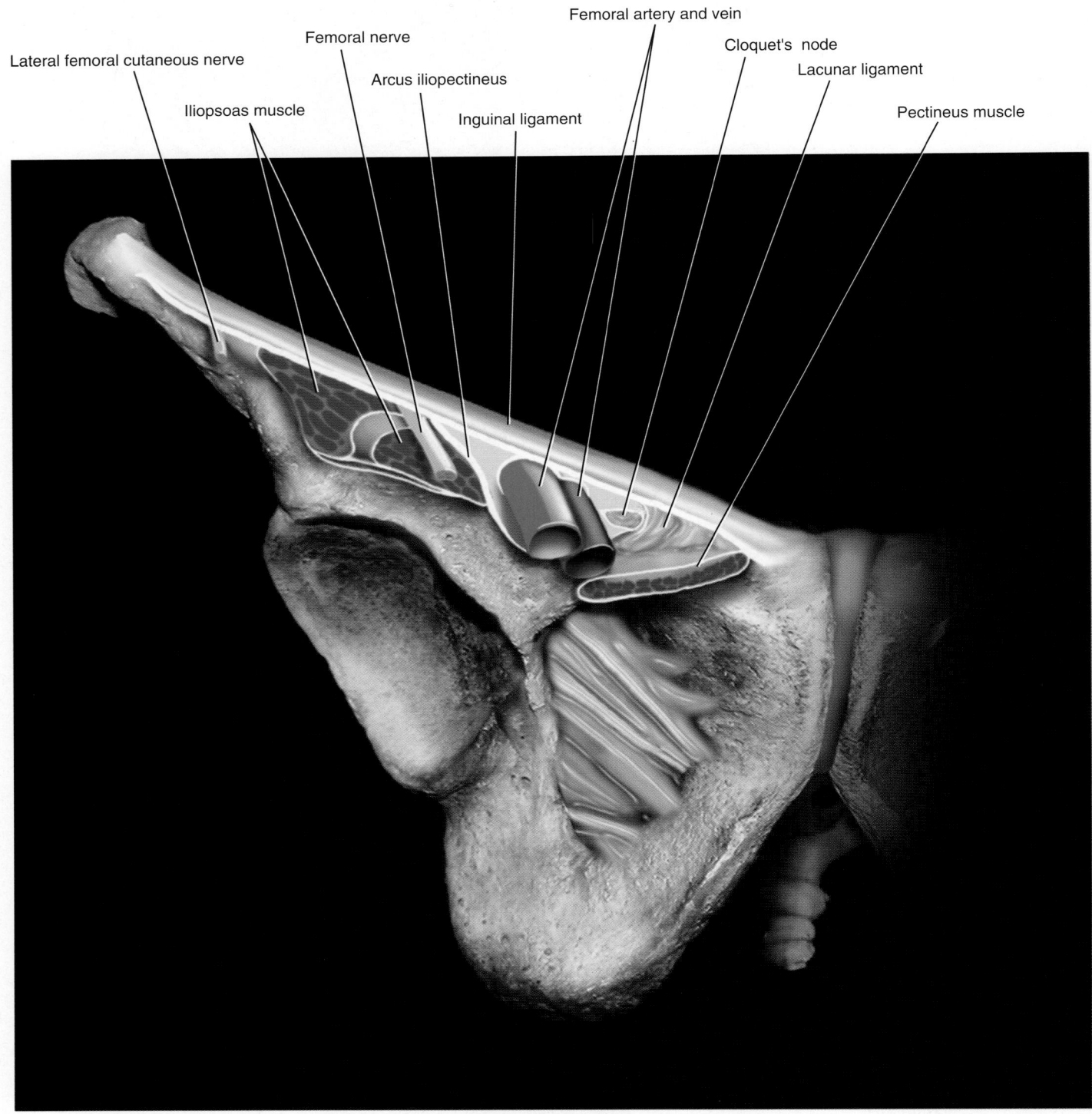

Lateral femoral cutaneous nerve

Femoral nerve

Femoral artery and vein

Cloquet's  node

Lacunar ligament

Iliopsoas muscle

Arcus iliopectineus

Inguinal ligament

Pectineus muscle

**FIGURE 1–50** This frontal view of the right hemipelvis shows, from medial to lateral, the femoral canal, Cloquet's lymph node, the femoral vein, the femoral artery, the femoral nerve, and lateral femoral cutaneous nerve. These major structures lie on the pectineus and iliopsoas muscles.

# CHAPTER 2

# Introduction to Pelvic Anatomy 2

*Michael S. Baggish*

## Autonomic Nervous System

The motor innervation of the intestines, ureter, urinary bladder, uterus, and adnexa is derived from the **autonomic nervous system** (Fig. 2–1).

The latter system in turn is divided into **sympathetic** and **parasympathetic** components.

The sympathetic cells are located within the lower thoracic and lumbar segments of the spinal cord; the parasympathetic cells are located in the sacral portion of the spinal cord. In general, the two systems work in opposition to each other (dual intervention) to maintain homeostasis. For example, the smooth muscles of the bronchioles relax under sympathetic mediation and constrict under parasympathetic stimulation.

Two types of cholinergic receptors are known: **nicotinic,** which are found on the postganglionic cells (postsynaptic) of both sympathetic and parasympathetic effectors, and **muscarinic,** which are found only in the parasympathetic portion of the autonomic nervous system.

**Adrenergic receptors** for **norepinephrine** and **epinephrine** are divided into $\alpha$ and $\beta$ and into further subtypes, which demonstrate sundry agonist and antagonist activities. For example, $\beta$ one ($\beta_1$) receptors are present in cardiac muscle, and $\beta$ two ($\beta_2$) receptors are present in the coronary arterioles.

Fibers that emanate from the central nervous system are designated as **preganglionic.** In the case of sympathetic preganglionic fibers, synapses occur in paravertebral and prevertebral ganglia, where **acetylcholine** is the transmitter. Parasympathetic fibers synapse near or within the effector organ, with acetylcholine as the neurotransmitter. **Postganglionic sympathetic** fibers travel from the ganglion to the effector (e.g., a blood vessel in which **norepinephrine** is the neurotransmitter). **Parasympathetic postganglionic** fibers are short and acetylcholine is the neurotransmitter at the postganglionic synapse. Additionally, **peptide neuromodulators** such as enkephalin and somatostatin are simultaneously released with acetylcholine or norepinephrine.

Figure 2–2 details three groups of nerves supplying the **autonomic input for female reproductive structures.** One group originates from the 9th through the **12th thoracic cord** segments, with preganglionic sympathetic fibers synapsing in the celiac and superior mesenteric ganglia, and postganglionic fibers following the ovarian vessels to synapse in the ovary and uterine tubes (oviducts). **Afferent sensory fibers** follow the same route in reverse. The second group, which is derived from **T12, L1,** and **L2** segments, supplies the oviducts and the great pelvic vessels and enters the pelvis via the **superior hypogastric plexus.** The third group emanates from **L2–L5** segments and synapses within the **inferior mesenteric plexus** and/or transmits via the **inferior hypogastric plexus** to the uterine and vagina plexuses. Postganglionic fibers in turn

synapse in the uterine body, cervix, vagina, and erectile structures within the vulva.

Parasympathetic preganglionic fibers arising from the **sacral nerve roots** follow the branches of the hypogastric vessels and synapse in the **uterovaginal plexus.**

As previously noted, the **hypogastric plexus** (nerves) descends into the pelvis over (anterior to) the aorta and the left common iliac vein, entering the presacral space.

The inferior hypogastric plexus descends deep into the pelvis of the periosteum of the sacrum, where it is dispersed with remnants of the uterosacral ligaments and fat and numerous small blood vessels at a 3 : 1 ratio of venules to arterioles.

The **bladder** and the **lower ureters** are innervated via the **pelvic plexuses** by the autonomic nervous system (Fig. 2–3). Sympathetic nerves emanate from **T10, T11, T12, L1, and L2.**

**Spinal cord segments** and **somatic motor neurons** controlling perivesical muscle and parasympathetic preganglionic neurons are located in **S2, S3, and S4 segments.**

**Sensory impulses** (visceral sensory) return to the spinal cord via similar pathways, transmitting via parasympathetic pathways and sacral cord segments. The latter transmit **pain** and **proprioception (e.g., distention).** Some sensory fibers from the trigone and the **urethrovesical junction** transmit pain via the pudendal nerves. Clearly, some sensory afferents reach the spinal cord via the hypogastric nerve plexus.

Parasympathetic postganglionic fibers synapse within the **bladder's detrusor muscle** and exit via the **postsynaptic muscarinic receptors,** resulting in muscle contraction.

Contemporary neuroanatomy data suggest a sparse number of sympathetic nerves in the bladder musculature, with the exception of the trigone, where greater numbers of sympathetic versus parasympathetic nerves are found.

During the **filling phase,** bladder volume increases while parasympathetic output is inhibited. At the same time, $\alpha$ **sympathetic discharge** causes the **urethral muscle** to contract, thereby retaining a high-pressure gradient that favors the urethra over the bladder. When the level of fullness transmits, via afferent sensors and fibers, a feeling of discomfort (associated with high bladder volume), **the brain in turn dispatches a release message,** which triggers a parasympathetic discharge. The bladder muscle contracts and empties. Concurrently, sympathetic synapses in parasympathetic ganglia **modulate ganglionic transmission,** resulting in urethral muscle relaxation (by blocking contraction). The pressure gradient shifts in such a way that bladder pressure exceeds urethral pressure, thereby allowing **micturition.**

Sympathetic and parasympathetic fibers supplying the large and small intestines emanate from the **celiac, superior** and **inferior mesenteric,** and **hypogastric plexuses** (Fig. 2–4). Preganglionic parasympathetic fibers likewise originate in **medullary nuclei (e.g., the medulla oblongata)** of the vagus nerve

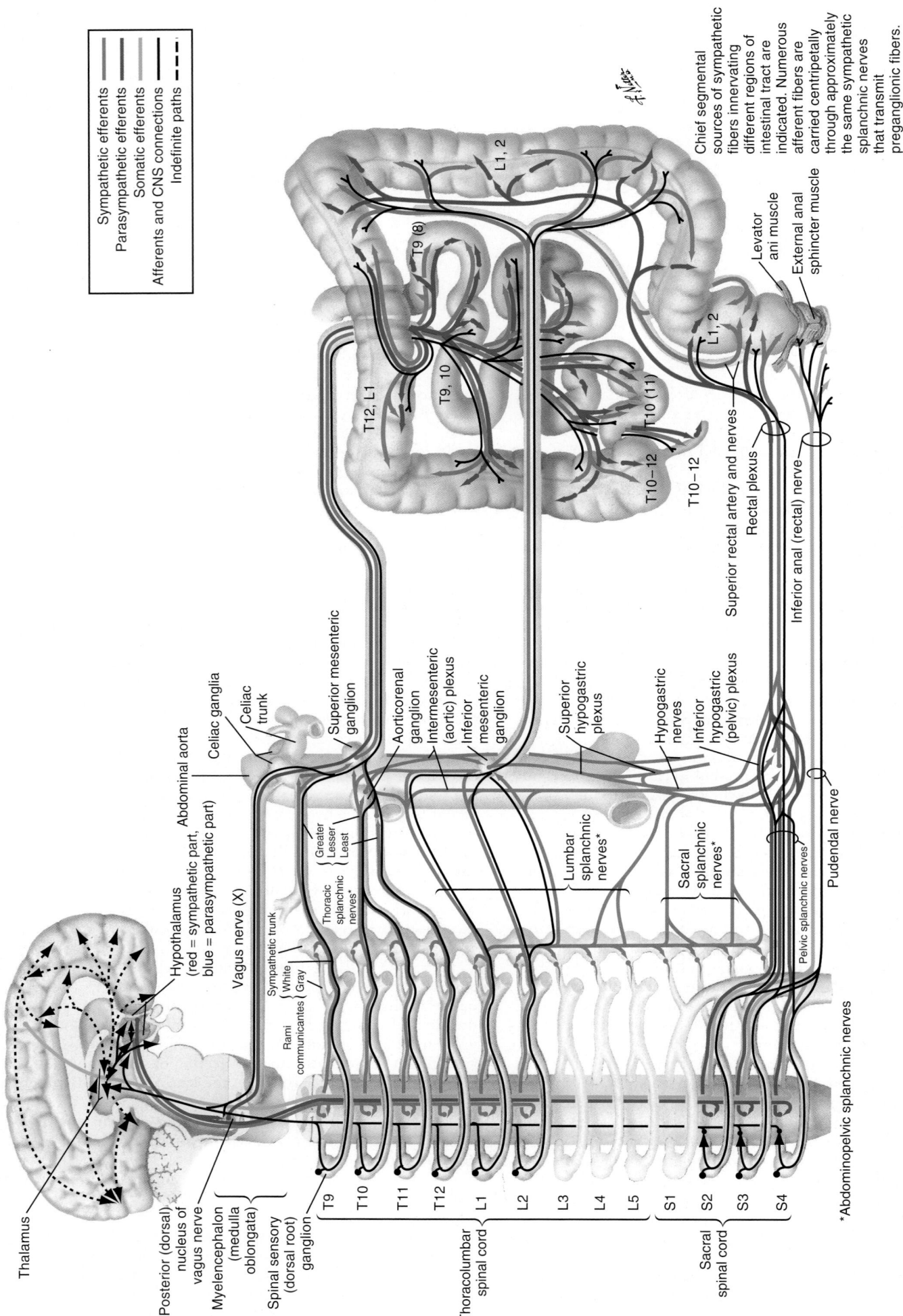

**FIGURE 2-1** Details of the autonomic nervous system. Sympathetic efferents are *red*, and parasympathetics (vagal and sacral) are blue. The autonomic nervous system, totally consisting of motor (efferent) somatic nerves that control voluntary muscle activity, is shown in green; sensory (afferent) organs and muscles are black and may share pathways with autonomic and somatic nerves. (By permission, Netter's Atlas of Human Anatomy.)

Sympathetic efferents
Parasympathetic efferents
Somatic efferents
Afferents and CNS connections
Indefinite paths

Chief segmental sources of sympathetic fibers innervating different regions of intestinal tract are indicated. Numerous afferent fibers are carried centripetally through approximately the same sympathetic splanchnic nerves that transmit preganglionic fibers.

L1, 2
T9 (8)
T12, L1
T9, 10
T10 (11)
T10-12
T10-12
L1, 2

Levator ani muscle
External anal sphincter muscle
Superior rectal artery and nerves
Rectal plexus
Inferior anal (rectal) nerve

Hypothalamus (red = sympathetic part, blue = parasympathetic part)
Abdominal aorta
Celiac ganglia
Celiac trunk
Superior mesenteric ganglion
Aorticorenal ganglion
Intermesenteric (aortic) plexus
Inferior mesenteric ganglion
Superior hypogastric plexus
Hypogastric nerves
Inferior hypogastric (pelvic) plexus

Vagus nerve (X)

Posterior (dorsal) nucleus of vagus nerve
Myelencephalon (medulla oblongata)
Spinal sensory (dorsal root) ganglion

Thalamus

Sympathetic trunk
Rami communicantes { White / Gray }
Thoracic splanchnic nerves*
Greater / Lesser / Least
Lumbar splanchnic nerves*
Sacral splanchnic nerves*
Pelvic splanchnic nerves
Pudendal nerve

Thoracolumbar spinal cord
T9
T10
T11
T12
L1
L2
L3
L4
L5

Sacral spinal cord
S1
S2
S3
S4

*Abdominopelvic splanchnic nerves

INNERVATION OF FEMALE REPRODUCTIVE ORGANS: SCHEMA

Note: Pain from intraperitoneal pelvic viscera (e.g., uterine contractions) goes via uterovaginal and pelvic plexuses, hypogastric nerves, superior hypo-gastric plexus, lower aortic plexus, lower lumbar splanchnic nerves, sympathetic trunk from L4 to L5 to spinal nerves T11, 12. Pain from subperitoneal pelvic viscera (e.g., cervical dilation and upper vagina) goes via pelvic splanchnic nerves to S2, 3, 4. Afferent fibers from lower vagina and perineum go via pudendal nerves to S2, 3, 4

| Sympathetic fibers { | Presynaptic ——— | Parasympathetic fibers { | Presynaptic ——— | Afferent fibers ——— |
| | Postsynaptic – – – | | Postsynaptic – – – | |

**FIGURE 2–2** The autonomic nerve supply to the female reproductive organs is shown here. Preganglionic fibers are shown as solid red (sympathetic) blue (parasympathetic) lines. Somatic (afferent) sensory nerves are shown as solid black lines. Sympathetic nerves arise from the lower thoracic and lumbar cord segments and synapse in outlying ganglia on the aorta or its main branches. Others enter the pelvis via the hypogastric nerves (plexuses). Postganglionic fibers travel along the ovarian vessels or the uterovaginal vessels. Parasympathetic input arises in the sacral cord and travels via pelvic splanchnic nerves to the various organs where synapses occur and short postganglionic fibers transmit impulses. (By permission, Netter's Atlas of Human Anatomy.)

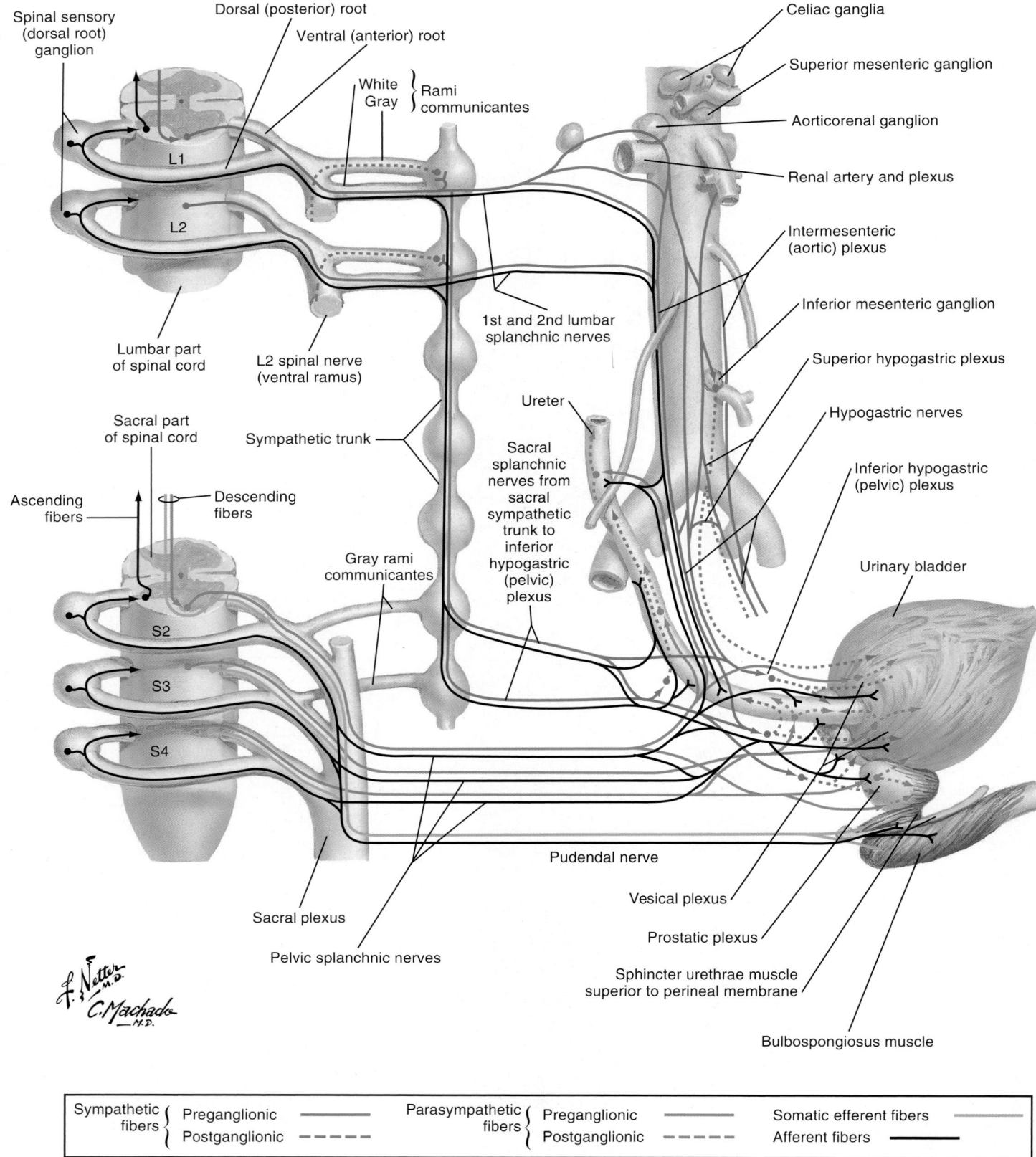

Spinal sensory (dorsal root) ganglion

Dorsal (posterior) root

Ventral (anterior) root

White / Gray } Rami communicantes

Celiac ganglia

Superior mesenteric ganglion

Aorticorenal ganglion

Renal artery and plexus

Intermesenteric (aortic) plexus

Inferior mesenteric ganglion

Superior hypogastric plexus

Hypogastric nerves

Inferior hypogastric (pelvic) plexus

Urinary bladder

L1

L2

Lumbar part of spinal cord

L2 spinal nerve (ventral ramus)

1st and 2nd lumbar splanchnic nerves

Ureter

Sacral splanchnic nerves from sacral sympathetic trunk to inferior hypogastric (pelvic) plexus

Sacral part of spinal cord

Symphathetic trunk

Ascending fibers

Descending fibers

Gray rami communicantes

S2

S3

S4

Pudendal nerve

Sacral plexus

Pelvic splanchnic nerves

Vesical plexus

Prostatic plexus

Sphincter urethrae muscle superior to perineal membrane

Bulbospongiosus muscle

| Sympathetic fibers { | Preganglionic | ——— | Parasympathetic fibers { | Preganglionic | ——— | Somatic efferent fibers | ——— |
| | Postganglionic | - - - - | | Postganglionic | - - - - | Afferent fibers | ——— |

**FIGURE 2–3** The bladder and the lower ureter are innervated via pelvic plexuses. Sympathetic fibers emanate from cord segments T10, T11, T12, L1, and L2. Parasympathetic preganglionic neurons are located in S2, S3, and S4 cord segments. Postganglionic parasympathetic neurons lie within the walls of the bladder and the ureter, whereas preganglionic sympathetic fibers are found in the vesical plexus (pelvic plexus). (By permission, Netter's Atlas of Human Anatomy.)

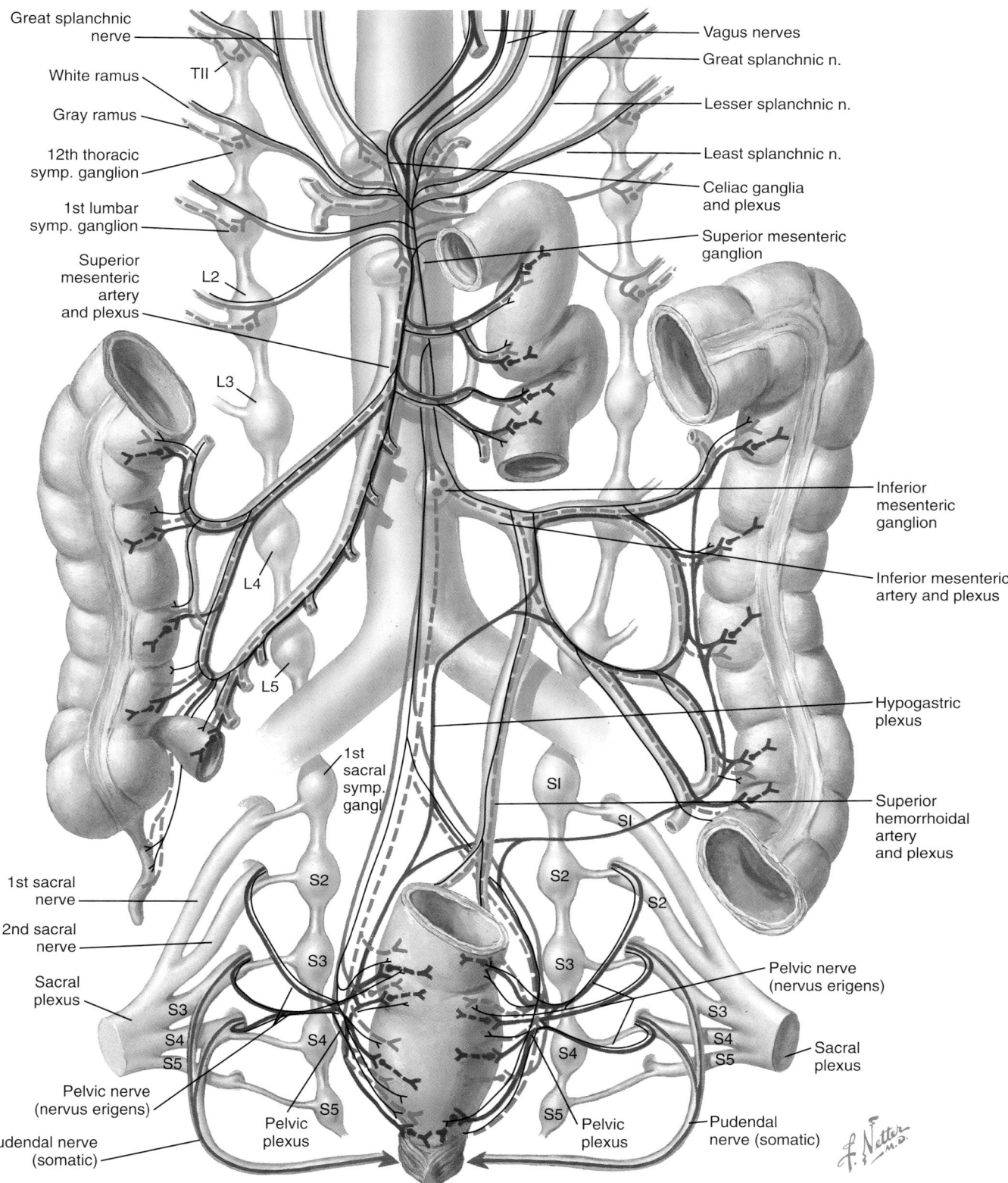

Great splanchnic nerve

White ramus

Gray ramus

12th thoracic symp. ganglion

1st lumbar symp. ganglion

Superior mesenteric artery and plexus

TII

L2

L3

L4

L5

1st sacral symp. gangl

1st sacral nerve

2nd sacral nerve

Sacral plexus

S2

S3

S3

S4

S5

Pelvic nerve (nervus erigens)

Pelvic plexus

Pudendal nerve (somatic)

S4

S5

Vagus nerves

Great splanchnic n.

Lesser splanchnic n.

Least splanchnic n.

Celiac ganglia and plexus

Superior mesenteric ganglion

Inferior mesenteric ganglion

Inferior mesenteric artery and plexus

Hypogastric plexus

Superior hemorrhoidal artery and plexus

SI

SI

S2

S2

S3

S4

S5

Pelvic nerve (nervus erigens)

Sacral plexus

Pelvic plexus

Pudendal nerve (somatic)

S3

S4

S5

**FIGURE 2–4** Large and small intestines are supplied with autonomic input via celiac, superior mesenteric, and inferior mesenteric plexuses, the vagus, and sacral nerves. The pelvic portion of the sigmoid colon, rectum, and anus receives sympathetic fibers via the superior and inferior hypogastric plexuses. The inferior hypogastric plexus receives parasympathetic fibers from S2, S3, and S4 nerve roots. The rectal plexus (pelvic plexus) is closely applied to the rectal connective tissue and carries sympathetic, parasympathetic, and afferent nerves. The pudendal nerve carries somatic efferent fibers to the levator ani and the external sphincter ani. (By permission, Netter's Atlas of Human Anatomy.)

and **sacral cord segments.** Vagally derived fibers supply the duodenum, jejunum, and ileum. Sympathetic preganglionic fibers are distributed from cord nuclei located at T8, T9, T10, T11, and T12, and at L1, L2, and L3; the latter relay within the ganglia of the sympathetic trunks and from there to plexuses, where synapses occur and postganglionic fibers distribute themselves to the intestines. **Afferent** and **efferent somatic fibers,** via the pudendal nerves, innervate voluntary (striated) muscles such as the levator ani and external sphincter ani. Because they are pelvic structures, innervation of the sigmoid colon, rectum, and anus is of special interest to gynecologists and obstetricians.

## Pelvic Plexus

The **inferior mesenteric plexus** receives fibers from the superior **mesenteric plexus** via the **lumbar splanchnic nerves.** Branches from the inferior mesenteric plexus accompany arteries to respective intestinal segments (e.g., **left colon, upper sigmoid colon**). The superior hypogastric plexus carries sympathetic preganglionic nerves and afferent nerves, which lie on either side of the **rectosigmoid** and **rectum** and become the **inferior hypogastric plexus (presacral)** (Fig. 2–5). This plexus receives parasympathetic preganglionic nerves, as well as somatic branches, from S2, S3, and S4 nerve roots via pelvic splanchnic nerves. The **rectal plexus** is a subdivision of the inferior hypogastric plexus and carries sympathetic preganglionic fibers, afferent sensory fibers, and parasympathetic preganglionic fibers. The **inferior hemorrhoidal branches** of the pudendal nerves receive sensory impulses from **anal receptors** located in the mucosa and the submucosa, especially in the **anal valves.** They transmit impulses via somatic efferents located in the sacral cord. The internal anal sphincter is supplied by sympathetic nerves originating in the L5 cord segment. The external anal sphincter is innervated by somatic efferent fibers via the **inferior hemorrhoidal nerves** and perianal branches (S4).

## Sigmoid Colon

The anatomic relationships of the sigmoid colon and the rectum to other pelvic viscera are critically important to the gynecologist. Figure 2–6 shows the entire sigmoid colon and its S configuration as it descends into the depths of the pelvis. Note that the sigmoid colon drapes over the left adnexa, virtually covering the tube and the ovary. The lower **sigmoid colon** then may be located at least partially posterior to the ovary and broad ligament. The entire sigmoid colon is attached to a mesentery and therefore is an intraperitoneal structure. Within the hollow of the sacrum, the sigmoid colon joins to the short straight **rectum.** The rectum becomes progressively extraperitoneal as it descends even deeper into the pelvis. The relationships to the draped-over sigmoid are anterior to the bladder and to the broad ligament as well as the anterior abdominal wall. The sigmoid colon is in contact with the posterior aspect of the uterine corpus, and the posterior leaf of the broad ligament at the midpelvis. The rectum and the rectosigmoid lie medial to the uterosacral ligaments. The rectum is directly posterior to the cervix where that structure connects to the uterosacral ligaments and to the posterior vaginal fornix. The rectum in fact is intimately close to the vagina and is susceptible to damage during hysterectomy (Fig. 2–7). Posterior to the rectum and the rectosigmoid are the middle sacral vessels and a large number of veins and venous sinuses.

The **sigmoid mesentery** receives branches of the inferior mesenteric vessels and crosses superficially over the left iliac vessels and the left ureter.

Venous drainage is frequently overlooked in anatomic drawings of the female pelvis. This is rather strange in that most bleeding encountered during surgical operations is venous in origin. Figure 2–8 details the relationship between the levator ani muscles and the anal sphincters. Venous drainage of the rectum and anus is detailed. Note the collateral circulation that exists between the **inferior mesenteric vein (portal system)** via the **superior rectal vein** and the **internal iliac veins (systemic system)** via the middle rectal and inferior rectal veins. Note the connectors between the internal pudendal veins via the inferior rectal veins and the middle rectal veins to the internal iliac veins.

The **rectal plexus** of the veins surrounds the rectum. Veins lie internal (submucosal) and external to the muscularis. Note the longitudinal pattern and the numerous venous sinuses.

Figure 2–9 shows a unique exposure that demonstrates critical muscular relationships between the levator ani and the anal sphincter in terms of topographic and deeper anatomy.

## Bladder and Pelvic Supports

The bladder neck (i.e., the urethrovesical junction) is located posteriorly to the lower margin of the pubic symphysis. Thus it is difficult to access and see under most circumstances. Most surgeons do not consider the extensive venous network of veins and sinuses surrounding the perivesical tissues, as well as the bladder wall and terminal ureter (Fig. 2–10). The support of the bladder neck can be readily seen in the anatomy laboratory by sawing through symphysis and tilting it forward. The posterior pubourethral ligaments can be seen to be the principle structures that anchor the urethra to the pubic bone (Fig. 2–11). The anterior pubourethral ligaments are less prominent but attach the urethra as it emerges under the symphysis to the anteroposterior margin of the symphysis pubis. The posterior aspect and bladder base are in close contact to the lower uterine corpus (anterior surface of the uterus) and are, in fact, attached to the cervix and vagina by the bladder pillars or vesicocervical and vesicovaginal pillars. These structures and their relationships are shown in Figure 2–12.

The urinary bladder, cervix, and vagina share common supporting structures (Fig. 2–12). Critical relationships exist between the distal ureter and branches of the anterior division of the hypogastric vessels, together with **cardinal ligaments** and **bladder pillars** (Fig. 2–13). The deeper portions of the cardinal ligaments are attached to the bladder base and the upper anterolateral vagina. The terminal ureter just cranial to entry into the bladder wall is intimately in contact with the **vesicocervical** and vesicovaginal ligaments (Fig. 2–14). To free the ureter from the cardinal ligament and vagina, the bladder pillars (vesicocervical and **vesicovaginal** ligaments) must be safely divided and ligated (Fig. 2–15). The most substantial supporting structures for the bladder base and the upper vagina are **deep parametrial structures (deep cardinal ligaments).** These substantial structures consist of fat, connective tissue (fibrous), and vascular channels. When these are severed, the bladder and the vagina may be more or less totally mobilized.

The only remaining support consists of common fibromuscular walls shared between the bladder, vagina, and rectum (Fig. 2–16).

A not-uncommon location for ureteral injury is the **ureterovesical junction,** which is intrinsically within the substance of the bladder. The course of the ureter within the bladder itself is oblique. This oblique course creates constriction and closure of the terminal ureter when the bladder contracts and empties. The ureteral closure aspect of bladder anatomy is important in that it prevents reflux of urine retrograde into the ureters when bladder pressure rises (e.g., during a detrusor contraction) (Fig. 2–17).

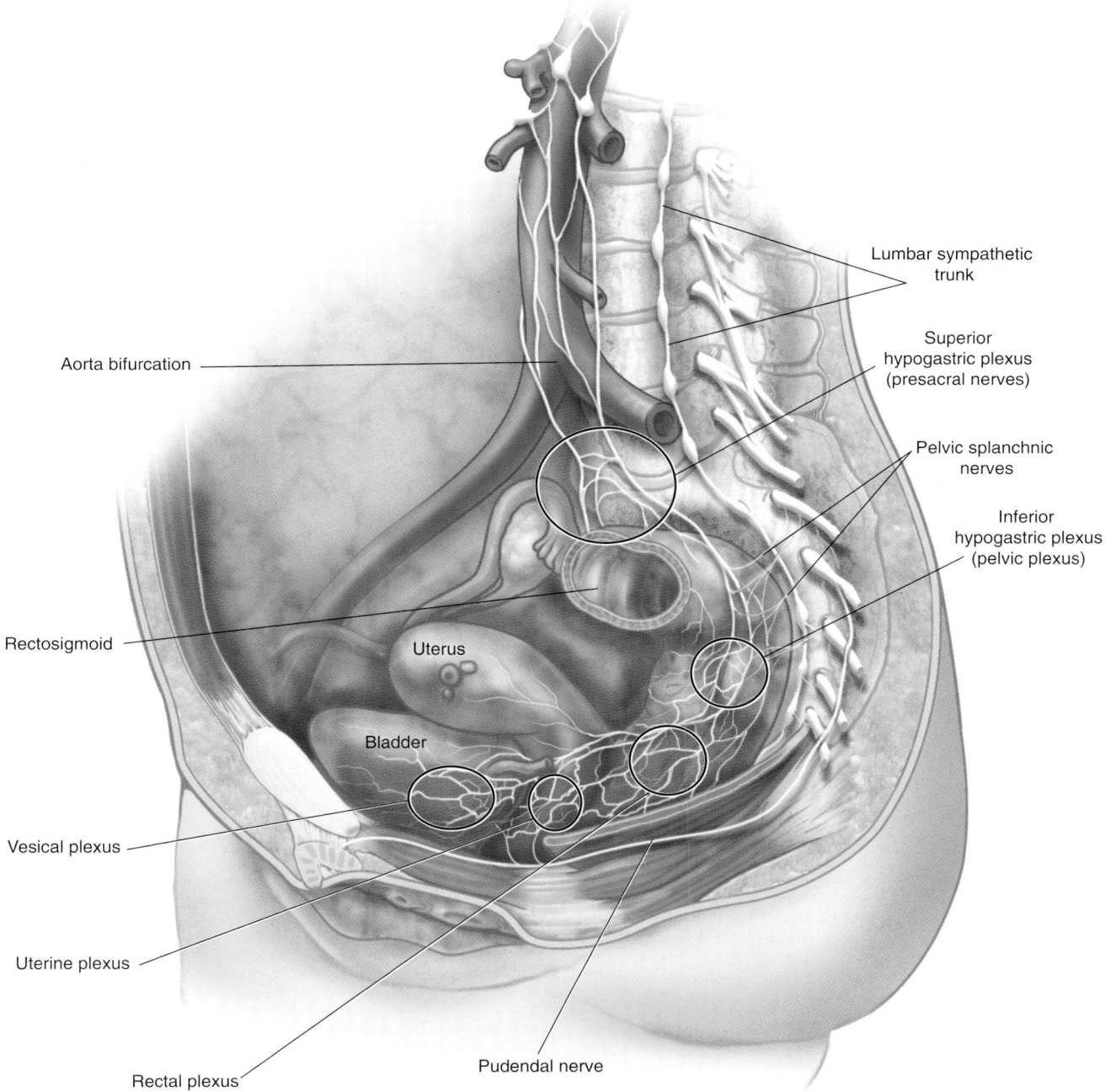

Lumbar sympathetic trunk

Superior hypogastric plexus (presacral nerves)

Pelvic splanchnic nerves

Inferior hypogastric plexus (pelvic plexus)

Aorta bifurcation

Rectosigmoid

Uterus

Bladder

Vesical plexus

Uterine plexus

Rectal plexus

Pudendal nerve

**FIGURE 2–5** Sagittal view of the hypogastric nerve plexus, which spawns several regional plexuses. The superior hypogastric plexus overlies the fifth lumbar and first sacral vertebrae. The plexus descends into the pelvis to the right or left side of the rectum. Sympathetic and parasympathetic nerves travel within the hypogastric plexus and the rectal plexus, both of which supply autonomic input to the rectum. These structures likewise supply the uterus (uterine plexus) and the bladder (vesical plexus). Sensory inferior afferent fibers traverse the same plexuses. Anal sensation is transmitted via the inferior rectal branch of the pudendal nerve. Motor innervation to the external sphincter ani and the levator ani is supplied by the pudendal nerve and its rectal branches.

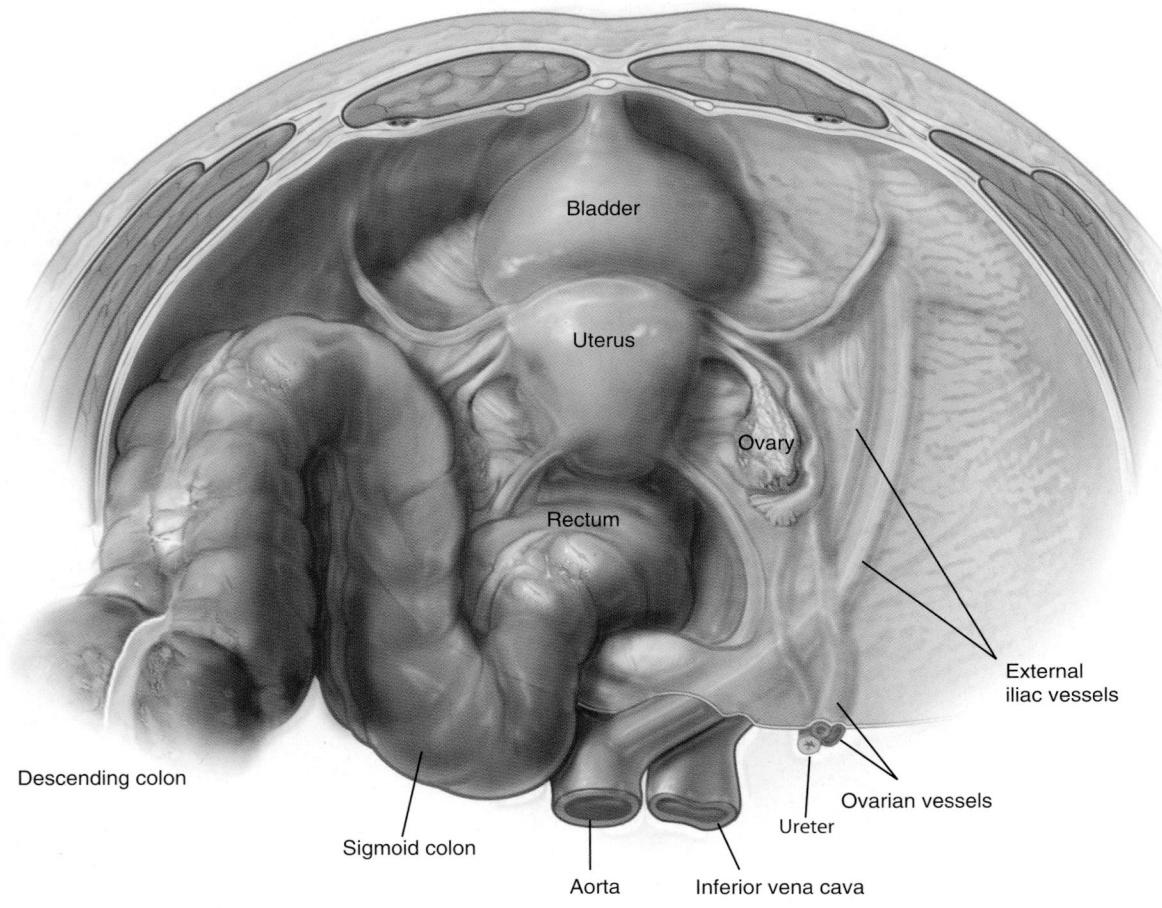

**FIGURE 2–6** The relationship of the sigmoid colon and the rectum to the reproductive organs is shown here. The sigmoid colon drapes over the left adnexa and rotates from left to right and then back to the midline, where it joins the rectum posterior to the cervix and the vagina; between the posterior vaginal fornix and the closely applied rectosigmoid is the pouch of Douglas. The mesentery of the sigmoid colon is best seen on the medial aspect of the colon and is attached to the posterior peritoneum covering the lumbar and sacral vertebrae.

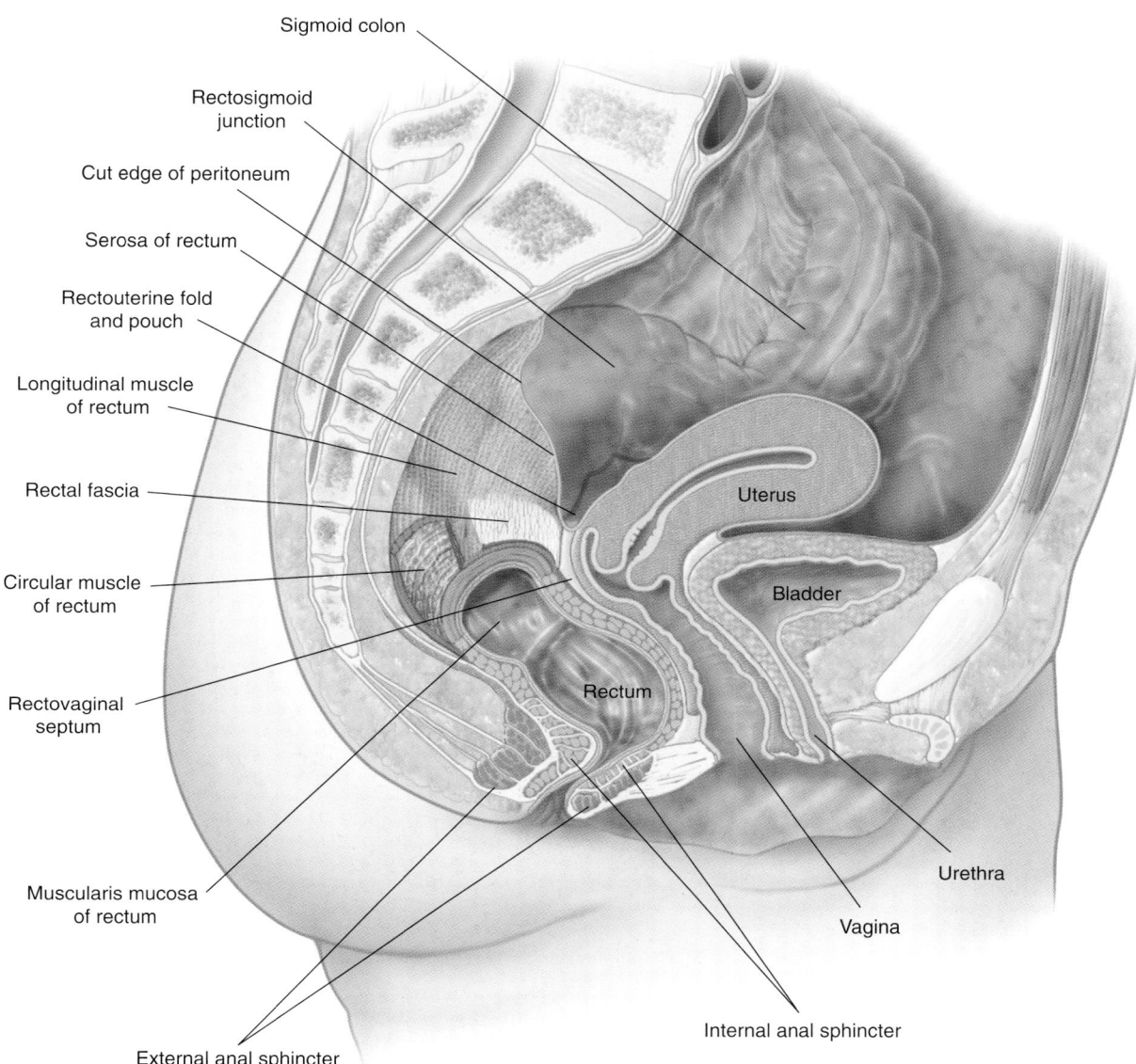

Sigmoid colon

Rectosigmoid
junction

Cut edge of peritoneum

Serosa of rectum

Rectouterine fold
and pouch

Longitudinal muscle
of rectum

Rectal fascia

Circular muscle
of rectum

Rectovaginal
septum

Muscularis mucosa
of rectum

External anal sphincter

Internal anal sphincter

Vagina

Urethra

Bladder

Uterus

Rectum

**FIGURE 2–7** The relationships of the sigmoid colon and the rectum from the perspective of a sagittal cut. This picture shows the extent of peritoneum covering relative to the sigmoid colon and rectum, as well as a cut-away depiction of the large bowel wall from mucosa to serosa. The course of the anus relative to the rectum and vagina is accurately depicted, including the positions of external and internal anal sphincters. Note the position of the rectovaginal septum, which is defined more cranially than caudally. The septum consists of shared components of the anterior rectal wall and the posterior vaginal wall. A similar relationship exists between the anterior vaginal wall and the posterior wall of the bladder and urethra.

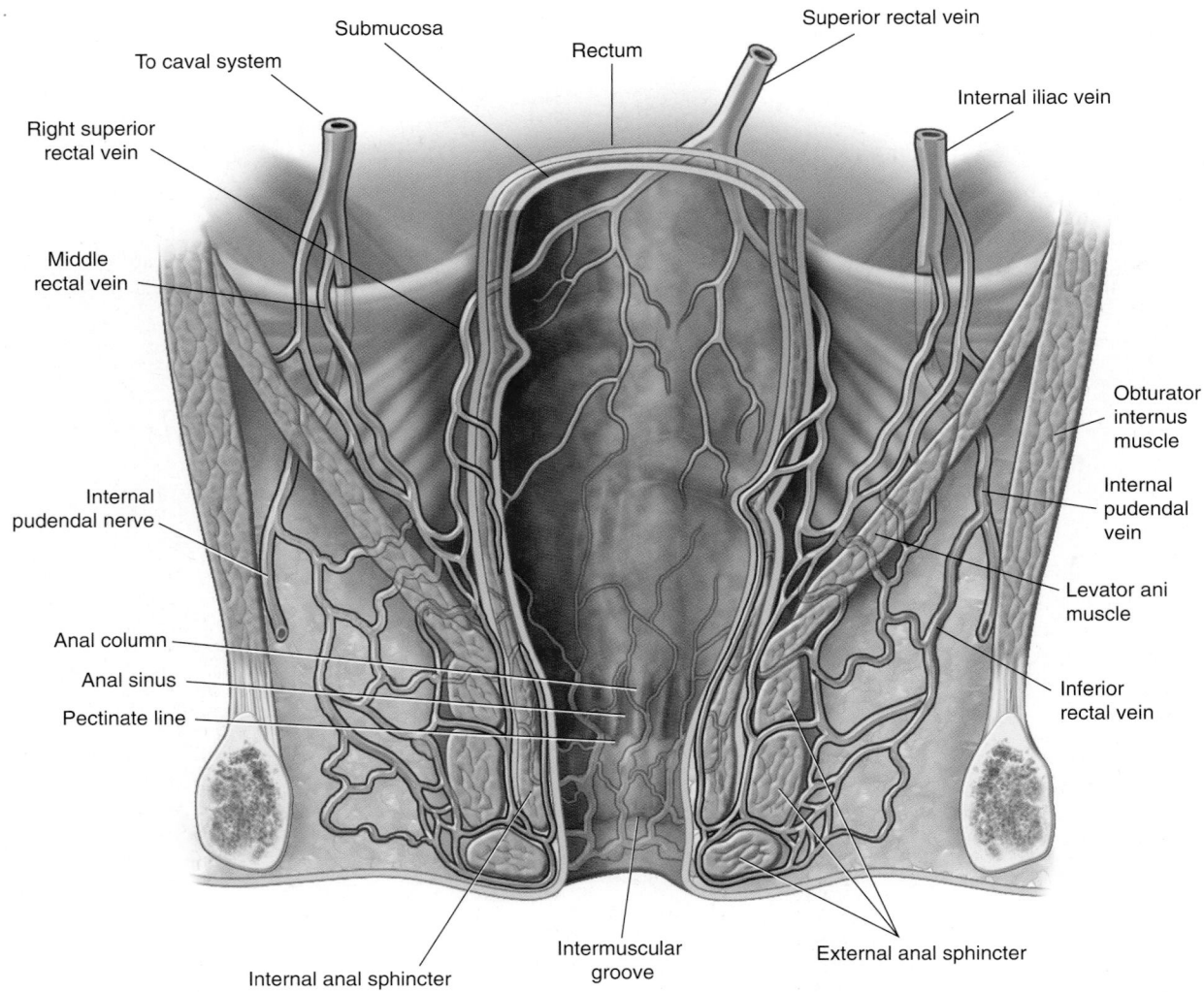

Submucosa
To caval system
Superior rectal vein
Rectum
Right superior rectal vein
Internal iliac vein
Middle rectal vein
Obturator internus muscle
Internal pudendal nerve
Internal pudendal vein
Anal column
Levator ani muscle
Anal sinus
Pectinate line
Inferior rectal vein
Internal anal sphincter
Intermuscular groove
External anal sphincter

**FIGURE 2–8** Venous drainage of the rectum is shown here. The arterial supply follows similar pathways but is more discrete. Within the muscularis and submucosa of the bowel wall are numerous anastomosing venules and sinuses. When cut or traumatized, these do not retract, as do arteries. Therefore, bleeding from the venous side may be relentless and difficult to stop. Two major systems drain rectal and perirectal tissues. The superior rectal venous system drains into the inferior mesenteric vein (portal system). The middle rectal vein drains into the internal iliac vein (systemic system), and the inferior rectal vein drains into the internal pudendal vein.

Increasing venous pressures that develop during pregnancy may lead to venous distention and stasis of outflow. Subsequent damage to the valves within the middle and inferior rectal veins by obstruction and congestion can lead to the development of internal and external hemorrhoids.

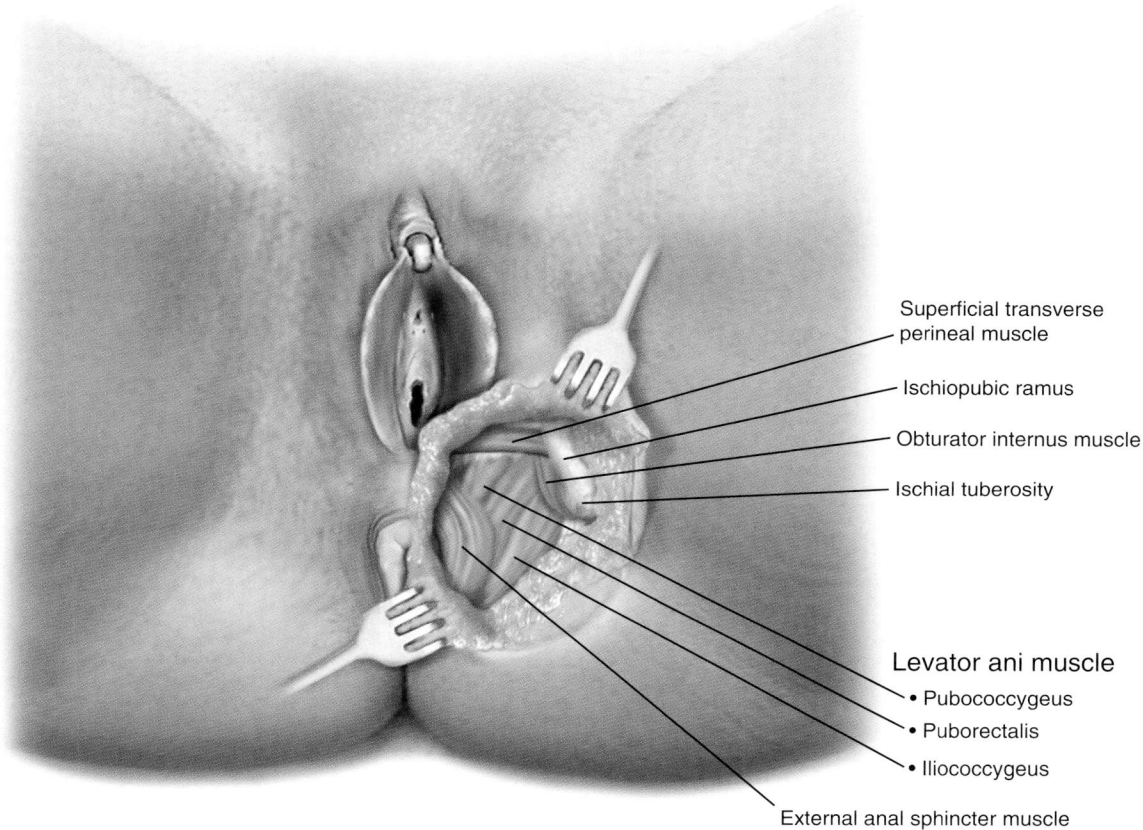

Superficial transverse perineal muscle

Ischiopubic ramus

Obturator internus muscle

Ischial tuberosity

Levator ani muscle
- Pubococcygeus
- Puborectalis
- Iliococcygeus

External anal sphincter muscle

**FIGURE 2–9** The topographic and deep anatomy of the perineum and the anal sphincter complex. Note the intermingling of the levator ani with the external sphincter ani. The levator ani plays a significant role in the mechanism of anal continence. When the sphincter ani muscle is injured, the levator ani may maintain continence (e.g., squeeze pressure). The levator action may be felt by the gynecologist during rectovaginal examination by having the patient contract her anal sphincter (and levator ani muscle).

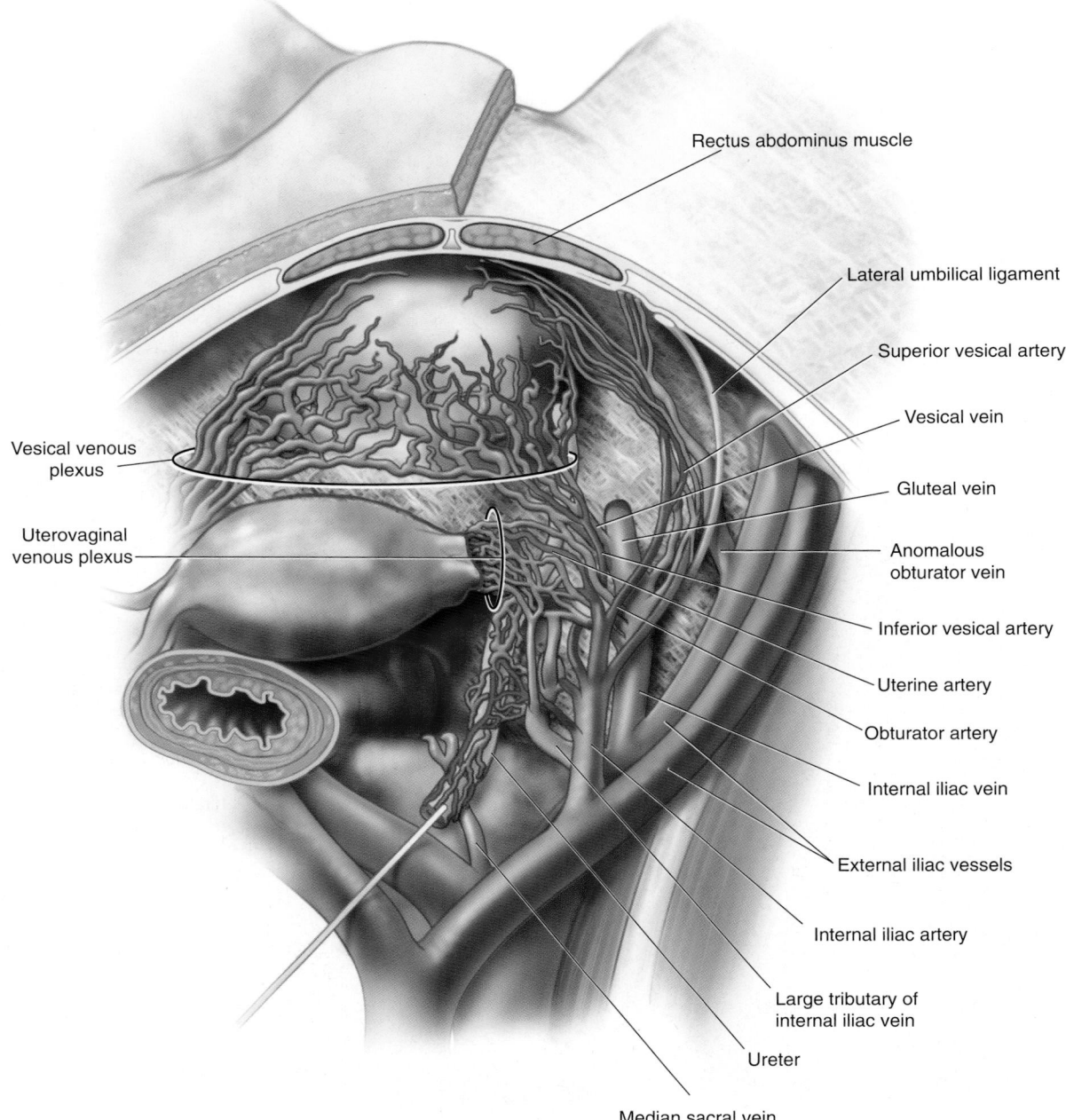

Rectus abdominus muscle

Lateral umbilical ligament

Superior vesical artery

Vesical vein

Gluteal vein

Anomalous obturator vein

Inferior vesical artery

Uterine artery

Obturator artery

Internal iliac vein

External iliac vessels

Internal iliac artery

Large tributary of internal iliac vein

Ureter

Median sacral vein

Vesical venous plexus

Uterovaginal venous plexus

**FIGURE 2–10** Blood supply to the urinary bladder is plentiful and emanates from several sources. Venous return may consist of a number of variable plexuses, which ultimately drain into the internal iliac vein. Extensive bleeding may be encountered as the result of disruption of these numerous venous channels during dissection of the perivesical space and paravaginal tissues. This figure shows the vasculature within the cardinal ligament after the round and broad ligaments have been removed. Note that the superior and inferior vesical arteries come off the anterior division of the hypogastric artery, as well as the lateral umbilical and uterine arteries, respectively. An anomalous obturator vein is shown. Venous drainage even for large vessels, including major internal iliac tributaries, may be anomalous. As shown in this drawing, two large internal iliac veins join with a single external iliac vein to form a short right common iliac vein.

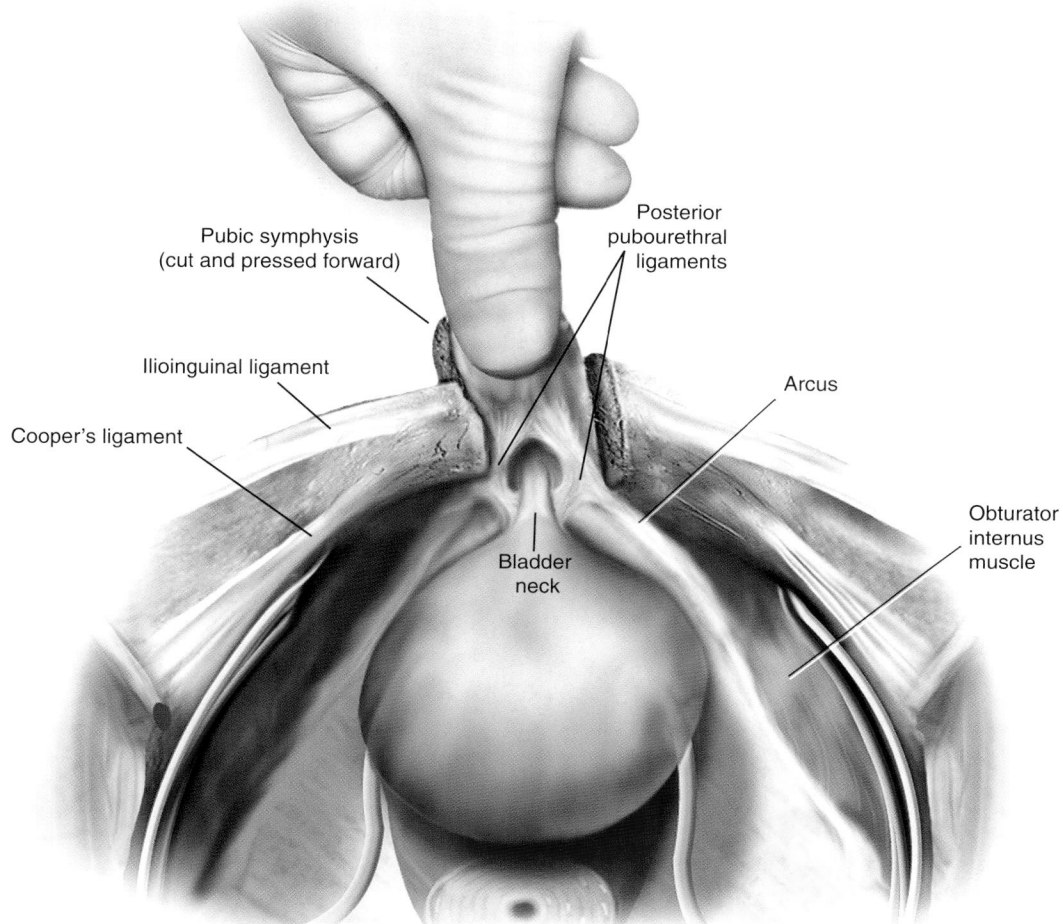

Pubic symphysis
(cut and pressed forward)

Posterior
pubourethral
ligaments

Ilioinguinal ligament

Arcus

Cooper's ligament

Obturator
internus
muscle

Bladder
neck

**FIGURE 2–11** The pubourethral (puboprostatic) ligaments extend from the proximal urethra to the posteroinferior and anteroinferior surfaces of the symphysis pubis. Note that the pubourethral ligament is a direct continuum of the arcus tendineus.

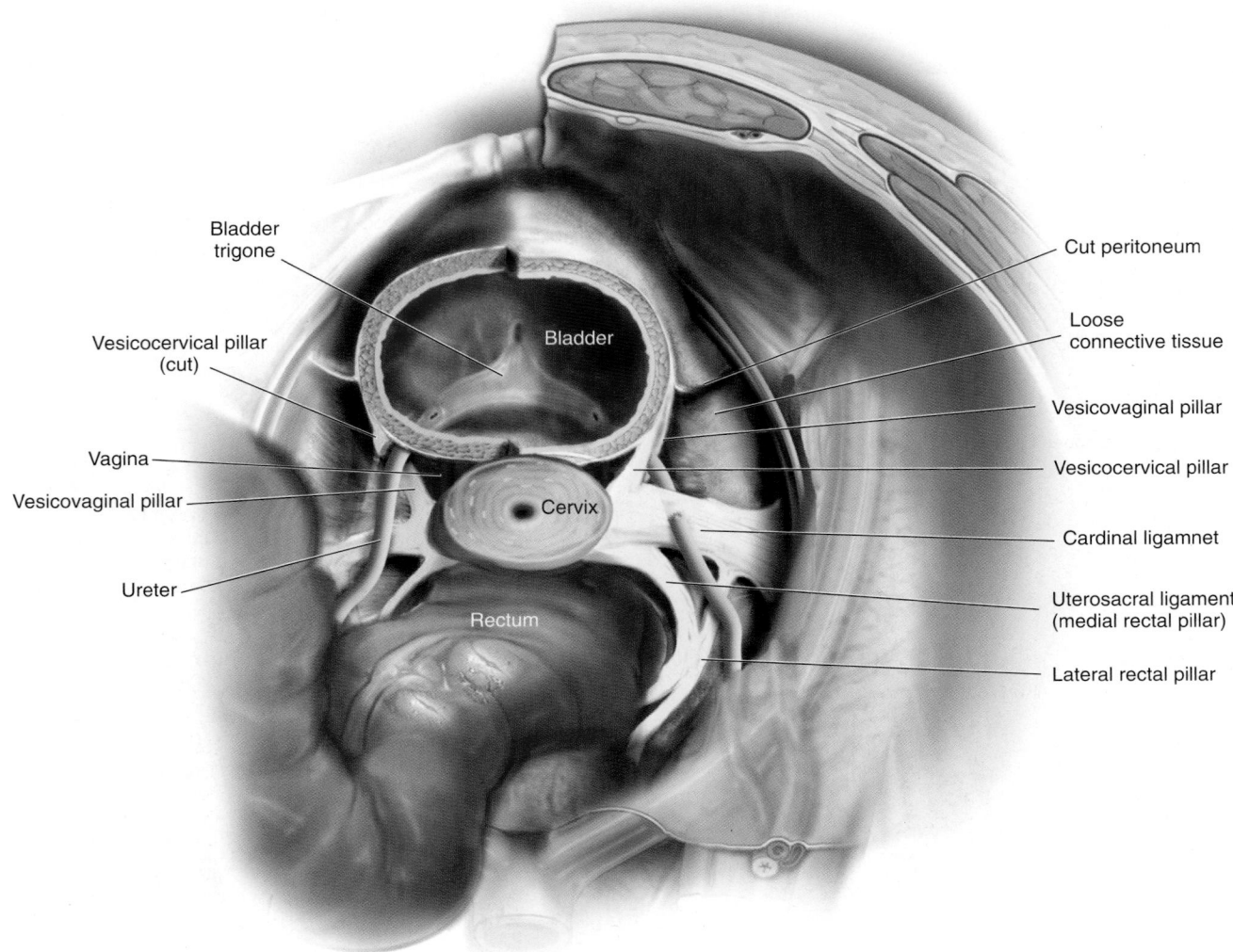

Bladder
trigone

Vesicocervical pillar
(cut)

Vagina

Vesicovaginal pillar

Ureter

Bladder

Cervix

Rectum

Cut peritoneum

Loose
connective tissue

Vesicovaginal pillar

Vesicocervical pillar

Cardinal ligamnet

Uterosacral ligament
(medial rectal pillar)

Lateral rectal pillar

**FIGURE 2–12** The bladder dome has been cut away, allowing viewers to peer into the depths of the bladder. The trigone is visible. The uterine corpus has also been removed, as in the case of the supracervical hysterectomy. The sigmoid colon and rectum are intact. Note the relationships of the bladder pillars to the cervix, vagina, and ureters.

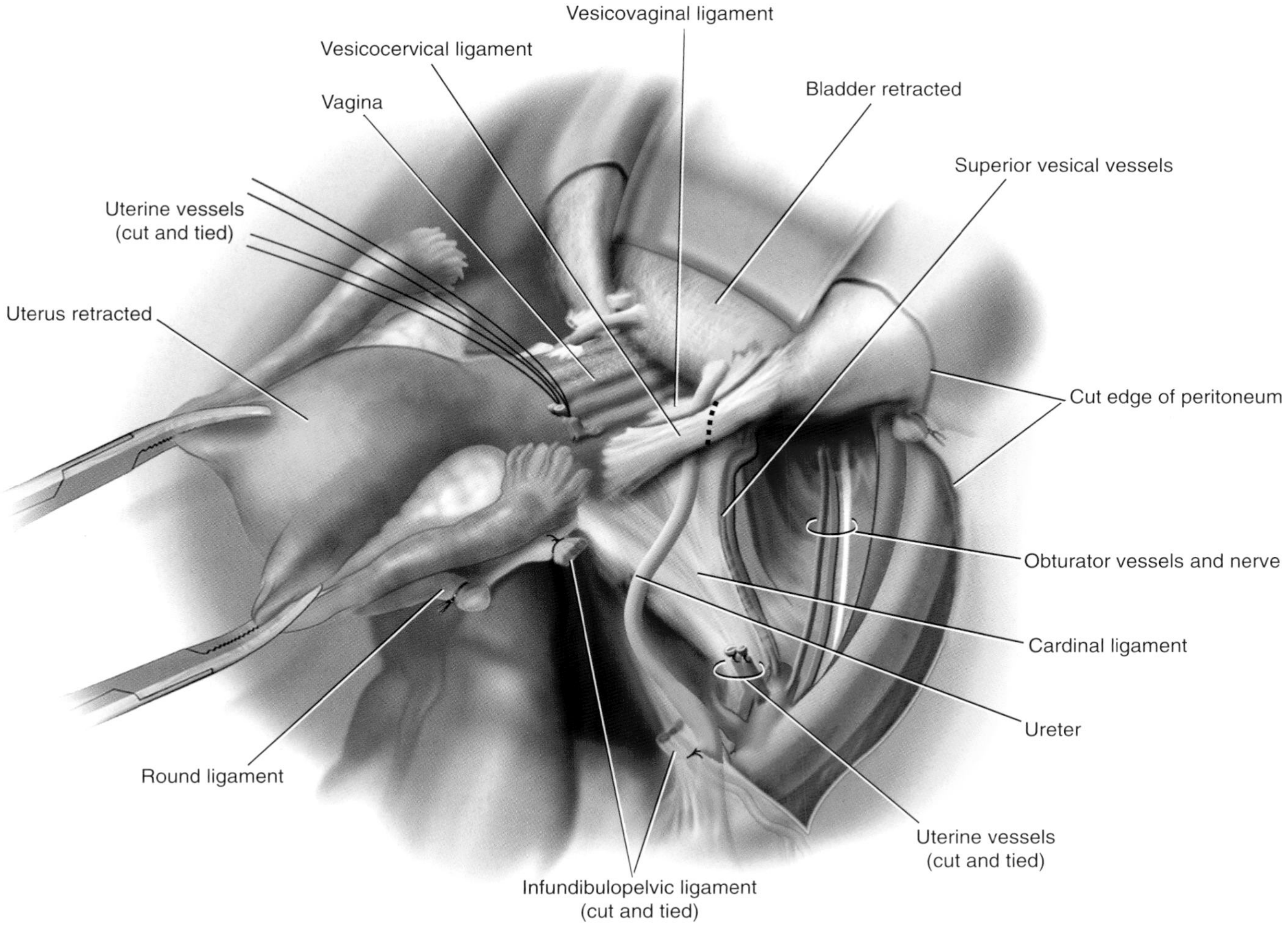

Vesicovaginal ligament

Vesicocervical ligament

Vagina

Bladder retracted

Superior vesical vessels

Uterine vessels
(cut and tied)

Uterus retracted

Cut edge of peritoneum

Obturator vessels and nerve

Cardinal ligament

Ureter

Uterine vessels
(cut and tied)

Round ligament

Infundibulopelvic ligament
(cut and tied)

**FIGURE 2–13** The central portion of the urinary bladder is retracted following incision of the vesicouterine peritoneal fold separation of the bladder from the cervix and vagina. Peripherally, the bladder remains attached to the cervix and vagina by the bladder pillars. Relationships of the vesical, uterine, and obturator vessels are seen here. The dotted line indicates where the vesicocervical ligament will be transsected.

Note that the ureter passes deep to the vesicocervical ligament (the anterior bladder pillar).

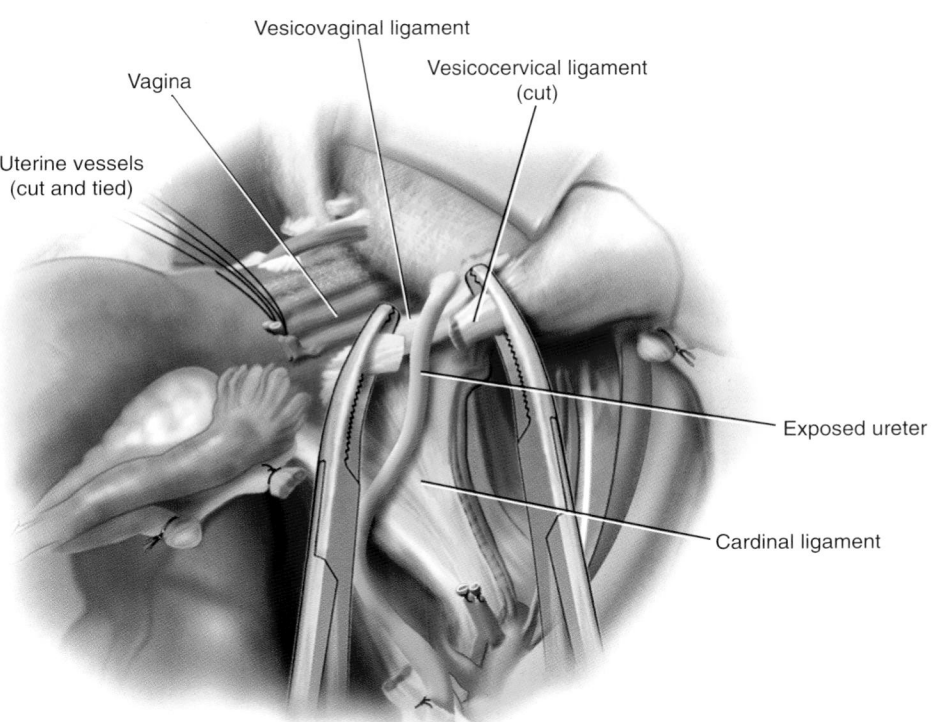

Vesicovaginal ligament

Vesicocervical ligament
(cut)

Vagina

Uterine vessels
(cut and tied)

Exposed ureter

Cardinal ligament

**FIGURE 2–14** The uterine vessels have been divided. The anterior bladder pillar (vesicocervical ligament) has been doubly clamped with tonsil clamps and has been divided. This fully exposes the ureter at the ureterovesical junction.

UNIT 1 ■ SECTION A

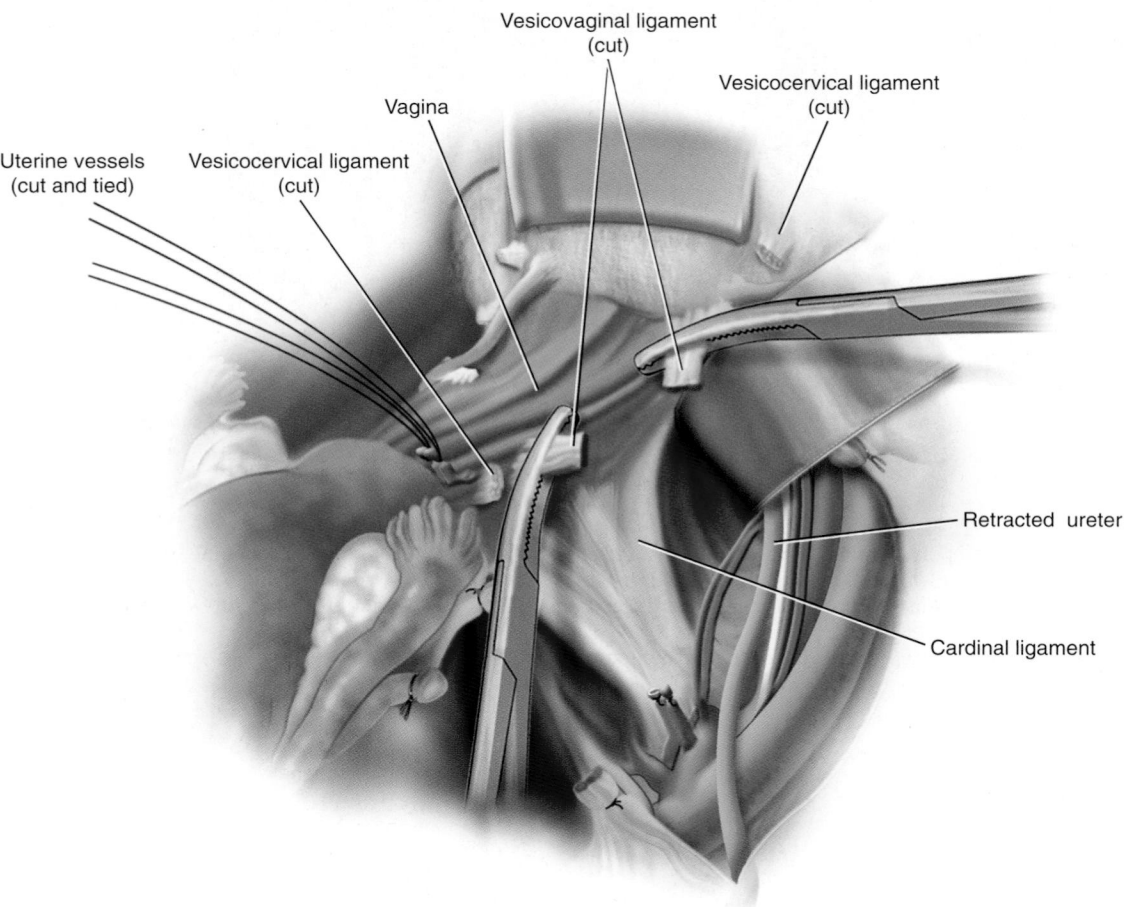

**FIGURE 2–15** The vesicovaginal ligament has been clamped and cut, which permits mobilization of the bladder and ureters. The upper vagina and the bladder base are held in place by the deep parametrium (deep cardinal ligaments) only.

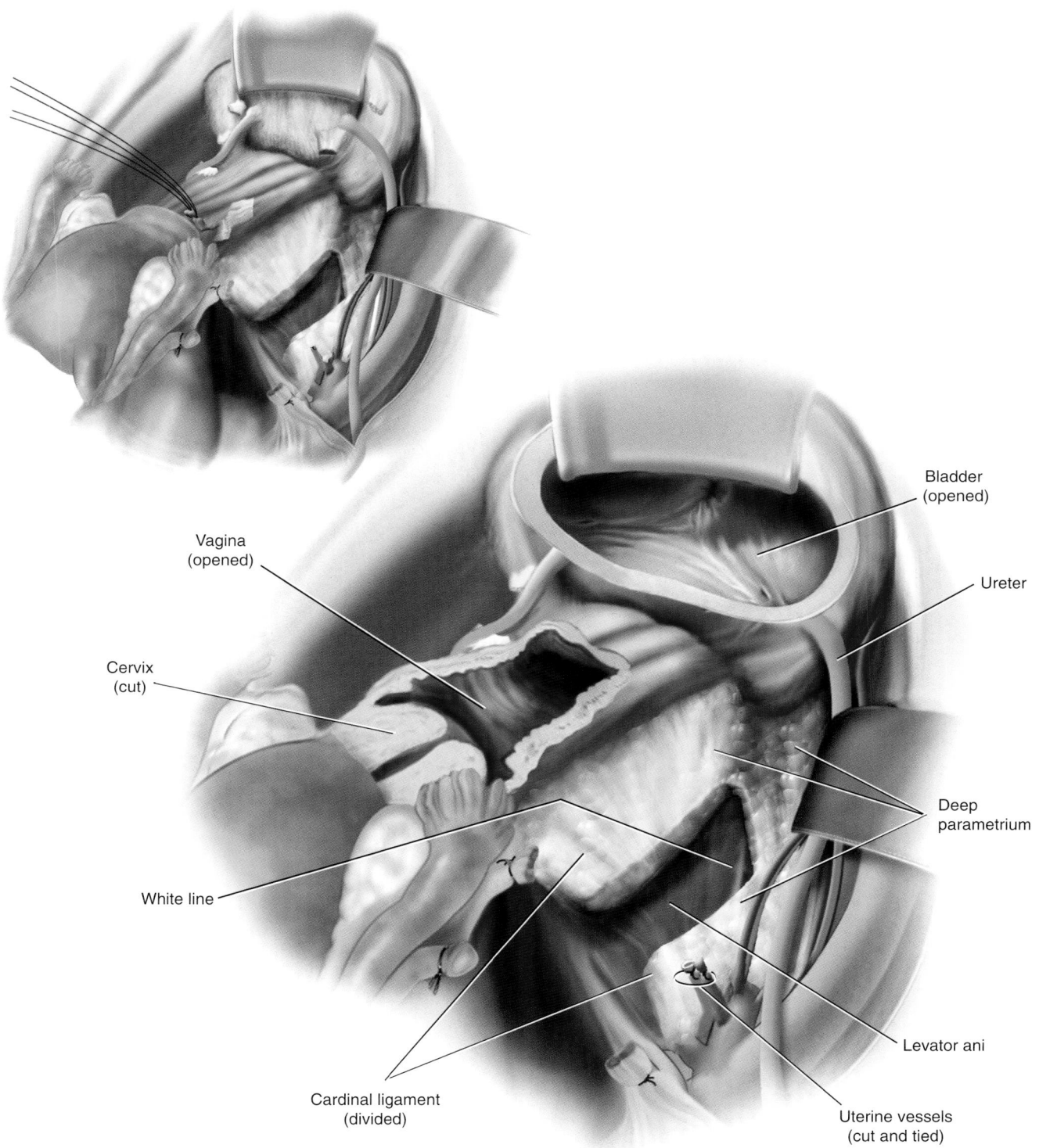

Bladder
(opened)

Ureter

Vagina
(opened)

Cervix
(cut)

Deep
parametrium

White line

Levator ani

Cardinal ligament
(divided)

Uterine vessels
(cut and tied)

**FIGURE 2–16** The upper vagina has been exposed and a portion of the anterior wall excised. The bladder dome has also been excised. The right cardinal ligament and a portion of the deep parametrium on the right have also been severed. Note that the deep parametrial attachment to the bladder base remains intact. This drawing illustrates the fibrofatty composition of these endopelvic "ligaments."

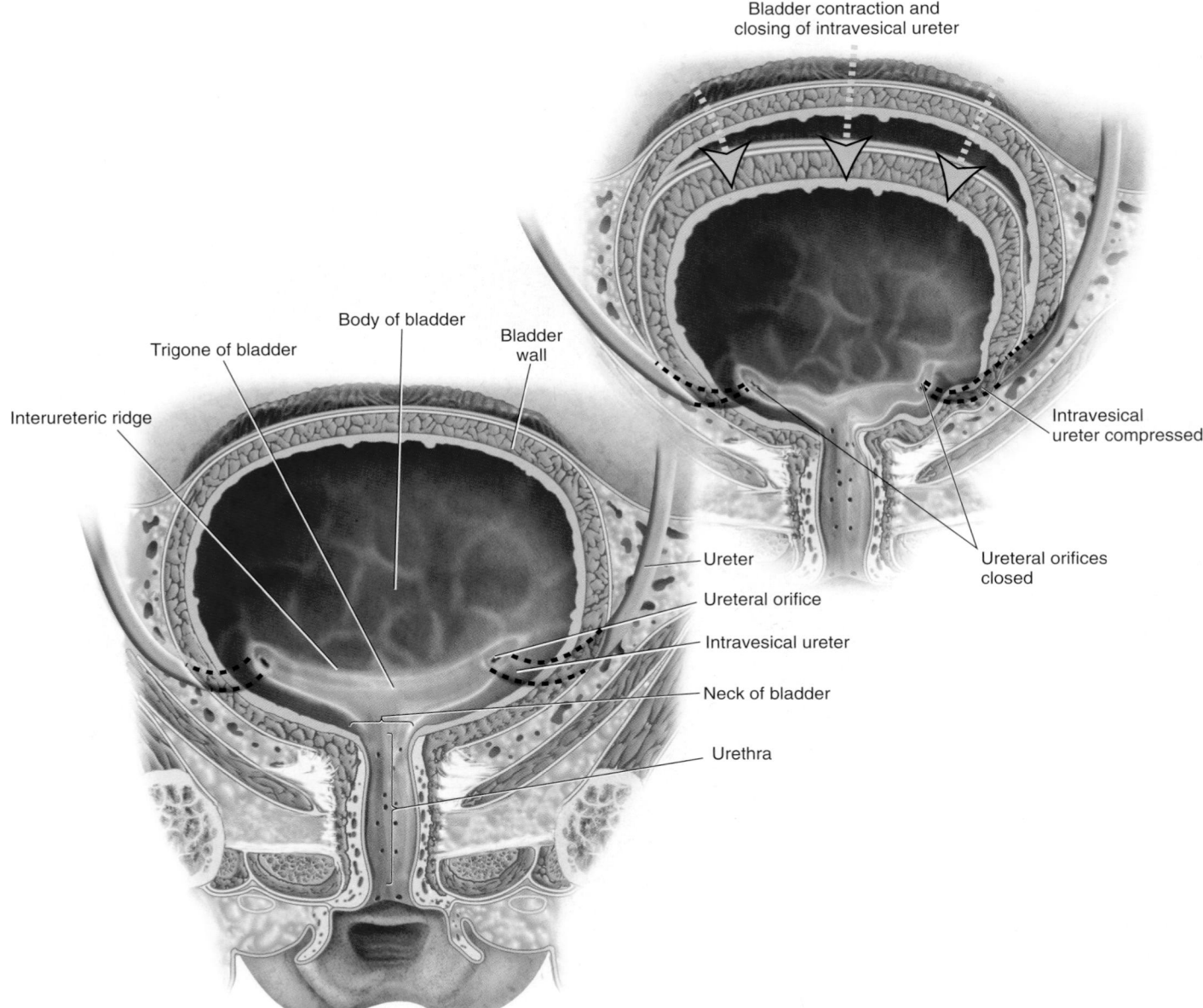

Bladder contraction and
closing of intravesical ureter

Body of bladder

Trigone of bladder

Bladder
wall

Interureteric ridge

Intravesical
ureter compressed

Ureteral orifices
closed

Ureter

Ureteral orifice

Intravesical ureter

Neck of bladder

Urethra

**FIGURE 2–17** The anterior portion of the bladder has been cut away to reveal the trigone and the full posterior wall, as well as the posterior wall of the urethra. The trigone and the intravesical course of the ureter can be seen (*dotted lines*).
    The upper right figure shows the bladder wall contracting and the intravesical ureter closing off. This picture is a frontal view.

# SECTION B

# Basic Foundations for Gynecologic Surgery

# CHAPTER 3

# Instrumentation

## *Michael S. Baggish*

A surgeon's tools are analogous to those of a carpenter, a mechanic, a research chemist, or an atomic physicist. High-quality instruments are required for the performance of precise and excellent surgery. Although a fine surgeon may overcome the deficits of inferior instruments, the real and potential difficulties presented by using second-rate tools make doing first-rate surgery harder. Good instruments coupled with good surgeons yield the best outcomes.

Throughout this book, reference is made to various instruments utilized in the performance of specific operations. For convenience, this section will codify the panoply of instruments commonly used in gynecologic surgery.

## Forceps

A number of forceps are available. Atraumatic forceps include the Adson and DeBakey instruments. For lymph node and fat dissection, for example, obturator fossa dissection, ring forceps are quite acceptable. Rat-tooth forceps are excellent for traction and for holding tissue securely; however, they may traumatize skin and other delicate tissues. Adson-Brown forceps are the best instruments for grasping skin edges during closure procedures (Fig. 3–1A–C). For fine work deep in the pelvis, for example, dissecting around the ureter or iliac vessels, the author prefers a bayonet forceps equipped with a brown-toothed tip (Fig. 3–1D, E).

## Clamps

Clamps may be subdivided into grasping and traction clamps, which include Allis and Ochsner clamps. Grasping clamps are relatively atraumatic, whereas traction clamps are best suited to specimens that will be excised or otherwise removed. Allis clamps are frequently required in vaginal and abdominal surgery. Babcock clamps are atraumatic instruments useful for grasping delicate structures, such as the oviducts, utero-ovarian ligaments, and other fragile tubular structures (Fig. 3–2A, B). Ochsner clamps, for example, may be applied to the cervix for traction during vaginal hysterectomy or on skin scars that are going to be cut out (Fig. 3–2C, D).

Dissecting or hemostatic clamps include standard and long tonsil clamps (Fig. 3–3A, B). These are excellent for fine dissection and for clamping bleeding vessels deep within the pelvis, particularly in strategic locations. The tips of these clamps are tapered and angled. One variety, the right-angle clamp, has a 90° angle (Fig. 3–3C). This is the instrument of choice for isolating large arteries from underlying veins, as occurs during hypogastric artery ligation.

Hemostatic clamps may be straight or curved. Mosquito clamps and the larger Kelly clamps are most commonly used to secure bleeding vessels. Additionally, the fine mosquito clamps may also be used as dissecting tools (Fig. 3–4A, B).

Large vascular pedicle clamps used for hysterectomy or radical hysterectomy should incorporate powerful, atraumatic jaws, a variety of curvatures, and suitable length to facilitate securing these large pedicles. These characteristics are exemplified by the Zeppelin clamps (Fig. 3–5A–C). Haney clamps of the straight and curved variety are the most common pedicle clamps used in the performance of vaginal hysterectomy (Fig. 3–5D).

## Scissors

Surgical scissors may be divided into fine dissecting instruments and heavy-duty mass-cutting devices. The first category includes Metzenbaum and Stevens scissors. The former are superior for dissection, whereas the latter are the superlative cutting tools (Fig. 3–6A, B). Large pedicles, vaginal cuffs, and ligaments are best cut with Mayo or Jorgenson scissors (Fig. 3–7A, B).

## Knives

Of course, the sharpest mechanical cutting tool is the scalpel. A variety of blade shapes are available for different applications. Scalpel handles may be a standard 6-inch length or an elongated 9- to 10-inch length (Fig. 3–8).

## Retractors

During contemporary abdominal surgery, a self-retaining retractor is essential. Several types are available, ranging from the frame type (Bookwalter and Kirschner) to the spreading type (O'Sullivan-O'Connor). The modern frame retractor has the advantage of remote location, that is, location outside of the abdominal cavity. Its varied blades may be placed within the abdomen and interchanged when necessary without compromising exposure or completely removing the retractor (Fig. 3–9A, B).

The O'Sullivan-O'Connor retractor and the Balfour retractor are the most commonly used devices for pelvic surgery. The O'Sullivan-O'Connor retractor is easy to use and has a sufficient variety of blades to satisfy most clinical conditions. This retractor is equally suitable for transverse and vertical incisions (Fig. 3–10A, B). The Balfour retractor is also a mainstay abdominal retractor in gynecologic and obstetric surgery. This device may

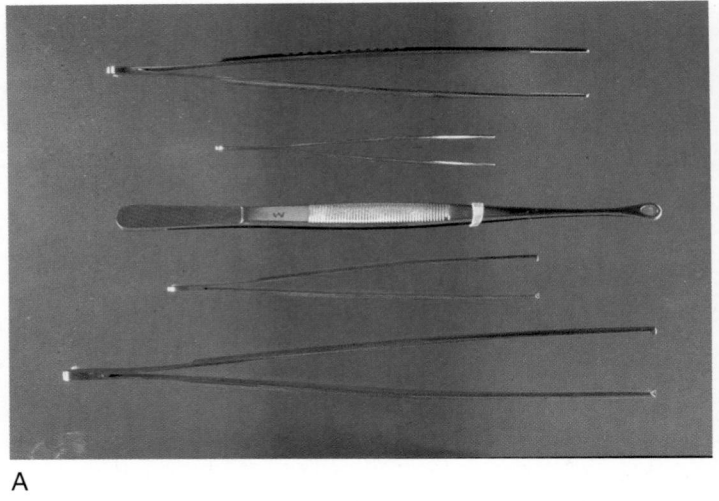

A

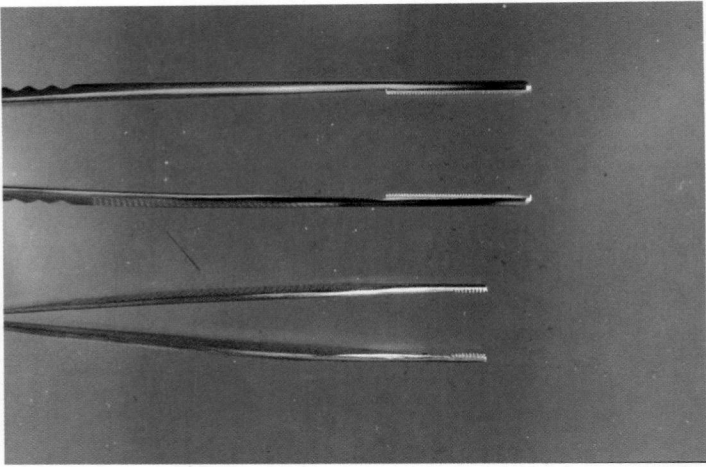

B

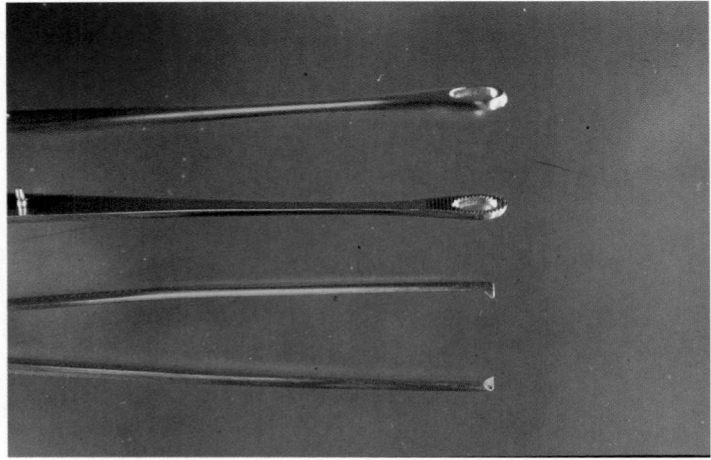

C

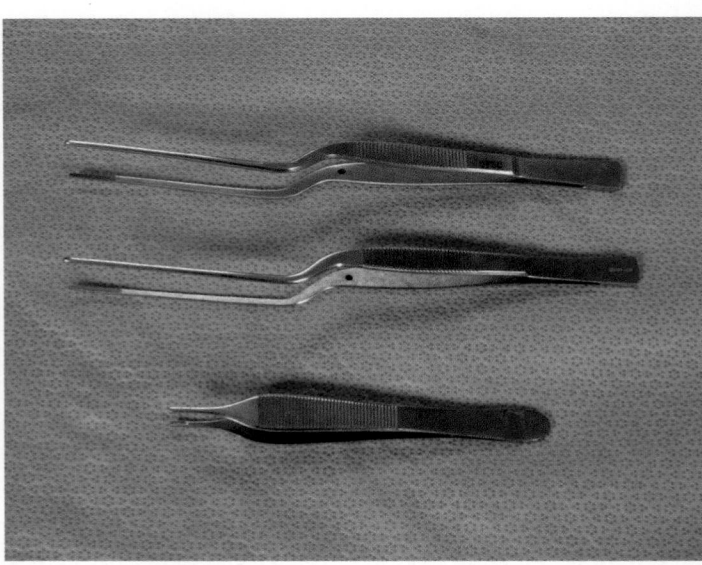

D

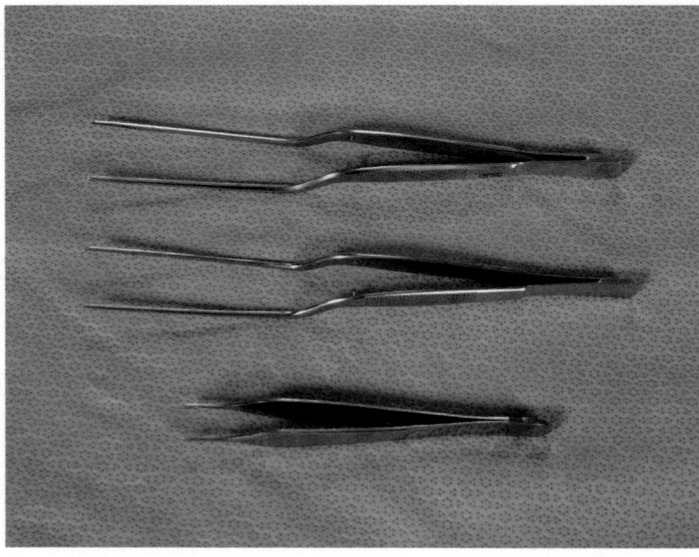

E

**FIGURE 3–1  A.** Five surgical forceps are shown. From the top: DeBakey, Adson-Brown, ring, rat-tooth, standard (6-inch), and medium (10-inch) tissue forceps. **B.** Close-up view of the atraumatic DeBakey (*top*) and Adson-Brown forceps (*bottom*). **C.** Close-up view of the ring forceps, which are ideal for clearing fatty tissue from the obturator fossa and between large vessels. Below is the grasping end of rat-tooth tissue forceps. **D.** Bayonet forceps (*top* and *center*) and Adson forceps (*bottom*) are ideal for fine tissue handling. **E.** Another view of the forceps shown in Figure 3–1D.

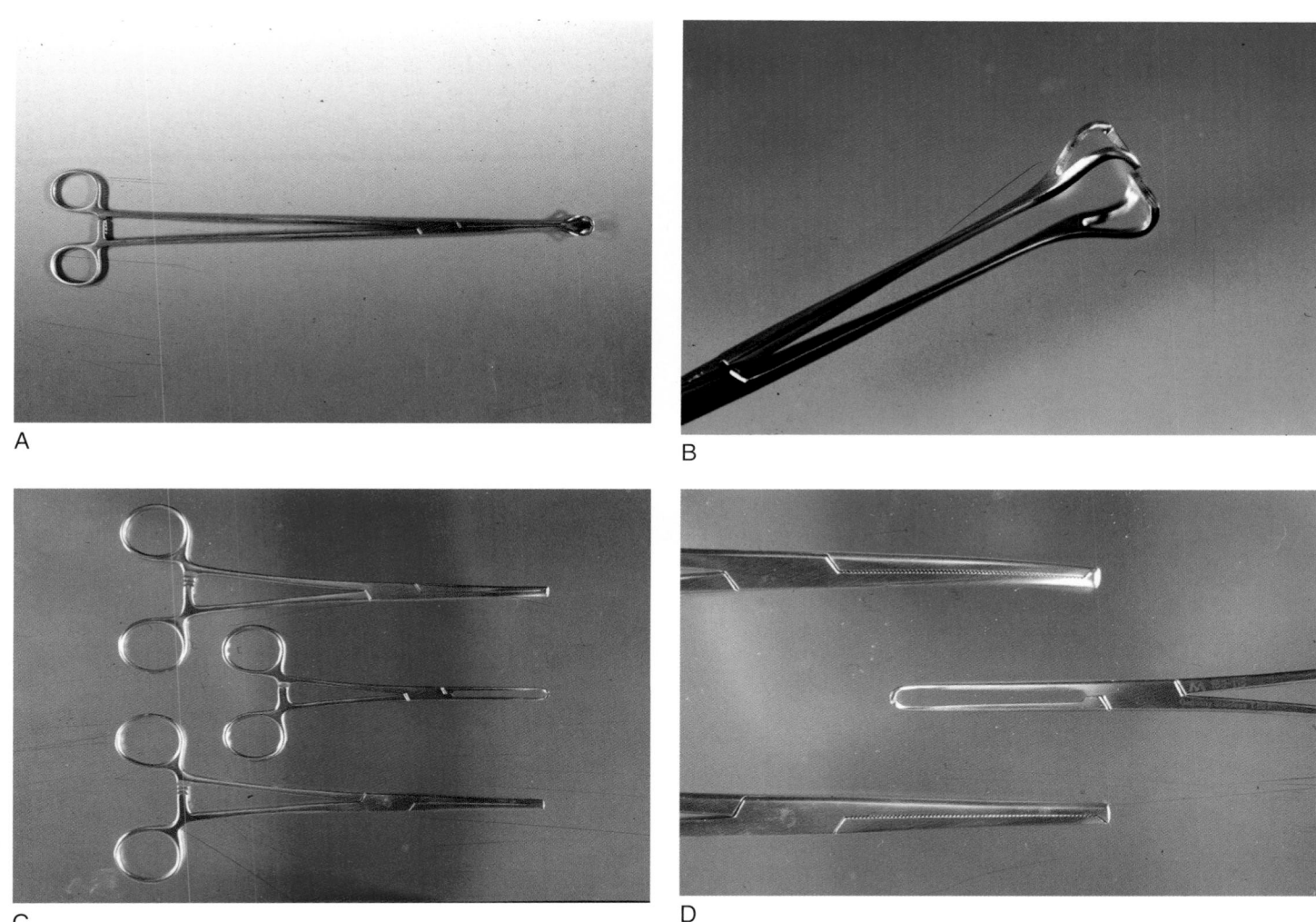

A

B

C

D

**FIGURE 3–2 A.** The Babcock clamp, which ranges in length from 8 to 14 inches, is an atraumatic grasping instrument ideal for placing traction on tubular structures while not crushing the tissue. **B.** Close-up of the shaft and terminus of the Babcock clamp. **C.** The three clamps illustrated here are curved Ochsner (*top*), Allis (*center*), and straight Ochsner clamps (*bottom*). **D.** Close-up view of Figure 3–2C. Note the toothed jaws of the Ochsner clamps (*top*), which grasps very securely but is rather rough on the tissue. In contrast, the Allis clamp (*center*) grasps tissue firmly but less aggressively than the Ochsner clamp, thereby avoiding crush trauma.

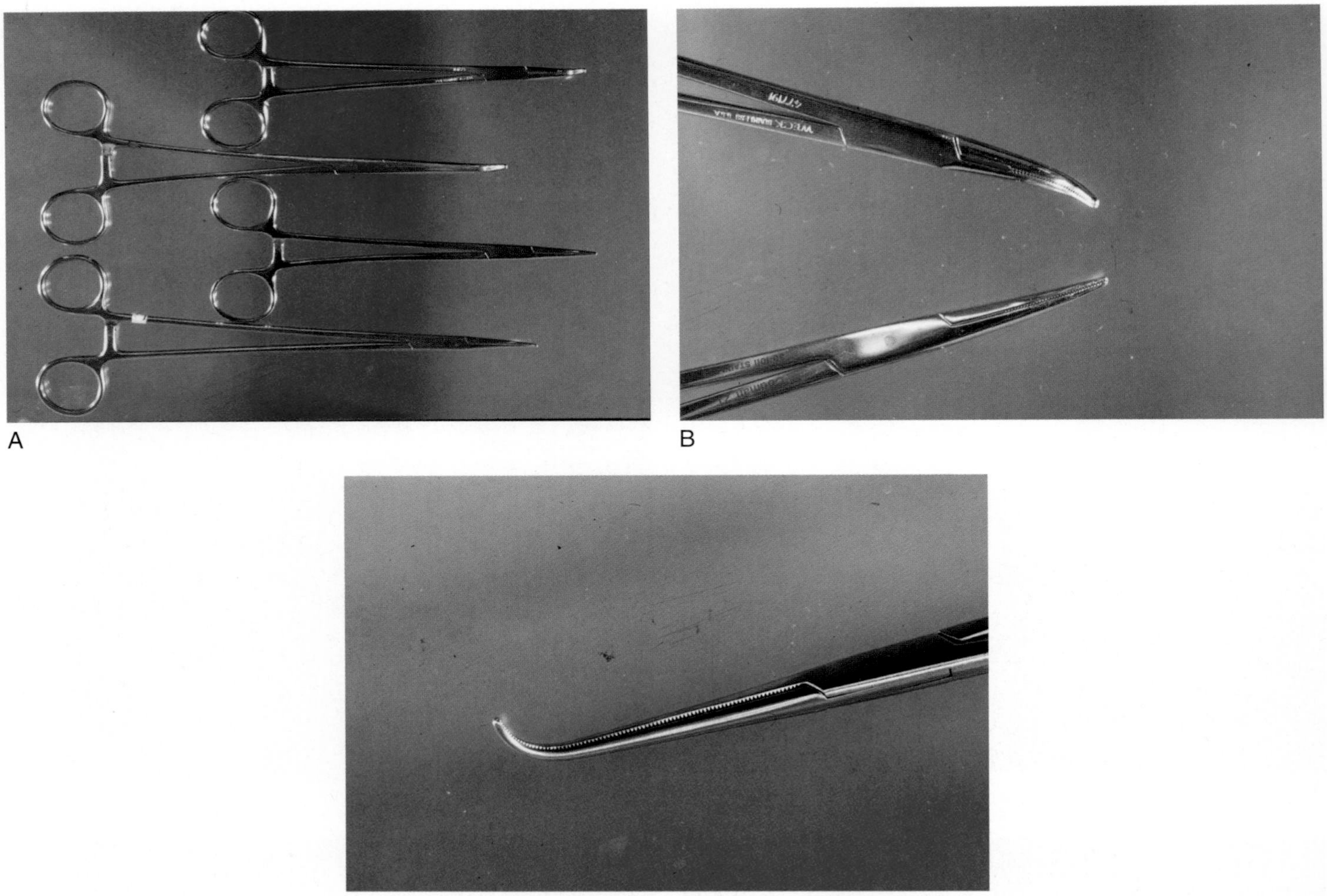

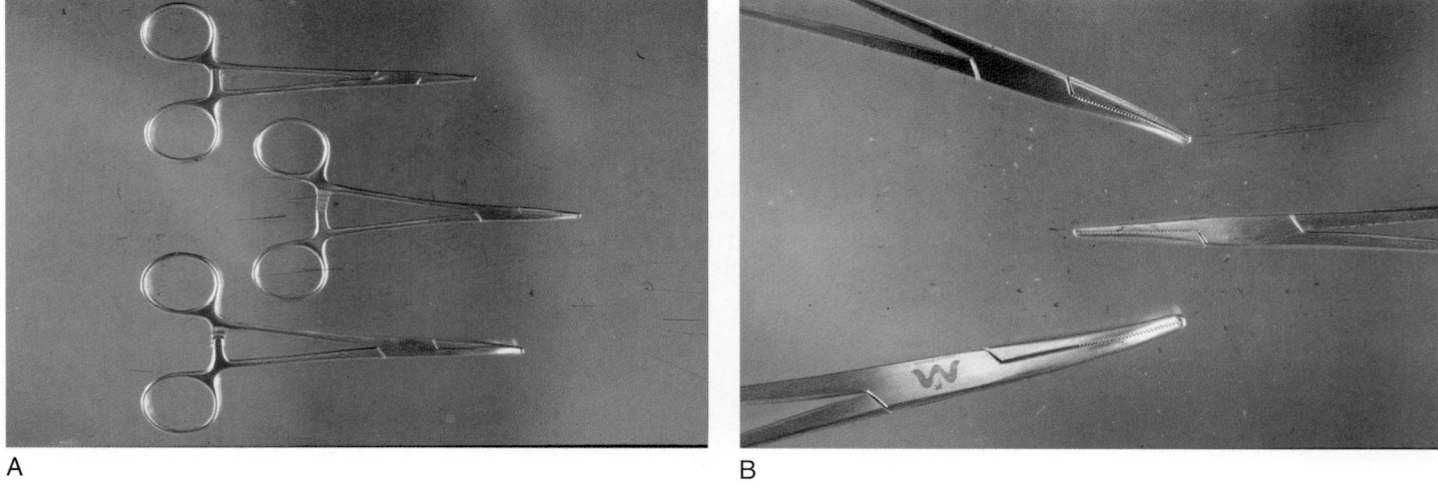

**FIGURE 3–3 A.** Tonsil dissection and hemostatic clamps are shown in standard and long variations. The two upper clamps are curved, and the lower two are straight. **B.** The fine, tapered tips of the tonsil clamp are well suited for fine dissection and for securing small bleeding vessels deep within the pelvis. **C.** The right-angle clamp is used to dissect around and to isolate the hypogastric artery. It is also useful for dissecting the ureter and receiving a traction tape or suture.

**FIGURE 3–4 A.** The two upper clamps are Halsted mosquito clamps. A curved Kelly clamp is pictured at the bottom. **B.** The detail in Figure 3–4A shows the heavier aspect of the Kelly hemostatic (*bottom*) compared with the finer, tapered Halsted mosquito clamp.

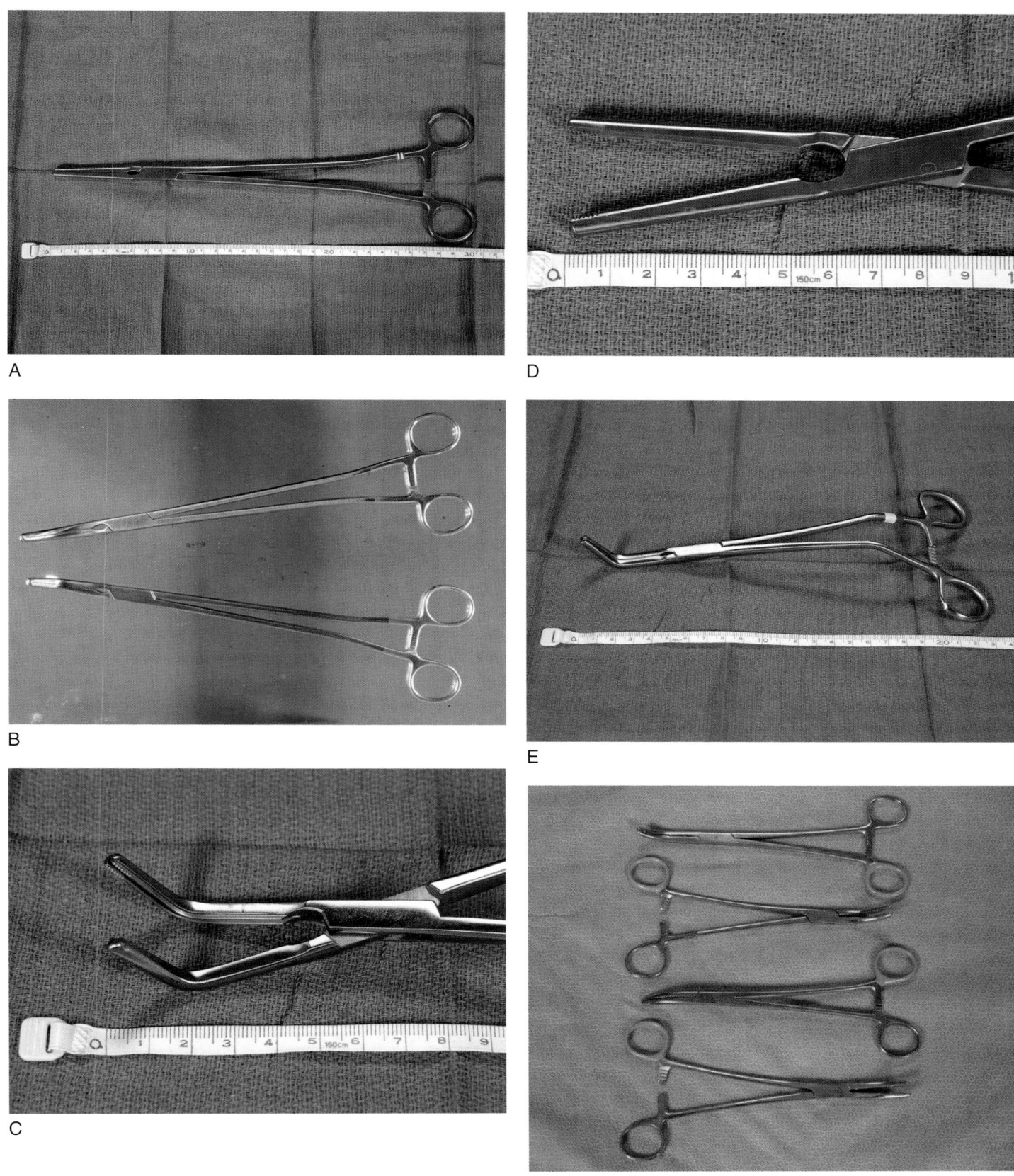

**FIGURE 3-5  A.** Straight Zeppelin clamp is shown here. Renditions of the same clamps in varying angles of curvature are also available. **B.** Two extra long Zeppelin clamps (14 inches) used for securing the vaginal angles in deep pelvises. **C.** Right angulated Zeppelin clamp is ideal for application at the vaginal angle and for clamping across the vaginal cuff. **D.** Detail of the jaw tip of a Zeppelin hysterectomy clamp. Note the longitudinal groove in one limb of the clamp and the machined ridge in the other limb. **E.** The grooved-out right jaw and interlocking teeth on the tip of the jaw prevent tissue slippage when the clamp is applied. **F.** Four Haney clamps are illustrated. These, like the Zeppelin clamps, are available in straight and curved variations. The instruments shown here are curved.

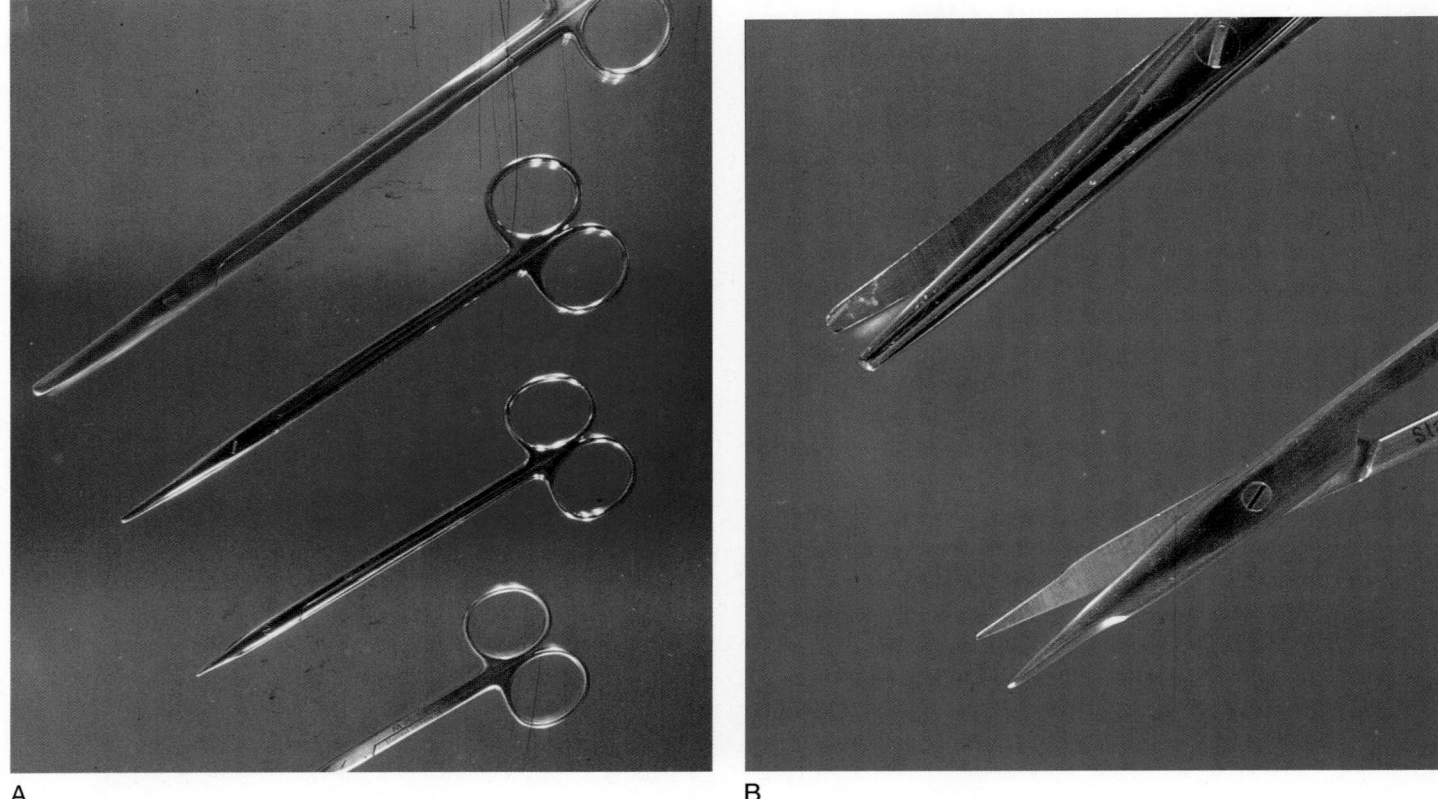

**FIGURE 3–6 A.** Two general types of dissecting scissors are shown here. The top two are long and standard Metzenbaum scissors. The bottom two are long and short Stevens tenotomy scissors. **B.** The differences between Metzenbaum and Stevens scissors are apparent. The latter are finer and are beveled for precision cutting.

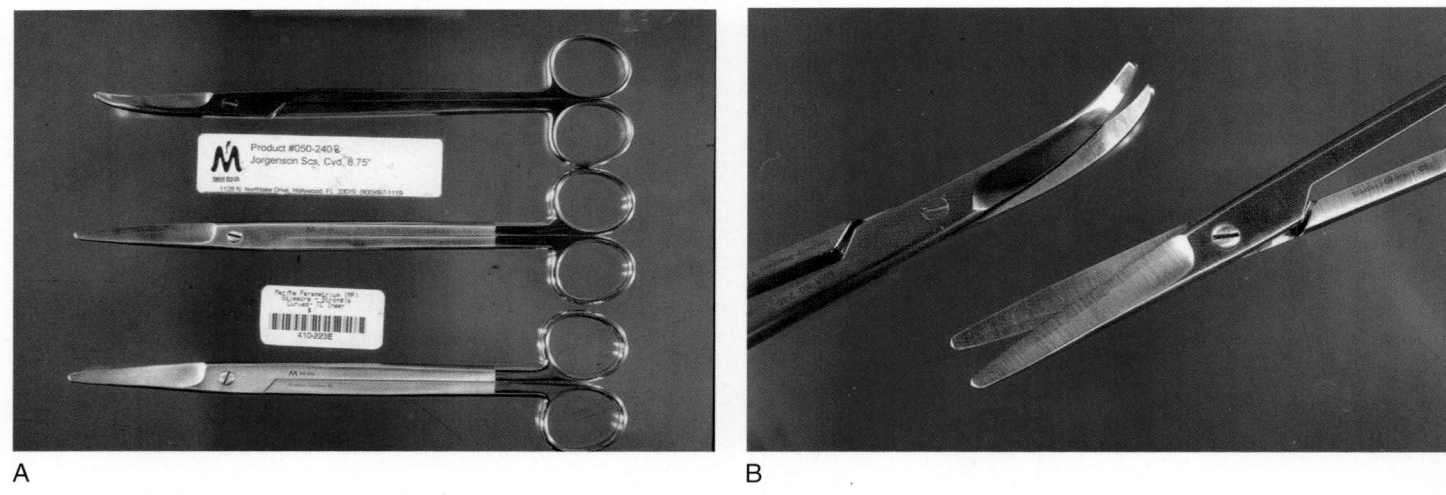

**FIGURE 3–7 A.** Mass tissue cutting (e.g., ovarian and parametrial pedicles) requires sharp, heavy-duty scissors as pictured. Mayo and Jorgenson scissors types are most commonly used for hysterectomy and radical hysterectomy. **B.** Angled Jorgenson scissors (*above*) are ideal for severing the cardinal ligaments and the vagina during hysterectomy operations.

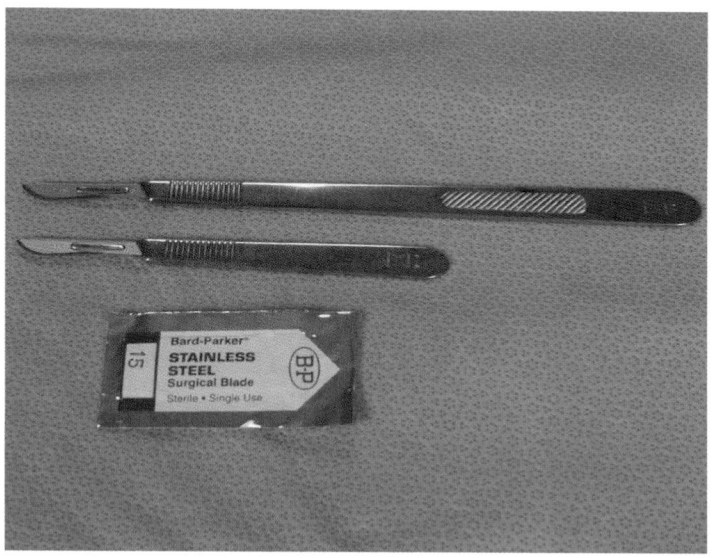

**FIGURE 3–8** Standard and long scalpel handles range from 6 inches to 10 inches in length.

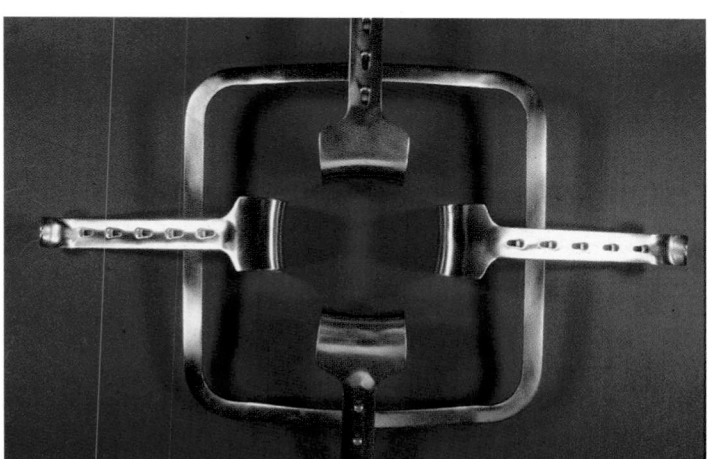

A

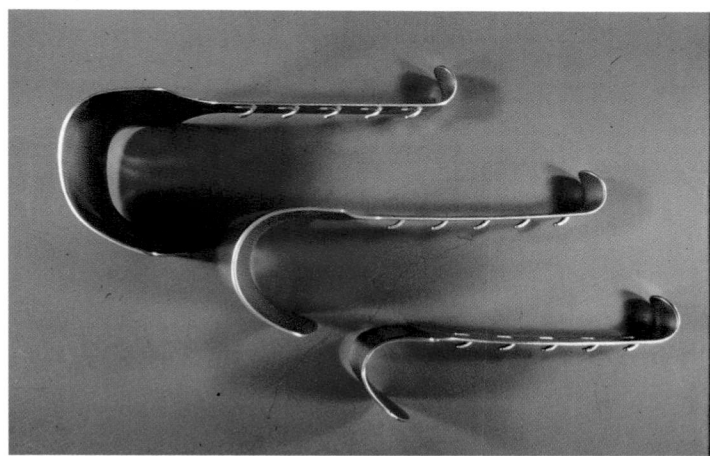

B

**FIGURE 3–9 A.** The frame retractor is placed over the open laparotomy incision. A wide selection of blades permits bladder and bowel retraction, as well as sidewall exposure. **B.** The ratchets on the undersides of the retractor blades are easily interlocked via a series of spaces located on the underside of the frame retractor.

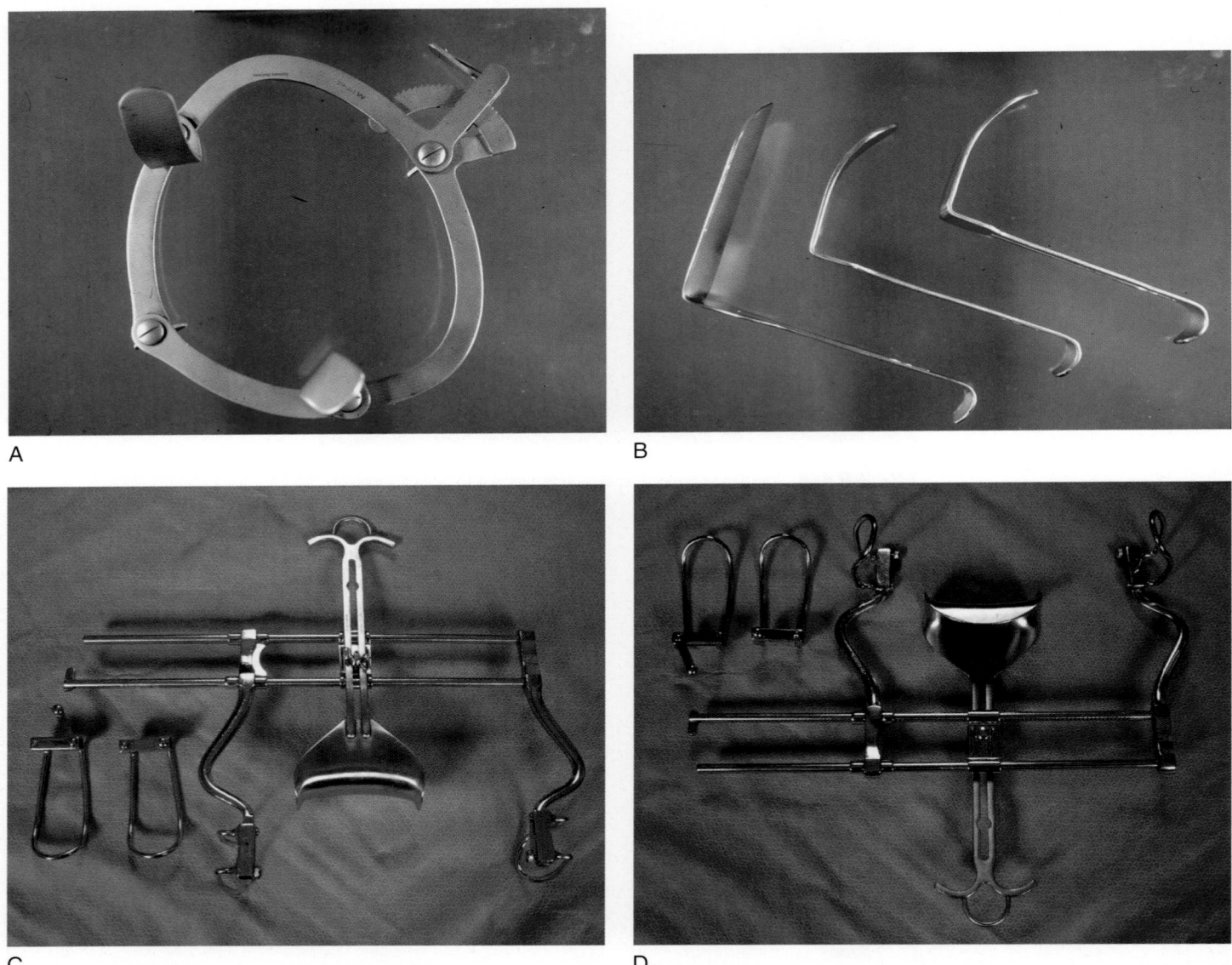

A

B

C

D

**FIGURE 3–10  A.** The O'Sullivan-O'Connor retractor is the most commonly used device of its kind for obstetric and gynecologic surgery. **B.** Several blades are attached to the retractor by wing nuts located fore and aft. **C.** The Balfour retractor is another self-retaining device. A bladder blade is shown here attached by a wing nut. **D.** The undersurface of the Balfour retractor is shown in this view. For obese patients, long retractor blades are postoperatively fitted to the frame.

be alternatively fitted with standard or deep lateral retractor pieces (Fig. 3–10C, D).

Among the many useful instruments for vaginal surgery are the weighted speculum and the Haney, Sims, Dever, and Breisky-Navratil retractors (Fig. 3–11A–D). The small Richardson retractor is particularly ideal for insertion beneath the anterior cervical circumcision (during vaginal hysterectomy) to facilitate entry into the vesicouterine space (Fig. 3–11E, F). Breisky-Navratil retractors are needed for deep vaginal work (e.g., paravaginal repair) (Fig. 3–11G).

Malleable retractors are well suited to protect the bladder, colon, and other structures during surgery. They are usually available in narrow or wide widths and can be bent to shape for more or less any specific intraoperative need (Fig. 3–11H).

The long-handled vein retractor is the instrument of choice for moving and retracting large vessels (e.g., the external iliac vein) during exposure of the obturator fossa or the hypogastric artery during ureteral dissection (Fig. 3–11I, J).

## Needle Holders

A variety of long and short needle holders are available for gynecologic surgery. Selection depends on the application for the device, the anticipated size of the needle and suture, and the anatomic location.

For fine needles, the long and short Ryder or fine bulldog instruments provide satisfactory options (Figs. 3–12 and 3–13). As an all-purpose needle holder, the long or medium bulldog device is an excellent choice (Figs. 3–14 and 3–15). For vaginal work, or when a curved instrument provides a strategic mechanical advantage, the Haney needle holder is the instrument the author prefers (Fig. 3–16).

As with any tool, correct usage provides the best overall results. The needle should be driven into the tissue perpendicularly and should traverse through the tissue in its natural arc. The action of needle holder movement is totally within the wrist. When suture ligatures are performed, for example during hysterectomy, the needle must be driven just below the toe of the pedicle clamps. If a transfixing stitch is to be placed, then the same stitch circles the pedicle and is driven toward the heel of the clamp (see Fig. 11–32 in Chapter 11).

## Dilators

The operation of dilatation and curettage (D & C) is one of the most often performed surgical procedures in both obstetrics and gynecology.

Cervical dilatation is a critical part of the D & C operation, as well as a necessary component of hysteroscopic examination of the uterus. Several types of cervical dilators are available, but the least traumatic are the graduated Hank's or Pratt devices (Figs. 3–17 and 3–18). For stenotic cervices, the author prefers to initiate dilatation with a baby Hegar dilator (Figs. 3–19 and 3–20).

A single-toothed tenaculum should always be used in conjunction with a dilator (Fig. 3–21).

## Curettes

The second critical instrument required for the D & C operation is the uterine curette. Several varieties of curettes, including sharp, serrated uterine, and sharp endocervical types, are available. As is the case for uterine dilators, the curette is required to stabilize the cervix with a tenaculum when a curettage is performed (Fig. 3–22A, B).

## Suction Curettes

Suction curettes are manufactured in a variety of sizes, shapes, and curvatures. Essentially, they are plastic cannulas with an offset terminal opening. They attach to a handpiece fitted with a suction control device. These are used principally for pregnancy termination, evacuation of incomplete or missed abortion, and hydatidiform mole evacuation (Fig. 3–23).

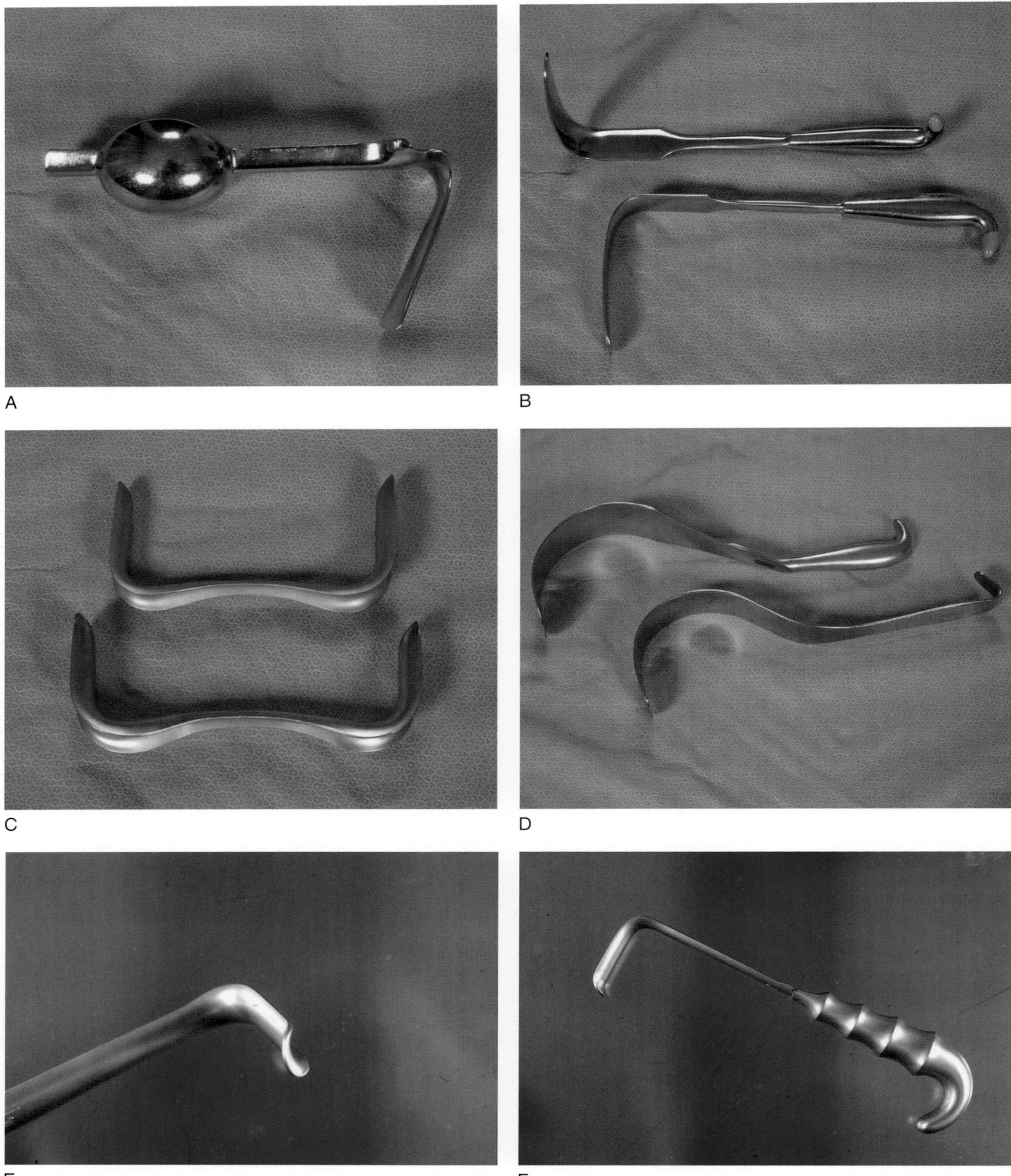

**FIGURE 3–11  A.** The weighted speculum is utilized as a self-retaining vaginal retractor. It is positioned along the posterior vagina and into the posterior fornix. **B.** The right-angled Haney retractor is placed into the anterior and posterior cul-de-sacs after the peritoneum is opened during vaginal hysterectomy. These retractors provide a barrier between the uterus and the rectum, as well as between the uterus and the bladder. **C.** Sims retractors may be used to examine the vagina as well as to retract it during surgery. A Sims retractor placed into the vagina along the posterior wall provides the easiest method of exposing the cervix to apply a tenaculum (to the cervix) for hysteroscopic and laparoscopic procedures. **D.** Dever retractors are utilized during abdominal operations to retract the intestines and occasionally the bladder. Narrow Dever retractors are ideal for lateral vaginal retraction during the performance of vaginal hysterectomy. **E.** The small, narrow Richardson retractor is an excellent device for retracting the anterior vagina during the initial phase of vaginal hysterectomy. **F.** The Richardson retractor is also useful for retracting the advanced bladder during the anterior colpotomy portion of vaginal hysterectomy.

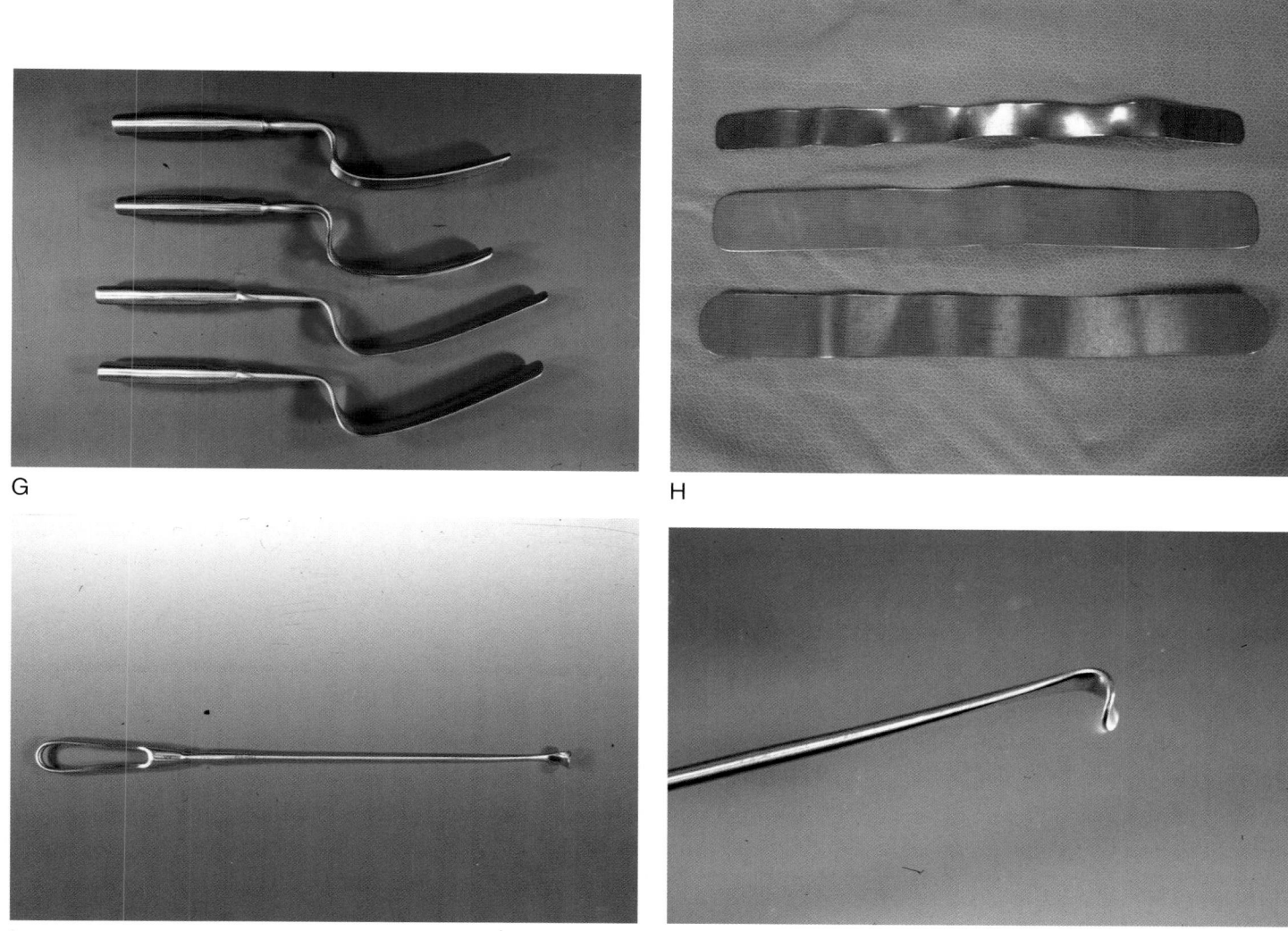

G

H

I

J

**FIGURE 3–11, cont'd  G.** Breisky-Navratil retractors pr vide excellent exposure during vaginal suspension procedures, such as sacrospinous ligament suspension operations. **H.** Malleable retractors can be bent and molded into many shapes. This allows them to be tailored to a specific clinical situation, whether the approach is abdominal or vaginal. The author favors the broad malleable retractor to place behind the uterus into the cul-de-sac of Douglas to protect the sigmoid colon and rectum. **I.** The vein retractor is used to retract delicate structures and should be handled gently. This device is the best instrument for retracting the external iliac vein when the obturator fossa is dissected. **J.** The vein retractor is also useful for retracting the ureter.

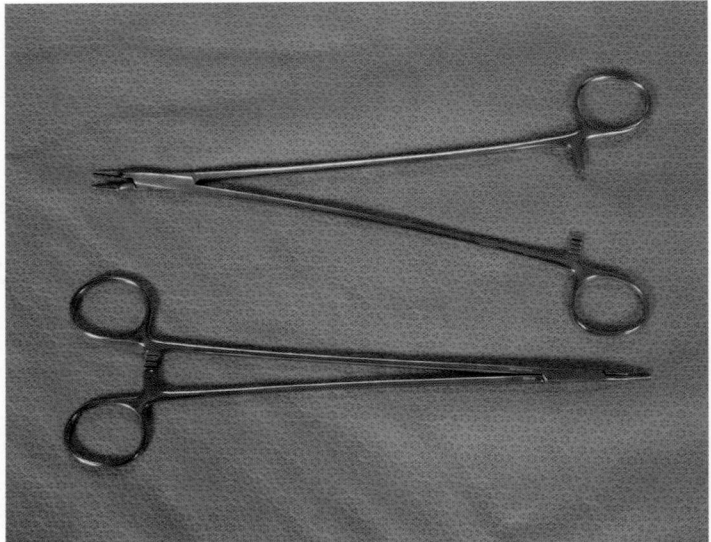

**FIGURE 3–12** The long Ryder needle holder is an excellent tool for deep suturing when fine needles and 3-0 or small-gauge suture material is required.

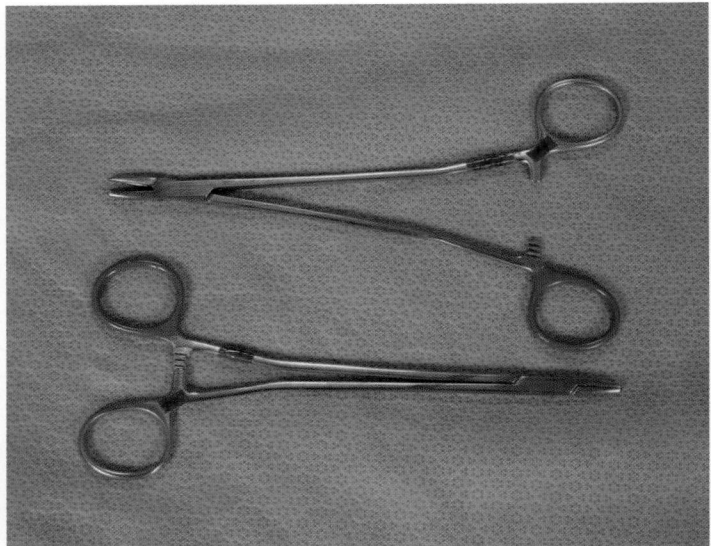

**FIGURE 3–13** This short, fine bulldog needle holder is used for fine suturing close to or on the surface, for example, in vulvar, lower vaginal, perianal, and urethral surgery.

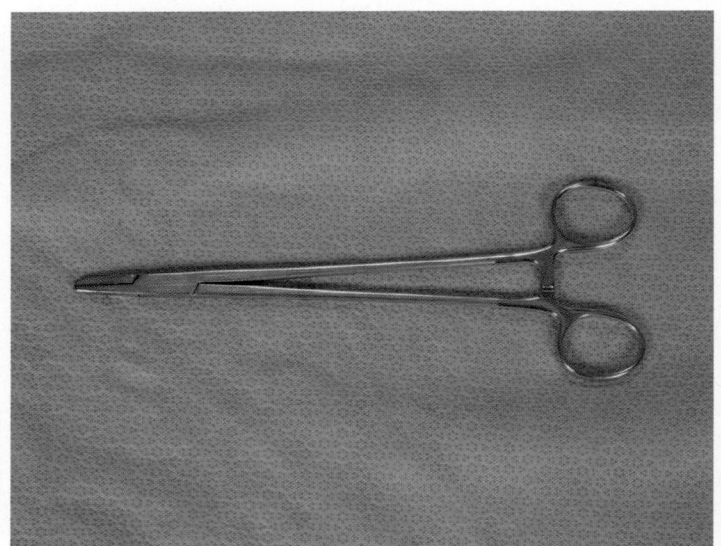

**FIGURE 3–14** The standard bulldog needle holder is a general-purpose needle holder.

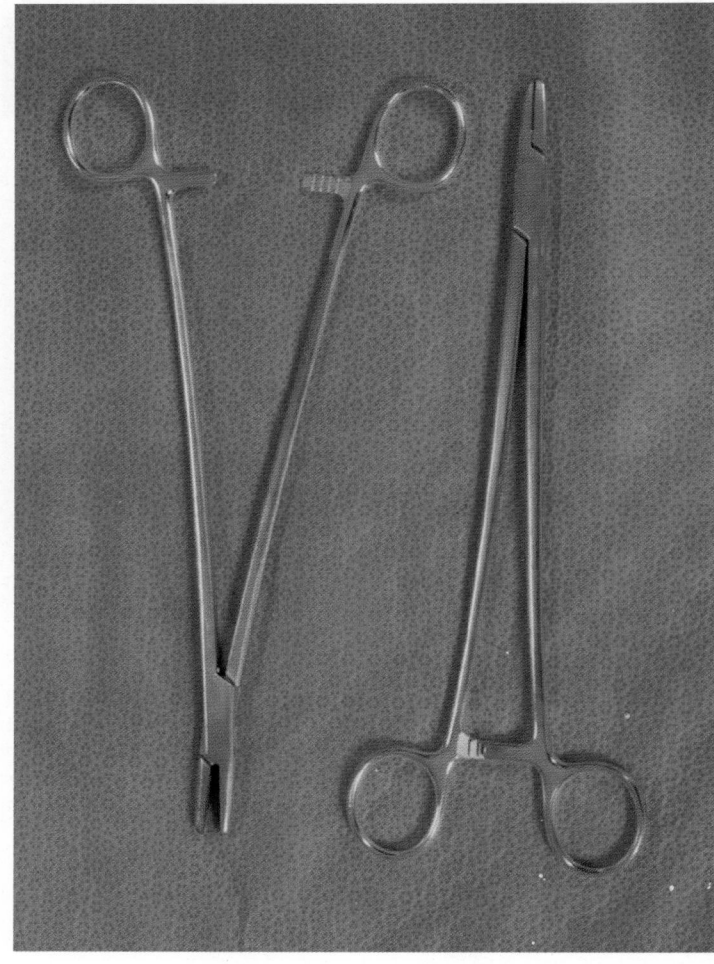

**FIGURE 3–15** Long bulldog needle holders are useful for suturing deep in the pelvis.

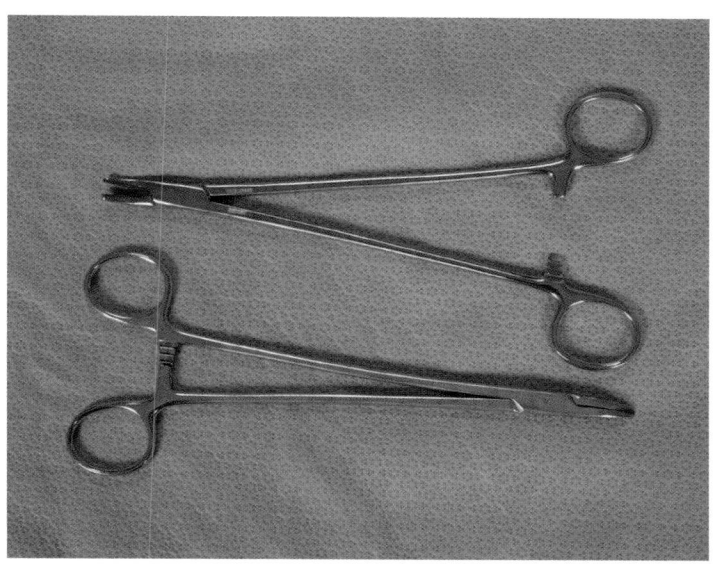

**FIGURE 3–16** The curved Haney needle holder offers a great mechanical advantage for driving and retrieving suture needles. The needle is driven with the convex curve of the jaws and is retrieved using the concave curve.

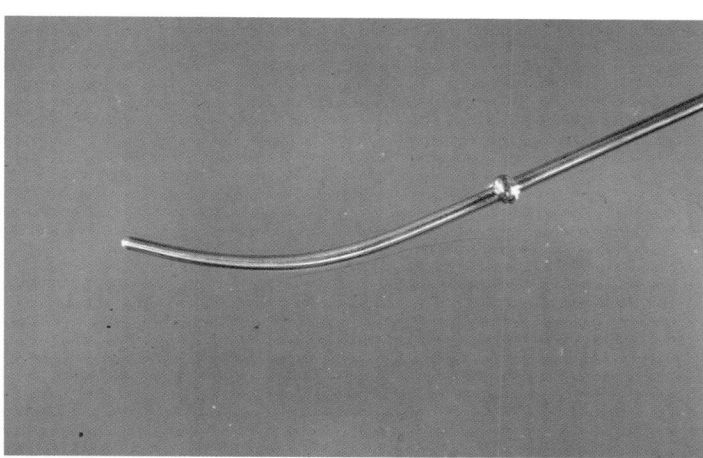

**FIGURE 3–17** Hank's dilator is gently tapered to permit the least traumatic type of cervical dilatation.

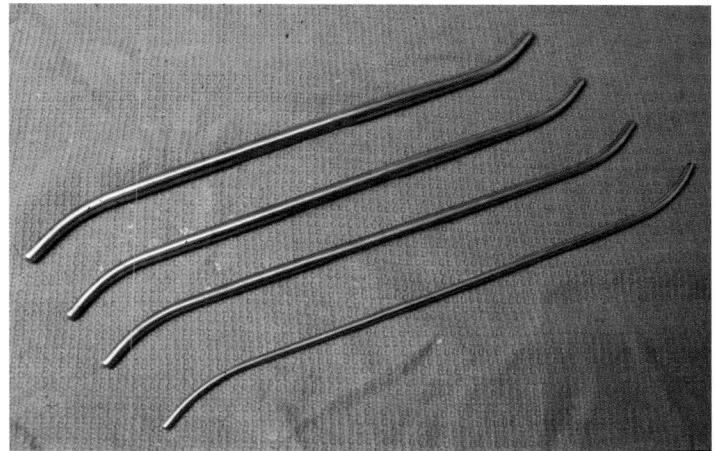

**FIGURE 3–18** This graduated set of Pratt dilators permits gradual, minimally traumatic cervical dilatation. The dilators are numbered using the French system (division by 3 equals the diameter in millimeters).

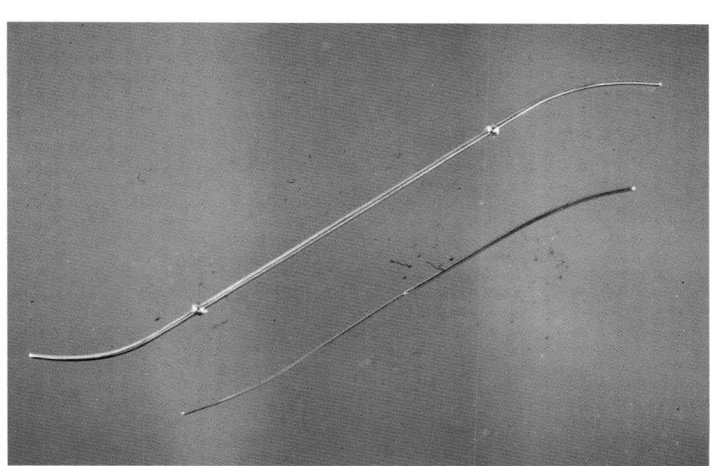

**FIGURE 3–19** Above is a Hank's dilator. Below is a baby Hegar dilator.

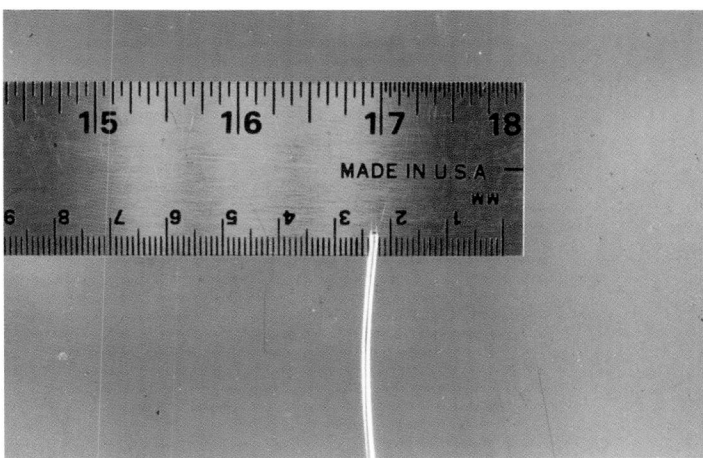

**FIGURE 3–20** The baby Hegar is 1.5 mm in diameter at one end and 2.5 mm on the opposite end. It is ideal for determining the axis of the cervical canal in cases of cervical stenosis.

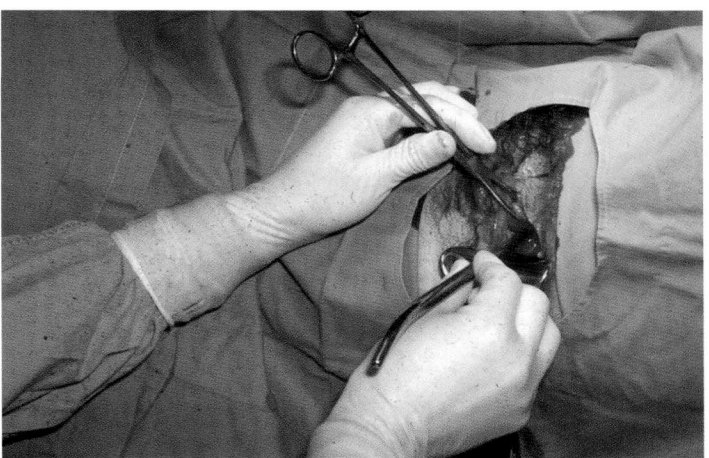

**FIGURE 3–21** A single-toothed tenaculum should be attached to the anterior lip of the cervix to provide countertraction during cervical dilation.

UNIT 1 ■ SECTION B

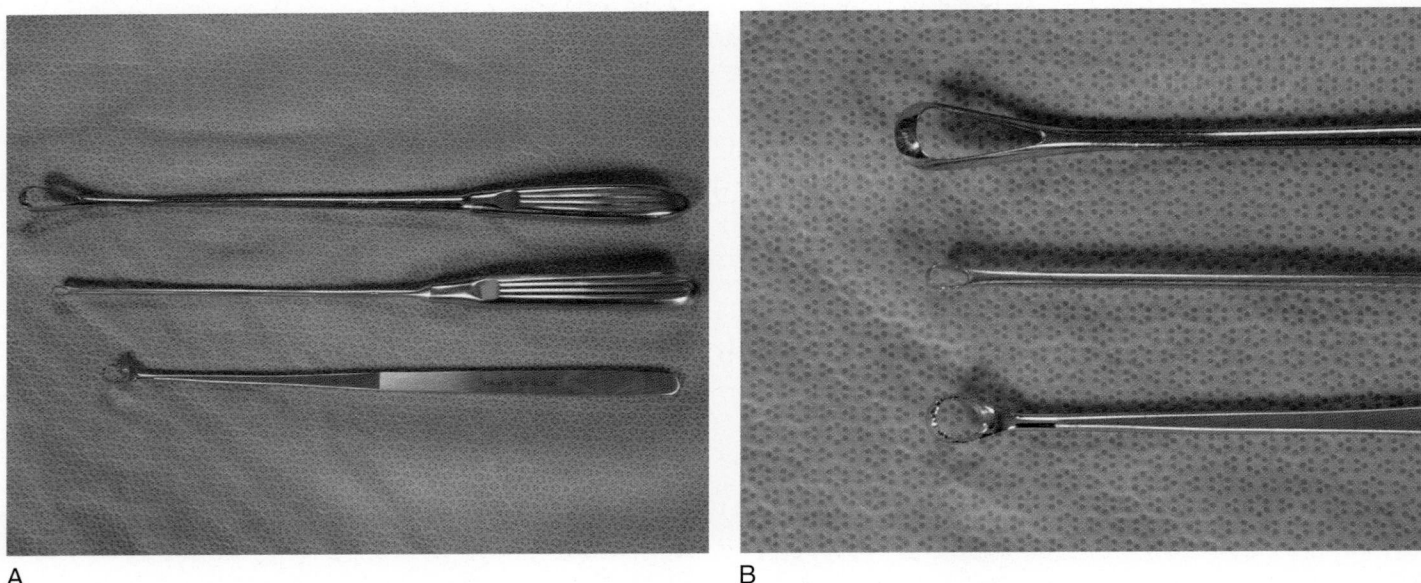

A    B

**FIGURE 3–22  A.** The bottom curette is a sharp, serrated curette (Haney type), which is ideally suited for curettage, principally in nonpregnant patients. The same can be said for the small, sharp curette (*middle*). The large, sharp curette at the top is well suited for curetting products of conception. **B.** Close-up view of the curettes illustrated in Figure 3–22A.

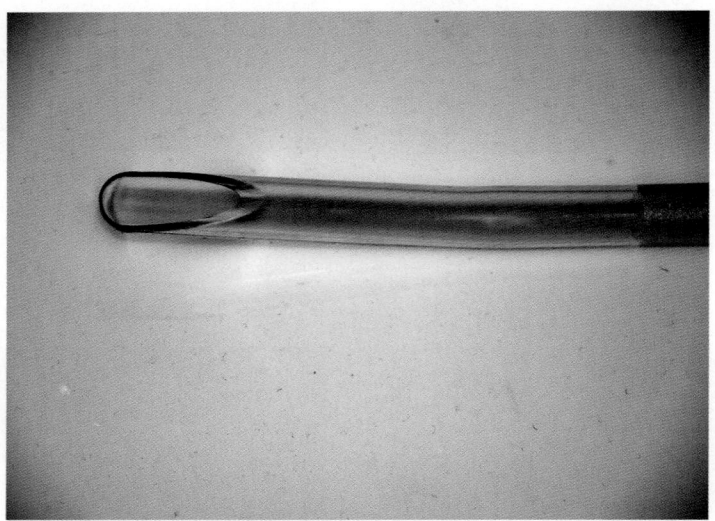

**FIGURE 3–23**  Suction cannulas are available in a variety of diameters, ranging from 6 to 14 mm. The device illustrated here is 12 mm in diameter.

# Suture Material, Suturing Techniques, and Knot Tying

*Michael S. Baggish*

## Suture Types

Sutures are utilized to close wounds, to secure bleeding vessels, and to seal off visceral structures. A wide variety of suture materials are available, which vary in terms of size, material, content, and consistency. For purposes of explanation, sundry sutures can be divided into **absorbable** and **nonabsorbable.** Absorbable materials are broken down by the body's enzyme systems and virtually disintegrate (Fig. 4–1). Nonabsorbable sutures resist enzymatic action and remain more or less permanently (with the exception of silk, which is gone within 2 years) in the body (Tables 4–1 and 4–2, Fig. 4–2). Tensile strength, particularly over time, is greater with nonabsorbable sutures. Sutures are sized on the basis of U.S. Pharmacopeia (USP)-equivalent diameters (Table 4–3). In infected tissues and otherwise dirty areas, absorbable sutures have an advantage in that they provide short-term tensile strength and then disappear. They are less likely to provide a foreign body nidus for continuous inflammation and infection, and for subsequent sinus formation. On the other hand, abdominal closure in the face of gross infection is an indication for the use of nonabsorbable suture material, to minimize the risk of dehiscence and/or evisceration. Almost all modern sutures are **swaged** onto a **needle** (Fig. 4–3). Needles generally may be divided into two overall groups: **cutting** and **tapered.** Cutting needles are used to penetrate denser and firmer tissues (e.g., fibrous tissue, periosteum, ligament fascia). Cutting needles have a **triangular point** (Fig. 4–4). If the additional cutting edge is on the inside curve of the needle, it is a standard cutting needle. If it is on the outside curvature of the needle, it is a reverse cutting needle. Tapered needles have a **cone-shaped tip** and are ideal for penetrating soft tissue and for producing the smallest hole (Fig. 4–5).

A variety of needle configurations accompany the suture to which they are swaged. **Straight needles** are ideal for subcuticular closures. Very fine sutures (e.g., 5-0, 6-0) are usually equipped with ¼ or ⅜ **circle needles**. Intermediate sutures (e.g., 2-0, 3-0) usually have ½ to ⅝ circle needles. Large sutures most often have ½ circle needles (Fig. 4–6).

## Suture Selection

Suture should be selected on the basis of several parameters: (1) the **volume of tissue** to be secured, (2) the **tensile strength** of the tissue to be sutured, and (3) the potential for **bacterial contamination.** A general guideline that can guide a gynecologic surgeon recommends that the smallest suture that can adequately accomplish the work at hand is the best suture for the job. For example, to select a 0 or 1 suture to secure a small bleeding arteriole deep in the pelvis makes no sense when a 3-0 or 4-0 stitch would suffice. On the other hand, attempting to secure a uterine vessel pedicle or infundibulopelvic ligament pedicle with a 3-0 suture rather than a 0 suture is equally foolhardy. **Braided suture** has a greater propensity to become contaminated with debris and bacteria within the interstices of the braid compared with **monofilament suture.** Silk suture is easy to handle and easy to tie down, hence it forms a secure knot. It should never be used in the urinary bladder, and for that matter, neither should any nonabsorbable suture material. Nylon suture is very strong but requires many throws to avoid unraveling. Polyester suture material has all the advantages of silk and better strength and integrity. Polypropylene (Prolene) does not adhere to tissue and is less reactive than nylon. It is ideal for situations in which tissues are infected or contaminated. A very new structure concept has been developed by Covidien (New Haven, CT). The unidirectional barbed technology does not slip and does not require knot tying (Fig. 4–6B).

#### TABLE 4–1 ■ Types of Suture Material

| Absorbable Suture | Degradation Time |
|---|---|
| Plain gut | 7 10 days |
| Chromic gut | 12 14 days |
| Vicryl (coated, braided, polyglactin) | 50% tensile strength at 3 weeks, all lost by 5 weeks |
| PDS II (polydioxanone monofilament) | 50% tensile strength at 4 weeks, 25% at 6 weeks |
| Maxon (monofilament polydioxanone) | 50% tensile strength at 4 weeks, 25% at 6 weeks |
| **Nonabsorbable Suture** | **Relative Tensile Strength** |
| Cotton | + |
| Silk | ++ |
| Nylon | +++ |
| Polyester and polypropylene | ++++ |
| Steel wire | +++++ |

**TABLE 4-2 ■ Ethicon Suture Characteristics**

| Ethicon Sutures | Material | Natural/ Synthetic | Construction | Coating (if applicable) | Material Color | Available Size Range | Strength Retention Profile | Absorption Time | Absorption Process |
|---|---|---|---|---|---|---|---|---|---|
| FAST-ABSORBING SURGICAL GUT suture | Beef serosa or sheep Submucosa | Natural | Monofilament (Virtual) | n/a | Yellowish-tan | 5/0-8/0 | 5-7 days* | 21-42 days | Proteolytic enzymatic digestion |
| SURGICAL GUT suture Plain | Beef serosa or sheep Submucosa | Natural | Monofilament (Virtual) | n/a | Yellowish-tan | 3-7/0 | 7-10 days* | 70 days | Proteolytic enzymatic digestion |
| SURGICAL GUT Chromic | Beef serosa or sheep Submucosa | Natural | Monofilament (Virtual) | Chromic salts | Brown Blue | 3-7/0 | 21-29 days* | 90 days | Proteolytic enzymatic digestion |
| Coated VICRYL RAPIDE[†] (polyglactin 910) suture | Polyglactin 910 | Synthetic | Braided | Polyglactin 370 Calcium stearate | Undyed (Natural) | 1-5/0 | 50% @ 5 days 0% @ 10-14 days | 42 days | Hydrolysis |
| Coated VICRYL[†] (polyglactin 910) suture | Polyglactin 910 | Synthetic | Braided | Polyglactin 370 Calcium stearate | Violet Undyed (Natural) | 3-8/0 | 75% @ 14 days 50% @ 21 days 25% @ 28 days[‡] | 56-70 days (63 day avg) | Hydrolysis |
| Coated VICRYL[†] (polyglactin 910) suture monofilament | Polyglactin 910 | Synthetic | Monofilament | n/a | Violet Undyed (Natural) | 9/0-10/0 | 75% @ 14 days 40% @ 21 days | 56-70 days (63 day avg) | Hydrolysis |
| Coated VICRYL PLUS (polyglactin 910) suture | Polyglactin 910 | Synthetic | Braided | Polyglactin 370 IRGACARE MP[§] (triclosan) | Violet Undyed (Natural) | 2-5/0 | 75% @ 14 days 50% @ 21 days 25% @ 28 days | 56-70 days (63 day avg) | Hydrolysis |
| MONOCRYL[†] (poliglecaprone 25) suture Undyed | Poliglecaprone 25 | Synthetic | Monofilament | n/a | Undyed (Natural) | 2-6/0 | 50%-60% @ 7 days 20%-30% @ 14 days | 91-119 days | Hydrolysis |
| MONOCRYL[†] (poliglecaprone 25) suture Dyed | Poliglecaprone 25 | Synthetic | Monofilament | n/a | Violet | 2-6/0 | 60%-70% @ 7 days 30%-40% @ 14 days | 91-119 days | Hydrolysis |

| Suture | Material | Type | Filament | Coating | Color | Sizes | Strength retention | Absorption | Mechanism |
|---|---|---|---|---|---|---|---|---|---|
| PDS† II (polydioxanone) suture | Polydioxanone | Synthetic | Monofilament | n/a | Violet Clear | 2-9/0 | 70 @ 2 weeks 50% @ 4 weeks 25% @ 6 weeks | 180-210 days | Slow hydrolysis |
| PERMA-HAND† SILK suture | Silk | Natural | Braided | Bees Wax | Black White | 5-9/0 | ≈1 year | n/a | n/a |
| SURGICAL STAINLESS STEEL suture | 316L Stainless Steel | Natural alloy | Monofilament | n/a | Metallic Silver | 7-10/0 | Indefinite | n/a | n/a |
| NUROLON† braided nylon suture | Nylon 6 | Synthetic | Braided | n/a | Black | 1-6/0 | 20% loss/yr | n/a | n/a |
| ETHILON† nylon suture | Nylon 6 | Synthetic | Monofilament | n/a | Black Green Clear | 2-11/0 | 20% loss/yr | n/a | n/a |
| MERSILENE† polyester fiber suture | Polyester/Dacron | Synthetic | Braided | n/a | Green White | 5-6/0 | Indefinite | | |
| MERSILENE† polyester fiber suture | Polyester/Dacron | Synthetic | Monofilament | n/a | Green | 10/0-11/0 | Indefinite | n/a | n/a |
| ETHIBOND† EXCEL polyester suture | Polyester/Dacron | Synthetic | Braided | Polybutilate | Green White | 5-7/0 | Indefinite | n/a | n/a |
| PROLENE† polypropylene suture | Polypropylene | Synthetic | Monofilament | n/a | Blue Clear | 2-10/0 | Indefinite | n/a | n/a |
| PRONOVA† poly(hexafluoropropylene-VDF) suture | Polymer blend of poly(vinylidene fluoride) and poly(vinylidene fluoride-cohexafluoropolypropylene) | Synthetic | Monofilament | n/a | Blue Clear | 2-10/0 | Indefinite | n/a | n/a |
| TOPICAL SKIN ADHESIVE | Material | | | | | | | | |
| DERMABOND† topical skin adhesive | 2-Octyl cyanoacrylate | Synthetic | Liquid topical adhesive | n/a | Very pale Violet | n/a | 5-10 days | n/a | n/a |

*Estimated strength retention.
†Trademark.
‡Sizes 6/0 and larger.
§Trademark of Ciba Specialty Chemicals Corp.

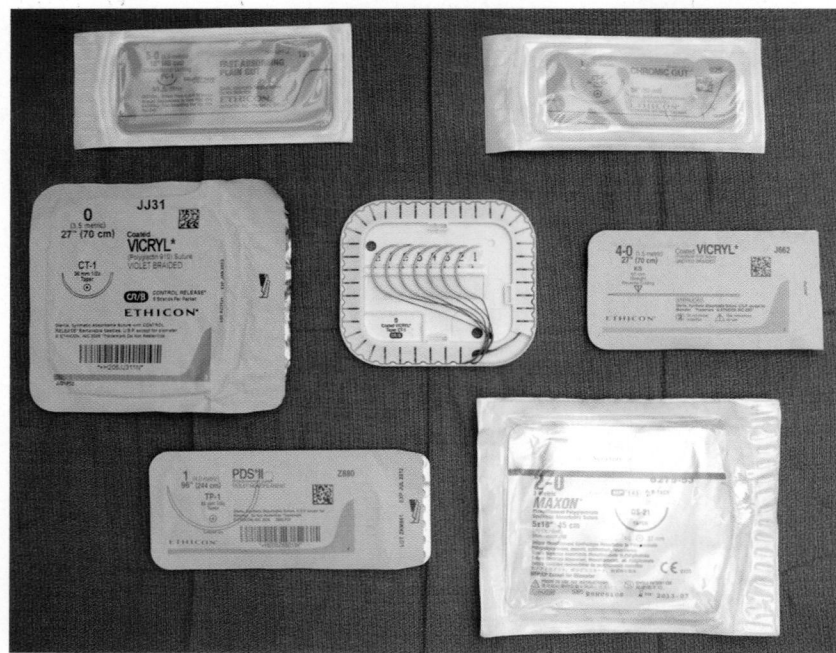

**FIGURE 4–1** A number of absorbable suture materials are illustrated: plain gut, chromic gut (*top row*), Vicryl (*middle row*), PDS, Maxon (*bottom row*).

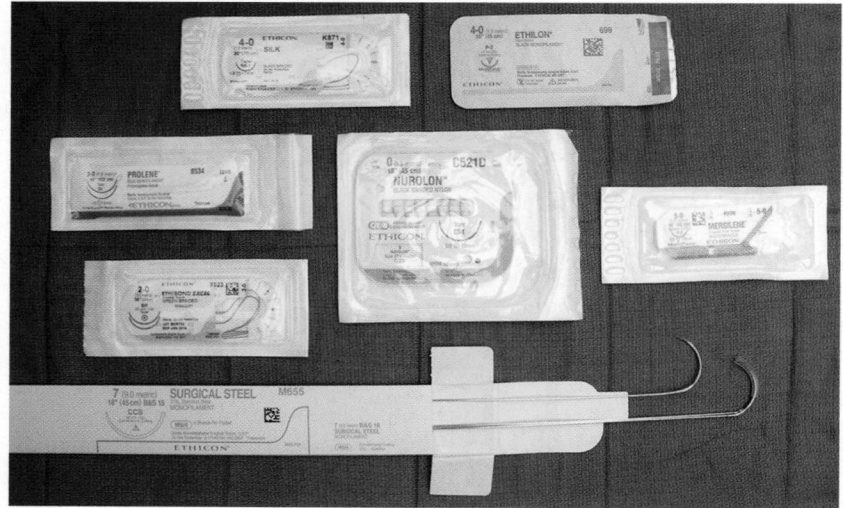

**FIGURE 4–2** Nonabsorbable sutures include silk, monofilament nylon (*top row*), polypropylene, braided nylon, Mersilene, polyester (*middle row*), steel wire (*bottom row*).

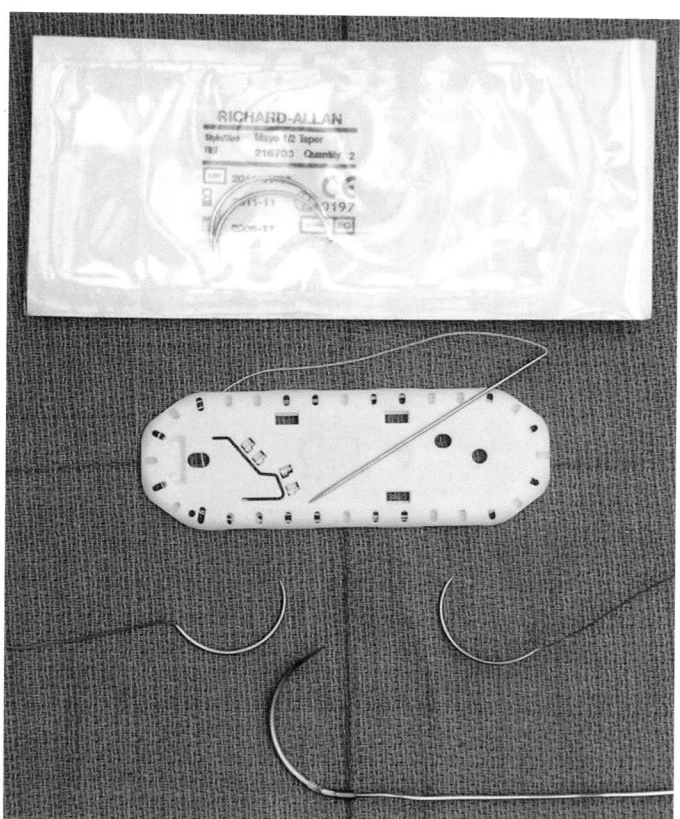

**FIGURE 4–3** Several needle types are shown here with the suture material swaged to the needle.

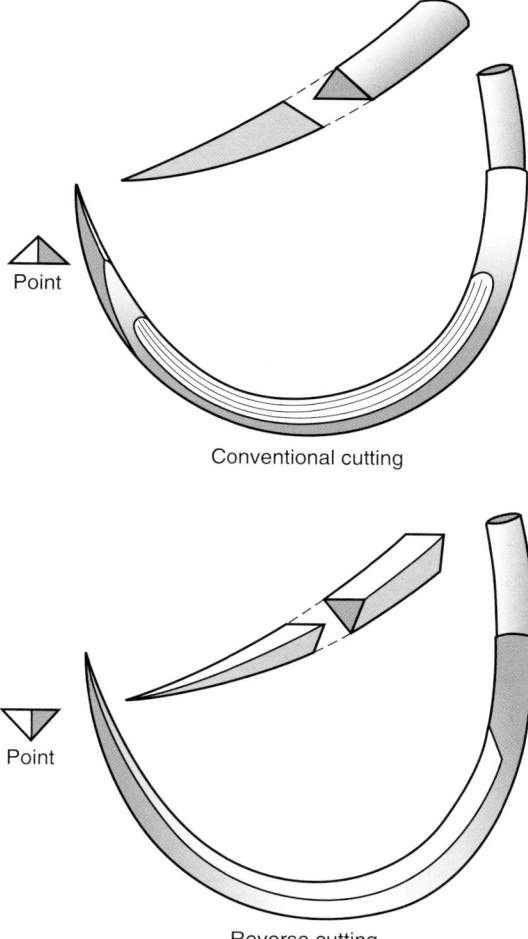

Conventional cutting

Reverse cutting

**FIGURE 4–4** The top figure shows a standard cutting needle with triangular tip and cutting edge located on the inside curve of the needle. At bottom is a reverse cutting needle with the cutting edge positioned on the outer curve of the needle.

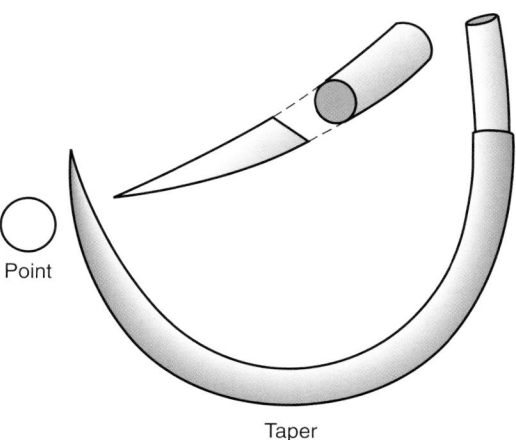

Taper

**FIGURE 4–5** The taper needle is seen to have a conical tip and creates a relatively smaller hole than does a cutting needle.

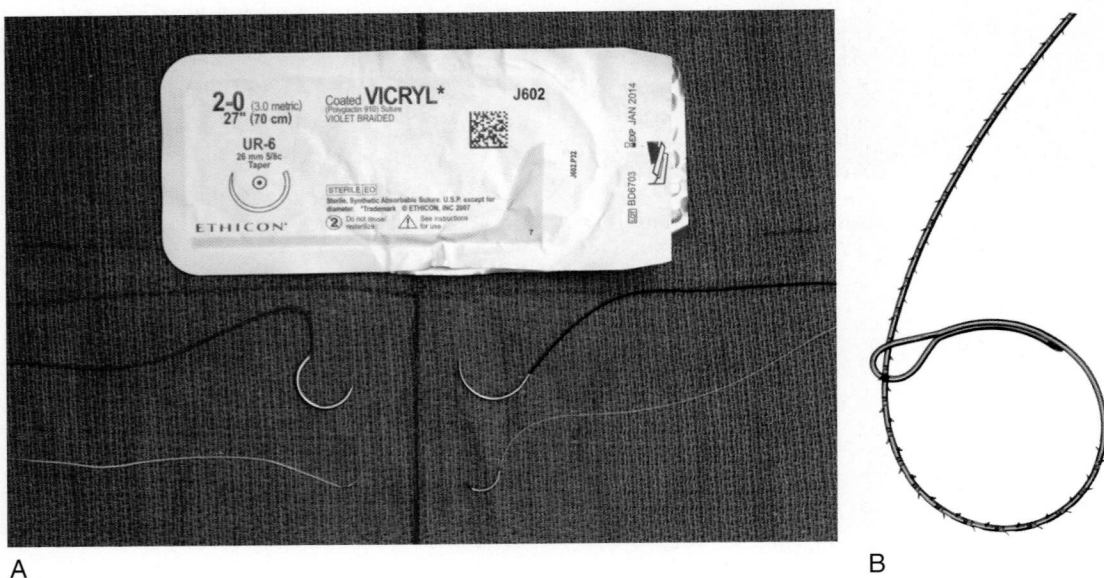

A

B

**FIGURE 4–6  A.** This picture illustrates several varieties of circular needles. Top, a package containing a $\frac{5}{8}$ circle. In the middle, a $\frac{5}{8}$ circle and a $\frac{1}{2}$ circle. Bottom, a $\frac{1}{4}$ circle and a $\frac{3}{8}$ circle. **B.** The V-Loc (polyglyconate) absorbable wound closure suture is barbed to prevent slippage and requires no terminal knot.

| TABLE 4–3 ■ Suture Size | |
|---|---|
| Suture | Mean Diameter, inch |
| 5-0 | .0056 |
| 4-0 | .0080 |
| 3-0 | .0100 |
| 2-0 | .0126 |
| 0 | .0159 |
| 1 | .0179 |

## Suture Techniques

Several suture techniques are useful for pelvic surgery. The fascia or skin may be closed by simple interrupted sutures (Fig. 4–7A) or alternatively by mattress sutures (Fig. 4–7B, C). Sub-cuticular skin closures are commonly utilized for transverse abdominal incisions and for episiotomy closures (Fig. 4–8A, B). Alternatively, skin, subcutaneous tissue, and peritoneum may be closed by a continuous running suture (Fig. 4–8C). Visceral peritoneum is usually closed by a continuous running suture (Fig. 4–9). Bladder lacerations are typically closed with a continuous through-and-through chromic suture (Fig. 4–10). Fascia may be closed securely with a running monofilament suture of PDS, or polypropylene (Prolene) (Fig. 4–11). In critical circumstances, stainless steel wire, nylon, or Prolene may be utilized as interrupted sutures taken widely through the fascia and peritoneum en masse (Fig. 4–12). The Smead-Jones far-near technique may be utilized for patients at risk for dehiscence (Fig. 4–13A, B). Mass ligature techniques may be indicated with the use of #1 Prolene to repair eviscerated abdomens (Fig. 4–14). Vascular pedicles are secured by suture ligatures (Fig. 4–15A through E). Large vessel pedicles and ligament pedicles are transfixed via Heaney-type suture ligatures (Fig. 4–15F, G). Bleeding vessels and uterine incisions are closed by hemostatic figure-of-8 ligatures (Fig. 4–16). Cul de sac obliteration, cervical cerclage, and vaginal peritoneal closure are implemented by purse string sutures (Fig. 4–17A, B). Open technique for a vaginal cuff hemostasis is referred to as a baseball or reefing stitch (Fig. 4–18). This continuous suture may be locked for additional hemostasis (Fig. 4–18). Exposed raw surfaces with sinus-type oozing can be best managed by a pleating suture (Fig. 4–19A through G). Intestines are anastomosed via a Connell continuous suture pattern (Fig. 4–20).

## Knot Tying

Every surgeon is required to tie a secure knot. New residents typically experience difficulty in tying a secure square knot. They end up not uncommonly tying granny knots, which tighten to such an extreme that the tissues strangulate. The first maneuver is to cross the suture to lay down a flat first throw. One of two techniques may be utilized: single-hand tie (Fig. 4–21A through I) or two-hand tie (Fig. 4–22A through I). Regardless of the technique selected, the sine qua non of a good tie-down is a square knot, which does not slip (i.e., the knot is tied under continuous tension).

## Surgeon's Knot

This knot is useful to prevent slippage (Fig. 4–23). New residents frequently use the technique. An extra loop is taken during the first throw of the tie. The two loops are tightened down and do not loosen during the maneuver of completing the second throw.

## Instrument Tie

This is a handy method for tying a fine suture (i.e., 5-0 and smaller) (Fig. 4–24). The short end is held with a long clamp (e.g., a tonsil clamp). The suture material is looped over the clamp, and the short end of the stitch is pulled through the loop. The maneuver is repeated, but the loop is reversed, thereby creating a square knot.

## Finishing a Continuous Stitch

At the termination of a running suture, the free end is held, as is a final loop of the suture material (Fig. 4–25). The two are tied together in a square knot.

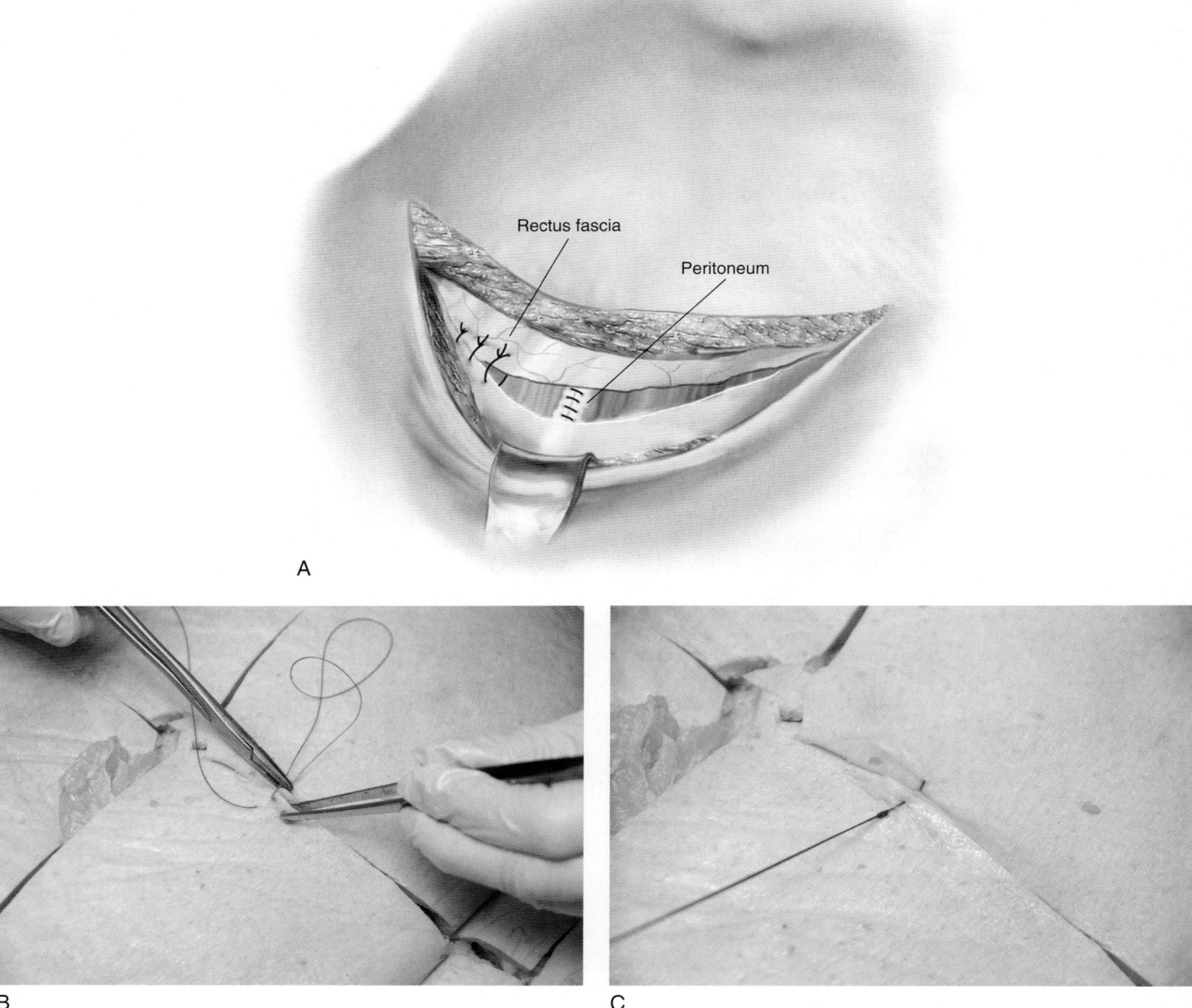

A

B                                                    C

**FIGURE 4–7  A.** Transverse incisions may be closed with simple interrupted sutures through the fascia. **B.** An everting mattress suture is illustrated here. The stitch is passed through the skin, existing on the opposite side. The needle is reversed and is passed back through the skin, exiting on the same side as the initial needle bite. **C.** The suture is tied on the initiating side of the skin.

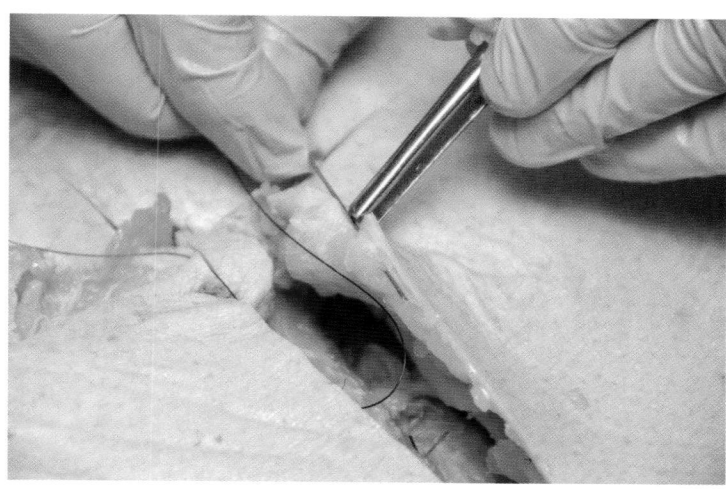

A

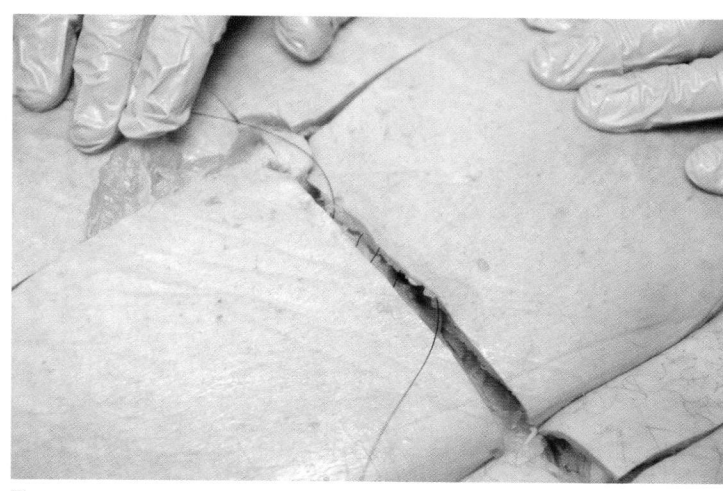

B

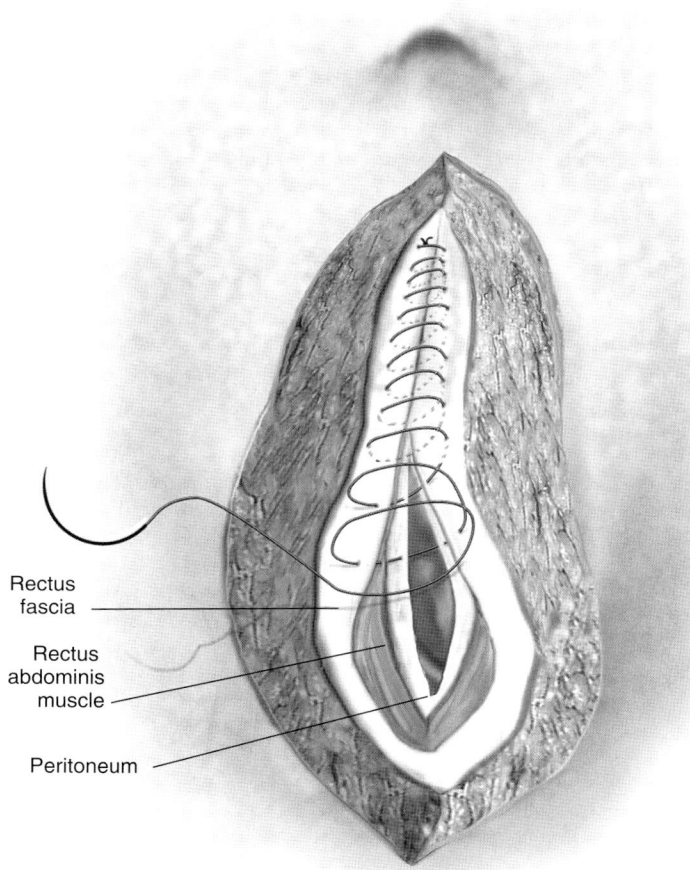

Rectus
fascia

Rectus
abdominis
muscle

Peritoneum

C

**FIGURE 4–8  A.** A straight cutting needle provides the best tool for placing a subcuticular stitch. **B.** Detail of the subcuticular suture line placement. **C.** Continuous closure with monofilament suture material, 0 or 1 (e.g., PDS II, Prolene).

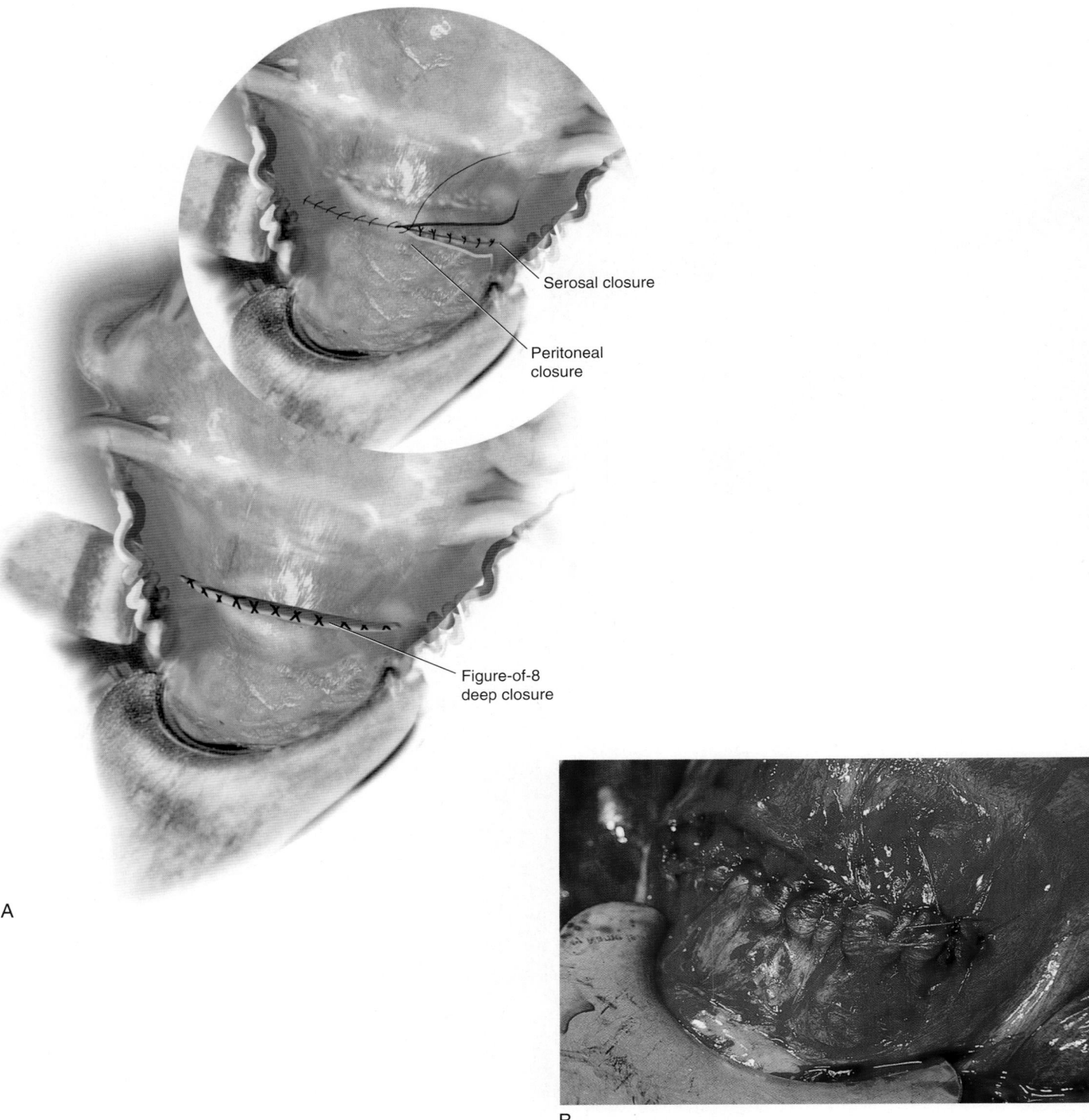

Serosal closure

Peritoneal
closure

Figure-of-8
deep closure

A

B

**FIGURE 4–9  A.** The superficial muscle and uterine serosae are closed with running or running lock sutures of 0 Vicryl. **B.** After the serosa is closed, the bladder peritoneum is sutured to the uterus at the upper margin of the incision.

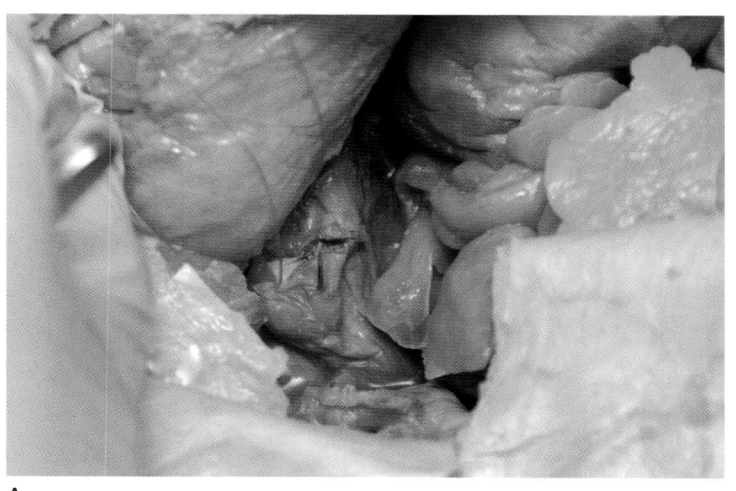

A

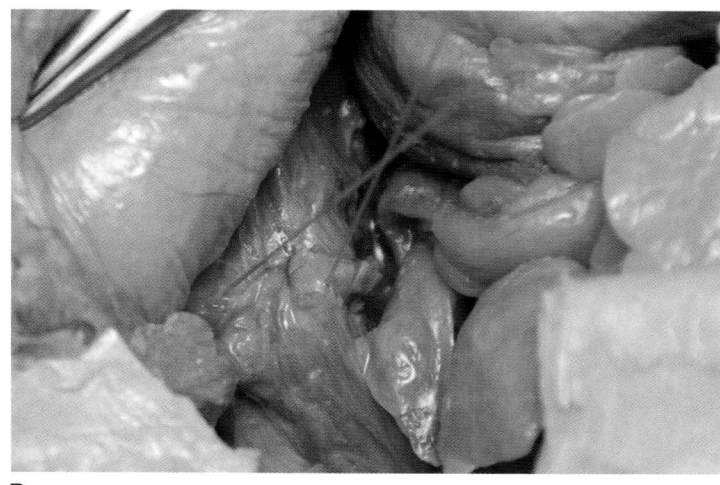

B

**FIGURE 4–10 A.** This bladder laceration is closed with a 2-0 running chromic suture, which is placed through all layers of the bladder dome. **B.** The laceration is closed.

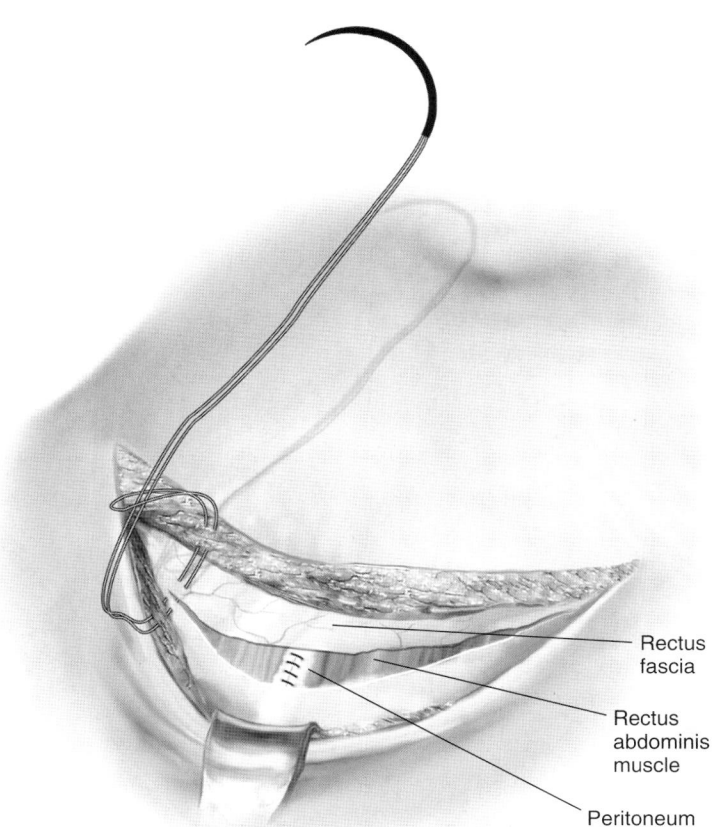

Rectus fascia

Rectus abdominis muscle

Peritoneum

**FIGURE 4–11** A looped PDS II or Prolene closure of a transverse incision is illustrated in this drawing.

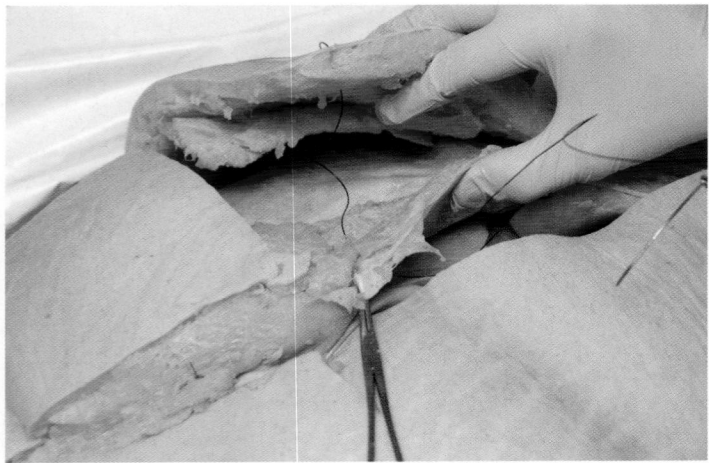

**FIGURE 4–12** A mass closure is performed using #4 nylon with a swaged surgeon's needle. The stitch penetrates skin, fat, fascia, and peritoneum.

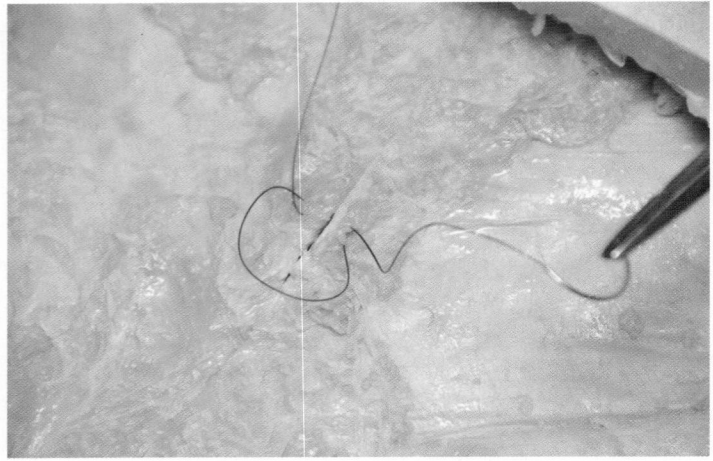

A

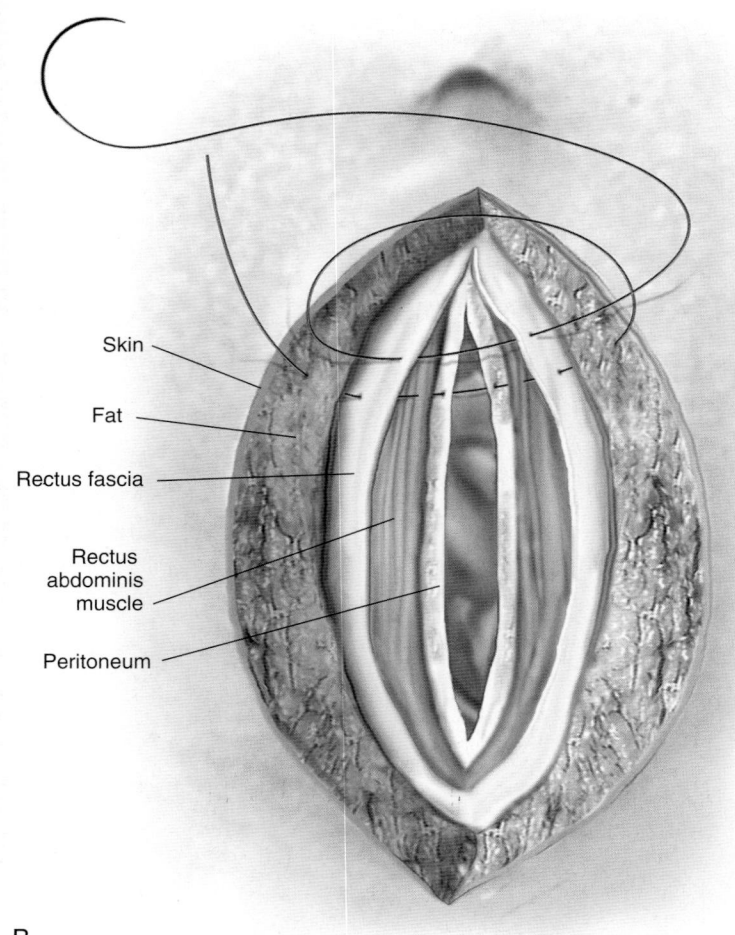

Skin

Fat

Rectus fascia

Rectus abdominis muscle

Peritoneum

B

**FIGURE 4–13  A.** The far-near fascial closure technique consists of an initial deep bite into the fascial margin, which protects against the suture cutting through the tissue. This is followed by fascial margin bites. The entire technique represents antidehiscence prophylaxis. **B.** A schematic view of the Smead-Jones closure.

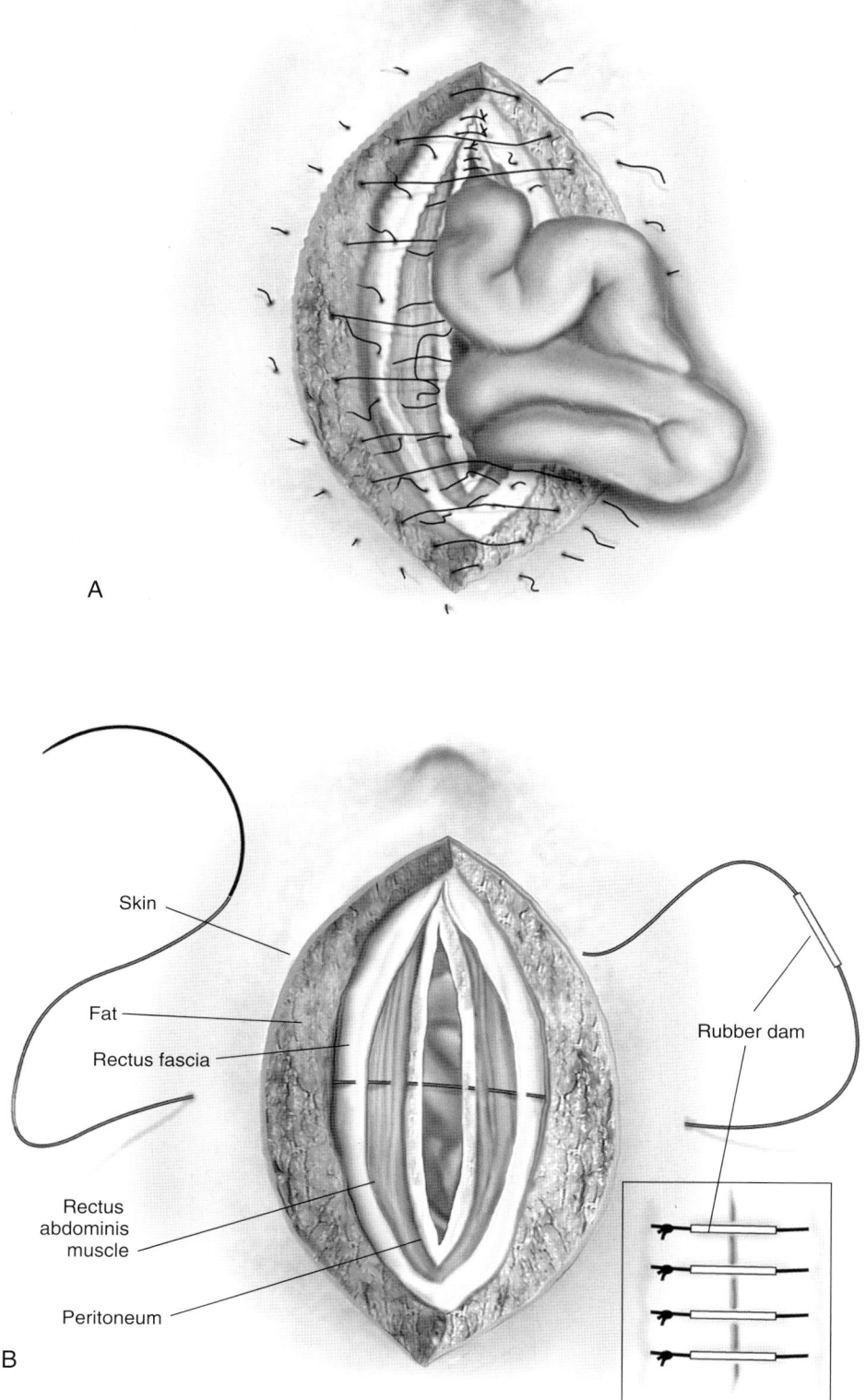

A

Skin

Fat

Rectus fascia

Rubber dam

Rectus
abdominis
muscle

Peritoneum

B

**FIGURE 4–14  A.** Burst abdomen with evisceration. Typically, the suture material exceeds
the tensile strength of the tissue, is tied too tightly, or is placed too close to the cut edge of the
fascia. The sutures can pull through the tissue. Alternatively, inadequately tied knots can unravel.
**B.** Closure of the burst abdomen is accomplished with #2 Prolene or #28 or grated steel wire as a
mass closure. The large surgeon's needle is placed with a wide margin lateral to the incision's edge
and is placed through all layers of the abdominal wall. The **inset** depicts rubber dams inserted
through the sutures to protect underlying skin.

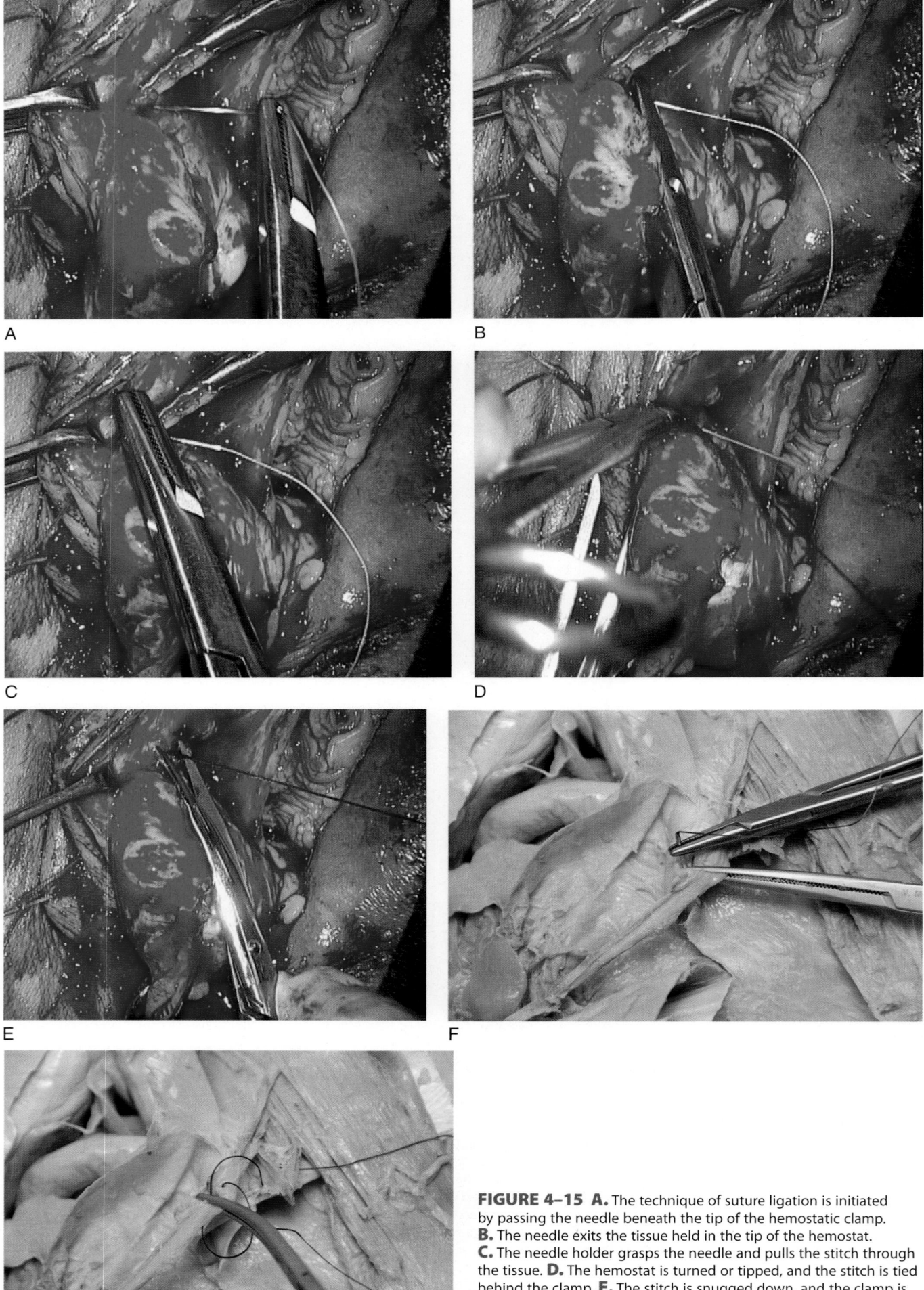

**FIGURE 4–15 A.** The technique of suture ligation is initiated by passing the needle beneath the tip of the hemostatic clamp. **B.** The needle exits the tissue held in the tip of the hemostat. **C.** The needle holder grasps the needle and pulls the stitch through the tissue. **D.** The hemostat is turned or tipped, and the stitch is tied behind the clamp. **E.** The stitch is snugged down, and the clamp is removed. The stitch is triply tied and is cut just above the knot. **F.** The transfixing suture is placed first through the tissue at the toe of the clamp. **G.** Then it is carried through the tissue held in the heel of the clamp.

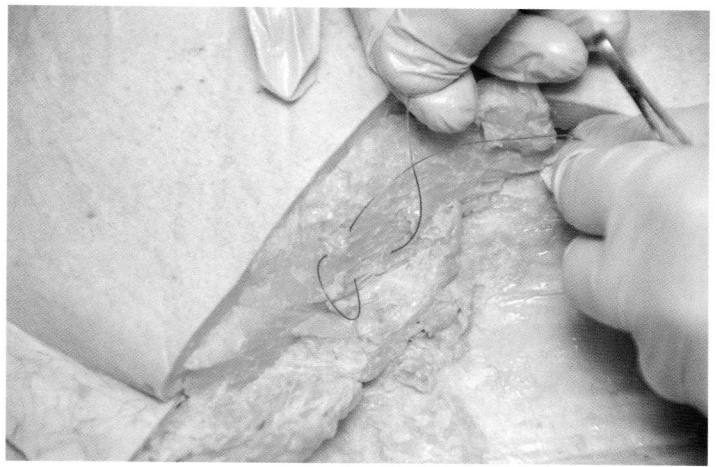

**FIGURE 4–16** The figure-of-8 stitch is a hemostatic measure designed to seal off bleeding vessels.

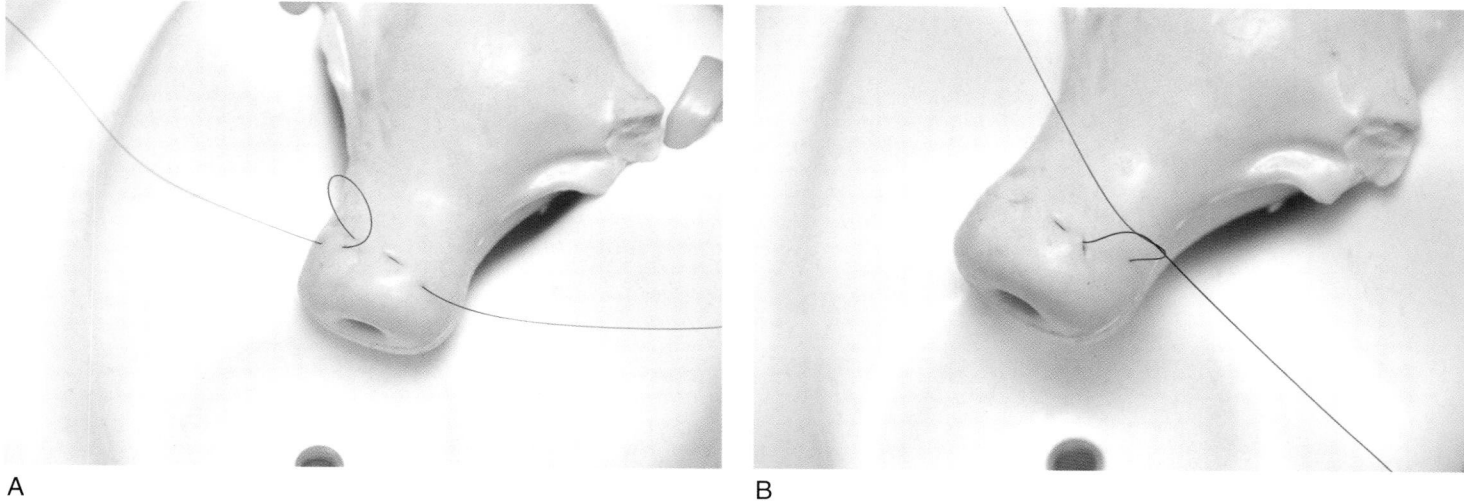

A                                                                        B

**FIGURE 4–17 A.** The purse string suture is illustrated on this uterine model. **B.** The circumference of the cervix will be included in this running stitch.

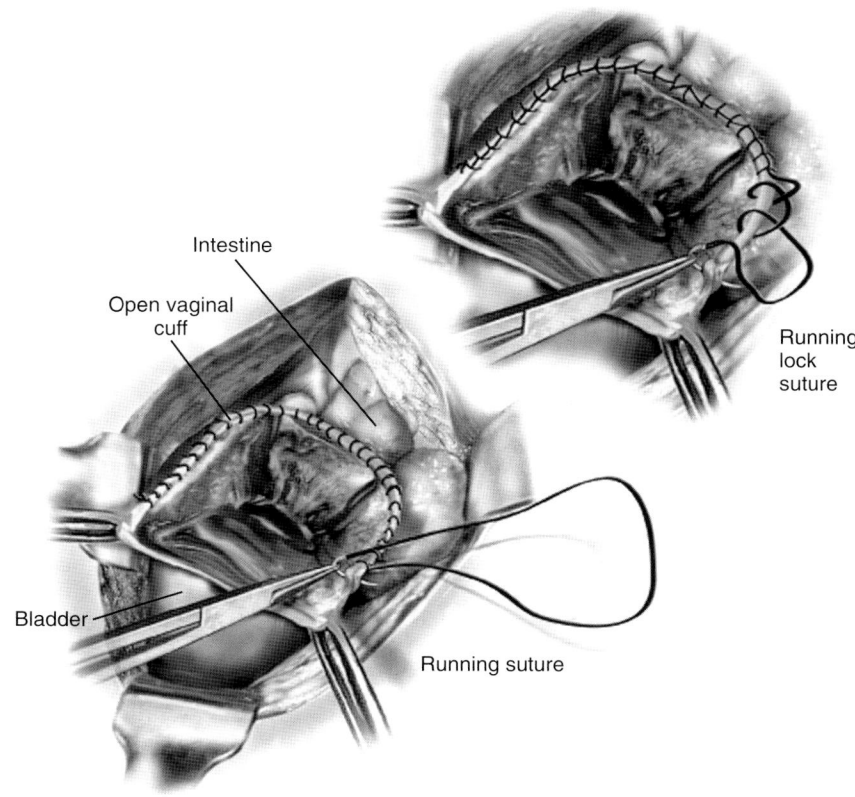

Intestine

Open vaginal cuff

Running lock suture

Bladder

Running suture

**FIGURES 4–18** The vaginal cuff may be left open or closed at the end of a hysterectomy operation. This drawing illustrates the baseball or reefing technique for securing hemostasis when the cuff remains opened. Above, a running lock stitch is shown; below, a simple continuous stitch.

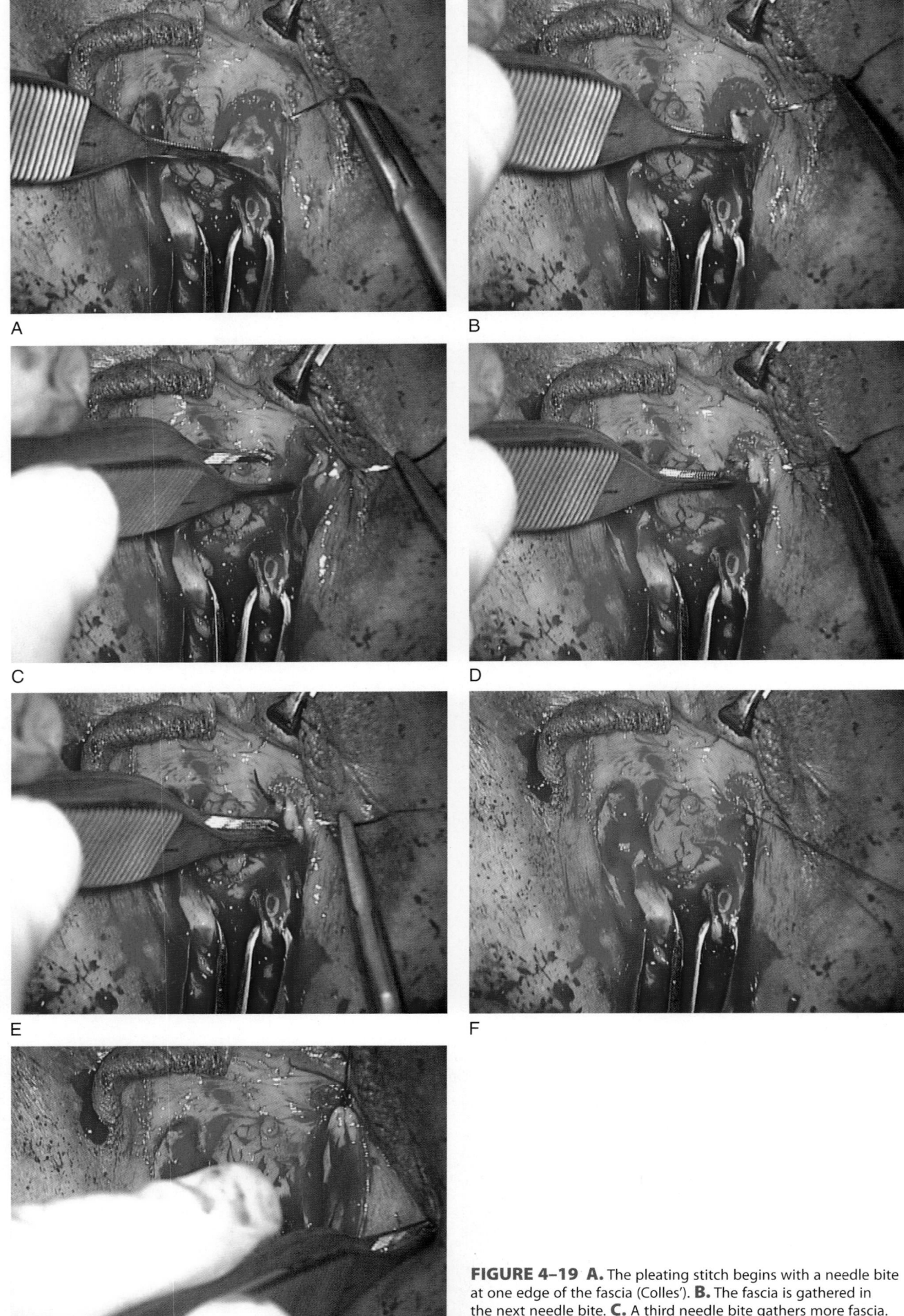

**FIGURE 4–19** **A.** The pleating stitch begins with a needle bite at one edge of the fascia (Colles'). **B.** The fascia is gathered in the next needle bite. **C.** A third needle bite gathers more fascia. **D.** A fourth bite is taken. **E.** Finally, a fifth bite is taken at the far edge of the incision. **F.** The two ends of the stitch are tightened and crossed. **G.** The suture is tied, with the edges of the fascia brought together and the small, oozing blood vessels sealed.

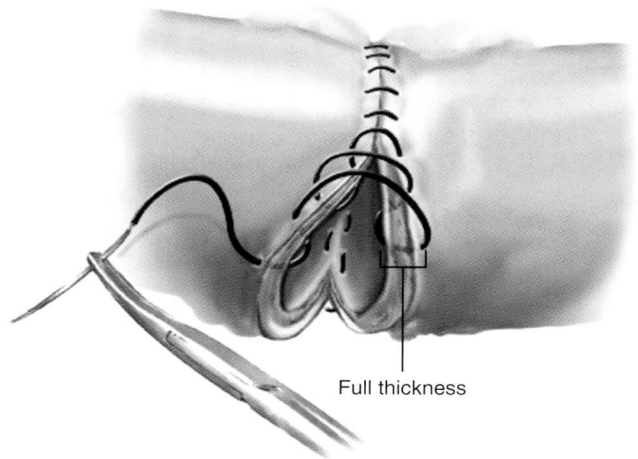

Full thickness

Connell suture pattern

**FIGURE 4–20** The Connell stitch enters from the serosal side, penetrates the full thickness of the intestinal wall, and exits through the mucosa. The stitch is carried back when a second needle stick is made in the opposite direction (i.e., through mucosa and bowel wall and through the serosa) then is carried to the opposite side, where the sequence is repeated.

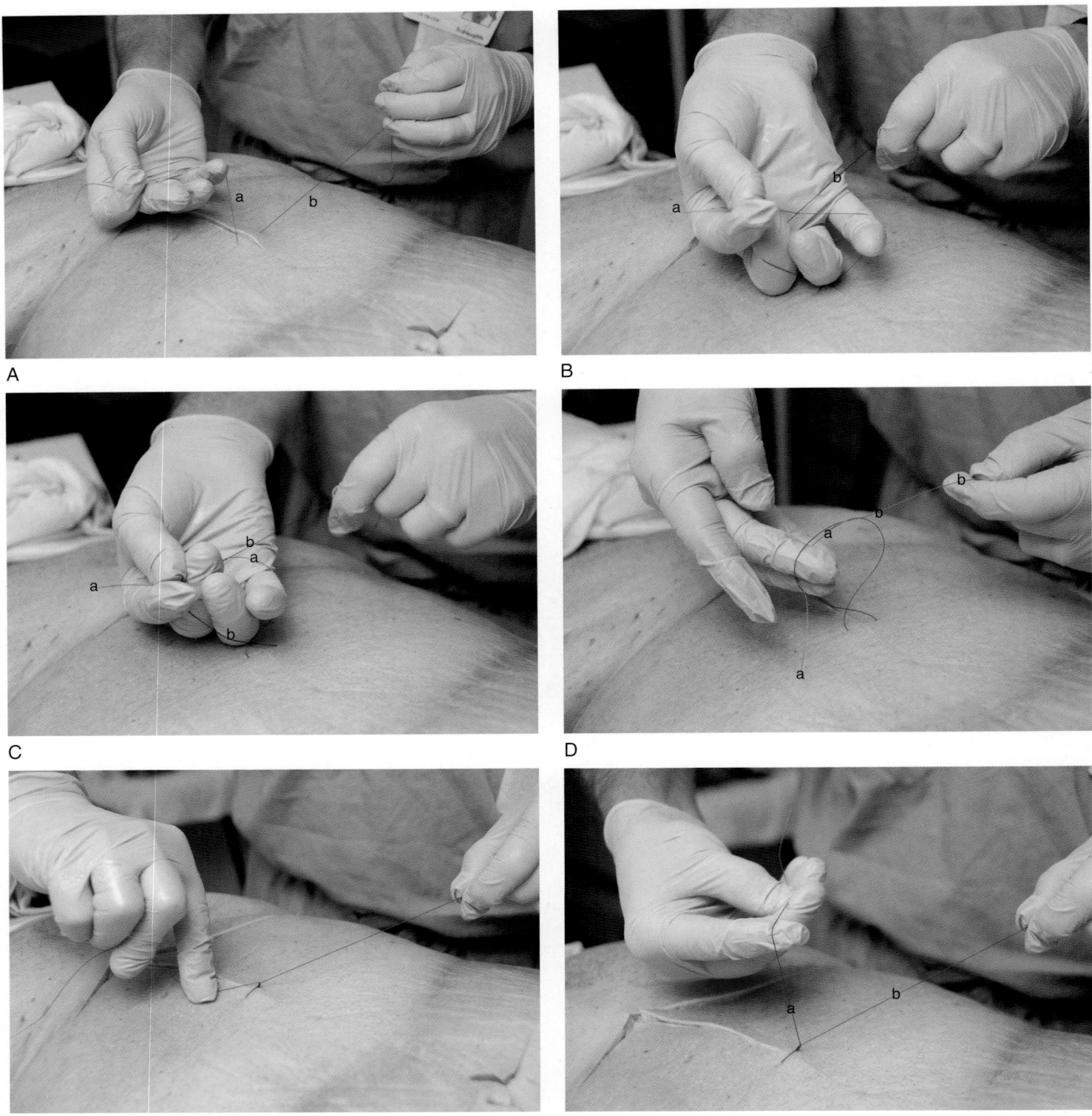

**FIGURE 4–21 A.** The single-hand tie is demonstrated. The first step is initiated by the surgeon laying the "a" limb of the suture across the palmar surface of the fingers of the dominant hand (in this case, right). The "a" suture is secured between the right thumb and index finger. The "b" portion of the suture is held under tension with the left hand. **B.** This magnified view of the "a" and "b" limbs of the suture illustrates the placement of fingers at the beginning of the tie. Note the "a" limb running across the palmar portion of the little finger, ring finger, and center finger and fixed by apposition of the index finger. The "b" limb crosses "a" in front of "a," behind the index, and in front of the center finger (between the index and center fingers). This begins the formation of a loop. **C.** At this point, the "b" limb role is entirely passive. The center and ring fingers flex back toward the palm, catching the "a" limb between these two fingers. **D.** While clasping the "a" limb suture tightly (between center and ring fingers), the loop is completed by drawing the fingers holding "a" backward, thereby withdrawing them from the loop while simultaneously completing the loop. **E.** The two ends of the stitch are pulled in opposite directions, snagging down the first loop (throw). **F.** The second portion (throw) of the one-hand tie is initiated by the right thumb and center finger opposing to secure suture "a," as the suture crosses the index finger between the crease of the distal joint and the end of the finger. Suture limb "b" is held taut and passively by the left hand.

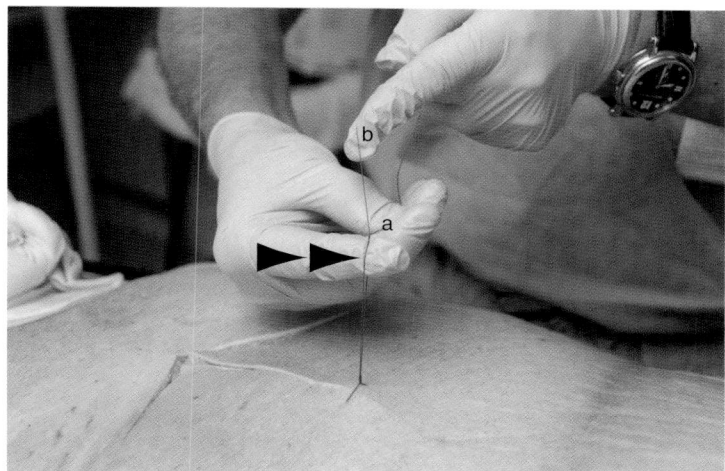

G

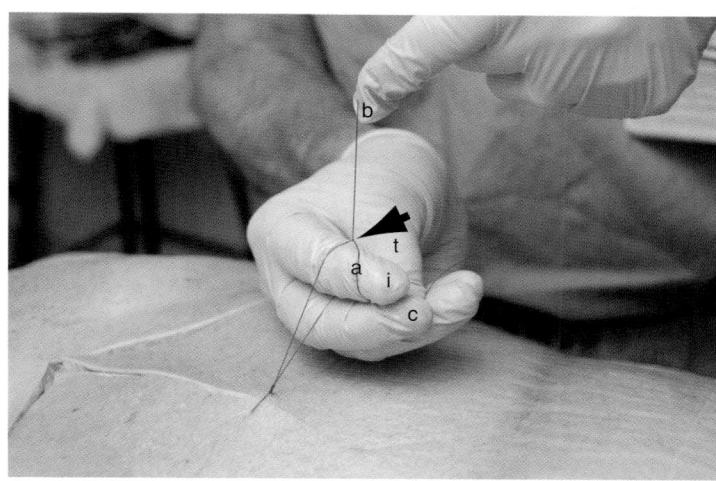

H

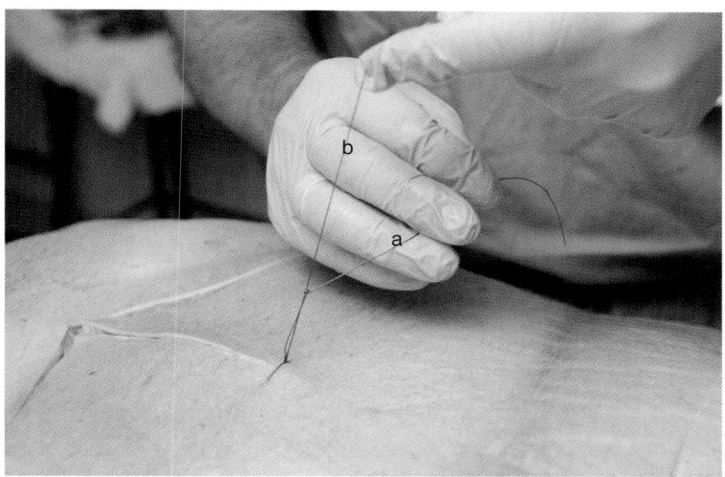

I

**FIGURE 4–21, cont'd G.** By utilizing the dorsal surface of the index finger to push upward on limb "a" to create tension, the next loop is created by moving limb "a" so as to cross over "b" at a 90° angle, with the index finger directed through the center of the incipient loop (*arrows*). **H.** The index finger (i) is flexed in a fashion analogous to pulling the trigger of a gun. It crosses under limb "b," while catching limb "a" between the point where "a" is held by the thumb (t) and the center finger (c), and the point where "a" and "b" cross each other (*arrow*). At this point, the index finger is flicked (straightened out from its previously flexed position), carrying with it the "a" suture limb and completing the second loop of the single-hand tie. **I.** The "a" and "b" limbs are pulled in opposite directions to cinch down the tie and complete the second portion of the single-hand tie.

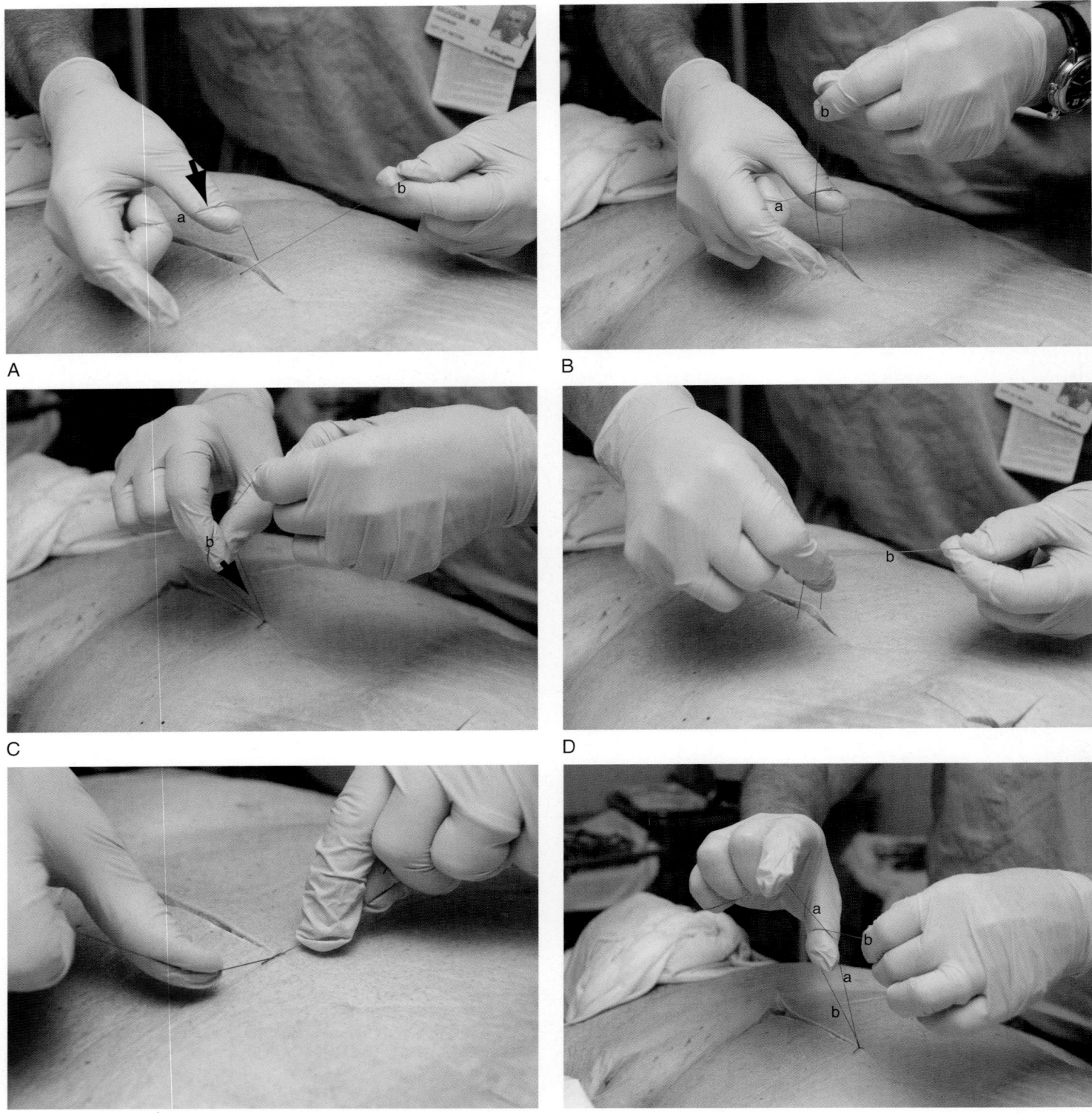

**FIGURE 4–22  A.** The two-handed tie begins with a tension grab of the suture limb "a," using the center ring and baby fingers, and allowing the thumb and index finger of the dominant hand free for manipulation. The "a" limb of the suture is placed across the dorsal dip of the thumb in a diagonal direction (*arrow*). **B.** Suture limb "b" is carried over the thumb so as to cross the thumb over limb "a" to initiate the loop. **C.** The index finger is moved into the loop pinching the thumb, thereby creating one side of the loop, with the right index finger holding loop "b" (between index and center fingers). The index finger points down through the loop (*arrow*). **D.** As the thumb is pulled from the loop, the index finger drops into the center of the loop. The thumb pushes limb "b" upward to the index finger, completing the loop. The left (nondominant) hand pulls limb "b" to close the loop. **E.** The squared loop is snugged down with the use of left or right index fingers. **F.** The second part begins when the "a" limb is grasped in the right hand, allowing the thumb and index finger to be free to move. The "b" limb is carried over the palmar (ventral) surface of the right thumb, and the thumb is flexed over "b," while the right hand holding "a" is rotated medially. This brings "a" across the thumb and carries "a" limb across "b" to form a loop.

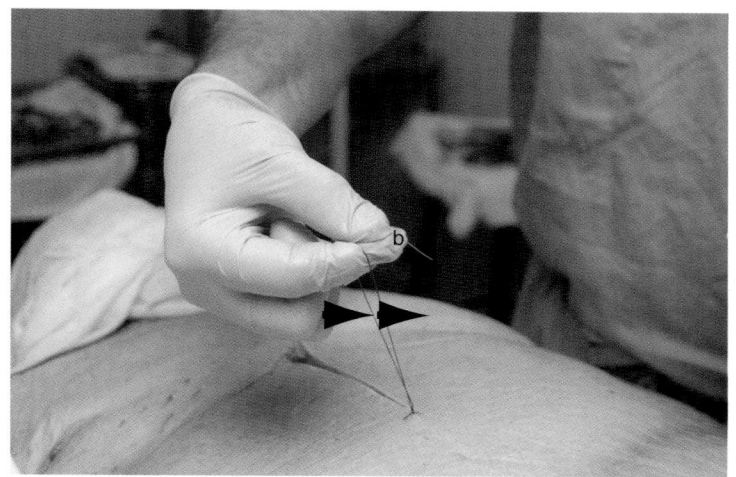

G

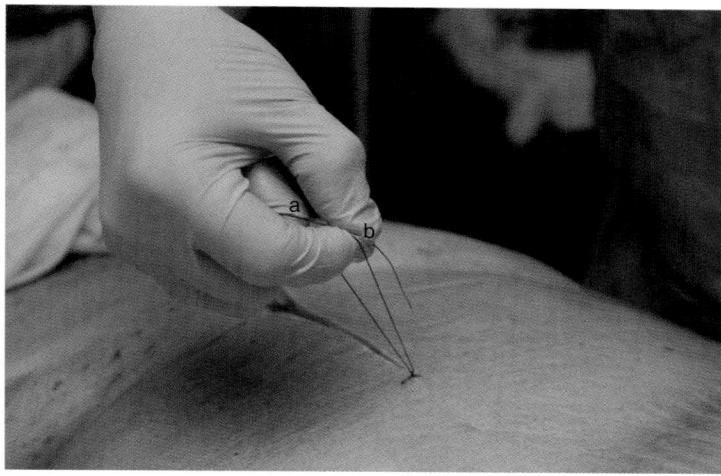

H

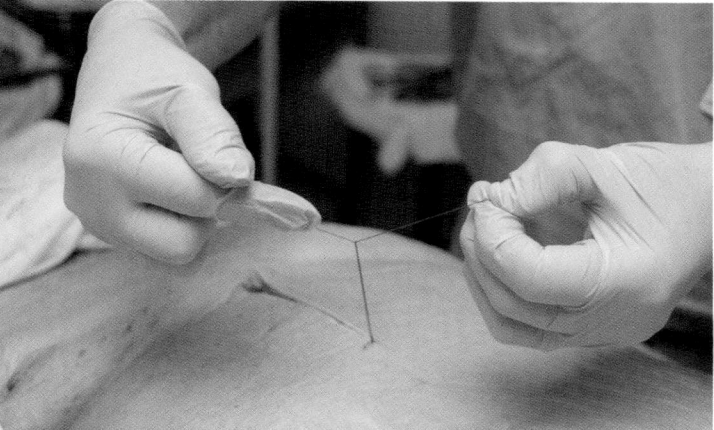

I

**FIGURE 4–22, cont'd  G.** Suture limb "b," which has been looped over "a," is now brought forward by the left hand so as to cross the ventral aspect of the thumb. Limb "b" is held in a pincer action between the right thumb and index finger. The right index finger actually pushes through the newly formed loop (*arrows*). **H.** View of Fig. 4-22G from the back. **I.** The limbs of the suture are now tightened down.

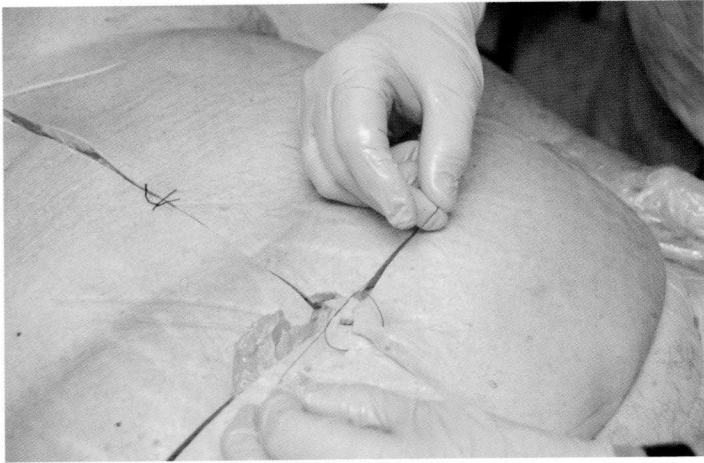

**FIGURE 4–23** A triple loop can be created to prevent slipping of the first tie-down. The technique is an alternative to a tension tie. This is called a "surgeon's knot."

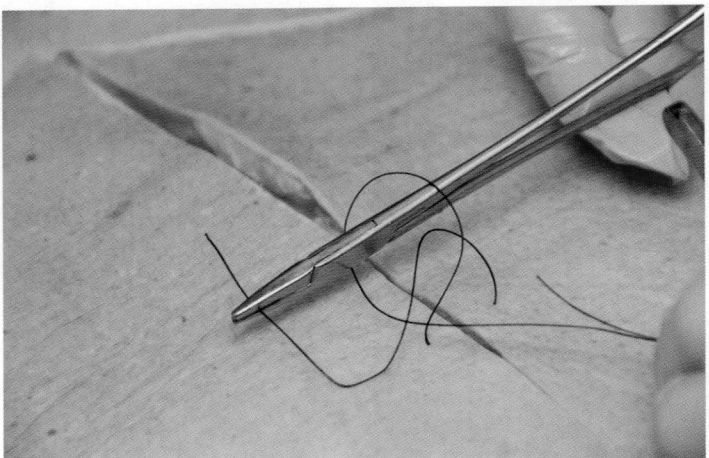

**FIGURE 4–24** An instrument tie is performed by circling the tip of the needle holder with the suture material, then grasping the short end of the stitch. This technique is well suited for fine sutures (e.g., 5-0, 6-0). The maneuver is repeated in the opposite direction to create a square knot.

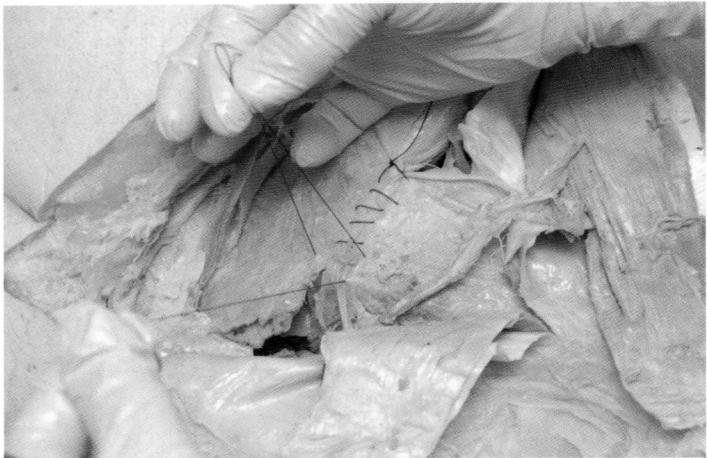

**FIGURE 4–25** A running (continuous) stitch is completed by securing the final loop, the needle end of the stitch.

# Energy Devices

*Michael S. Baggish*

## Electrosurgery—Laser—Harmonic Scalpel

Energy-releasing devices have been used in the past and currently are employed in pelvic surgery. The raison d'être for such tools consists of hemostasis and speed.

Compared with cold knife or scissor cutting, energy devices create a greater degree of surrounding tissue damage, usually in the form of thermal injury leading to necrosis, devitalization, subsequent fibrosis, and scar formation. Because of the aforesaid events, tissues neighboring the operative site are vulnerable to injury by a variety of mechanisms. The surgeon, his or her assistants, and supporting nursing staff must be fully acquainted with these devices and with the mechanisms by which each device produces desired and undesired actions. The aforesaid exercise is intended to protect a patient from unintended injury.

## Electrosurgery

Two terms misused relative to electrosurgery are *cautery* and *bovie*. A cautery is rarely used in a modern operating room. It refers to heating of a conducting metal (e.g., an iron poker, a branding iron, an electric stove top heating element) until it has reached sufficient temperature such that the iron glows red. The heat of the device makes direct contact (e.g., severed limb stump), thereby cauterizing open vessels and quenching the flow of blood. In 1928, William Bovie, a physicist, and Harvey Cushing, a neurosurgeon, developed an electrosurgical unit capable of cutting and coagulating.

The Bovie unit was thus an early spark gap generator, which has been for many years obsolete. Contemporary microprocessor-controlled electrosurgical units are not Bovie units.

The following four terms are of key import for understanding the physics and tissue interactions of electrosurgery units:

  current
  voltage
  resistance
  power

*Current* refers to the flow of electrical charges. Without current flow, no electrosurgical action would happen. It is measured in amps (Amperes). The action of the electric generator produces a current within a complete electrical circuit. Current flows in the direction of positive charges.

For work to be accomplished, electrical charges must be moved from one point to another (i.e., the **difference in potential** between two points is expressed as **volts** [a potential force]). **Impedance** to the conduction of electrical current through a given medium is referred to as its **resistance** and is expressed

in **ohms.** The relationship of current, potential, and resistance is expressed as **Ohm's law:**

$$V = IR \text{ or } R = \frac{V}{I}$$

$$1\,OHM = \frac{1\,VOLT}{1\,AMPERE}$$

**Power** is equivalent to work performed over a period of time and is expressed in **watts.**

$$P = I^2 R$$

$$or$$

$$P = VI$$

Two major types of current flow are described: **direct** and **alternating.** In the United States, electrosurgery utilizes **radiofrequency (RF)** (>100,000 Hertz or cycles per second) alternating current to **cut** or **coagulate** tissue.

A **monopolar circuit** travels from the **electrosurgical unit (ESU)** via a copper wire to an electrode, where vaporization (100°C) [i.e., cutting or coagulation] (60°C) occurs.

The current is then conducted through the patient's body, usually via the great blood vessels, and is returned to the ESU via a **neutral electrode** (ground plate), which is also connected by a copper wire to the ESU (Fig. 5–1).

A **bipolar circuit** consists of two wires leaving the ESU; the first wire is connected through a two-part electrode to the portion that serves as the active electrode. The second portion, which serves as the return or neutral electrode, is connected to the second wire, which returns the current to the ESU. The advantage of the bipolar system is obvious. Electrical current flows only between active and neutral electrodes. Tissue action is observed only between the electrodes. Thus no current will traverse the patient's entire body, as is the case with monopolar circuits (Fig. 5–2).

**Cutting** versus **coagulation waveforms** can be visualized on an oscilloscope (Fig. 5–3). Cutting is distinguished by (unmodulated) sine wave form characterized by high current flow, low peak-to-peak voltage, and rapid attainment of high tissue temperatures (e.g., 100°C) with attendant **cellular vaporization.** The best cutting and least coagulation artifacts occur with peak voltages ranging from 200 to 600 volts (Fig. 5–4A, B).

In contrast, electrocoagulation is modulated and exhibits lower current flow and higher voltages (Fig. 5–5). During coagulation, heating occurs less rapidly and at lower temperatures (60°C–70°C), rendering the cell dried or **desiccated,** because ions and water are driven out of the cells; resistance to flow

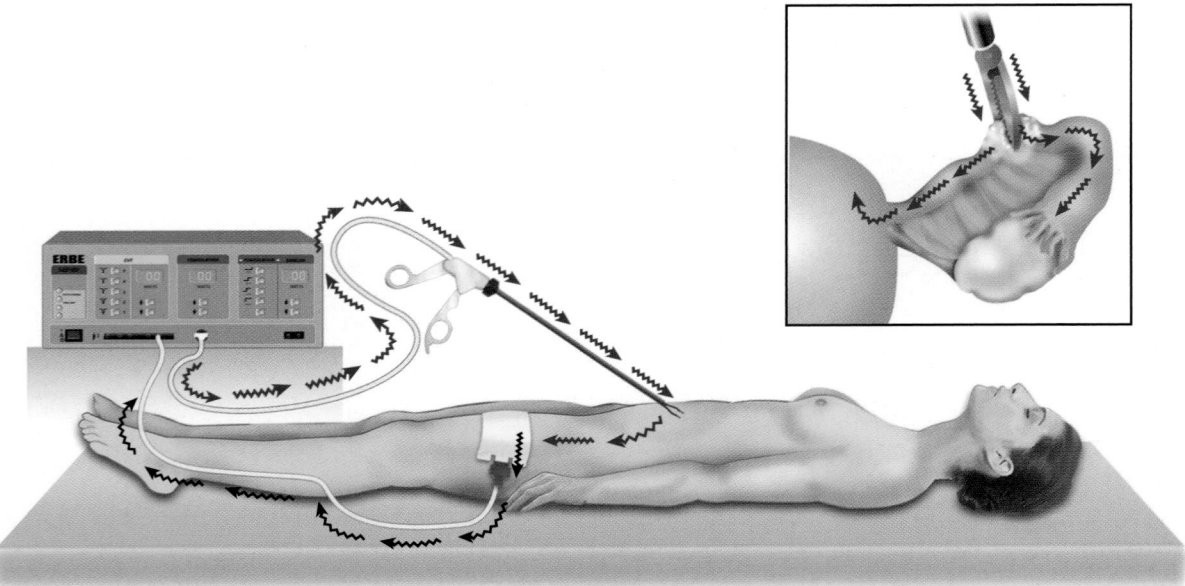

**FIGURE 5–1** This illustration shows the electrical current flow with a monopolar circuit. Active current leaves the electrosurgical unit (ESU) and flows through the grasping forceps to create high current density where the forceps jaws close on the tissue (**inset**). The current is conducted through the patient's body to exit over a large surface area (ground plate) and return to the ESU.

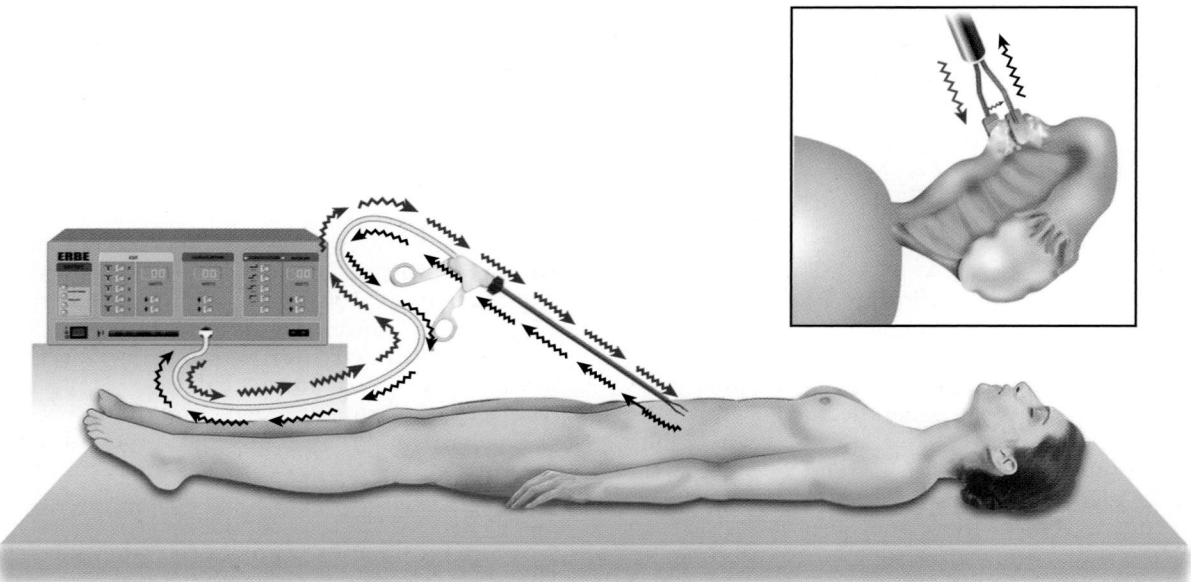

**FIGURE 5–2** This illustrates a bipolar circuit. The current form in the electrosurgical unit (ESU) flows through an insulated conductor of the bipolar forceps to exert its thermal action on the tissue (**inset**). The current flows from the active jaw (electrode) to the inactive (neutral) jaw of the electrode. The current flows back to the ESU via the insulated neural limb of the bipolar forceps. Note that current flow to tissue is limited to that which is enclosed between active and neutral electrodes (forceps jaws).

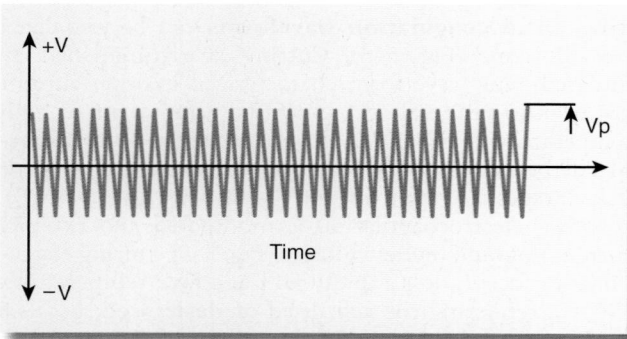

**FIGURE 5–3** A typical oscilloscopic pattern for "cutting current." Note that the peak-to-peak voltage is relatively low and there is no modulation of amplitude. Current flow is high.

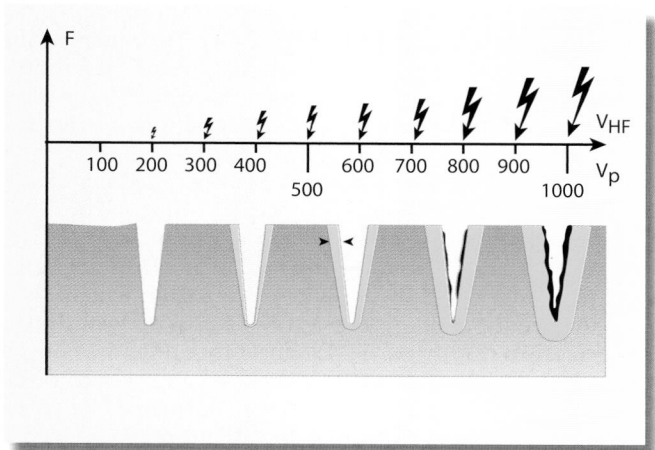

A

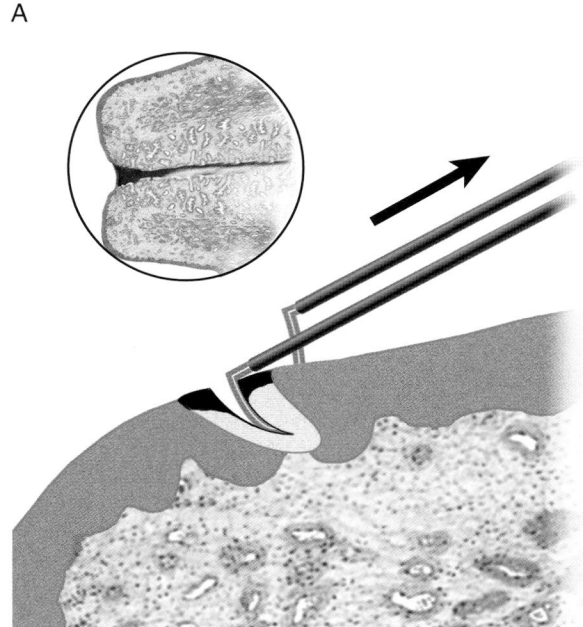

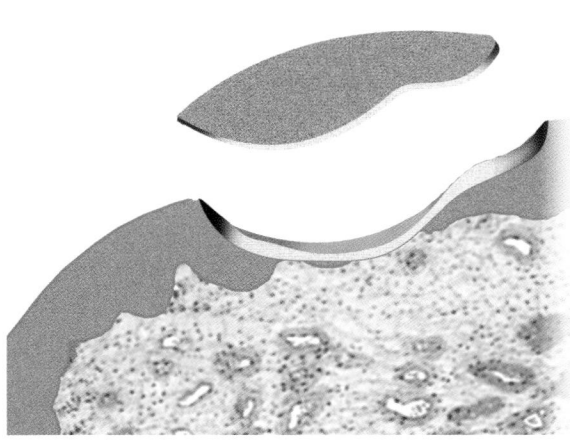

B

**FIGURE 5–4 A.** As voltage increases, the relative size of the electrical spark also increases. The effect on tissue of increased voltage is an increase in the area of coagulation artifact. **B.** A cutting loop electrode is illustrated here cutting into the cervix. The electrosurgical unit (ESU) foot pedal is activated just before the loop makes contact with the cervix. This creates an open circuit. Relatively high voltages are created as the electrode encounters the cervix. This is notable by high resistance and high thermal temperatures, thereby creating carbon formation (*black*). As voltage is diminished, current flow is picked up and the tissue is vaporized with little coagulation artifact. When the electrode exits, high temperatures again create thermal artifact.

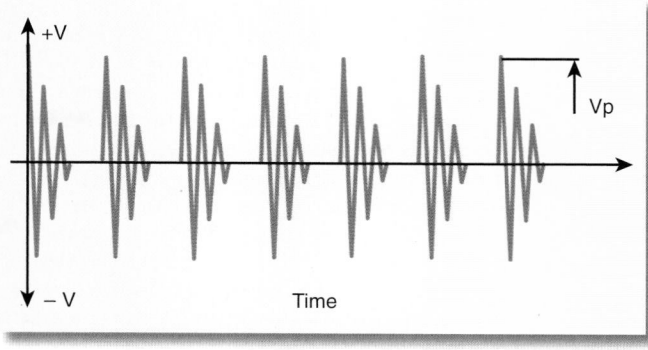

A

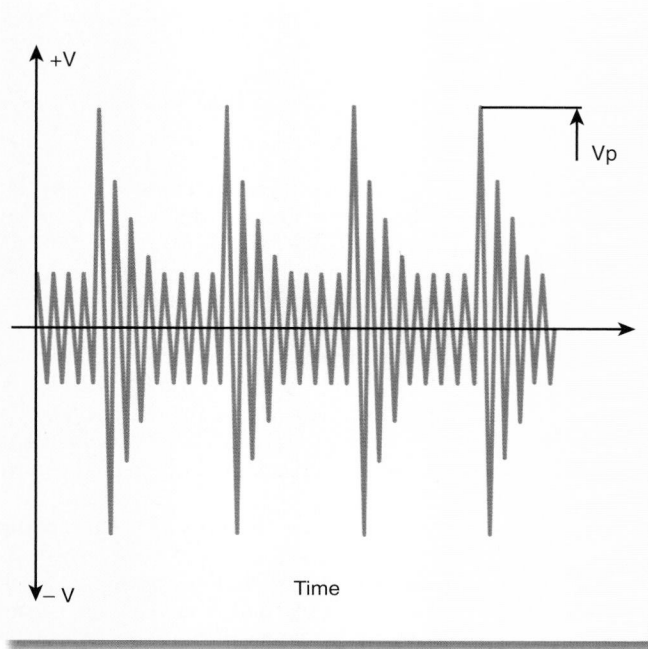

B

**FIGURE 5–5** Frequency modulation produces high-voltage (peak-to-peak) intermittent bursts (i.e., noncontinuous output). This results in less current flow and higher resistance. Temperatures are elevated more slowly and are at subvaporization levels (i.e., coagulating).

increases as the cells lose conducting ions. Fulguration (spray coagulation) occurs when the coagulating electrode is held close to the tissue target but does not touch the tissue. Here very high voltages are required to allow the spark to jump across the air space and coagulate the cells. Typically, **fulguration** creates superficial coagulation as opposed to deeper penetrating contact coagulation (Fig. 5–6).

During the coagulation cycle, high temperatures are reached within close proximity to the electrode. Thermal conductivity spreads the heat action peripheral to the electrode-tissue interface. This is an important concept that surgeons must understand because structures in proximity to the coagulation target may be thermally damaged by spreading conductive heat (Figs. 5–7 and 5–8).

Several hazards related to electrosurgery are illustrated in the chapters that discuss endoscopic complications (laparoscopic and hysteroscopic).

## Laser Surgery

A laser is a device that generates an energized light beam (light amplification by stimulated emission of radiation). This **stimulated radiation** in turn is utilized for surgery. Laser action on tissue is the result of conversion to heat (thermal), shock waves (fracture of tissue), or photochemical reactions (interaction with a dye or chemical compound).

Many actions of a laser depend on the ability of the light beam to be **absorbed.** Some beams are **reflected** from a tissue interface and exert no action. Depending on the energy of the **incident laser beam,** it will penetrate tissue to variable depths and will be stopped only when the incident energy has been fully absorbed.

Because laser beams are produced across the **electromagnetic spectrum,** they may be absorbed selectively; this in turn is based on wavelength (Fig. 5–9A). For example, argon and KTP/532 lasers emit in the visible bands at 0.51 micron and will be selectively absorbed by hemoglobin-containing areas (e.g., varicosities, hemangiomas) (Fig. 5–9B), whereas a **carbon dioxide ($CO_2$)** laser (10.6 microns) emitting in the far infrared is absorbed by water very efficiently and likewise by all tissues, regardless of color. The **neodymium (Nd)-yttrium aluminum garnet (YAG)** laser actually penetrates water (i.e., is not absorbed and principally coagulates tissue via front scatter). Several lasers are efficiently transmitted by flexible fibers (e.g., **argon, KTP,** Nd:YAG, **holmium [Ho]-YAG**). The $CO_2$ laser is not transmitted well by fiber but traverses air and exerts its actions without directly touching the tissue (Fig. 5–10A, B).

The $CO_2$ laser has been used as a cutting, vaporizing coagulation tool for gynecologic surgery (Fig. 5–11). Through use of its property of being effectively absorbed by even small amounts of water, the penetration of a $CO_2$ laser beam can be precisely controlled **(heat sink action).** The tissue actions of this laser depend on several variables.

The diameter of a laser beam may be controlled by focusing it through a lens. A tightly focused beam (<1 mm) will be rapidly absorbed by tissue cells. Light energy is instantaneously converted to heat energy, causing intracellular water to boil at 100°C; this is followed by conversion to steam, which causes the cell to literally blow up (Fig. 5–12). **Explosive evaporation** or **vaporization** results in the disappearance of a mass of cells. Moving the linear laser beam will produce an incision or cut. When the laser beam is out of focus (i.e., **defocused** or >2 mm in diameter), the absorbed beam is spread out over a larger area, which creates temperatures of 60°C to 80°C, thus (desiccating) coagulating tissues, rather than vaporizing them (Fig. 5–13). The $CO_2$ laser may be delivered to tissue via a handpiece, a wave guide, or a micromanipulator (Fig. 5–14A, B).

The concept of expressing laser tissue effects in terms of **power density (PD)** is desirable:

$$PD = Watts/cm^2 = Power (watts) Beam diameter (\pi r^2)$$

A simple empirical formula allows close and rapid calculation of the PD:

$$PD = \frac{Watts \times 100}{diam\ mm^2} (express\ as\ watts/cm^2)$$

As the reader can readily understand, the most efficient way to raise the power density is to diminish laser beam diameter or **spot size** (see Fig. 5–13). Conversely, the most effective way to reduce penetration and decrease power density is by increasing the spot size (increasing beam diameter).

The Nd:YAG laser (10.6 microns) is commonly utilized for hysteroscopic and laparoscopic surgery because it penetrates water and other fluids, is a very effective coagulating device, and is efficiently transmitted by flexible fibers (e.g., quartz), which range from 0.5 mm to 1 mm or more in diameter (Fig. 5–15A, B). This allows the laser to be delivered through the operating channels of even small endoscopes. The same may be said for the Ho-YAG laser, which is an efficient cutting device.

Lasers are desirable tools because they do not conduct through tissues (e.g., electrosurgery) and are not dependent for fluid penetration/absorption on hypotonic fluids. There is no danger of electroshock. Clearly, lasers can accomplish certain things that other tools cannot.

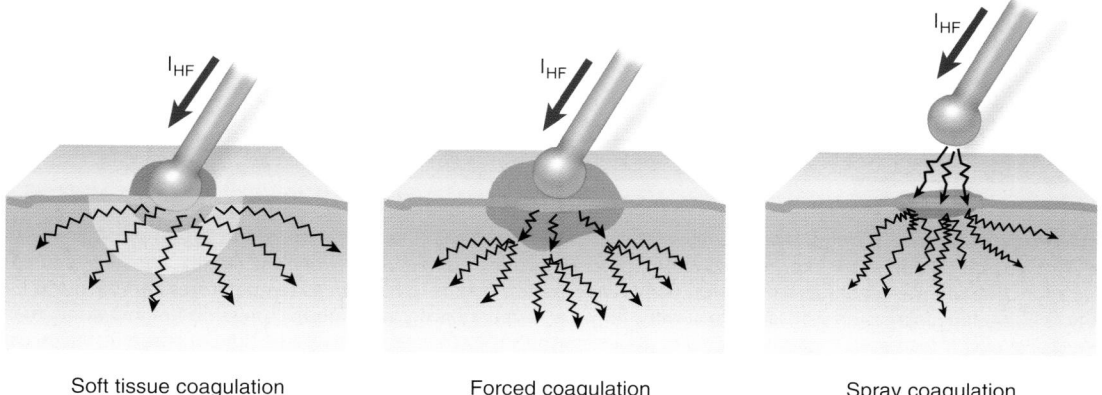

Soft tissue coagulation        Forced coagulation        Spray coagulation

**FIGURE 5–6** Constant-voltage electrosurgical units (ESUs) can precisely vary peak-to-peak voltages, thereby allowing a variety of coagulation modalities. Soft coagulation occurs at peak-to-peak voltages ≤200 volts. Deeper coagulation may be achieved at peak-to-peak voltages ≥600 volts (i.e., forced coagulation). Spray coagulation creates superficial coagulation. The electrical spark must transverse the air space between the electrode and the tissue. This requires peak-to-peak voltages ≥100 volts.

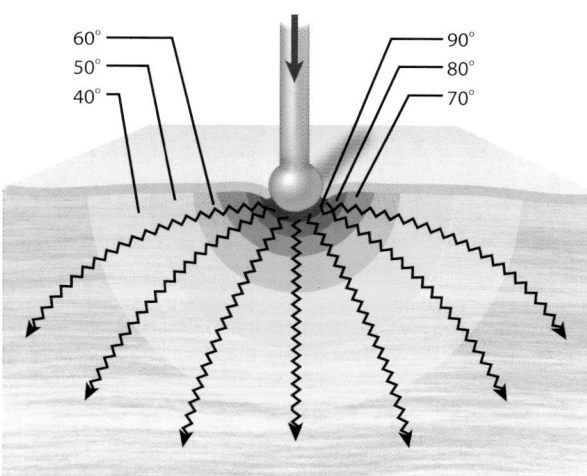

**FIGURE 5–7** Every surgeon must be cognizant that heat spreads via conductivity through tissue. The highest temperatures are recorded in the immediate vicinity of the electrode-tissue interface. As thermal energy spreads concentrically, the temperature decreases. Time of electrode contact is a critical factor relative to the distance to which harmful heating action affects tissues.

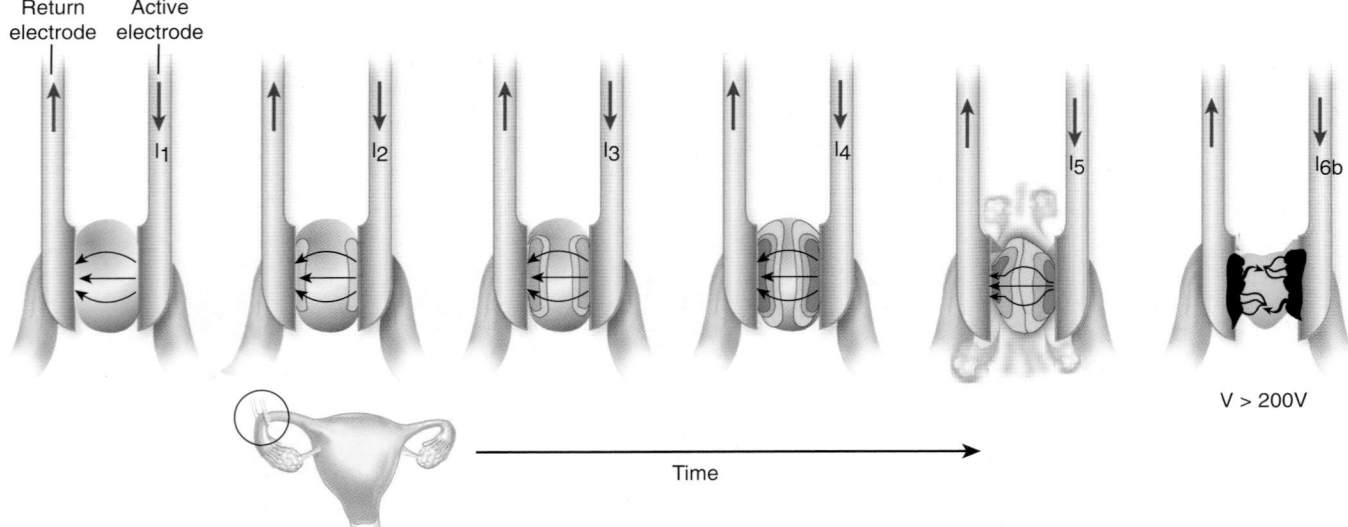

**FIGURE 5–8** This illustration details the thermal action of bipolar electrodes. The tissue between the forceps arms heats to coagulation temperatures as a function of time-on-tissue. As a critical point, vaporization begins to happen as temperatures approach 100°C. Ions are driven out of the cells, thereby increasing resistance to current flow (i.e., a vapor barrier is created). If power is not increased, then electronic conduction ceases. If power is increased to permit sparks to penetrate the vapor barrier, then superheating of tissue results in carbonization when temperatures approach or exceed 400°C.

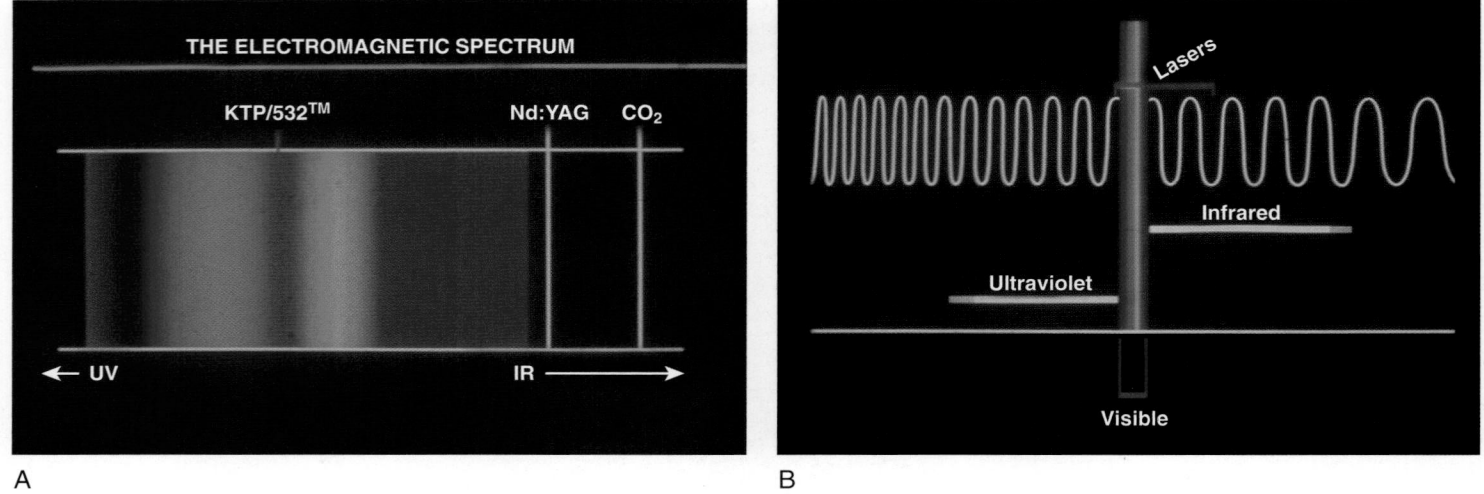

**FIGURE 5–9 A.** A schema of visible and invisible parts of the electromagnetic spectrum is shown here. Note that the KTP/532 laser emits in the visible green. The helium-neon laser emits in the visible red. The neodymium-yttrium aluminum garnet (Nd:YAG) laser and the carbon dioxide ($CO_2$) laser emit in the infrared (near and far, respectively) and are not visible. **B.** This picture details the wavelengths of light within the spectrum. Note the very small visible band, which was magnified in Figure 5–9A.

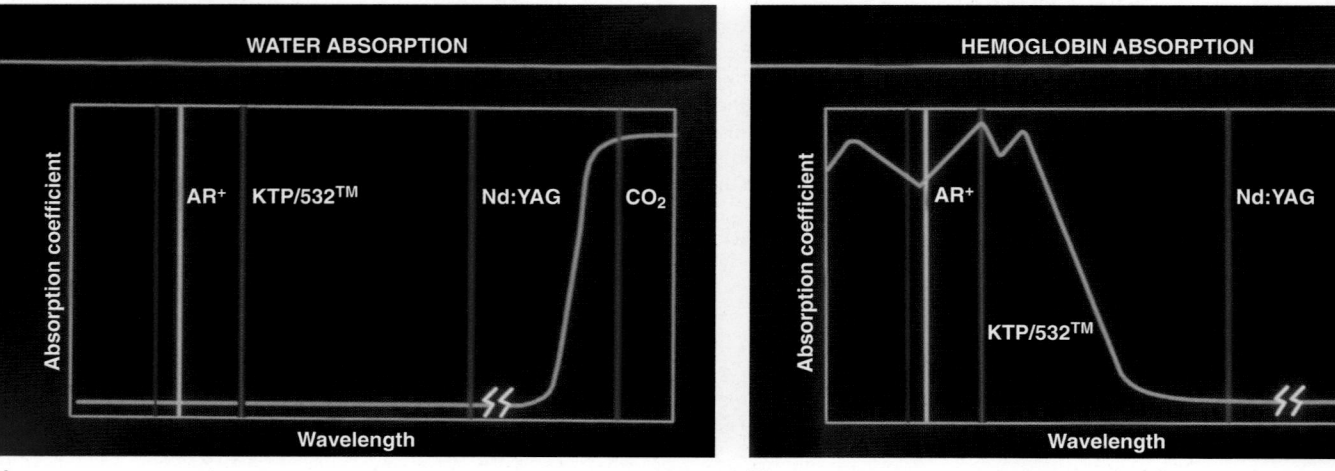

**FIGURE 5–10 A.** Water absorption according to laser wavelength is detailed here. Note the high level of absorption for the carbon dioxide ($CO_2$) laser. **B.** Selective absorption for hemoglobin occurs at the wavelengths where argon lasers and KTP/532 lasers operate.

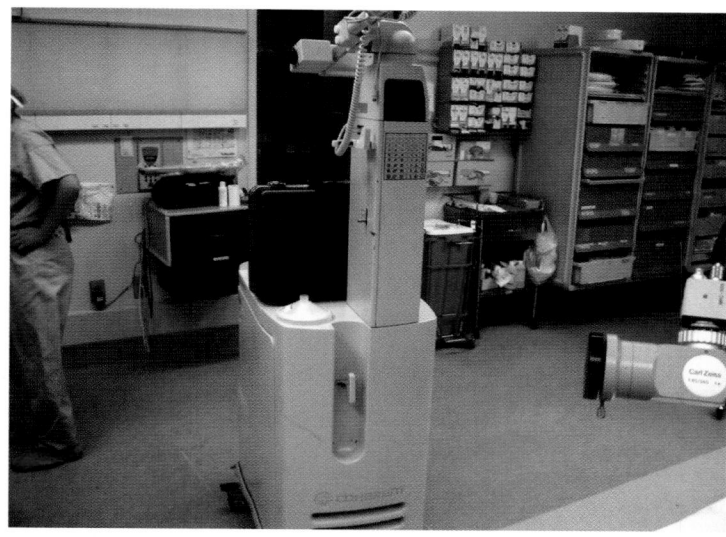

A

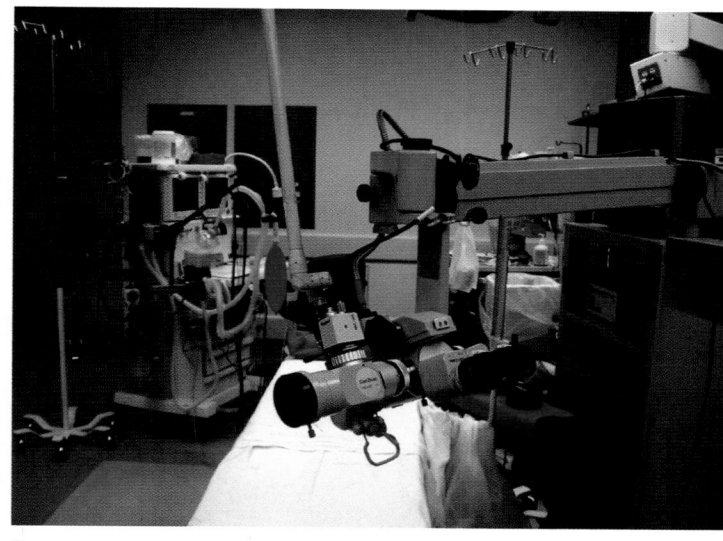

B

**FIGURE 5–11 A.** A high-power output carbon dioxide ($CO_2$) laser is shown here. The vertical structure contains the $CO_2$ laser tube. This laser is capable of superpulse and continuous modes. **B.** The laser arm couples to the operating microscope. The laser beam is precisely controlled via a micromanipulator. Note the cube-sized three-chip video cameras mounted to the beam splitter on the left side of the microscope.

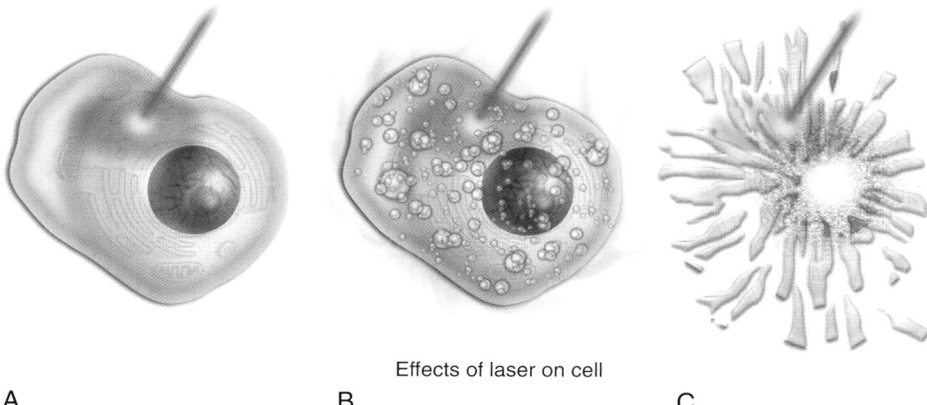

Effects of laser on cell

A                    B                    C

**FIGURE 5–12** The schematic pictures depict laser tissue interaction. The laser light beam is absorbed by the cell(s). **A.** Light energy is instantaneously converted to thermal energy. Cell water heats rapidly and begins to boil at 100°C. **B.** The water converts to a gaseous state (steam), which expands and explodes the cell and its contents. **C.** This process is referred to as explosive evaporation (vaporization).

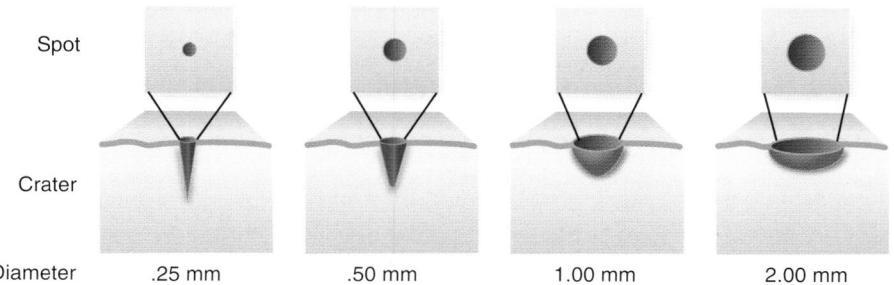

Spot

Crater

Diameter     .25 mm        .50 mm        1.00 mm        2.00 mm

**FIGURE 5–13** The depth of a laser wound is controlled by a series of factors. The power setting of the laser beam is a clear factor. More important is the laser beam diameter or spot size. A tightly focused laser beam will create a deep conical crater because the power density is high. A defocused beam or spot will create a wider, shallower, bowel-shaped crater. The latter has a lower power density. The sharply focused beam creates less coagulation, whereas the defocused beam creates more coagulation.

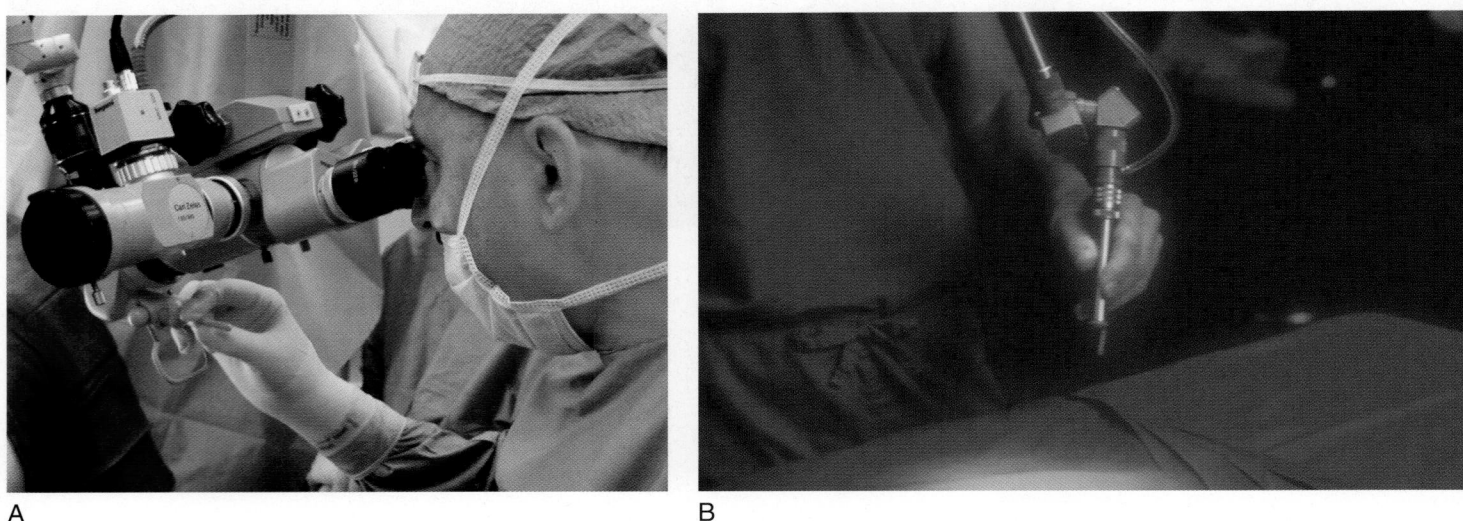

A                                                                    B

**FIGURE 5–14 A.** This magnified view shows the surgeon controlling the laser beam by means of a micromanipulator. **B.** The laser handpiece provides the surgeon with an alternative delivery system for a carbon dioxide ($CO_2$) laser beam.

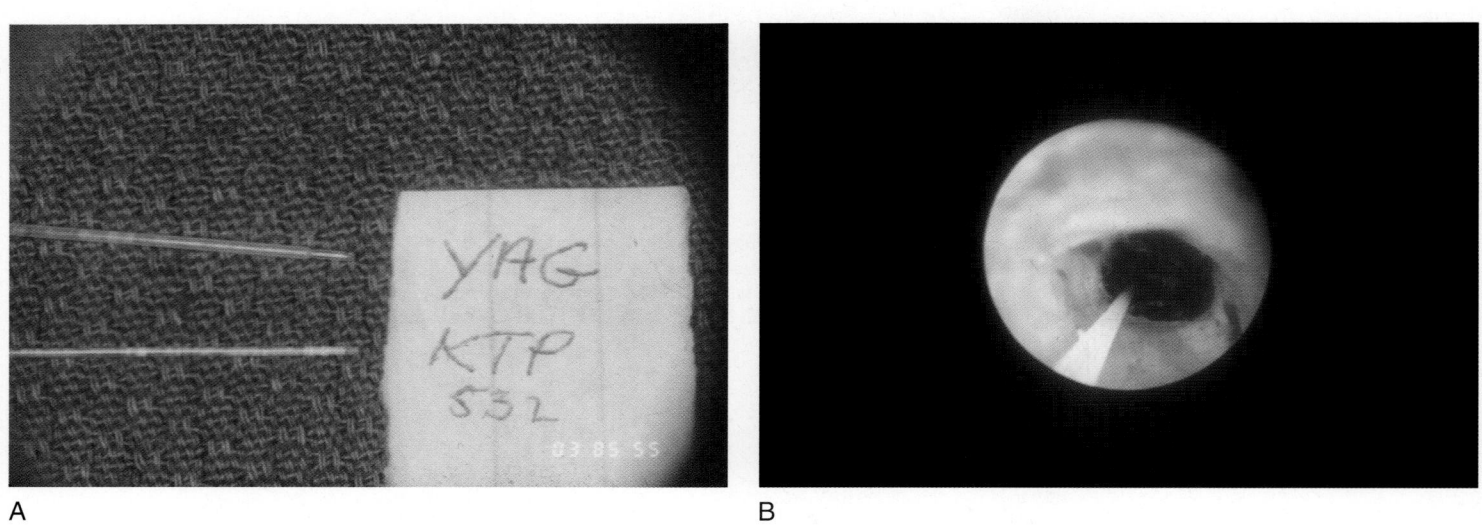

A                                                                    B

**FIGURE 5–15 A.** Neodymium (Nd)-yttrium aluminum garnet (YAG), KTP/532, holmium-YAG, and argon laser beams may be delivered to tissue by means of fine optical fibers. These lasers will penetrate water rather than being absorbed by it. **B.** This hysteroscopic photo shows an Nd:YAG laser fiber, which is delivered via the operating channel of a hysteroscope to the interior of the uterus. The result of an endometrial ablation is clearly visible.

## Ultrasonic Surgery

Ultrasonic radiation results in energy outputs, which may be applied to diagnosis (sonography) and to surgery. The latter requires much higher power density compared with the former.

Two techniques and devices of surgical usage have been described: the **cavitron ultrasonic surgical aspirator (CUSA)** and the **harmonic scalpel.**

The ultrasonic aspirator has been used extensively for radical oncology surgery. This device dissects and creates hemostasis by coagulating vessels of up to 1 mm in diameter and atraumatically exposing vessels of larger diameter. Typically, tissues with higher water composition are selectively removed, whereas fibrous collagen, elastin-bearing tissues are not damaged. The CUSA simultaneously irrigates and suctions away debris, thereby maintaining a clear operative field. Unlike with electrosurgery or laser surgery, smoke vapor is not produced. However, a mist of fine particulate matter is produced, and the surgeon must take precautions to avoid contamination via contact or inspiration. Ultrasonic devices act on tissue by three mechanisms:

**Viscous stress:** Creates microbubbles, which may lead to cellular membrane disruption.

**Thermal conversion:** The sound wave is absorbed with conversion to heat. Fibrous, collagenous tissues absorb the waves more efficiently and demonstrate greater thermal coagulation effects. Additionally, the vibrating surgical tip of the transducer becomes hot as the result of friction (Fig. 5–16).

**Cavitation:** Fluid motion and shear stress perpetuate and reinforce ultrasonic wave absorption, creating progressively greater acoustic energy dissipation. This action results in alternate expansion and collapse of bubbles with similarly alternating conversion of liquid to gas (vapor) and back from gas to liquid. Because of the coinciding acute variance in pressure gradients, cellular cavities are created with an end point of cell disruption. The aforesaid events are clearly affected by increased exposure time to the sound waves (Fig. 5–17).

Both CUSA and harmonic scalpel utilize a piezoelectric crystal as the source of sound waves. The CUSA vibrates at 23 kHz, and the harmonic scalpel vibrates at 55.5 kHz with a linear blade motion of 50 to 100 microns (Fig. 5–18). Several variables determine the speed and action of the device (Fig. 5–19). These include the following:

**Power setting** (the highest power setting is associated with the greatest vertical excursion of the blade and the sharpest cutting effect).

**Blade thinness** (a honed or beveled blade surface will produce the most effective cutting action; in contrast, a thicker, nonsharp surface will result in inefficient cutting).

**Tissue stretch** (taut tissue is cut faster and with reduced coagulation artifact).

**Grip pressure** (the greater the grip pressure on a scissors-like device, the less the coagulation action).

As with electrosurgery and laser surgery, ultrasonic surgery is increasingly applied to endoscopic techniques. The harmonic scalpel tends to perform more slowly than comparable electrosurgery and laser devices. Nevertheless, it is an alternative energy device that has its peculiar set of advantages.

**UNIT 1 ■ SECTION B**

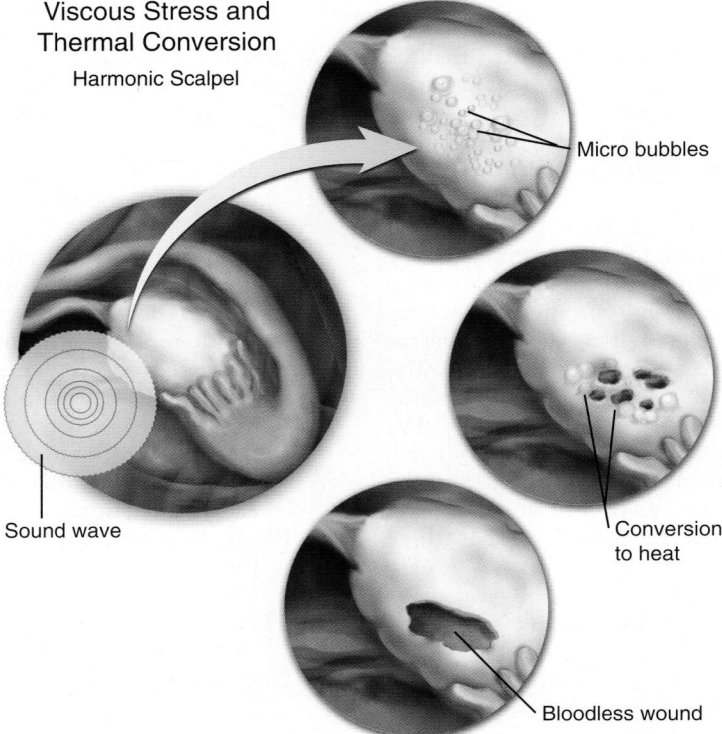

**FIGURE 5–16** The harmonic scalpel delivers high-frequency sound waves to tissue. The effects of these sound waves are to cut tissue and coagulate small blood vessels. The actions of viscous stress and friction leading to heat (thermal) conversion are illustrated.

Cavitation

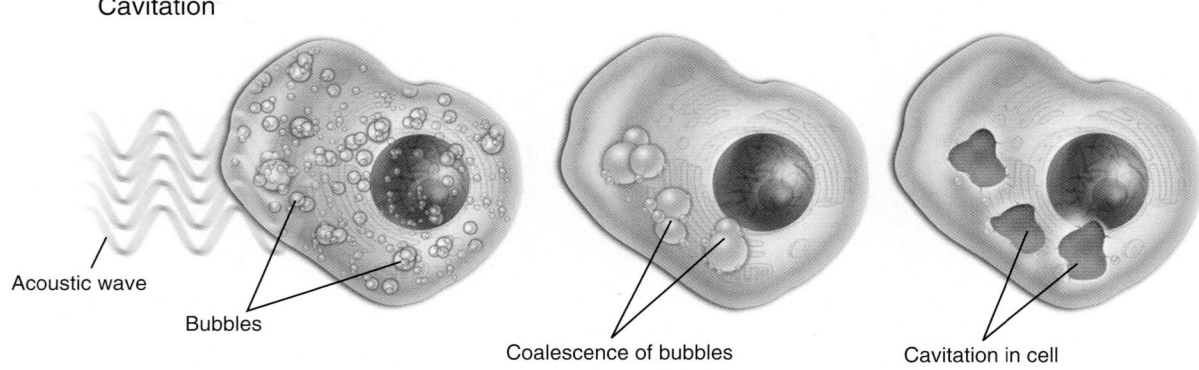

**FIGURE 5–17** Cavitation is created by sound waves impinging on cells and creating microbubbles, which in turn coalesce into larger bubbles. The latter collapse and create holes or cavitation artifacts within the cell.

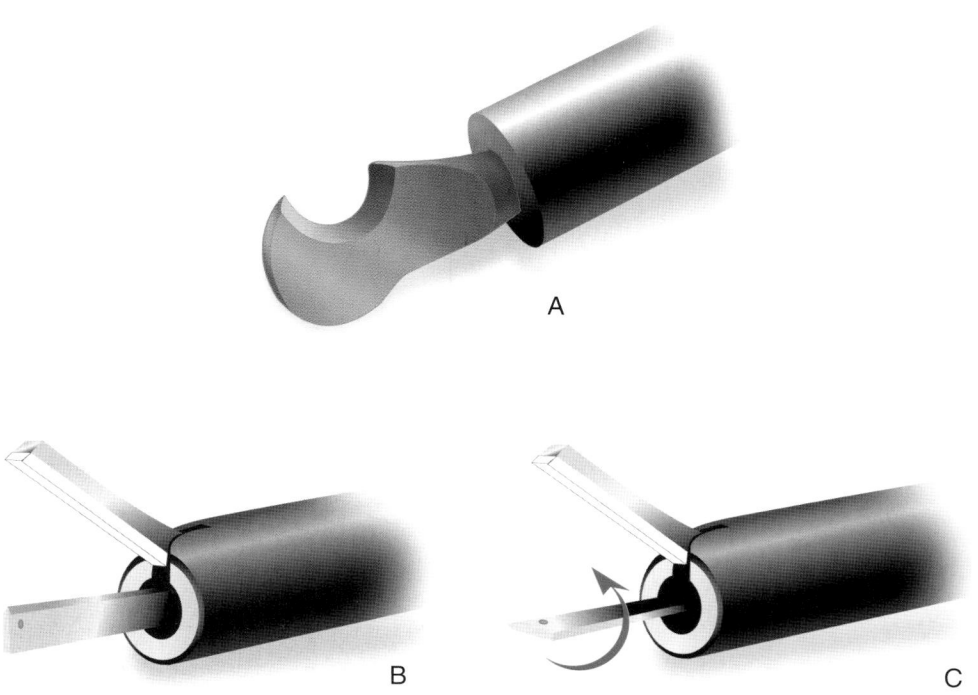

A

B

C

**FIGURE 5–18 A.** A harmonic scalpel hooked blade. The beveled surface is utilized for cutting. The convex, thicker, outer surface will coagulate tissue. **B.** The scissors-like device cuts tissue with the lower blade on edge. **C.** When the blade is rotated flat, the device coagulates tissue.

### Harmonic scalpel blade

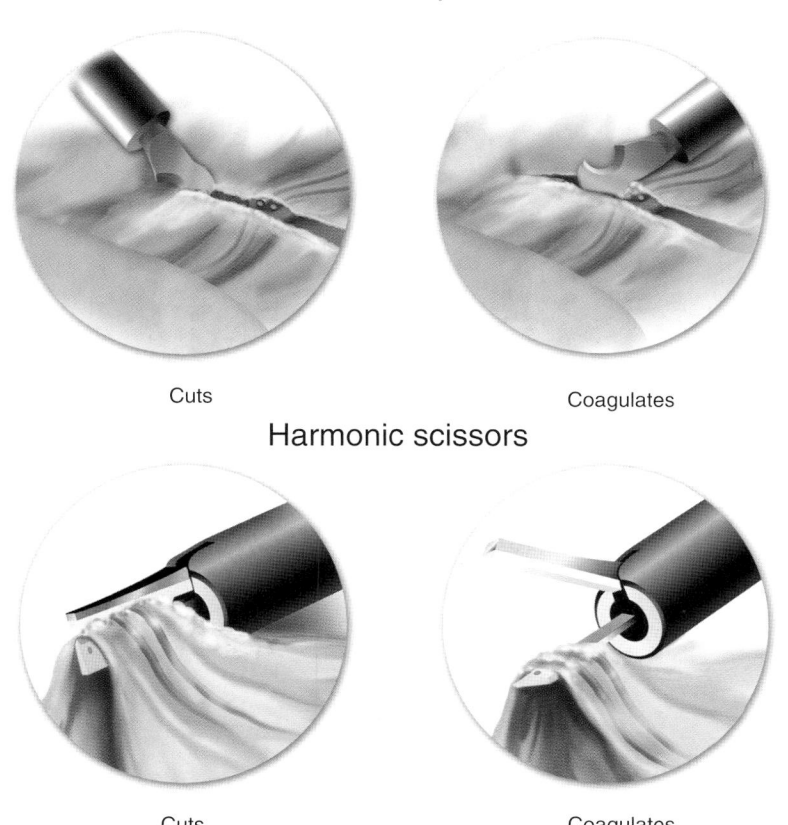

Cuts

Coagulates

### Harmonic scissors

Cuts

Coagulates

**FIGURE 5–19** The tissue actions of the harmonic scalpel are illustrated here. Tissue stretch is an important factor for efficient cutting action and reduction of friction-generated heat.

# CHAPTER 6

# Positioning and Nerve Injury

*Michael S. Baggish*

## Positioning the Patient

Proper care in positioning patients for cervical, vulvar, vaginal, anal, uterine, and endoscopic surgery is of vital interest for the gynecologic surgeon. The **dorsal lithotomy position** regardless of whether it is implemented with a candy cane or Allen, or knee-crutch leg supports remains an unnatural state Figs. 6–1 through 6–3. When lithotomy position is coupled with the **Trendelenburg position,** additive abnormalities may ensue. Improper positioning can and will result in neurologic injury. Table 6–1 illustrates the frequency, causative factor(s), and specific locations of nerve injuries associated with obstetric and gynecologic surgery. The proper lithotomy position includes thighs and legs gently flexed; ankles and feet evenly supported; and avoidance of dorsiflexion of the foot, minimal abduction at the hip, buttocks firmly seated on the operating table, avoidance of overhanging buttocks, and knees (lateral) free from contact with leg support devices. Several lithotomy positions are acceptable. A low lithotomy position is quite satisfactory for dilation and curettage, hysteroscopy, and cystoscopy (see Fig. 6–1). A mid to high lithotomy position provides the best exposure for vulvar and vaginal surgery (Fig. 6–4). Although Allen leg supports are satisfactory for laparoscopic procedures, they are not advantageous or for that matter desirable for most vulvar and vaginal procedures. They may be indicated for radical vulvectomy surgery.

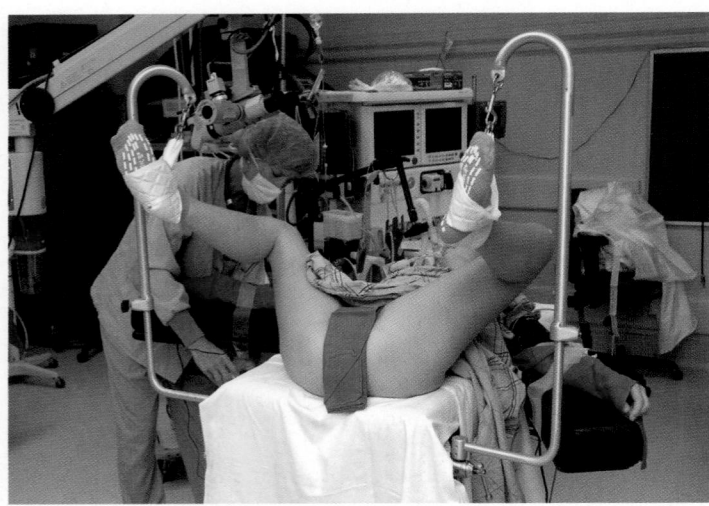

**FIGURE 6–1** This patient illustrates the low lithotomy position. Her legs are suspended in candy cane supports.

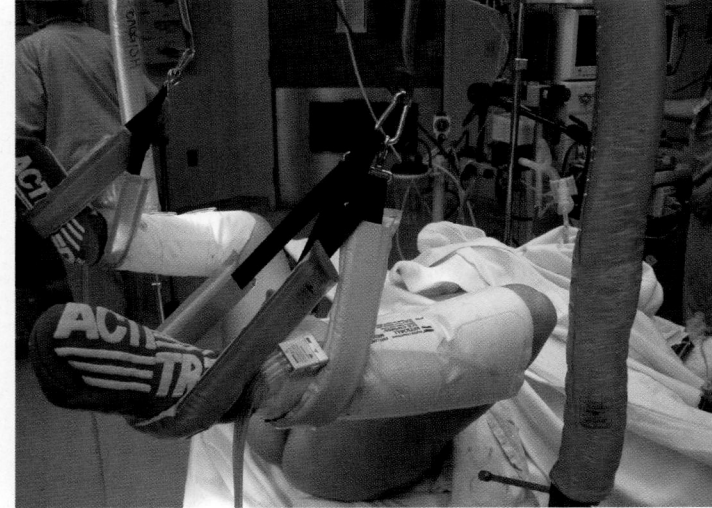

**FIGURE 6–2** This leg support incorporates a gel padding to protect the legs and feet.

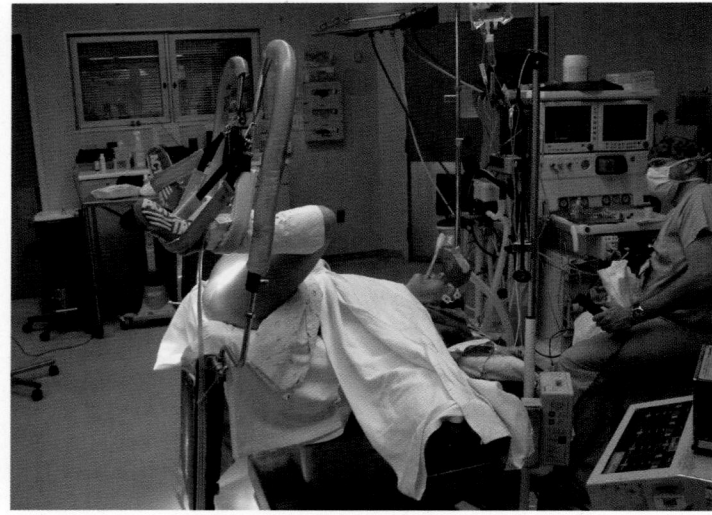

**FIGURE 6–3** The Trendelenburg (head-down) position adds to the risk of nerve injury when the patient is in the lithotomy position. The inferior extremities are further deprived of blood flow.

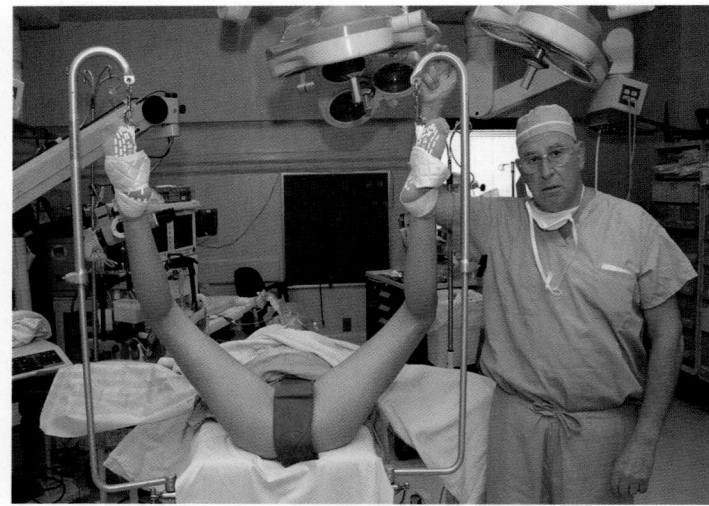

**FIGURE 6–4** The high lithotomy position requires that the legs are flexed at the knee. Extension at the knee joint adds to the risk of sciatic or lumbosacral trunk injury.

**TABLE 6–1 ■ Nerve Injuries Associated With Positioning and Pelvic Surgery**

| Symptom/Sign | Relative Frequency | Causative Factor | Affected Nerve(s) |
| --- | --- | --- | --- |
| (1) Sharp, cutting pain, chronic, burning pain (late) lower abdomen | 7% | Scar formation with entrapment; cutting suturing | Ilioinguinal<br>Iliohypogastric |
| (2) Numbness, lateral thigh<br>- Paresthesia<br>- Hyperesthesia | 6% | Compression with retractor<br>Injury to nerve with energy device<br>Rare, positioning | Lateral<br>Femoral<br>Cutaneous |
| (3) Numbness, burning pain, upper labia, thigh | 17% | Incision or tearing of the nerve<br>Retractor compression | Genitofemoral |
| (4) Numbness, anteromedial thigh<br>- Weakness with external rotation<br>- Adductor weakness | 20%-30% | Direct injury by cutting, clamping, suturing<br>Needle injury (TVT)<br>Pressure (e.g., obturator hernia) | Obturator |
| (5) Numbness, anteromedial thigh<br>- Weakness with leg extension<br>- Weakness with flexion at the hip<br>Absent knee jerk | 11%-30% | Compression by the inguinal ligament<br>Compression by retractors<br>Rare, direct injury | Femoral |
| (6) Buttock pain<br>- Posterior pain and posterolateral leg pain<br>- Numbness foot and leg<br>- Foot-drop<br>- Pain with straight-leg raising | 10% | Suture<br>Stretch<br>Compression (peroneal) | Lumbosacral trunk<br>Sciatic |

## Peripheral Nerve Injury

Hyperflexion at the hip will render the patient susceptible to **femoral nerve injury** (Fig. 6–5). The mechanism of injury relates to the fact that the rigid inguinal ligament compresses the femoral nerve trunk as the latter passes beneath it in its course from the abdomen into the thigh.

Hyperextension at the knee joint and hip can produce stretch injuries to the **lumbosacral trunk** and/or **sciatic nerve.** Short periods of leg extension with the feet in candy cane supports are tolerable, but after 30 minutes, the risk of injury is increased. Excessive abduction (>45°) over 2 hours will endanger the **obturator, genital femoral,** and/or **femoral nerves** (Fig. 6–6). The latter nerve is particularly vulnerable when external rotation is added to abduction >45°. Compression at the head of the fibula will injure the peroneal division (Fig. 6–7) of the **sciatic nerve,** leading to paresis and pain in the leg following distribution of that nerve. Other causes of neuropathies associated with gynecologic surgery in patients who are not in the **lithotomy position** include self-retaining abdominal retractors, radical surgery, compression related to tight and prolonged packing, hematomas, tumors, and direct injury (e.g., incising the nerve). Figure 6–8A, B shows the key

nerves and plexuses that supply innervation to the pelvis and inferior extremities. The relationships of the large nerve roots and trunks to the bony pelvis and to the ligamentous structures are detailed in the drawing. The largest nerves include (1) the sciatic nerve, which lies deep within the pelvis and exits the pelvis via the greater sciatic foramen (the nerve is in close proximity to the ischial spine and sacrospinous ligament [Fig. 6–9]); (2) the lumbosacral trunk, which contains elements of the lumbar and sacral plexuses and lies on the sacroiliac joint; and (3) the femoral nerve, which is embedded within the psoas major muscle. The nerve is exposed as it crosses beneath the inguinal ligament and exits via a groove between the iliacus muscle and the psoas major muscle (iliopsoas). After draping, it is wise to change the position of the suspended inferior extremities when surgery extends beyond 2 hours. Additionally, relief of pressure from retractor blades should be carried out every hour or two. Care must be taken with assistants leaning or resting on a patient's inferior extremities in the lithotomy position (Fig. 6–10). The latter can result in strain on nerves caused by iatrogenically induced excessive abduction and external rotation.

Figures 6–11 through 6–17 illustrate the mechanisms involved in various nerve injuries.

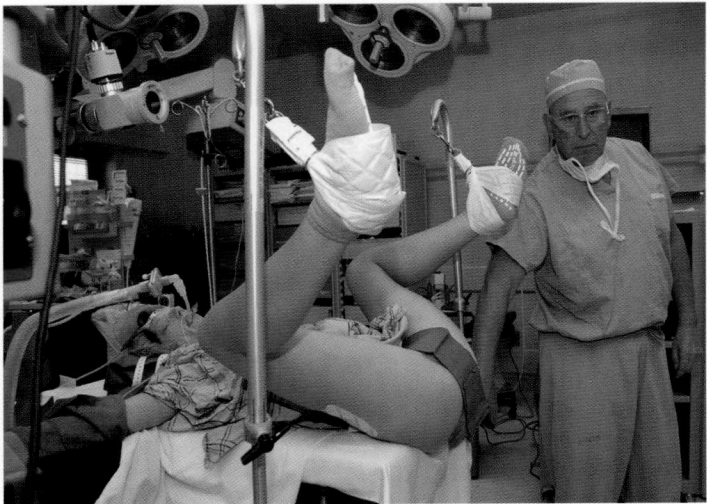

**FIGURE 6–5** Hyperflexion at the hip exposes the patient to femoral nerve injury. The point of risk is located beneath the rigid inguinal ligament, where compression of the exposed nerve occurs.

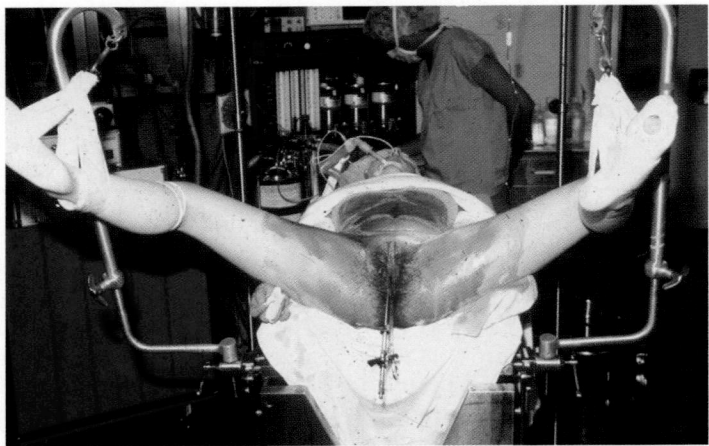

**FIGURE 6–6** Extreme abduction combined with external rotation exposes several nerves to the risk of injury, especially with prolonged operative time.

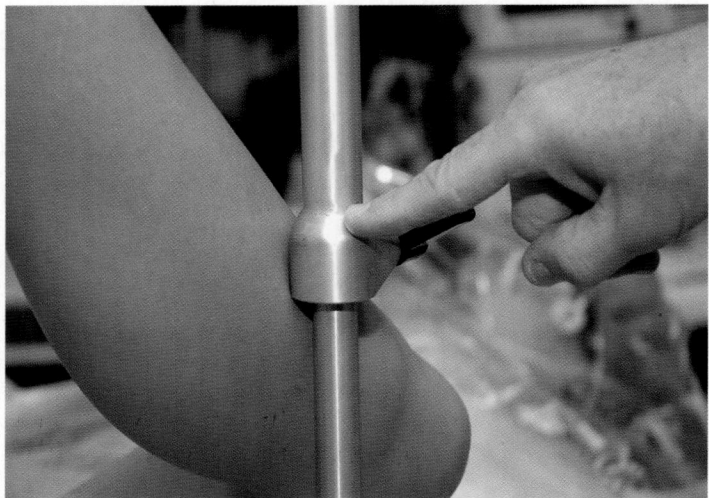

**FIGURE 6–7** Lateral pressure at or below the knee will result in compression injury to the peroneal division of the sciatic nerve.

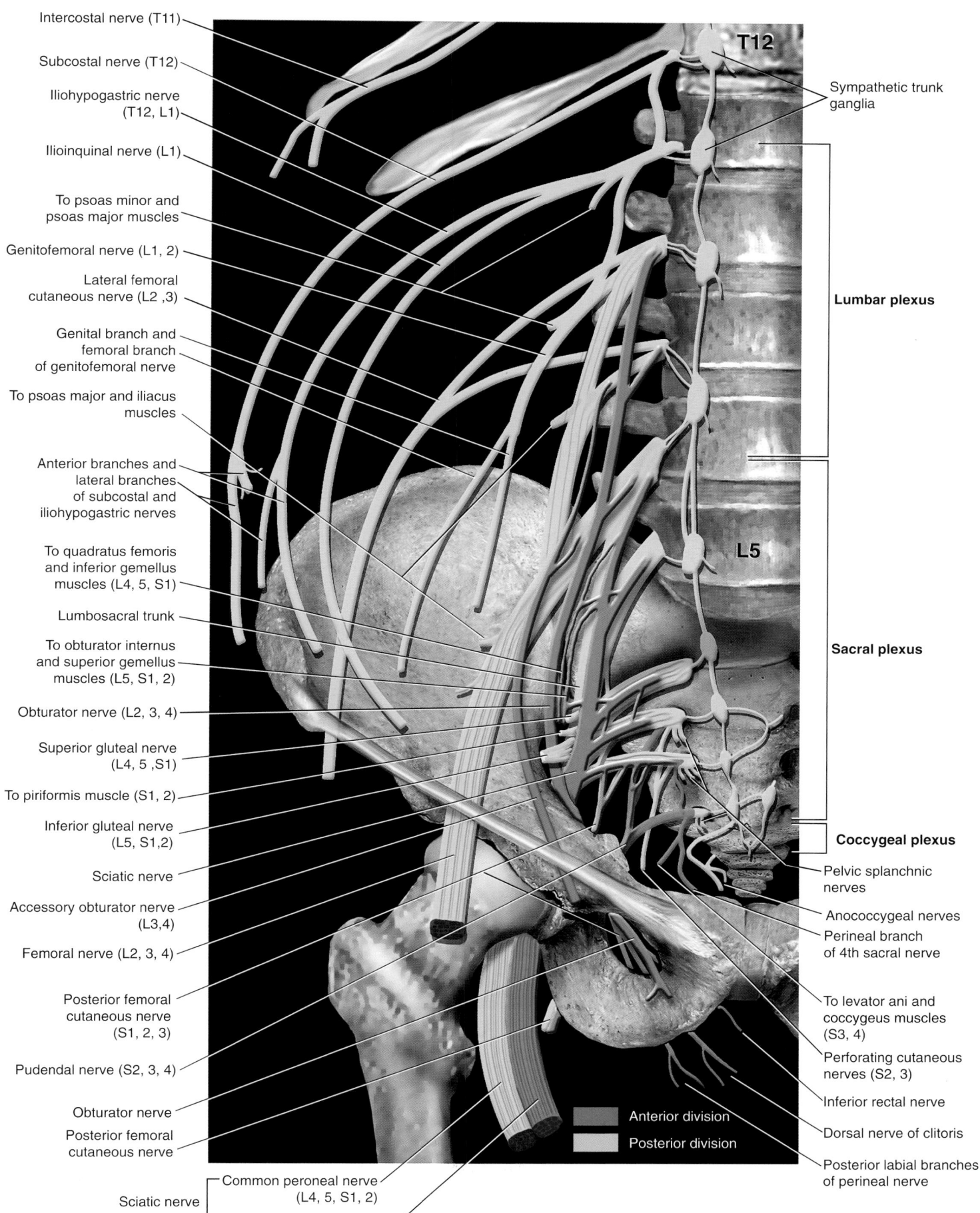

Intercostal nerve (T11)

Subcostal nerve (T12)

Iliohypogastric nerve
(T12, L1)

Ilioinquinal nerve (L1)

To psoas minor and
psoas major muscles

Genitofemoral nerve (L1, 2)

Lateral femoral
cutaneous nerve (L2 ,3)

Genital branch and
femoral branch
of genitofemoral nerve

To psoas major and iliacus
muscles

Anterior branches and
lateral branches
of subcostal and
iliohypogastric nerves

To quadratus femoris
and inferior gemellus
muscles (L4, 5, S1)

Lumbosacral trunk

To obturator internus
and superior gemellus
muscles (L5, S1, 2)

Obturator nerve (L2, 3, 4)

Superior gluteal nerve
(L4, 5 ,S1)

To piriformis muscle (S1, 2)

Inferior gluteal nerve
(L5, S1,2)

Sciatic nerve

Accessory obturator nerve
(L3,4)

Femoral nerve (L2, 3, 4)

Posterior femoral
cutaneous nerve
(S1, 2, 3)

Pudendal nerve (S2, 3, 4)

Obturator nerve

Posterior femoral
cutaneous nerve

Sciatic nerve

Common peroneal nerve
(L4, 5, S1, 2)

Tibial nerve (L4, 5, S1, 2, 3)

T12

Sympathetic trunk
ganglia

Lumbar plexus

L5

Sacral plexus

Coccygeal plexus

Pelvic splanchnic
nerves

Anococcygeal nerves

Perineal branch
of 4th sacral nerve

To levator ani and
coccygeus muscles
(S3, 4)

Perforating cutaneous
nerves (S2, 3)

Inferior rectal nerve

Dorsal nerve of clitoris

Posterior labial branches
of perineal nerve

Anterior division

Posterior division

UNIT 1 ■ SECTION B

A

**FIGURE 6–8 A.** This schema details the various nerves and their roots of origin, which innervate pelvic and inferior extremity structures. The divisions of the nerve trunks are color-coded and superimposed on an actual pelvis (after Netter).

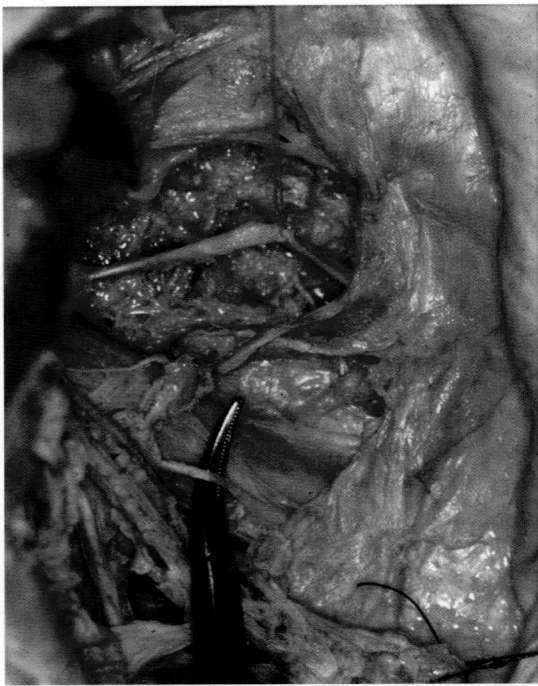

B

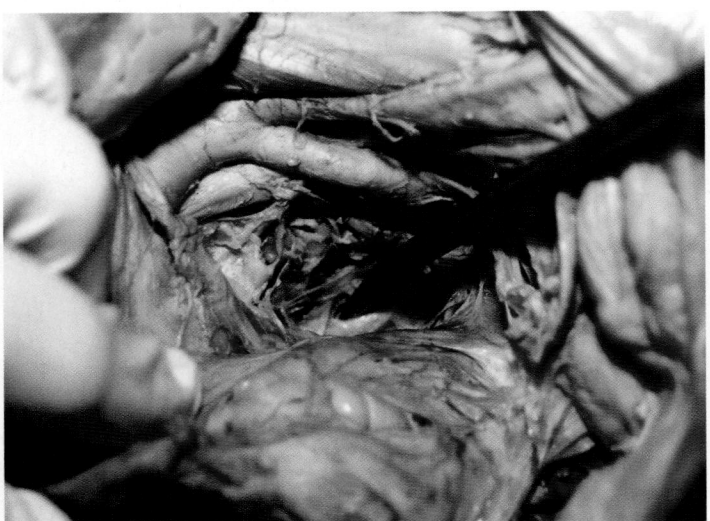

**FIGURE 6–9** This dissection follows the posterior division of the left hypogastric artery deep into the pelvis to the level of the ischial spine. The scissors points to the large white nerve trunk of the sciatic nerve. Note the surrounding "wormlike" complex of large venous structures.

**FIGURE 6–8, cont'd  B.** Actual dissection shows a tonsil clamp resting on the left psoas major muscle. The nerve that is tented up by the clamp is the genital femoral nerve. Lateral to the psoas major muscle and partially covered with fat is the iliacus muscle. The nerve crossing that muscle is the lateral femoral cutaneous nerve.

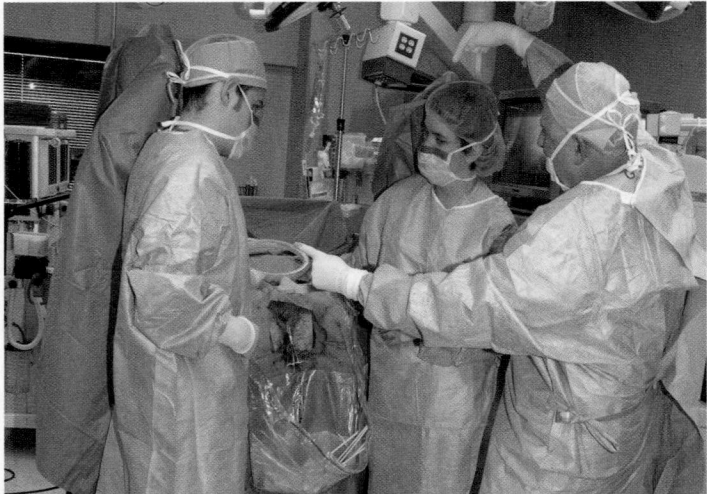

**FIGURE 6–10** The draped patient in lithotomy position may suffer nerve injury as a result of assistants leaning on the suspended inferior extremities.

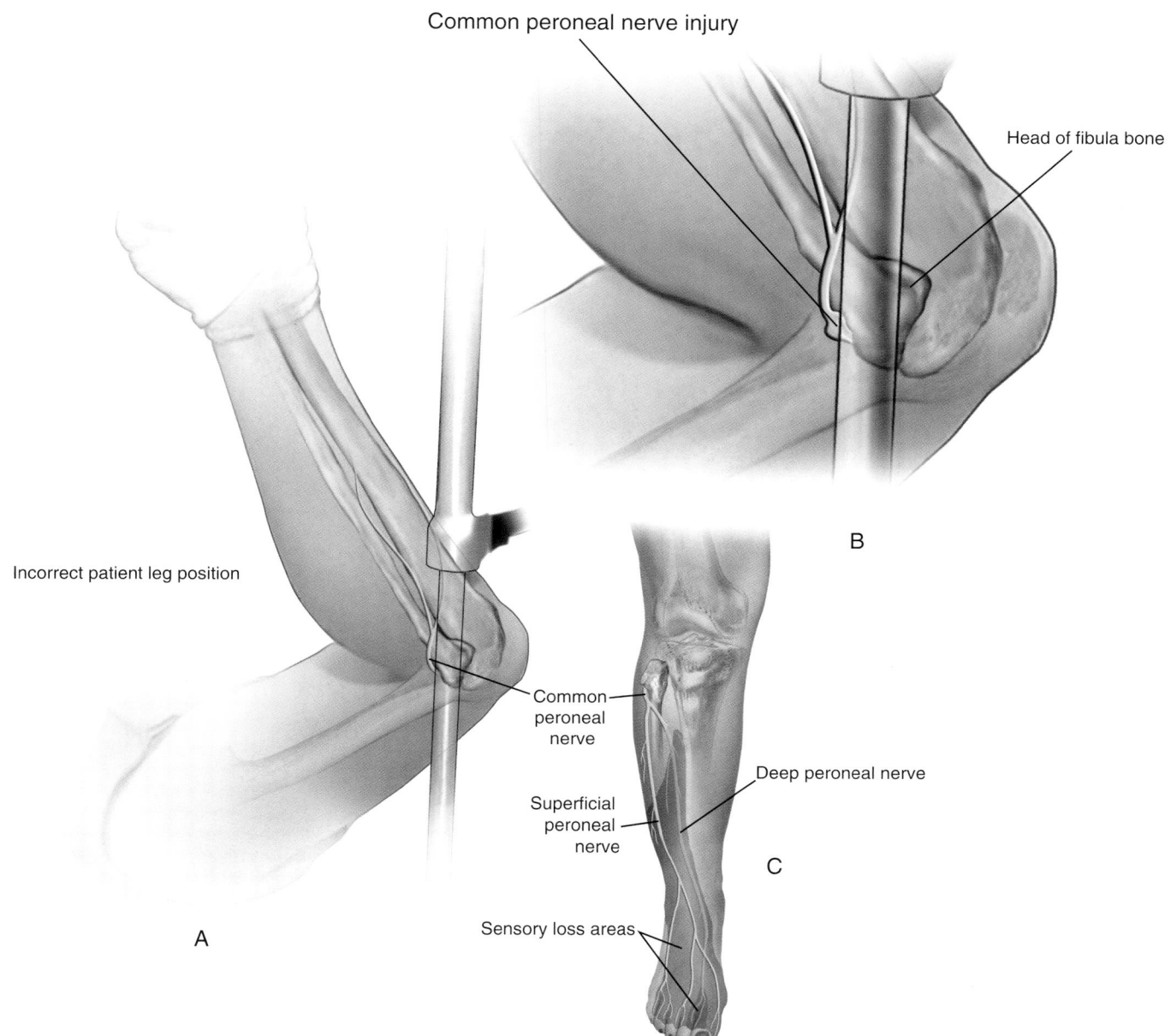

**FIGURE 6–11 A.** The peroneal division of the sciatic nerve is shown lateral to the head of the fibula. **B.** Close-up shows compression of the nerve between the fibula bone and the metal candy cane stirrup support. **C.** The neurologic deficit caused by compression injury is shown here.

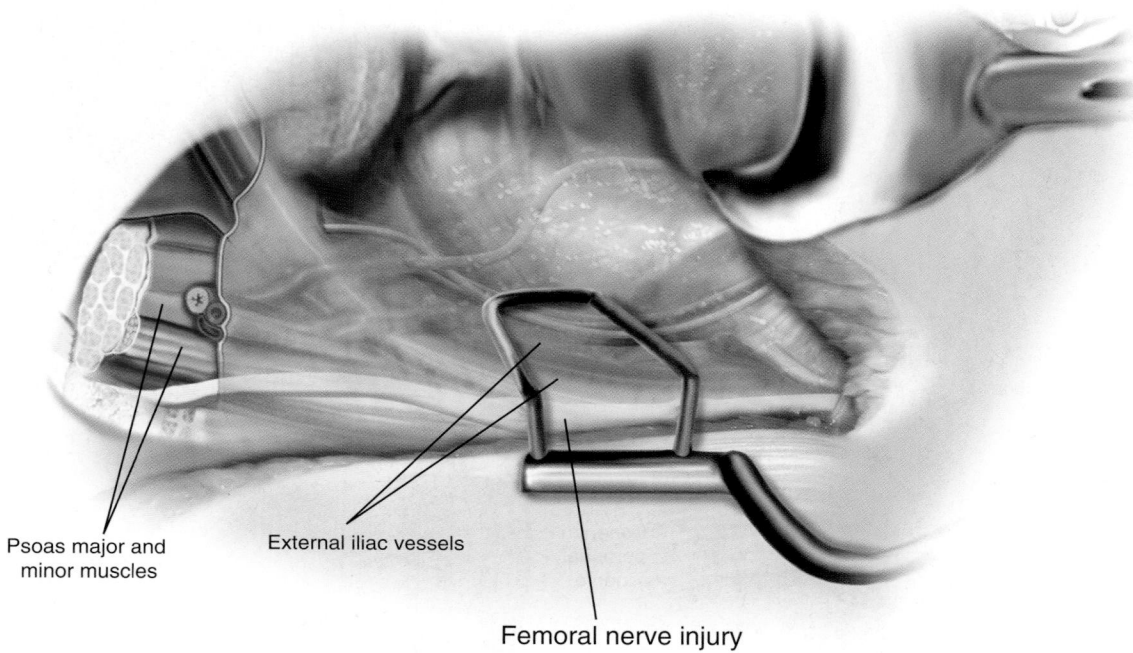

Psoas major and
minor muscles

External iliac vessels

Femoral nerve injury

**FIGURE 6–12** A common cause of postoperative femoral neuropathy is abdominal self-retaining retractor compression. Here the retractor blade compresses the psoas major muscle and the femoral nerve, which transmits within the belly of the muscle. Deep blades are particularly prone to cause femoral nerve ischemia, especially when the pressure applied is unrelieved over a long time.

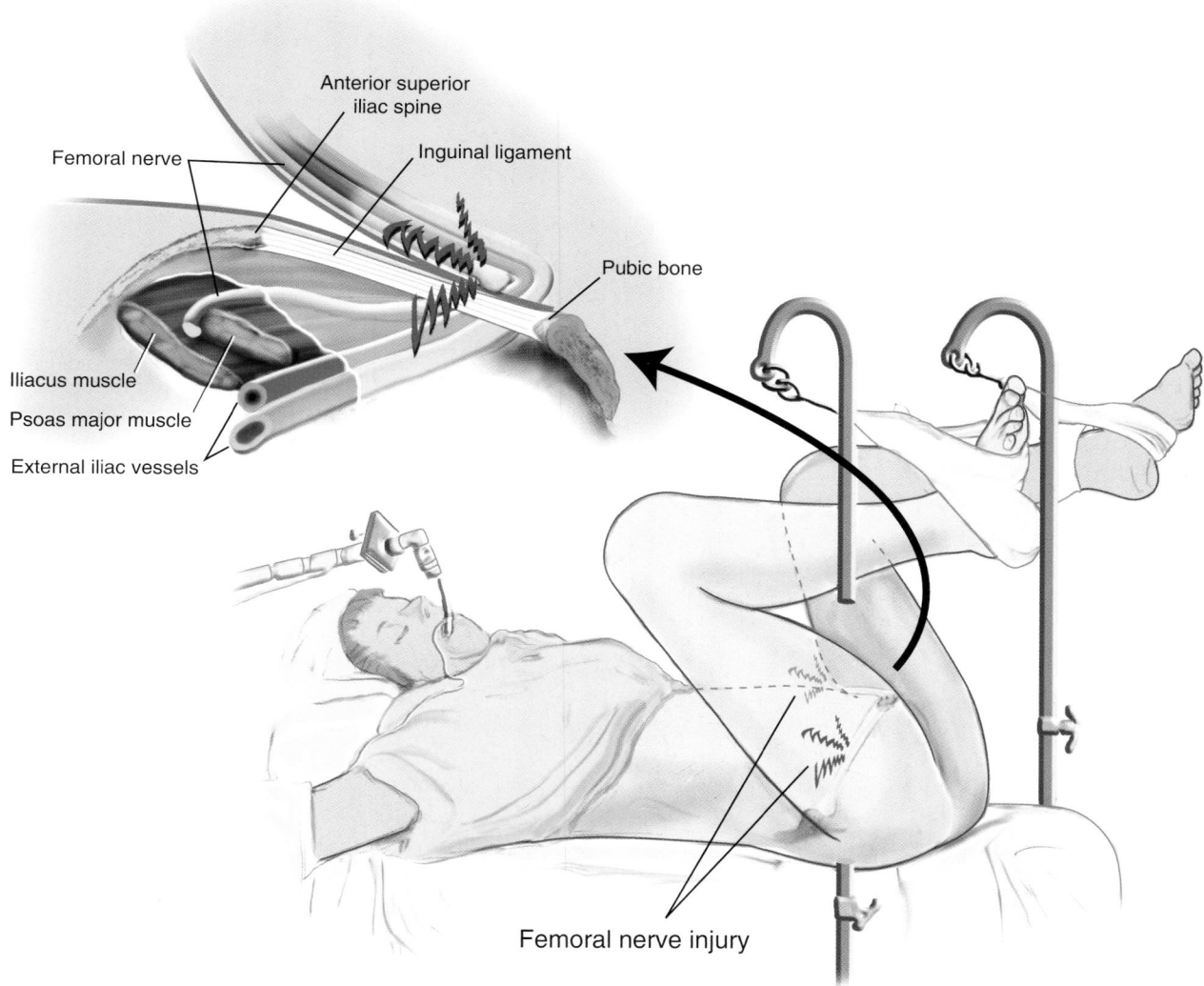

Anterior superior
iliac spine

Inguinal ligament

Femoral nerve

Pubic bone

Iliacus muscle

Psoas major muscle

External iliac vessels

Femoral nerve injury

**FIGURE 6–13** The lithotomy position associated with hyperflexion at the thigh, especially for operations lasting longer than 2 hours, places the femoral nerve at risk. In the aforesaid circumstances, the femoral nerve is compressed between the inguinal ligament and the pubic ramus. Ischemia is the result of prolonged compression.

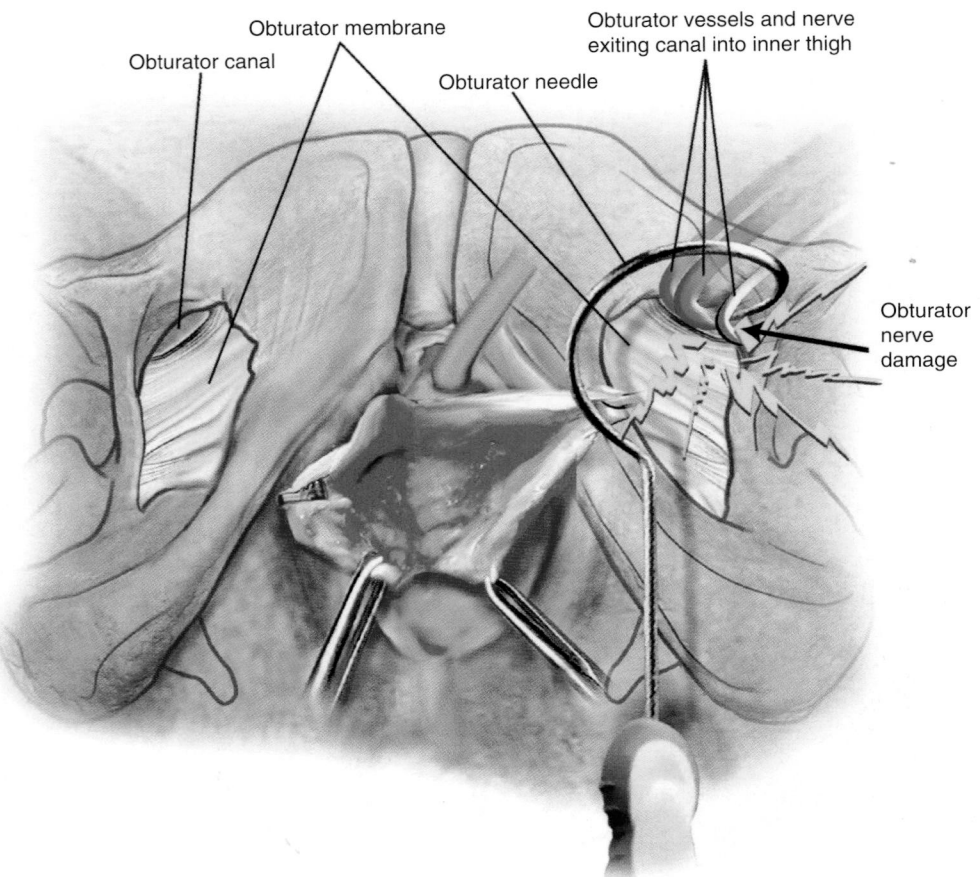

**FIGURE 6–14** The obturator nerve may sustain injury as it exits the obturator canal and enters the thigh. Here a transobturator needle is shown hooking the neurovascular bundle.

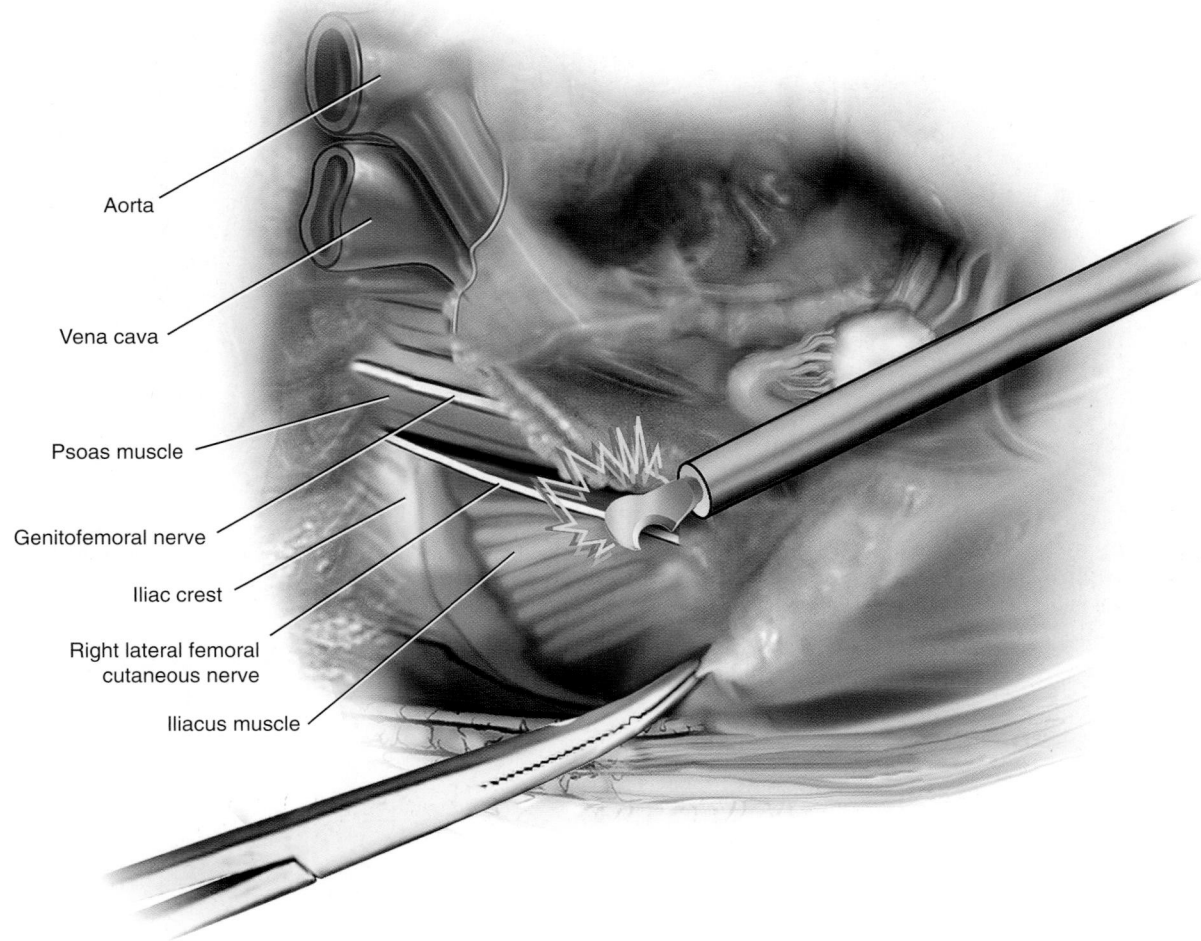

**FIGURE 6–15** Energy devices employed for adhesiolysis may cause inadvertent injury to pelvic nerves. This illustration demonstrates a cutting device (harmonic scalpel) incising peritoneal attachments lateral to the psoas major muscle and cutting the lateral femoral cutaneous nerve.

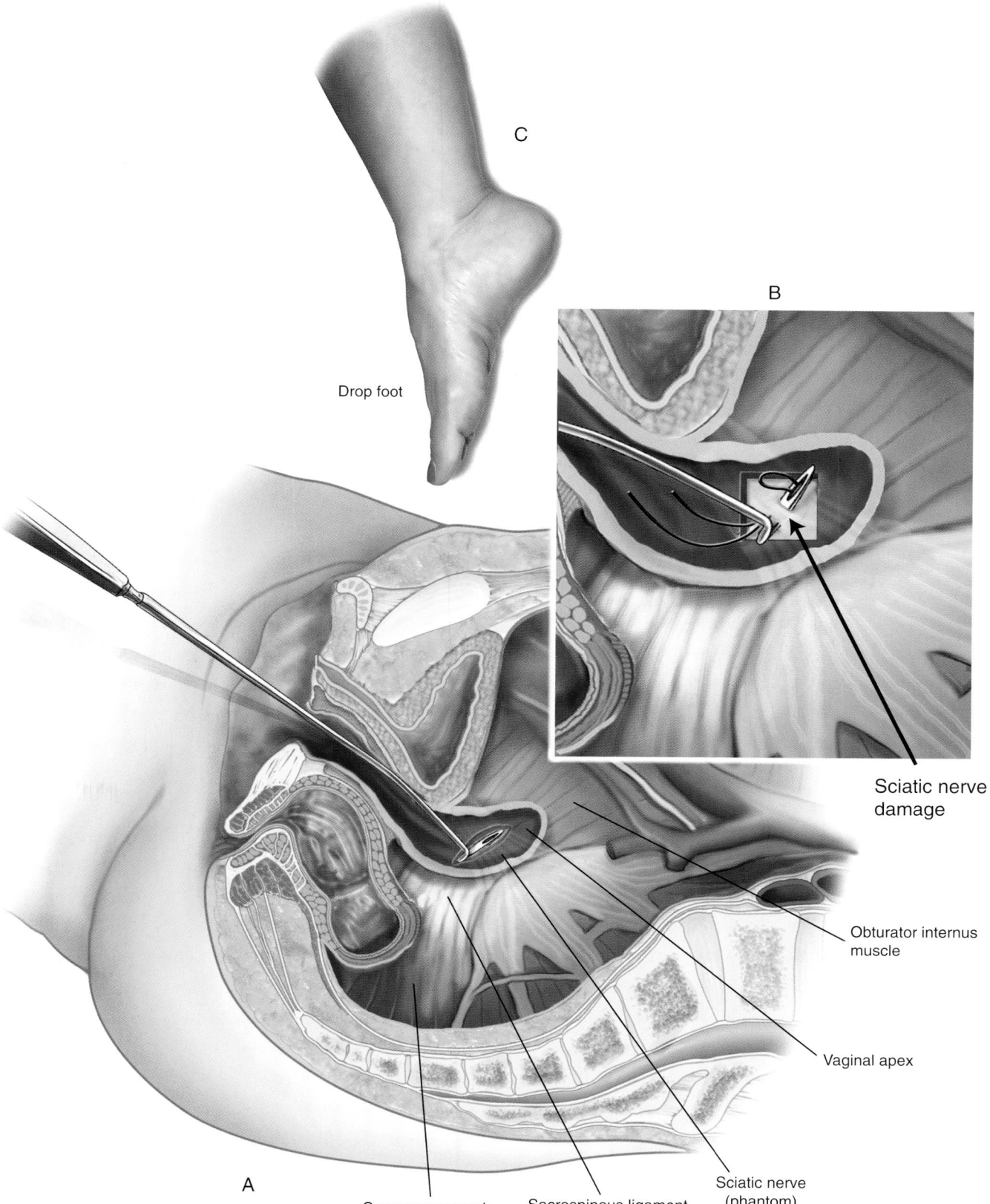

C

Drop foot

B

Sciatic nerve
damage

Obturator internus
muscle

Vaginal apex

A

Coccygeus muscle    Sacrospinous ligament    Sciatic nerve
(phantom)

**FIGURE 6–16** Transvaginal sacrospinous colpopexy may result in suture injury to the sciatic nerve or to one of the sacral nerve roots. Severe buttock pain and/or foot-drop should alert the gynecologist to rule out sciatic neuropraxia.

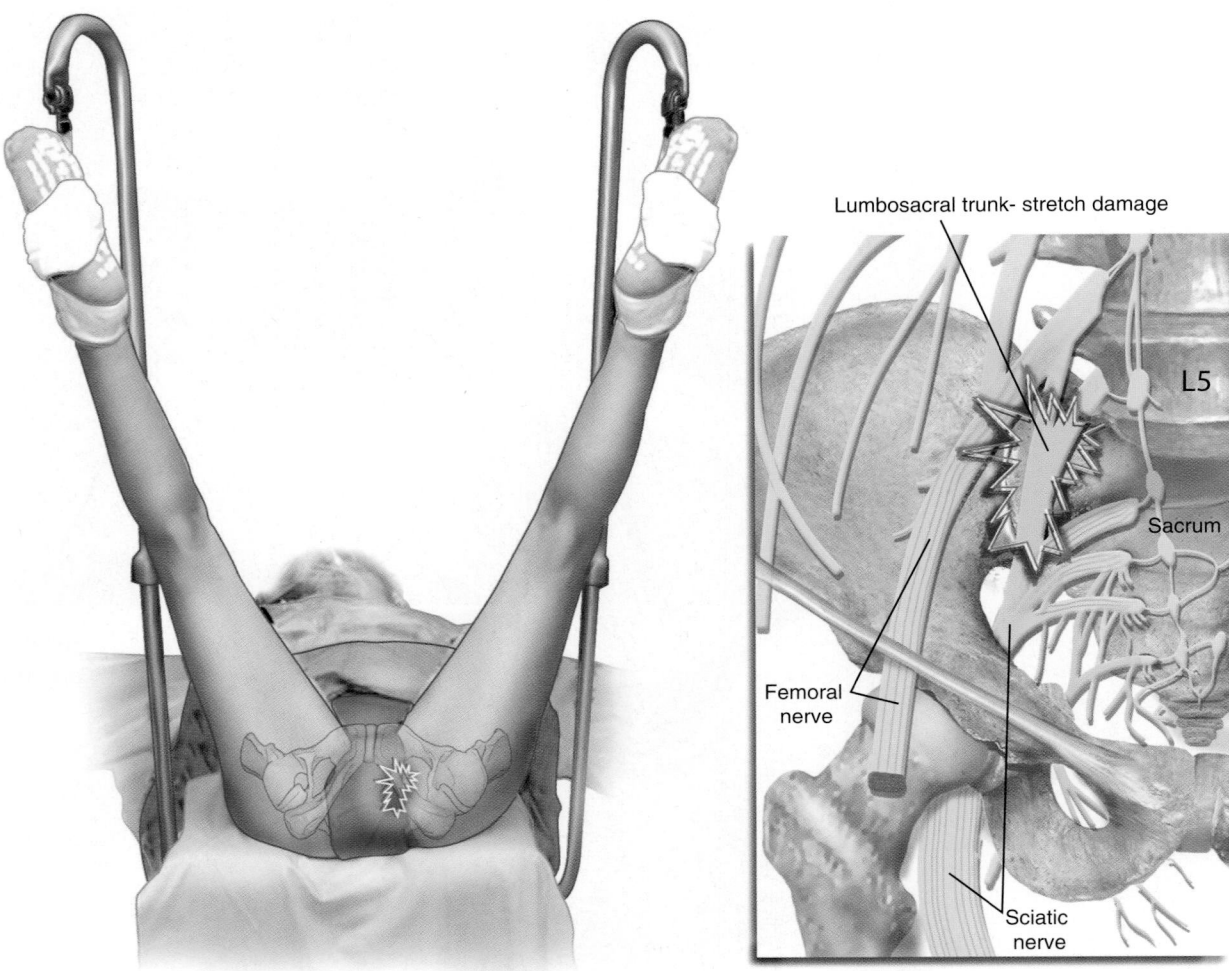

Patient leg position—stretch injury

**FIGURE 6–17** Extended inferior extremities in the lithotomy position can create a stretch injury to the lumbosacral trunk. The patient will exhibit a combination of lumbar and sacral distribution symptoms.

## Compartment Syndrome

Compartment syndrome affecting the extremities is a particularly disabling condition that occurs when the lithotomy position is combined with **leg support,** producing **calf compression** or **ankle dorsiflexion. Impaired circulation** to the inferior extremities (most frequently caused by hypovolemia and hypotension) is another key instigating factor. The Trendelenburg position creates additive risk for the development of vascular compromise. Postoperative patients who develop inordinate pain, hyperesthesia, and/or paresis in the legs and feet should trigger the gynecologist to include compartment syndrome high up in differential diagnosis considerations. Tense shins and calves are created by increased intracompartmental pressure (Fig. 6–18).

Compartment syndrome may be associated with pelvic vascular injury (e.g., during laparoscopic surgery, following postpartum hemorrhage), traumatic injury (e.g., fracture of leg/thigh bones), hematomas, cellulitis, vascular thrombosis, necrotizing fasciitis, prolonged lithotomy position, and compression stockings. Dorsiflexion at the ankle joint significantly increases compartment pressure.

The pathophysiology of compartment syndrome is related to increasing volume and increasing pressure within unyielding fascial compartments (i.e., limited anatomic spaces). The initiating factor is **diminished blood flow** to contents within the compartment, thereby creating **muscle ischemia.** The ischemia in turn increases vascular resistance and further decreases blood flow to the muscles. As a result of continuing ischemia, hemorrhage and edema are additive to **intrafascial pressure.** The aforesaid happens because of sievelike leakage from venules within the compartment. When the extremities are lowered from lithotomy to supine position, improved flow is established at heart level. The (initiating) hypovolemia, once ameliorated, will result in **reperfusion** of the extremity. If vascular permeability persists, then further leakage and edema into the fascial space will continue, resulting in still greater intrafascial pres-sure. Tissue pressure in the compartments ranges on average from 4 to 10 mm Hg but should not exceed 20 mm Hg. **Fasciotomy** should be performed for pressures of 30 to 40 mm Hg. Neglected compartment syndrome can lead to extensive muscle necrosis, nerve injury, myoglobinemia, cardiac arrhythmia, and myoglobinuric renal damage.

**Abdominal compartment syndrome** may be defined as a condition that arises from elevated intra-abdominal pressure, leading to visceral injury, as well as to renal, cardiac, and respiratory dysfunction. The abdominal cavity is essentially a closed space, containing viscera and encircled by muscular walls. Acute increases in volume within the abdominal cavity can translate to increases in intra-abdominal pressure. Although normal intra-abdominal pressure ranges from 3 to 10 mm Hg, pressures greater than 25 mm Hg require timely treatment. Gynecologic conditions associated with risk of abdominal compartment syndrome include massive hemorrhage, large hematoma formation, peritonitis and sepsis, intestinal perforation, uterine/ovarian tumors, ascites, and abdominal or tubal pregnancy (Fig. 6–19).

The pathophysiologic ramifications of abdominal compartment syndrome include decreased venous return to the heart with decreased cardiac output, renal dysfunction caused by compression of renal veins, and hepatic abnormality related to pressure on the portal circulation. Intestinal ischemia will eventuate and progress to bowel necrosis because of reduced visceral blood flow and thrombosis (Fig. 6–20). Respiratory function may be compromised as the result of elevation of the diaphragm and transmission of higher intrathoracic pressure, causing reduced lung capacity.

Intra-abdominal pressure may be conveniently measured by placing 100 mL of water into the bladder via a Foley catheter, then connecting the catheter via tubing to a pressure transducer.

The management of abdominal compartment syndrome requires performing laparotomy to reduce pressure and treating the inciting cause(s).

UNIT 1 ■ SECTION B

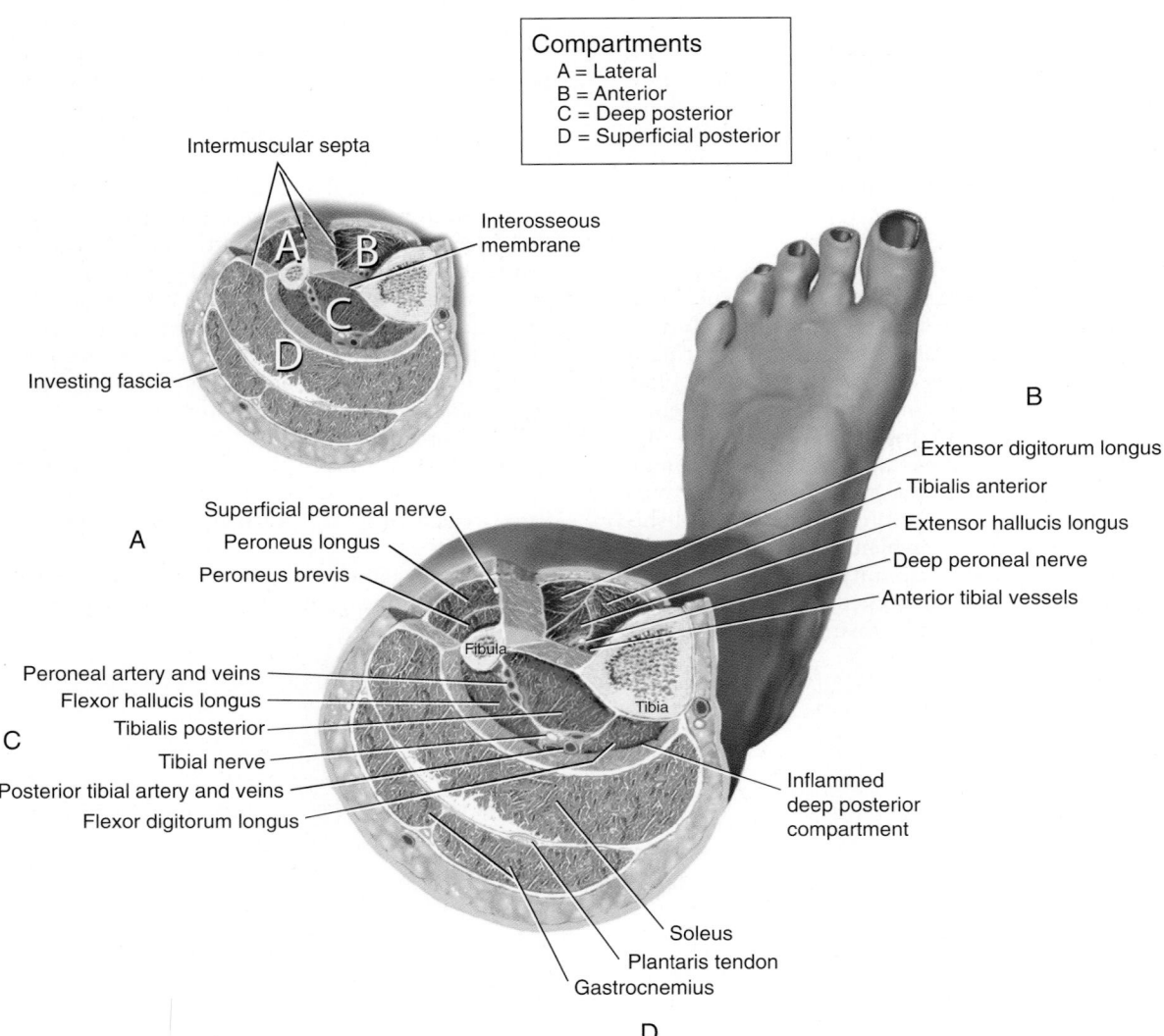

Compartments
A = Lateral
B = Anterior
C = Deep posterior
D = Superficial posterior

Intermuscular septa

Interosseous membrane

Investing fascia

B

Extensor digitorum longus

Tibialis anterior

Extensor hallucis longus

Deep peroneal nerve

Anterior tibial vessels

A

Superficial peroneal nerve
Peroneus longus
Peroneus brevis

Fibula

Peroneal artery and veins
Flexor hallucis longus
Tibialis posterior
Tibial nerve
Posterior tibial artery and veins
Flexor digitorum longus

C

Tibia

Inflammed deep posterior compartment

Soleus
Plantaris tendon
Gastrocnemius

D

**FIGURE 6–18** Cut-away of the leg illustrates the tight fascial compartments bounded by the leg bones and the fascial sheaths. The three compartments are lateral, anterior, and posterior.

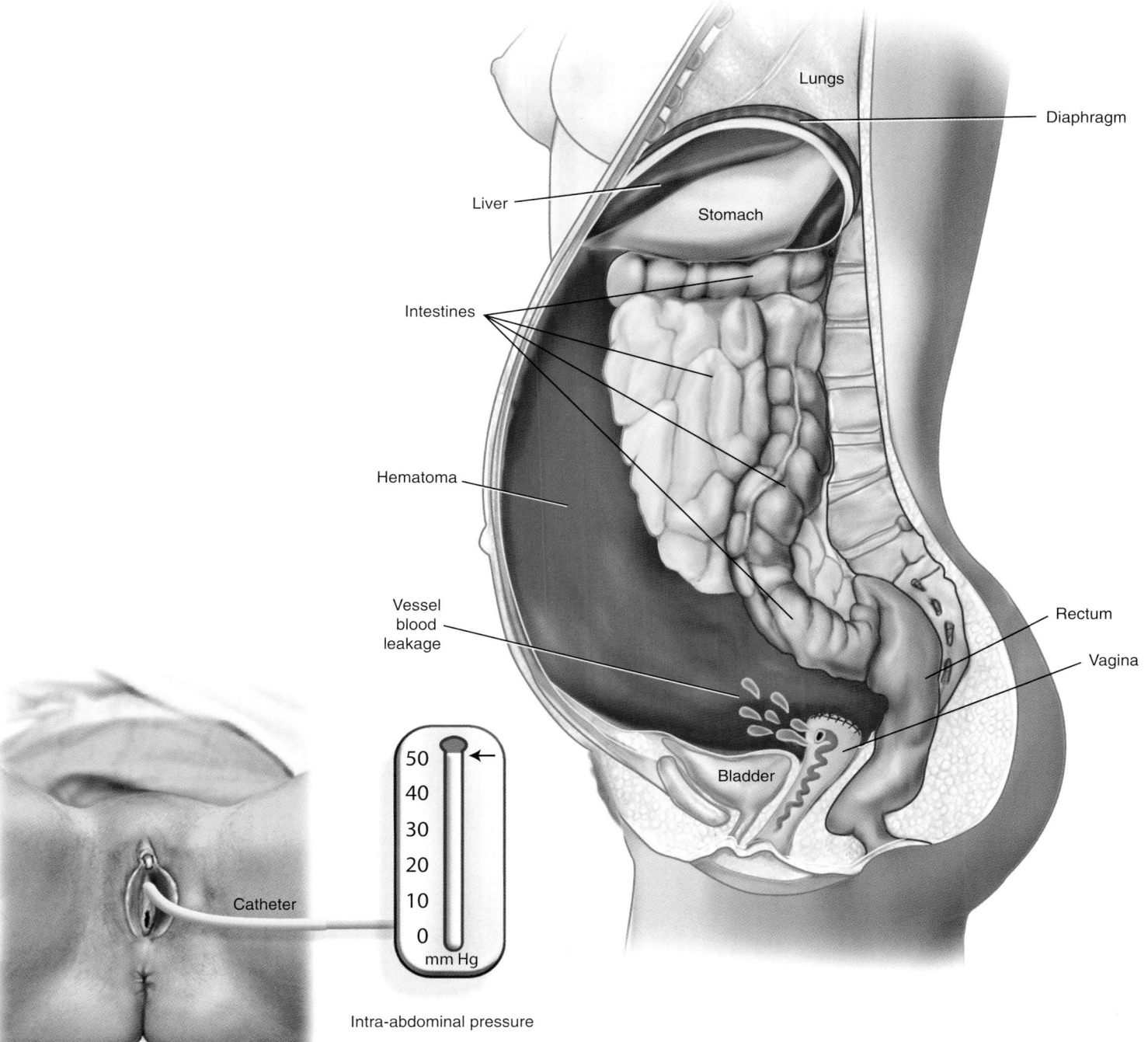

**FIGURE 6–19** This picture illustrates the formation of a large intra-abdominal hematoma. In this case, the hematoma occurred as the result of a leaking blood vessel, which had not been secured during a hysterectomy. Abdominal compartment syndrome is a possible sequel of the increased intra-abdominal pressure created by the large accumulation of blood within closed space. Intra-abdominal pressure measurements can be obtained by placing a catheter into the bladder and attaching it to a pressure transducer. Pressures greater than 25 mm Hg are diagnostic of significant abdominal compartment syndrome.

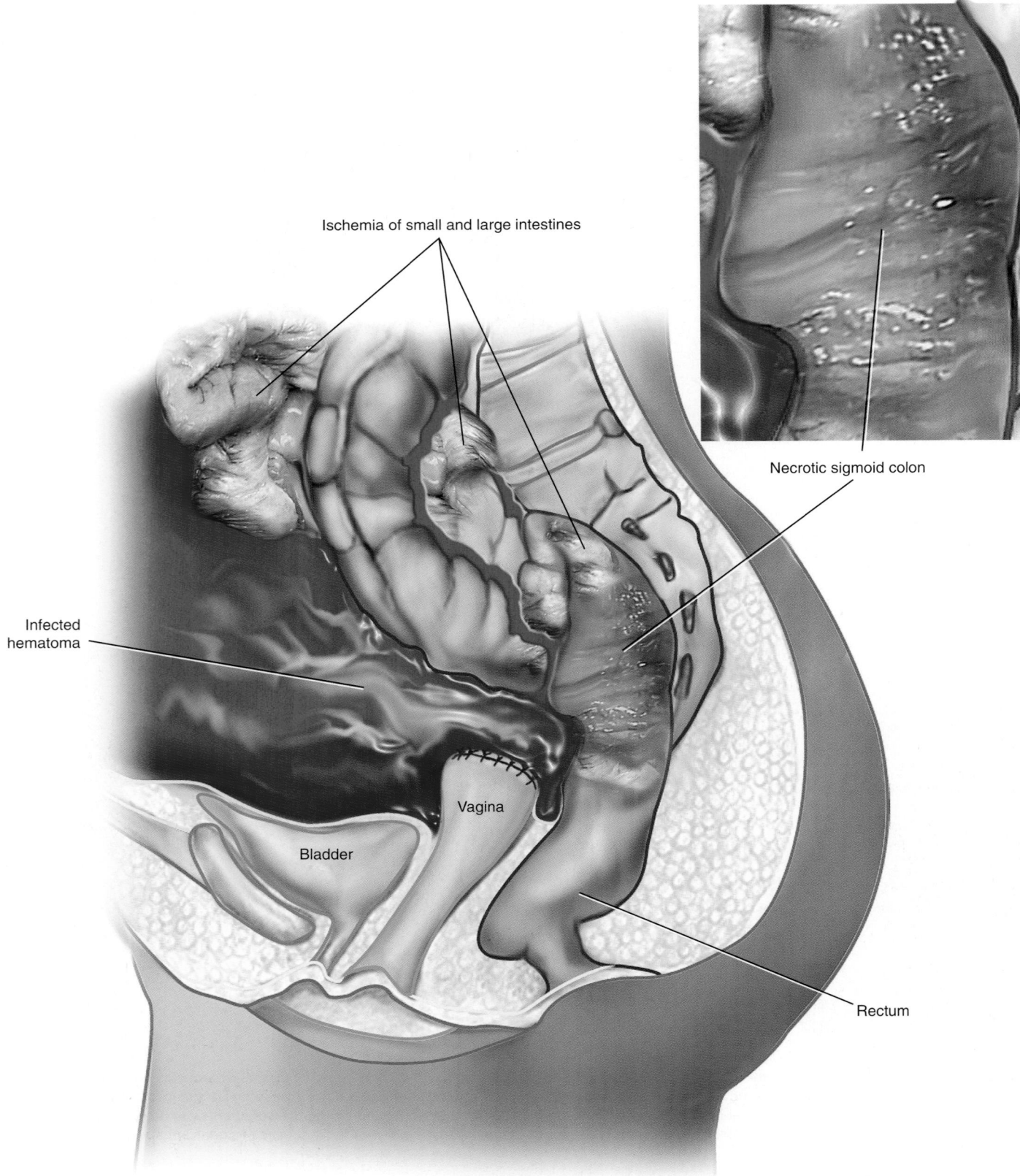

Ischemia of small and large intestines

Necrotic sigmoid colon

Infected hematoma

Vagina

Bladder

Rectum

**FIGURE 6–20** As a result of abdominal compartment syndrome, capillary and small vessel circulation to visceral structures is compromised. This drawing shows the results of prolonged increases in intra-abdominal pressure. The sigmoid colon is necrotic. Additional areas of the small and large intestines show signs of ischemia. The **inset** details the diffusion of coliform bacteria throughout the necrotic large bowel wall, causing infection of the hematoma.

# Abdominal Surgery

# Anterior Abdominal Wall

# CHAPTER 7

# Anatomy of the Lower Abdominal Wall

*Michael S. Baggish*

The pelvic surgeon is mainly involved with the abdomen below or at the level of the umbilicus. The abdominal wall below the level of the umbilicus consists of skin, fat, fascia, and several relatively thin muscles.

Specific skin and bony landmarks should be noted (e.g., the umbilicus roughly overlies the bifurcation of the aorta) (Fig. 7–1). The anterior superior iliac spine marks the origin of the inguinal ligament and of the sartorius muscle. The upper surfaces of the pubic bone and symphysis mark the terminus of the inguinal ligament and the insertion of the rectus abdominis muscle (Fig. 7–2).

The cadaver is typically in the supine position (see Fig. 7–1). The abdominal wall from superficial to deep consists of skin, subcutaneous fat, fascia, muscle, properitoneal fat, and peritoneum. Once the skin and fat are dissected away, the gray-white glistening fascia comes into view (see Fig. 7–2). This is the superficial investment layer of the underlying muscle (Fig. 7–3). When all layers have been traversed, the peritoneal cavity is entered. The peritoneum of the anterior wall is called the *parietal peritoneum*, and the peritoneum investing the viscera is known as the *visceral peritoneum*. The large and small intestines are directly beneath the parietal peritoneum of the anterior abdominal wall (Fig. 7–4).

The strength of the otherwise thin layer of muscle and fascia derives from the crisscrossing of various muscle fibers. The external oblique muscles are vectored downward (caudally) and medially. The rectus muscles run straight up and down (vertically) from the xiphoid to the symphysis pubis (Figs. 7–5 and 7–6). It is interesting to note that the tough fascial sheath of the rectus muscles is formed by contributions of other muscles of the anterior abdominal wall (i.e., the external oblique, internal oblique, and transversus abdominis muscles [Fig. 7–7]).

At the point where the two rectus muscles join in the midline, a white line, aptly called the *linea alba*, is visible (see Fig. 7–5B).

The fibers of the internal oblique muscle cross those of the external oblique. Similarly, the transversus abdominis muscle crosses both the internal and external oblique muscles as it vectors in an almost horizontal direction. Throughout, the posterior rectus sheath contains transversalis fascia (Fig. 7–8).

The inguinal ligament and canal are seen in the lowest portion of the abdomen. Actually, the ligament is an anatomic boundary between the abdomen and the thigh (Figs. 7–9A–C and 7–10). As the external iliac vessels cross between the pubic ramus and the inguinal ligament, they become the femoral artery and vein. The inguinal ligament and the sartorius muscle of the thigh originate at the anterior superior iliac spine (Fig. 7–11A). The length of the inguinal ligament may be accurately estimated by placing one finger on the iliac spine and another finger on the pubic tubercle (Fig. 7–11B) and measuring the distance between these fingers. The internal inguinal ring is the point of entry (into the inguinal canal) for intra-abdominal structures, such as the round ligament. They exit the canal onto the abdominal wall via the superficial inguinal ring (Fig. 7–12A–E).

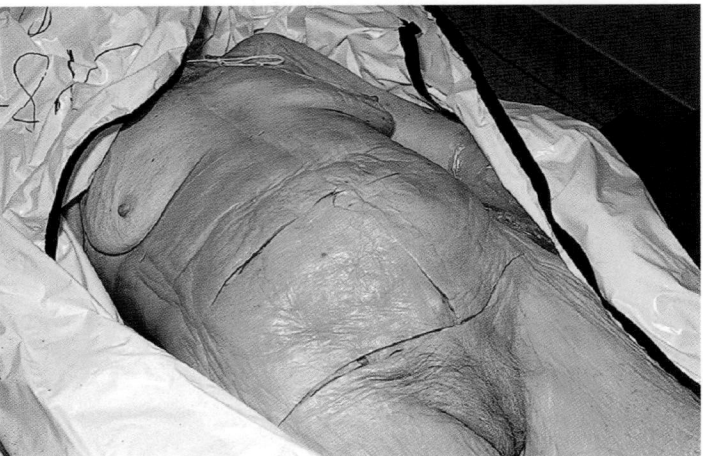

**FIGURE 7–1** Important skin surface landmarks include the umbilicus, the anterior superior iliac spines, the pubic symphysis, and the xiphoid process.

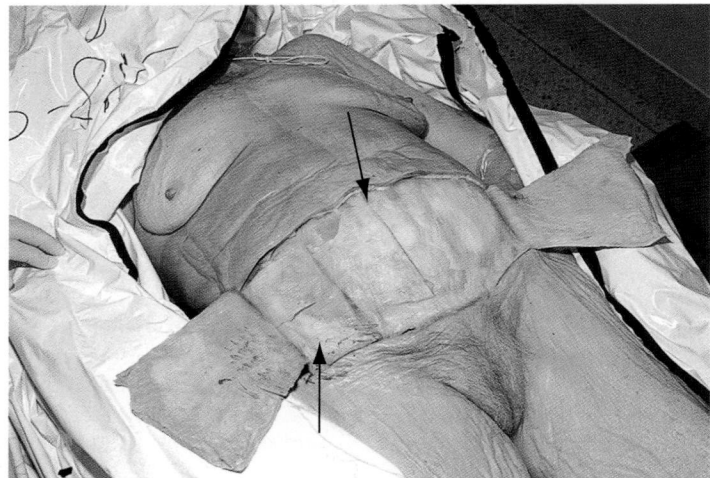

**FIGURE 7–2** After the lower abdominal flaps have been retracted, the gray-white fascia (aponeurosis) of the external oblique and rectus abdominis muscles is in clear view. The arrows indicate surface landmarks (umbilicus [*upper arrow*], anterior superior iliac spine [*lower arrow*], and upper margin of the pubic symphysis).

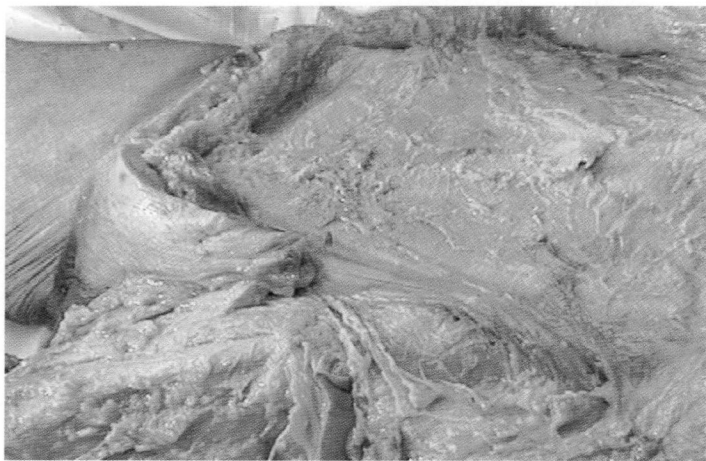

**FIGURE 7–3** Skin and fat have been retracted except for the area of the mons. The fascia of the external oblique and rectus abdominis is intact.

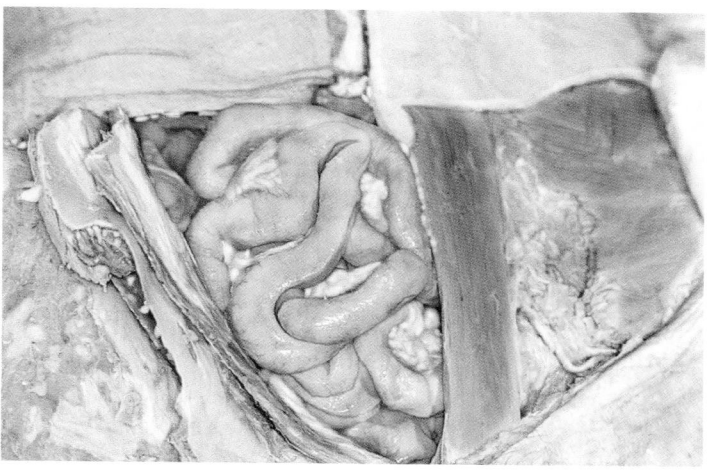

**FIGURE 7–4** The peritoneal cavity has been entered. The small and large intestines occupy the entire space within the lower abdomen. They constitute the most superficial viscus encountered in the abdominal cavity.

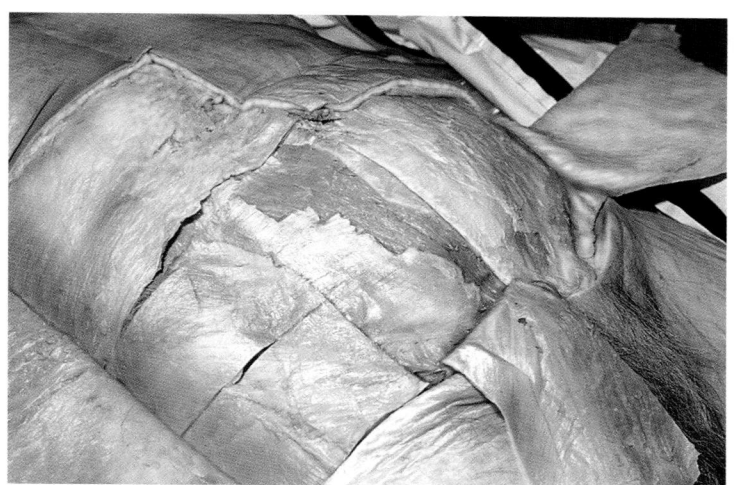

A

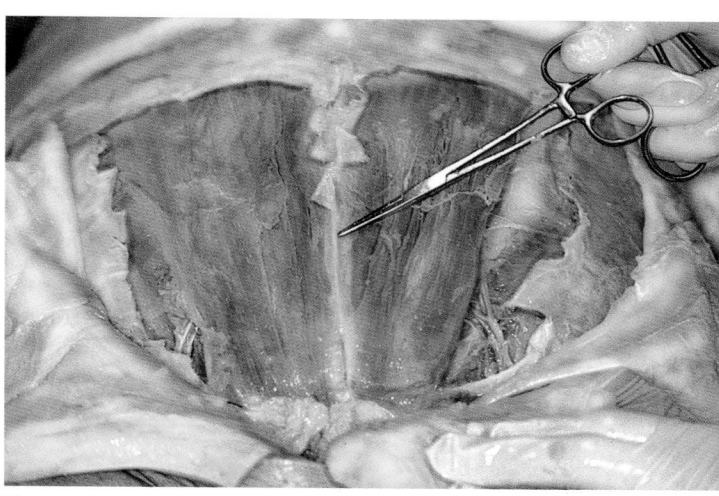

B

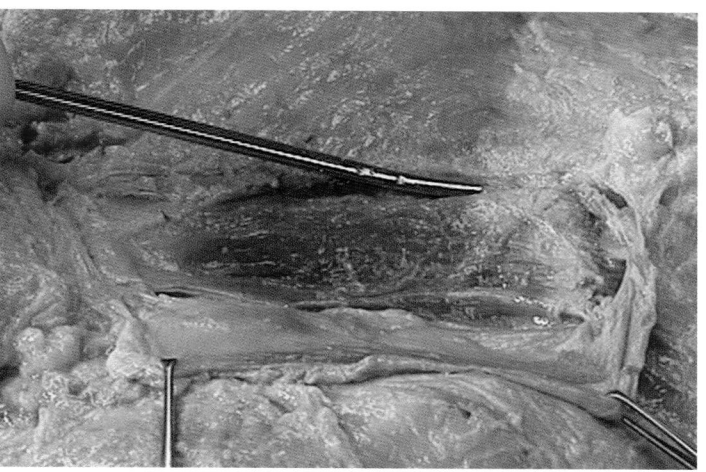

C

**FIGURE 7–5 A.** The anterior portion of the rectus abdominis muscle sheath has been incised and retracted, exposing the vertical fibers of the muscle. **B.** It is clear from this photograph how the name of the linea alba originated. **C.** The scissors point to the diastasis recti.

UNIT 2 ■ SECTION A

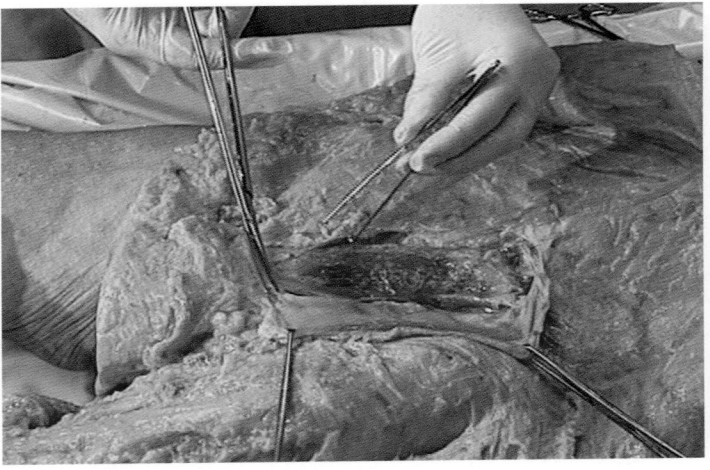
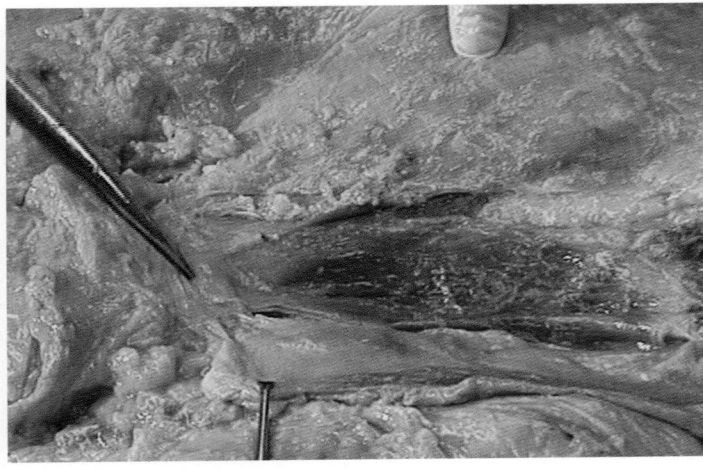

A

B

**FIGURE 7–6  A.** The left rectus abdominis muscle has been exposed. **B.** Enlarged view of the left rectus abdominis muscle. The scissors point to the pubic tubercle.

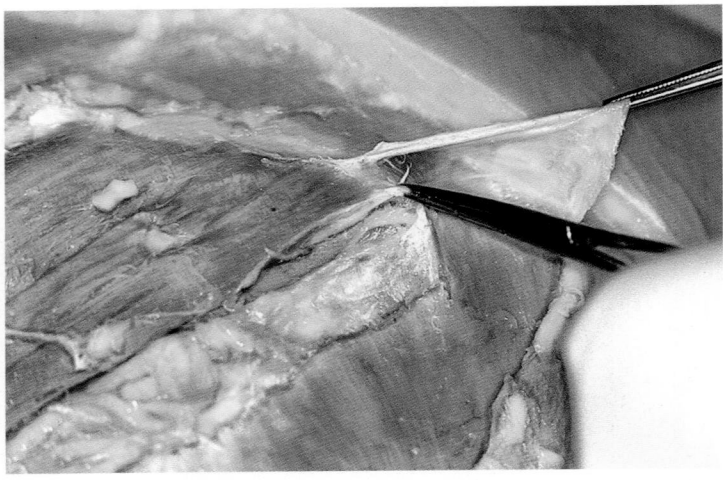

A

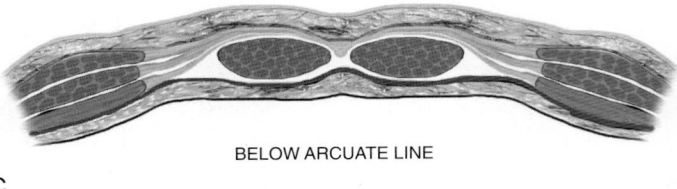

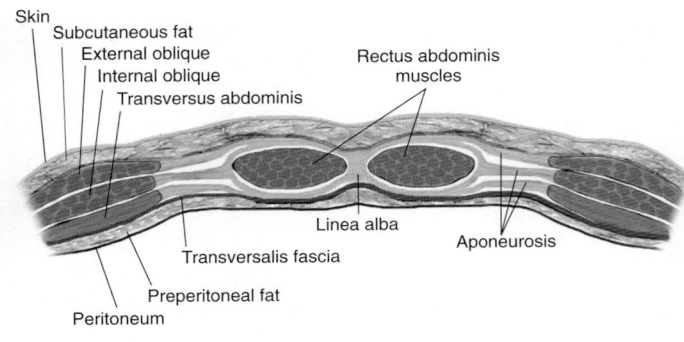

Skin
Subcutaneous fat
External oblique
Internal oblique
Transversus abdominis
Rectus abdominis muscles
Linea alba
Aponeurosis
Transversalis fascia
Preperitoneal fat
Peritoneum

ABOVE ARCUATE LINE

BELOW ARCUATE LINE

C

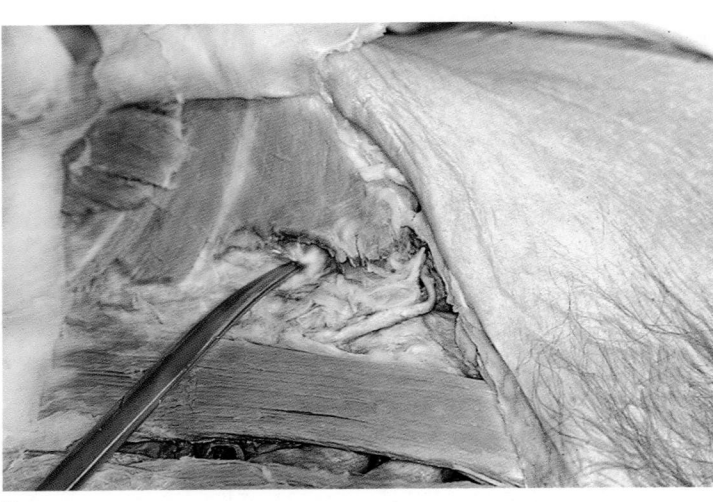

B

**FIGURE 7–7  A.** The external oblique muscle has been retracted. Part of the rectus sheath has been removed (*left-center*), exposing the rectus muscles. The contribution of the internal oblique fascia to the rectus sheath is demonstrated (*clamps*). **B.** The tip of the clamp rests on the fascia of the transversus abdominis muscle (transversalis fascia), which in turn constitutes the posterior rectus sheath. **C.** Cross-sectional drawings of the anterior abdominal wall show the formation of the rectus sheath above and below the arcuate line (one-third the distance from the umbilicus to the symphysis pubis). Note that below the line, the anterior sheath receives components from the external and internal oblique muscles and the transversus. The posterior sheath is thin and consists only of transversalis fascia.

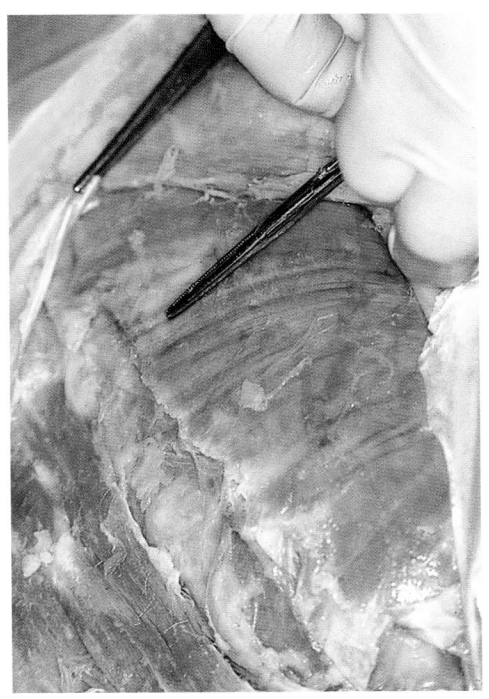

**FIGURE 7–8**  The transversus muscle fibers are directed straight (horizontally) across the abdomen rather than obliquely.

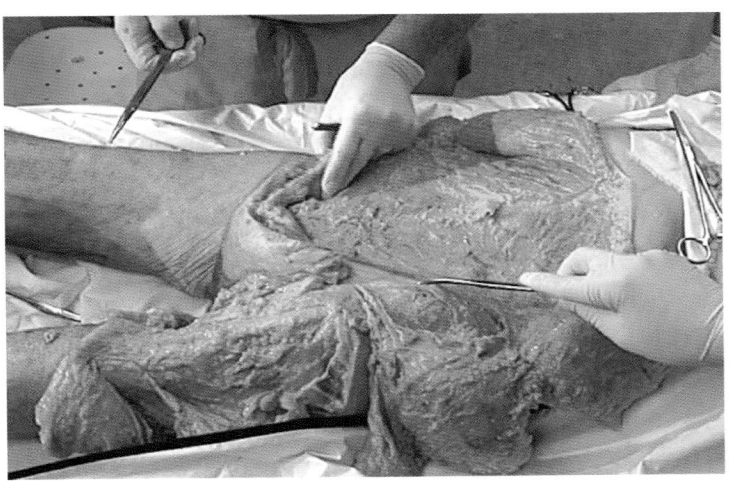

A

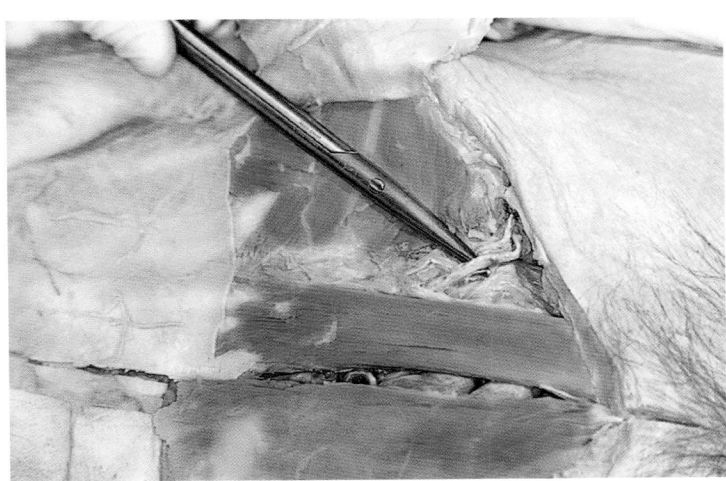

B

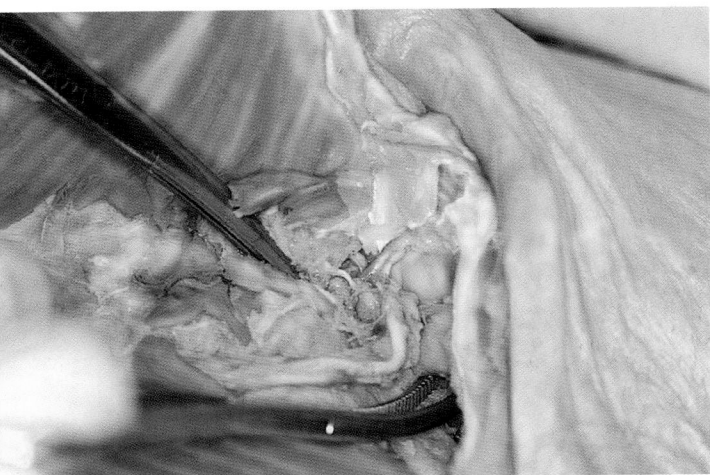

C

**FIGURE 7–9  A.** The scissors tip points to the left anterior superior iliac spine. The dissector's hand is placed in the crural area beneath the inguinal ligament on the right. **B.** The scissors tip is beneath the left inferior epigastric vessels. These vessels originate from the external iliac vessels at a point immediately cranial to their passage beneath the inguinal ligament. **C.** The lower (opened) clamp lies on the transversalis fascia and under the left external iliac vein as it crosses beneath the inguinal ligament.

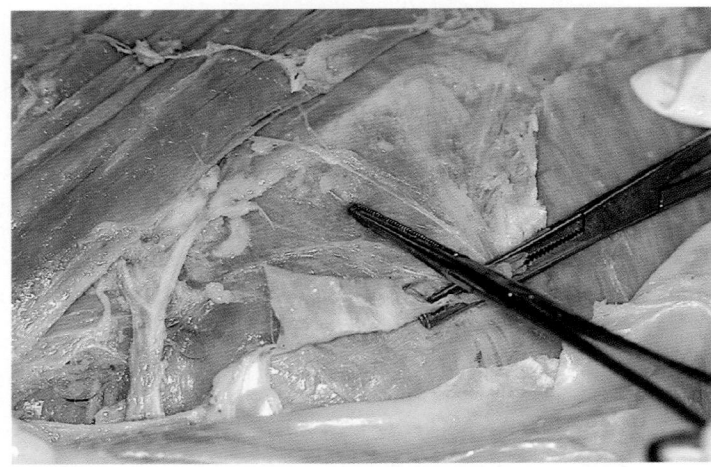

**FIGURE 7–10** The clamp points to the transversus muscle.

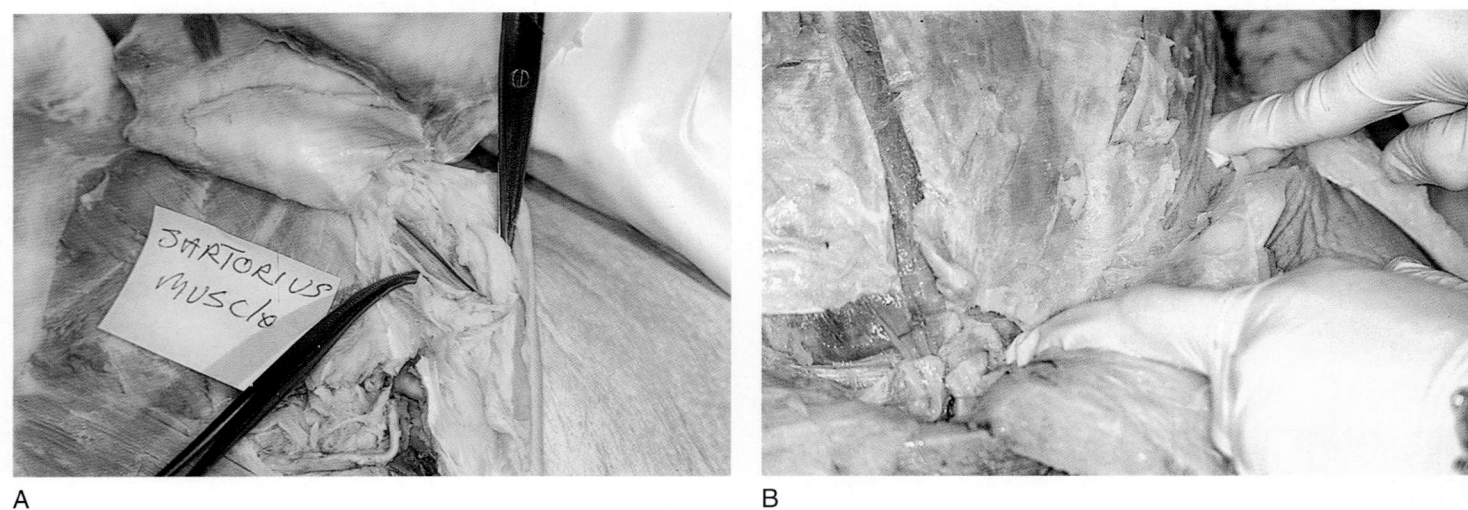

A

B

**FIGURE 7–11  A.** The curved clamp points to the sartorius muscle. This muscle has a common origin with the inguinal ligament from the anterior superior iliac spine and forms the lateral margin of the femoral triangle (in the thigh). **B.** The course of the inguinal ligament is marked by the surgeon's fingers. Note the intact but dissected rectus sheath.

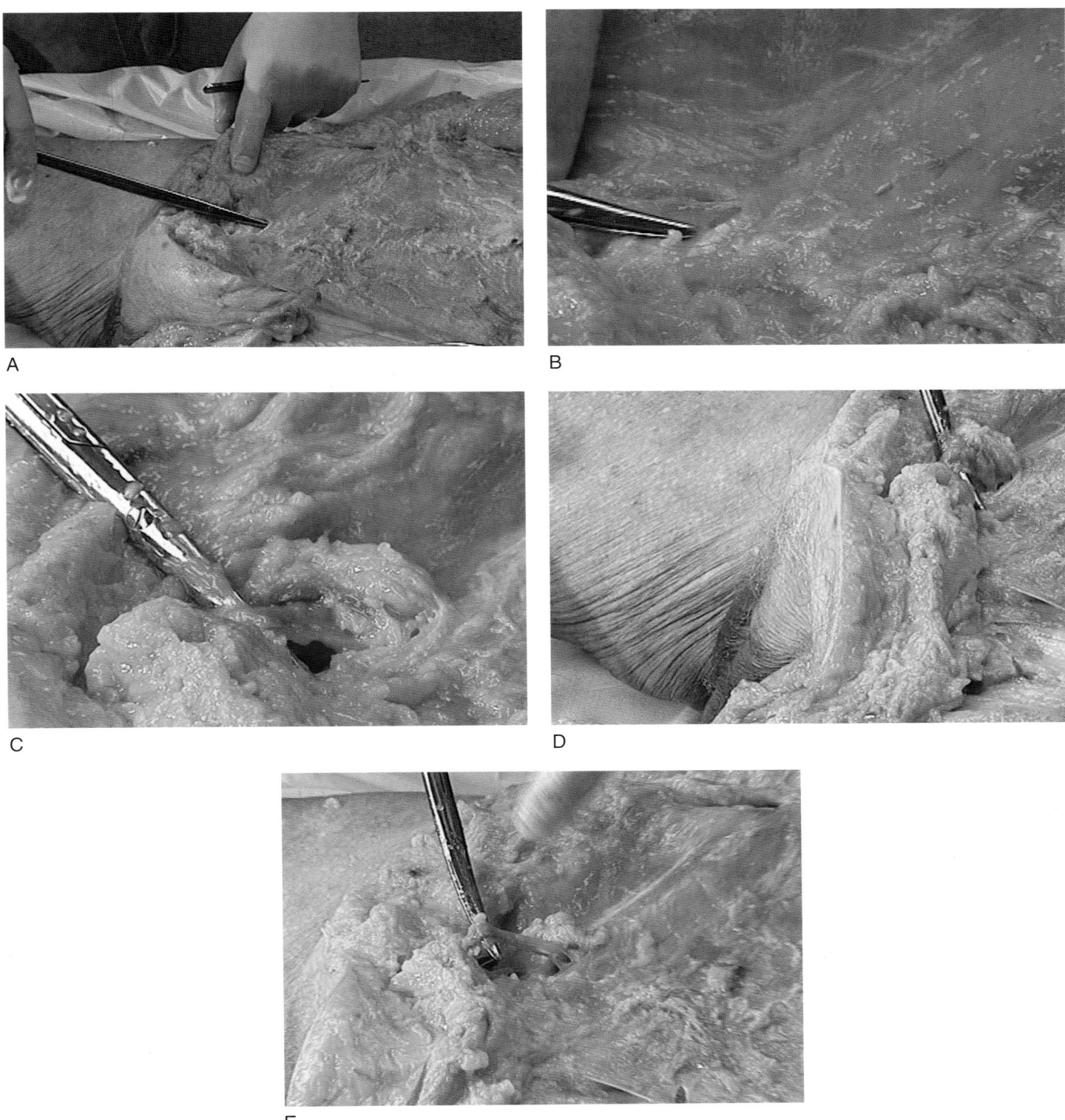

A

B

C

D

E

**FIGURE 7–12** **A.** The scissors tip is placed into the right superficial inguinal ring. **B.** Magnified view of the superficial inguinal ring. Note the inguinal ligament, which is a deeper pink color. **C.** The round ligament (*above scissors*) emerges from the superficial inguinal ring. **D.** The round ligament descends into the fat of the mons, then into the fat of the labium majus. **E.** The ilioinguinal nerve also exits via the superficial inguinal ring. Note the white-pink inguinal ligament in the background.

## Vessels

The inferior epigastric vessels take their origin from the external iliac vessels at a point cranial to the inguinal ligament. The inferior epigastric vessels pierce the transversalis fascia and run across the transversus muscle to enter a space between the rectus muscle and the posterior sheath (Fig. 7–13). The external oblique is reflected laterally to demonstrate the inferior epigastric vessels, ascending cranially at the lateral margin of the left rectus abdominis muscle. The left inferior epigastric vessels are shown crossing the abdominal wall toward the edge of the left rectus abdominis muscle (Fig. 7–14). Hesselbach's triangle, which is formed by the inguinal ligament, the inferior epigastric, and the lower lateral margin on the rectus muscle, is shown in Figure 7–15. The inferior epigastric artery can be traced to the external iliac artery and crosses over the external iliac vein (Fig. 7–16A, B). The external iliac vessels cross into the thigh under the inguinal ligament. The femoral canal and Cloquet's lymph node lie just medial to the external iliac vein (Fig. 7–17A–E). The superior pubic ramus and the lateral portion of the iliopectineal line and ligament (Cooper's ligament) are in close proximity to the iliac and inferior epigastric arteries. Figure 7–18 illustrates the typical course of the inferior epigastric vessels relative to lower abdominal landmarks. Figure 7–19 details the cadaver dissection data that were used to compile the quantitative aspects of Figure 7–18. Two fingers were placed above the upper margin of the symphysis pubis. The ruler indicates that the distance from midline to the inferior epigastric vessels is 6 to 7 cm.

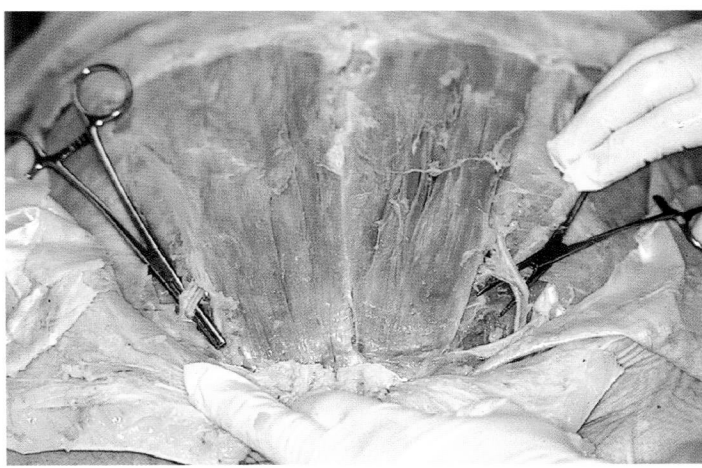

FIGURE 7–13  The inferior epigastric vessels run from lateral to medial and ascend between the lateral margin of the rectus muscle and the posterior sheath (transversus fascia).

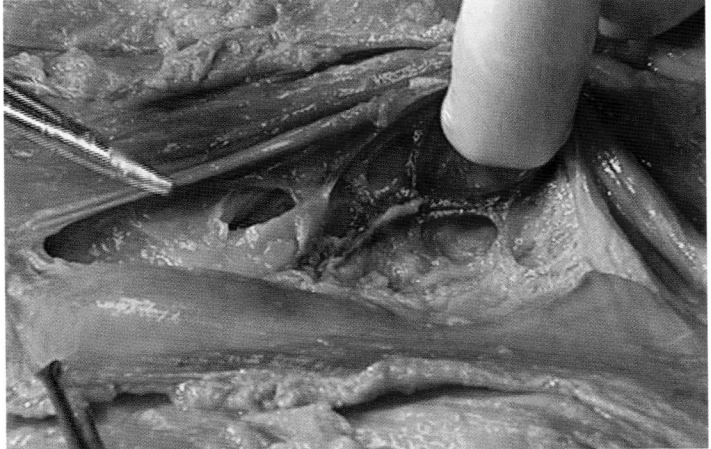

FIGURE 7–14  The left rectus abdominis muscle is elevated. The inferior epigastric vessels have been dissected at the lateral margin of the muscle. The Allis clamp holds the opened anterior rectus sheath.

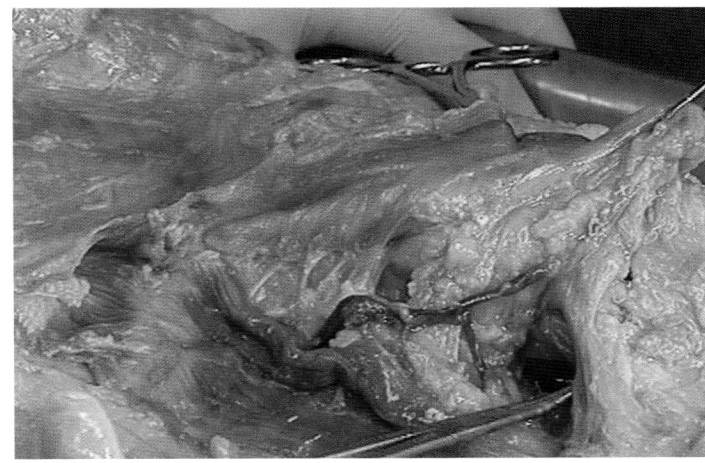

A

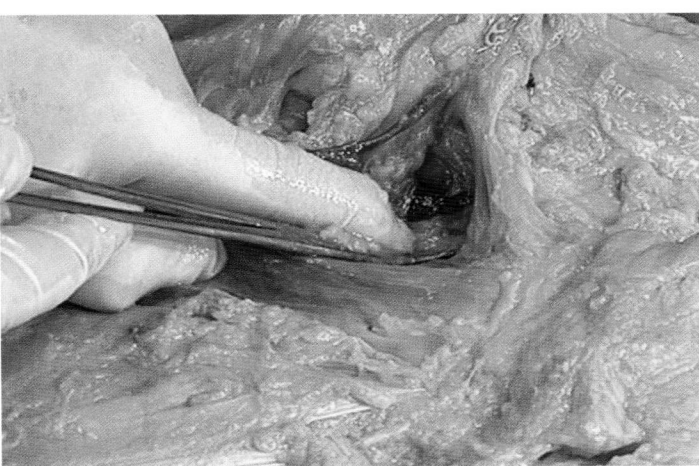

B

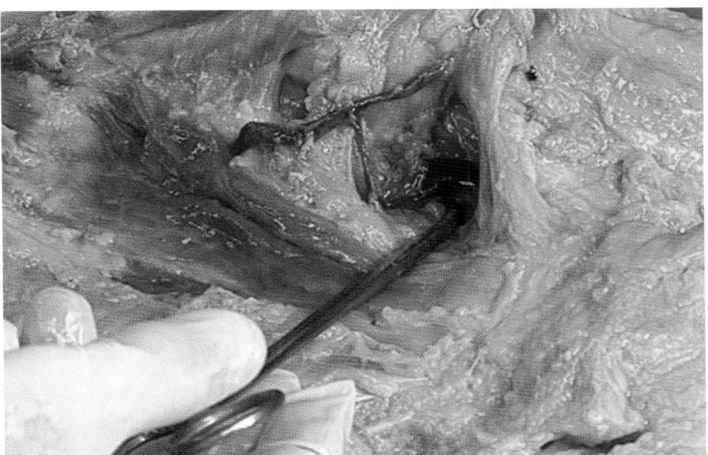

C

FIGURE 7–15  A. The inferior epigastric vessels have been dissected laterally and inferiorly in the direction of the inguinal ligament. The clamp points to the external iliac vein. B. The clamp has been moved medially and rests on the pubic bone and points directly to the distal inguinal ligament. C. This magnified view shows the external iliac vein at a point immediately cranial to the inguinal ligament.

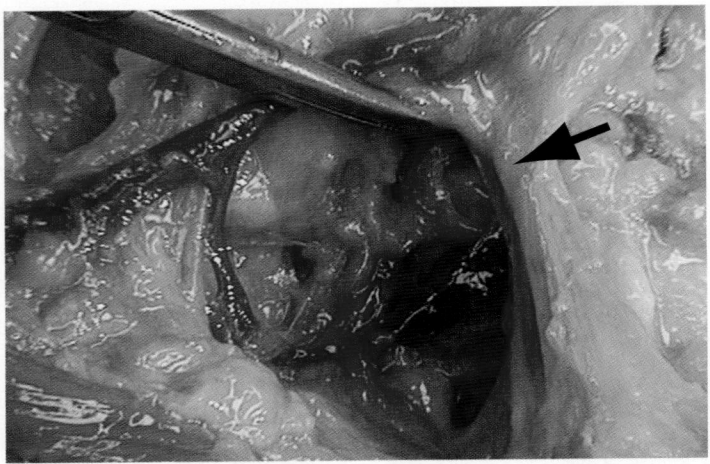

A

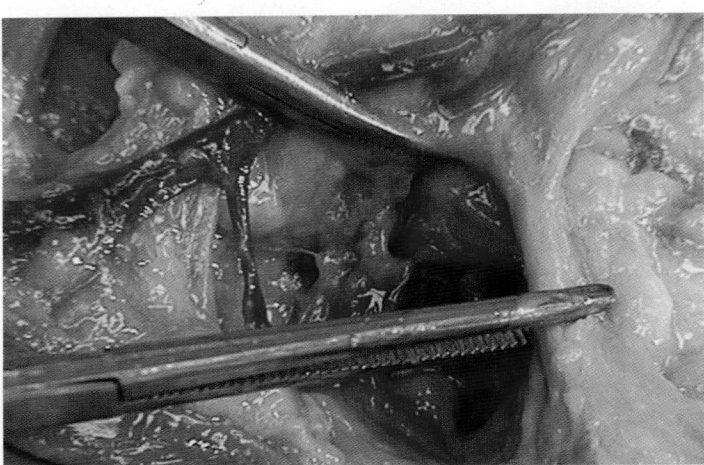

B

**FIGURE 7–16  A.** The clamp points to the origin of the inferior
epigastric artery from the external iliac artery. This point is located just
above the inguinal ligament (*arrow*). **B.** Magnified view of the external
iliac vessels crossing into the thigh sandwiched between the pubic bone
and the inguinal ligament (Kocher clamp holds the inguinal ligament).
The tonsil clamp rests on the external iliac artery.

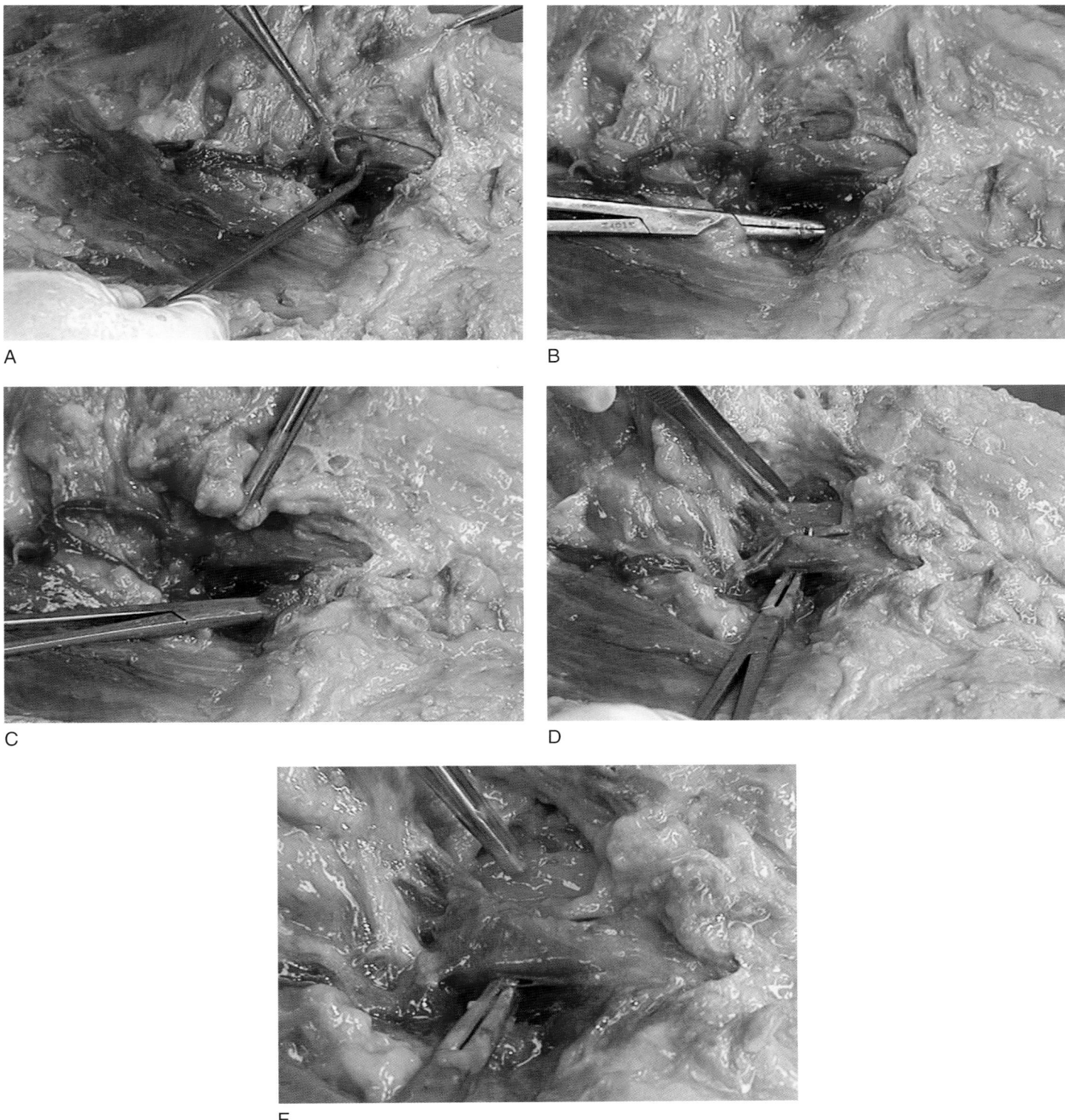

**FIGURE 7–17  A.** The inguinal ligament has been cut. The external iliac (femoral) artery is exposed by the tonsil clamp. **B.** The Kelly clamp is just beneath Cloquet's lymph node (the lowest node in the external iliac chain). Note the location is immediately medial to the iliac (femoral) vein. **C.** The clamp has been advanced through the femoral canal. Note the tip of the Kelly clamp within the fat of the thigh. The Kocher clamp holds the superior cut margin of the inguinal ligament. Immediately lateral to the femoral canal is the external iliac (femoral) vein, followed still further laterally by the external iliac (femoral) artery. **D.** The clamp has been positioned under the external iliac artery. The forceps rest on the psoas major muscle. **E.** Magnified view of part D showing the light pink psoas major muscle (forceps).

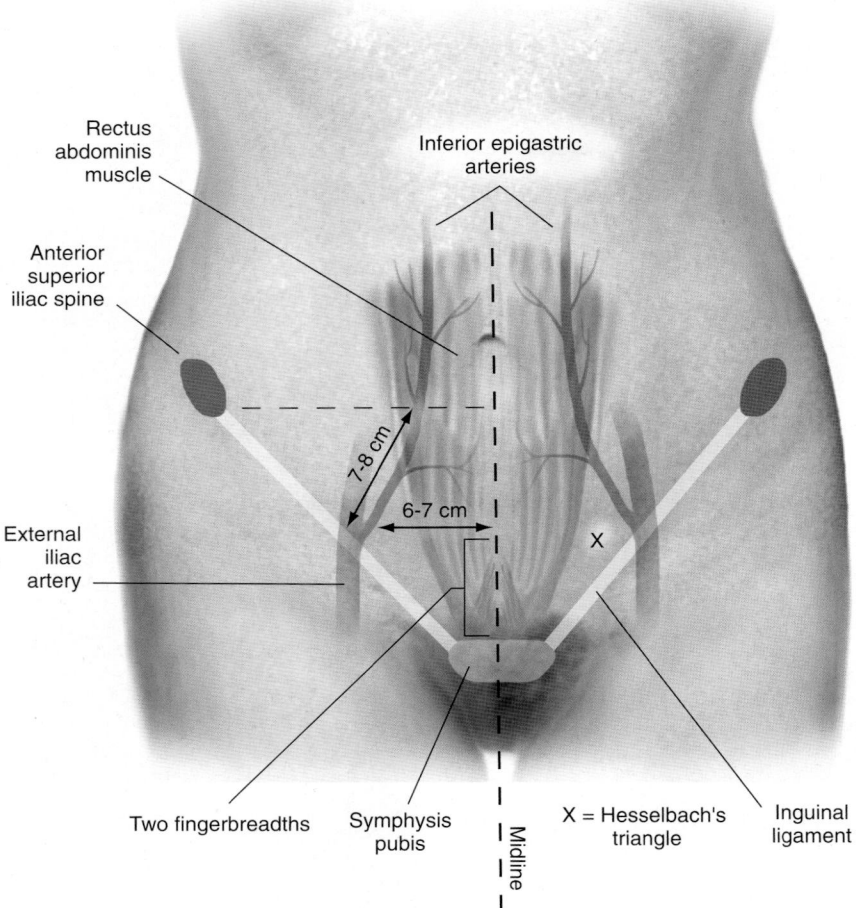

Rectus abdominis muscle

Inferior epigastric arteries

Anterior superior iliac spine

External iliac artery

7-8 cm

6-7 cm

X

Two fingerbreadths

Symphysis pubis

Midline

X = Hesselbach's triangle

Inguinal ligament

**FIGURE 7–18** A point two fingerbreadths (4 cm) above the upper margin of the pubic symphysis in the midline serves as a useful landmark for demarcating the origin of the inferior epigastric artery. By measuring 6 to 7 cm from this point in a straight line laterally, one reaches the point where the inferior epigastric penetrates the fascia of the transversus abdominis muscle. The vessel proceeds upward obliquely for 7 cm to enter the posterior rectus sheath.

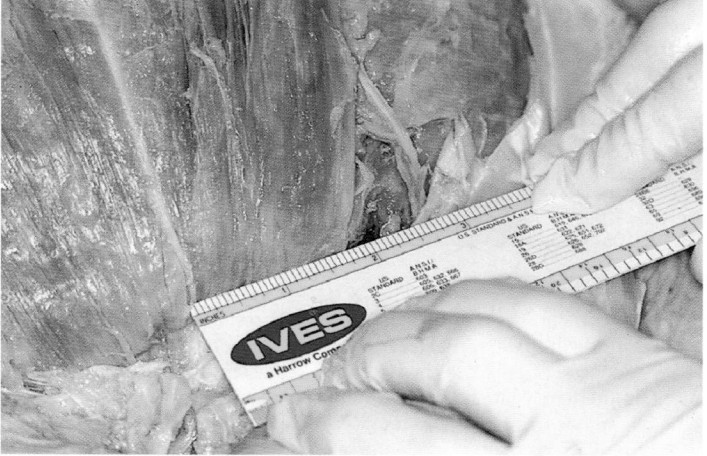

**FIGURE 7–19** The ruler measures from the linea alba laterally to the inferior epigastric vessels, a distance of exactly 6.4 cm.

# CHAPTER 8

# Abdominal Incisions

## *Michael S. Baggish*

Before performing an incision in the abdominal wall, the gynecologic surgeon should have anticipated the type(s) of surgical procedure that will be done and possible complicating aspects associated with the operation. Consideration should be given to how far cephalad from the pelvis the operative exposure will need to be. Additionally, the surgeon should weigh the cosmetic desire(s) of the patient, the urgency of the surgery, the patient's history of previous laparotomies, and the risk of postoperative wound dehiscence.

Knowledge of pelvic anatomy of the anterior abdominal wall is essential to avoid or secure major vessels, to enhance appropriate repair so as to reduce the risk of incisional hernia or wound dehiscence, and to facilitate smooth entry. Practically, incisions may be categorized as midline or transverse. Transverse incisions may be further subdivided into muscle-splitting and muscle-cutting varieties.

## Transverse Incisions

### Maylard Incision

The Maylard incision is made two fingerbreadths above the symphysis pubis (i.e., approximately 3–4 cm) (Fig. 8–1A, B). It is carried down through the subcutaneous fat and through Scarpa's fascia (Fig. 8–2). The fascia overlying the abdominal wall muscles is identified (Fig. 8–3). Scarpa's fascia covers the sheath of the rectus abdominis muscles and the aponeurosis of the external oblique. The operator should, of course, be familiar with the course of the inferior epigastric vessels, which lie on the transversalis fascia. After taking their origin deeply at the lowest portion of the external iliac artery and vein, the inferior epigastric vessels range anteriorly, cephalad, and medially to cross the lower abdominal wall and locate alongside the rectus abdominis muscles. The fascia overlying the rectus abdominis muscles is cut transversely, and the incision is continued laterally to include a greater or lesser portion of the external oblique aponeurosis (depending on the planned width of the incision) (Fig. 8–4). Next, the fascia is cut in the midline between the two recti (Fig. 8–5A–C). The operator inserts one or two fingers under the rectus muscle from the midline to the right or left, depending on which muscle is to be cut first. The finger(s) emerges from the lateral border under the rectus muscle above the inferior epigastric vessels (Fig. 8–6). The muscle is carefully cut over the operator's finger(s) or a sterile tongue blade (Fig. 8–7). A similar procedure is carried out on the opposite side (Fig. 8–8A). If the incision is to be extended, the inferior epigastric vessels are isolated, doubly clamped, cut, and suture ligated with 3-0 Vicryl or 2-0 silk. Finally, the peritoneum is elevated, incised, and opened along the length of the incision transversely (Fig. 8–8B).

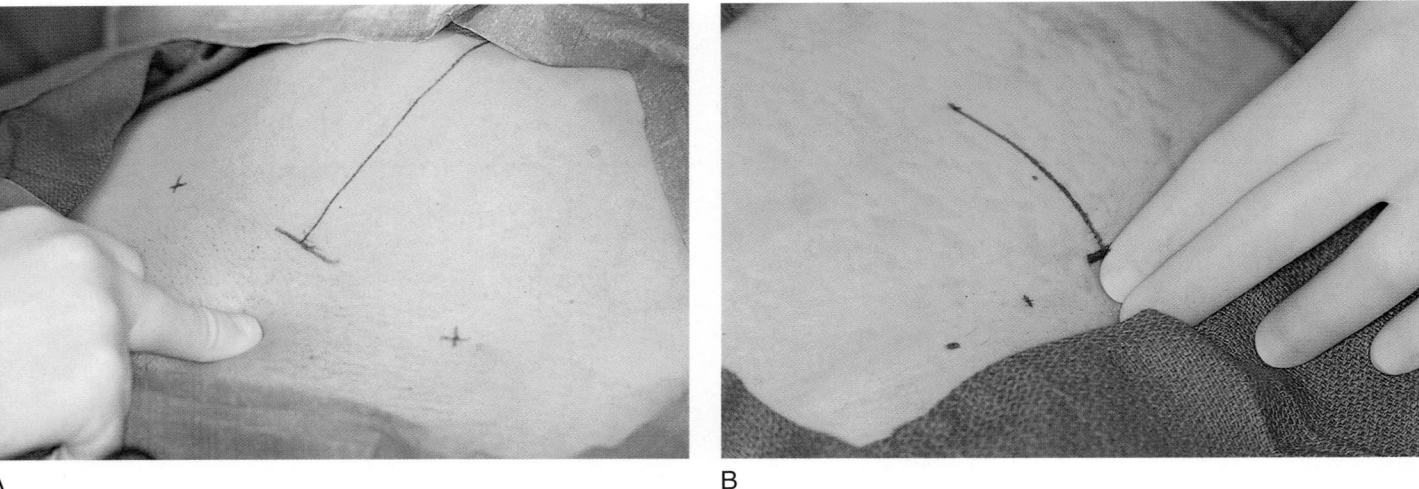

A                                                                    B

**FIGURE 8–1  A.** The midline is marked with a solid vertical line. **B.** The Maylard incision is made 4 cm (two fingerbreadths) above the superior margin of the pubic symphysis, indicated by the dotted line.

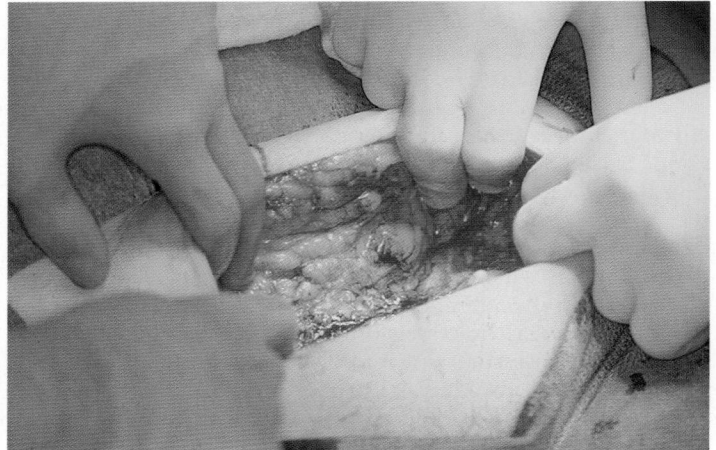

**FIGURE 8–2**  The transverse incision is carried deep through the thick fat to Scarpa's fascia.

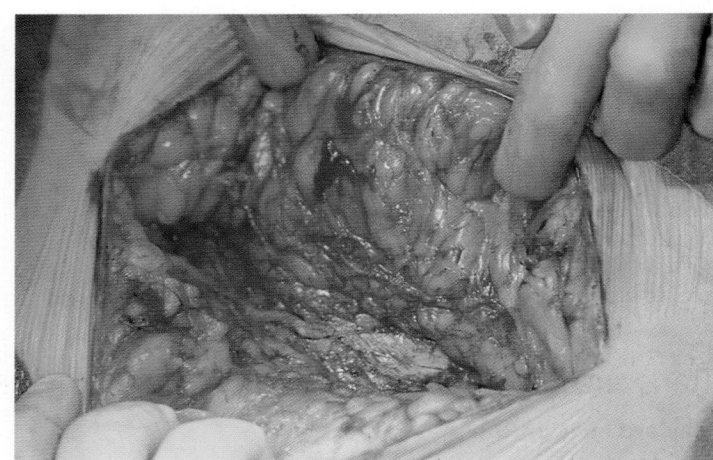

**FIGURE 8–3**  The underlying fascia of the rectus sheath is visible at the depth of the incision.

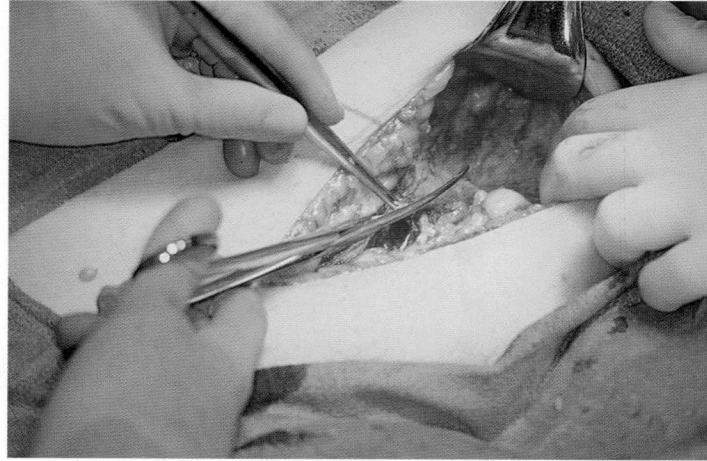

**FIGURE 8–4**  The fascia of the anterior rectus sheath is incised transversely with curved Mayo scissors.

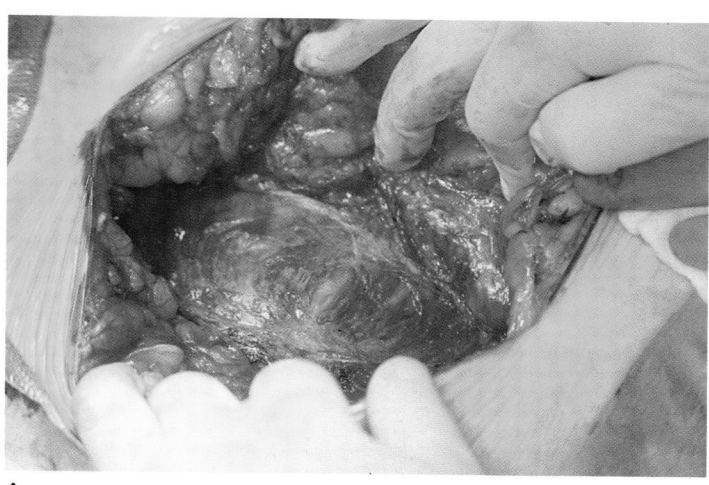

A

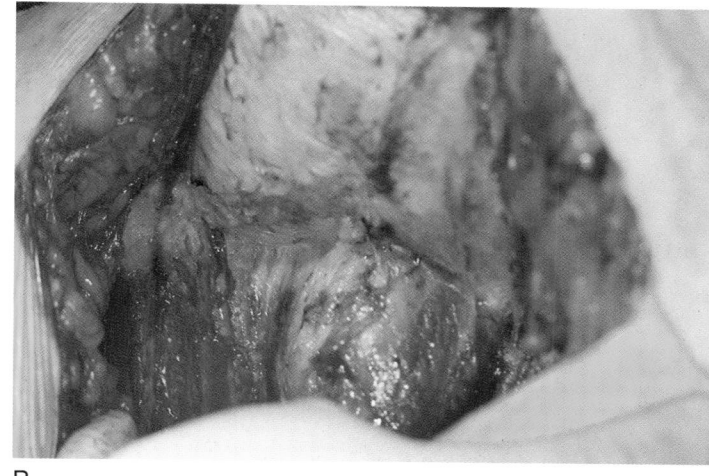

B

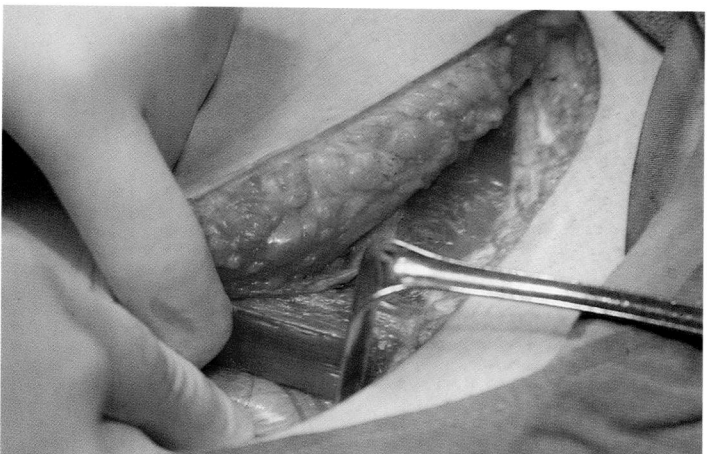

C

**FIGURE 8–5 A.** The rectus muscle is now clearly in view. **B.** The lower portion of the rectus fascia (sheath) is dissected from the muscle belly. **C.** The inferior epigastric vessels are identified.

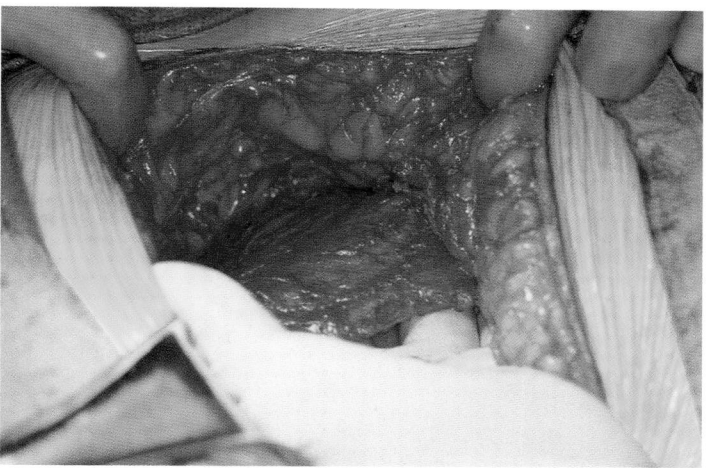

**FIGURE 8–6** The linea alba has been incised, and the fingers of the operator's hand bluntly dissect the muscle from the posterior sheath/peritoneum.

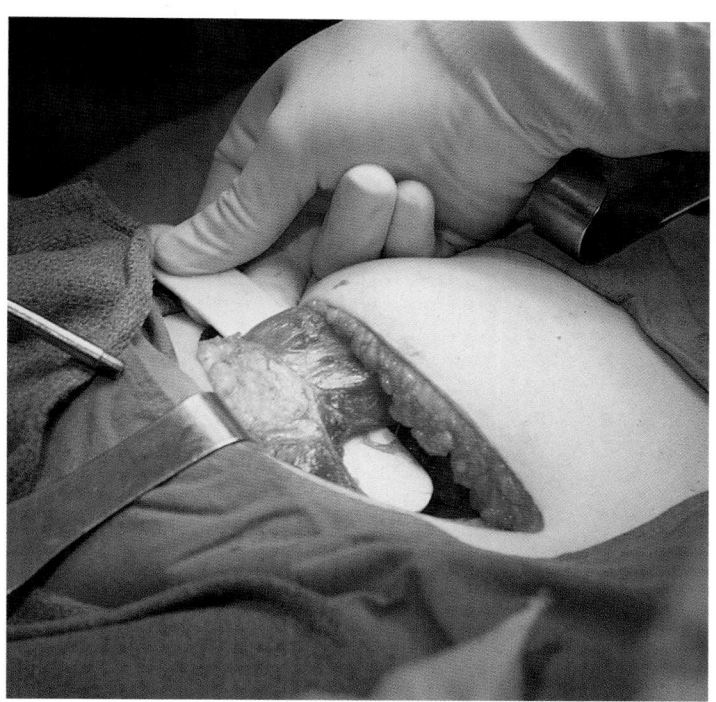

**FIGURE 8–7** The belly of the rectus sheath is isolated before it is cut.

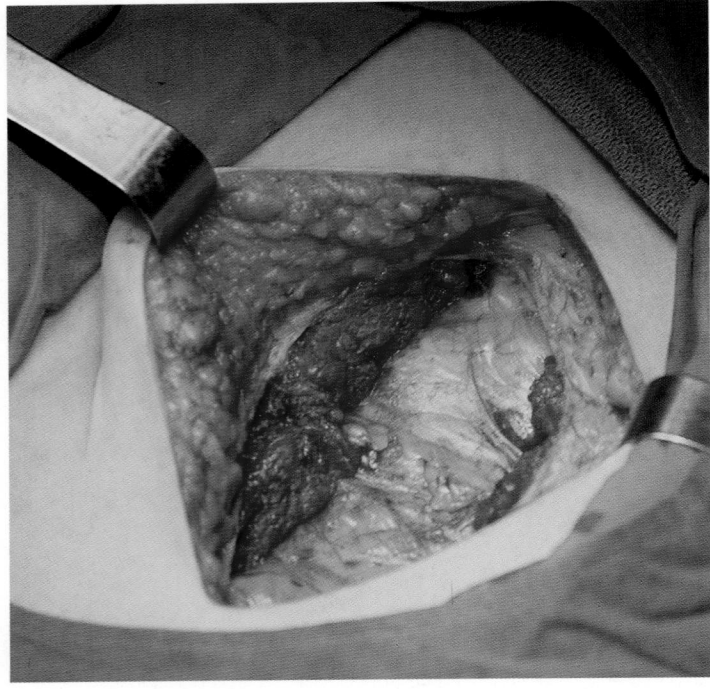

A

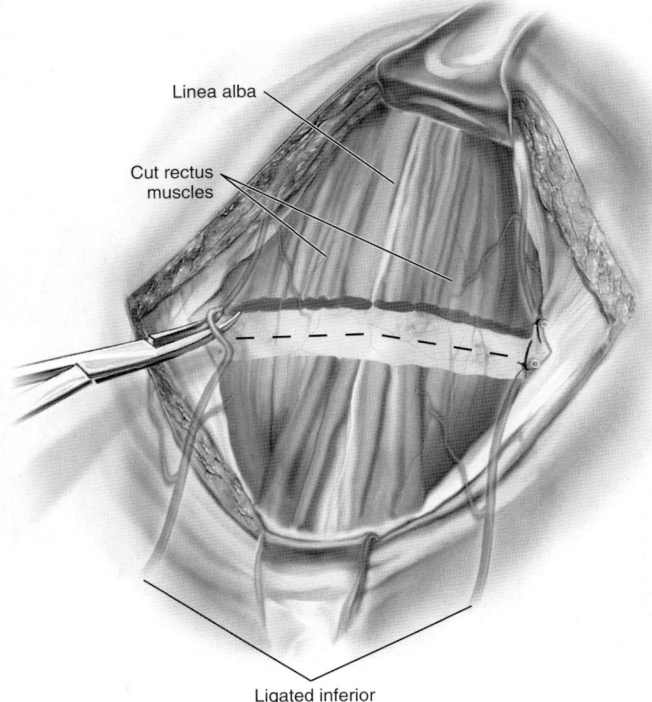

Linea alba

Cut rectus
muscles

Ligated inferior
epigastric arteries

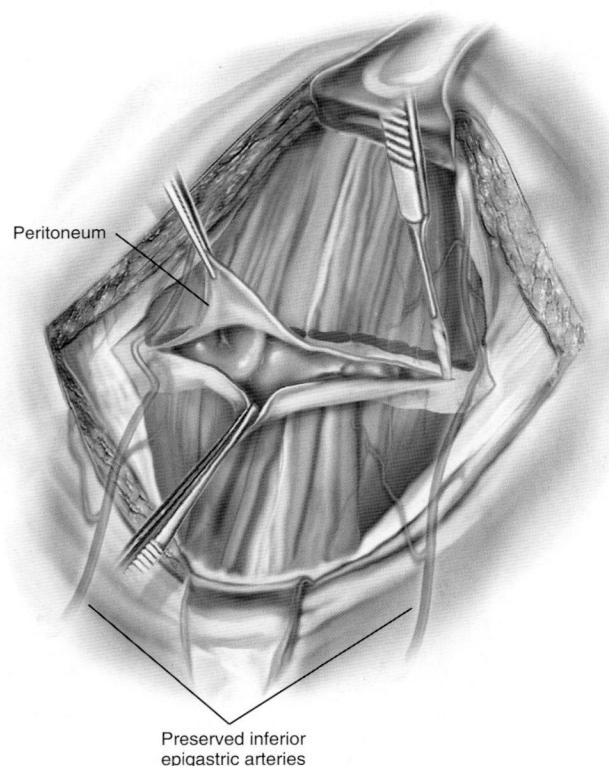

Peritoneum

Preserved inferior
epigastric arteries

B

**FIGURE 8–8  A.** The rectus muscles have been fully divided. Note how dry the field and muscles are even in the absence of any ligatures.
**B.** The schematic view (*upper figure*) shows the isolation and division of the inferior epigastric vessels and the transverse sectioning of the rectus muscles. The lower figure shows the incision through the peritoneum (in this case preserving the inferior epigastric vessels).

## Pfannenstiel Incision

This incision is made transversely in a manner similar to the Maylard incision, although some surgeons may prefer to curve the incision upward toward the anterior superior iliac spine to gain more exposure (the "smile" incision) (Fig. 8–9A, B). The cut traverses the skin, the fat, Scarpa's fascia, and the rectus sheath (i.e., to the lateral margin of the rectus sheath). Typically, the incision through the fascia is superficial and therefore is unlikely to impinge on the inferior epigastric vessels (Fig. 8–10A). The sheath is clamped and elevated to allow dissection of the sheath cranially and to free it from the underlying rectus abdominis muscles (Fig. 8–10B, C). This plane can be accentuated by the operator's spread fingers, creating countertraction via pressure on the rectus muscles (Fig. 8–11). The dissection is continued upward for several centimeters (Fig. 8–12) and may be continued to the level of the umbilicus (Fig. 8–13). The rectus muscles are separated vertically in the midline, and the peritoneum is entered. The properitoneum and peritoneum are opened together vertically in the midline (Fig. 8–14). The pyramidalis muscles are similarly cut in the midline down to the level of the symphysis pubis (Fig. 8–15A–C). The peritoneum is carefully dissected inferiorly to the level of the bladder reflection (Fig. 8–16).

## Cherney Incision

This incision is made approximately 1 cm lower than the Maylard incision. The incision is carried through the skin, fat, subcutaneous tissue, and Scarpa's fascia. The rectus sheath is opened transversely. The rectus muscles are divided transversely from their insertion onto the symphysis pubis. The incision may now be extended laterally through the aponeurosis of the external oblique by isolating, ligating, and cutting the inferior epigastric vessels. The rectus muscles may likewise be freed upward to enhance the space for surgical exposure (Fig. 8–17A–E).

## Kustner Incision

This hybrid incision is a transverse incision through the skin and subcutaneous tissue only (i.e., it is used for cosmetic rather than structural reasons). From this point on the exposure is identical to that of a vertical incision. The fascia is opened in the midline, along the linea alba. The rectus muscles are separated vertically by sharp dissection. The pyramidalis muscles are cut. The peritoneum is entered and opened vertically in the midline (Fig. 8–18A, B).

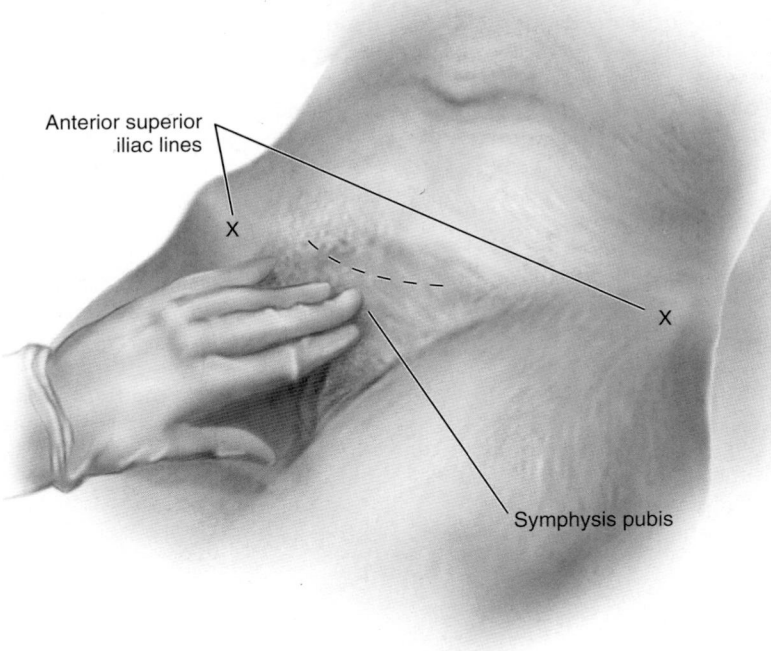

A

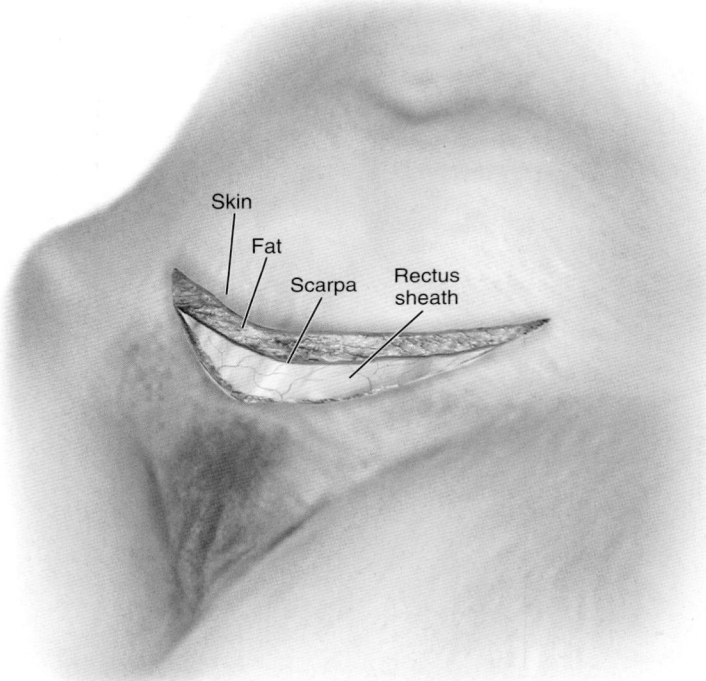

B

**FIGURE 8–9  A.** Preparation is made for the curvilinear Pfannenstiel incision (smile incision) at the level of the pubic hair line. **B.** The incision is carried down through the skin, fat, and Scarpa's fascia to the fascia overlying the rectus sheath.

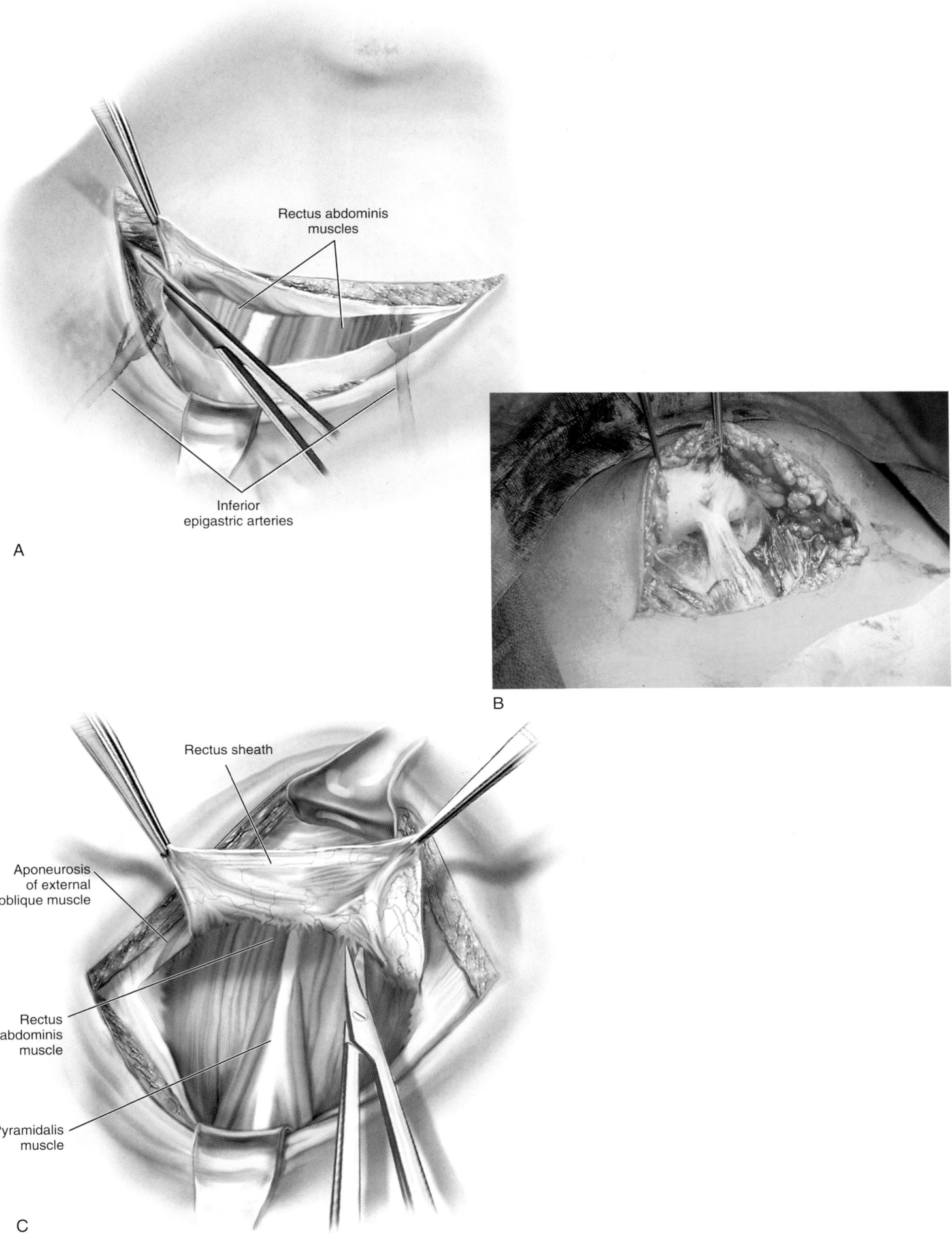

**FIGURE 8–10 A.** The rectus fascia is incised, with care taken to avoid injuring the underlying inferior epigastric vessels. **B** and **C.** The cranial (*upper*) flap of the fascia is sharply dissected upward, exposing the underlying rectus muscles.

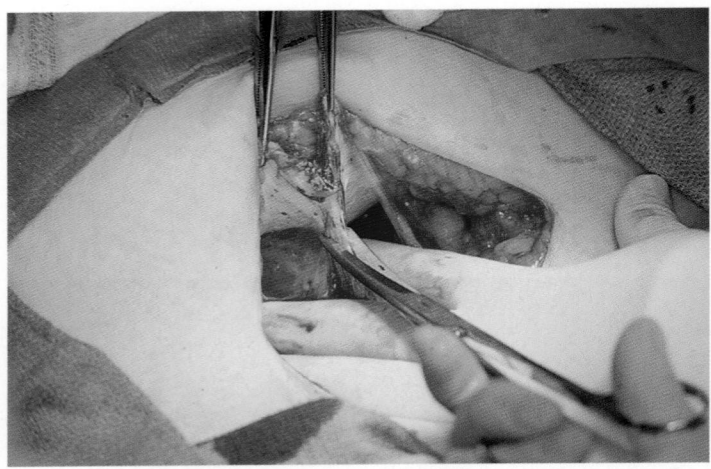

**FIGURE 8–11** Scissors are needed to cut the rectus sheath in the midline, whereas the sheath on either side can be easily dissected with the operator's fingers.

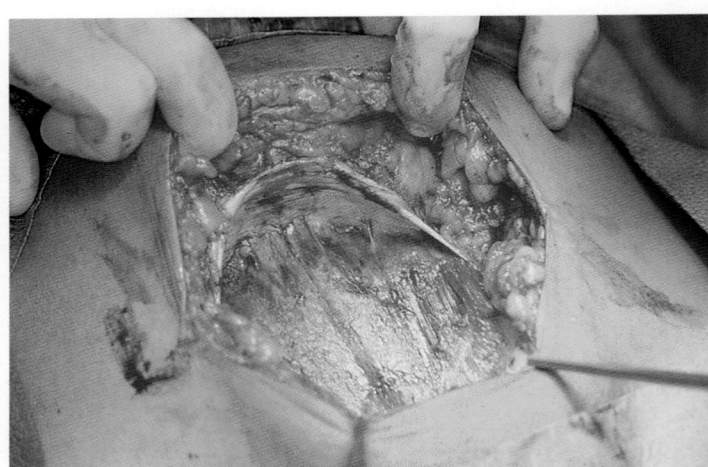

**FIGURE 8–12** The sheath is freed both cranially and caudally.

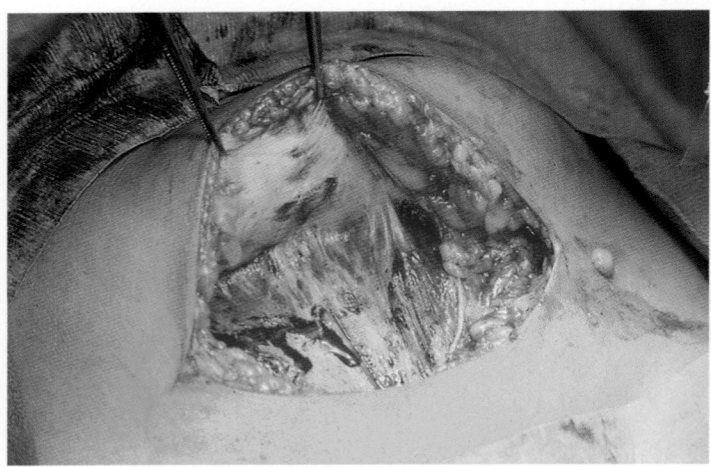

**FIGURE 8–13** The linea alba is clearly exposed for a distance of 8 cm.

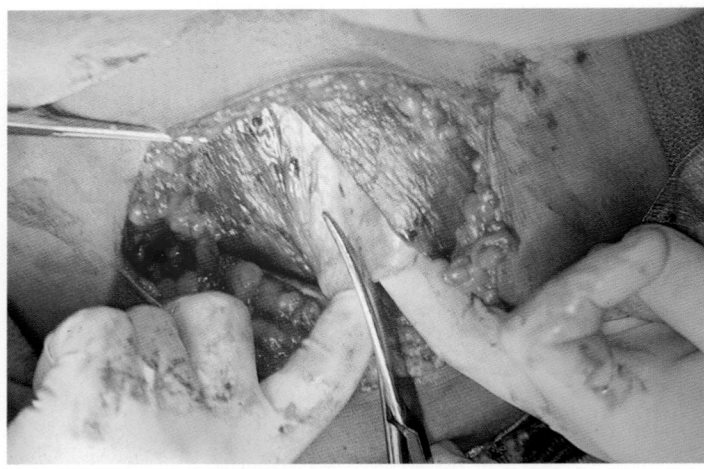

**FIGURE 8–14** The peritoneum is entered and opened by a midline incision.

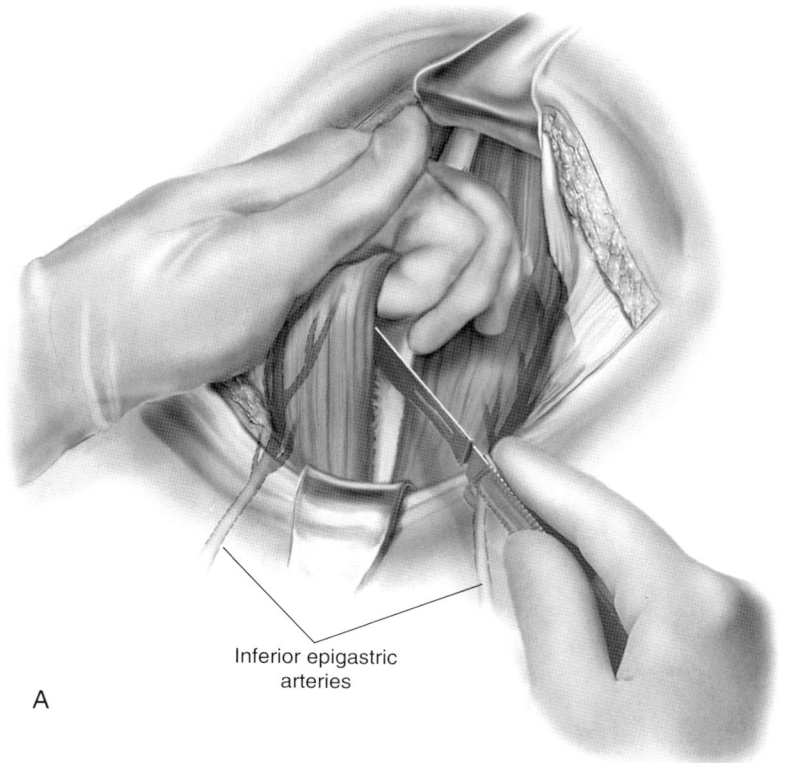

Inferior epigastric
arteries

A

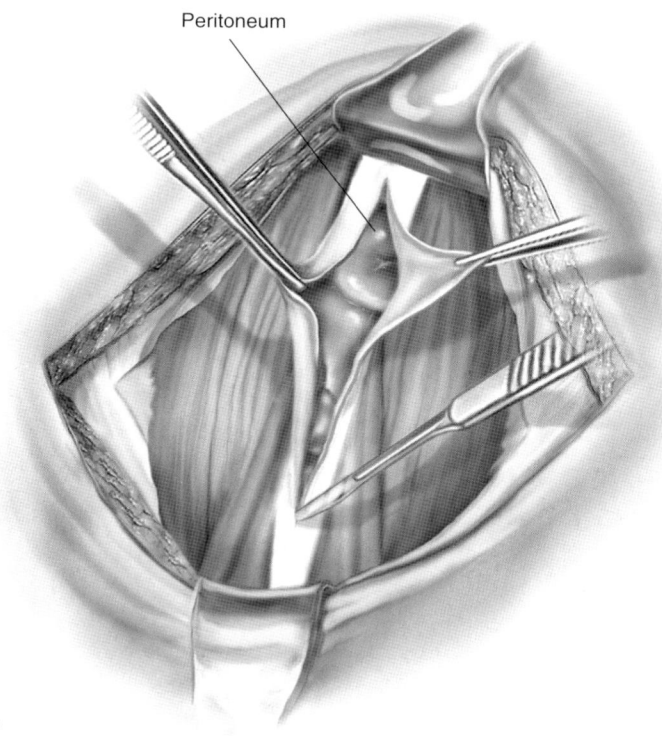

Peritoneum

B

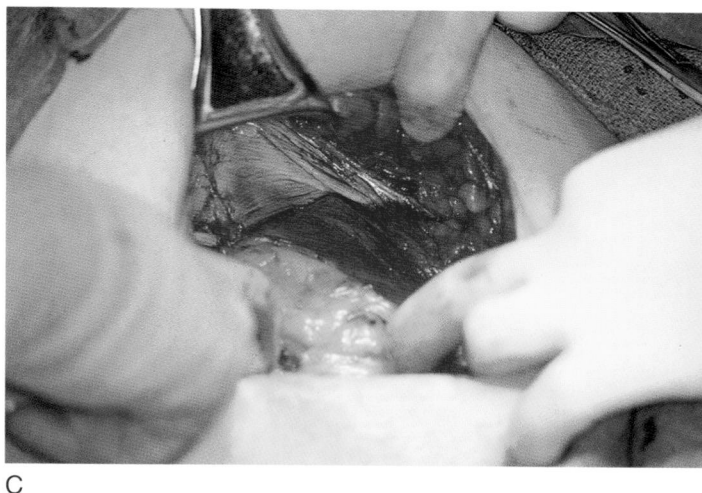

C

**FIGURE 8–15 A.** The rectus muscles are sharply separated from each other before the incision is made into the peritoneum, as shown in Figure 8–14.
**B.** The peritoneum may be opened vertically with scissors or a scalpel. **C.** The omentum is clearly visible underlying the peritoneum.

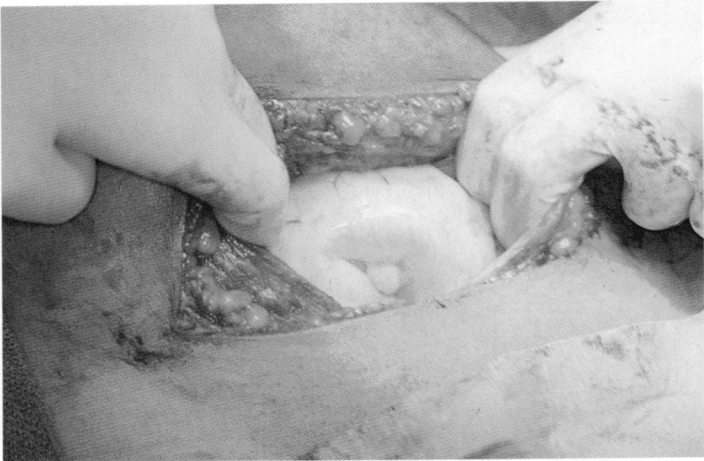

**FIGURE 8–16** The underlying small intestine fills the wound as the omentum is pushed away.

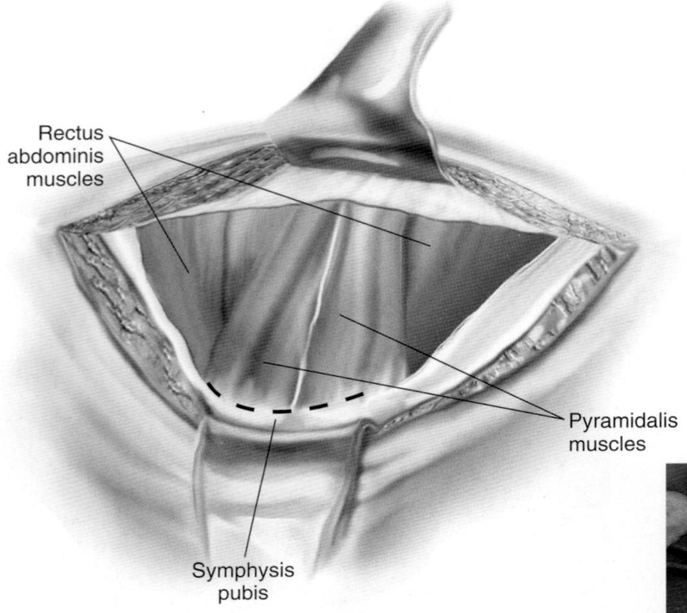

Rectus abdominis muscles

Pyramidalis muscles

Symphysis pubis

A

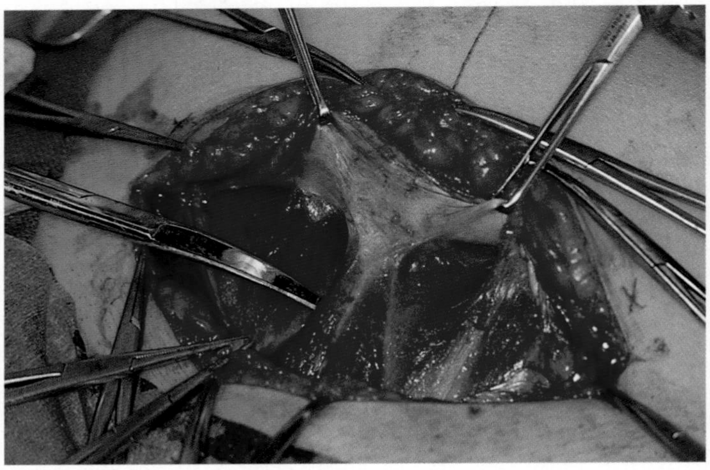

B

**FIGURE 8–17 A.** The Cherney incision is made immediately above the symphysis pubis and is carried down to the rectus sheath, which is opened transversely. The inferior epigastric vessels are sectioned and the insertion of the muscle(s) onto the pubic bone is separated and reflected upward (cranially). The peritoneum is incised laterally, thereby creating excellent exposure of the abdominal cavity and pelvis. **B.** The rectus sheath has been opened transversely. The Allis clamps hold the cranial portion of the sheath. The scissors point to the pyramidalis muscle.

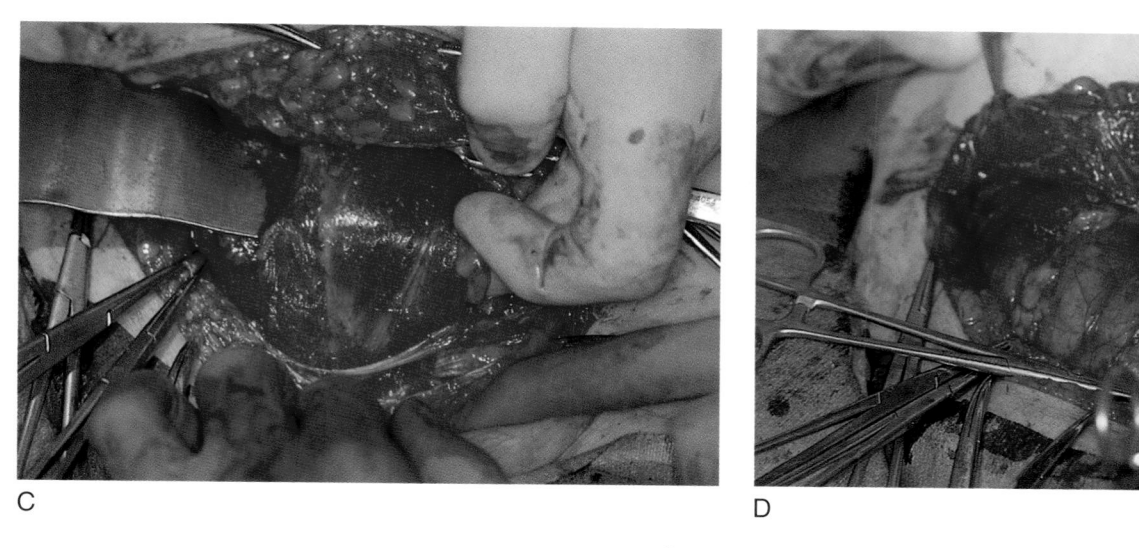

C

D

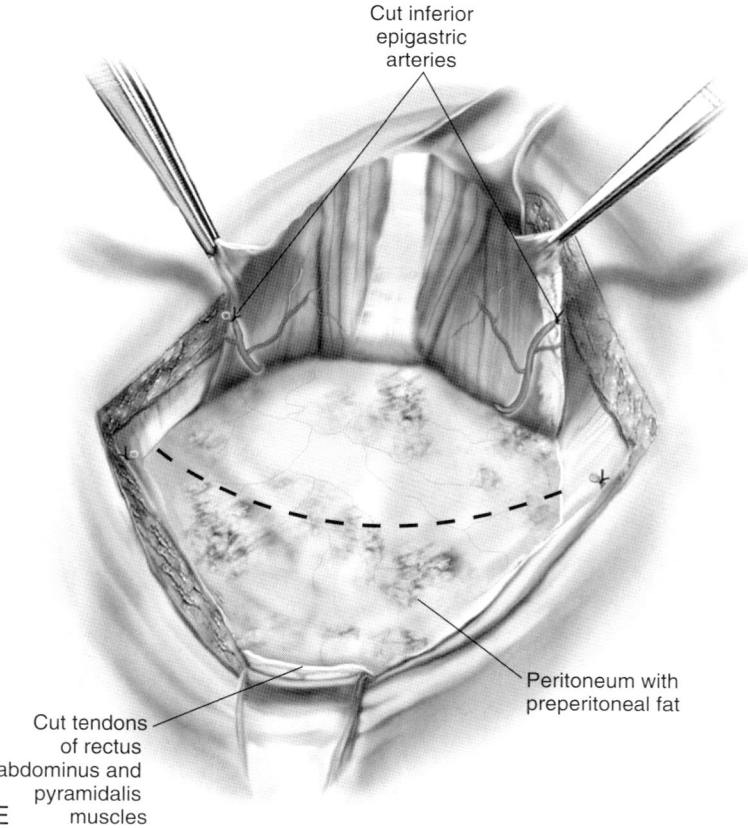

Cut inferior
epigastric
arteries

Peritoneum with
preperitoneal fat

Cut tendons
of rectus
abdominus and
pyramidalis
E muscles

**FIGURE 8–17, cont'd   C.** The rectus muscle (*left*) has been dissected from the underlying fascia. The operator's finger is at the lateral margin. The assistant's hand marks the attachment of the muscle to the symphysis pubis. **D.** The muscles have been cut free from the symphysis pubis. Note the excellent and wide exposure. **E.** The transversus fascia/peritoneum is widely exposed and may be opened transversely (*dashed line*) to provide excellent pelvic exposure. (See previous page for illustration.)

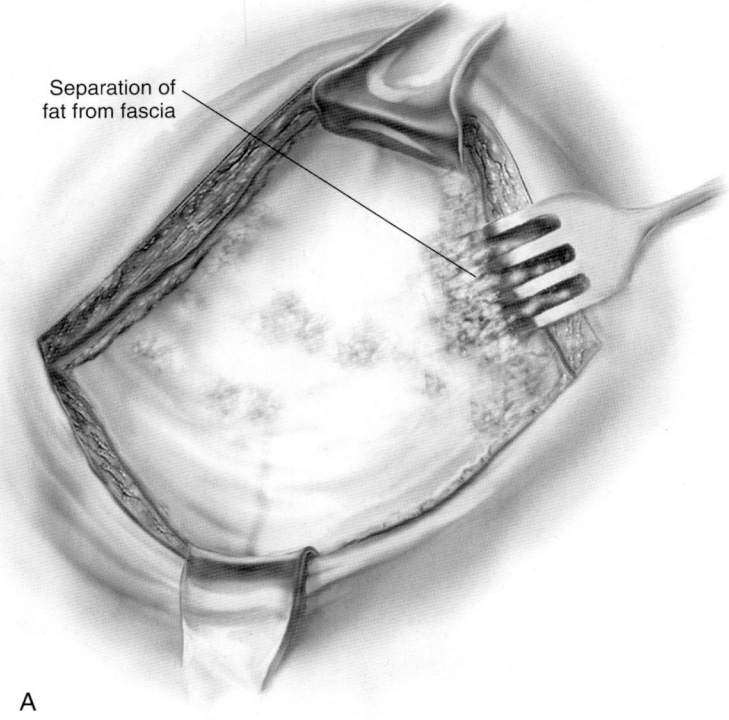

Separation of
fat from fascia

A

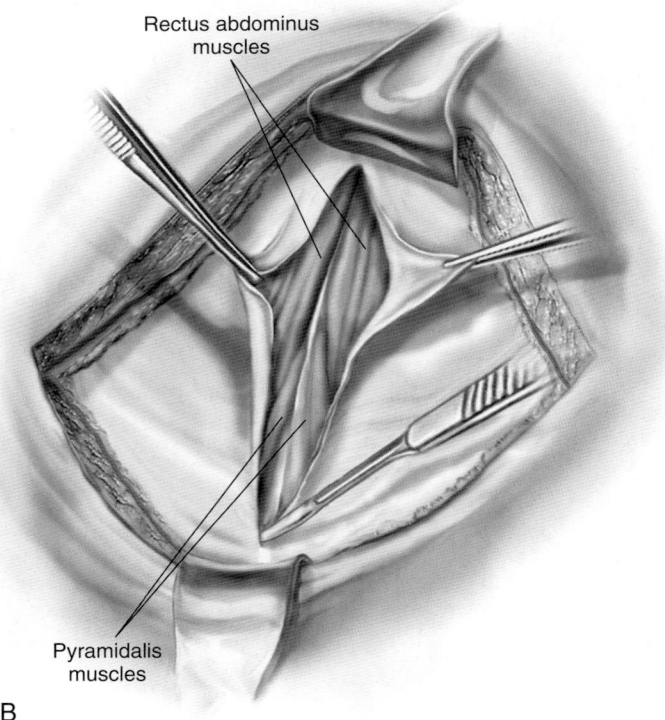

Rectus abdominus
muscles

Pyramidalis
muscles

B

**FIGURE 8–18 A.** The skin and fat have been opened transversely. The dissection now extends vertically to separate the fascia overlying the muscles from the fatty tissue. **B.** The rectus sheath is opened vertically in the midline. The posterior rectus sheath and the peritoneum will be likewise cut in the midline.

## Midline Incision

The midline incision is commonly used for lower abdominal operative procedures in obstetric, gynecologic, and general surgery cases. For emergencies it has the advantages of offering the most rapid entry and the least amount of incisional bleeding. The greatest deficiency of the midline incision is its diminished postoperative tensile strength compared with that of transverse fascial incisions. Therefore, a greater propensity is observed for wound dehiscence as well as ventral hernias with the midline vertical approach. Specific closure techniques have been designed principally to decrease the risk of dehiscence with midline incisions.

The incision starts at the level of the umbilicus and is carried as a *straight line* to the symphysis pubis (Fig. 8–19). Although Howard Kelly was said to have routinely opened the belly via a single vertical cut through all the layers of the abdominal wall, this method is not recommended by the authors of this book. The initial cut is, however, typically carried down through the skin, subcutaneous fat, and Scarpa's fascia (Fig. 8–20). Next, the rectus sheath is opened vertically along the entire length of the incision (Fig. 8–21). The right and left rectus muscles are identified and, by means of sharp and blunt dissection, the muscles are separated in the midline caudad to the level of the pyramidalis muscles (Fig. 8–22). The pyramidalis muscles are cut with Mayo scissors or a scalpel in the midline down to the upper edge of the symphysis pubis.

Next the properitoneal fat is pushed to the right or left at the upper level of the incision between the rectus abdominis muscles (Fig. 8–23A–C). The peritoneum is grasped with two forceps or two clamps and elevated. A sharp knife incision opens into the peritoneal cavity (Fig. 8–23C). Using a Metzenbaum scissors or Mayo scissors, the peritoneum is opened for the length of the incision over the operator's index and center fingers or a wide malleable retractor (Fig. 8–24) so as to protect the underlying intestine from injury. The lower portion of the incision should be opened with great care to avoid injury to the urinary bladder. Typically, the fatty tissue around the bladder demonstrates significantly greater vascularity when compared with the midline peritoneum and fat.

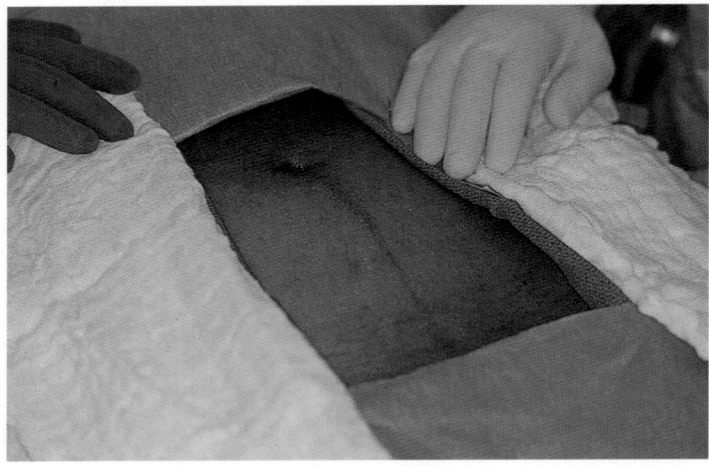

**FIGURE 8–19** The linea nigra is clearly shown in this patient and is an excellent reference point for initiating a vertical incision.

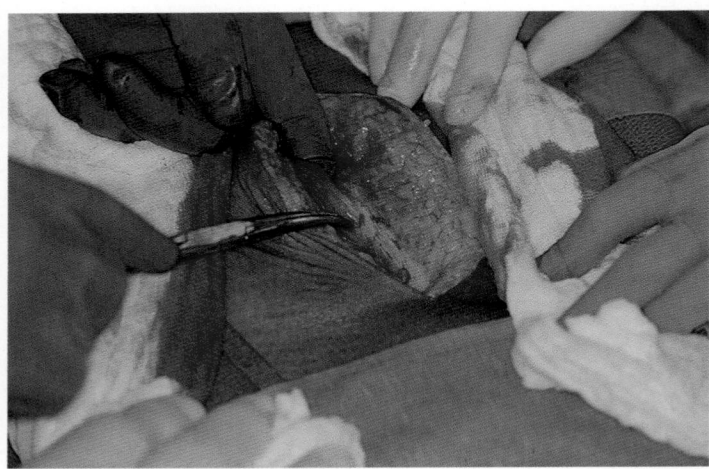

**FIGURE 8–20** The midline incision is carried down to the level of the rectus sheath.

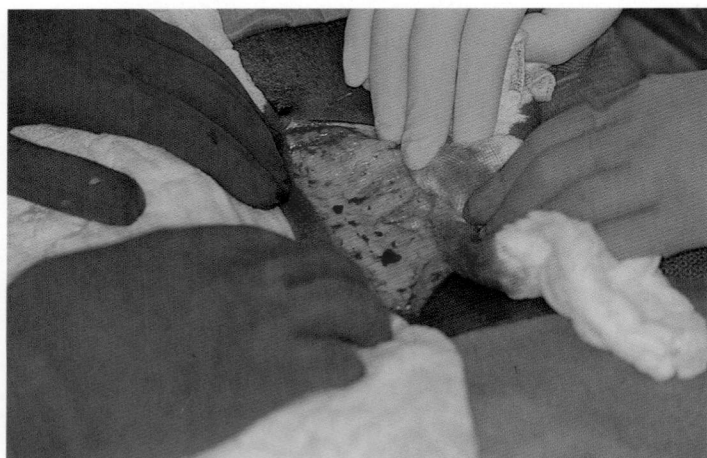

**FIGURE 8–21** The fat is sharply dissected from the silvery gray sheath.

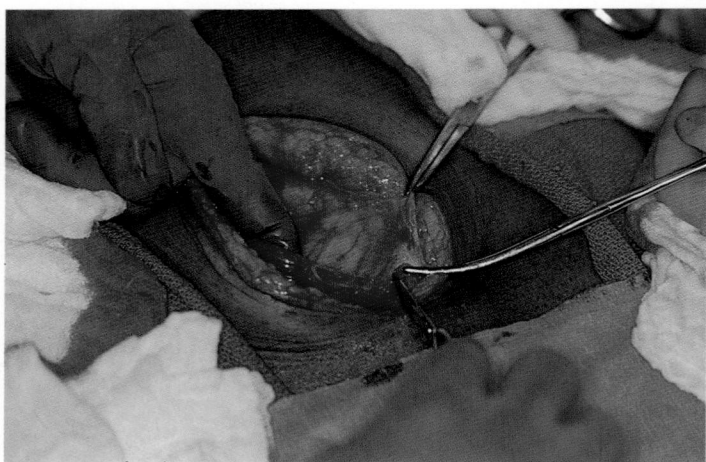

**FIGURE 8–22** The sheath has been opened and the two rectus abdominis muscles are separated from each other.

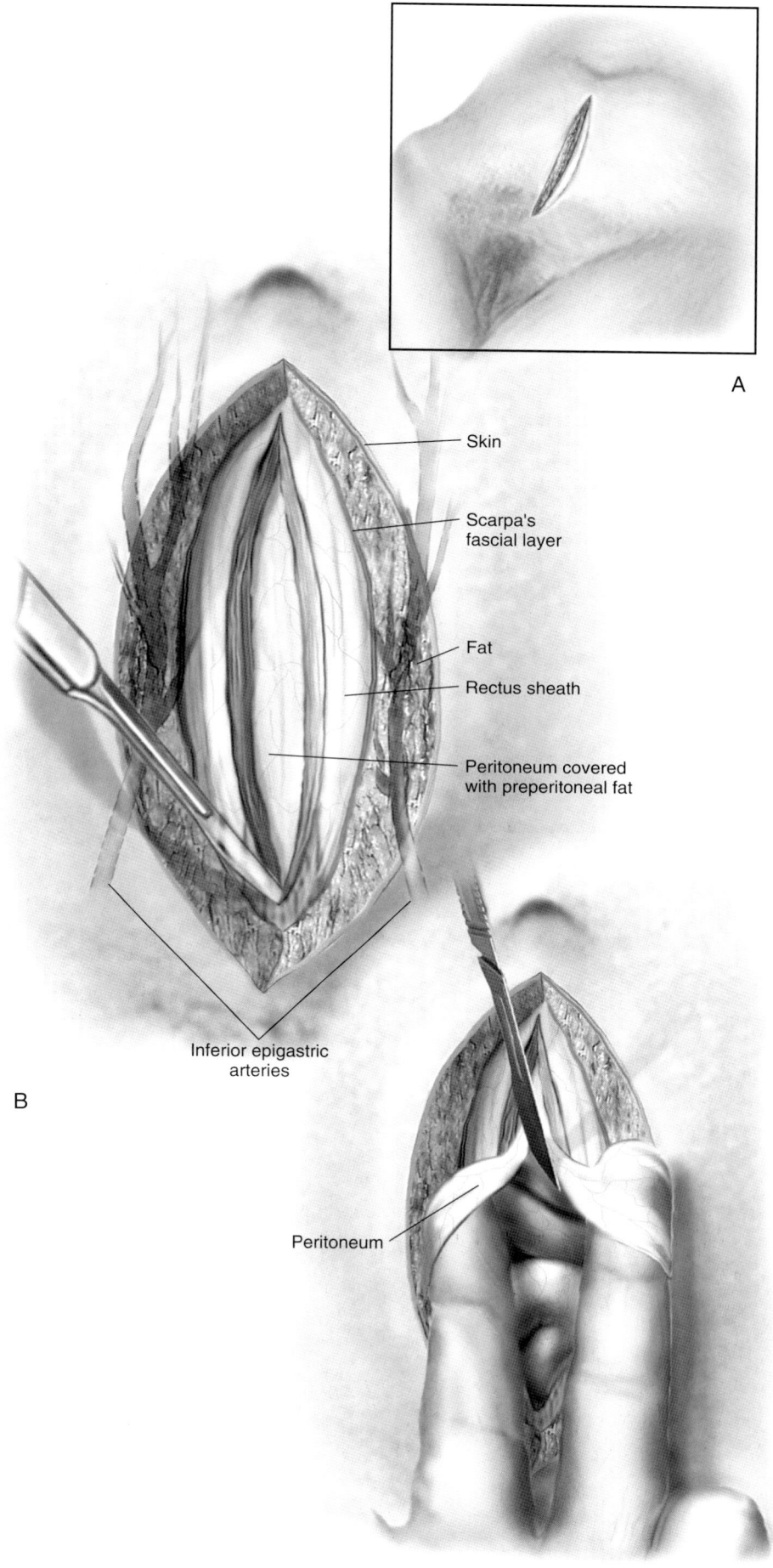

**FIGURE 8–23  A.** Schema for the vertical midline incision. The cut is made below the umbilicus and is carried caudad to the upper margin of the symphysis pubis. **B.** The underlying posterior sheath and the peritoneum are brought into view between the separated rectus muscles (*middle*). **C.** The peritoneum is opened in the midline sharply, with care taken to shield the underlying intestines from injury (*lower*).

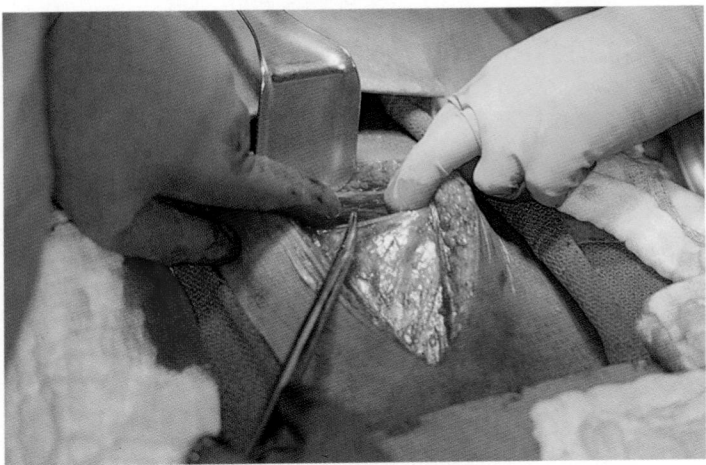

**FIGURE 8–24** The peritoneum is entered at the upper extremity of the incision and is "tented-up" to allow safe incision (i.e., well away from the underlying intestine).

# SECTION B

# Uterus

# Intra-abdominal Pelvic Anatomy

*Michael S. Baggish*

The anatomy pertinent to surgery of the uterus, adnexa, and neighboring pelvic structures is not only intraperitoneal but, perhaps more important, extraperitoneal.

## Uterine Support

The main uterine support is provided by the cardinal ligaments, which extend from roughly the level of the cervicoisthmic junction peripherally in a fanlike fashion laterally and posteriorly, where it blends with the fat and fascia of the pelvic sidewall (Fig. 9-1). This ligamentous structure divides the pelvis into right and left paravesical spaces anteriorly and pararectal spaces posteriorly (Fig. 9-2A, B). The cardinal ligament can be divided into an upper portion at the junction of the uterus and cervix and a lower portion at the juncture of the cervix and vagina (Fig. 9-3).

The uterosacral ligaments connect to the cardinal ligaments at the cervical attachment of the latter and extend posteriorly and inferiorly toward the ischial spines and sacrum. However, these terminal attachments may be difficult to identify precisely (see Figs. 9-2 through 9-4). Between the uterosacral ligaments and covered by a peritoneal reflection onto the posterior aspect of the uterus is the top of the rectovaginal septum. This is the portal of entry to the rectouterine space.

The round ligaments arise from the anterolateral fundus and extend ventrally and laterally to the anterior abdominal wall, entering the inguinal canal and terminating in the fat of the labium majus on either side (Fig. 9-5). The round ligaments, in contrast to the other "ligaments," are mainly composed of smooth muscle. The infundibulopelvic ligaments are in reality peritoneal vascular conduits, which carry the ovarian vessels from the posterolateral pelvic brim in an anteromedial direction to gain attachment to the uterus at the level of the cornua.

The broad ligament is a tentlike structure that comprises anterior and posterior peritoneum containing areolar fat (see Fig. 9-5). The "ligament" begins anteriorly at the round ligament and finishes posteriorly at the infundibulopelvic ligament.

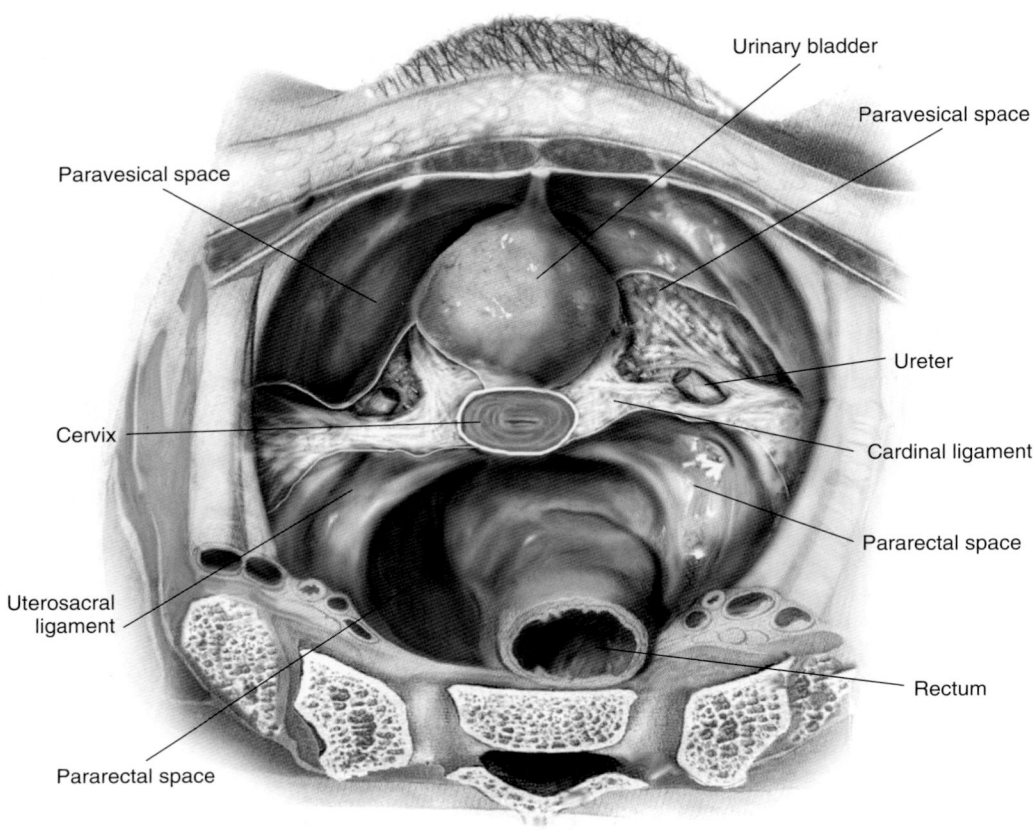

**FIGURE 9–1** The uterine fundus has been excised. The cardinal ligaments stretch from the cervix to the sidewall and are contiguous with the uterosacral ligaments and the paravesical, pararectal, and paravaginal fascia. Note the course of the ureters as they penetrate the cardinal ligaments.

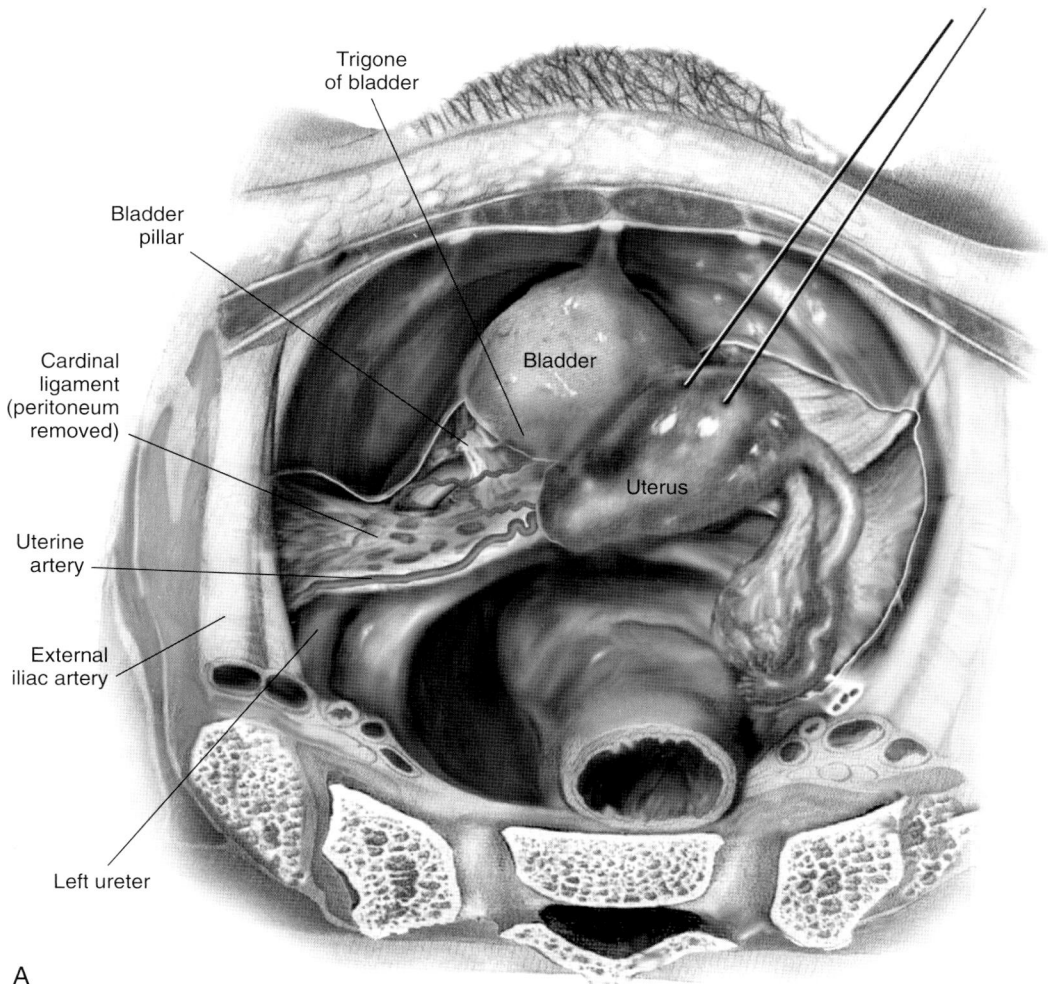

Trigone
of bladder

Bladder
pillar

Cardinal
ligament
(peritoneum
removed)

Uterine
artery

External
iliac artery

Left ureter

Bladder

Uterus

A

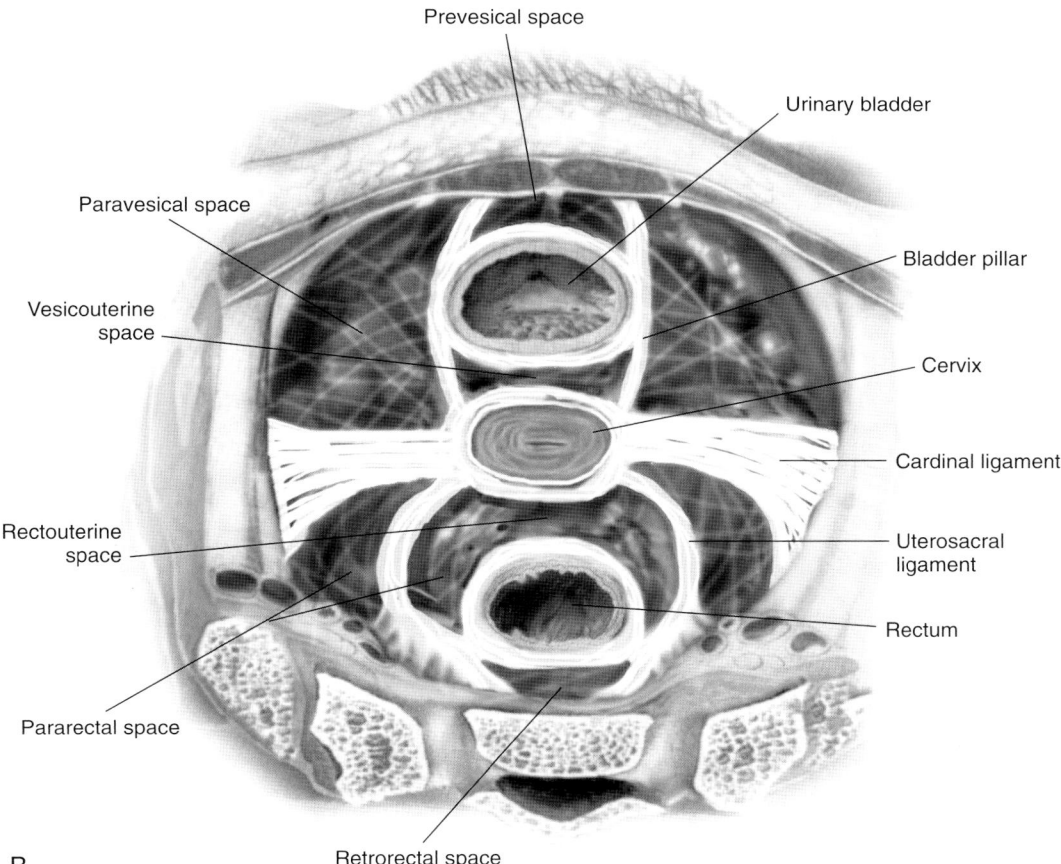

Prevesical space

Urinary bladder

Paravesical space

Bladder pillar

Vesicouterine
space

Cervix

Cardinal ligament

Rectouterine
space

Uterosacral
ligament

Rectum

Pararectal space

Retrorectal space

B

**FIGURE 9–2 A.** The cardinal ligament may be divided into an upper portion at the junction of the uterine body and cervix and a lower portion at the junction of the cervix and vagina. **B.** The various anatomic spaces within the pelvis are schematically demonstrated.

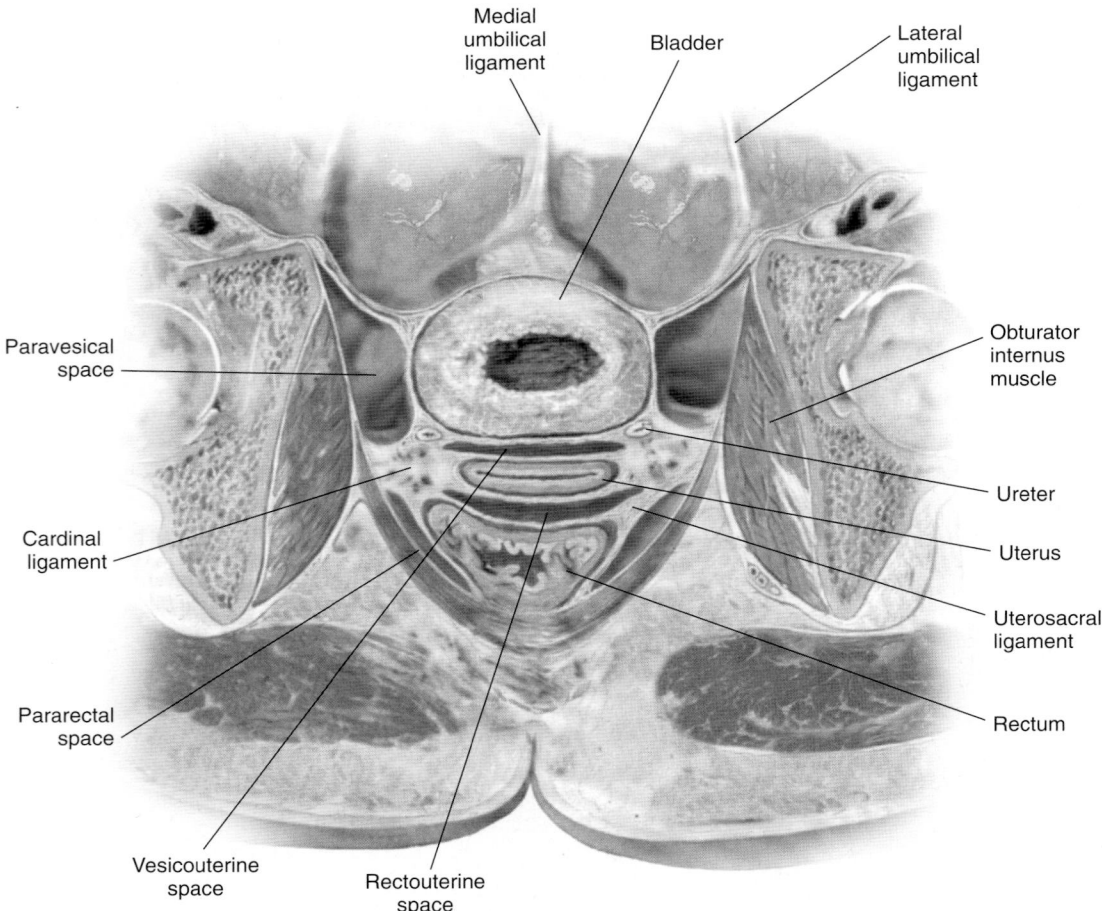

**FIGURE 9–3** The sagittal view demonstrates the relationships between the cardinal ligaments and the various anatomic spaces. Note that the sidewall largely consists of the obturator internus muscle mass and its fascia.

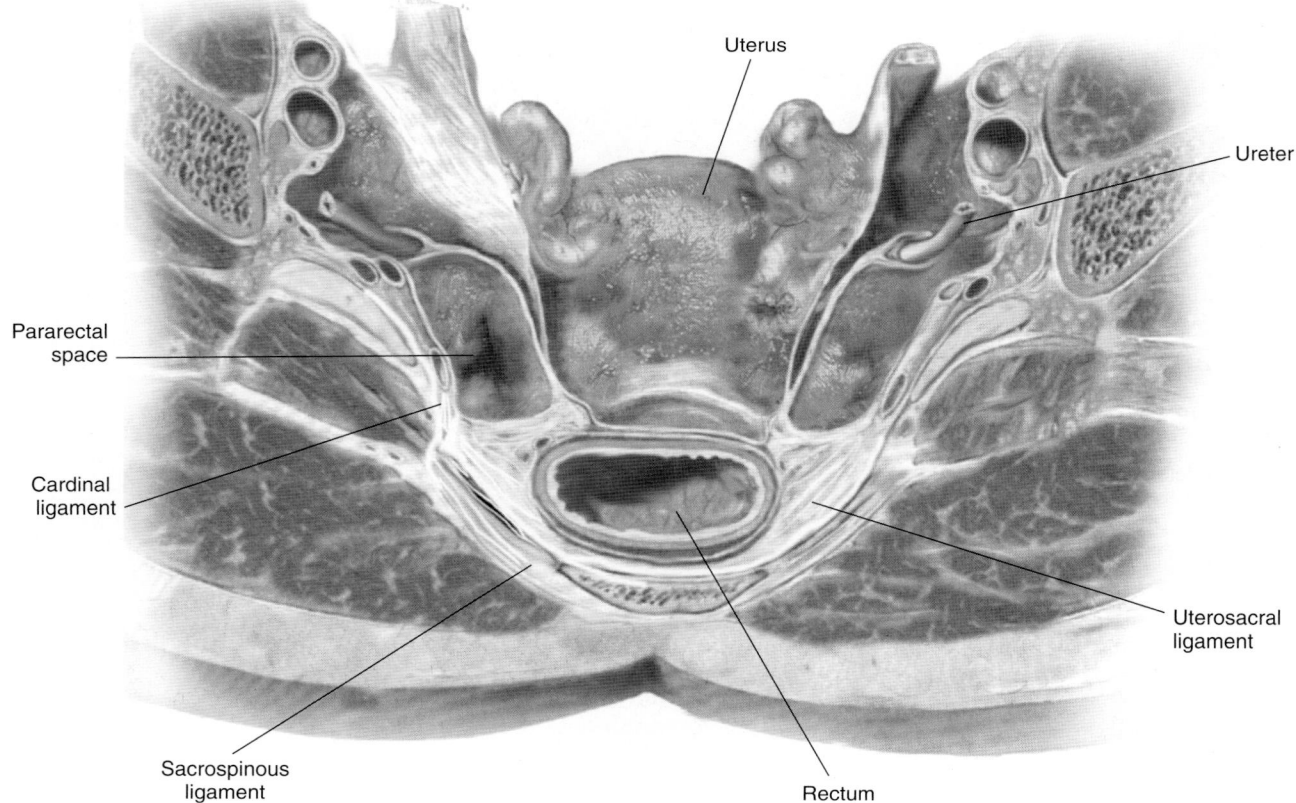

**FIGURE 9–4** Sagittal view of the posterior pelvis shows the uterosacral ligaments, sacrospinous ligaments, and cardinal ligaments and their relationships to the viscera. Note the position of the ureter from this perspective.

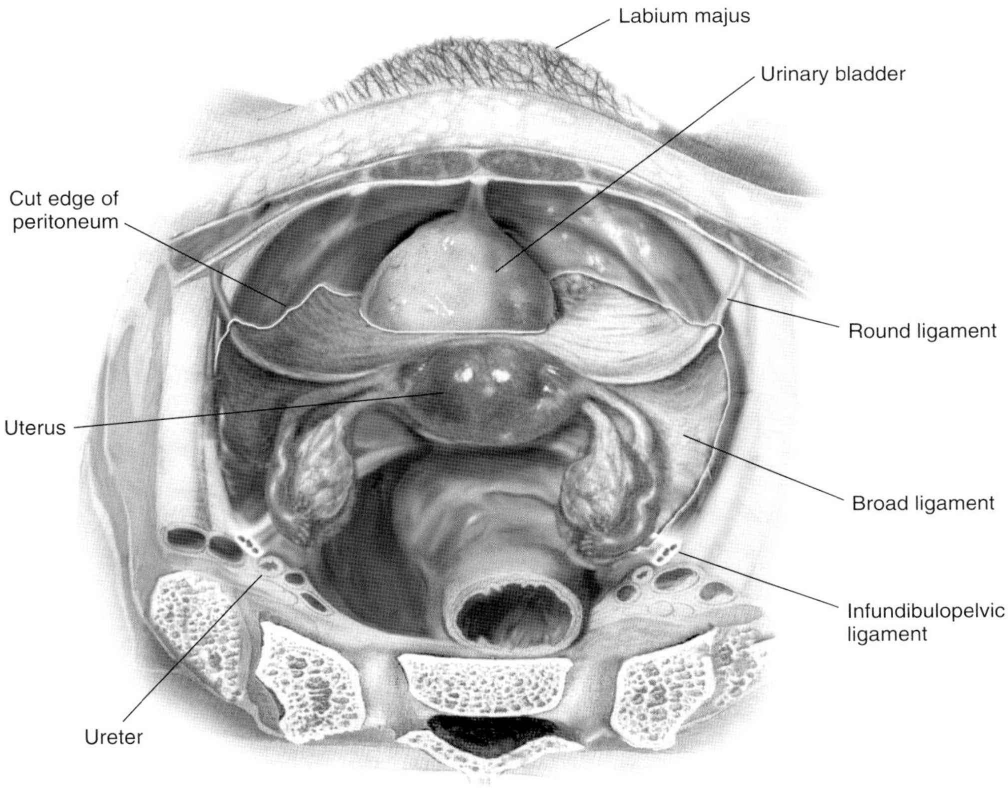

**FIGURE 9–5** The peritoneum has been opened, exposing the broad ligaments. This is the easiest portal of entry into the retroperitoneal space and the pelvic sidewall structures. The weblike fat contents are easily and bloodlessly dissected.

## Pelvic Anatomy

Exposure of extraperitoneal structures must be accomplished safely and expeditiously. Access to the left ureter, left iliac vessels, and left ovarian vessels can be gained by sharply incising the peritoneal sidewall attachment of the sigmoid colon; more extensive exposure is offered by continuing the separation of the descending colon from the psoas major muscle (Fig. 9–6A, B). Similarly, opening the top of the broad ligament between the round and infundibulopelvic ligaments lateral to the pulsation of the external iliac artery (i.e., over the psoas major muscle) provides easy access to both right and left sidewall/retroperitoneal spaces (Fig. 9–7A–C). After entry to the retroperitoneum is gained, exposure of the pelvic ureter and uterine vascular supply requires incision of the broad ligament (Fig. 9–8A–D).

The course of the ureter from the point where it enters the pelvis to the point where it enters the bladder consists of anatomic landmarks that every obstetrician-gynecologist must know. The greatest number of surgery-related injuries to the ureter happens to the segment between the uterine artery crossing point and bladder entry. The uterine artery crosses the lower third of the pelvic ureter obliquely lateral and cephalad to the uterus. The ureter may be crossed again by the inferior vesical artery as it enters the bladder. The vaginal artery lies behind the ureter. The distal ureter is exceedingly close to anterolateral fornix of the vagina (Fig. 9–9A–I).

The ureters gain entry to the pelvis by crossing lateromedially over the psoas muscle; they cross the common iliac vessels at the point where the external and internal iliac arteries bifurcate (Fig. 9–10). The ureter descends into the pelvis medial to the internal iliac artery (hypogastric artery) and obturator fossa (Fig. 9–11). Its course is consistently one of deep descent and medial swing, particularly after the uterine artery crosses over it (superior and anterior). The entire course of the right ureter can be seen in Figure 9–12.

The left ureteral course is complicated by the position of the sigmoid colon overlying it and the presence of the inferior mesenteric vessels that supply the left colon (see Fig. 9–7A, B). The left ureter crosses the common iliac artery in concert with the ovarian arteries and descends into the pelvis, following a similar course to the right ureter. The ovarian vessels cross the common iliac in concert with the ureter. The ureter is behind the ovarian vascular pedicle and slightly medial to it (Figs. 9–13A–D and 9–14A).

The arterial blood supply to pelvic structures emanates from the abdominal aorta, which branches into right and left common iliac vessels at the L4–L5 vertebral level (Figs. 9–14B and 9–15 through 9–18A). To the right of the aortic bifurcation lies the origin of the inferior vena cava. The cava is formed by the union of left and right common iliac veins (Fig. 9–18B). The left common iliac veins cross in front of (anterior to) the sacrum within the bifurcation of the aorta and under the right common iliac artery to join the right common iliac vein, which lies posterior to the right common iliac artery (Figs. 9–18C, D). The inferior mesenteric artery arises from the *lower* left side of the abdominal aorta, giving off numerous branches to the left colon and sigmoid.

Following bifurcation, the external iliac artery assumes a relatively superficial position just medial to the psoas major muscle (Fig. 9–19). The external iliac vein is considerably larger than the artery and lies beneath (posterior to) it. The vein covers the entrance to the obturator fossa, which can be exposed by carefully retracting the vein upward (Fig. 9–20). The fossa is demarcated by the obturator nerve and artery, which cross through this fat-laden space whose lateral boundary is the obturator internus muscle (see Figs. 9–20A–C and 9–21). The obturator neurovascular bundle leaves the pelvis and enters the thigh medially via the obturator foramen (Fig. 9–22A, B).

The major portion of the pelvic blood supply is derived from the hypogastric vessels (internal iliac arteries and veins), which branch within the obturator fossa (Fig. 9–23). Curiously, the major risk in dissecting the fossa is related to the numerous and anomalous veins that occupy the lateral floor of the fossa (Fig. 9–24). The hypogastric artery branches into anterior and posterior divisions. The posterior division plunges down into the deep recesses of the pelvis toward the ischial spine, in turn branching into a large superior gluteal artery and a smaller lateral sacral artery (Fig. 9–25). These are important sources for collateral pelvic circulation. The anterior division gives branches to the bladder, uterus, vagina, obturator, and internus and pectineus muscles, and terminates in the inferior gluteal and internal pudendal arteries.

During simple or radical hysterectomy, an understanding of the relationships of the structures mentioned earlier is vital to avoiding unnecessary blood loss and injury (Figs. 9–26 and 9–27).

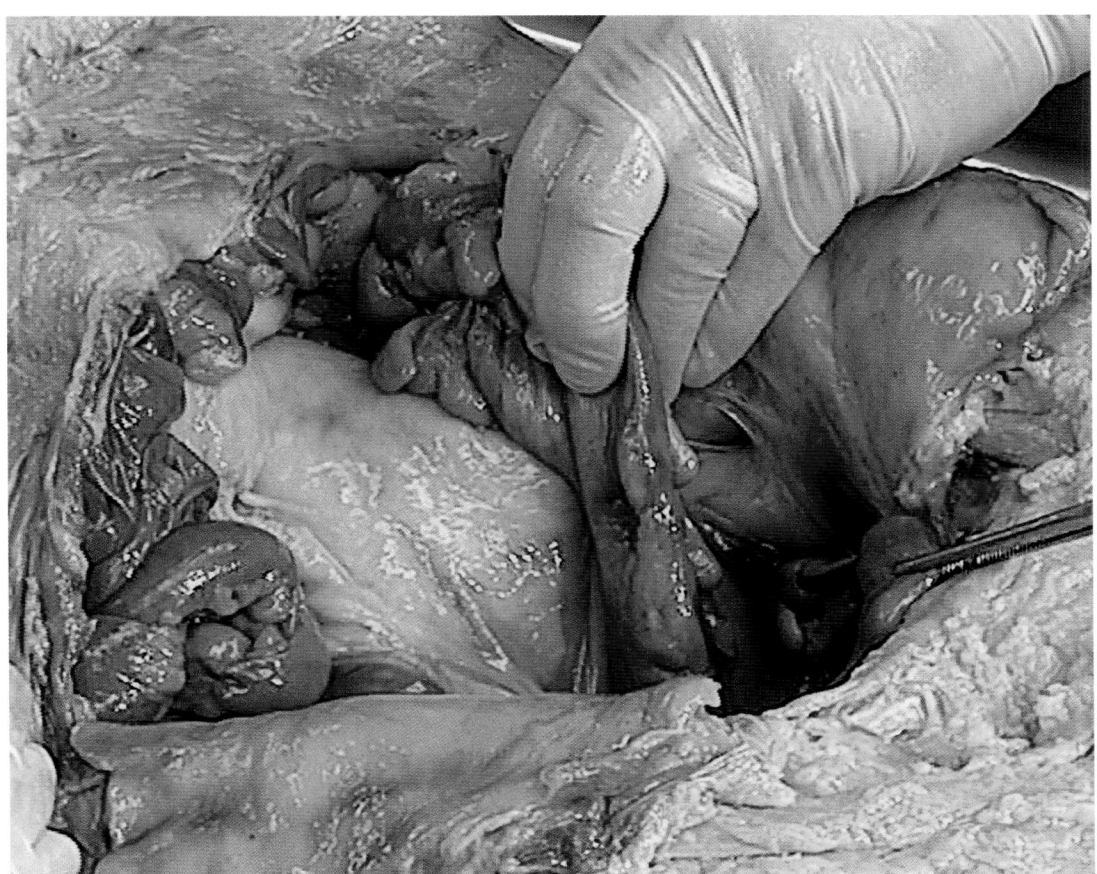

A

B

FIGURE 9–6 A. The uterus is pulled up and forward with a long Kocher clamp. The left tube and ovary are seen to lie deep in the pelvis. The sigmoid colon has been elevated and pulled medially to expose the left adnexa. B. The attachments of the sigmoid colon to the parietal peritoneum of the left abdominal wall and gutter are clearly in view as traction is placed on the sigmoid colon in the direction of the midline. Typically, the sigmoid colon overlies the left adnexa, which is attached to the parietal peritoneum via the ovarian vascular pedicle (infundibulopelvic ligament).

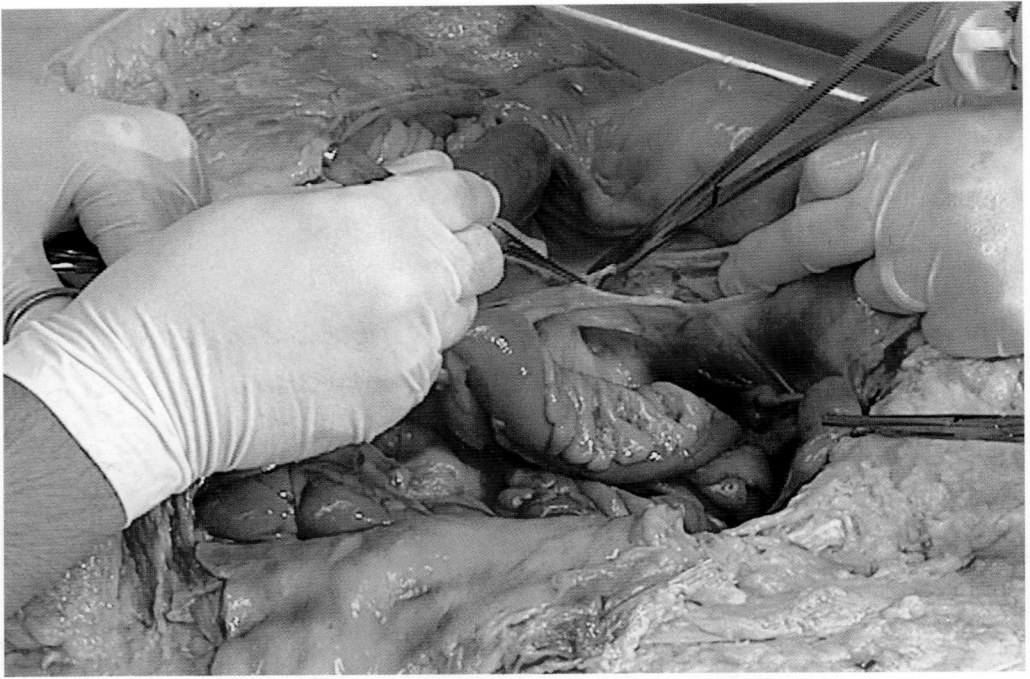

A

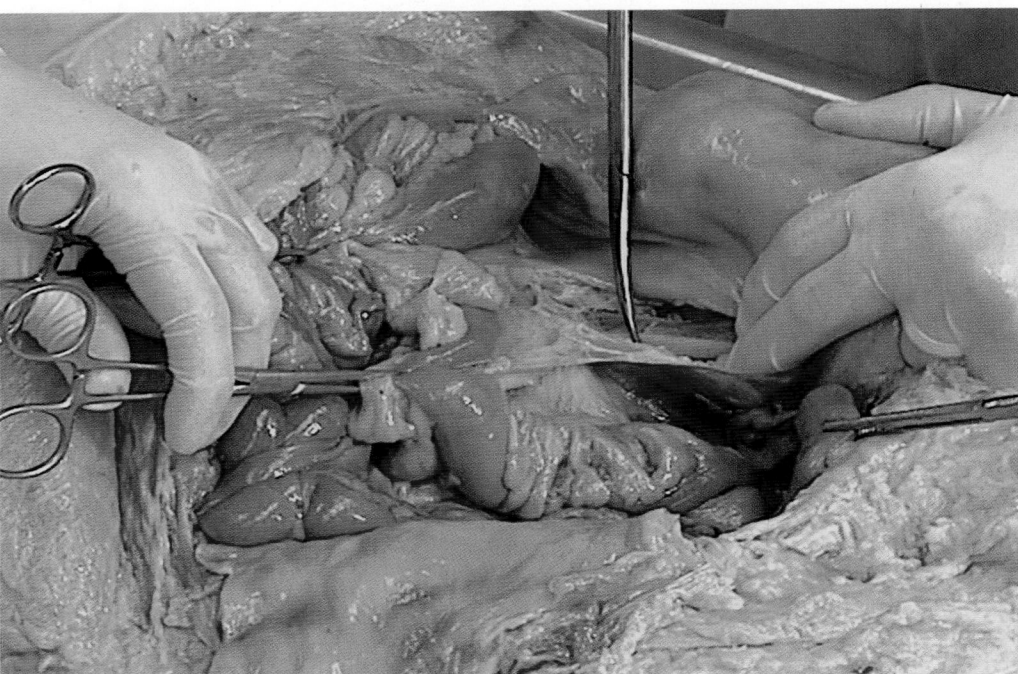

B

**FIGURE 9–7** **A.** The peritoneal attachments of the sigmoid and descending colon have been cut. The retroperitoneal space has been entered on the left side. **B.** Further dissection permits mobilization of the sigmoid colon, and excellent exposure of the psoas major muscle intersects with the sigmoid colon to create an almost perfect 90° angle.

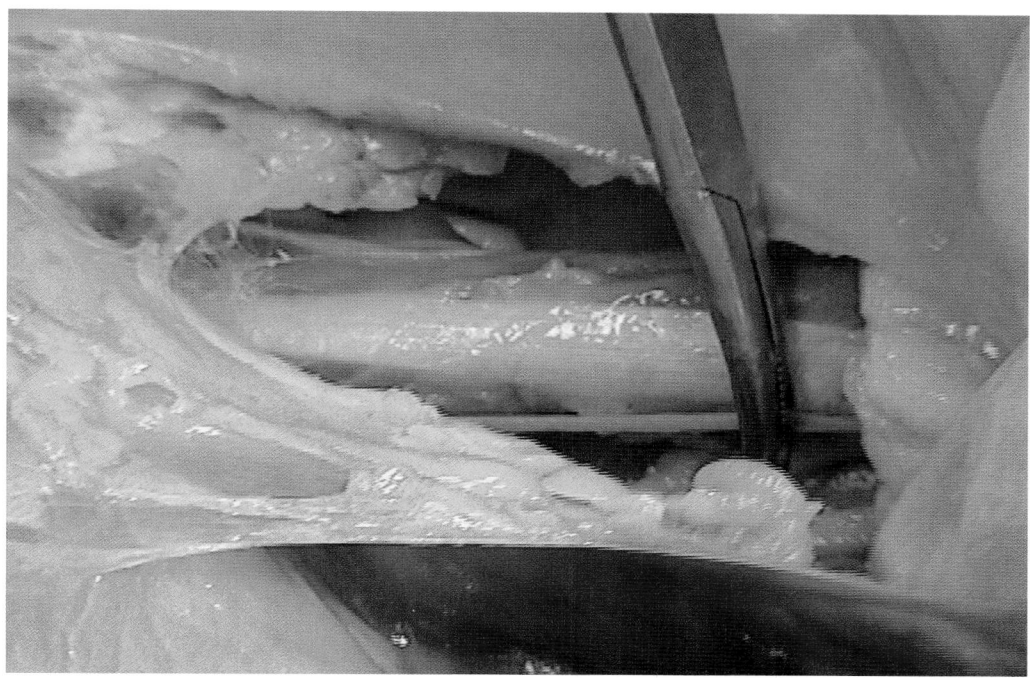

C

**FIGURE 9–7, cont'd  C.** The psoas major muscle and the psoas minor tendon as well as the genitofemoral nerve are exposed as a result of incising and dissecting the sigmoid colon peritoneal attachments.

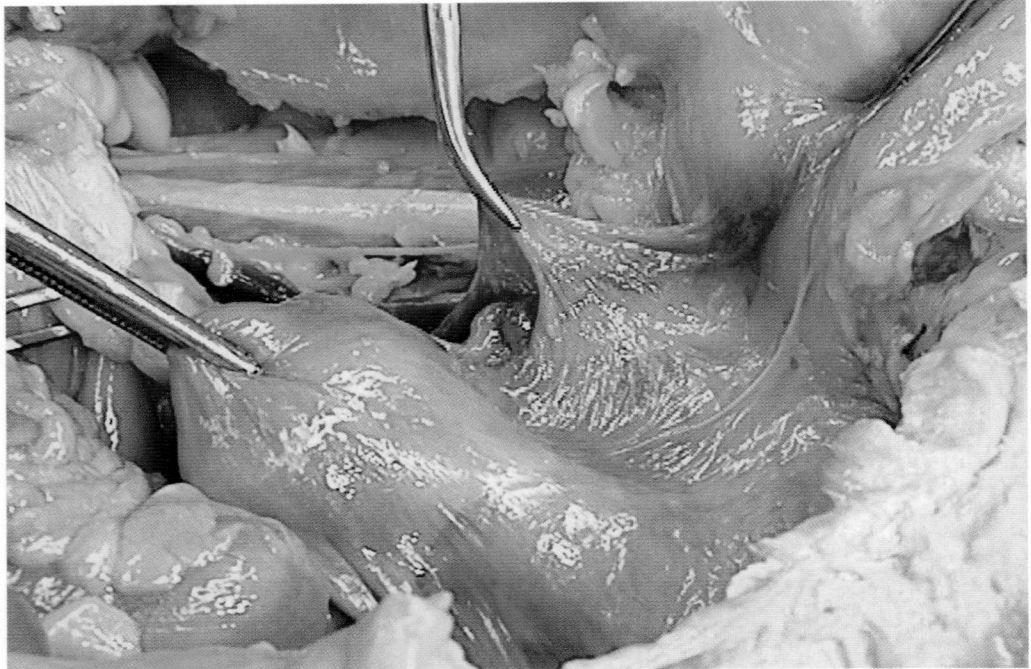

A

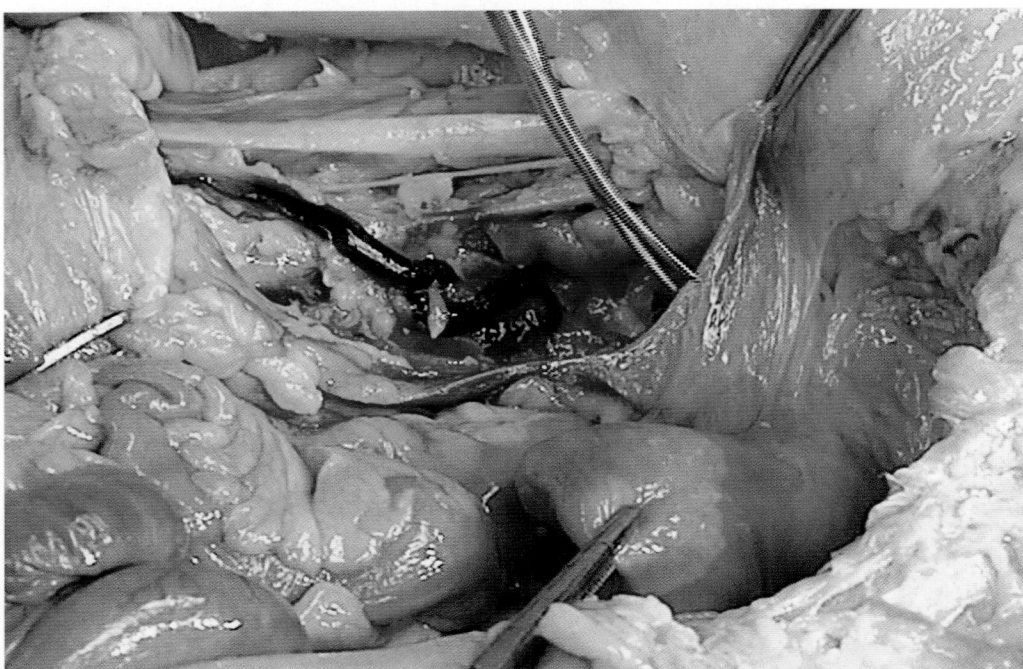

B

**FIGURE 9–8 A.** The uterus has been placed on traction by elevating the fundal clamp and pulling cranially. The tonsil clamp to the left exposes the left broad ligament. **B.** The left ureter (hemorrhagic) crosses the common iliac artery and descends into the pelvis medial to the internal iliac (hypogastric) artery. The uterus is pulled to the right and the left broad ligament is likewise placed on traction for subsequent incision.

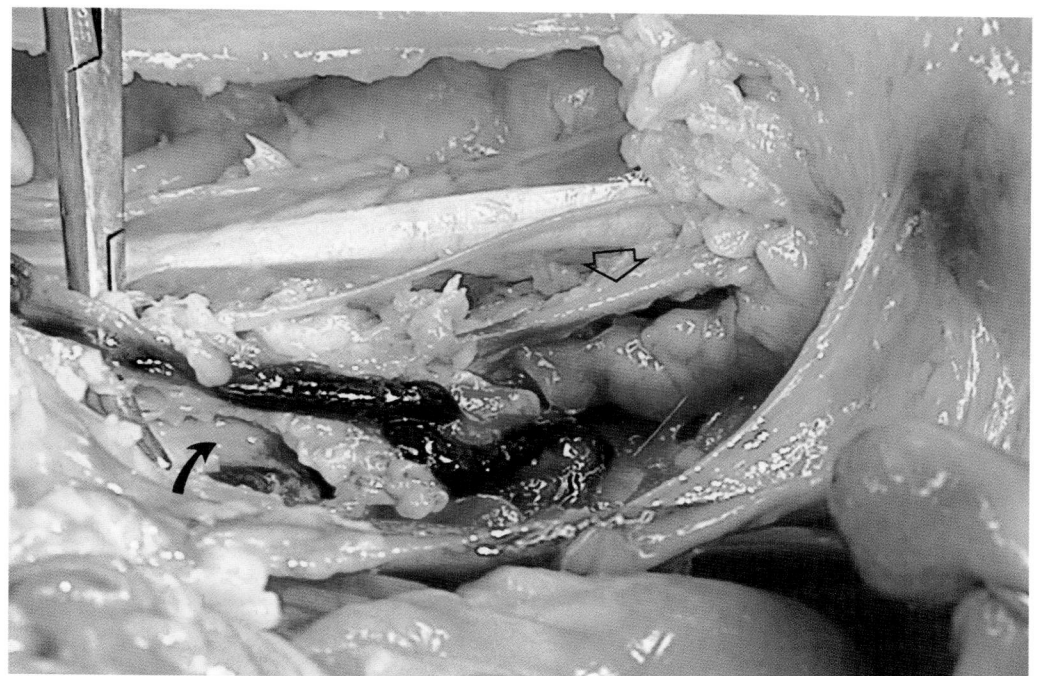

C

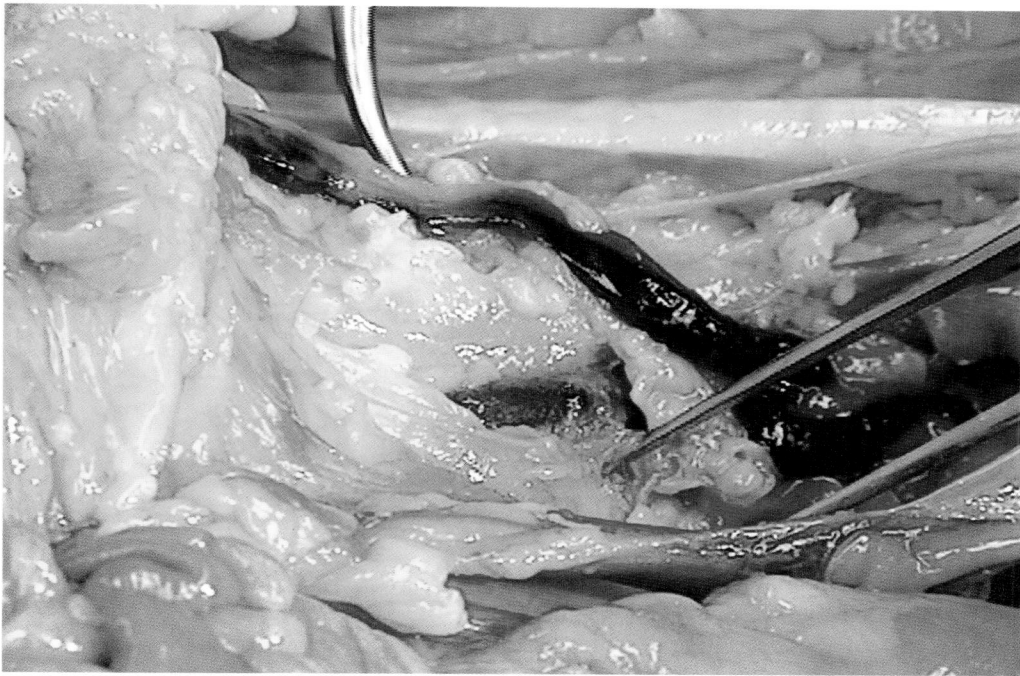

D

**FIGURE 9–8, cont'd  C.** Close-up view of the left ureter (above the clamp and hemorrhagic) crossing the left common iliac artery (*arrow*). Note the left external iliac artery just medial to the psoas major muscle (*open arrow*). **D.** Immediately above the forceps, the dark blue common iliac vein is visible. It lies below the common iliac artery.

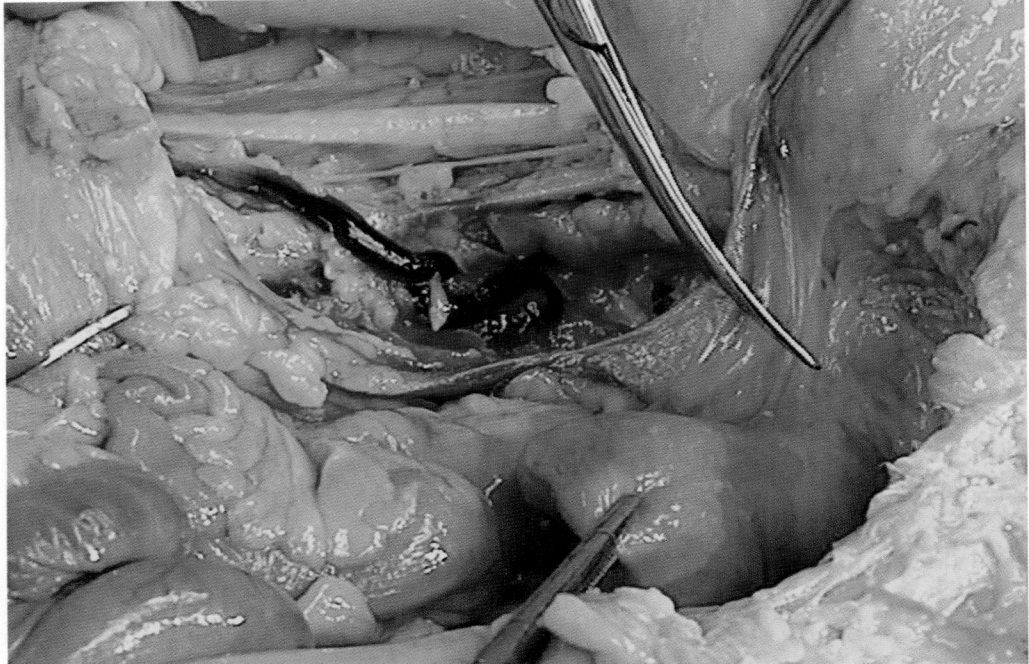

A

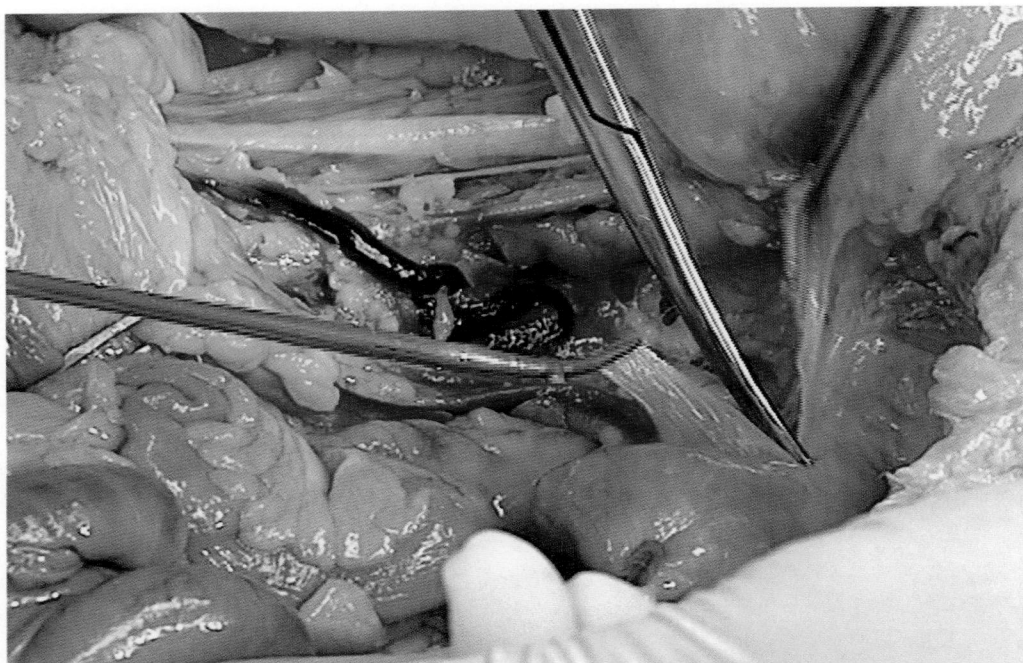

B

**FIGURE 9–9  A.** The broad ligament is cut with Metzenbaum scissors. **B.** The incision is carried downward to the cervicocorporal junction of the uterus.

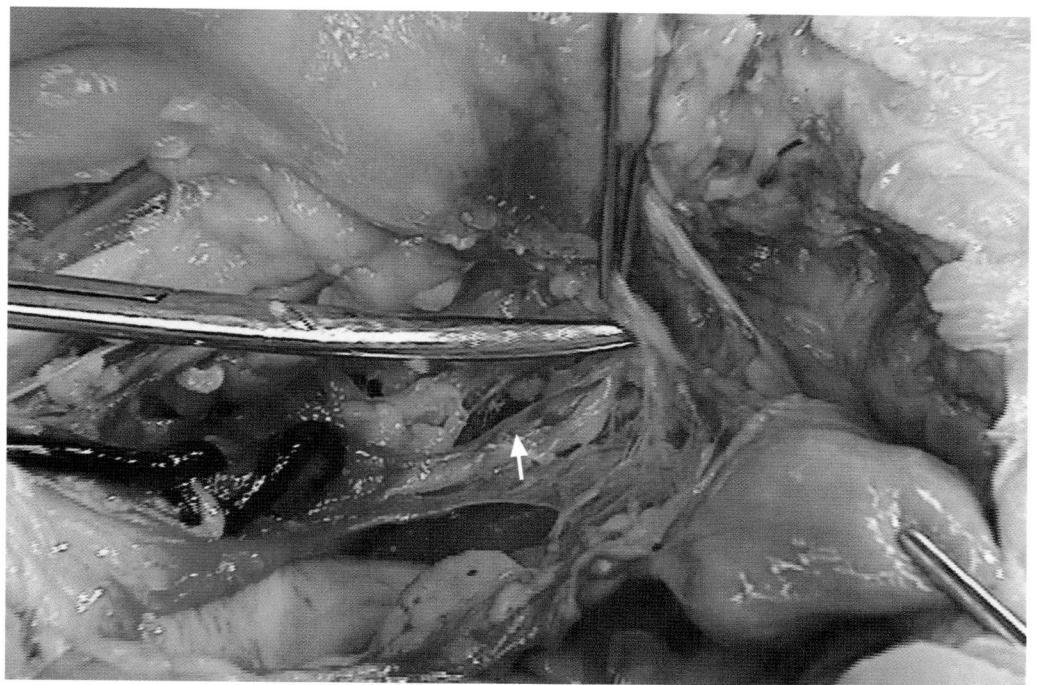

C

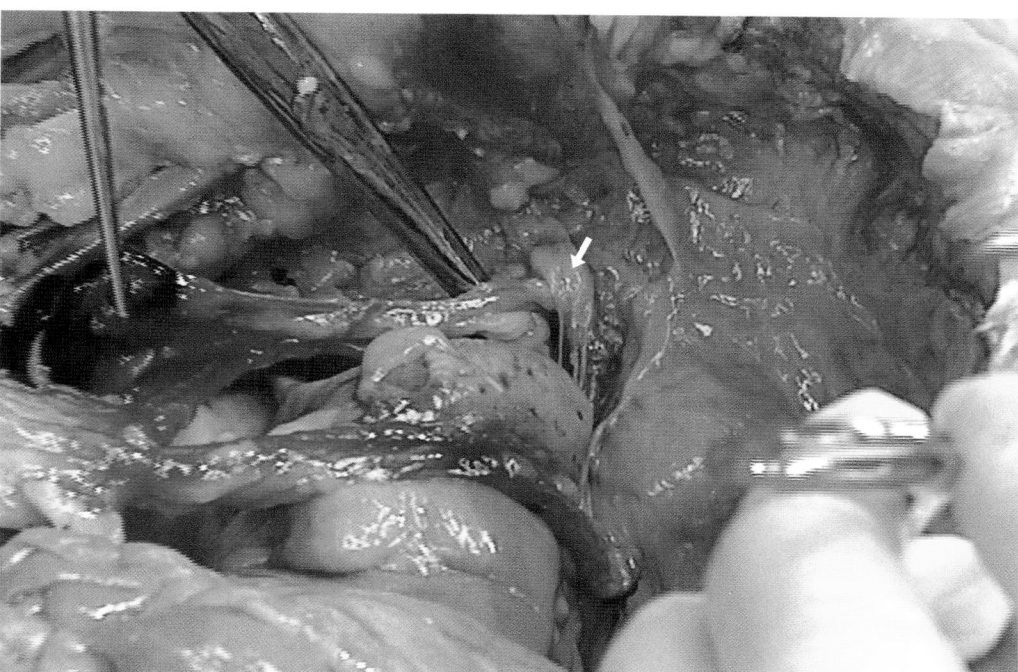

D

**FIGURE 9–9, cont'd   C.** The uterine vessels are exposed and isolated with the use of Metzenbaum scissors. The ureter is crossing beneath the uterine vessels (*arrow*). The uterus is twisted to the right and is held in a Kocher clamp (*lower right corner of the photograph*). **D.** The broad ligament is completely opened. The view is from directly above looking down. The scissors are beneath the left ureter. The ureter is crossing under the uterine vessels (*arrow*).

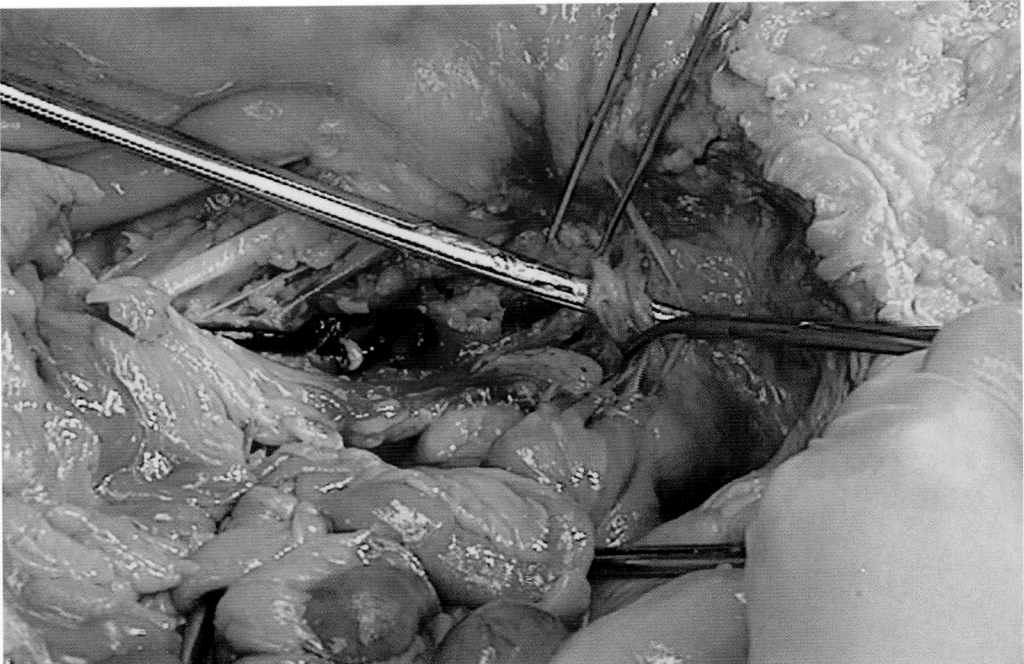

E

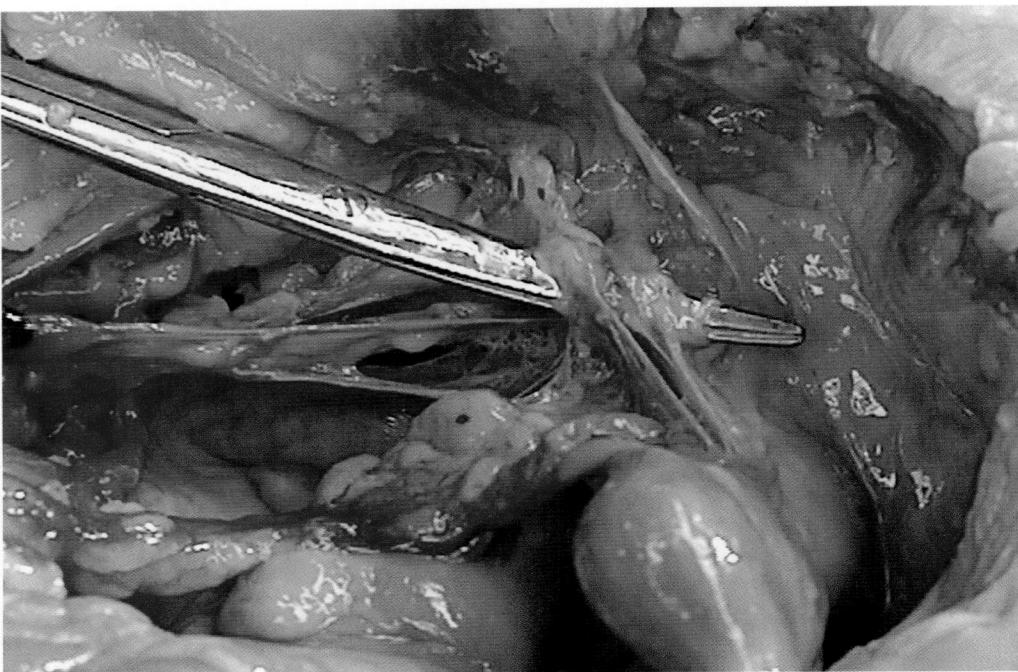

F

**FIGURE 9–9, cont'd   E.** The uterine vessels are isolated. The Metzenbaum scissors have dissected a space between the uterine vessels and the ureter. The tonsil clamp has been placed across the vessels at the side of the uterus. **F.** Detail of the dissection shown in Figure 9–9E. The ureter is directly under the blades of the scissors.

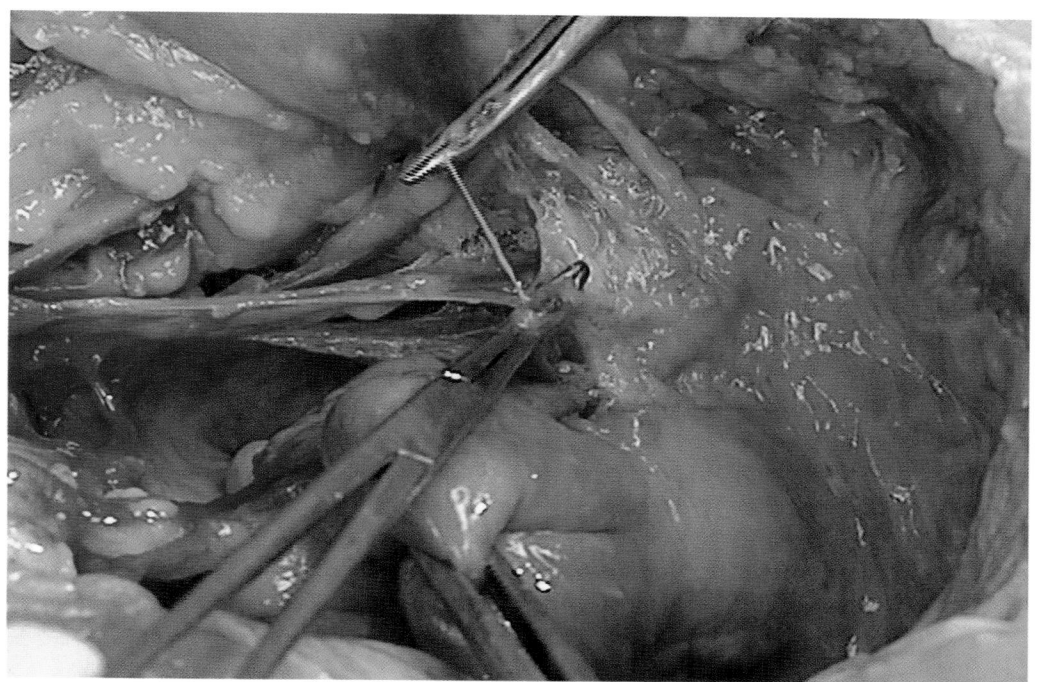

G

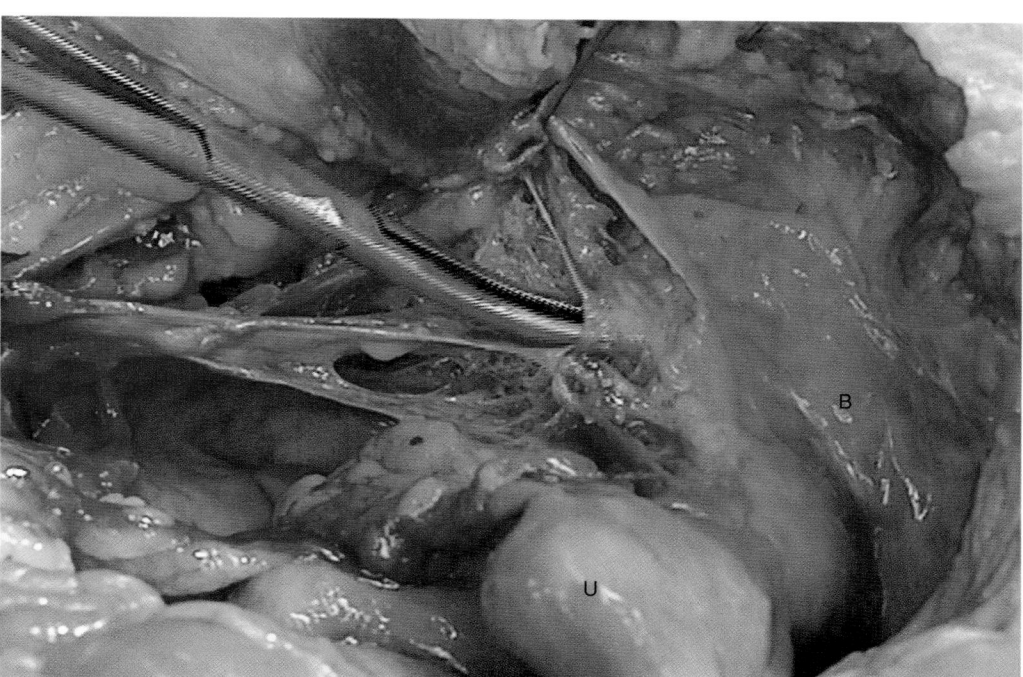

H

**FIGURE 9–9, cont'd   G.** The uterine vessels have been clamped with tonsil clamps and cut to expose the underlying ureter. **H.** The ureteral dissection is continued to the point where it enters the urinary bladder (B). The uterus is labeled U.

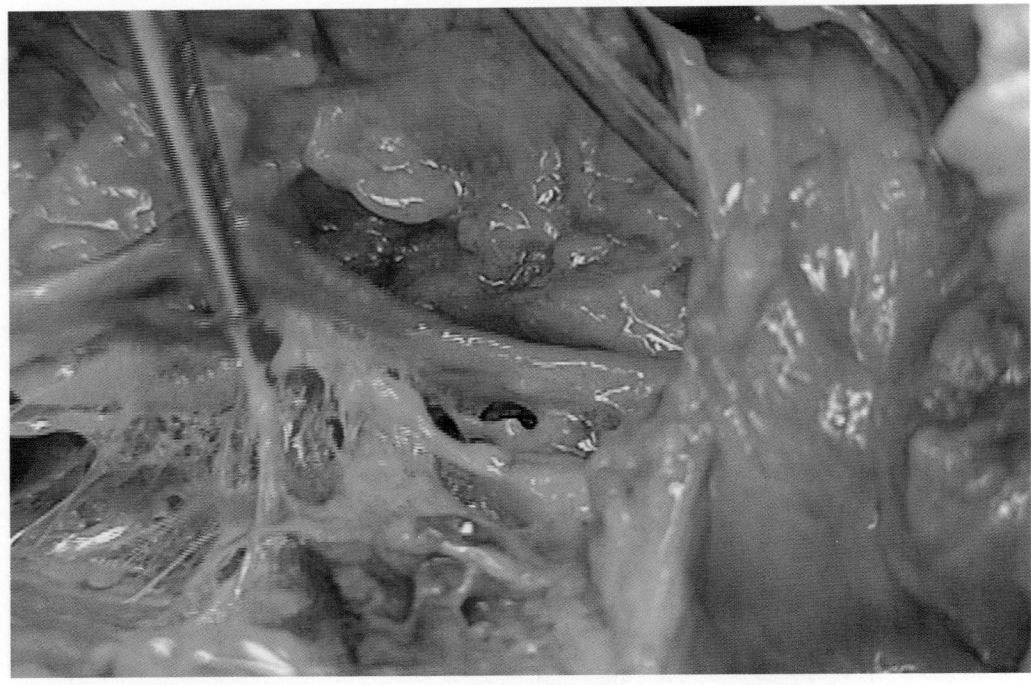

I

**FIGURE 9–9, cont'd  I.** Magnified view of the ureter entering the bladder. The forceps is grasping the ureter at the point where the uterine vessels had previously crossed above.

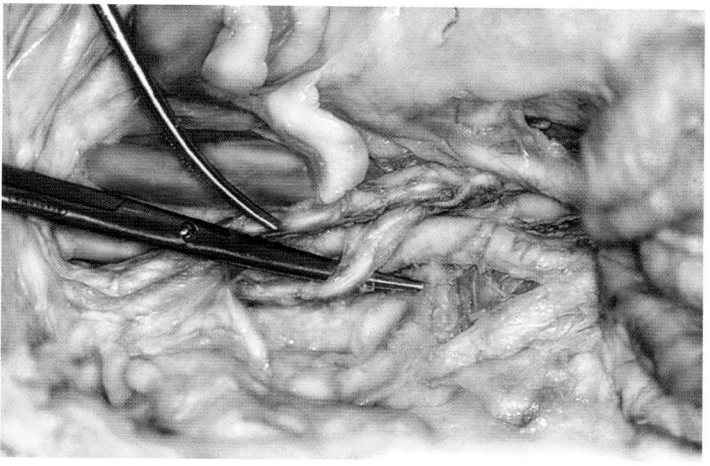

FIGURE 9–10 The scissors separate the right ureter from the ovarian vessels (grasped by the clamp). Both structures cross the common iliac vessels to enter the pelvis. Note that the tip of the scissors points to the left common iliac vein as it crosses the sacrum. It will unite with the right common iliac vein to form the inferior vena cava, which is seen to the right of the bifurcation of the aorta.

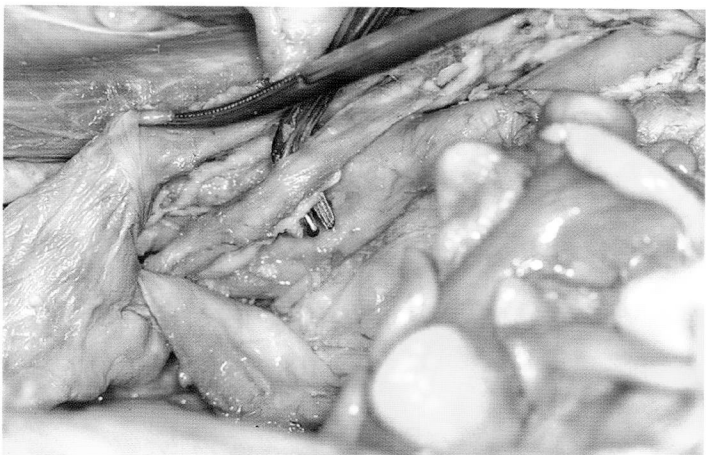

FIGURE 9–11 A right-angle clamp retracts the ureter to expose the bifurcation of the right common iliac artery into external (*above*) and internal (*below*) iliac arteries. Note the blue vena cava to the right of the common iliac artery (*upper right corner of photograph*).

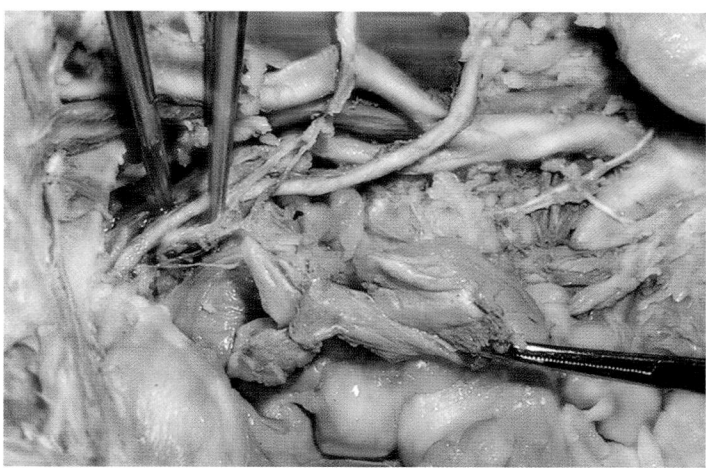

FIGURE 9–12 The entire course of the right ureter is seen from the point where it crosses the common iliac artery to its entry into the urinary bladder. The lateral clamp points to the vaginal artery. The medial clamp is directly in front of the uterine artery, where it crosses over the ureter. The sigmoid colon is covering the small uterus.

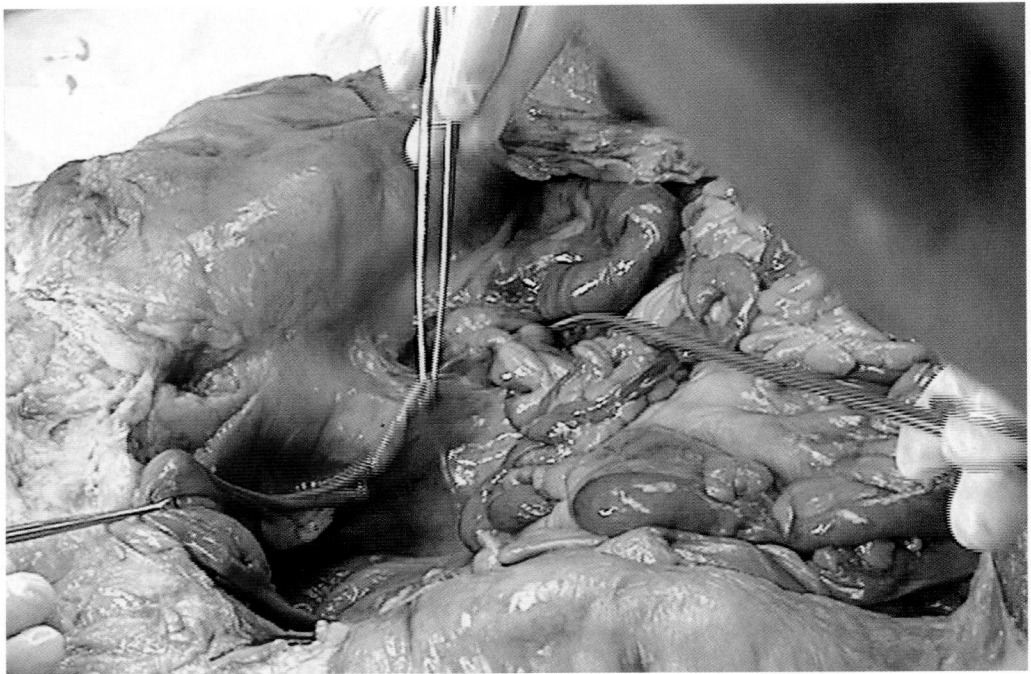

A

B

**FIGURE 9–13  A.** The uterus is held on traction with a clamp. The forceps elevate the extension of the ovarian vascular pedicle to the retrocecal area. The tonsil clamp rests on the cecum. **B.** The enlarged view details the method by which the surgeon can extend the location of the ovarian pedicle into the retroperitoneum. Because the ureter is closely applied to the ovarian vessels (i.e., posterior and slightly medial), the surgeon can anticipate how a safe dissection to locate the ureter should proceed.

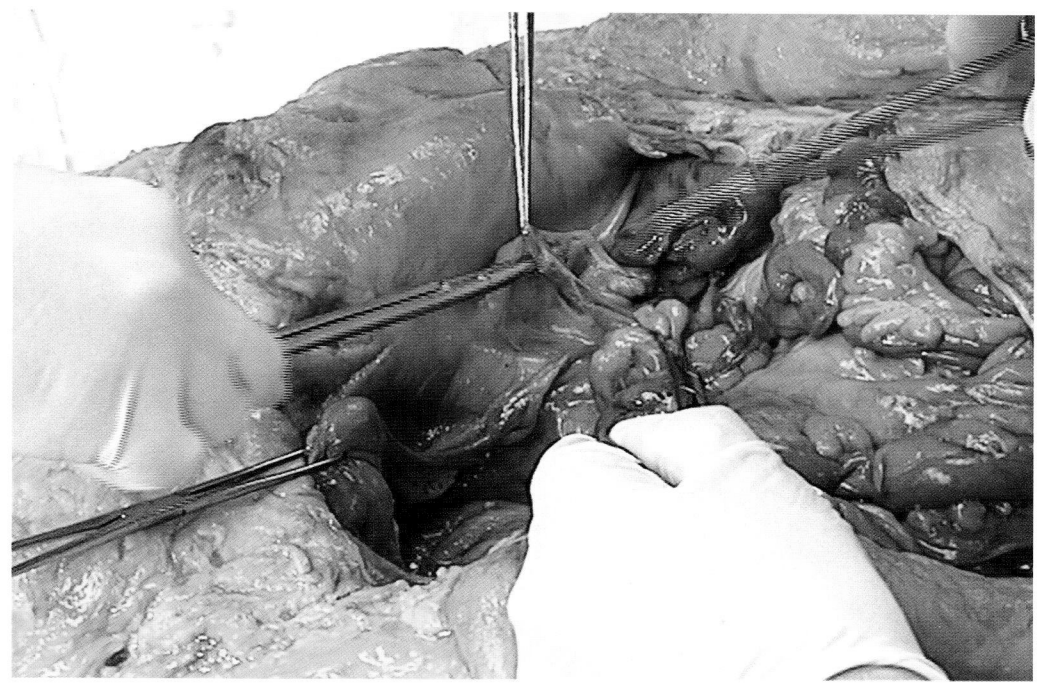

C

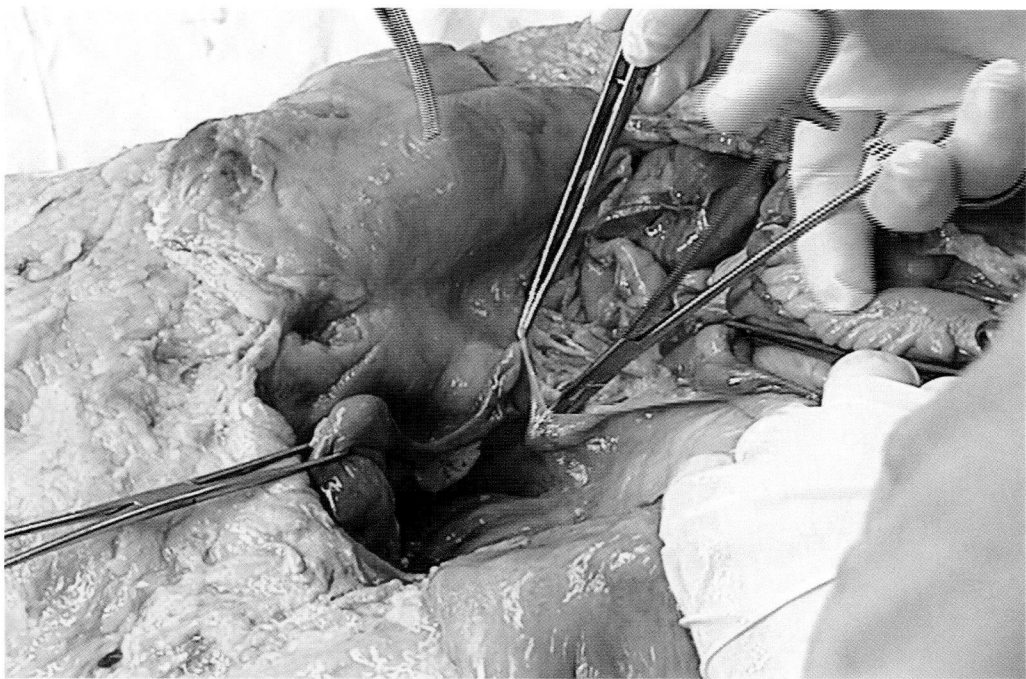

D

**FIGURE 9–13, cont'd  C.** The cecum is mobilized by cutting its peritoneal attachments and extending the incision cranially via the right gutter. The ureter and ovarian vessels cling together at the pelvic brim. **D.** The incision is carried carefully to the medial aspect of the ureter.

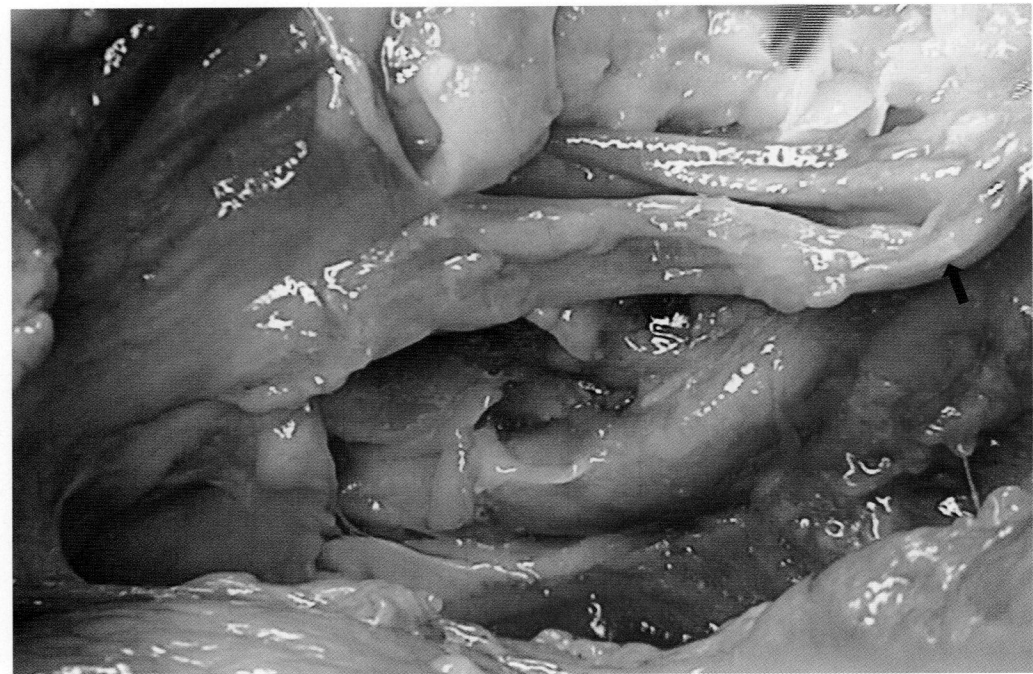

A

B

**FIGURE 9–14  A.** The ureter is traced caudally to the point where it crosses the common iliac artery. This picture shows the ureter (*arrow*) and the common iliac bifurcation. **B.** The ureter (*white arrow at top of photo*) has been retracted above the common iliac bifurcation. The tip of the tonsil clamp rests on the external iliac artery. The hypogastric artery (H) is quite large. At the "crotch" between the iliac arteries lies the external iliac vein (V), which is joined by the internal (hypogastric) iliac vein (located deep to the hypogastric artery) to form the common iliac vein.

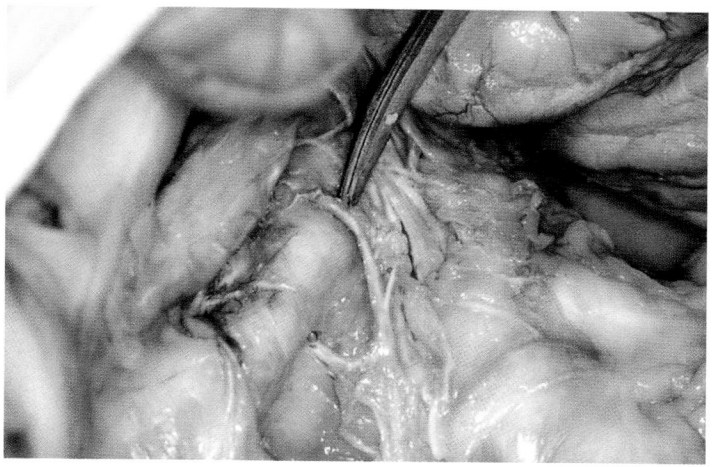

**FIGURE 9–15** The clamp rests on the aorta at its bifurcation. The hypogastric nerves are draped over the vessels.

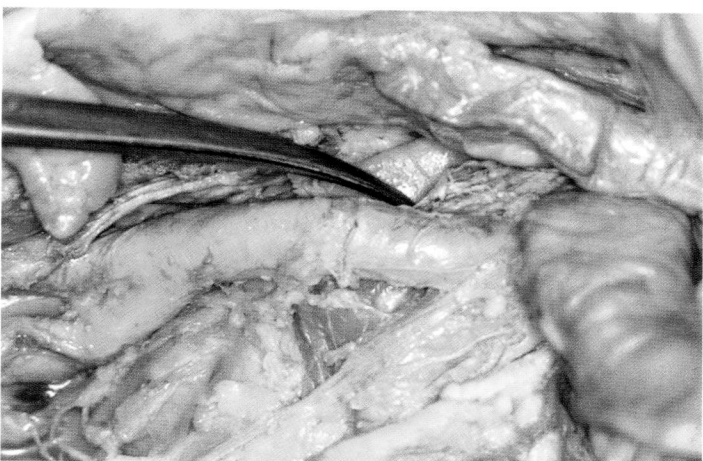

**FIGURE 9–16** The scissors rest on the inferior vena cava. The large left common iliac vein crosses the sacrum to join the right common iliac vein (barely seen lateral to the artery) to form the inferior vena cava.

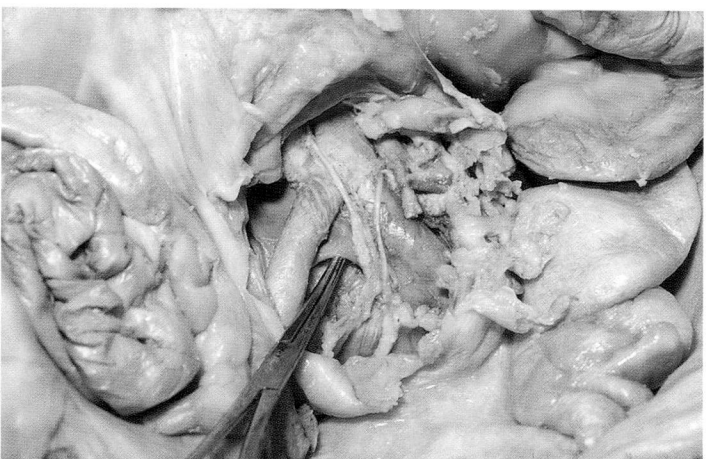

**FIGURE 9–17** A view from the foot of the table. The clamp is under the left common iliac vein. Note the middle sacral vessels partially obscured by the hypogastric plexus. The vena cava is seen to the right of the aorta and the right common iliac artery. The sacrum is just beneath the clamp.

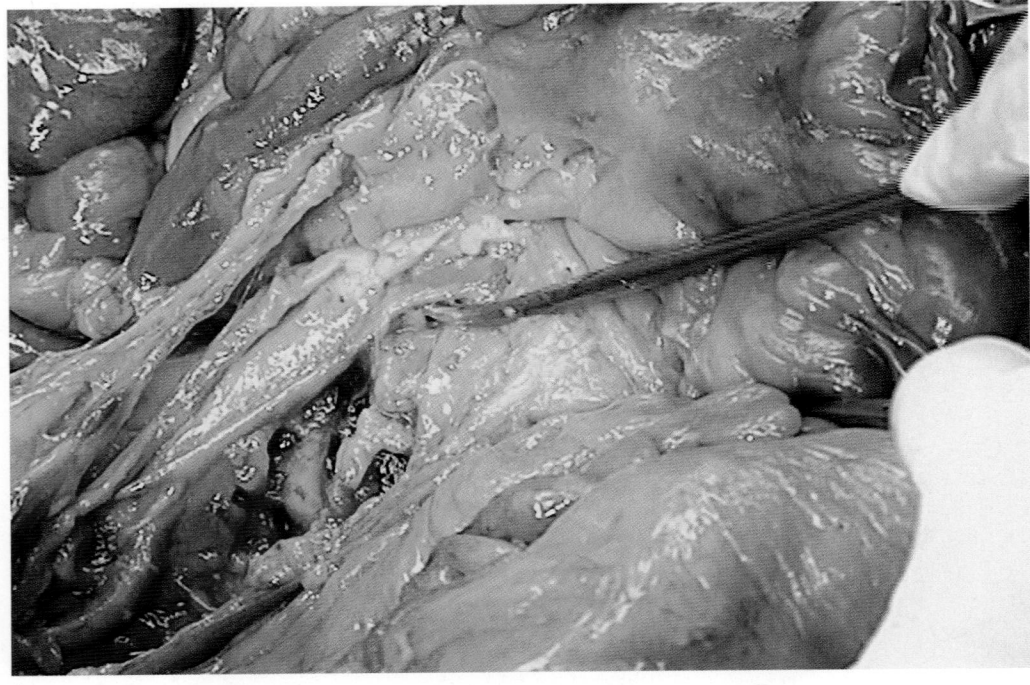

A

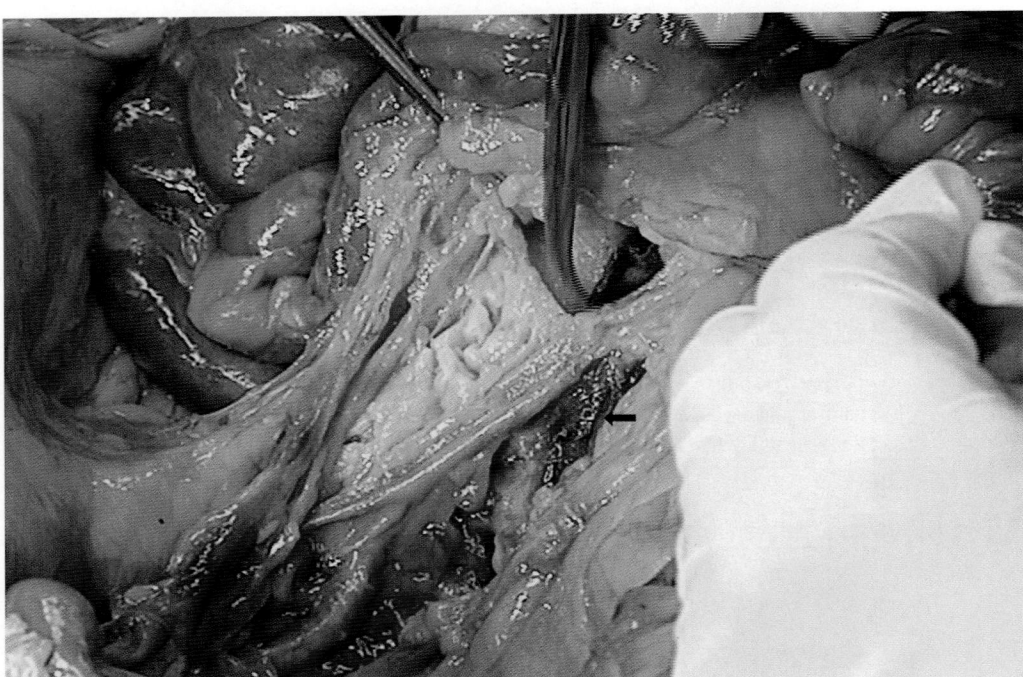

B

**FIGURE 9–18  A.** The clamp rests on the bifurcation of the aorta. The right common iliac artery is lifted up by the tonsil clamp. **B.** The inferior vena cava lies to the right of the aortic bifurcation. The arrow points to the left common iliac vein. Note whether the presacral space has been exposed by incising the peritoneum and retracting the sigmoid colon to the left. The clamp points to the inferior vena cava.

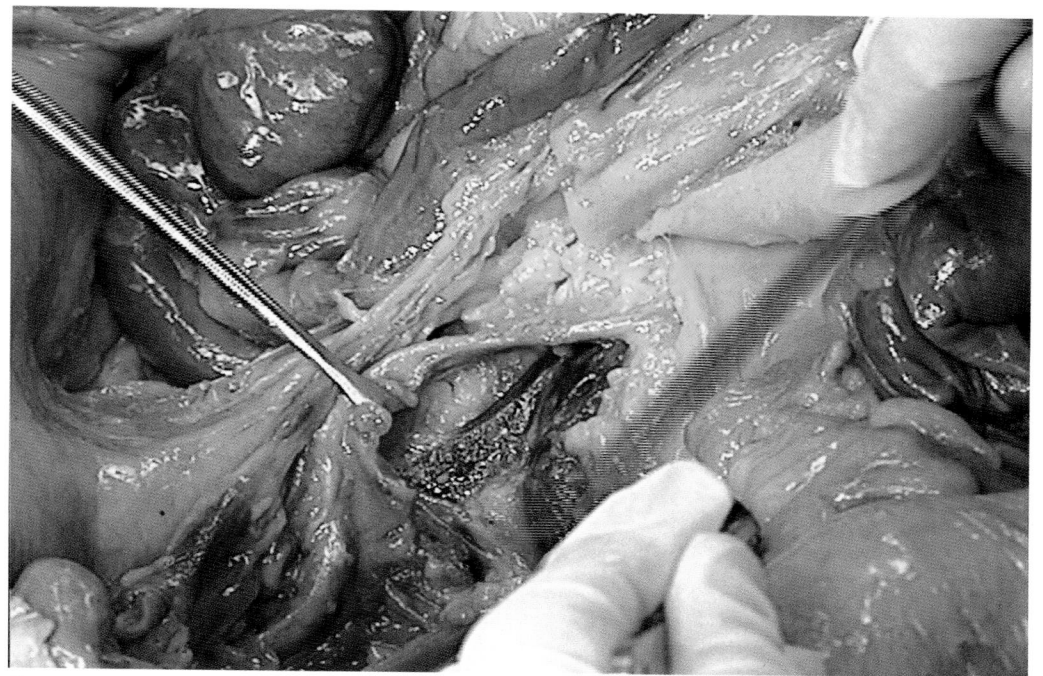

C

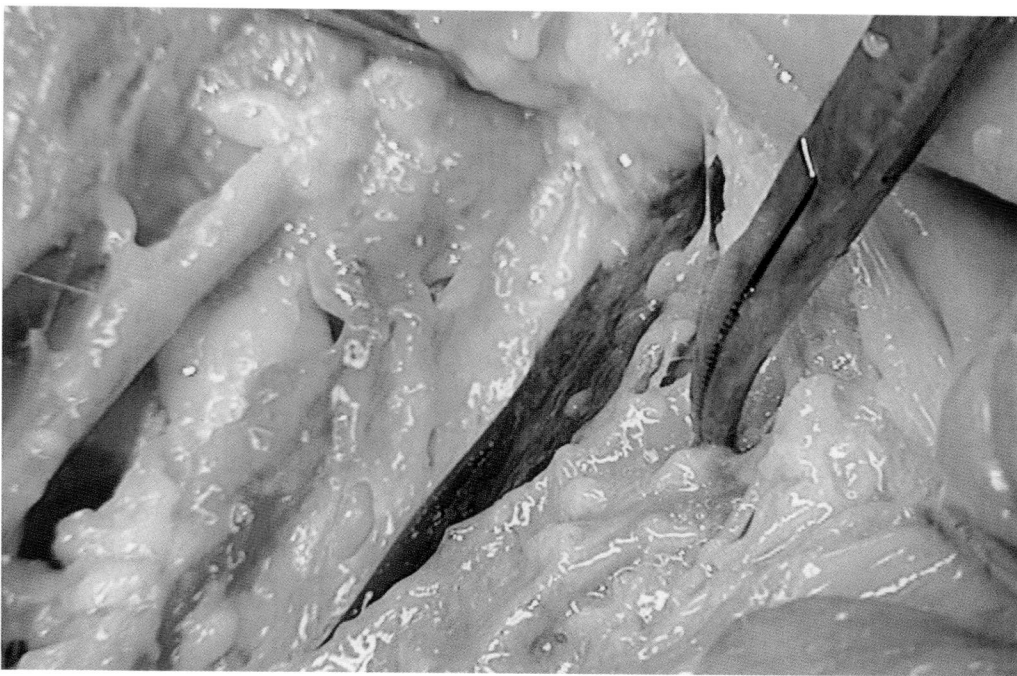

D

**FIGURE 9–18, cont'd  C.** The Allis clamp grasps the edge of the posterior parietal peritoneum as the presacral space is entered. The left common iliac vein is the first structure that must be identified. The left iliac vein joins the right to form the vena cava, as is shown here. **D.** The clamp points to the aorta immediately cranial to the bifurcation. The inferior vena cava is to the right of the aorta.

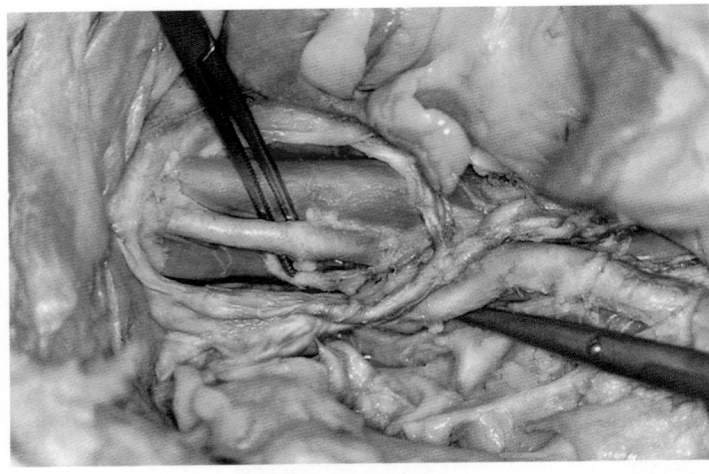

**FIGURE 9–19** The clamp dissects the right external iliac artery and lies between the artery and the blue right external iliac vein. The tip of the scissors lies beneath the right common hypogastric artery. The ureter, together with the infundibulopelvic ligament, crosses the vessels.

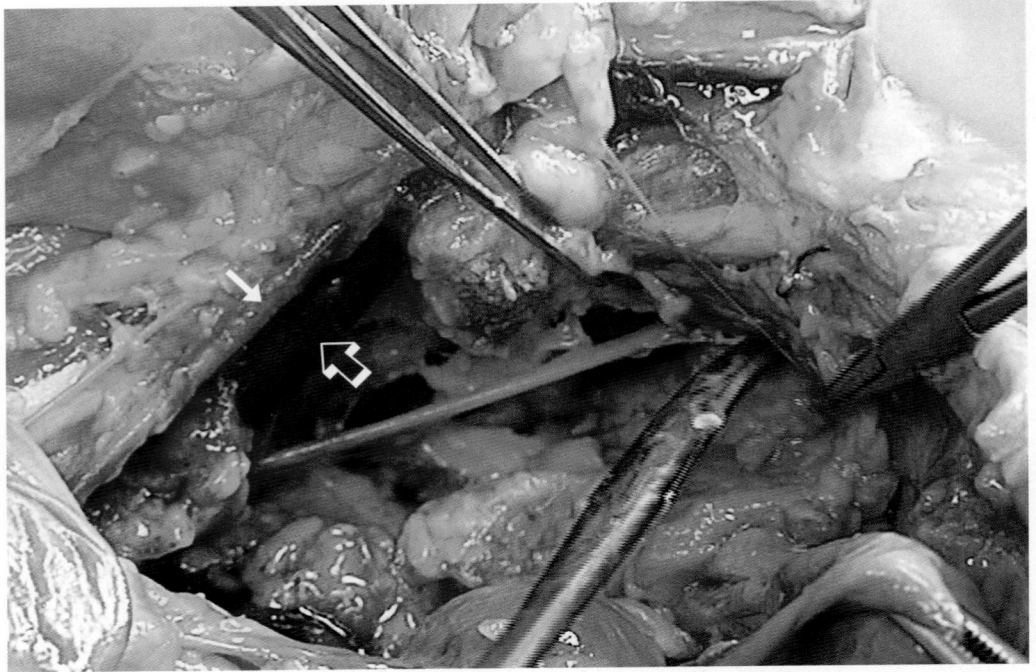

A

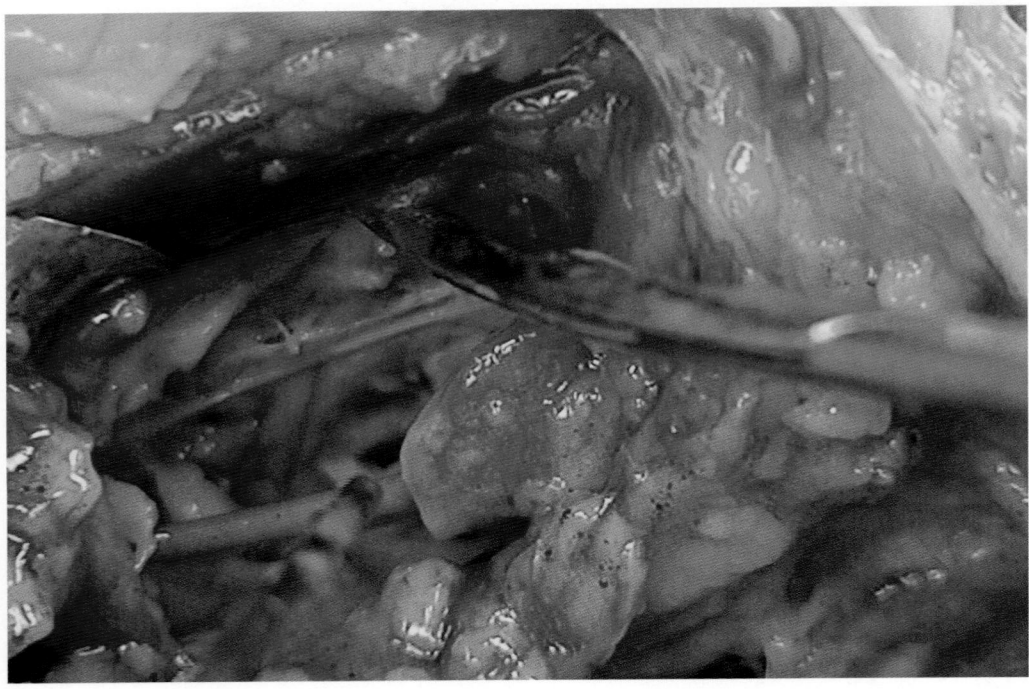

B

**FIGURE 9–20  A.** The obturator fossa has been cleared of fat. The external iliac artery (*white arrow*) and vein (*open arrow*) are seen in the background. The obturator nerve stretches across the fossa. **B.** The external iliac vein is held by a vein retractor. The scissors tip is directly under the vein. The obturator nerve and artery cross the space (fossa).

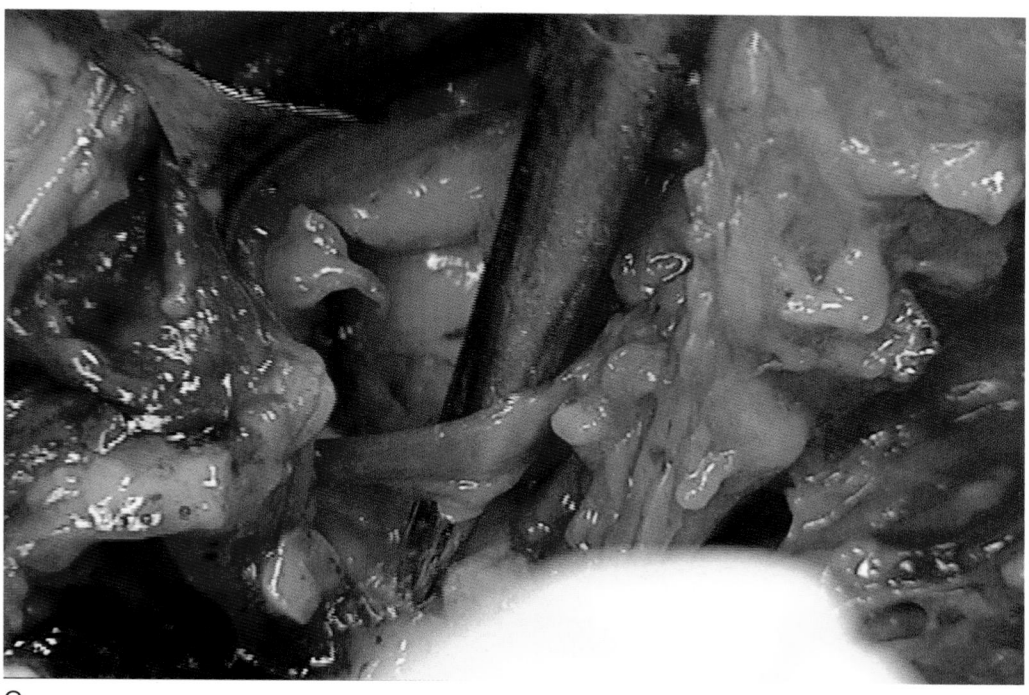

C

**FIGURE 9–20, cont'd  C.** Magnified view of vein held in the retractor (*upper left*) and scissors dissecting the obturator nerve.

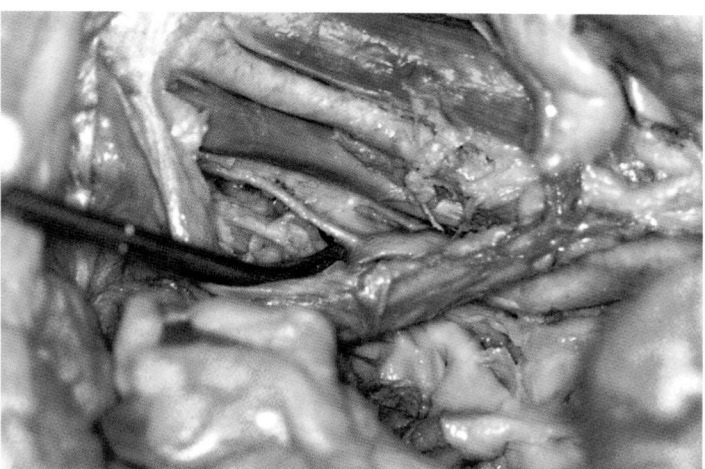

**FIGURE 9–21** The right obturator fossa has been exposed. Under most circumstances, the external iliac vein would require upward traction via a vein retractor. The clamp rests under the obturator artery, which is a branch of the anterior division of the hypogastric artery.

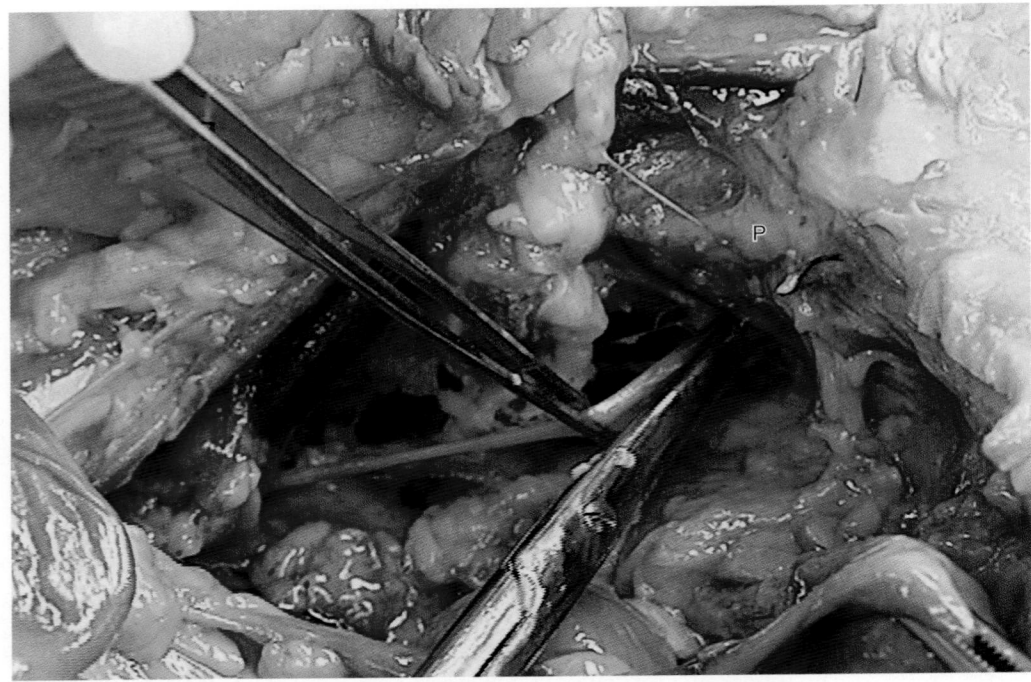

A

B

**FIGURE 9–22  A.** The nerve and vessels leave the obturator fossa via the obturator foramen (tip of scissors). The pubic bone (P) can be seen above the foramen. **B.** Magnified view of the nerve exiting the pelvis via the obturator foramen. The pubic bone (P) is seen in the background.

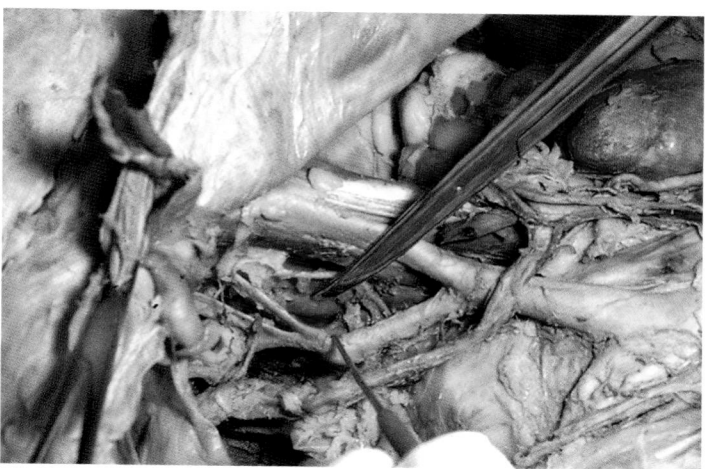

**FIGURE 9–23** The scissors point to the obturator internus muscle. This forms the lateral boundary of the obturator fossa and the "pelvic sidewall." The hypogastric artery (anterior division) is retracted medially with the hook.

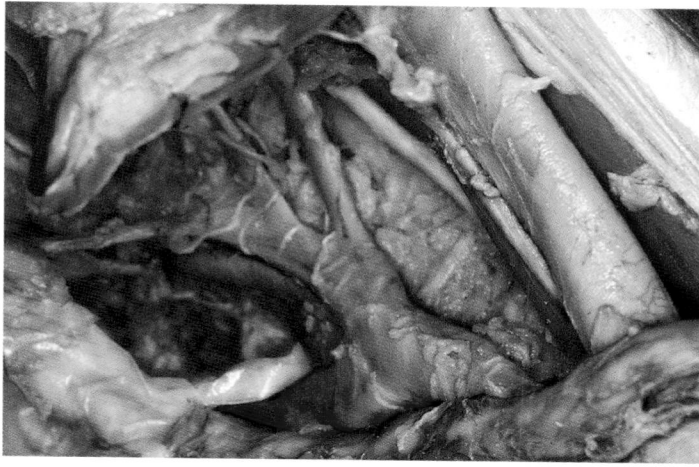

**FIGURE 9–24** The posterior division of the hypogastric artery is viewed clearly. The internal iliac vein is just below and slightly lateral to the artery.

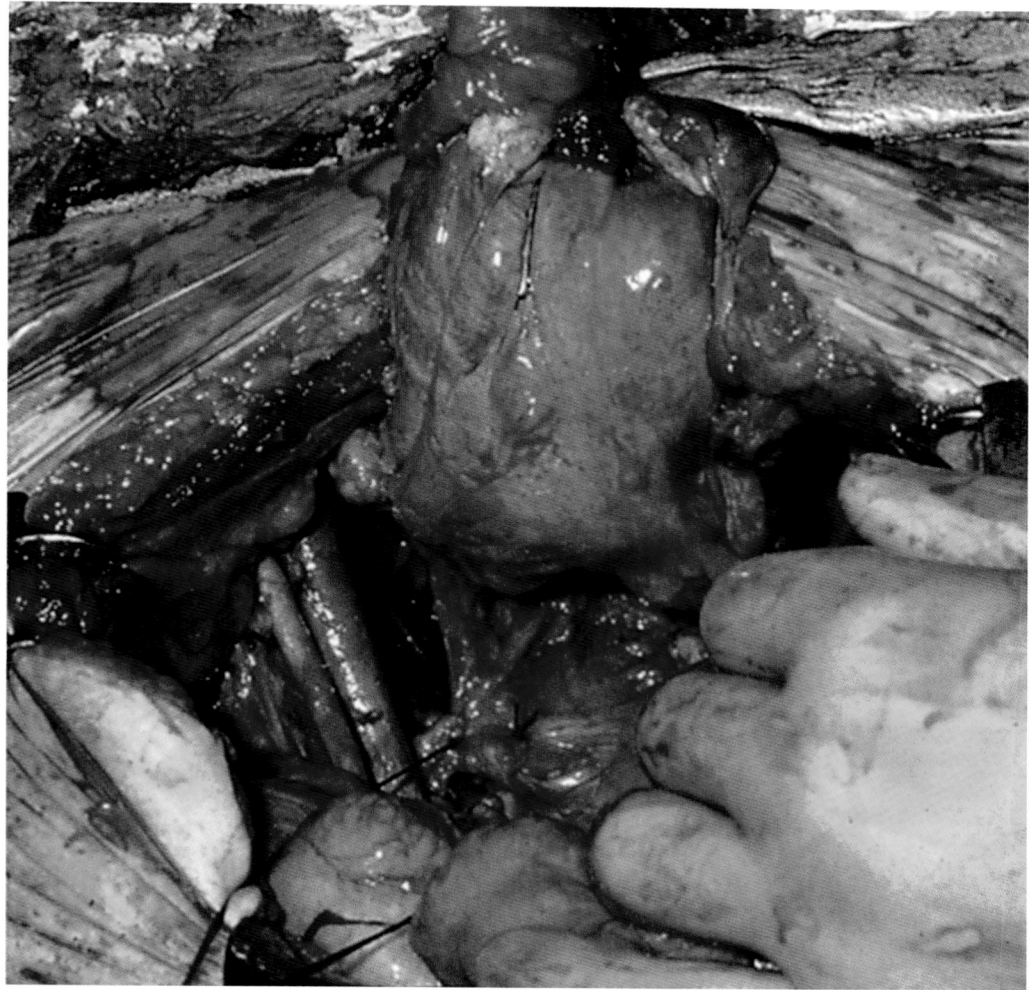

**FIGURE 9–25** View of the obturator fossa obtained during a pelvic lymphadenectomy. The uterus is pulled anteriorly and to the right for exposure.

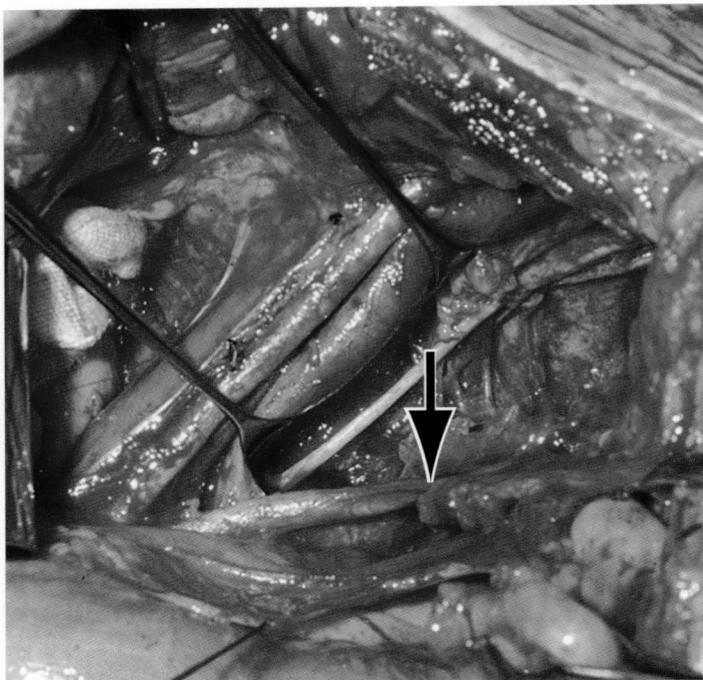

**FIGURE 9–26** A vein retractor is positioned beneath the large external iliac vein, exposing the obturator fossa. The fat-containing lymph nodes have been cleared from the fossa. The obturator nerve has been exposed. The arrow points to the hypogastric artery. The ureter is medial to the hypogastric artery (traction ligature).

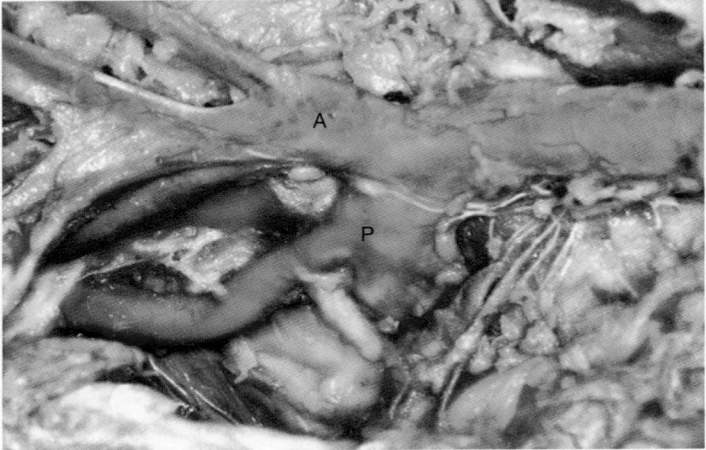

**FIGURE 9–27** The entirety of the right hypogastric vessels is exposed. The two main divisions of the hypogastric artery (anterior and posterior), as well as their branches, are seen. A, anterior division; P, posterior division.

# CHAPTER 10

# Dilatation and Curettage

*Michael S. Baggish*

Dilatation and curettage (D & C) is one of the most commonly performed operations in the world. The most informative method for performing this procedure is to combine it with a diagnostic hysteroscopy. No data support the contention that hysteroscopy spreads endometrial cancer cells to any extent greater than other diagnostic studies (e.g., D & C, endometrial biopsy). Furthermore, no evidence suggests that the cells will metastasize.

A standard instrument table is set up and includes diagnostic hysteroscopic equipment (Fig. 10-1A–C). Before the D & C is performed, an examination under anesthesia (EUA) is done to demarcate the position and size of the uterus, as well as the presence or absence of adnexal masses. After the vulva and vagina have been prepared, the patient is draped while in the lithotomy position. A Sims retractor or weighted speculum is placed along the posterior wall of the vagina. The anterior lip of the cervix is grasped with a single-toothed tenaculum (Fig. 10-2). The uterus is carefully sounded. The passed sound stops when it encounters resistance to forward movement, which occurs when the tip of the sound comes in contact with the uterine fundus. Next, with the use of tapered dilators (Pratt or

Hanks), the cervix is progressively dilated (Fig. 10-3). Dilatation should be limited to the amount required for the widest portion of the curette to pass easily into the uterine cavity (Fig. 10-4). Systematic curettage is carried out by scraping the endometrium from fundus to cervix starting at 12 o'clock on the anterior uterine wall, working around to 3 o'clock, then 6 o'clock on the posterior uterine wall, and via 9 o'clock, making it back to 12 o'clock again (Fig. 10-5A–C). A nonadherent sponge is placed into the posterior vaginal fornix to catch the curettings as they emit from the cervix (Fig. 10-6). When the surgeon judges that the uterine cavity has been completely curetted, the procedure stops.

If a diagnosis of endometrial or endocervical cancer is suspected, a fractional curettage should be performed. The appropriate order of this operation is to curette the endocervical canal first; this is followed by curettage of the endometrial cavity (Fig. 10-7A, B). The individual specimens are separately placed into individually labeled bottles.

At the terminus of the case, the uterus can be resounded or directly viewed by hysteroscopy. The purpose of the preceding exercise is to determine whether the uterus has been perforated.

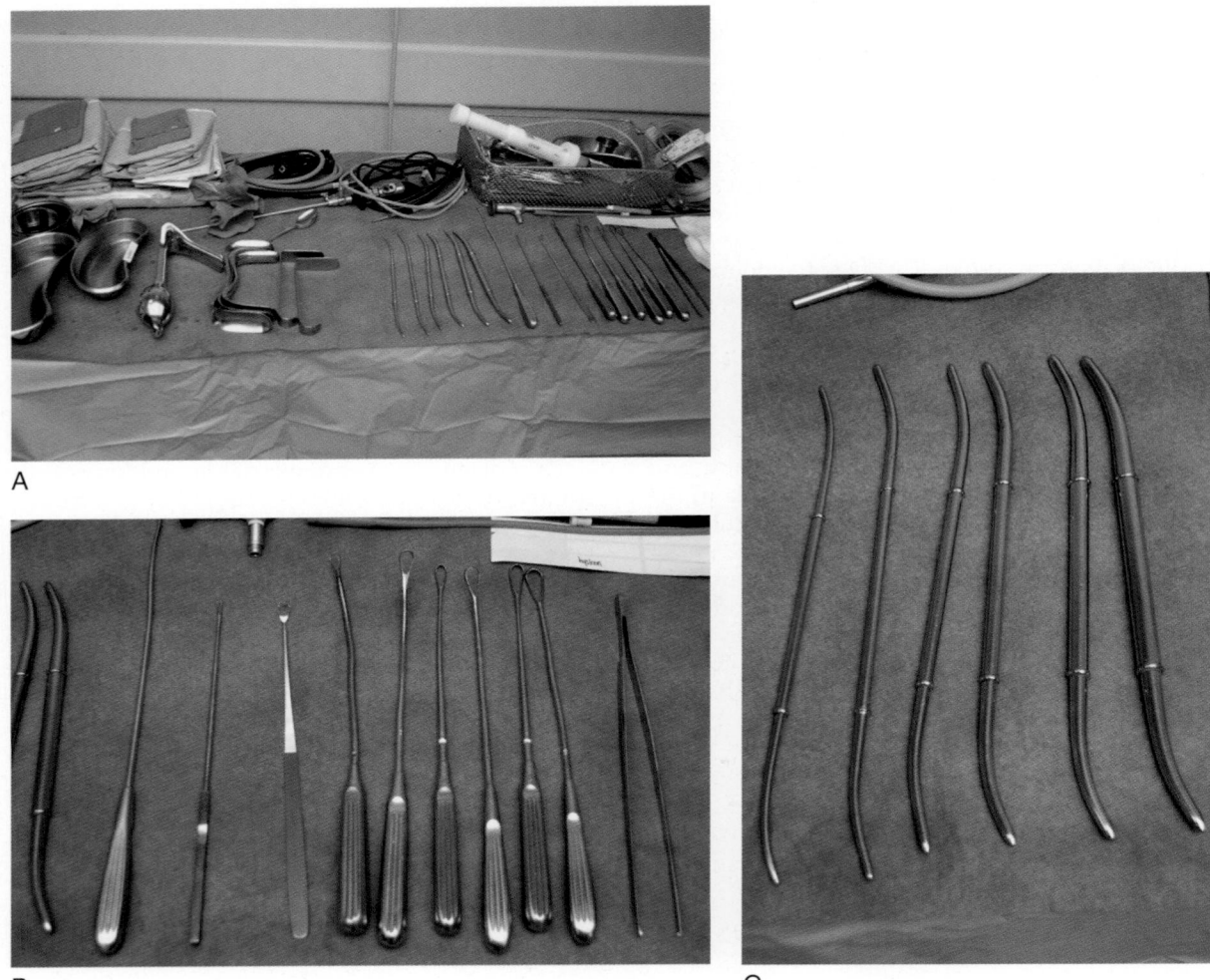

A

B                                                    C

**FIGURE 10–1  A.** The instruments required for dilatation and curettage are shown here. The equipment in the background is hysteroscopic and includes the Baggish Hyskon hand pump (in the basket) (Cook OB/GYN). **B.** A variety of sharp curettes are available; however, the serrated curette in the center is the most effective device. To the left of the serrated curette is an endocervical canal curette (Kevorkian). To the left of the Kevorkian curette is a malleable uterine sound. **C.** Hanks or Pratt dilators are tapered and produce the least trauma in cervical dilatation.

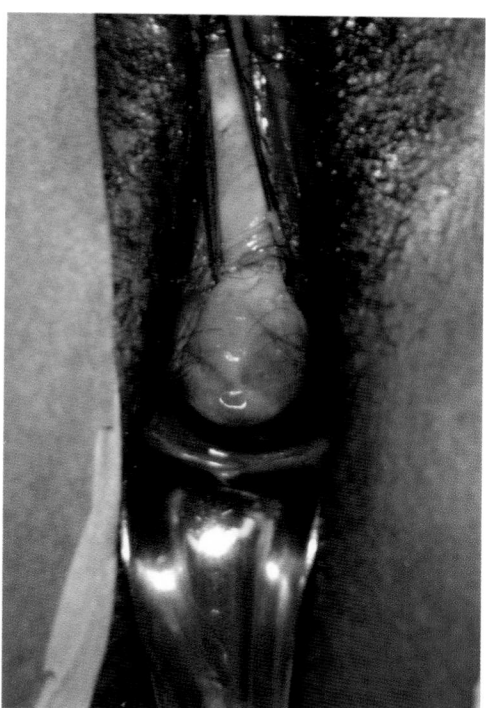

**FIGURE 10–2** A Sims retractor is placed along the posterior wall of the vagina. The cervix is held with a single-toothed tenaculum.

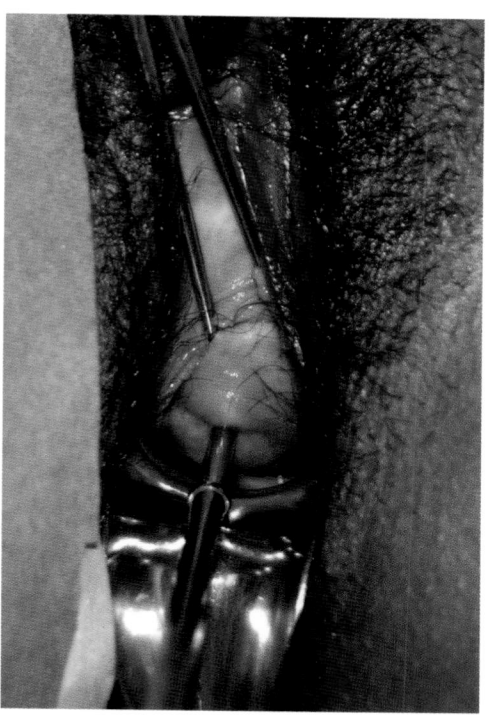

**FIGURE 10–3** The cervix is systematically dilated.

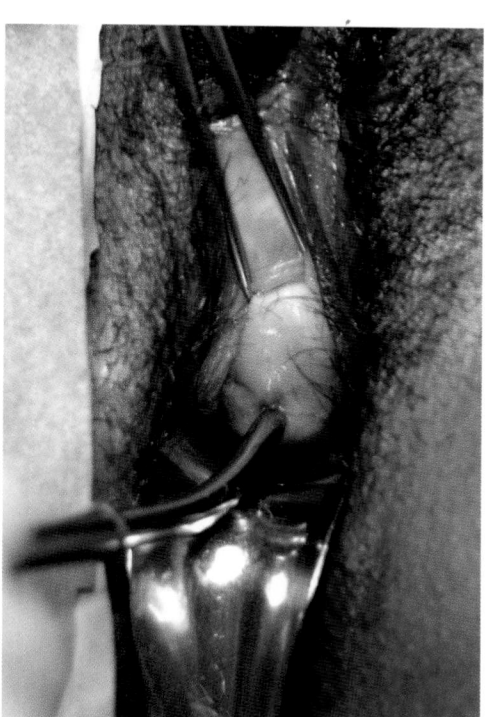

**FIGURE 10–4** Dilatation should be continued until the cervical canal has been sufficiently enlarged to accommodate the head of the curette.

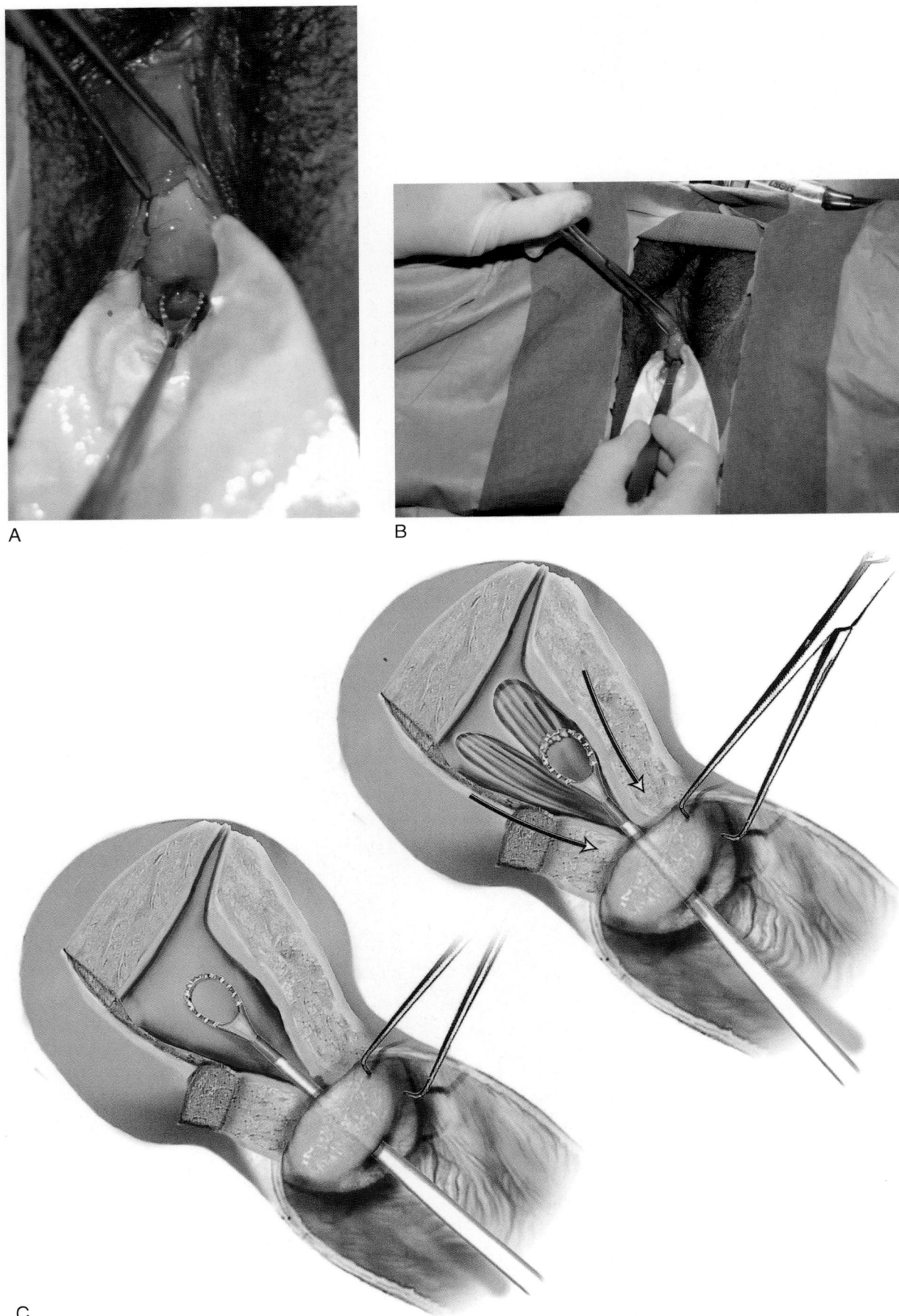

A

B

C

**FIGURE 10–5  A.** A sponge is placed into the posterior fornix and the sharp curette is introduced into the cervix. **B.** The curette is gently placed into the uterine cavity to reach sufficient depth so as to encounter fundal resistance. The curette is pulled down to the cervix along the anterior wall, continuing clockwise until the entire cavity is covered. **C.** *Lower,* The sharp edge of the curette is placed in contact with the endometrial surface. *Upper,* As the curette is pulled downward, it cuts a swath through the endometrium, thereby obtaining a strip of tissue for histopathologic evaluation. As the curette is pushed forward and rotated, only light pressure should be applied to the instrument. The hazard of perforation is always present during this in-stroke phase. If perforation is suspected, the procedure should be terminated immediately.

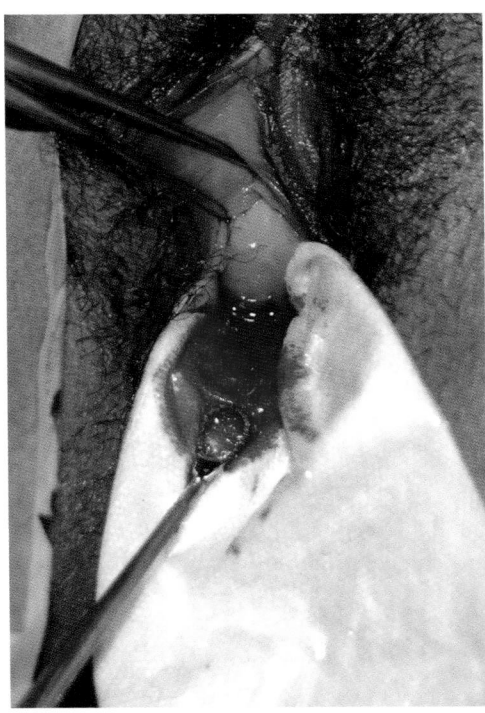

**FIGURE 10–6** The curette may be pulled from the endometrial cavity intermittently. The specimen is collected on the nonadherent sponge.

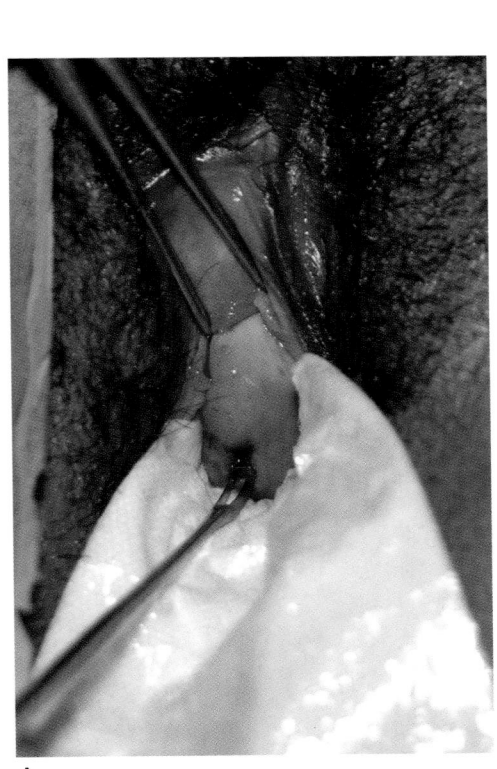

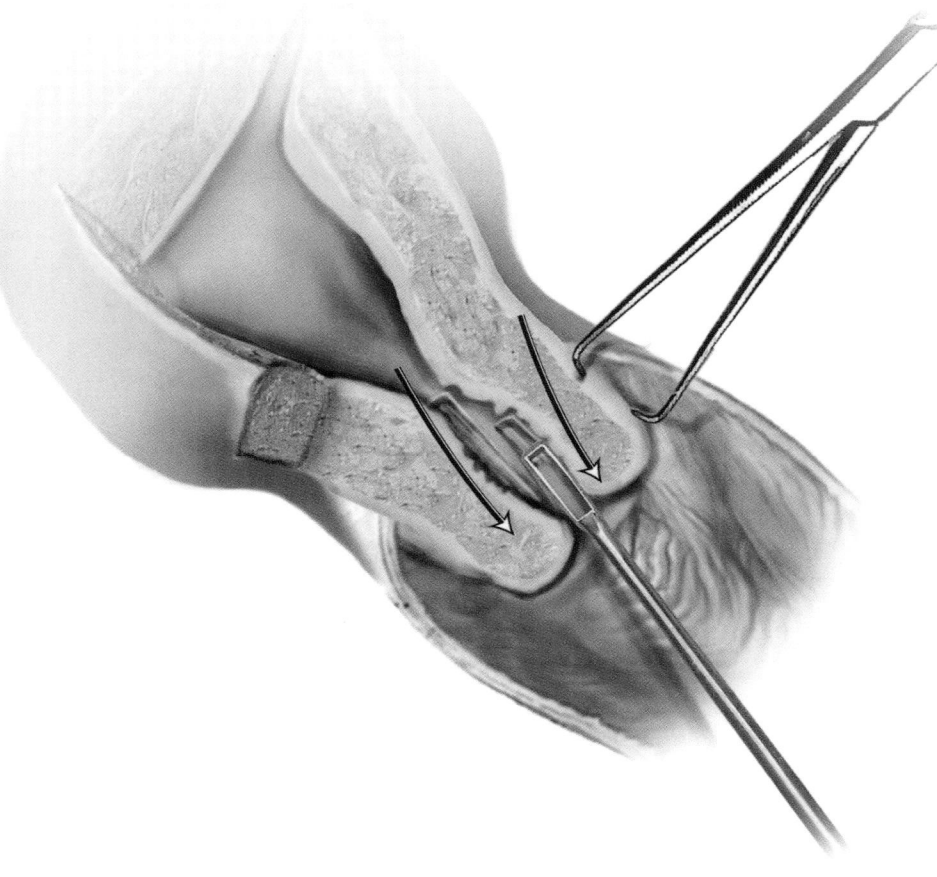

A                                    B

**FIGURE 10–7 A.** When a fractional curettage is indicated (e.g., suspected carcinoma of the endometrium), the endocervical component should be done first and the curettings collected. The specimen containing endocervical curettings is placed in a separate container and sent to pathology in the company of the jar containing the endometrial curettings. **B.** Endocervical curettage is performed with a Kevorkian curette. A tenaculum is always applied for countertraction. The curettage is initiated at the level of the internal os, and each stroke is taken in a downward direction, terminating just inside the external os. Mucus and curettings are collected on a sponge. A Kelly clamp may be needed to twirl and remove the mucus-laden specimen from the cervical os.

## Suction Curettage

The technique of vacuum or suction curettage is an outgrowth of the other methods for evacuating uterine contents, such as dilatation and sharp curettage (Fig. 10–8). During the late 1950s and early 1960s, suction curettage attained popularity in the Iron Curtain countries of Eastern Europe and the USSR as a rapid method for first-trimester induced abortion. Coupled with its rapidity was the advantage of diminished blood loss. It is unclear whether this technique was first used in Eastern Europe or China. Nevertheless, by 1963 the technique had been transplanted to the United States and was being used for first-trimester terminations of pregnancy. Soon this same technique was also applied to the evacuation of spontaneous incomplete abortion, as well as to missed abortion. Soon vacuum curettage was the instrument of choice in the Far East for the evacuation of hydatidiform mole, regardless of the gestational size of the uterus. Malaysia, Indonesia, China, Hong Kong, and Singapore were regions where trophoblastic disease, a relative rarity in Western countries, was a common disorder and in fact a public health problem.

Local or general anesthesia is required for this operation. A pelvic examination is a prerequisite to determine the size and the position of the uterus. Next, a careful sounding of the uterus is carried out. A concentrated oxytocin solution is infused continuously. Fluid volume must be carefully monitored, particularly in cases of hydatidiform mole in which overzealous fluid infusion can easily trigger pulmonary edema. The technique of suction or vacuum curettage requires the uterine cervix to be dilated to accommodate the suction curette, and obviously the degree of dilatation depends on the anticipated diameter of the curette, which ranges from 8 mm to 16 mm, with the average device measuring 10 mm (Fig. 10–9). The cervix is stabilized with a single-toothed tenaculum attached to the anterior lip of the cervix. Following cervical dilatation, for example, a 30-French (10-mm) suction curette is placed into the uterine cavity. The purpose of overdilatation is to permit unimpeded free sliding of the curette into and out of the uterine corpus. This technical point is crucial because a tight fit between cannula and cervix can produce "grabbing" on the in-stroke, which in turn can increase the risk of perforation.

The suction machine is turned on after one end of the hose is attached to the curette and the opposite end to the intake port of the specimen collection jar (container). Similarly, a cotton mesh collection bag is applied to the inner aspect of the collection container and is secured in place with a rubber O ring. The suction curette (cannula) is inserted into the uterus and gently advanced to the point where the operator feels the fundus of the uterus. **No suction is applied yet.** Next, a finger is placed over the hole at the base of the suction cannula (curette), thereby creating suction. The curette is drawn down toward the cervix with a twisting motion to the curette in its downward course (Fig. 10–10). The activated curette is not pulled through the cervix because the force of the suction could strip away the endocervical epithelium. Thus, at the location of the internal cervical os, the operator's finger is lifted from the hole in the curette, which immediately relieves the created suction (Fig. 10–11A, B). The device is pulled from the cervix and is completely cleared of tissue. The process is repeated several times while the cannula (curette) is turned in different directions to encompass the entire uterine cavity. Suction is **never activated** during the **in-thrust phase.** It is applied only when the curette is moving in a downward or outward direction. When no further tissue is seen within the tubing, the procedure is stopped. The uterus is carefully resounded to ensure that *no* perforation has occurred. Optionally, sharp curettage may be done to check for any retained tissue.

The collection bag is detached, placed in formalin, and sent to the pathology laboratory for microscopic diagnosis (Fig. 10–12). A 0.2-mg dose of methylergonovine (Methergine) is administered to the patient, who is given an order for pad counts and 24 hours of oral Methergine (0.2 mg every 4–6 hours for 24 hours only). If the procedure is performed to evacuate a septic abortion, then antibiotics should be administered after cultures have been obtained.

The greatest risks of this procedure are uterine perforation and blood loss. Perforation with the suction applied is very dangerous and can lead to bowel or major vessel injury, either of which requires prompt diagnosis and emergency intervention. If the uterus is not contracting (i.e., by infusion of oxytocin), then it serves as a sponge filled continuously with blood. Applying a suction cannula to this "sponge" is akin to squeezing the sponge dry; however, this sponge quickly refills from its reservoir of body blood. A noncontracted uterus can therefore be the model for massive blood loss sucked up and collected in the suction bottle.

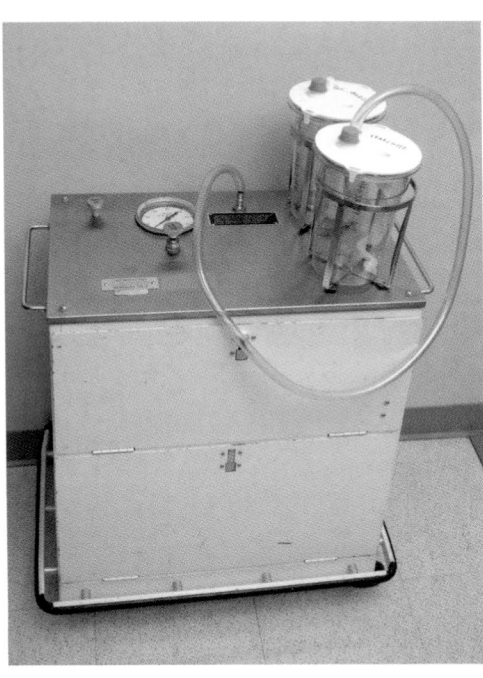

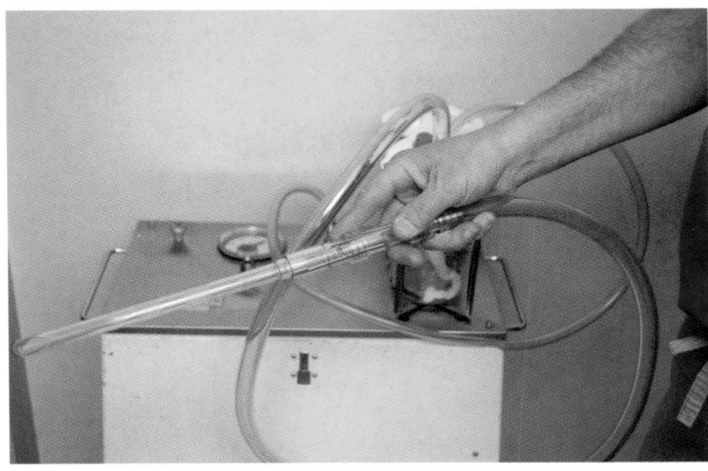

**FIGURE 10–9** Thick-walled plastic suction tubing of 2 to 2.5 cm diameter is attached to a vacuum jar with a specimen collection trap. The other end of the hose is fitted with a handle to which a plastic cannula plugs in. As noted, several sizes of cannulas (vacuum curettes) are available, ranging from 8 to 16 mm.

**FIGURE 10–8** A suction curettage vacuum pump requires a high flow rate to move sufficient air volume to create enough negative pressure to suck up intrauterine contents rapidly.

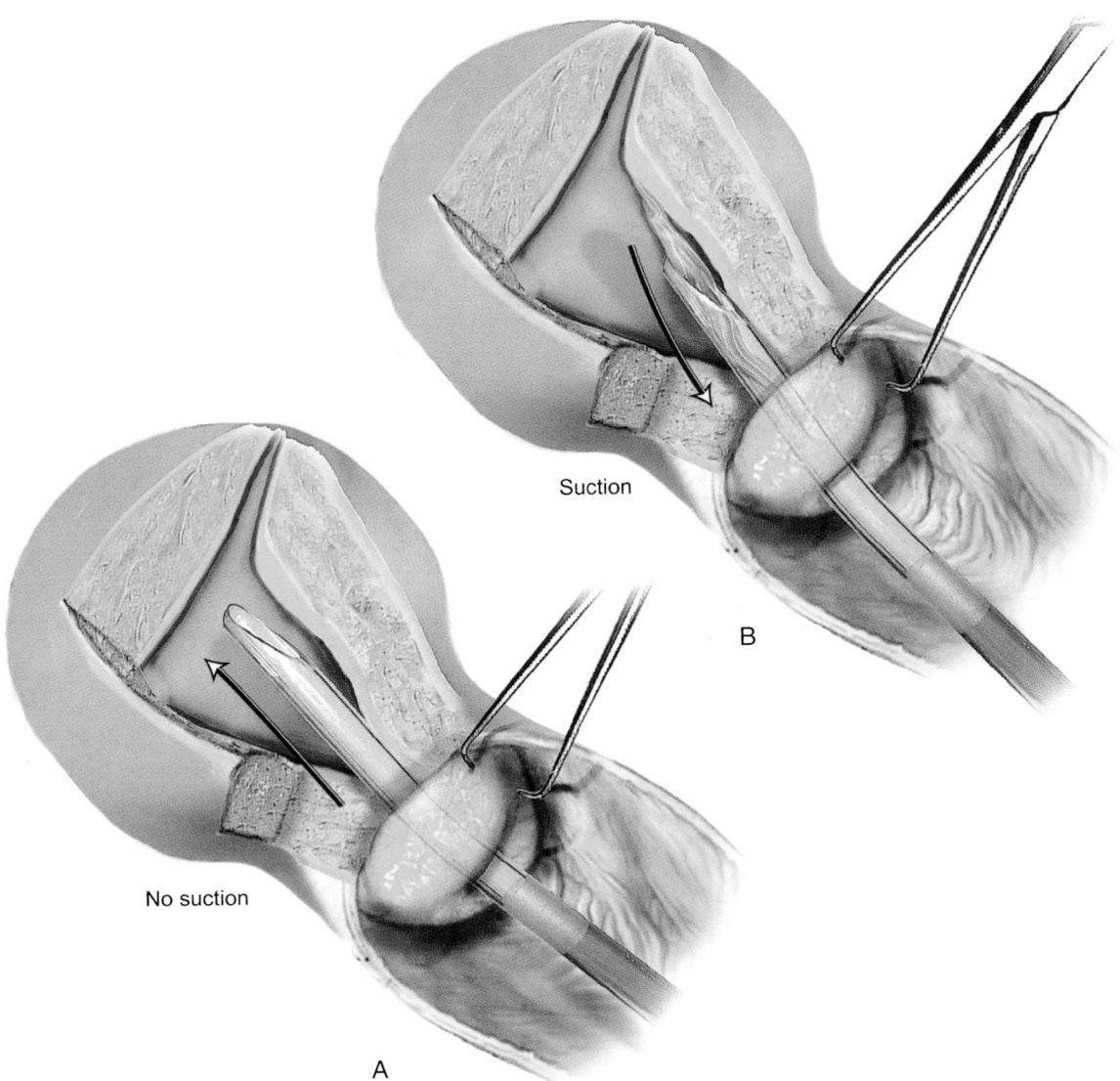

Suction

B

No suction

A

**FIGURE 10–10 A.** The vacuum (suction) cannula is gently placed into the uterus until fundal resistance is felt. No suction is applied until the curette has been properly positioned. **B.** As the curette is pulled back, suction is applied. The endometrium is sucked into the cannula and thence into the connecting tubing. Suction is relieved at the level of the internal cervical os.

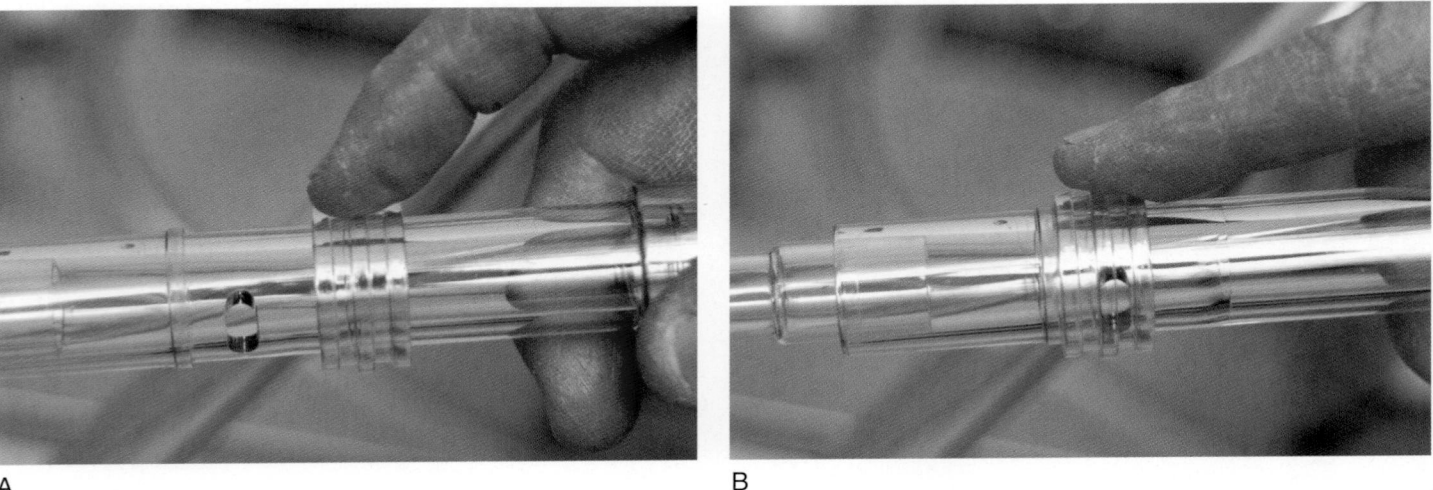

A                                                                                                                                    B

**FIGURE 10–11 A.** A sliding ring on the vacuum handle controls the suction. The ring is in the open position, and no suction is created. **B.** The ring has been pushed forward to close off the opening in the handle of the apparatus, thereby creating a substantial suction.

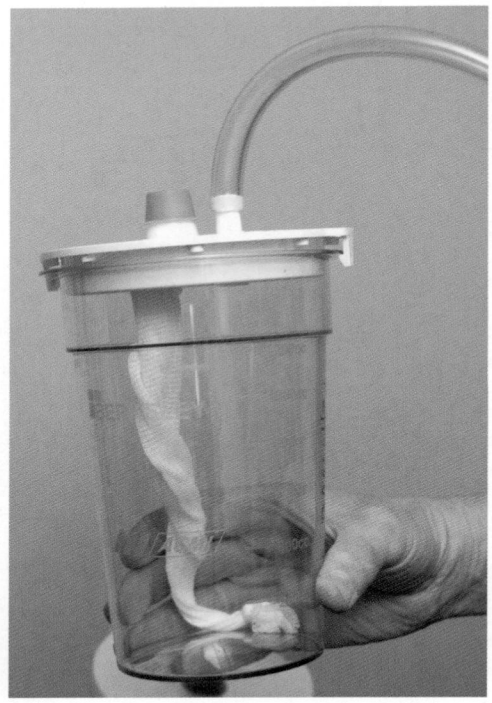

**FIGURE 10–12** The specimen is caught in the gauze bag attached to the vacuum input port (blue cap) by a rubber O ring. Blood and fluid flow through the bag and are collected in the jar. For large evacuations (e.g., hydatidiform mole), the two jars should be connected by plastic tubing in series to avoid entry of fluid into the pump mechanism (see Fig. 10–8).

# CHAPTER 11

# Abdominal Hysterectomy

## *Michael S. Baggish*

Abdominal hysterectomy is one of the most frequently performed surgical procedures in the United States. The basis for this operation is an open abdomen (laparotomy), which provides adequate exposure for isolation of the uterus and adnexa from surrounding structures to allow cutting and securing of support structures that attach the uterus to the pelvic floor and sidewalls.

These supporting structures include (1) vascular pedicles together with their peritoneal and connective tissue investments (e.g., infundibulopelvic ligament, uterine artery and veins); (2) muscular supports (e.g., the round ligaments); (3) connective tissue–vascular/neural condensations (e.g., cardinal, uterosacral ligaments); and (4) fat and peritoneum (e.g., broad ligament, uterovesical, uterorectal folds).

Strategic surrounding structures include the bladder anteriorly, the rectum posteriorly, and the ureters and great vessels laterally.

The blood supply to the uterus emanates from the hypogastric arteries and via the ovarian arteries from the aorta. The venous drainage enters the hypogastric veins, the vena cava (right ovarian), and the left renal vein (left ovarian). The uterine artery crosses from the anterior division of the hypogastric artery obliquely above the ureter to join the uterus at the junction of the corpus and cervix. The artery divides into a larger, ascending branch and a smaller, descending branch that supplies the cervix and anastomoses with the vaginal artery. The latter also takes origin from the anterior division of the hypogastric artery.

## Total Abdominal Hysterectomy With Bilateral Salpingo-oophorectomy

After the abdomen has been opened and the intestine *carefully* packed, a self-retaining retractor is placed (Fig. 11–1A, B). The abdomen has been previously explored. The pelvic contents in the operative field are identified, and any pathology or anatomic distortion is noted (Fig. 11–2).

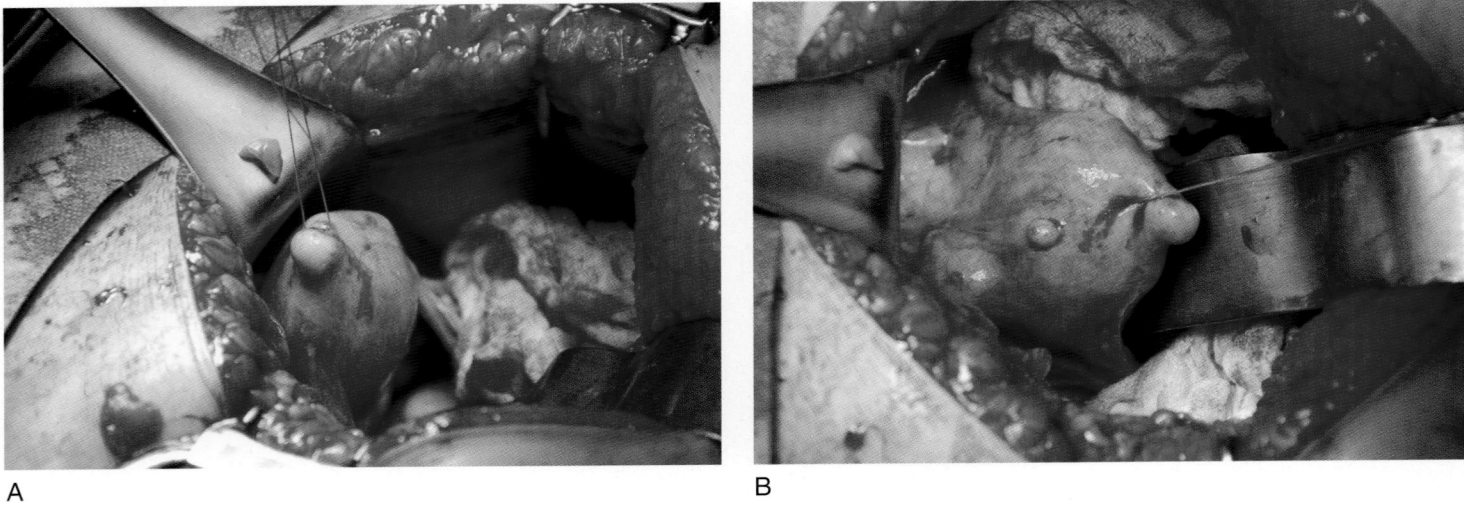

A                                                                                  B

**FIGURE 11–1  A.** The myomatous uterus in situ, the Balfour self-retaining retractor is in place. A Richardson retractor is positioned between the bladder and the uterus. **B.** A 0 Vicryl stitch placed into the uterine fundus pulls the uterus posteriorly, exposing the vesicouterine peritoneum. A malleable retractor has been placed between the uterus and the sigmoid colon.

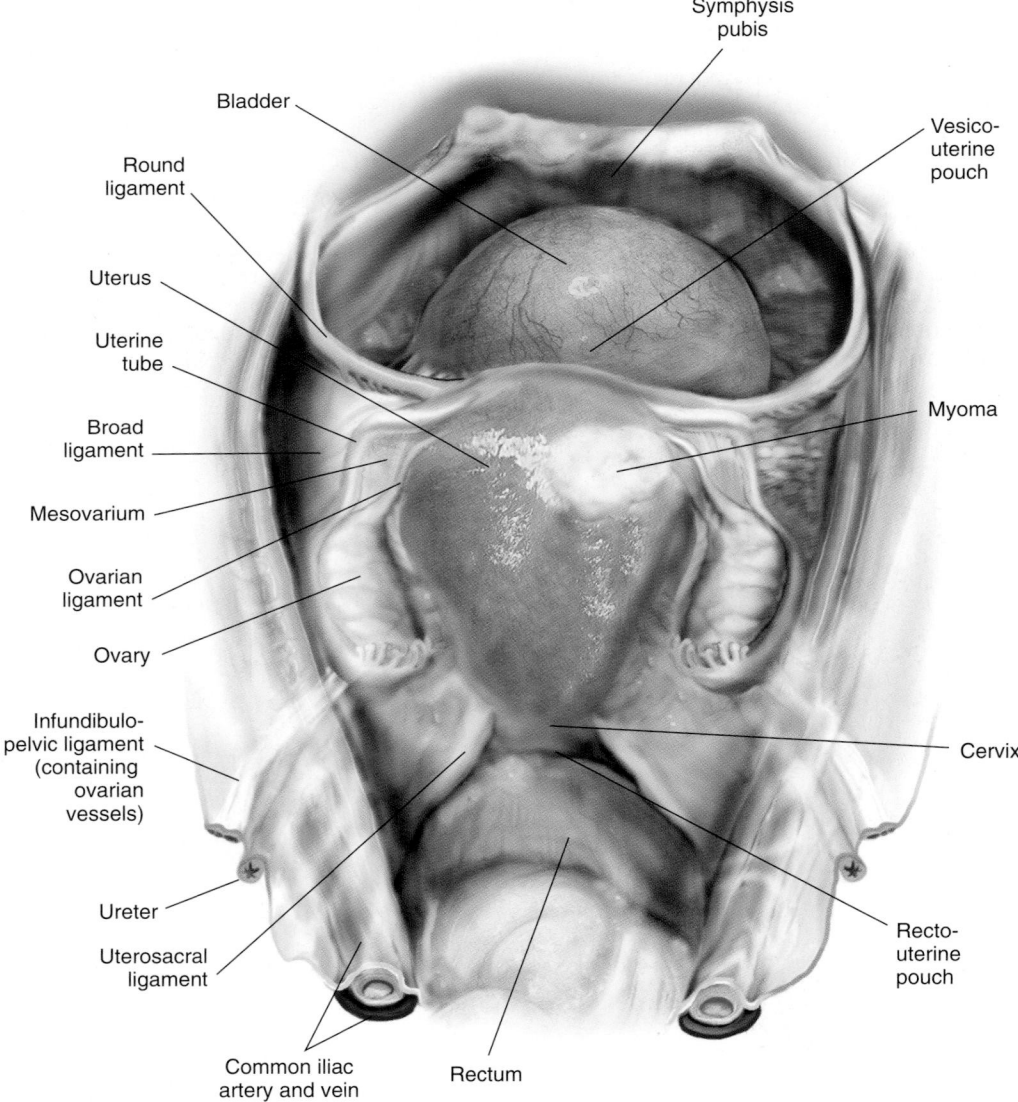

**FIGURE 11–2** Schematic topographic view of the pertinent anatomy encountered during hysterectomy.

Thus, surgery is performed in a logical stepwise fashion.

1. The round ligaments are clamped, divided, and suture-ligated with 0 Vicryl (Fig. 11–3A, C).
2. The bladder flap is cut by grasping the peritoneum of the vesicouterine fold just below its reflection onto the uterus (Figs. 11–4 and 11–5A–D). Steps 1 and 2 are repeated on the opposite sites (Fig. 11–6).
3. With the use of a sponge forceps, the bladder is gently pushed inferiorly from the cervix. Care is taken to stay in the midline, pushing onto the cervix (Figs. 11–7A, B and 11–8). If the patient has had previous surgery (e.g., a cesarean section), the bladder should be separated from the uterus by sharp dissection.
4. The infundibulopelvic ligaments (ovarian arteries and veins) are isolated from the ureter and triply clamped (Fig. 11–9A–E). The ligament is divided between the first and second clamps. The vessels are doubly ligated with the tissue beneath the lowermost clamp simply ligated or suture-ligated. The tissue beneath the second (middle) clamp is suture-ligated with 0 Vicryl (Fig. 11–10).

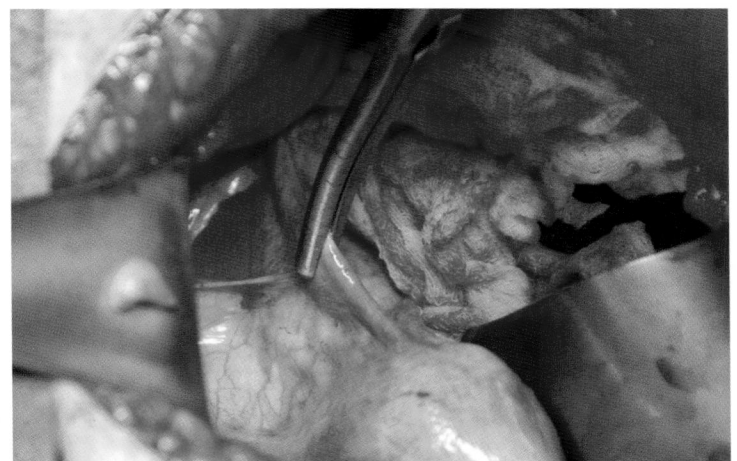

A

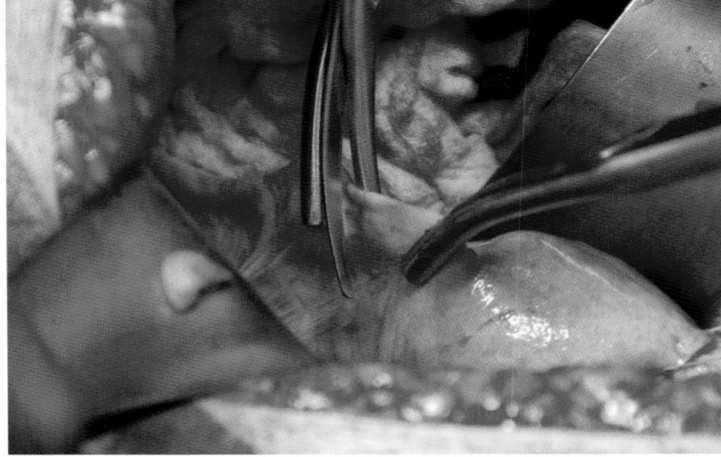

B

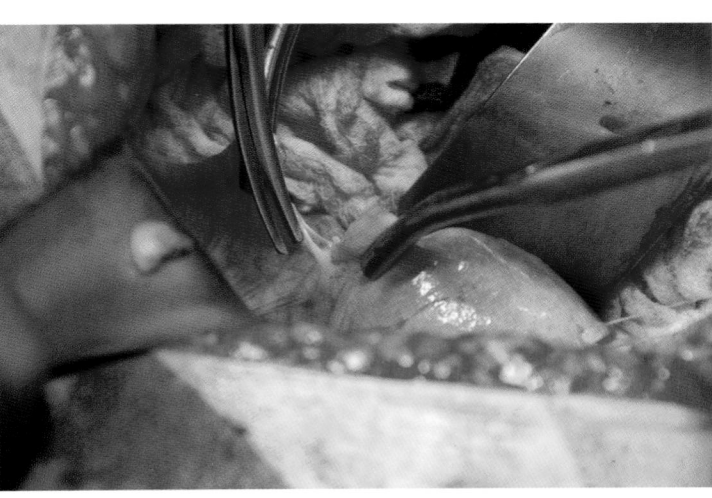

C

**FIGURE 11–3 A.** The round ligament is clamped with a Zeppelin clamp. **B.** A second clamp is placed on the round ligament at the point where it attaches to the uterus and the ligament is divided. **C.** The cut is extended into the upper portion on the anterior leaf of the broad ligament.

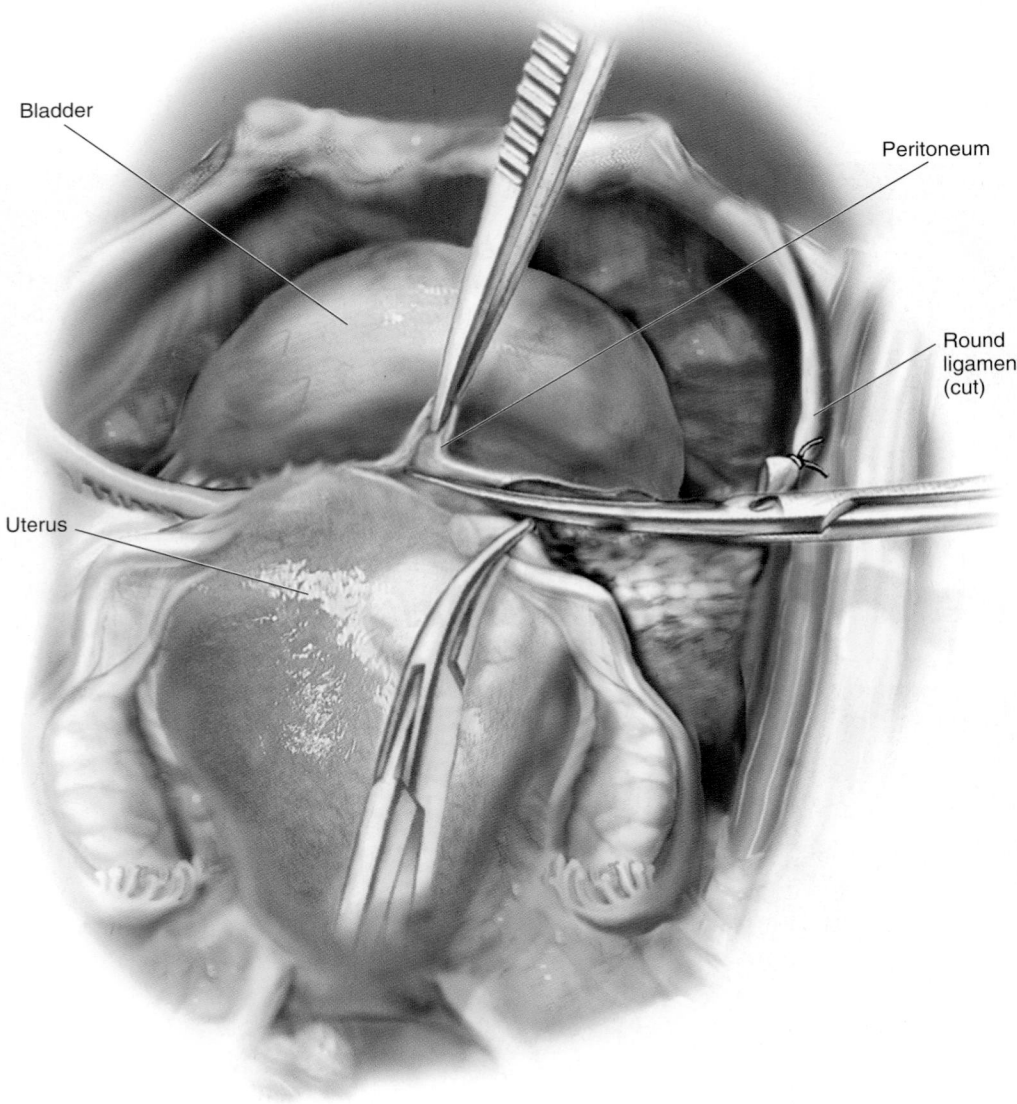

Bladder

Peritoneum

Round
ligament
(cut)

Uterus

**FIGURE 11–4** The round ligament is cut, and the peritoneal reflection between the bladder and
the uterus is dissected by slipping the scissors beneath the peritoneal edge and spreading the scissors
repeatedly as the scissor is advanced. Next, the dissected peritoneum is cut.

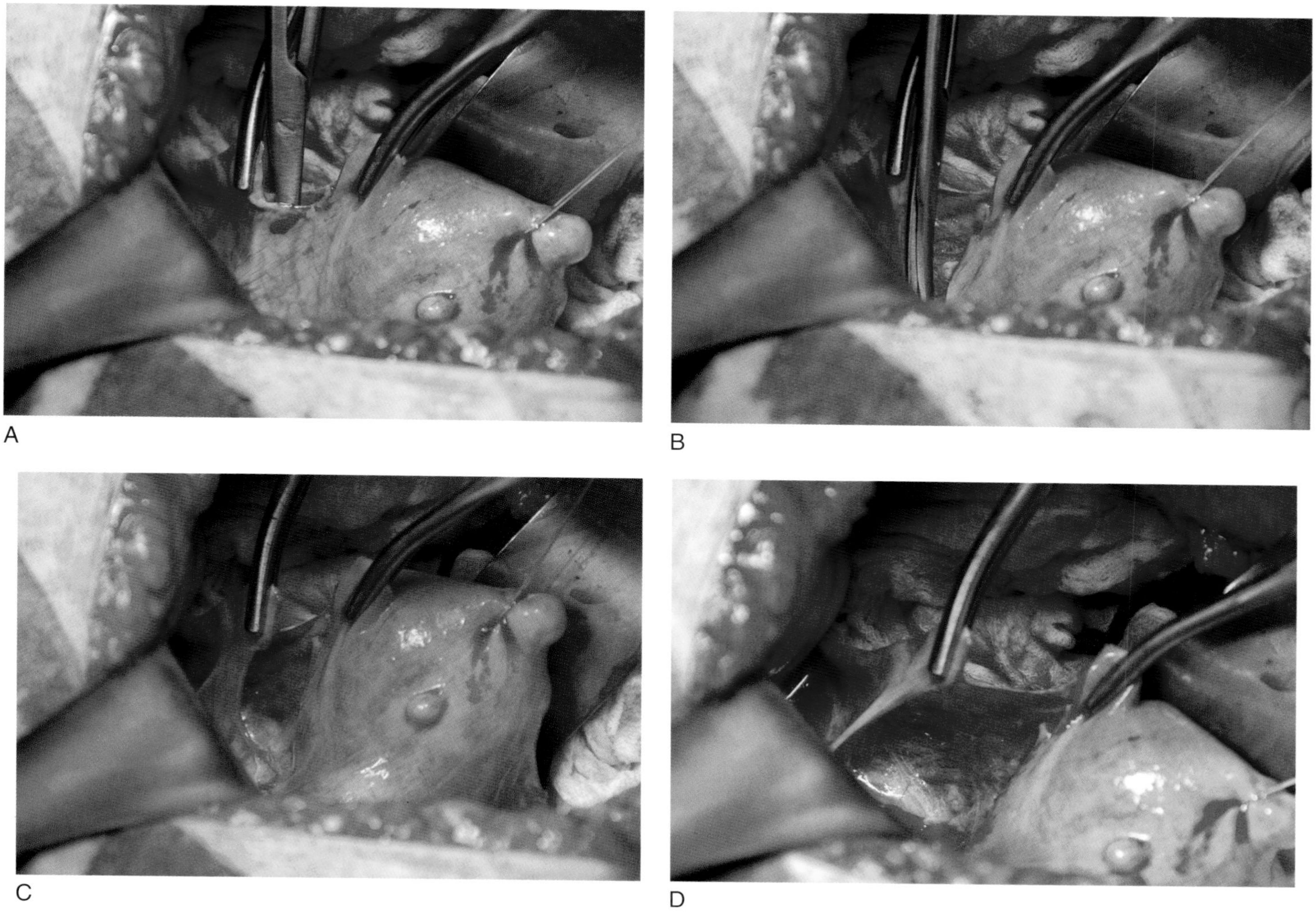

A

B

C

D

**FIGURE 11–5  A.** The scissor is slipped under the vesicouterine peritoneum within a bloodless space, in preparation for cutting the peritoneum. **B.** The bladder peritoneum is cut, thereby severing the attachment between the bladder and the uterus. **C.** The loose areolar tissue deep within the anterior leaf of the broad ligament is dissected. **D.** The pelvic ureter lies at the floor of the dissected broad ligament.

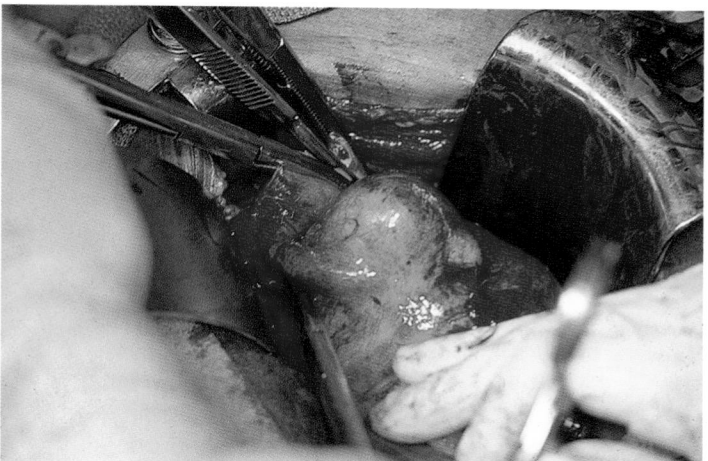

**FIGURE 11–6**  The left round ligament is divided similarly to the procedure performed on the right side.

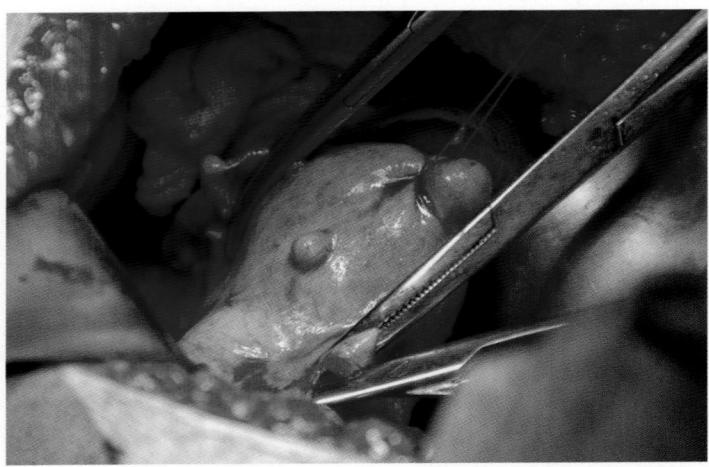

A

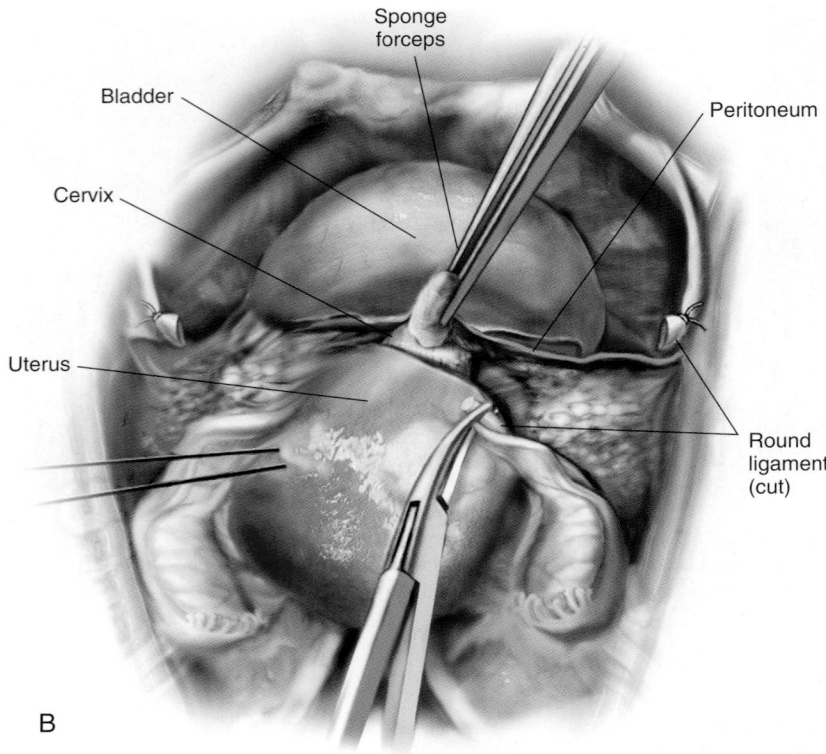

Sponge
forceps

Bladder

Peritoneum

Cervix

Uterus

Round
ligament
(cut)

B

**FIGURE 11–7  A.** The left round ligament has been cut. The left side of the vesicouterine peritoneum is dissected with scissors and cut so as to join up with the severed peritoneum on the right side. **B.** The bladder is pushed inferiorly by applying pressure on the cervix and bladder with a sponge stick. The pressure should mainly be applied to the cervix.

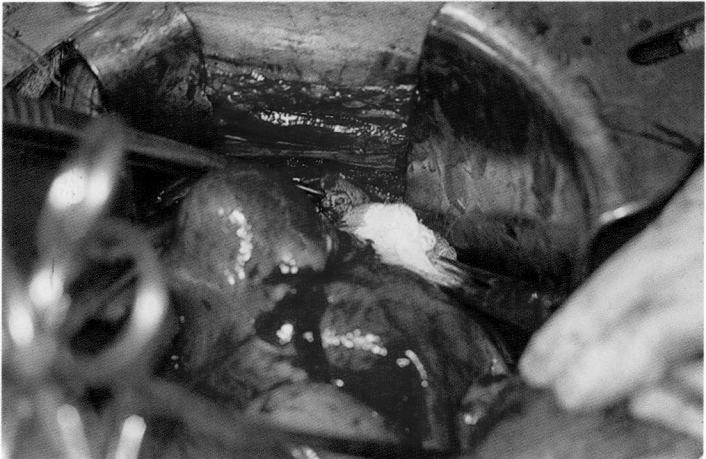

**FIGURE 11–8** When sponge forceps are applied to the bladder, care must be taken to stay in the midline; straying to the right or left will invariably tear the surrounding vesical (vesicle) and uterine vessels.

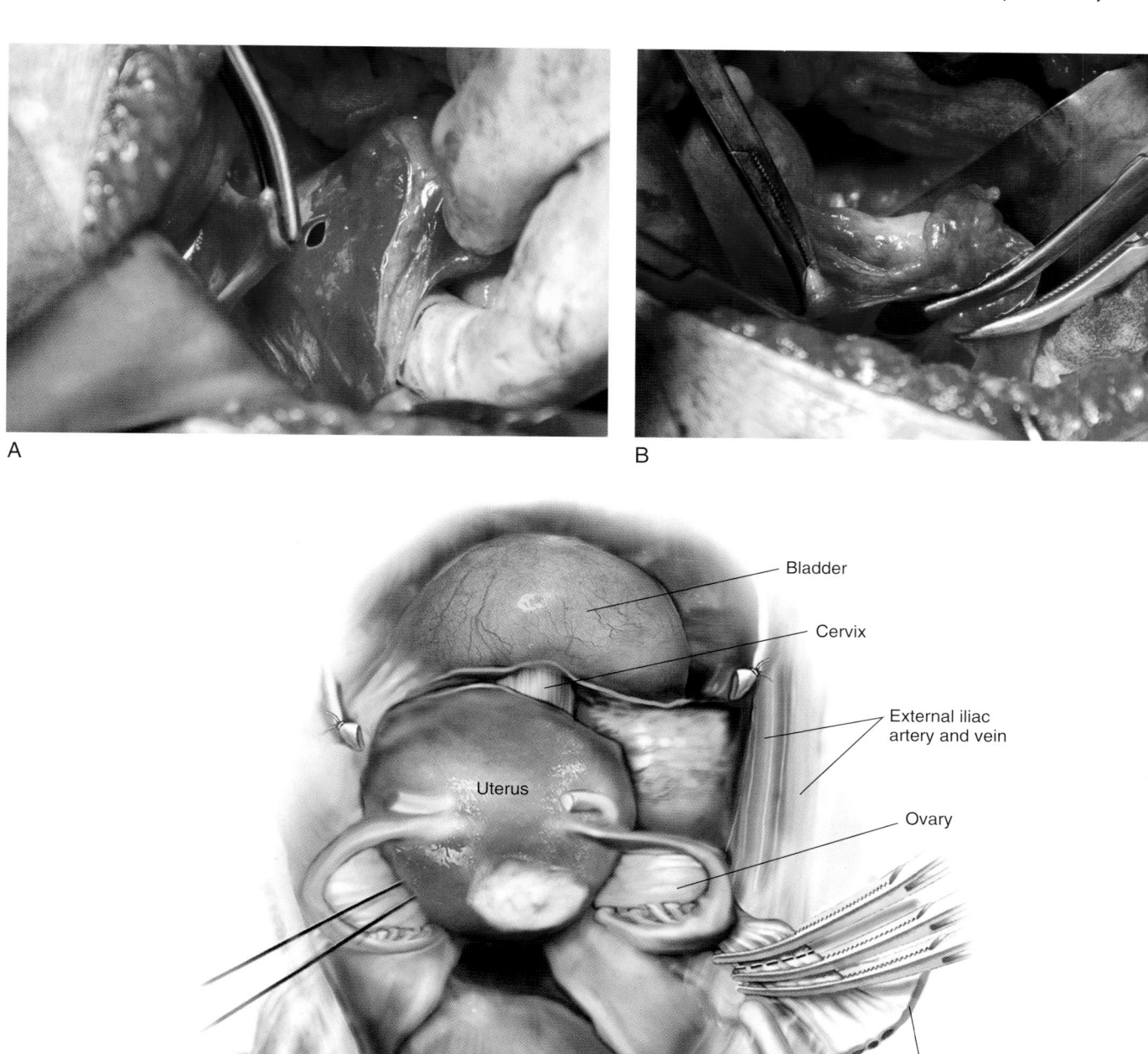

A

B

C

Bladder

Cervix

External iliac
artery and vein

Uterus

Ovary

Infundibulo-
pelvic ligament
(containing
ovarian
vessels)

Ureter

Common iliac
artery and vein

**FIGURE 11–9  A.** The posterior leaf of the broad ligament is isolated and opened. **B.** The ovarian vessels (infundibulopelvic ligaments) are clamped with Zeppelin clamps with identical curvature. **C.** The infundibulopelvic ligament is triply clamped with Zeppelin clamps and divided along the dashed line between the clamp closest to the ovary and the two clamps farthest from the ovary.

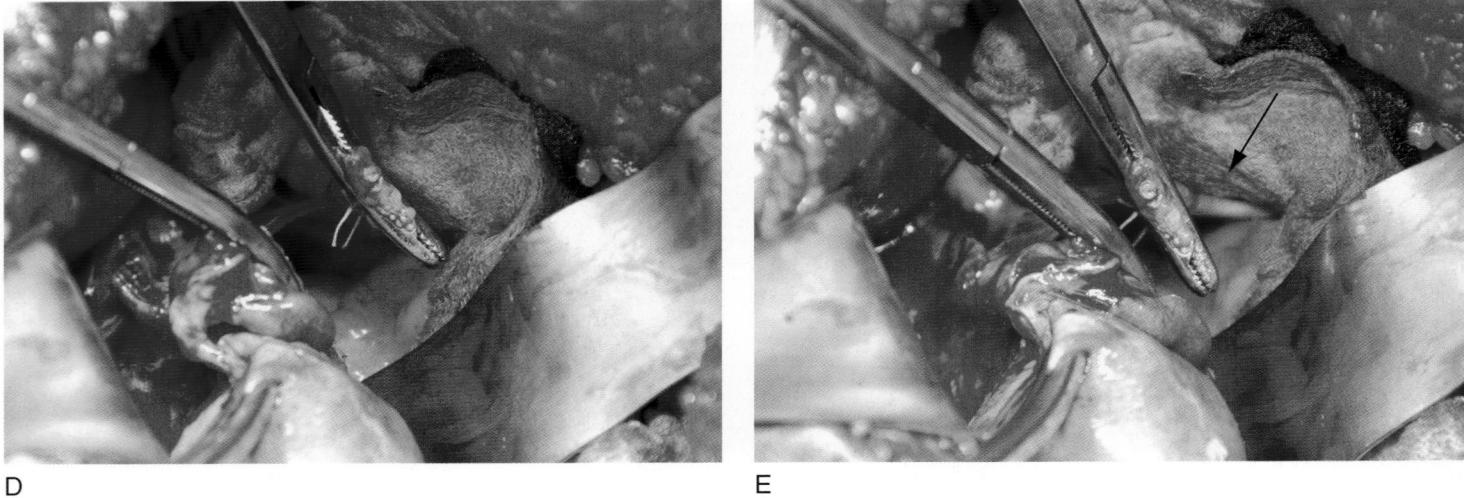

D                                                                                    E

**FIGURE 11–9, cont'd  D.** The ovarian vessels have been cut free from the adnexa, and one suture ligature has been placed and tied. **E.** The two portions of the cut infundibulopelvic ligament are shown here. A second suture ligature will be placed midway and below the clamp to which the arrow points. The suture ligature will be tied "fore and aft."

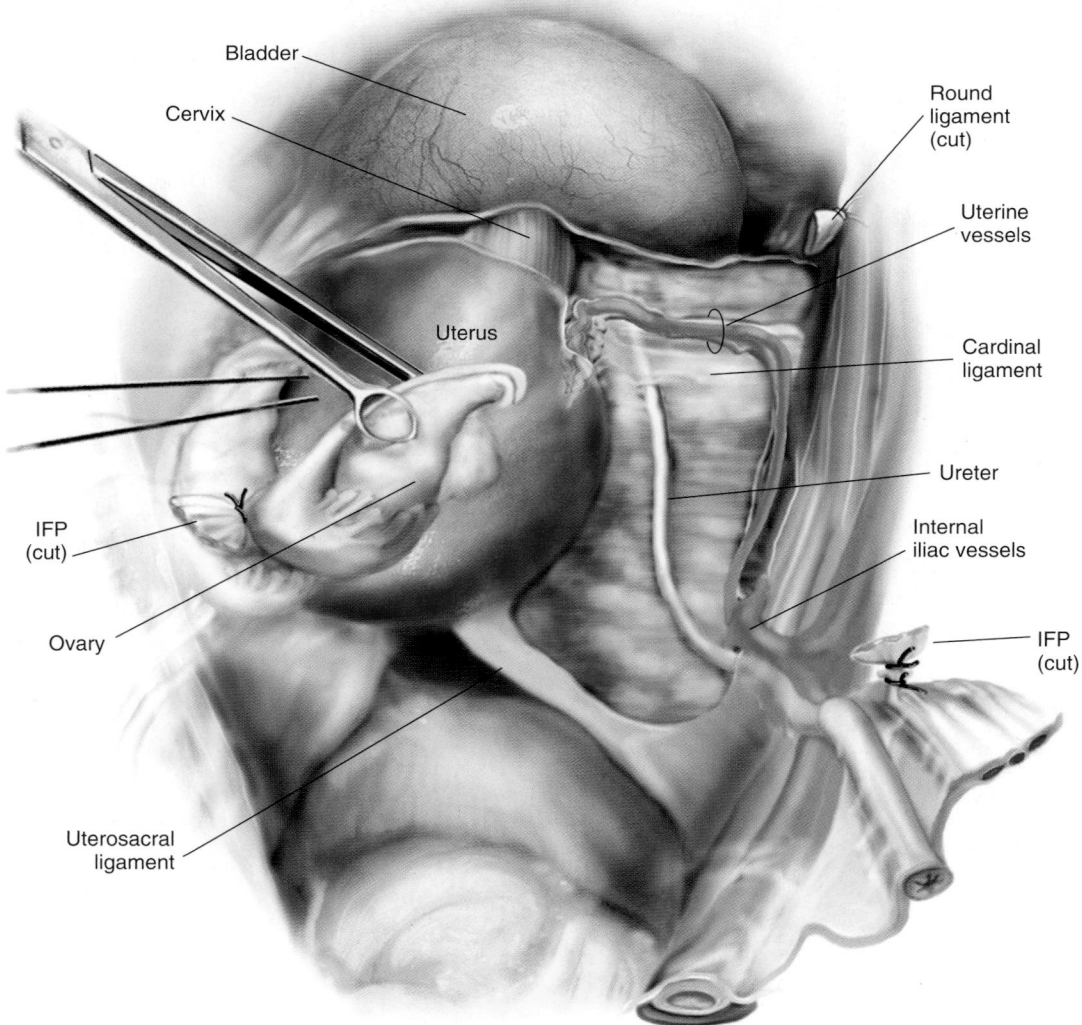

**FIGURE 11–10** The lowest clamp on the infundibulopelvic ligament is tied with 0 Vicryl. The remaining clamp is removed after a suture is passed under the clamp and is tied fore and aft (around the tip and heel of the clamp). The ligament, thus doubly secured, is then divided. A similar procedure is performed on the right and left sides. The ureter is identified to the point where it is crossed over by the uterine vessels.

5. The uterine vessels are skeletonized (i.e., excessive connective tissue is trimmed away, denuding the vessels) (Fig. 11–11A, B). The vessels are clamped, with this first clamp applied tightly to the uterus (Fig. 11–11C, D). A second clamp is applied directly above, never below, the first uterine vessel clamp (Fig. 11–12). Finally, a third clamp is applied above the second to secure back-bleeding (Fig. 11–13A, B). The uterine vessels are cut with scissors or scalpel (Fig. 11–14A, B). Next, the uterine vessels are doubly suture-ligated with 0 Vicryl, with care taken to pass the needle immediately beneath the tip of the clamp (Fig. 11–15A, B). The clamps (with the exception of the uppermost clamp) are removed after suture placement (see Fig. 11–14B). The procedure is identical for the right and left sides.

6. The cardinal ligaments are clamped in juxtaposition to the uterus, with care taken to avoid infringement of the ureter, which is very close to the uterine cervical junction. The upper portion of the cardinal ligament is then cut (Fig. 11–16A–E). The procedure is carried out on either side. The ligaments are sutured with 0 Vicryl with a transfixing stitch.

7. The uterosacral ligaments on either side are clamped, cut, and suture-ligated. This again is carried out close to the uterus, because farther back (posteriorly), the ligaments are intimately associated with the ureters. In fact, definite identification of the ureter once again is advised at this point in the procedure. Finally, the cervix is palpated and is confirmed to be separate from the vagina. A clamp is placed across the vagina after it has been confirmed that the margin of the urinary bladder is free and clear. The specimen is removed and the vagina is closed (Fig. 11–17A–J).

8. Alternatively, particularly if the corpus is bulky, the uterus may be "subtotaled" (i.e., the body of the uterus is amputated from the cervix). The uterus is elevated (the remaining clamps are those applied to prevent back-bleeding clamps during step 5) (Fig. 11–18). A sharp scalpel cuts the cervix free from the corpus (Fig. 11–19).

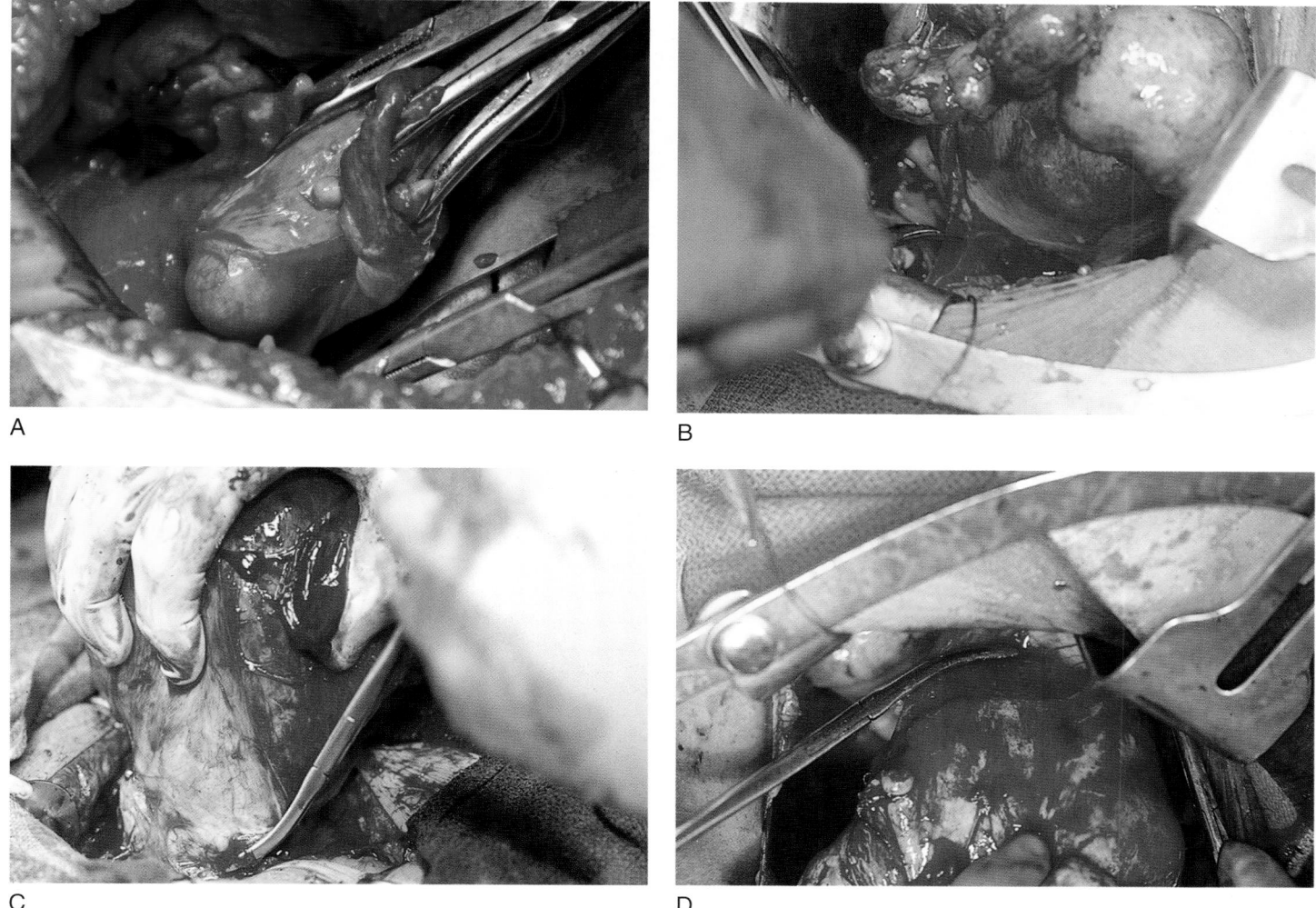

A

B

C

D

FIGURE 11–11 A. The uterus is pulled upward and the uterine vessels are prepared for clamping. Note that the bladder has been pushed down from the cervix (see Figs. 11–7B and 11–8A). B. The uterine vessels are skeletonized from the surrounding connective tissue, permitting the ureters to drop away laterally. The uterine vessels can now be identified as they ascend laterally onto the uterus and rise upward to anastomose with the ovarian vessels at the level of the uterotubal junction. C. The first clamp to secure the uterine vessels is applied above the bladder reflection and intimately close to the uterus. D. The clamp should extend inward to the cervicouterine junction such that the tip of the clamp glances off the solid uterine tissue while grabbing the vessels and their accompanying connective tissues securely. The next two clamps will be applied above this sentinel first clamp.

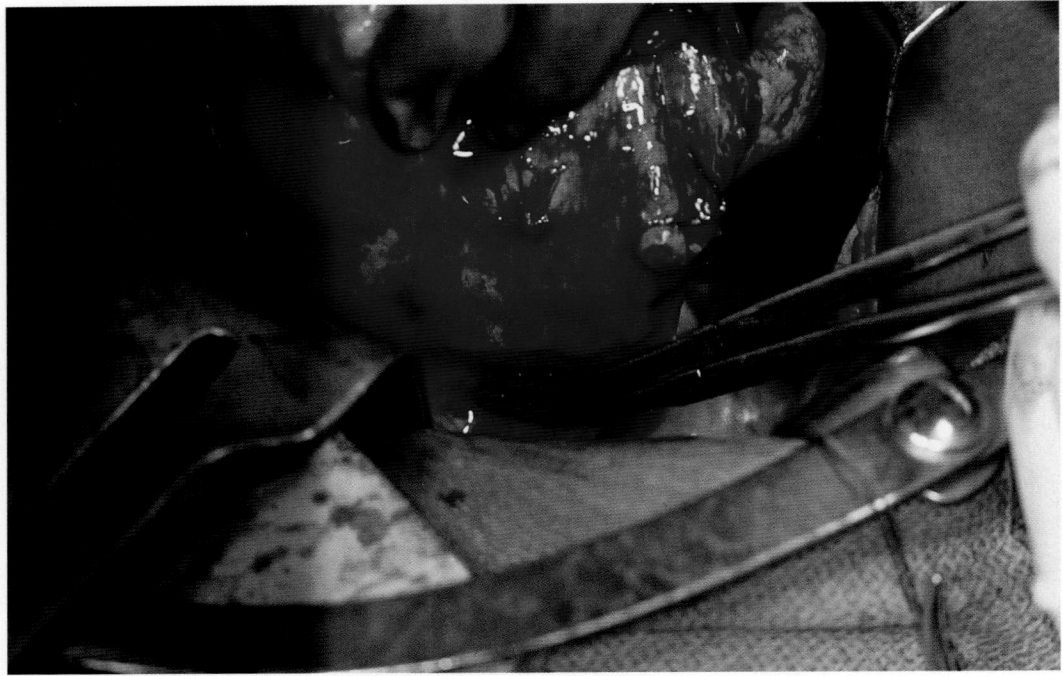

**FIGURE 11–12** The second clamp has been placed close above the first clamp. The clamp itself should have an identical curve to the first clamp applied.

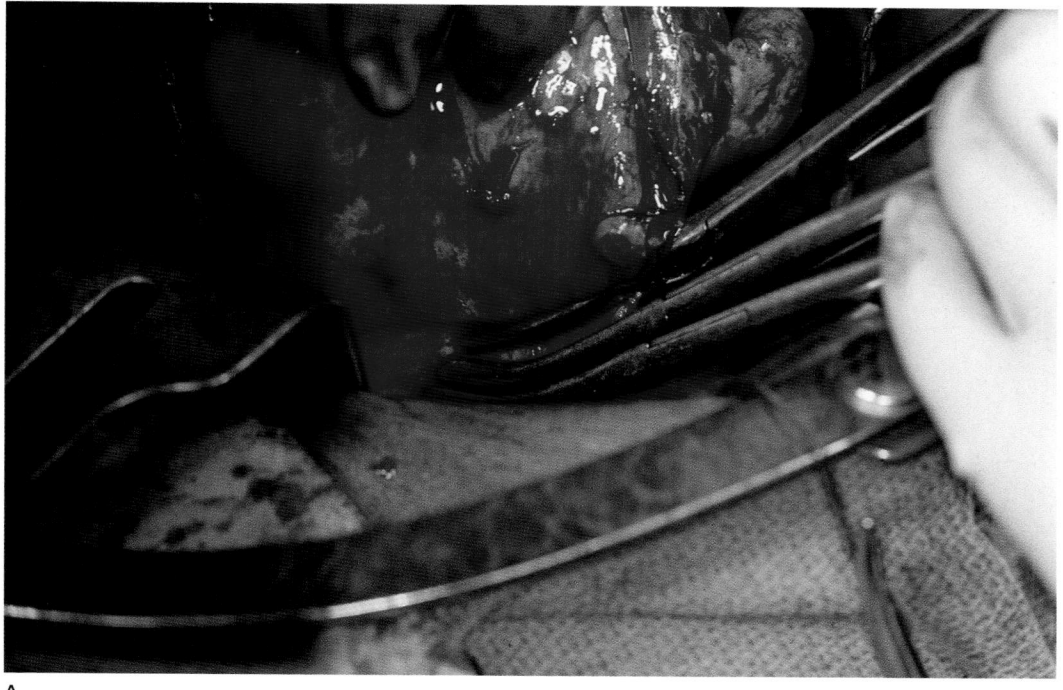

A

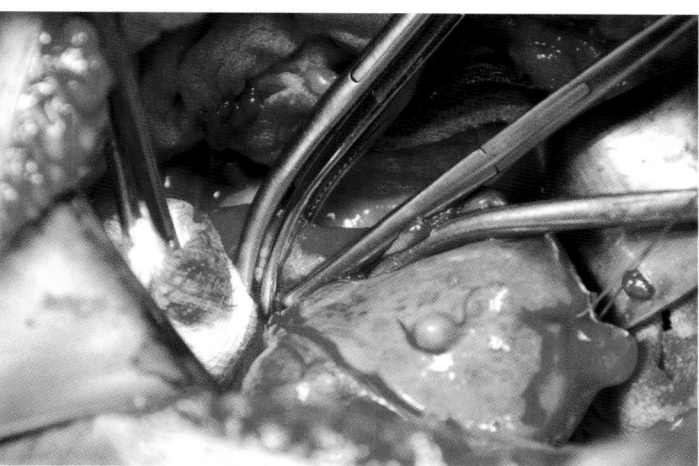

B

**FIGURE 11–13 A.** A third clamp is applied for the purpose of controlling back-bleeding. **B.** Two curved Zeppelin clamps are placed across the uterine vessels. A straight clamp is placed close to the corpus for back-bleeding. The cut will be made between the second applied curved clamp and the straight clamp.

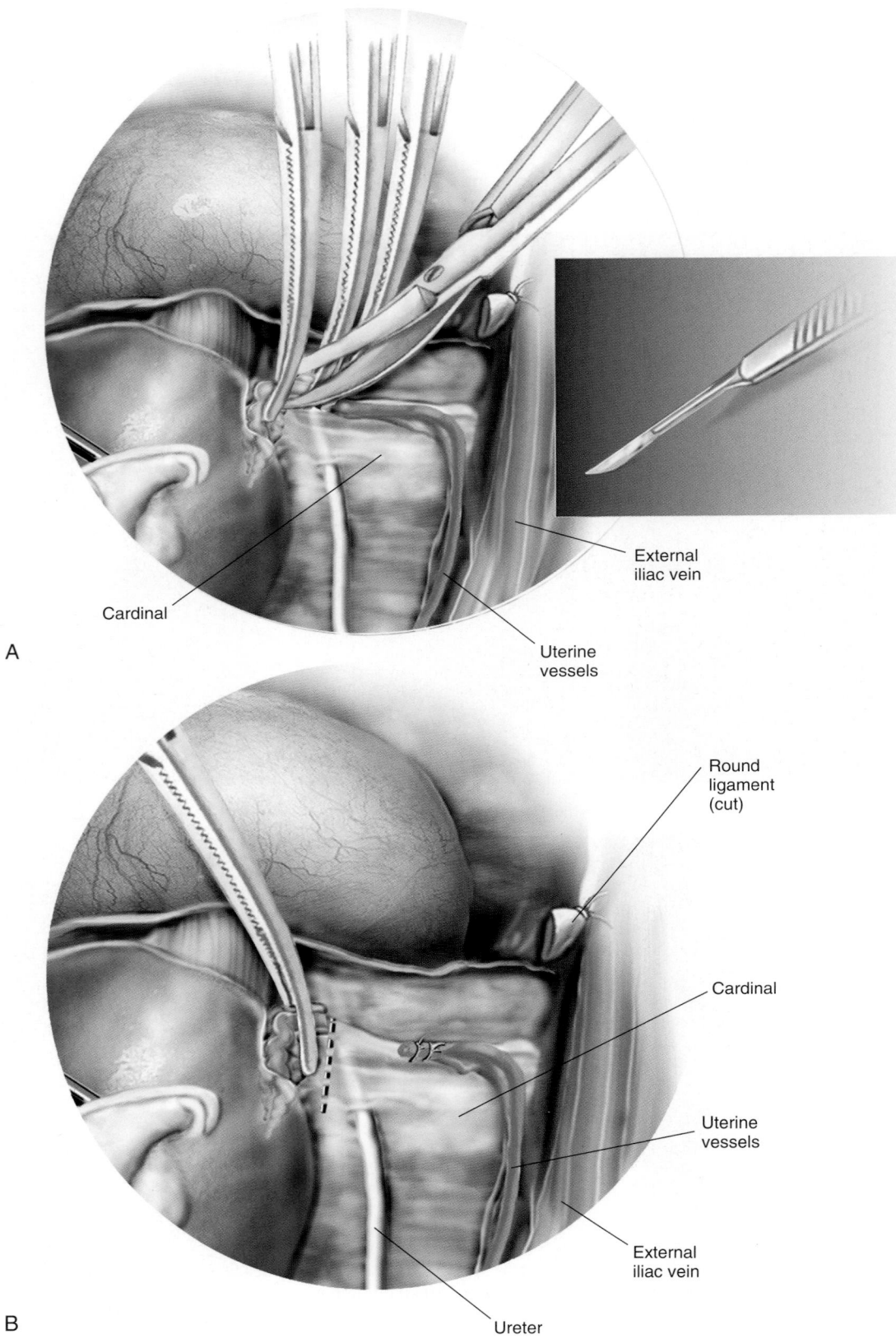

Cardinal

A

External
iliac vein

Uterine
vessels

Round
ligament
(cut)

Cardinal

Uterine
vessels

External
iliac vein

Ureter

B

**FIGURE 11–14 A.** The uterine vessels are cut between the second and third clamps applied. This may be accomplished with either scissors or a knife. The incision should not extend beyond the tip of the clamp. **B.** Suture ligatures of 0 Vicryl are placed just below the tip of each clamp and tied. The uterine vessels are thus doubly suture-ligated. Again, the location of the ureter should be checked. At this point, the ureter traverses the cardinal ligament to reach the bladder base. The dashed line indicates where the cardinal ligament will subsequently be clamped and cut.

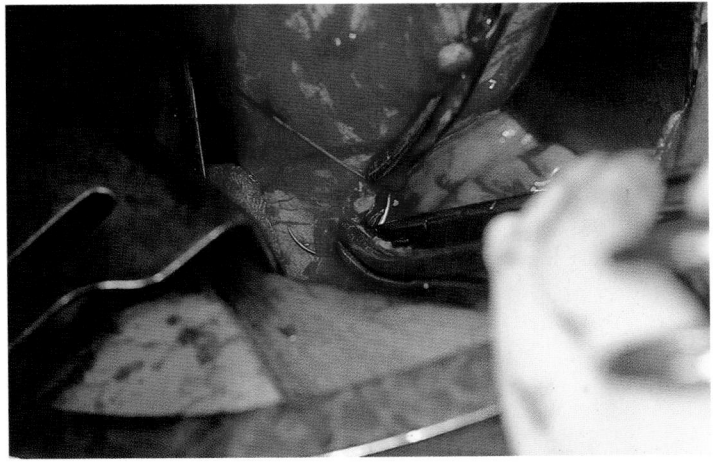
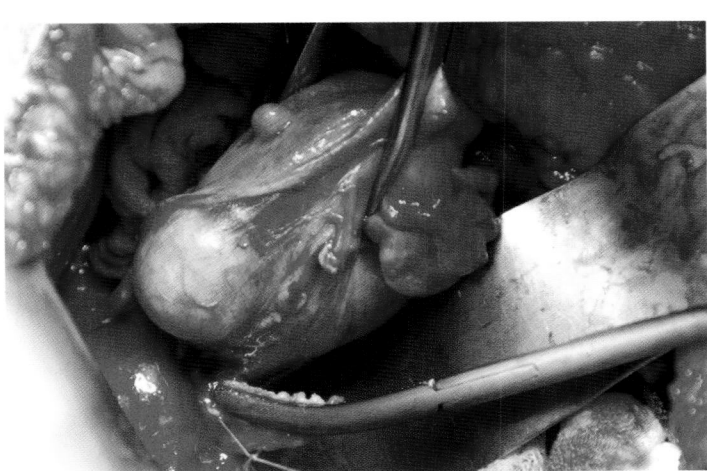

A

B

**FIGURE 11–15 A.** Technique for suturing the uterine artery pedicle. Note that the needle passes directly beneath the tip of the uterine artery clamp. The back-bleeding clamps can be removed after both uterine arteries have been divided and suture-ligated, because by this point the ovarian and uterine vessels have been ligated. **B.** The uterine vessels have been cut. A suture ligature has been placed and is being tightened and tied. A second suture ligature will be placed beneath the remaining clamp.

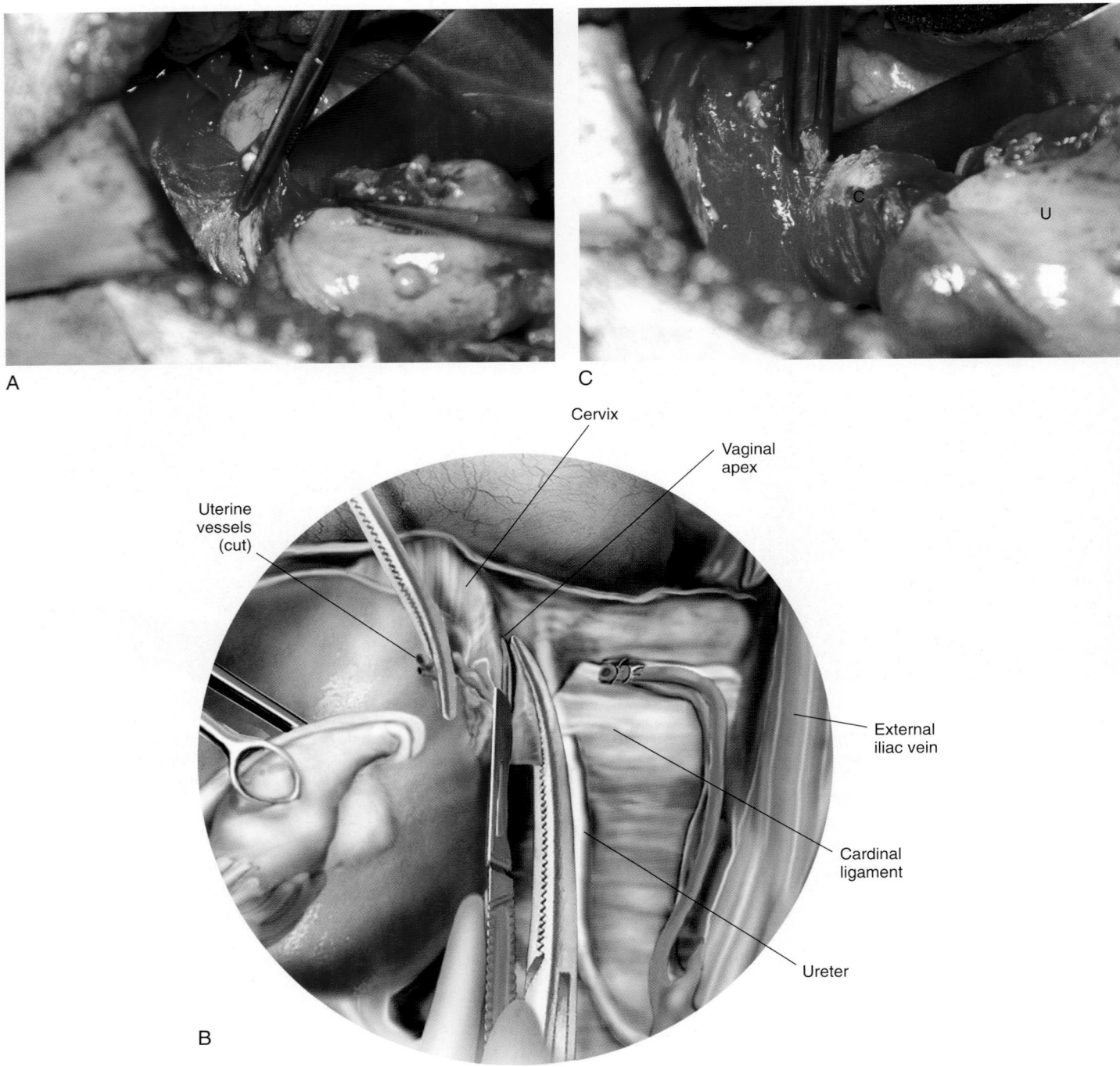

Cervix

Vaginal apex

Uterine vessels (cut)

External iliac vein

Cardinal ligament

Ureter

A

C

B

**FIGURE 11–16  A.** The cardinal ligament is clamped. **B.** The upper portion of the cardinal ligament may now be clamped close to the upper portion of the cervix. **C.** The cut edge of the cardinal ligament is held within the clamp. The cervix is seen at C with the body of the uterus above U.

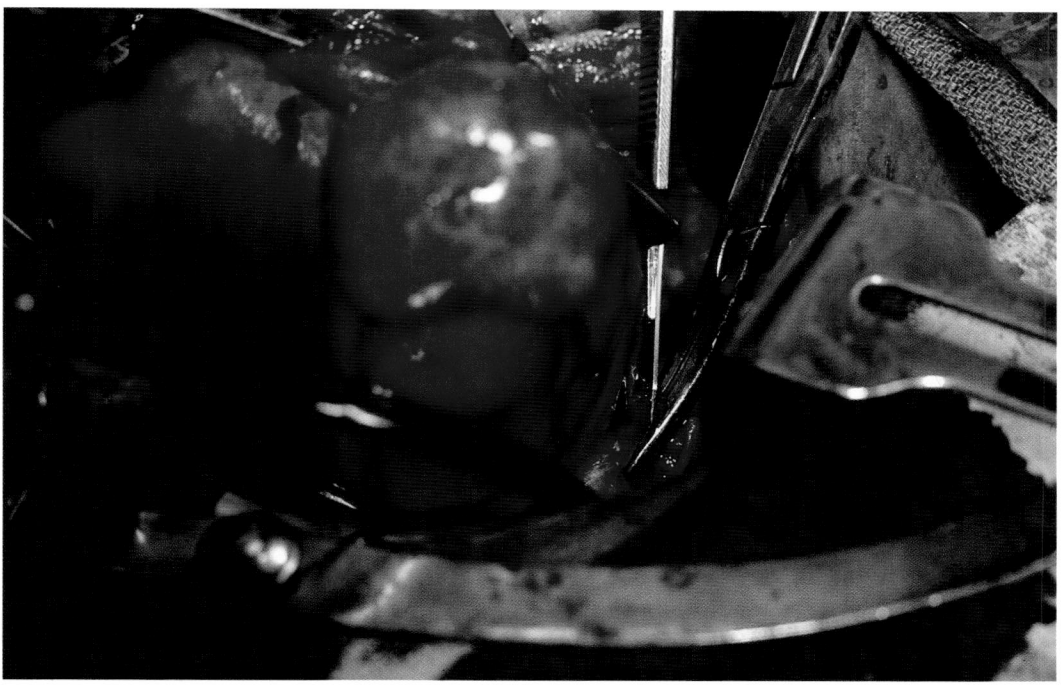

D

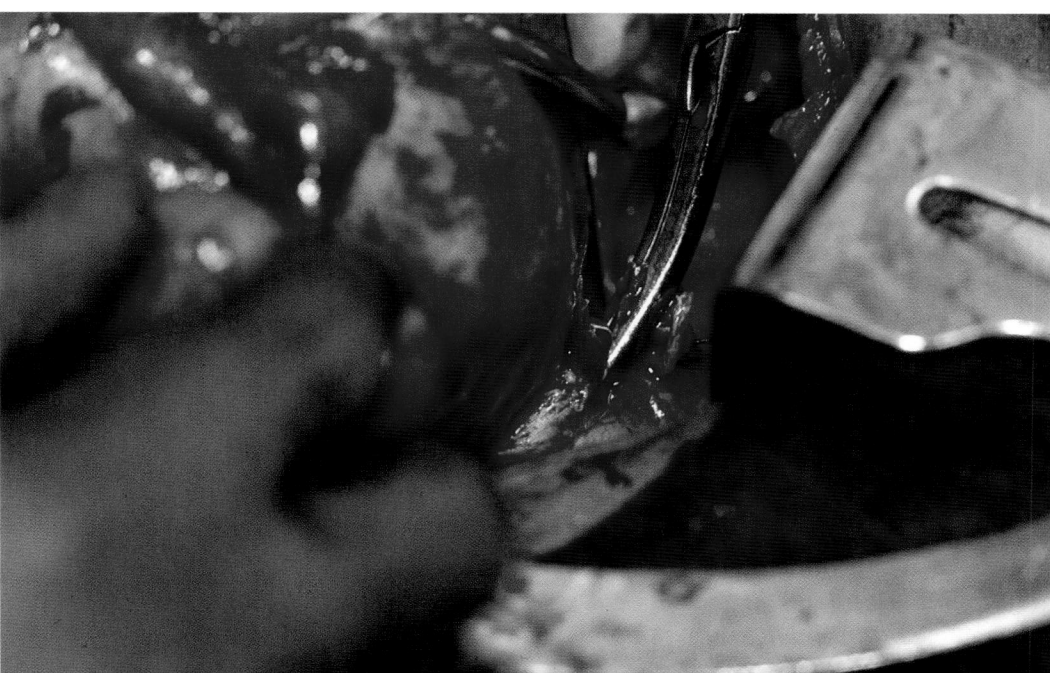

E

**FIGURE 11–16, cont'd D.** The clamped upper cardinal ligament is incised. **E.** The cardinal ligament is now free at the cervicouterine junction.

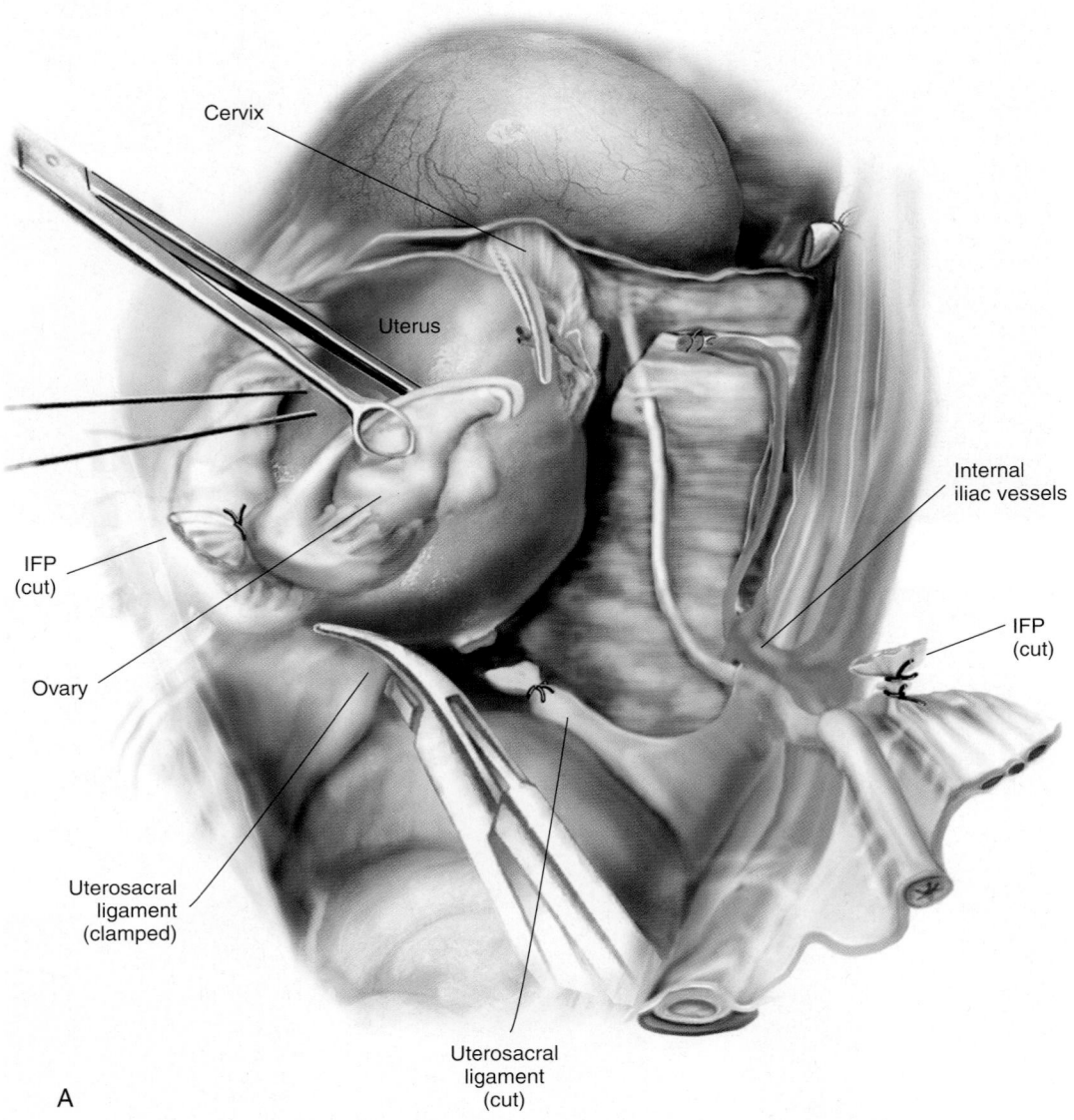

Cervix

Uterus

Internal
iliac vessels

IFP
(cut)

Ovary

IFP
(cut)

Uterosacral
ligament
(clamped)

Uterosacral
ligament
(cut)

A

**FIGURE 11–17  A.** Next, the uterosacral ligaments are clamped close to the uterus and incised. The clamped uterosacral ligament is suture-ligated by means of a transfixing suture. Similarly, the cut upper cardinal ligament is ligated by a transfixing suture.

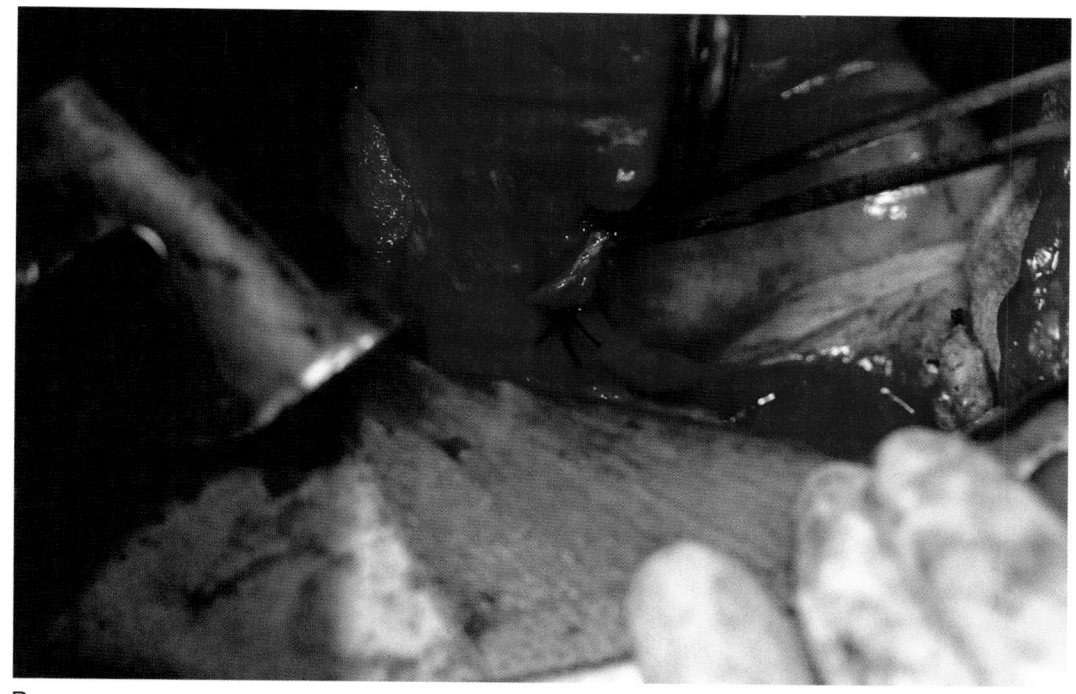

B

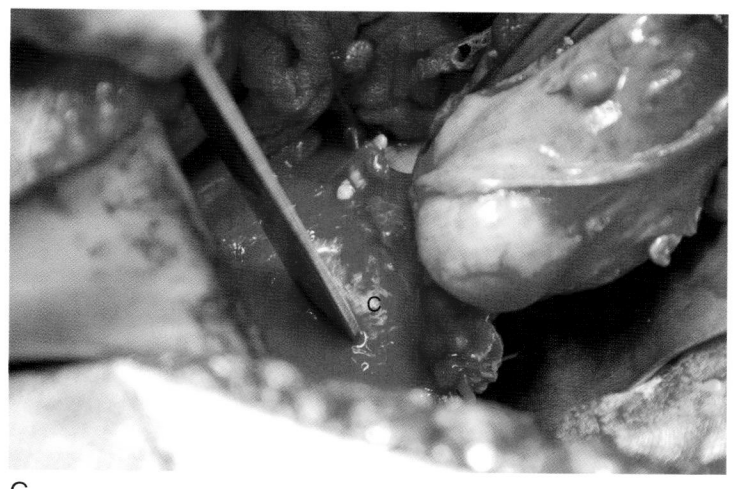

C

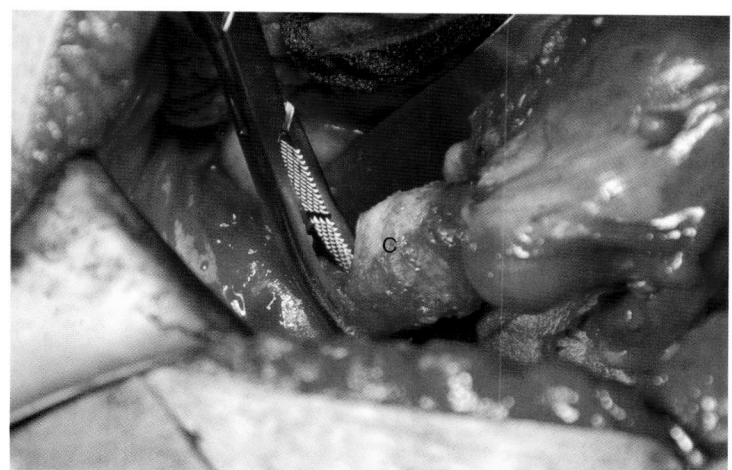

D

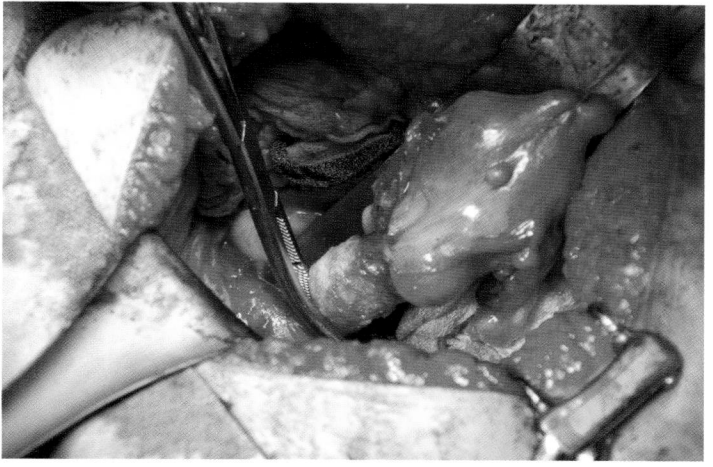

E

**FIGURE 11–17, cont'd  B.** The uterosacral ligaments are bilaterally cut and sutured (as in Fig. 11–17A). The forceps is holding the cut end of the left uterosacral ligament. **C.** The pubocervical fascia covering the cervix (C) has been cut transversely with a scalpel. With the handle of the scalpel, the fascia is pushed inferiorly. **D.** The edge of the vagina below the cervix (C) is isolated from the bladder, and a clamp is placed across the vagina. **E.** The clamp is closed.

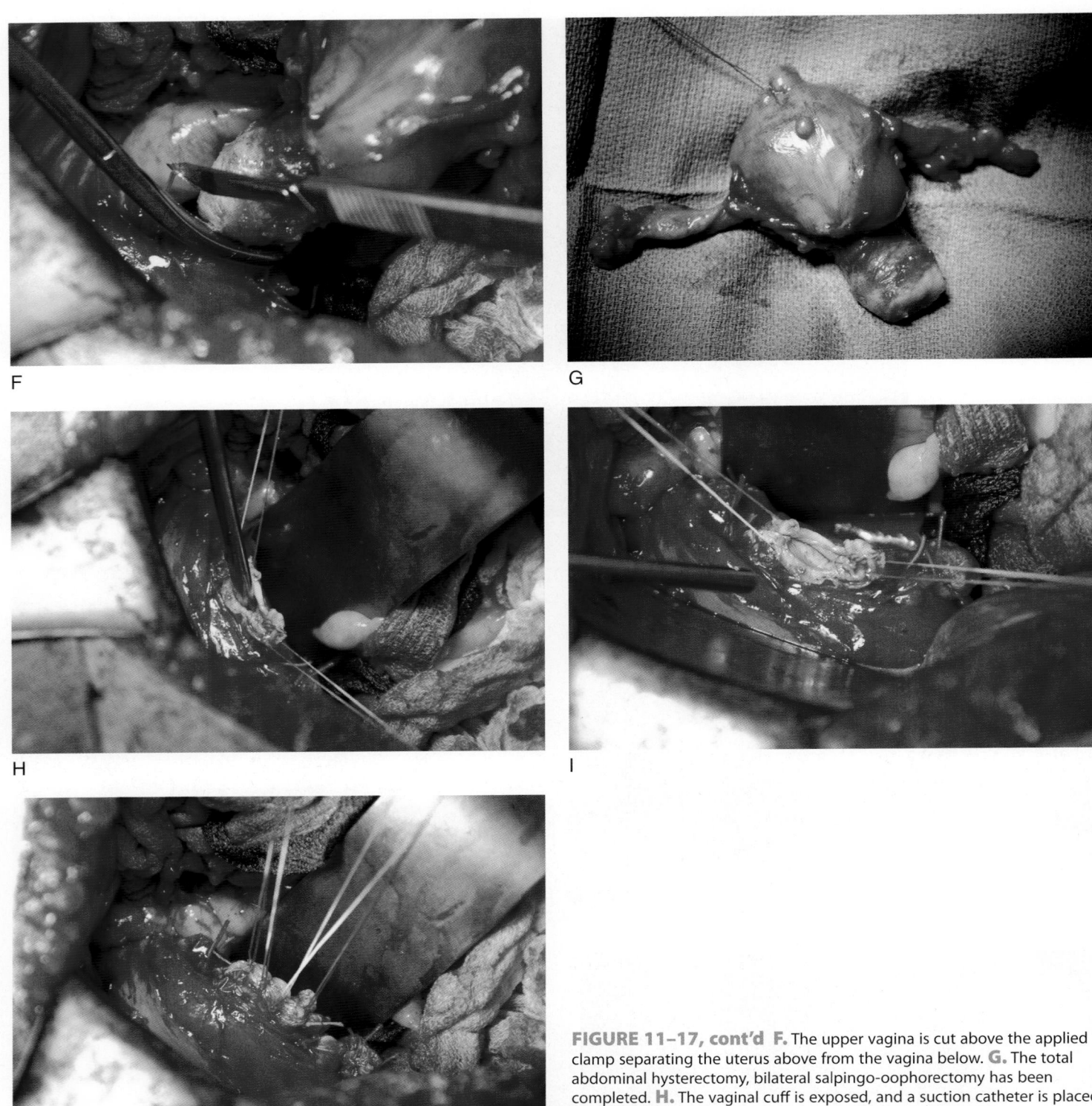

**FIGURE 11–17, cont'd  F.** The upper vagina is cut above the applied clamp separating the uterus above from the vagina below. **G.** The total abdominal hysterectomy, bilateral salpingo-oophorectomy has been completed. **H.** The vaginal cuff is exposed, and a suction catheter is placed into the vagina. **I.** The anterior and posterior walls of the vagina are inspected. **J.** The vagina has been closed with interrupted 0 Vicryl sutures. Note that the sigmoid colon is protected by the malleable retractor.

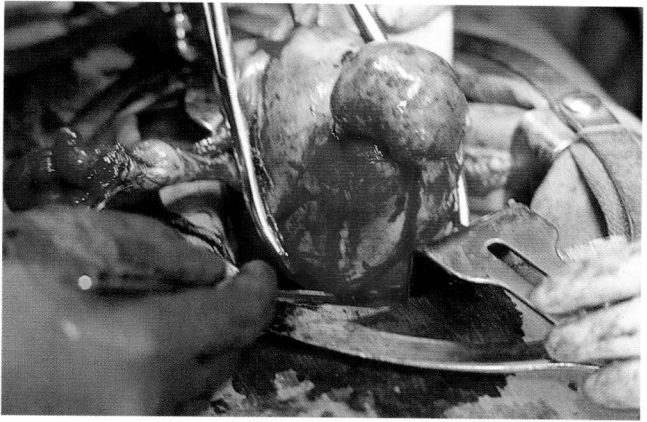

**FIGURE 11–18** In the case of a large, bulky uterus the body of the uterus may be separated from the cervix to provide better viewing within the pelvis. A scalpel cuts between the corpus and the cervix.

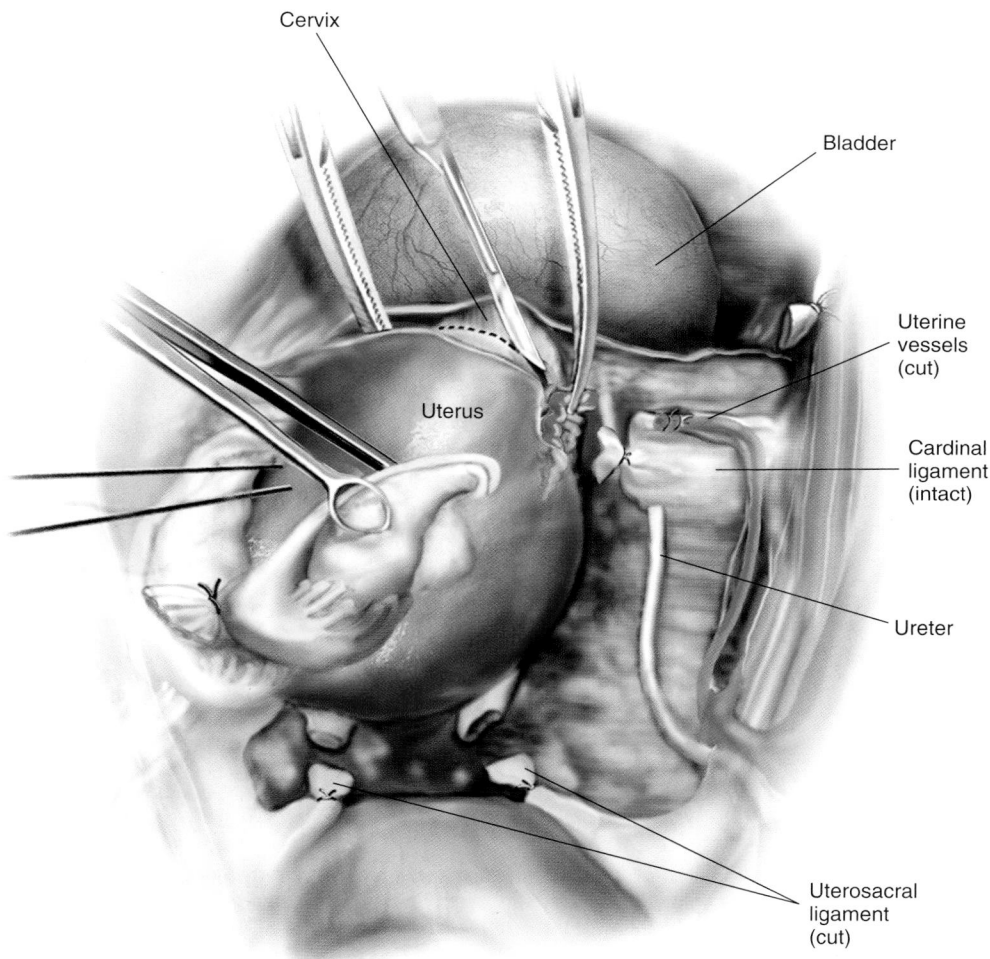

**FIGURE 11–19** The dashed line shows the plane through which the scalpel will cut the uterine body free relative to performing a temporary subtotal procedure (see Fig. 11–18). No bleeding should be encountered during the maneuver.

9. The cervix is grasped with two tenacula, and the superficial portion of the lower part of the cardinal ligament is clamped on each side. Note that the clamp is applied close to the sides of the cervix away from the ureter (Fig. 11–20A, B). The pubovesical cervical fascia is incised and pushed inferiorly, creating a plane between the bladder base and the cervix (Fig. 11–21). Finally, straight clamps are placed along the lowest portion of the cardinal ligaments, with the tips of the clamps within the peeled down pubovesical cervical fascia (Fig. 11–22). The ligaments are cut with a sharp scalpel and sutured with a 0 Vicryl transfixing stitch (Fig. 11–23).

10. The bladder is pushed farther inferiorly, with use of the established infrafascial plane within the pubovesical cervical fascia. Note that the vagina is behind and the bladder and ureters are in front of the plane. Clamps are applied within the pubovesical cervical fascial plane to secure the vaginal angles (Fig. 11–24). The cervix is cut away from the top of the vagina, and a small margin of vagina is incorporated with it (Fig. 11–25). The vaginal angles are secured, and the vagina is closed with interrupted figure-of-8 sutures of 0 Vicryl (Figs. 11–26 and 11–27A). Alternatively, the vaginal cuff may be left open by suturing the edges with a continuous running lock suture of 0 Vicryl (Fig. 11–27B). The wound should be irrigated to facilitate identification of bleeding sites.

11. Next the vagina is suspended by suturing the stumps of the cardinal and uterosacral ligaments to the vaginal vault (Fig. 11–28).

12. Finally, the peritoneum is carefully closed. The position of the ureter must be definitely identified so as not to ligate it during this phase of peritoneal closure.

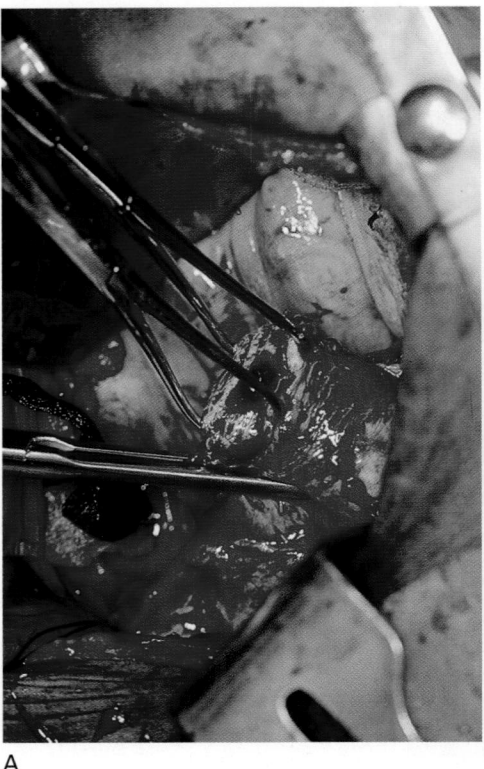
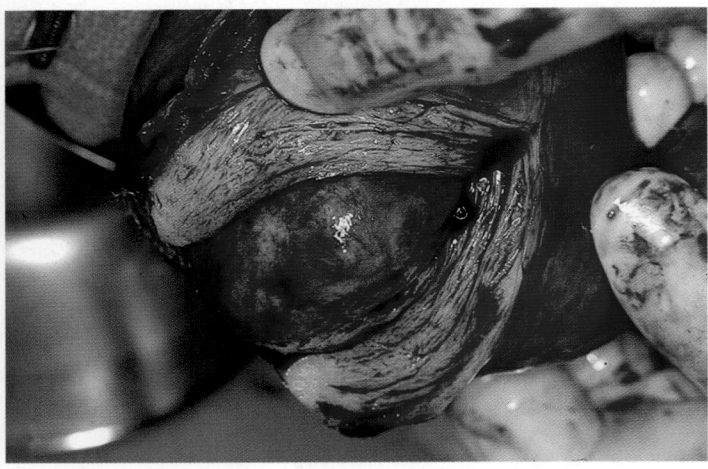

A

B

**FIGURE 11–20 A.** The corpus of the uterus has been separated and removed from the field. Two tenacula have been placed through the cervical stump. The right cardinal ligament has been cut and sutured by a transfixing ligature. A Zeppelin clamp has been placed on the left cardinal ligament close to the cervix (view from head looking toward feet). **B.** The separated corpus is cut, demonstrating a large submucous myoma.

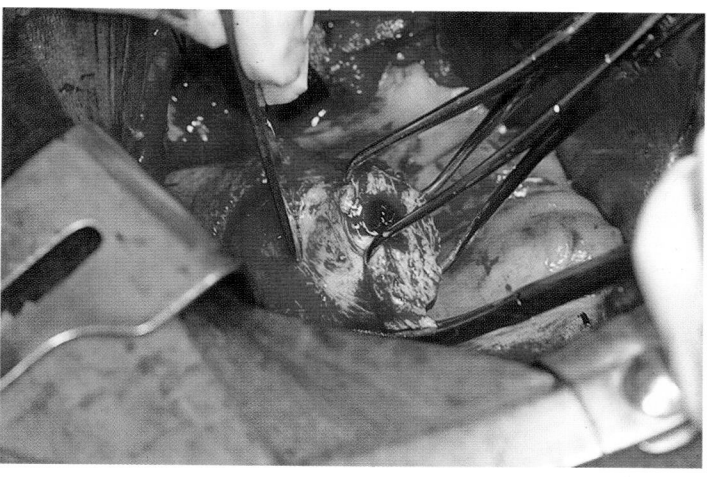

**FIGURE 11–21** The pubovesical cervical fascia is cut transversely with a scalpel and is dissected inferiorly.

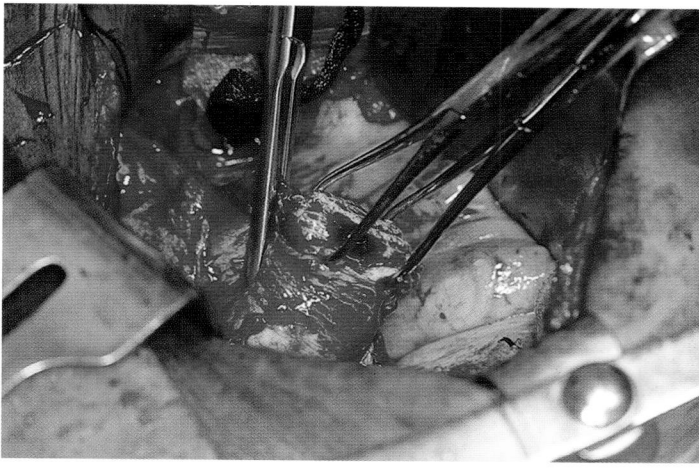

**FIGURE 11–22** A straight Zeppelin clamp is placed across the bottom of the cardinal ligament with the point of the clamp angled within the pubovesicocervical fascia. Clamping within the fascial layer prevents injury to the bladder and ureters.

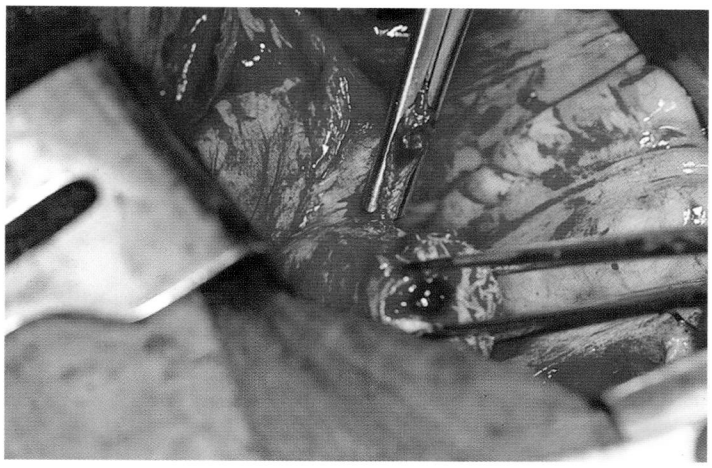

**FIGURE 11–23** The lower portion of the cardinal ligament is cut.

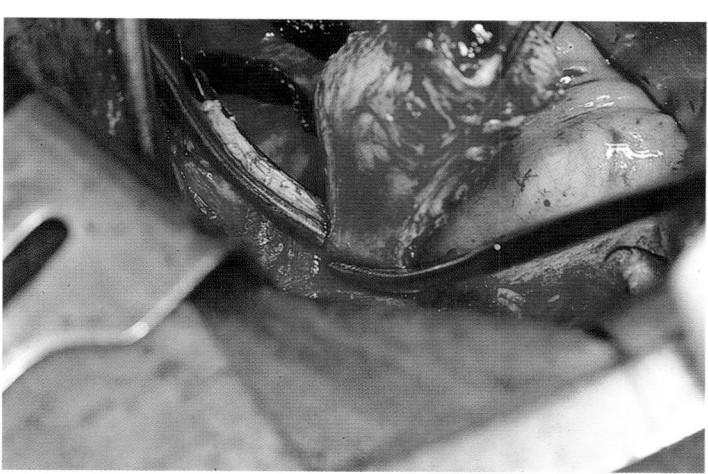

**FIGURE 11–24** Zeppelin clamps are placed at the angles of the vagina as the cervix is cut away from the top of the vagina.

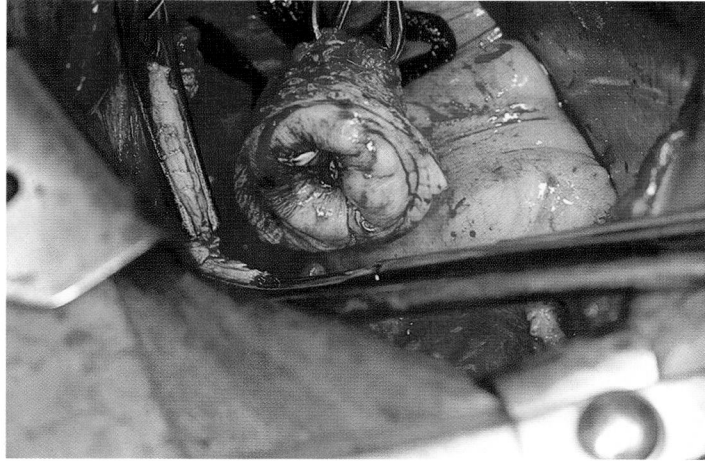

**FIGURE 11–25** The excised cervix is shown with its peripheral "cuff" of vagina. Below, the Zeppelin clamps are across the vaginal vault.

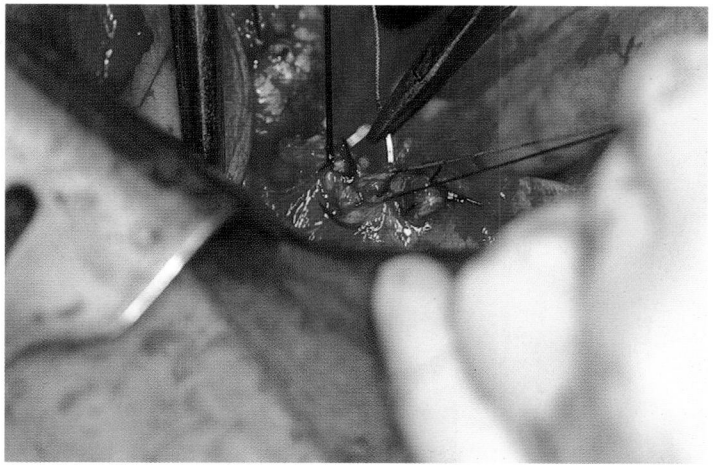

**FIGURE 11–26** The top of the vagina may be closed with figure-of-8 (hemostatic) sutures as pictured here or, alternatively, may be left open by running a continuous locking stitch completely around the upper margin of the vagina.

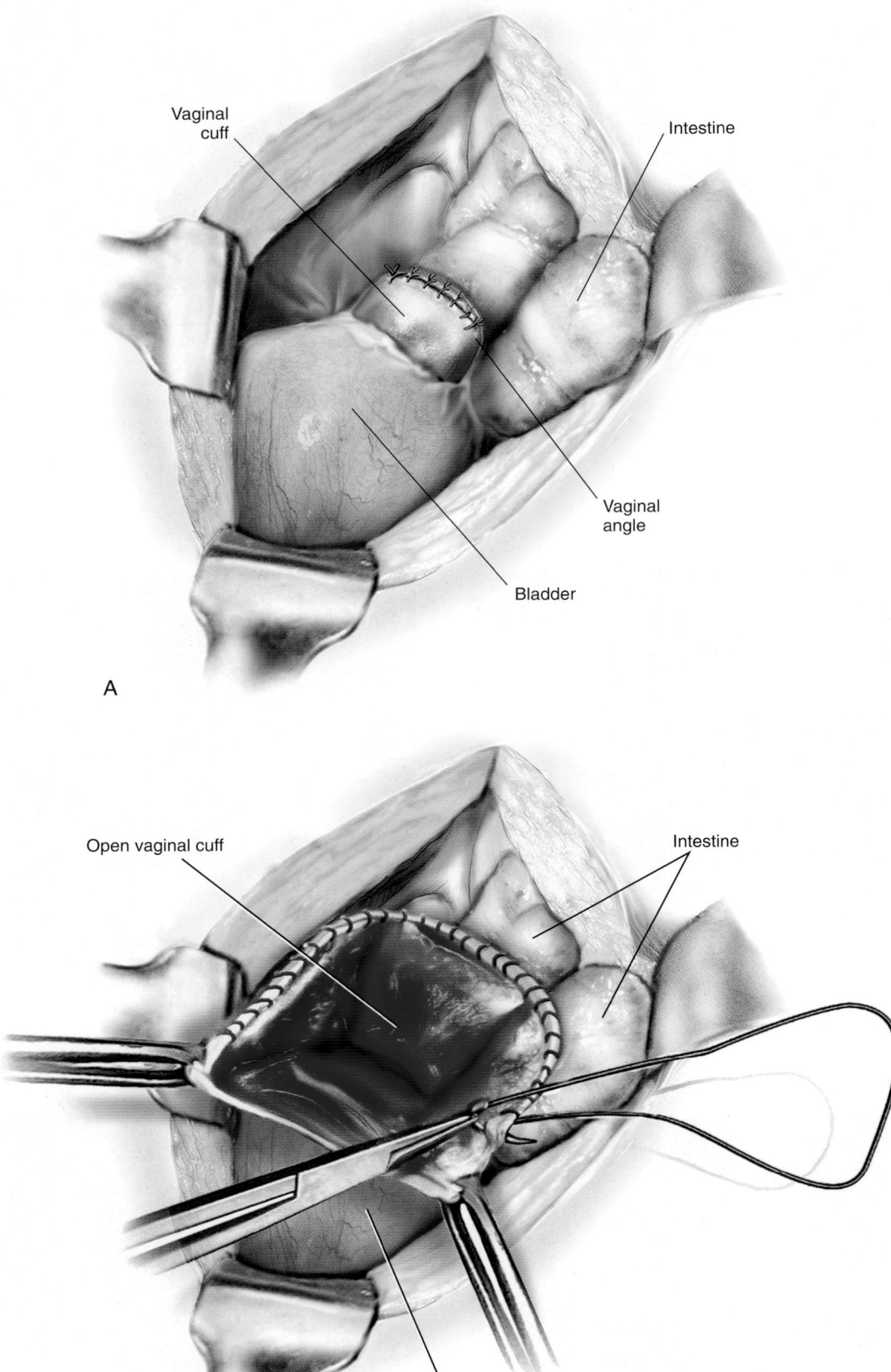

**FIGURE 11–27  A.** This view is taken from the front perspective. The uterus is gone. The top of the vagina is neatly separated from the bladder and has been sutured closed. **B.** The uterus has been removed. The edges of the vagina have been grasped with Allis clamps. The upper margin (cuff) of the vagina is reefed with a running or running lock stitch. Following closure, the vagina is suspended (see Fig. 11–28).

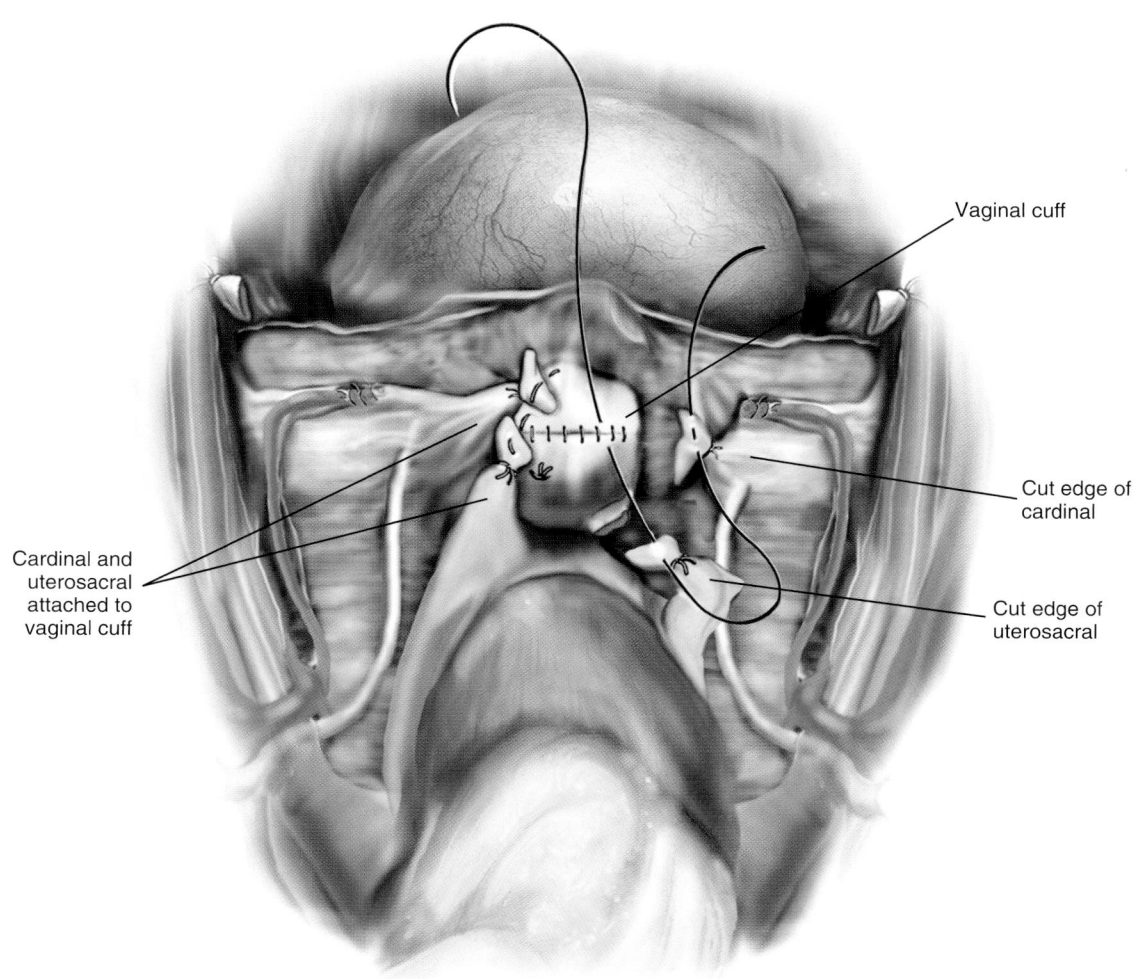

Vaginal cuff

Cut edge of
cardinal

Cut edge of
uterosacral

Cardinal and
uterosacral
attached to
vaginal cuff

**FIGURE 11–28** The final steps to complete the hysterectomy are to suspend the vaginal vault by suturing the cardinal and uterosacral ligament stumps into the vagina. In this picture, the suspension has been completed on the left side, and the right side has been sutured but not yet tied into place. Finally, the cut edges of the perineum are approximated by a running suture of 3-0 Vicryl.

## Subtotal Hysterectomy

This procedure is not frequently done, although during the 1940s, 1950s, and even early 1960s, its performance was commonplace. The advantages of the operation are principally speed and a diminished risk of ureteral injury because the cardinal ligaments are not taken down. For emergency obstetric surgery (e.g., nonresponsive uterine atony, massive rupture), the operation is ideal.

Subtotal hysterectomy concludes after step 5 of the total hysterectomy (described in the previous subsection and depicted in Figs. 11–18 and 11–19). When the corpus is severed and removed from the field, operative exposure is always positively affected. The descending or cervical branch of the uterine artery is left intact if possible. If this branch is clamped with the larger ascending branch, no difficulty relative to vascular supply to the cervix is encountered because anastomotic branches of the

vaginal artery provide ample collateral circulation. Typically, the uterosacral and cardinal ligaments are intact; therefore, no suspension is required. The top of the exposed cervix should be closed; this can be accomplished by suturing the posterior surfaces to the anterior surfaces with the use of interrupted simple sutures or figure-of-8 sutures of 0 Vicryl (Fig. 11–29). Upon completion of cervical closure, the wound is irrigated to check for bleeding points. Next, the peritoneum from the earlier bladder reflection (see Fig. 11–4) is sutured to the posterior leaf of the previously incised peritoneum with a running stitch of 3-0 Vicryl (Fig. 11–30). The author recommends, before the top of the cervical stump is sutured, that the surgeon cut a thin disc from the exposed cervix at the point of separation from the body of the uterus to ensure that no functioning endometrium remains. The removed sample should be sent to pathology for frozen section. This procedure will eliminate the 7% risk of subsequent cyclic bleeding.

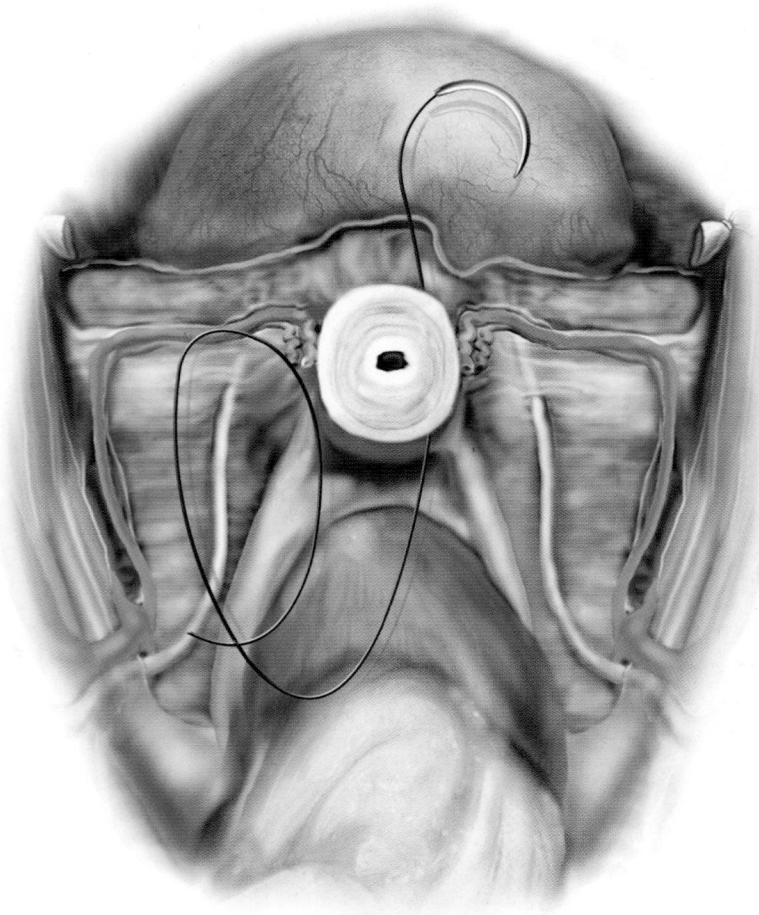

**FIGURE 11–29** In this picture, a subtotal hysterectomy is illustrated. The body of the uterus has been amputated (see Figs. 11–18 through 11–20). The cervix with its attached ligaments will be left in place. The intra-abdominal portion of the cervix is closed by a row of interrupted simple or figure-of-8 sutures.

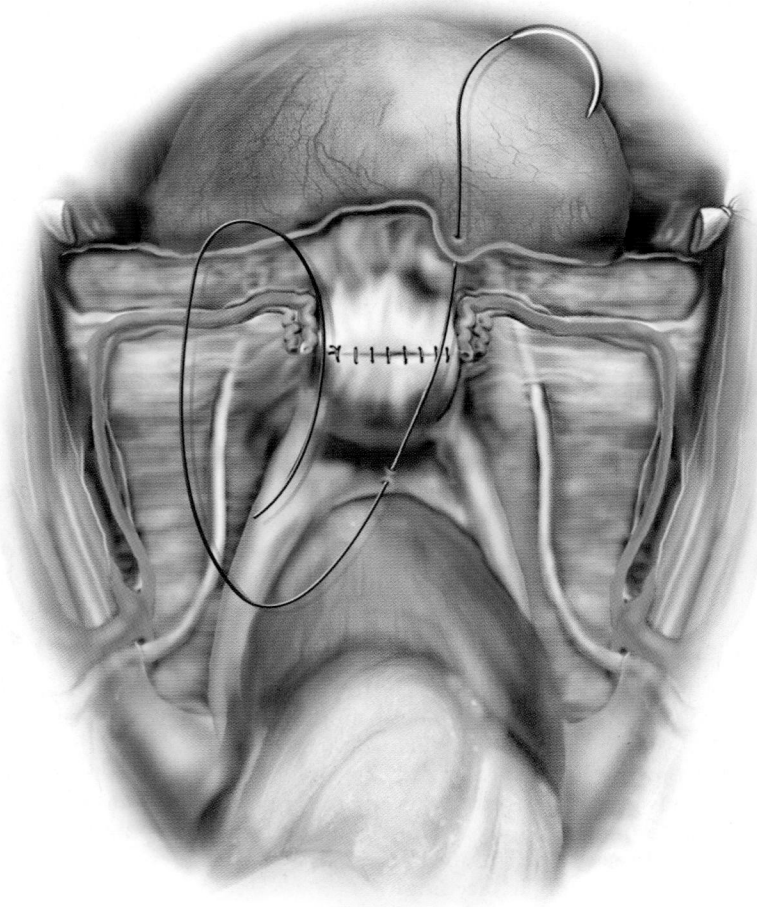

**FIGURE 11–30** The top of the cervix has been closed. The peritoneum (visceral) is closed over the operative site.

## Simple Abdominal Hysterectomy

Another variant of the abdominal hysterectomy is preservation of the adnexa at the time of uterine extirpation. In this instance, the utero-ovarian ligament and the oviduct are triply clamped close to the uterine fundus. The incision is made with scissors or knife between the clamp closest to the uterus and the second clamp. Transfixing suture ligatures of 0 Vicryl are placed behind the third (most distant from the uterus) and second clamps. A simple tie or suture ligature can be placed under the first clamp to prevent back-bleeding as an alternative to keeping the clamp attached until the uterine vascular supply is secured (Fig. 11–31). The three suturing techniques described herein and in preceding paragraphs are illustrated in Figure 11–32.

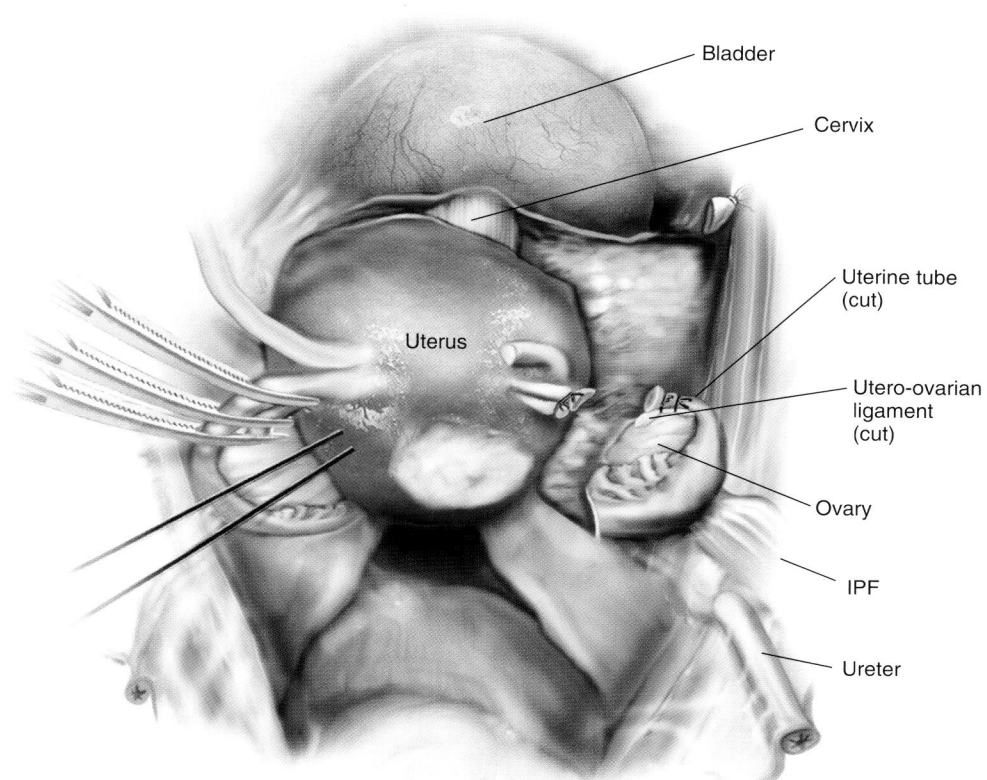

Bladder

Cervix

Uterine tube
(cut)

Uterus

Utero-ovarian
ligament
(cut)

Ovary

IPF

Ureter

**FIGURE 11–31** The technique of simple hysterectomy without excision of the tubes and ovaries. On the right side, the round ligament has been divided and sutured. The tube and utero-ovarian ligament have been cut and doubly suture-ligated. On the left side, three clamps have been placed across the tube and utero-ovarian ligament. Note that a traction stitch has been placed into the uterine fundus.

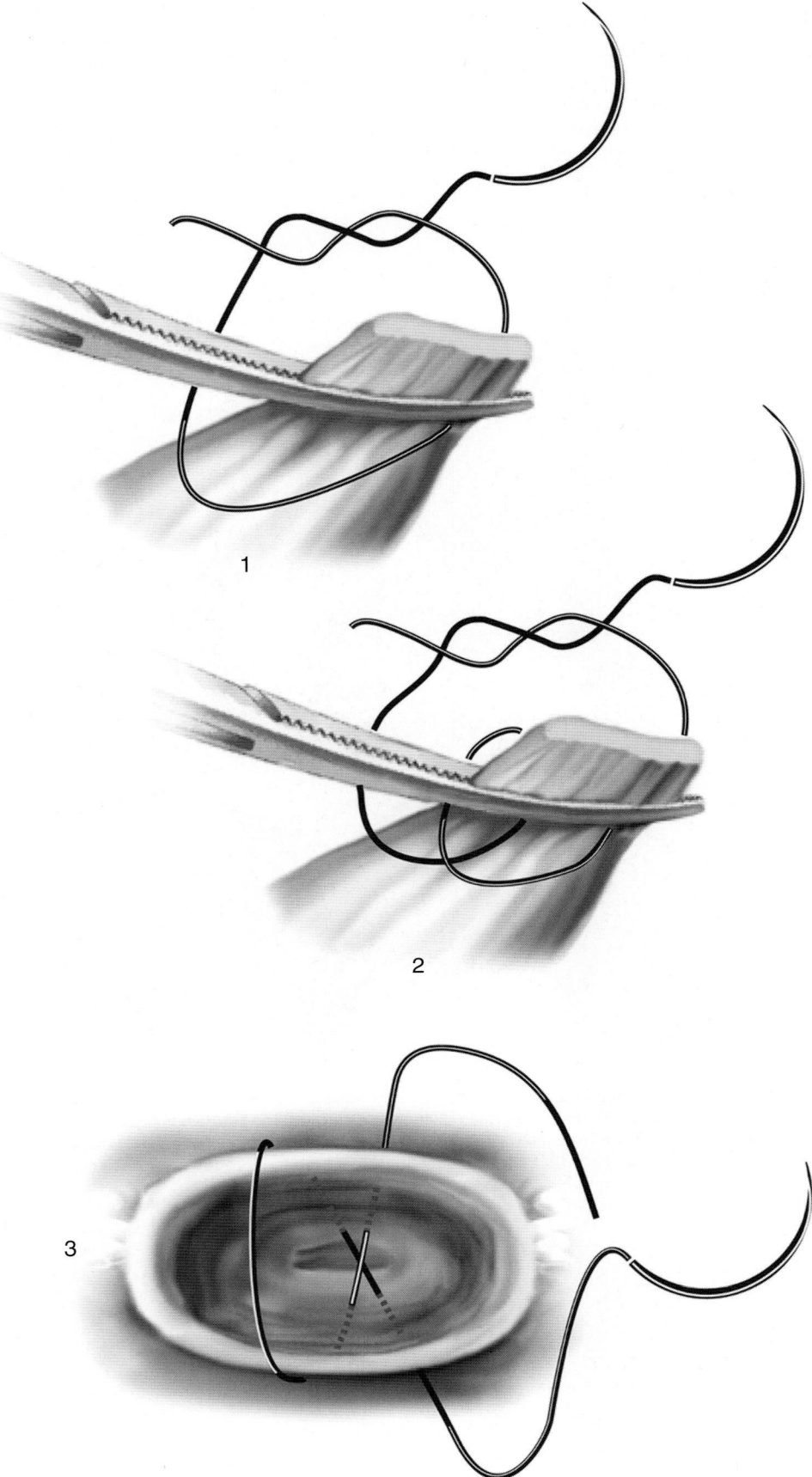

**FIGURE 11–32** Three types of sutures are used for hysterectomy: (1) simple suture ligature, (2) transfixing suture ligature, and (3) figure-of-8 suture ligature.

# CHAPTER 12

# Radical Hysterectomy

*Helmut F. Schellhas* ■ *Michael S. Baggish*

## Supplemental Anatomy for Radical Hysterectomy and Pelvic Lymphadenectomy

An understanding of the anatomy of the retroperitoneal space is required to initiate lymphadenectomy and exposure of the great vessels (Fig. 12–1A–C). Although the course of the ureter was covered earlier in this section, additional anatomic dissection views are needed to help the reader understand the operative steps necessary to perform radical hysterectomy (Fig. 12–2). In truth, radical hysterectomy and lymphadenectomy are exer-

cises in anatomic dissection. It is therefore imperative to have precise knowledge of the retroperitoneum, particularly the relationships of the ureter to the great vessels and of the vessels to one another (Fig. 12–3A–L).

The structures most vulnerable to injury and most difficult to repair are the veins accompanying the large pelvic arteries (Fig. 12–4). The precise location of these veins and their careful retraction are crucial to the safe performance of the surgery (Fig. 12–5A, B). All of these anatomic relationships come together during the dissection of the obturator fossa (Fig. 12–6).

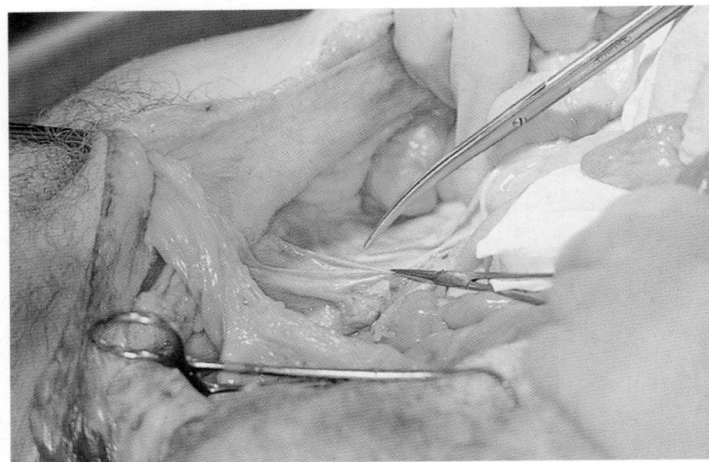

A

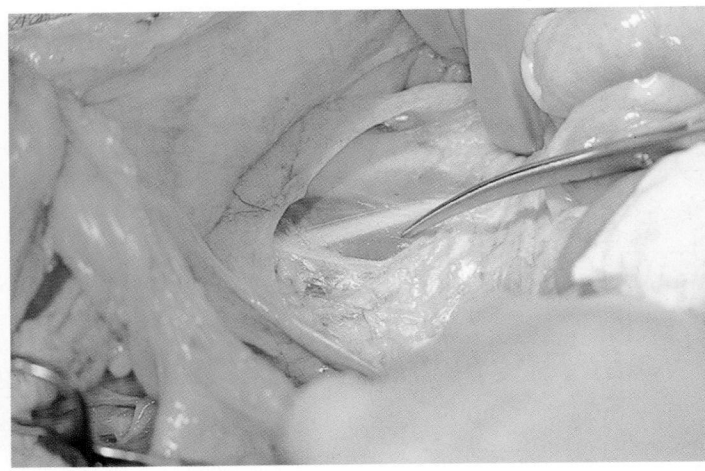

B

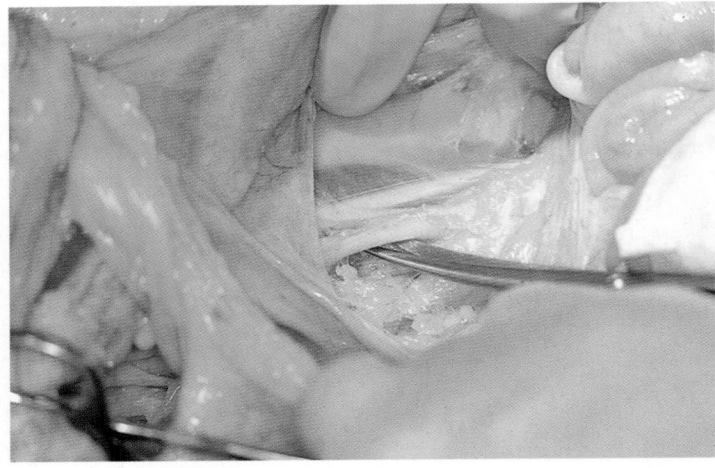

C

**FIGURE 12–1 A.** The retroperitoneum is entered by grasping the round ligament and cutting the peritoneum at the top of the broad ligament in a linear and foot-to-head direction. **B.** The scissors point to the belly of the psoas major muscle, which is lateral to the external iliac artery. **C.** The external iliac artery has now been exposed and lies above the spread tips of the scissors.

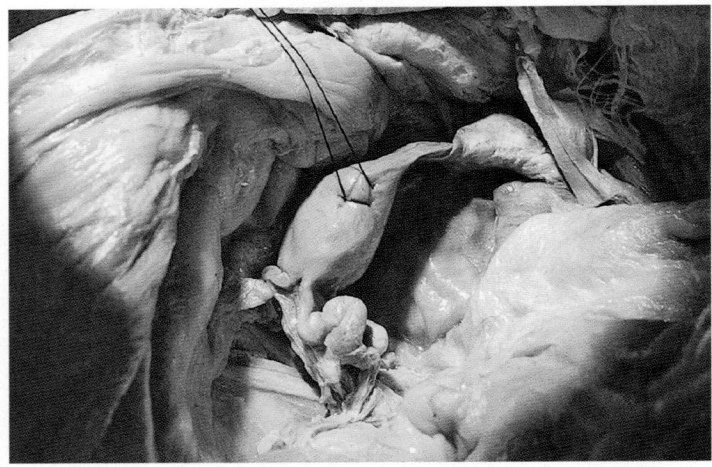

**FIGURE 12–2** Orientation view of the uterus in situ with a ligature placed into the fundus for traction.

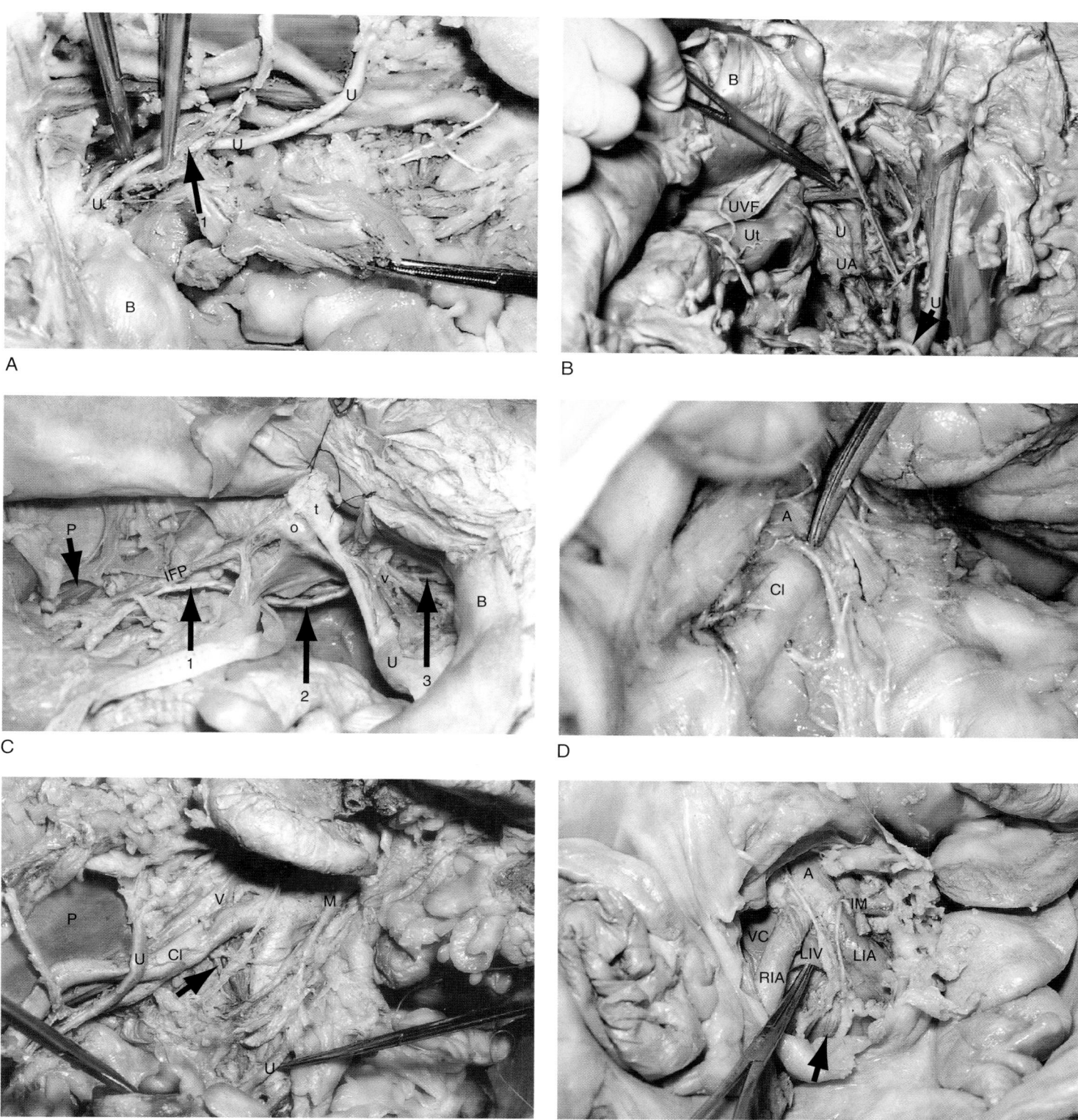

A        B

C        D

E        F

**FIGURE 12-3  A.** The entire course of the right ureter is shown here. U, ureter; 1, uterine artery; B, bladder (view from left side). **B.** The entire course of the right ureter viewed from overhead. Ut, uterus; U, ureter; B, bladder; UVF, uterovesical fold; UA, feeding vessel to ureter. The clamp points to the uterine artery. **C.** The entire course of the left ureter is shown. U, uterus; arrows 1, 2, and 3 point to the ureter; IFP, infundibulopelvic ligament; O, ovary; t, tube; B, bladder; P, psoas major muscle; V, uterine vessels. **D.** The scissors point to the aorta (A) and fibers of the hypogastric nerve plexus. CI, common iliac artery. **E.** The large vessels within the retroperitoneal space are well visualized in this photograph. The iliac veins and vena cava are also shown. A, aorta; M, inferior mesenteric artery; CI, common iliac artery; U, ureter; P, psoas major muscle. **F.** The presacral space is exposed. The arrow points to the middle sacral vessels. The clamp elevates the left internal iliac vein (LIV). A, aorta; RIA, right common iliac artery; LIA, left common iliac artery; IM, inferior mesenteric artery; VC, vena cava.

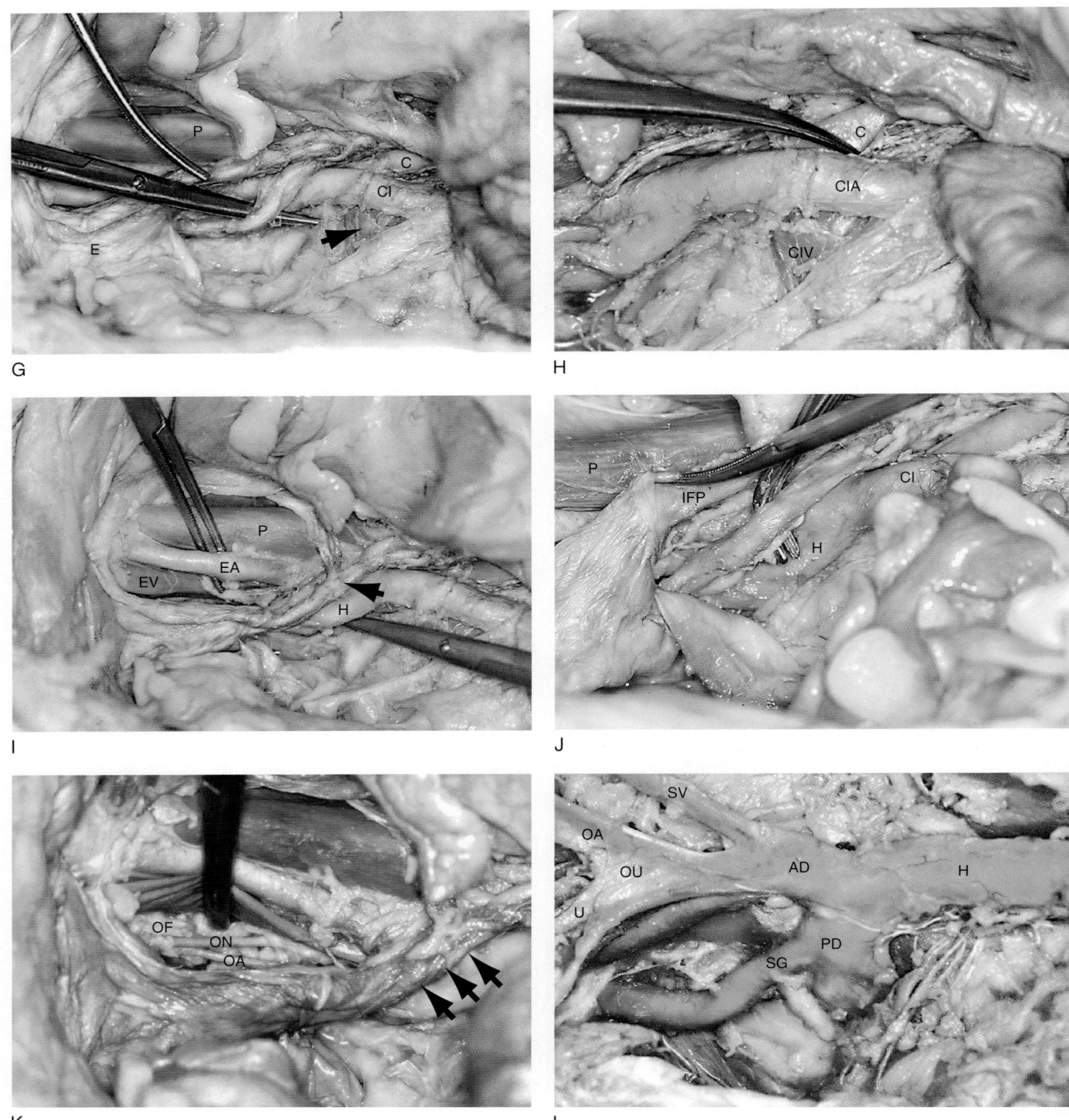

**FIGURE 12–3, cont'd  G.** The right ureter is elevated by the scissors. The clamp points to the ovarian vessels. The arrow points to the left common iliac vein. CI, common iliac artery (right); C, inferior vena cava; E, external iliac vein; P, psoas major muscle. **H.** Detail at presacral space. CIA, common iliac artery (right); CIV, common iliac vein (left); C, vena cava. **I.** The arrow points to the right ureter and the infundibulopelvic ligament. H, hypogastric artery; EV, external iliac vein; EA, external iliac artery; P, psoas major muscle. **J.** The ureter above the right-angle clamp has been separated from the ovarian vessels (infundibulopelvic ligament [IFP]). P, psoas major muscle; H, hypogastric artery; CI, common iliac artery. **K.** The arrows point to the right ureter. The clamp elevates the right external iliac vein to expose the obturator fossa (OF), the obturator nerve (ON), and the obturator artery (OA). **L.** Detailed dissection of the hypogastric artery (H) shows the anterior division (AD), the posterior division (PD), the common trunk with the obliterated umbilical and superior vesical artery (OU, SV), the obturator artery (OA), and the uterine artery (U). The superior gluteal artery (SG) branches from the posterior division (PD).

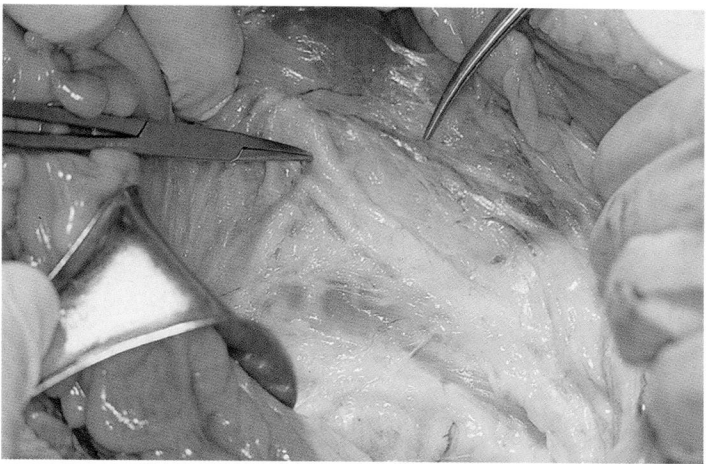

**FIGURE 12–4** The peritoneum has been opened over the terminus of the abdominal aorta (clamp). Both right and left common iliac arteries are clearly seen. The large vein is the left common iliac vein.

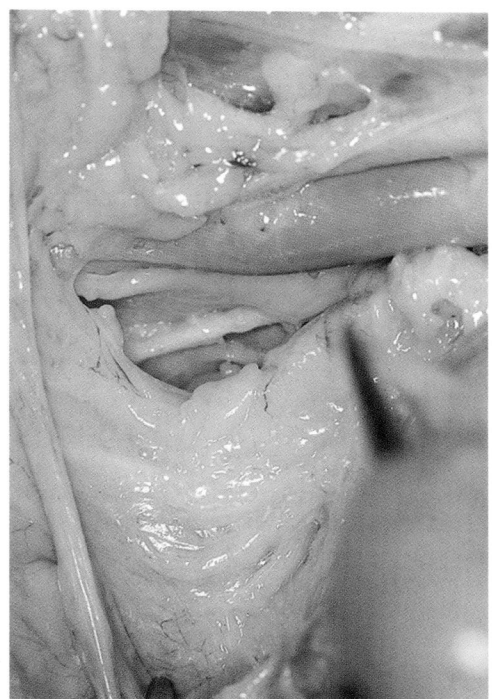

A

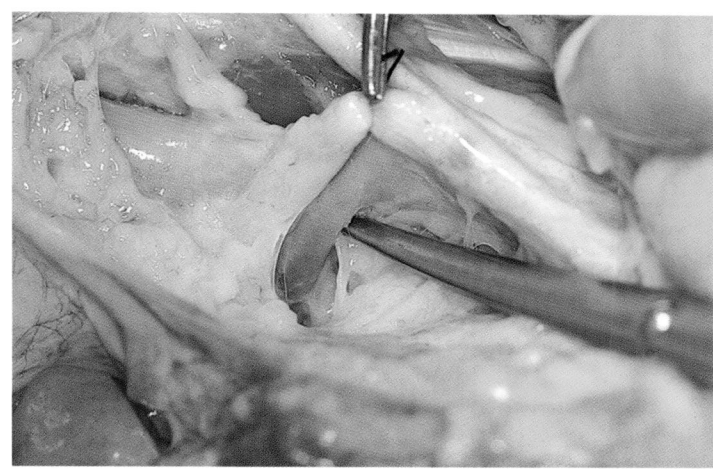

B

**FIGURE 12–5 A.** The external iliac artery and vein (*blue*) cross above the obturator fossa. Removal of some fat and lymph nodes partially exposes the obturator nerve (*white*) and the obturator artery (*pink*). **B.** The anterior division of the hypogastric artery has been ligated. A clamp elevates the hypogastric artery to expose the hypogastric vein. The tip of the scissors is just beneath the junction of the hypogastric and external iliac veins.

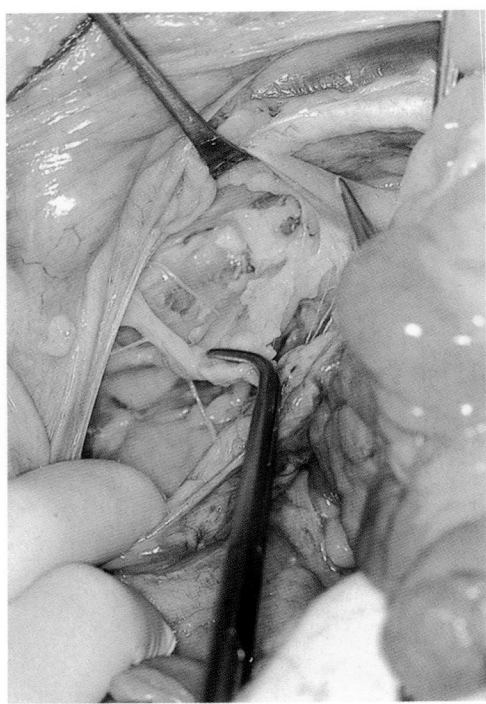

**FIGURE 12–6** A vein retractor elevates the external iliac vein. The lymph node–bearing fat is being dissected from the obturator fossa with the clamp. The obturator internus muscle is visible behind the fat.

## Radical Hysterectomy and Pelvic Lymphadenectomy

Radical hysterectomy and pelvic lymphadenectomy differ from simple abdominal hysterectomy in two major aspects.

First, the parametria are widely excised, as is the vagina. This requires the ureter to be dissected free for its entire course within the pelvis to the point where the ureter enters the bladder. Additionally, the bladder and the rectum must be separated from the vagina for a distance of 2 to 5 cm below the level of the cervicovaginal junction. Second, the tissues containing fat and lymph nodes are dissected and excised from the external iliac vessels, the obturator fossa, the internal iliac vessels, and the common iliac vessels to the level of the aorta. On occasion, the nodal dissection may expand upward around the aorta to the level of the renal arteries.

The operation is essentially an anatomic exercise.

As with simple abdominal hysterectomy (described in Chapter 11), the round ligaments are clamped and divided, and a bladder flap is developed on either side. The top of the broad ligament is incised in a cranial direction. The infundibulopelvic ligament is clamped, transsected, and doubly suture-ligated. If the ovaries are to be saved, the utero-ovarian ligament is clamped, divided, and doubly suture-ligated (Fig. 12–7).

At this point, the peritoneum on the lateral aspect of the broad ligament is dissected further laterally to expose the psoas major muscle. The external iliac artery is then identified and cleared of fat, as is the external iliac vein (Figs. 12–8 and 12–9).

During the course of the dissection, the ureter is identified and dissected free at the point where it crosses the common iliac artery to enter the pelvis (Fig. 12–10). The ureter is located posterior to (beneath) the ovarian vascular complex. As the external iliac node dissection proceeds toward the iliac bifurcation, the internal iliac artery is identified and cleared of fat (Fig. 12–11). Care is taken to protect the thin-walled external and internal iliac veins.

A vein retractor is placed under the external iliac vein and the vein is gently elevated (Fig. 12–12). This exposes the obturator fossa, which is filled with fat and lymph nodes (Fig. 12–13). The fat is dissected out of the fossa, and the obturator nerve and artery are cleaned of fat and lymph tissue (Fig. 12–14). The dissection is carried laterally until the fascia of the obturator internus muscle is reached (Fig. 12–15). Great care must be taken to not tear or otherwise injure the tributaries of the internal iliac veins because they bleed profusely and are very difficult to secure. When the obturator dissection is finished, the operator turns attention to the common iliac node dissection (Fig. 12–16). Again, great care must be taken to not injure the left common iliac vein.

Next, the ureter is dissected inferiorly, with the encompassing fibrofatty tissue removed and medially reflected to be removed with the uterus. The uterine arteries and veins are clamped far laterally, just distal to their origin from the anterior division of the hypogastric artery. If the hypogastric artery is to be clamped, this should be done distal to the origin(s) of the superior and inferior gluteal arteries (Fig. 12–17A–D).

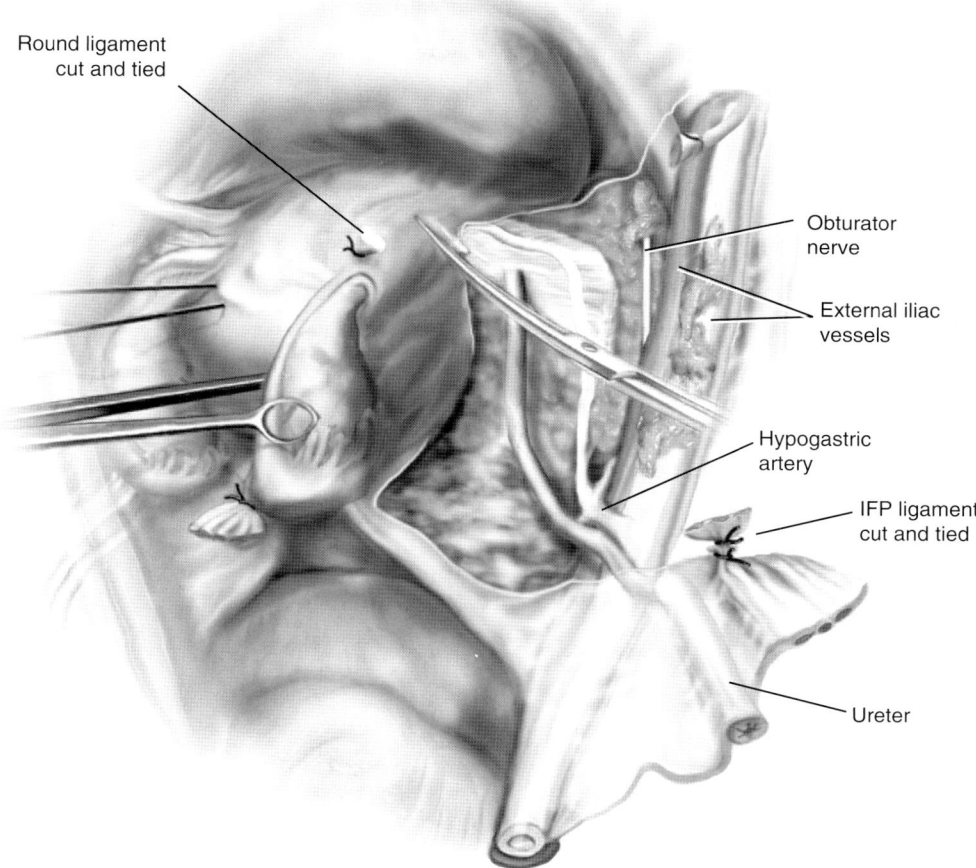

Opening of
broad ligament and
paravesical space

Round ligament
cut and tied

Obturator
nerve

External iliac
vessels

Hypogastric
artery

IFP ligament
cut and tied

Ureter

**FIGURE 12–7** The round ligament has been clamped, cut, and suture-ligated. The top of the broad ligament has been opened. The psoas muscle under external iliac artery and fat (FAT), external iliac vessels, and ureter have been identified. The upper portion of the paravesical space has been entered lateral to the superior vesical artery. IFP, infundibulopelvic.

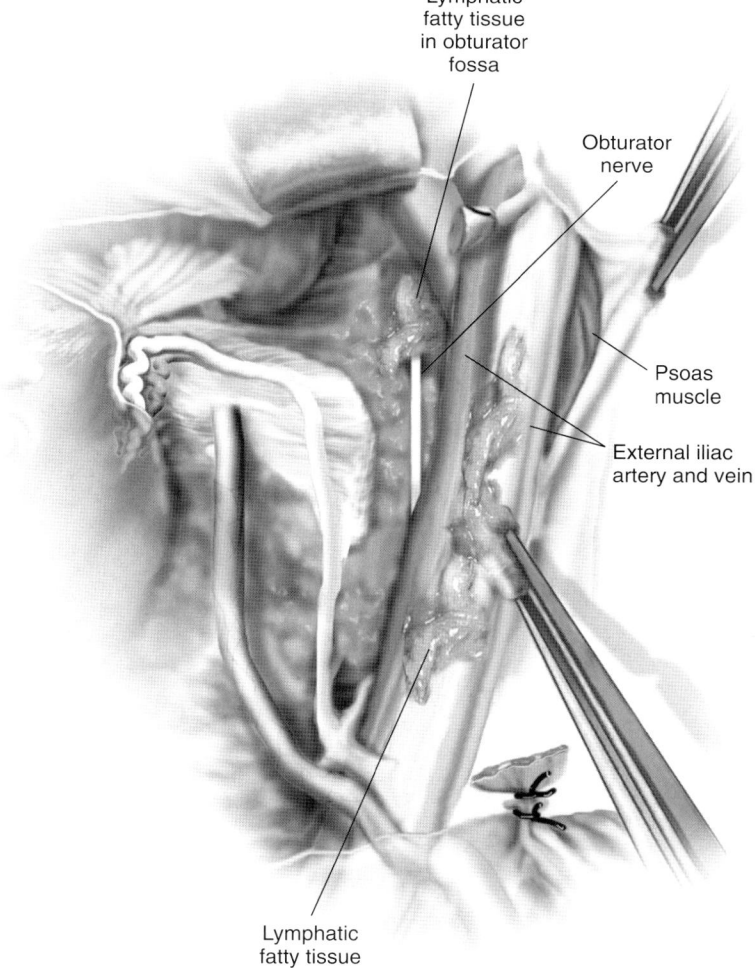

Lymphatic
fatty tissue
in obturator
fossa

Obturator
nerve

Psoas
muscle

External iliac
artery and vein

Lymphatic
fatty tissue

**FIGURE 12–8** Fat and lymph nodes have been dissected from the external iliac artery and vein. The obturator nerve has been partially exposed.

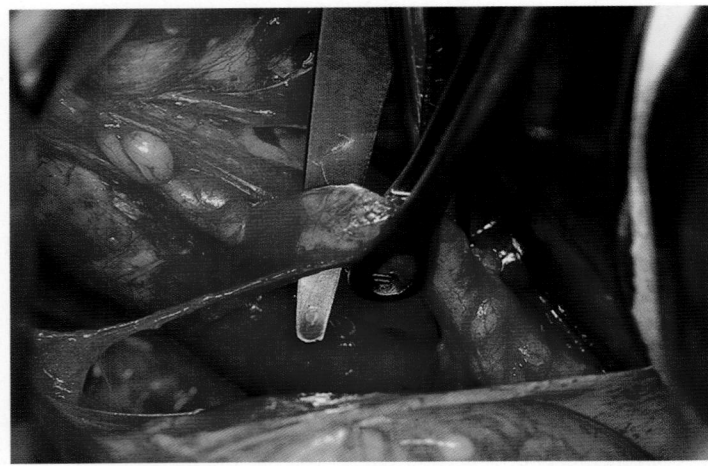

**FIGURE 12–9** In the background is the large, blue external iliac vein. The lymph node–bearing fat is grasped with a ring pick-up, while the surgeon sharply dissects the fatty tissue from the vessels.

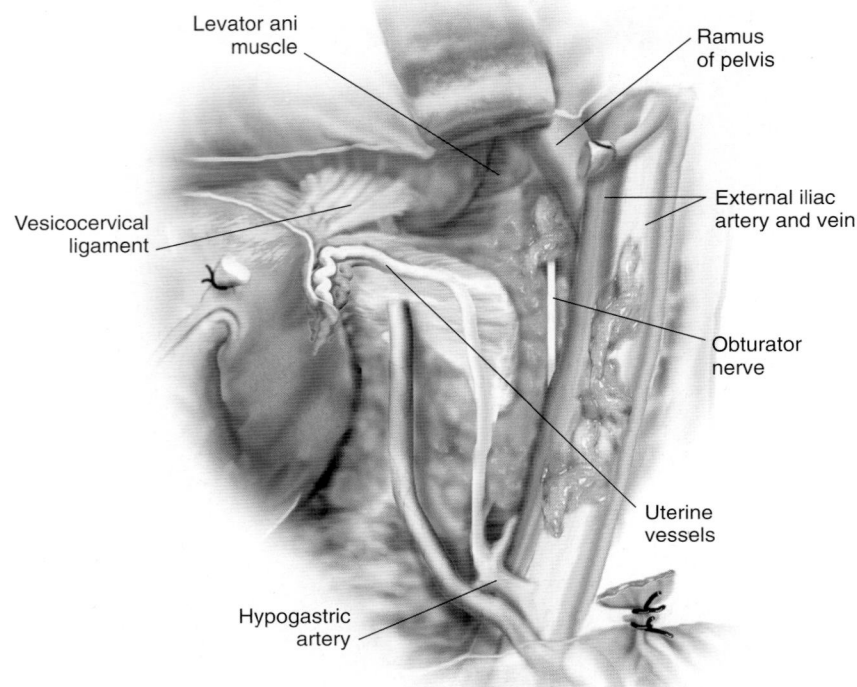

Levator ani
muscle

Ramus
of pelvis

Vesicocervical
ligament

External iliac
artery and vein

Obturator
nerve

Uterine
vessels

Hypogastric
artery

**FIGURE 12–10** The ureter is dissected inferiorly into the pelvis to the level of the point where the uterine artery crosses over it.

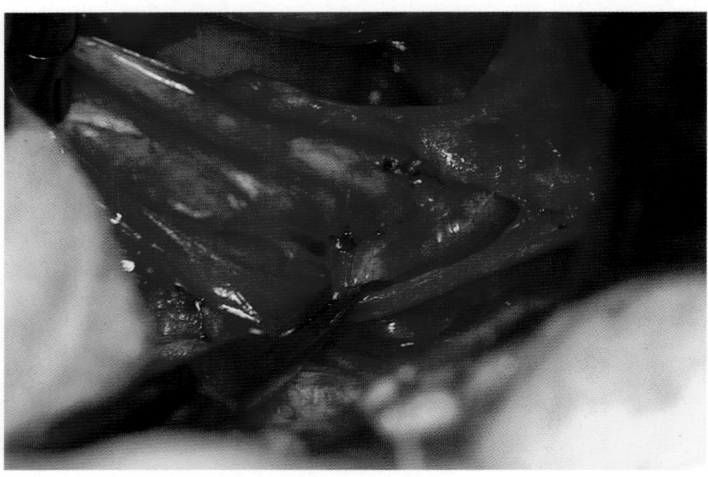

**FIGURE 12–11** Medial to the ureter and posterior and inferior to the external iliac artery lies the internal iliac (hypogastric) artery. Nodes and fat are cleared from this vessel.

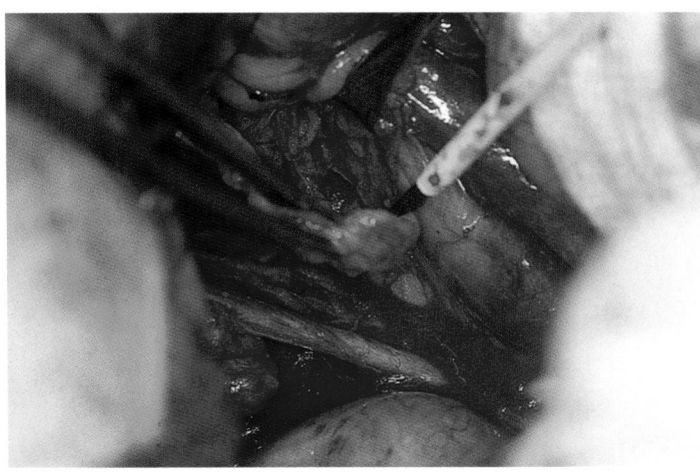

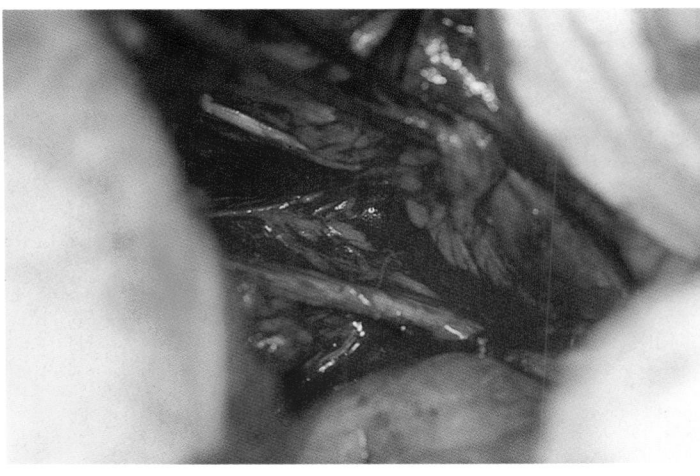

**FIGURE 12–12** Nodal tissue is extracted from the hypogastric artery and vein. The ureter is noted slightly inferior (below) and medial. The vein retractor is seen to the left and above the yellow electrosurgical pencil. The retractor gently elevates the slate blue external iliac vein.

**FIGURE 12–13** Fat and nodes are now pulled from the obturator fossa. This is done by gently teasing the tissue from the space using ring pick-ups. The external iliac vein is retracted upward by means of gentle traction on a vein retractor.

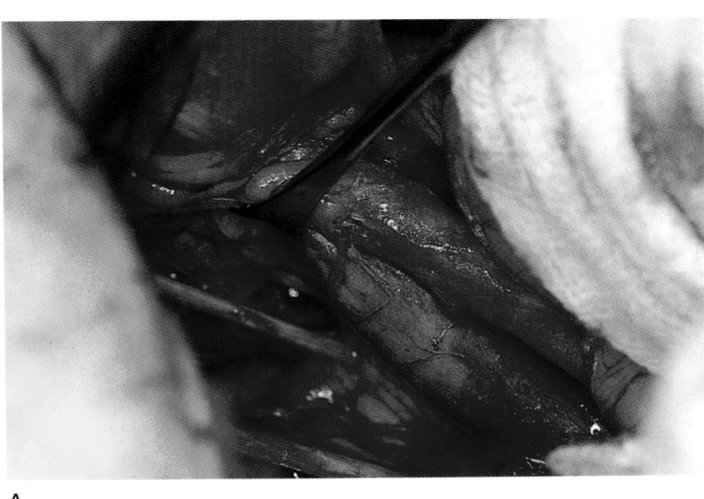

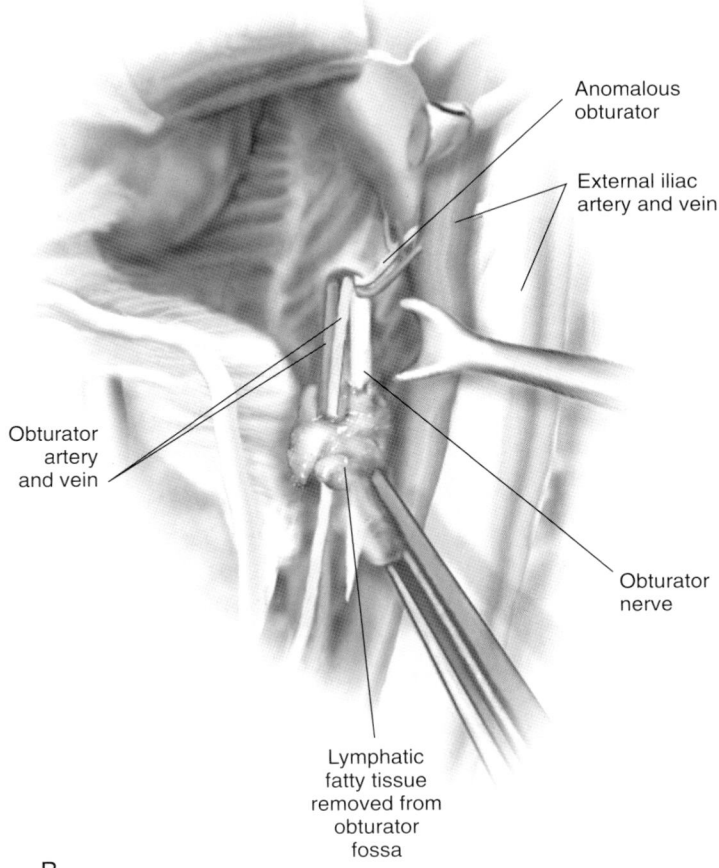

A

B

**FIGURE 12–14 A** and **B.** The obturator nerve is in clear view. Note the ureter at the lower margin of the picture. Its course parallels the obturator fossa structures with the exception that the obturator nerves and vessels assume a somewhat elevated course as they leave the pelvis via the obturator foramen. The ureter, on the other hand, descends deeper into the pelvis, vectoring toward the bladder base.

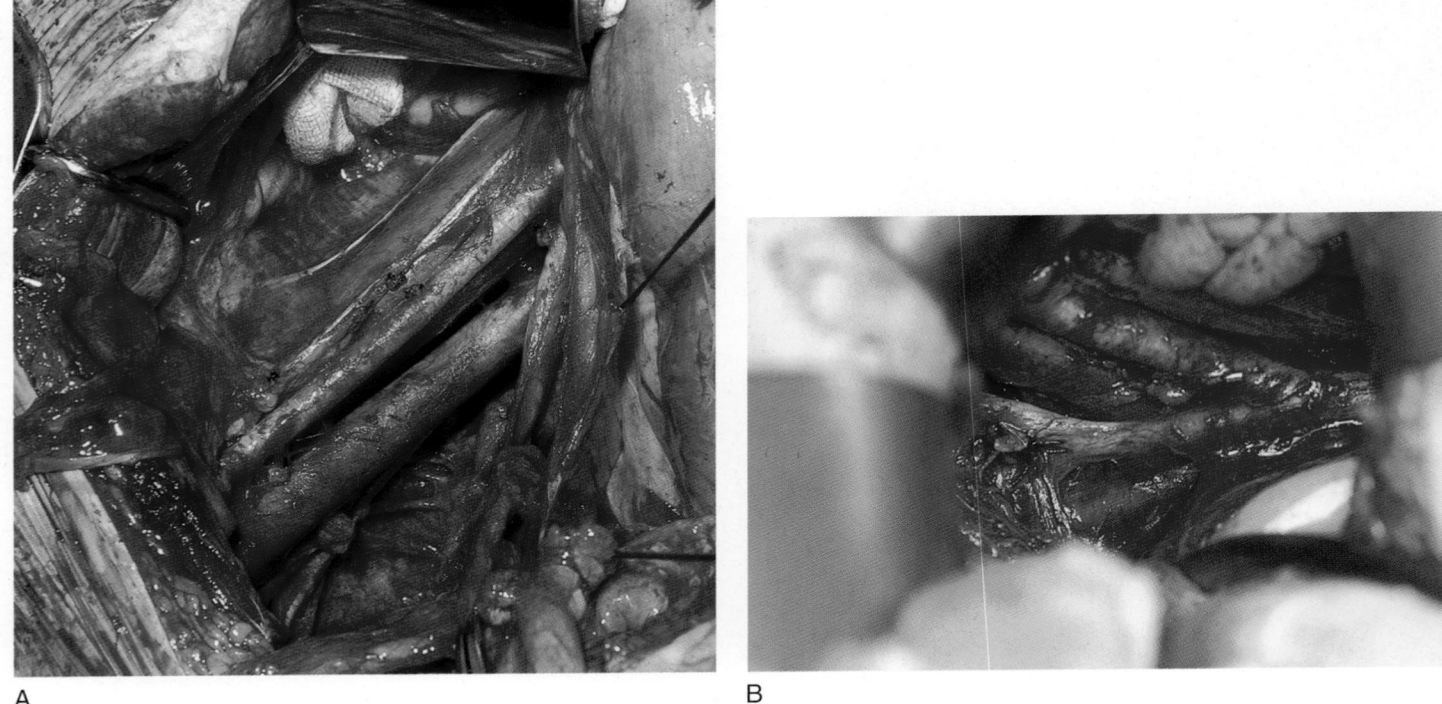

A

B

**FIGURE 12–15  A.** The node dissection of the obturator fossa is complete, as is the dissection of the external iliacs. Beneath the external iliac vein and deeply lateral is the obturator internus muscle. **B.** The internal iliac (hypogastric) artery and vein have been cleaned of fat and lymph nodes. Note the location of the vein (hypogastric).

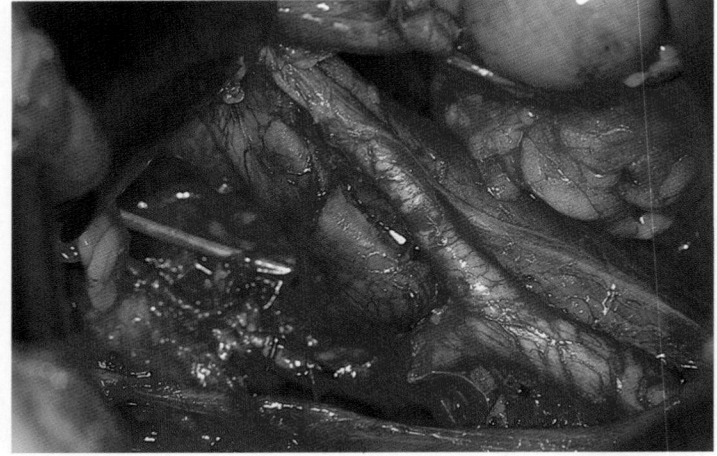

**FIGURE 12–16**  The common, external iliac, and internal iliac arteries and veins have been dissected. The obturator nerve marks the dissected obturator fossa. The ureter is visible at the lower margin of the figure.

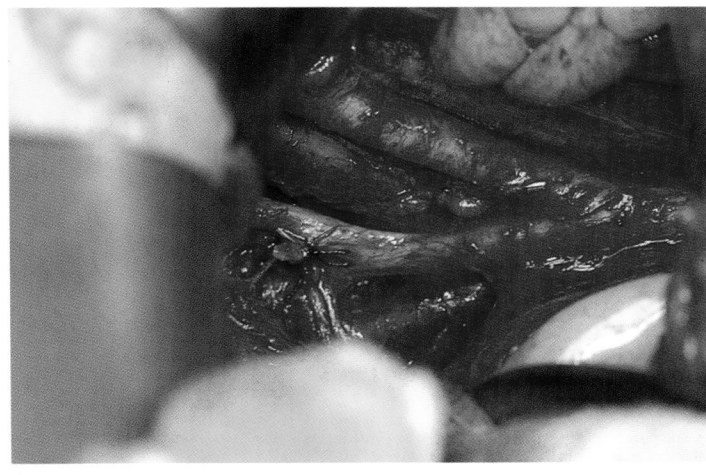

A

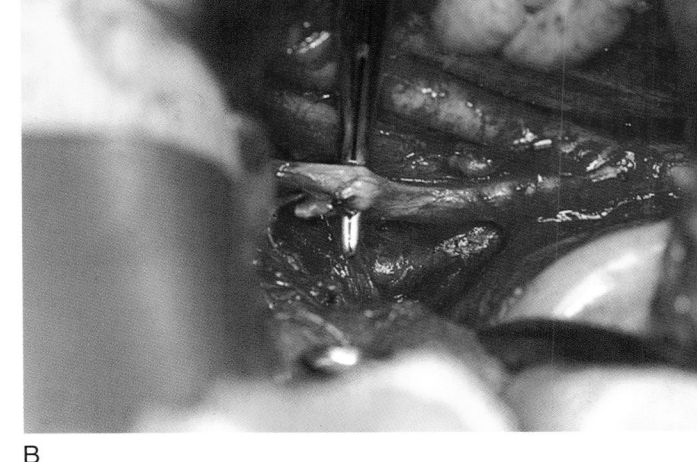

B

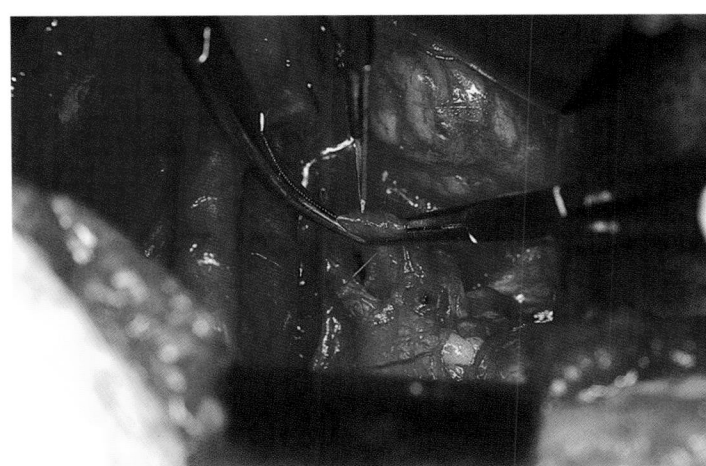

D

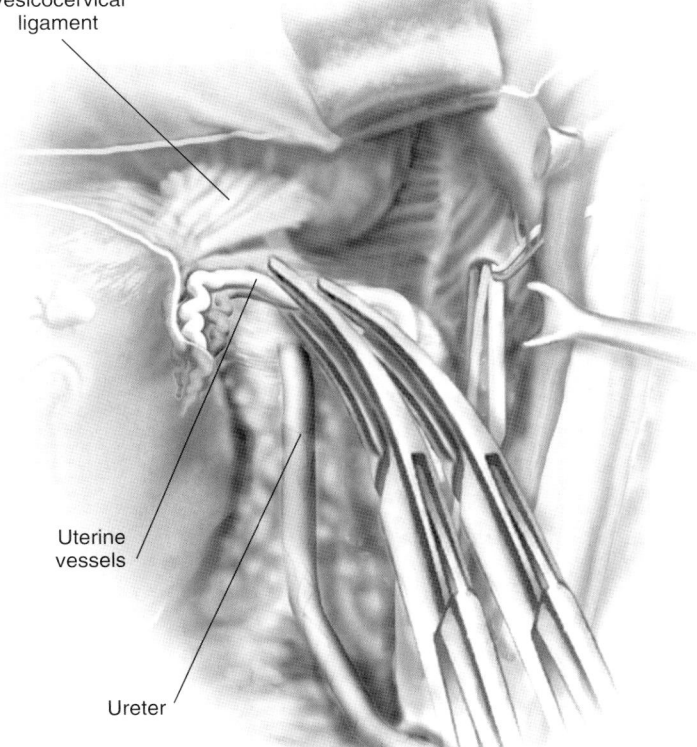

Vesicocervical
ligament

Uterine
vessels

Ureter

C

**FIGURE 12–17 A.** The posterior division of the hypogastric artery has been exposed. **B.** The origin of the uterine artery from the anterior division of the hypogastric artery is isolated above the tonsil clamp. **C.** The uterine artery is clamped lateral to the pelvic ureter. **D.** The uterine artery is cut and doubly ligated. The veins are typically ligated with the artery but may be separately clamped, divided, and tied.

At this point, the ureter is entering its tunnel through the cardinal ligament just cephalad to where it enters the wall of the bladder (Fig. 12–18A, B). The tunnel is unroofed by means of right-angle and tonsil clamps and Metzenbaum scissors (Fig. 12–19A–C). The pedicles are secured with 3-0 Vicryl suture ligatures (Fig. 12–20A). The ureter is now free of the parametria (Fig. 12–20B). Next, the bladder pillars are identified, cut, and secured (Fig. 12–21). The vesicouterine space is dissected downward well below the uterine cervix.

The peritoneum between the uterosacral ligaments is divided and the rectouterine space is developed and dissected down-

ward below the cervix. The uterosacral ligaments are cut and suture-ligated (Fig. 12–22).

The lower cardinal ligament, deep parametrial (paravaginal) fat, and fascia are clamped and cut medial to the ureter (Fig. 12–23). The vagina is clamped approximately 4 cm below the cervix, and the specimen is removed (Figs. 12–24 through 12–26). The anterior and posterior peritonei are closed with 3-0 Vicryl. The retroperitoneum is drained (Fig. 12–27). A suprapubic catheter is placed and the abdomen closed by means of the Smead-Jones technique or a suitable substitute (Figs. 12–28 through 12–31).

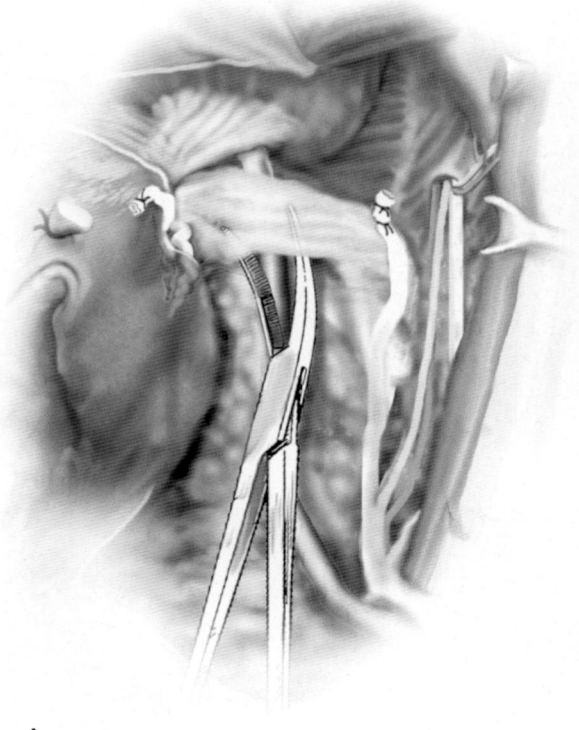

A

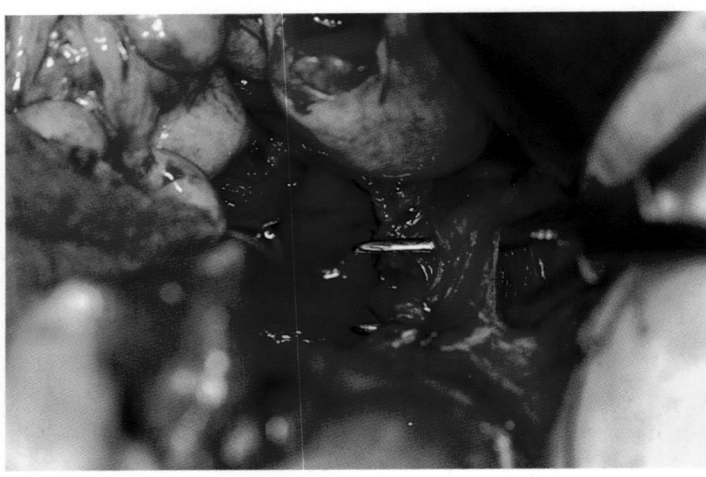

B

**FIGURE 12–18 A.** The ureter is dissected to the level of the cardinal ligament. At this point, the ureter penetrates the cardinal ligament in its short course to the bladder. The "tunnel" is dissected by inserting a right-angle clamp between the ureter and the roof of the tunnel (cardinal ligament). **B.** The roof of the ureteral tunnel is stretched with tonsil clamps before the edges of this tissue are clamped.

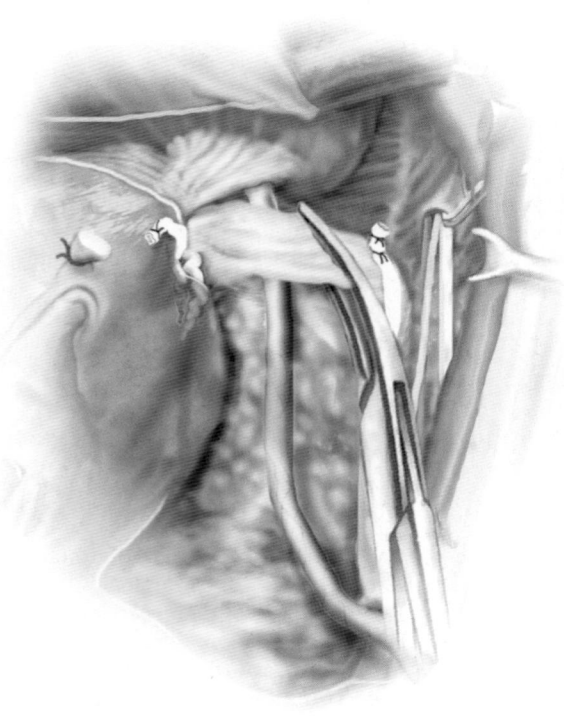

A

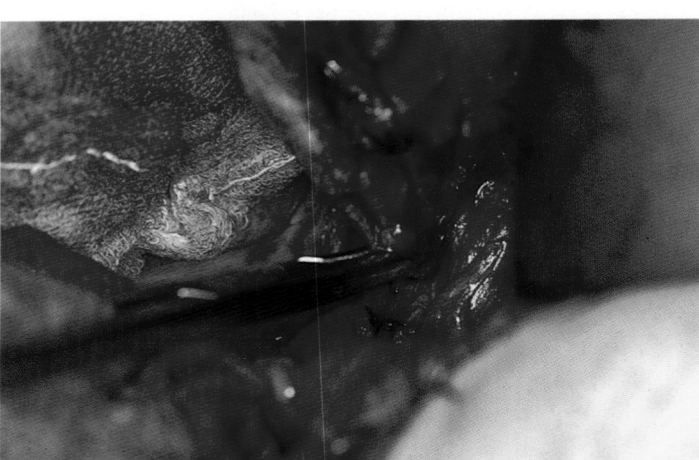

B

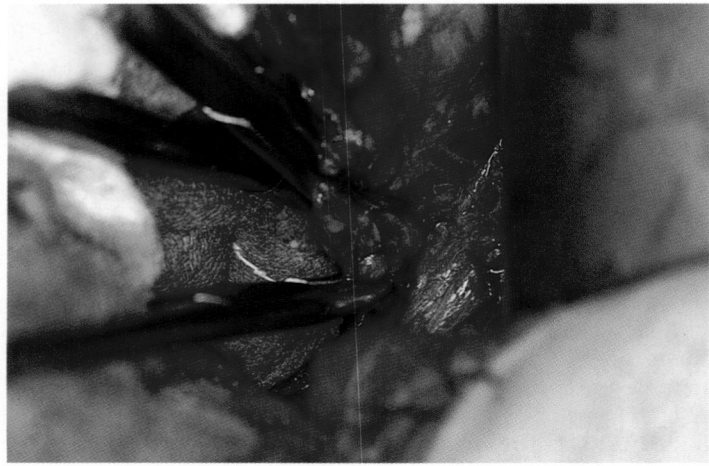

C

**FIGURE 12–19 A.** When the ureter is clearly freed from the roof of the tunnel, the ligament margins above the ureter are clamped with tonsil clamps. **B.** A tonsil clamp is placed at the lateral edge of the tunnel before it is cut. **C.** The tunnel is being cut with Metzenbaum scissors. A knife can be used if the ureter is covered by the closed right-angle clamp.

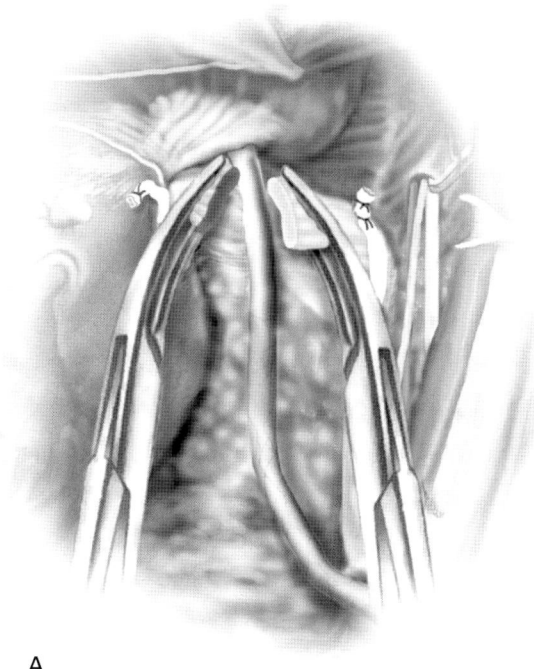

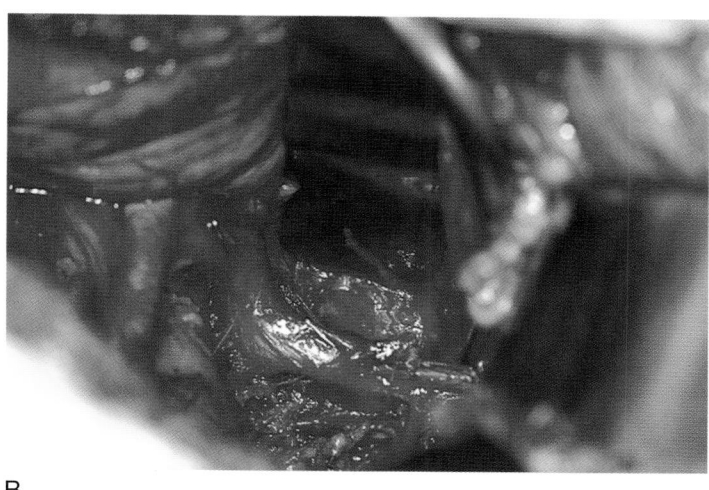

B

A

**FIGURE 12–20 A.** The cut edges of the cardinal ligament are suture-ligated with 0 Vicryl, and the ureter is freed from the posterior bed of the ligament. **B.** The ureter is entirely free and mobile as it makes its way under the bladder pillar to enter the urinary bladder.

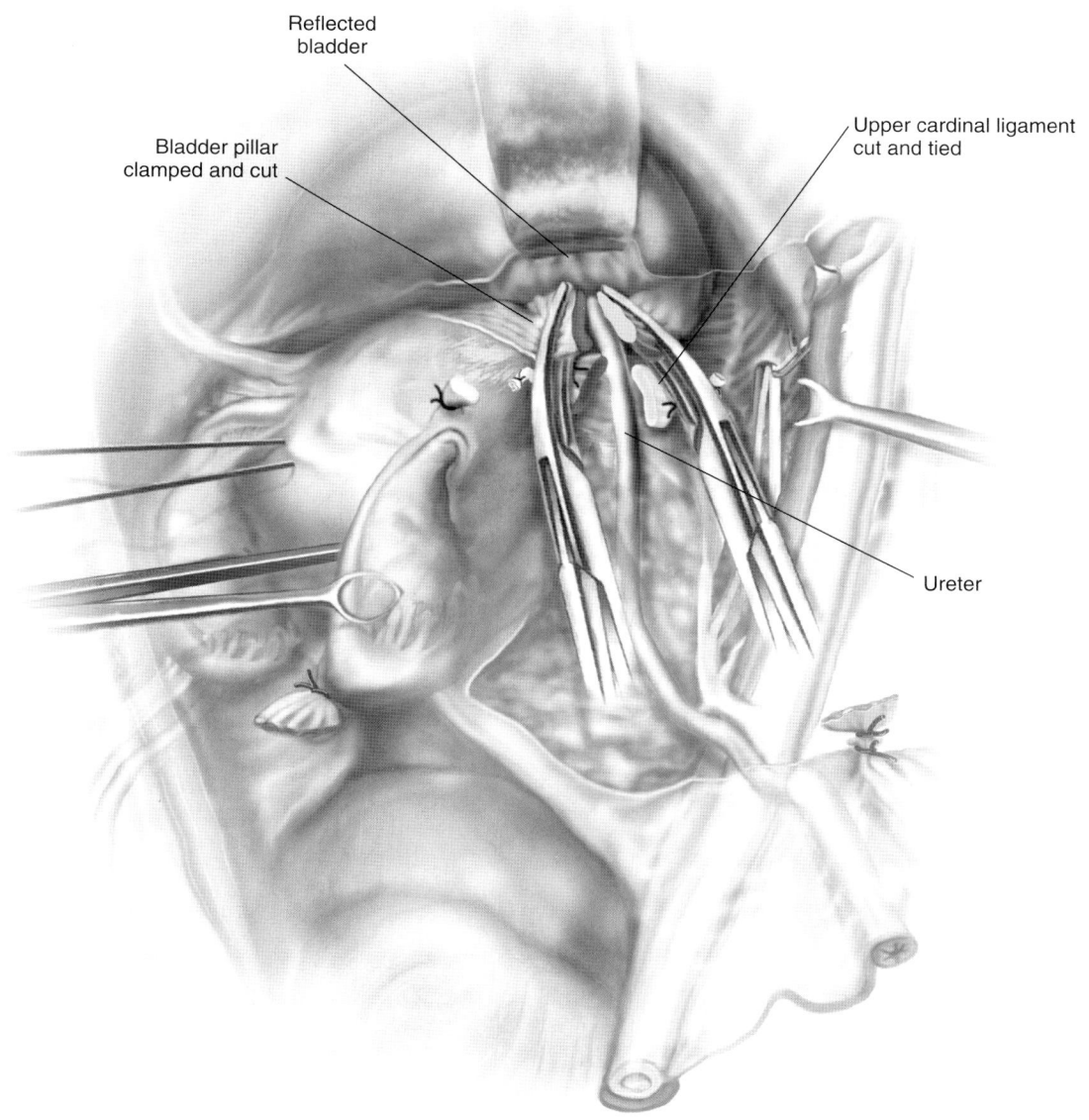

Reflected
bladder

Upper cardinal ligament
cut and tied

Bladder pillar
clamped and cut

Ureter

**FIGURE 12–21** The bladder pillar has been divided. Each portion will be suture-ligated with 0 Vicryl.

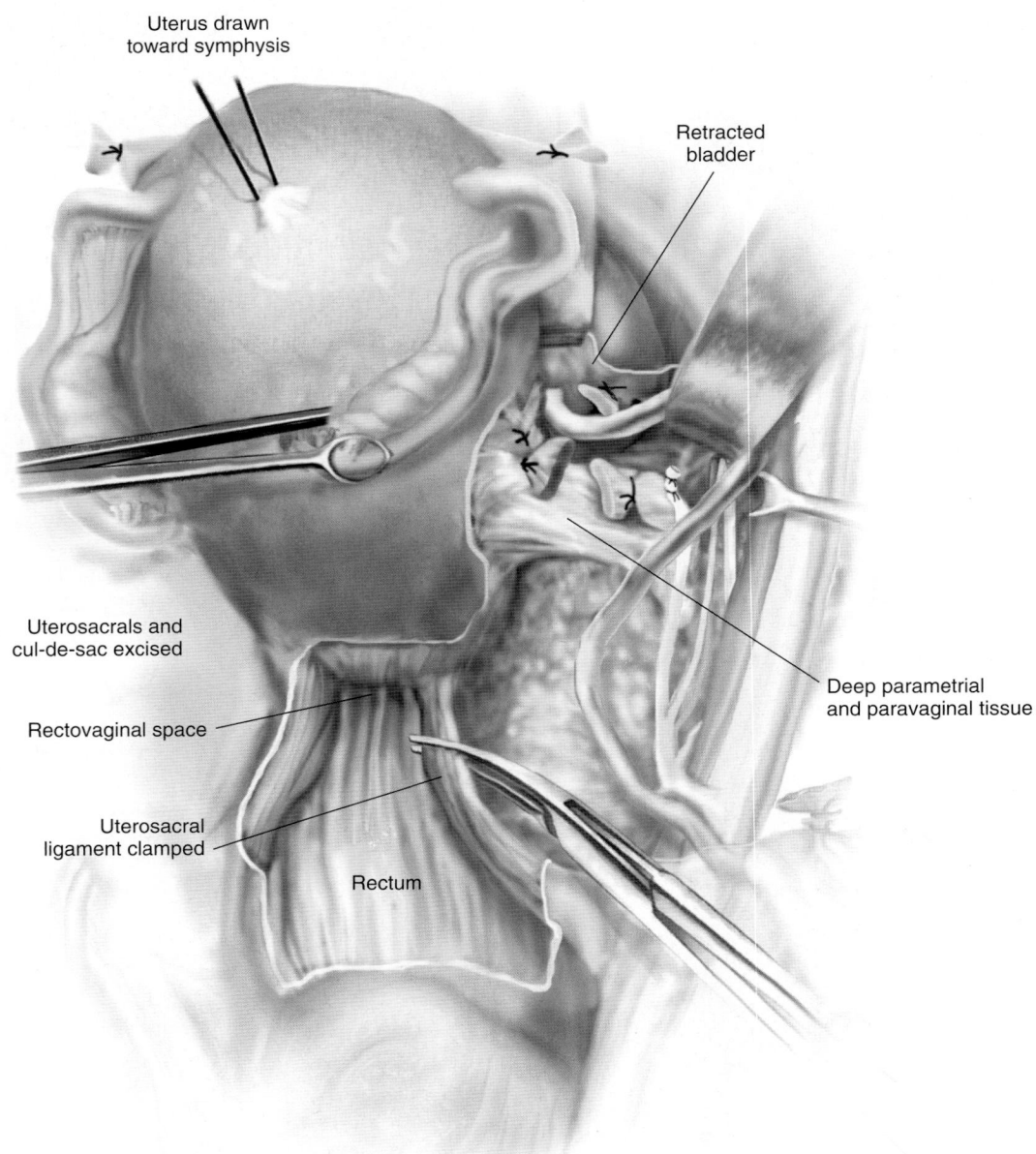

Uterus drawn
toward symphysis

Retracted
bladder

Uterosacrals and
cul-de-sac excised

Rectovaginal space

Uterosacral
ligament clamped

Rectum

Deep parametrial
and paravaginal tissue

**FIGURE 12–22** The uterosacral ligaments are clamped. The peritoneum between the two uterosacral ligaments is cut, and the rectovaginal space is dissected. The uterosacral ligaments are cut, and the stumps are suture-ligated with 0 Vicryl.

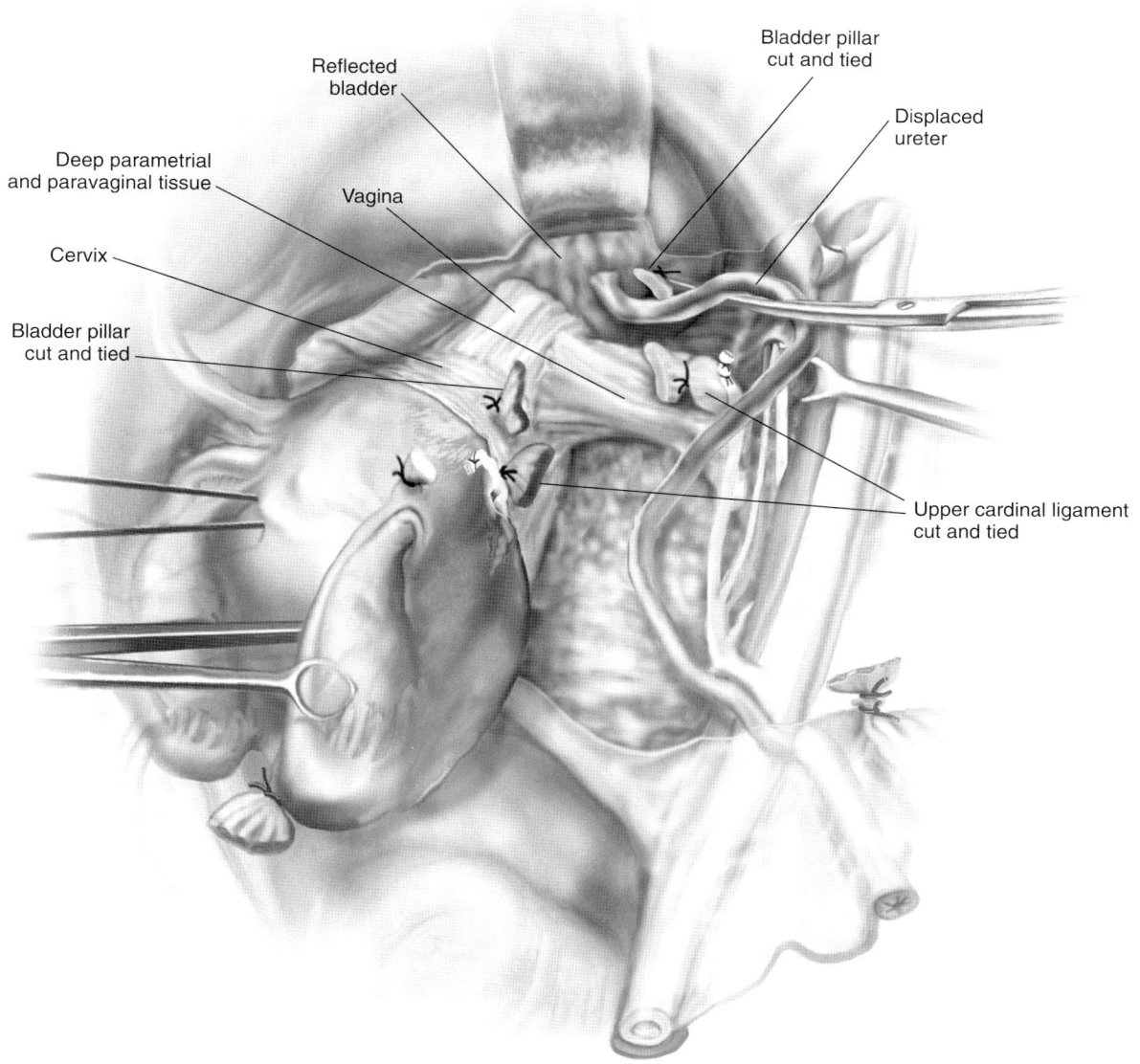

**FIGURE 12–23** The lateral parametrial tissue is located below the cervix and is attached to the lateral walls of the vagina. The ureter is retracted to permit the surgeon to expose this tissue.

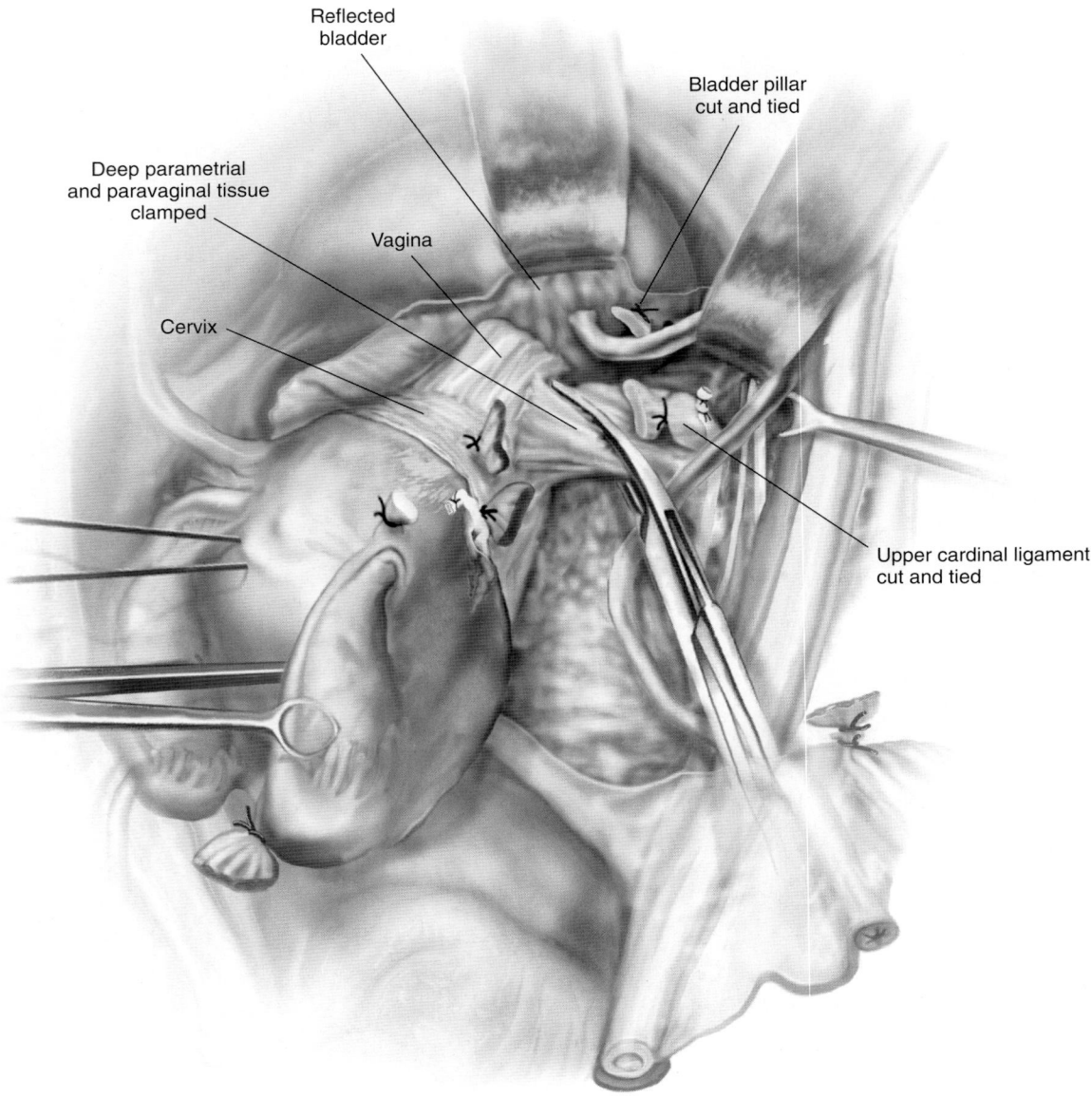

**FIGURE 12–24** A long, curved Zeppelin clamp grasps the tissue. Long Mayo scissors are utilized to cut the tissue medial to the applied clamp. The final clamp will be placed across the vagina.

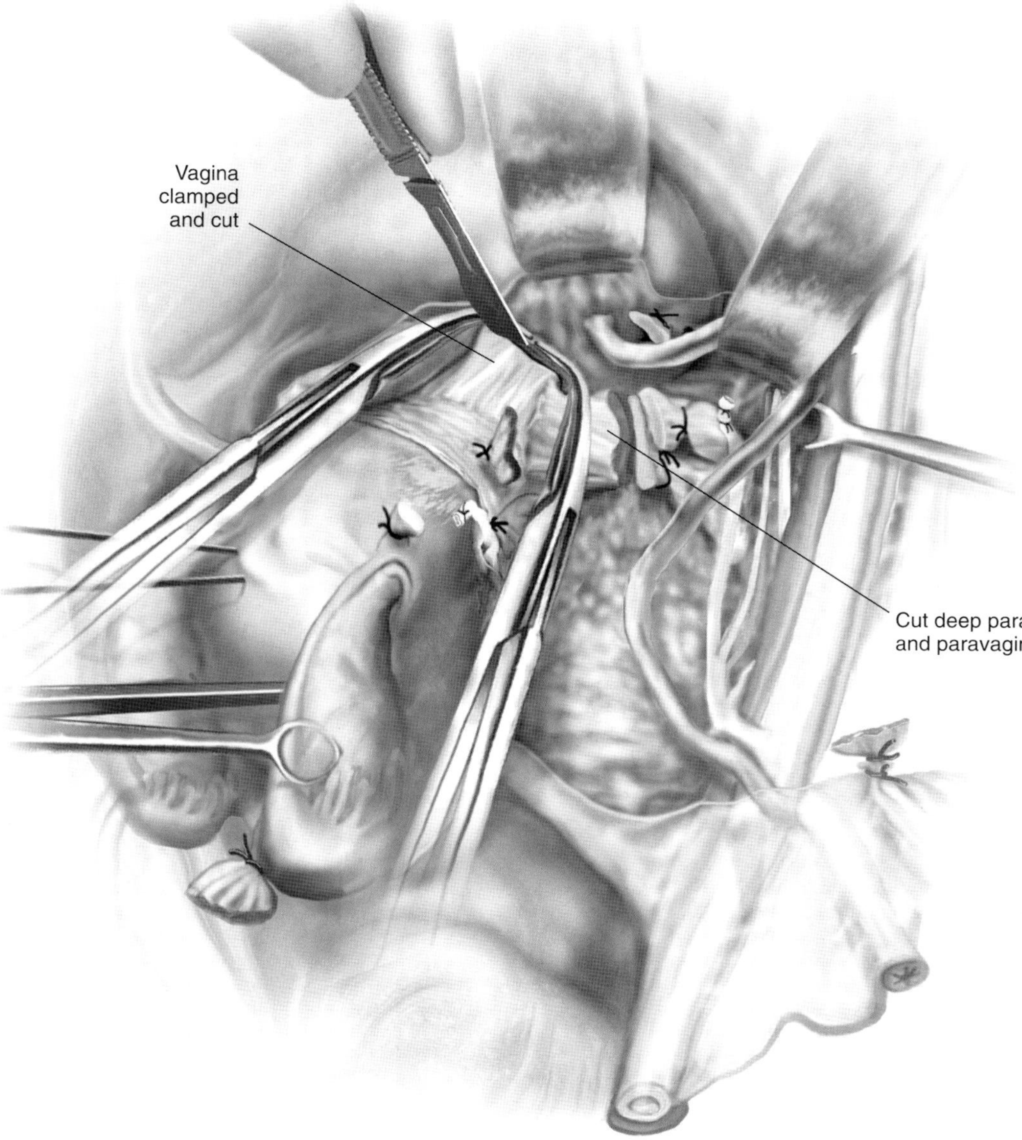

Vagina
clamped
and cut

Cut deep parametrial
and paravaginal tissue

**FIGURE 12–25** Zeppelin clamps are placed across the vagina approximately 4 cm inferior to (below) the fornices. The vaginal attachment is severed, and the uterus, together with the attached parametria, is removed.

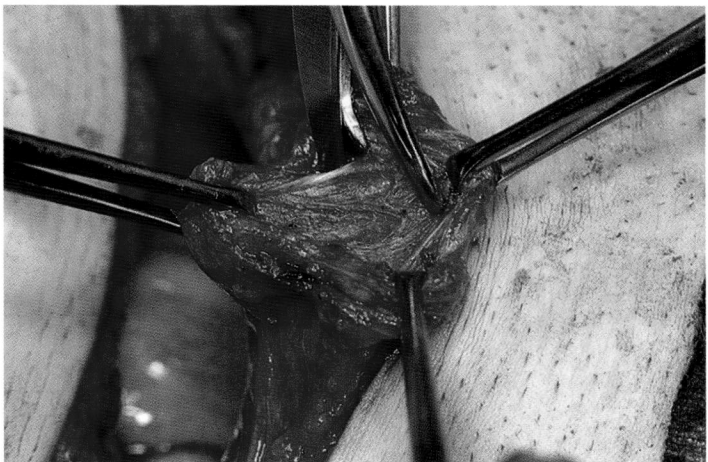

**FIGURE 12–26** The bladder dome is grasped and a small cystotomy is created.

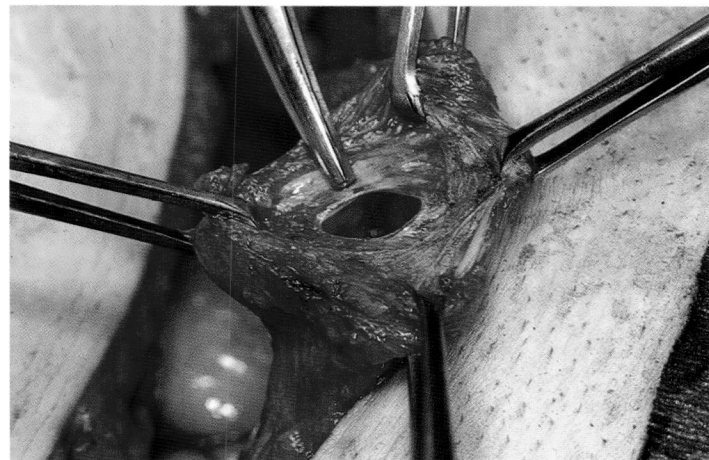

**FIGURE 12–27** Through this small opening, a Foley (suprapubic) catheter will be introduced.

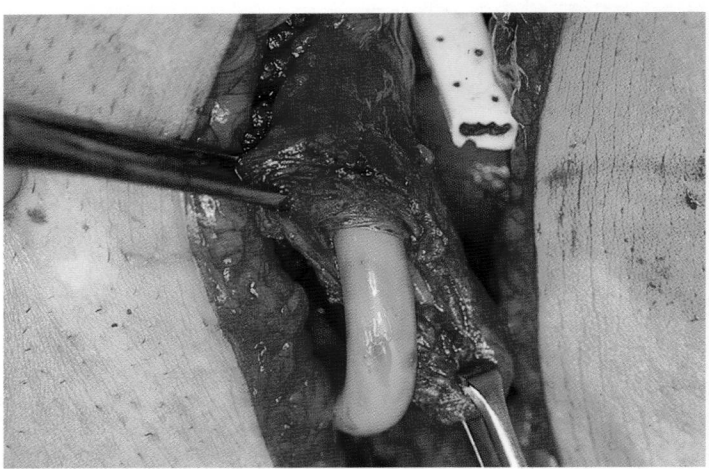

FIGURE 12–28  The catheter is secured by a purse-string suture. The upper edge of the incision shows the tip of the drain, which is placed retroperitoneally before the peritoneum is closed.

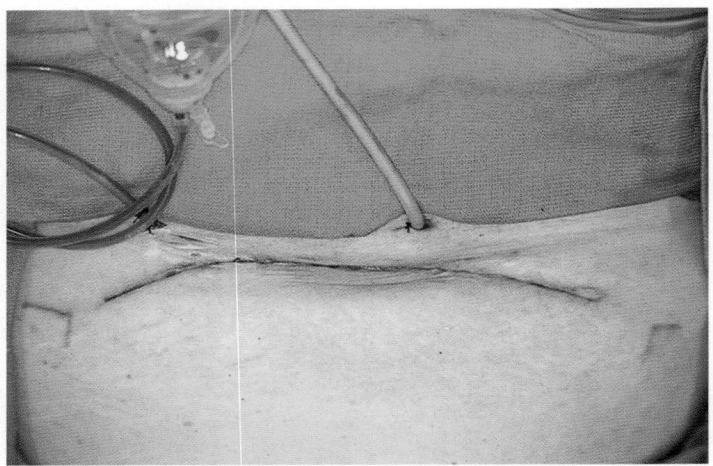

FIGURE 12–29  The abdominal incision is closed. The suprapubic catheter and Jackson-Pratt drains are brought out via separate stab wounds.

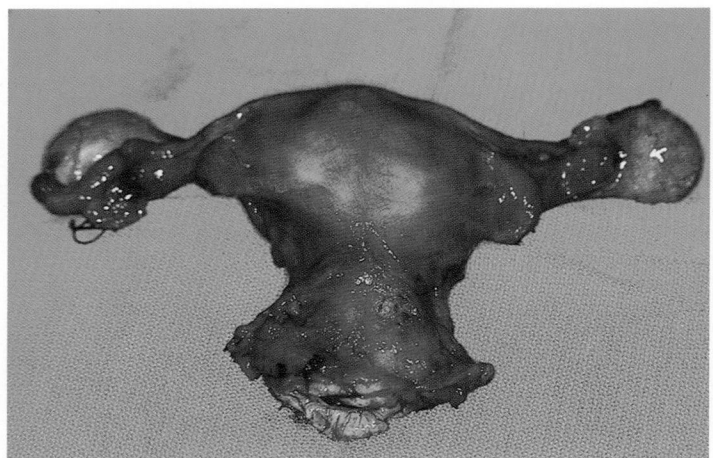

FIGURE 12–30  The excised specimen includes parametria, paravaginal tissue, and an adequate vaginal margin of tissue.

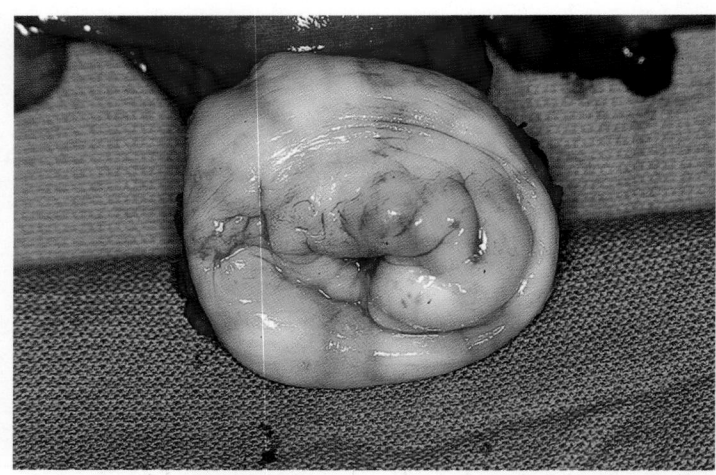

FIGURE 12–31  The cervix and attached 4-cm vaginal cuff.

# CHAPTER 13

# Endometrial Carcinoma With Lymph Node Sampling

*James Pavelka* ■ *Jack Basil*

Endometrial cancer is the most common gynecologic malignancy in the United States. Since 1988, endometrial cancer has been regarded by the International Federation of Gynecology and Obstetrics (FIGO) as a surgically staged disease. Despite this, at present only a minority of women with endometrial cancer undergo formal surgical staging. The considerable heterogeneity in surgical care for women with endometrial cancer is due to multiple factors: limited access to gynecologic oncologists in some regions, a generally favorable prognosis—particularly with histologic grade 1 disease (Fig. 13–1), and fundamental disagreement regarding the role of pelvic and aortic lymphadenectomy in women with endometrial cancer.

A full staging procedure for most endometrial cancer consists of a total (extrafascial) hysterectomy with bilateral salpingo-oophorectomy, as well as pelvic and aortic lymphadenectomy and pelvic washings. In available literature, oncologic outcomes are similar for open, laparoscopic, and robotic approaches; the route of the procedure therefore may be individualized to the needs of each patient and surgeon. In some select cases of endometrial cancer that is preoperatively identified to be metastatic to the cervix (stage II), a radical hysterectomy may be chosen by the surgeon. Although the role of surgical cytoreduction is not as well established for endometrial cancer as it is for ovarian cancer, data suggest a survival benefit in cases of metastatic disease when optimal cytoreduction is achieved.

For a pelvic lymphadenectomy (Figs. 13–2 to 13–4) the generally accepted boundaries are as follows: cephalad—mid common iliac artery; caudal—circumflex iliac vein; lateral—pelvic sidewall and mid-psoas muscle; medial—circumflex iliac vein; and dorsal—obturator nerve. Ideally, all nodal and fatty tissue in this anatomically defined region is removed, with hemostasis maintained via cautery or clips. Although additional nodal tissue is present medial to the superior vesical artery and deep to the obturator nerve, this is not routinely sampled in endometrial cancer surgery.

Aortic lymphadenectomy (Fig. 13–5) is less commonly performed than pelvic lymphadenectomy because of a somewhat lower risk of isolated aortic nodal metastases and a more difficult dissection around major vascular structures. Typical boundaries of this dissection include the following: cephalad—ovarian vein on the right and inferior mesenteric artery on the left; caudal—mid common iliac artery; lateral—psoas muscle; medial—mid aorta; and dorsal—spine. Some centers advocate routinely removing the high aortic nodes as well, and continuing this dissection up to the renal veins.

Some authors, both historically and recently, have argued that lymphadenectomy has no therapeutic role in endometrial cancer, and given the potential for morbidity, this phase of the operation should be omitted, except in the presence of grossly metastatic disease. Others will selectively perform lymphadenectomy if the uterine features include deep myometrial invasion or a high-grade tumor (Figs. 13–6 and 13–7). Another perspective is that routine lymphadenectomy allows individualization of care, and when performed systematically and competently, offers a low risk of complications. It is our belief and practice that when combined with the features of the primary tumor, routine and systematic pelvic and aortic lymphadenectomy on nearly every patient with endometrial cancer is the most accurate and cost-effective available means of assigning or withholding postoperative adjuvant therapy, with very low attendant morbidity.

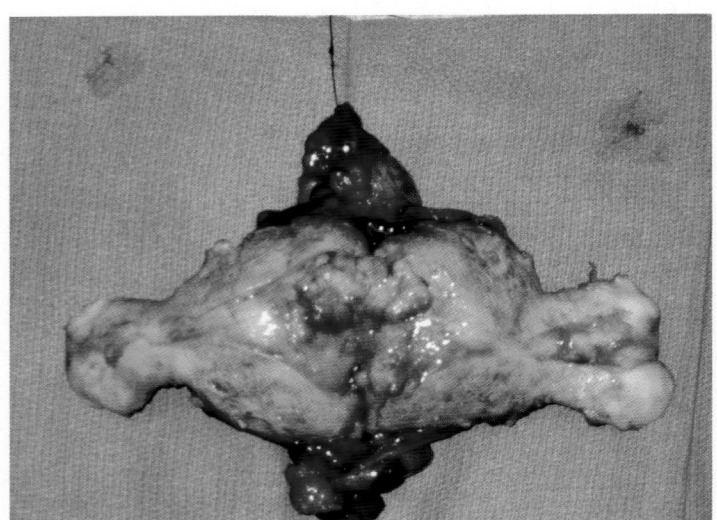

**FIGURE 13-1** The uterus has been bivalved to demonstrate a relatively small, exophytic grade 1 endometrioid tumor. The risk of lymph node involvement of such a tumor can range from 3% to 6%.

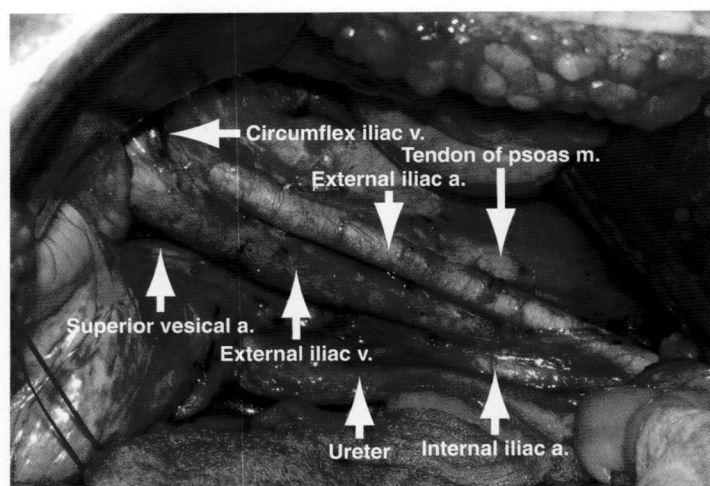

**FIGURE 13-2** Pictured is a typical view from the patient left side perspective of a right pelvic lymph node dissection. Most of the anatomic landmarks, including the iliac vessels, ureter, and psoas muscle, can be readily observed.

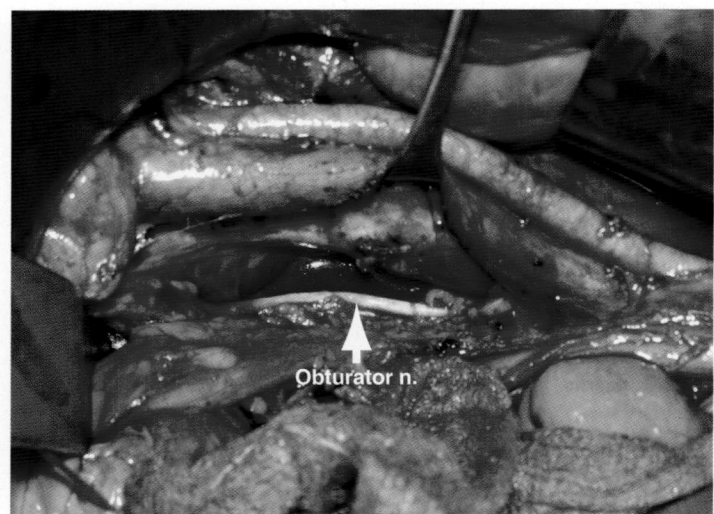

**FIGURE 13-3** This is the same dissection as is shown in Figure 13-2, with the external iliac vein elevated with a vein retractor to expose the obturator space. The obturator nerve and the pelvic sidewall are apparent.

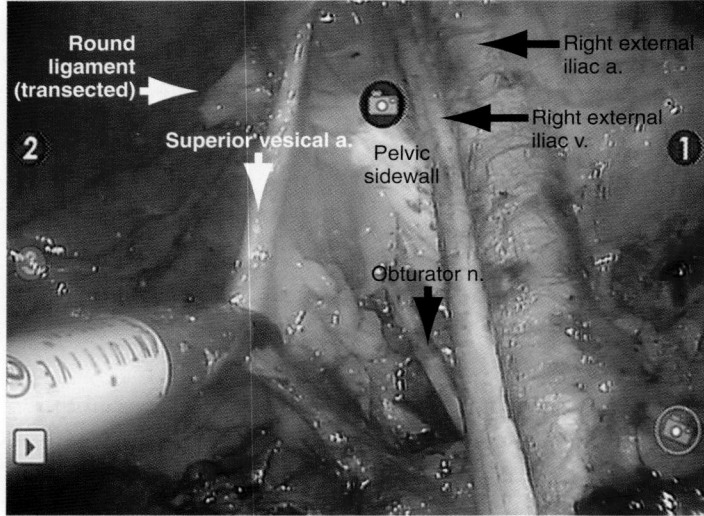

**FIGURE 13-4** This laparoscopic image was obtained during robotic right pelvic lymphadenectomy. The definitions of anatomy and quality of dissection are equivalent to those used in an open approach.

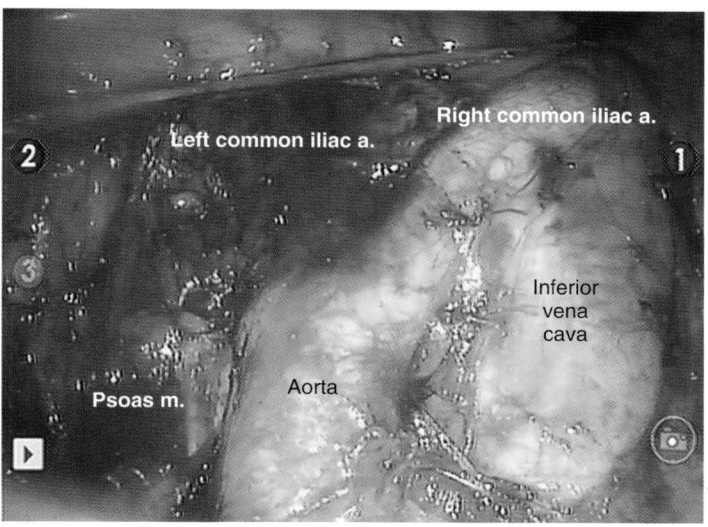

FIGURE 13–5 The duodenal reflection and the right ovarian vein are just cephalad to the bottom of this image obtained during robotic bilateral aortic lymphadenectomy. Additional nodal tissue can be seen between the great vessels and at the lateral margin of the vena cava, and it will be removed before the procedure is completed.

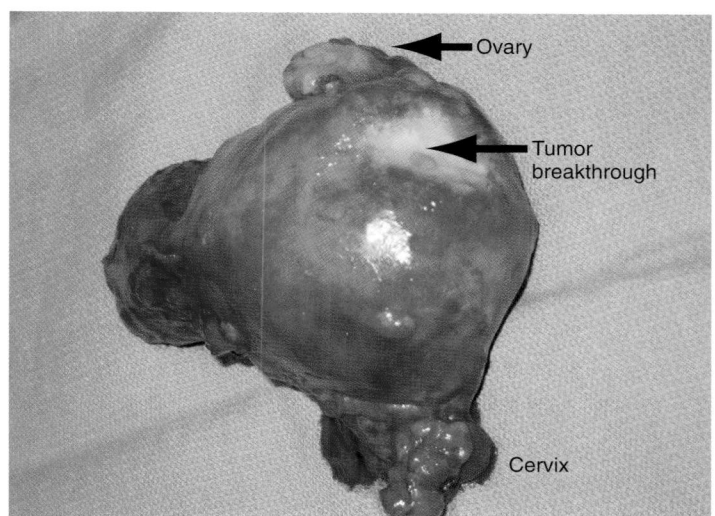

FIGURE 13–6 The dimpling on the posterior fundus of this uterus is indicative of full-thickness invasion of a poorly differentiated endometrial tumor, as can be appreciated in Figure 13–7.

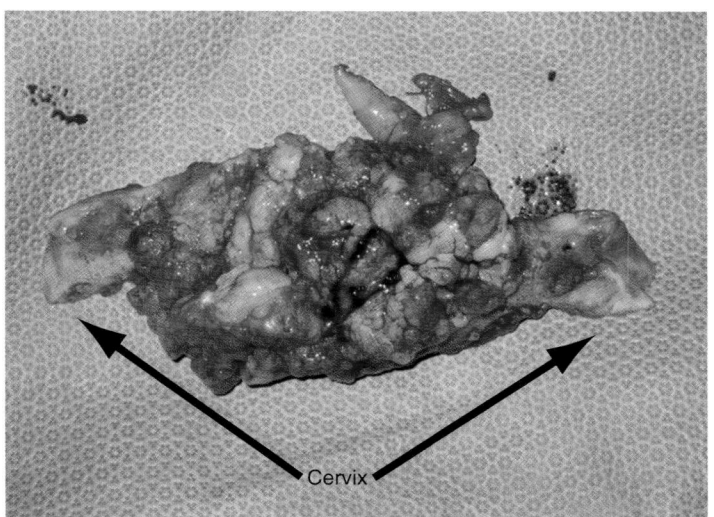

FIGURE 13–7 This was a poorly differentiated tumor that had almost completely replaced the myometrium. Such tumors have a very high rate of metastatic spread.

# CHAPTER 14

# Myomectomy

*Michael S. Baggish*

Abdominal myomectomy is performed as an alternative to hysterectomy. The indications for myomectomy are collateral and consist of the desire to preserve the uterus together with the presence of symptomatic intramural or subserosal myomata uteri. Typical symptoms experienced by women in whom *no* submucous component exists are pressure on the bladder or bowel, partial obstruction of the ureters, and pain. Although this operation has been performed laparoscopically, most surgeons consider laparotomy to be the route of choice.

The uterus is typically distorted (Fig. 14–1). Although the arterial supply to myomata is relatively sparse, the venous return is large, thin-walled, and anomalous (Figs. 14–2 through 14–4). The surgeon must cut through the capsule to reach the core of the myoma to remove it, and must traverse tissue planes that contain these venous sinuses. Because of the increased vascularity, many surgeons prefer to use an energy source to diminish bleeding (e.g., carbon dioxide [$CO_2$] laser, electrosurgical needle electrode). The author additionally uses a 1:200 solution of vasopressin (20 units). Approximately 20 to 30 mL of this solution is injected just beneath the capsule (Fig. 14–5A). The anesthesiologist should be alerted to monitor the patient's blood pressure and pulse during injection of vasopressin. Next, an outline is made for the incision. This may be performed with cold steel, $CO_2$ laser, or needle electrode (Fig. 14–5B). The author prefers to limit the posterior extent of the incision to diminish subsequent adhesion formation (Fig. 14–5C). In the case illustrated, a slightly defocused $CO_2$ laser handpiece is utilized with power set at 50W and a laser spot 1.5 to 2.0 mm in diameter (power density 1250–2200 $W/cm^2$) (Fig. 14–6). The edges of the capsule are retracted, and the myoma is dissected peripherally off the capsule (Fig. 14–7). The operator's index finger can actually be used to separate the myoma from the capsule. The laser, needle electrode, or scissors may be used to cut away adhesions (Fig. 14–8). Care should be taken to carry out the dissection gently and carefully to avoid entry into the uterine cavity and injury to the interstitial portion of the oviduct (Fig. 14–9A–C).

When the base of the myoma is reached, the arterial pedicle should be clamped and suture-ligated (Fig. 14–9D, E). The specimen is then removed. Typically, the author cuts the myoma to determine whether there is any gross suspicion of sarcoma or infection. A pulpous, rotting interior suggests the need for a frozen section or at least a careful postoperative histologic assessment. Some excess capsule may be trimmed away (Fig. 14–9F). The uterus is reconstructed by bringing muscle to muscle together with interrupted 0 Vicryl (Fig. 14–10A, B). This may require a two-layered closure. Next, the serosa is closed with running or interrupted 2-0 or 3-0 Vicryl sutures. At the completion of closure, the author prefers to cover the exposed suture line with a parietal peritoneal graft or a patch of Interceed absorbable adhesion barrier or other suitable material. Typically, the surgeon measures and cuts the specimen (Fig. 14–11A, B). Submucous myomata are responsible for 90% of the bleeding associated with these common tumors and should be treated hysteroscopically. If the myoma is too large for hysteroscopic extirpation, even after 3 to 4 months of gonadotropin-releasing hormone (GnRH) agonist suppression, the patient should undergo a hysterectomy (Fig. 14–12).

Occasionally, a myomectomy is performed and no suspicion of malignancy is evidenced (Fig. 14–13A–D), but it is surprising to note that the permanent histopathologic sections reveal leiomyosarcoma (Fig. 14–14A, B). In this circumstance, the patient must be promptly notified of these findings and strongly advised to undergo total abdominal hysterectomy (Fig. 14–15A, B).

Cervical myomata may be excised via the vaginal route with the use of a microscope-mounted $CO_2$ laser. Essentially, the anterior or posterior wall or both walls of the cervix are divided to afford exposure. The myoma is then cut out from the respective wall to which it is attached. The cervix is repaired in layers with 2-0 or 3-0 Vicryl. The split walls are closed with 3-0 Vicryl (Fig. 14–16A–E). Occasionally, a cervical myoma is so large and so vascular that an abdominal hysterectomy is indicated. In this circumstance, the size of the cervical myoma would make the abdominal route a safer choice than vaginal hysterectomy (Fig. 14–17A–C).

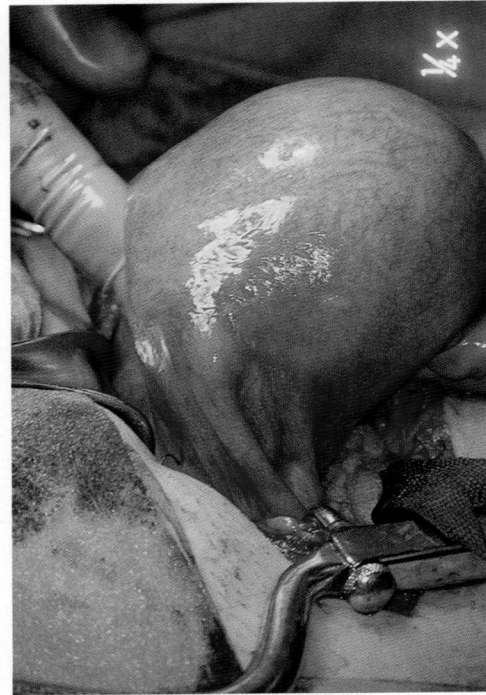

**FIGURE 14–1** The uterus is lifted out of the pelvis so any anatomic alterations created by the myomatous mass can be identified.

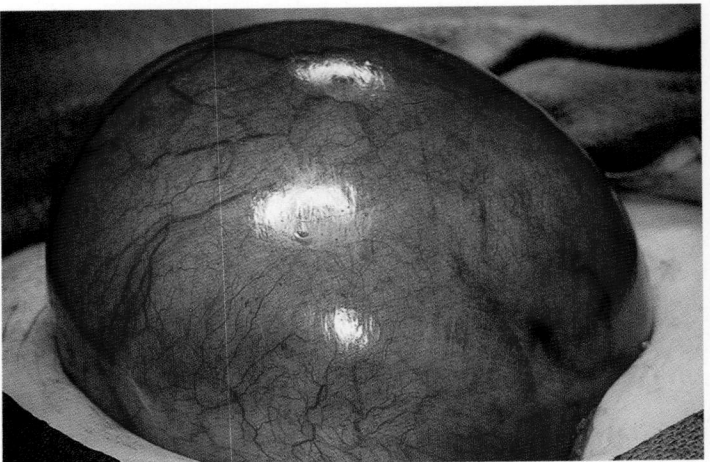

**FIGURE 14–2** The myoma is a large 6- to 8-cm solitary lesion.

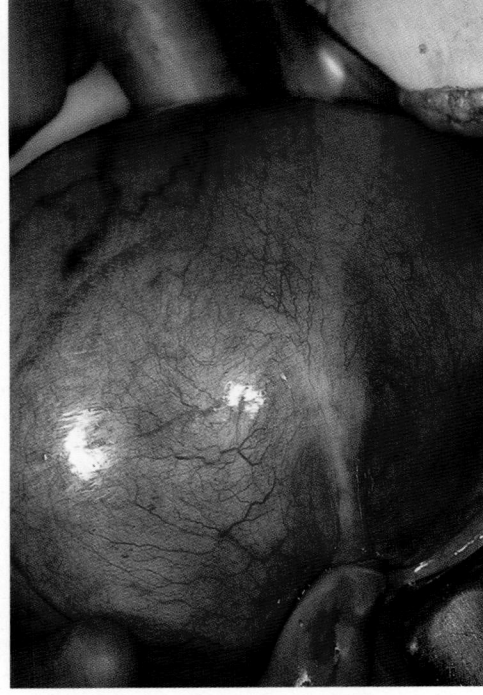

**FIGURE 14–3** Venous return from the myomatous uterus is large and anomalous. Large, sinusoidal vessels are seen in the subserous location.

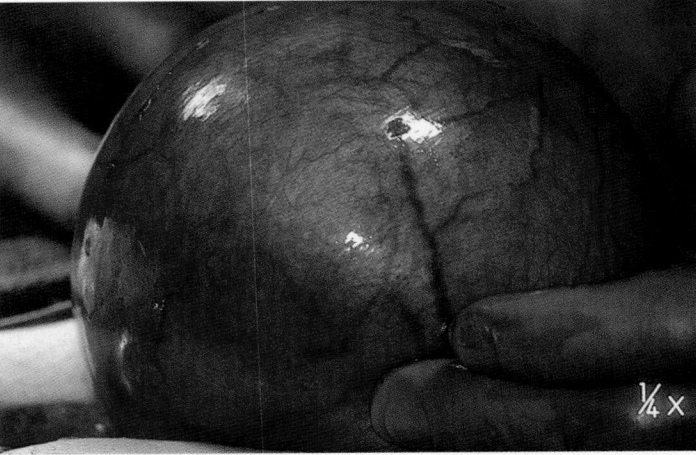

**FIGURE 14–4** The course of the large vessels should be carefully identified before a uterine incision is made.

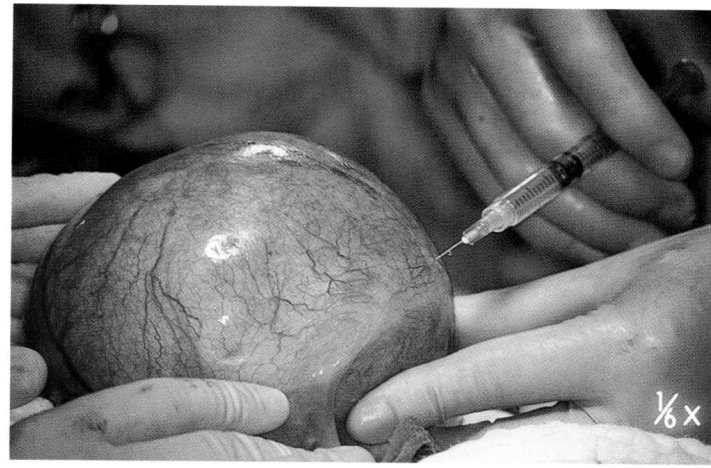

A

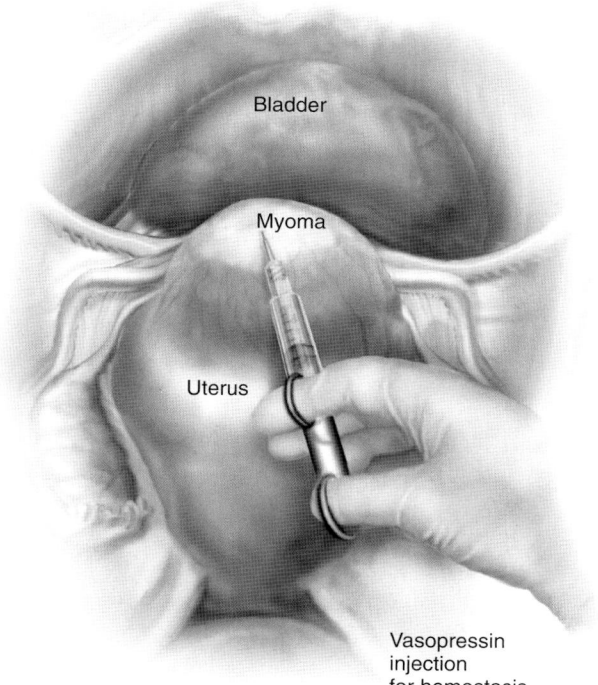

B

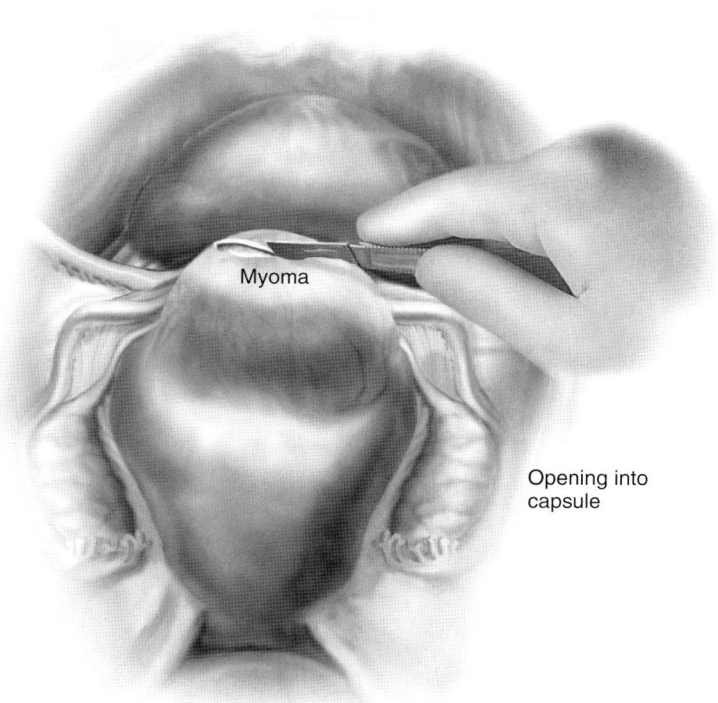

C

**FIGURE 14–5  A.** A 1:200 solution of vasopressin is injected into the uterus for hemostasis. Care should be taken to avoid intravascular injection. **B.** The injection is performed with the use of a 10-mL triple-ring syringe and a 1½-inch, 25-gauge needle. The subserosa is first injected. The tissue immediately blanches white. The needle is advanced into the substance of the myoma, and the solution is injected. Typically, 20 to 25 mL is injected. **C.** A transverse or vertical incision is made into the myoma. If possible, an anterior or anterofundal cut is made.

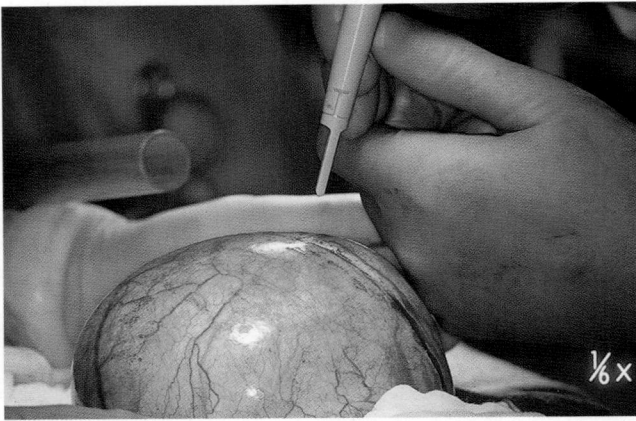

**FIGURE 14–6** Alternatively, a carbon dioxide ($CO_2$) laser (handpiece delivery system) may be used to open the uterus. The laser is a precise energy device that offers additional hemostasis.

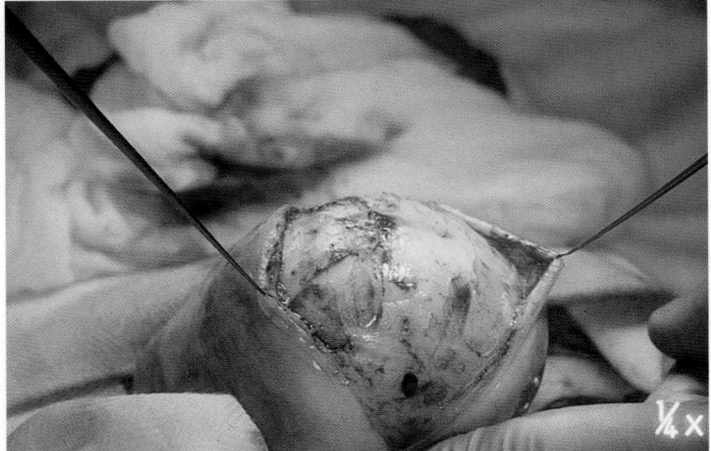

**FIGURE 14–7** When the capsule of the myoma is reached, deeper incising should cease. The myoma is now dissected peripherally.

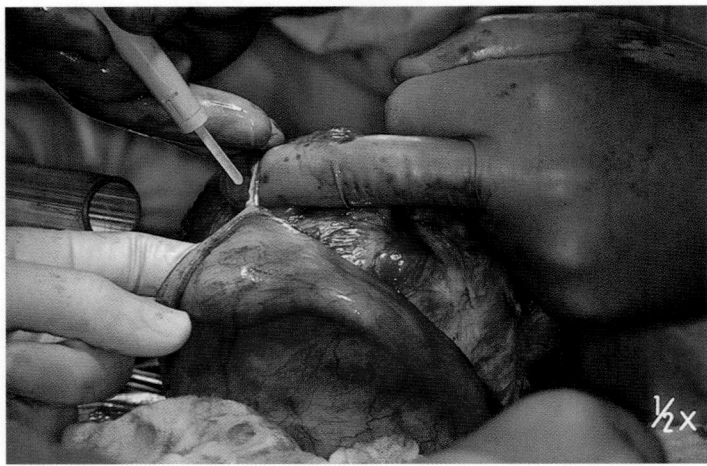

**FIGURE 14–8** Small adhesions may be encountered between the uterine wall and the myoma capsule. These adhesions should be cut sharply.

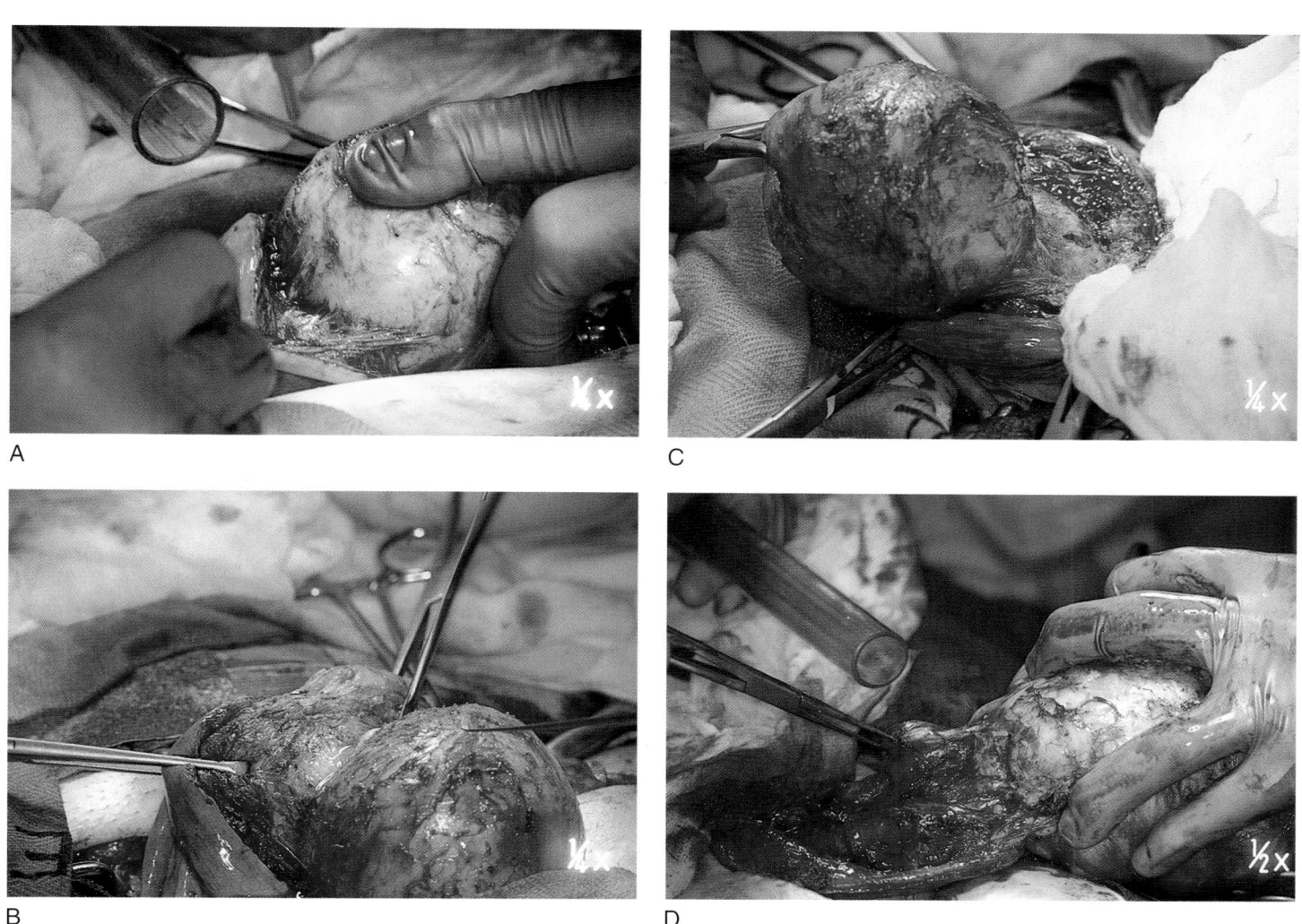

**FIGURE 14–9  A** and **B.** With a combination of sharp and blunt dissection, the myoma is separated from the normal myometrium. **C** and **D.** The dissection is carried to its basal attachment (the tumor) to the uterine wall.

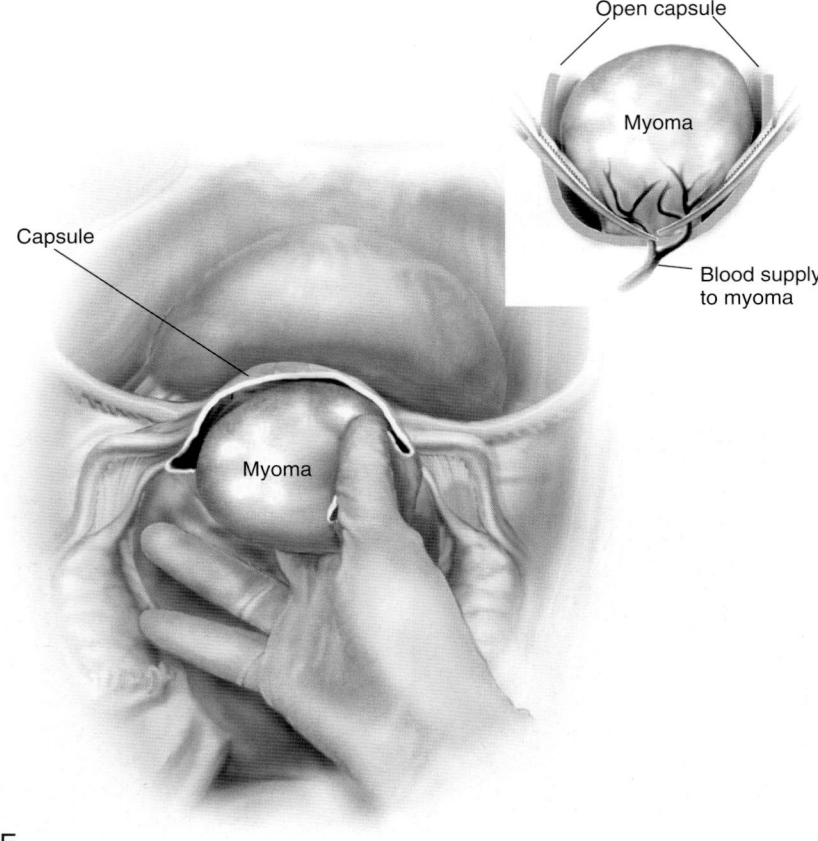

Open capsule

Myoma

Blood supply
to myoma

Capsule

Myoma

E

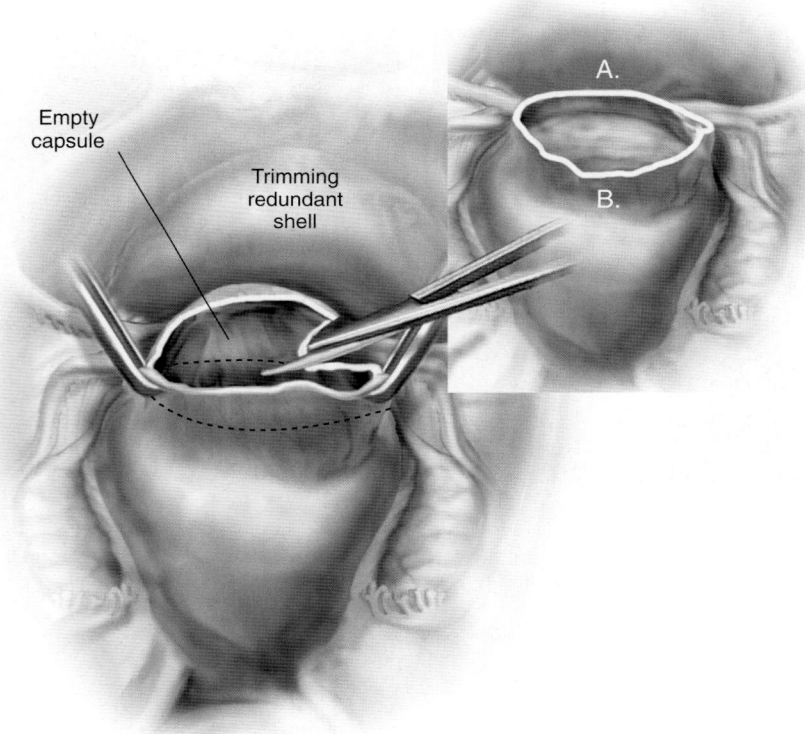

Empty
capsule

Trimming
redundant
shell

A.

B.

F

**FIGURE 14–9, cont'd  E.** The feeding artery is clamped and suture-ligated with
0 Vicryl. **F.** Excess uterine serosa is trimmed away. The anterior wall (*A*) will be closed
to approximate and overlap the posterior wall (*B*).

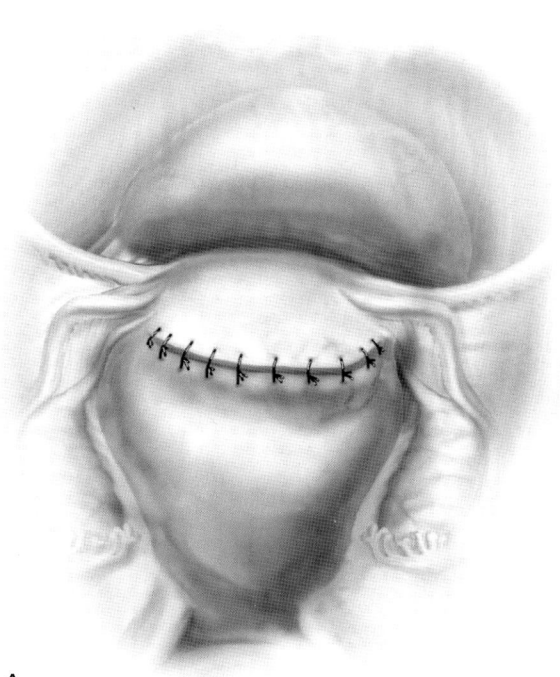

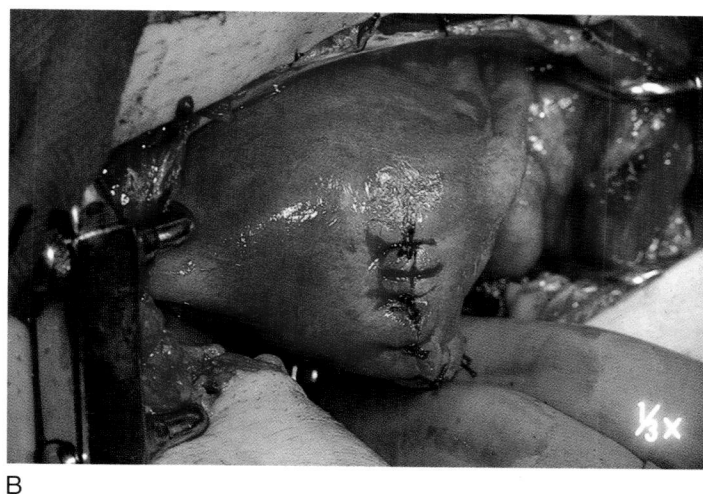

B

A

**FIGURE 14–10  A.** Closure is implemented by suturing the anterior margin over the posterior margin to strengthen the wound integrity. This illustrates a transverse closure. **B.** The interrupted-suture technique for vertical incision closure will be completed by tacking peritoneum or Interceed over the incision.

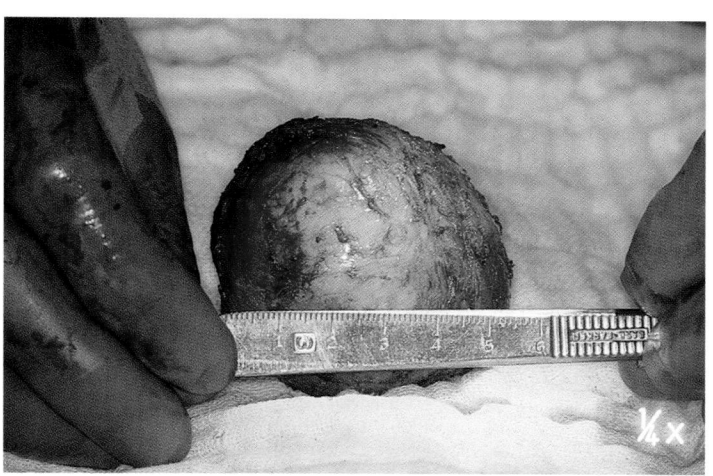

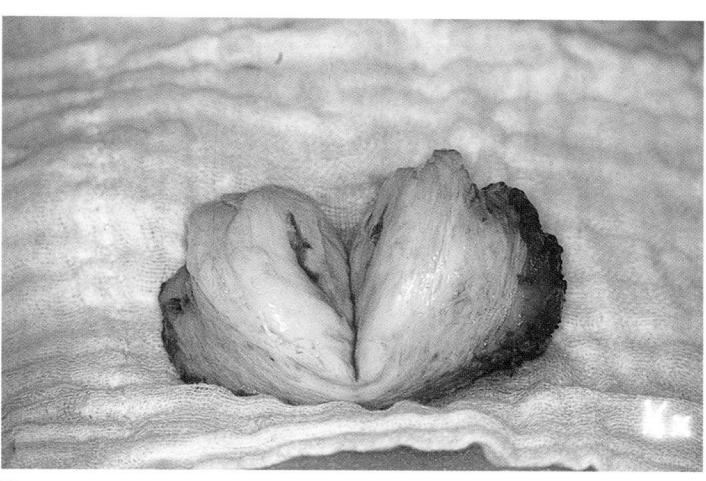

A                                                            B

**FIGURE 14–11  A.** The extracted myoma is grossly studied and measured. **B.** The myoma is bisected to allow examination of its interior. The specimen is then placed in formalin and sent to pathology. If the myoma has undergone purulent degeneration, a culture should be taken before the tumor is placed in fixative. If sarcoma is suspected, a sample on the interior may be sent for frozen section analysis.

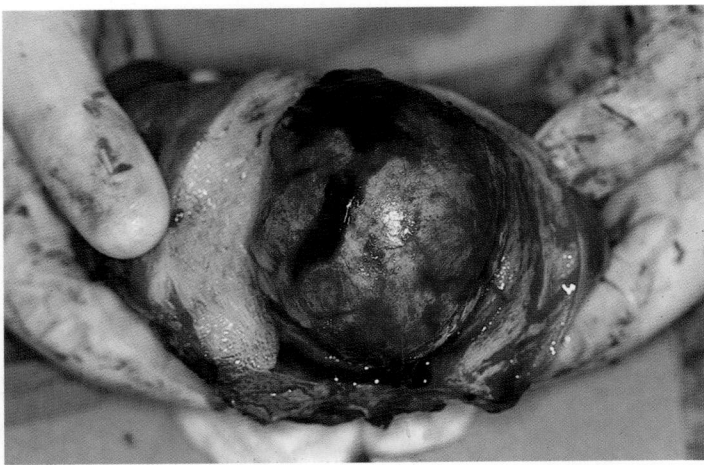

**FIGURE 14–12**  Bleeding symptoms and anemia suggest the presence of a submucous myoma. The submucous myoma should be treated by hysteroscopy or hysterectomy.

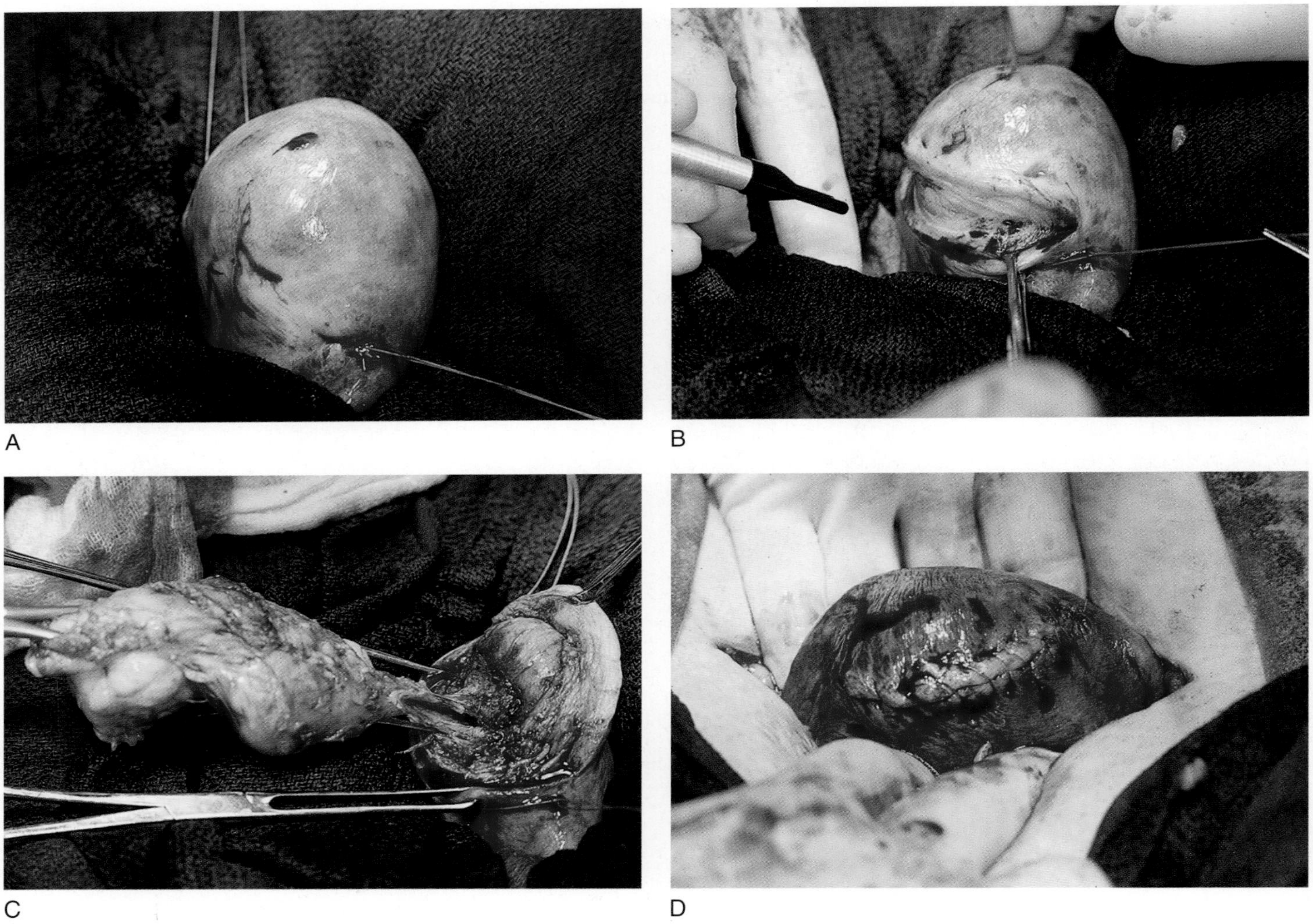

A

B

C

D

**FIGURE 14–13  A.** This large myomatous uterus has been injected with a 1:200 vasopressin solution. **B.** An anterior transverse incision is made into the uterus above the urinary bladder peritoneal reflection. **C.** The myoma is dissected free from the uterine wall; unfortunately, the uterine cavity is entered. **D.** After removal of the myomatous mass, the uterus is closed in layers with 0 Vicryl. The serosa is closed with 2-0 Vicryl. Note that the uterus has been reduced to a normal size.

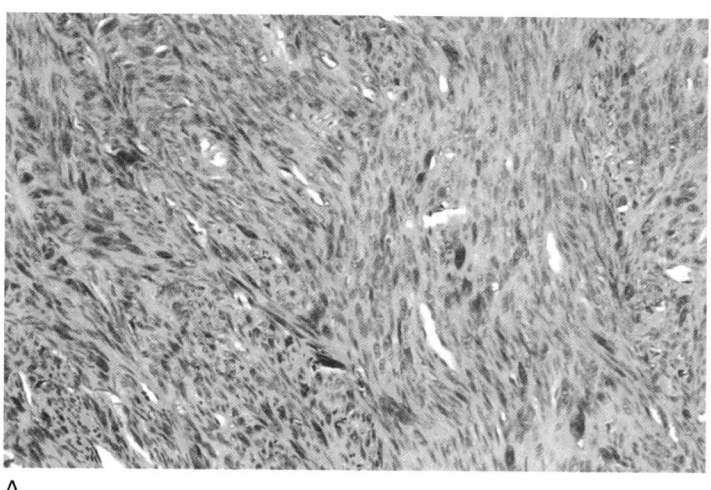

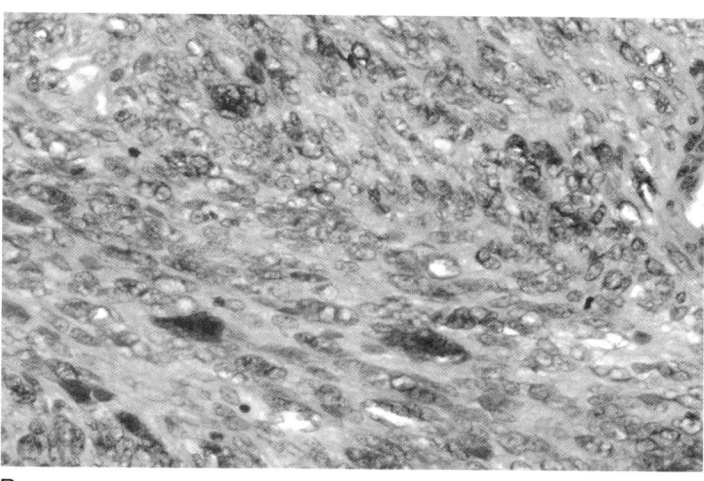

A

B

**FIGURE 14–14 A.** Histologic section from the uterus pictured in Figure 10–13A–C. The hematoxylin and eosin (H&E)-stained section (×10) shows increased cellularity, nuclear pleomorphism, and hyperchromatism. **B.** Histologic section (×20) clearly confirms the diagnosis of leiomyosarcoma. Four mitotic figures are seen in this single field. The stromal (muscle) cells are clearly malignant. (From Baggish MS, Barbot J, Valle V: *In* Diagnostic and Operative Hysteroscopy, 2nd ed. Mosby, St Louis, 1999.)

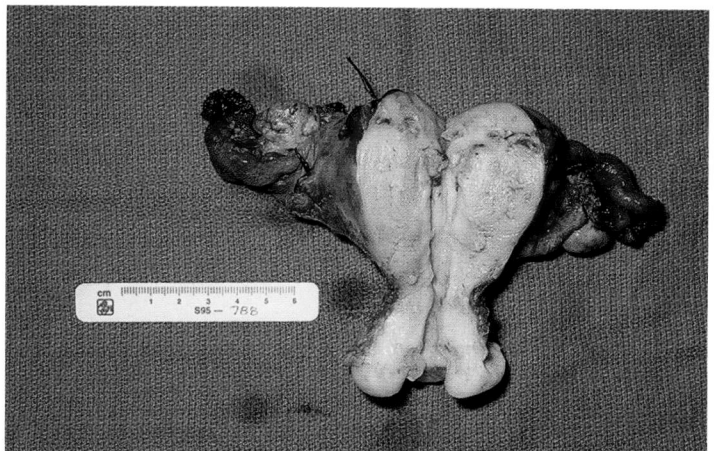

A

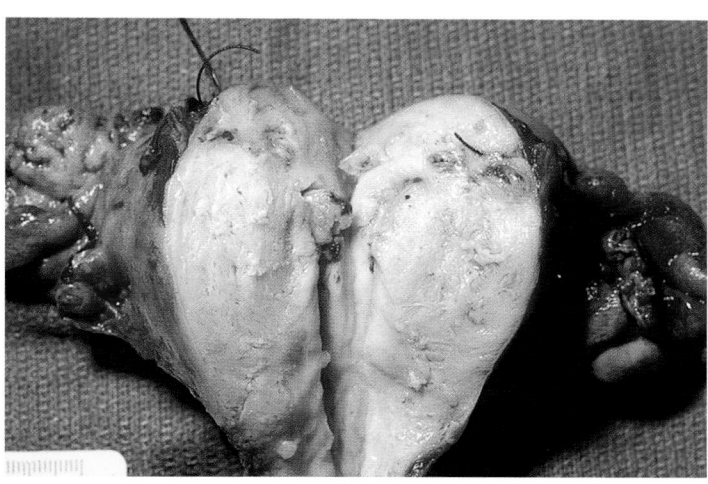

B

**FIGURE 14–15 A.** Hysterectomy specimen from the patient depicted in Figures 14–13 and 14–14. The normal-sized uterus has been removed. **B.** The cut wall of the uterus appears to be normal. Microscopic sections were benign (i.e., no residual sarcoma).

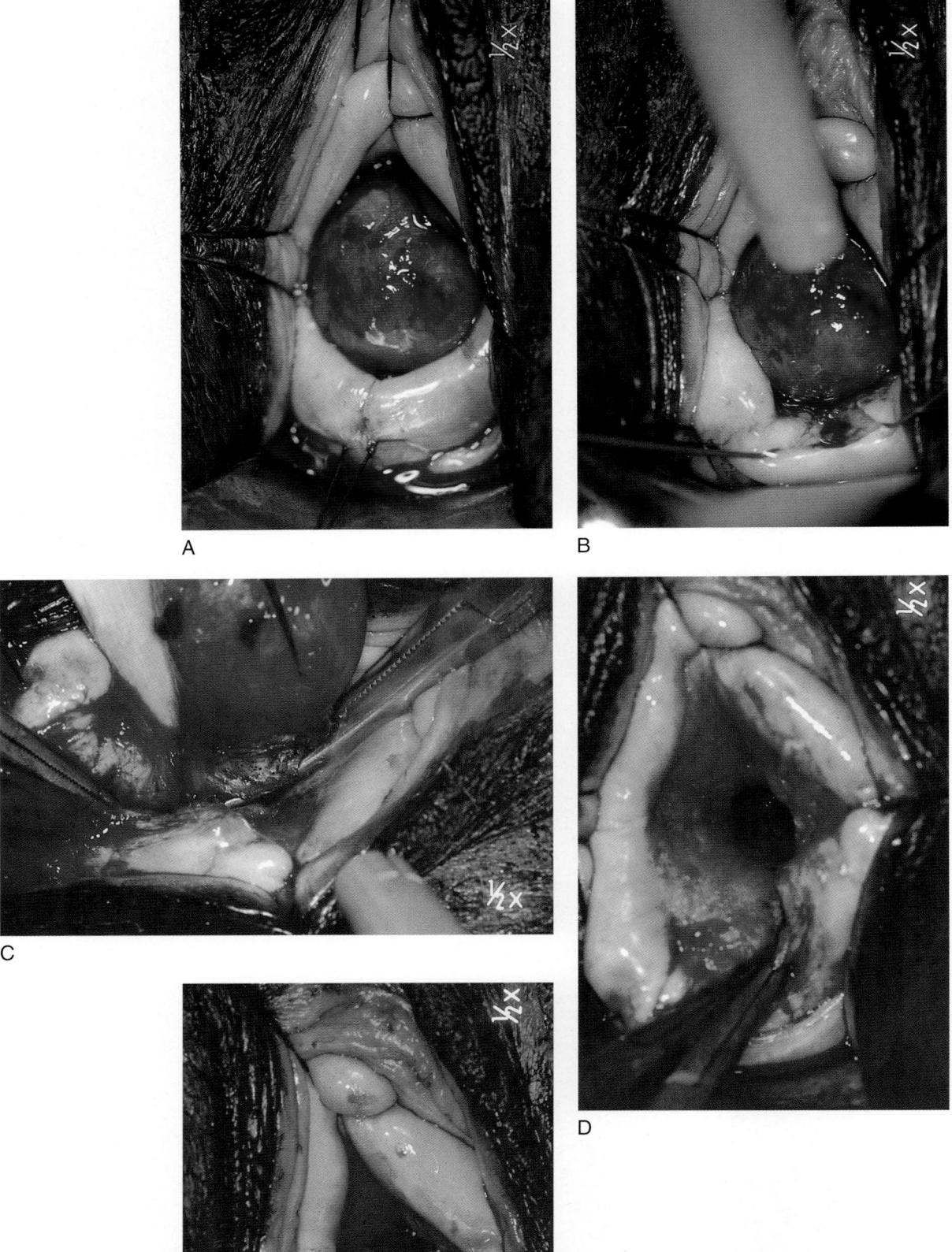

**FIGURE 14–16** **A.** A cervical myoma is present, but the pedicle location is not visible. Traction sutures have been placed anteriorly and laterally. **B.** The posterior lip of the cervix has been injected with a 1:100 solution of vasopressin. The carbon dioxide ($CO_2$) laser beam (microscope-coupled) has begun to cut the cervix posteriorly to gain access to the myoma pedicle. Titanium hooks place traction on either side of the incision. The red helium-neon aiming beam is visible. **C.** The pedicle has been clamped with a Kelly clamp. A moist tongue depressor has been placed between the myoma and the interior of the cervix. The laser beam has partially cut through the base of the myoma. **D.** The myoma has been removed. The stump of the pedicle will be sutured with 3-0 Vicryl. **E.** The surgery has been completed. The cervix has been sutured with 3-0 Vicryl. (From Baggish MS, Barbot J, Valle V: *In* Diagnostic and Operative Hysteroscopy, 2nd ed. Mosby, St Louis, 1999.)

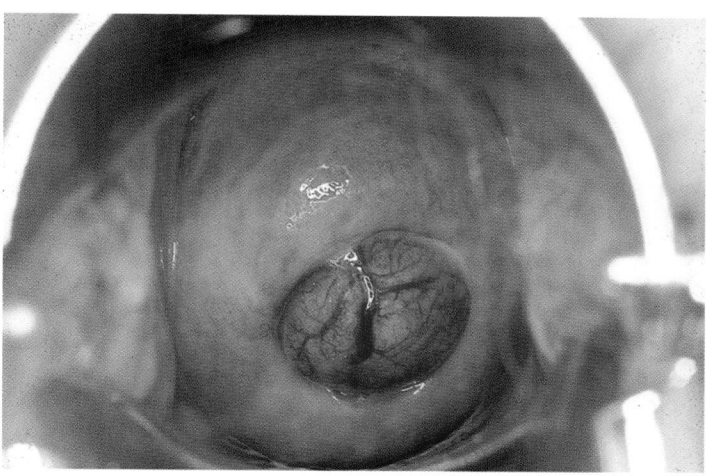

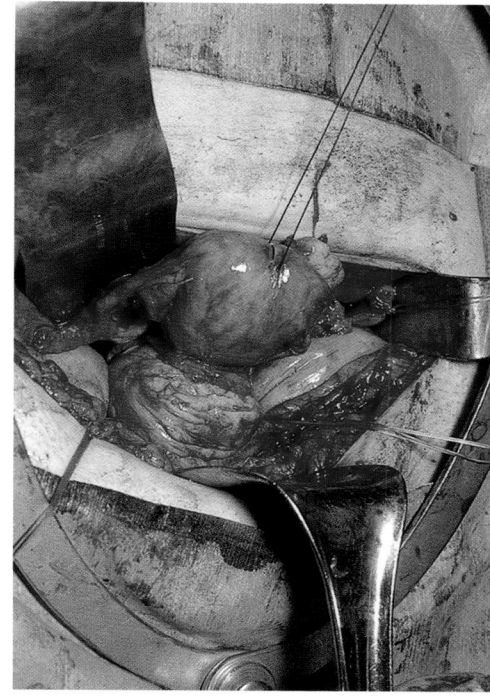

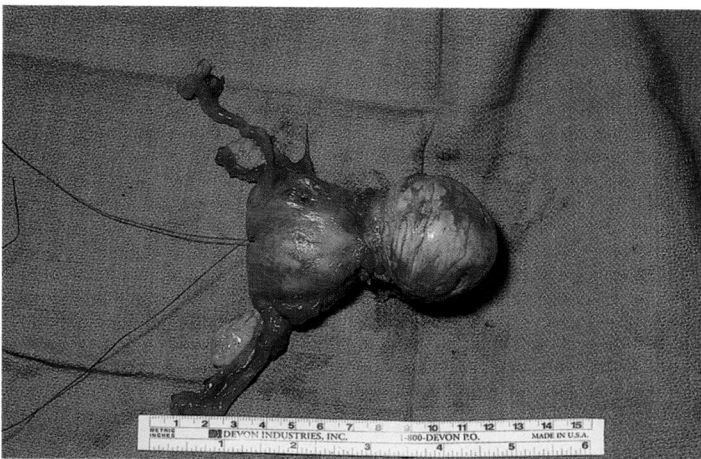

**FIGURE 14–17  A.** This patient has a large cervical myoma. The thin-walled vessels are subject to rupture. These vessels will not retract and will bleed heavily for a prolonged period. **B.** The patient opted for hysterectomy rather than myomectomy. **C.** The total volume of this tumor was much greater than anticipated, in fact, even bigger than the body of the uterus. In this case, hysterectomy was the best choice because the large size of the myoma would preclude use of the vaginal-cervical route of removal.

# CHAPTER 15

# Surgical Treatment of Unusual Myoma Conditions

*Michael S. Baggish*

Several bizarre variants of myoma may be encountered. Benign metastasizing myoma (leiomyomatosis peritonealis disseminata) consists of multiple intraperitoneal benign tumors and even distant myoma metastasis, typically to the lungs (Fig. 15–1). These cases may have a propensity for occurrence during pregnancy. Symptoms include paroxysmal attacks of dyspnea and hemoptysis. Myomas may regress after the pregnancy terminates (see Fig. 15–1).

Intravenous leiomyomatosis is associated with smooth muscle tumors extending into venous channels (Fig. 15–2). This condition illustrates clinically the enigma about the origins of uterine leiomyomata in general: Do these tumors arise from a smooth muscle cell from the myometrium or from a smooth muscle cell within the media of the blood vessel itself? This unusual phenomenon represents a dissociation between clinical and histologic malignancy in which benign uterine myomas may propagate via blood vascular channels, although the condition rarely kills the patient.

The uterus is typical of one containing irregularly enlarged myomata uteri (Fig. 15–3). The venous pattern over the uterus and within the broad ligament is unusually prominent, and an indurated, woody texture may be found. As the pedicles are cut, glistening, white extensions (Fig. 15–4), some as wide as 2 to 3 cm in diameter, may be seen (Fig. 15–5). As veins separate, the intravascular tumor may ooze out of the involved vessels in a wormlike fashion (Fig. 15–6). Microscopically, the vessel wall contains plugs of typical benign smooth muscle lying free within the lumen (Fig. 15–7) or attached to the wall of the vein (Fig. 15–8A, B).

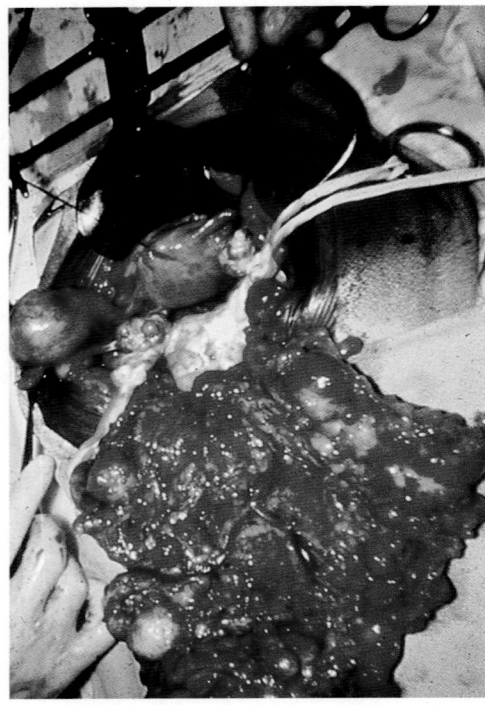

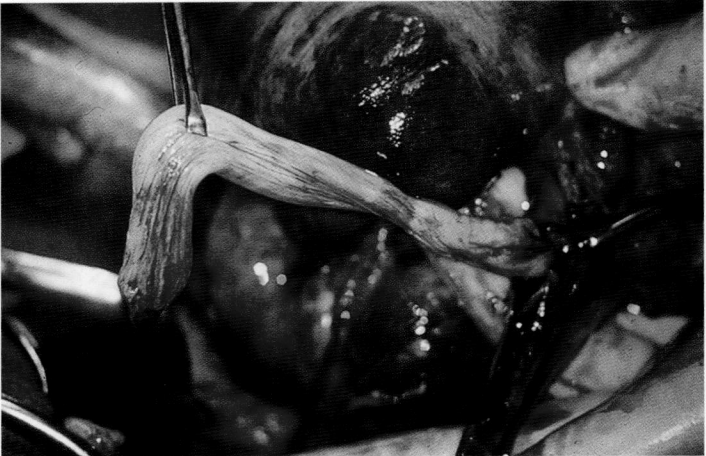

**FIGURE 15–2**  A large intravenous myoma extension is teased out of a distended vein.

**FIGURE 15–1**  Leiomyomatosis peritonealis disseminata. The omentum is filled with myomata of various sizes.

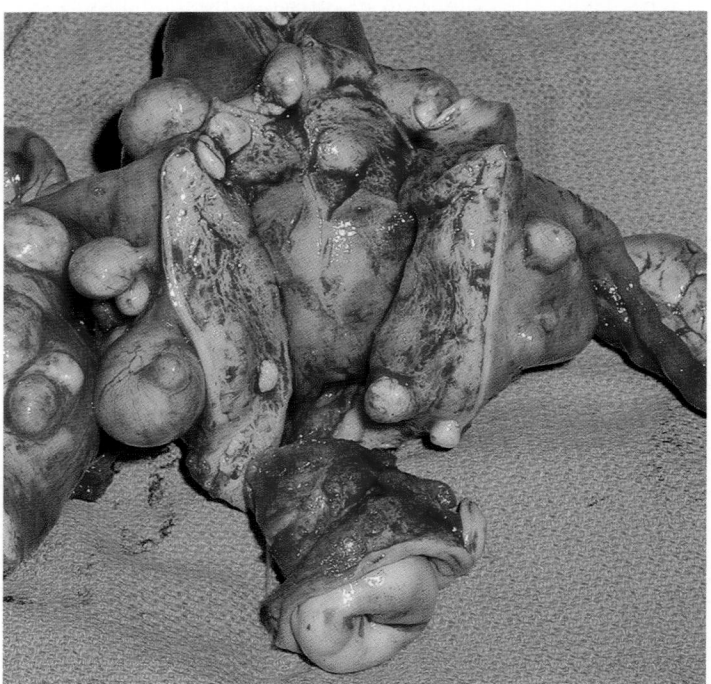

**FIGURE 15–3**  An enlarged irregular uterus filled with myomata. Note the submucous, intramural, subserous varieties within this single uterus.

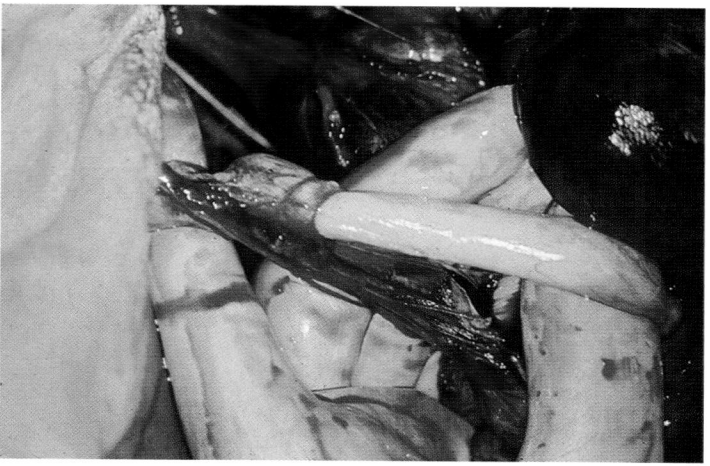

**FIGURE 15–4** A glistening white serpentine myoma is seen to enter a thin-walled venous sinus. Note that the color of the intravenous myoma is very close to the color of the surgeon's gloves.

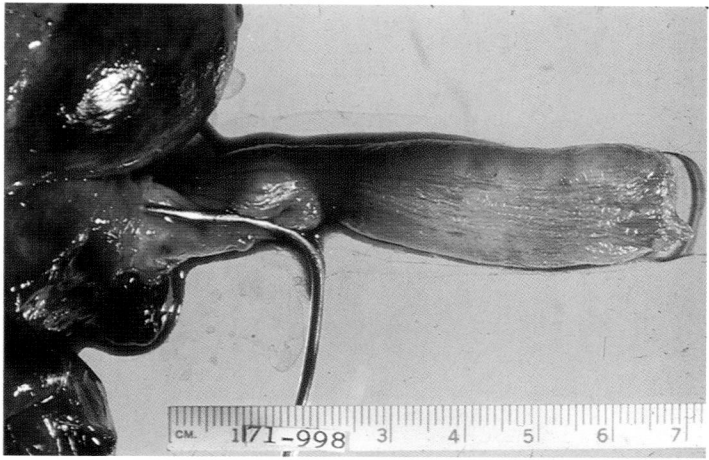

**FIGURE 15–5** An intravenous leiomyoma extension 2 cm in diameter fills the uterine vein, giving a woody feeling to the distended uterine, parauterine, and bladder vessels.

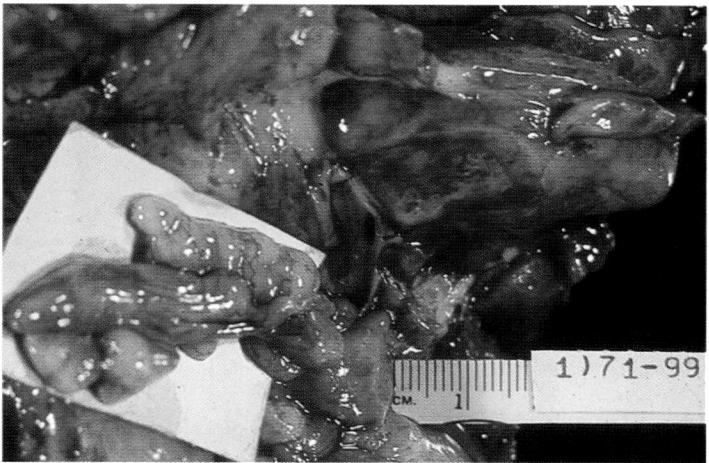

**FIGURE 15–6** As vascular pedicles are cut, the myoma oozes out of the vessels in a wormlike fashion. The differential diagnosis is between intravenous leiomyomatosis and endolymphatic stromal myosis (stromatosis).

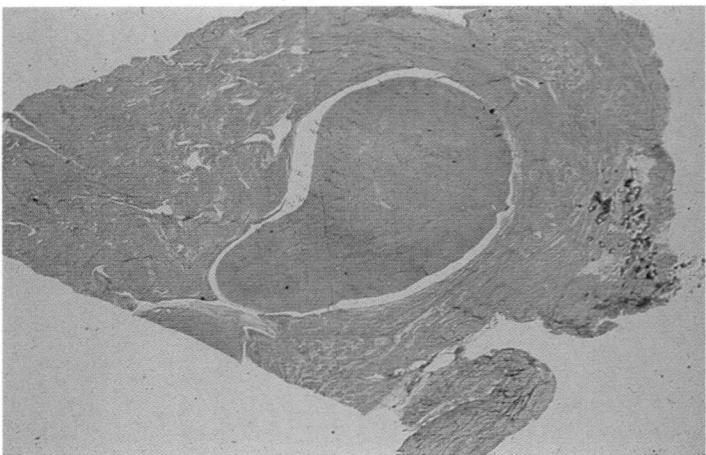

**FIGURE 15–7** Elastic tissue stain shows a microscopic plug of myoma within a venous space.

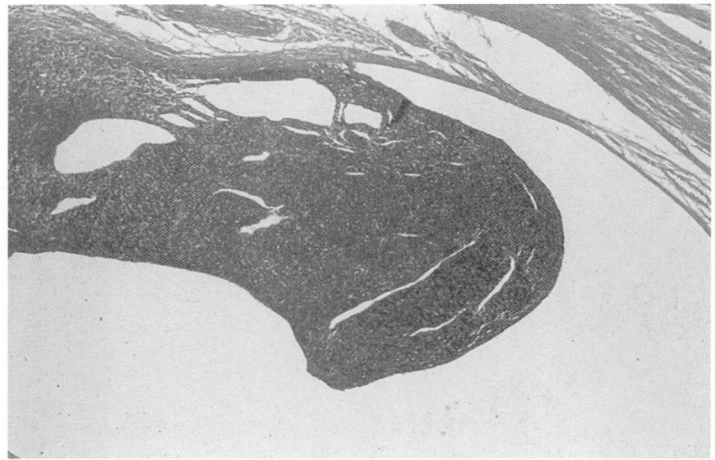

A

B

**FIGURE 15–8  A.** Benign myoma with a venous space and attached to the wall of the vein. **B.** High-power view of a benign myoma within a uterine vein.

# CHAPTER 16

# Unification of Bicornuate Uterus

## Michael S. Baggish

Incomplete fusion of the müllerian ducts leads to a variety of disorders, ranging from subseptate uterus to complete failure of fusion with uterus didelphys (Fig. 16–1). The subseptate uterus is treated hysteroscopically by sectioning the septum with a scissors, laser, or electrosurgical device. The uterus didelphys requires no treatment other than section of the vaginal septum to prevent traumatic tears (Fig. 16–2).

The bicornuate uterus may require a unification procedure to enhance the size of the uterine cavity if reproductive outcome problems are demonstrated (e.g., abortion, preterm labor) (see Figs. 16–1 and 16–3).

Diagnostic differentiation between a septate and a bicornuate uterus cannot be accomplished by hysteroscopy or by hysterosalpingography (Fig. 16–4). The diagnosis is made laparoscopically by observing the broad and indented fundus, the typical heart-shaped configuration. A hysterogram is performed to gain some insight into the size and configuration of the divided cavities (Fig. 16–5A–C).

At laparotomy traction, sutures are placed at each fundal extreme away from the site of transection. A 1:200 vasopressin solution is injected into the uterus along and within the lines of resection (Fig. 16–6). A wedge-shaped incision is made through the body and fundus of the uterus in the vertical plane (Figs. 16–7A, B). The resultant tissue removed includes the heart-shaped defect (Fig. 16–7C). The two separate cavities are now ready to be joined to form a single uterine cavity (Figs. 16–7D, E). Closure is made beginning on the posterior wall with simple or figure-of-8 stitches placed submucosally and carried intramuscularly (Figs. 16–8A, B). The closure is carried over the fundus and is completed on the anterior surface (Fig. 16–8C). The author typically uses 0 Vicryl for the intramuscular layer (Fig. 16–8D). Next, with 2-0 or 3-0 Vicryl, the superficial muscle and serosa are closed with a running or running lock suture (Fig. 16–9).

Shadow of bicornuate
uterine cavities

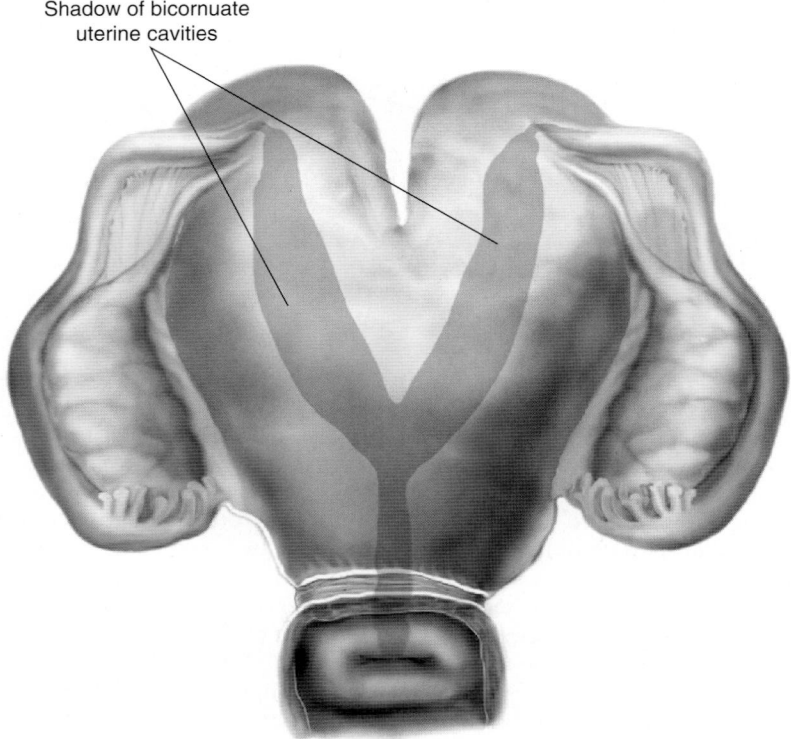

**FIGURE 16–1** External view of heart-shaped bicornuate uterus. Note the schema of a hysterogram superimposed on the uterus.

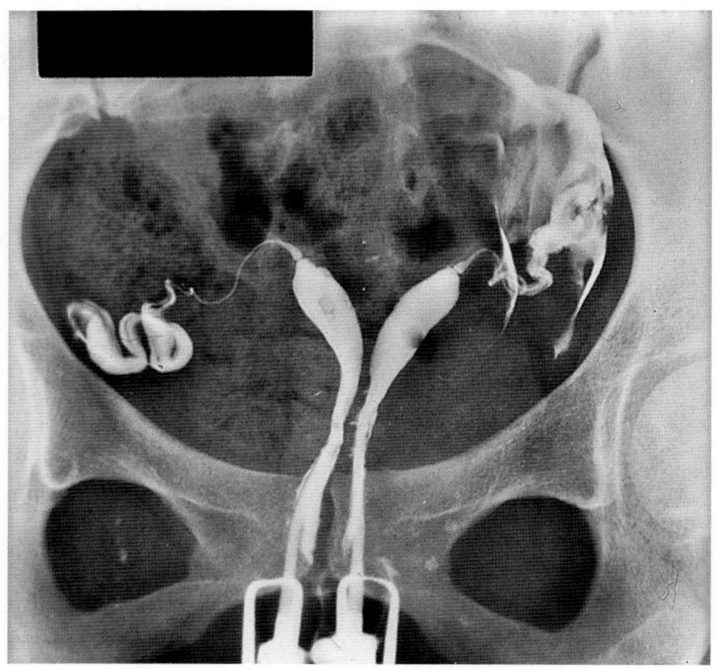

**FIGURE 16–2** Hysterosalpingogram of a complete fusion defect illustrating duplication of the uterus and cervix. The vagina was septate.

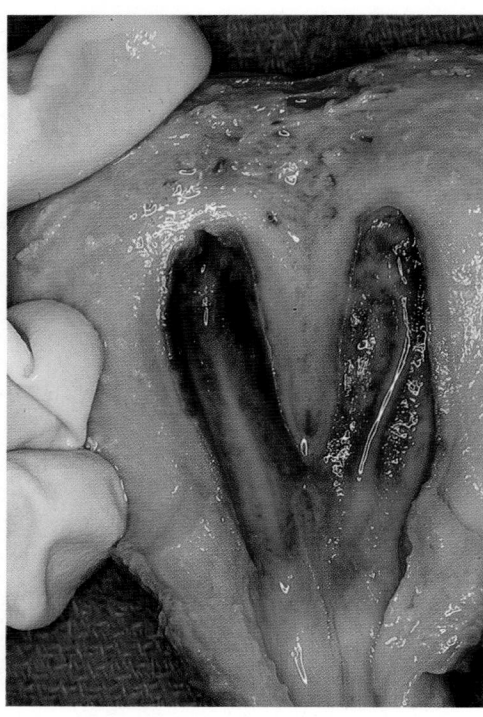

**FIGURE 16–3** Specimen of an extirpated uterus showing a septated cavity and a single cervix.

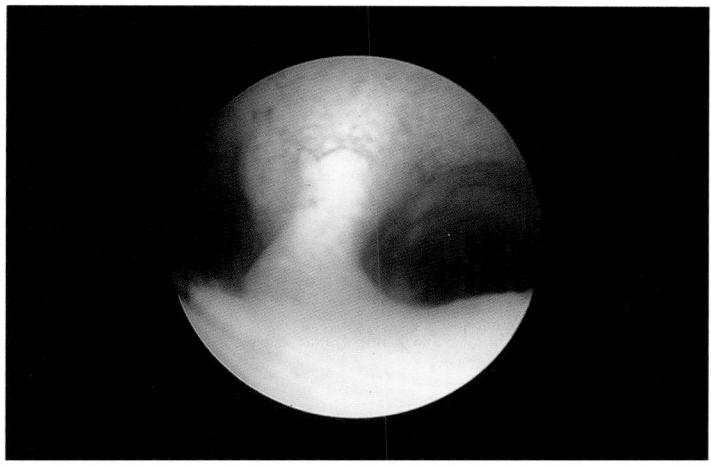

**FIGURE 16–4** Hysteroscopic view of bicornuate uterus.

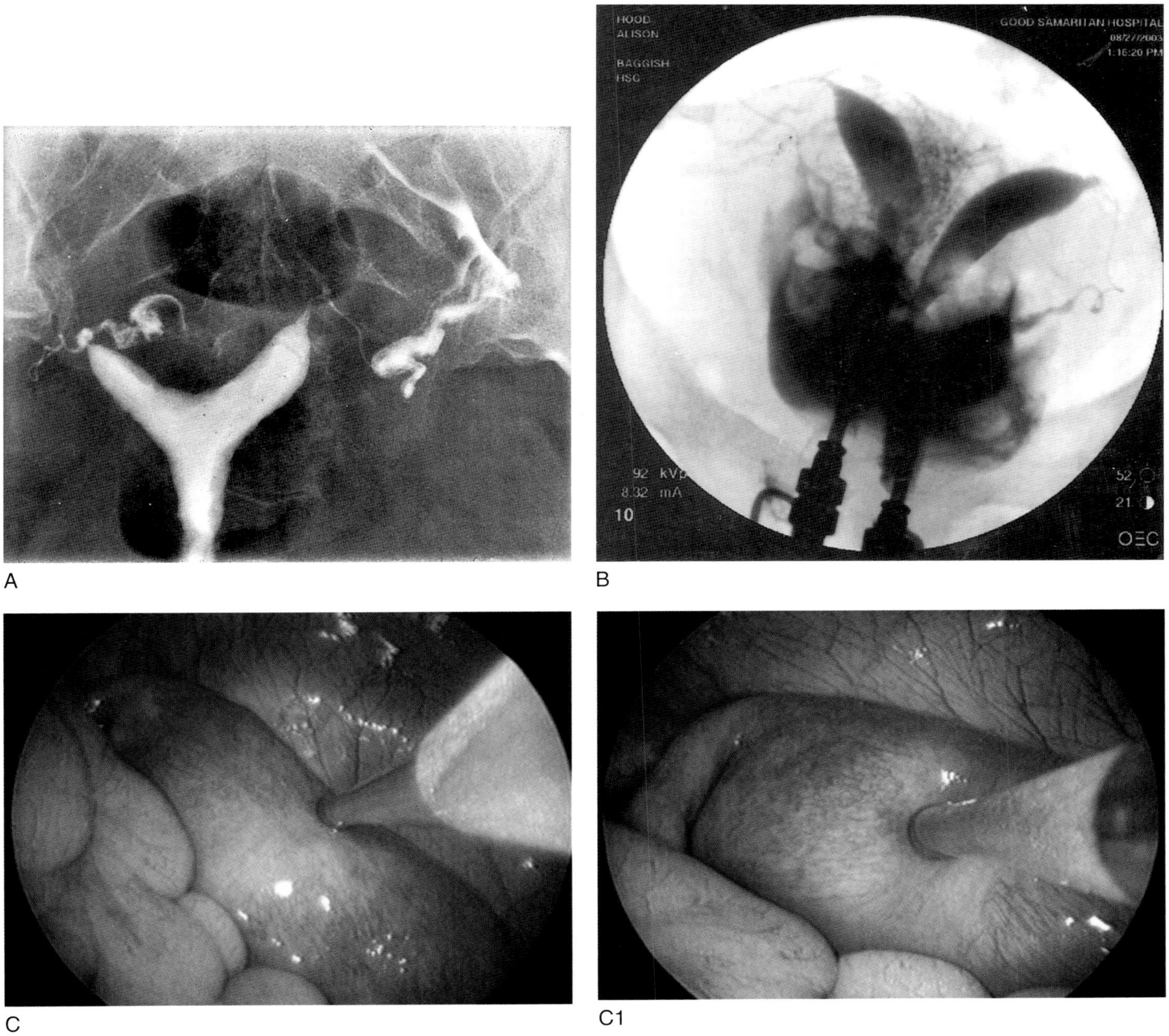

A

B

C

C1

**FIGURE 16–5 A.** Hysterosalpingogram showing a bicornuate uterus. In actuality, the diagnosis was established laparoscopically. **B.** Hysterogram of what was considered to be a complete fusion defect. Note the two cervices and the two distinctly separate uterine horns. **C.** Laparoscopic photographs of Figure 16–5B show a single, broad structure that has the appearance of a bicornuate uterus.

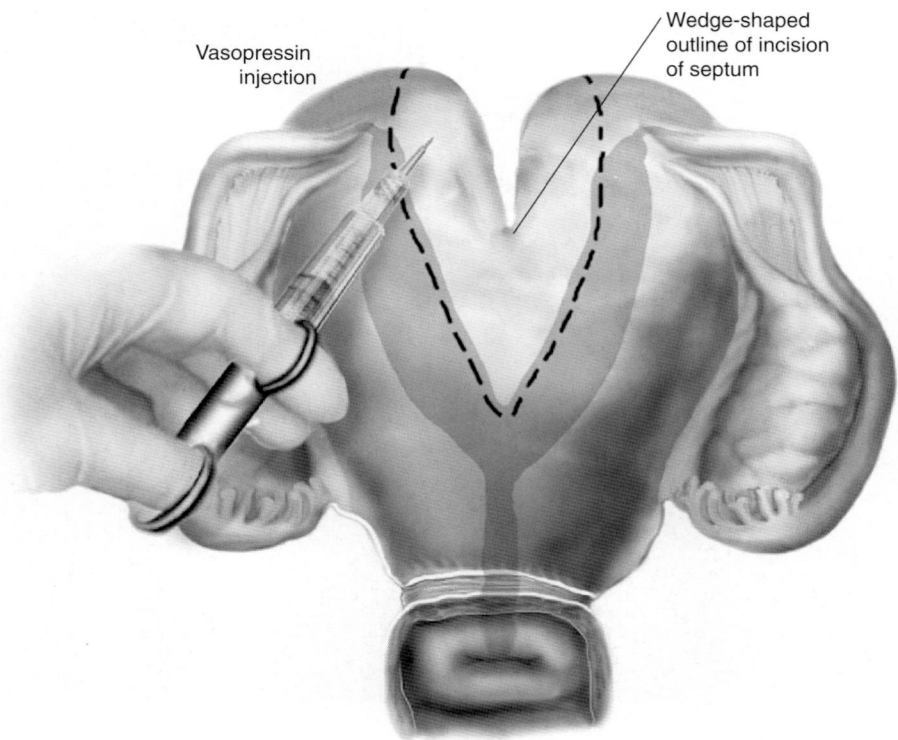

Vasopressin injection

Wedge-shaped outline of incision of septum

**FIGURE 16–6** In preparation for unification of the two uterine cavities, a 1:200 solution of vasopressin is injected along the lines of intended resection.

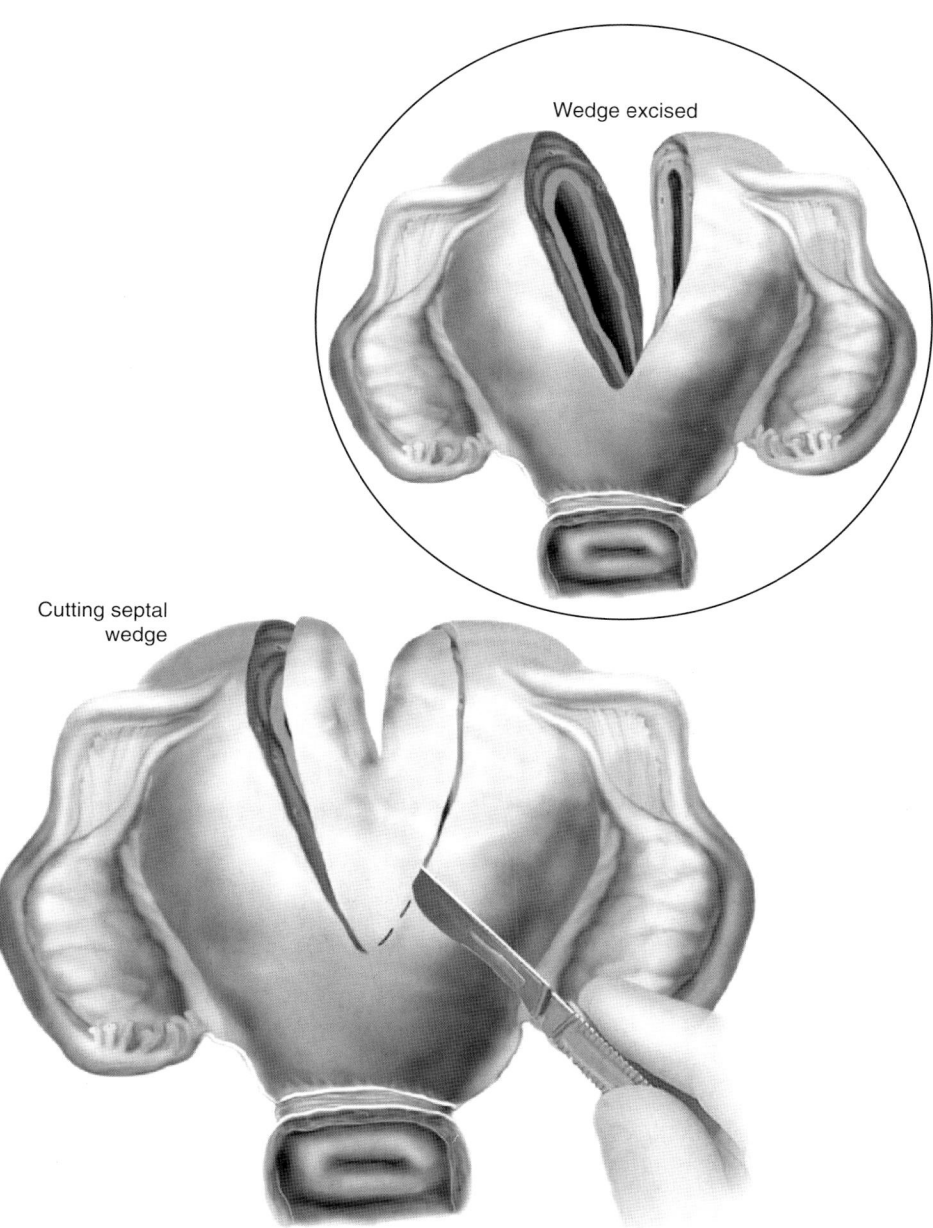

Wedge excised

Cutting septal
wedge

A

**FIGURE 16–7  A.** With the use of a knife, a carbon dioxide ($CO_2$) laser, or an electrosurgical needle electrode, the septum and defect are wedged out. The **inset** shows the cavities after excision. Hemostasis is attained with 3-0 Vicryl figure-of-8 suture ligatures.

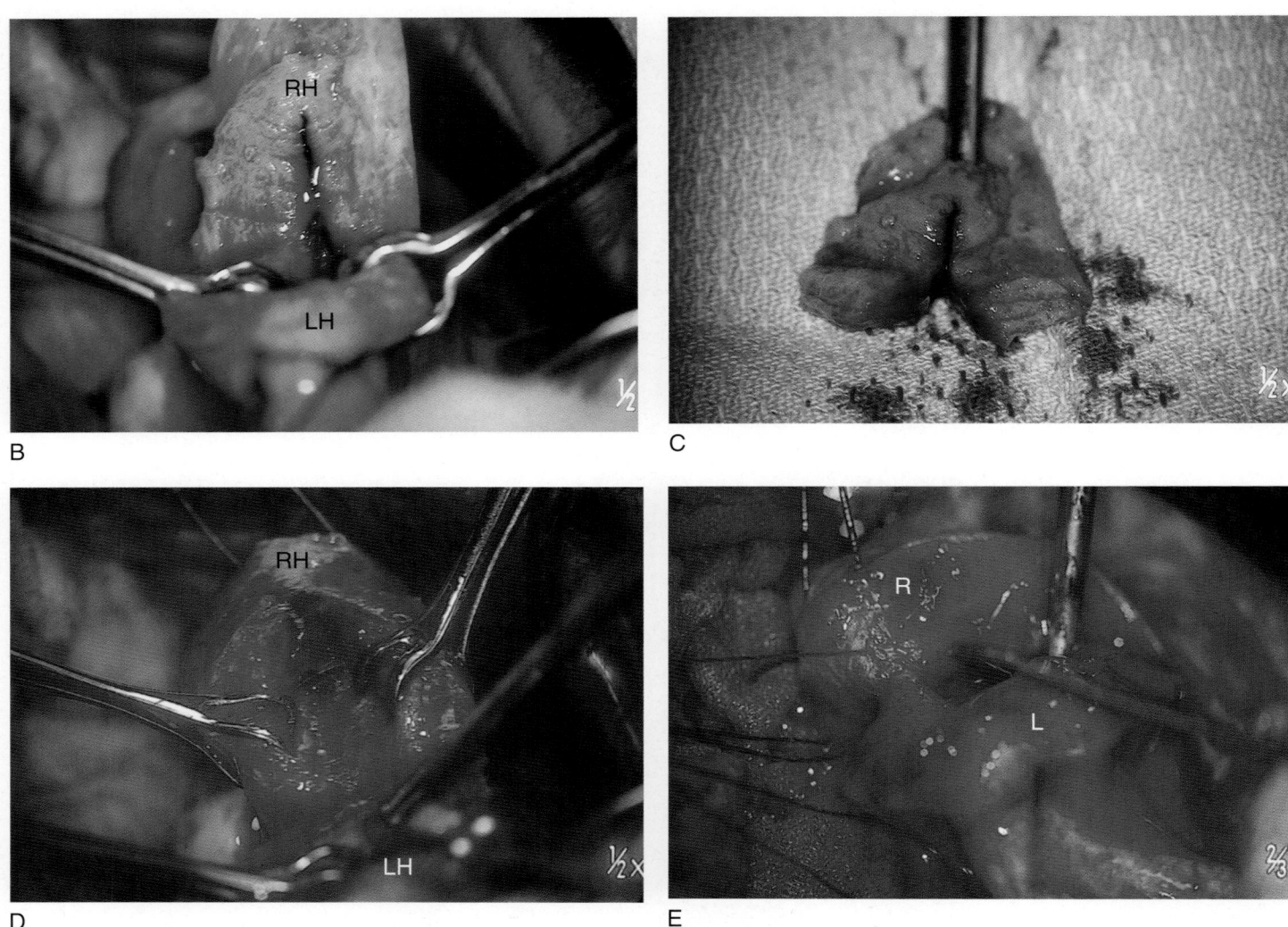

B

C

D

E

**FIGURE 16–7, cont'd   B.** The right horn (RH) of the uterus is exposed in the center of the photograph. The wedge has been removed. The left horn (LH) is held in Babcock clamps. **C.** The heart-shaped (inverted) wedge of uterus is held in the Kocher clamp. **D.** Each uterine horn is held with Babcock clamps and will be drawn together for the placement of myometrial stitches, which will unite the two horns (RH and LH) into a new single-cavity uterus. **E.** The figure-of-8 stitch is begun from the inside (submucosal) and through the inner two thirds of the myometrium (L), then is carried into the right myometrium (R) and out the right submucosa.

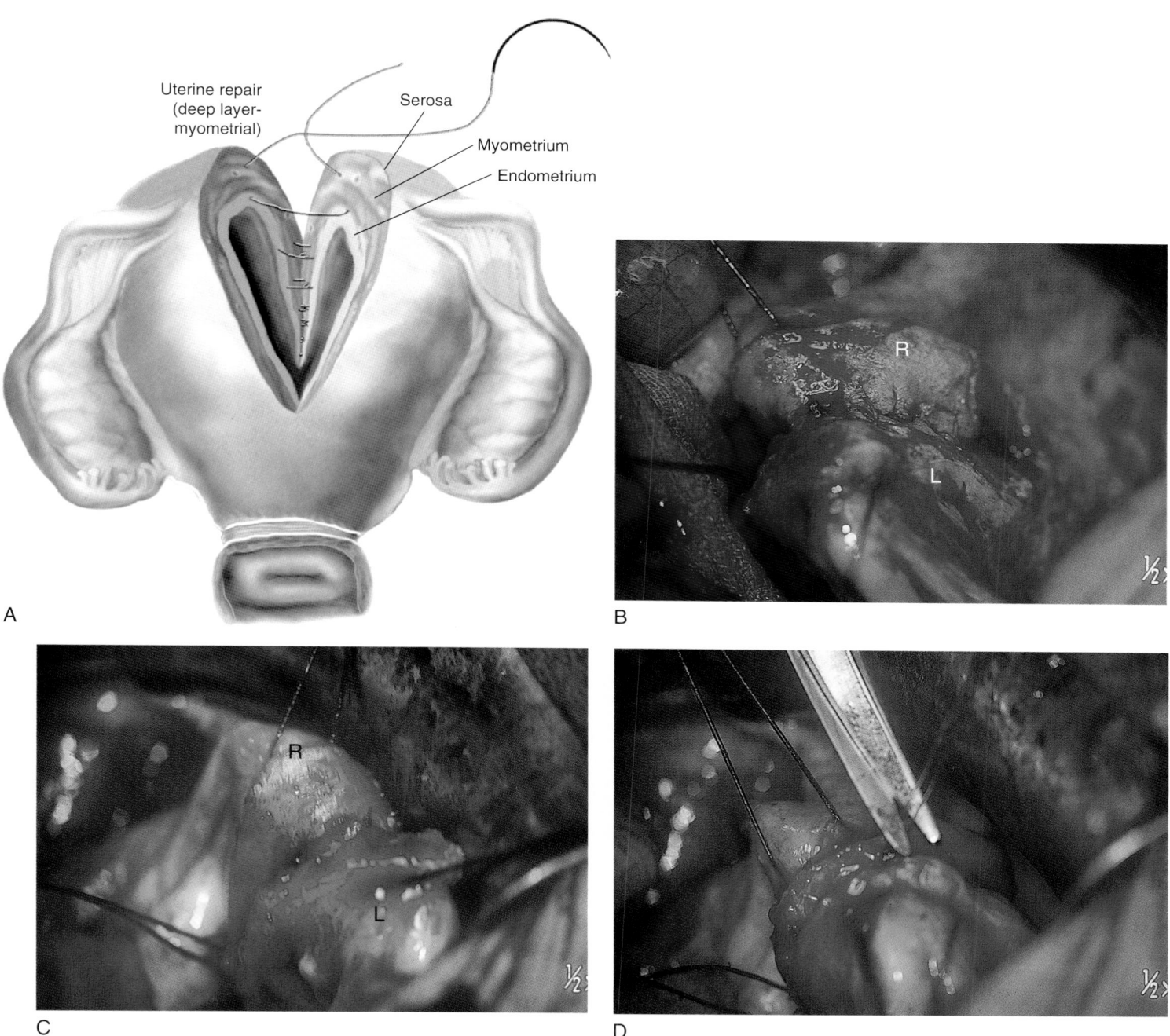

**FIGURE 16–8  A.** The uterine cavity is closed by placing subendometrial intramyometrial 0 Vicryl simple or figure-of-8 sutures, beginning on the posterior wall and terminating on the anterior uterine wall. **B.** Zero Vicryl sutures have been placed into the posterior uterine wall, uniting right (R) and left (L) horns. **C.** The closure is carried over the uterine fundus. **D.** The myometrial closure is complete. The somewhat blurred left oviduct is seen in the foreground.

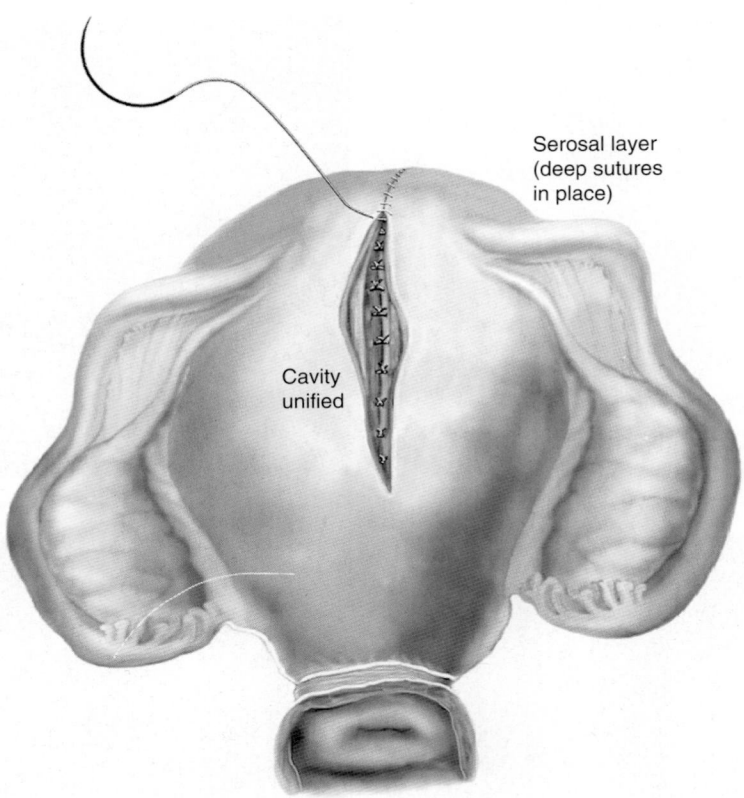

Serosal layer
(deep sutures
in place)

Cavity
unified

**FIGURE 16–9** The operation is finished by closing the serosal surface of the uterus with a running 3-0 Vicryl or PDS suture.

# SECTION C

# Abdominal Surgery During Pregnancy

# CHAPTER 17

# Abdominal Cerclage of the Cervix Uteri

*Michael S. Baggish*

Typically, cervical cerclage is performed via the vaginal route. The simple purse-string McDonald closure and the submucosal Shirodkar closure are accomplished with a low level of bleeding and relatively little pain, and within a short time.

When the cervix is extremely short as a result of obstetric injury, deep conization, multiple excisional/ablative procedures, or virtual amputation, vaginal placement of a constricting suture or band may be difficult or impossible to perform. In fact, anecdotal accounts about ureteral ligation have been reported in conjunction with McDonald suture placement.

Clearly, the observed lengthening of the cervix following cerclage cannot be accounted for by narrowing the cervical canal. It is obvious that the increased cervical length is attributable to inclusion of the uterine isthmus within the suture.

A laparotomy is required for this technique. Five steps are critical for the successful and safe performance of abdominal cerclage: (1) elevation of the uterus to expose the isthmus and cervix, (2) identification of the uterine vessels, (3) precise identification of the position of the ureters, and (4) placement of the cerclage band above the uterosacral ligaments by (5) location of an avascular plane between the uterine vessels and the isthmus.

This operation is performed during the second trimester at approximately 14 to 16 weeks' gestation. The fundus is grasped between the operator's thumb and forefinger over a lap pad. A space is opened in the vesicouterine and rectouterine peritoneum (Fig. 17-1). The bladder is gently pushed inferiorly. The peritoneum will be advanced at the end of the operation to cover the strap. The job of holding the uterus is transferred to an assistant once proper traction and positioning have been achieved.

The uterosacral ligaments are identified. The uterine vessels are felt pulsating as they ascend the side of the uterus (Fig. 17-2). The pelvic ureter is identified relative to the uterine vessels and the uterosacral ligament. An avascular space is identified between the uterine vessels and isthmus. If this cannot be seen, then the peritoneum should be opened over the uterine artery similar to skeletonization so that a space can be seen.

The needle or carrier is passed anteroposteriorly above the uterosacral ligament and posteroanteriorly again above the uterosacral ligament on the opposite side (Fig. 17-3). The strap of Mersilene mesh is gently tightened and tied into place (Fig. 17-4). The anterior and posterior surfaces are anchored to prevent migration up or down with 0 Vicryl sutures (Fig. 17-5). The vesicouterine and rectouterine peritoneum is folded over the strap and sutured closed with 3-0 Vicryl.

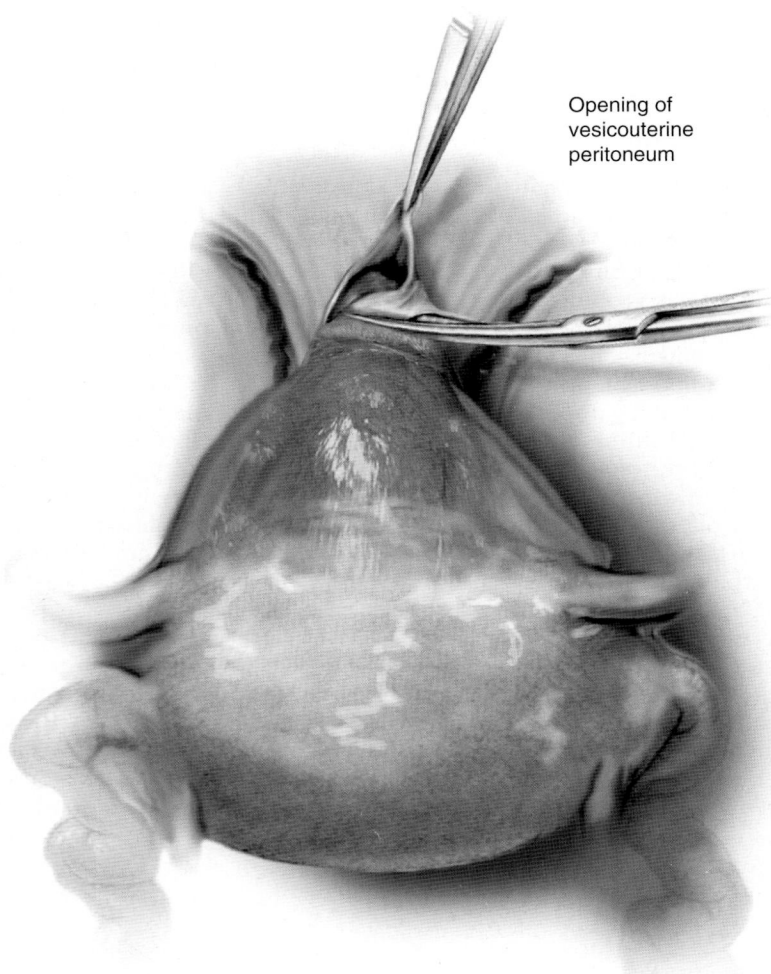

Opening of
vesicouterine
peritoneum

**FIGURE 17–1** The vesicouterine and rectouterine folds are incised. The bladder is pushed down with a sponge stick to expose the cervicocorporal junction of the uterus.

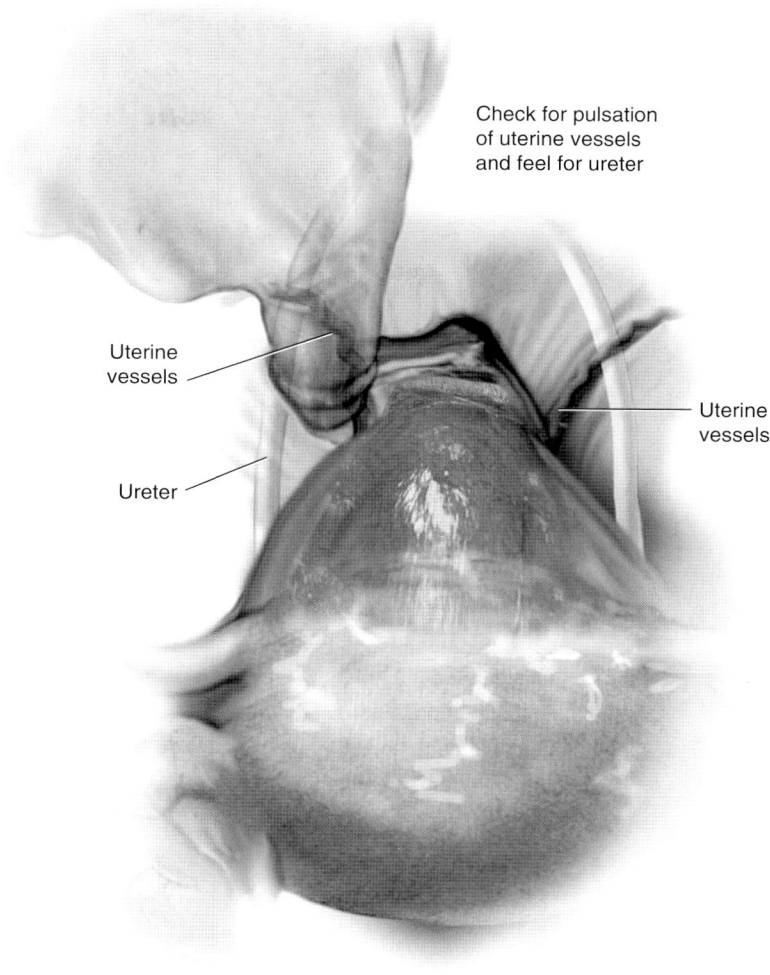

Check for pulsation
of uterine vessels
and feel for ureter

Uterine
vessels

Uterine
vessels

Ureter

**FIGURE 17–2** The uterine vessels are palpated at the side of
the uterus, and an avascular space is identified between these
vessels and the uterus.

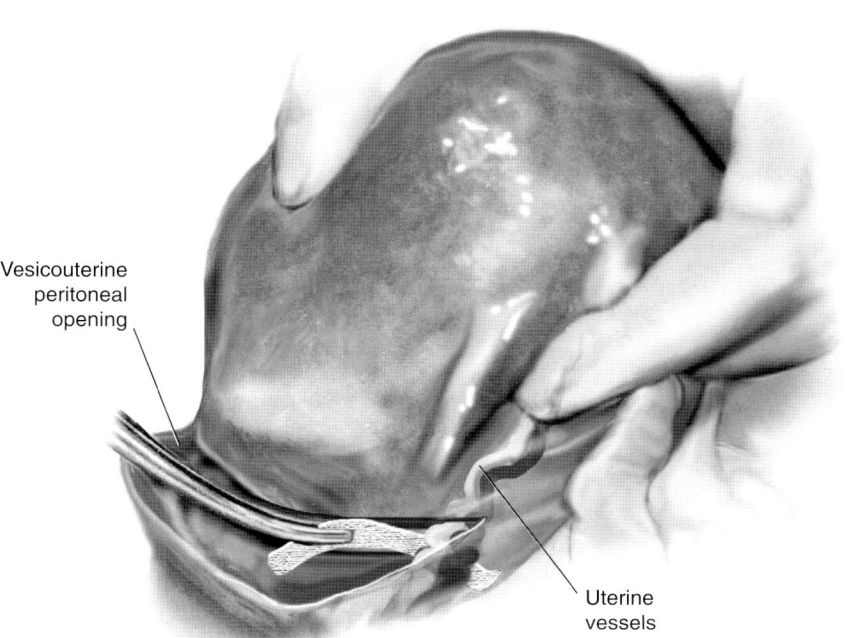

Vesicouterine
peritoneal
opening

Uterine
vessels

**FIGURE 17–3** A Mersilene strap is placed under the
vessels via a needle or carrier and brought out posteriorly
above the uterosacral ligaments.

Mersilene strap
passed anteriorly
under uterine vessels

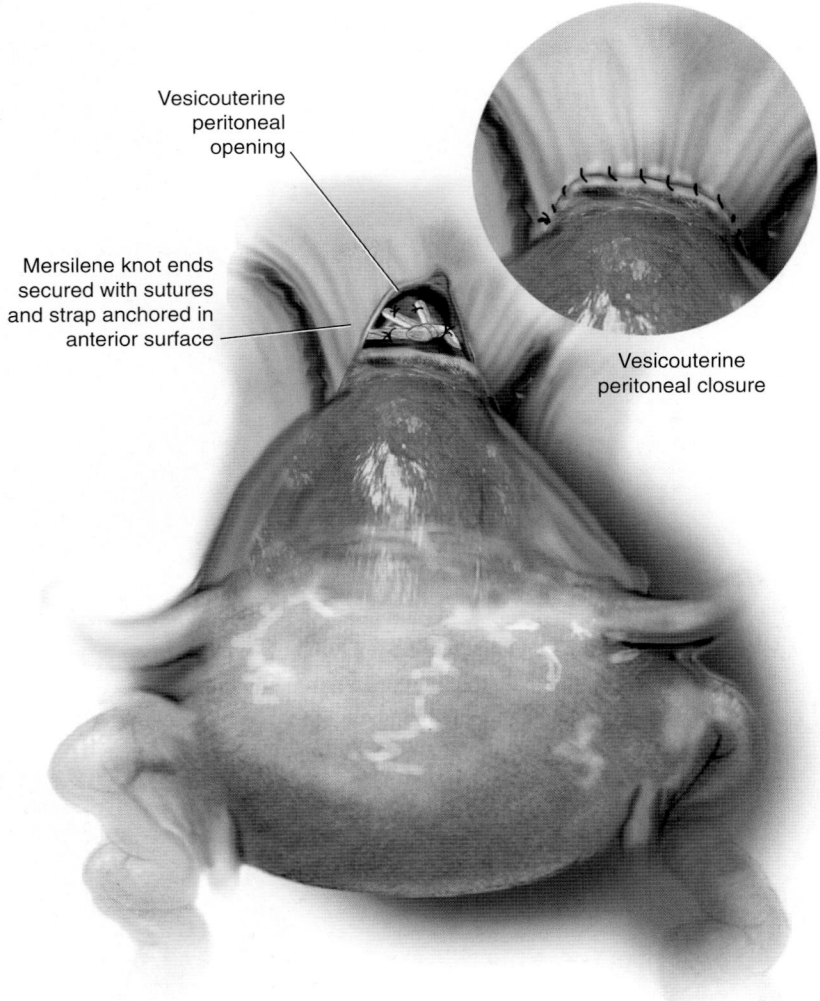

Vesicouterine
peritoneal
opening

Mersilene knot ends
secured with sutures
and strap anchored in
anterior surface

Vesicouterine
peritoneal closure

**FIGURE 17–4** The Mersilene is tied anteriorly and closes the cervix. The operator's finger in the cervix determines the tightness of the suture. The Mersilene is then suture-anchored with 3-0 Vicryl to the uterine wall to prevent slippage. The peritoneum is replaced between the bladder and the uterus and closed with a 3-0 running Vicryl stitch.

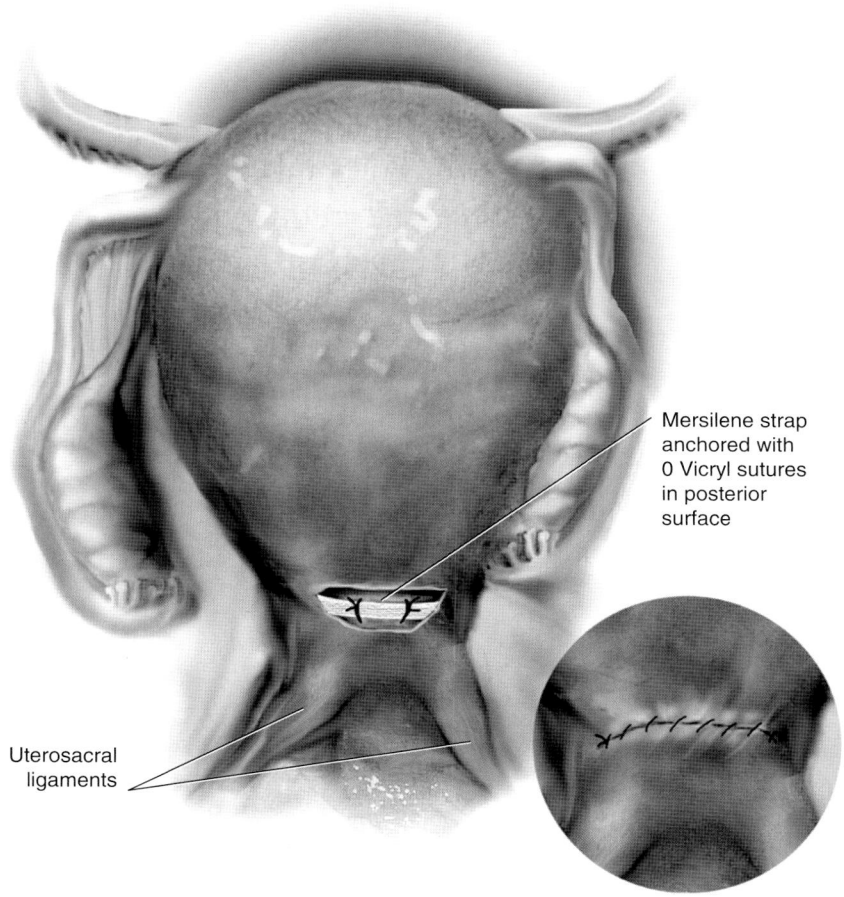

Mersilene strap
anchored with
0 Vicryl sutures
in posterior
surface

Uterosacral
ligaments

Rectouterine
peritoneal
closure

**FIGURE 17–5** The posterior portion of the strap is sutured to the uterine wall with 3-0 Vicryl and the rectouterine peritoneum is replaced. It is sutured closed with a running 3-0 Vicryl suture.

# CHAPTER 18

# Cesarean Section

## *Michael S. Baggish*

Cesarean section is one of the most commonly performed operations in the United States. A transverse or vertical entry laparotomy is performed. A transverse incision is selected more frequently (by a ratio of 10 to 1). The uterus may be left in situ within the abdominal cavity, or it may be exteriorized.

The technique of low transverse cesarean section is performed as follows. The bladder is emptied by the insertion of a Foley catheter. First, a bladder blade is inserted anteriorly (Fig. 18–1). The small and large intestines are packed away with moistened abdominal (laparotomy) pads, which should be carefully counted and tagged. The round ligaments should be identified so the degree and direction of uterine rotation can be determined. Identification of enlarged or aberrant vessels should be documented.

The reflection of peritoneum from the bladder dome to the uterus is grasped with a Kelly clamp (Fig. 18–2). The peritoneal reflection is elevated. With a Metzenbaum scissors, the bladder peritoneal reflection is sharply divided and is extended transversely for the length of the proposed uterine incision, typically 8 to 10 cm (Figs. 18–3 and 18–4). The bladder is gently pushed inferiorly away from the lower uterine segment. This not uncommonly results in small-vessel disruption and light bleeding (Fig. 18–5).

A trace incision is made into the uterus above the bladder reflection (Fig. 18–6). With the use of a scalpel, a deeper central cut, approximately 4 cm in length, is carried down to the amniotic sac, which bulges through the wound (Fig. 18–7A, B). Alternatively, the sharp incision is stopped just short of entry into the uterine cavity. At this point, the muscle may be spread with the surgeon's index fingers and the cavity entered bluntly (Fig. 18–8A, B).

In either case, once the bulging membranes have been identified, the incision may be extended to right and left by using scissors or by spreading with fingers (Fig. 18–9). The location of the uterine arteries should be ascertained to avoid inadvertent extension of the incision through them. The membranes are opened, and amniotic fluid is suctioned as it pours out into the wound.

The head of the infant (cephalic presentation) appears beneath the incision (Fig. 18–10). It is grasped beneath the chin and occiput and is gently delivered. It is rotated to facilitate delivery of the shoulders, and this is followed by delivery of the breech. The umbilical cord is clamped (doubly) and cut. The placenta is now seen in the depths of the wound (Fig. 18–11). It is separated and extracted. The uterine cavity is manually explored and clots are evacuated. The edges of the incision are grasped with Babcock clamps. A 10-mm Hegar dilator is passed through the cervix. Alternatively, a 36-French Pratt dilator may be passed through the cervix to facilitate lochial drainage. The incision is inspected for any extensions. The uterine vessels and bladder are checked for any injuries.

The incision is closed in layers. The deep muscle is approximated with interrupted figure-of-8 suture ligatures of 0 Vicryl (Figs. 18–12 and 18–13A). The superficial muscle and the uterine serosa are closed by a running 0 Vicryl (see Fig. 18–13A, **Inset,** and 18–13B). The bladder flap peritoneum is sutured over the incision with running 3-0 Vicryl or PDS suture.

The uterus is massaged and replaced into the abdominal cavity. Retractors and packs are removed and carefully counted to ensure that each and every implement has been accounted for.

A low vertical section may be performed by incising vertically through the lower uterine segment. Care must be taken to avoid extension of this incision into the bladder. The only advantage of this incision is that it permits further extension superiorly into the active portion of the uterus to gain greater space to manipulate the fetus (e.g., in the delivery of a transverse presentation).

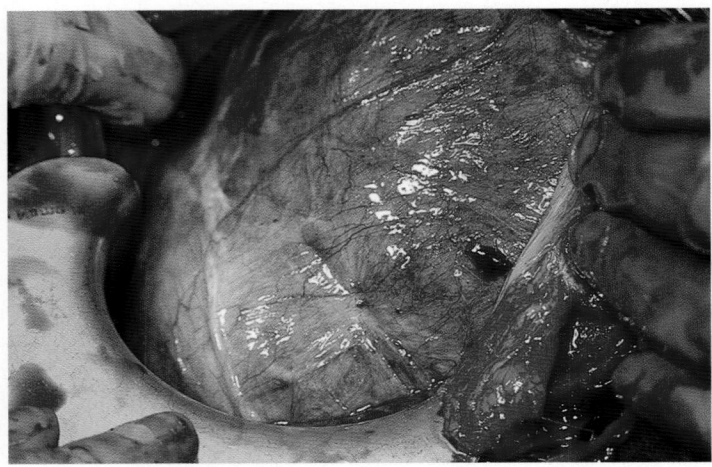

**FIGURE 18–1** Full-term pregnant uterus exposed and exteriorized. A bladder retractor is seen in the foreground. The edges of the entry incision are beneath the obstetrician's hands.

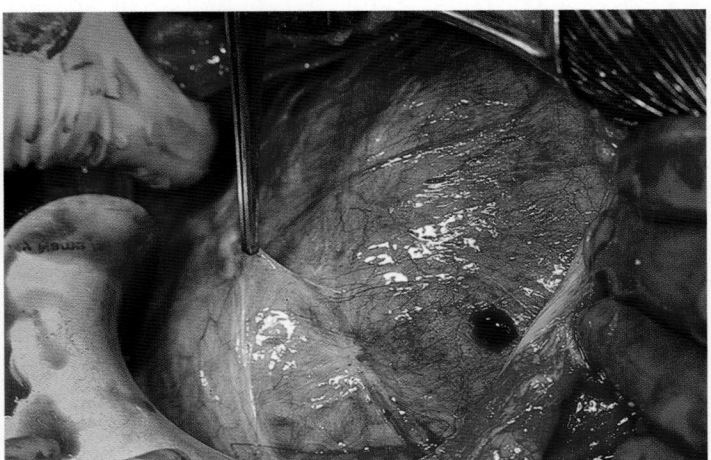

**FIGURE 18–2** The peritoneal reflection between the bladder and the uterus is elevated.

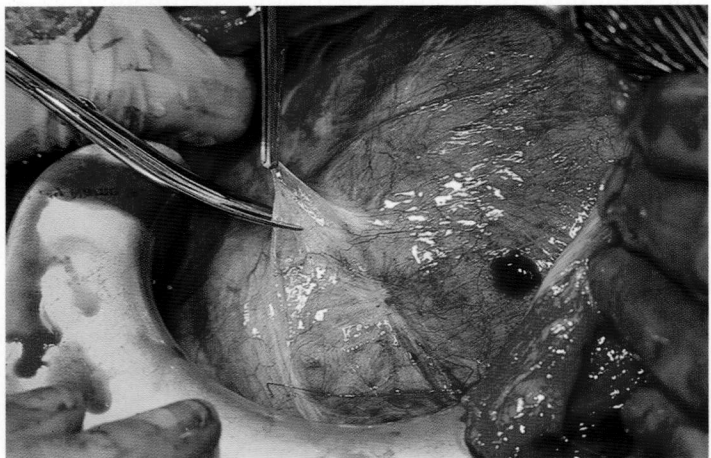

**FIGURE 18–3** The bladder peritoneum is incised sharply in an avascular plane. Vascularization of this peritoneum may be seen in cases of placenta previa or accreta.

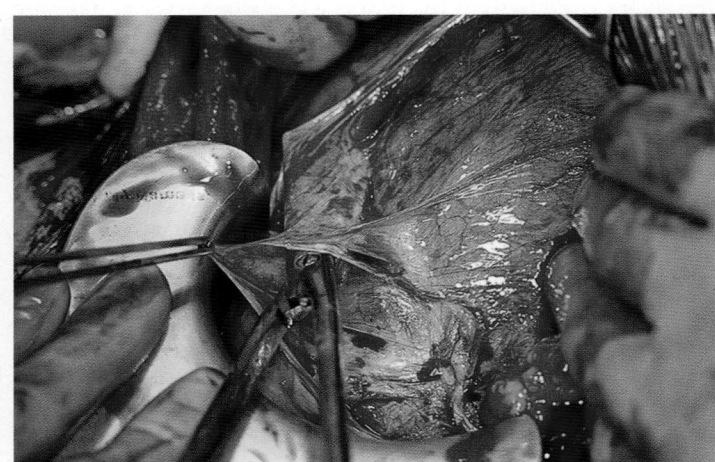

**FIGURE 18–4** The dissection is completed along the length of the anticipated deeper uterine incision.

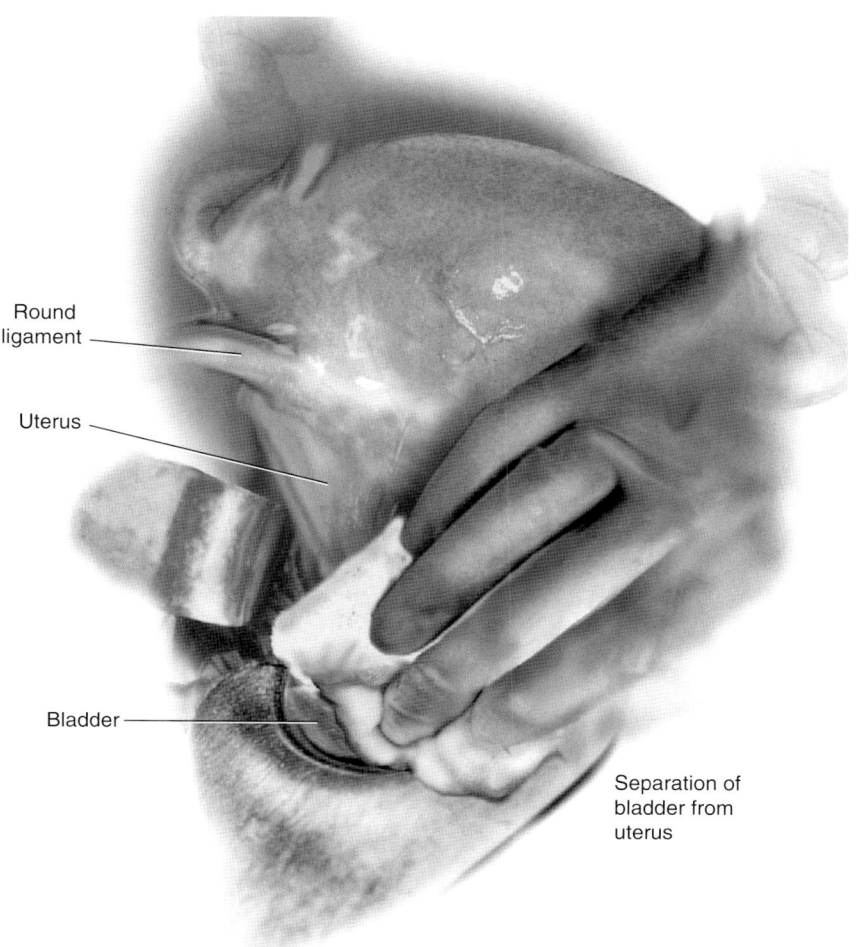

Round ligament

Uterus

Bladder

Separation of bladder from uterus

**FIGURE 18–5** The operator gently pushes the bladder inferiorly, detaching it from the lower uterine segment.

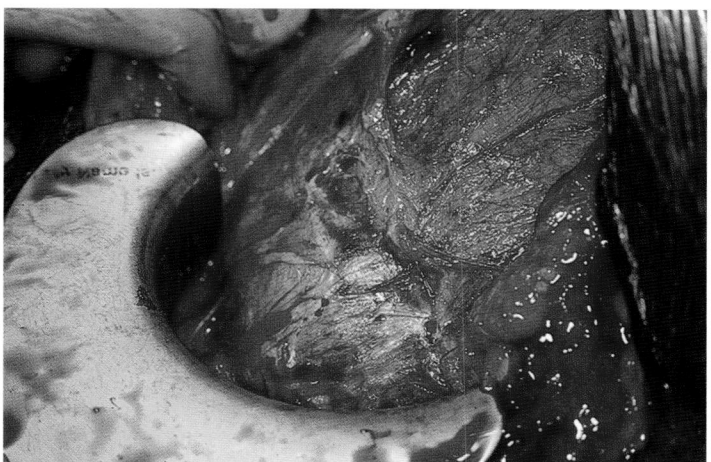

**FIGURE 18–6** The lower uterine segment is now exposed. The uterine arteries are palpated to determine the lateral extreme of the uterine incision.

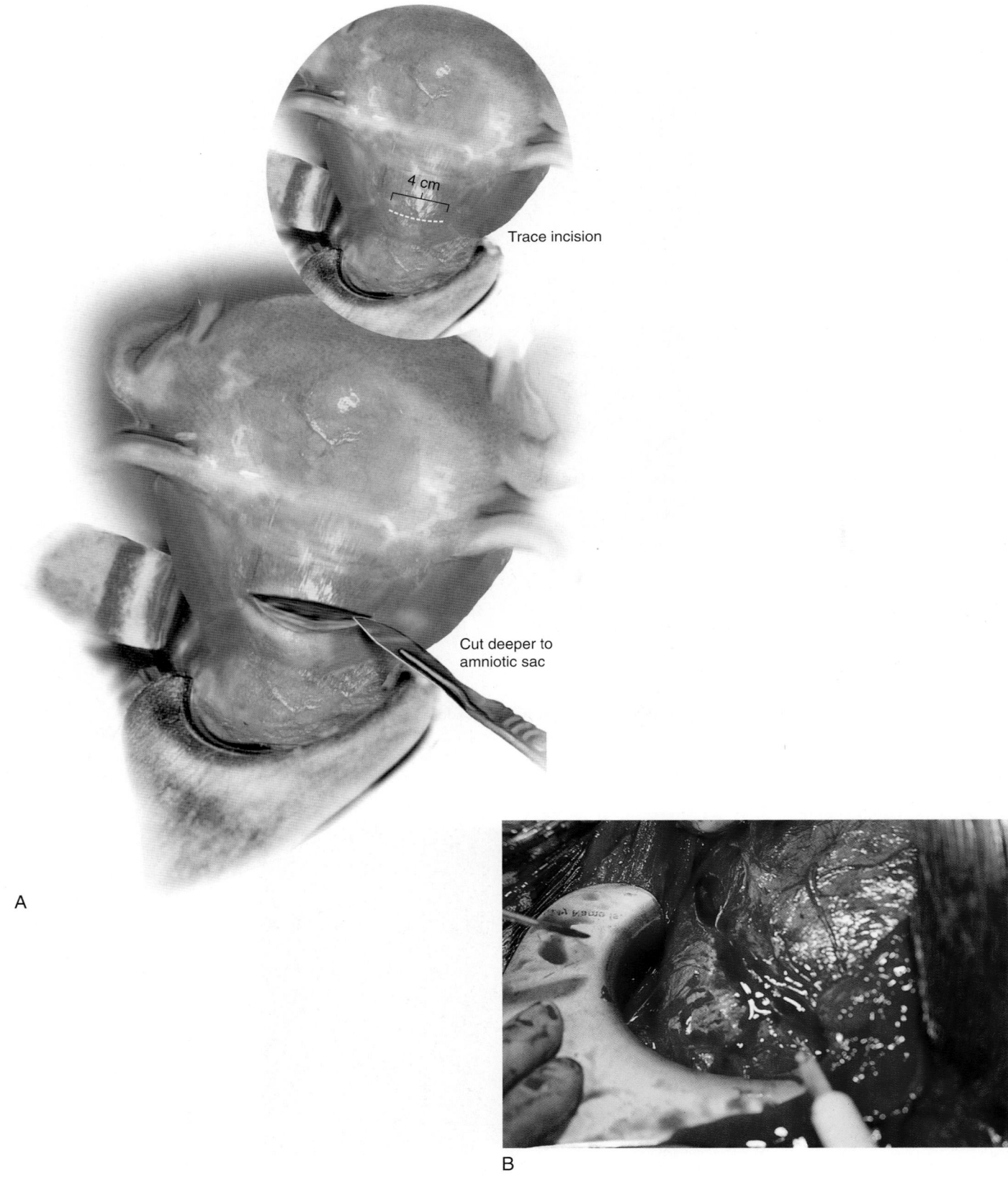

4 cm

Trace incision

Cut deeper to
amniotic sac

A

B

**FIGURE 18–7  A.** A small (3- to 4-cm) trace incision is made, then is extended deeper through the myometrium. **B.** At this point, bleeding is brisk, and suctioning is essential to detect when the uterine cavity has been entered.

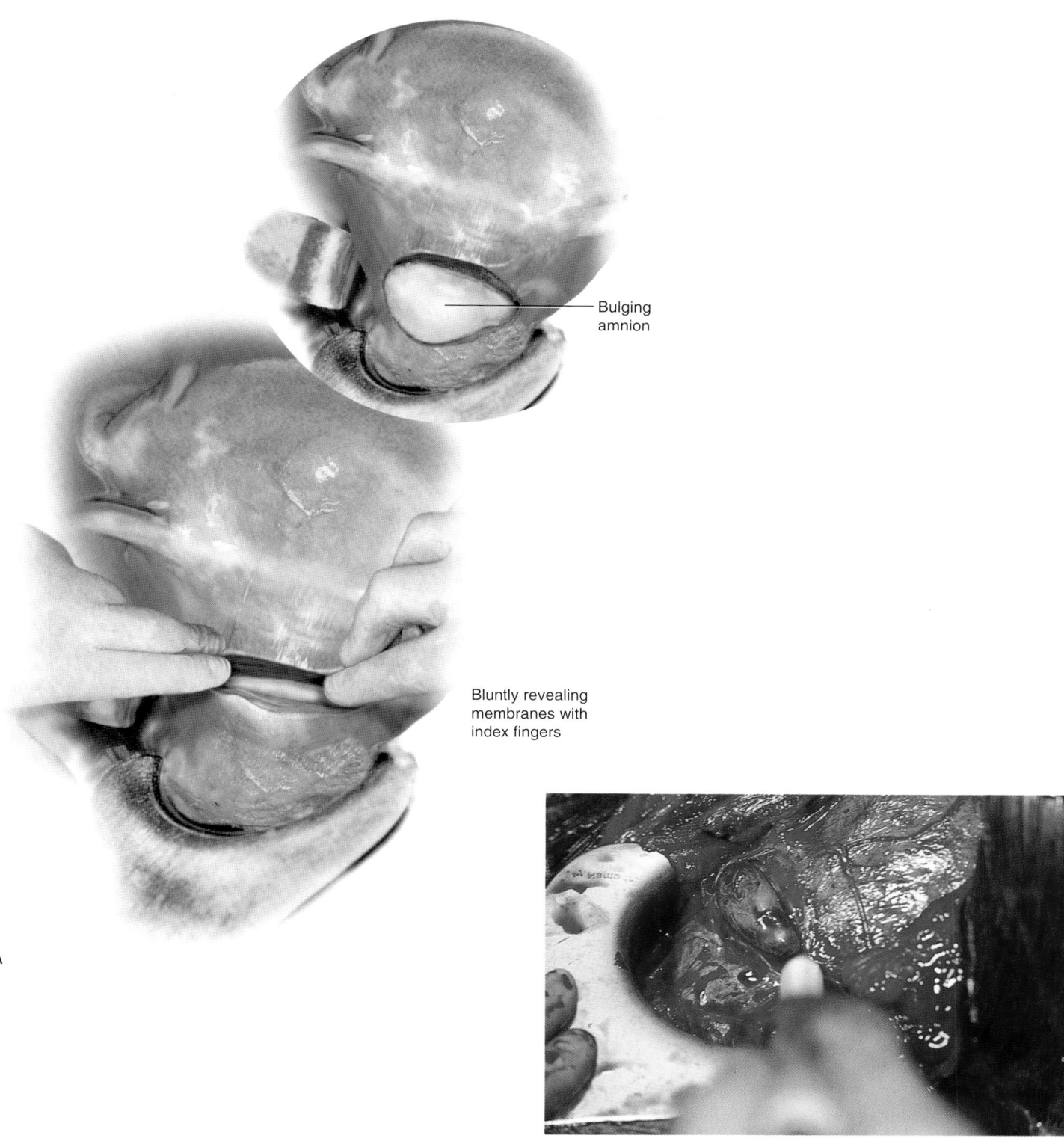

Bulging amnion

Bluntly revealing membranes with index fingers

A

B

**FIGURE 18–8  A.** Alternatively, the cavity may be entered bluntly by spreading the index fingers through the last thin layer of myometrium. **B.** The appearance of bulging membranes signals entry into the endometrial space.

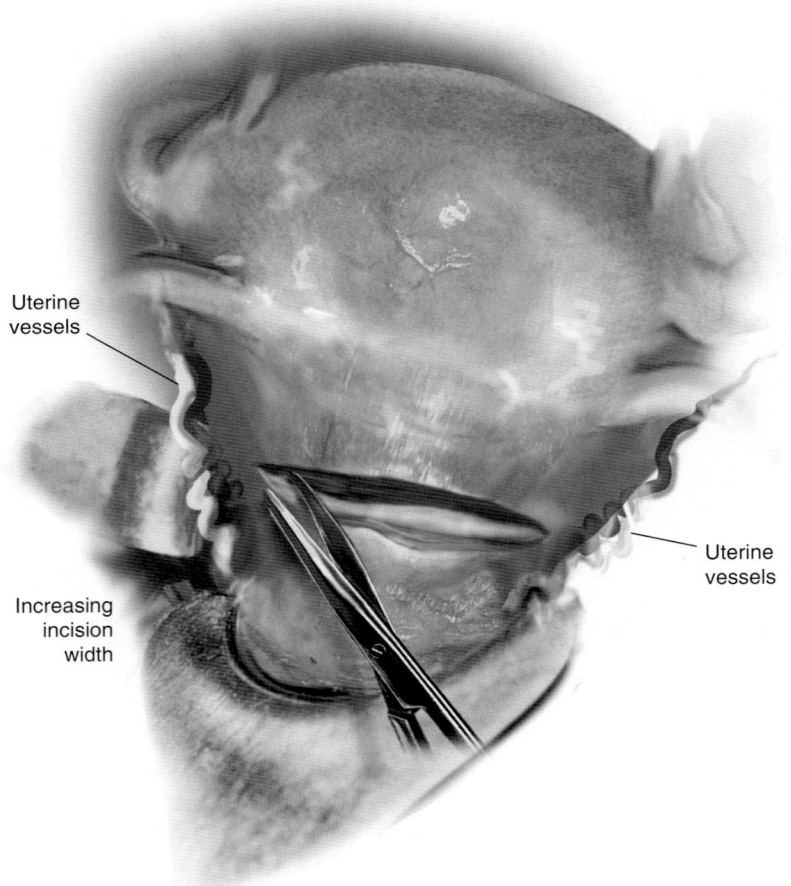

Uterine
vessels

Uterine
vessels

Increasing
incision
width

**FIGURE 18–9** With the membranes intact, the small entry incision may be widened laterally.

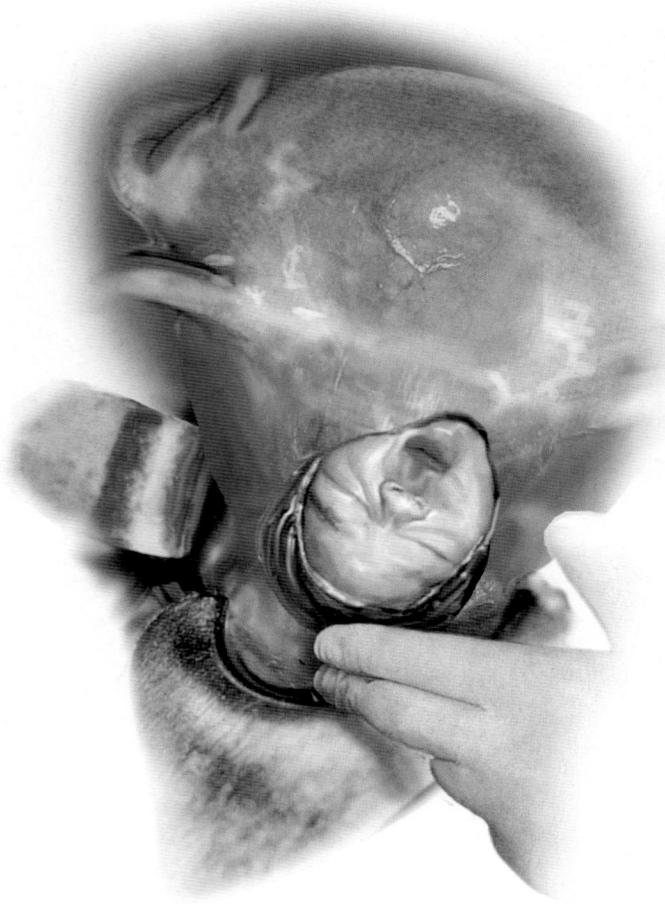

**FIGURE 18–10** The membranes are now ruptured and widely opened. The infant's head comes into view, and delivery is implemented.

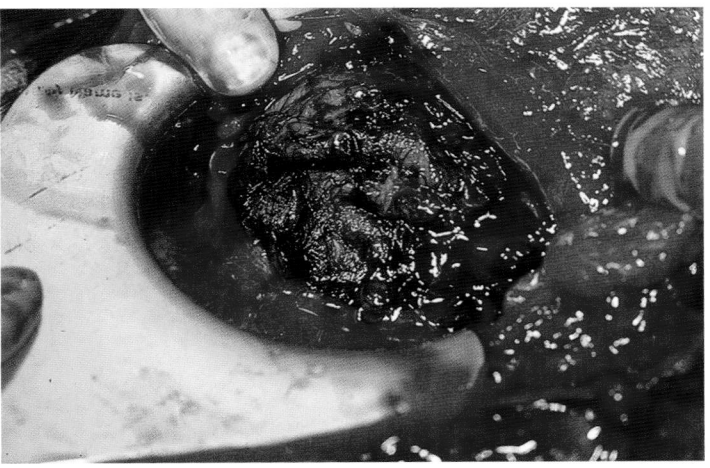

FIGURE 18–11 The placental location is observed and recorded. Next, the placenta is manually removed. The uterine cavity is explored and cleared of any adherent membranes.

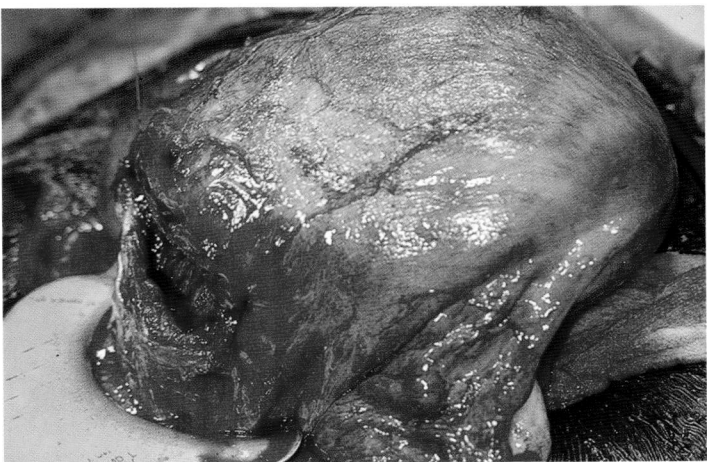

FIGURE 18–12 The deeper muscle is closed with interrupted 0 Vicryl figure-of-8 sutures.

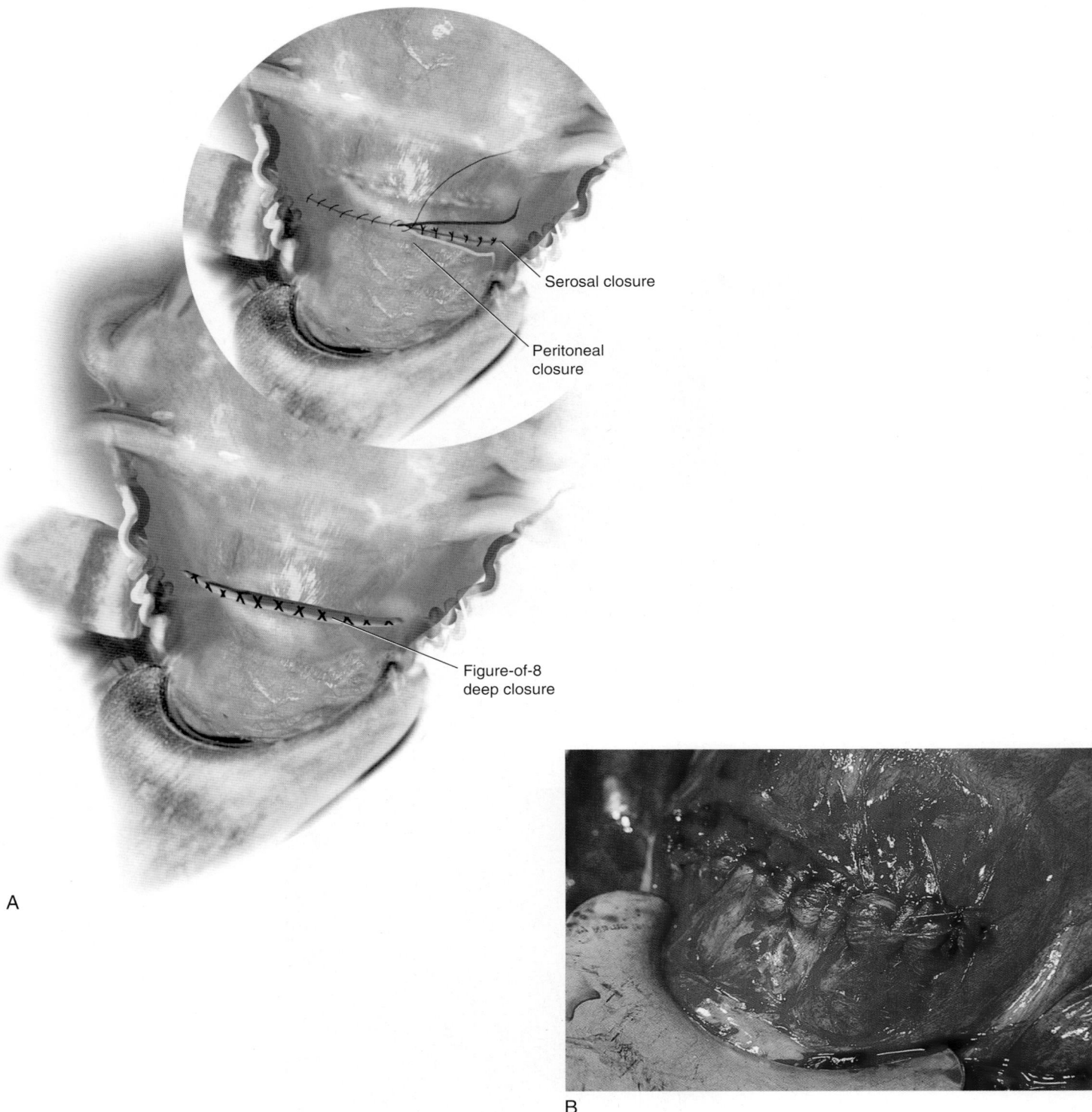

Serosal closure

Peritoneal closure

Figure-of-8 deep closure

A

B

**FIGURE 18–13  A.** The superficial muscle and uterine serosa are closed with running or running lock sutures of 0 Vicryl. **B.** After the serosa is closed, the bladder peritoneum is sutured to the uterus at the upper margin of the incision.

# CHAPTER 19

# Cesarean Section Hysterectomy

*Michael S. Baggish*

The distinguishing features of an abdominal hysterectomy performed on a pregnant patient, whether associated with cesarean section or performed after a vaginal delivery, are (1) the greater vascularity compared with the nonpregnant patient, (2) the close association of a dilated cervix and vagina with the greatly distended ureters, and (3) a tendency for the postpartum patient to form blood clots. Most hysterectomies in this setting are performed as an emergency operation, typically to treat bleeding difficulties (Figs. 19–1A–C).

The ureters must be identified on the right and left sides of the pelvis. They are best located as they cross the common iliac vessels and descend into the pelvis. The best operation to perform under these circumstances is a subtotal hysterectomy (Fig. 19–2). The cervix can be removed months or years later, via the vaginal or the abdominal route, if necessary. The subtotal hysterectomy is least likely to result in ureteral injury and is completed most rapidly.

First, if a cesarean section has been performed, the uterus is closed with a running lock stitch of 0 Vicryl. Next, the round ligaments are clamped, sutured, and cut close to the uterus. Then, if the ovaries are to be retained, the utero-ovarian ligaments and oviducts are triply clamped, cut, and suture-ligated with 0 Vicryl.

The ureters must be dissected and traced under *direct* vision inferiorly to the level of the uterine arteries.

The bladder peritoneum has already been pushed inferiorly as part of the cesarean section. The uterine vessels are skeletonized. Three clamps (Zeppelin) are placed on the uterine arteries at the cervicouterine junction and above the cardinal and uterosacral ligaments (Fig. 19–3). The fundus is then sharply cut away from the cervix (see Fig. 19–3, **Inset**). The cervical stump is closed with figure-of-8 sutures using 0 Vicryl. The uterine vessels are doubly secured with 0 Vicryl transfixing sutures. The peritoneum is closed with a running 3-0 Vicryl continuous suture. No suspension is required because the major supporting ligaments have been left intact (Fig. 19–4).

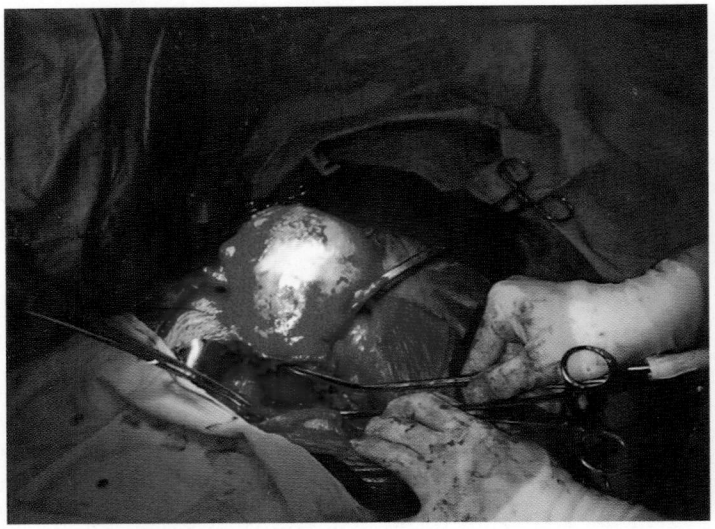

A

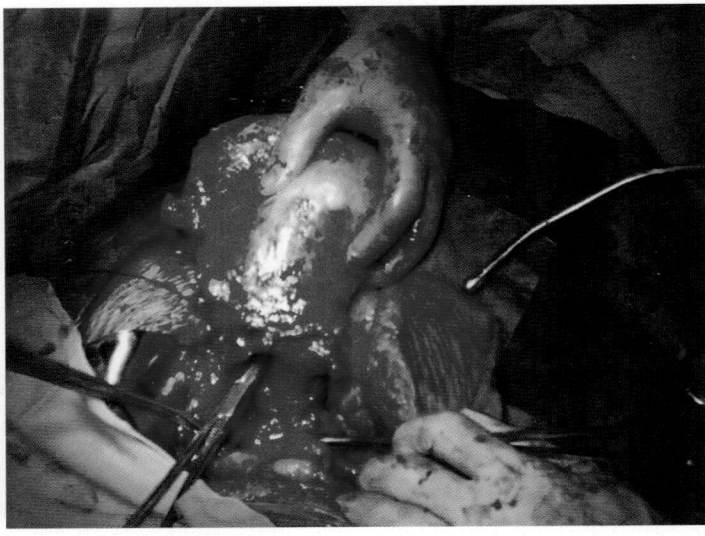

B

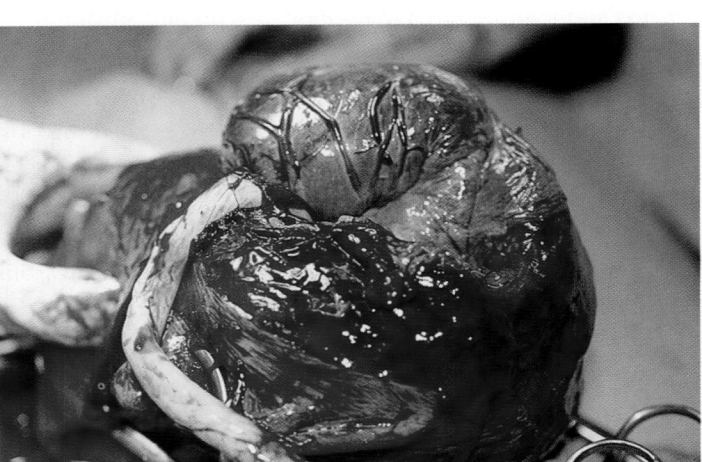

C

**FIGURE 19–1 A.** This uterus ruptured at the site of a previous transverse cesarean section scar. **B.** Enlarged view of the lower segment rupture. Note that the Kelly clamp points to the site of the rupture. **C.** The uterus has been opened somewhat irregularly because of a rupture. The placenta is being delivered before hysterectomy is performed.

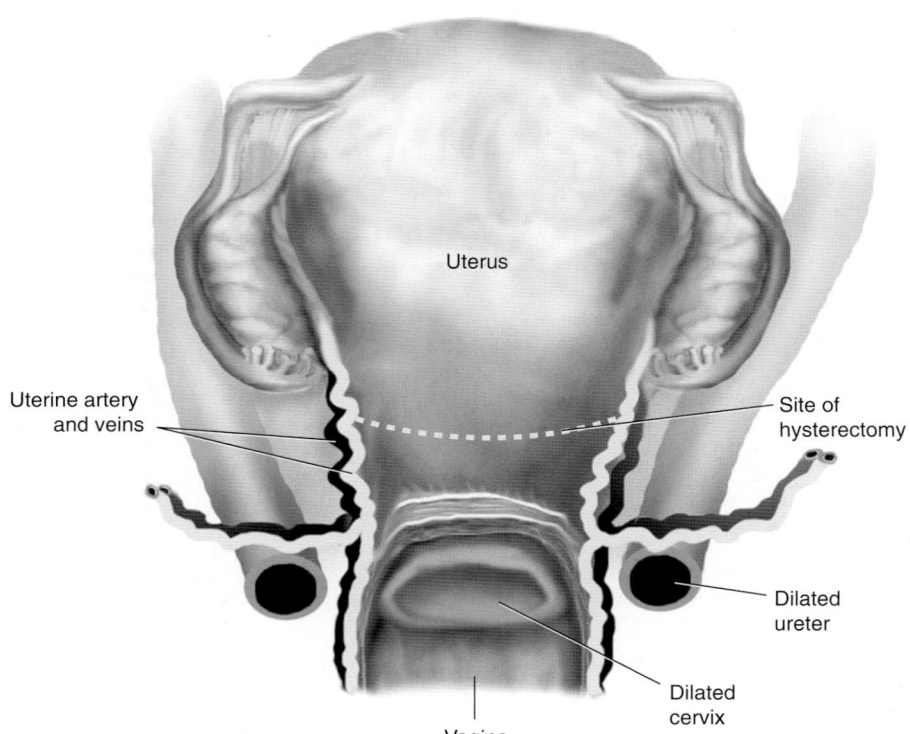

Uterus

Uterine artery and veins

Site of hysterectomy

Dilated ureter

Dilated cervix

Vagina

**FIGURE 19–2** Anterior view of the uterus. Note the positions of the greatly dilated ureters and their close proximity to the dilated cervix. A trace has been placed indicating the site for subtotal hysterectomy.

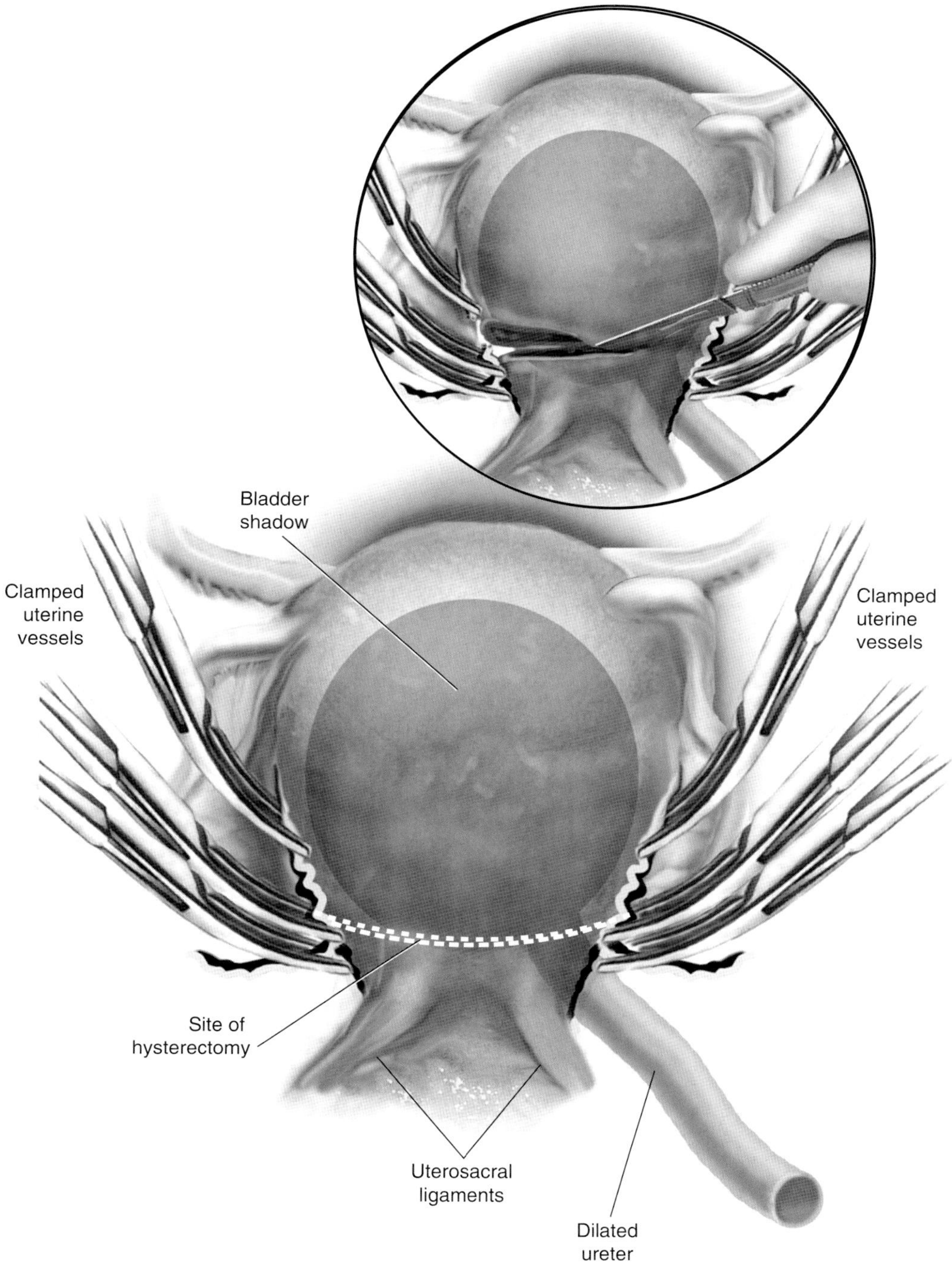

Bladder
shadow

Clamped
uterine
vessels

Clamped
uterine
vessels

Site of
hysterectomy

Uterosacral
ligaments

Dilated
ureter

**FIGURE 19–3** Posterior view of the uterus. The uterine arteries have been doubly clamped, and the third clamp is placed on the uterine vessels higher up to control back-bleeding. **Inset,** A scalpel cuts the uterus, separating the corpus from the cervix. The line of incision is between the upper clamp and the lower two clamps.

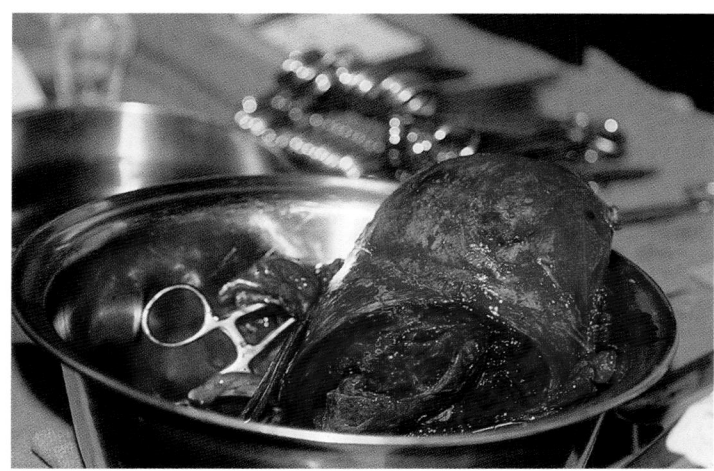

**FIGURE 19–4** The operation is quickly completed and the specimen is removed from the operative field.

# CHAPTER 20

# Hypogastric Artery Ligation

*Michael S. Baggish*

This operation is usually performed as an emergency procedure for postpartum hemorrhage in lieu of hysterectomy. It also may be performed for nonobstetric uncontrolled bleeding (e.g., post-irradiation hemorrhage, vaginal laceration bleeding, cervical bleeding, posthysterectomy bleeding). Hypogastric ligation affects clotting by reducing ipsilateral pulse pressure (85% decrease) and blood flow (50% decrease).

The operation requires a laparotomy. The retroperitoneum is entered by opening the peritoneum above the external iliac artery over the psoas major muscle (Fig. 20–1). The external iliac artery and vein are exposed in the direction of the bifurcation of the common iliac artery (Fig. 20–2). As the dissection proceeds cranially, the ovarian vessels and the ureter are encountered as they cross the common iliac artery (Fig. 20–3). The external iliac artery is retracted with a vein retractor to expose the hypogastric artery (Fig. 20–4). A long right-angle clamp is used to carefully dissect a plane between the common hypogastric artery and its underlying vein (Fig. 20–5). Injury to the hypogastric vein(s) must be avoided at all costs because these large veins, deeply located in the pelvis, are exceedingly difficult to suture. By spreading and closing the clamp, the dissection can be quickly completed. A ligature of 0 Vicryl is passed through the tip of the right-angle clamp and pulled under the hypogastric artery (Fig. 20–6). The ureter is reidentified and observed not to be caught in the ligature. The ligature is then tied with three or four throws and cut (Figs. 20–7 and 20–8). The common and external iliac arteries are rechecked to ensure that only the correct vessel (i.e., the hypogastric artery) has been tied off. Additionally, it is advisable to examine the integrity of the hypogastric vein (Fig. 20–9). The peritoneum is closed with a 3-0 Vicryl running stitch. The procedure is repeated on the contralateral side.

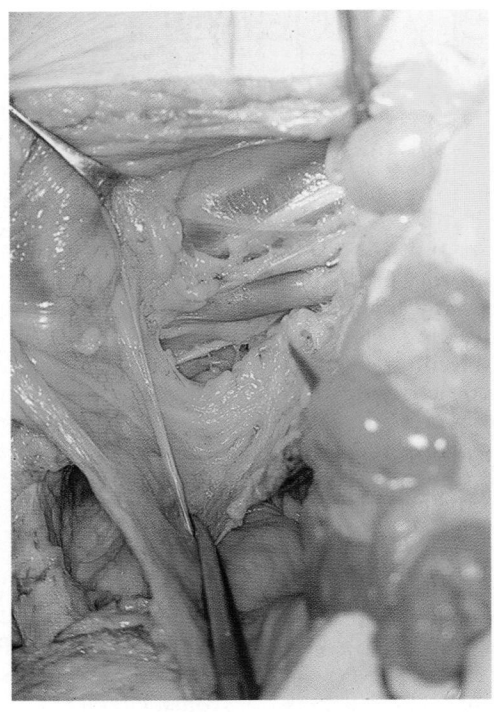

**FIGURE 20–1** The peritoneum overlying the external iliac artery and the psoas major muscle has been opened, exposing the external iliac artery and vein.

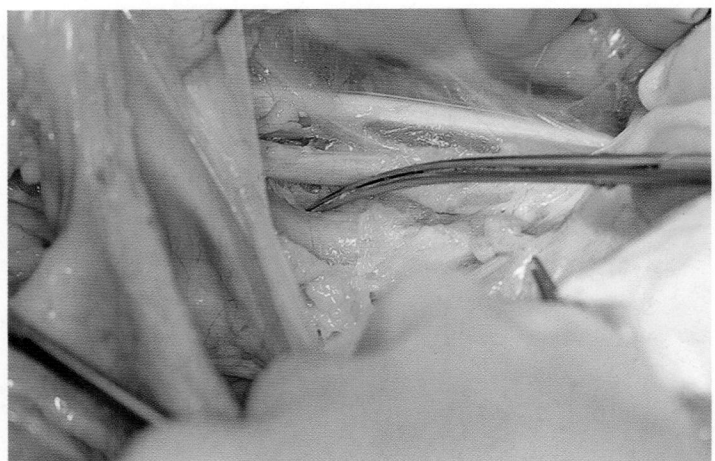

**FIGURE 20–2** The scissors are resting on the right external iliac vein.

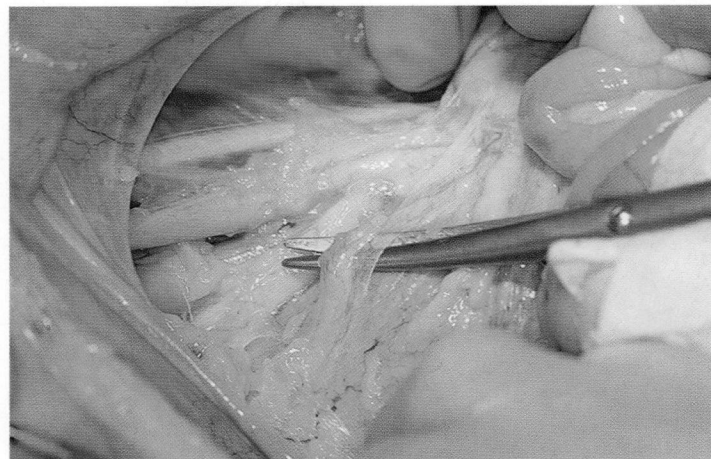

**FIGURE 20–3** The right ureter is identified as it crosses over the pelvic brim and the right common iliac artery.

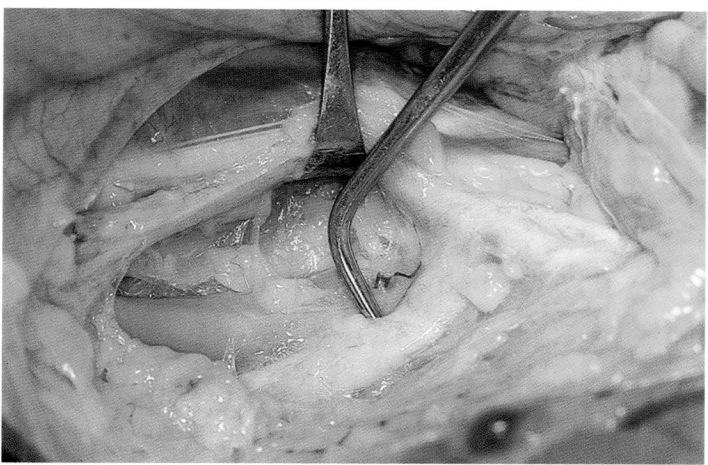

**FIGURE 20–4** Dissection is begun between the right hypogastric artery and vein with the use of a right-angle clamp. Care must be taken not to injure the underlying hypogastric vein.

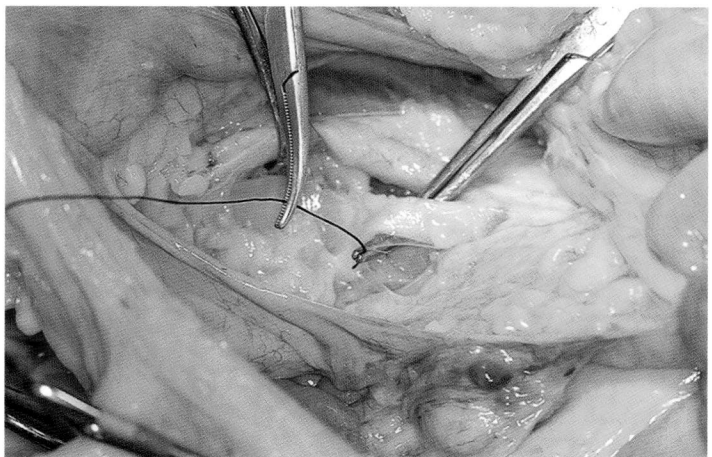

**FIGURE 20–5** The clamp has created a plane between the hypogastric artery and vein. A ligature of 0 Vicryl is passed to the tip of the right-angle clamp.

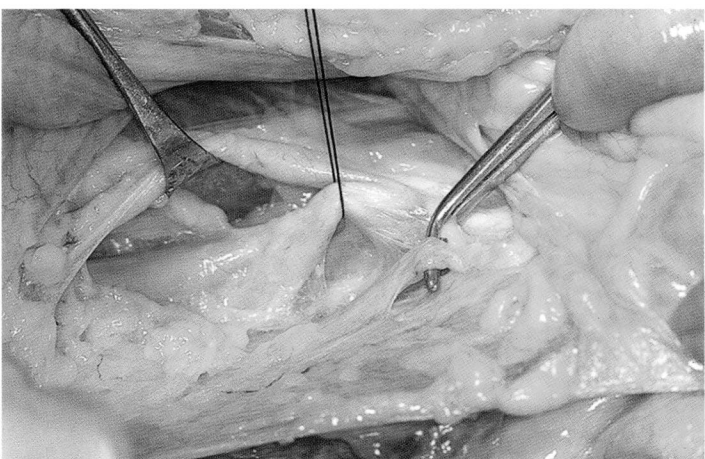

**FIGURE 20–6** The ligature has been completely passed beneath the common hypogastric artery. The ends of the ligature have been grasped and traction applied to gently elevate the vessel. The right ureter is reidentified.

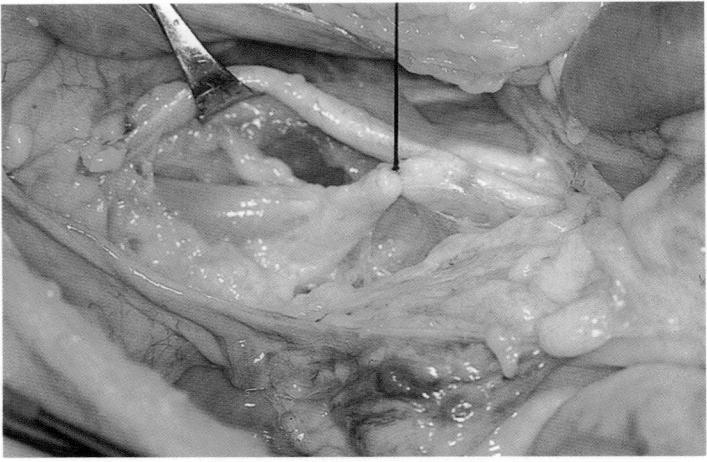

**FIGURE 20–7** The ligature is secured with three throws. Each throw is tied down squarely. The external iliac artery is retracted with a vein retractor.

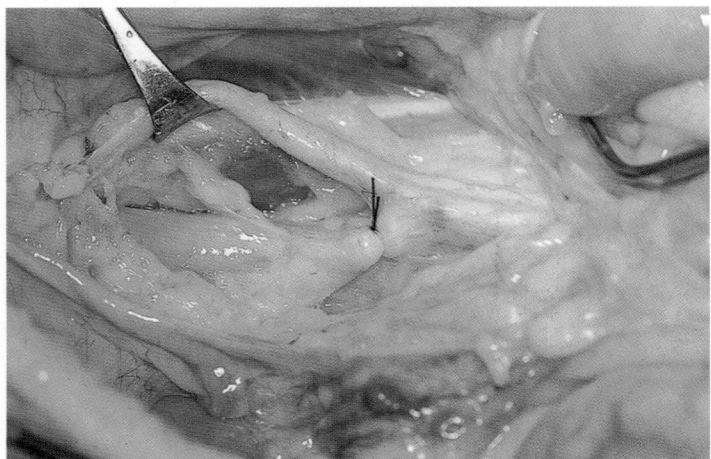

**FIGURE 20–8** The ligature is cut.

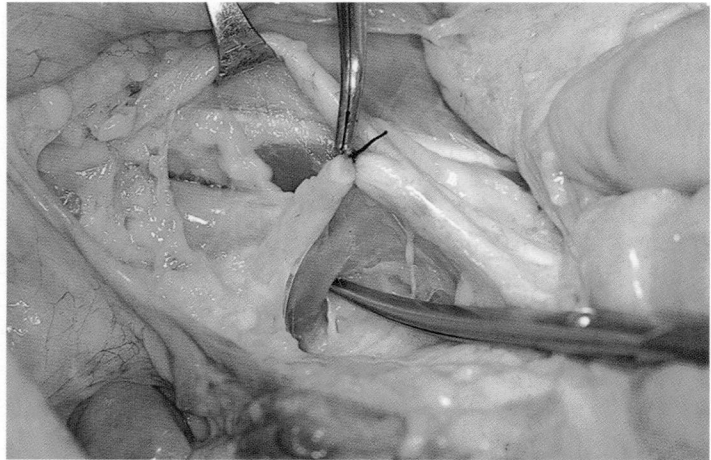

**FIGURE 20–9** A final inspection is carried out to ensure that the common and external iliac arteries were not inadvertently ligated. Similarly (tip of scissors), the hypogastric vein is checked to ensure that it is intact.

# CHAPTER 21

# Trophoblastic Disease

*Michael S. Baggish*

Understanding the process of normal implantation and the development of villi together with the role played by the trophoblast is essential for similarly comprehending aberrations caused by abnormal trophoblastic generation (Figs. 21–1 through 21–3). Anatomic, microanatomic, and physiologic changes create a spectrum of disorders referred to as trophoblastic disease.

Trophoblastic disorders may be divided into benign and malignant categories (Table 21–1). In developed countries (e.g., North America, United Kingdom, Western Europe), the incidence of hydatidiform mole is 1:1000 pregnancies, and choriocarcinoma is seen in 1 in 30,000 pregnancies. In the Far East, the number of molar pregnancies is 3 to 10 times greater, and the risk for choriocarcinoma is 10 to 60 times greater. Moles are subdivided into complete or partial. Complete moles are characterized by extreme villous swelling (hydropic change),

trophoblastic hyperplasia, and paucity of fetal blood vascular channels (Figs. 21–3 through 21–6). Complete moles result from a single 23 X sperm fertilizing a defective ovum that contains no maternal genes. As a result of subsequent endoreduplication, the mole contains 46 XX chromosomes. In the case of partial mole, two sperms fertilize an egg with 23 X chromosomes, creating a triploid mole containing 69 XXX chromosomes (Fig. 21–7).

Diagnosis is considered by a high index of suspicion based on clinical signs and symptoms of vaginal bleeding, hyperemesis, excess uterine size for gestational age, early-onset preeclampsia, hyperthyroidism, and intrauterine infection. The diagnosis is confirmed by viewing a passed molar vesicle, by pelvic ultrasound, by obtaining serial rising levels of serum and urine human chorionic gonadotropin (hCG), and by the presence of theca-lutein cysts (Fig. 21–8).

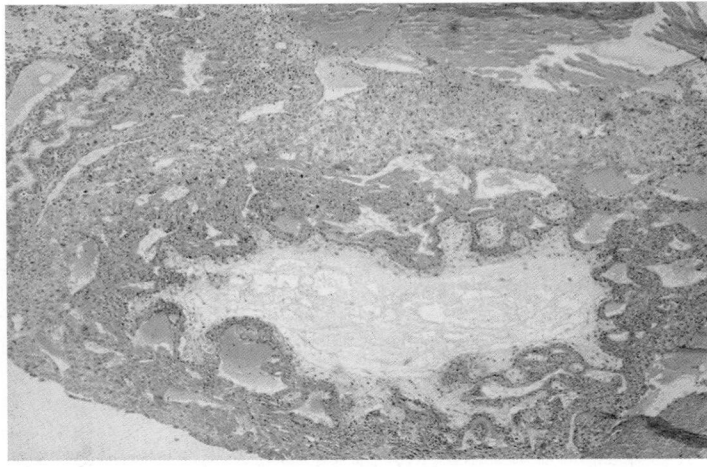

**FIGURE 21–1** Early implantation site. The deeper pink tissue is trophoblast, which is invading the decidua (*light pink*). Note the endometrial gland to the far left.

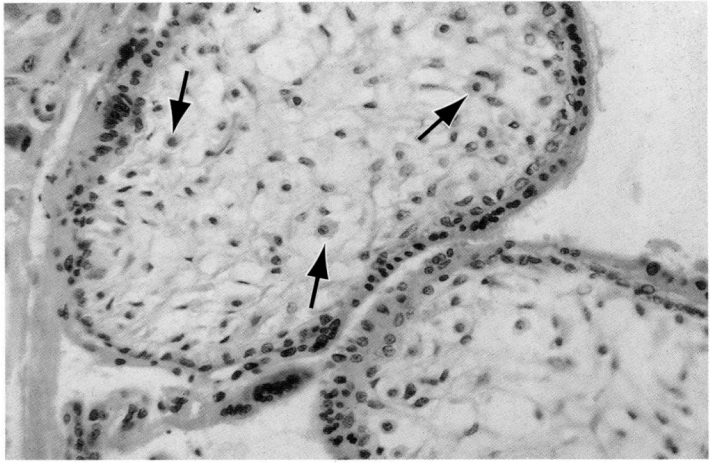

A

**FIGURE 21–2 A.** Immature villi have two layers of trophoblast surrounding the villous connective tissue core. The outer, deep pink layer is syncytiotrophoblast, whereas the inner layer is cytotrophoblast. Note the open villous vascular channels and the Hofbauer cells (*arrows*).

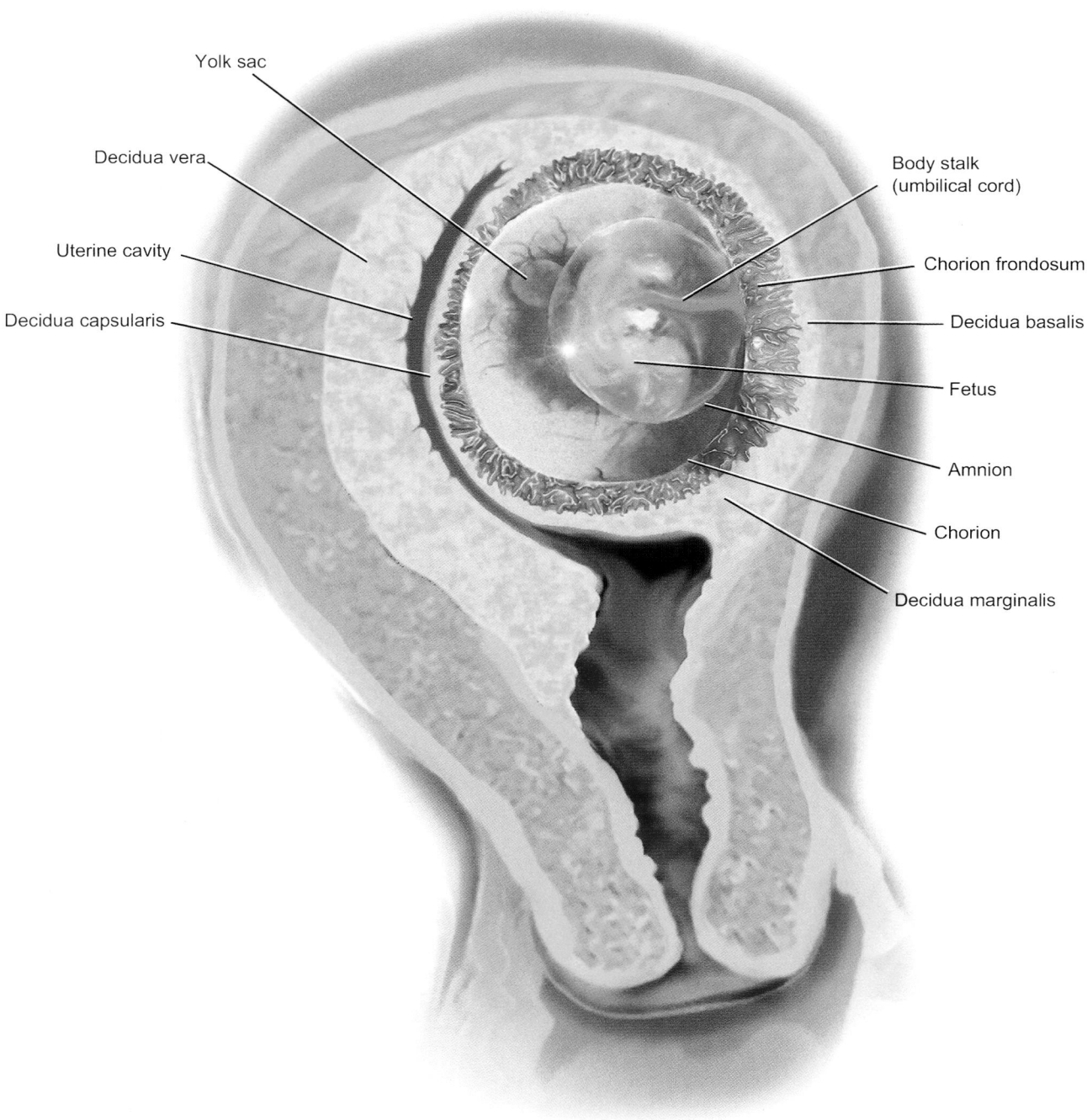

B

**FIGURE 21–2, cont'd  B.** Trophoblastic cells make up the chorion and the villi, that is, the major part of the placenta. In this picture, the chorionic tissues are shown encapsulating the developing embryo and amnion. Major invasion and development of villi occur at the decidua basalis. The peripheral chorion frondosum will atrophy to form the bald chorion (chorion laeve).

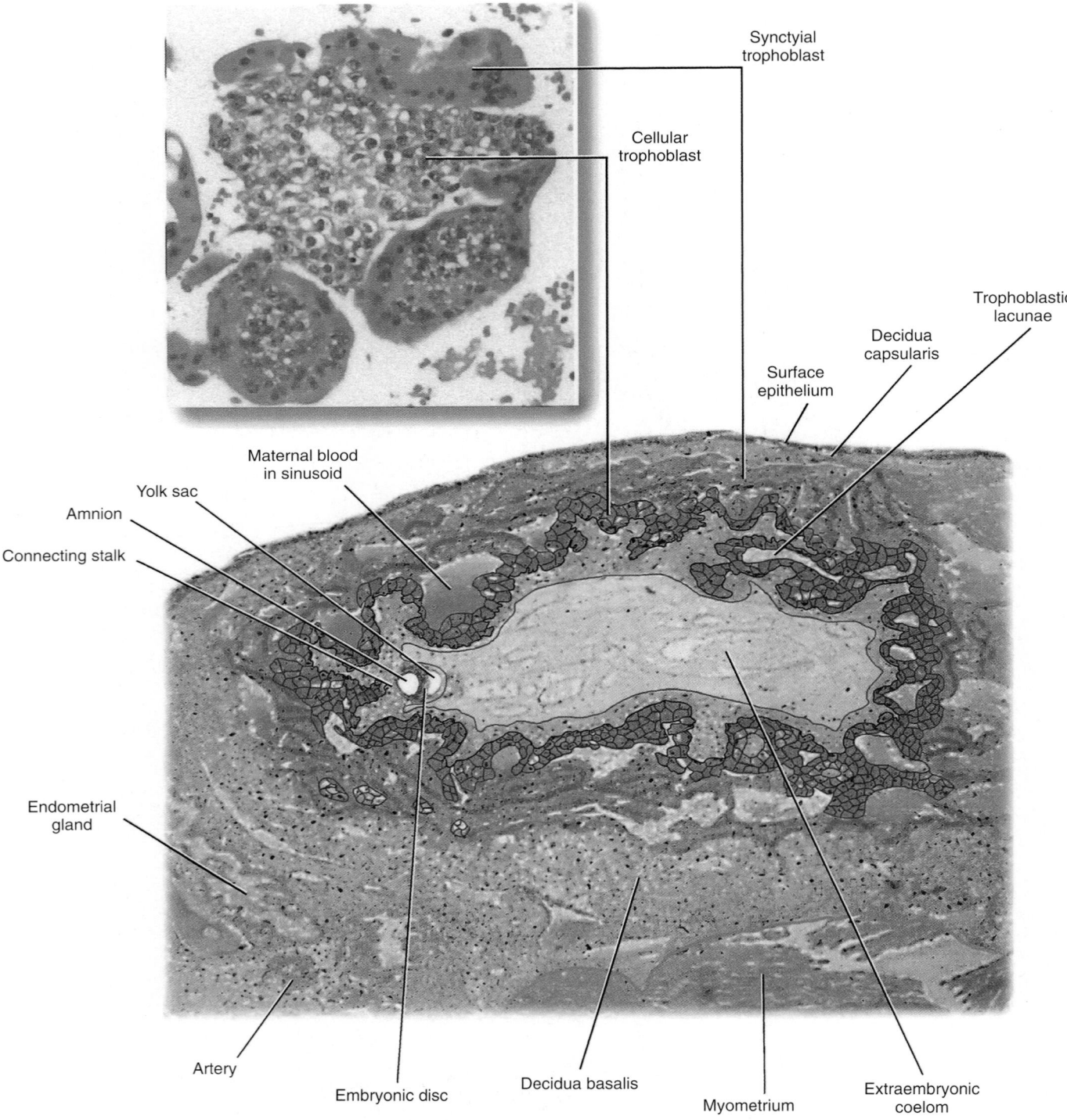

Synctyial
trophoblast

Cellular
trophoblast

Trophoblastic
lacunae

Decidua
capsularis

Surface
epithelium

Maternal blood
in sinusoid

Yolk sac

Amnion

Connecting stalk

Endometrial
gland

Artery

Embryonic disc

Decidua basalis

Myometrium

Extraembryonic
coelom

C

**FIGURE 21–2, cont'd  C.** Physiologic trophoblast exhibits many of the characteristics of the premalignant and the malignant trophoblast. In this illustration, a trophoblast is shown to invade the maternal endometrium, open up maternal blood sinuses, create vacuoles, form blood lakes, and form primitive villi. The **inset** shows cores of cytotrophoblast being surrounded by syncytiotrophoblast. Strikingly normal trophoblast does not destroy the maternal tissues during the invasive process, whereas malignant trophoblast creates widespread necrosis.

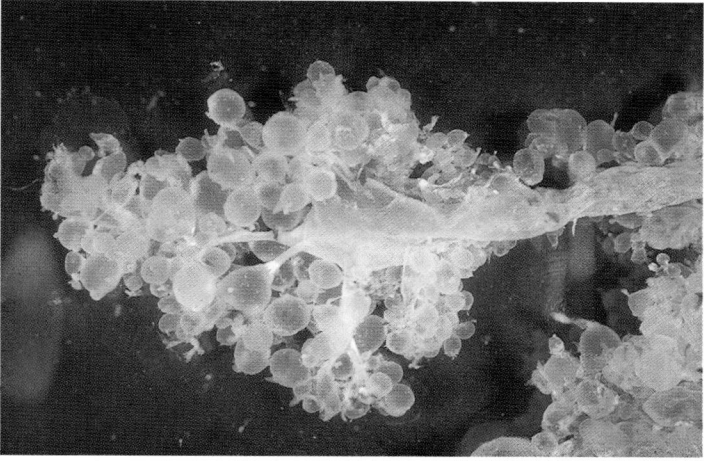

**FIGURE 21–3** Well-developed, magnified view of a complete hydatidiform mole. The molar vesicles are fluid-filled distended villi. They can break off the main stem and be passed to the outside via the vagina, in which case the diagnosis of mole can be made with certainty. In the case of hydatidiform mole, no amnion is formed; therefore, direct entry and egress between the vagina and the uterine cavity exist.

**TABLE 21–1 ■ Classification of Trophoblastic Disorders**

| Benign | Malignant |
|---|---|
| Complete hydatidiform mole | Invasive mole |
| Partial hydatidiform mole | Choriocarcinoma |
| | Placental site trophoblastic tumor |

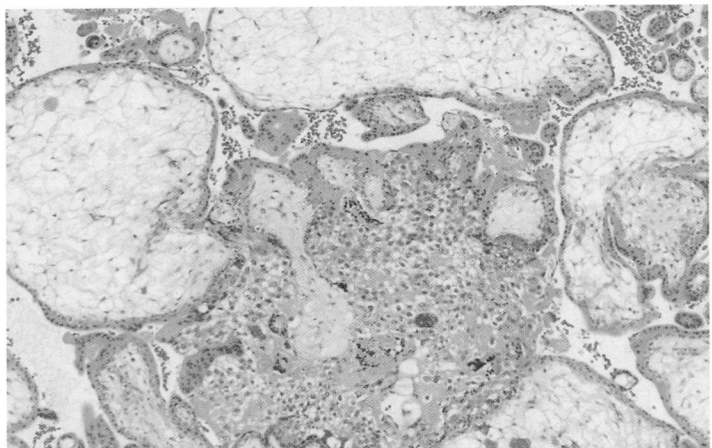

**FIGURE 21–4** Low-power view of distended, hydropic villi clustered around masses of trophoblastic cells.

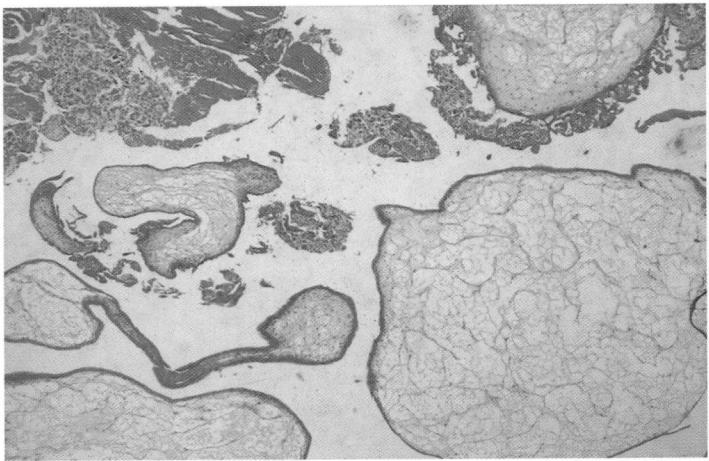

**FIGURE 21–5** Higher-power photomicrograph shows hydropic villi, absence of fetal vessels, and trophoblastic hyperplasia—three elements necessary to diagnose hydatidiform mole.

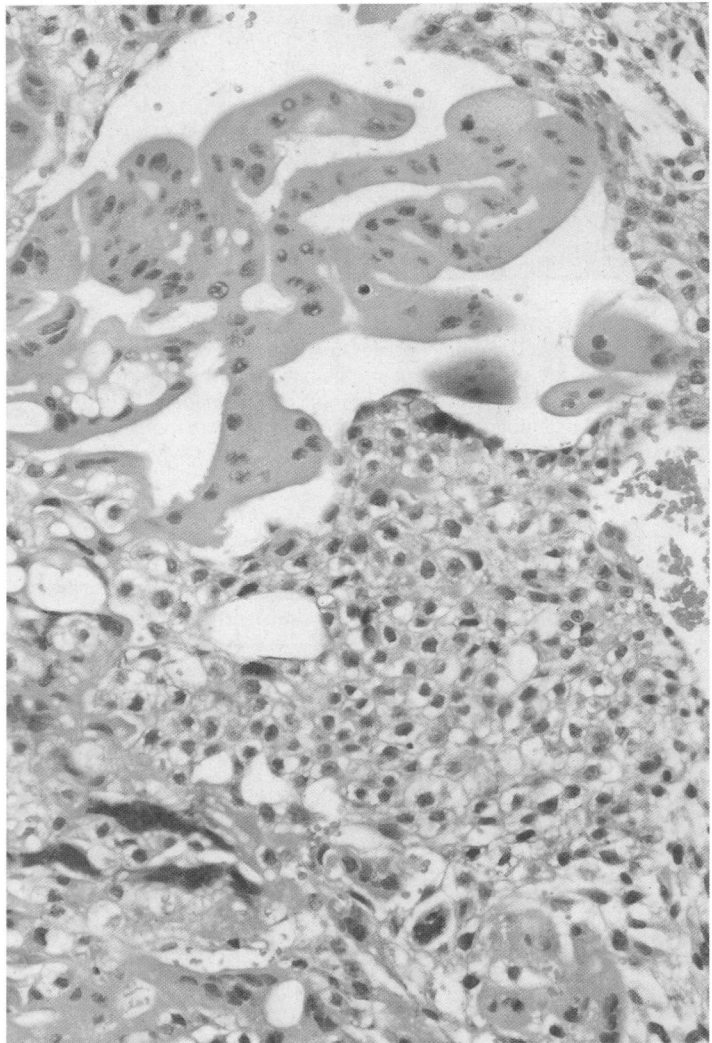

**FIGURE 21–6** High-powered view of trophoblast shown in Figure 21–4. Note the proliferation of the cytotrophoblast that represents the immature, dividing trophoblast cells. Cytotrophoblasts are small cells with well-developed cell membranes. Syncytiotrophoblasts are mature cells comprising a number of cytotrophoblast cells melding to form the multinucleate syncytium. Note that individual cell membranes have been lost. Vacuole formation is commonly seen with trophoblastic proliferation and harkens back to a property of the primitive trophoblastic cells observed during normal implantation.

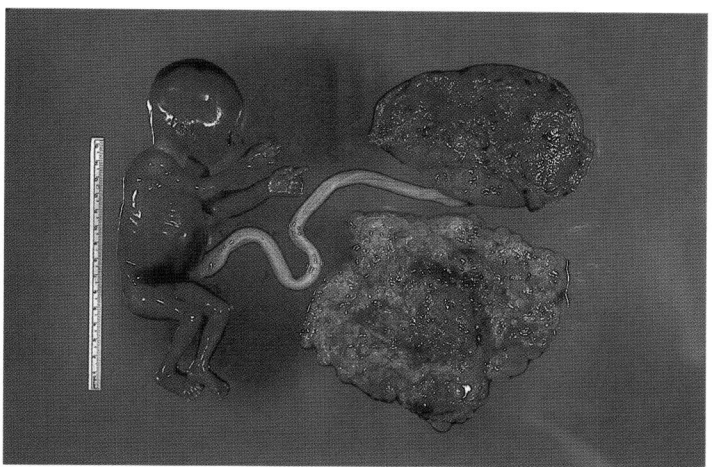

**FIGURE 21–7** The rare occurrence of a twin gestation is shown, in which one entity is a mole and the other a relatively normally developed fetus.

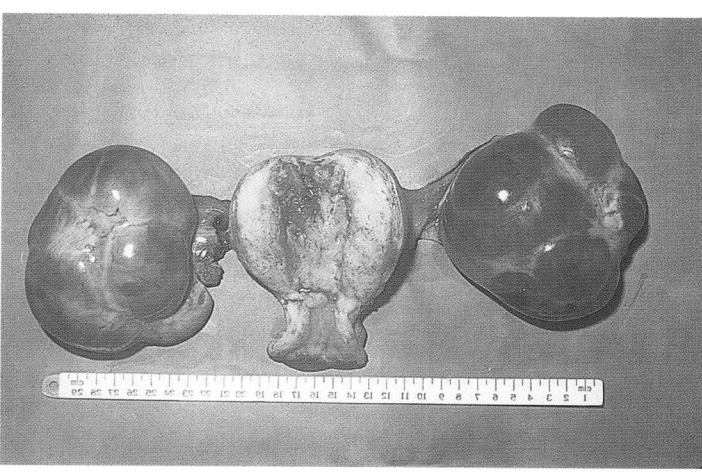

**FIGURE 21–8** Theca-lutein cysts are associated with all forms of trophoblastic disease. The theca cells of the ovarian cortex grow in response to chorionic gonadotropin, which is elaborated by both types of trophoblastic cells.

When the diagnosis has been made and confirmed, a plan should be made to evacuate the mole in a timely fashion. Hysterectomy with the mole in situ has a definite place in the management of the disorder (Fig. 21–9). The technique differs from routine hysterectomy in the following ways: The ovarian blood supply is secured before uterine manipulation; only minimal uterine manipulation is required to enable the uterine vessels to be clamped. If the blood supply is secured first, molar villous transportation will be minimized (Fig. 21–10). If future fertility is desired, then the most appropriate technique for elimination of the mole is suction curettage. Oxytocin must be flowing intravenously during this procedure; otherwise, very large volumes of blood can be lost in very short periods of time. Because most patients with hydatidiform mole have previously hemorrhaged and are suffering from anemia, additional blood loss can precipitate sudden shock. Very gentle, careful sounding should be performed before dilatation. The utmost care is required to avoid perforation. As with the sounding, cervical dilatation must be performed in the axis of the uterine position and with great care so as not to perforate. Pratt dilators are best for this stage of the procedure. A 10- or 12-mm suction curette should be utilized, and dilatation should exceed the diameter of the cannula by at least 2 mm, to allow easy movement of the suction cannula into and out of the uterus. Obviously, suction is applied only during the withdrawal movement of the cannula. Uterine size, that is, cervical/fundal height, should be frequently rechecked because it rapidly changes as the molar tissue is suctioned up. The author prefers not to follow suction with sharp curettage because this maneuver introduces the greatest risk for uterine perforation and deportation of molar villous products.

Fluid management is a key factor in the safe care of such patients because they are prone to fluid overload and pulmonary edema. Therefore, the gynecologist is well advised to limit infusions of water, lactated Ringer's, or saline solutions. Oxytocin should be concentrated in 500 mL $D_5S$ with 20 to 50 units. Beta-blockers should be available for administration if signs of thyroid storm are observed. The patient's hemoglobin, hematocrit, and white cell count should be checked before and after the procedure, together with electrolytes. Additionally, the patient's intake and output should be monitored by obtaining daily weights.

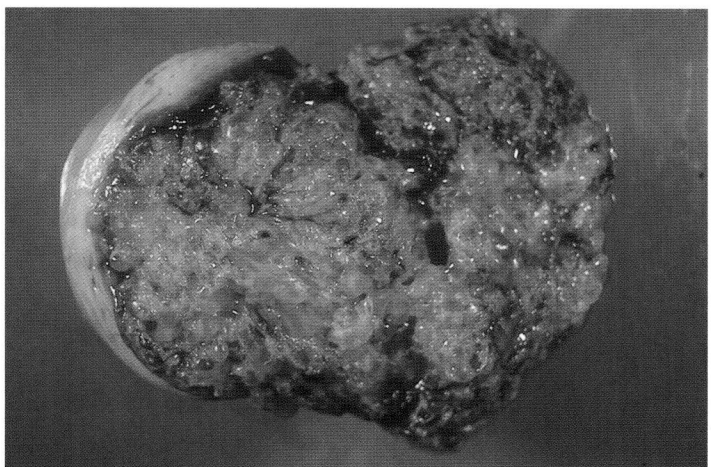

**FIGURE 21–9** Complete moles in high-risk women (e.g., women >40 years of age or of high parity) should be treated by hysterectomy with the mole in situ if future fertility is not a consideration.

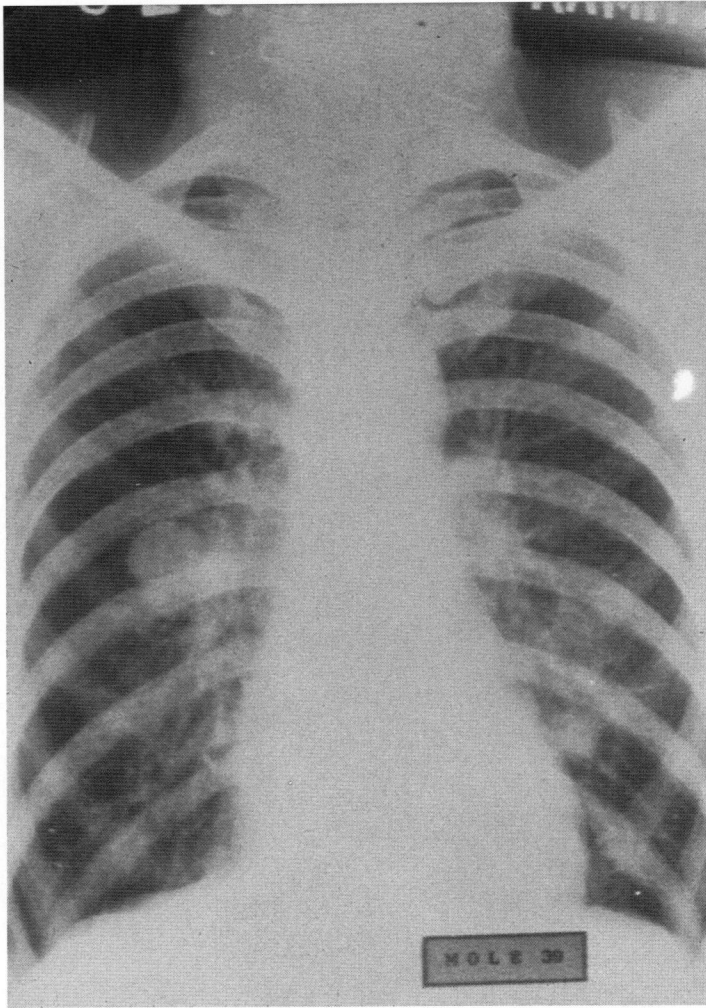

**FIGURE 21–10** During hysterectomy procedures for the treatment of hydatidiform mole, it is wise to secure the vascular supply at the initiation of the operation to avoid villous deportation. This radiograph shows several nodules. When sampled, the pulmonary lesions revealed benign, hydropic villi together with fibrosis. During 12-month follow-up, the pulmonary lesions spontaneously regressed.

Complete and partial moles should be followed up by serial hCG levels and chest radiographs. Pregnancy should be postponed during follow-up, and the author prefers administration of oral contraceptives because these are both effective and easy to administer. The advantages of oral contraceptives outweigh any theoretical disadvantages.

Following hysterectomy or weekly suction evacuation, hCG titers should be obtained (urine and serum) until three negative hCG titers are obtained. Then, two to four weekly hCG assays should be obtained for 3 months, followed by monthly titers for 1 year. Chest radiographs should be obtained monthly.

Invasive mole or choriocarcinoma is suspected with recurrence of vaginal bleeding, amenorrhea, rising or plateauing hCG titers, or pulmonary lesions on radiograph. Hysteroscopy with sampling will permit a tissue diagnosis for intrauterine lesions. Occasionally, an invasive mole will present with symptoms and signs more or less identical to those of a ruptured ectopic pregnancy (Fig. 21–11). In these cases, the invading trophoblast erodes through the uterine muscle and with attendant heavy bleeding (Figs. 21–12 and 21–13) ruptures into the peritoneal cavity (Fig. 21–14). Choriocarcinoma represents the most

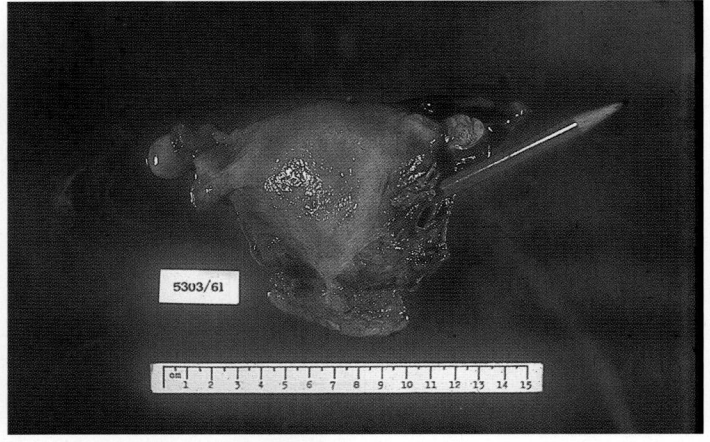

**FIGURE 21–11** This invasive mole (penetrating mole) presented with signs and symptoms of a ruptured ectopic pregnancy. At laparotomy, a massive hemoperitoneum was observed. The trophoblastic tissue had, in fact, eroded through the full thickness of the uterine wall.

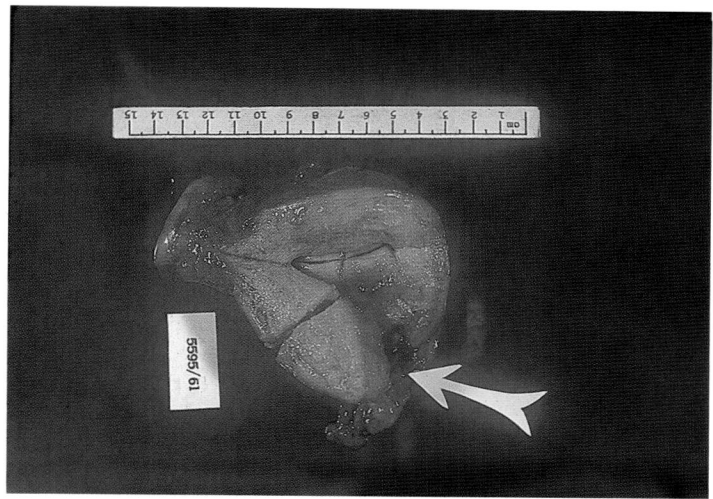

**FIGURE 21-12** Cut view of a uterus containing an invasive mole. The arrow points to fundal destruction caused by invading trophoblastic cells.

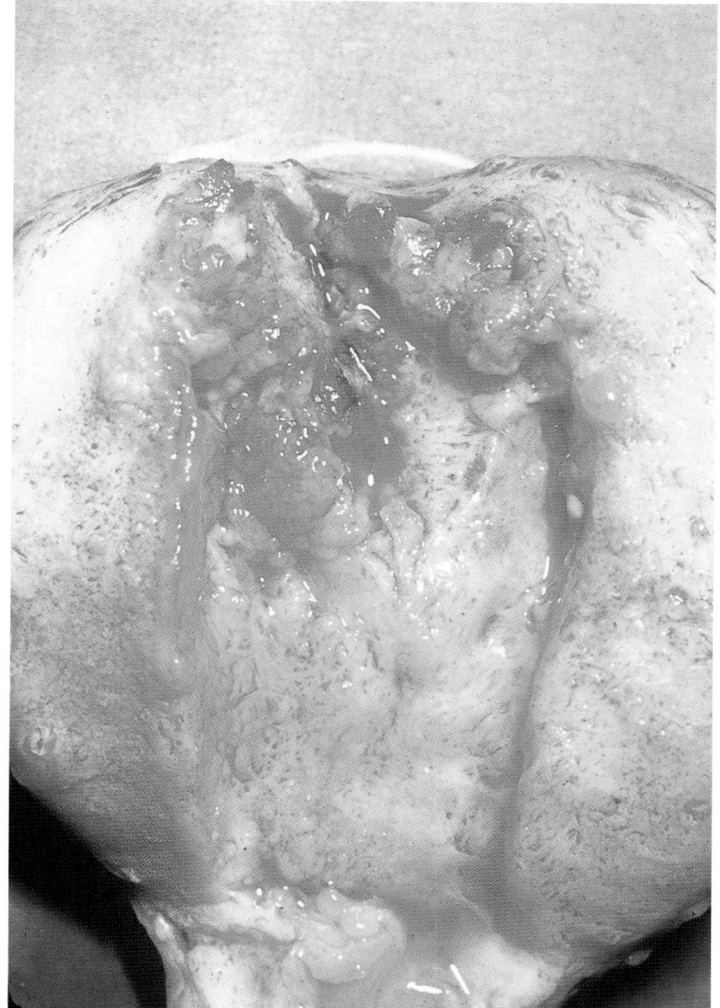

**FIGURE 21-13** High-power view of invasive molar tissue that necrosed the myometrium.

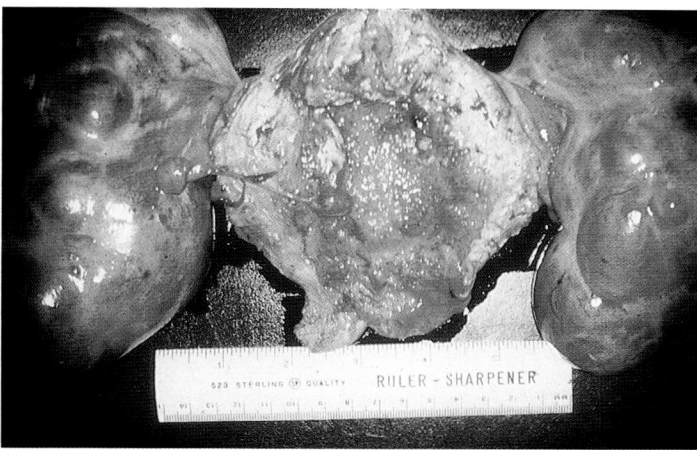

**FIGURE 21-14** Theca-lutein cysts associated with an invasive mole (hysterectomy specimen). The ovaries could have been preserved because the cysts will regress after the molar tissue has been eradicated.

dedifferentiated aspect of trophoblastic disease and the most malignant phase of the disorder. The disease invades the uterine wall early (Fig. 21–15). As with hydatidiform and invasive mole, choriocarcinoma is associated with the formation of theca-lutein cysts (Fig. 21–16).

In fact, choriocarcinoma may not present with any local signs or symptoms. The first hint of its presence may be pulmonary, hepatic, or cerebral symptoms created by metastatic disease (Figs. 21–17 through 21–25). Every gynecologist should be warned about performing a biopsy of vaginal metastatic choriocarcinoma because these lesions are apt to bleed profusely and are difficult to control with suture or electrocoagulation (Fig. 21–26).

Surgery plays a significant role in the treatment of invasive mole and choriocarcinoma. Hysterectomy coupled with chemotherapy may offer the best chances of cure. Chemotherapy will create side effects. Particularly vulnerable are rapidly growing cell populations, such as bone marrow, gastrointestinal epithelium, skin, and hair.

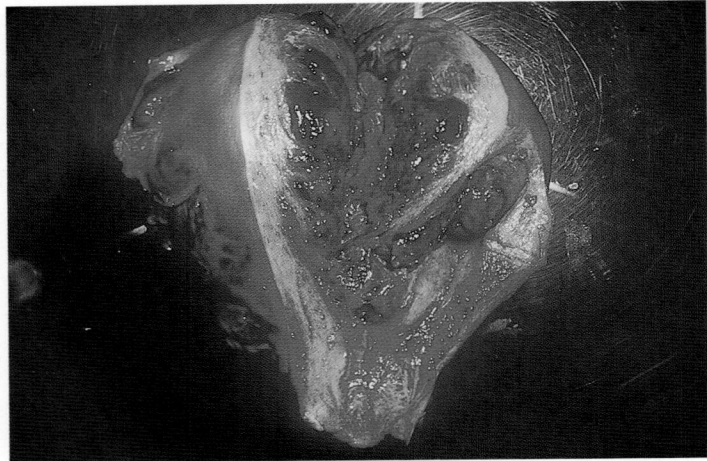

**FIGURE 21–15** Cut surface of the uterus that is riddled with choriocarcinoma. Note the extensive hemorrhage. Because trophoblastic cells have the propensity to invade blood vessels, hemorrhage is usually extensive and severe in cases of choriocarcinoma.

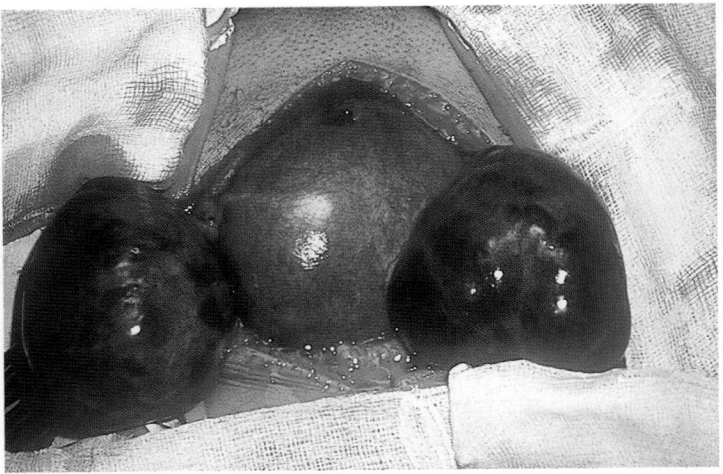

**FIGURE 21–16** Large theca-lutein cysts are also associated with choriocarcinoma involving the uterus.

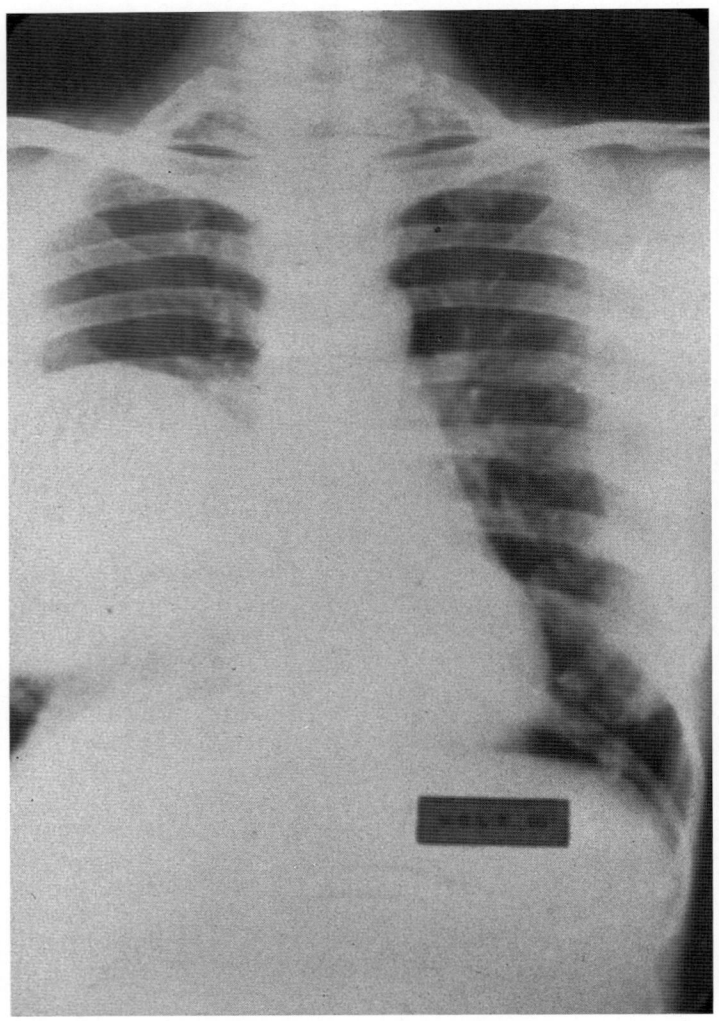

**FIGURE 21–17** The most common metastatic site associated with choriocarcinoma is the lung. This radiograph shows a large, cannonball lesion occupying the greater part of the right lung.

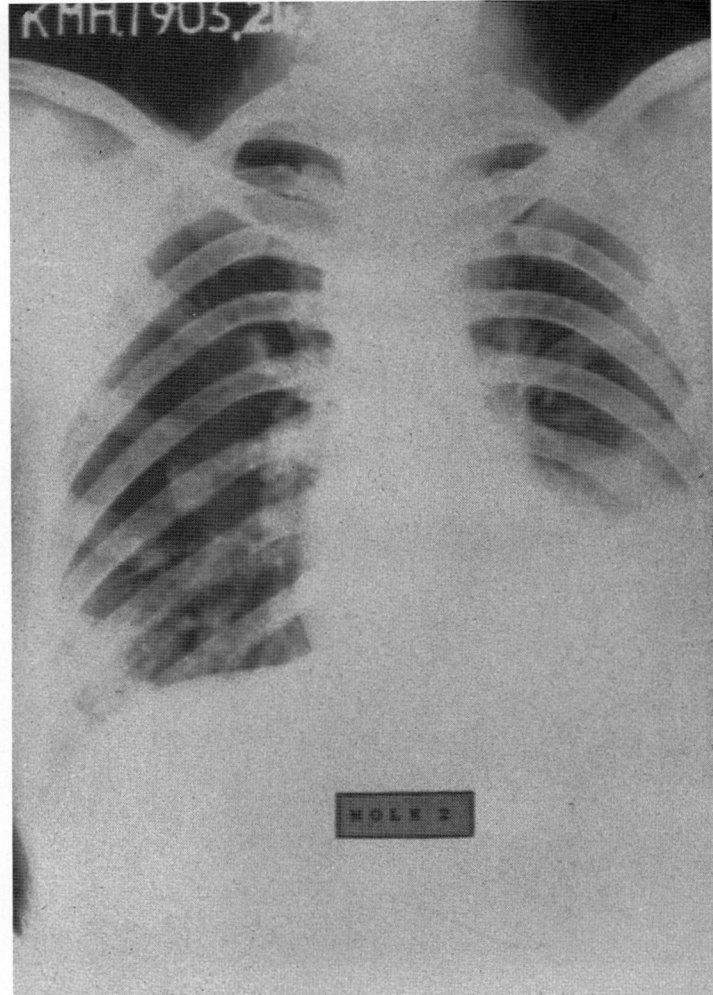

**FIGURE 21–18** Numerous pulmonary and rib metastases are seen in this case of metastatic choriocarcinoma.

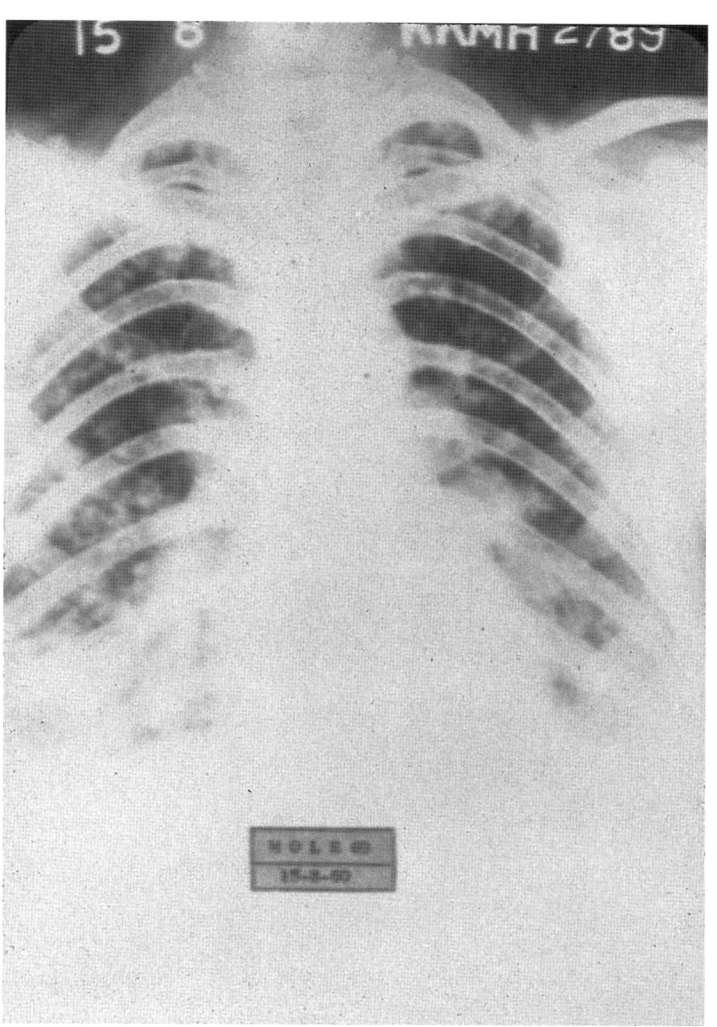

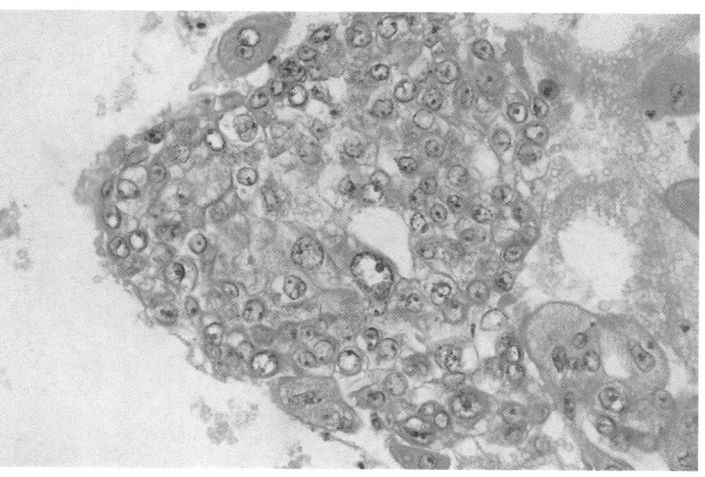

**FIGURE 21–20** Choriocarcinoma is the most undifferentiated of the trophoblastic disease entities. The trophoblast cannot differentiate to form villi. Here, solid masses of mainly cytotrophoblasts are present.

**FIGURE 21–19** Metastatic choriocarcinoma with miliary pattern on radiograph.

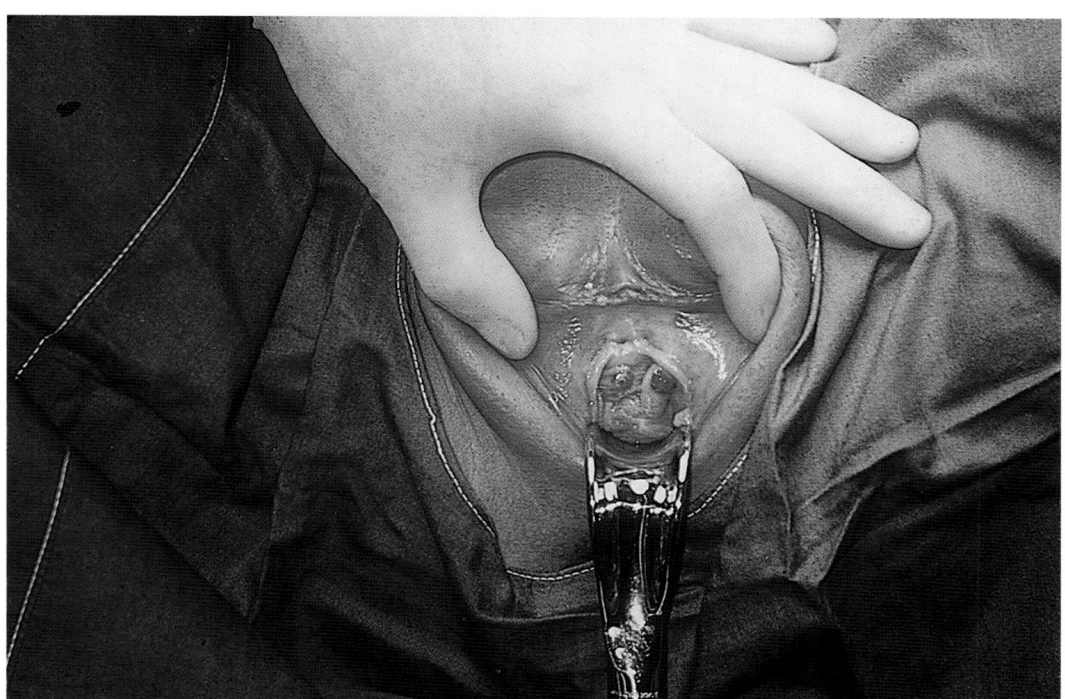

**FIGURE 21–21** One of the more common metastatic sites for choriocarcinoma is the vagina. Because these lesions are exceedingly vascular, great care should be exercised when a biopsy is performed.

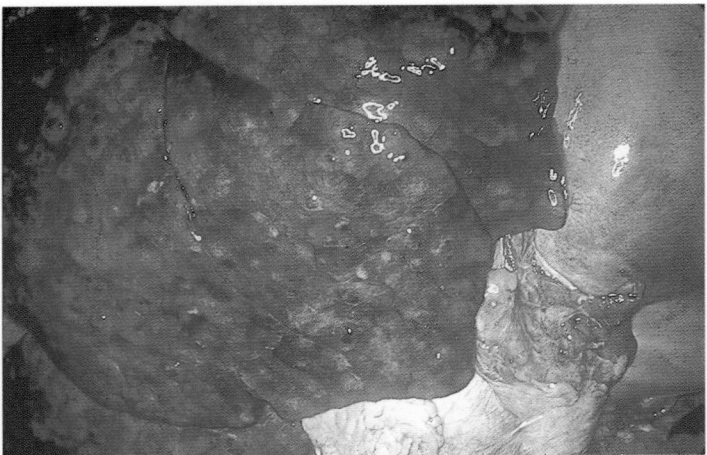

**FIGURE 21–22** Postmortem specimen of the lung of a patient who died of metastatic choriocarcinoma. The lung is congested and red because of extensive hemorrhage within the lung parenchyma.

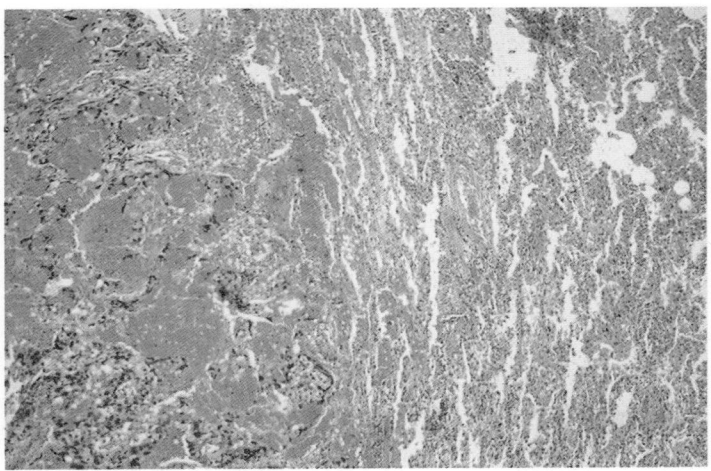

**FIGURE 21–23** Histopathologic section of the lung shown in Figure 21–22. To the left is invading trophoblastic tissue surrounded by hemorrhage. To the right are congested alveoli.

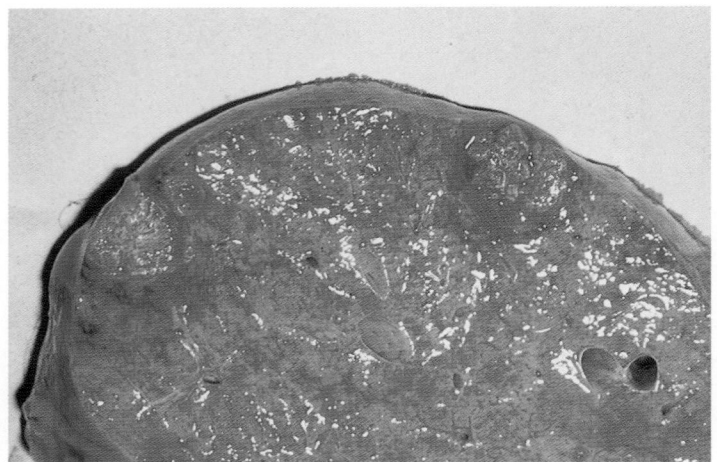

**FIGURE 21–24** Section of the liver showing subcapsular nodules of metastatic choriocarcinoma.

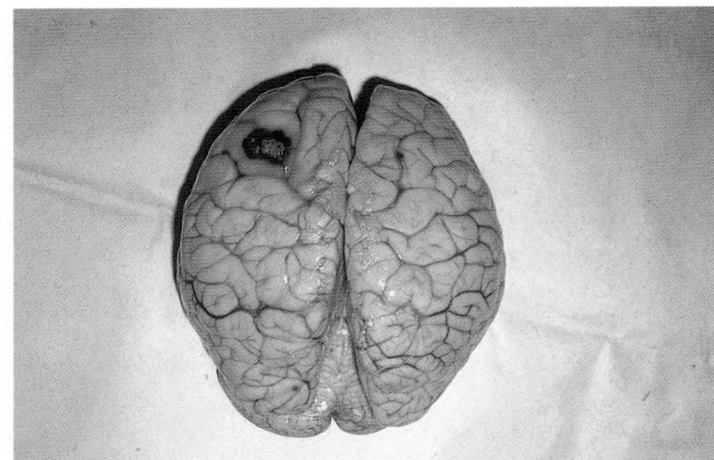

**FIGURE 21–25** A metastatic trophoblastic nodule is seen on the surface of the left cerebral hemisphere.

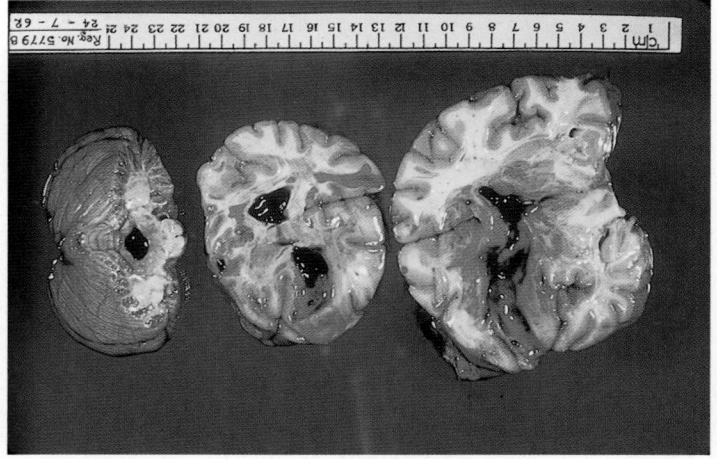

**FIGURE 21–26** Cut sections of the brain show much greater damage than is perceived in Figure 21–25. Note the very large intraventricular hemorrhage, which, in fact, was the terminal event for this patient.

# SECTION D

# Adnexa

# CHAPTER 22

# Ovarian Cystectomy and Cystotomy

*Michael S. Baggish*

Any cystic mass of the ovary has the potential for malignancy. A frozen section should be performed when a conservative treatment plan has been selected. Cystectomy permits the cystic structure to be selectively removed while the residual ovarian tissue is preserved. Cystectomy may be performed for functioning cysts (follicular and corpus luteum), benign cystic teratomas, and endometriotic cysts.

The technique for cystectomy is similar for all of the preceding conditions. The ovary is stabilized with placement of a Babcock clamp on the utero-ovarian ligament (Fig. 22-1). If the procedure is performed by laparotomy, then 3-0 Vicryl traction sutures may be placed into the ovarian tissue outside of the cystic area. The stitches are clamped with mosquito clamps and held by an assistant. A 1:200 vasopressin solution is injected into the stretched-out capsule of the ovary, which overlies the cyst (Fig. 22-2). An incision is made into the capsule with an energy device (laser or electrosurgical) or knife (Figs. 22-3 and 22-4).

The incision between the cyst wall and the ovarian capsule provides a plane that can be dissected on either side of the initial incision (Figs. 22-5 and 22-6). The incision may be extended at will to facilitate separation of the cyst from the ovarian capsule (Fig. 22-7A, B). The dissection continues to completely circumscribe the ovary (Fig. 22-7C). Finally, the base of the cyst is clamped or coagulated, and the cyst is removed intact and sent to pathology (Fig. 22-7D). Any ovarian cyst other than an obvious corpus luteum cyst should be sent for frozen section. The remaining capsular tissue is folded upon itself, and no sutures are placed. Alternatively, the excess capsule may be trimmed away and the ovary closed with 4-0 Vicryl.

In some circumstances, particularly with endometriomas, difficulty may be encountered in stripping away the ovarian capsule from the cyst wall (Fig. 22-8). In these cases, the author has preferred to resect a portion of the ovary that includes approximately 50% of the cyst and then to vaporize the cyst lining from the inside. The technique is described as follows.

The utero-ovarian ligament is grasped with Babcock clamps. Stabilizing sutures of 3-0 Vicryl are placed into the periphery of the ovary outside the field of proposed resection (Fig. 22-9). A carbon dioxide ($CO_2$) laser or other suitable energy device is selected to cut the ovary. Alternatively, 1:200 vasopressin can be injected and a knife utilized (Fig. 22-10). The cyst is opened linearly and drained (Fig. 22-11A–C). A hemisphere of ovary is cut away (Fig. 22-12). The interior lining of the cyst is then vaporized (Fig. 22-13). The char is irrigated away (Fig. 22-14A–C). The edges of the ovary are grasped and approximated by suturing the obliterated cyst wall together with 3-0 Vicryl and then approximating the wound margin with 3-0 or 4-0 Vicryl (Fig. 22-15). The reconstituted ovary now has been reduced to normal size (Fig. 22-16).

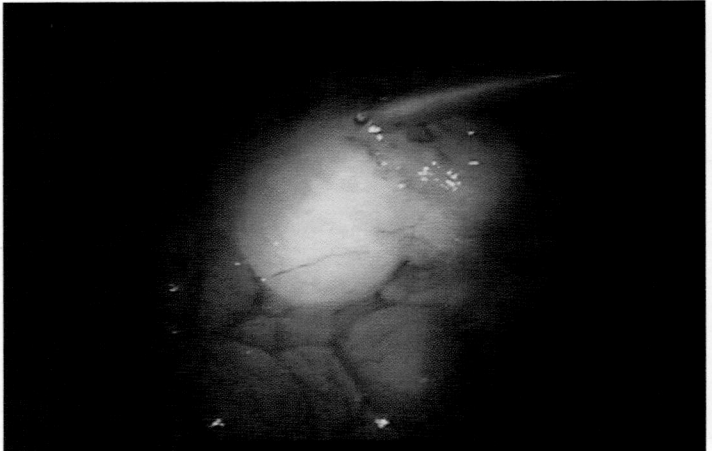

**FIGURE 22-1** The ovary is enlarged by a benign cystic teratoma.

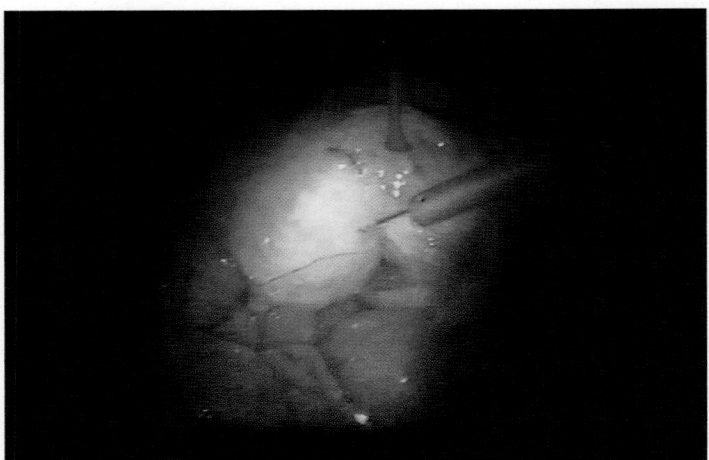

**FIGURE 22-2** The cyst is injected with a 1:200 vasopressin solution before the cystectomy is begun.

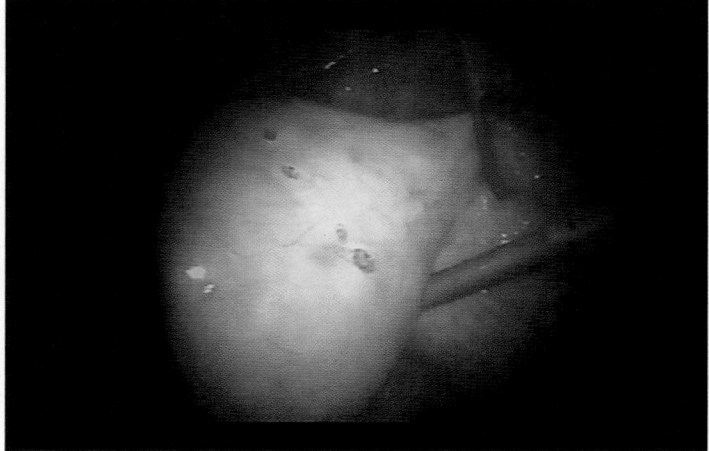

**FIGURE 22-3** Carbon dioxide ($CO_2$) laser trace spots are placed into the ovary to indicate the direction or extent of the incision. This may be done with a bipolar needle or by scoring the tissue with a shallow knife incision.

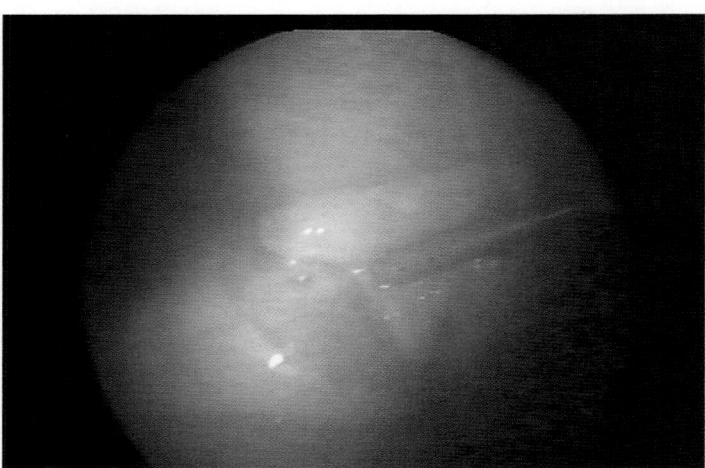

**FIGURE 22-4** A cut has been created along the previously marked incision line. Note that the ovarian capsule partially retracts from the underlying cyst wall. A haze is created by the smoke of the energy source vapor.

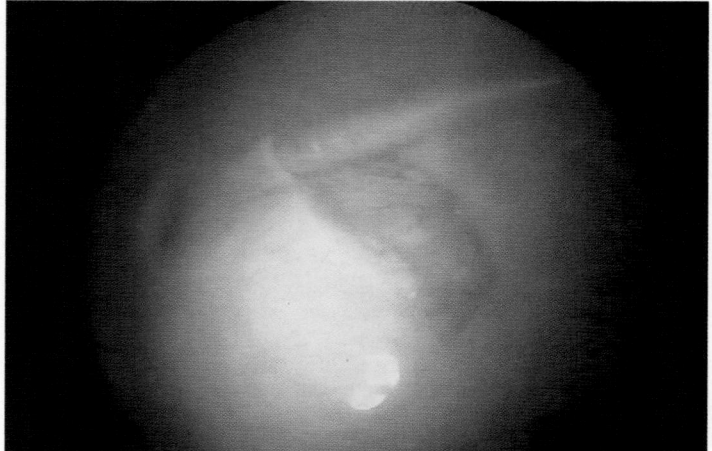

**FIGURE 22-5** An irrigating cannula dissects a space between the capsule and the cyst wall with pressurized saline injection.

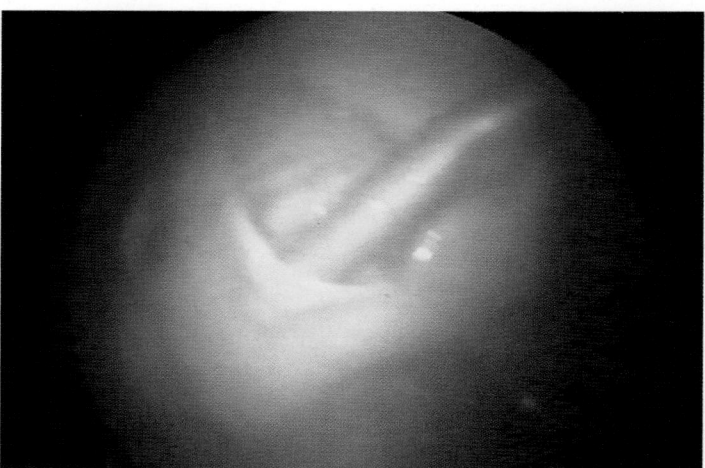

**FIGURE 22-6** Dissection of the cyst wall continues circumferentially around the ovary.

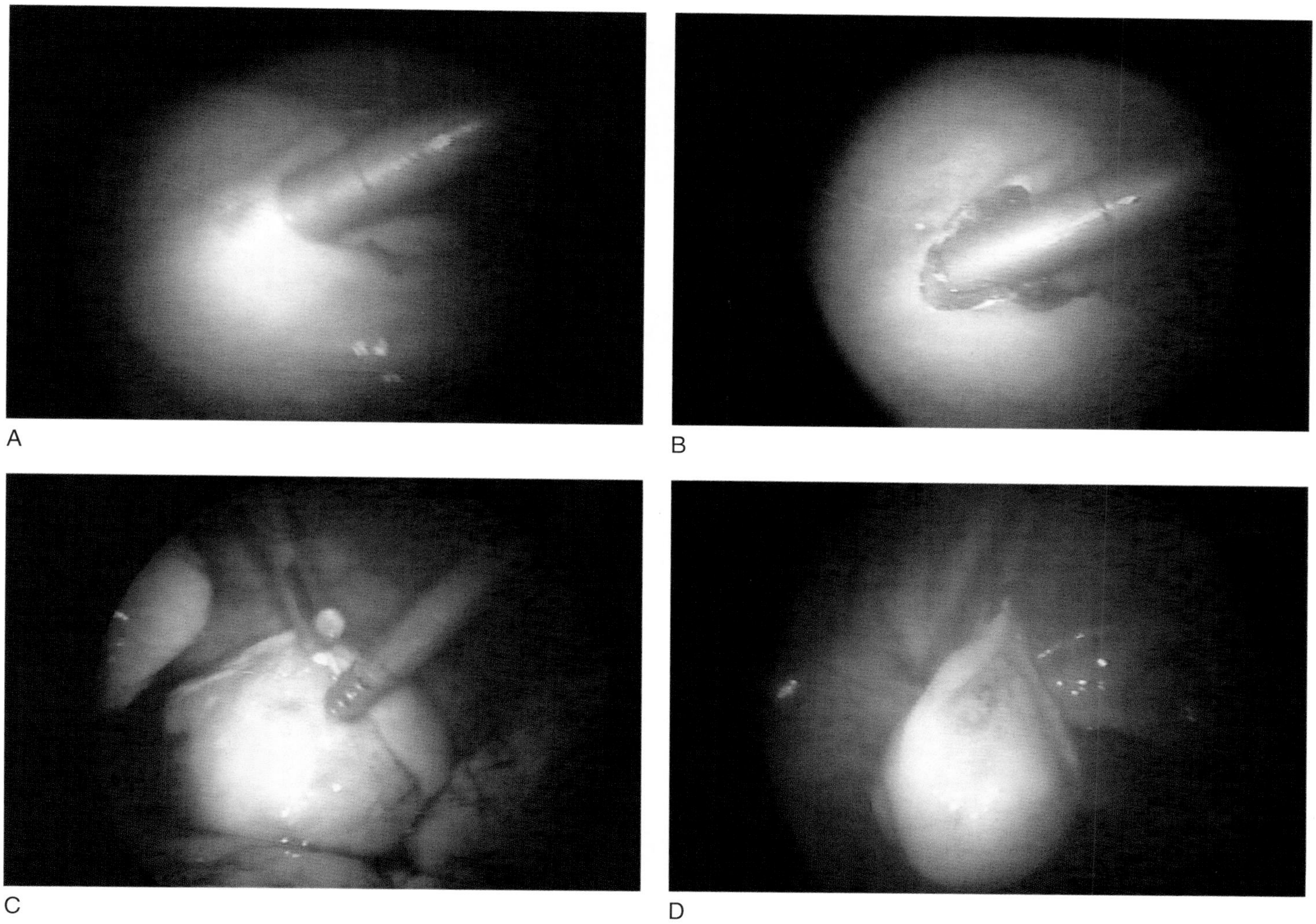

A

B

C

D

**FIGURE 22–7 A.** The initial incision is extended to facilitate mobilization of the cyst. **B.** When the incision extension has been completed, further hydrodissection continues. **C.** The cyst has been 90% separated from the ovarian wall. **D.** The cyst has been completely separated from the ovary and is being removed from the abdominal cavity. In this case, the second laparoscopic puncture incision is lengthened to create a microlaparotomy.

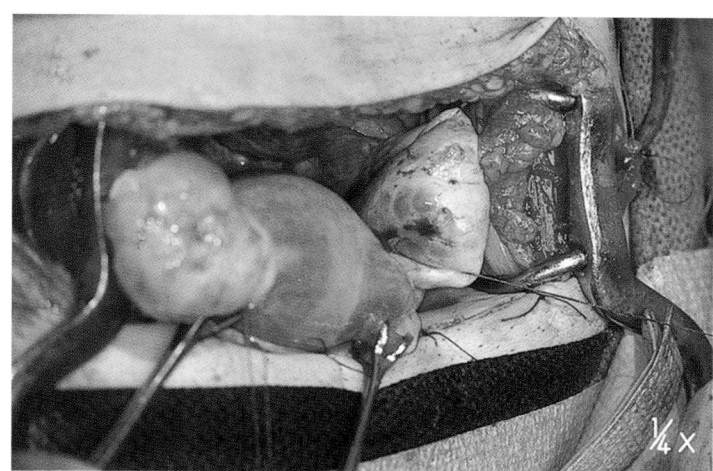

**FIGURE 22–8** Bilateral, large endometriomas. The endometrial cysts are approximately as large as the uterus.

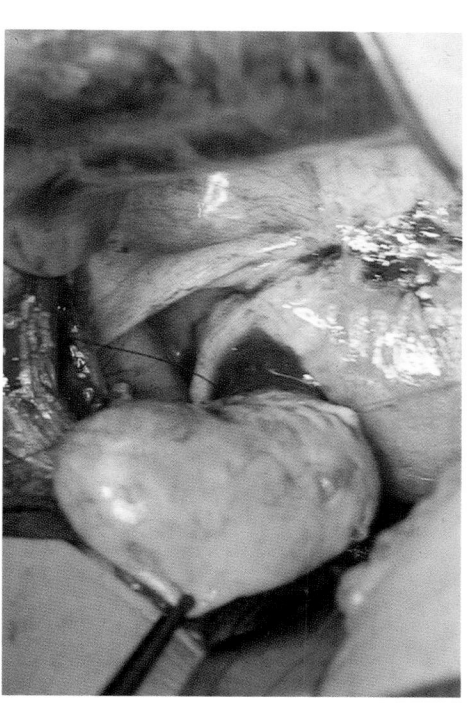

**FIGURE 22–9** Stay sutures are placed into the ovary for traction.

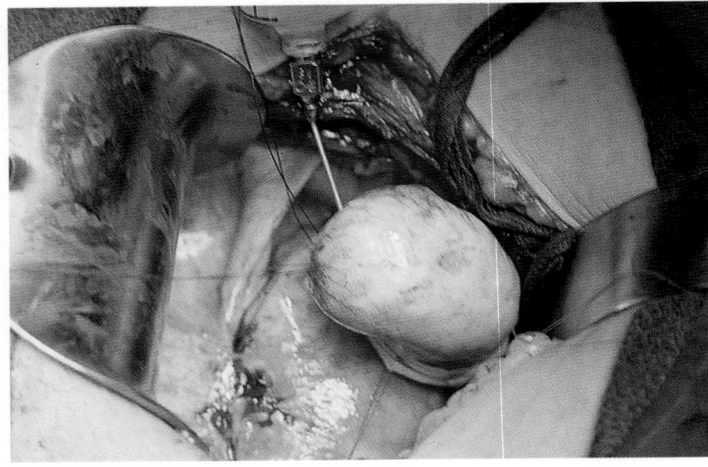

**FIGURE 22–10** A 1:200 vasopressin solution is injected into the ovary for hemostasis before the cystic structure is opened.

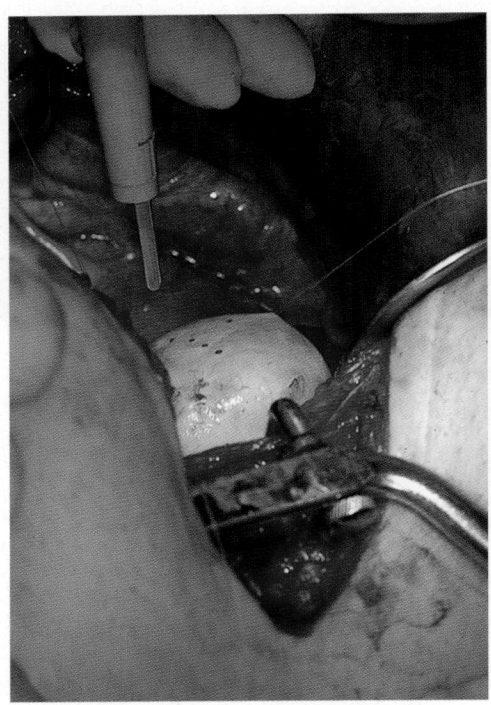

A

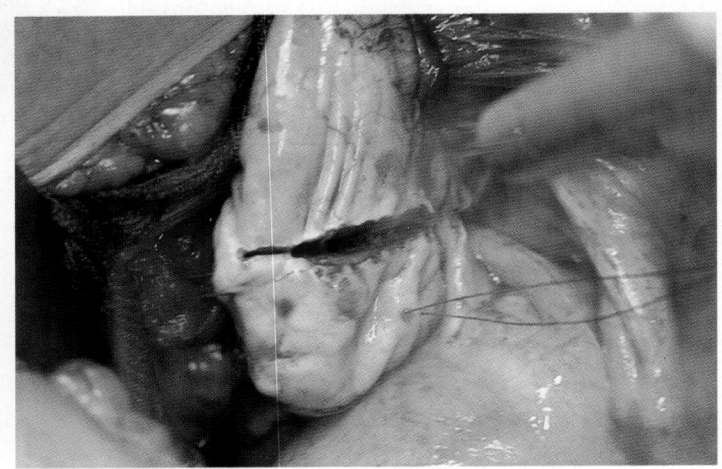

B

C

**FIGURE 22–11 A.** Laser trace spots (carbon dioxide [$CO_2$] laser) made with a superpulse mode trace the extent of the incision to be made. **B.** As the incision cuts into the interior of the cyst, dark brown bloody fluid escapes from the ovary and is suctioned away from the field. **C.** Approximately half of the enlarged ovary is resected. The interior of the remaining half containing a portion of the interior cyst wall is irrigated to clean out any residual bloody contents.

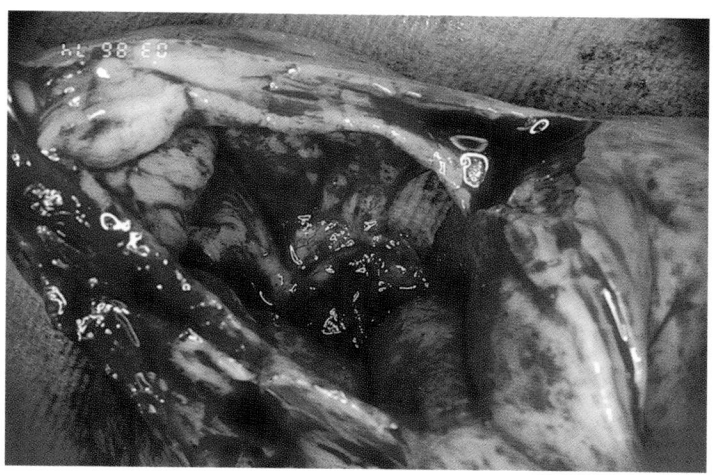

**FIGURE 22–12** The excised cyst is examined and sent to pathology.

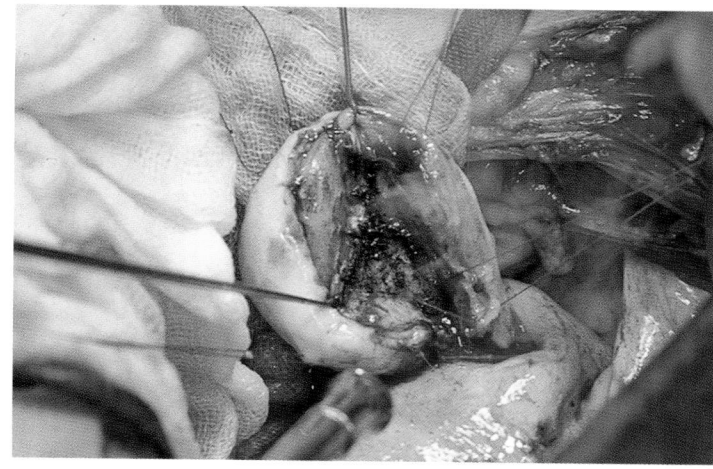

**FIGURE 22–13** The carbon dioxide ($CO_2$) laser is targeted to the interior of the remaining half of the ovary. The lining of the endometrioma is vaporized.

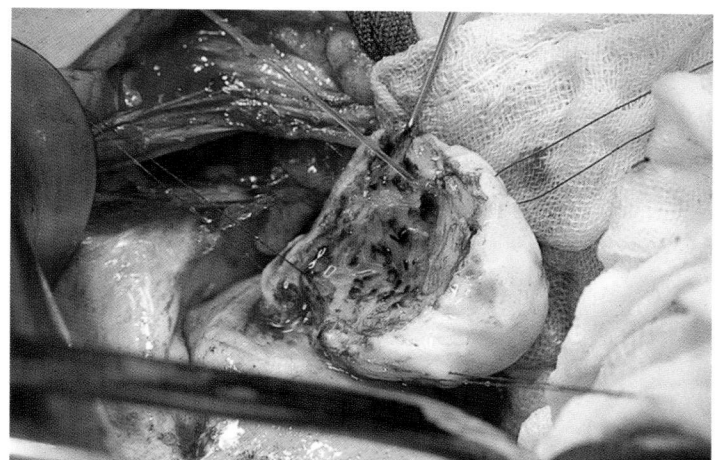

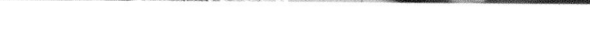

A

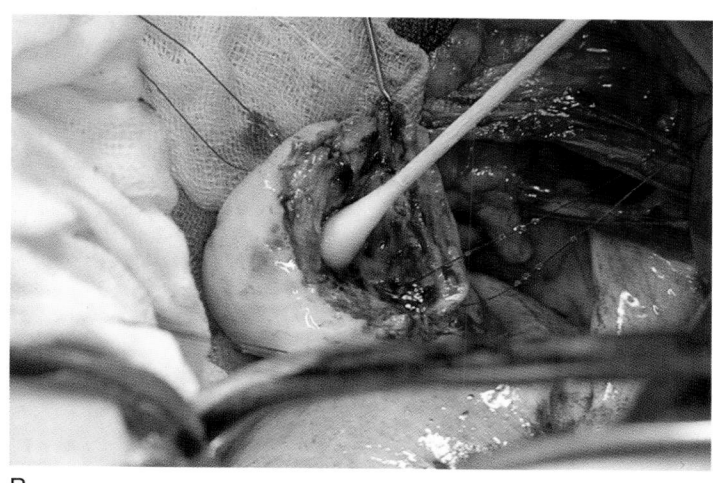

B

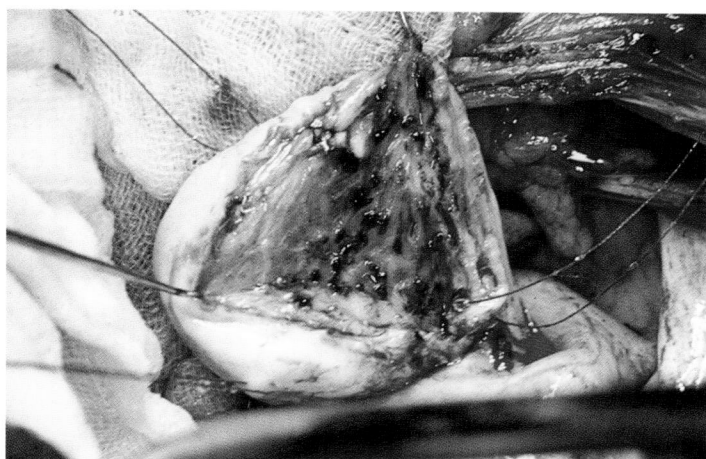

C

**FIGURE 22–14 A.** The char is irrigated with copious amounts of sterile normal saline injected under pressure. **B.** A saline-soaked cotton-tipped applicator further facilitates removal of devitalized tissue. **C.** The remaining ovarian tissue without cyst wall is ready for closure.

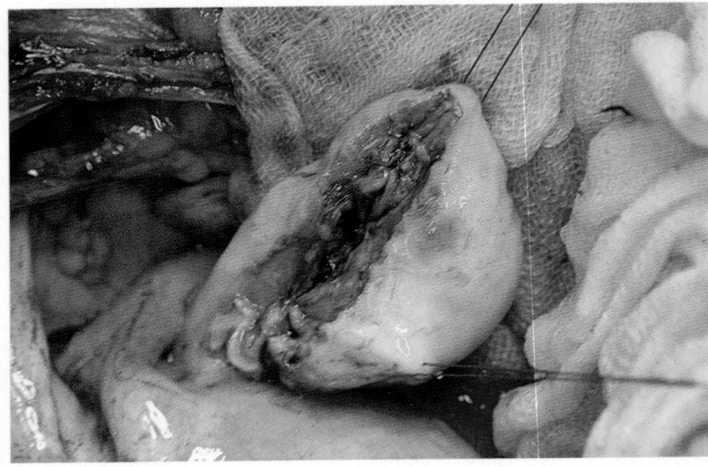

**FIGURE 22–15** The cyst cavity is obliterated as 4-0 Vicryl sutures bring the opposing walls together. The vaporized surfaces will naturally adhere to each other.

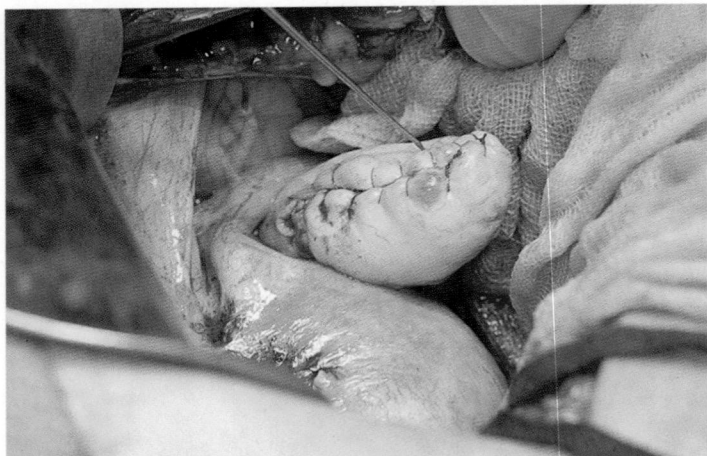

**FIGURE 22–16** The capsule of the ovary is closed with a 4-0 Vicryl running suture. The net effect of the operation is elimination of the cyst with restoration of a normal-sized ovary.

# CHAPTER 23

# Surgery for Pyosalpinx, Tubo-ovarian Abscess, and Pelvic Abscess

## Michael S. Baggish

Infections emanating from the tube may result in a variety of abscesses that may require surgical intervention. With the exception of a pelvic abscess, which is typically managed by incision and drainage, tubal abscesses are excised if intensive antibiotic treatment fails to elicit a response.

Operative management of these infections utilizes a combination of techniques, including adhesiolysis, salpingectomy, salpingo-oophorectomy, and even hysterectomy.

The criteria for drainage of a pelvic abscess are (1) walling-off of the pus (i.e., creation of a pyogenic membrane), and (2) fluctuance (i.e., "pointing" of the abscess just before an anticipated spontaneous rupture). Typically in this location, the pointing process is manifested as the leading edge of the pyogenic membrane dissecting a space within the rectovaginal septum (i.e., between the rectum and vagina). This, of course, is best demonstrated by performance of a rectovaginal examination and palpation of the bulge in the septum.

Drainage is performed transvaginally. The cervix is grasped with a single-toothed tenaculum. The vagina has been carefully and gently prepared with povidone-iodine (Betadine) or another suitable surgical preparatory solution. A weighted or Sims retractor is placed along the posterior vaginal wall.

Just before incising into the lower cul-de-sac (septum), the surgeon double-gloves and performs a rectovaginal examination to establish the exact position of the rectum relative to the contemplated incision site (Fig. 23–1). Next, an incision is cut into the cul-de-sac. This may be facilitated by careful insertion of an 18-gauge needle attached to a syringe into the abscess and withdrawal of a sample of pus, followed by cutting directly along the track of the needle with a scalpel (Fig. 23–2).

As soon as a 1- to 1.5-cm incision is made, the operator's index finger is inserted into the abscess cavity to (1) provide a guide for enlarging the incision, and (2) break up fibrous septa to enhance drainage (Fig. 23–3). After appropriate culture samples have been obtained and a large rubber drain or two have been inserted into the abscess cavity, and its edges are sutured to the incision edges with 2-0 chromic catgut, a large safety pin is attached to the exposed end of the drain(s) (Figs. 23–4 and 23–5).

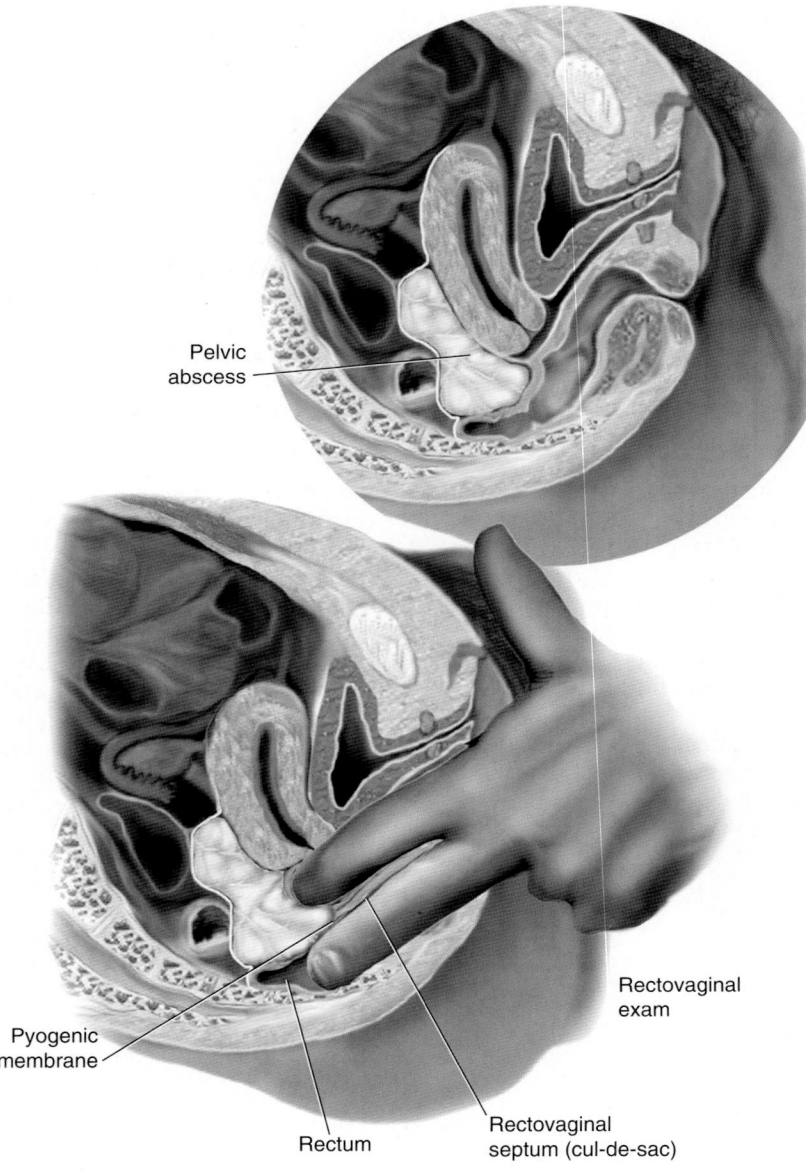

Pelvic
abscess

Pyogenic
membrane

Rectum

Rectovaginal
septum (cul-de-sac)

Rectovaginal
exam

**FIGURE 23–1** A pelvic abscess is illustrated via a hemisection through the pelvis. Fluctuance is identified by performing a rectovaginal examination and verifying that the abscess has begun to dissect the rectovaginal septum.

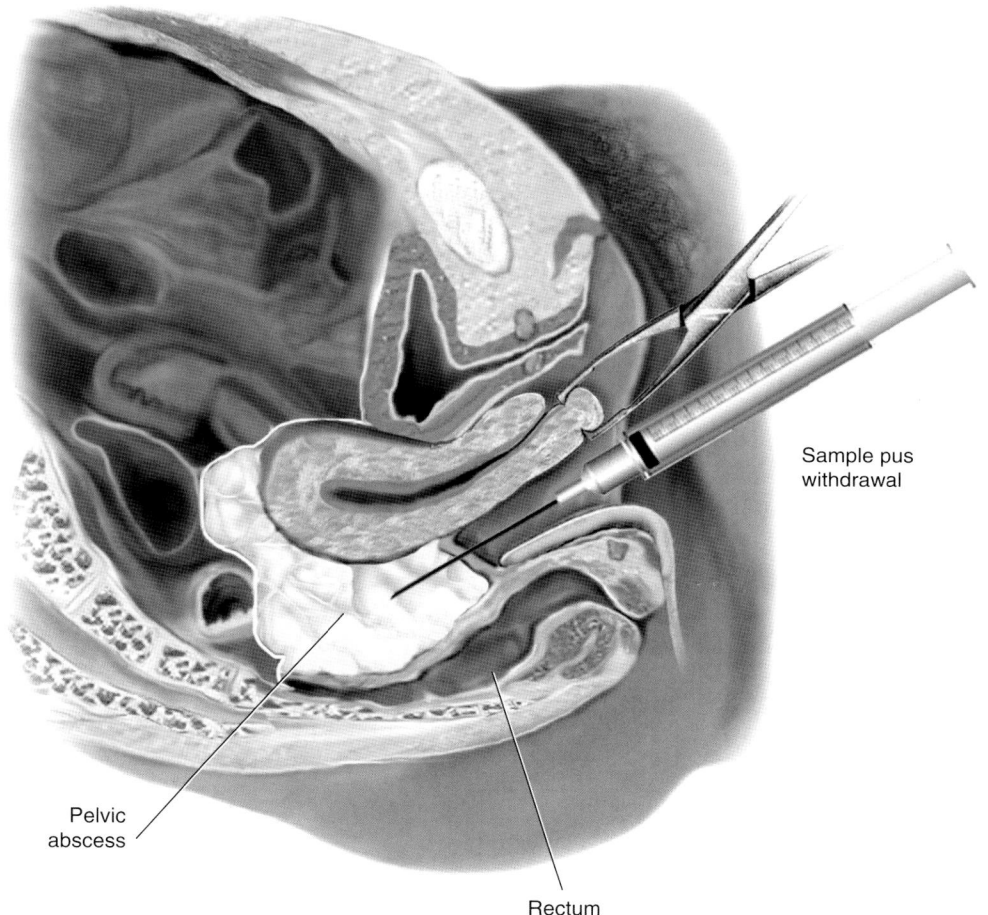

Sample pus
withdrawal

Pelvic
abscess

Rectum

**FIGURE 23–2** The posterior lip of the cervix is grasped with a tenaculum. The cervix and the uterus are pulled downward and anteriorly. An 18-gauge needle is inserted into the bulging cul-de-sac mass. The plunger on the syringe is withdrawn and pus is sucked into the syringe.

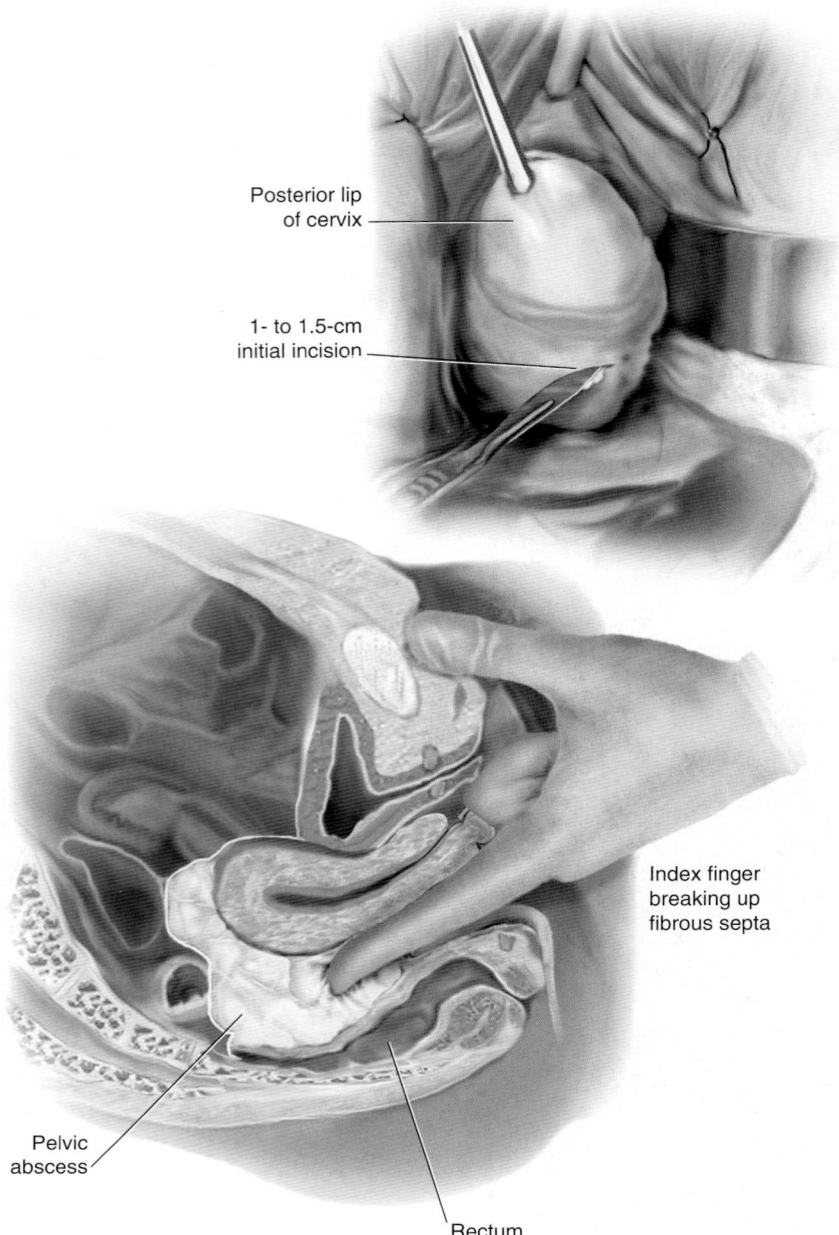

Posterior lip
of cervix

1- to 1.5-cm
initial incision

Index finger
breaking up
fibrous septa

Pelvic
abscess

Rectum

**FIGURE 23–3** With the needle track used as a guide, a scalpel cuts into the abscess cavity. Flow of pus signals entry through the pyogenic membrane. The surgeon's index finger is inserted into the abscess cavity. Fibrous septa are broken up.

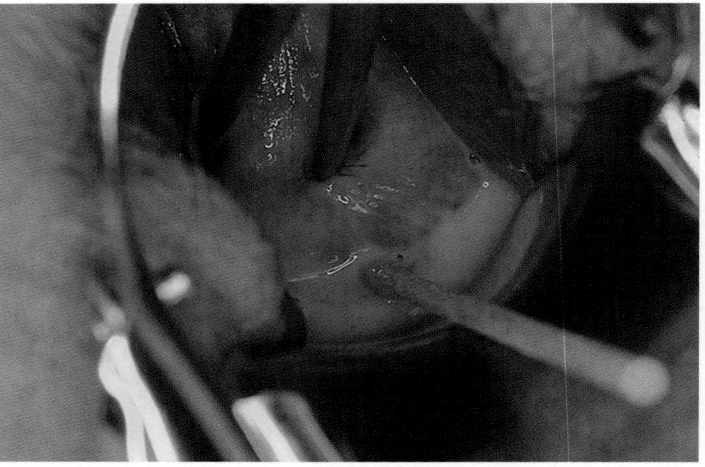

**FIGURE 23–4** Pus drained from a pelvic abscess fills the posterior vaginal fornix. A cotton-tipped applicator is inserted into the abscess cavity.

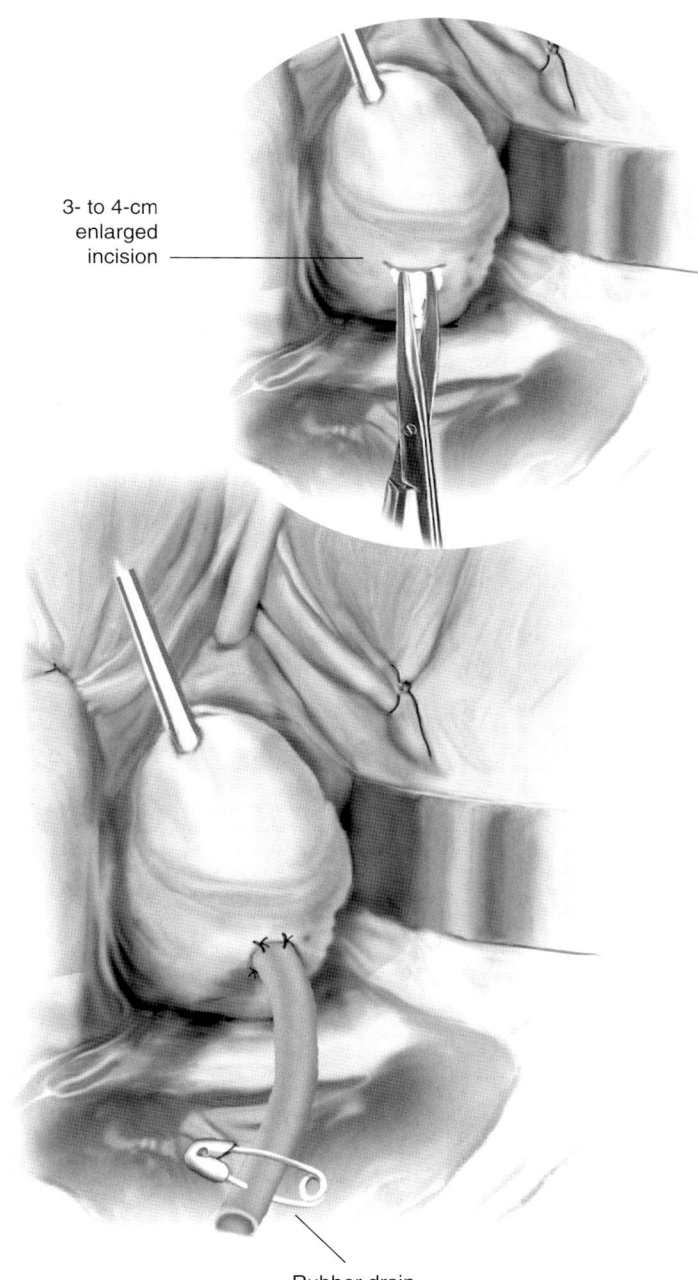

3- to 4-cm
enlarged
incision —

Rubber drain
with large safety pin

**FIGURE 23–5** The initial incision is enlarged to 3 to 4 cm to permit better drainage. A large drain is placed into the abscess cavity and is anchored with two or three 2-0 chromic catgut stitches. It is advised that the total length of the drain be measured and recorded before it is placed, and that the drain length be remeasured and recorded when it is removed. A safety pin should always be inserted into the outside extremity of the drain.

A tubo-ovarian abscess that does not "point" (localize) into the inferior portion of the pelvis but instead enlarges into the upper abdomen may rupture intraperitoneally. This results in spreading of peritonitis from the lower abdomen and pelvis into the upper abdomen, creating an emergency situation. An enlarging tubo-ovarian abscess is a hazard for rupture because the ovary, in contrast to the oviduct, does not have the capacity to expand when pus collects within its substance. Hence, an enlarging tubo-ovarian mass is unpredictable and should be excised (Fig. 23–6).

The tube is grasped at its distal extreme with a Babcock clamp. The infundibulopelvic ligament is grasped with a Babcock clamp, and a traction suture of 0 or 1-0 Vicryl is placed through the utero-ovarian ligament. Dissection is carried upward and retroperitoneally to separate the ovarian vessels from the ureter above the point where the two structures cross into the pelvis over the common iliac artery (Fig. 23–7). The

infundibulopelvic ligament is triply clamped and sectioned. The dissection is carried inferiorly to facilitate separation of the tubo-ovarian complex from surrounding structures. The mass is invariably stuck to the intestine, which must be sharply separated from the abscess (Fig. 23–8).

Next, the distal tube and the utero-ovarian ligament are together triply clamped (Fig. 23–9). The tubo-ovarian abscess now is isolated and can be excised (Fig. 23–10A, B). Hemostasis is secured by doubly suture-ligating beneath the two clamps left on the infundibulopelvic and utero-ovarian pedicles.

The ureter, small and large intestines, and opposite adnexa are carefully examined for any disease or injury. Vascular pedicles are rechecked for bleeding (Fig. 23–11). Copious irrigation is performed. Drains are inserted into the cul-de-sac and lateral gutter. These are brought out of the abdomen through separate stab wounds.

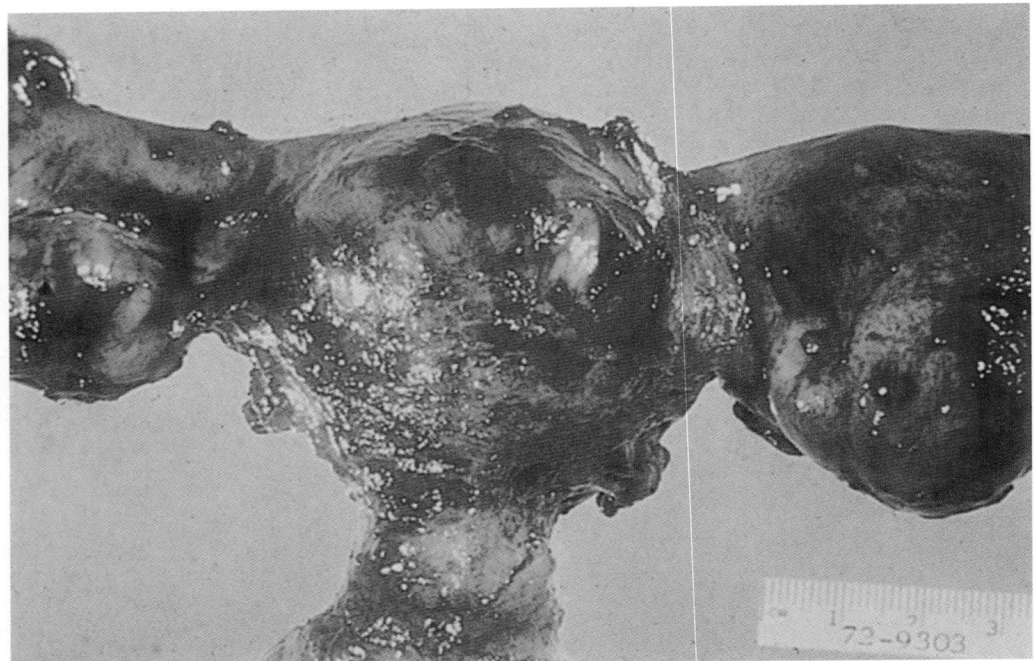

**FIGURE 23–6** The right adnexa is involved in a common infectious mass: a tubo-ovarian abscess.

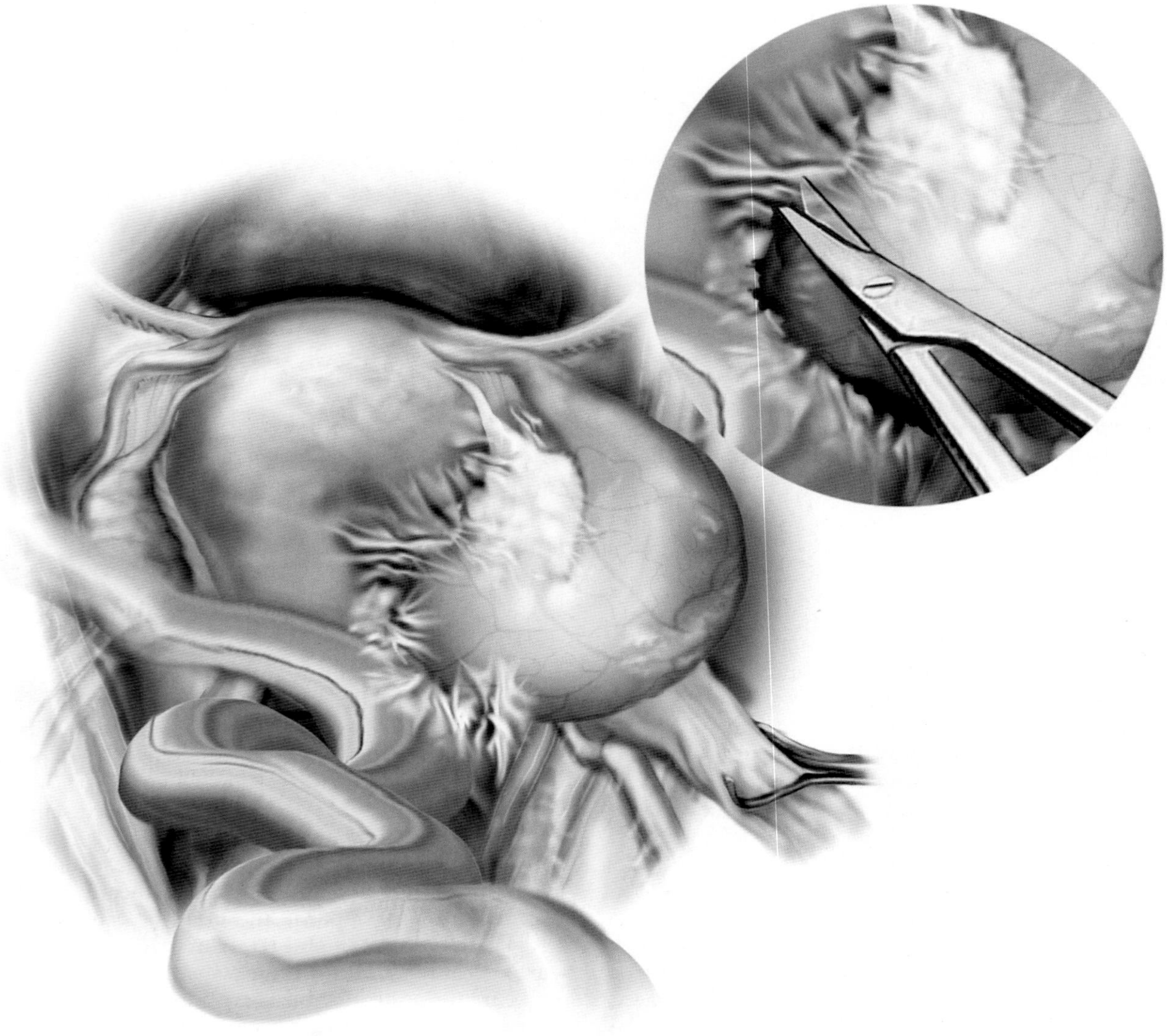

**FIGURE 23–7** The infundibulopelvic ligament is grasped with a Babcock clamp for traction. The utero-ovarian ligament, if visible, likewise may be grasped for traction. Adhesions between the mass and neighboring structures (in this figure, intestine) are sharply divided.

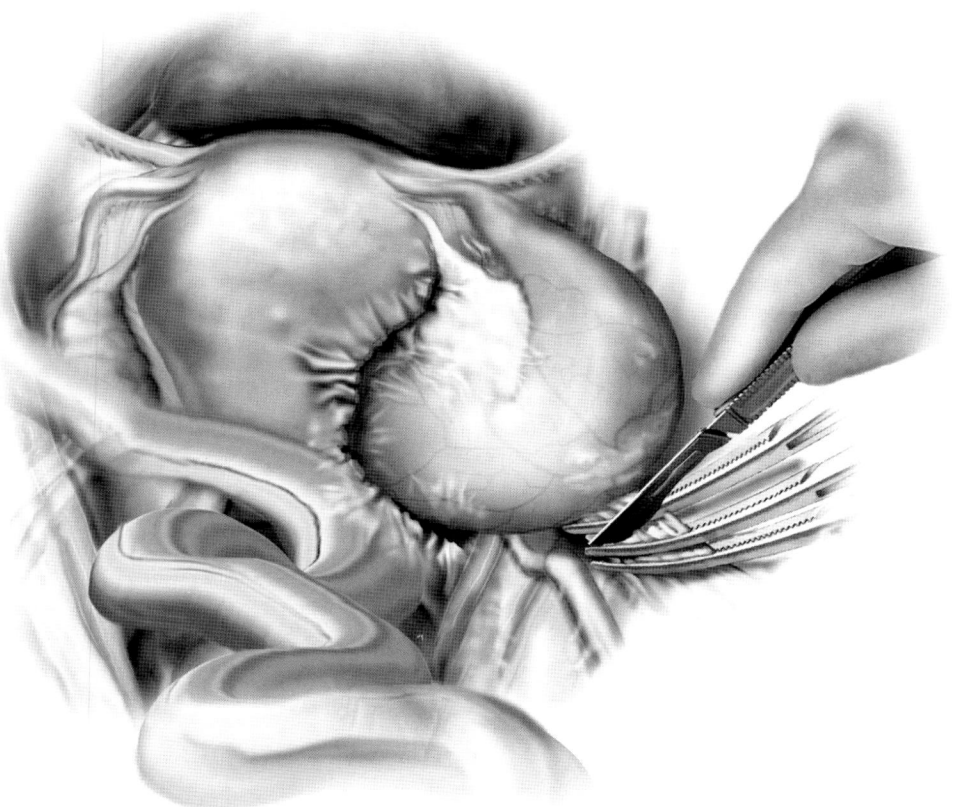

**FIGURE 23–8** The infundibulopelvic ligament is secured from its close neighbor, the ureter. The ligament containing the ovarian vessels is triply clamped, divided, and doubly suture-ligated with 0 Vicryl.

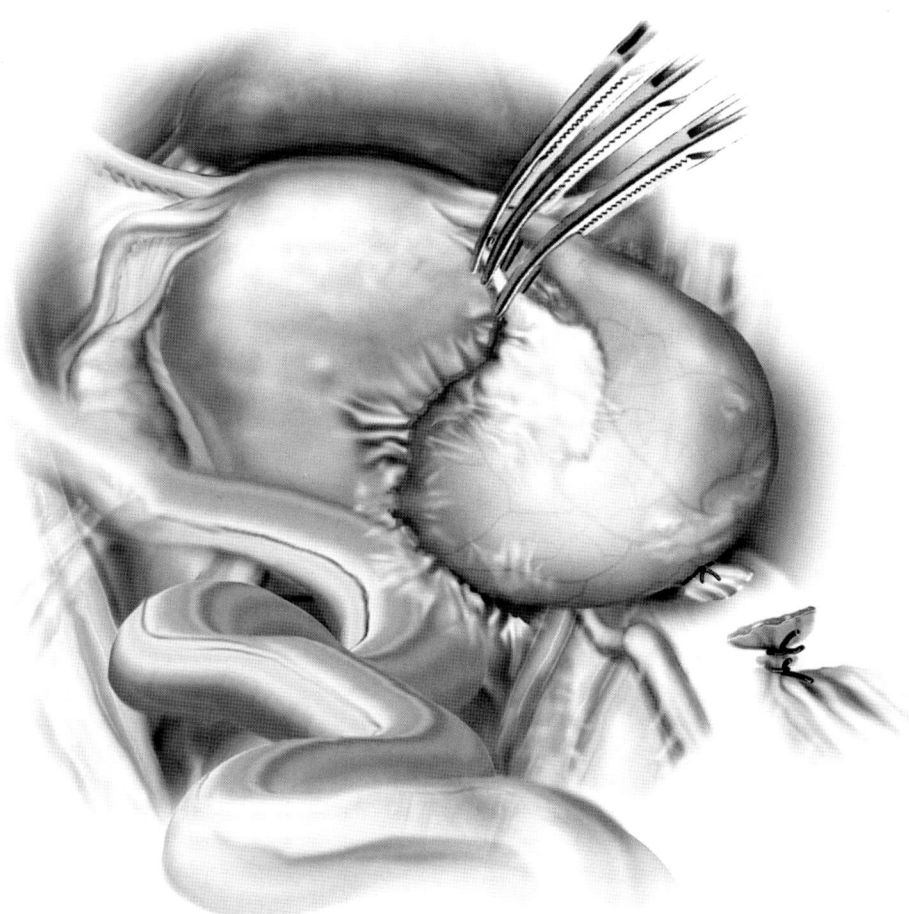

**FIGURE 23–9** The oviduct and the utero-ovarian ligament are likewise triply clamped, cut, and doubly suture-ligated.

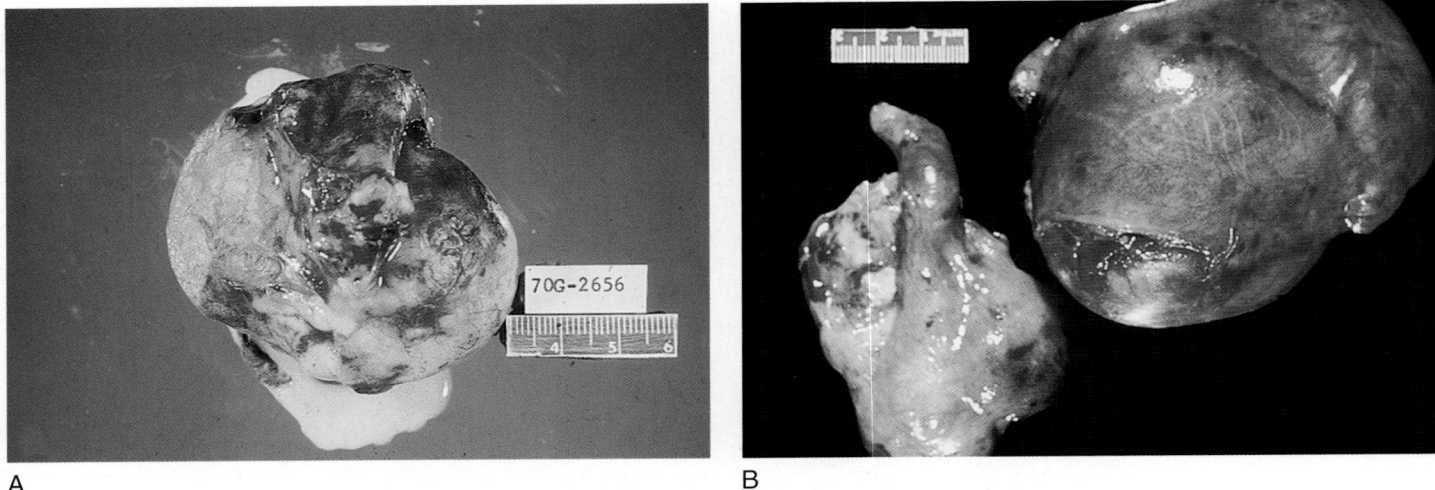

A                                                                    B

**FIGURE 23–10  A.** The large, pus-filled mass is excised en masse. The mass should be cut open while fresh, and a variety of cultures obtained. The specimens should be immediately sent to bacteriology. **B.** On occasion, a hysterectomy may be performed together with the salpingo-oophorectomy. Depending on the patient's clinical condition, this may be a total or a subtotal hysterectomy.

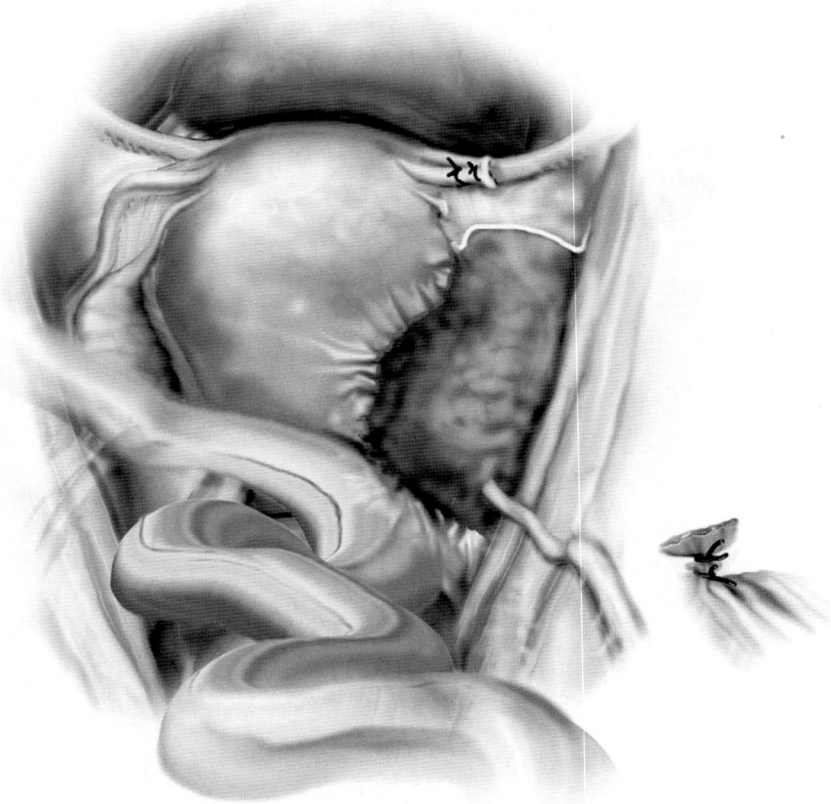

**FIGURE 23–11**  After the diseased adnexa have been excised, the ureter is carefully inspected for its integrity before the peritoneum is closed. Gutter drains should also be placed before closure.

# CHAPTER 24

# Adhesiolysis

*Michael S. Baggish*

Adhesions create anatomic difficulties because they blur normal tissue planes and boundaries. Adhesions may range from thin and filmy to thick and fleshy. Fibrosis may simply agglutinate one structure to another. The key points in separating adhesions are to utilize sharp dissection whenever possible and to avoid blunt dissection, because the latter frequently results in the tearing of one or both adhesed structures during dissection (e.g., when separating adhesed intestine from the uterus, it is better to err in the direction of leaving extra tissue attached to the bowel and to dissect closer to the uterus) (Fig. 24–1A–E). The author avoids energy sources when the adhesions are proximate to bowel, bladder, ureter, or larger blood vessels. The initial cut should attempt to reverse the original attachment sequence rather than create new tissue planes.

Careful and detailed inspection of visceral structures closely involved in adhesiolysis surgery is vitally important to avoid missing an iatrogenic bowel or bladder, or ureteral injury. Tubo-ovarian adhesiolysis may require magnification to avert heavy, obscuring hemorrhage. In this location, carbon dioxide ($CO_2$) laser and bipolar electrosurgery are vital tools to prevent or reduce bleeding (Fig. 24–2A–C).

Adhesions covering or enveloping the ovary are better treated by careful laser vaporization rather than by sharp dissection (Fig. 24–3A–C). Omental adhesions may require the omentum to be doubly clamped, cut, and suture-ligated to facilitate takedown. Sidewall adhesions deserve some special considerations. Ovary and tube may be "plastered" to the pelvic peritoneum (Fig. 24–4A, B). The surgeon must identify the anatomy behind the adhesions. In this instance, entry into the retroperitoneal space facilitates identification. The external iliac vein, hypogastric artery and vein, ureter, and ovarian vessels must be identified and secured from injury during adhesiolysis. Injection of sterile water with a fine needle may facilitate the development of a safe dissection plane between adhesions involving the bladder, bowel, and sidewall structure (Fig. 24–5A–D).

Adhesiolysis cannot be optimally accomplished without the use of traction and countertraction (see Fig. 24–5). The latter technique helps the clinician to identify the plane of attachment of the adhesion to a visceral structure and in turn permits the least bloody and least traumatic separation. Adhesions are obviously always best dissected from superficial (first cut) to deep (last cut). Similarly, the tip of the scissors must always be in view. If an energy device (e.g., a $CO_2$ laser) is to be used, a backstop should be placed behind the adhesion. Similarly, in this circumstance, water can serve as a backstop because it will absorb laser light (Fig. 24–6A–J).

The technique used by the author for adhesions that are layered consists of making a small, careful nick at the edge of the adhesion, insinuating a fine dissection scissors into the adhesion, and alternately spreading and closing the scissors blade to expose any structure within the adhesion before cutting it. This can also be done with a laser coupled to an adjustable backstop (Fig. 24–7). In this manner, a plane of safe dissection is established, allowing the adhesions to be transected sharply. Similarly, one can use a Touhy needle (18 or 22 gauge) to inject saline into the adhesion to facilitate separation.

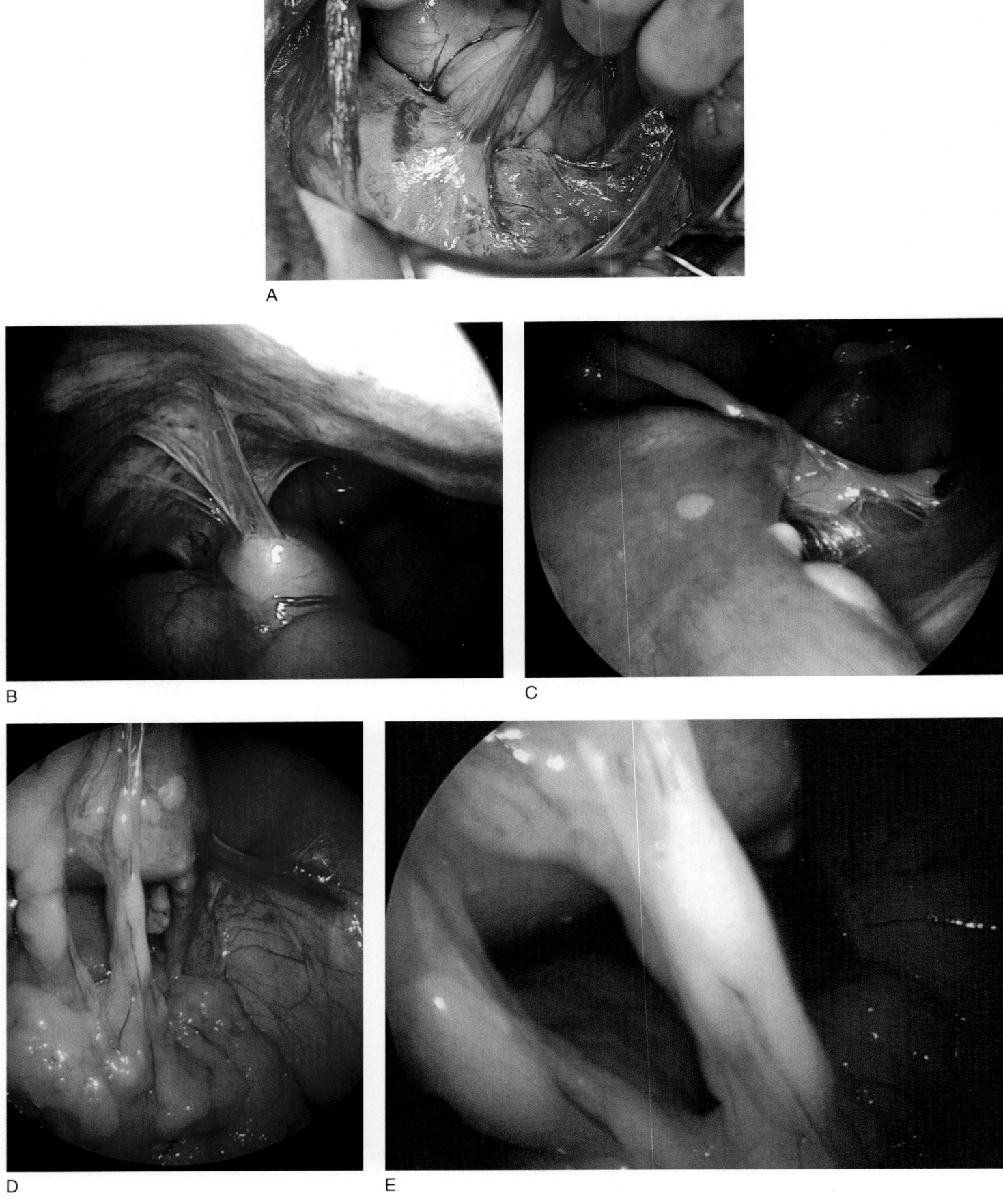

A

B

C

D

E

**FIGURE 24–1** **A.** Typical adhesions formed between the sigmoid colon and uterus, as well as between the small bowel and uterus. Note that traction produced by the surgeon's hand clearly demonstrates the attachments of the adhesions, as well as their vascularity. **B.** A thick adhesion is clearly visible in this picture. When cut, this type of adhesion may bleed because of the infiltration of parasitic and thin-walled blood vessels. **C.** Filmy and vascularized adhesions between the uterine fundus and the small intestine. **D.** Extensive vascularized adhesions between the posterior surface of the uterus and the colon. **E.** Close-up of fleshy adhesions between the uterus and the sigmoid colon.

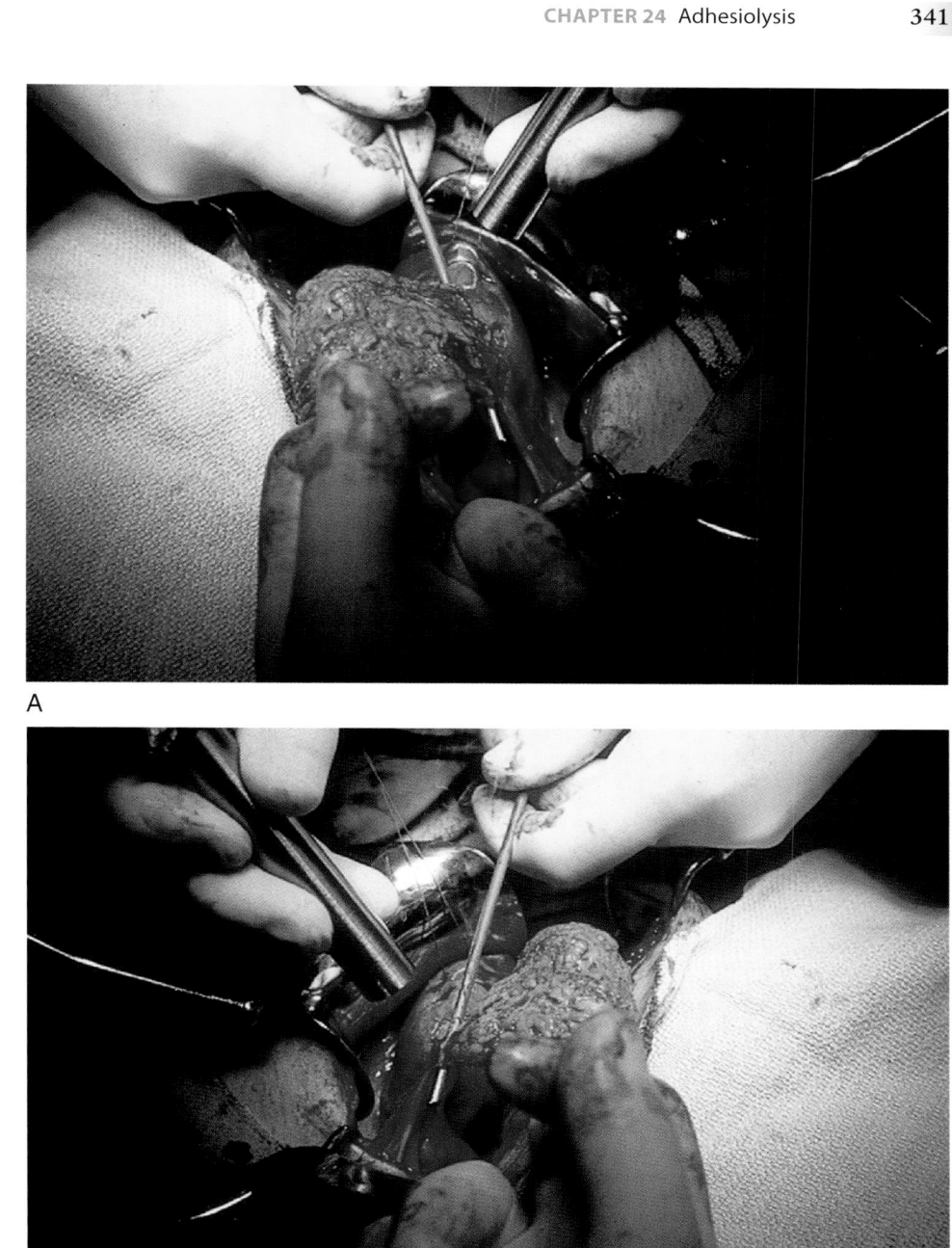

A

B

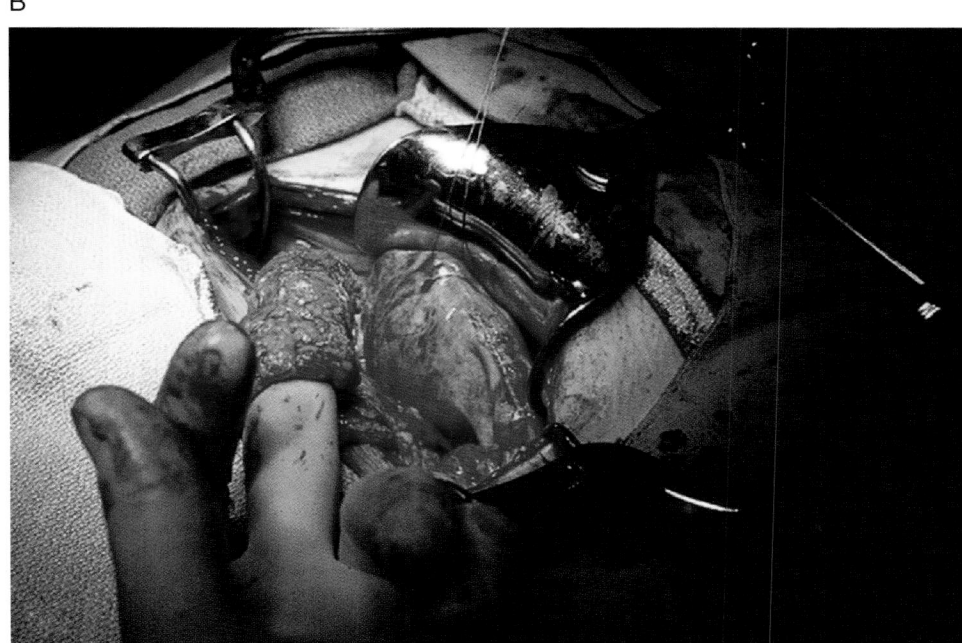

C

FIGURE 24–2 **A.** Omentum-to-uterus adhesion has been placed in traction and backstopped with a metal probe. **B.** The adhesion is divided with use of the carbon dioxide ($CO_2$) laser. The underlying colon is protected from laser beam injury by the backstop. **C.** The adhesed omentum has been neatly and atraumatically separated.

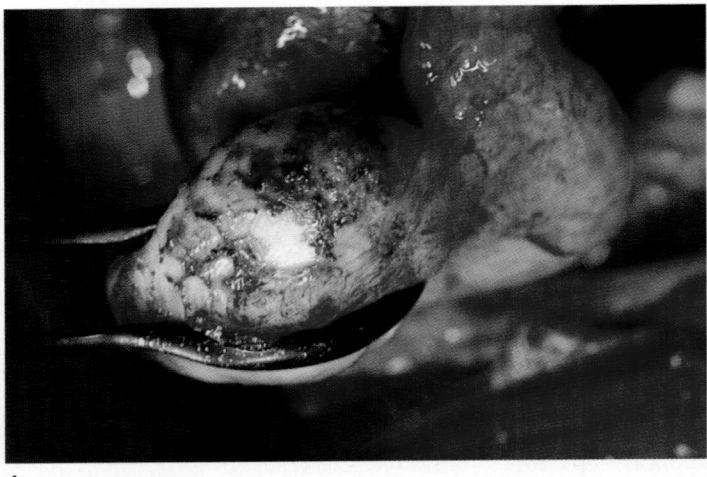

A

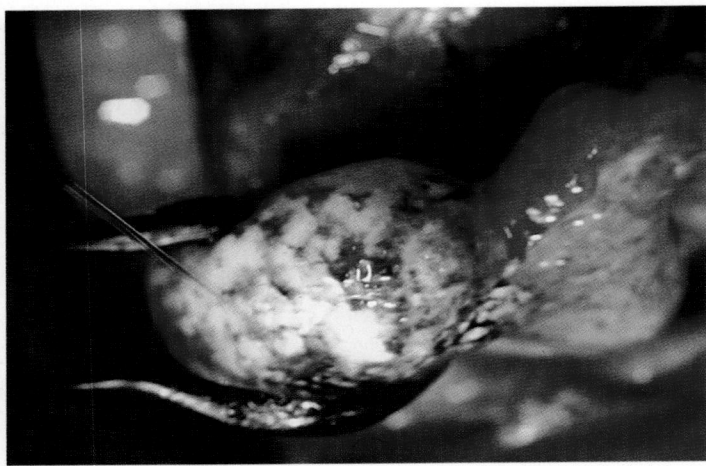

B

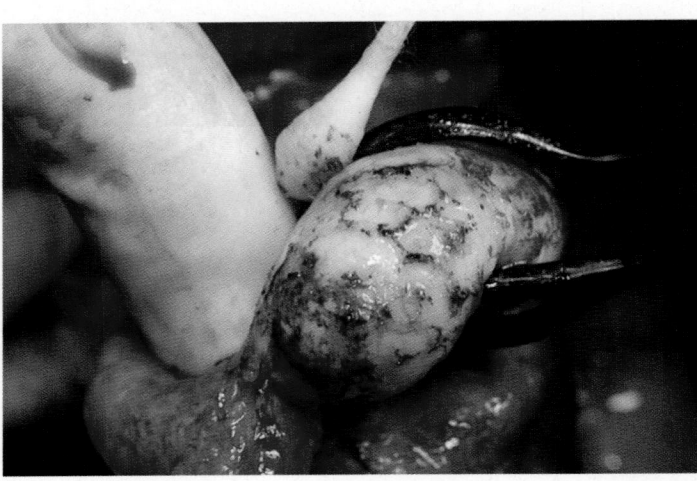

C

**FIGURE 24–3 A.** Encapsulation of the ovary by adhesions is best dealt with by tightly controlled carbon dioxide ($CO_2$) laser vaporization. **B.** Vaporization of the adhesion is virtually complete. Note that this technique preserves the (white) capsule of the ovary. A jet of the irrigation stream is seen as char is washed away. **C.** Larger pieces of the vaporized adhesions are debrided with a moistened cotton-tipped applicator.

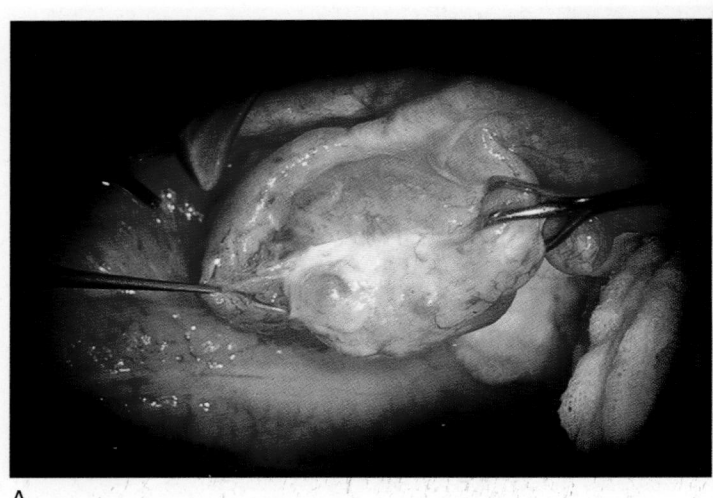

A

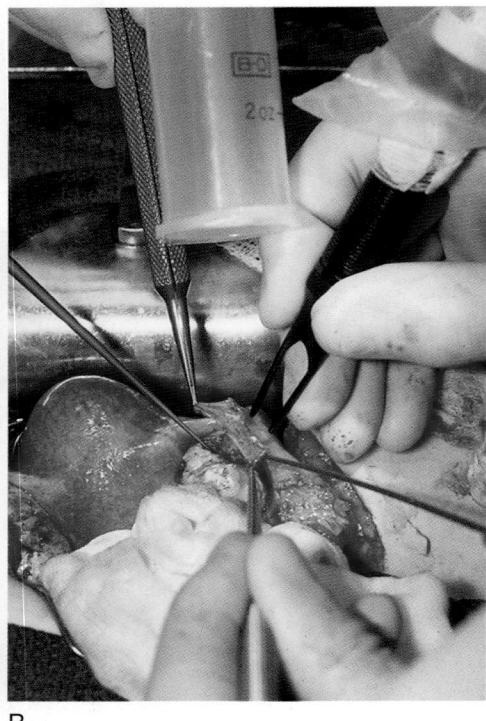

B

**FIGURE 24–4 A.** Dense tubo-ovarian adhesions are best lysed by injecting sterile water or saline beneath the adhesions to develop a plane for dissection. **B.** An energy device may be used, but it must be capable of fine incisions and minimal thermal spread. Alternatively, sharp dissection with fine scissors and fine suture-ligature to control bleeding may be used.

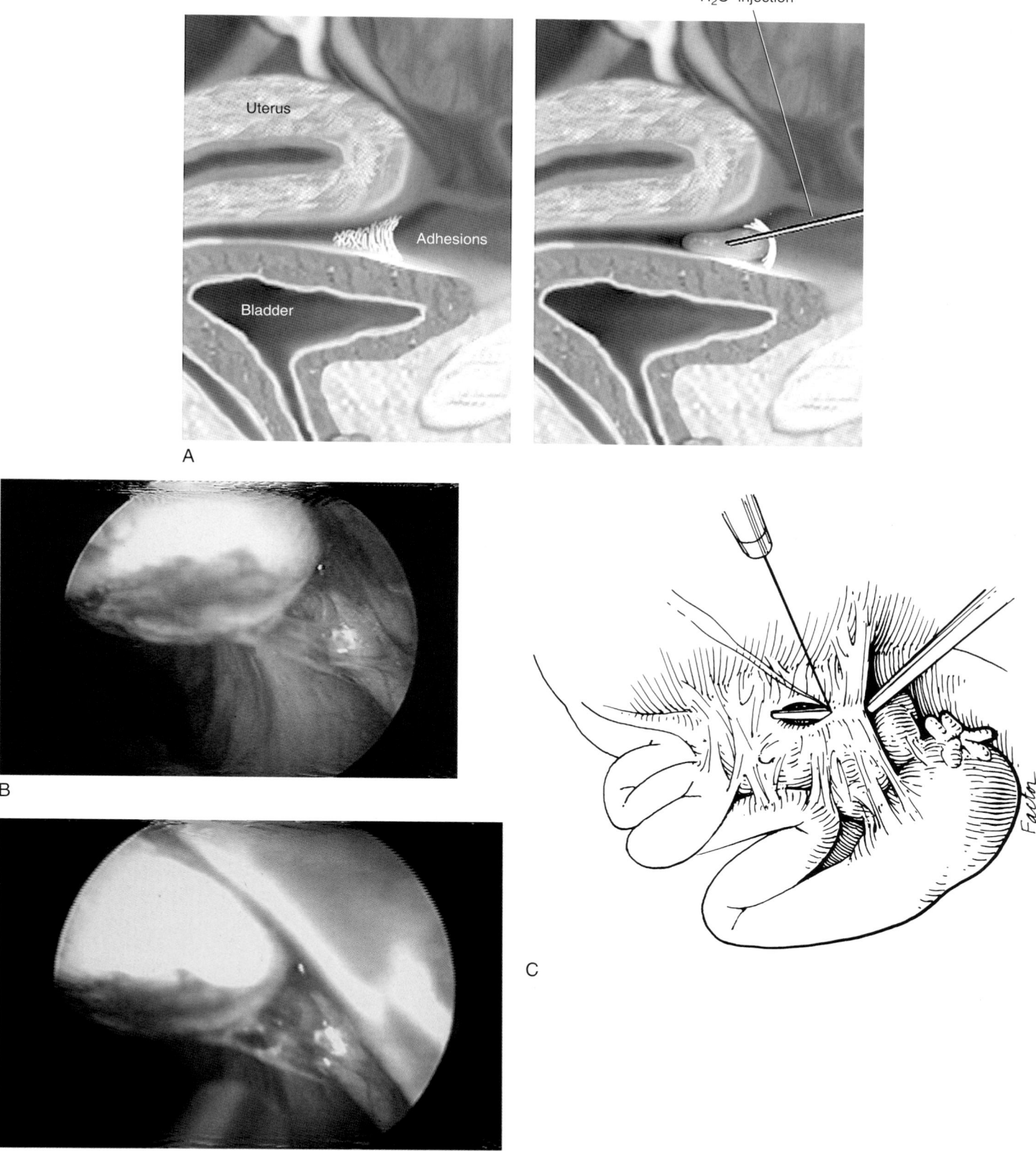

**FIGURE 24–5  A.** Sterile water is injected between dense uterine and urinary bladder adhesions to provide both a plane of dissection and a heat sink. **B.** The ovary is held down in its fossa by an adhesive band. **C.** Adhesions are cut between tube and ovary with a focused carbon dioxide ($CO_2$) laser beam with a manipulating backstop in place. **D.** The $CO_2$ laser sharply cuts the adhesion with the use of a wave guide inserted via the operating channel of the laparoscope.

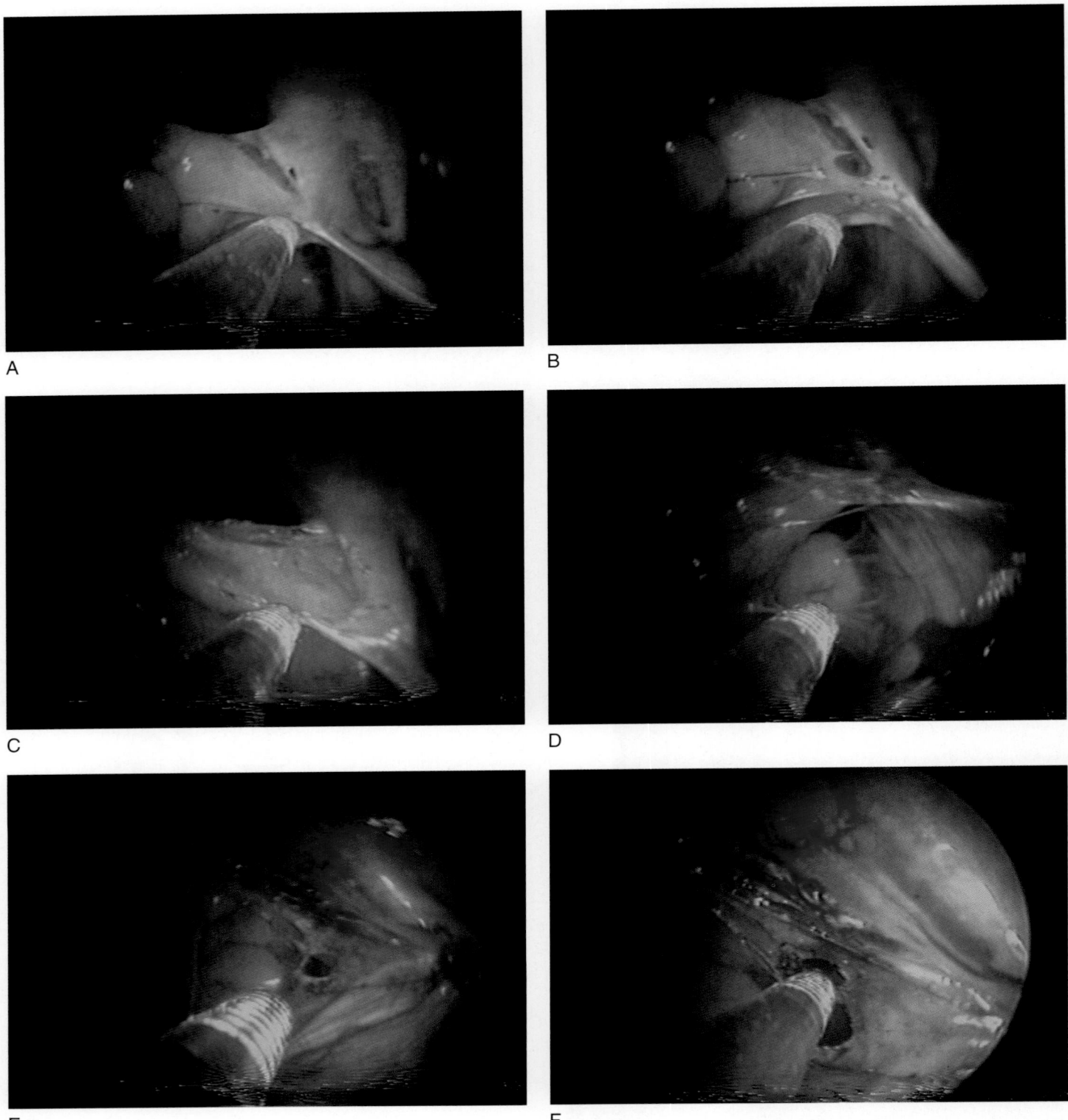

A

B

C

D

E

F

**FIGURE 24–6** **A.** Layer adhesions are identified between the sigmoid colon and the lateral pelvic wall. The tube and the infundibulopelvic ligament are seen on the far right. Traction permits the surgeon to identify the plane of cleavage. **B.** Initial cuts are made by the carbon dioxide ($CO_2$) laser beam, which is delivered by a wave guide (foreground). **C.** The adhesion (first layer) is cut close to the tube. **D.** A second layer of less dense adhesions is identified as the upper layer of adhesions is cut. **E.** The second layer is penetrated by the laser beam. The pelvic floor is protected by the infusion of water beneath the adhesions. **F.** A large hole is created in the adhesions as they are vaporized.

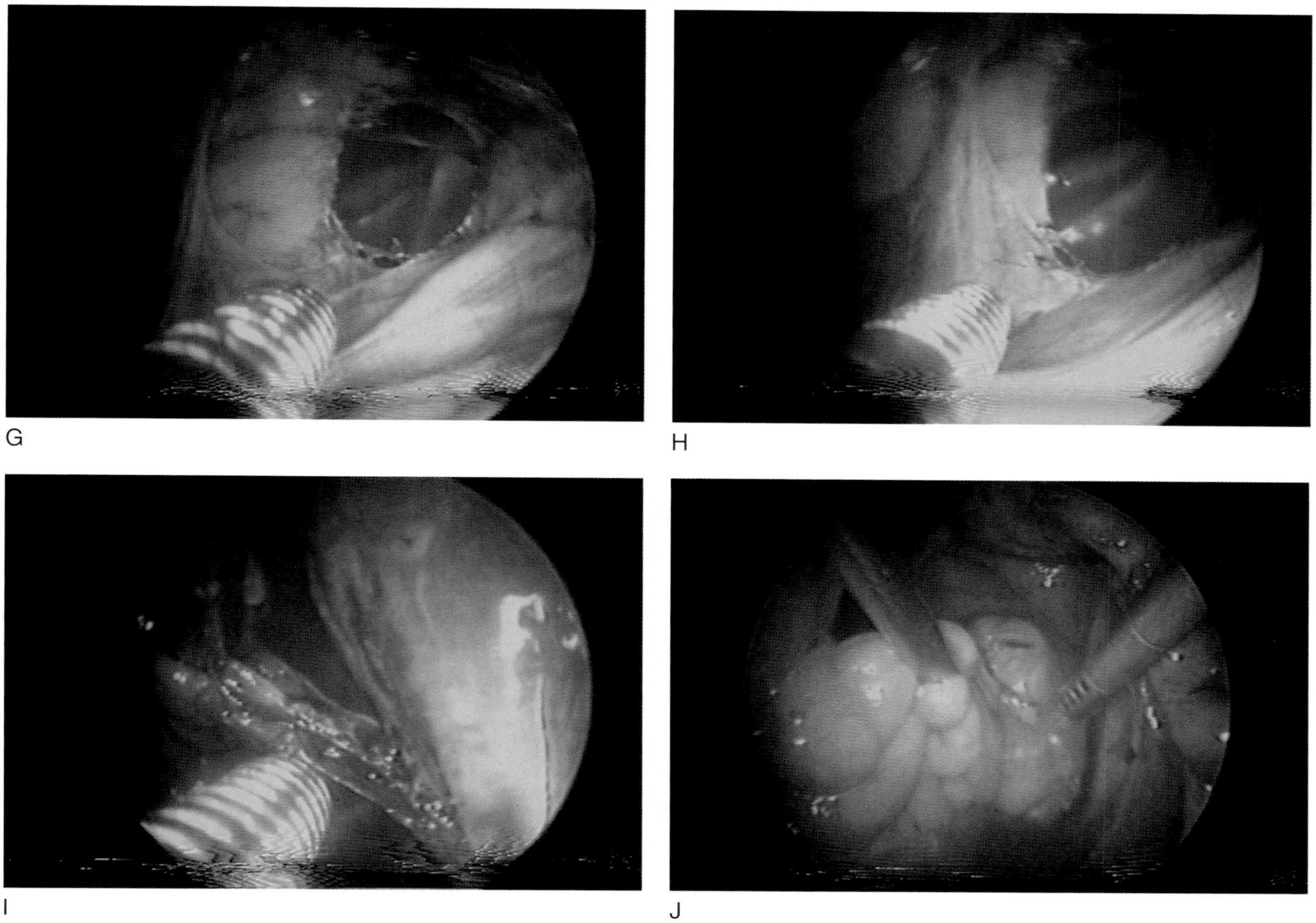

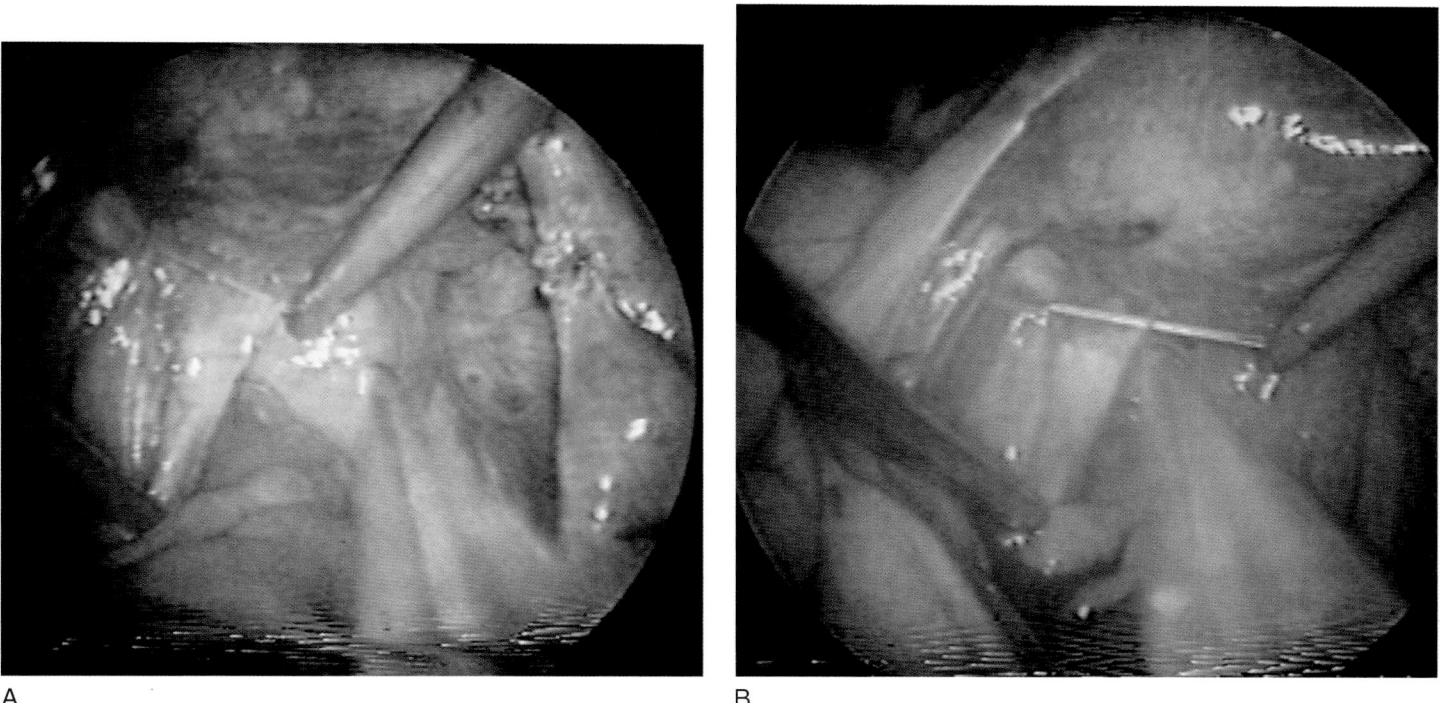

FIGURE 24–6, cont'd  G. The pelvic floor is viewed through the hole in the adhesion. H. The dissection is virtually complete. I. A final strand of an adhesion between the bowel and the bladder is cut. J. The sigmoid colon is completely free from the reproductive organs. The intestine and the uterus are awash in irrigation fluid.

FIGURE 24–7  A. The posterior surface of the uterus is adhesed to the cul-de-sac. An adjustable backstop is placed behind the adhesions. B. The adhesions are sharply cut over the backstop.

# CHAPTER 25

# Surgical Management of Pelvic Endometriosis

*Michael S. Baggish*

Endometriosis can produce cysts within the ovary as well as reactive adhesions. Endometriosis produces inflammation, sometimes exceedingly severe, in the vicinity of implants (Fig. 25-1). It is curious that the inflammatory response does not necessarily coincide with the severity of endometriosis. The appearance of pelvic endometriosis may likewise assume a variety of patterns, ranging from brownish spots to colorless microcysts (Fig. 25-2A-E).

Endometriosis surgery is performed after attempts at medical therapy have failed to resolve symptoms and eliminate visible lesions. The surgery discussed in this chapter is conservative (i.e., preserves the reproductive organs). The radical treatment strategy is removal of the reproductive organs via hysterectomy, as illustrated in Chapter 11 in Section B. A rather confusing term used indiscriminately is "definitive treatment at surgery." This phrase typically is used in reference to hysterectomy, but in fact could mean conservative management. Therefore this term would be better eliminated from usage. Surgical removal of the endometriosis with preservation of the uterus and adnexa is accomplished by sharp excision or laser surgery. The best laser for this purpose is the superpulsed carbon dioxide ($CO_2$) laser. Another acceptable laser is the KTP-532 fiberoptic laser. The least preferred device is the neodymium yttrium-aluminum-garnet (Nd:YAG) laser because it produces the greatest degree of thermal artifact (coagulation necrosis). Unless otherwise specified, the laser referenced herein will be a superpulsed $CO_2$ laser delivered laparoscopically or directly via handpiece. In strategic areas of endometriosis involvement, injection of sterile water or saline beneath implants creates a heat sink as well as a plane for dissection and serves to protect normal underlying tissue from damage (Fig. 25-3A, B).

Vaporization of implants is performed at a setting of 5 to 10 W at 100 to 300 pulses/sec and 0.1 to 0.5 msec width with a beam diameter of 1 to 2 mm (Fig. 25-4A-G). When peritoneal or tubal surfaces are to be "brushed" (i.e., very superficially vaporized), power (power density) is reduced sufficiently to permit a single cell layer or a few cell layers to be selectively eliminated (Fig. 25-5A-E). Deeper vaporization or excision may be required. The depth is determined by magnified observation of the wound. As long as siderophagic blood is emitted from the site, endometriosis is present (Fig. 25-6A-G). The most severe cases of endometriosis (stage 4) will require combinations of treatment strategies, including vaporization, excision, adhesiolysis, cystectomy, and possible partial organ excision followed by pelvic reconstruction (Fig. 25-7A-F).

Endometriosis may extend deeply into underlying tissue. In the cul-de-sac, penetration may reach the rectovaginal septum. In these instances, the tissue should be sharply resected by using a combination of laser and scissors (Fig. 25-8A, B).

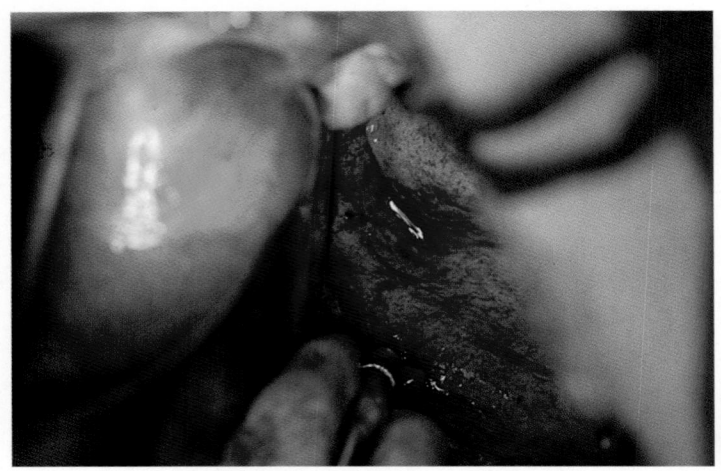

**FIGURE 25–1** Foci of endometriosis deep in the ovarian fossa. Note the extensive inflammatory reaction in the peritoneum surrounding the overt endometrial implants.

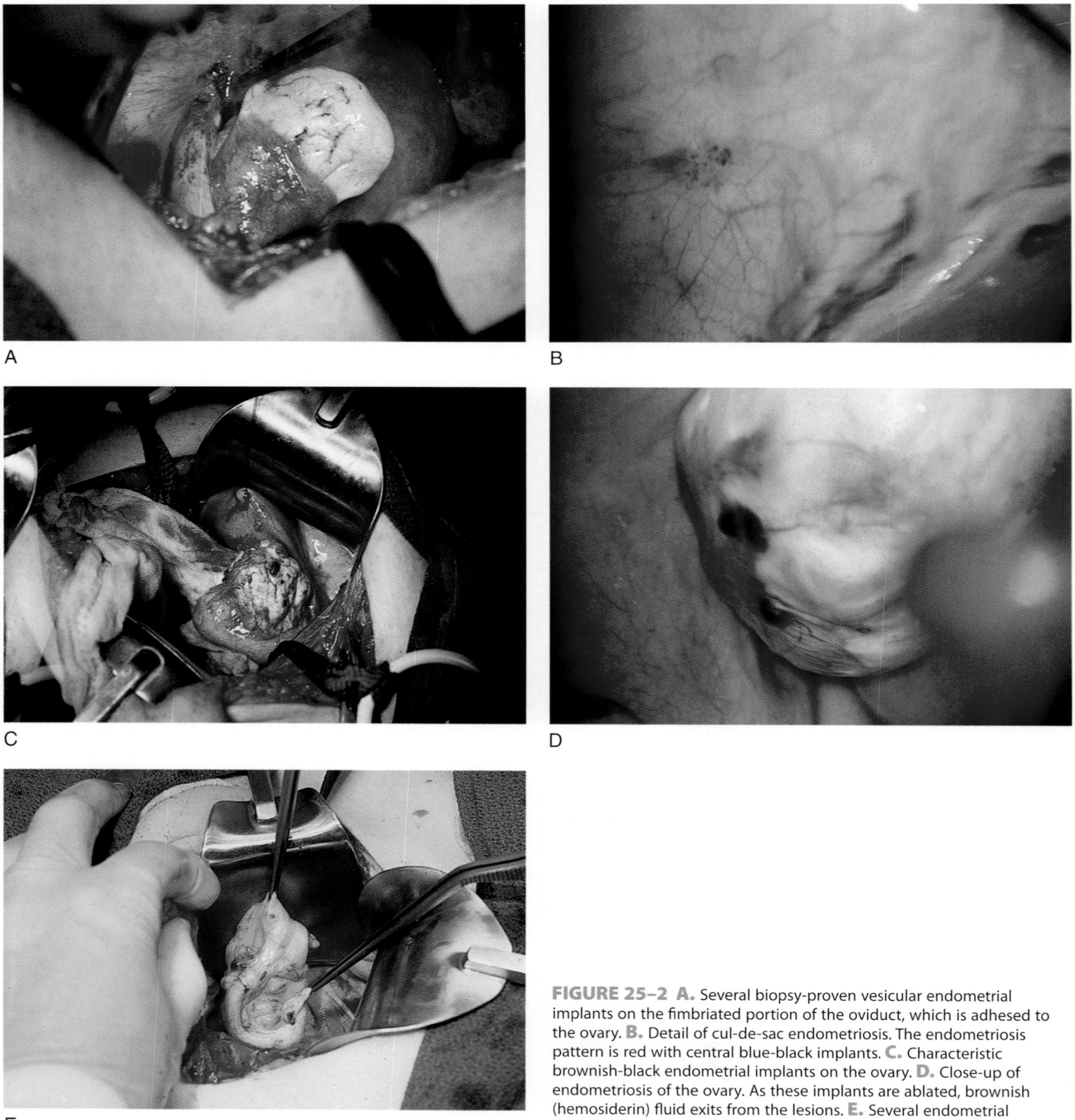

A

B

C

D

E

**FIGURE 25–2** **A.** Several biopsy-proven vesicular endometrial implants on the fimbriated portion of the oviduct, which is adhesed to the ovary. **B.** Detail of cul-de-sac endometriosis. The endometriosis pattern is red with central blue-black implants. **C.** Characteristic brownish-black endometrial implants on the ovary. **D.** Close-up of endometriosis of the ovary. As these implants are ablated, brownish (hemosiderin) fluid exits from the lesions. **E.** Several endometrial implants on the sigmoid colon create dyschezia.

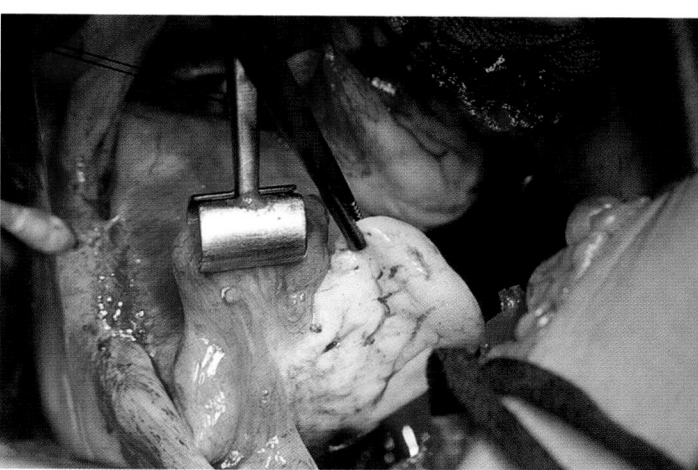

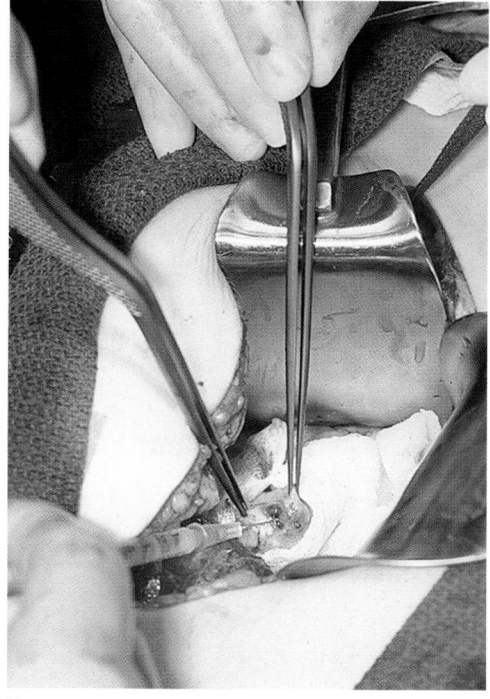

A

B

**FIGURE 25–3 A.** The left adnexa is held in the foreground. To the left, extensive endometriosis involves the urinary bladder. Scar formation resulting from the endometriosis distorts the uterus and the round ligaments, which appear to be inserted into the bladder. **B.** Sterile water is injected beneath sigmoid colonic endometrial implants with use of a 27-gauge needle. The water creates a heat sink to protect the underlying muscularis and mucosa of the intestine. The same technique is used for bladder endometriosis (see Fig. 25–3A).

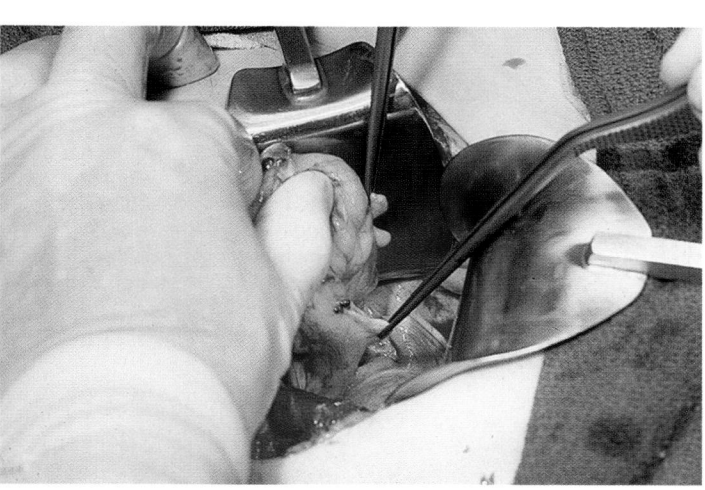

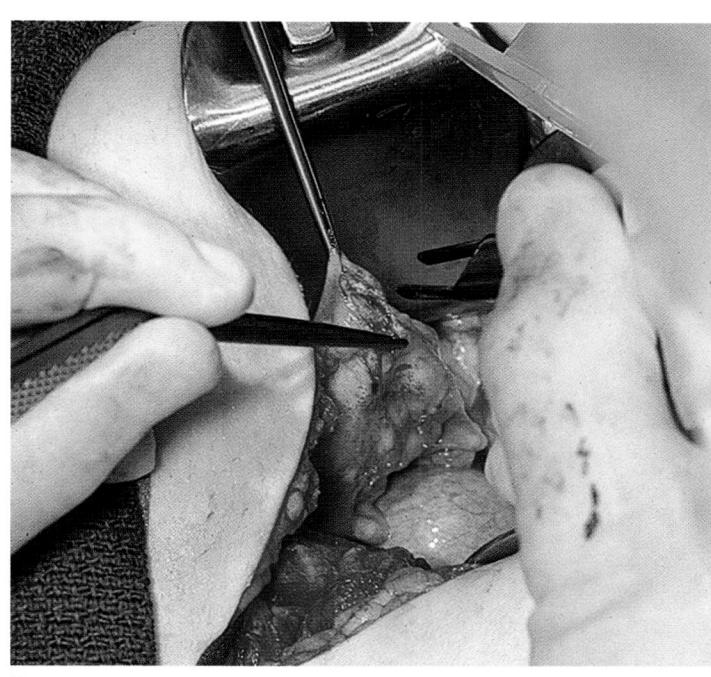

A

B

**FIGURE 25–4 A.** The colon is held in preparation for ablation (in this case) or excision of the endometriosis. **B.** The endometriosis has been vaporized from the colon (see Figs. 25–2E, 25–3B, and 25–4A).

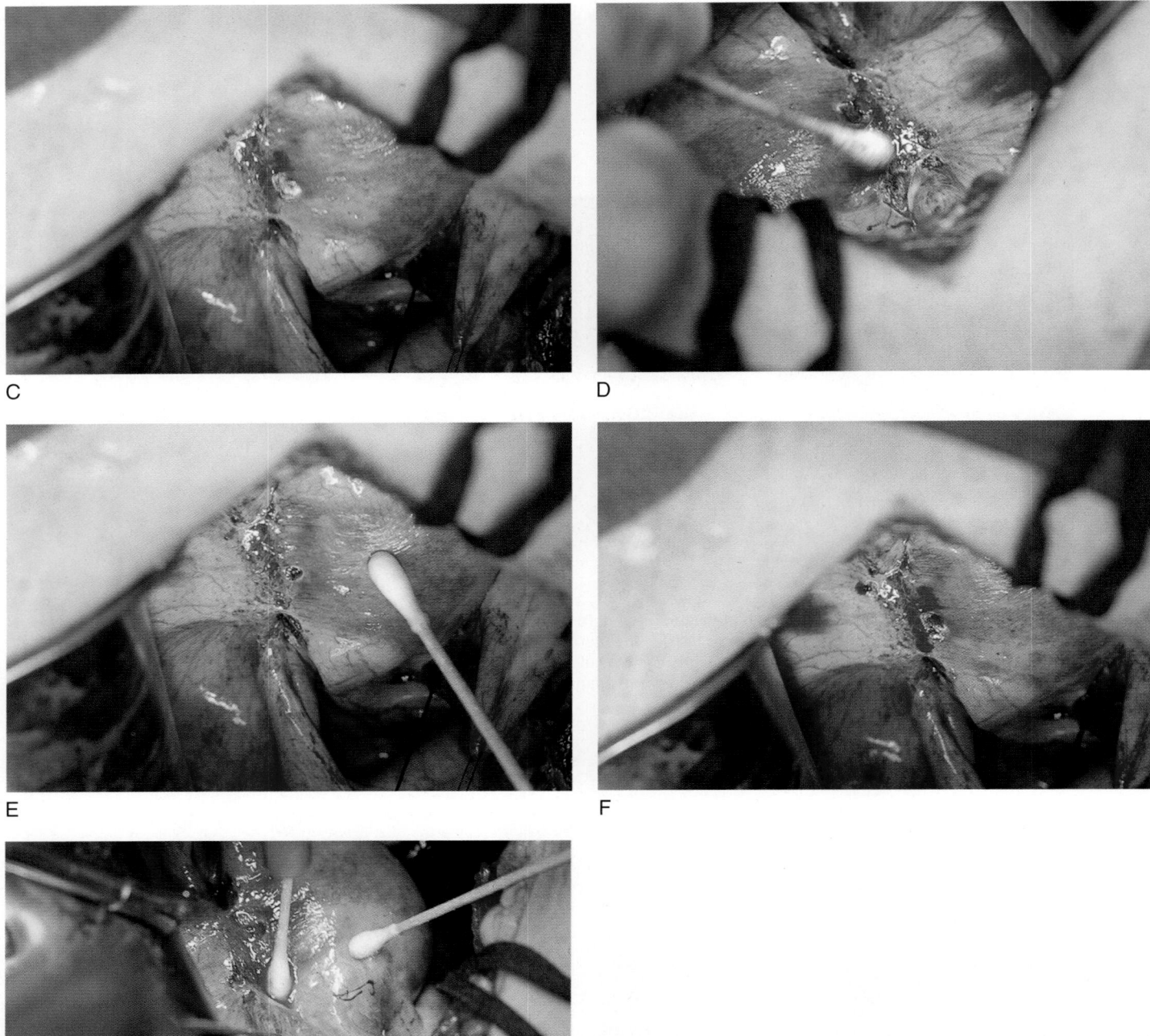

C

D

E

F

G

**FIGURE 25–4, cont'd  C.** The endometriosis of the bladder has been vaporized. Some char is present where the laser altered the implant. Note the right round ligament and the uterus, which are adhesed to the bladder (see Fig. 25–3A). **D.** Multiple bladder implants have been vaporized. **E.** Neighboring uterine endometrial implants are vaporized. **F.** Note the hemosiderin-laden fluid streaming from the round ligament implant. **G.** The bladder and the uterus are copiously irrigated upon completion of the destruction of all endometriotic implants. The wet cotton-tipped swab extricates any residual char.

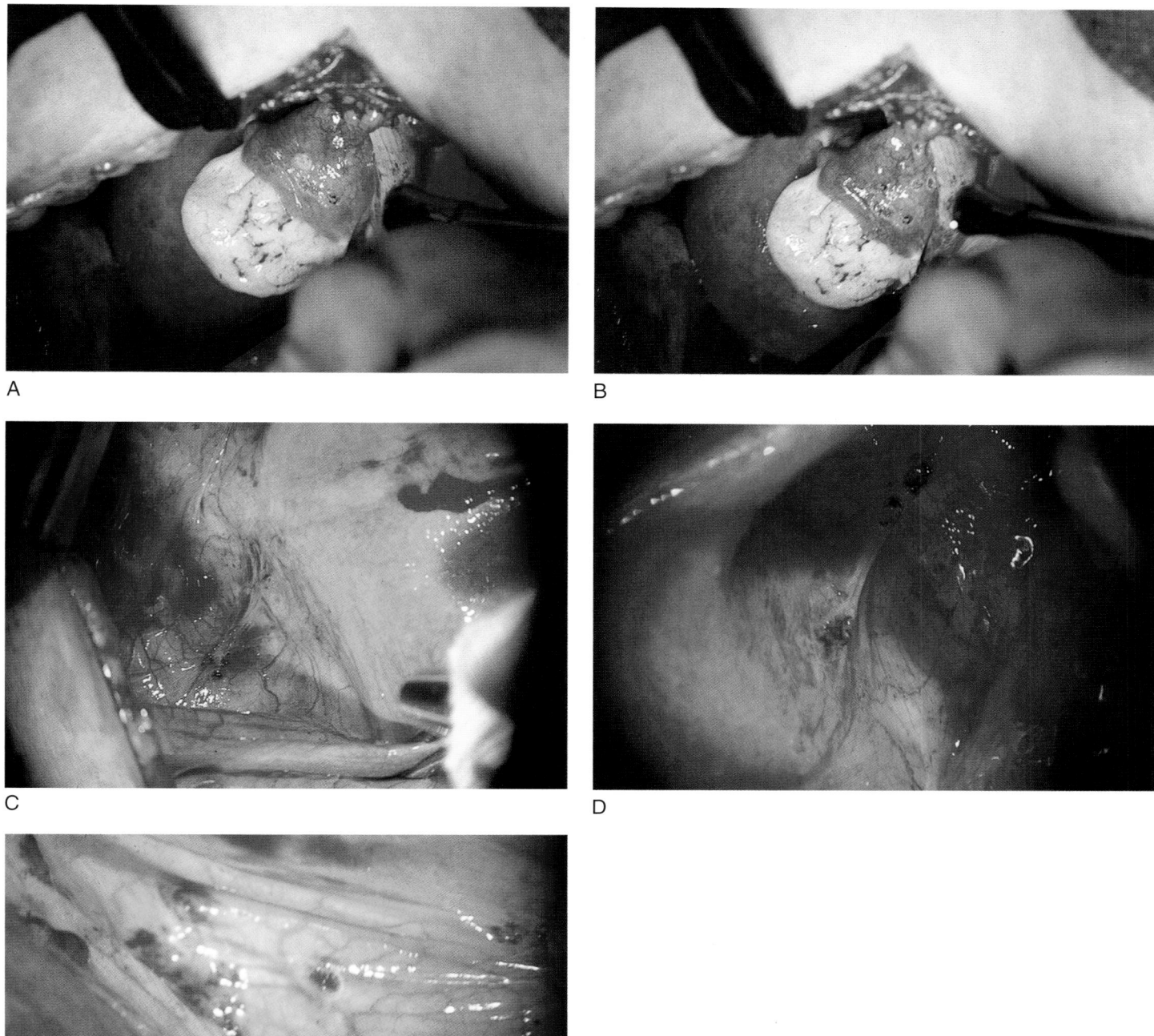

**FIGURE 25–5 A.** The vesicular (pattern) implants on the fimbrial portion of the oviduct have been carefully vaporized (see Fig. 25–2A). **B.** Upon completion of vaporization, the tube is thoroughly irrigated with normal saline or heparinized Ringer's lactate. **C.** Cul-de-sac endometriosis located in close proximity to the ureter. Injection of sterile water beneath the implants will create a plane of dissection and a heat sink. **D.** The foci of endometriosis have been vaporized (see Fig. 25–5C). **E.** Close-up view of the vaporization of the implants. The char is irrigated away as the next step in treatment of this disorder.

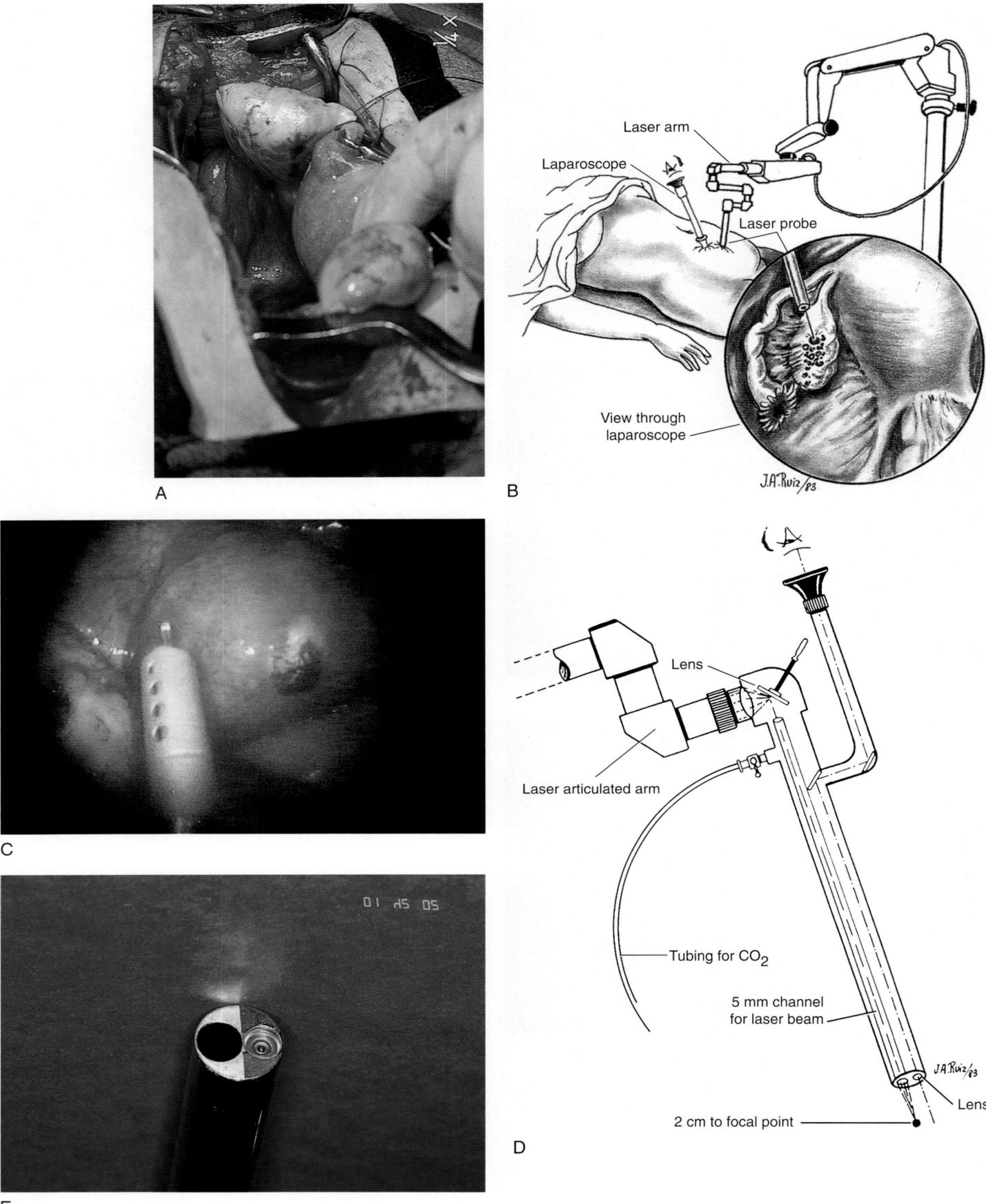

**FIGURE 25–6  A.** The left ovary not only has surface implants but also is enlarged, suggesting the presence of an endometrial cyst. **B.** Schema for a second-puncture laser probe and the laparoscopic technique for treating endometriosis. The laser may also be delivered via a wide channel built into the operating laparoscope (so-called single-puncture delivery) (see Fig. 25–6E). **C.** Laparoscopic view of second-puncture delivery of a fiber laser beam. The laser fiber is placed through an irrigating probe. Thus, irrigation and vaporization are carried out with the same device and require the use of only one of the surgeon's hands. **D.** Schema for delivering the carbon dioxide ($CO_2$) laser beam through the operating channel of the laparoscope. In this case, single-puncture delivery integrates the operating tool within a single instrument that is also used to provide light and an optical view of the operative field. **E.** The terminus of an operating laparoscope for $CO_2$ laser delivery. Note the relative size of the laser channel (*left*) compared with the optic (*right*).

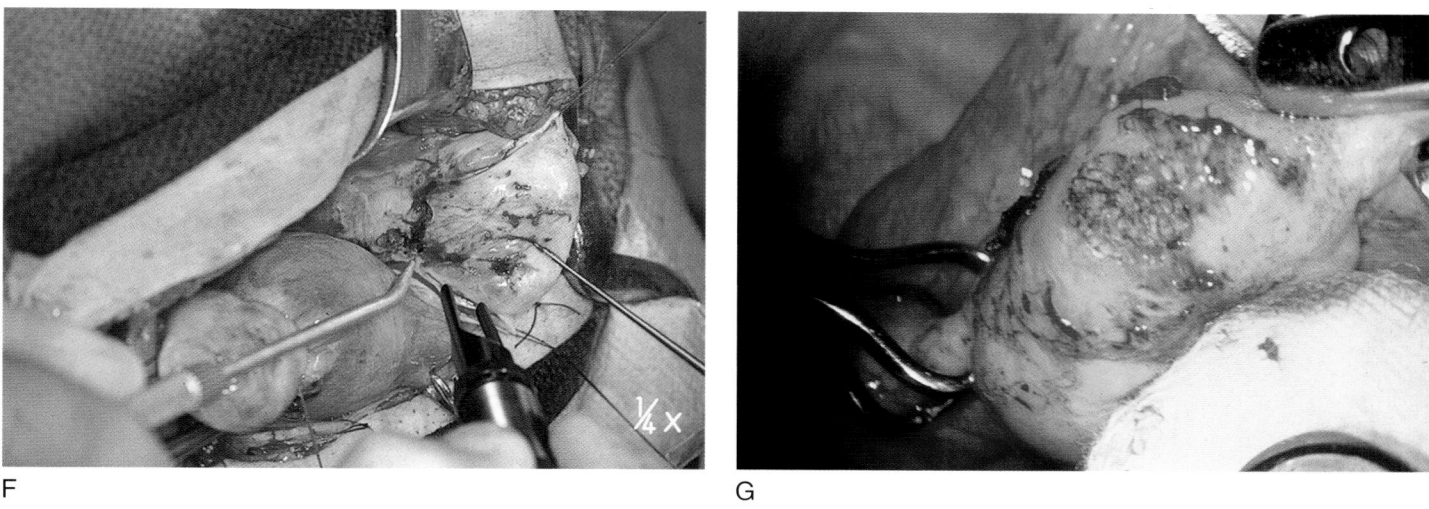

F    G

**FIGURE 25–6, cont'd  F.** Endometriosis of the ovary is vaporized by a laser handpiece. The probe points to fluid exiting a vaporized implant.
**G.** Close-up of the completed vaporization of ovarian endometriosis.

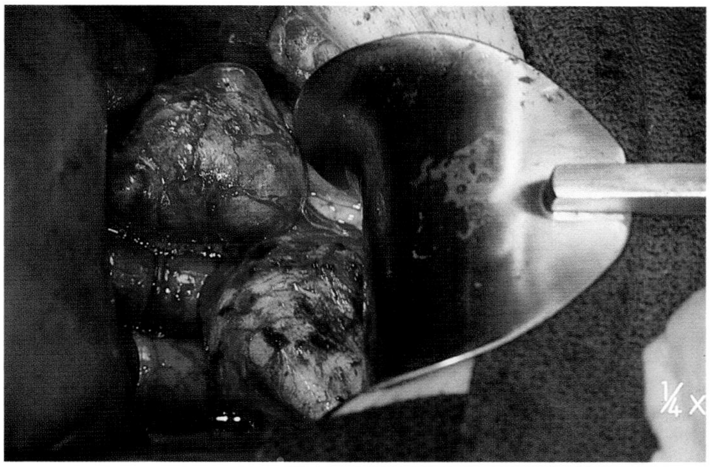

A 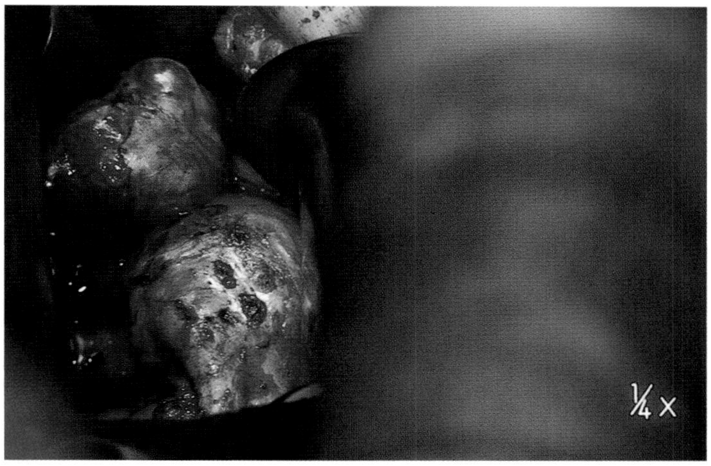    B

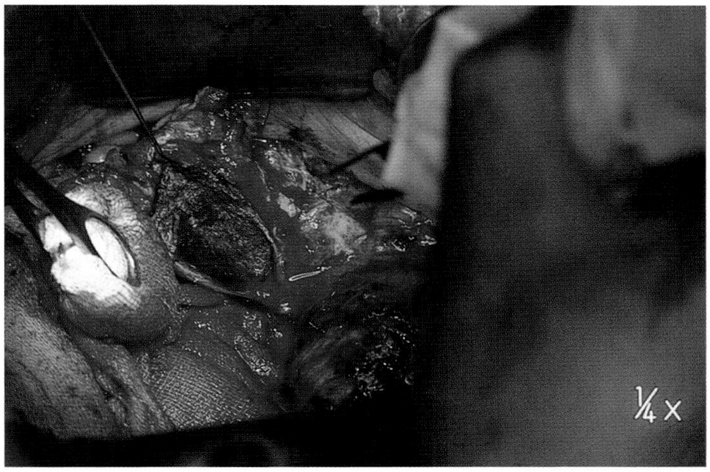

C 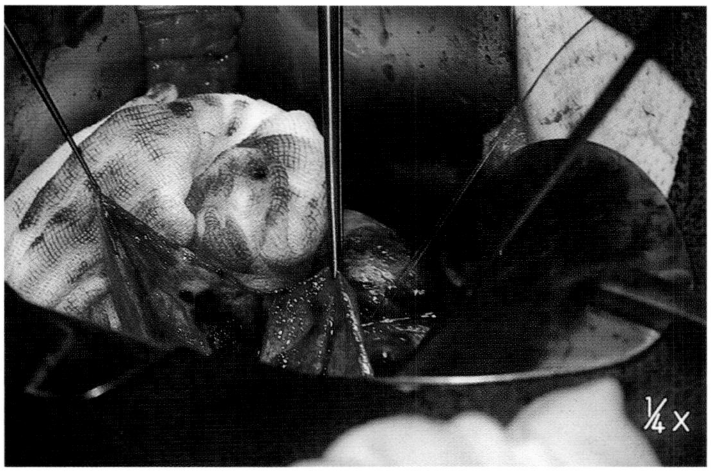    D

**FIGURE 25–7  A.** Stage 4 endometriosis. The uterus exhibits multiple implants. The ovaries have bilateral endometrial cysts. The uterus and sigmoid were densely adhesed to the cul-de-sac (these have been dissected free). **B.** The uterine endometriosis has been vaporized. **C.** Ovarian deep implants are vaporized. **D.** An endometrioma has been opened and drained. The walls of the cyst will be resected.

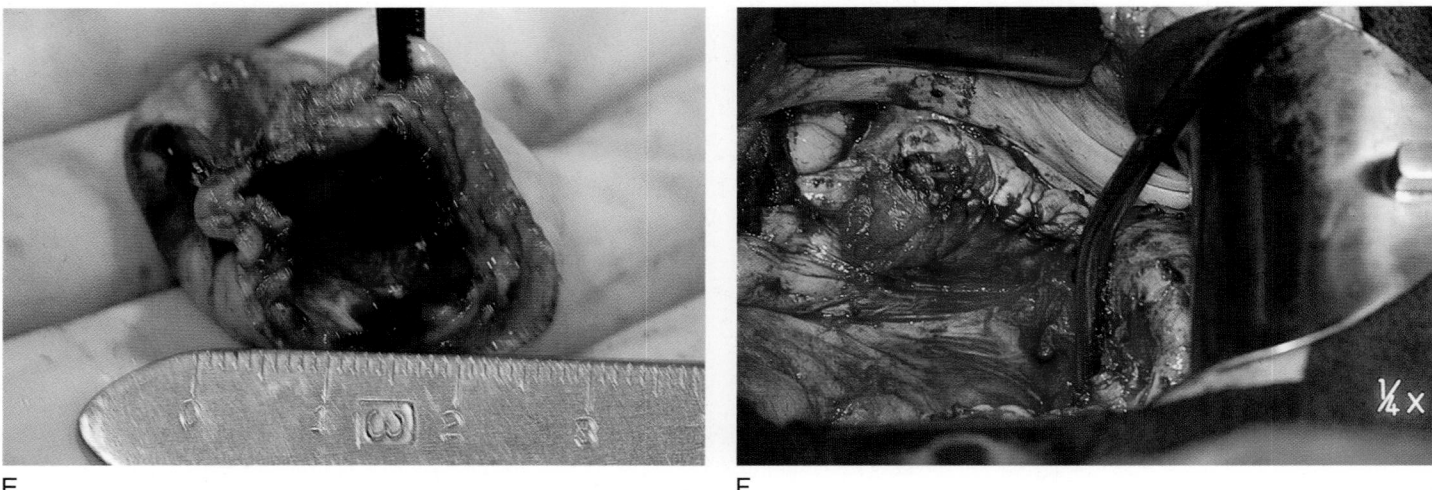

E

F

**FIGURE 25–7, cont'd  E.** The resected cyst is held in the surgeon's hand before it is sent to pathology. **F.** Approximately half of the treated ovary is conserved. The wound is closed in two layers with 3-0 and 4-0 polydioxanone (PDS) sutures.

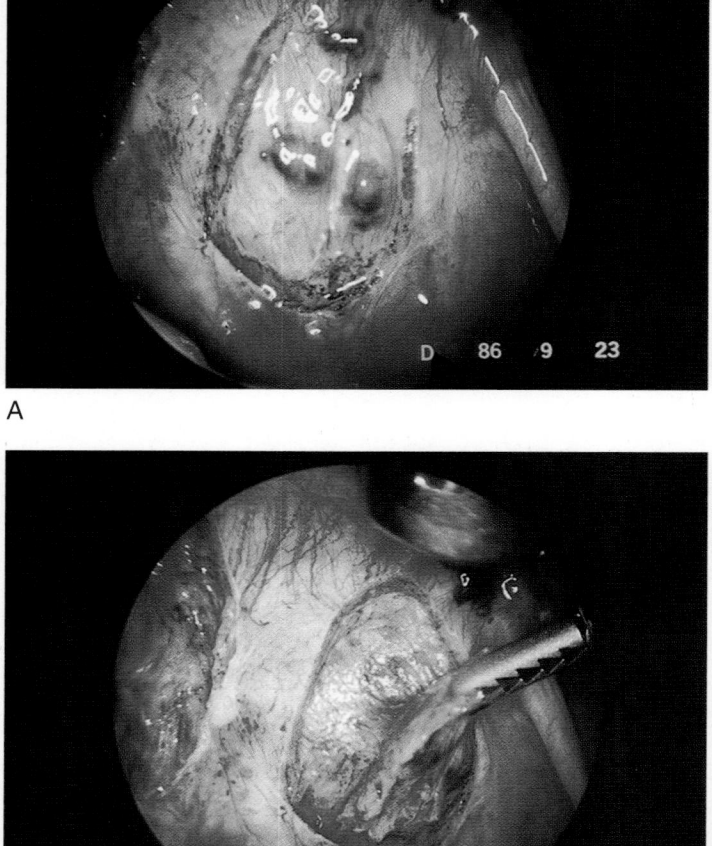

A

B

**FIGURE 25–8  A.** Deeply infiltrating endometriosis. The endometriosis has been outlined by a carbon dioxide ($CO_2$) laser. (Courtesy Dan Martin, MD.) **B.** The endometriosis has been sharply excised from the cul-de-sac. (Courtesy Dan Martin, MD.)

# Surgical Management of Ectopic Pregnancy

*Michael S. Baggish*

## Linear Salpingostomy for Tubal Ectopic Pregnancy

Ectopic pregnancy may occur in a variety of locations. A vast majority of these occur within some part of the oviduct (Fig. 26–1). The goal of early diagnosis and prompt therapy is prevention of rupture and severe internal hemorrhage (Fig. 26–2). Although most tubal ectopic pregnancies are managed laparoscopically, certain circumstances may require laparotomy. These include large tubal pregnancies, rupture with substantial hemorrhage and hypovolemia, and cornual pregnancies. The open procedure for treating a leaking or unruptured tubal pregnancy is identical to the laparoscopic procedure. A linear salpingostomy is performed as the operation of first choice. If the tube has been severely damaged or if bleeding cannot be controlled, then a salpingectomy should be done.

The affected tube is identified, as is the ipsilateral ovary (Fig. 26–3). Any blood in the abdominal cavity is evacuated. The contralateral tube and ovary are likewise examined for pathol-ogy. Next, the tube containing the tubal pregnancy is isolated via abdominal packs. A 1:100 vasopressin solution is injected (Fig. 26–4). It is wise to place traction (untied) stitches at either extreme of the bulging tube; alternatively, Babcock clamps may be applied. A trace incision is made on the antimesenteric edge of the tube with the use of an energy device (laser or electrosurgical) (Figs. 26–5 and 26–6). The incision is extended transmurally until the products of conception are contacted (Fig. 26–7).

At this point, the pressure of the blood and clot expands the opening in the tube (Figs. 26–8 and 26–9). An irrigating probe is placed into the incision to facilitate separation of the products from the wall of the oviduct (Fig. 26–10). Traction is placed on the products, and the entire mass of blood, placenta, and embryo is removed (Fig. 26–11). The bed is irrigated (Fig. 26–12). The tube may be closed in one layer using 3-0 or 4-0 Vicryl, or the wound edges may be simply approximated and allowed to seal spontaneously (Figs. 26–13 through 26–17).

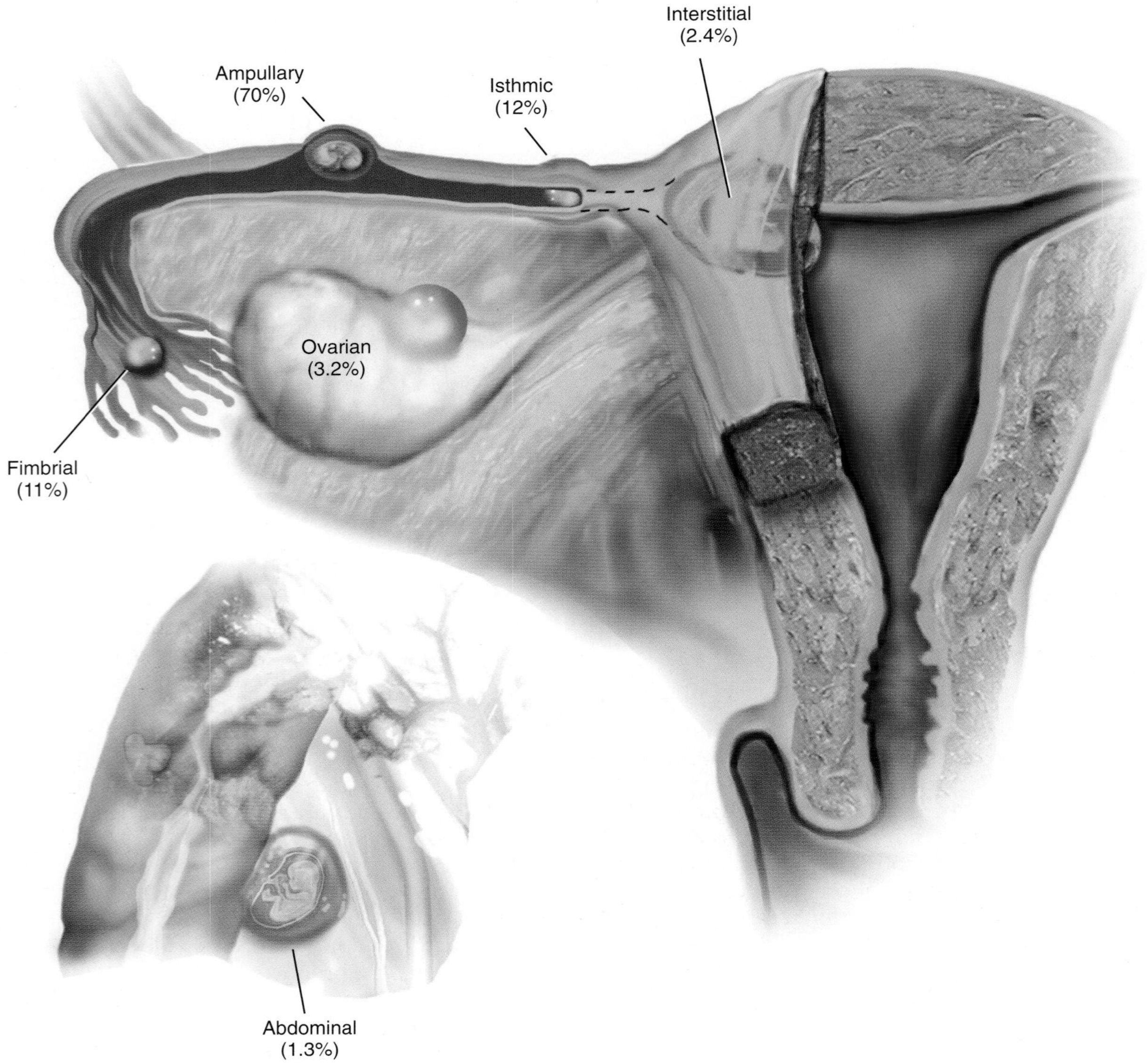

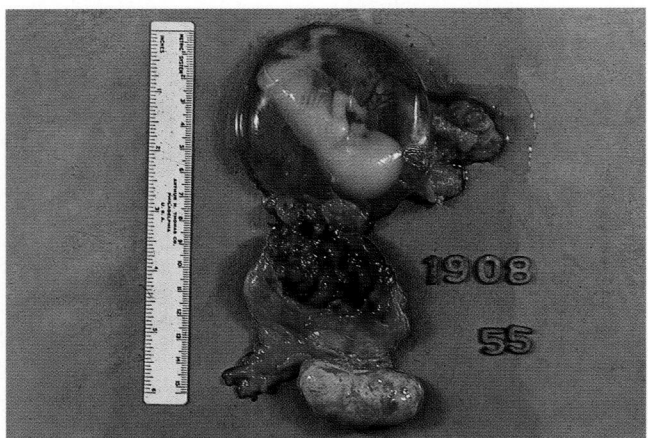

**FIGURE 26–1** This schematic drawing illustrates the various intra-abdominal sites and their relative frequencies for ectopic pregnancy.

Ampullary
(70%)

Isthmic
(12%)

Interstitial
(2.4%)

Ovarian
(3.2%)

Fimbrial
(11%)

Abdominal
(1.3%)

**FIGURE 26–2** This ruptured ectopic pregnancy implanted on the mesentery of the ileum. When the abdominal pregnancy was diagnosed, the fetus had grown to 14 weeks' gestational size.

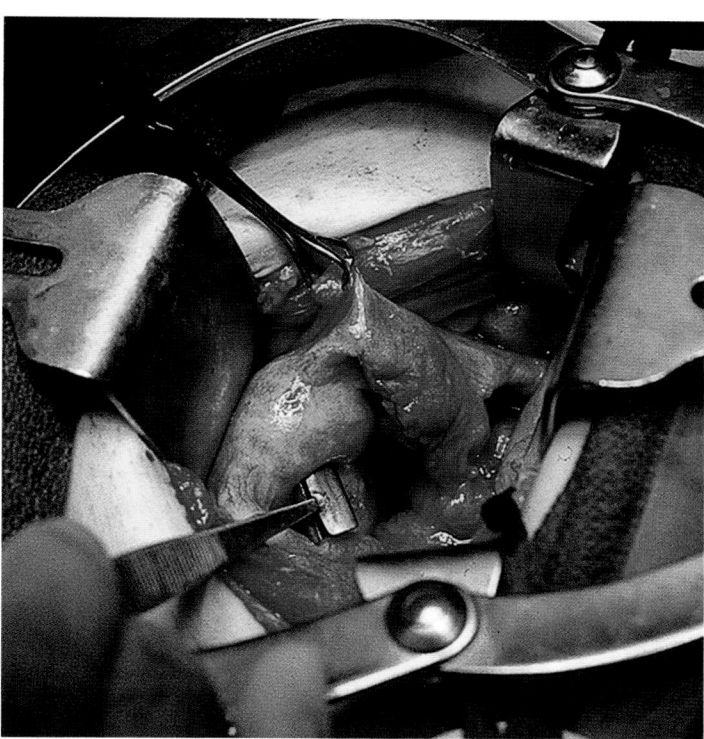

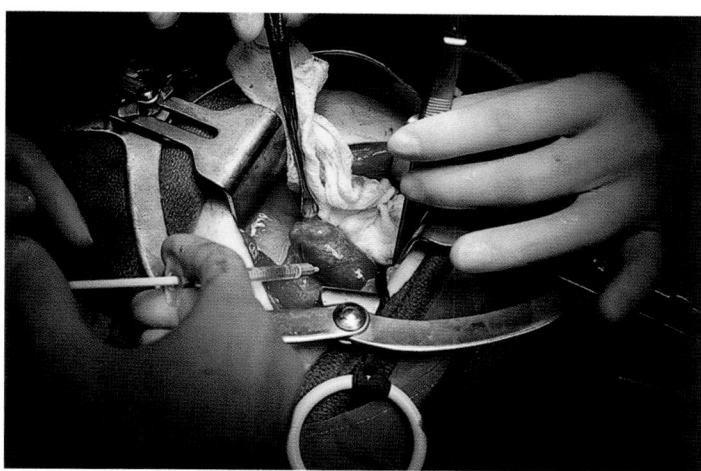

**FIGURE 26-4** The oviduct is injected with 1:100 vasopressin solution. The surgical site is injected to induce vasoconstriction.

**FIGURE 26-3** The right oviduct is grasped and elevated to reveal a swollen ampullary portion of the tube.

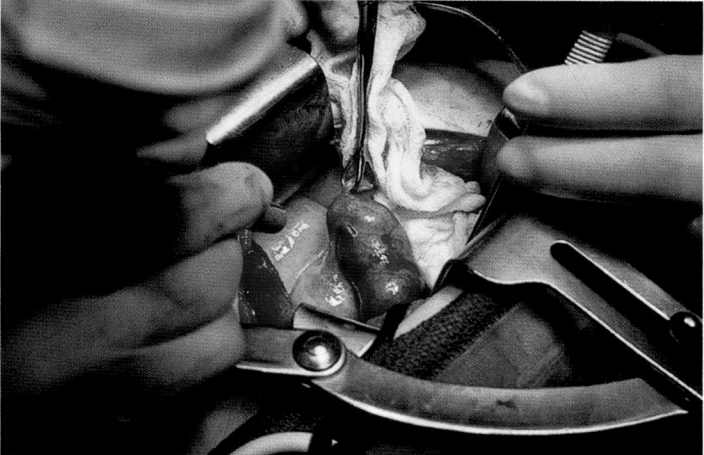

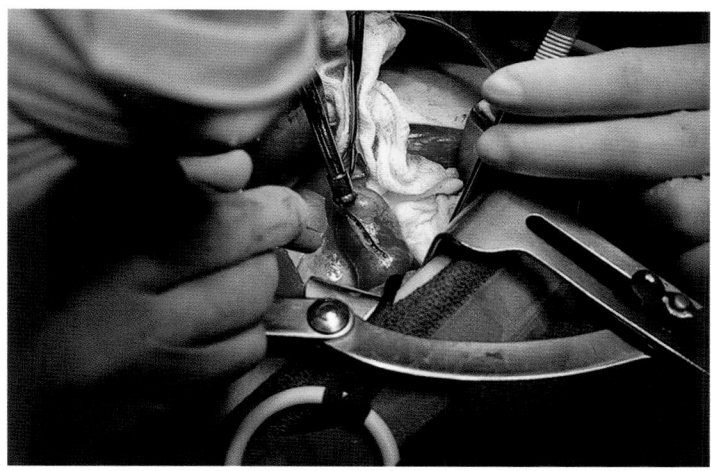

**FIGURE 26-5** The antimesenteric surface is opened with an energy device (laser or electrosurgical) for purposes of hemostasis. In this case, a carbon dioxide ($CO_2$) laser is used.

**FIGURE 26-6** The incision is linear and measures between 1 and 2 cm in length.

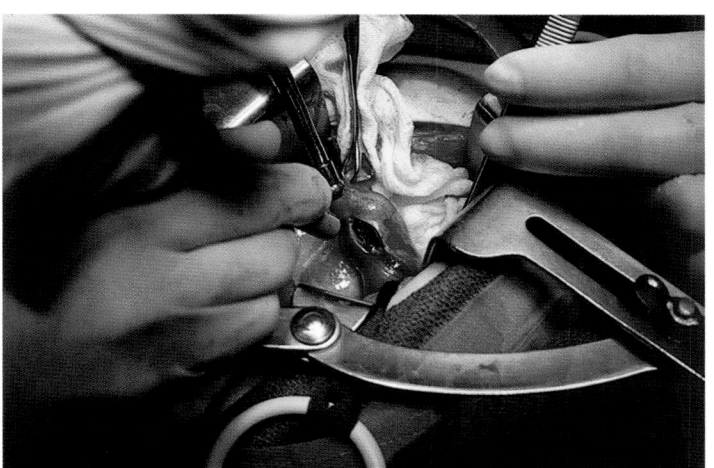

**FIGURE 26-7** As the tubal lumen is encountered, the pressure of the blood spreads the incision.

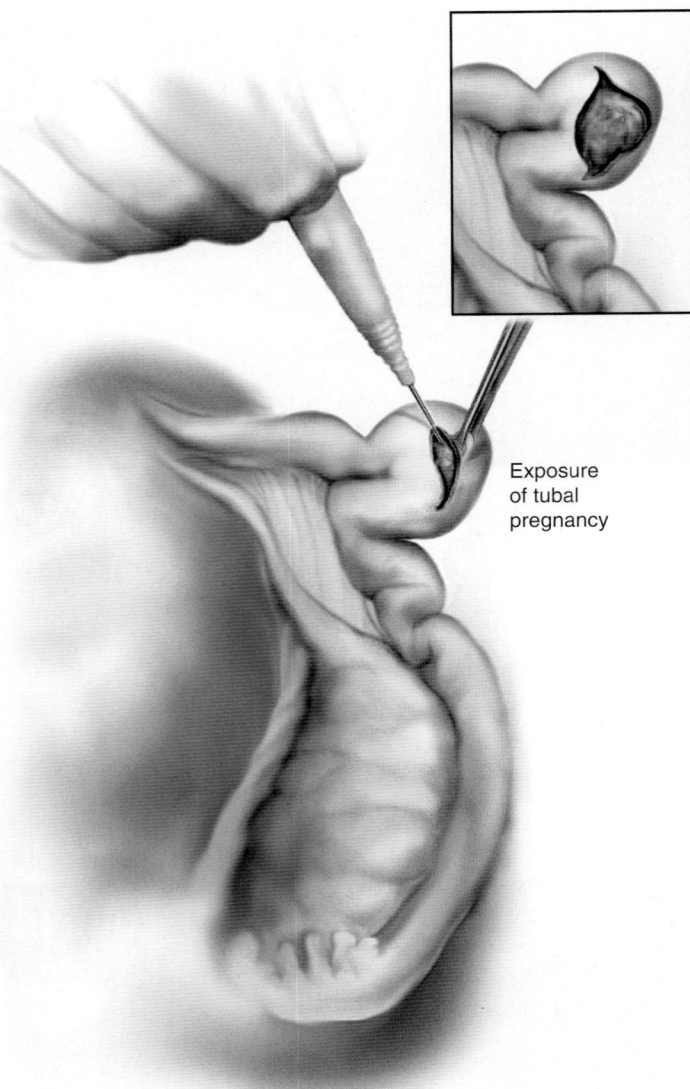

Exposure
of tubal
pregnancy

**FIGURE 26–8** Alternatively, an electrosurgical handpiece equipped with a needle electrode may be used to perform the salpingostomy. The net effect is similar to that produced by the carbon dioxide ($CO_2$) laser.

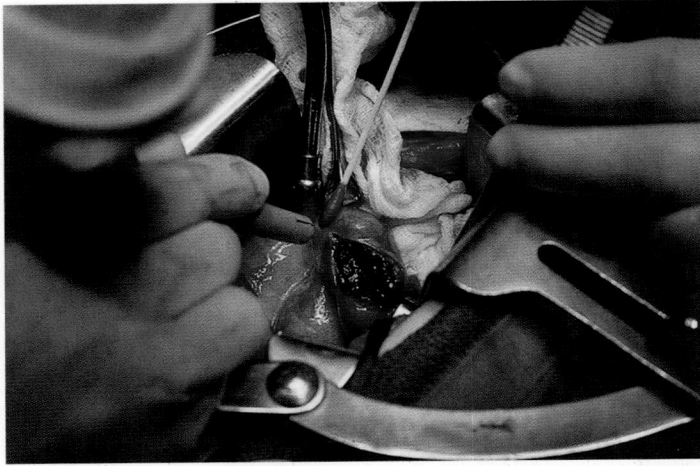

**FIGURE 26–9** Typically, the tubal pregnancy presents as a large blood clot within the lumen.

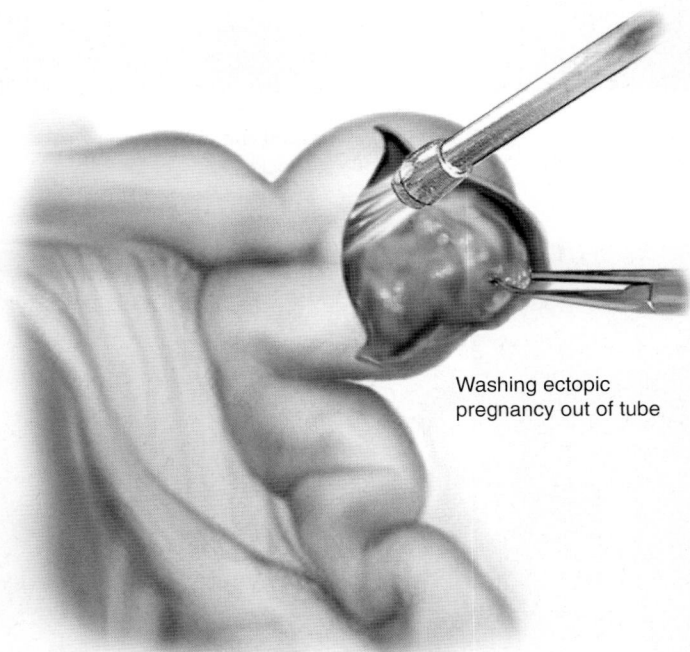

Washing ectopic
pregnancy out of tube

**FIGURE 26–10** A small cannula is inserted into the incision, and the pressure of the irrigating solution dislodges the products of conception from the tube wall.

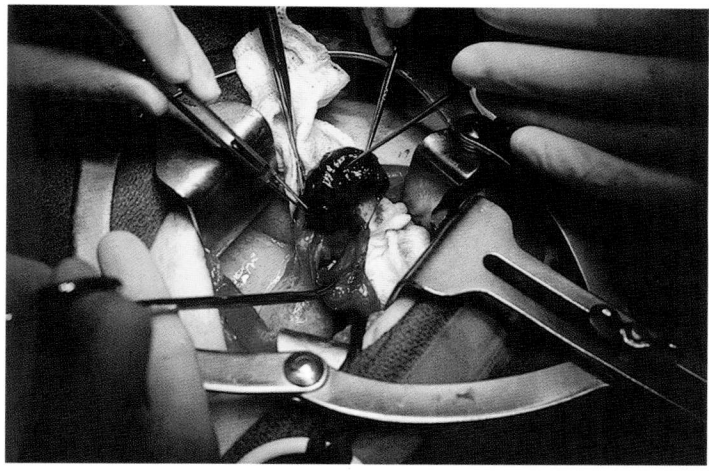

**FIGURE 26–11** With the use of fine manipulating hooks or forceps, the entire ectopic pregnancy is removed en masse.

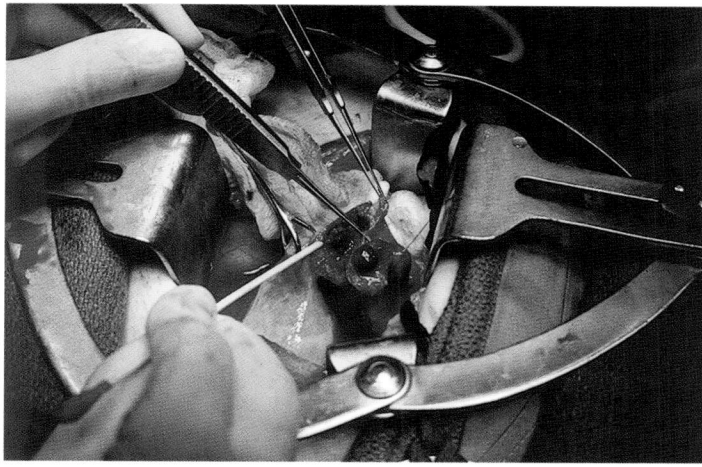

**FIGURE 26–12** The tubal bed is typically dry but should be irrigated with saline to check for bleeding. The repair may be initiated.

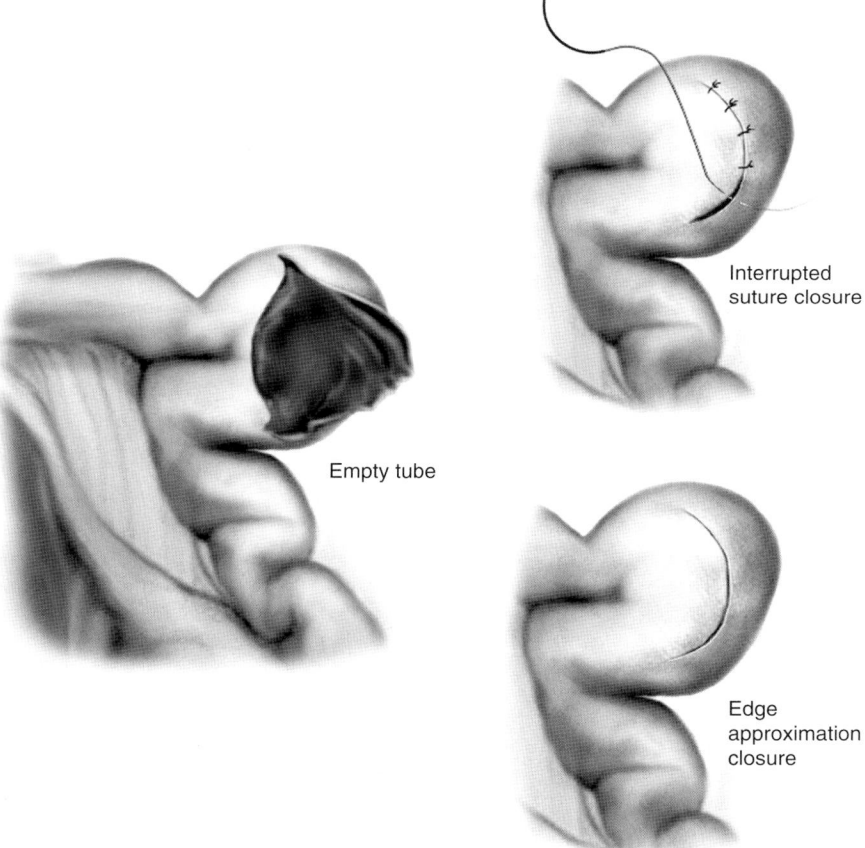

Empty tube

Interrupted suture closure

Edge approximation closure

**FIGURE 26–13** The incision may be closed with 4-0 Vicryl, interrupted through-and-through, simple sutures, or the edges of the incision may be simply pulled together and allowed to seal spontaneously.

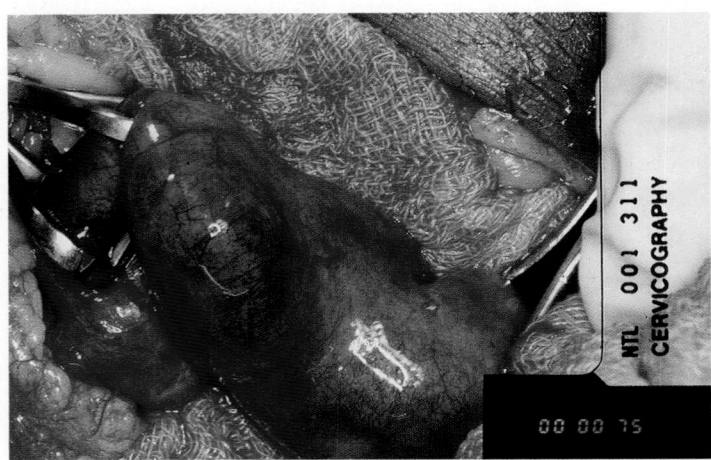

**FIGURE 26–14** Unruptured ectopic pregnancy within the ampullary portion of the tube. Two Babcock clamps isolate the affected tubal segment.

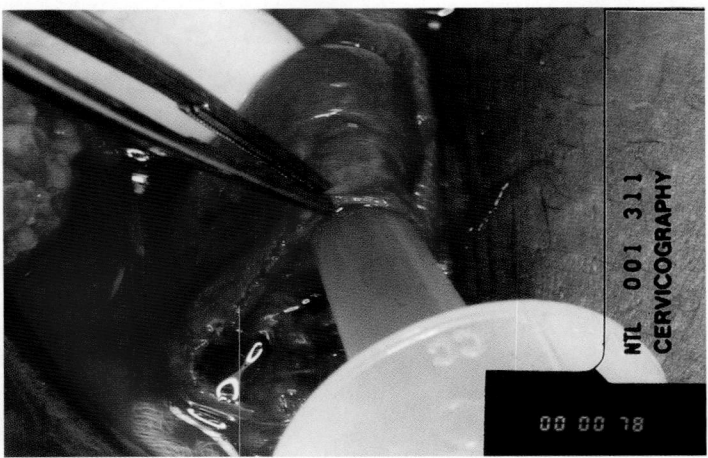

**FIGURE 26–15** A salpingostomy has been performed, and the products have been extracted. The tube and the ectopic bed are irrigated with warmed saline.

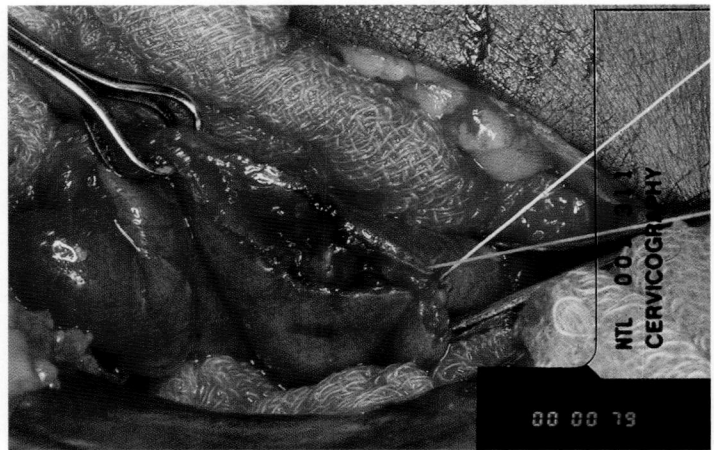

**FIGURE 26–16** The linear incision in the oviduct will be closed, in this case with the use of 4-0 Vicryl.

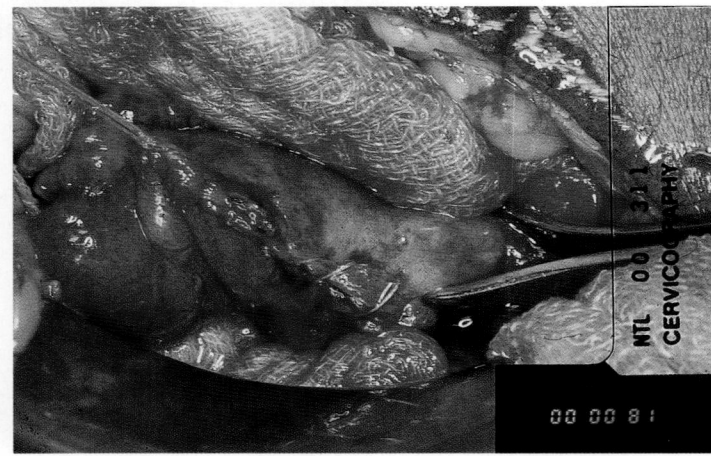

**FIGURE 26–17** The incision has been closed with simple interrupted stitches.

## Cornual Excision and Salpingectomy for Cornual Ectopic Pregnancy

This abnormal implantation occurs in the interstitial portion of the oviduct and has a high potential for very serious hemorrhage related to the greater size of the ectopic pregnancy, the rich vascular network formed by the anastomosis of the uterine and ovarian arteries, and the later gestational age of the conceptus at the time of diagnosis (Fig. 26–18A, B). Cornual pregnancies account for 2.6% of all ectopic pregnancies and present a five times greater risk for fatality (i.e., 2.5% maternal mortality) (Fig. 26–19).

The affected tube is grasped with Babcock clamps. The mesosalpinx is doubly clamped and incised between the two clamps along its entire length. The clamped pedicles are suture-ligated on either side with 0 Vicryl. The ovary may be preserved by avoiding the infundibulopelvic and utero-ovarian ligaments (Fig. 26–20).

When the tubouterine junction is reached, a figure-of-8 suture of 1 Vicryl or polydioxanone (PDS) is placed so as to encompass the bulging mass of the cornual pregnancy.

A 1:200 vasopressin solution (10 to 15 mL) is injected into the cornua.

With a scalpel or energy device, the cornual pregnancy is wedged out of the uterus (Fig. 26–21). Simultaneously, the previously placed figure-of-8 suture is tightened to control bleeding. When the entire tubal mass has been excised, several pumping arterioles will have to be secured by clamping and suture ligatures. The large figure-of-8 suture is then tied (Fig. 26–22). The cornual portion of the uterus is further secured by placing three or four additional figure-of-8 sutures through the serosa and myometrium (Fig. 26–23).

The uterus is peritonized and supported by placement of a U-shaped stitch from the cornual resection site through the ipsilateral round ligament. As the suture is tightened and tied into place, a knuckle of round ligament and peritoneum is pulled over to cover the operative site (see Fig. 26–23).

Rudimentary horn pregnancy occurs rarely, that is, in 1 of 100,000 pregnancies. This condition is attributed to pregnancy occurring in a noncommunicating horn of a bicornuate uterus. Rupture risk is high, and outcomes are similar to those for ruptured cornual pregnancy (Figs. 26–24 and 26–25).

UNIT 2 ■ SECTION D

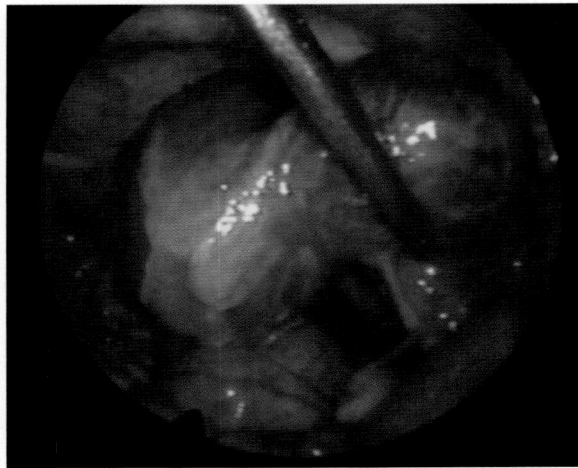

A

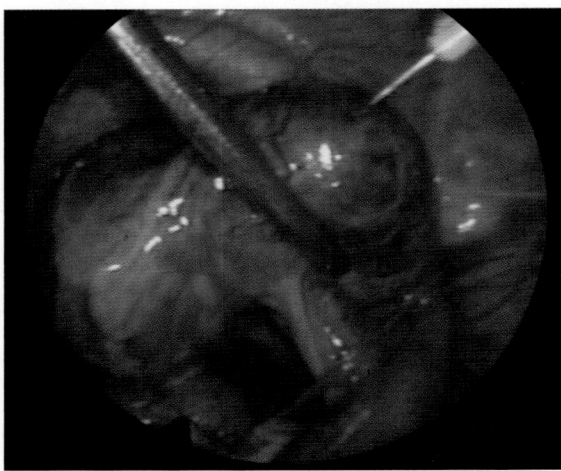

B

**FIGURE 26–18  A.** An interstitial pregnancy presents as a bulge in the cornual region of the uterus. **B.** Laparoscopic view of an unruptured right cornual pregnancy.

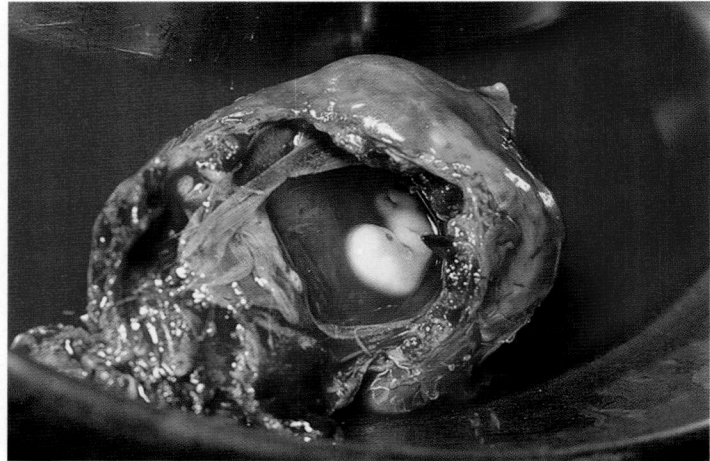

**FIGURE 26–19**  This large cornual pregnancy clearly shows the site of rupture.

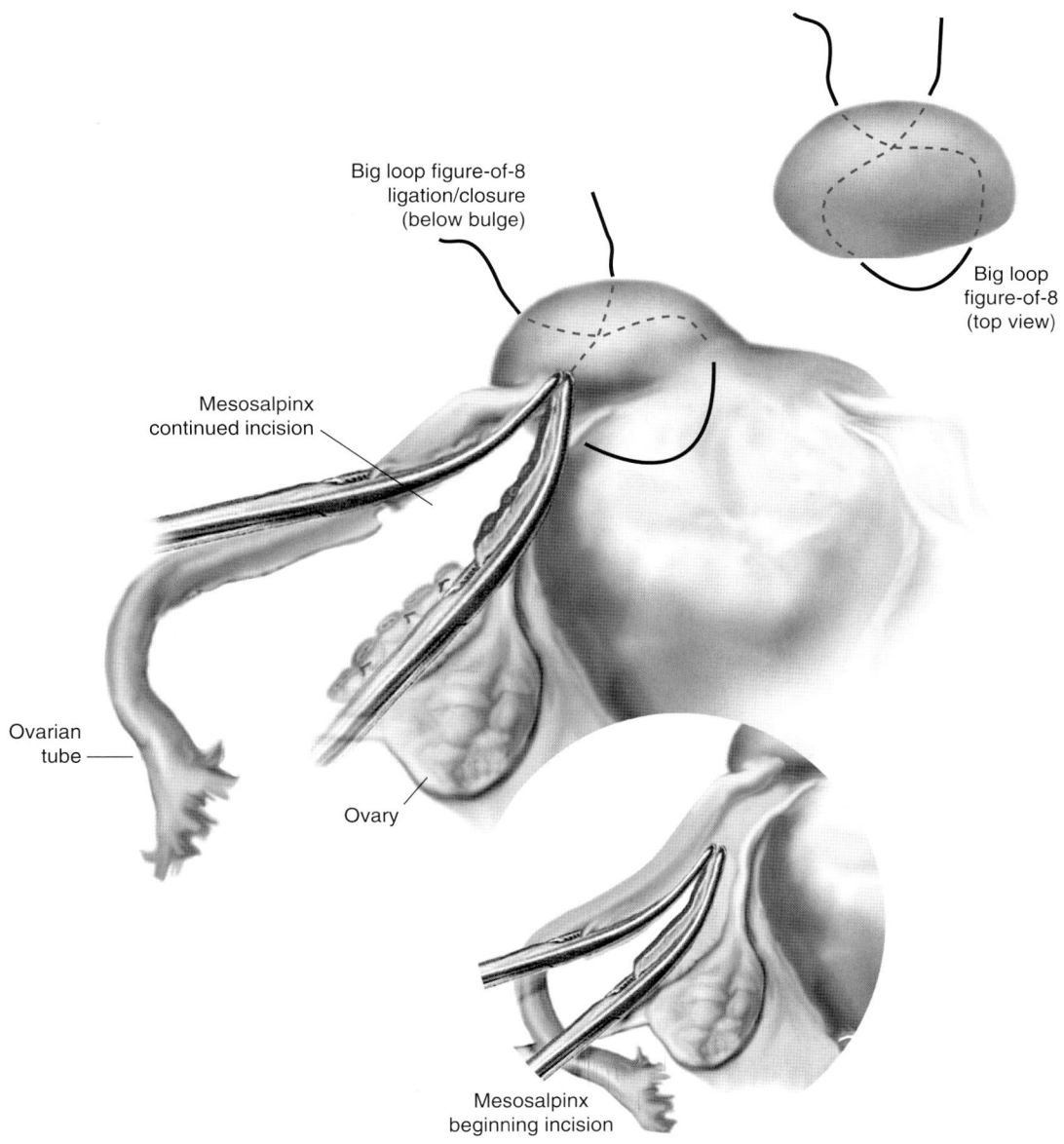

Big loop figure-of-8
ligation/closure
(below bulge)

Big loop
figure-of-8
(top view)

Mesosalpinx
continued incision

Ovarian
tube

Ovary

Mesosalpinx
beginning incision

**FIGURE 26–20** The mesosalpinx on the affected side is serially double-clamped with Kelly clamps and incised with Metzenbaum scissors. Each vascular pedicle is suture-ligated in transfixing fashion with 0 Vicryl. When the cornu is reached, a 0 or 1 Vicryl suture is placed deeply beneath the ectopic mass in figure-of-8 fashion. The suture is tagged with a mosquito clamp and left untied.

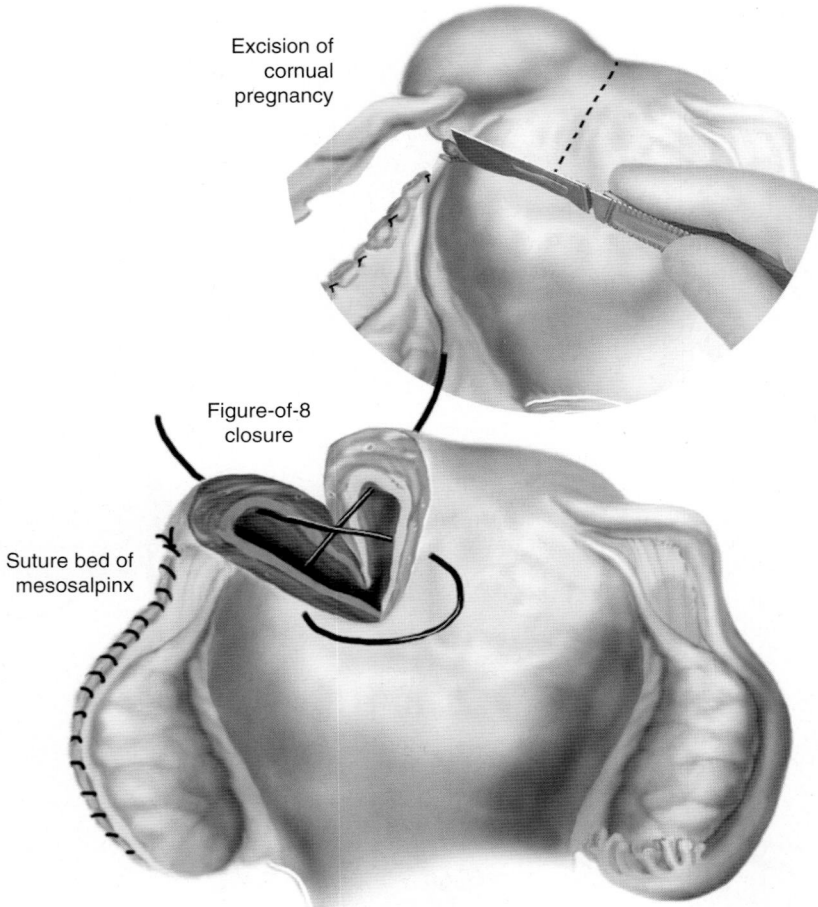

**FIGURE 26–21** The cornual pregnancy is excised after injection with a 1:100 or 1:200 vasopressin solution. The previously placed figure-of-8 suture is triply tied, producing immediate hemostasis.

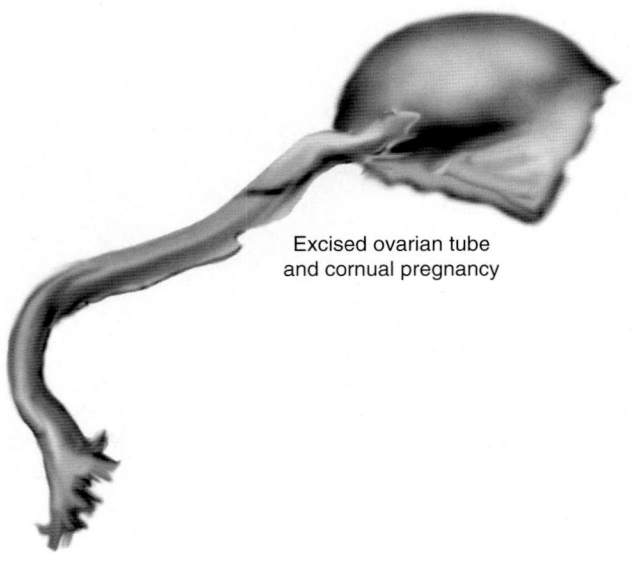

**FIGURE 26–22** The en bloc excised cornual pregnancy is examined, then is handed off to the nurse.

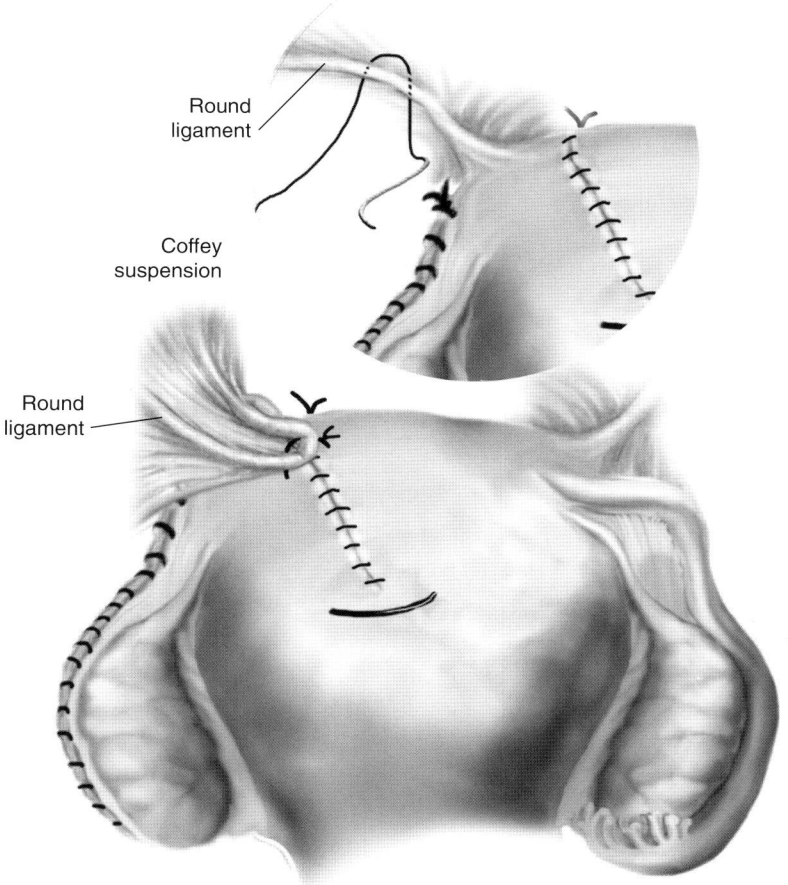

Round
ligament

Coffey
suspension

Round
ligament

**FIGURE 26–23**  Additional but shallower figure-of-8 sutures are placed linearly to gain additional hemostasis and to close the remainder of the incision. A U-shaped suture of 0 Vicryl is placed through the uterine wall at the cornual incision and is brought through the ipsilateral round ligament at its junction with the broad ligament. The net effect of this stitch when tied is to cover the incision with peritoneum and to suspend the uterus on that side.

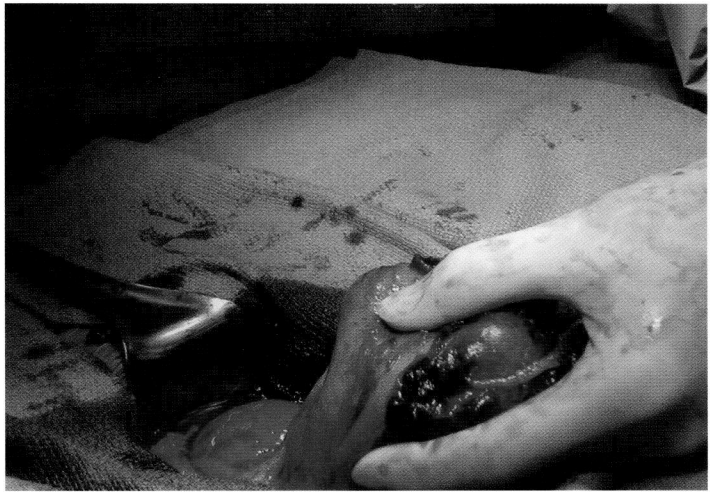

**FIGURE 26–24**  Preoperative diagnosis of a ruptured or leaking cornual ectopic pregnancy was made. At laparotomy, a bicornuate uterus with a noncommunicating and ruptured unicornuate uterus was found.

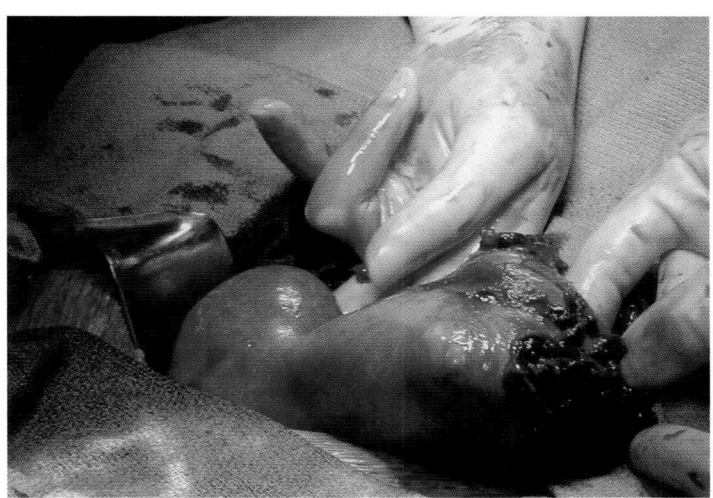

**FIGURE 26–25**  This view shows the site of rupture to be in the thinned cornu of the unicornuate portion of the bicornuate uterus.

## Salpingectomy for Isthmic Ectopic Pregnancy

Isthmic as well as ampullary ectopic pregnancy may be treated by linear salpingostomy, or alternatively by salpingectomy, or even by segmental resection.

Salpingectomy is performed by elevating the oviduct and ovary and serially clamping and suture-ligating the mesosalpinx. The tube can be clamped and cut off at the uterine terminus (Figs. 26–21 through 26–33). The decision to resect the interstitial remnant offers both advantages and disadvantages (Figs 26–34 through 26–36). Resection will eliminate the risk that a future cornual ectopic pregnancy may occur as the result of transmigration of a fertilized ovum but will greatly increase the risk of uterine rupture if a future intrauterine pregnancy should occur.

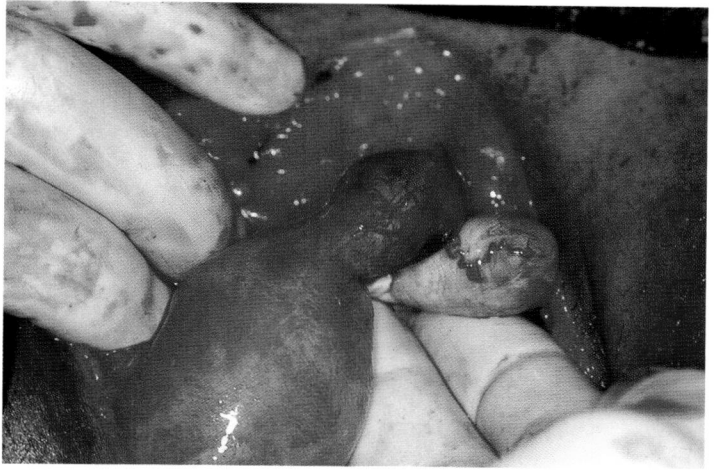

**FIGURE 26–26** The tubal pregnancy site is isolated in the isthmus close to the cornual portion of the oviduct.

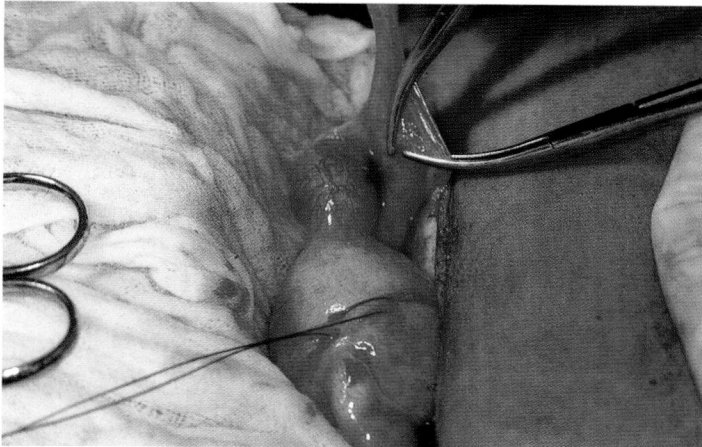

**FIGURE 26–27** The mesosalpinx is grasped at the fimbrial end of the tube and is doubly clamped with Kelly clamps.

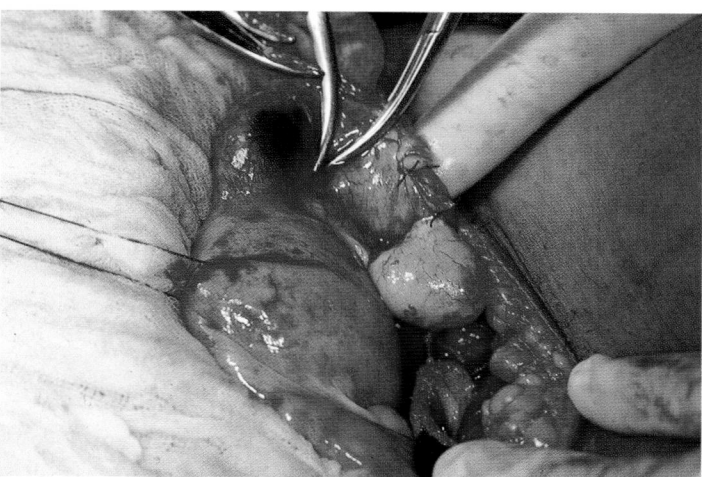

**FIGURE 26–28** The maneuver shown in Figure 26-27 is repeated until the tubouterine junction is reached.

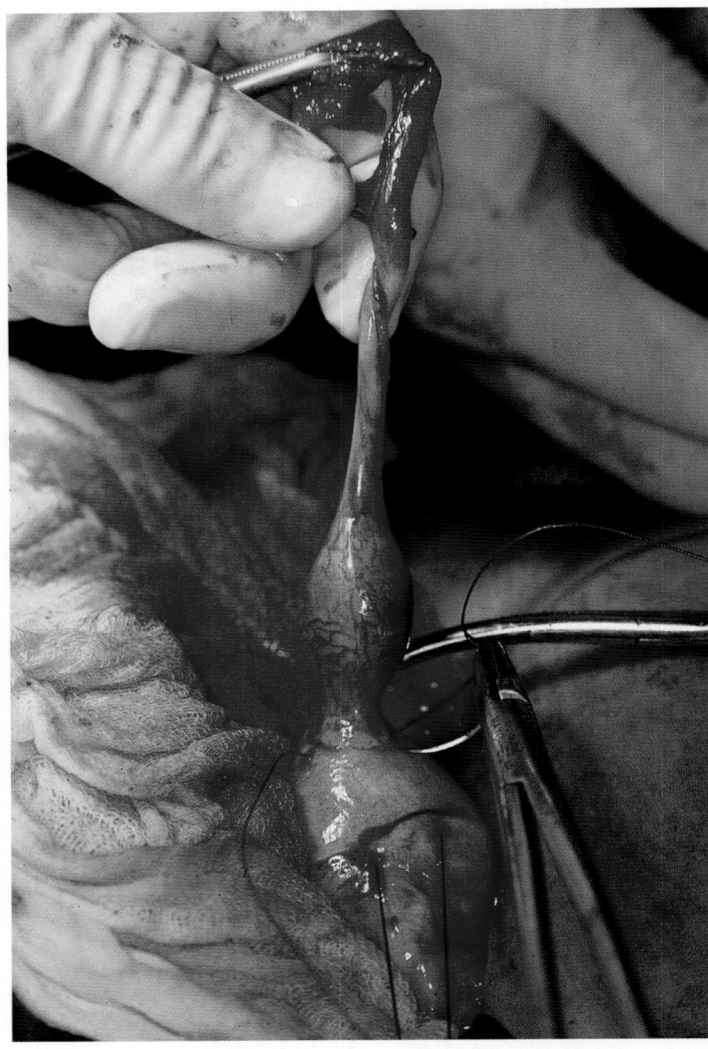

**FIGURE 26–29** If the cornu is to be resected, a 0 Vicryl figure-of-8 stitch is placed widely and deeply into the area to be resected.

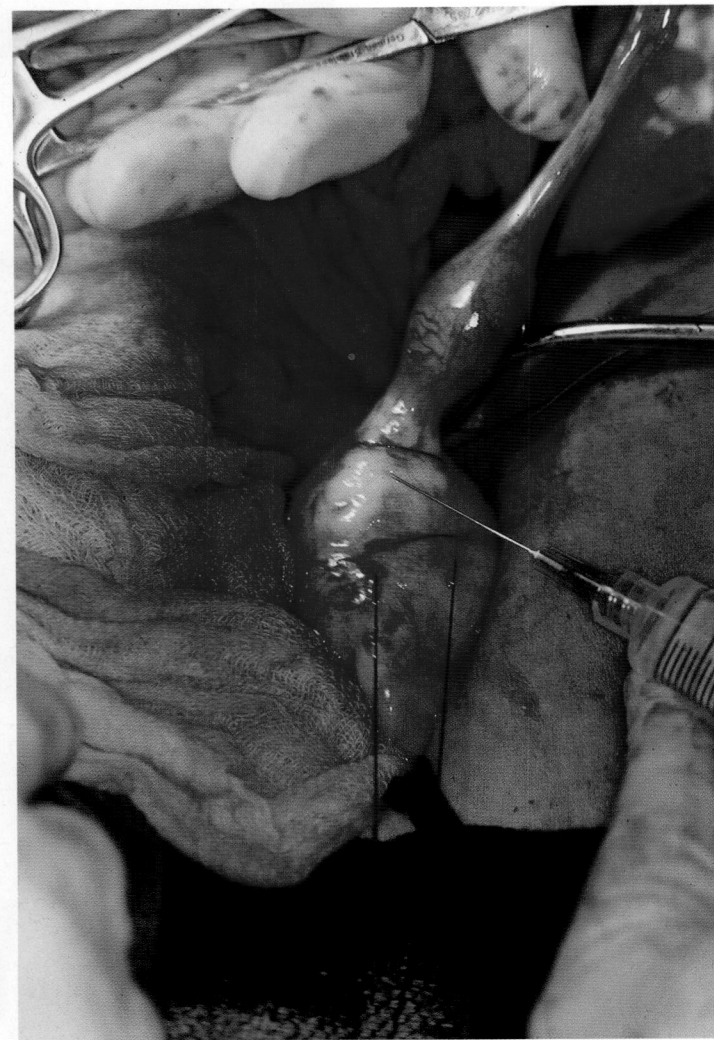

**FIGURE 26–30** Vasopressin 1 : 100 solution is injected into the cornua via a 25-gauge needle.

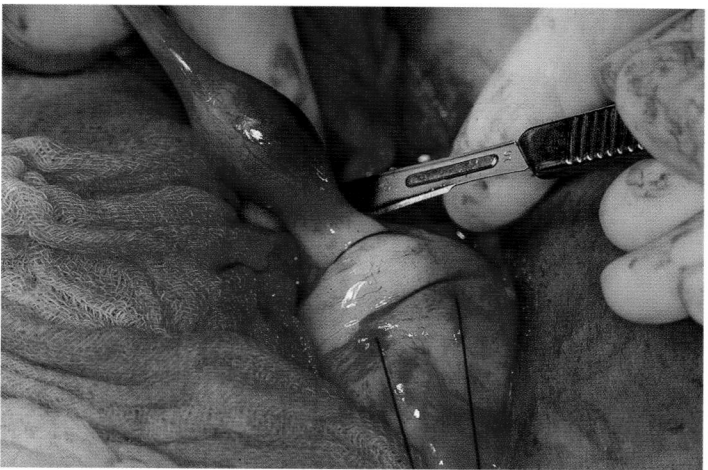

**FIGURE 26–31** The tube is cut by a wedging-type excision.

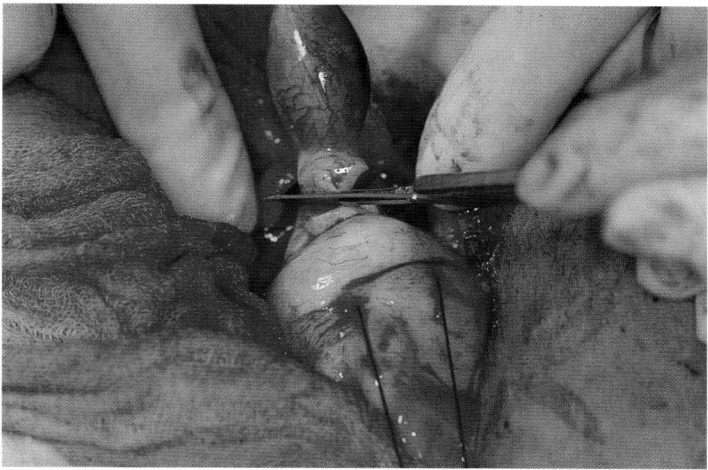

**FIGURE 26–32** As the wedge is removed from the cornual portion of the uterus, the figure-of-8 stitch is tightened.

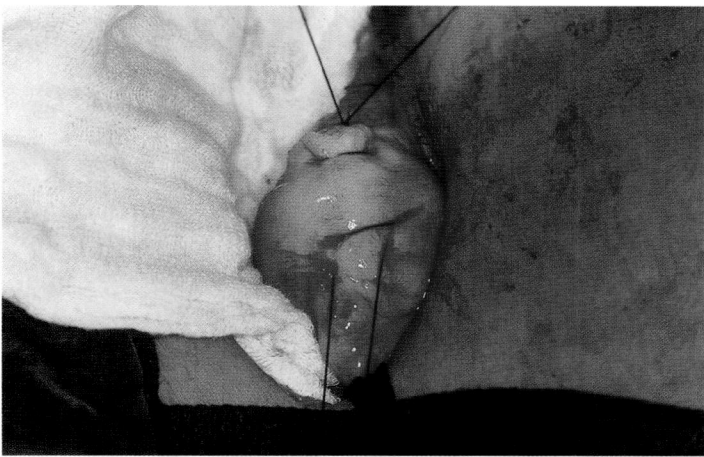

**FIGURE 26–33** The figure-of-8 suture is tightened into place, and good hemostasis is seen.

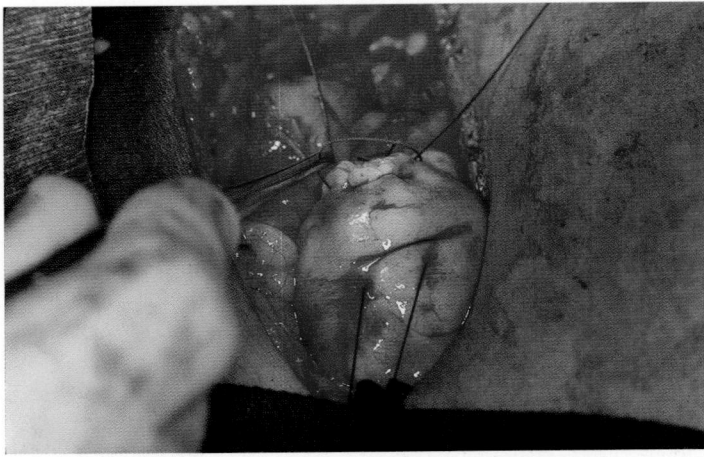

**FIGURE 26–34** Additional 0 Vicryl sutures may be placed if needed.

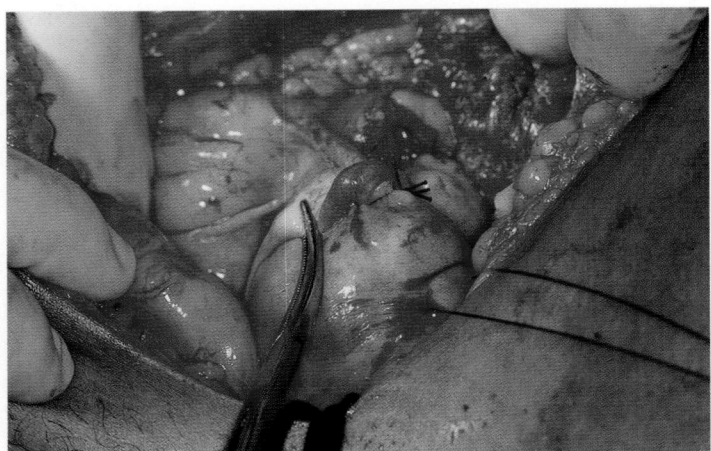

**FIGURE 26–35** A knuckle of round ligament is pulled over the incision; it covers the suture line and suspends the operative side of the uterus.

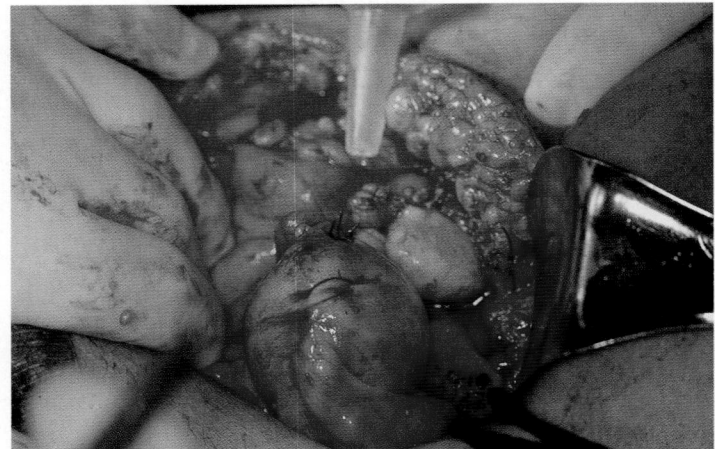

**FIGURE 26–36** On completion of the surgical site, ovary, ovarian vessels, ureter, and surrounding intestine are carefully examined while the field is irrigated with sterile saline.

# CHAPTER 27

# Surgical Management of Ovarian Residual and Remnant

*Michael S. Baggish*

After hysterectomy without salpingo-oophorectomy (bilateral or unilateral), the residual adnexa not uncommonly becomes symptomatic in the form of chronic abdominal pain. The reasons for this pain are myriad but frequently involve adhesions between the residual adnexa attached to the intestines, the bladder, or the peritoneum. The adnexa itself may be completely invested in fibrous tissue and may be densely bound to the pelvic wall in the region of the obturator fossa. Surgery to remove the residual requires careful, gentle, sharp dissection and contemporaneous, compulsive hemostasis. Obviously, precise knowledge of pelvic anatomy is requisite to a successful, noncomplicated outcome. Figure 27-1 illustrates the above points in that distinguishing between hydrosalpinx and intestine may be challenging (Fig. 27-2).

The remnant ovary represents a portion of an ovary that ostensibly had been completely removed at the time of the previous oophorectomy. Obviously, the premise was incorrect because the retained piece of ovarian tissue provides testimony to the fact that the excision of the ovary was not complete.

Pieces of ovarian tissue remaining behind after an incomplete removal of the ovary create significant problems for the unfortunate patient. Typically, these remnants are encased in adhesions, are subjected to a variable blood supply, and create pain.

The remnant tissue tends to be plastered to the pelvic sidewall in close proximity to portions of the infundibulopelvic ligament, the ureter, and the external iliac vessels (Fig. 27-3). Not frequently, the large intestine is also tightly adhesed to the ovary. Dissection is performed by gaining retroperitoneal entry to (1) free the intestine from the ovarian tissue, (2) free the ovary from the sidewall structures (above) without damaging those structures, and (3) remove the fragments of ovary and repair the peritoneal defect (Fig. 27-4). The surgeon should **not** hesitate to consult a urologist to pass a retrograde catheter into the ureter on the affected side.

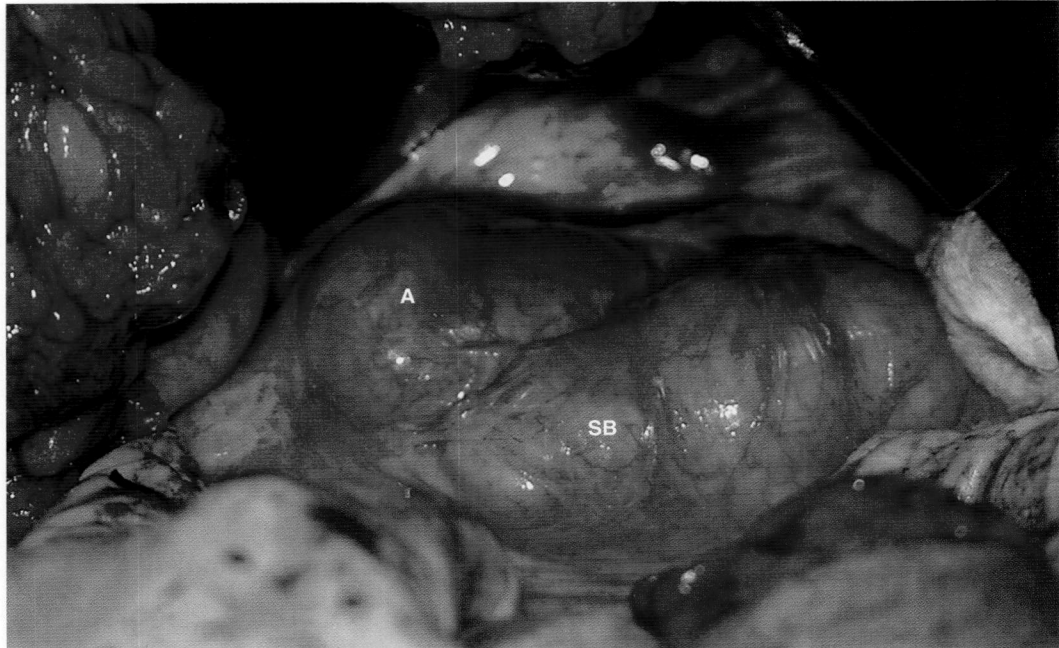

**FIGURE 27-1** Residual ovary and tube seen during laparotomy in a woman with three previous cesarean sections and two subsequent procedures, including a total abdominal hysterectomy. Following extensive adhesiolysis, the right adnexa (A) was exposed deep to the adhesed small intestines (SB). A similar state of affairs was noted on the left. Note the similarity of appearance between the hydrosalpinx and the adhesed small intestine.

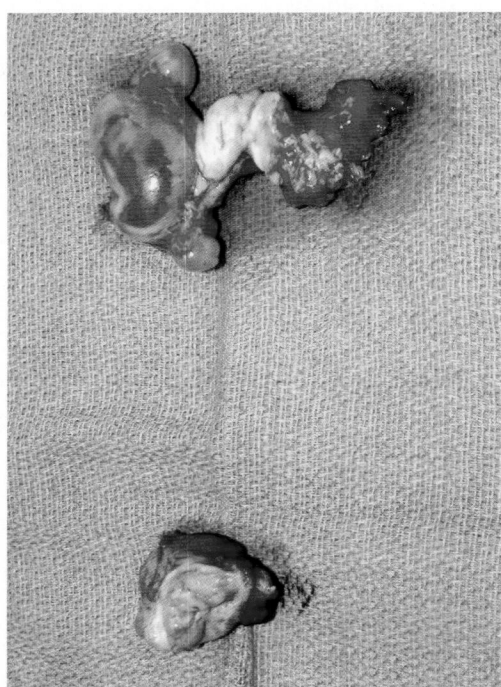

**FIGURE 27-2** The retroperitoneal spaces were entered over the psoas major muscle, and the right and left ureters were identified. The right and left tubes and ovaries were dissected free of surrounding structures and were removed. Hemostasis was obtained and long tonsil clamps with 3-0 Vicryl suture ligatures were used. The patient had a history of pulmonary embolism; therefore she was given 40 mg of Lovenox 2 hours postoperatively. The removed specimens are seen here. The hydrosalpinx on the left side leaked out when a Babcock clamp was placed onto the tube.

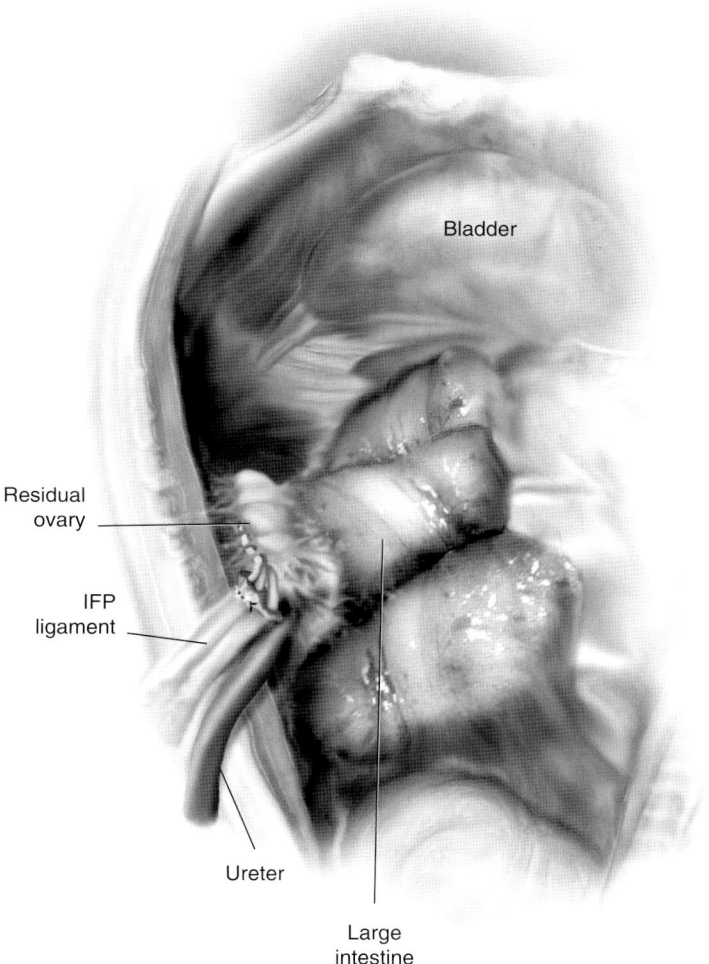

**FIGURE 27–3** The remnant ovary is seen adhesed to the colon and sidewall of the pelvis. Note the relationship of the ovarian vessels and ureter to the ovarian mass. IFP, infundibulopelvic ligament.

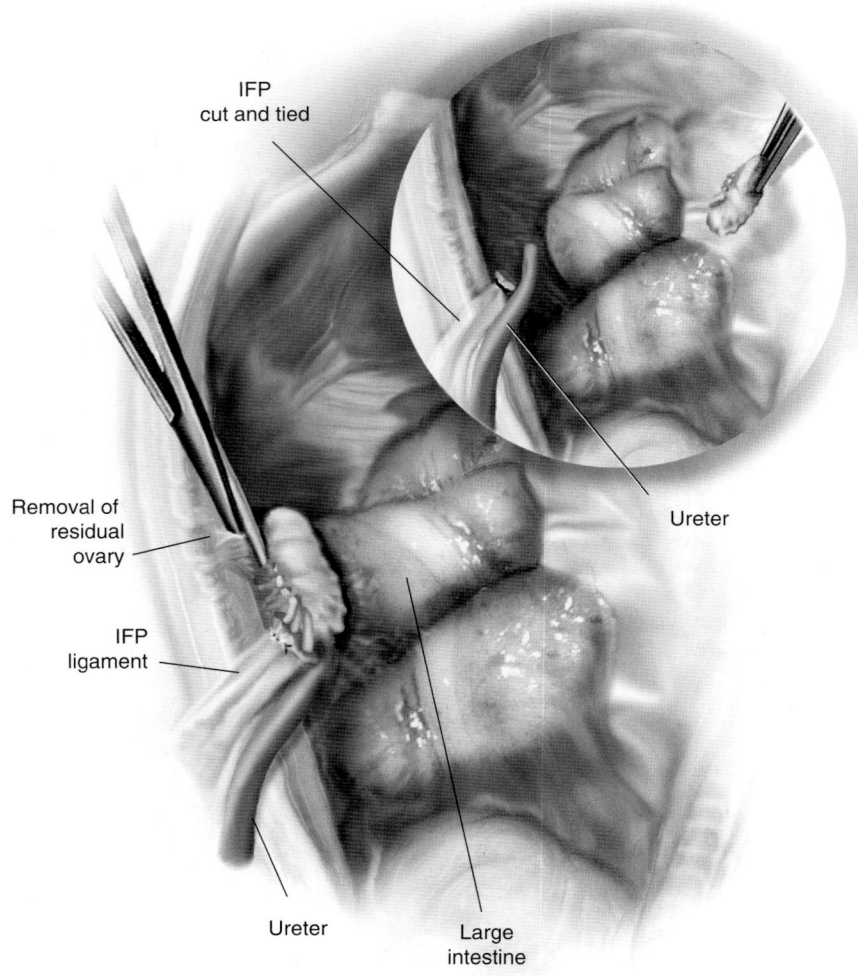

IFP
cut and tied

Removal of
residual
ovary

IFP
ligament

Ureter

Ureter

Large
intestine

**FIGURE 27–4** The sigmoid colon has been separated from the remnant by sharp dissection coupled with assiduous hemostasis. The ovary is dissected free from the sidewall structure. **Inset:** The remnant is removed. The course of the ureter is checked and the ureter is carefully examined for any sign of injury. IFP, infundibulopelvic ligament.

# CHAPTER 28

# Ovarian Tumor Debulking

## *Jack Basil*

Ovarian cancer is a surgically staged disease, and most cases are advanced stage III or IV at the time of initial diagnosis. The cornerstone of therapy for ovarian cancer is maximal surgical cytoreduction, or tumor debulking, surgery. Ovarian cancer is thought to spread by contiguous growth and by dissemination through the lymphatics. Once the cancer has reached the external surface of the ovary, the cells exfoliate and implant inside the abdominal-pelvic cavity, causing peritoneal disease. Once ovarian cancer has disseminated, it tends to grow on the lining of the peritoneum and on the outside of the viscera in the abdomen and pelvis. Once outside the ovary, this malignancy has a predilection to metastasize to the deep portions of the anterior and posterior cul-de-sacs, the surface of the diaphragm (especially the right side), and the omentum, including both infracolic and gastrocolic portions. Additionally, ovarian cancer is found to involve the surfaces of the large and small bowel and its mesentery, the spleen, the liver, and the stomach. Approximately one fourth of cases of ovarian cancer are confined to the ovary. It is of paramount importance to completely surgically stage these cases at the time of diagnosis so that the appropriate treatment can be given. Surgery for an undiagnosed pelvic mass or a presumed ovarian cancer customarily begins with a vertical midline skin incision (Fig. 28–1A–D). This approach allows for removal of the mass or ovary (especially if it is large) and, more important, for maximal exposure of the abdominal-pelvic cavity, so that a thorough exploration can be performed. The incision usually is started at the level of the pubic symphysis and is extended cephalad. It can be extended all the way to the xyphoid process if necessary.

In a minority of cases, ovarian cancer can be confined to the ovary, and a "conservative staging procedure" can be performed (Fig. 28–2A, B). A conservative staging procedure consists of unilateral adnexectomy, pelvic washings, peritoneal biopsies, omentectomy, and lymph node dissection (usually to include pelvic and para-aortic areas; Fig. 28–3A, B). This conservative staging technique should be limited to children, adolescents, and women of childbearing years whose malignancy is grossly confined to one ovary.

To date, no accurate screening test has been developed for ovarian cancer; therefore most ovarian cancers have spread into the abdominal-pelvic cavity by the time of diagnosis (Fig. 28–4A–D). The goal of surgical treatment in these cases is maximal tumor debulking, also termed *surgical cytoreduction*. This usually consists of total abdominal hysterectomy, bilateral salpingo-oophorectomy, omentectomy, and tumor debulking. Additionally, ascites, if present, is removed as a component of this surgery. When gross bulky disease is found outside the abdomen, removal of lymph node tissue is usually reserved for those cases in which lymph nodes contain bulky disease. Often the omentum is a site of metastatic disease (Fig. 28–5). Commonly, most cases of metastatic disease for ovarian cancer are found in the omentum (Figs. 28–6A, B and 28–7A, B).

Optimal tumor debulking (defined as no residual disease = 1 to 2 cm at the conclusion of the surgery) provides a survival advantage to patients with ovarian cancer. Optimal tumor debulking often can involve surgery on such organs as bowel, bladder, liver, and spleen (Fig. 28–8). The concept of decreasing residual tumor burden is thought to make postoperative adjuvant therapy most effective. This correlates with a survival advantage in patients who undergo optimal tumor debulking for ovarian cancer.

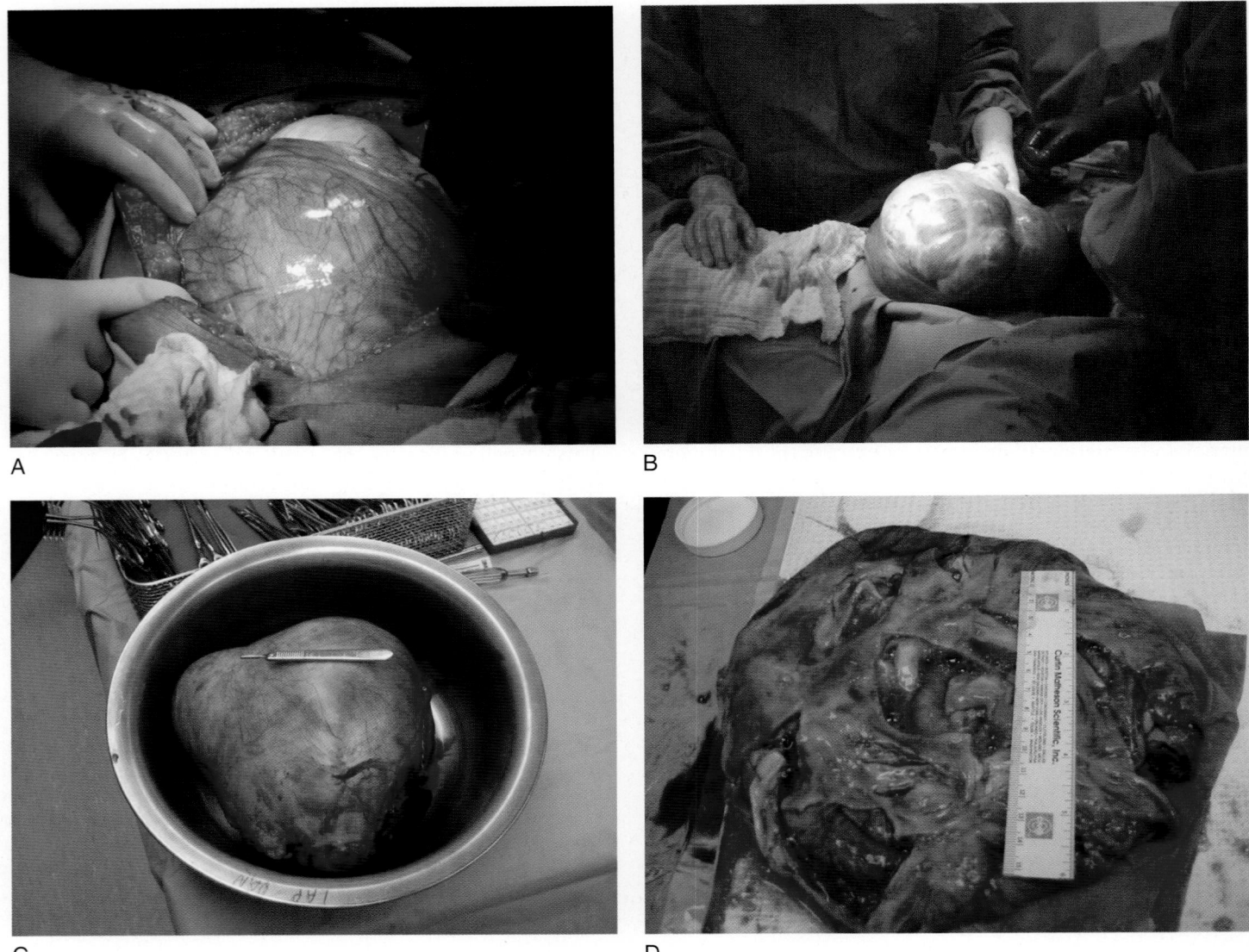

A

B

C

D

**FIGURE 28–1  A.** The right ovary is markedly enlarged and contains an adenocarcinoma. The right fallopian tube and mesosalpinx can be seen draping over the lower three quarters of the ovary. The vertical midline skin incision extends from the symphysis pubis to up above the umbilicus and provides adequate exposure in this case. **B.** The large ovarian mass has been delivered through the vertical midline skin incision. **C.** The adenocarcinoma of the right ovary measures 20 × 15 × 8 cm. **D.** Most of the right ovary was fluid-filled, but it did contain multiple thick septations and the adenocarcinoma of the ovary, which consisted of mixed serous and mucinous subtypes.

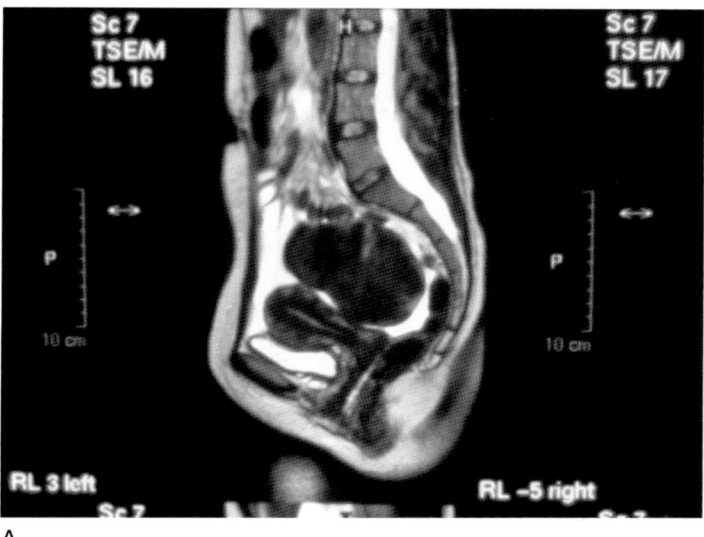
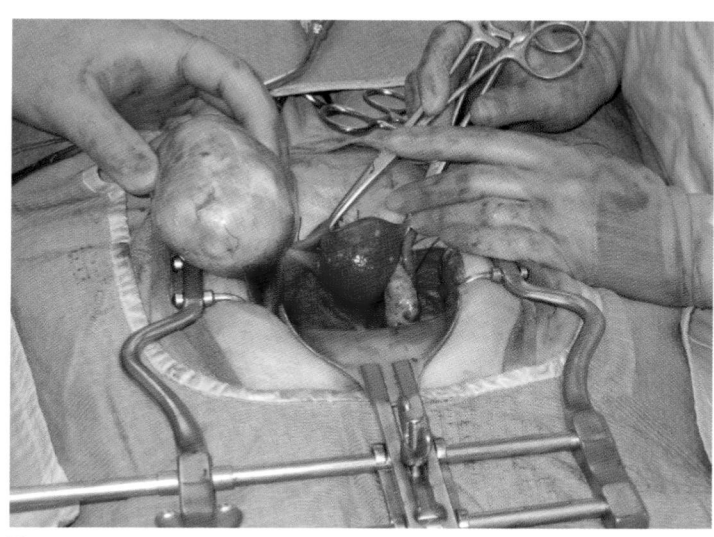

A

B

**FIGURE 28–2  A.** This preoperative magnetic resonance image (MRI) of the pelvis shows an ovarian mass clearly distinct from the bladder, the uterus, and the rectosigmoid colon. **B.** Ovarian cancer is confined to the left ovary, and a normal uterus and right ovary can be seen. Conservative staging can be employed in this case.

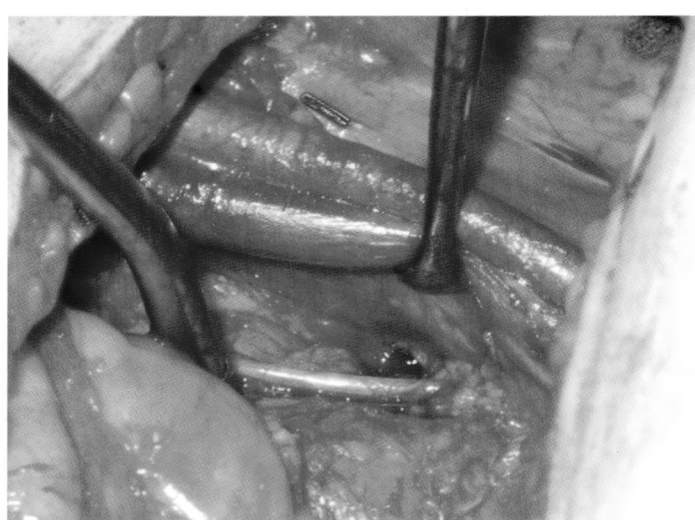
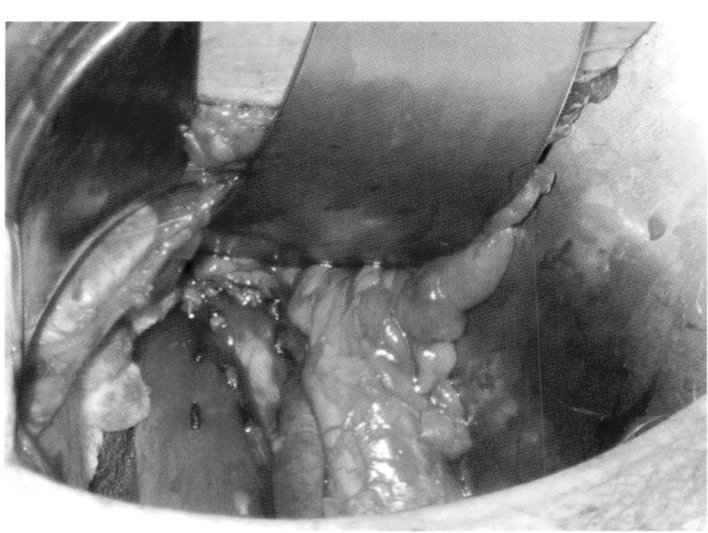

A

B

**FIGURE 28–3  A.** A pelvic lymph node dissection has been performed. The external iliac artery and vein have been stripped of all lymph node tissue and are being gently retracted by a vein retractor to expose the obturator nerve. The obturator lymph node pad has also been removed to expose the obturator internus muscle and the pelvic sidewall. **B.** A right-sided para-aortic lymph node dissection has been performed. Surgical clips can be seen on the surface of the psoas major muscle and the inferior vena cava. Medial to the inferior vena cava, the aorta can be seen as well as the ureter.

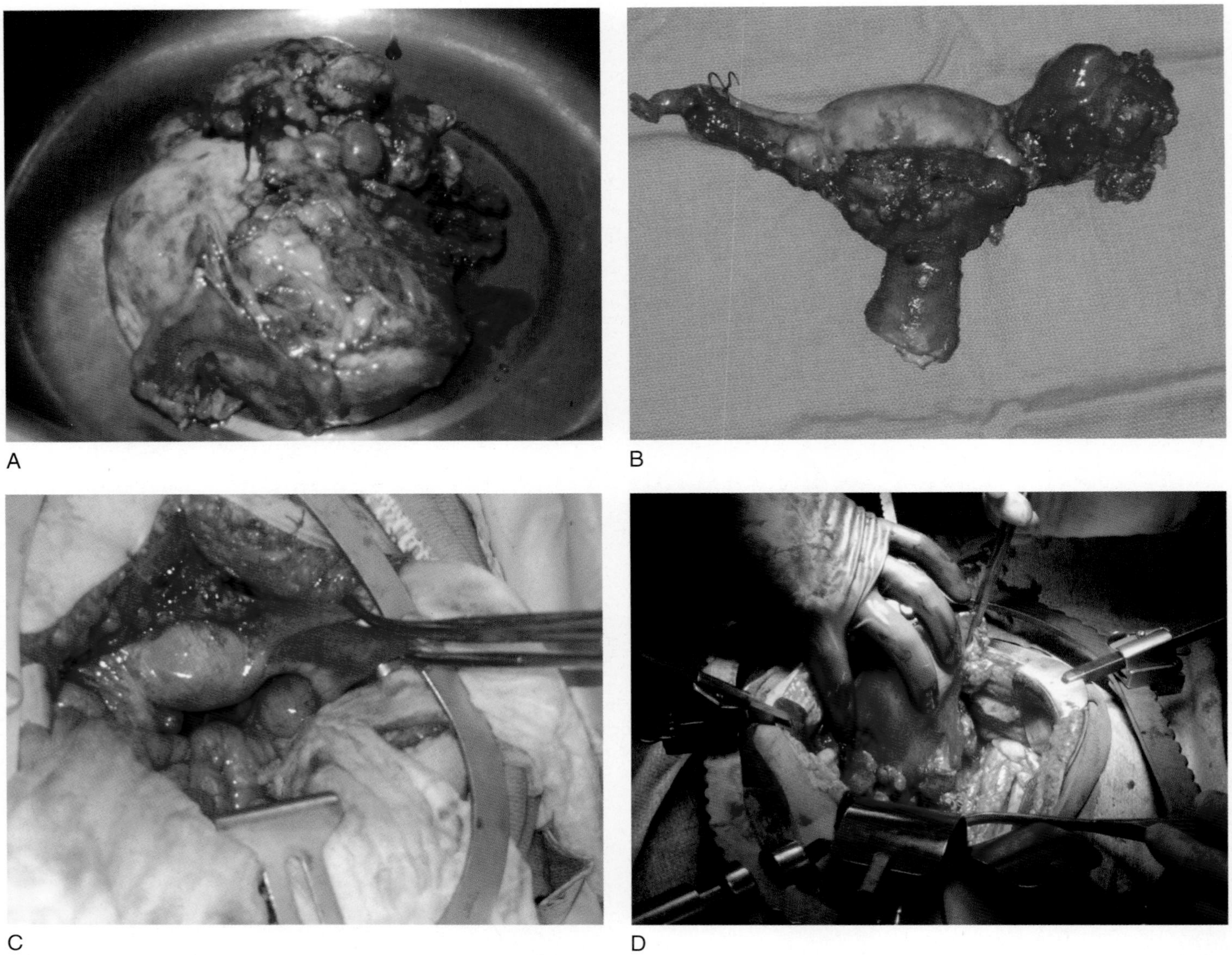

A

B

C

D

**FIGURE 28–4  A.** A cancerous ovary with extensive gross disease on its surface. **B.** The contralateral ovary and posterior uterine serosa contain gross metastatic disease. **C.** Extraovarian disease along the vesicouterine peritoneum causing obliteration of the anterior cul-de-sac. **D.** Extraovarian disease involving the posterior cul-de-sac.

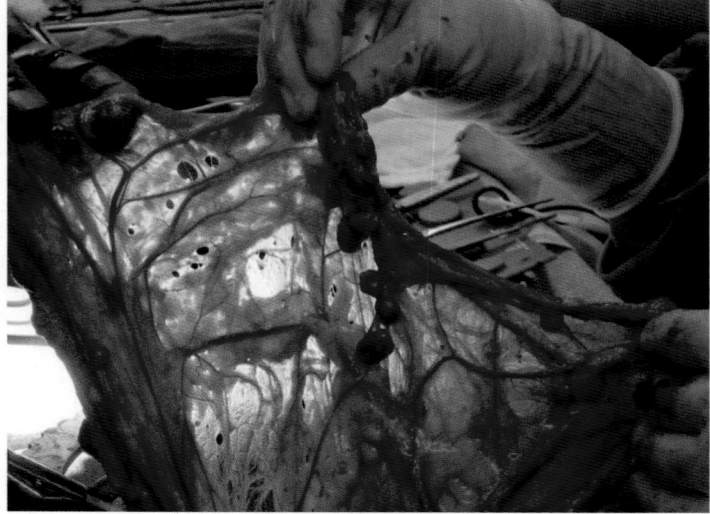

**FIGURE 28–5**  Small metastatic implants of an ovarian malignancy can be seen throughout the omentum.

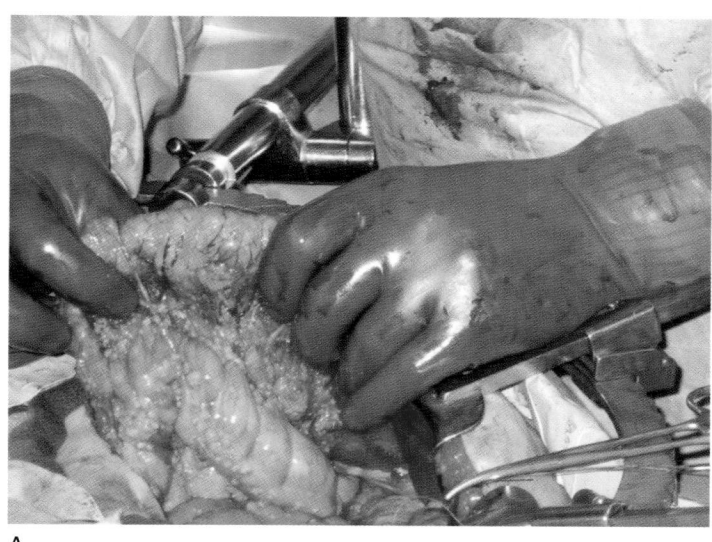

A

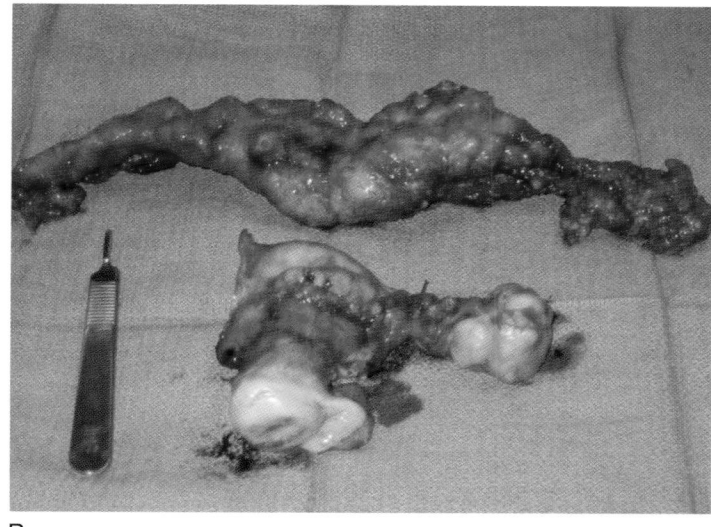

B

**FIGURE 28–6 A.** Metastatic ovarian cancer with omental caking involving the infracolic omentum. Metastatic tumor implants can be seen along the tinea coli of the transverse colon. **B.** A left ovary, uterus, cervix, and omentum depicting a left-sided ovarian cancer with metastatic disease along the anterior uterine serosa and in the omentum. Most of the disease is contained in the omentum.

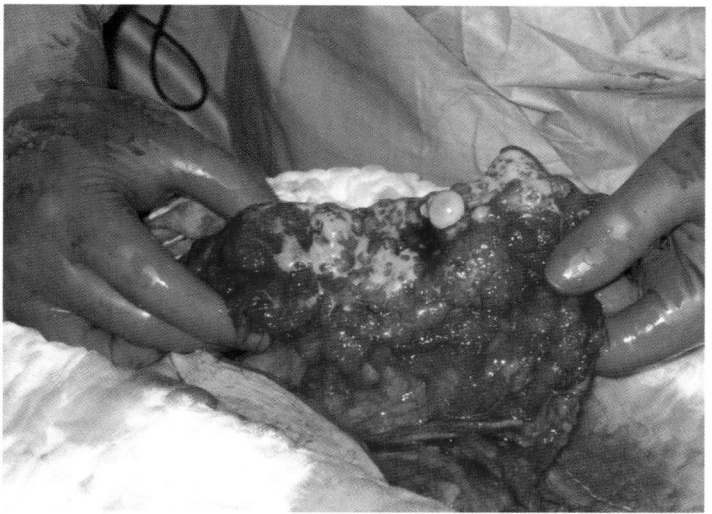

A

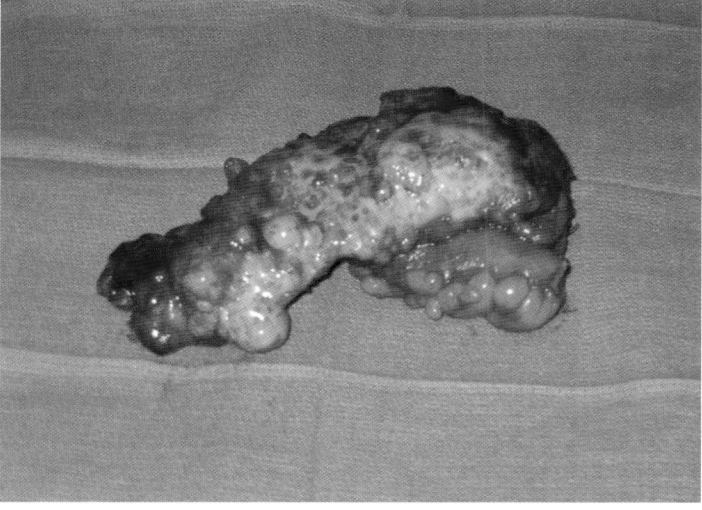

**FIGURE 28–8** A portion of omentum with metastatic ovarian cancer that was firmly adherent to a portion of small bowel. To accomplish optimal tumor debulking, the portion of small bowel adherent to the omental cake was resected and a bowel reanastomosis was performed.

B

**FIGURE 28–7 A.** A case of metastatic ovarian cancer replacing the omentum. **B.** An omental cake is shown firmly adherent to the transverse colon.

UNIT 2 ■ SECTION D

# CHAPTER 29

# Tuboplasty

## *Michael S. Baggish*

The oviducts may be obstructed principally at three locations: (1) at the cornua; (2) at the fimbriated end; and (3) at any point between these two locations. The causes of oviductal obstruction are myriad and include infection, ectopic pregnancy, endometriosis, intentional tubal ligation, and partial salpingectomy. Before surgery is performed, a thorough diagnostic survey should be done, including laparoscopy, chromotubation, and hysterosalpingography. Several of the techniques described here can be performed by laparoscopy, laparotomy, or microsurgery. Similarly, the incisional portions of these procedures may be performed with conventional mechanical devices, superpulsed carbon dioxide ($CO_2$) lasers, or electrosurgical tools. The author prefers to utilize a variety of instruments, basing selection on the circumstances of the pathology and the relative advantages of a particular device for a specific circumstance. These surgical techniques use fine instruments, gentle tissue manipulation, small-gauge suture material, and needles. Compulsive hemostasis is required for successful outcomes.

## Fimbrioplasty (Hydrosalpinx)

A hydrosalpinx connotes a damaged tube (Fig. 29–1). Methylene blue dye should be injected transcervically to determine whether the tube fills. If the tube distends with the dye, then a fimbrioplasty may be attempted (Fig. 29–2). Traction sutures of 4-0 Vicryl are placed to permit gentle tissue manipulation and to obtain good stability of the oviduct during surgery (Fig. 29–3). A $CO_2$ superpulsed laser (Lumenis, Santa Clara, California) set at 12 W at 300 pulses/sec is focused to deliver a 1-mm-diameter spot (Fig. 29–4). A hole is drilled into the central point of the fimbrial adhesion (Fig. 29–5). Blue dye spews forth as the oviductal canal is entered. A lacrimal probe is inserted into the opening. Four radial cuts are made from the central point and are carried into the tubal lumen (Fig. 29–6). These may range from 3 to 10 mm in length.

The edges of each radial cut are then sutured back to the tubal serosa or are laser brushed to create a cuff (Fig. 29–7). The preferred suture material is 5-0 polydioxanone (PDS)/Vicryl. The cuff exposes to the ovary a large surface area of tubal ciliated cells. Patency is again checked by retrograde injection of methylene blue dye (Fig. 29–8).

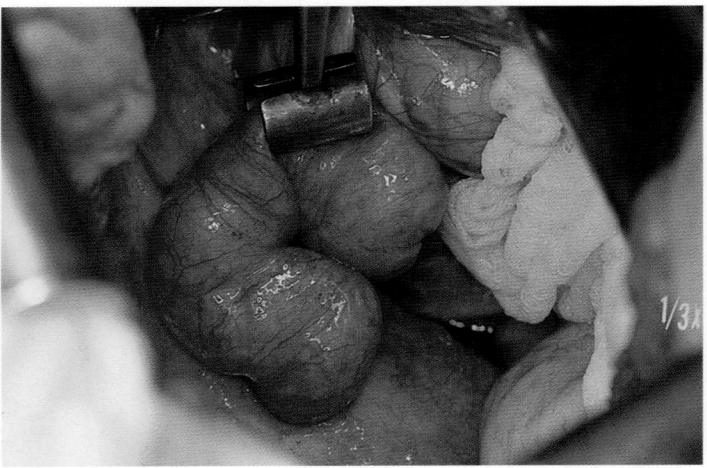

**FIGURE 29–1** The distended oviduct is secured for inspection with a tube clamp. This figure demonstrates a classic hydrosalpinx.

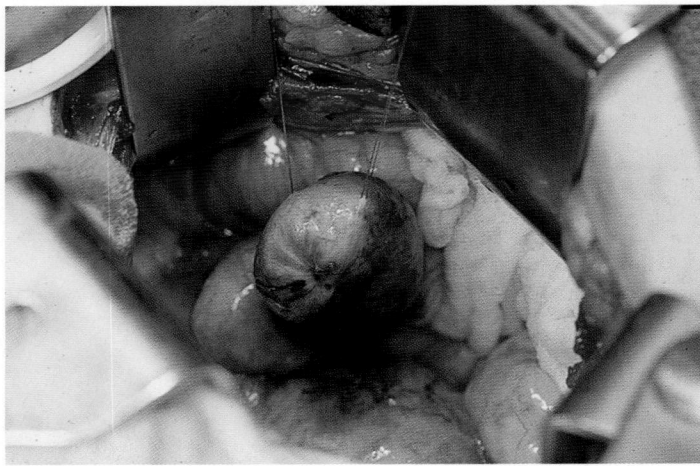

**FIGURE 29–2** The oviduct is filled with methylene blue injected retrogradely through a transcervical Cohen-Eder cannula.

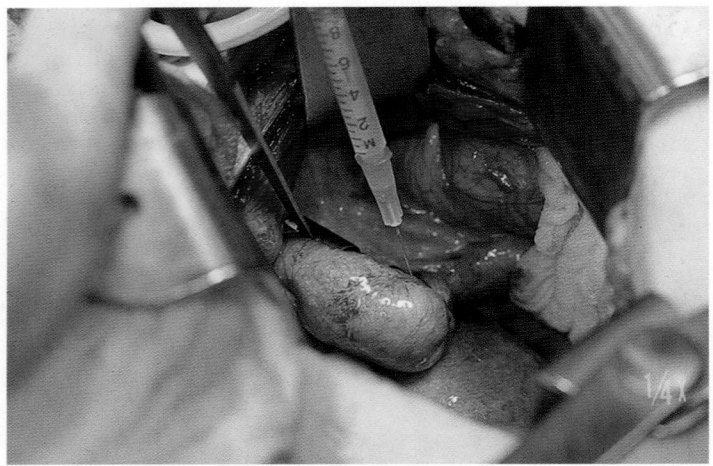

**FIGURE 29–3** A 1:200 solution of vasopressin is injected into the planned operative site with a 25-gauge needle.

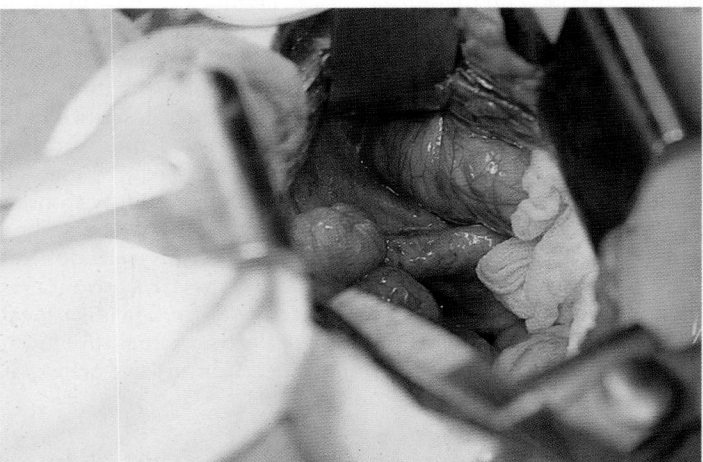

**FIGURE 29–4** The helium-neon aiming beam of a carbon dioxide ($CO_2$) superpulsed laser is aimed at the dimple in the fimbriated end of the hydrosalpinx. This represents the site of central agglutination of the fimbria.

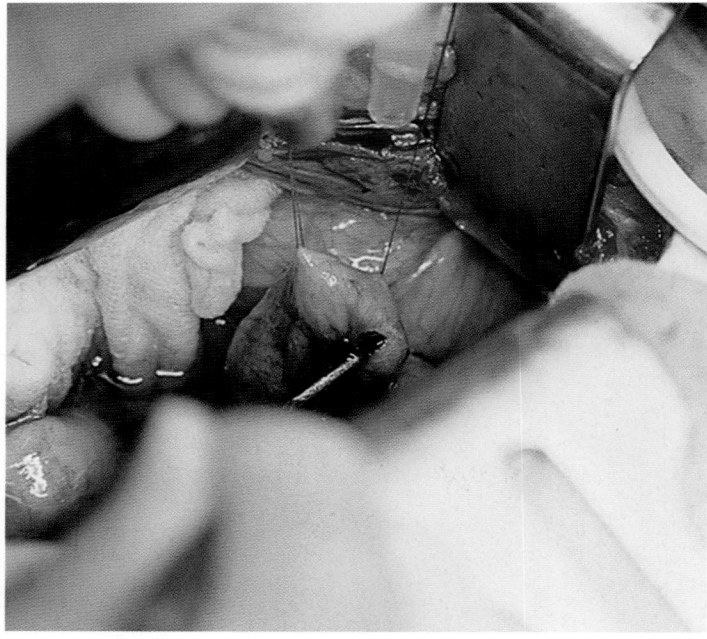

**FIGURE 29–5** Entry into the tubal lumen is signified by the leakage of methylene blue–tinged fluid. A metal probe is inserted into the lumen.

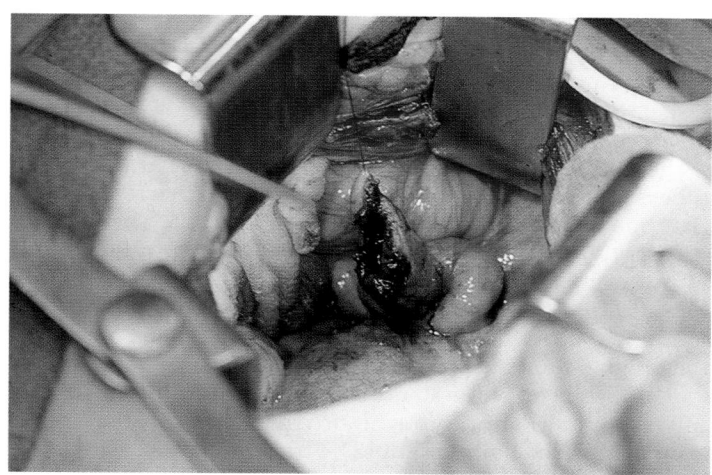

**FIGURE 29–6** The tube is opened widely by cutting four flaps.

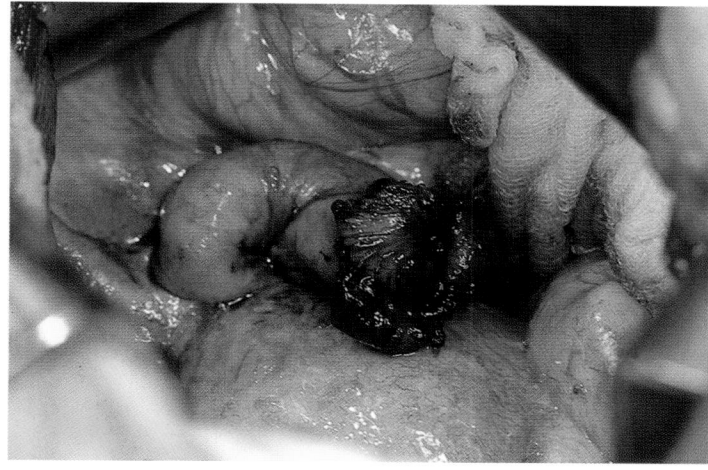

**FIGURE 29–7** The flaps are sutured back through the tubal serosa, creating an open cuff.

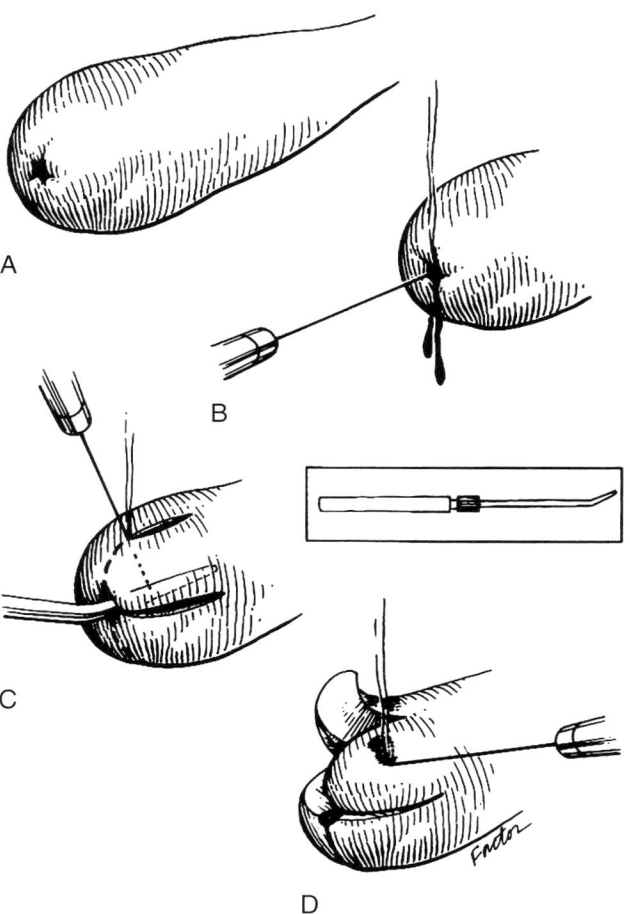

**FIGURE 29–8** The entire process is illustrated schematically. Instead of suturing the flaps, a cuff is created by lasering the flap serosa at low power (brushing), thus creating a slow, mild serosal coagulation and resultant retraction of the tubal mucosa.

## Midtubal Anastomosis

Midtubal obstruction (e.g., as produced by previous tubal ligation) may be treated by segmental resection followed by anastomosis over a stent.

Methylene blue dye is injected retrogradely, filling the nonoccluded portion of the distal (uterine end) oviduct (Fig. 29–9). A 1:200 solution of vasopressin is then injected just beyond the obstruction (Fig. 29–10). The tube is cut with a scalpel to the level of the mesosalpinx (i.e., a circumferential cross-sectional cut). Blue dye emits from the opened lumen of the oviduct. A fine probe is inserted in the direction of the uterine cavity. Four 5-0 Vicryl sutures are placed clockwise, full thickness through the cut edge of the tube, and are held with mosquito clamps.

Attention is drawn to the fimbriated end of the tube. A probe is placed through the fimbria and is advanced until it meets the obstruction (Fig. 29–11). This marks the point where the scar tissue begins. A 1:200 vasopressin solution is injected into the tube at this point. The knife cuts the oviduct as mentioned earlier until the tip of the probe is exposed (see Fig. 29–11). The obstructed segment is cut away and the mesosalpinx sutured with a 4-0 Vicryl running lock stitch. A fine plastic or Silastic tube is threaded through the newly opened oviduct (Fig. 29–12). Care should be taken to avoid kinking the tube. The previous stitches (placed from outside in) are now taken up and sutured into the proximal segment through an inside-out technique (Fig. 29–13). The four stitches may now be tied over the stent. If additional stitches are desired, they should be placed before the original four sutures are secured.

The distal end of the stent tube is fed into the uterine cavity. All suture lines are thoroughly irrigated. The portion of the stent exiting the fimbria should be trimmed (Fig. 29–14).

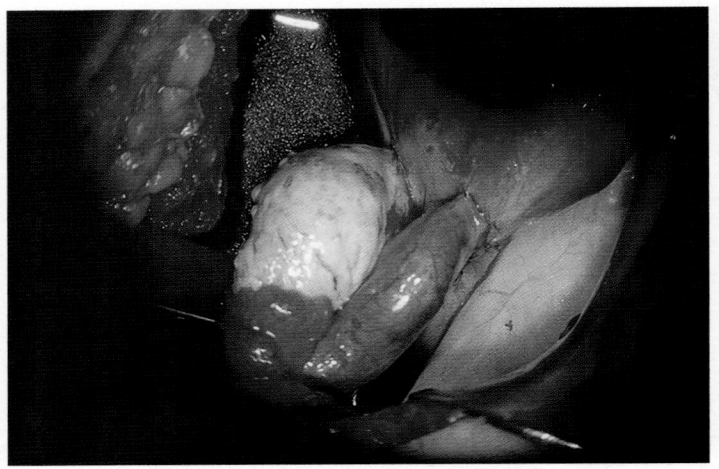

**FIGURE 29–9** Methylene blue dye injected transcervically distends the distal oviduct to the point of ampullary obstruction.

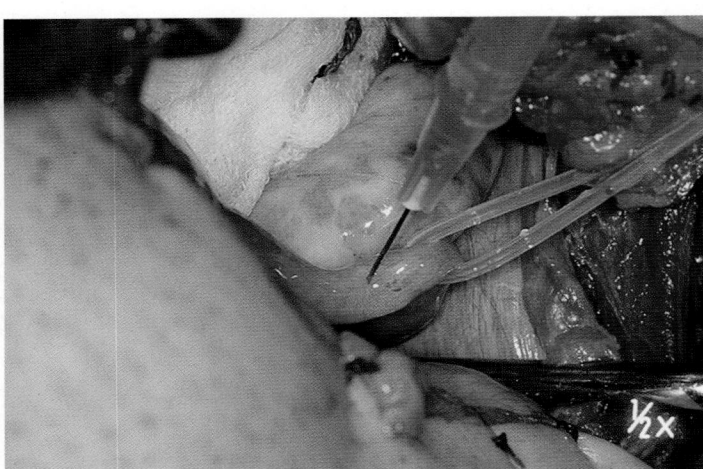

**FIGURE 29–10** The tube is manipulated with polyethylene tubing placed through the mesosalpinx. A 1:200 vasopressin solution is injected into the distal oviduct at the point of the obstruction.

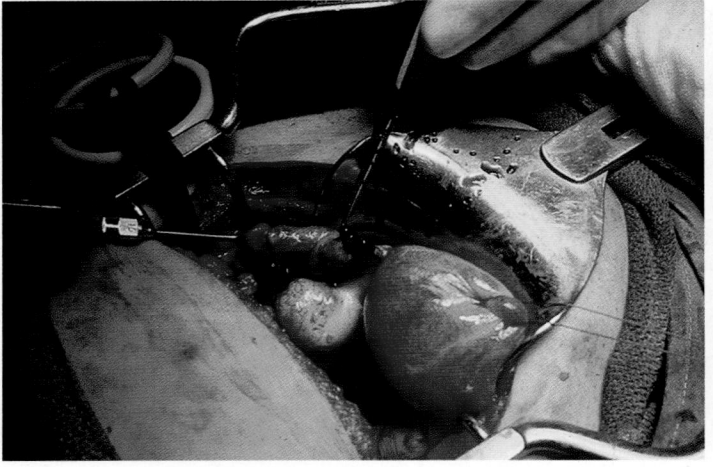

**FIGURE 29–11** A cannula is fed through the fimbria to the point of proximal obstruction. As the obstructed area is cut away, blue dye spills forth.

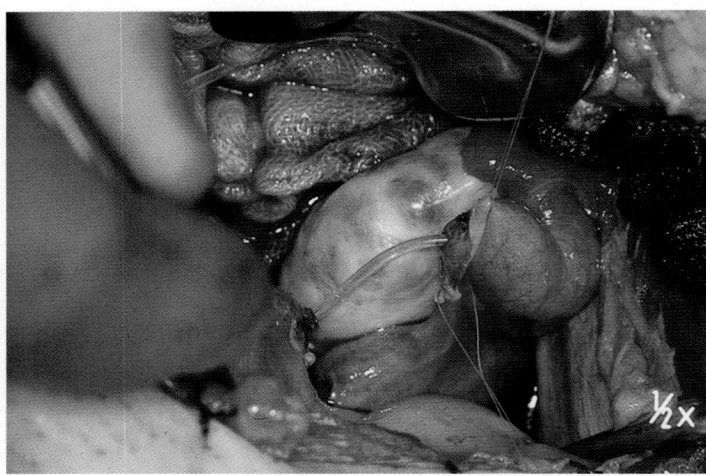

**FIGURE 29–12** The proximal (fimbriated) and distal (uterine) patent segments of the oviduct are cannulated with polyethylene tubing, which acts as a stent to facilitate the anastomosis.

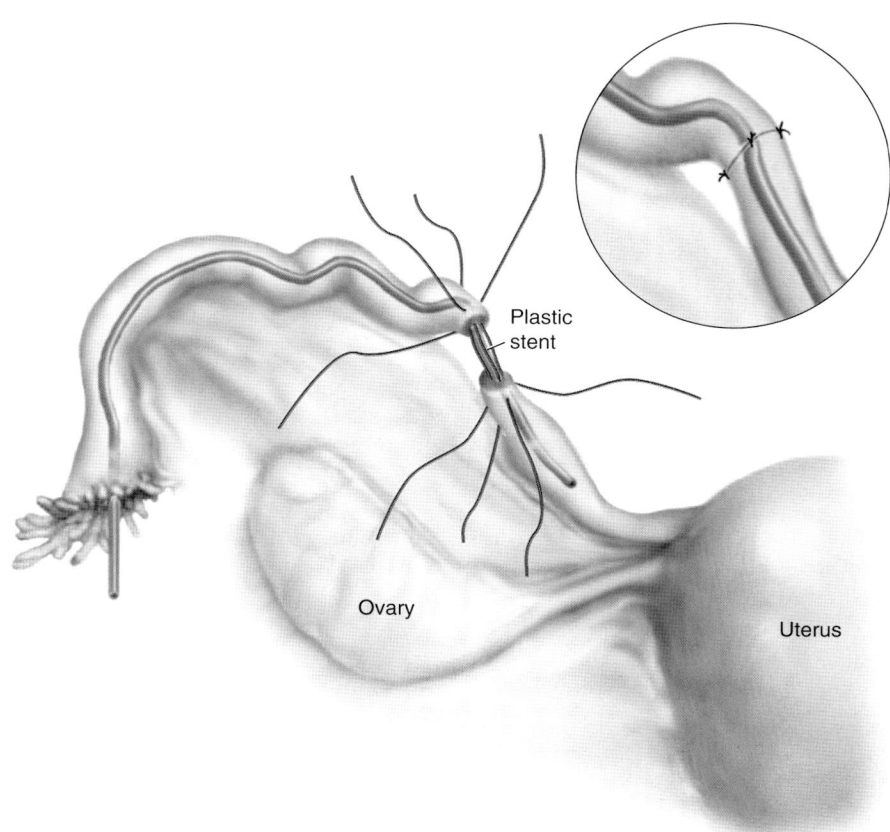

**FIGURE 29–13** Fine Vicryl (5-0) sutures are placed full thickness into the oviduct, with care taken to avoid stitching the stent. Entry into one tubal segment extends from serosa to mucosa. The other segment is sutured from inside (mucosa) out (serosa). The stitches are tied on the serosa and cut on the knot.

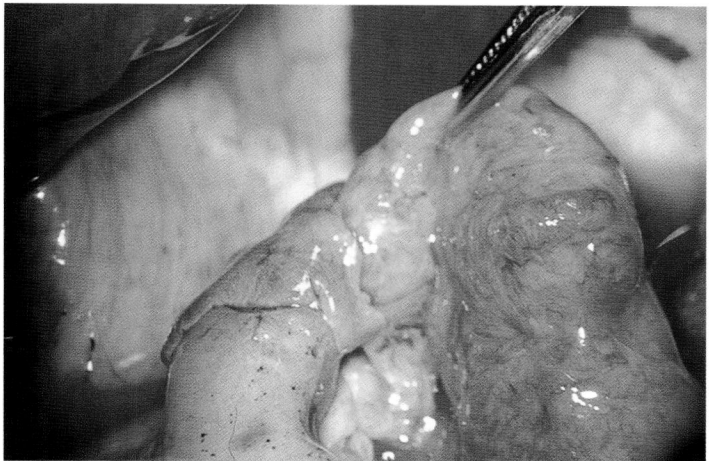

**FIGURE 29–14** The tube has been anastomosed and has been demonstrated to be open. The 5-0 Vicryl sutures are barely visible. It is obvious that this anastomosis has been performed with the use of the operating microscope.

## Cornual Anastomosis

The fimbriated end of the tube is probed by means of a polyethylene cannula inserted into the tube. Dye (methylene blue) is injected. The tube is injected with 1:200 vasopressin and is cut just proximal to the obstruction. All bleeding points are secured. The remaining obstructed segment of tube is excised and the mesosalpinx suture-ligated with 3-0 Vicryl (Fig. 29–15).

The cornual portion of the uterus is injected with 1:200 vasopressin (Fig. 29–16). Serial sharp cuts are made into the cornua (Fig. 29–17). At the same time, methylene blue is injected retrogradely through the cervix. When the open portion of the interstitial portion of the oviduct is transected, blue dye squirts forth. A lacrimal probe is inserted into the interstitial tube lumen and is advanced into the uterine cavity. The probe is withdrawn, and the polyethylene stent described earlier is fed through the distal tube lumen into the uterine cavity (Fig. 29–18).

Anastomosis of the two segments of tube is carried out with 5-0 or 6-0 Vicryl interrupted sutures (Fig. 29–19). The serosal portion of the oviduct then is anchored to the uterine serosa with 5-0 Vicryl. The cornual defect is closed simultaneously with 4-0 Vicryl (Fig. 29–20).

The abdomen is thoroughly irrigated before closure is performed. The stent is recovered via hysteroscopy 3 to 4 weeks postoperatively.

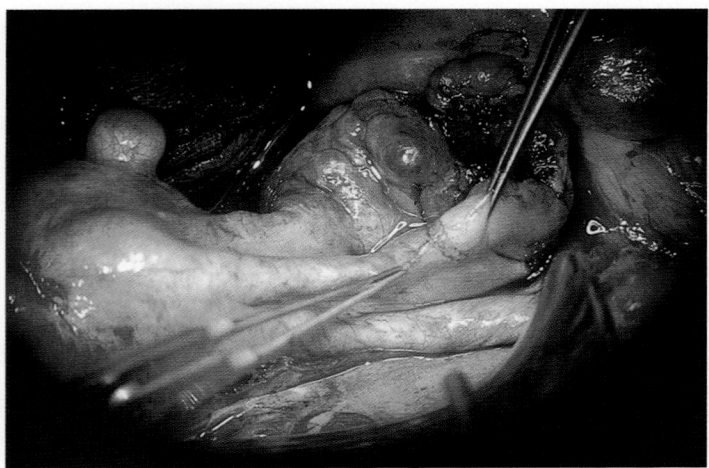

**FIGURE 29–15** The proximal tube has been injected via fimbrial cannulation to demonstrate the area of obstruction. The tube will be cut open at the scored area. The entire segment of cornual and isthmic oviduct is obstructed.

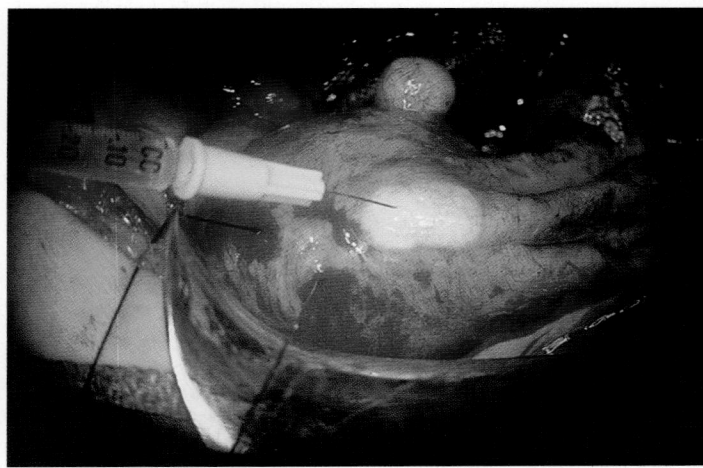

**FIGURE 29–16** A 1:200 vasopressin solution is injected into the cornua with a fine (25-gauge) needle.

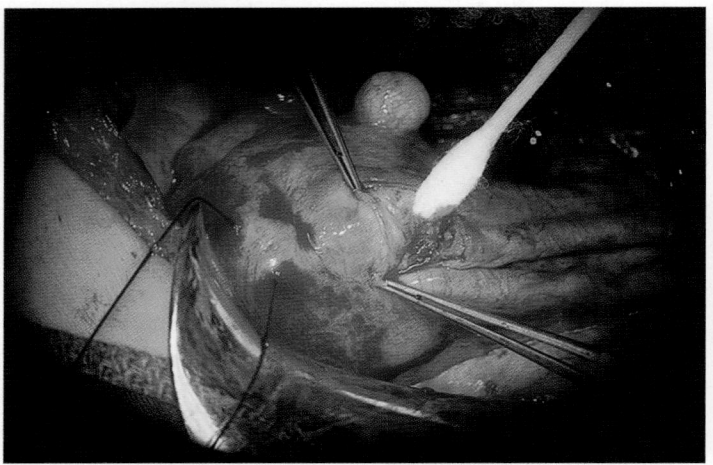

**FIGURE 29–17** The cornua is serially sliced until the transcervically injected methylene blue dye flows freely from the opened interstitial portion of the tube.

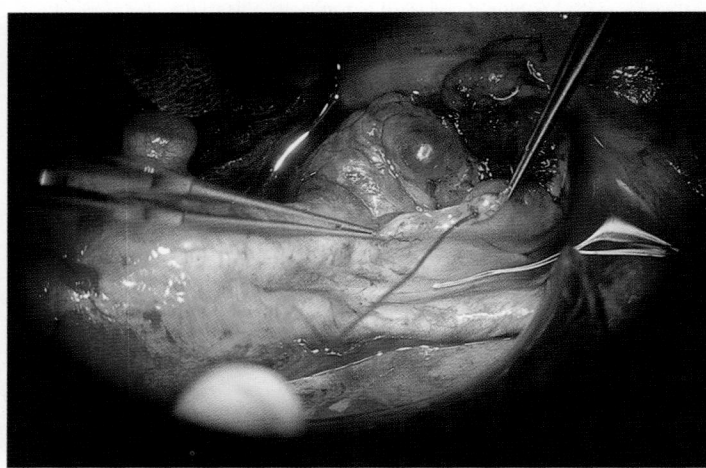

**FIGURE 29–18** The two open ends of the oviduct are approximated at the cornua after the obstructed segment is removed.

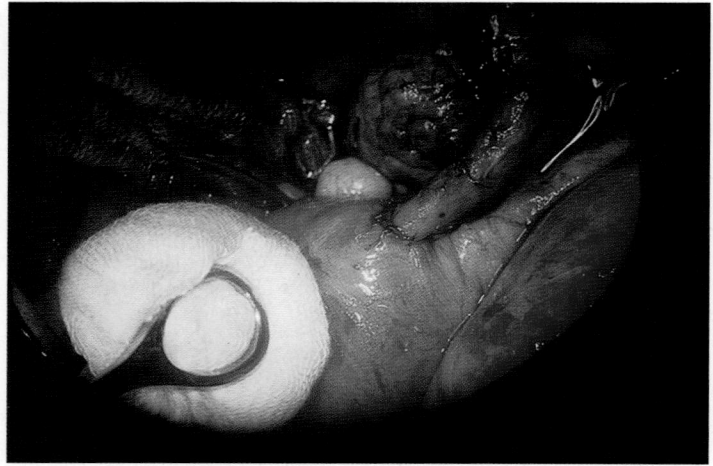

**FIGURE 29–19** The tube is anastomosed into the cornua in a two-layered closure.

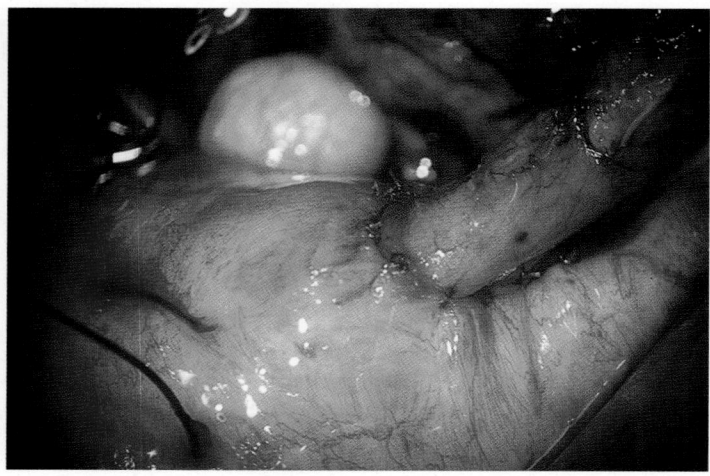

**FIGURE 29–20** The cornual incision is closed with 4-0 Vicryl. The serosa of the tube is sutured to the serosa of the uterus with 5-0 Vicryl.

# CHAPTER 30

# Tubal Sterilization

## *Michael S. Baggish*

Tubal interruption, or bilateral partial salpingectomy, is a relatively easy and direct method of accomplishing surgical sterilization. Typically, this operation is performed at the time of cesarean section, or immediately postpartum in the case of vaginal delivery. Two operations are especially well suited for these particular circumstances. Modified Irving and Pomeroy techniques are enhanced as further tubal separation may be anticipated as the result of rapid regression of the uterine mass to a nonpregnant size and shape. Most interval sterilizations are performed via laparoscopy (Fig. 30–1A–H). The Uchida operation can be performed as a postpartum or an interval operation. Simple fimbriectomy or ampullary-isthmus excision is well suited as an interim operation.

Whatever method is selected for tubal sterilization, certain precepts must be followed. First, an executed sterilization permit must be obtained for each and every patient, and each patient must be informed that the operation is a permanent sterilization procedure, and that there is no possibility of pregnancy in the future. Paradoxically, patients also must be told that a failure rate is associated with each operation. Second, the tube must be carefully distinguished from the two other structures located at the top of the broad ligament: most anteriorly, the round ligament, and most posteriorly, the utero-ovarian ligament (Fig. 30–2). Next the tube should be traced from the uterus to the fimbriated end and then secured with a Babcock clamp or stay suture-ligature. Finally, the location of the ipsilateral ovary should be viewed relative to the tube. The proximal and distal ends of the tube are grasped with Babcock clamps, and the stretched tube is held straight and elevated upward so as to clearly expose the mesosalpinx.

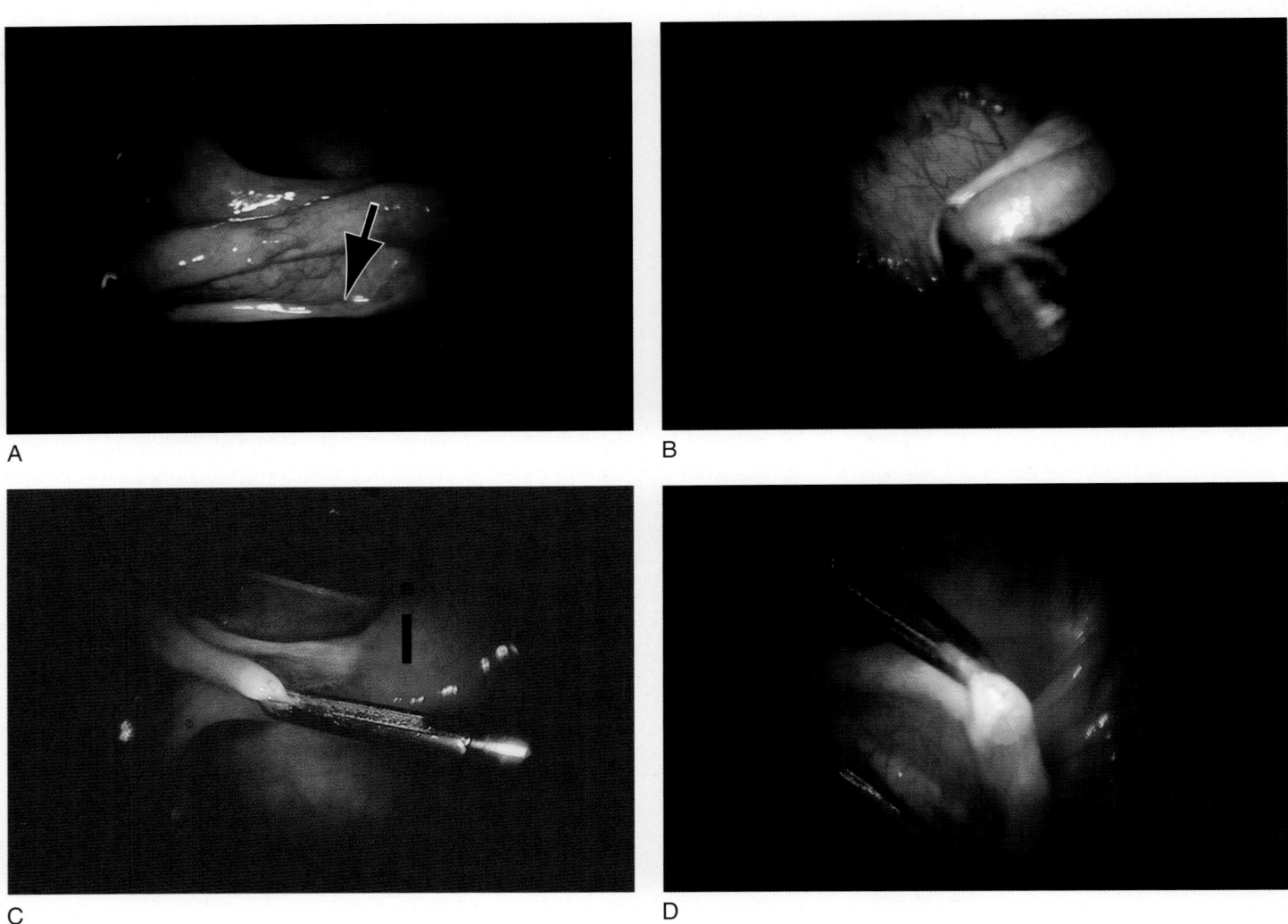

**FIGURE 30–1  A.** Endoscopic view of the oviduct. Note anteriorly the curving round ligament and below (*arrow*) the whitish utero-ovarian ligament. **B.** The close-up of the tube grasped by the forceps. **C.** Panoramic view from the front (anterior) detailing the three tubular structures emanating from the top of the uterus (*dark line*). Grasped within the forceps is the tube. Anteriorly is the round ligament and posteriorly the utero-ovarian ligament. **D.** Electric current is applied via the grasping forceps. White blanching (coagulation) occurs above and below the point where the tube is held by the forceps.

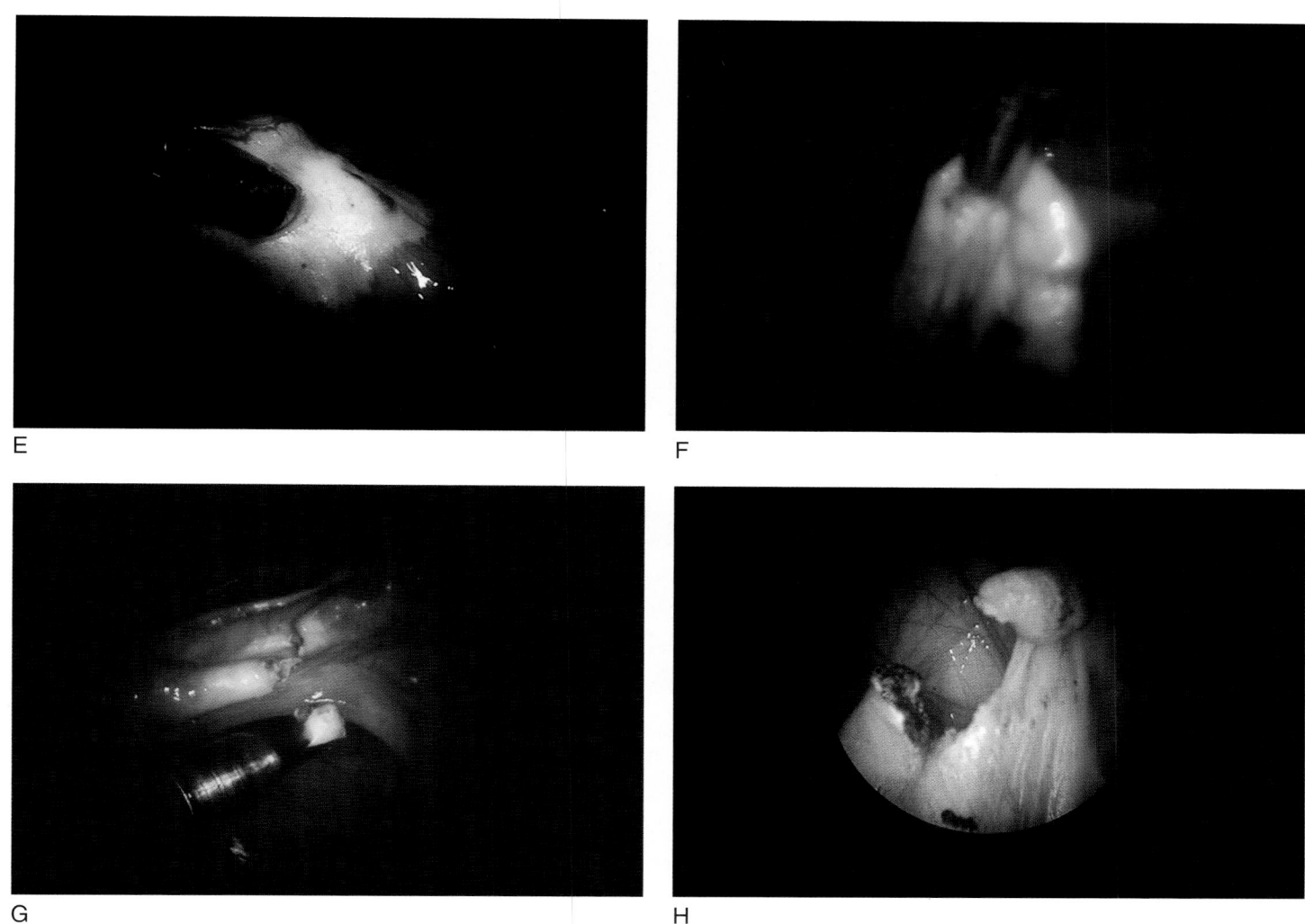

E

F

G

H

**FIGURE 30–1, cont'd  E.** Close-up view of the extensive coagulation. **F.** To achieve satisfactory hemostasis, coagulation continues until the mesosalpinx is coagulated. **G.** A coagulated segment of the oviduct is removed and sent to pathology. **H.** Completed laparoscopic bilateral partial salpingectomy performed by electrosurgical coagulation.

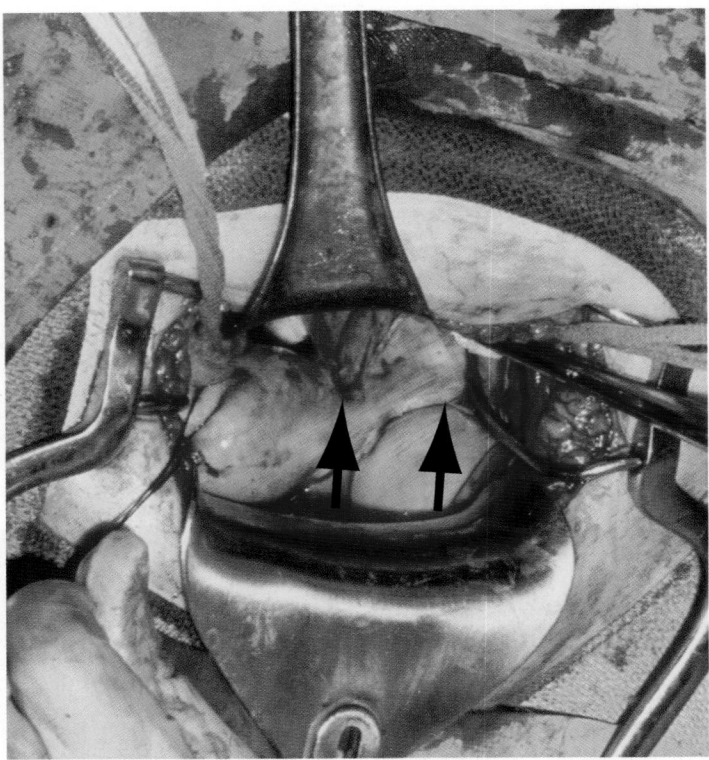

**FIGURE 30–2** Laparotomy performed on a woman who had a failed bilateral partial salpingectomy. The failure was caused by bilateral ligation of the round ligaments rather than ligation of the oviducts (*arrows*).

## Modified Irving Procedure

A window is made under a 3-cm segment of tube with the use of fine, straight mosquito clamps, thus securing fat and vessels within the mesosalpinx (Fig. 30–3A). Next, Kelly clamps are applied to the uterine end and to the fimbriated end of the isolated tubal segment (Fig. 30–3B). The tube is ligated and then is suture-ligated on each end with 3-0 Vicryl or polydioxanone (PDS) double-armed sutures. The segment of tube is cut out and sent to pathology for diagnosis. The sutures are cut close to the knot on the distal (fimbriated) end. The two sutures are held with needles on the uterine end (Fig. 30–3C). A needle guide or mosquito clamp is pushed into the posterior aspect of the uterus after the distance that the tied proximal tubal segment will stretch without tension is measured. Each needle is sutured via the guide through the hole created in the posterior wall of the uterus. As the needle guide is removed, the ends of the suture (after the needles have been cut free) are tightened, securing the proximal tubal stump into the myometrium of the posterior uterine wall. The ends of the suture are tied, and not only are the proximal and distal ends of the tubes widely separated, but the uterine end is also sealed off inside the wall of the uterus (Fig. 30–3D).

## Pomeroy Operation

In the Pomeroy operation, a knuckle of the ampullary portion of the tube is pulled up with a mosquito hemostat or Allis clamp (Fig. 30–4A). A Kelly clamp is placed across the base of the pulled-up knuckle of tube (Fig. 30–4B). Scissors are used to excise the knuckle of tube by cutting along the superior marginal surface above the Kelly clamp application. Next, a 0 chromic catgut suture ligature is placed below the center of the Kelly clamp and is secured fore and aft (Fig. 30–4C). The clamp is removed as three knots are tied into place. Hemostasis is checked and the suture ligature is cut just above the knot (Fig. 30–4D).

## Fimbriectomy

This operation may be performed by minilaparotomy (abdominally) or by posterior colpotomy (vaginally) or by laparoscopy. The oviduct is located and secured close to the uterus with a Babcock or Allis clamp. The fimbriated portion of the tube is clamped with a Kelly clamp; a second Kelly clamp is placed across the tube at the ampullary-fimbrial junction. The tube is cut between the first and second Kelly clamps, and the fimbriated end sent to pathology. The tube is ligated and suture-ligated with 2-0 silk or 3-0 nylon (Fig. 30–5).

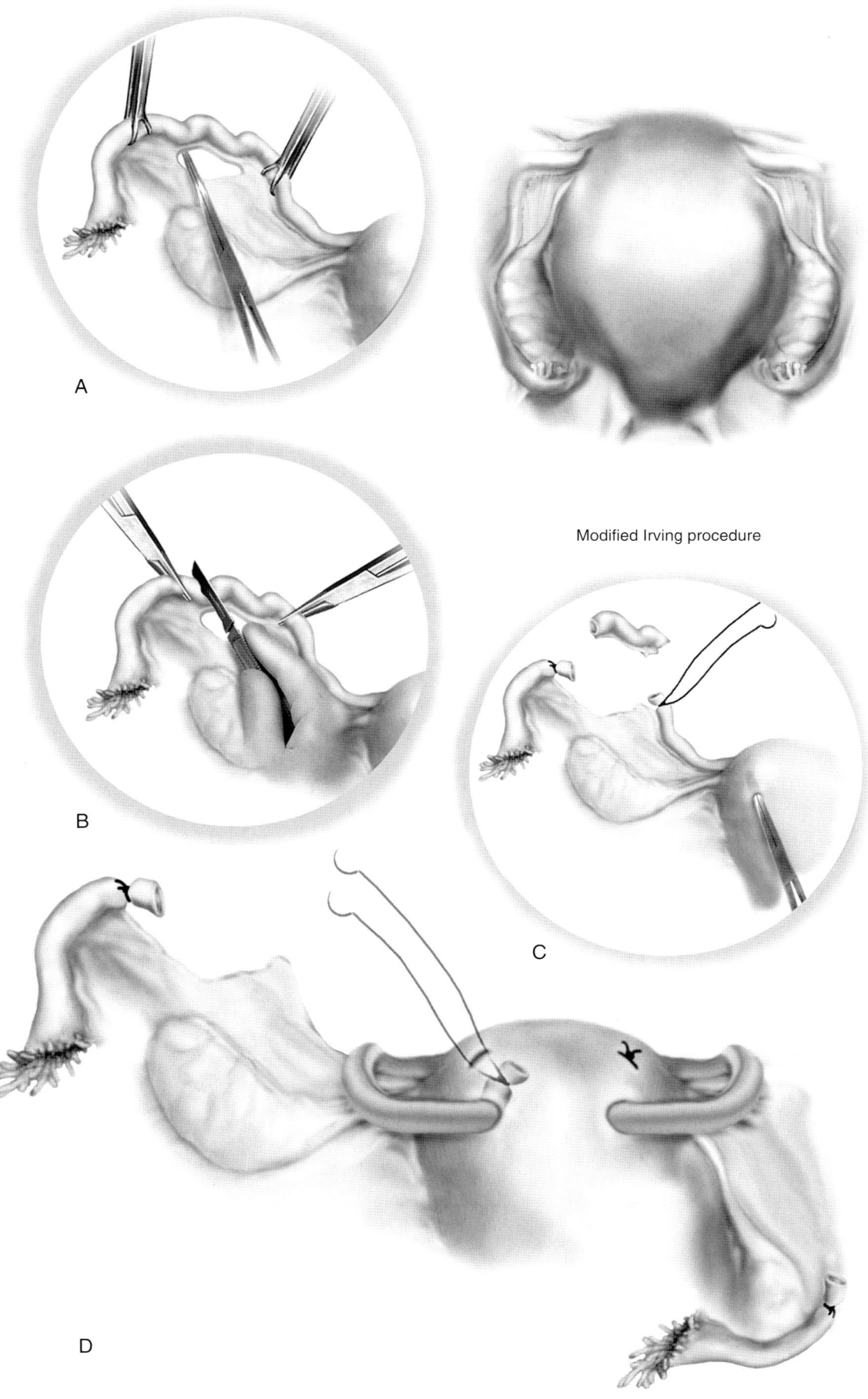

A

B

Modified Irving procedure

C

D

**FIGURE 30–3** The modified Irving procedure. **A.** A mosquito clamp is used to create a window in the mesosalpinx beneath the tube segment that is to be removed. **B.** Two mosquito or Kelly clamps are placed at each extreme of the isolated segment, and the segment is cut out. **C.** Suture-ligatures are placed through each end of the remaining oviduct and tied under the clamps, which are then removed; however, the double-armed suture attached to the uterine oviductal remnant is held. A grooved director or mosquito clamp is used to burrow a hole into the posterior aspect of the uterus. **D.** The sutures are fed through the tract and into the uterine wall. The uterine oviductal segment is buried in the uterine wall as the suture ends are pulled snugly and tied into place.

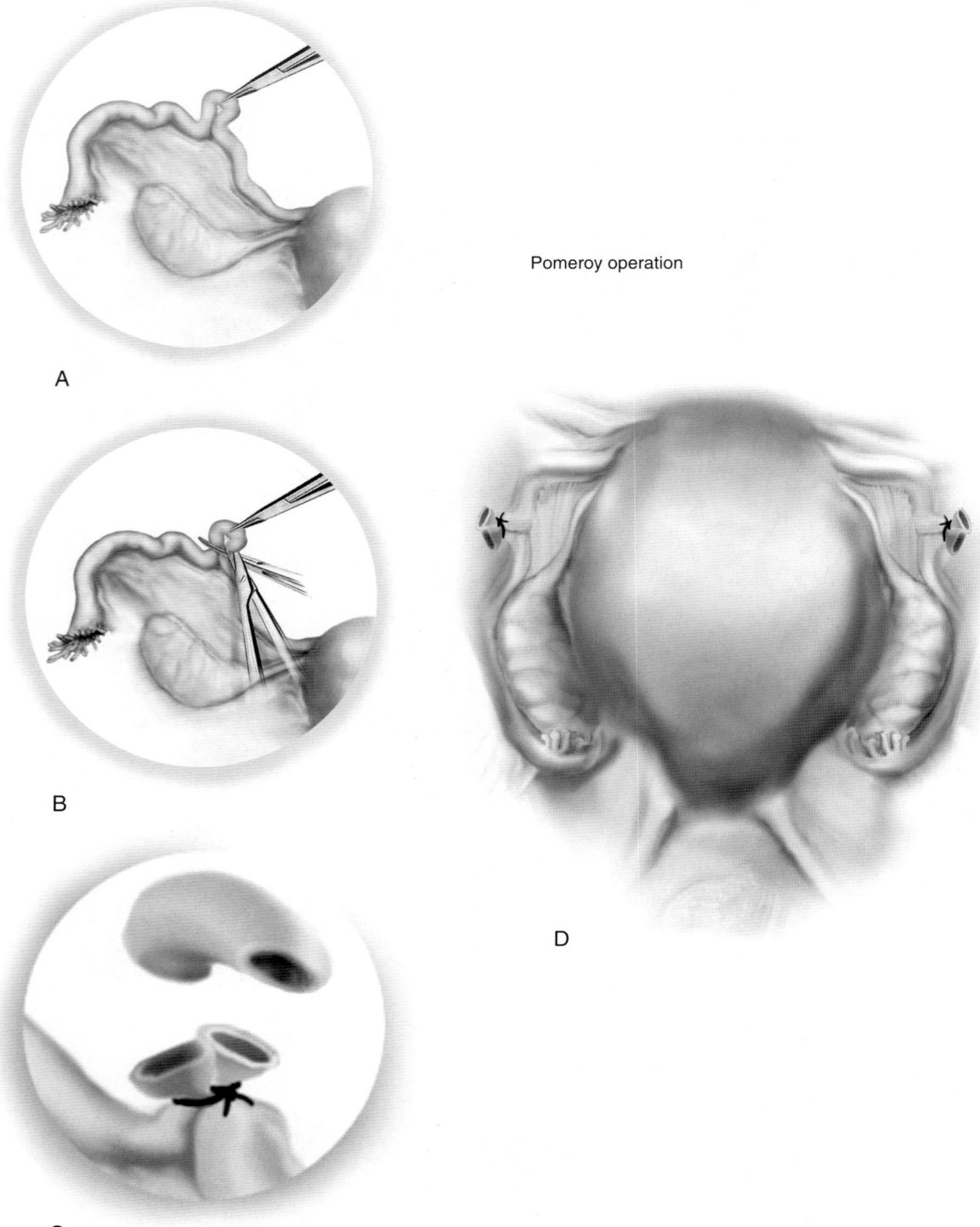

Pomeroy operation

A

B

C

D

**FIGURE 30–4** The Pomeroy operation. **A.** A clamp is used to grasp a knuckle of ampulla and pull it upward. **B.** A second Kelly clamp is placed across the base of the knuckle, and the tube above the Kelly clamp is cut off and sent to pathology. **C.** Next, a 0 chromic catgut ligature is placed around the Kelly clamp and is tied snugly into place. **D.** As the pregnant uterus involutes and the tensile strength of the chromic catgut weakens, the cut tube segments are pulled apart.

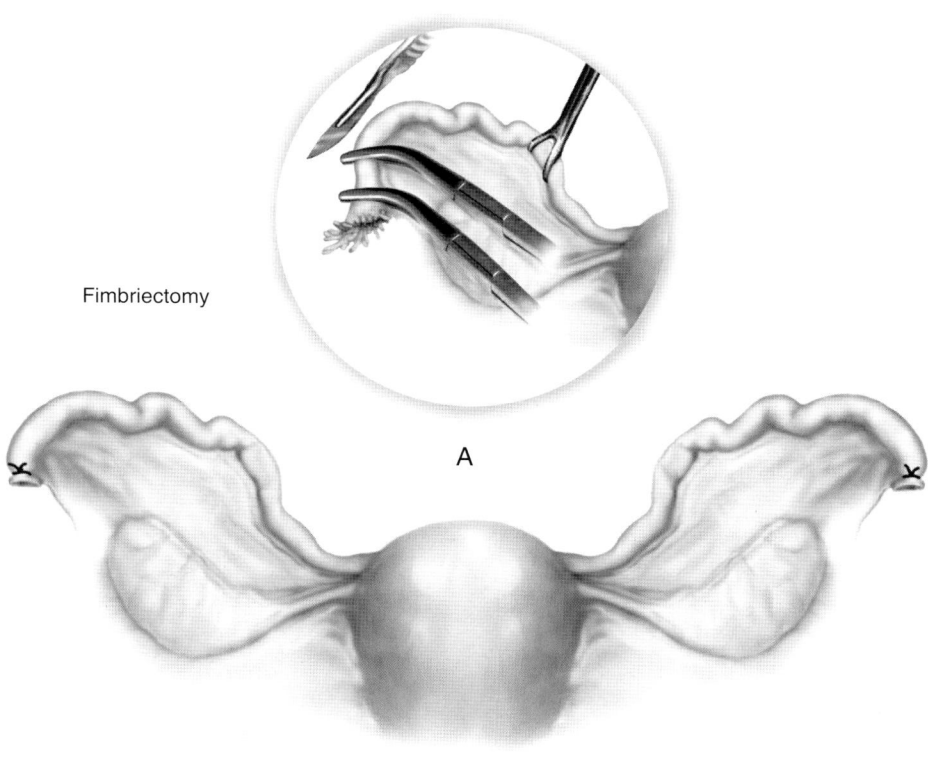

Fimbriectomy

A

B

**FIGURE 30–5** Fimbriectomy is a simple operation. **A.** The fimbriated ends of the tube are clamped with Kelly clamps, and the fimbriae are amputated. **B.** The ends are suture-ligated with 2-0 silk or 3-0 nylon.

## Simple Bilateral Partial Salpingectomy

This is an interval operation and may be performed by mini-laparotomy or by laparoscopy. The tube is grasped with an Allis clamp at midpoint in its length. A hole is made with a mosquito clamp in the mesosalpinx directly below the elevated portion of the oviduct. The hole measures approximately 1.5 to 2 cm. The tube is clamped at either pole above the mesosalpingeal opening. Scissors are used to cut out the segment of tube, and either end is suture-ligated with 2-0 or 3-0 silk or nylon (Fig. 30–6). Alternatively, the ends of the tube may be coagulated with bipolar forceps rather than clamped and ligated with suture.

## Uchida Operation

The Uchida operation may be performed postpartum or as an interval procedure. The principles of the operation are similar to those of the Irving operation (i.e., not only is the oviduct divided, but one end is also physically isolated from the other by a barrier).

The tube is grasped at the ampullary-isthmic junction. The serosa of the 2-cm segment of tube is infiltrated with 5 to 10 mL of a 1:200 vasopressin/saline solution (Fig. 30–7A, B). With a sharp scalpel, the dorsum (antimesenteric side) of the tube is shallowly incised in a parallel fashion to the axis of the oviduct. An Allis clamp is used to grasp the tube beneath the serosa and strip it from the surrounding serosa by moving the clamp forward and backward along the length of the incision (Fig. 30–7C). Either pole of the tubal segment is clamped with mosquito clamps, and the segment (1.5 cm) of tube is cut out. Each end is suture-ligated with 2-0 silk or nylon (Fig. 30–7D). The uterine end of the tube is buried in the mesosalpinx as it is closed with 3-0 Vicryl. The other ligated end remains outside of the reconstituted mesosalpinx (Fig. 30–7E).

## Silastic Band Operation

This technique typically is performed by laparoscopy; however, it may be utilized at laparotomy as well. The procedure requires a special tool: the band applicator. This is a tong forceps with two cylindrical tubes in which the outer cylinder moves over the inner cylinder as the tongs grasper pulls a knuckle of tube into the inner cylinder. Essentially, the tube is grasped at the thinnest portion of the ampulla. Before the start of the procedure, a Silastic band is loaded onto the terminal inner cylinder (Fig. 30–8A). The tube segment is held in the tongs and is slowly drawn up into the hollow inner cylinder (Fig. 30–8B). The trigger mechanism at the same time causes the outer cylinder to push the Silastic band onto the intercepted knuckle of tube and the proximal mesosalpinx in a fashion analogous to the Pomeroy technique, except that no portion of tube is cut (Figs. 30–8C and 30–9). The tube simply necroses slowly because its blood supply is compromised by the tight Silastic band.

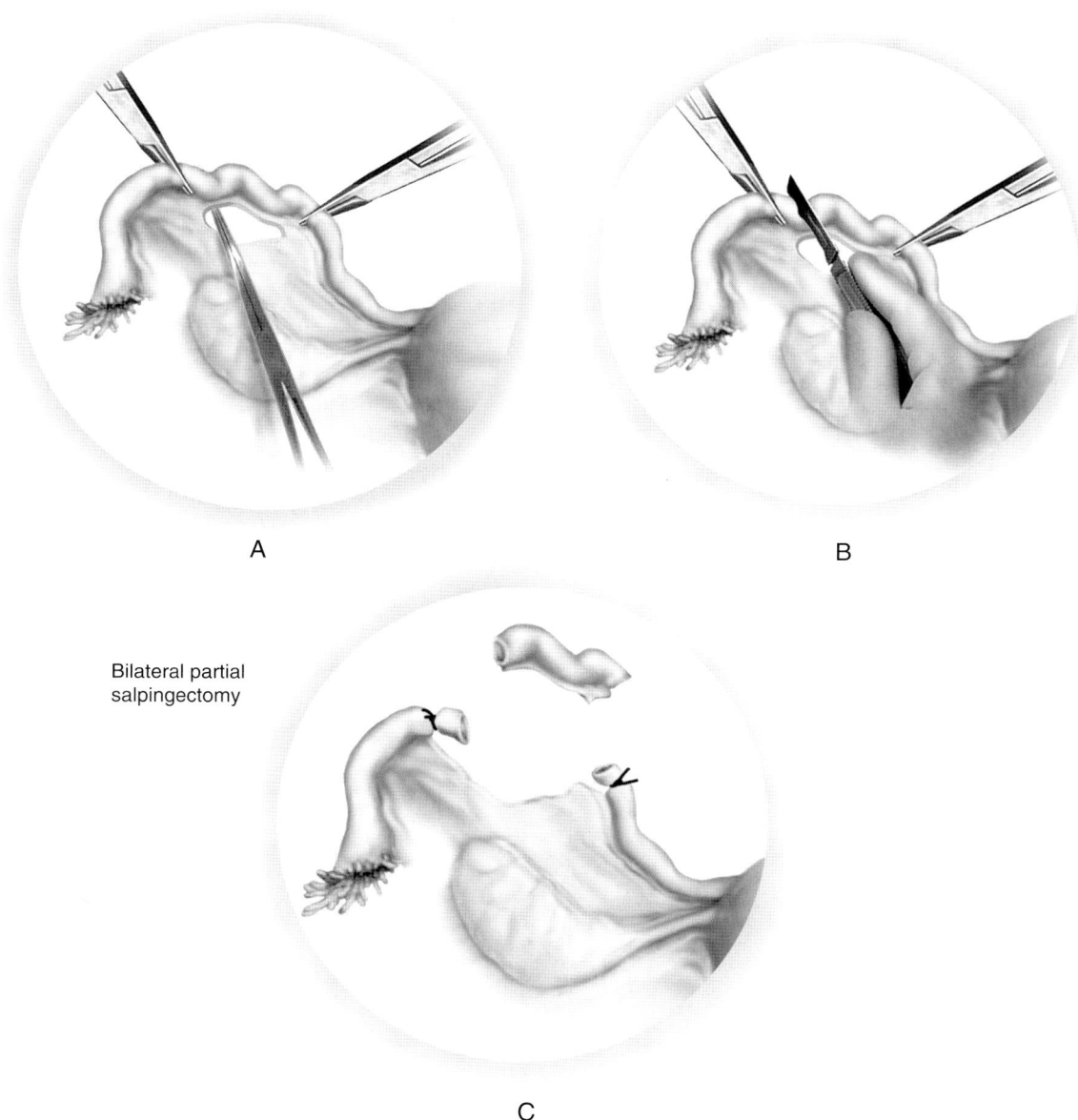

A

B

Bilateral partial
salpingectomy

C

**FIGURE 30–6 A-C.** Bilateral partial salpingectomy is performed in exactly the same manner as the Irving operation; however, neither tubal segment is isolated from the other. The ends are simply ligated with permanent suture material.

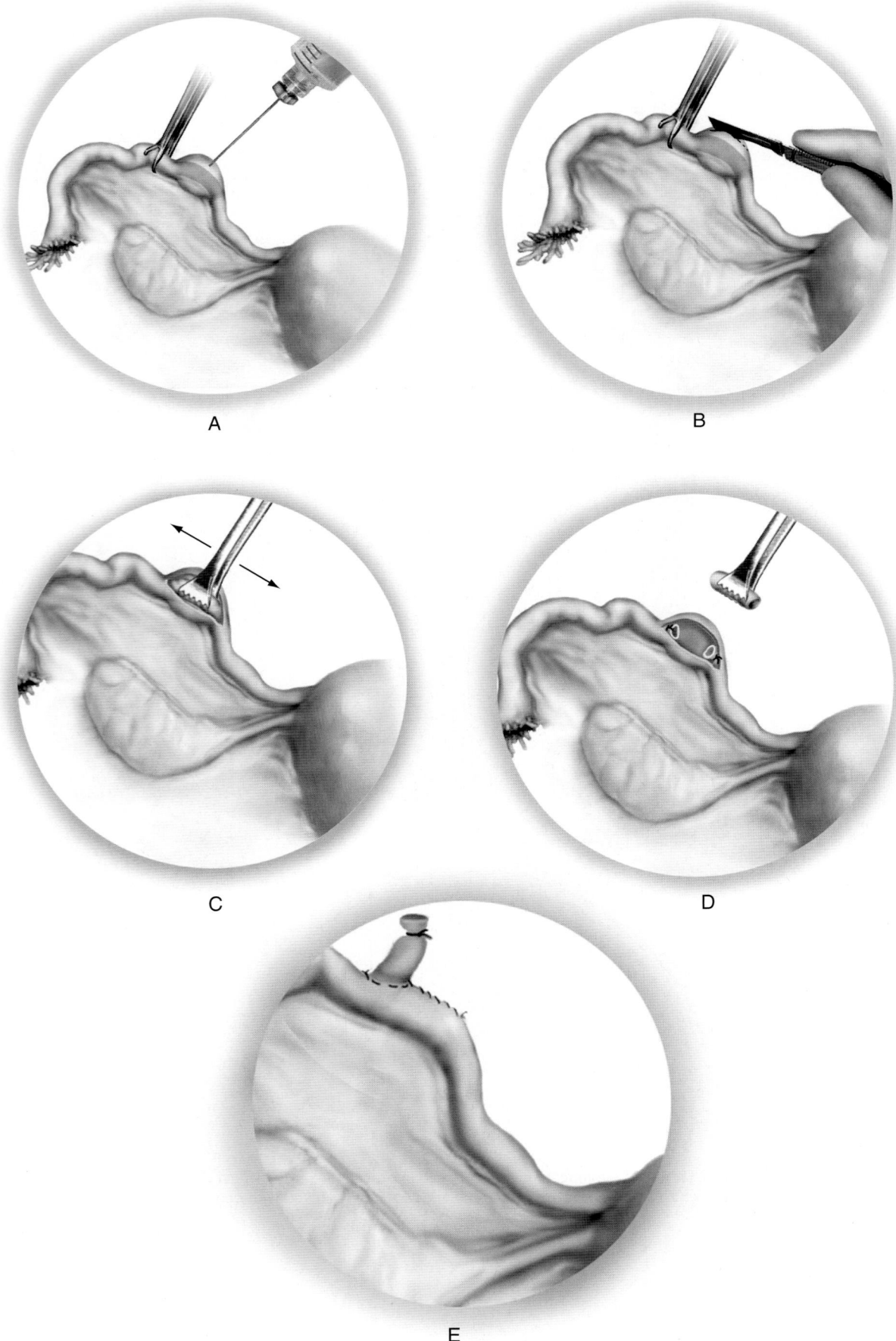

**FIGURE 30–7 A.** The Uchida operation utilizes an injection of 1:200 vasopressin into the mesosalpinx for the dual purpose of hemostasis and creation of a dissection plane. **B.** A linear incision is made above the oviduct in the ballooned-out segment that has followed vasopressin injection. **C.** With a Uchida clamp or a loosely applied Allis clamp, the oviduct is freed from the mesentery by moving the clamp back and forth within the mesosalpinx. The freed segment is ligated at either end with 2-0 silk or nylon, and the segment is cut out. **D** and **E.** The fimbriated end of the tube remains out of the mesosalpinx during closure of the mesentery, whereas the uterine end of the tube is buried in the mesosalpinx.

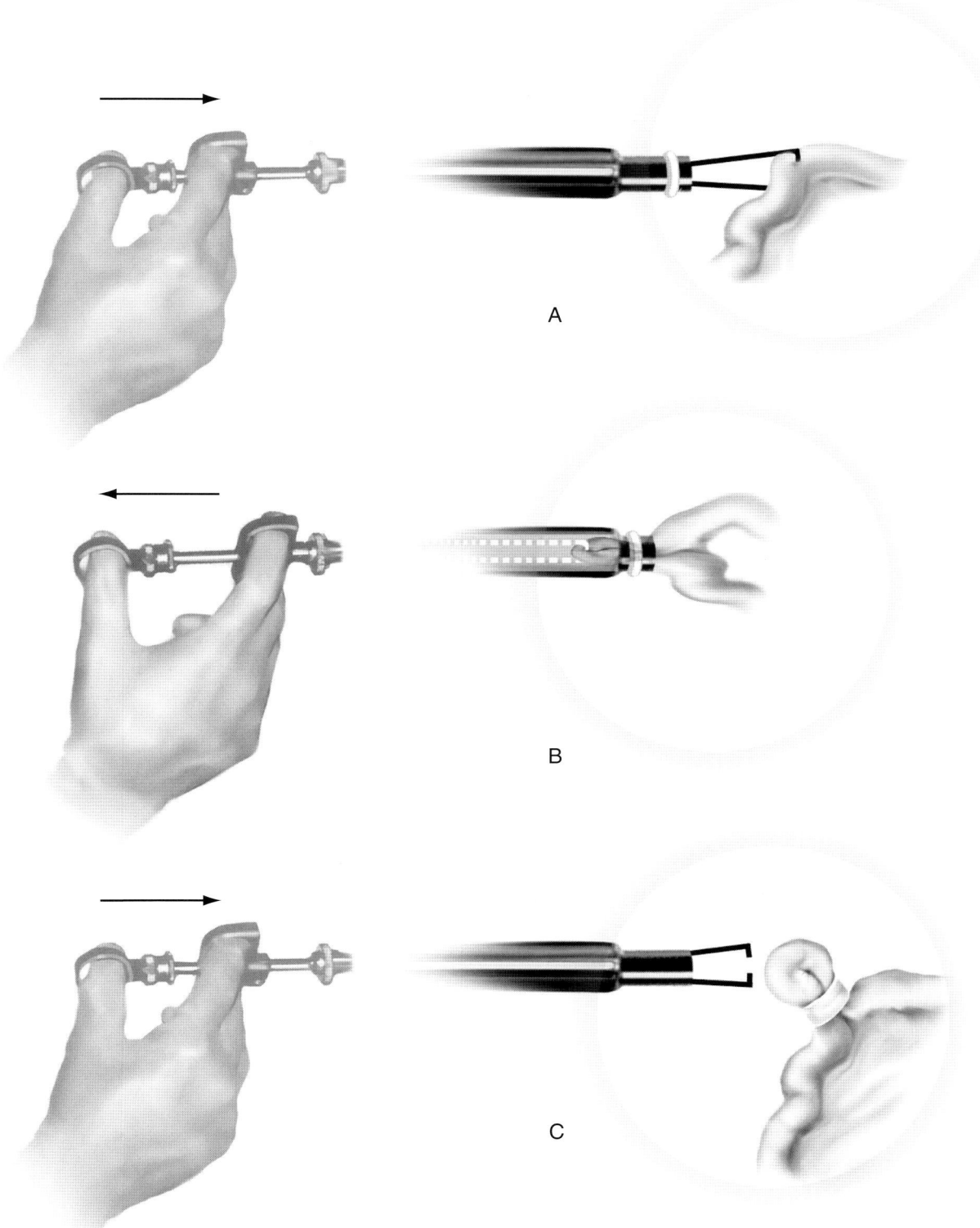

A

B

C

**FIGURE 30–8** The Silastic banding of the oviducts requires a special tongs forceps. **A.** An isthmic segment of the tube is grasped with the tongs. Note that a Silastic band has been loaded onto the inner cylinder of the forceps at its terminal portion. **B.** Next, the tongs containing a knuckle of tube are drawn into the inner cylinder of the tongs forceps. At the same time, the spring-loaded inner cylinder is pulled back against the fixed outer cylinder, causing the band to be pushed onto the base of the knuckle of oviduct. **C.** The tongs are released (i.e., extended outward), freeing the banded tube.

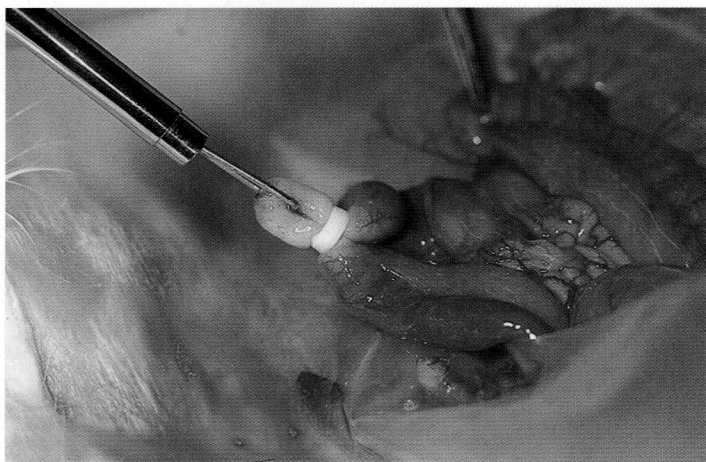

**FIGURE 30–9** The Silastic banding technique performed upon a rabbit uterine horn. Note the white color of the banded knuckle of oviduct, which is the result of its blood supply being cut off.

# SECTION E

# Retropubic Space

# CHAPTER 31

# Anatomy of Retropubic Space

*Michael S. Baggish* ■ *Mickey M. Karram*

The boundaries of the retropubic space (space of Retzius) are the symphysis pubis anteriorly, the pubic rami laterally, and the sidewalls composed of pubic bone and obturator internus muscle. The anterior aspects of the proximal urethra and extraperitoneal portions of the bladder are seen upon exposure of the retropubic space. Figure 31–1 illustrates the view from above the retropubic space. Note that the floor of the retropubic space is formed by the fibrofatty outer lining of the vaginal wall termed *endopelvic fascia*, the perivesical fascia, and fibers from the levator ani muscle. This trapezoid structure provides support for the proximal urethra and bladder. Figure 31–2 shows a sagittal section of the normal anatomy of the pelvis. Figures 31–3, 31–4, and 31–5 demonstrate the relationship of the space to the urinary bladder, pelvic sidewall, upper thigh, and uterus.

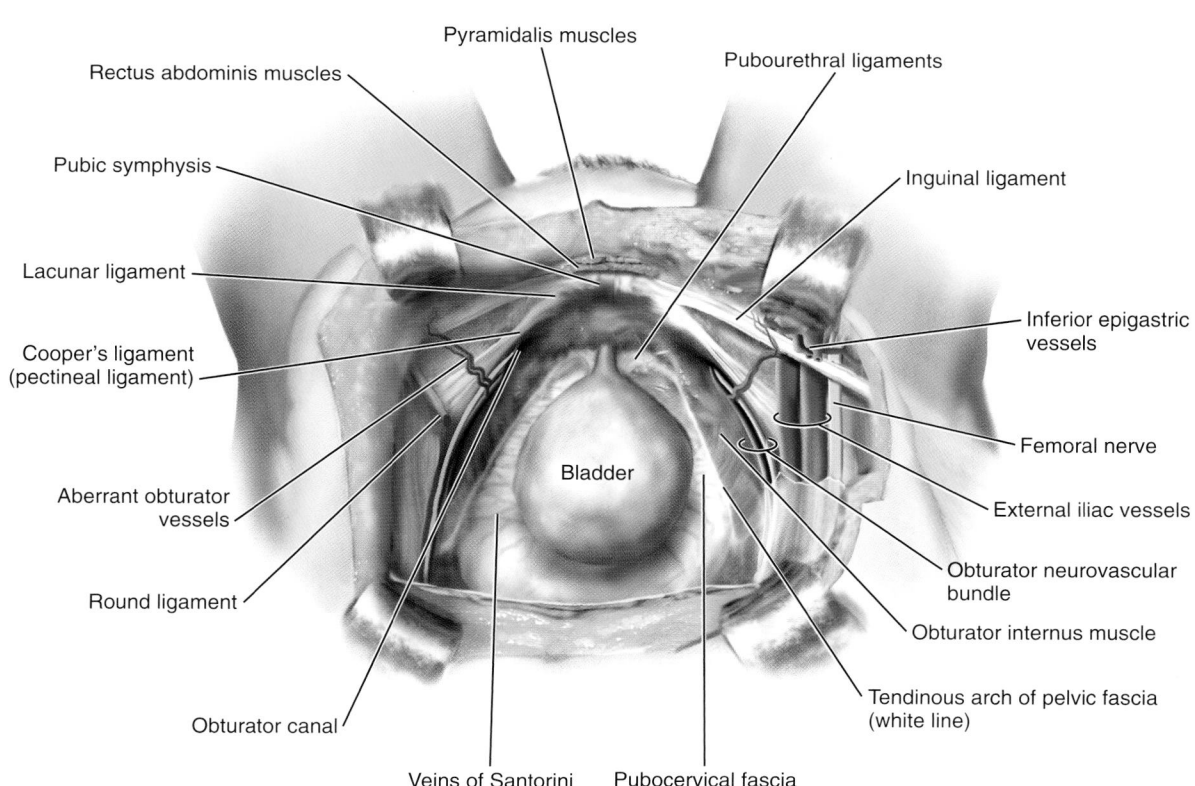

Pyramidalis muscles
Rectus abdominis muscles
Pubourethral ligaments
Pubic symphysis
Inguinal ligament
Lacunar ligament
Cooper's ligament (pectineal ligament)
Inferior epigastric vessels
Aberrant obturator vessels
Femoral nerve
Round ligament
Bladder
External iliac vessels
Obturator neurovascular bundle
Obturator internus muscle
Obturator canal
Tendinous arch of pelvic fascia (white line)
Veins of Santorini
Pubocervical fascia

**FIGURE 31–1** Normal anatomy of the pelvis viewed from above. Note how the proximal urethra and extrapertioneal portions of the bladder are exposed through the retropubic space. Note the trapezoid-shaped endopelvic fascia or inside lining of the muscular portion of the vaginal wall. The fascia provides the support for the anterior wall.

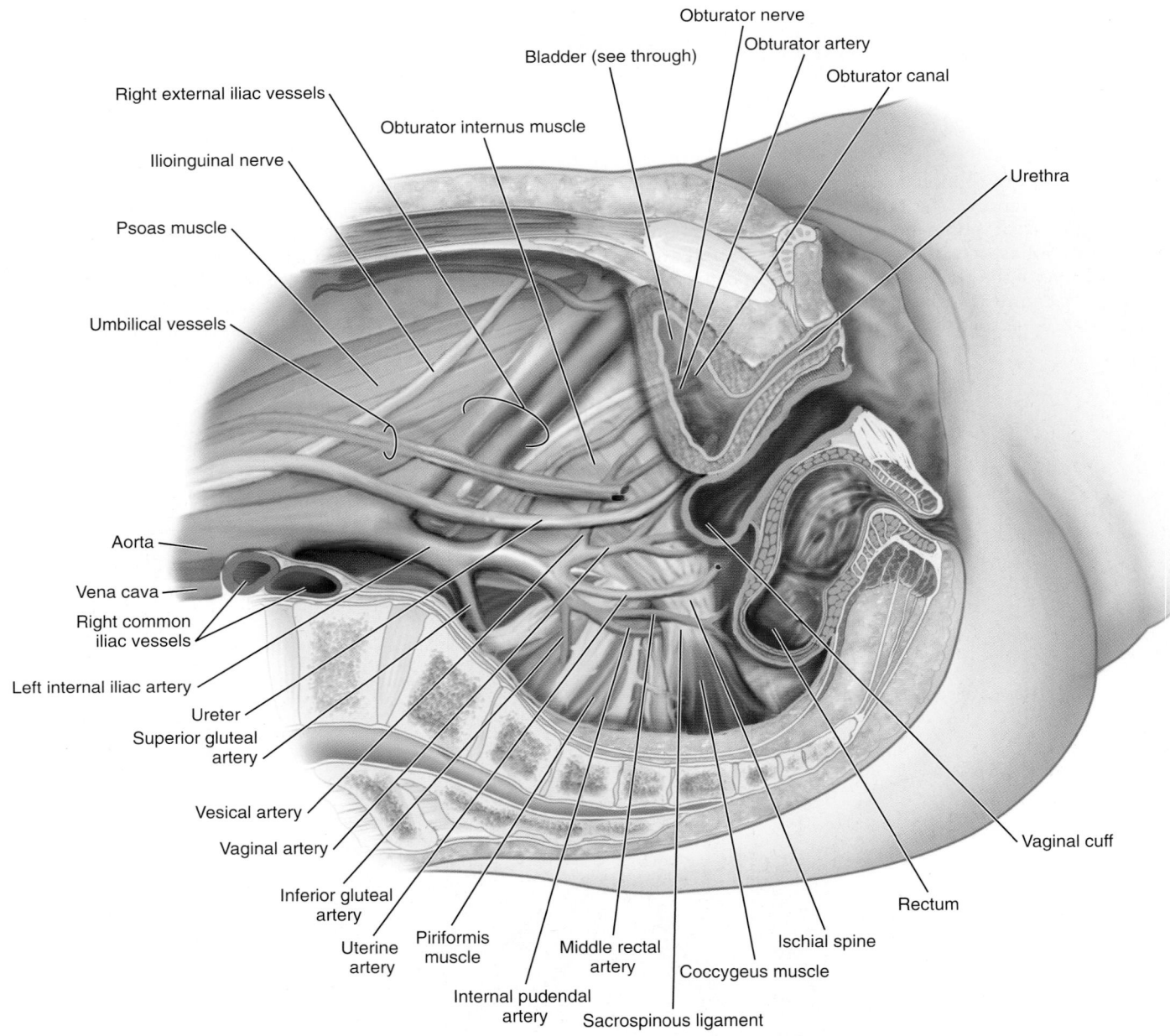

Obturator nerve

Bladder (see through)    Obturator artery

Obturator canal

Right external iliac vessels

Obturator internus muscle

Ilioinguinal nerve

Urethra

Psoas muscle

Umbilical vessels

Aorta

Vena cava

Right common iliac vessels

Left internal iliac artery

Ureter

Superior gluteal artery

Vesical artery

Vaginal artery

Vaginal cuff

Inferior gluteal artery

Rectum

Uterine artery    Piriformis muscle    Middle rectal artery    Ischial spine

Coccygeus muscle

Internal pudendal artery    Sacrospinous ligament

**FIGURE 31–2** Sagittal section of the normal anatomy of the pelvis. Note how the various vessels, nerves, and muscles relate to the bladder and retropubic space. Note now the external iliac vessels exit the pelvis underneath the inguinal ligament just lateral to the uppermost portion of the retropubic space, while the obturator neurovascular bundle passes through the retropubic space to exit the pelvis through the obturator canal.

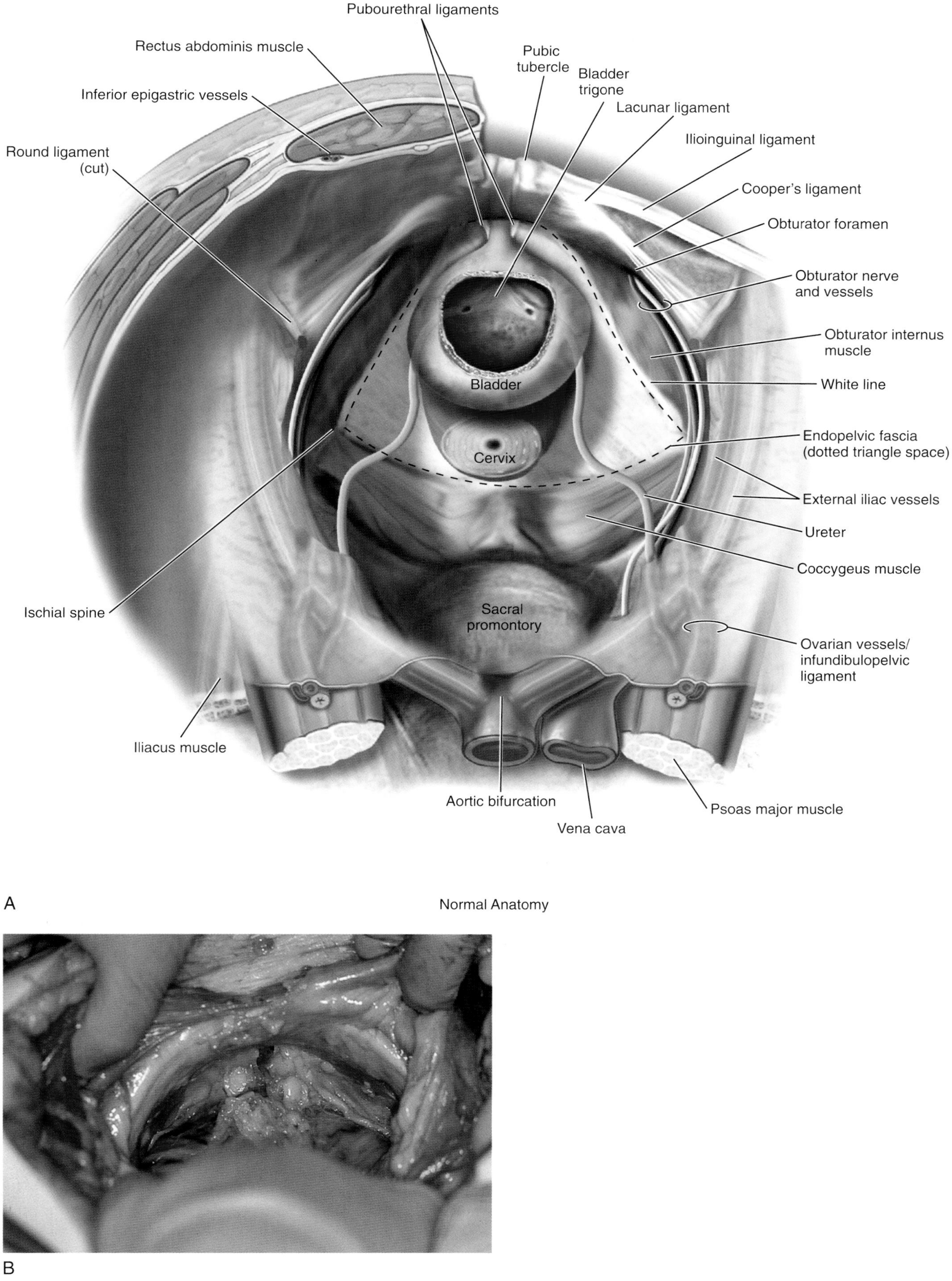

Pubourethral ligaments

Rectus abdominis muscle

Inferior epigastric vessels

Round ligament (cut)

Pubic tubercle

Bladder trigone

Lacunar ligament

Ilioinguinal ligament

Cooper's ligament

Obturator foramen

Obturator nerve and vessels

Obturator internus muscle

White line

Bladder

Cervix

Endopelvic fascia (dotted triangle space)

External iliac vessels

Ureter

Coccygeus muscle

Ischial spine

Sacral promontory

Ovarian vessels/ infundibulopelvic ligament

Iliacus muscle

Aortic bifurcation

Vena cava

Psoas major muscle

A

Normal Anatomy

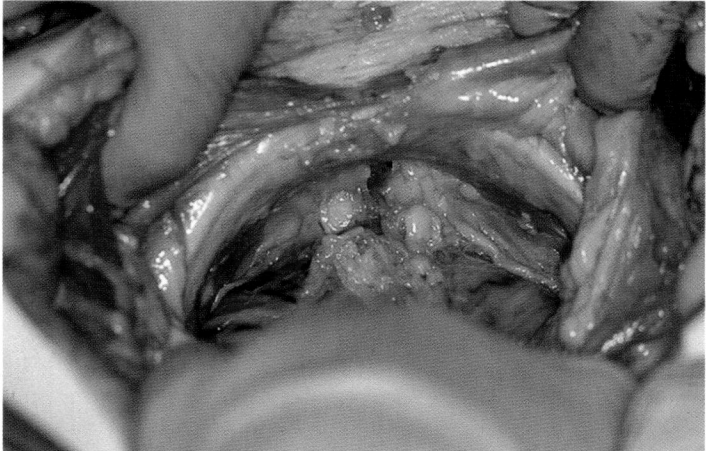

B

**FIGURE 31–3 A.** Surgical anatomy of the retropubic space. Note that the proximal urethra and bladder rest on the anterior vaginal wall with its underlying muscular component, or pubocervical fascia. The vagina attaches laterally to the white line, or arcus tendineus fasciae pelvis. The veins of Santorini run within the vaginal wall and are commonly encountered during colposuspension procedures. Other important vascular structures that may be encountered in this space include the obturator neurovascular bundle, the aberrant obturator artery and vein, and the external iliac artery and vein. **B.** Retropubic space in a female cadaver. Note that abundant retropubic fat is usually encountered upon initial dissection into the space.

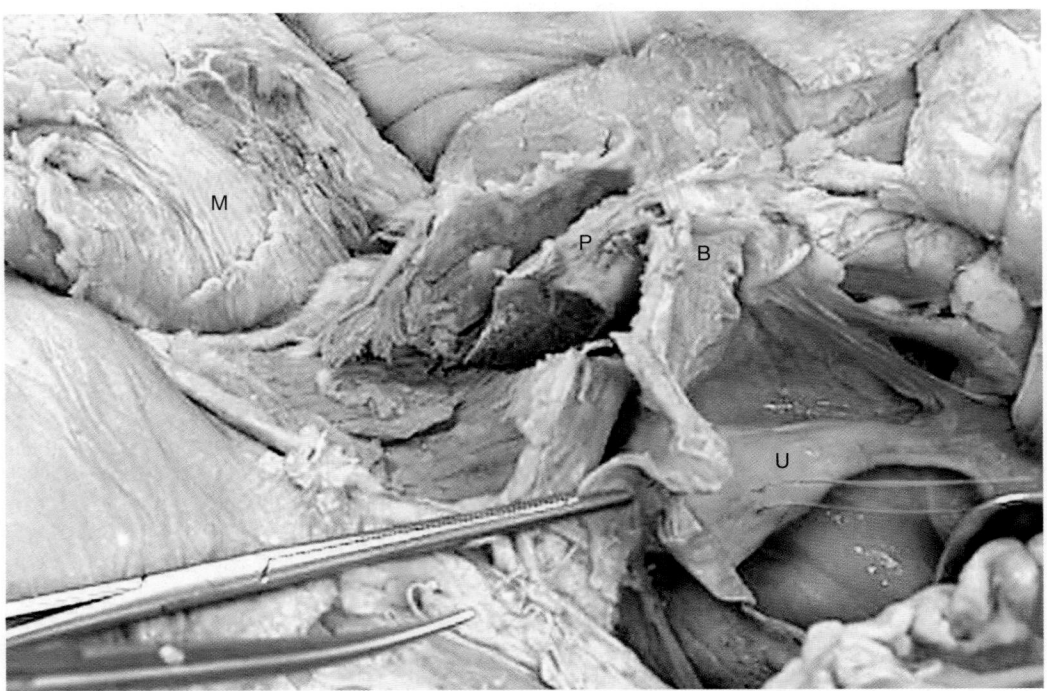

**FIGURE 31–4** The uterus (U) is elevated via a fundal (blue) suture. The bladder (B) is held straight upward via a white stitch. The sawed pubic symphysis (P) is most forward (anterior). The mons veneris (M) has been cut and flapped forward anteriorly.

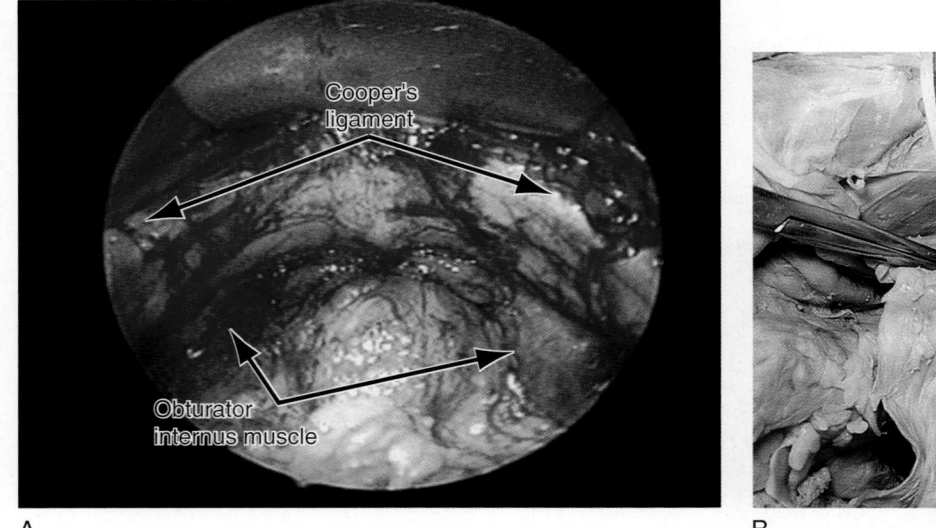

A

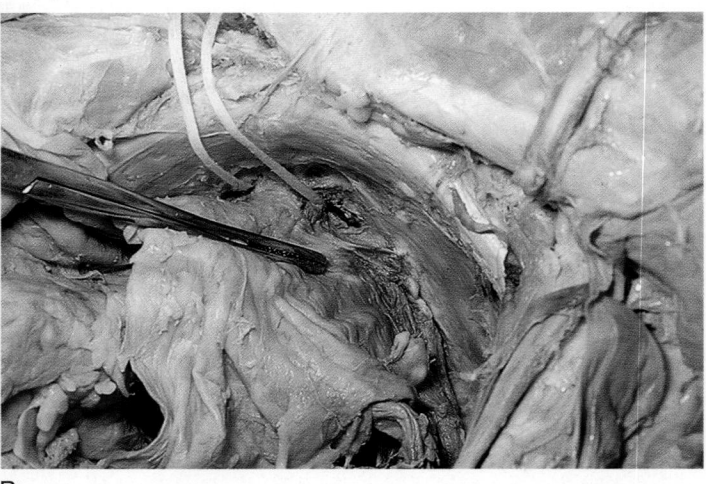

B

**FIGURE 31–5 A.** Retropubic space in a live patient. The arrows point to the top lateral portions of the space noting Cooper's ligament. Below this, the obturator internus muscle is seen on each side. Note again the abundant retropubic fat commonly seen in this space. **B.** The retropubic space has been totally exposed. A large straight clamp is placed across the urinary bladder. An umbilical tape has been placed just above the urethrovesical junction. The tip of a probe placed in the vagina protrudes through the internal projection of the right anterolateral fornix.

The adipose tissue behind the symphysis between the bladder and the pubic bones can be gently separated by blunt finger dissection. The space is progressively developed from the superior to the inferior margin of the pubic symphysis (see Figs. 31–4, 31–5, and 31–6). The lateral development of the retropubic space extends to the perivesical space and terminates at the pelvic sidewall or, more precisely, at the obturator internus muscle (Fig. 31–7A–C and 31–8A, B). The lateral aspects of the retropubic space are demarcated in the dissections shown in Fig. 31–9A–F. The arcus tendineus originates from the obturator internus fascia. This whitish thickening of the obturator fascia can vary in its configuration from a single line to a wishbone or double-line structure. The pubococcygeus muscle (levator ani) in turn takes its origin from the arcus tendineus. The broad levator ani funnels downward into the depths of the pelvis. A portion of the levator ani arises from the inferior margin of the pubic ramus on either side in close proximity to the urethra, where it plays a key role in the sphincter mechanism to maintain urinary continence (see Fig. 31–8A, B). At the inferior extent of the space are located the urethrovesical junction, the anterolateral vaginal fornices, and the levator ani muscles (see Figs. 31–8A, B; 31–9A, and 31–10). The urethrovesical junction and the greater mass of the urinary bladder are exposed within the space of Retzius. Specifically, these structures lie on the floor of the retropubic space (Figs. 31–11A, B and 31–12A, B). At the level of the proximal urethra, the pubourethral (puboprostatic) ligaments are noted; these are stylized in Figure 31–3. The actual structures run from the posterior symphysis pubis to the pubocervical fascia (endopelvic fascia) in contact with the proximal urethra on each side and are thought to be key structures for the maintenance of continence (Figs. 31–13A–D). The arcus tendineus fasciae pelvis, or white line, stretches from the posterior aspect of the symphysis pubis and continues in a downward sloping direction along the fascial margin of the obturator internus muscle to terminate at the ischial spine. The attachment of the pubocervical fascia (endopelvic fascia) to the white line partially maintains the support of the lateral vaginal wall. Detachments of the pubocervical fascia from the white line will lead to paravaginal defects. The arcus tendineus can be seen clearly (see Fig. 31–9A–F). It is a fascial landmark (see Figs. 31–11 and 31–12). From the point where the levator ani takes origin from the arcus, the muscle swings downward toward the midline, thus composing a portion of the pelvic floor (see Fig. 31–8B). The levator ani muscles envelop the urethra, vagina, and rectum as the latter two (2) traverse and penetrate the diaphragm into the perineum. If the symphysis pubis is cut in the midline with a saw, the levator ani muscle can be followed inferiorly as it inserts into the lateral walls of the vagina and urethra deep to the vestibular bulb and clitoral crura.

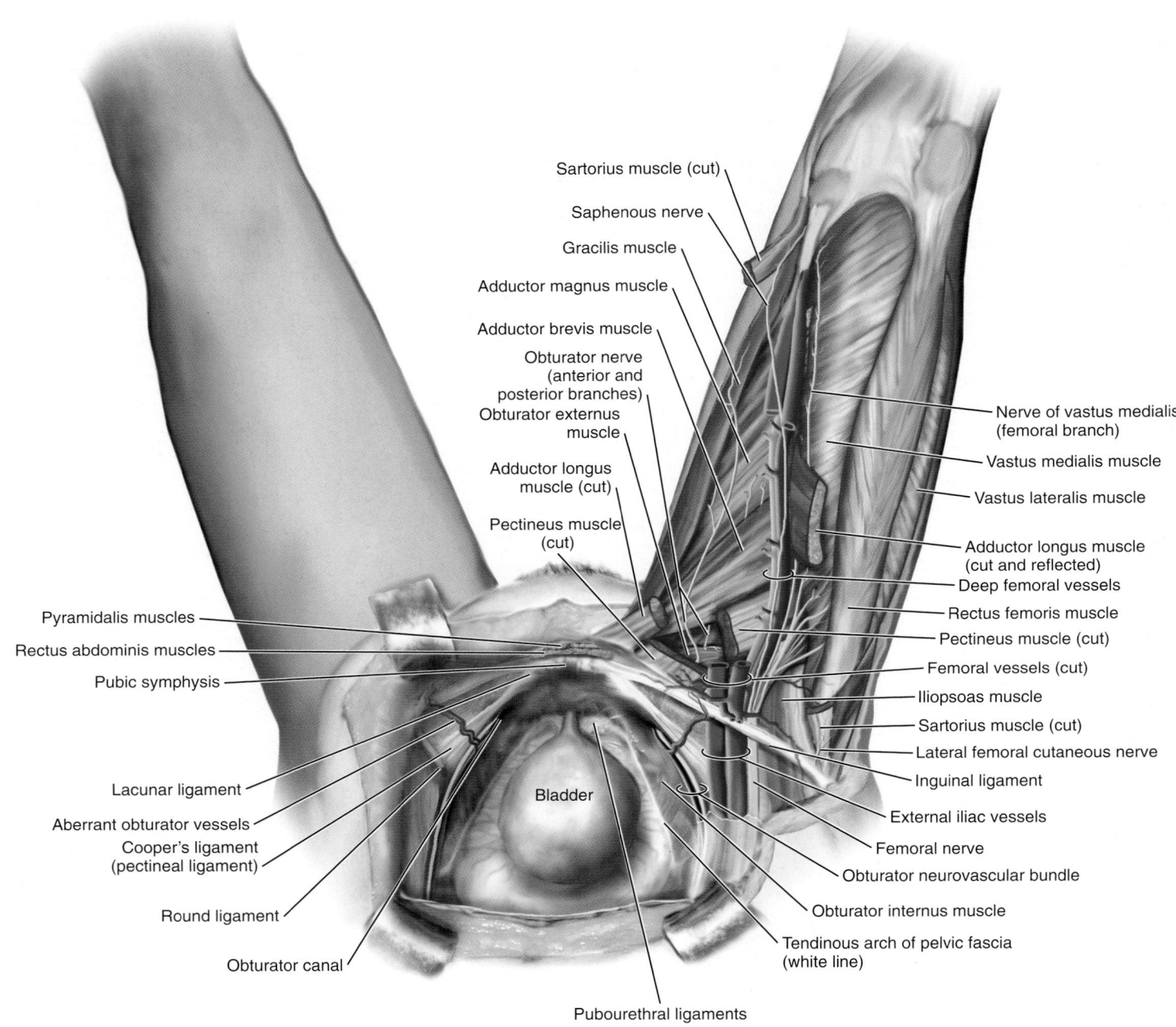

**FIGURE 31–6** Anatomy of the retropubic space as it relates to the thigh.

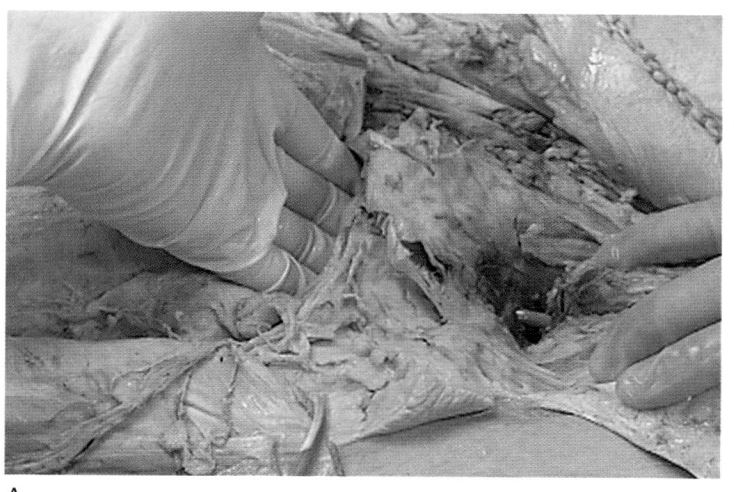

A

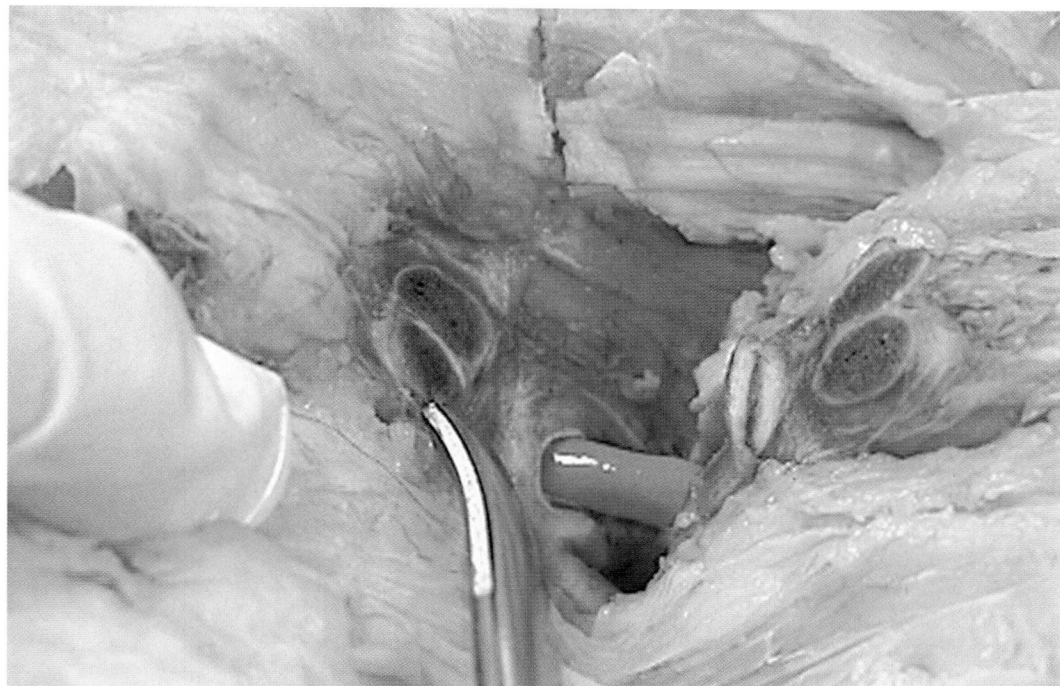

B

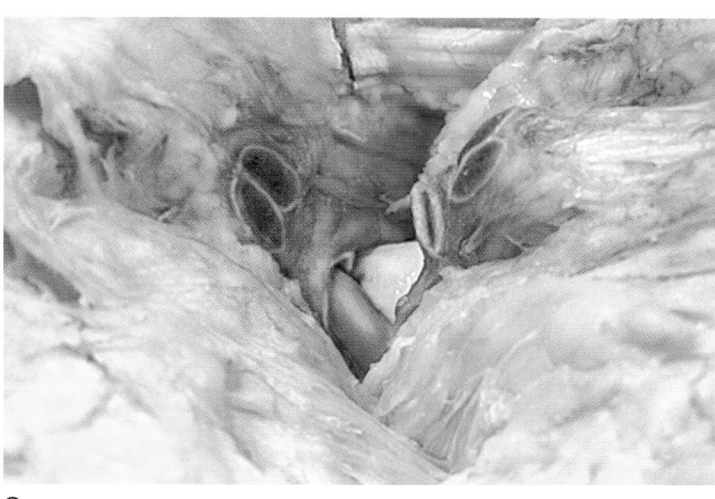

C

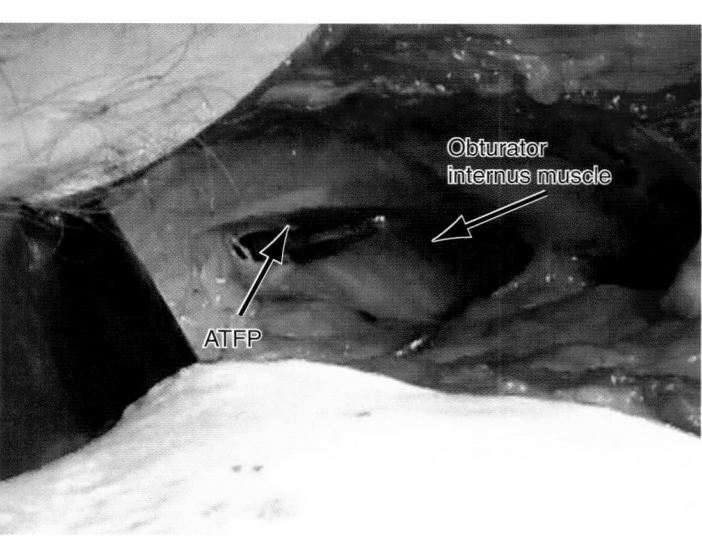

D

FIGURE 31–7 **A.** The operator's hand lies in the retropubic space. The mons has been cut so as to create a flap that is held forward by the assistant. A red rubber catheter had been placed into the urethra. **B.** Detail at the point where the urethra crosses under the symphysis pubis. The scissors points to the cavernous corpora cavernosa of the clitoris. **C.** A gloved finger has been placed in the vagina. The vestibular bulb lies above the urethra. **D.** A retropubic view is a cadaver. Note that the tips of Mayo scissors have been passed through the urogenital diaphragm and are entering the right inferolateral portion of the retropubic space. This is the area that commonly is penetrated during performance of a suburethral sling procedure. The scissors penetrate the fascial attachment to the arcus lateral to the urethra and medial to the arcus tendineus fasciae pelvis (ATFP). Also note the obturator internus muscle.

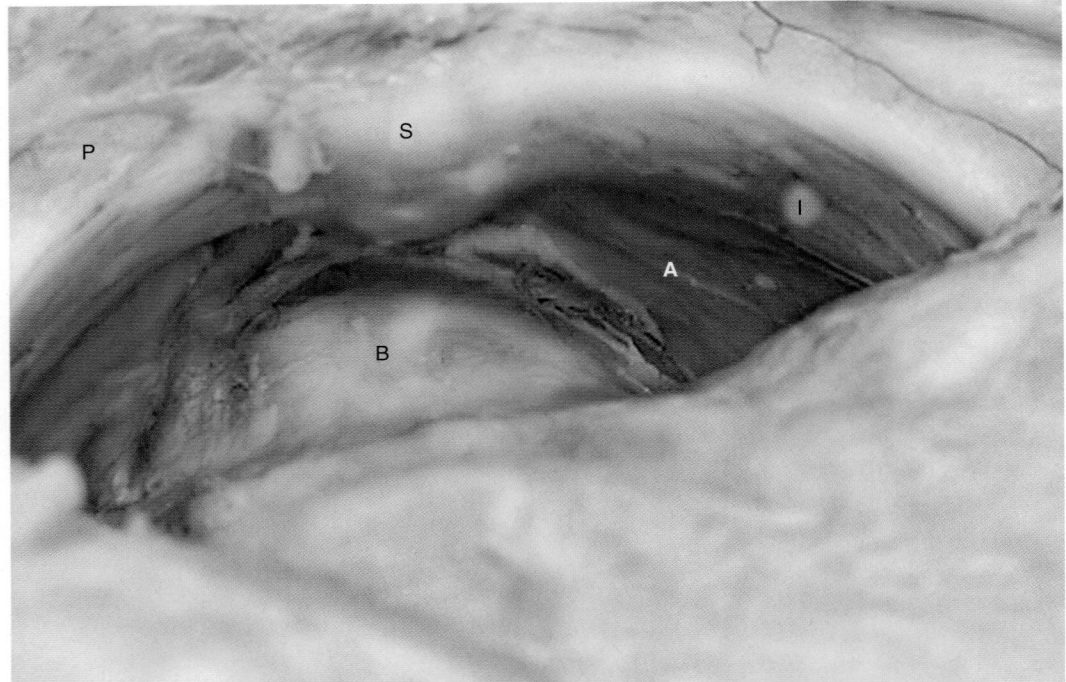

A

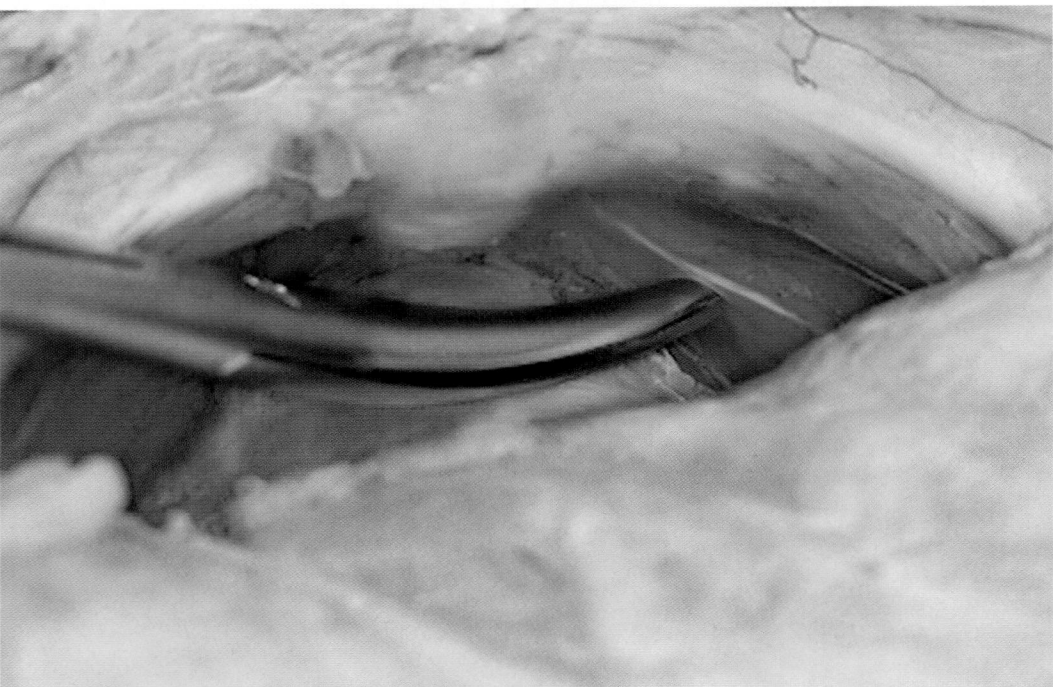

B

**FIGURE 31–8 A.** The entirety of the retropubic space is exposed. The symphysis (S) and pubic rami (P) occupy the anterior boundaries. The fascia of the obturator internus muscle (I) and the arcus (A) are clearly seen on the right side. The bladder (B) fills the posterior portion of the space. **B.** The scissors points to the white line (arcus). Below this point is the takeoff, or origin, of the levator ani muscle.

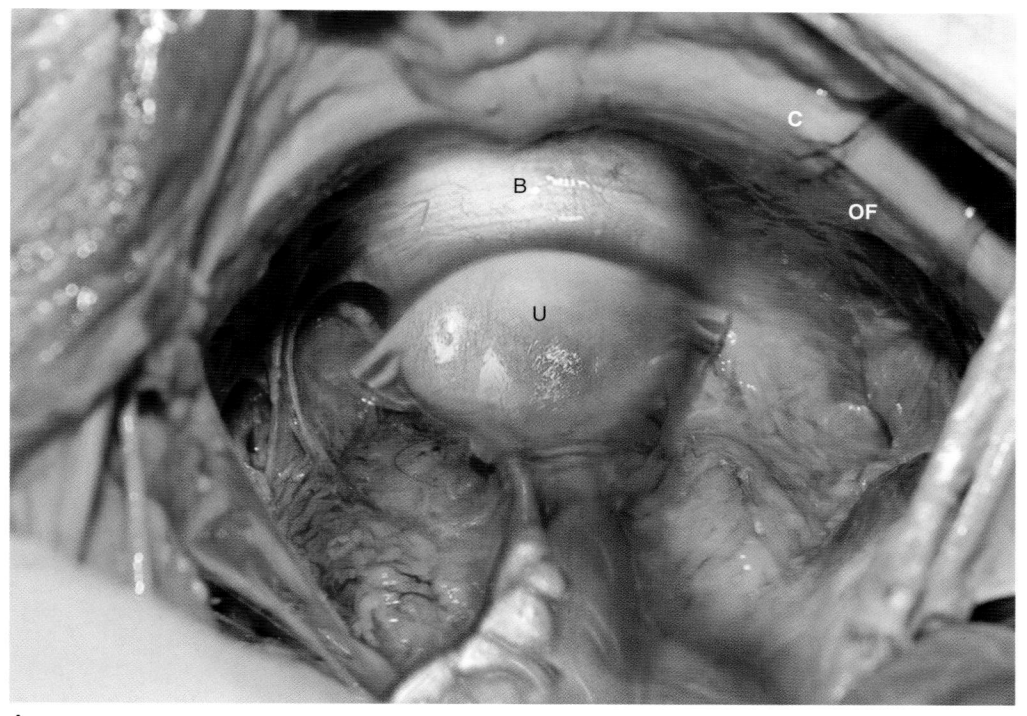

A

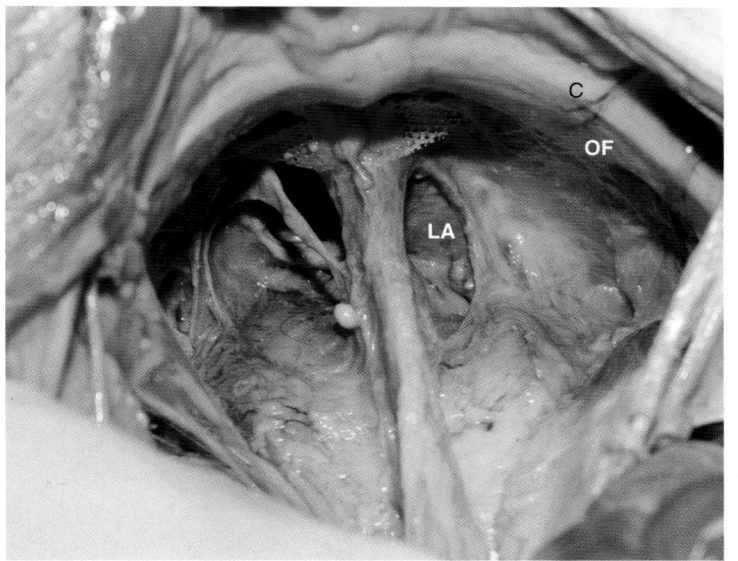

B

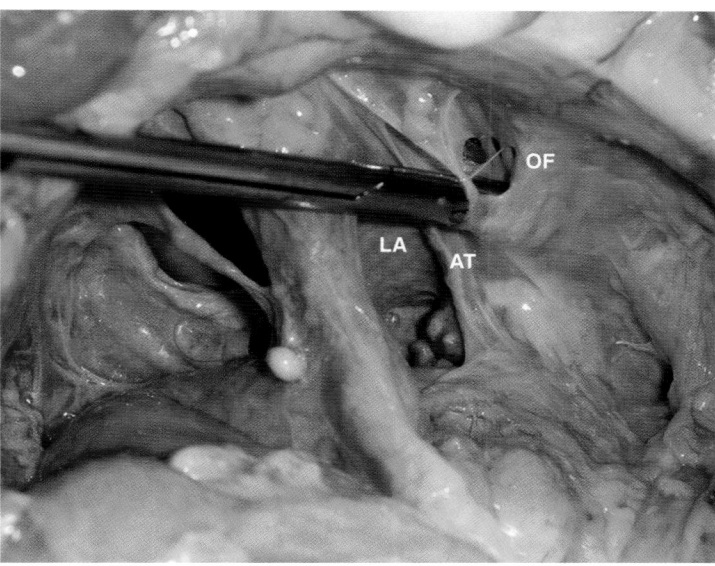

C

**FIGURE 31–9 A.** Fresh cadaver dissection exposing the retropubic space and exposure of the perivesical space. Cooper's ligament (C) occupies a forward area on the ileopecineal line. The fascia covering the obturator internus muscle and the levator ani muscle is labeled (OF). The uterus (U) and the urinary bladder (B) are supported by the endopelvic fascia as well as by various "ligaments". **B.** Close-up view of the opened retropubic space. The uterus, bladder, and proximal urethra have been excised. Cooper's ligament is identified on the iliopectineal line of the pubic bones (C). The obturator fascia forms the lateral boundary of the space (OF). The margin of the levator ani (pubococcygeus) is seen (LA). **C.** A scissors has dissected between the obturator fascia (OF) and the underlying obturator internus muscle. The arcus tendineus is in fact formed by the obturator fascia (AT). The levator ani (LA) is clearly seen beneath the arcus tendineus.

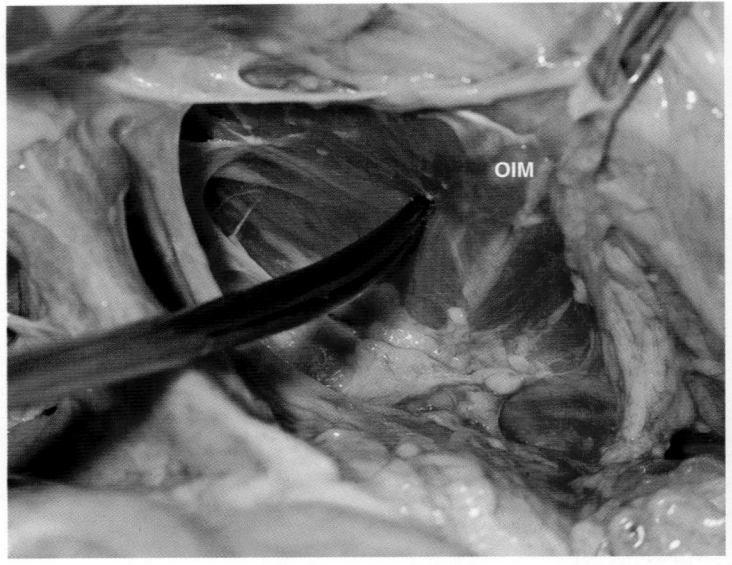

D

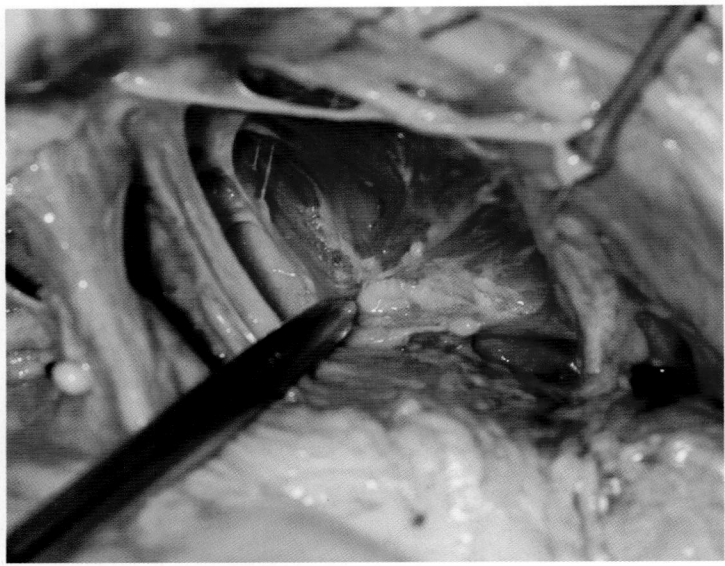

E

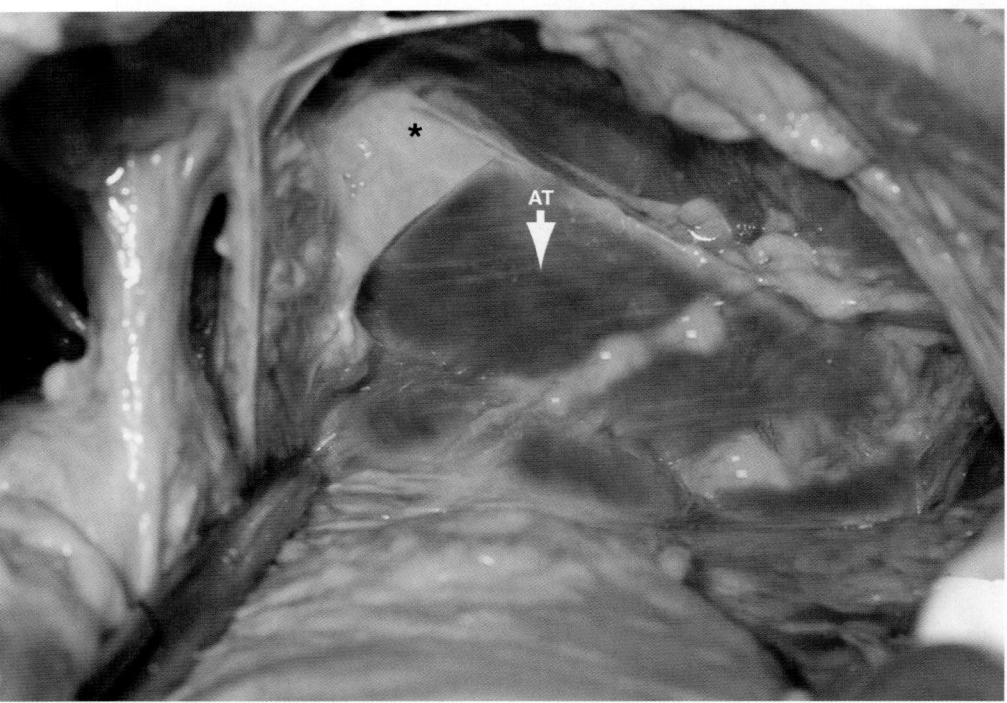

F

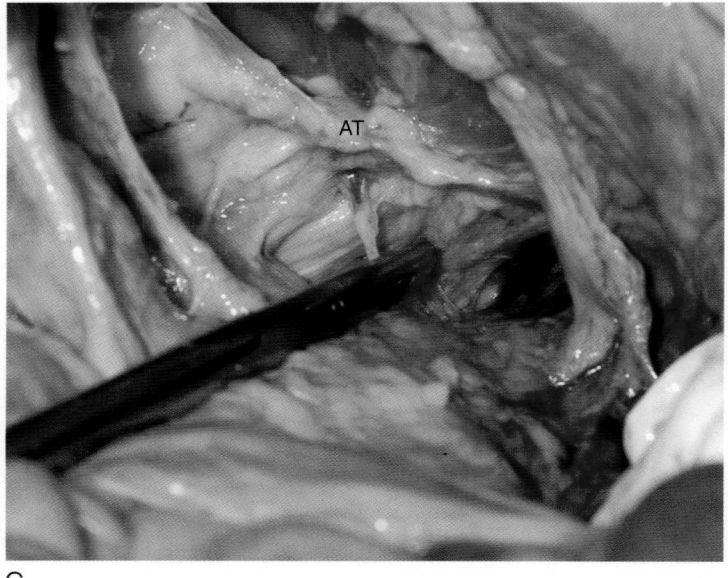

G

**FIGURE 31–9, cont'd   D.** The obturator fascia has been removed. The scissor tip points to the obturator internus muscle (OIM). **E.** The scissors depresses the arcus tendineus. **F.** The levator ani (pubococcygeus) is exposed as it sweeps downward into the depths of the pelvis (at the *arrow*). Note the muscle(s) originates from the arcus tendineus (AT). The obturator internus muscle lies above the white line (AT). The asterisk marks the remnant of the fascia that overlies the levator ani muscle (superior fascia LA). **G.** The white line (arcus tendineus) terminates 2 cm distal at the ischial spine (*dark space*). The slop of the arcus is a smooth line from its superficial point downwards and deep.

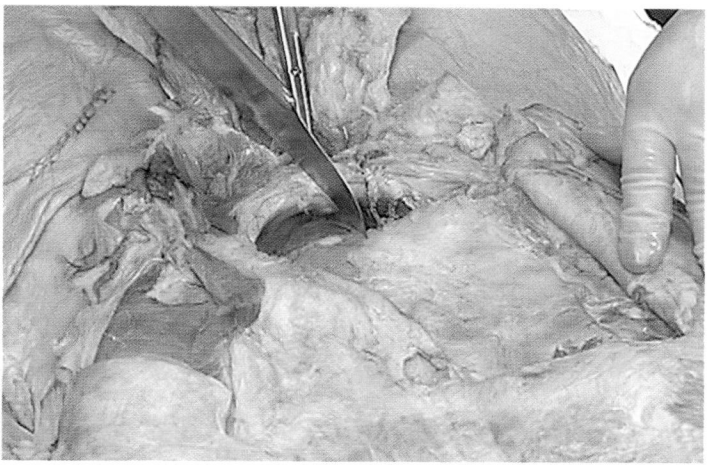

FIGURE 31–10 The pubic bone is being sawed to expose the structures passing beneath the symphysis.

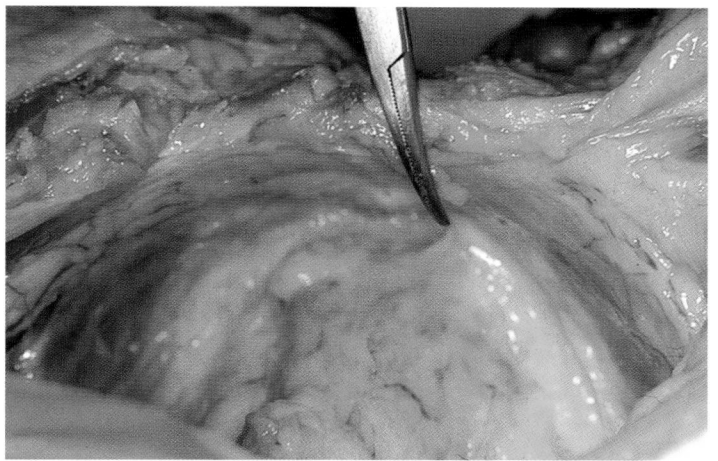

A

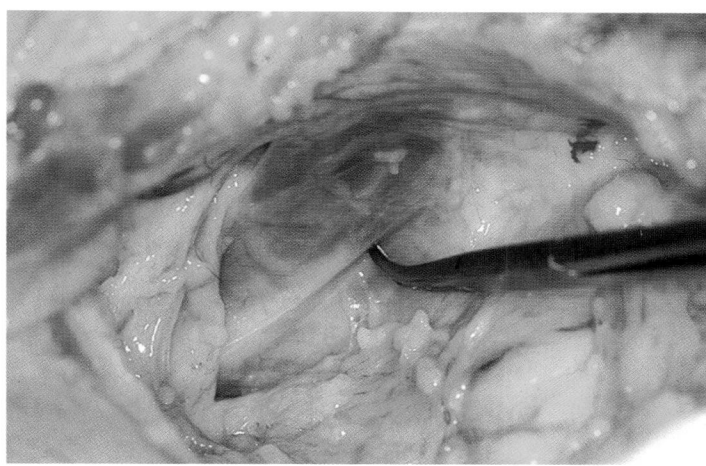

B

FIGURE 31–11 A. Fresh cadaver dissection exposing right and left white lines. The clamp tip is located just to the right of the symphysis pubis. B. Close-up detail of the left obturator internus muscle above the arcus tendineus (tip of clamp).

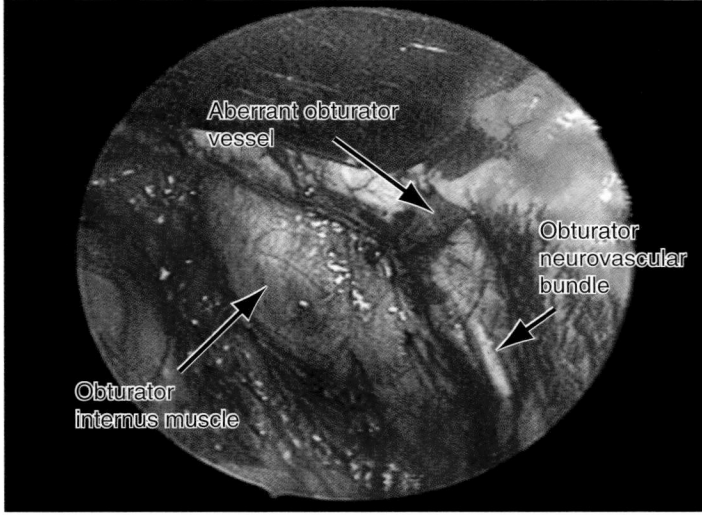

FIGURE 31–12 Laparoscopic view of the right sidewall of the retropubic space in a live patient. Note the aberrant obturator vessel seen draping over Cooper's ligament. Also note the obturator neurovascular bundle as it exits the pelvis through the obturator canal and the obturator internus muscle with its overlying fascia.

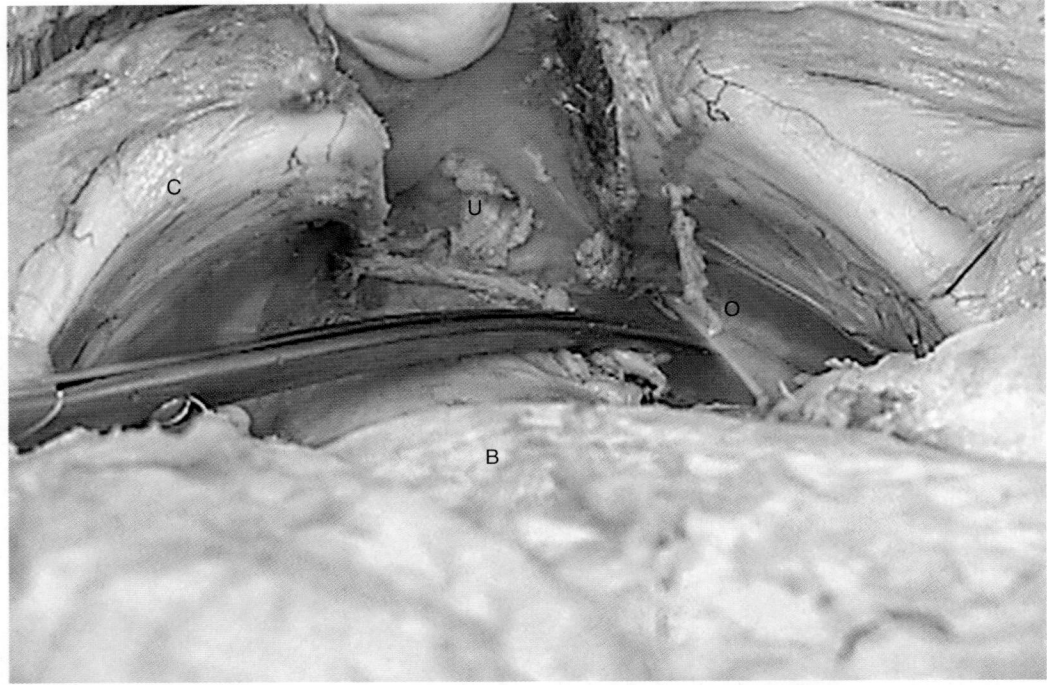

A

B

**FIGURE 31–13  A.** The scissors is placed just beneath the arcus tendineus. The operator's thumb pressed the sawed symphysis forward. The arcus leads directly to the posterior puboprostatic (pubourethral) ligaments. The urethra (U) passes beneath the posterior margin of the symphysis, and the obturator internus muscle (O) makes up the pelvic sidewall. Cooper's ligament (C) and the bladder dome (B) are labeled. **B.** The blade of the scissors tenses the right posterior puboprostatic ligament (PP) attached to the urethra at its junction with the bladder. The obturator fascia (O) lies below the pubic rami (P).

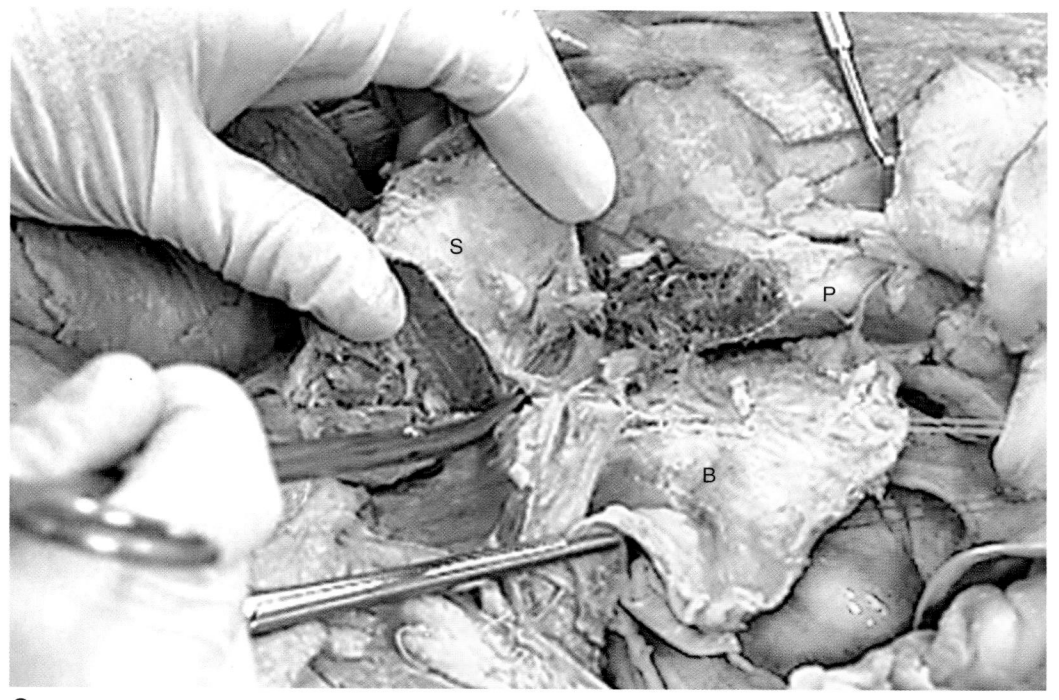

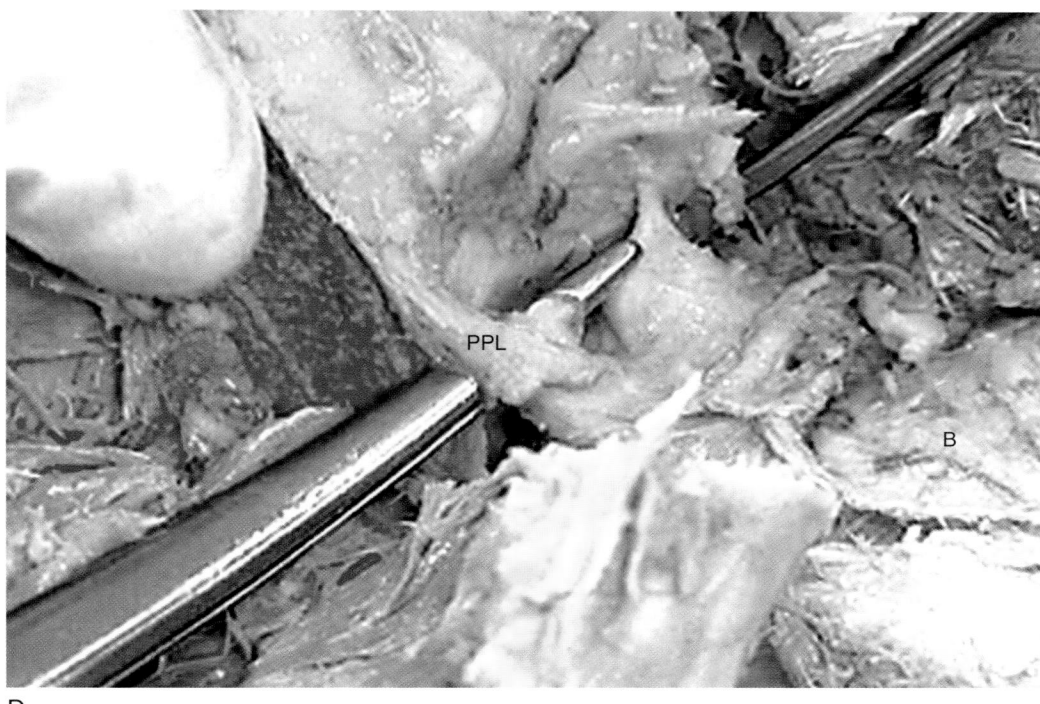

**FIGURE 31–13, cont'd C.** The sawed symphysis (S) is pushed farther forward. The clamp tip is under the left puboprostatic ligament, bladder (B), and pubic bone (P). **D.** Close-up of Figure 31–13C: puboprostatic ligament (PPL) and bladder (B).

A ridge of bone and ligamentous tissue is observed just beneath the superior margin of the superior pubic ramus. These are the iliopectineal line and Cooper's ligament, respectively (Fig. 31–14). As the dissection of the superior pubic ramus continues laterally and posteriorly, the external iliac artery and vein are identified as they pass under the inguinal ligament and into the thigh to become the femoral artery and vein (Fig. 31–15A, B). Other important vascular structures in this space include the veins of Santorini (see Fig. 31–3), which run within the vaginal wall at right angles to the sidewall, as well as the obturator neurovascular bundle, which exits the pelvis through the obturator foramen (Figs. 31–15C and 31–16A, B). Frequently an anomalous vessel crosses the pubic bone just forward of the external iliac vessels. This is known as the aberrant, or anomalous, obturator artery and vein (Fig. 31–17). Injury to these vessels can result in heavy bleeding when a Burch urethropexy is performed. Special care must be taken to avoid vascular injury during retraction of the anterior abdominal wall to expose Cooper's ligament at the time of retropubic urethropexy.

The vagina, bladder, and urethra are supported as a unit by structures within the retropubic space. As noted, these struc-tures share some connective tissue walls (Fig. 31–18A, B). Perivesical and perivaginal fascial structures provide the major pelvic support for the upper vagina and bladder base. Clearly, the most impressive and concretely defined support is the deep parametrium (i.e., the deep cardinal ligament [pictured in Fig. 31–19A]). More pictures and discussion relative to upper vaginal support are included in Chapter 51 ("Anatomy of the Vagina"). The deep cardinal ligament attaches to the pelvic sidewall in an arcing fashion and more specifically attaches to the obturator internus fascia deep within the retropubic space (Fig. 31–20A–C).

Injuries to the structures constituting the natural support of the bladder and urethra, including the endopelvic fascia, levator ani muscles (including the investing fascia enveloping these muscles), perivesical fascia, puboprostatic (pubourethral) ligaments, and deep parametrium, will result in recognizable defects. The most notable of these tissue injuries results in the creation of a cystourethrocele. Atrophy and diminution of vascular structures around and within the proximal urethra in conjunction with the above defects will lead to urinary incontinence.

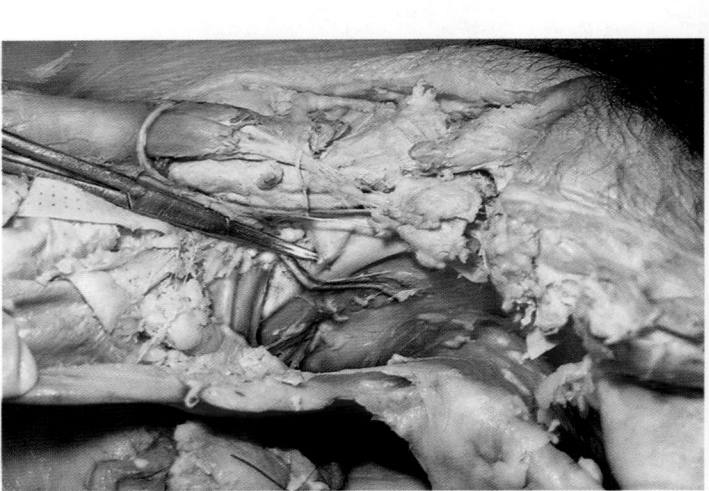

A

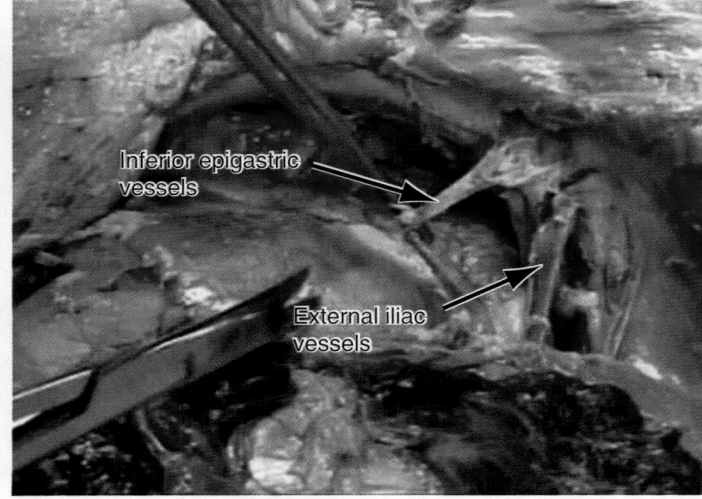

B

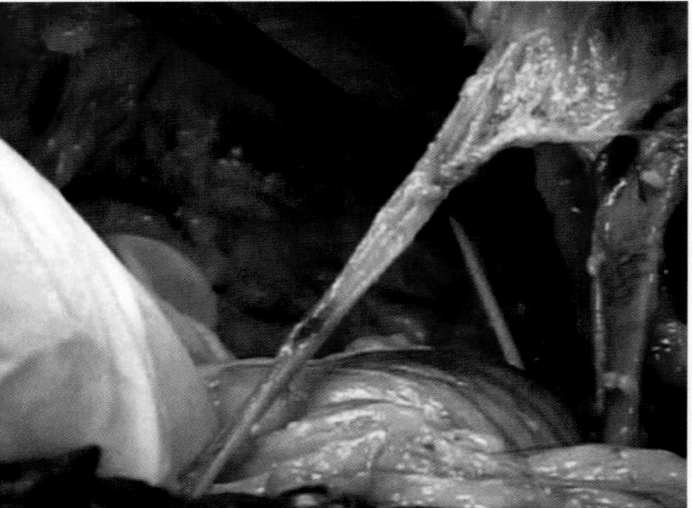

C

**FIGURE 31–14  A.** The connective tissue has been cleaned away from the left superior pubic ramus. The clamp has been inserted into Cooper's ligament. Note the skin and hair of the mons in the upper right quadrant. **B.** Note the lowest portion of the external iliac vessels. Also noted are the inferior epigastric vessels as they rise from the external iliac vessels and pass in a cephalad direction. **C.** A close-up view of the external iliac vessels and origin of the inferior epigastric vessels. Also seen is the obturator neurovascular bundle as it passes through the retropubic space.

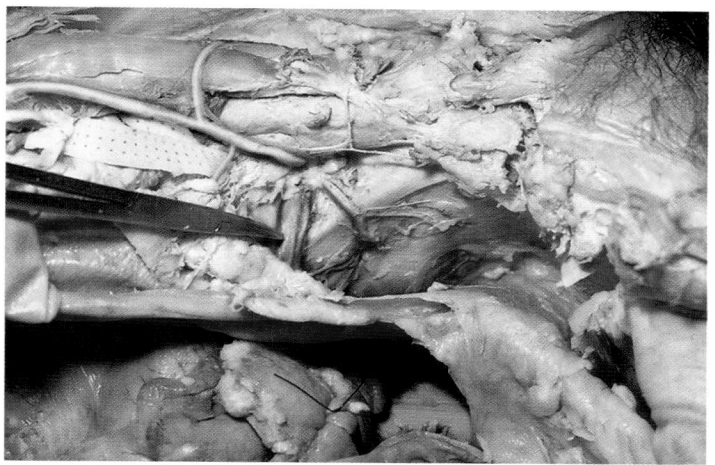

A

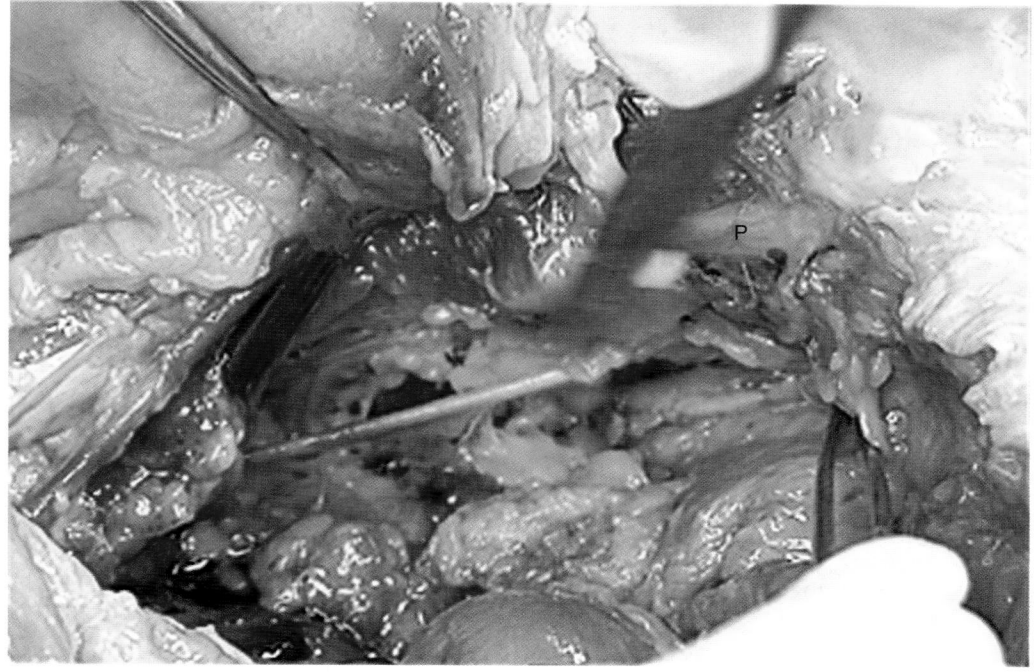

B

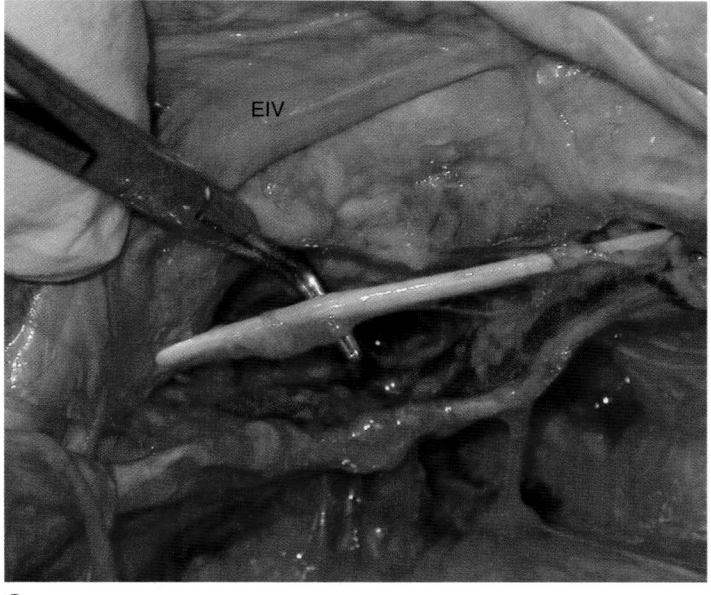

C

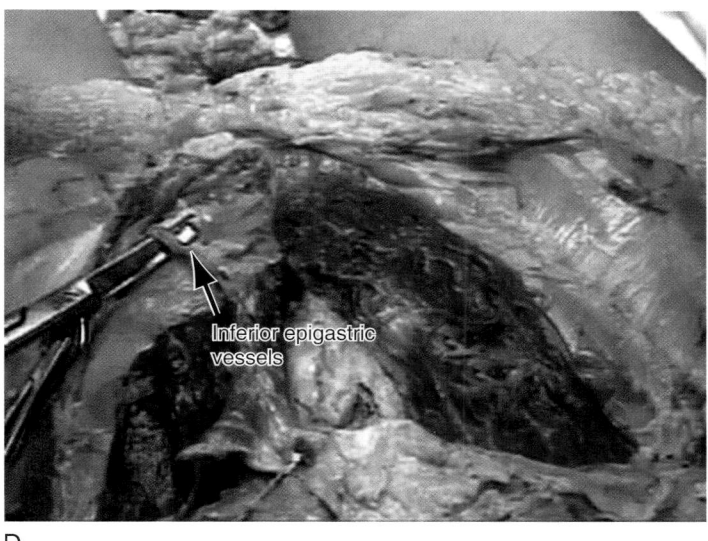

D

**FIGURE 31–15  A.** The lateral and posterior portions of the pubic ramus are crossed by the external iliac vessels. The clamp points to the external iliac vein. **B.** The left external iliac vein is held via a vein retractor. The pubic ramus (P) has been dissected clear of fat. The obturator nerve is seen crossing the retropubic space. **C.** The right-angle clamp tenses the left obturator nerve. The nerve and artery can be seen entering the short obturator canal beneath the left pubic ramus. The external iliac vein (EIV) is seen crossing over the ramus laterally. **D.** A cadaveric dissection notes the origin of the inferior epigastric vessels from the right external iliac.

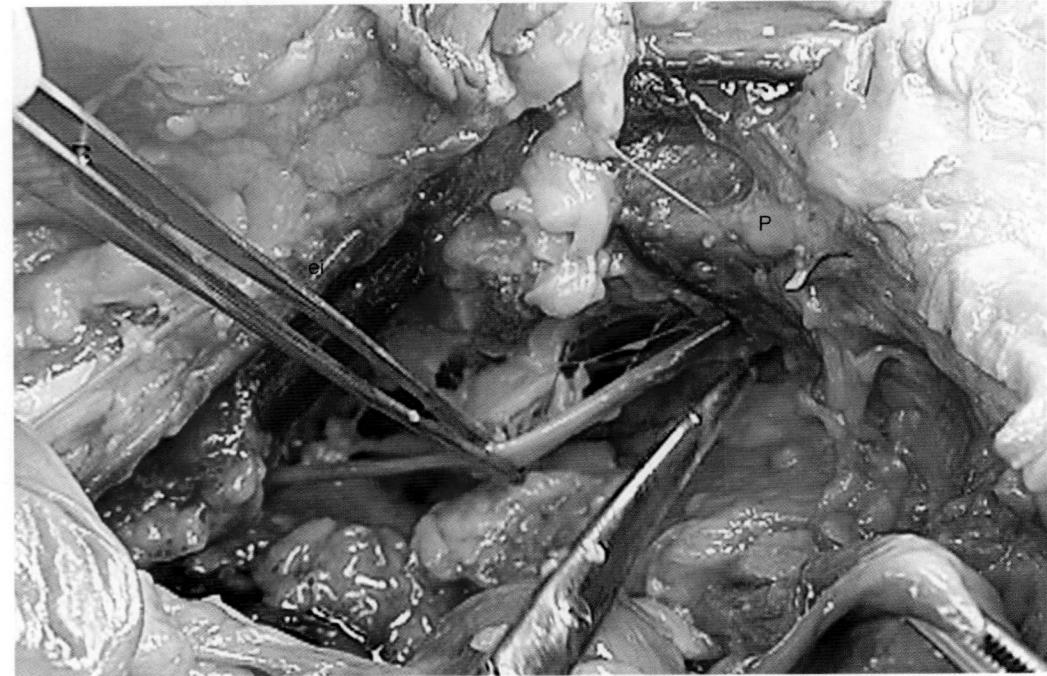

A

B

**FIGURE 31–16** The external iliac artery (ei) and vein are crossing over the pubic bone (P) into the thigh. The forceps grasps the obturator nerve, which is exiting the retropubic space via the obturator foramen. **B.** Close-up view of Figure 31–16A. The tip of the scissors is poking into the obturator foramen. Immediately above is the pubic ramus (P) covered in Cooper's ligament (*pink*).

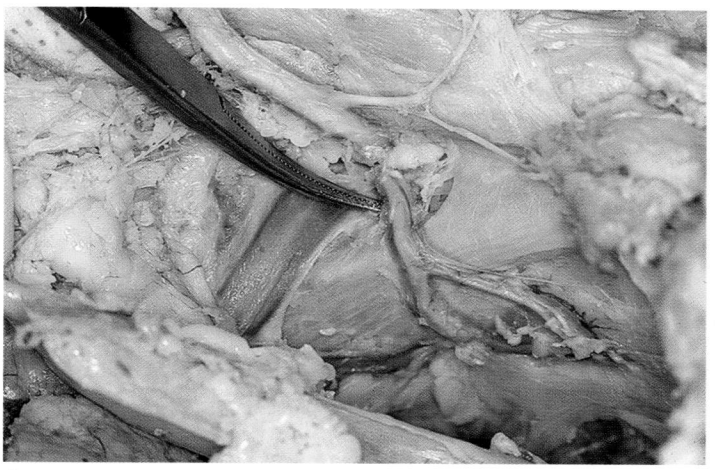

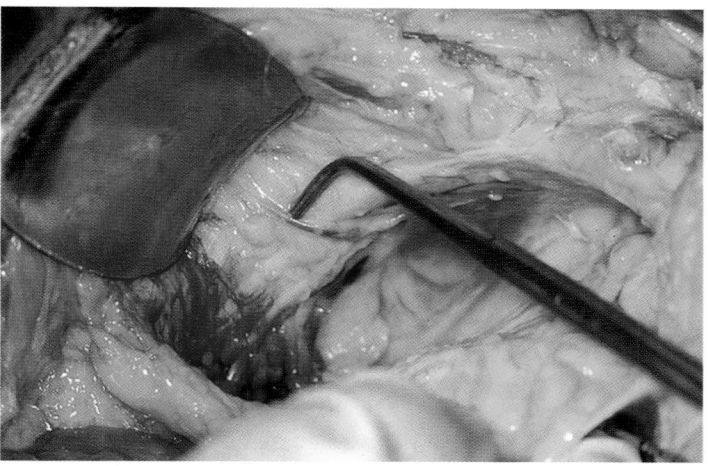

**FIGURE 31–17 A.** Not infrequently, an anomalous obturator vessel will cross the lateral superior pubic ramus and the iliopectineal line. Inadvertent severing of this vessel results in heavy bleeding that is difficult to control because the artery retracts. Note that the direction of a potential retraction intersects with the course of the external iliac vein. **B.** Still another variation of anomalous obturator vessels is located just above the right-angle clamp. A small portion of the left external iliac vein is seen beneath the edge of the retractor blade.

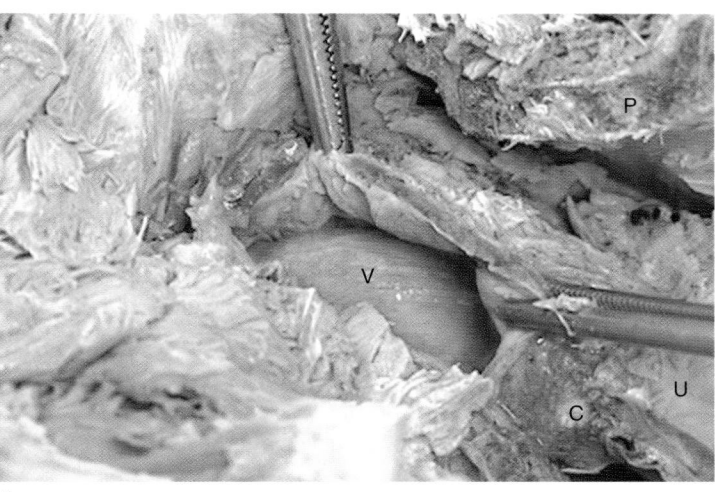

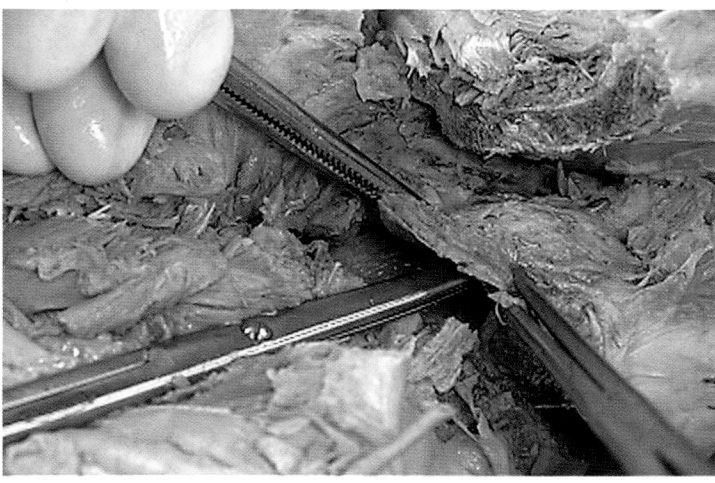

**FIGURE 31–18 A.** Beneath the sawed out pubic symphysis (P), the bladder (with the exception of the base) has been cut away to expose the upper vagina (V). The cut edges (anterior wall) are held by Kocher clamps. Sagittal sections of the cervix (C) and uterus (U) are seen to the lower right. **B.** A long scissors had pierced the lateral vaginal fornix. Note that it enters the retropubic space.

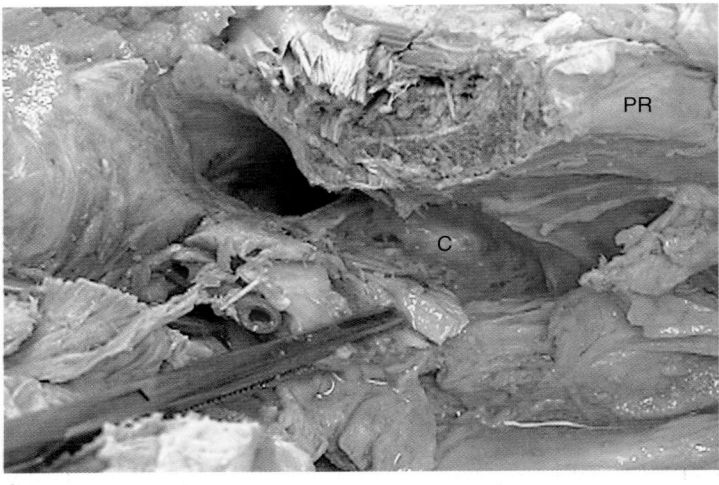

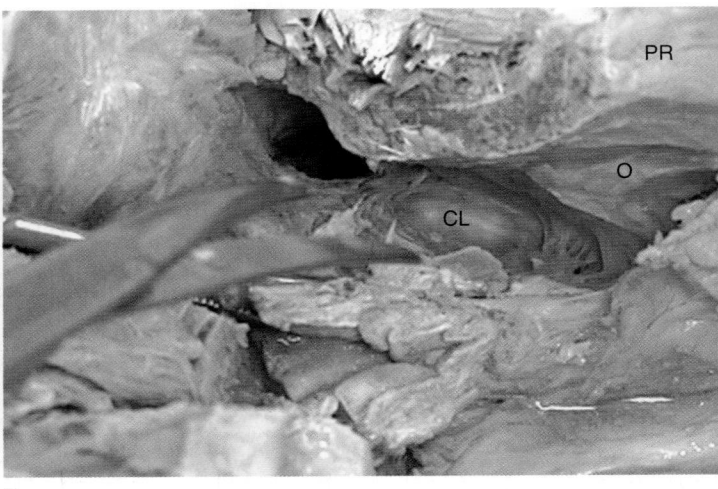

A

B

**FIGURES 31–19  A.** The anterior urethral wall has been cut open. The bladder base and the posterior wall of the urethra are densely attached to the anterior vagina. The perivesical and perivaginal support consists most notably of the deep cardinal ligament (C), which arcs back and attaches to the obturator internus fascia. Note the pubic ramus (PR) above. **B.** The scissor is poised to cut the deep parametrium (cardinal ligament) (CL). After this ligament, the unit consisting of the vagina, urethra, and bladder is virtually free and can be easily mobilized. Note the pubic ramus (PR) and the obturator internus muscle (O).

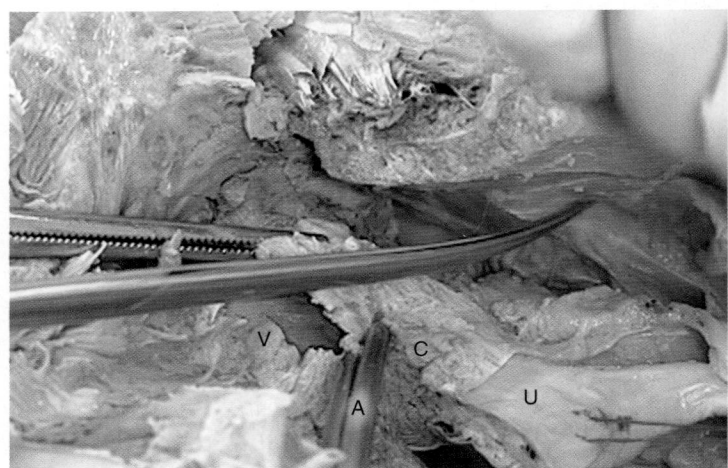

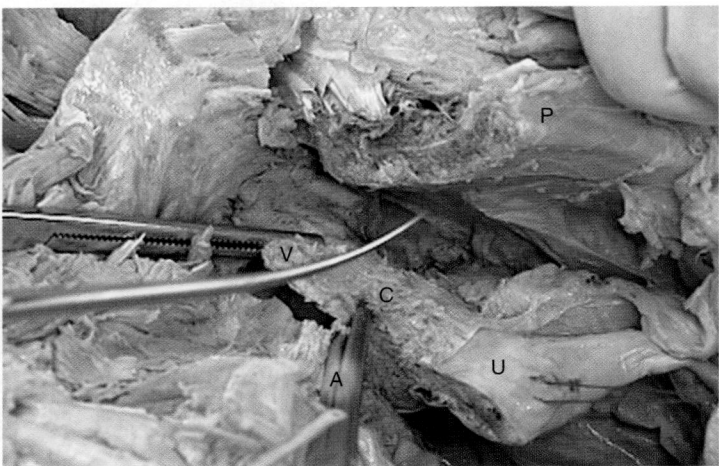

A

B

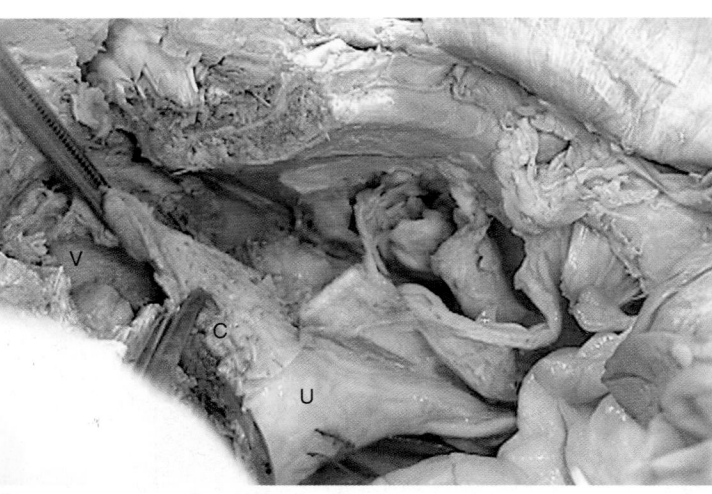

**FIGURE 31–20  A.** The scissors points to the obturator internus muscle. The Kocher clamps hold the cut anterior vaginal wall. The opened vagina (V) is visible. The hemisected cervix (C) and uterus (U) attach to the vagina at the Kocher clamp. The fundus of the uterus is held by a Vicryl (blue) suture. **B.** Similar view to Figure 31–17A, but taken in the panoramic mode. The pubic bone (P) is cut. The scissors rests on the fascia of the obturator internus muscle (I). The vagina (V) is attached to the hemisected cervix (C) and uterus (U). **C.** View from above the retropubic space. The bladder and urethra have been cut out. Also, the deep cardinal ligament has been incised. The cervix (C), uterus (U), and vagina (V) are the only major structures left. Note their relationship to the pubic bone (P) and the missing symphysis pubis.

C

# CHAPTER 32

# Operative Setup and Entry Into the Retropubic Space

*Mickey M. Karram*

Operations involving the retropubic space are best done with the patient in the supine position and the patient's legs in a frogleg position or, preferably, in low Allen stirrups. Many of these operations are best performed with a hand in the vagina, which allows easy access to the vaginal area. The vagina, perineum, and abdomen are all sterilely prepped and draped in a fashion that permits easy access to the lower abdomen and the vagina. We prefer to use a three-way Foley catheter with a 30-mL balloon that is inserted sterilely into the bladder and kept in the sterile field. This allows easy palpation of the bladder neck, and in situations where the edges of the bladder are not clearly delineated, one can easily fill the bladder in a retrograde fashion to help in dissection or to help diagnose a small cystotomy or inadvertent suture placement in the bladder. The drainage port of the catheter is left to gravity drainage, and the irrigation port is connected to sterile water that is placed on an IV pole. One perioperative IV dose of an appropriate prophylactic antibiotic is given for retropubic operations.

A Pfannenstiel or Cherney incision (Figs. 32–1 and 32–2) (also see Chapter 8) is used to gain entry to the retropubic space.

If intraperitoneal surgery is also being performed, the peritoneum is left open until the retropubic repair is completed. Routine assessment and, if appropriate, obliteration of the cul-de-sac are performed in these situations (see Chapter 41). The retropubic space is exposed by staying close to the back of the pubic bone (Fig. 32–3). The surgeon's hand is used to gently displace the bladder and urethra downward (Fig. 32–4). As was previously mentioned, the presence of a large Foley balloon helps facilitate this dissection (Fig. 32–5). Sharp dissection usually is not necessary in primary cases. If a previous retropubic or needle suspension procedure or suburethral sling procedure has been performed, or in rare situations when pelvic surgery has led to dense suprapubic adhesions, sharp dissection should be utilized to enter the space. Adhesions should be dissected sharply from the pubic bone until the anterior bladder wall, urethra, and vagina are free of adhesions and are mobile. If identification of the urethra or lower border of the bladder is difficult, one may perform a high cystotomy, which, with a finger inside the bladder, helps to define the bladder's lower limits for easier dissection, mobilization, and subsequent elevation of the paravaginal tissue (see Chapter 30).

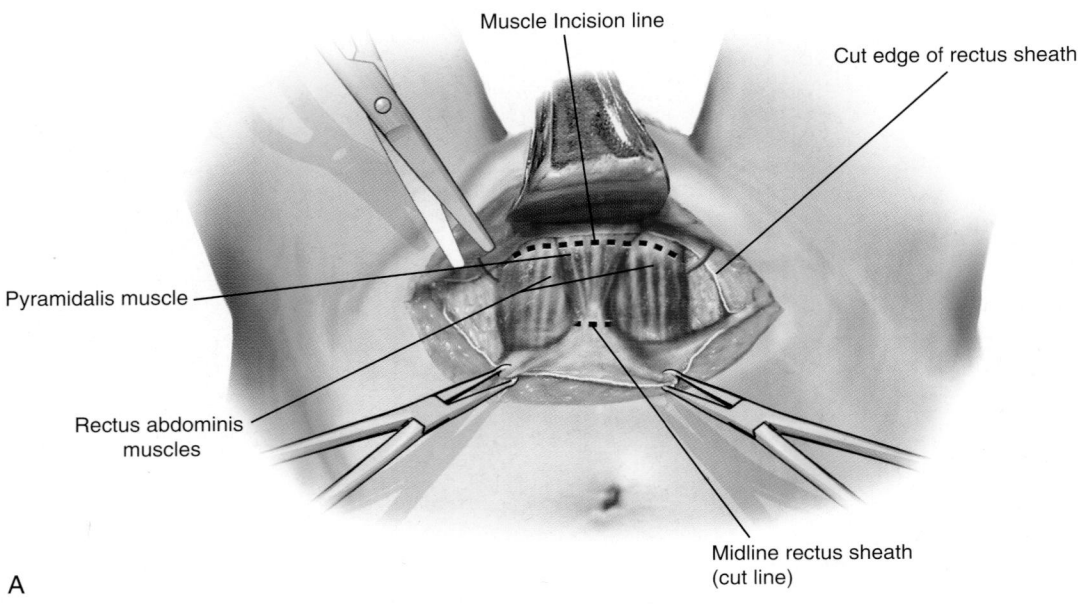

Muscle Incision line

Cut edge of rectus sheath

Pyramidalis muscle

Rectus abdominis
muscles

Midline rectus sheath
(cut line)

A

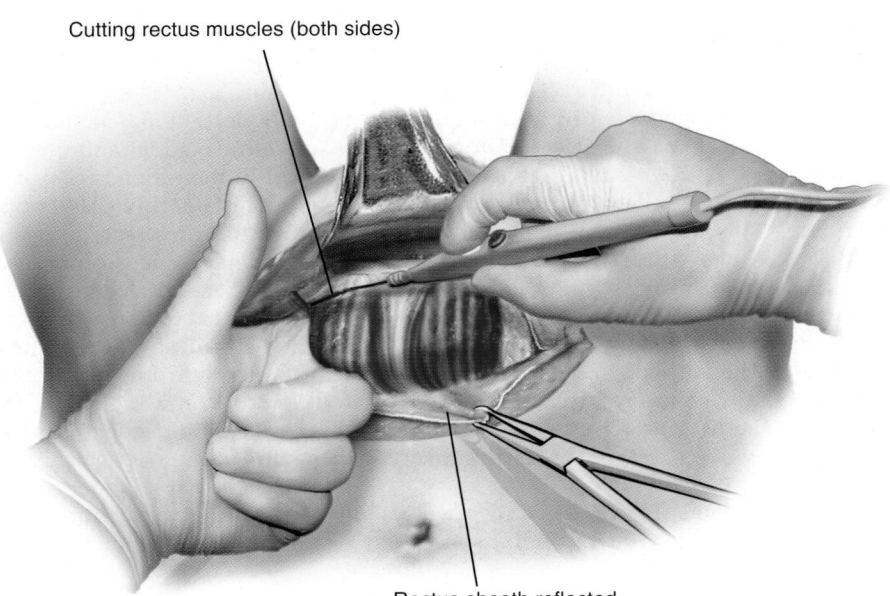

Cutting rectus muscles (both sides)

Rectus sheath reflected

B

**FIGURE 32–1** Technique of performing a Cherney incision to facilitate entrance into the retropubic space.
**A.** Rectus muscle isolated and exposed very low near its insertion into the pubic bone. **B.** Monopolar cautery
is used to cut through the lowest portion of the rectus muscle.

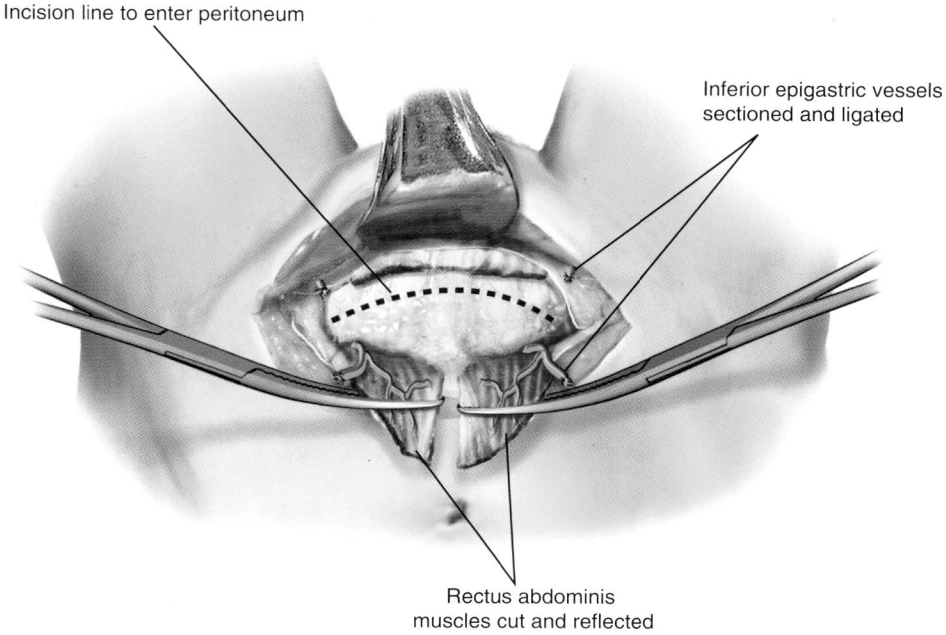

Incision line to enter peritoneum

Inferior epigastric vessels
sectioned and ligated

Rectus abdominis
muscles cut and reflected

C

**FIGURE 32–1, cont'd  C.** The rectus muscle is reflected back, allowing easy access to the retropubic space. Note that if the peritoneum is going to be entered, it should be opened with a transverse incision.

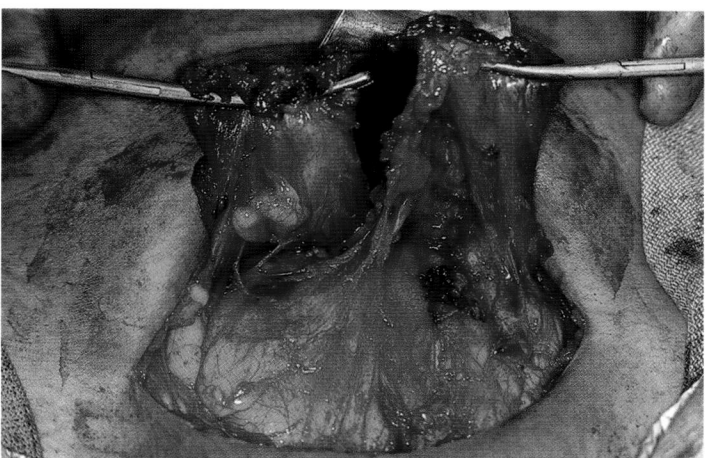

**FIGURE 32–2** A Cherney incision is commonly utilized for retropubic procedures, especially if lower abdominal or retropubic scarring is encountered. Note that the rectus abdominis muscles have been detached from the back of the symphysis pubis, very near their insertion. The muscles are then carefully dissected off the anterior peritoneum. Care must be taken to avoid the inferior epigastric vessels.

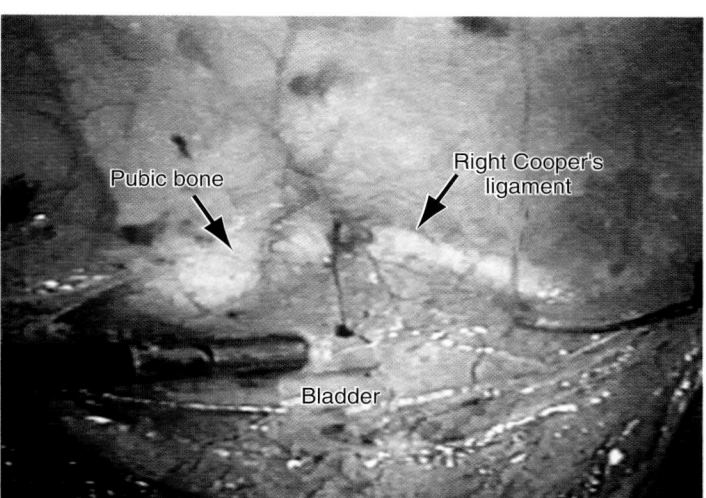

Pubic bone

Right Cooper's
ligament

Bladder

**FIGURE 32–3** This figure demonstrates the upper portion of the retropubic space viewed laparoscopically. *Note:* In a patient who has not had any previous retropubic surgery, an avascular plane of dissection is initiated at the level of the pubic bone. The bladder is displaced in a downward direction, and the dissection instrument or finger is maintained in direct contact with the back of the pubic bone at the midline.

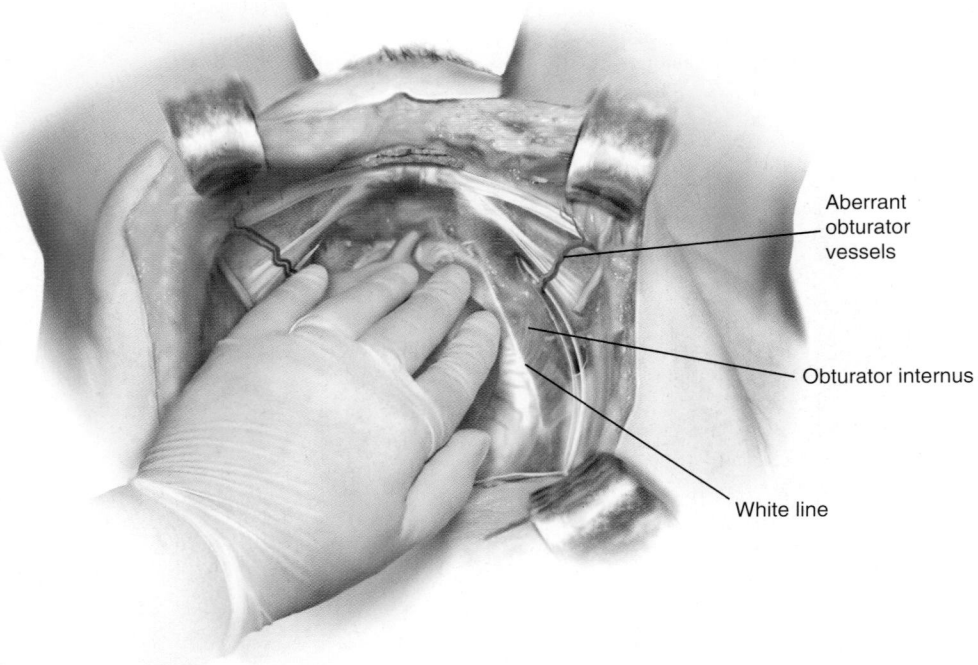

Aberrant obturator vessels

Obturator internus

White line

**FIGURE 32–4** Technique used to expose the retropubic space. The surgeon's hand is used to gently displace the bladder and urethra downward.

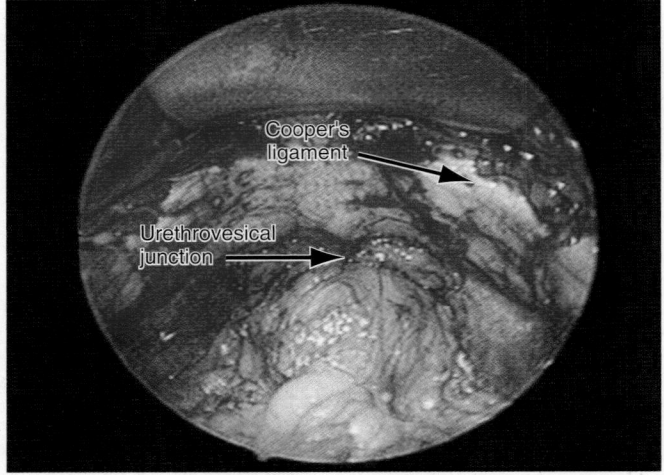

Cooper's ligament

Urethrovesical junction

**FIGURE 32–5** A view of the completely dissected retropubic space. A large Foley balloon facilitates this dissection, which can easily be done bluntly in the patient who has not had any previous retropubic procedures. Ideally, the dissection should be done down to the level of the urethrovesical junction at the midline and to the level of the arcus tendineus fasciae pelvis on each side.

# CHAPTER 33

# Retropubic Urethropexy for Stress Incontinence

*Mickey M. Karram*

## Modified Burch Colposuspension

After the retropubic space is entered, the urethra and anterior vaginal wall are depressed. Dissection at the midline is avoided, thus protecting the delicate musculature of the urethra and urethrovesical junction from surgical trauma. Attention is directed to the tissue on either side of the urethra. The surgeon's nondominant hand is placed in the vagina with the index and middle fingers on one side of the proximal urethra. Two sponge sticks are utilized to gently mobilize the bladder to the opposite side (Figs. 33–1 through 33–3). Most of the overlying fat can be cleared away with the use of a swab mounted on a curved forceps. This dissection is accomplished with forceful elevation of the surgeon's vaginal finger until glistening, white periurethral fascia and vaginal wall are seen (see Figs. 33–1, 33–4, and 33–5). This area is extremely vascular, with a rich, thin-walled venous plexus, and should be avoided if possible. The positions of the urethra and the lower edge of the bladder are determined by palpating the Foley balloon, or by partially distending the bladder if necessary to find the rounded lower margins of the bladder as it meets the anterior vaginal wall.

Dissection lateral to the urethra is completed bilaterally, and vaginal mobility is judged to be adequate by using the vaginal finger to lift the anterior vaginal wall upward and forward (see Figs. 33–1 and 33–5). Either 0 or 1 delayed-absorbable or nonabsorbable sutures are then placed lateral in the anterior vaginal wall. We apply two sutures of graded polyester on an SH needle (Ethibond by Ethicon, Inc., Somerville, NJ) bilaterally, using double bites for each suture. These sutures are double-armed so that each end of the suture can subsequently be brought up through Cooper's ligament (see Figs. 33–4, 33–6, and 33–7). Proper placement of these sutures is important to provide adequate support and to avoid undue urethral kinking or elevation leading to postoperative voiding dysfunction or retention. We prefer to place the sutures in the lateral portion of the vagina just lateral to the tip of the vaginal finger, which should be elevating the most mobile and pliable portion of the vagina lateral to the bladder neck (see Figs. 33–1 through 33–8). The distal suture is placed 2 cm lateral to the proximal third of the urethra, and the proximal suture is placed approximately 2 cm lateral to the bladder wall or slightly proximal to the level of the urethrovesical junction (see Figs. 33–4 and 33–7). In placing the sutures, one should take a full-thickness bite of the vaginal wall, excluding the epithelium. This maneuver is accomplished

by suturing over the surgeon's vaginal finger at appropriate selected sites (see Figs. 33–4 and 33–5). On each side after the two sutures are placed, they are passed through the pectineal or Cooper's ligament, so that all four suture ends exit above the ligament (see Figs. 33–4 and 33–7). The retropubic space can be extremely vascular, and visible vessels should be avoided if possible. When excessive bleeding occurs, it can be controlled by direct pressure, sutures, or vascular clips. Severe bleeding usually stops with direct pressure, or after the fixation sutures are tied. After all four sutures are placed in the vagina and through Cooper's ligament, the assistant ties first the distal sutures and then the proximal ones while the surgeon elevates the vagina with the vaginal hand (see Fig. 33–8). If desired, a suprapubic catheter is placed through the extraperitoneal portion of the dome of the bladder. In tying the sutures, one does not have to be concerned about whether the vaginal wall meets Cooper's ligament.

## Marshall-Marchetti-Krantz Procedure

The retropubic space is exposed as previously described. Again, the surgeon's nondominant hand is placed in the vagina, and dissection of the periurethral fat is performed as previously described for the Burch colposuspension. Some surgeons routinely perform a cystotomy to aid in periurethral dissection and suture placement.

Delayed-absorbable or permanent sutures are used and are placed at right angles to the urethra and parallel to the vesical neck. A single suture is placed bilaterally at the urethrovesical junction. A double bite is taken over the surgeon's finger, incorporating the full thickness of the vaginal wall and excluding the epithelium. After placement of the sutures, the point of fixation of the urethra to the symphysis pubis can be determined by elevating the two vaginal fingers to the point where the vesical neck comes in contact with the pubic symphysis and noting the position at which the sutures will be placed into the pubic periosteum. The needle is placed medially to laterally against the periosteum and is turned with a simple wrist action. This may involve the cartilage in the midline, depending on the width, thickness, and availability of the periosteum. The sutures on each side are placed accordingly and are tied with the vaginal finger elevating the urethrovesical junction (Fig. 33–9).

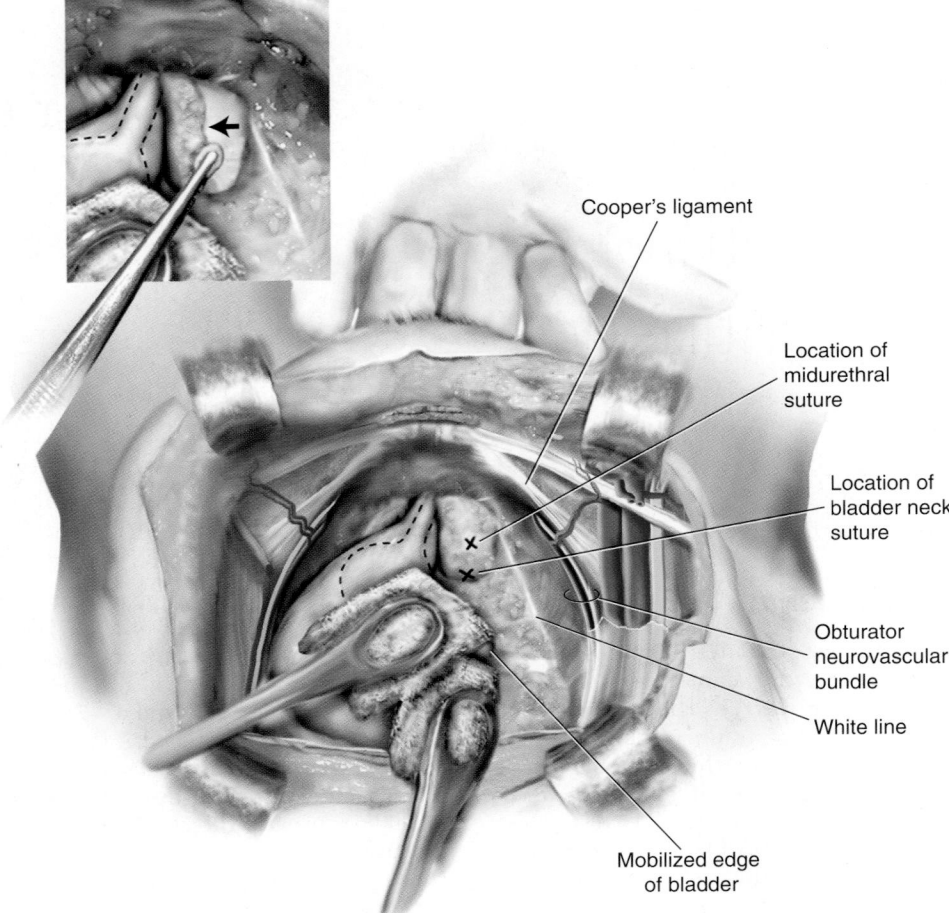

Cooper's ligament

Location of
midurethral
suture

Location of
bladder neck
suture

Obturator
neurovascular
bundle

White line

Mobilized edge
of bladder

**FIGURE 33–1** Burch colposuspension. The bladder is gently mobilized to the opposite side with sponge sticks. The anterior vaginal wall is elevated by the middle finger of the surgeon's nondominant hand, and fat is mobilized medially (see **inset**) with a swab mounted on a curved forceps or suction tip. The position of the sutures (indicated with an *X*) ideally should be at least 2 cm lateral to the proximal urethra and bladder neck, usually on the lateral downslope of the tissue elevated by the vaginal finger.

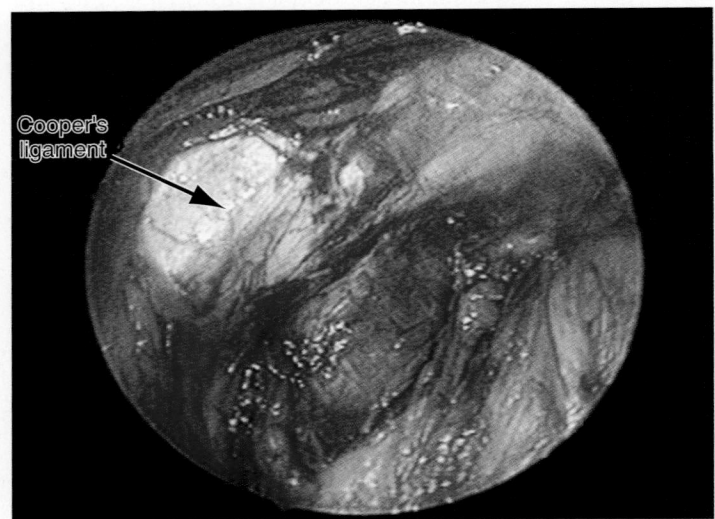

Cooper's
ligament

**FIGURE 33–2** Lateral view of the retropubic space in a live patient. *Note:* The tissue has been cleaned off over Cooper's ligament on the left side. This is the area through which the suspension sutures will be passed during performance of a Burch colposuspension.

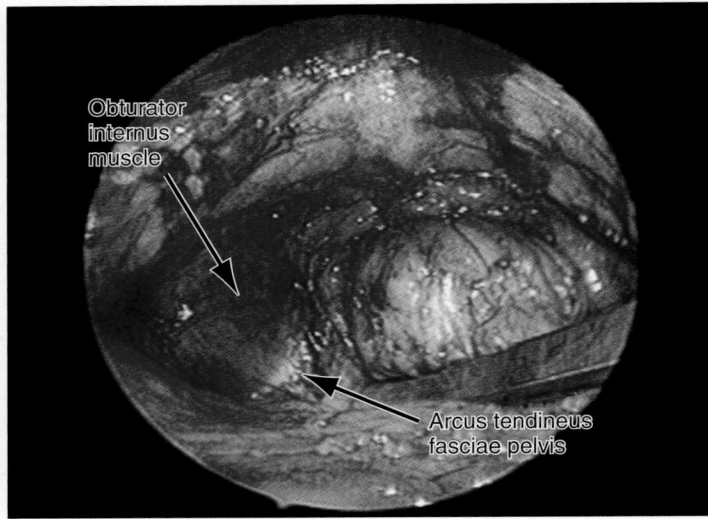

Obturator
internus
muscle

Arcus tendineus
fasciae pelvis

**FIGURE 33–3** The lateral retropubic space on the left side is shown. Note the obturator internus muscle, which inserts into the arcus tendineus fasciae pelvis.

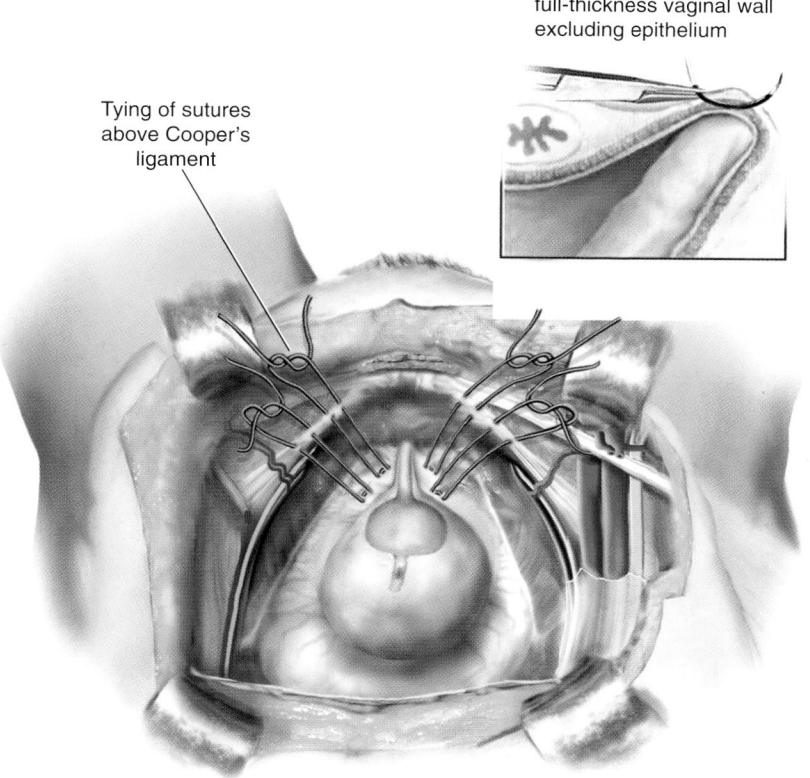

Needle passed through
full-thickness vaginal wall
excluding epithelium

Tying of sutures
above Cooper's
ligament

**FIGURE 33-4** Sutures have been appropriately placed on each side of the proximal urethral and bladder neck. Note that figure-of-8 bites are taken through the vagina. Double-armed sutures are used so that the end of each suture can be brought up through the ipsilateral Cooper's ligament, thus allowing the sutures to be tied above the ligament.

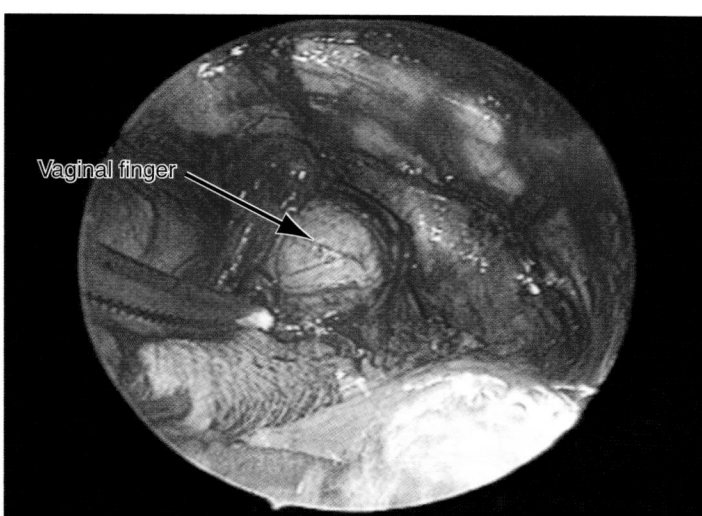

Vaginal finger

**FIGURE 33-5** The first step of the Burch colposuspension is to elevate the vagina and mobilize the fat in a medial direction. *Note:* A sponge stick is used to initially mobilize the bladder medially, and then the fat is cleaned off with a small Kitner-type instrument. Elevating the vagina reveals the muscular lining of the vaginal wall through which sutures will be passed lateral to the midurethra and lateral to the bladder neck.

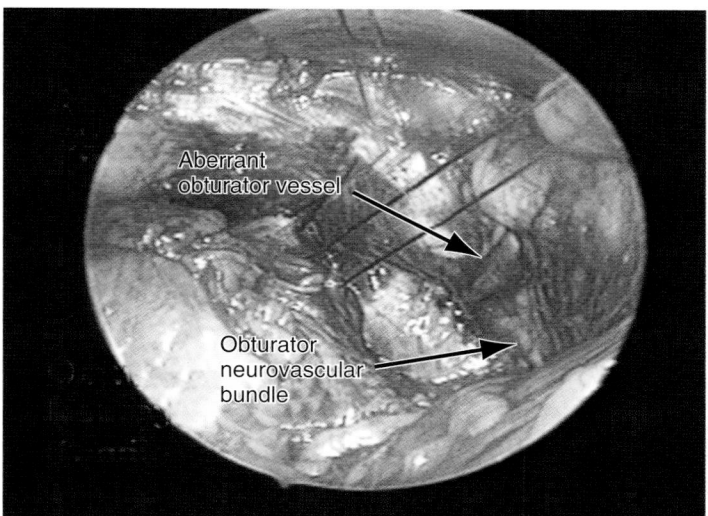

Aberrant
obturator vessel

Obturator
neurovascular
bundle

**FIGURE 33-6** Two Burch colposuspension sutures have been passed through the full thickness of the vaginal wall on the patient's right side. The suture lateral to the midurethra has also been passed through Cooper's ligament on that side. Noted in this picture is an aberrant obturator vessel draping down over the most lateral aspect of Cooper's ligament. Also noted is the obturator neurovascular bundle as it exits the pelvis through the obturator canal.

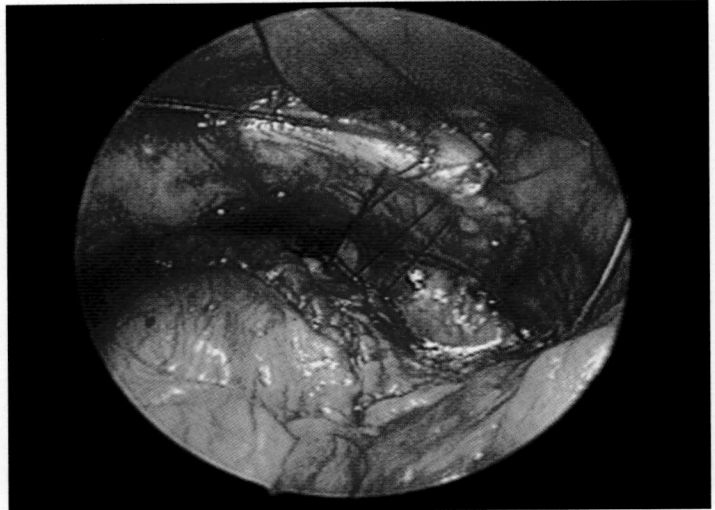

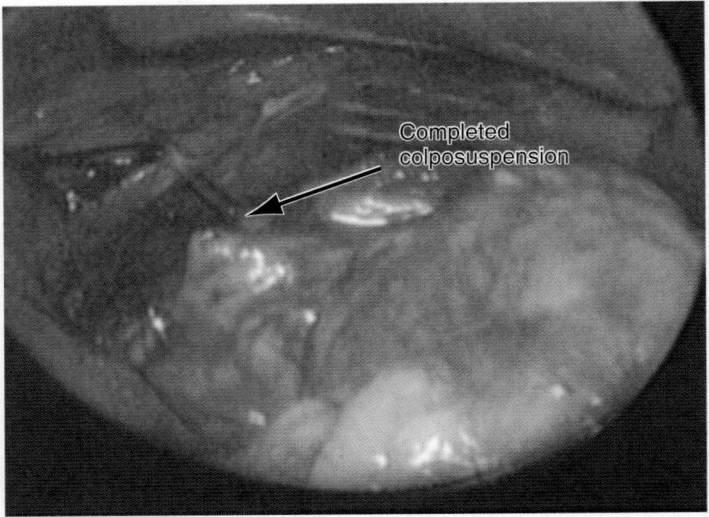

FIGURE 33–7 Both Burch colposuspension sutures have been passed on the right side. Again note that each end of the suture has been brought up through Cooper's ligament and the knots tied above the ligament, completing the colposuspension on the right side.

FIGURE 33–8 The completed colposuspension is shown on the patient's left side. Again note that the knot is tied above Cooper's ligament, and sutures are elevated just until the slack or tension is taken out of the suture. It is very common to see, as in this photograph, a suture bridge that exists between the elevated vagina and Cooper's ligament.

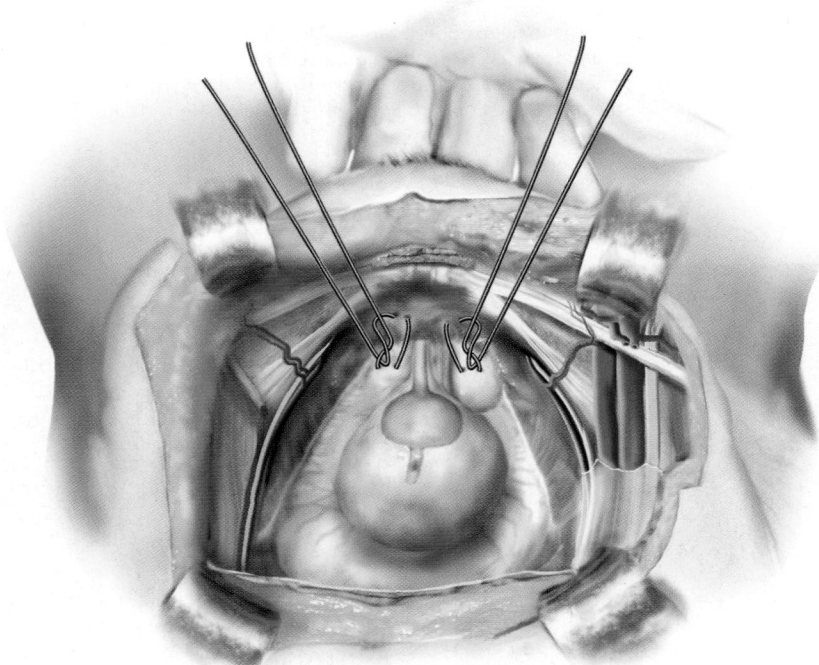

FIGURE 33–9 Marshall-Marchetti-Krantz procedure. One suture is placed bilaterally at the level of the bladder neck and then into the periosteum of the pubic symphysis.

# CHAPTER 34

# Retropubic Paravaginal Repair

*Mickey M. Karram*

Anterior vaginal wall prolapse may be the result of detachment of the vagina from its normal lateral attachment. The object of the paravaginal defect repair is to reattach bilaterally the anterior lateral vaginal sulcus with its overlying fascia to the lateral sidewall at the level of the arcus tendineus fasciae pelvis, which is its normal attachment.

The retropubic space is entered, and the bladder and vagina are depressed and retracted medially to allow visualization of the lateral retropubic space and the lateral pelvic sidewall, including the obturator internus muscle and the fossa containing the obturator neurovascular bundle (Figs. 34–1 through 34–3; also see Chapter 31 on Retropubic Anatomy). Blunt dissection can be carried dorsally from this point until the ischial spine is palpated. The arcus tendineus fasciae pelvis, or white line, is often visualized as a white band of tissue running from the back of the symphysis pubis to the ischial spine (see Figs. 34–2 and 34–3). It is the anatomic separation between the lower edge of the obturator internus muscle and the beginning of the iliococcygeal portion of the levator ani muscle. A paravaginal defect represents avulsion of the vagina with its muscular layer or pubocervical fascia off the arcus tendineus fasciae pelvis or possibly an avulsion of the arcus as well as the fascia off the obturator internus muscle (see Figs. 34–1 through 34–3). Figure 34–1C depicts various anatomic defects that can be encountered when a paravaginal defect is present. It should be noted that at times the white line can be so attenuated that it may not be anatomically identifiable.

A retropubic paravaginal defect repair is performed as follows: The surgeon's nondominant hand is inserted into the vagina. While gently retracting the bladder medially with sponge sticks (as shown in Fig. 33–1 in Chapter 33), the surgeon elevates the anterior lateral vaginal sulcus. Starting near the vaginal apex, a suture is placed first through the full thickness of the vagina excluding the epithelium. This suture should be in the lateral edge of the underlying muscular tissue of the vagina, or the pubocervical fascia. The needle then is passed into the obturator internus fascia or, if visualized, the arcus tendineus fasciae pelvis, 1 to 2 cm anterior to its origin at the ischial spine. After this first stitch is tied, four or five additional sutures are placed through the vaginal wall and then into the arcus tendineus fasciae pelvis or obturator internus fascia (see Fig. 34–1B). These stitches are placed at 1-cm intervals toward the pubic ramus. Tying of the sutures reapproximates the vagina with its fascia to the lateral pelvic sidewall (Figs. 34–1, 34–4, and 34–5). The most distal suture should be placed as close as possible to the pubic ramus into the pubourethral ligament. Usually 2-0 or 3-0 nonabsorbable sutures on a medium-sized tapered needle are utilized for this repair.

In patients who have genuine stress incontinence plus a paravaginal defect, a combined Burch colposuspension and retropubic paravaginal repair should be performed. This has been termed a *paravaginal plus procedure* (see Figs. 34–4 and 34–5).

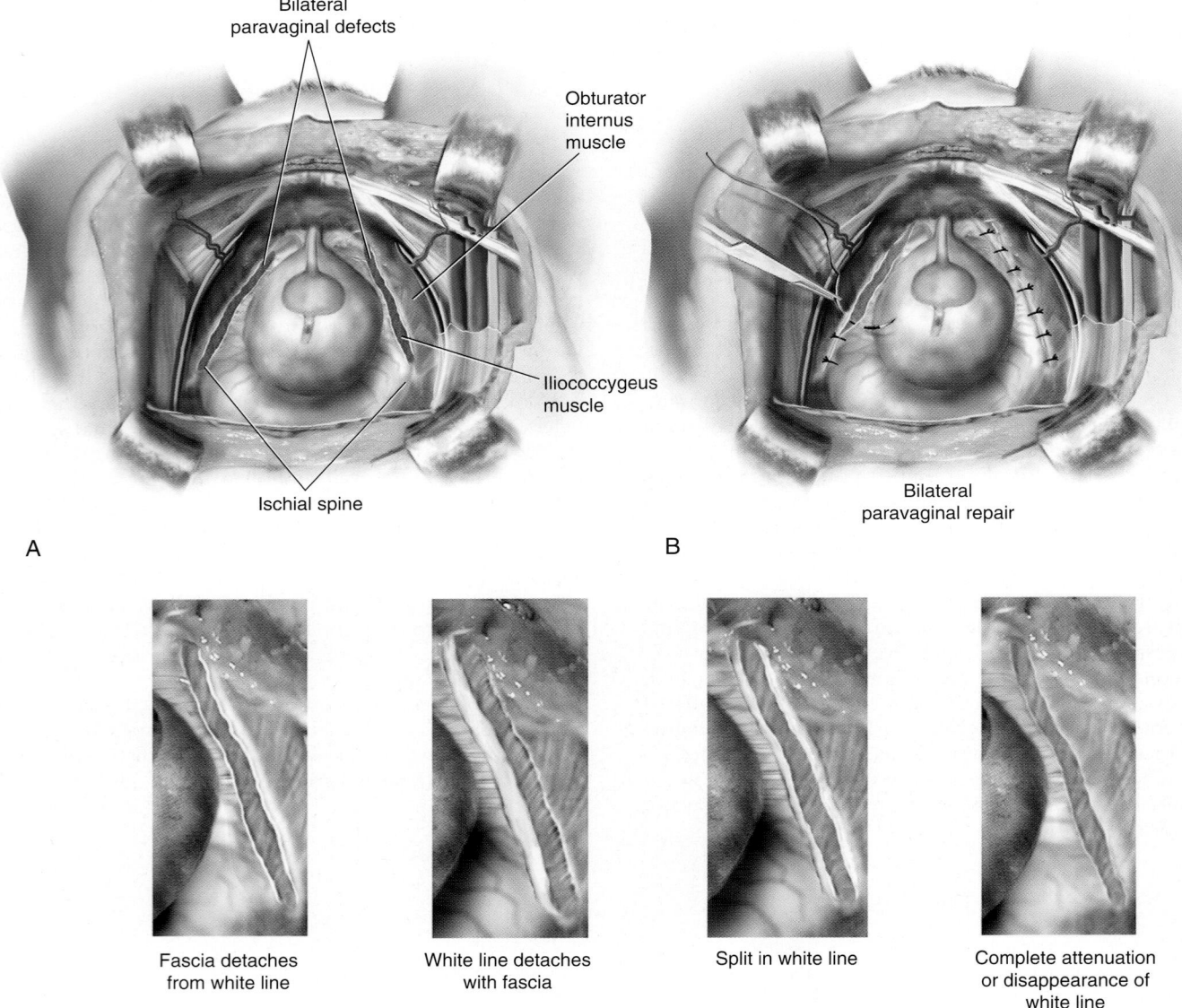

A

B

C

**FIGURE 34–1** Retropubic paravaginal defect repair. **A.** Bilateral paravaginal defects are illustrated. **B.** The defect on the right has been completely repaired, and the defect on the left is being repaired from just distal to the ischial spine and working toward the pubic symphysis. **C.** Four potential anatomic findings in patients with paravaginal defects are illustrated. Note that all result in falling away of the vagina with its underlying fasciae from the lateral pelvic sidewall.

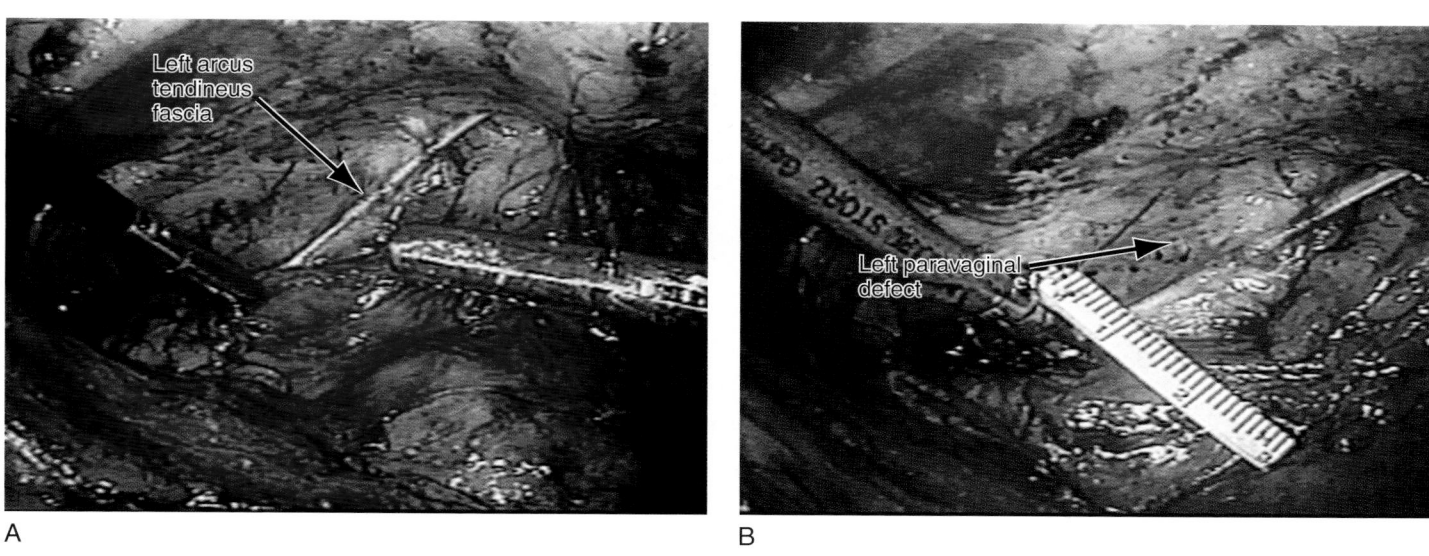

A                                                      B

**FIGURE 34–2** Demonstrates a patient with a left paravaginal defect repair. **A.** Note that the arcus tendineus fasciae pelvis has been detached. **B.** A 2-cm paravaginal defect is noted.

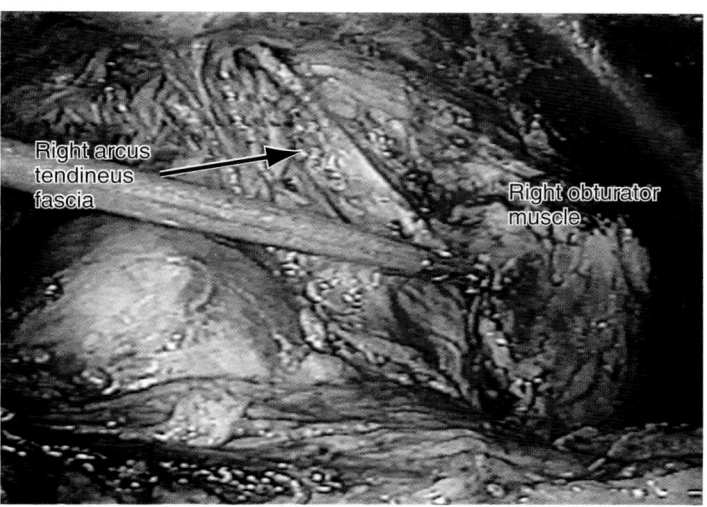

**FIGURE 34–3** Demonstrates a right paravaginal defect on the same patient as in Figure 34–2. Again note the detached arcus tendineus fasciae pelvis.

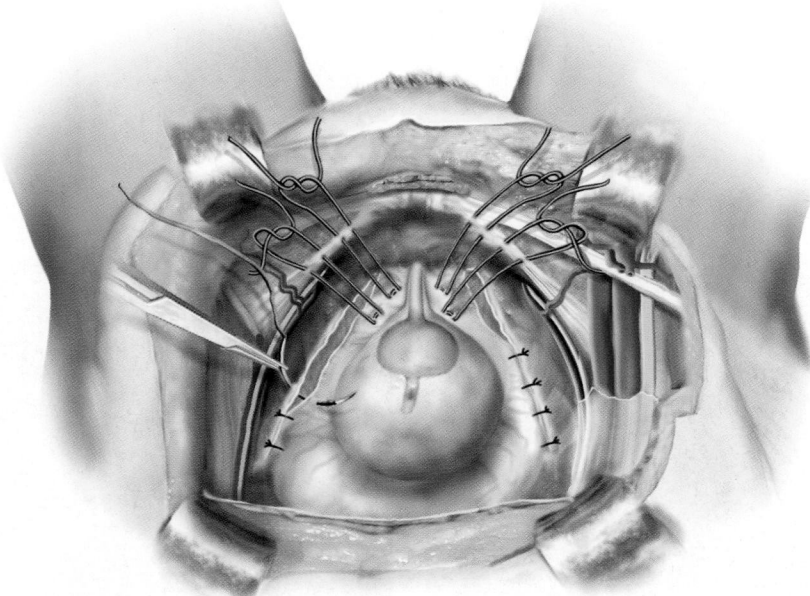

**FIGURE 34–4** Paravaginal defect plus repair. Combined Burch colposuspension and retropubic paravaginal defect repair.

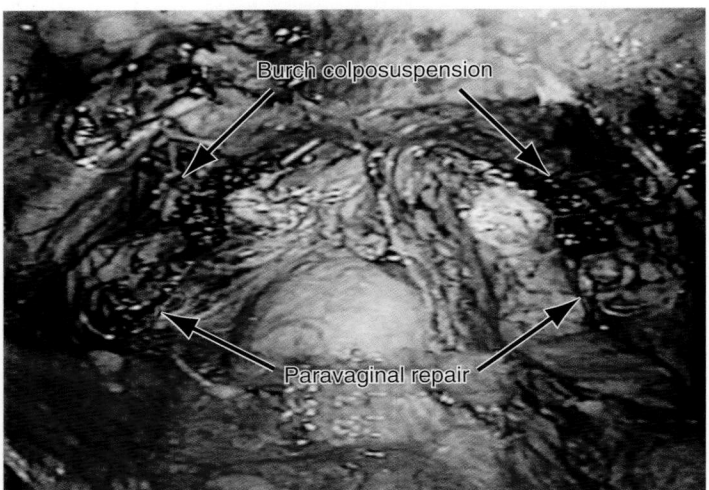

**FIGURE 34–5** Completed paravaginal prep plus procedure. Note that the Burch colposuspension stitches have been placed to pass to Cooper's ligament, and the paravaginal stitches have reattached the detached arcus to the obturator internus fascia.

# CHAPTER 35

# Retropubic Vesicourethrolysis

## *Mickey M. Karram*

The technique of retropubic or abdominal vesicourethrolysis has been described as a takedown of a retropubic repair that has resulted in urinary retention or significant voiding dysfunction. The goal of the operation is to free and mobilize the bladder and the proximal urethra. The procedure is performed as follows.

A large Foley catheter with a 30-mL balloon is placed inside the bladder. A transverse muscle–cutting incision, usually a Cherney incision (Fig. 35–1), is performed to facilitate exposure into the retropubic space. The bladder then is taken down sharply over the back of the symphysis pubis all the way down to the proximal urethra. It is best to make a high cystotomy to help in this dissection (Figs. 35–2 and 35–3). It is important to completely mobilize the bladder as well as the proximal urethra from the back of the symphysis. Very commonly, sutures or bone anchors from a previous suspension are encountered (Fig. 35–4). Dissection is extended laterally toward the pelvic sidewall and is taken down to the level of the arcus tendineus fasciae pelvis (white line) or the lower margin of the obturator internus fascia (Figs. 35–5 and 35–6). With the concern of rescarification in this area, it is at times beneficial to make a window in the peritoneum and bring in a piece of omentum to be placed between the back of the symphysis and the proximal urethra (Fig. 35–7). Usually resuspension is not necessary in these patients. If a high cystocele is noted following a paravaginal defect, a retropubic paravaginal repair is performed simultaneously.

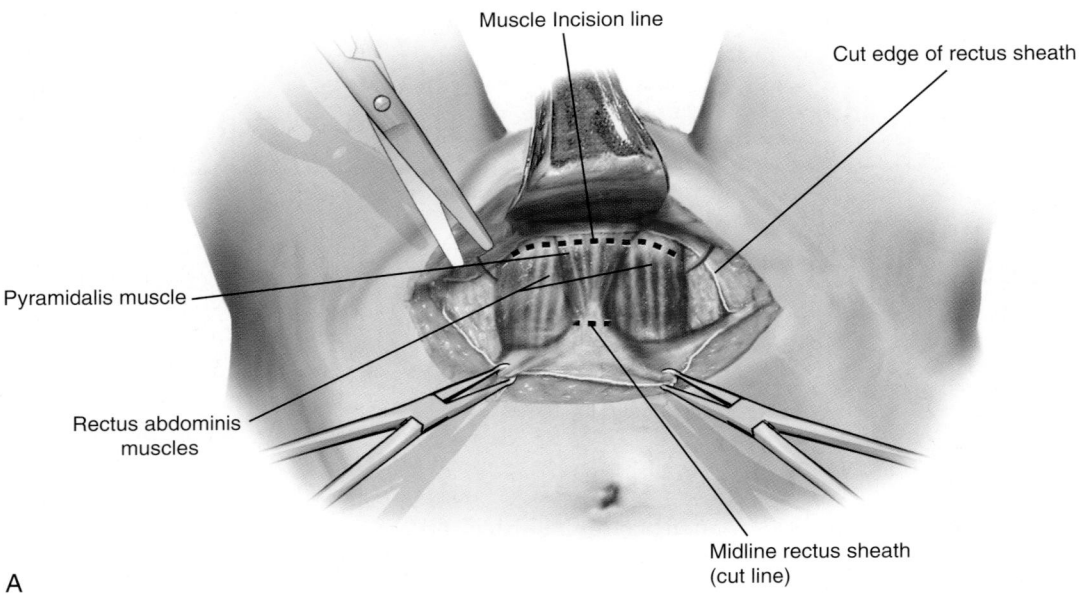

Muscle Incision line

Cut edge of rectus sheath

Pyramidalis muscle

Rectus abdominis muscles

Midline rectus sheath (cut line)

A

Cutting rectus muscles (both sides)

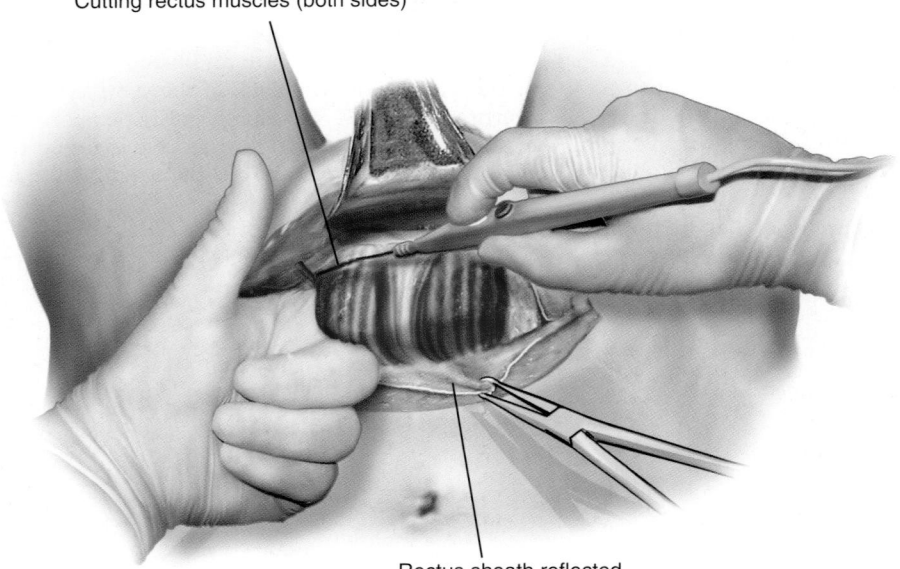

Rectus sheath reflected

B

Incision line to enter peritoneum

Inferior epigastric vessels sectioned and ligated

Rectus abdominis muscles cut and reflected

C

**FIGURE 35–1** Technique for a Cherney muscle-cutting incision. **A.** A finger is taken around the entire belly of the rectus muscle. The finger should be behind the rectus muscle and in front of the peritoneum. The insertion of the muscle is then taken off the back of the symphysis by means of electrocautery. **B.** The muscle has been completely detached from its insertion. **C.** Easy access to the retropubic space is apparent once both rectus muscles have been cut.

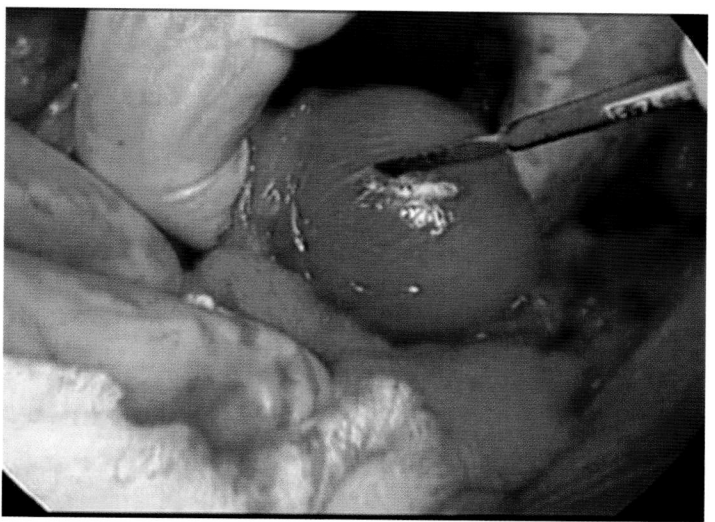

**FIGURE 35-2** Demonstrates the technique for a high extraperitoneal cystotomy, which is commonly performed during a retropubic vesicourethrolysis. A large Foley balloon has been placed in the bladder. The balloon is mobilized into the dome of the bladder. With an electrocautery pencil, the wall of the bladder is cut, creating the cystotomy.

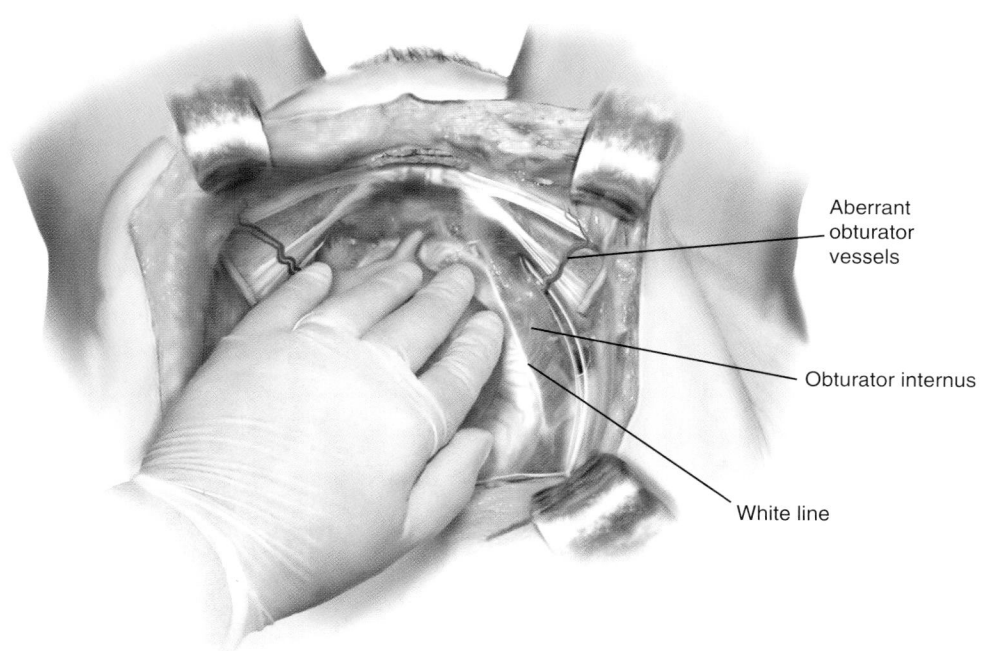

Aberrant obturator vessels

Obturator internus

White line

**FIGURE 35-3** The technique of retropubic vesicourethrolysis involves sharp dissection, where the tissue is cut away from the back of the pubic bone.

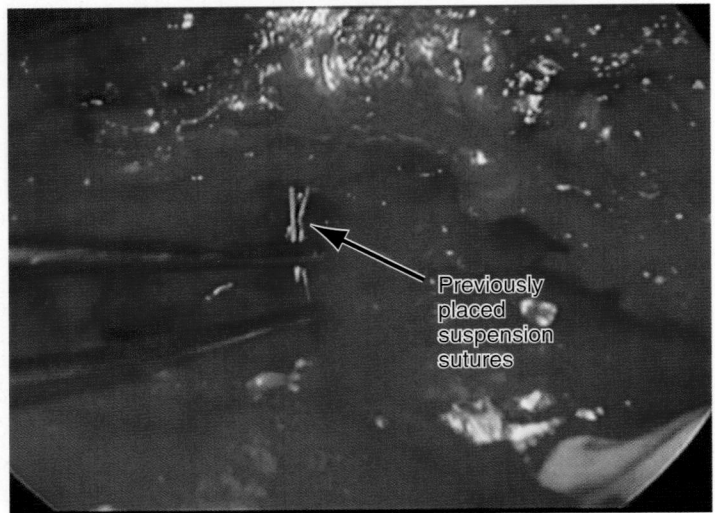

**FIGURE 35–4** Previously placed suspension sutures are encountered and commonly are taken down during a retropubic vesicourethrolysis.

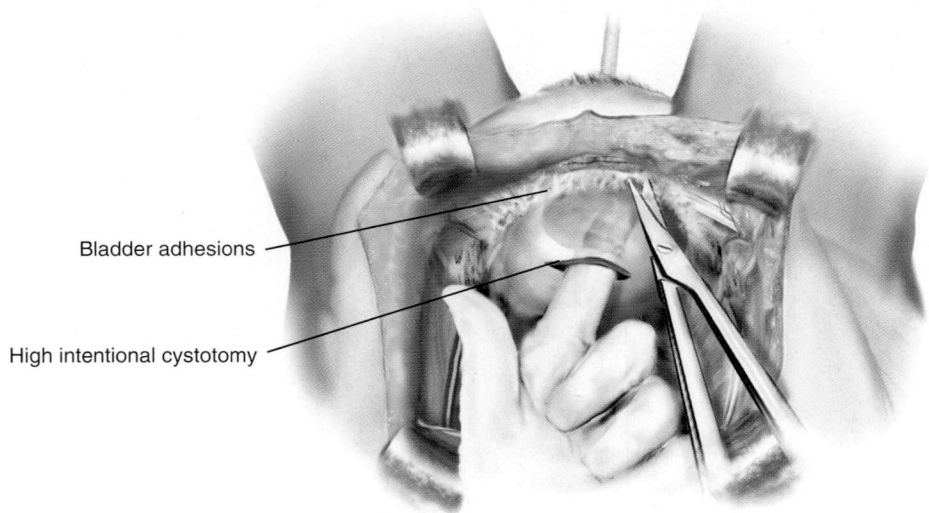

Bladder adhesions

High intentional cystotomy

**FIGURE 35–5** Retropubic vesicourethrolysis. A high extraperitoneal cystotomy has been made to facilitate sharp dissection of the bladder of the back of the symphysis pubis.

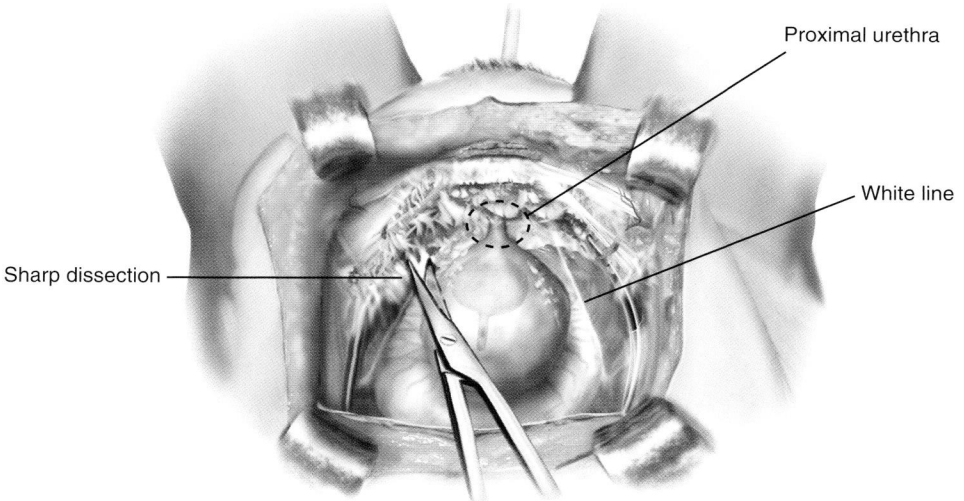

Proximal urethra

White line

Sharp dissection

**FIGURE 35–6** Sharp dissection is continued down in the midline until the proximal one third of the urethra has been mobilized off the symphysis. The dissection is extended laterally down to the level of the paravaginal attachment at the arcus tendineus fasciae pelvis (*white line*).

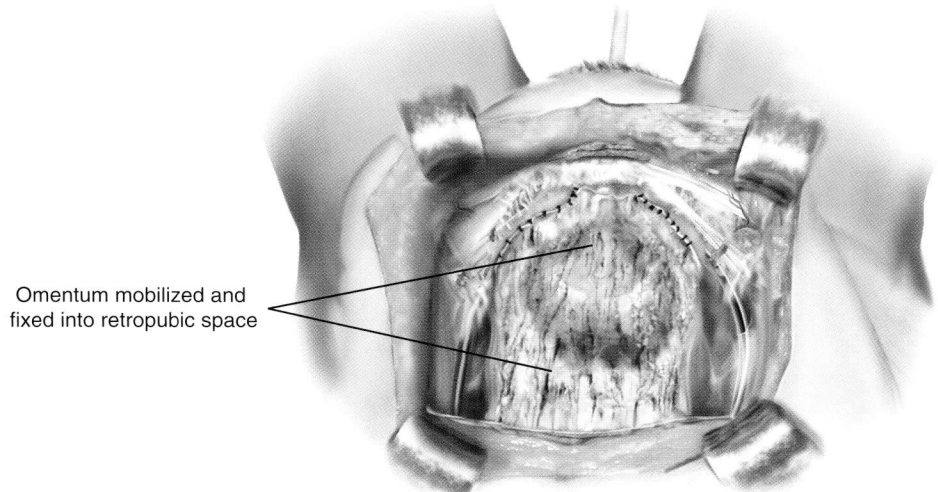

Omentum mobilized and fixed into retropubic space

**FIGURE 35–7** To prevent rescarification in this area, a piece of omentum can be brought through a window in the peritoneum. The omentum then is sutured at the midline to the lower aspect of the symphysis and laterally to the obturator fascia with numerous delayed-absorbable sutures.

# SECTION F

# Retroperitoneum and Presacral Space

# CHAPTER 36

# Anatomy of the Retroperitoneum and the Presacral Space

*Michael S. Baggish*

The retroperitoneal space may be entered at several points in a safe and easy manner. The broad ligament may be entered by grasping and tenting up the round ligament. The ligament may be suture-ligated and cut, or simply grasped in a clamp. The peritoneum posterior to the ligament is cut vertically back in the direction of the ovarian vessels and ureter. The author recommends **always** first palpating the pulse of the external iliac artery and **always** opening lateral to that vessel over the psoas major muscle. The muscle is identified (as is the genitofemoral nerve). Next, the external iliac artery is identified just medial to the muscle edge (Figs. 36–1 through 36–4).

The sigmoid colon joins the rectum posterior to the uterus. Above this junction, the sigmoid proceeds upward and swings to the left, where it is attached to the peritoneum reflected over the psoas major muscle and iliacus muscle. This is not an adhesion but rather a normal physiologic attachment and corresponds to the area beneath the peritoneum where the left ovarian artery and veins, as well as the left ureter, are located. This is the general area where these structures cross the left common iliac artery. Cutting the peritoneum over the psoas muscle and reflecting the colon medially represents still another method of safely gaining entry into the left retroperitoneum. Further extending the cut into the broad ligament opens the retroperitoneal space wider and permits an excellent view of the course of the ureter (Figs. 36–5 through 36–9).

The peritoneal incision and dissection proceed superiorly (upward), extending from the round ligament over the psoas muscle and the external iliac artery. The uterus is pulled sharply to the left or right side of the pelvis. This places the structures to be identified on traction. The ovarian vessels and ureter are identified as they cross over the common iliac artery (Figs. 36–10 through 36–12). Immediately posterior to (beneath) the external iliac artery is the large (bluish) external iliac vein. This thin-walled vessel follows a course identical to that of the external iliac artery. Retracting the vein and removing or pushing aside the fatty tissue surrounding the vessel brings into view the obturator internus muscle. This muscle is often referred to as the pelvic sidewall (Fig. 36–13).

Entry into the presacral space may be achieved by pulling the rectosigmoid to the left side of the pelvis and incising the peritoneum vertically just to the right side of the sigmoid peritoneal attachment to the posterior pelvis (Fig. 36–14). This dissection will begin at the aortic bifurcation and will proceed inferiorly over the presacral space (Figs. 36–15 and 36–16A, B).

The most vulnerable structure exposed to real or potential injury in this location is the left common iliac vein, which crosses the sacral promontory from left to right. It must be identified immediately (Figs. 36–17 and 36–18).

The middle sacral vessels and the middle hypogastric plexus are identified descending over the sacrum into the depths of the sacral hollow. The vessels emerge beneath the left common iliac vein, whereas the nerves cross over the vein (Fig. 36–19A–G).

The hypogastric nerve plexus descends into the pelvis over the anterior surface of the aorta and enters the presacral space between the iliac arteries. The plexus crosses over the left common iliac vein and lies anterior to the middle sacral vessels (Figs. 36–19 through 36–21). To the left and lateral lie the inferior mesenteric artery and its branches (Fig. 36–22). To the right and lateral lies the right ureter (see Fig. 36–22). If one were to extend the dissection above the pelvis and broaden the exposure laterally, the ureters would lead the dissector to the kidney, the ovarian arteries to the aorta, and the ovarian veins to the vena cava and left renal vein (Figs. 36–23 and 36–24).

The common iliac artery bifurcation is an excellent point of reference to ensure differentiation between the external and internal (hypogastric) iliac arteries (Fig. 36–25A, B). The pelvic ureter is always medial to the internal iliac artery (Fig. 36–26). The internal iliac artery itself quickly divides into two sections (anterior and posterior) (Fig. 36–27A, B). Of particular importance are the numerous and frequently anomalous pelvic veins lying posterior and deep to the internal iliac artery (Fig. 36–28). If one were to follow the posterior division of the hypogastric artery into the depths of the pelvis and through the treacherous venous field to the area of the ischial spine and the lateral edge of the sacrum, large sacral nerve roots would be encountered (Fig. 36–29).

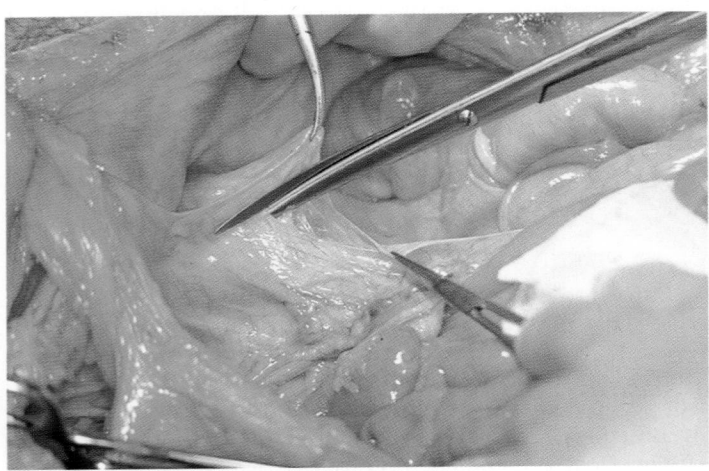

**FIGURE 36–1** The retroperitoneal space may be entered by elevating the peritoneum at the top of the broad ligament between the round and infundibulopelvic ligaments. The peritoneum is incised and opened parallel to the psoas major muscle. This dissection is performed on the right side.

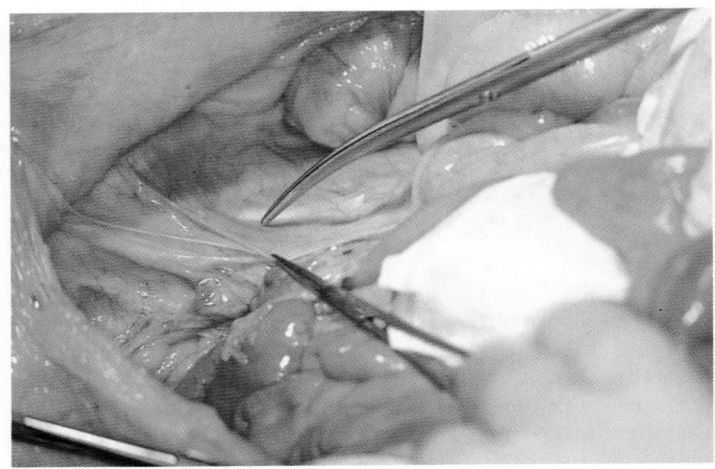

**FIGURE 36–2** The medial edge of the opened peritoneum is held with a forceps. The tip of the scissors points to the medial margin of the right psoas major muscle.

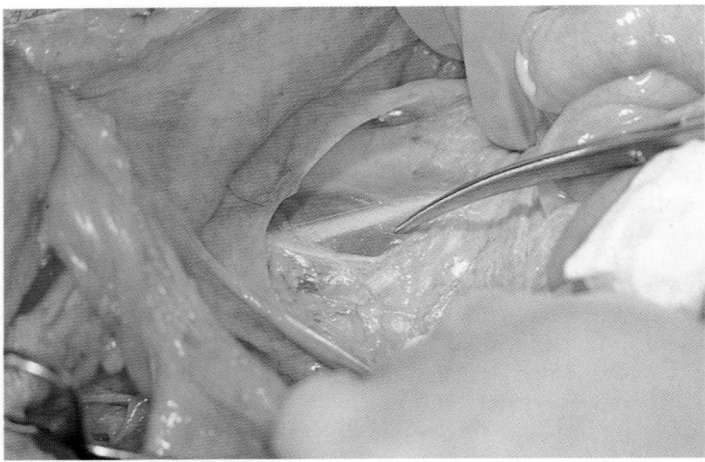

**FIGURE 36–3** The fat has been cleared away from the right psoas major muscle, and the tip of the scissors rests on the belly of the muscle.

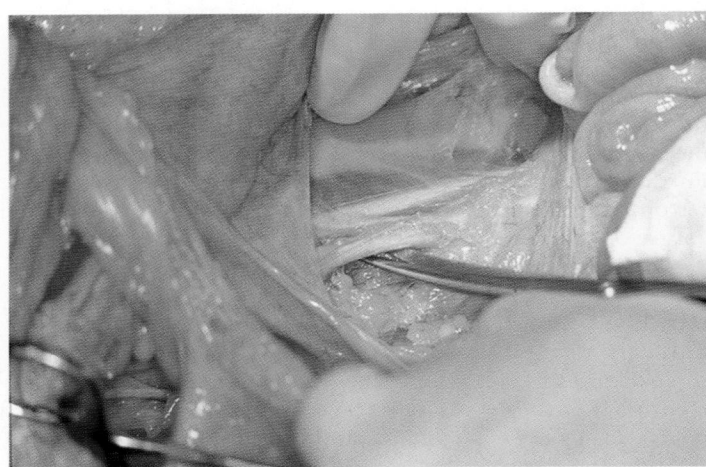

**FIGURE 36–4** The right external iliac artery has been identified just medial and slightly inferior to the psoas major muscle. The spread scissors are under the artery.

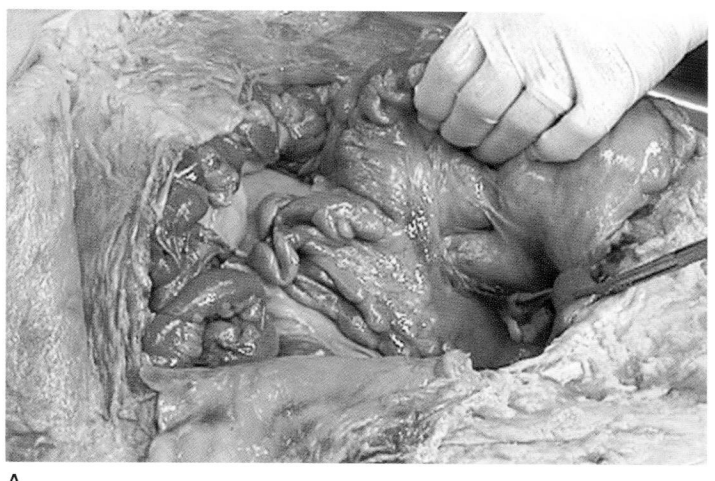

A

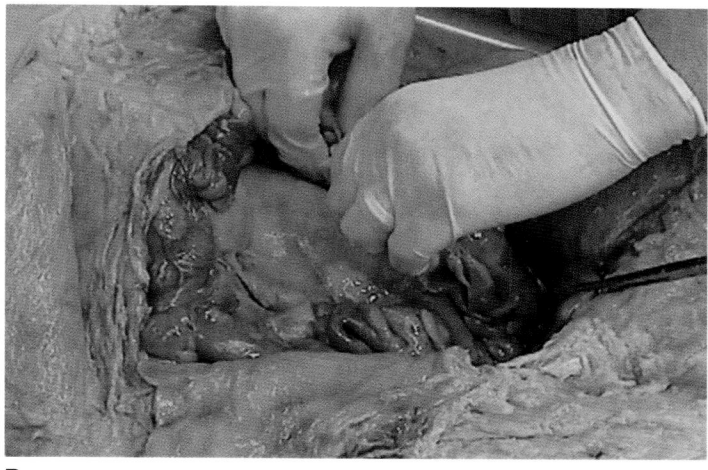

B

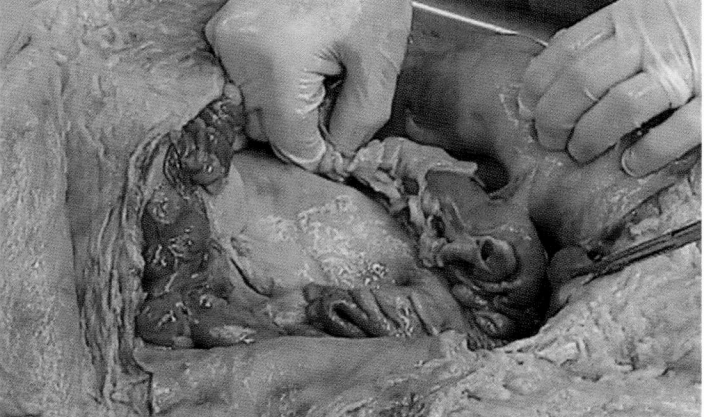

C

FIGURE 36–5  A. The sigmoid has been pulled out of the pelvis. Note the extension of the infundibulopelvic ligament toward the root of the sigmoid mesentery. The colon covers the uterus and left adnexa in its in situ position. The mesentery of the colon is exposed and reveals that the sigmoid colon is an intraperitoneal structure. The sigmoid colon initially lies to the left of the midline. The S configuration can be seen here as well. The colon swings to the right and joins the rectum posterior to the uterus (held up in the Kocher clamp). B. This view shows the somewhat redundant sigmoid colon covering the left adnexa. The uterus can be seen because it is being pulled forward and upward by the applied clamp. C. The sigmoid colon is pulled to the right, exposing the attachments to the laterally disposed parietal peritoneum. This is a very convenient location from which to enter the left retroperitoneal space.

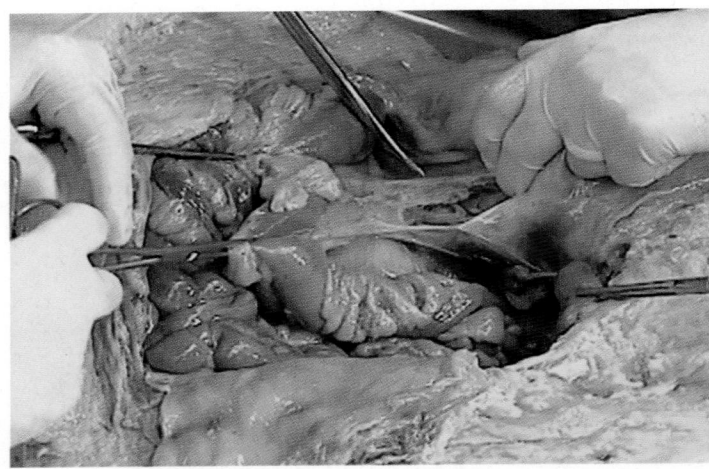

A

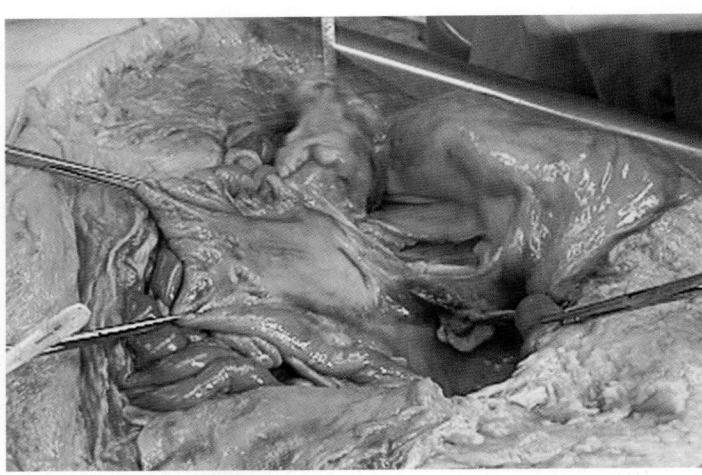

B

**FIGURE 36–6  A.** The peritoneal attachments of the sigmoid colon have been cut, allowing the large bowel to be mobilized to the right. The attachments of the lower portion of the descending colon are about to be cut. **B.** The left retroperitoneal space has been opened lateral to the point where the ovarian vessels and ureter enter the pelvis. The psoas major muscle is seen vectoring at a 90° angle to the sigmoid colon.

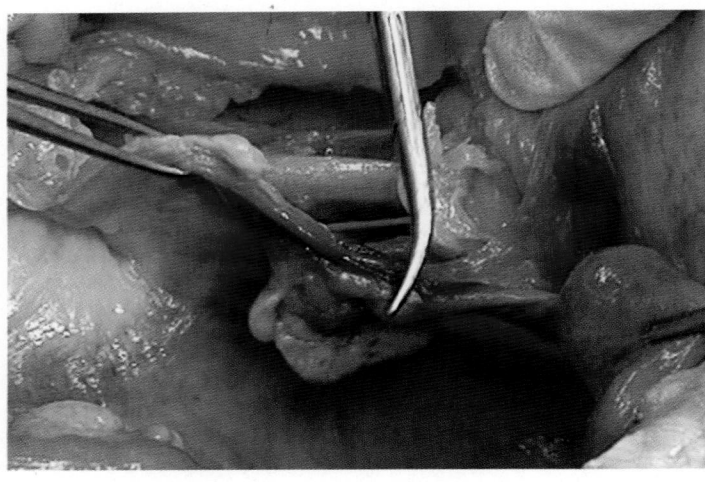

A

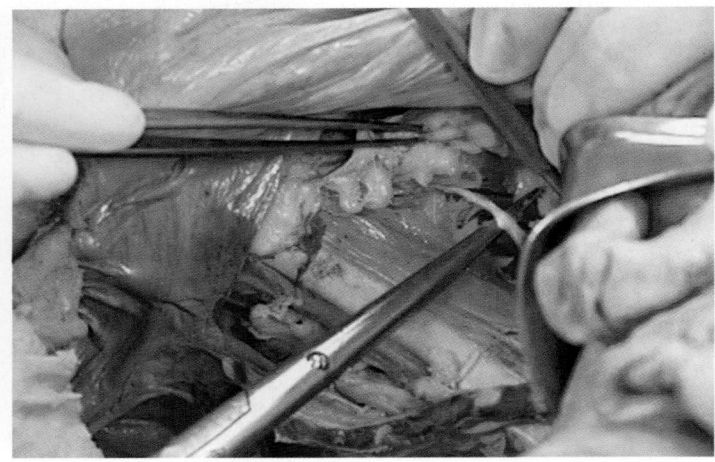

B

**FIGURE 36–7  A.** Detail of the left retroperitoneal space. The clamp holds the left oviduct and the left ovary. The forceps holds the ovarian blood supply (infundibulopelvic ligament). The ureter (unseen) lies immediately posterior to the ovarian vessels. The psoas major muscle is seen in the background. The genitofemoral nerves (on the psoas) can be seen posterior to the tendon of the psoas minor muscle. **B.** This dissection has been carried lateral to the psoas major muscle and to the iliacus muscle. The scissors elevate the lateral femoral cutaneous nerve.

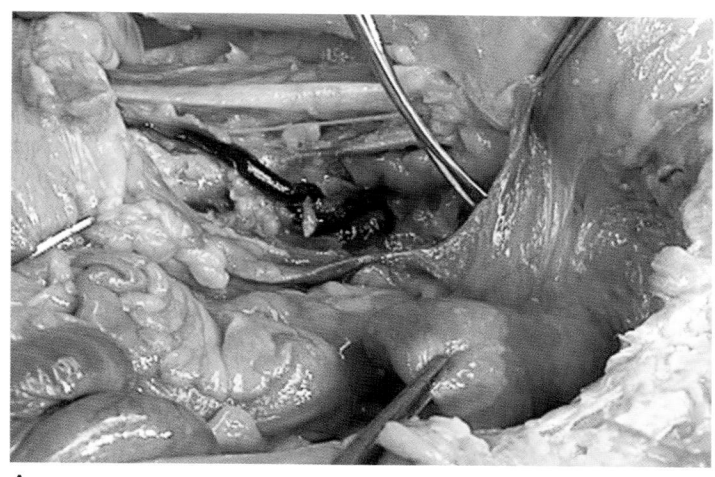

A

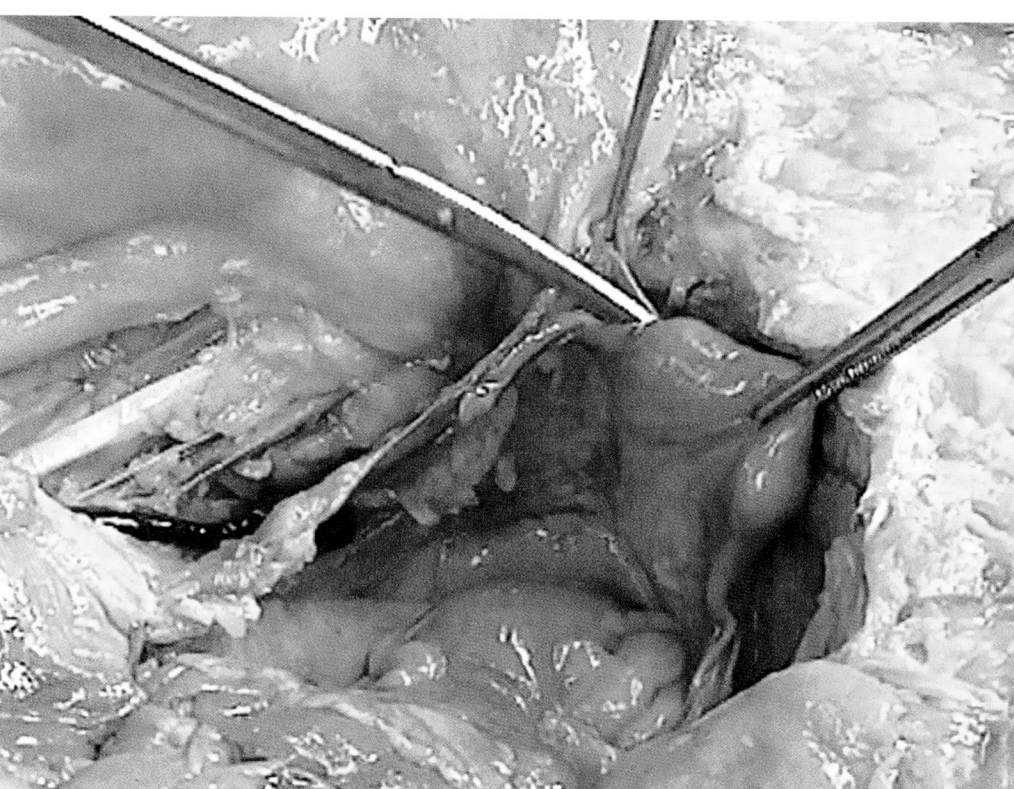

B

FIGURE 36–8  **A.** The uterus has been grasped with a Kocher clamp and pulled upward and to the right. The broad ligament on the left is held upward on tension. The scissors will cut the broad ligament to further expose the left retroperitoneal space. The ureter has been dissected from the ovarian vessels. A thrombosed supply vessel marks the ureter. In the background are the external iliac artery, the genitofemoral nerve, and the psoas major muscle. **B.** The broad ligament has been cut. The uterovesicle peritoneum is being incised. The entire left retroperitoneal space is opened. The sigmoid-rectal junction is behind the cervix and posterior vagina. The cul-de-sac is filled with redundant colon. **C.** The sigmoid colon is pulled out of the cul-de-sac, exposing the entire cul-de-sac. Note the more prominent left uterosacral ligament.

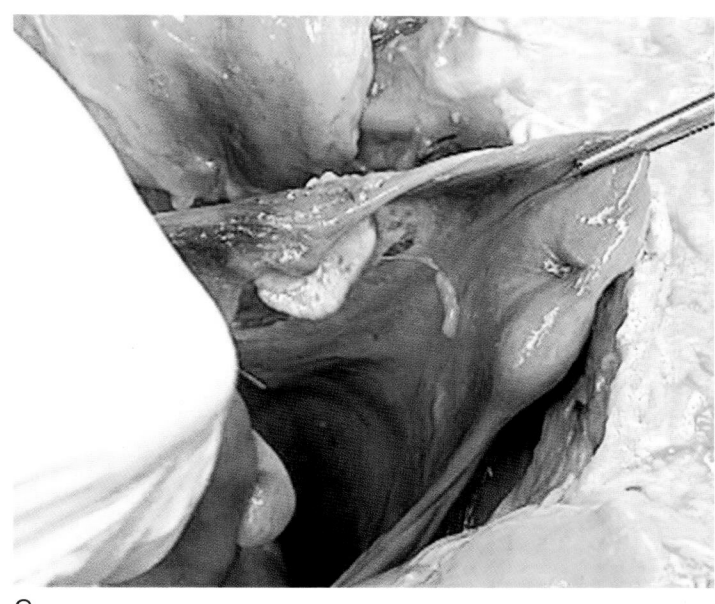

C

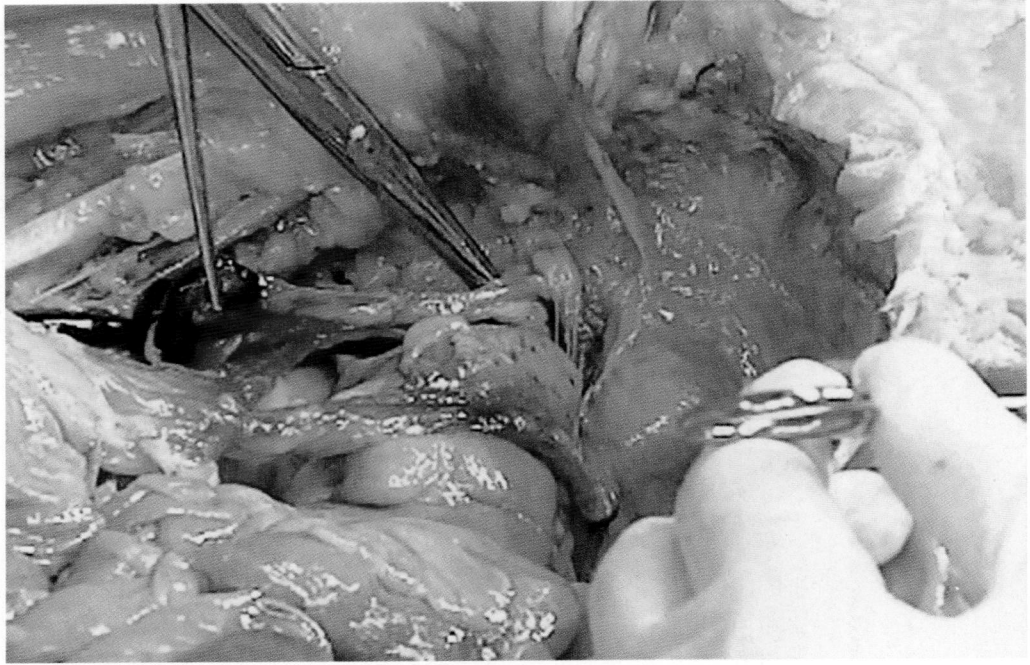

A

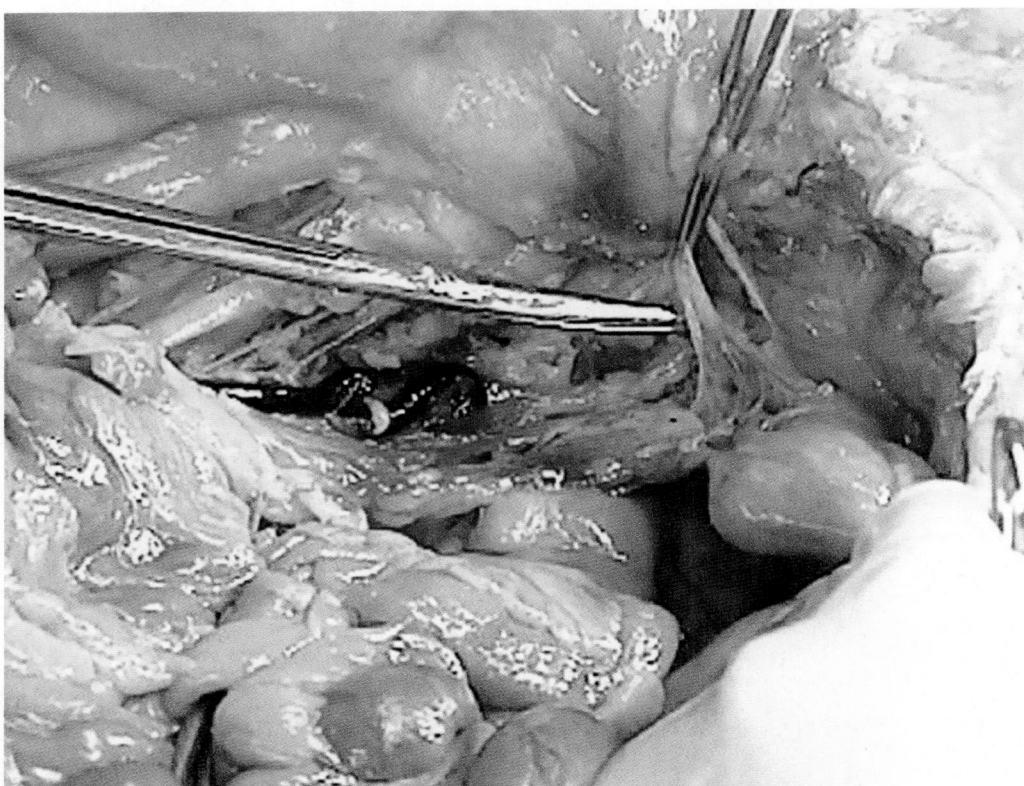

B

**FIGURE 36–9  A.** A length of ureter is shown. Proximally, the ureter is held with forceps (at the termination of the thrombosed feeding vessel). Distally, the scissors are slipped under the ureter at the point where the uterine vessels cross over it. **B.** The uterine vessels are tented-up by the forceps. The scissors tip begins to dissect them free of the ureter. The surgeon's gloved finger points to the uterine fundus.

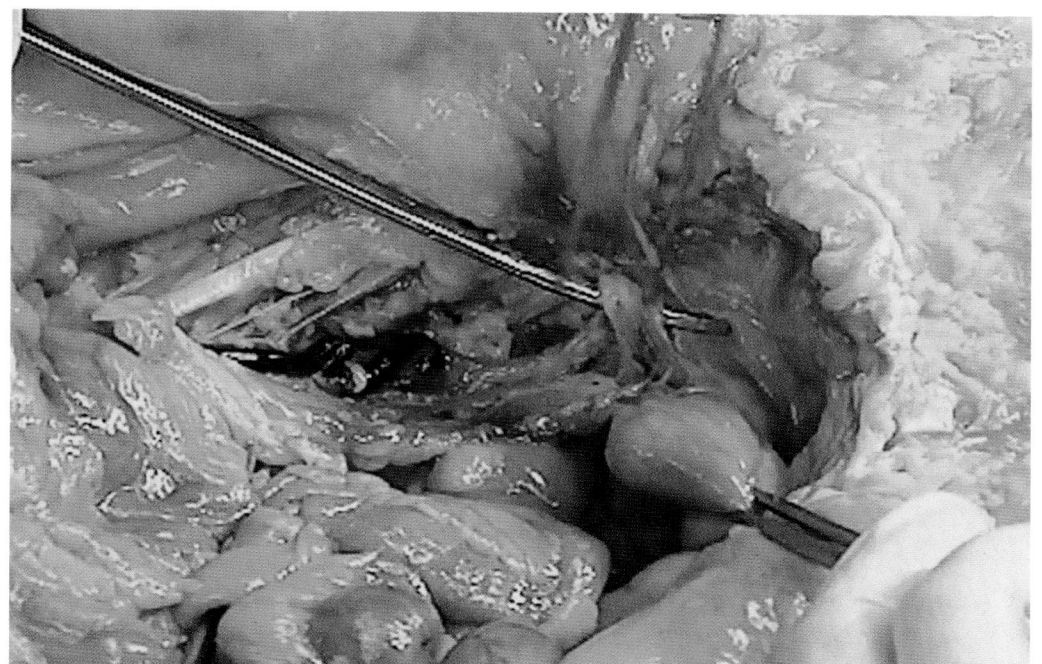

C

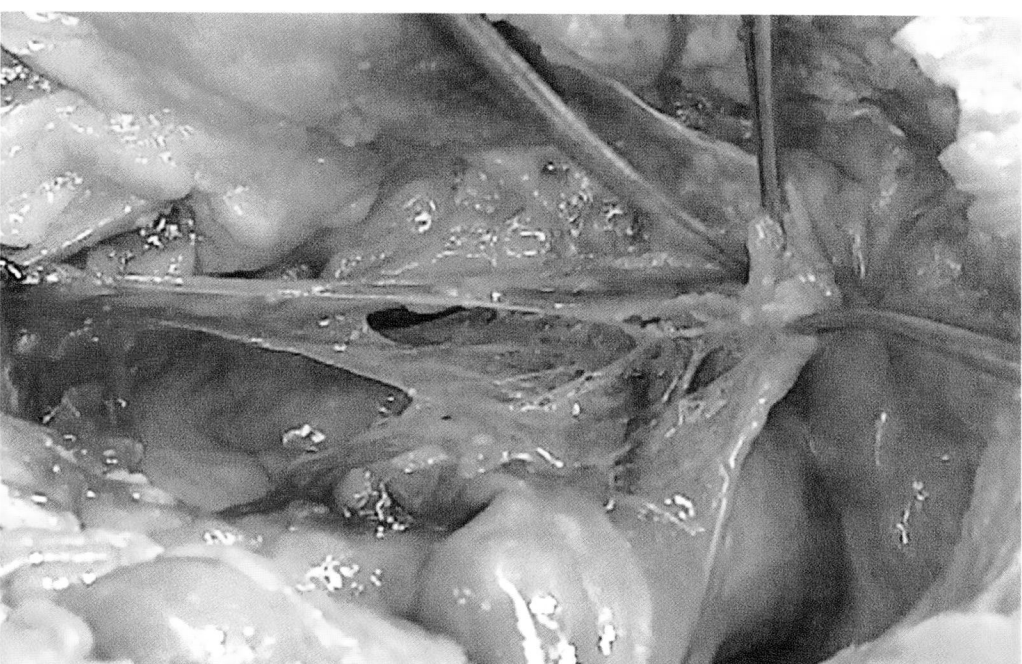

D

**FIGURE 36–9, cont'd  C.** The uterine vessels have been dissected free from the underlying ureter. The scissor tip rests on the urinary bladder. The Kocher clamp applies traction to the uterus. **D.** Close-up view of the ureter entering the bladder. The uterine vessels have been cut. The near (*right*) tonsil clamp holds half of the severed vessels. The scissors are dissecting the bladder wall.

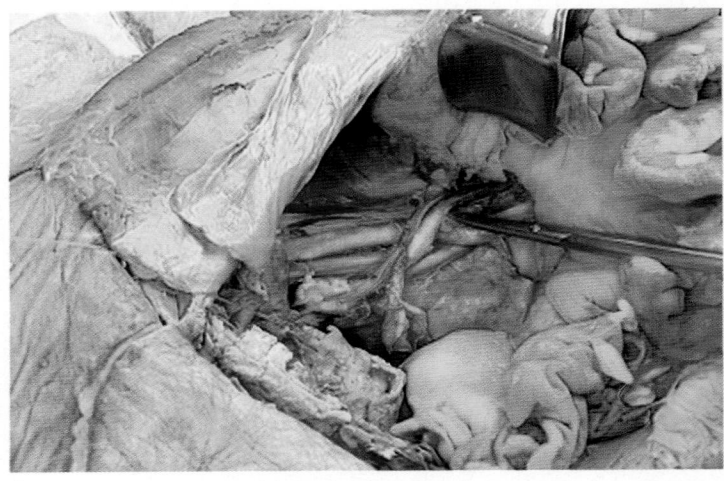

A

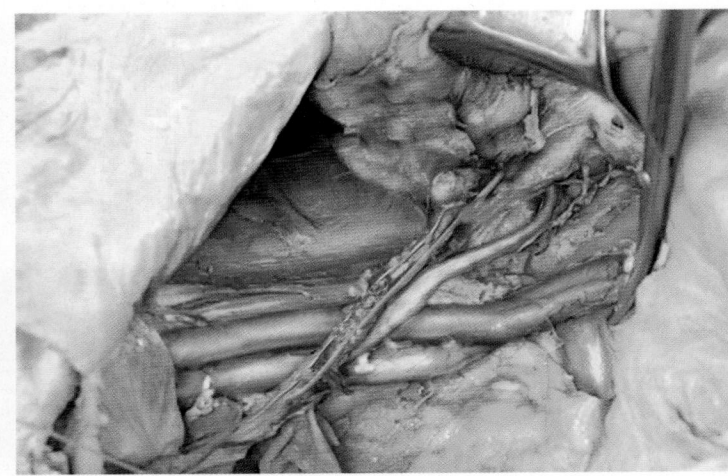

B

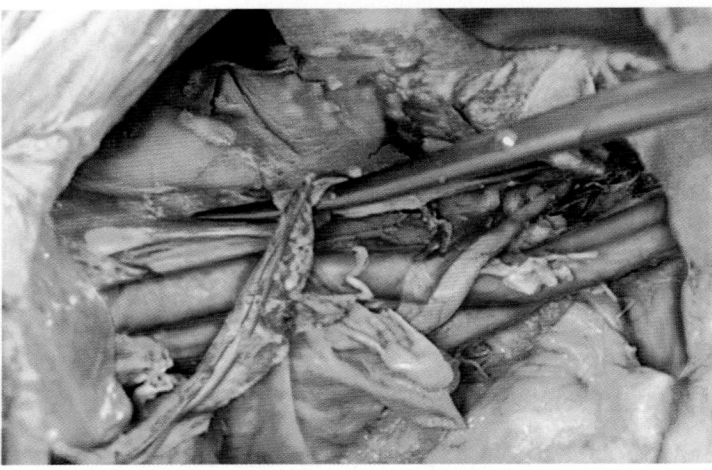

C

**FIGURE 36–10 A.** The right retroperitoneal space has been opened by cutting the peritoneal attachments of the cecum and ascending colon. The ureter (posterior and medial) descends into the pelvis with the ovarian vessels over the common iliac artery. **B.** The ovarian vessels are stretched. The ureter lies medial to the infundibulopelvic ligament and slightly posterior to it. The scissors rest on the left common iliac vein. The ureteral crossover is slightly caudad to the iliac artery bifurcation. **C.** Close-up view of the ovarian vessels, which are held upward by the scissors. The ureter crossover is seen medial and posterior to the ovarian vessel crossover. The ovarian vessels have been artificially advanced forward.

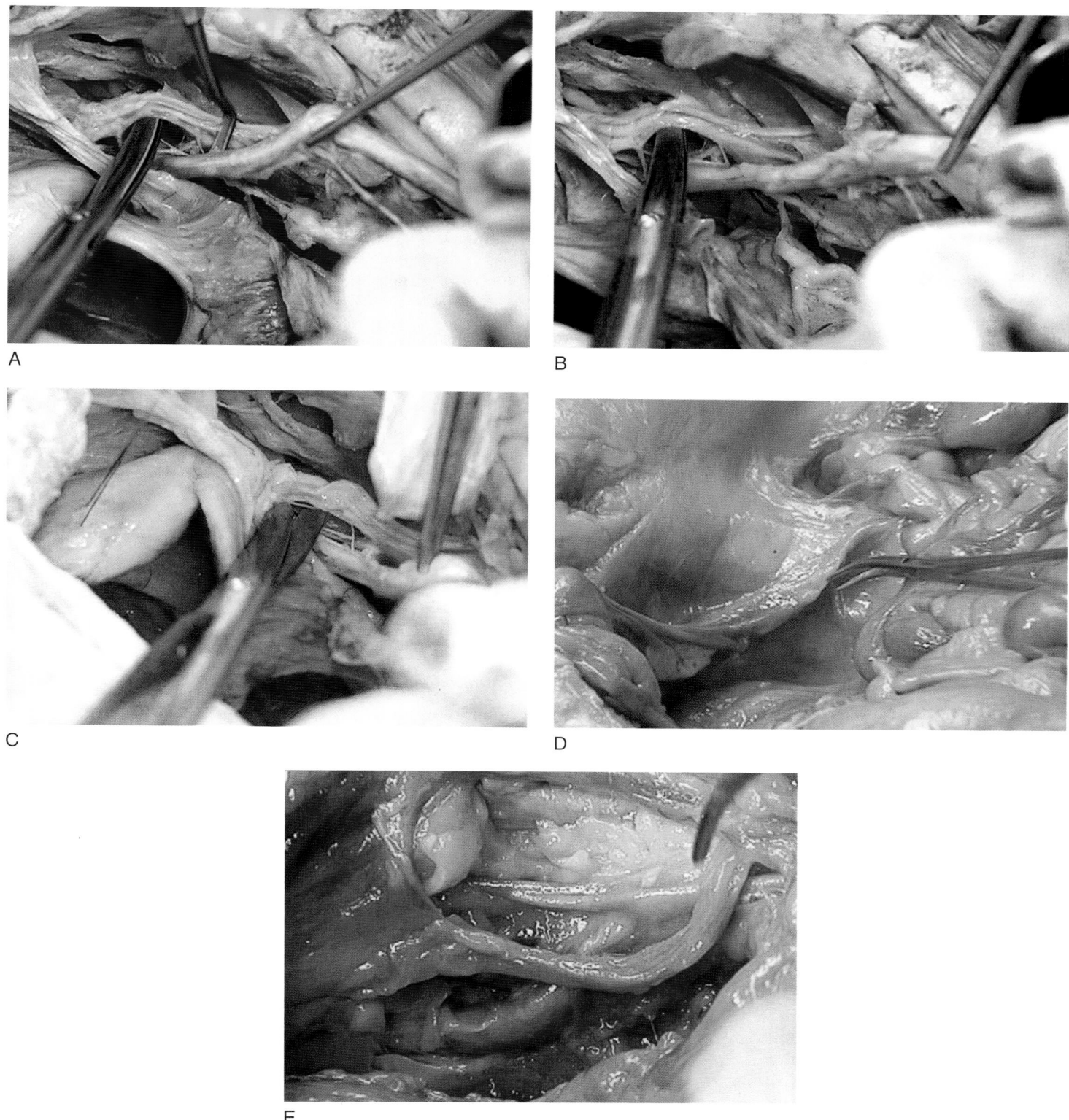

**FIGURE 36–11 A.** Close-up dissection of the right ureter as it crosses beneath the right ovarian artery (held upward by the scissors). The ureter is held by the forceps and is pointed to by the right-angle probe. The uterus lies in front of the scissors shaft, and the right uterosacral ligament is below the shaft. **B.** Close-up view of the ureter crossing under the right uterine vessels. **C.** The scissors are spread under the uterine artery. The stitch places traction on the uterus. The adnexa are retracted beneath the blades of the scissors. **D.** The clamp points to the ovarian vessels as they enter the retroperitoneum beneath the peritoneum and at the root of the ileocecal mesentery. The cecum is above. The uterine fundus is (sutured) to the far left. **E.** The right retroperitoneum has been opened. The ureter has been dissected free from the ovarian vessels. The ureter crosses over and lies medial to the right iliac artery bifurcation. The clamp points to the right common iliac artery.

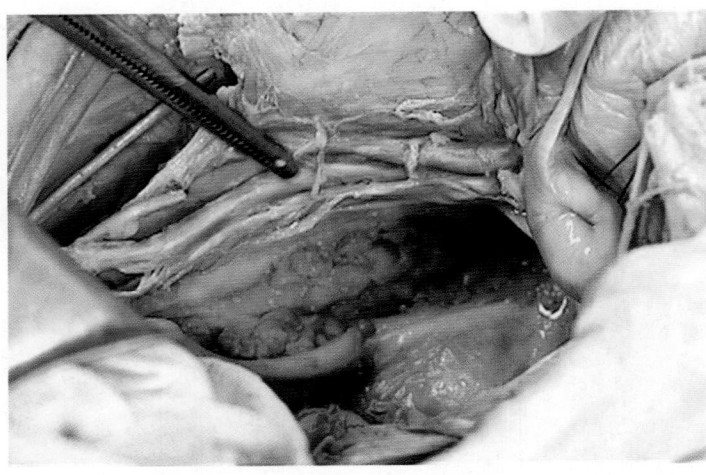

**FIGURE 36–12** The blue-tinged left uterine artery is shown. The adnexa are retracted out of the picture. The clamp points to the left ureter. The ovarian vessels have been cut.

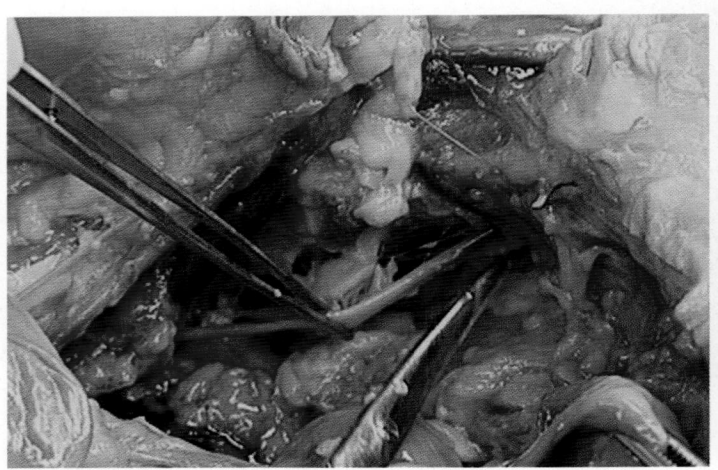

A

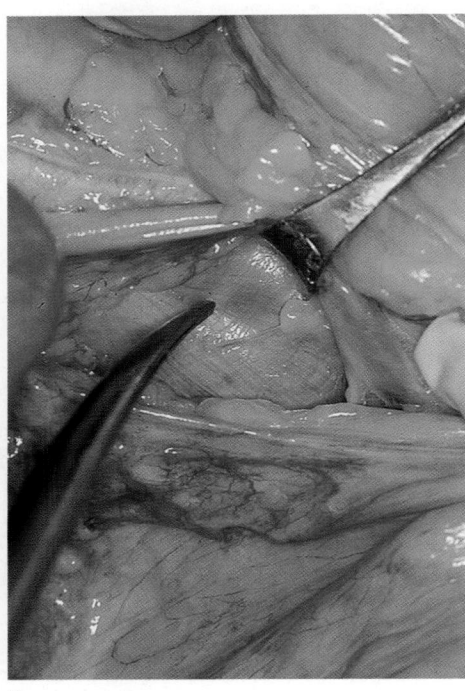

B

**FIGURE 36–13  A.** The obturator space (fossa) has been dissected. The left obturator nerve is held by the forceps. The external iliac artery and vein are seen above. **B.** The external iliac vein is retracted to show the upper margin of the obturator internus muscle.

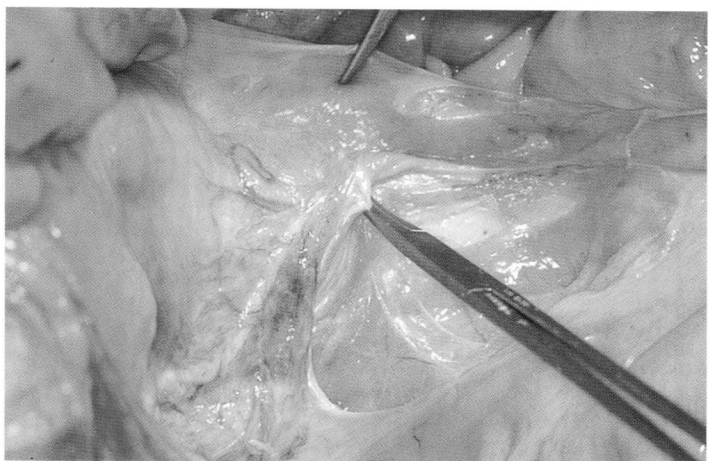

**FIGURE 36–14** The sigmoid colon has been retracted to the right. The peritoneum overlying the sacrum and aortic bifurcation is elevated and incised.

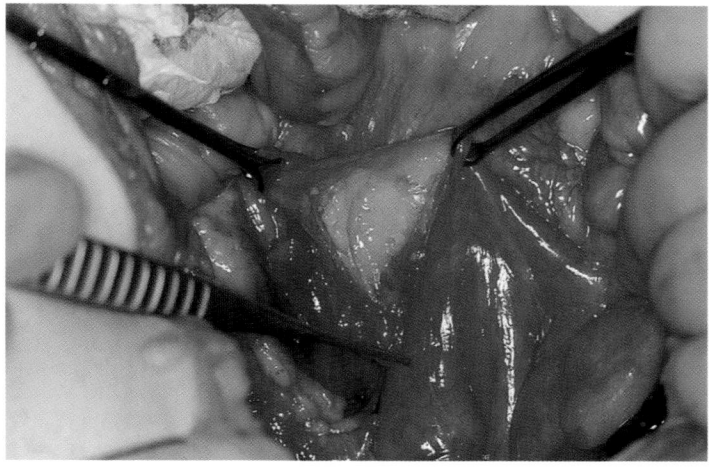

A

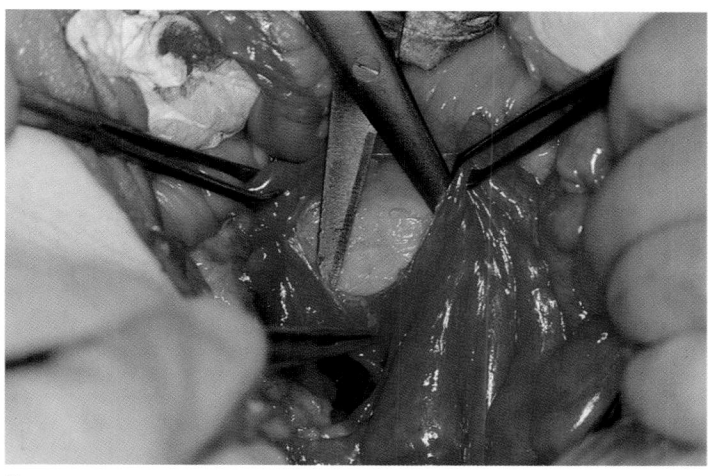

B

**FIGURE 36–15 A.** The edges of the peritoneum are held with two Allis clamps. The presacral space is opened, exposing the underlying properitoneal fat. **B.** The dissecting scissors carefully expose the underlying sacral bone, middle sacral vessels, and hypogastric nerve trunks.

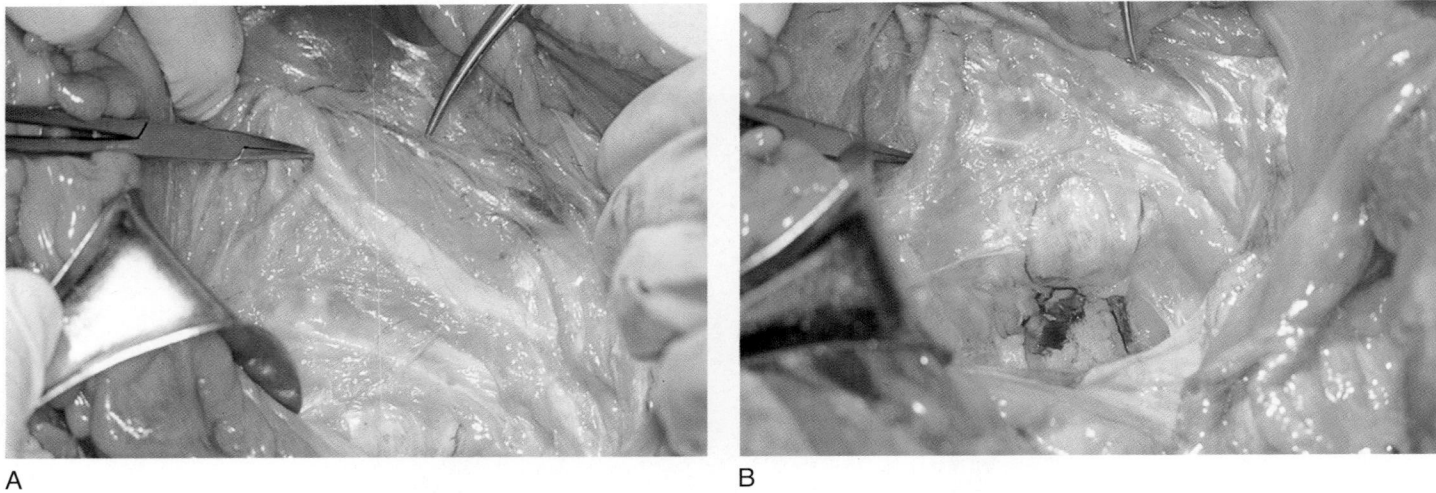

A                                                                              B

**FIGURE 36–16 A.** The straight clamp points to the aorta. Below the bifurcation, the left common iliac vein can be seen extending from the left to the right side of the pelvis. The scissors point to the left ovarian vascular pedicle. **B.** The sacral promontory and the presacral space are exposed.

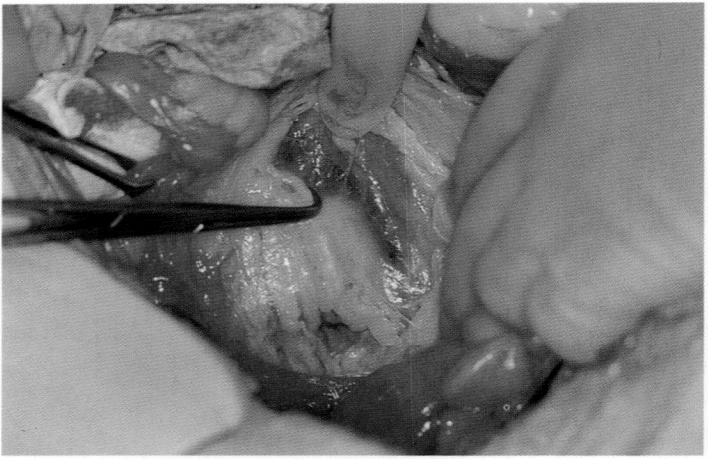

**FIGURE 36–17** A tonsil clamp dissects the presacral space. The tip of the clamp points to the left common iliac vein where it crosses the sacrum from left to right.

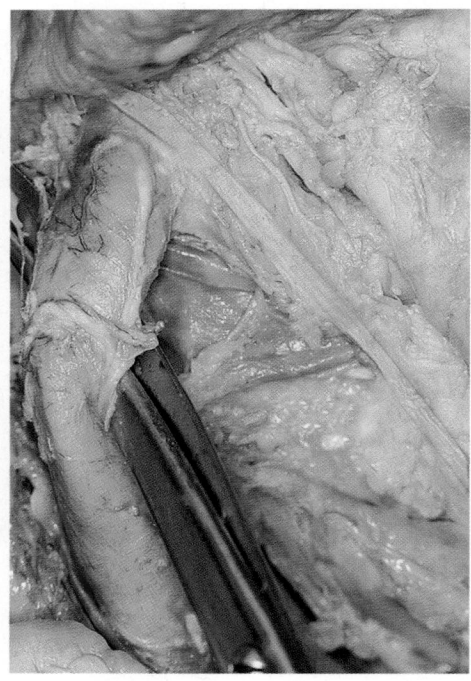

**FIGURE 36–18** The right common iliac artery is elevated with scissors to show the left common iliac vein crossing under it.

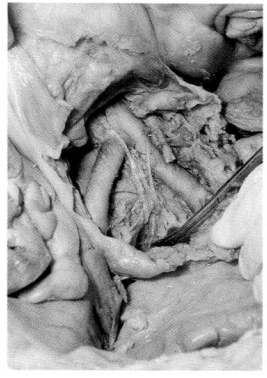

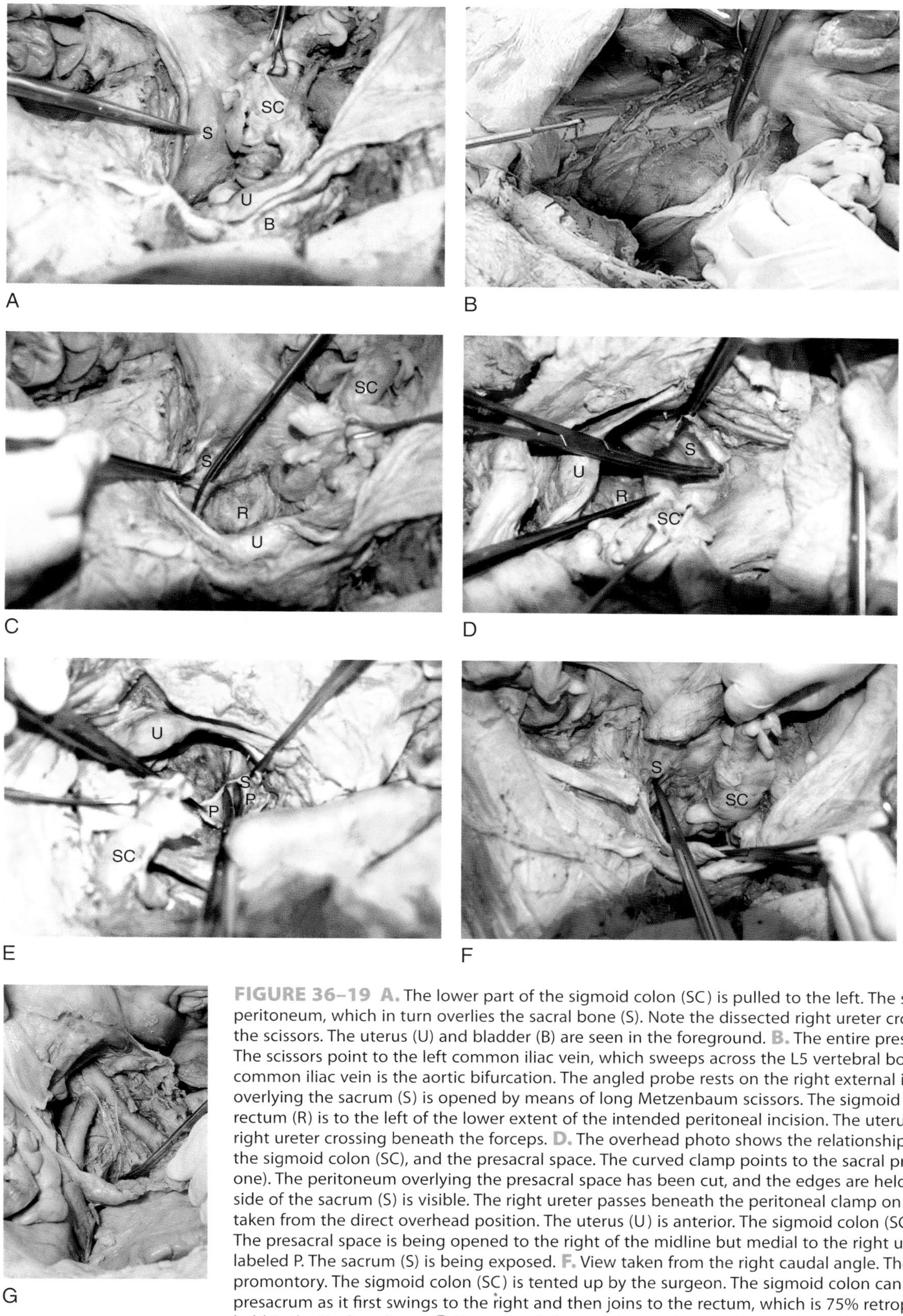

**FIGURE 36–19 A.** The lower part of the sigmoid colon (SC) is pulled to the left. The scissors lie on the posterior parietal peritoneum, which in turn overlies the sacral bone (S). Note the dissected right ureter crossing beneath the closed blades of the scissors. The uterus (U) and bladder (B) are seen in the foreground. **B.** The entire presacral space has been opened up. The scissors point to the left common iliac vein, which sweeps across the L5 vertebral body. Above (cranial to) the left common iliac vein is the aortic bifurcation. The angled probe rests on the right external iliac artery. **C.** The peritoneum overlying the sacrum (S) is opened by means of long Metzenbaum scissors. The sigmoid colon (SC) is pulled to the left. The rectum (R) is to the left of the lower extent of the intended peritoneal incision. The uterus (U) is in the foreground. Note the right ureter crossing beneath the forceps. **D.** The overhead photo shows the relationships of the uterus (U), the rectum (R), the sigmoid colon (SC), and the presacral space. The curved clamp points to the sacral promontory (sacral vertebral body one). The peritoneum overlying the presacral space has been cut, and the edges are held in the straight clamps. The right side of the sacrum (S) is visible. The right ureter passes beneath the peritoneal clamp on the right side. **E.** This picture is taken from the direct overhead position. The uterus (U) is anterior. The sigmoid colon (SC) is in the foreground, out of focus. The presacral space is being opened to the right of the midline but medial to the right ureter. The peritoneal edges are labeled P. The sacrum (S) is being exposed. **F.** View taken from the right caudal angle. The scissors point to the sacral promontory. The sigmoid colon (SC) is tented up by the surgeon. The sigmoid colon can be easily followed down over the presacrum as it first swings to the right and then joins to the rectum, which is 75% retroperitoneal. Note that the uterus is held in the Kocher clamp. **G.** The curved clamp points to the middle sacral vessels. Above, two strands of the hypogastric plexus descend into the presacral space.

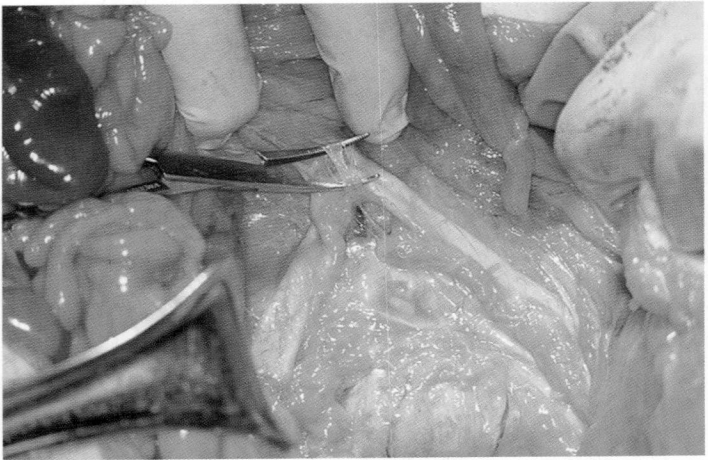

**FIGURE 36–20** The spread tip of the clamp exposes the hypogastric plexus over the aorta.

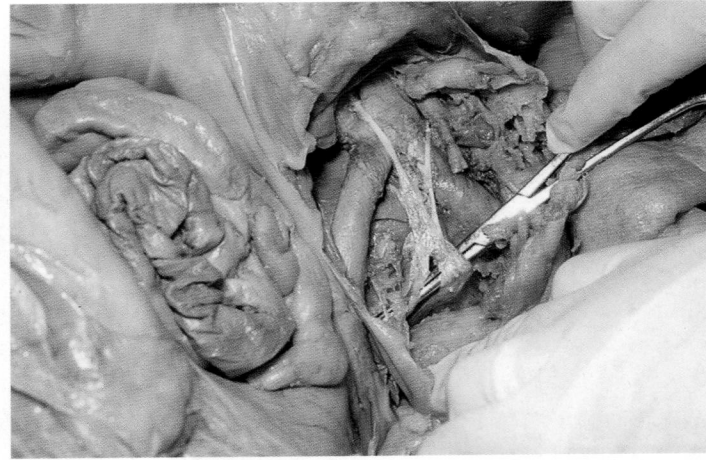

**FIGURE 36–21** The main mass of the hypogastric plexus is displayed above the underlying clamp.

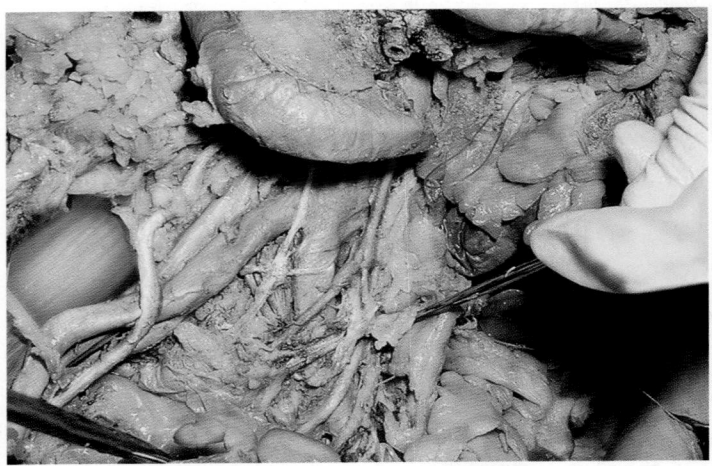

**FIGURE 36–22** Panoramic view of the bifurcation and the hypogastric nerve. To the immediate left is the inferior mesenteric artery arising from the aorta and branching to supply the colon. Farther to the left (clamp) is the left ureter crossing over the left common iliac artery. To the right is the right common iliac artery. The right ureter crosses over the lower portion of the iliac just cranial to (above) the point where the ureter crosses.

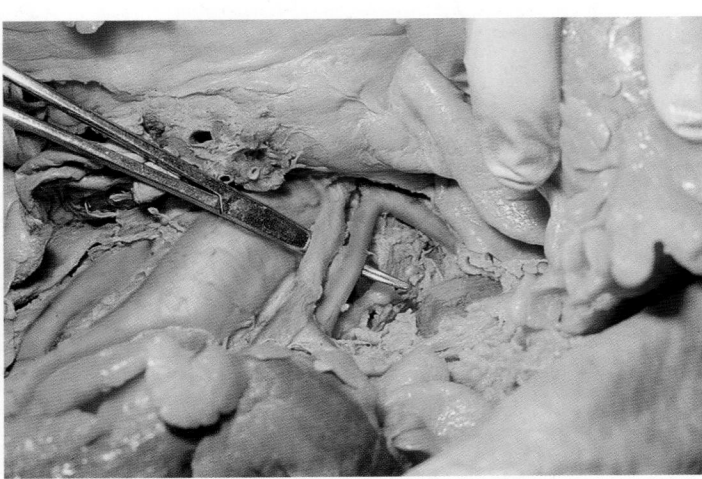

**FIGURE 36–23** The left ovarian vessels are shown at the point where the vein enters the left renal vein and the artery enters the aorta.

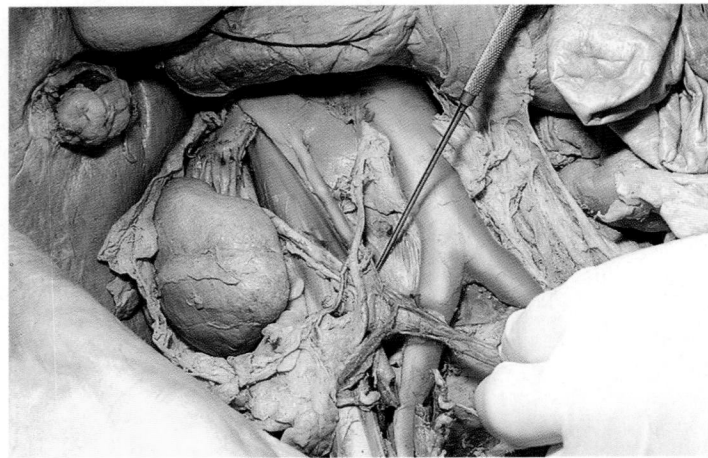

**FIGURE 36–24** Panoramic view of the right ovarian vein entering the vena cava (hook) and the artery entering the aorta.

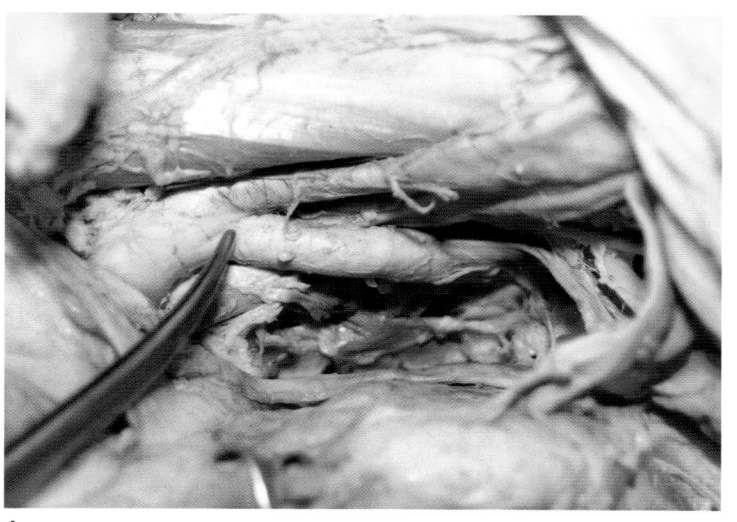

A

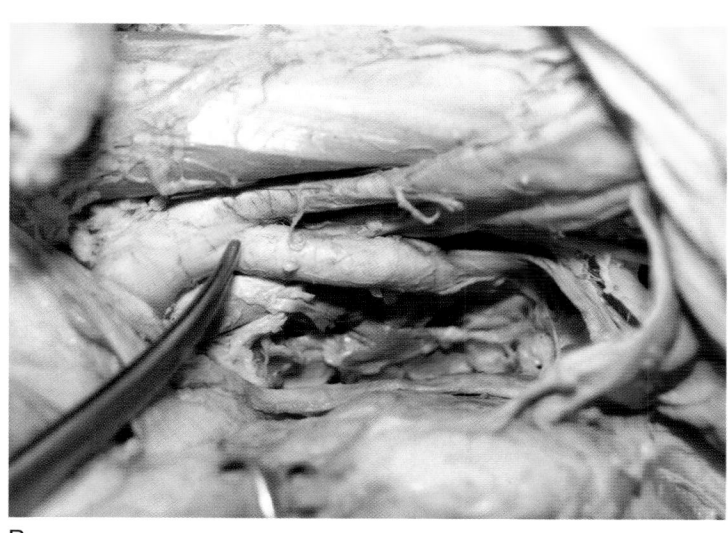

B

**FIGURE 36–25 A.** The scissors point to the iliac artery bifurcation. Below are the numerous and frequently anomalous deep pelvic veins. Above is the psoas major muscle. **B.** Magnified view of Figure 36–25A. The external iliac artery is above and the internal iliac just forward of the scissors.

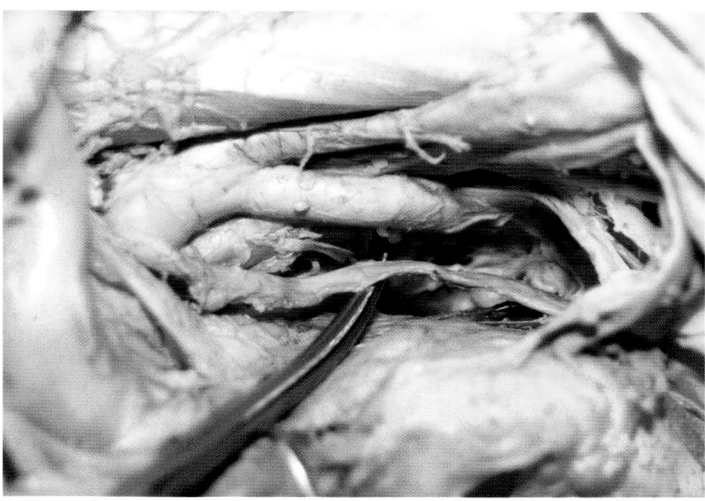

**FIGURE 36–26** The ureter is shown elevated by the scissors.

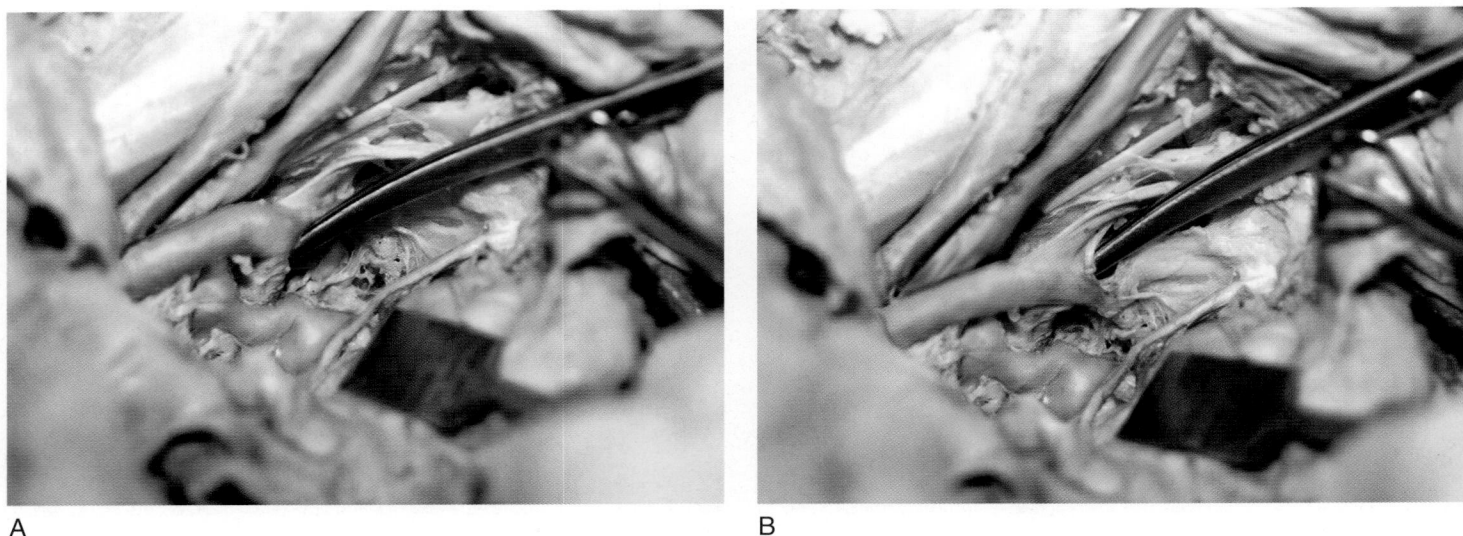

A                                                          B

**FIGURE 36–27  A.** (Magnified) The scissors point to the posterior division of the hypogastric (internal iliac) artery. **B.** (Magnified) The scissors point to the internal iliac vein. The anterior division of the hypogastric artery is above the scissors.

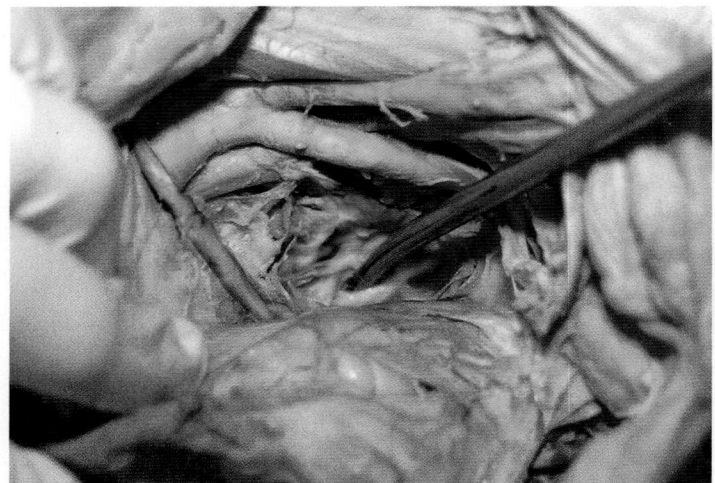

**FIGURE 36–28** (Magnified) The scissors dissect one of the large sacral roots that contribute to the sciatic nerve.

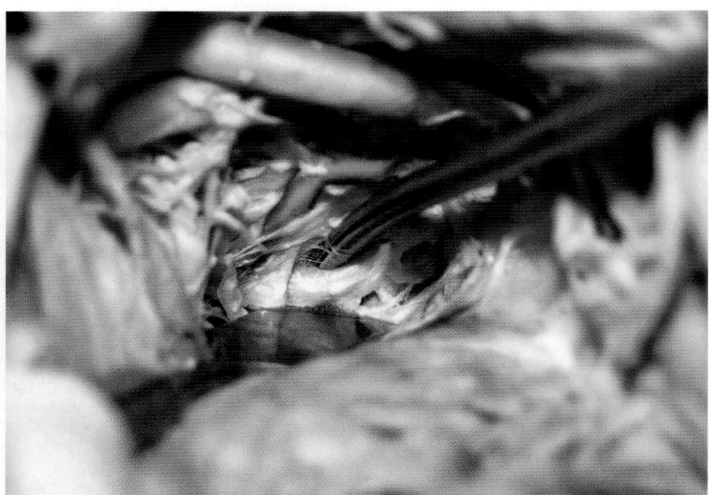

**FIGURE 36–29** Magnified view of the sciatic nerve, which is surrounded by a large mass of pelvic veins.

# CHAPTER 37

# Identifying and Avoiding Ureteral Injury

*Michael S. Baggish*

The ureter is covered by an anastomotic network of small arteries and veins. Several larger vessels feed and drain this network. Generally, above the ureteral crossover of the common iliac vessels, the arterial blood supply emanates from the medial aspect (e.g., aortic, ovarian, renal). Within the pelvis, the arterial supply to the ureter enters from the lateral direction (e.g., hypogastric, uterine, vesical, vaginal) (Fig. 37–1).

Although circulation is good, stripping the ureter of its adventitial sheath where its anastomotic network is located will result in segmental devitalization.

Ureteral length ranges between 22 and 30 cm and extends from the renal pelvis to the ureteral orifice located at either extremity of the trigonal, ureteric ridge. The lumen of the muscular ureter is approximately 3.0 to 4.0 mm in diameter (9- to 12-French).

The course of the ureter may be divided into three anatomic zones (Fig. 37–2).

Zone 1: Between the renal pelvis and iliac arteries
Zone 2: Between the ureteral crossover of the iliac arteries and the point where the uterine arteries cross over the ureter
Zone 3: Between the uterine artery crossover of the ureter and the point where the ureters enter the urinary bladder

The ureter is naturally narrowed at the ureteropelvic junction, at the iliac vessel crossover, and at the ureterovesical junction. The ureter is narrowed in its intramural passage through the bladder wall. During pregnancy, hypertrophied ovarian vessels may create obstruction of the ureter above the point where they cross it. The resulting hydroureter and hydronephrosis may cause pain and urinary infection. The right ureter is more frequently and more significantly obstructed than the left.

## Exposing the Ureter

Three techniques may be used to directly expose the pelvic ureter. These procedures require the surgeon to gain entry into the retroperitoneal space.

The first and most direct entry point is reached by grasping the posterior parietal peritoneum overlying the psoas major muscle (lateral to the external iliac artery) and cutting the peritoneum in a parallel direction to the external iliac artery (Fig. 37–3). The latter artery is easily palpated at the medial edge of the psoas major muscle (Fig. 37–4). The external iliac artery is dissected cranially to the iliac bifurcation, where the ureter crosses into the pelvis superficial to the common iliac vessels and medial to the hypogastric vessels (Fig. 37–5). The ureter is smaller in diameter and is lighter (white) in color than the iliac artery. The ureter does not pulsate; however, it does demonstrate peristaltic activity.

The second approach divides the round ligament so as to gain entry into the interior of the broad ligament (Fig. 37–6). The loose areolar tissue between the anterior and posterior leaves of the ligament is easily dissected with the tip of the Metzenbaum scissors or via a long tonsil clamp. As the dissection progresses deep to the floor of the broad ligament (i.e., passes the external iliac artery and vein), a white tubular structure comes into view, clinging to the medial leaf of the peritoneal edge. This is the ureter, which can be observed to undergo peristalsis (Fig. 37–7).

The third approach requires the surgeon to grasp the right or left adnexa and gently create traction by stretching the infundibulopelvic ligament. This is accomplished by pulling the ovary and tube anteriorly and in a slightly caudal direction.

The surgeon follows the infundibulopelvic ligament to the point where it enters the retroperitoneum (Fig. 37–8A). The peritoneum is picked up with a bayonet or other suitable toothed forceps and incised in a parallel direction to the ovarian vessels (Fig. 37–8B). The ureter lies posterior and medial to the ovarian vascular pedicle and in fact is attached to the ovarian vessels (one artery; two veins) at this location (Fig. 37–9). As in the other instances the ureter tends to be paler that the ovarian vessels and will be seen to undergo peristaltic activity.

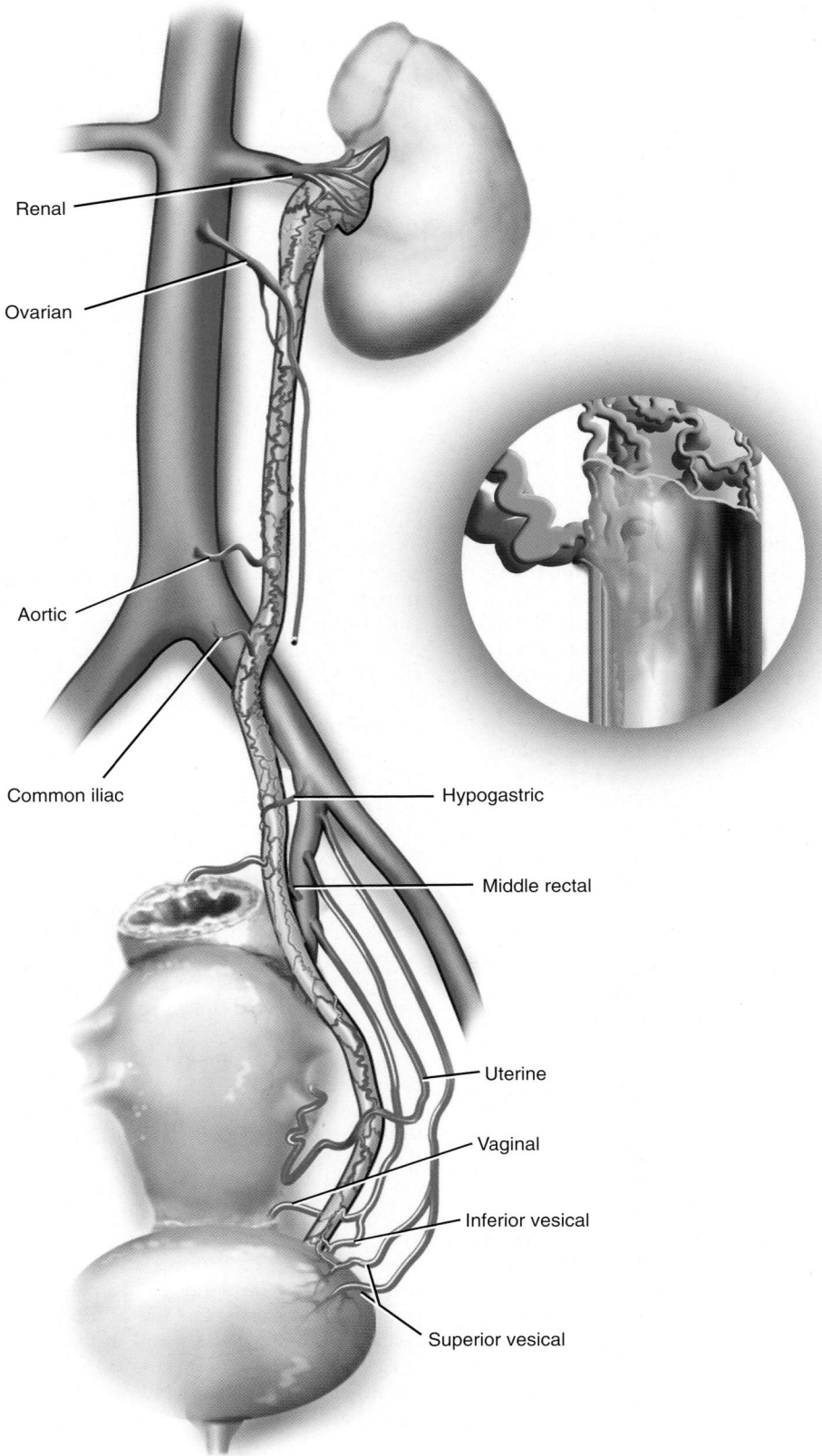

Renal

Ovarian

Aortic

Common iliac

Hypogastric

Middle rectal

Uterine

Vaginal

Inferior vesical

Superior vesical

**FIGURE 37–1** The ureter has its own vascular supply, which emanates from several neighboring vessels. These vessels include renal, ovarian, aortic, iliac, rectal, uterine, and vaginal. The network of anastomotic vessels supplies the ureter from the renal pelvis to the bladder and lies in the adventitia of the ureter.

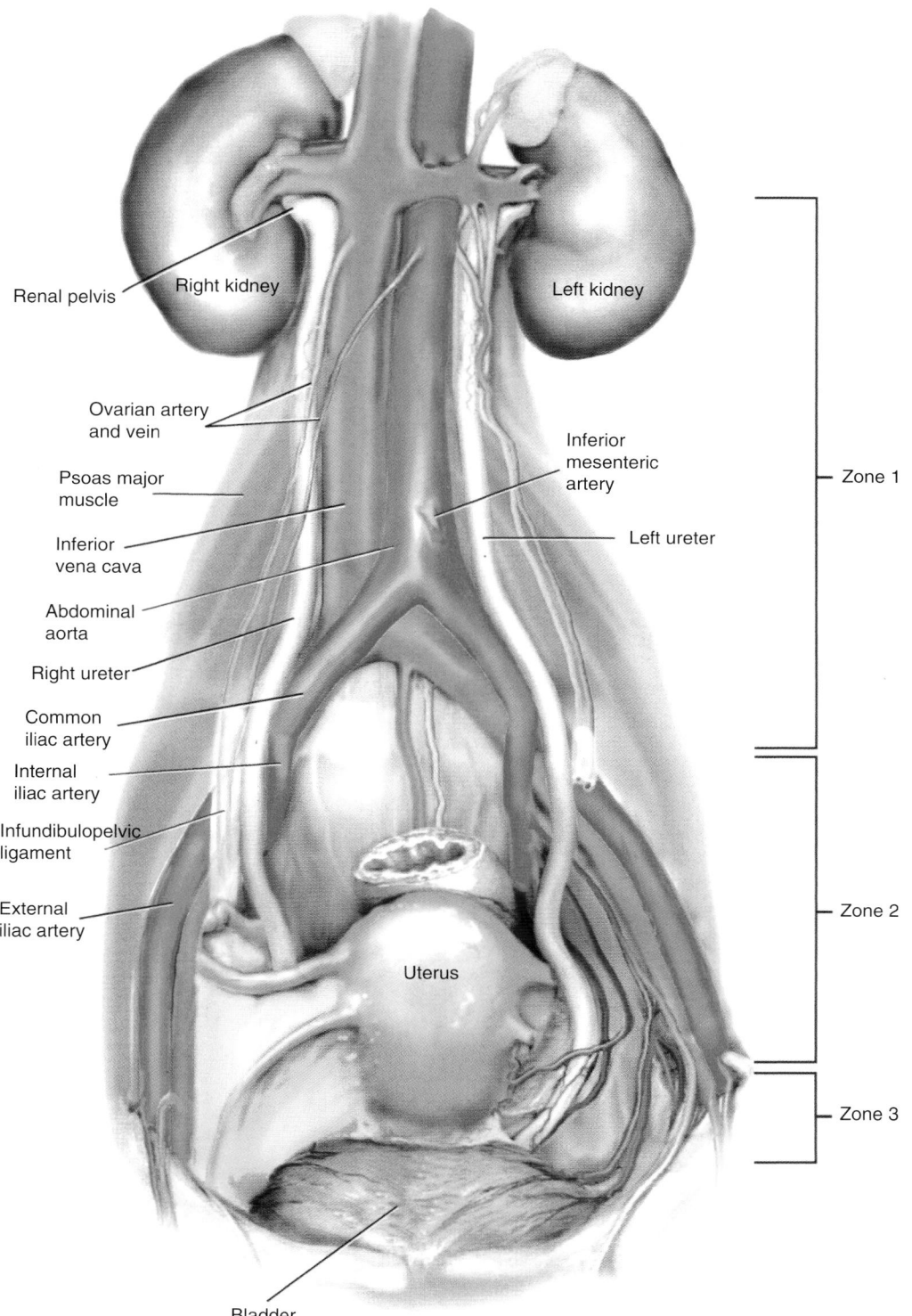

Renal pelvis
Right kidney
Left kidney
Ovarian artery and vein
Inferior mesenteric artery
Psoas major muscle
Left ureter
Inferior vena cava
Abdominal aorta
Right ureter
Common iliac artery
Internal iliac artery
Infundibulopelvic ligament
External iliac artery
Uterus
Bladder
Zone 1
Zone 2
Zone 3

**FIGURE 37–2** The three zones of ureteral anatomy. Although the shortest zone is zone 3, this is where most injuries occur. Note the anatomic differences between the right and left ureters. The left ureter is a bit more lateral in zones 1 and 2 and is lateral and to the left of the blood supply of the sigmoid colon (see Fig. 37–5).

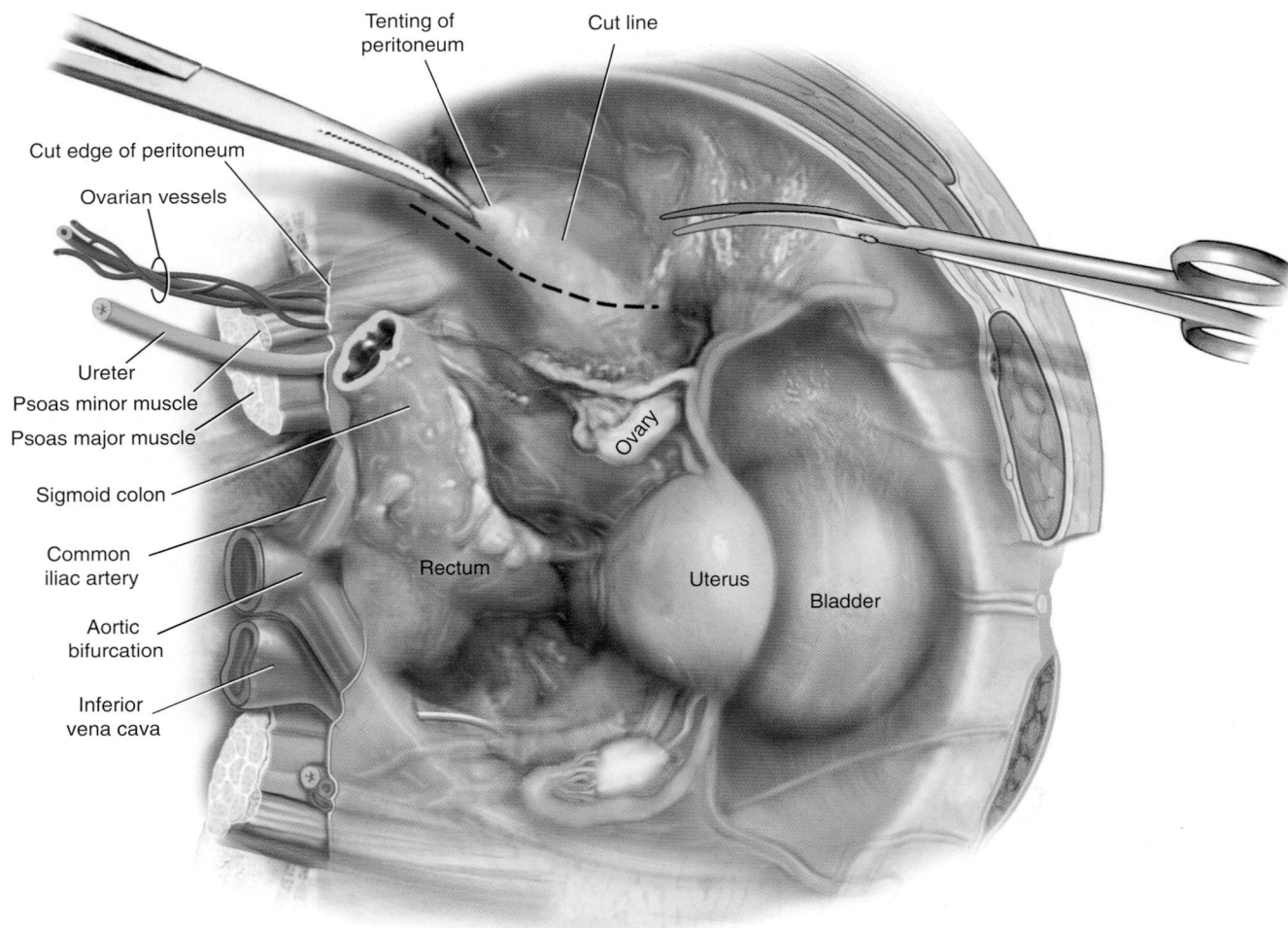

Tenting of
peritoneum

Cut line

Cut edge of peritoneum

Ovarian vessels

Ureter

Psoas minor muscle

Psoas major muscle

Sigmoid colon

Common
iliac artery

Aortic
bifurcation

Inferior
vena cava

Rectum

Ovary

Uterus

Bladder

**FIGURE 37–3** The parietal peritoneum overlying the psoas major muscle is grasped with forceps and opened by cutting with Metzenbaum scissors. The cut is linear and parallel to the course of the muscle.

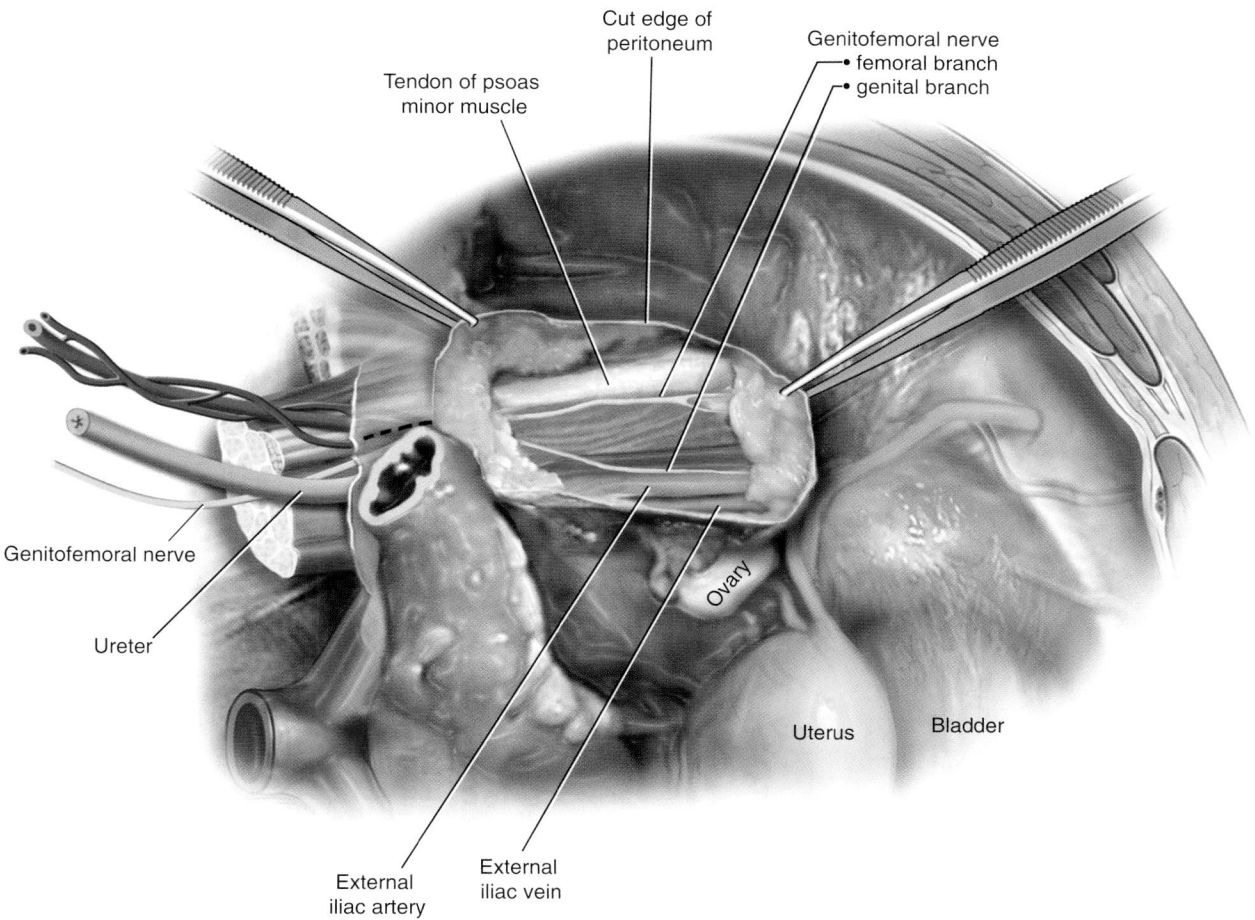

**FIGURE 37–4** The tendon of the psoas minor muscle and the genitofemoral nerve is identified. At the medial margin of the psoas major muscle, the pulsations of the external iliac artery may be felt. The external iliac vein is immediately posterior and slightly medial to the artery.

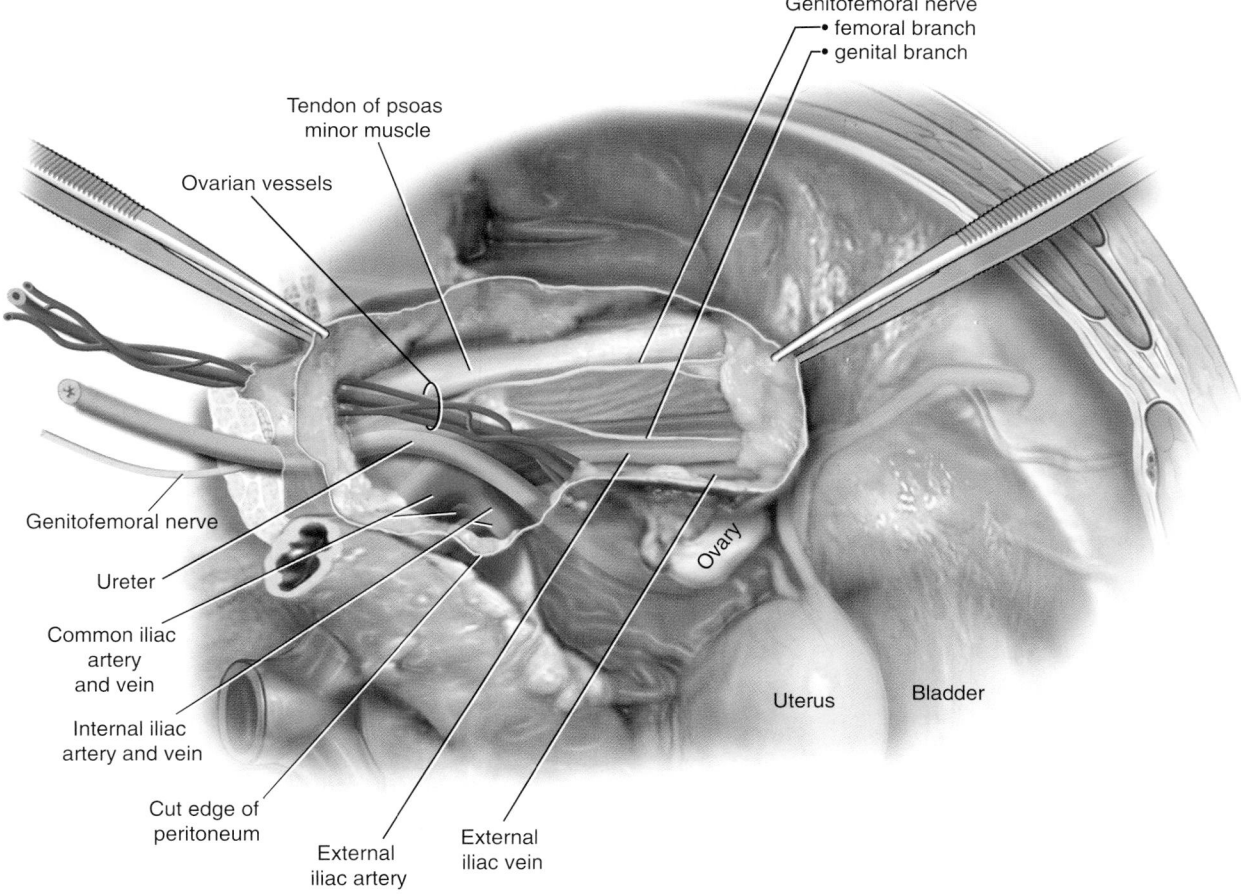

**FIGURE 37–5** Following the external iliac artery cephalad will lead the surgeon to the ureter, where it courses superficial to the common iliac vessels. Note that the ovarian vessels are anterior and slightly lateral to the ureter.

UNIT 2 ■ SECTION F

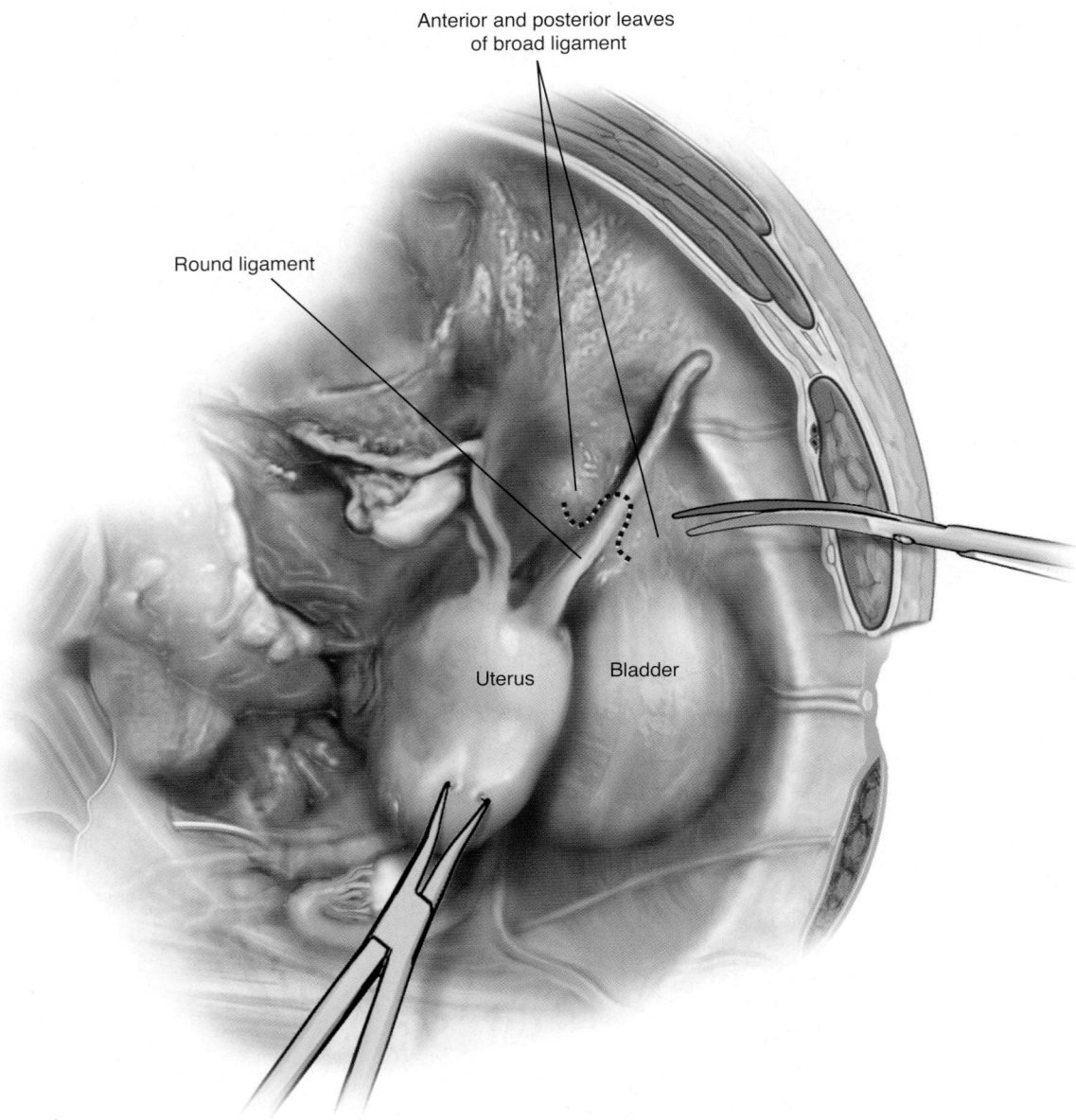

**FIGURE 37–6** The round ligament is grasped with a Kelly or tonsil clamp and tented up. The ligament is divided between the two clamps (*dotted line*). This in fact opens the anterior and posterior leaves of the broad ligament.

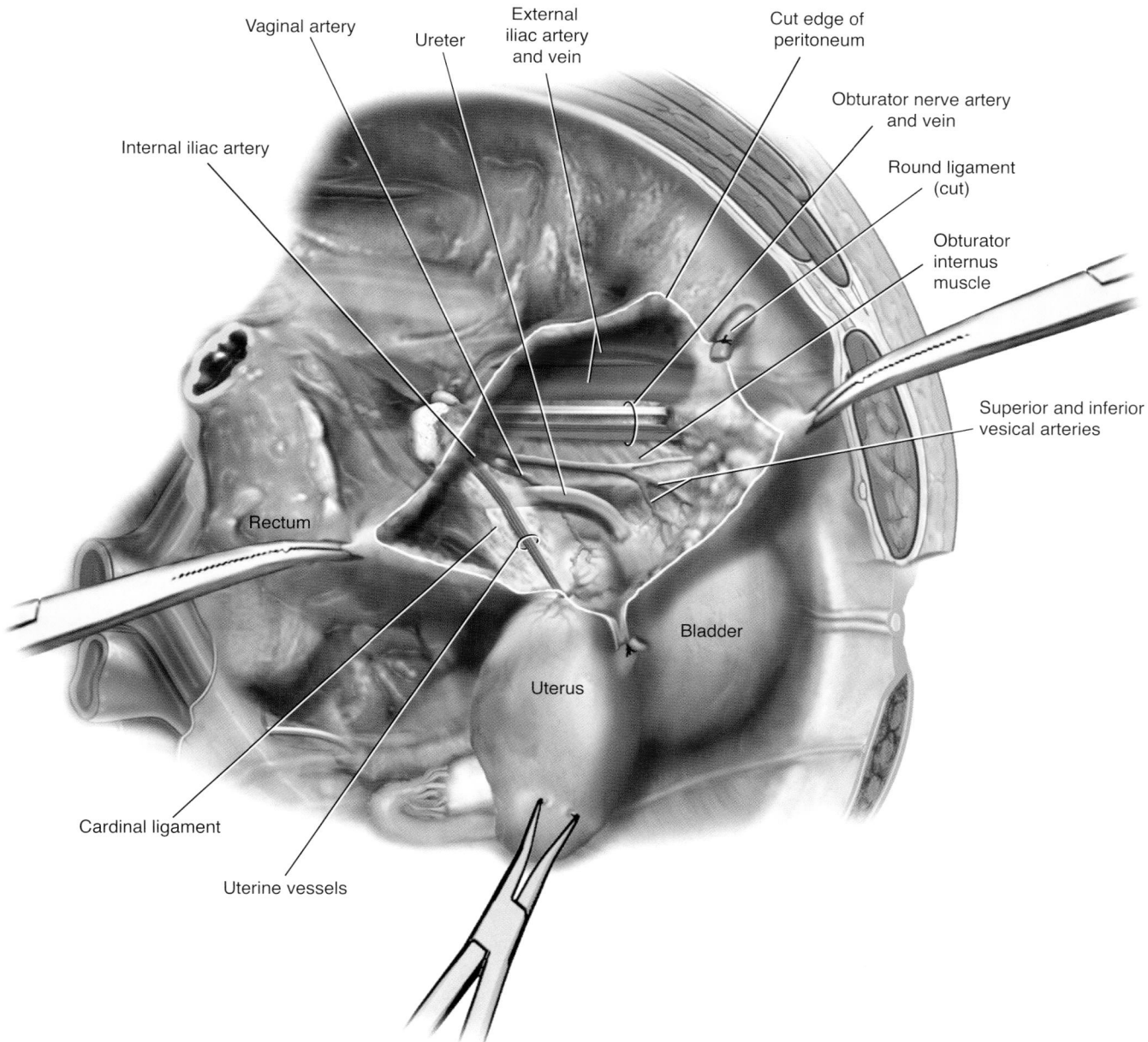

**FIGURE 37–7** The psoas major muscle and the external iliac vessels are identified first by palpation, then by dissection. The loose areolar tissue within the broad ligament is separated by spreading the tonsil clamp. Deep to the external iliac vessels, the surgeon can feel the hypogastric artery. Medial to it lies the ureter.

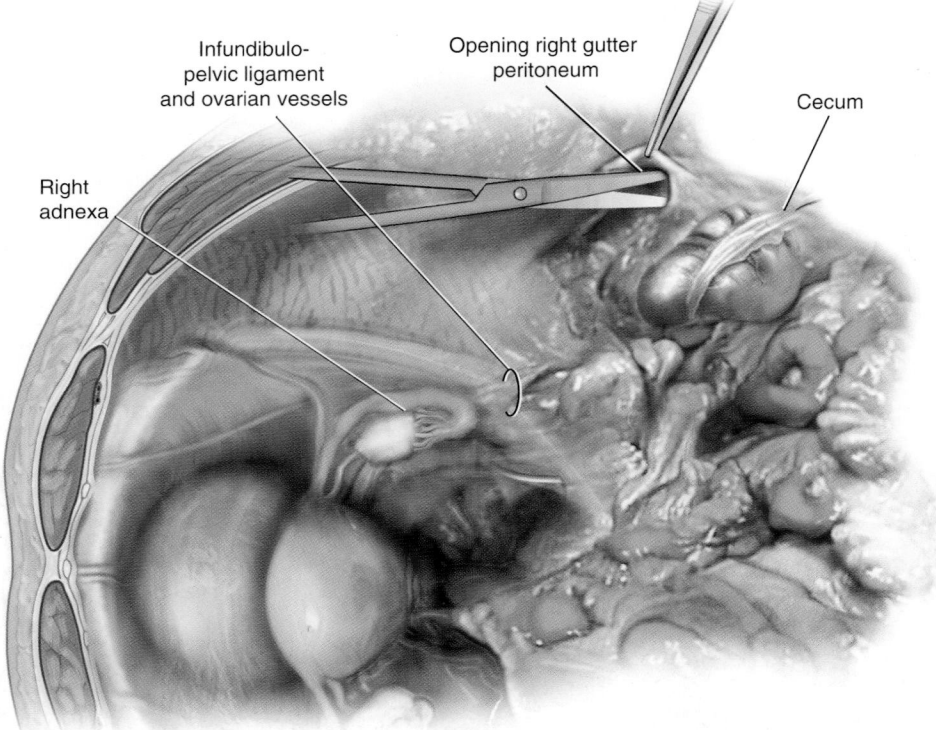

A

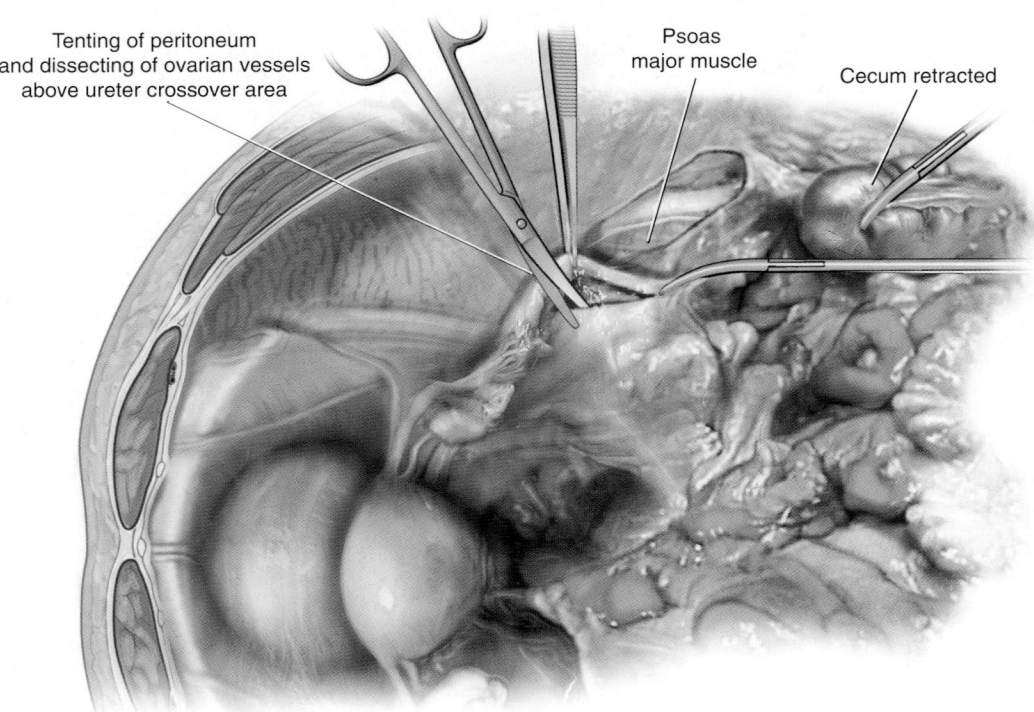

B

**FIGURE 37–8  A.** Traction is placed on the infundibulopelvic ligament, and it is followed to its retroperitoneal point of origin. **B.** The peritoneum is sharply opened lateral to the infundibulopelvic ligament and directly over the psoas major muscle.

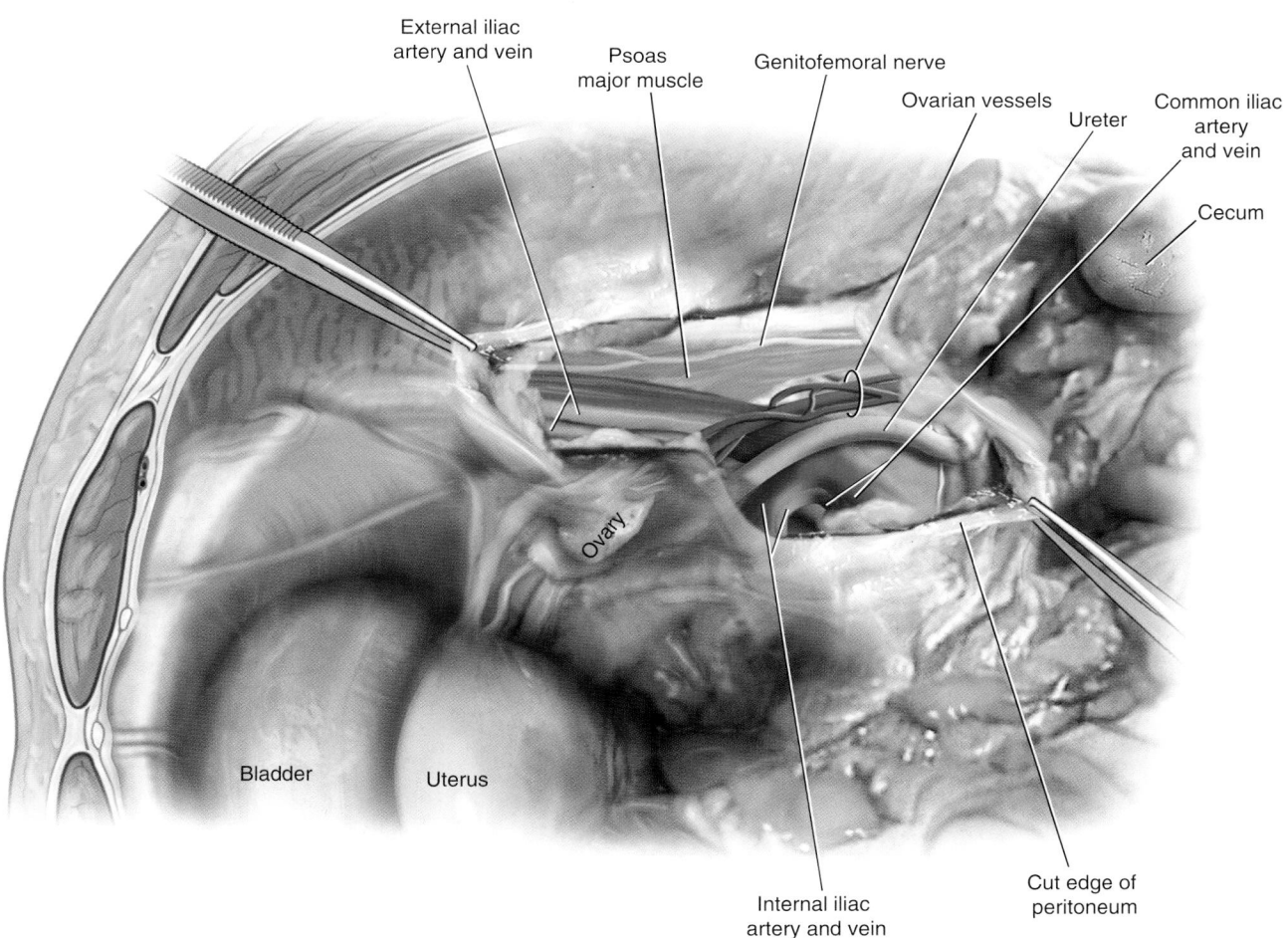

**FIGURE 37–9** The ureter is located just medial and slightly posterior to the ovarian vessels.

## Anatomic Relationships of Right and Left Ureters

Clearly, differences should be noted between right and left ureteral anatomic relationships.

Because zone 1 is out of the pelvis, gynecologists uncommonly dissect in this area. However, the relationships will be described (see Fig. 37–2). The ureter leaves the renal pelvis and is located lateral to the ovarian artery and vein, as well as to the inferior vena cava. The ureter lies on the psoas major muscle. At approximately one third of the distance between the kidney and the iliac vessels, the ovarian vessels cross over and lie anterolateral to the ureter. As the ureter crosses the common iliac artery at its bifurcation into external and internal iliac arteries, it is posterior to the ovarian vessels but is encompassed in a common peritoneal sheath (Fig. 37–10). This is a common site for iatrogenic ureteral injury, which typically happens at the time of infundibulopelvic ligament clamping, cutting, suturing, and coagulation. Special care must be taken when a laparoscopic stapling device is applied to secure the infundibulopelvic ligaments (Fig. 37–11).

The right ureter is easier to isolate than the left because of the position of the sigmoid colon and its accompanying mesentery (Fig. 37–12). The space between the ureter and the left common iliac artery is occupied by the inferior mesenteric artery, which transverses the sigmoid mesentery to supply the large intestine (Fig. 37–13). This is a large vessel that emanates from the lower left side of the aorta just cephalad to the common iliac artery bifurcation of the aorta. Similarly, the primary branches from the inferior mesenteric artery are large vessels. These vascular channels may be confused with the ureter on the left side.

Both right and left ureters descend into the pelvis and occupy a position medial and parallel to the hypogastric arteries. The ureter is in close relationship to the obturator fossa. Again, the ureter is medial and is roughly parallel to the fossa at the level of the obturator artery and nerve. At the caudal end of the obturator fossa, the ureter sinks deeper into the pelvis and is crossed from lateral to medial obliquely by the uterine vessels. The uterine vessels continue medially to reach the lateral margin of the uterus at the cervicocorporal junction (Fig. 37–14).

Ninety percent of ureteral injuries occur within zone 3. Not only is the 2.5-cm distance between uterine artery crossover and bladder entry a difficult area for exposure of the ureter, it is also replete with numerous and anomalous vascular channels.

The medial aspect of the ureter is sandwiched between the uterine artery (anteriorly) and the vaginal artery (posteriorly). Additionally, the ureter is crossed by the vesical arteries (Fig. 37–15).

The ureter enters the upper portion of the cardinal ligament, which consists of condensed fat and fibrous tissue, honeycombed with venous sinuses. The ureter passes beneath the bladder pillar (vesicouterine ligament) to enter the base of the urinary bladder obliquely (trigone) (Fig. 37–16A, B).

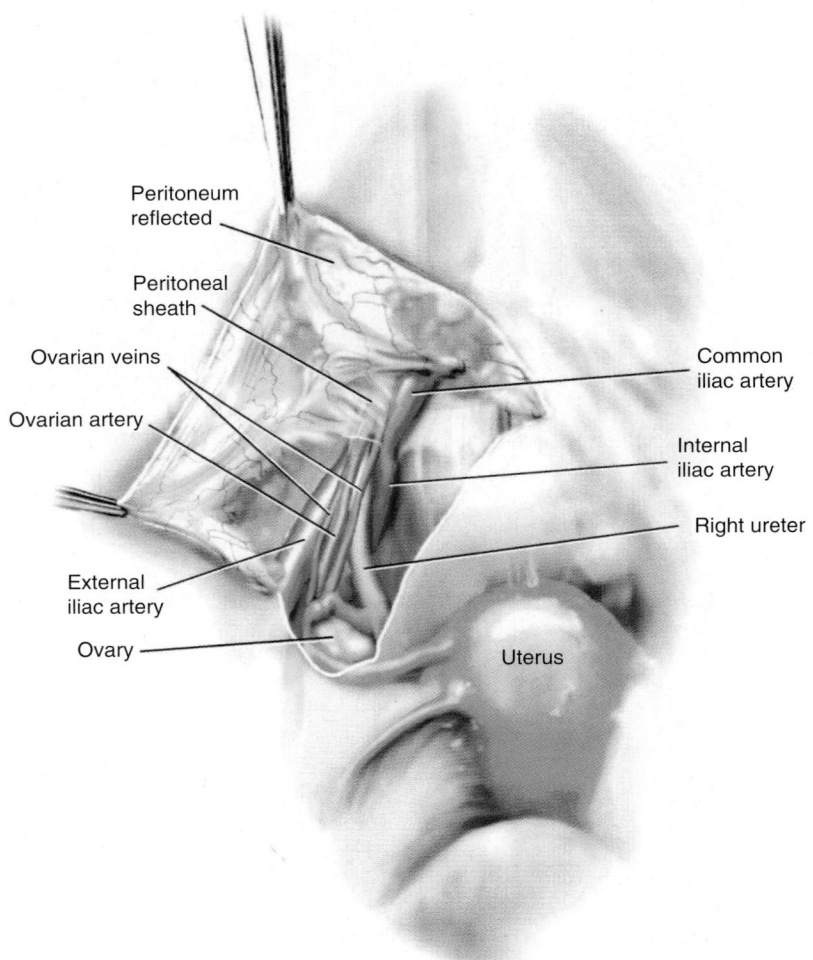

**FIGURE 37–10** The ureter leaves the renal pelvis and is located lateral to the ovarian artery and vein, as well as to the inferior vena cava. The ureter lies on the psoas major muscle. At approximately one third of the distance between the kidney and the iliac vessels, the ovarian vessels cross over and lie anterolateral to the ureter. As the ureter crosses the common iliac artery at its bifurcation into external and internal iliac arteries, it is posterior to the ovarian vessels but is encompassed in a common peritoneal sheath.

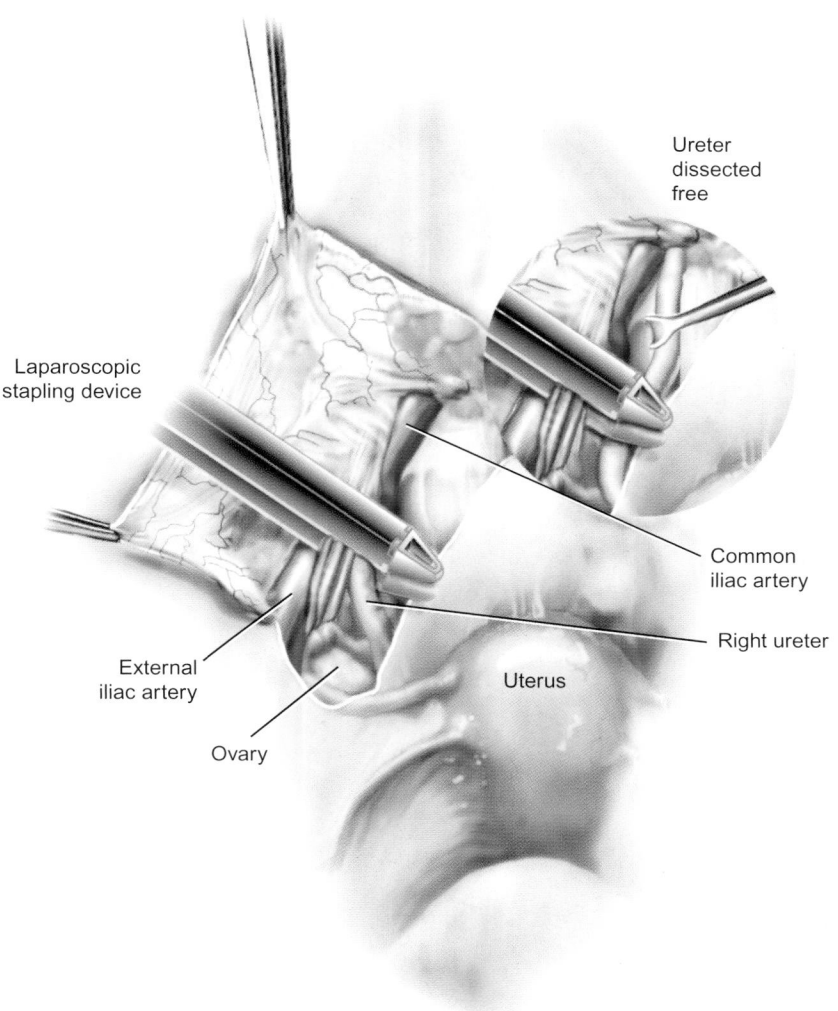

**FIGURE 37–11** This is a common site for iatrogenic ureteral injury, which typically happens at the time of infundibulopelvic ligament clamping, cutting, suturing, and coagulation. Special care must be taken when a laparoscopic stapling device is applied to secure the infundibulopelvic ligaments.

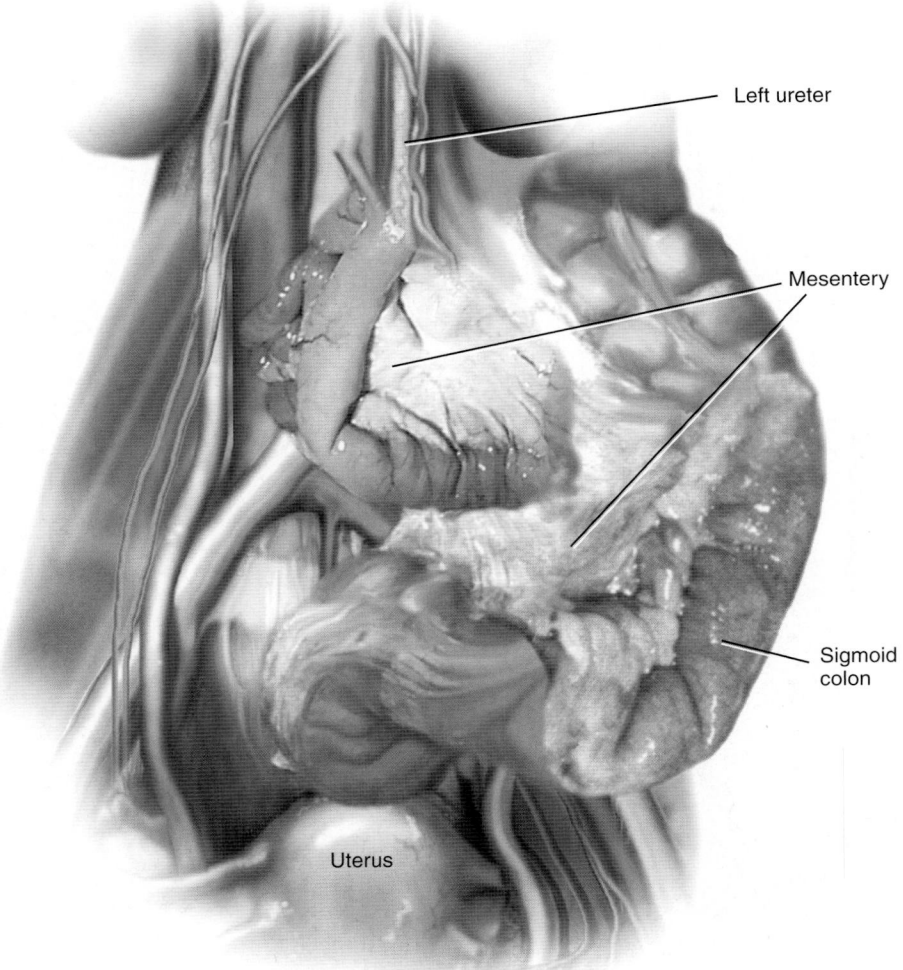

Left ureter

Mesentery

Sigmoid colon

Uterus

**FIGURE 37–12** The right ureter is easier to isolate than the left because of the position of the sigmoid colon and its accompanying mesentery.

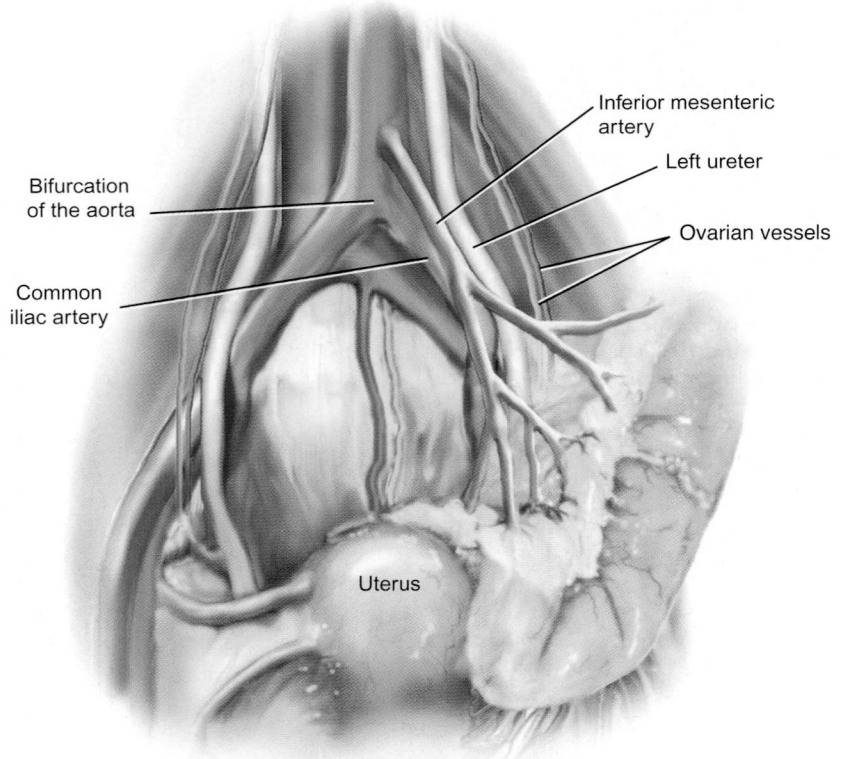

Inferior mesenteric artery

Left ureter

Bifurcation of the aorta

Ovarian vessels

Common iliac artery

Uterus

**FIGURE 37–13** The space between the ureter and the left common iliac artery is occupied by the inferior mesenteric artery, which traverses the sigmoid mesentery to supply the large intestine.

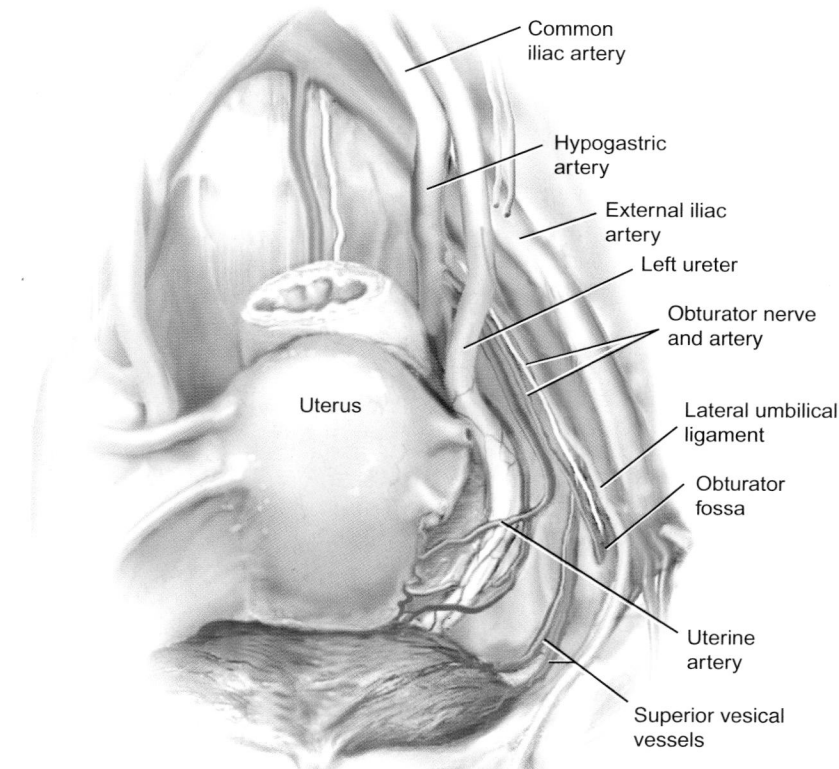

**FIGURE 37–14** This large vessel emanates from the lower left side of the aorta just cephalad to the common iliac artery bifurcation of the aorta. Similarly, the primary branches from the inferior mesenteric artery are large vessels. These vascular channels may be confused with the ureter on the left side. Both right and left ureters descend into the pelvis and occupy a position medial and parallel to the hypogastric arteries. The ureter is in close relationship to the obturator fossa. Again, the ureter is medial and roughly parallel to the fossa at the level of the obturator artery and nerve. At the caudal end of the obturator fossa, the ureter sinks deeper into the pelvis and is crossed from lateral to medial obliquely by the uterine vessels. The uterine vessels continue medially to reach the lateral margin of the uterus at the cervicocorporal junction.

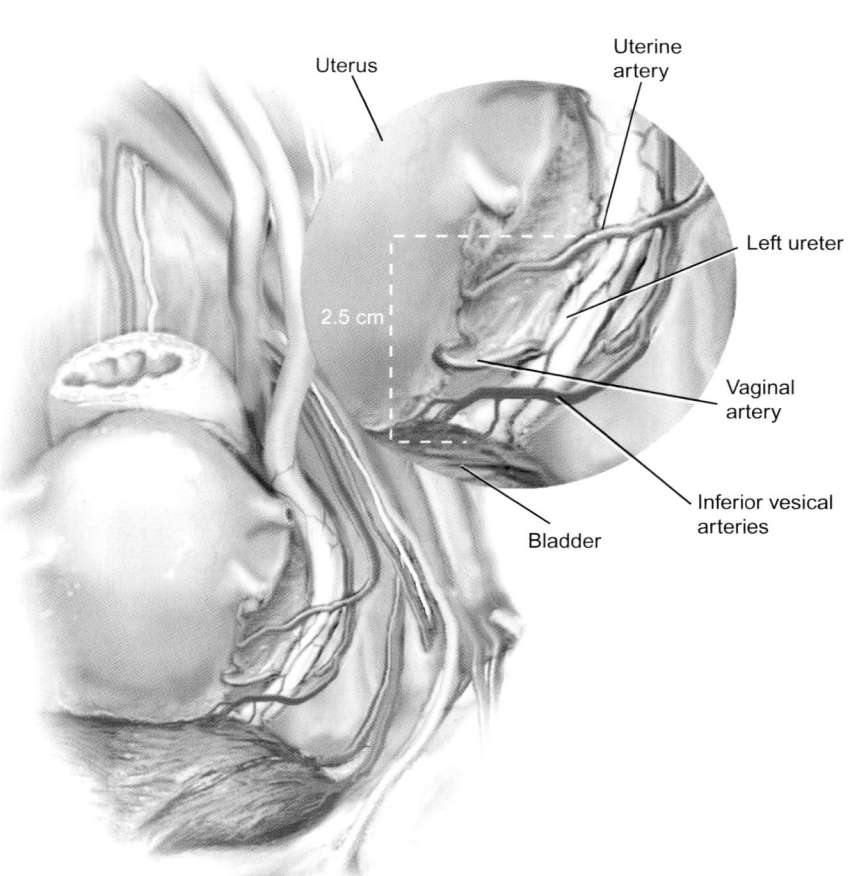

**FIGURE 37–15** Ninety percent of ureteral injures occur within zone 3. Not only is the 2.5-cm distance between uterine artery crossover and bladder entry a difficult area for exposure of the ureter, it is also replete with numerous and anomalous vascular channels. The medial aspect of the ureter is sandwiched between the uterine artery (anteriorly) and the vaginal artery (posteriorly). Additionally, the ureter is crossed by the vesical arteries.

UNIT 2 ■ SECTION F

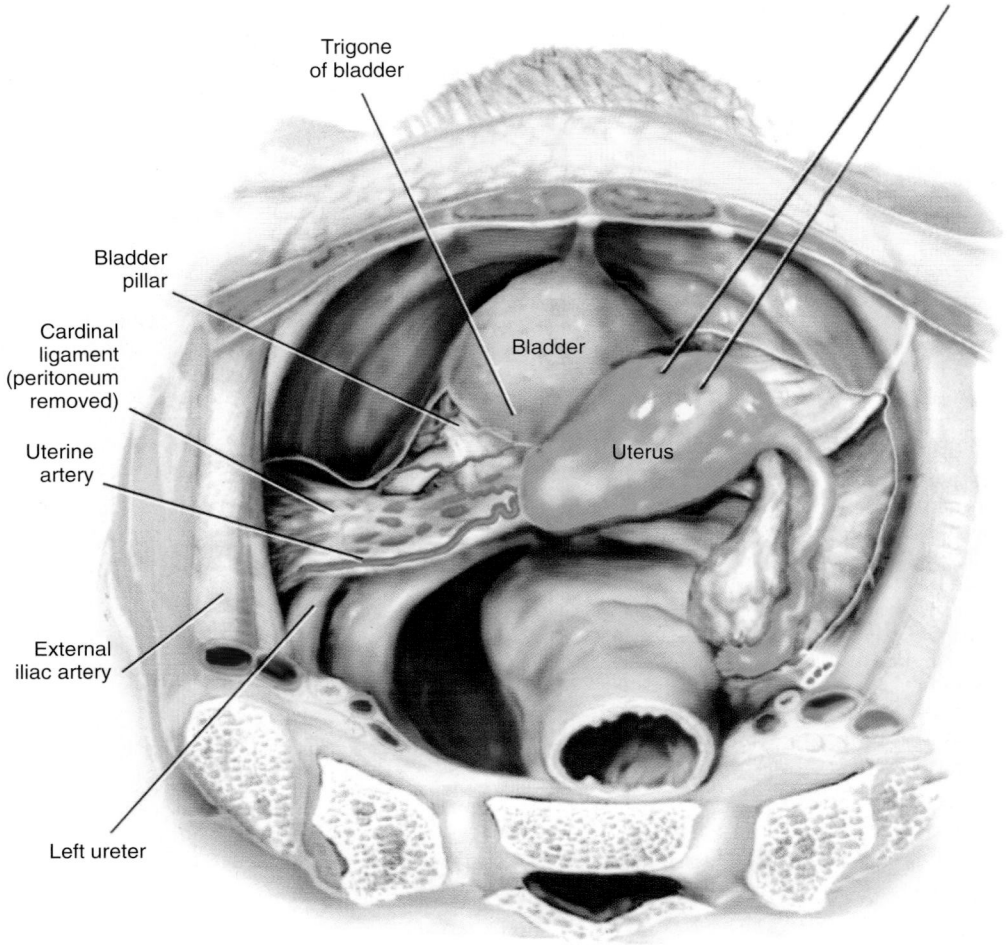

Trigone
of bladder

Bladder
pillar

Cardinal
ligament
(peritoneum
removed)

Uterine
artery

External
iliac artery

Left ureter

Bladder

Uterus

A

Opening of
left ureter

Bladder
opened

Neck of
bladder

Trigone
of bladder

Left ureter

Uterus

B

**FIGURE 37–16  A** and **B.** The ureter
enters the upper portion of the cardinal
ligament, which consists of condensed
fat and fibrous tissue, honeycombed
with venous sinuses. The ureter passes
beneath the bladder pillar (vesicouterine
ligament) to enter the base of the
urinary bladder obliquely (trigone).

The lowest portion of the ureter as it enters the bladder can be exposed only by deeply dissecting the vesicouterine space. This is not difficult to accomplish. The pubovesicocervical fascia overlying the anterior surface of the uterine cervix is incised superficially and transversely with a sharp scalpel blade (Fig. 37-17). The space between the fascia and the substance of the outer wall of the cervix is dissected bluntly with the back of the scalpel handle to develop the initial plane (Fig. 37-18). Next, with a long scissors or the operator's index finger, the dissection proceeds inferiorly to develop a wide space between the bladder and the vagina (Fig. 37-19). As with the rectouterine space, this can be extended all the way down to the level of the vaginal introitus (Fig. 37-20).

After the operator enters the retroperitoneal space (see Chapter 36), the most convenient point at which the ureter can be identified is where it crosses lateral to and medial above the common iliac artery. By careful dissection with a long tonsil clamp and with the use of an untied hammock of umbilical tape to provide counteraction, the ureter can be clearly viewed to the point of uterine artery crossover (Fig. 37-21A, B).

Any procedure performed on or around the uterosacral ligaments must take into account the position of the ureter relative to the operative site. In other words, the location must be precisely known (Fig. 37-22). Palpation of what the operator believes to be the ureter is not accurate. The ureter is relatively closer to the ligament posteriorly and laterally (Fig. 37-23).

At the level of the cardinal ligament, the ureter passes obliquely toward the bladder base and is closely applied to the lateral angle of the vagina (Fig. 37-24). Dissection of the ureter through the cardinal ligament is difficult because the ligament is honeycombed with thin-walled vessels. The ureter can be unroofed by clamping above and excising that portion of the cardinal ligament.

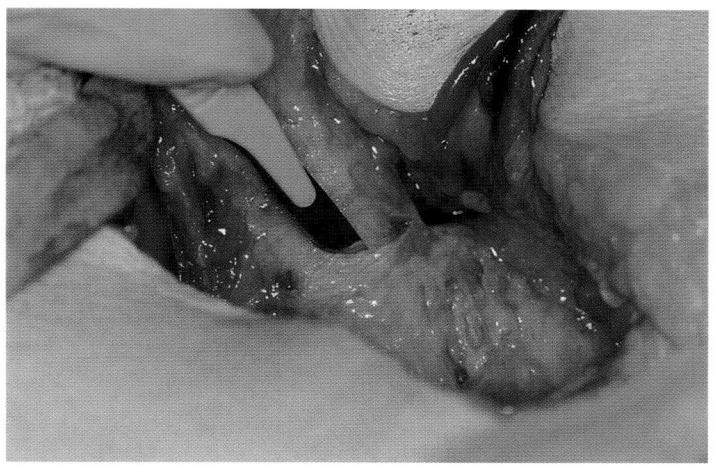

**FIGURE 37-17** The lowest portion of the ureter as it enters the bladder can be exposed only by deeply dissecting the vesicouterine space. This is not difficult to accomplish. The pubovesicocervical fascia overlying the anterior surface of the uterine cervix is incised superficially and transversely with a sharp scalpel blade.

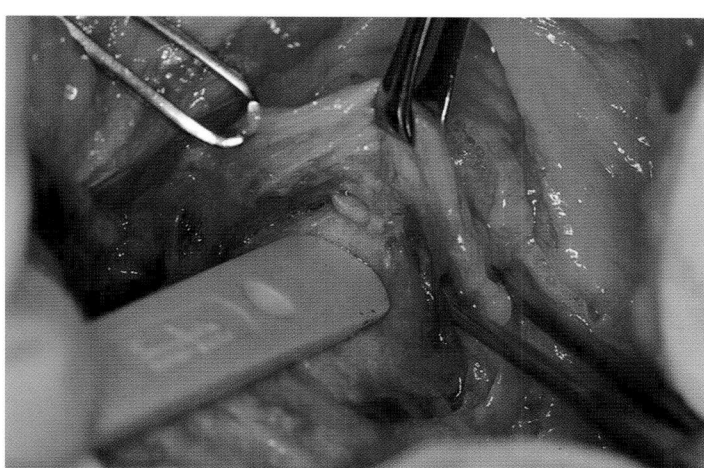

**FIGURE 37-18** The space between the fascia and the substance of the outer wall of the cervix is dissected bluntly with the back of the scalpel handle to develop the initial plane.

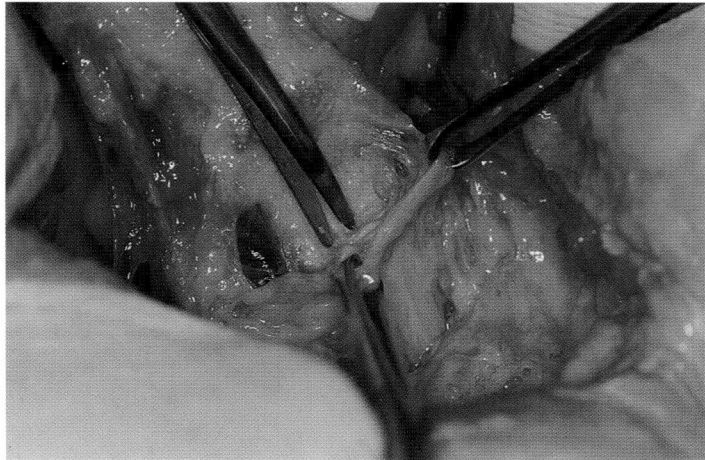

**FIGURE 37-19** Next, with the use of long scissors or the operator's index finger, the dissection proceeds inferiorly to develop a wide space between the bladder and the vagina.

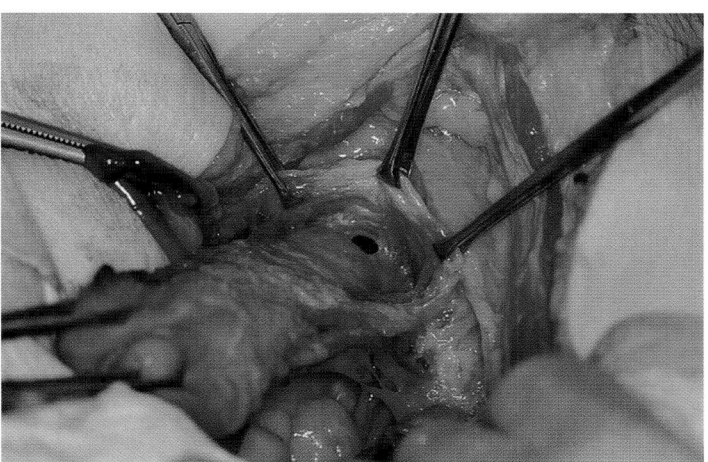

**FIGURE 37-20** As with the rectouterine space, this can be extended all the way down to the level of the vaginal introitus.

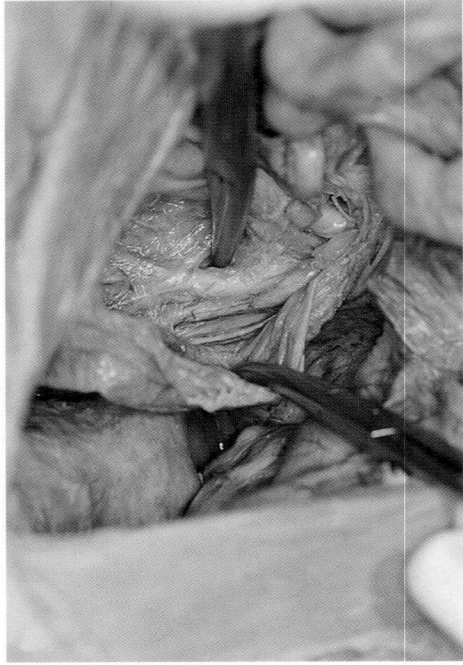

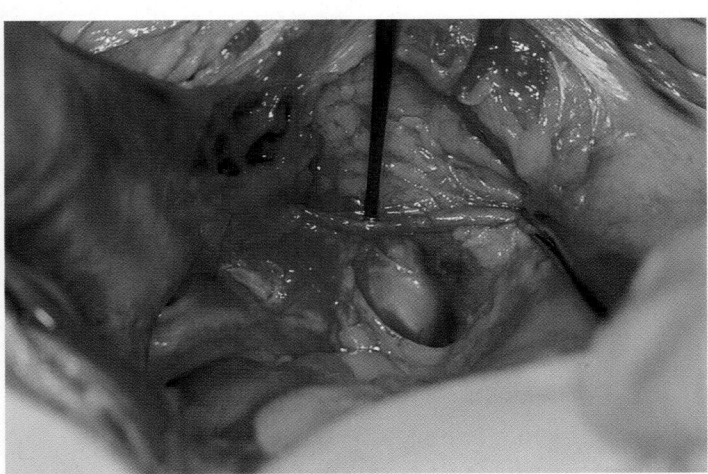

A                                    B

**FIGURE 37–21 A** and **B.** After the operator enters the retroperitoneal space (see Chapter 36), the most convenient point at which the ureter can be identified is where it crosses lateral to medial above the common iliac artery. By careful dissection with a long tonsil clamp and with the use of an untied hammock of umbilical tape to provide counteraction, the ureter can be clearly viewed to the point of uterine artery crossover.

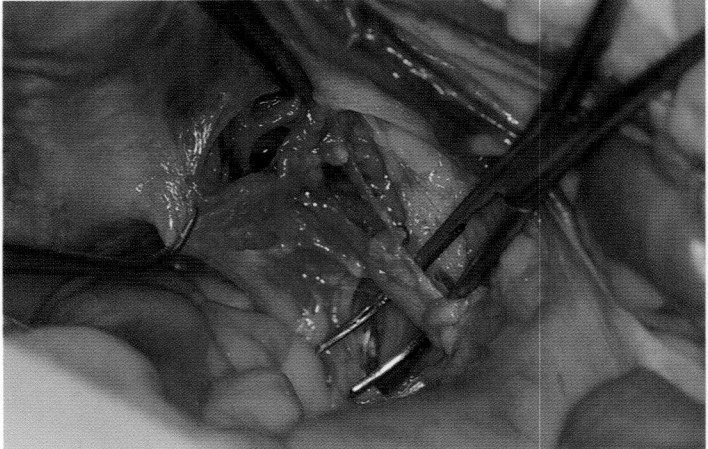

**FIGURE 37–22** Any procedure performed on or around the uterosacral ligaments must take into account the position of the ureter relative to the operative site. In other words, the location must be precisely known.

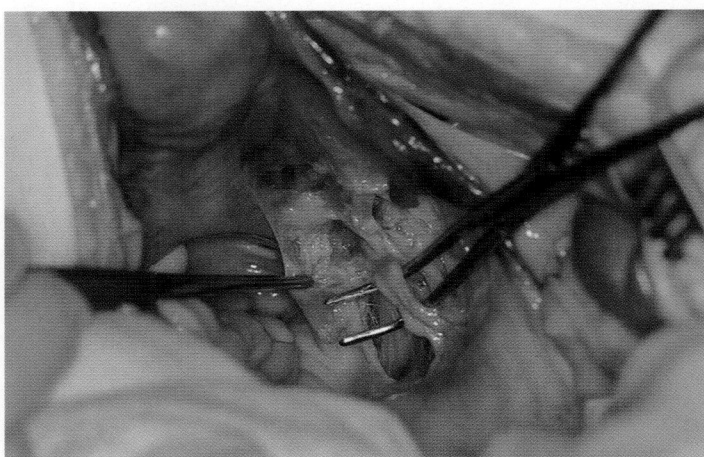

**FIGURE 37–23** Palpation of what the operator believes to be the ureter is not accurate. The ureter is relatively closer to the ligament posteriorly and laterally.

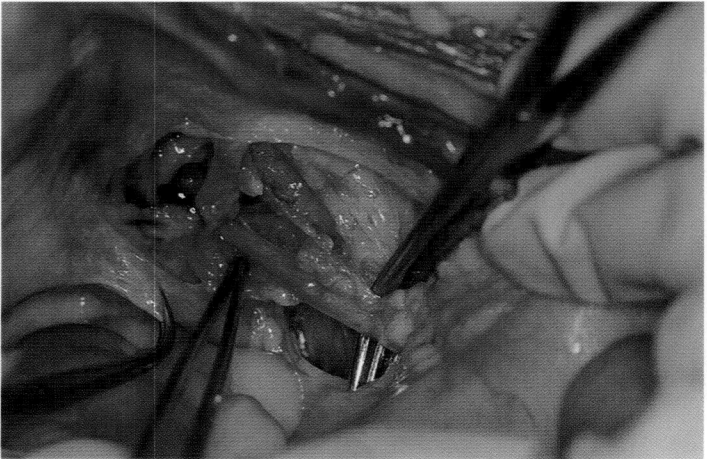

**FIGURE 37–24** At the level of the cardinal ligament, the ureter passes obliquely toward the bladder base and is closely applied to the lateral angle of the vagina.

# CHAPTER 38

# Presacral Neurectomy

## Michael S. Baggish

Pain fibers are transmitted from the uterus via the hypogastric plexus. The hypogastric plexus of nerves cascades downward as a continuation of the celiac plexus on the anterior aspect of the distal portion of the abdominal aorta (Fig. 38–1). The hypogastric plexus is variable in configuration but can be rather loosely separated into superior, middle, and inferior divisions. The middle hypogastric plexus typically divides into two main nerve trunks coursing inferiorly within the presacral space. The nerves are always medial to the common iliac arteries but cross over (anteriorly) the left common iliac vein (Fig. 38–2). The middle sacral vessels are located posterior (deep) to these nerves. The inferior hypogastric plexus continues to descend into the lower pelvis and joins with the pelvic plexus, receiving rectal, vesical, and uterine afferents and carrying sympathetic efferents.

The middle hypogastric plexus is accessed by reflecting the sigmoid to the left and anteriorly (Fig. 38–3). The peritoneum overlying the sacrum is grasped and incised vertically toward the sacral promontory (Fig. 38–4). Care is taken to identify the left common iliac vein, the left ureter, and the inferior mesenteric artery (and vein) (Fig. 38–5A, B).

The hypogastric nerves are dissected with a long tonsil clamp or right-angle clamp, with care taken to avoid injuring the middle sacral vessels (Fig. 38–6). A 3- to 4-cm segment of nerve is isolated. At the upper and lower extremes of the dissection, a permanent ligature is passed beneath the dissected hypogastric nerve and is tied tightly (Fig. 38–7). The segment of nerve between the two ligatures is dissected from its loose attachments to the underlying sacral bone. With long curved Mayo scissors, the nerve segment is cut out and is placed in fixative for subsequent pathologic diagnosis (Fig. 38–8).

The operative site is examined for bleeding and is irrigated with normal saline. The cut edges of the peritoneum are grasped and closed with running or interrupted 3-0 Vicryl sutures (Fig. 38–9).

If the middle sacral vessels are injured, significant bleeding will occur. This hemorrhage is difficult to control because these vessels are difficult to clamp or suture. The author recommends pushing a sterile stainless steel thumb tack into the sacrum, thereby compressing the vessels.

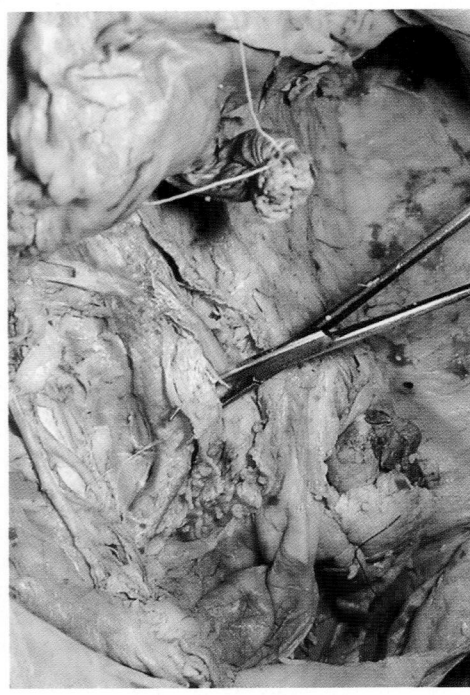

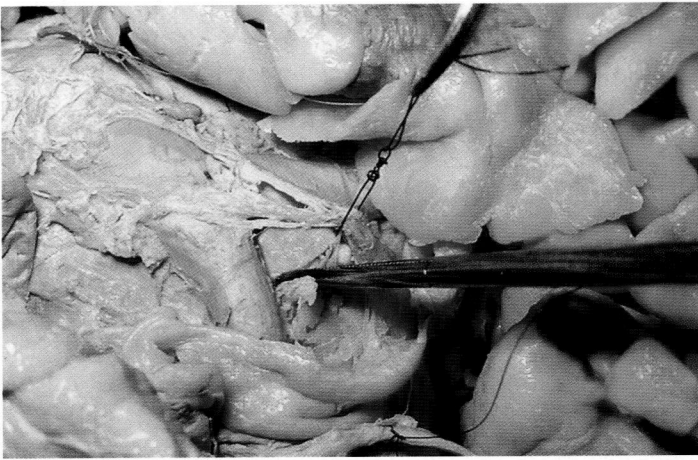

**FIGURE 38–2** The tip of the clamp points to the left common iliac vein. The elevated ligature encircles the middle hypogastric plexus as it descends into the pelvis over the presacral space.

**FIGURE 38–1** The curved clamp lies on the abdominal aorta just cranial to its bifurcation. The clamp has dissected free and lies beneath the hypogastric nerve (plexus). The view is from below, looking into the pelvis. Note the inferior vena cava to the right of the aorta.

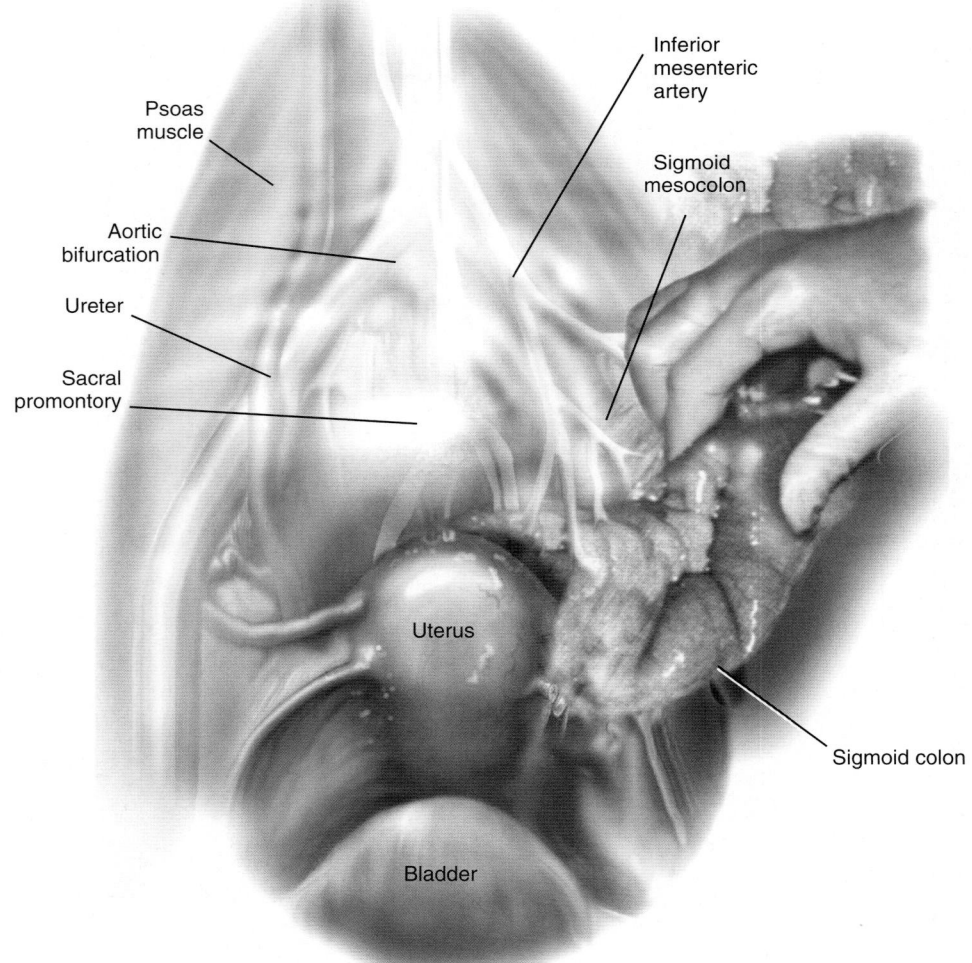

Psoas muscle

Aortic bifurcation

Ureter

Sacral promontory

Inferior mesenteric artery

Sigmoid mesocolon

Uterus

Bladder

Sigmoid colon

**FIGURE 38–3** The operator has retracted the sigmoid colon to the left. The peritoneum covering the presacral space remains intact.

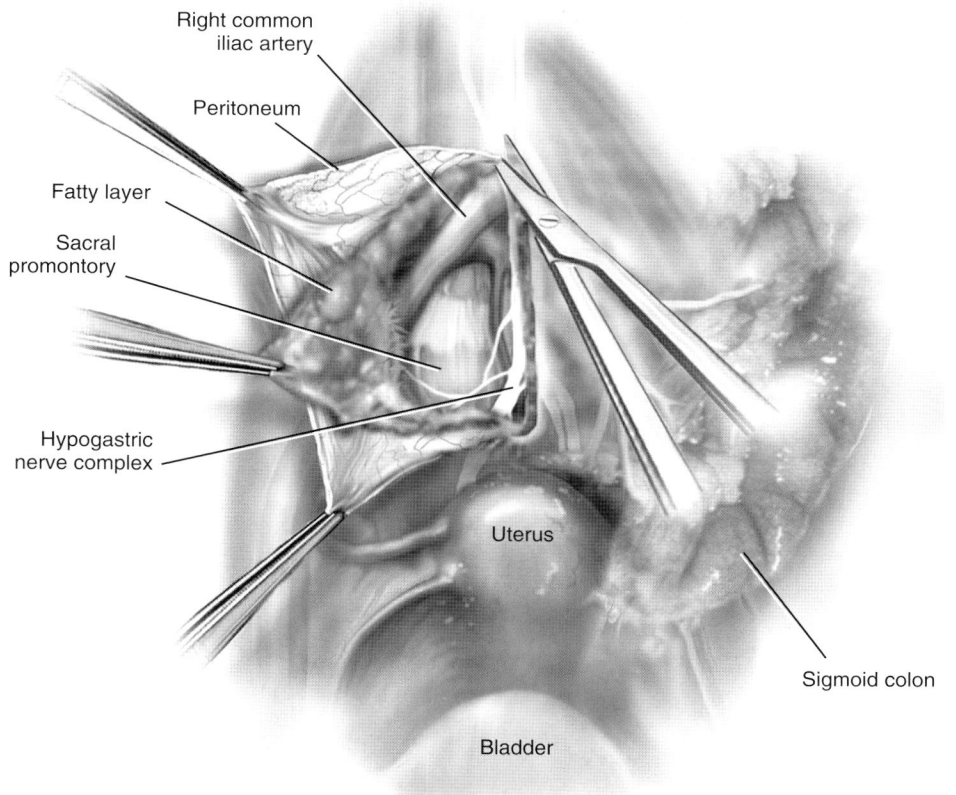

Right common
iliac artery

Peritoneum

Fatty layer

Sacral
promontory

Hypogastric
nerve complex

Uterus

Sigmoid colon

Bladder

**FIGURE 38–4** The peritoneum has been excised upward toward the sacral promontory. The structures overlying the anterior surface of the sacrum and the L5 vertebra are visualized.

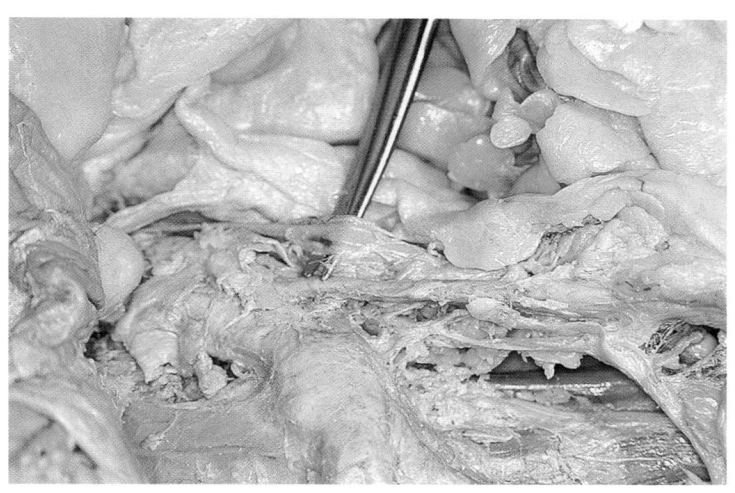

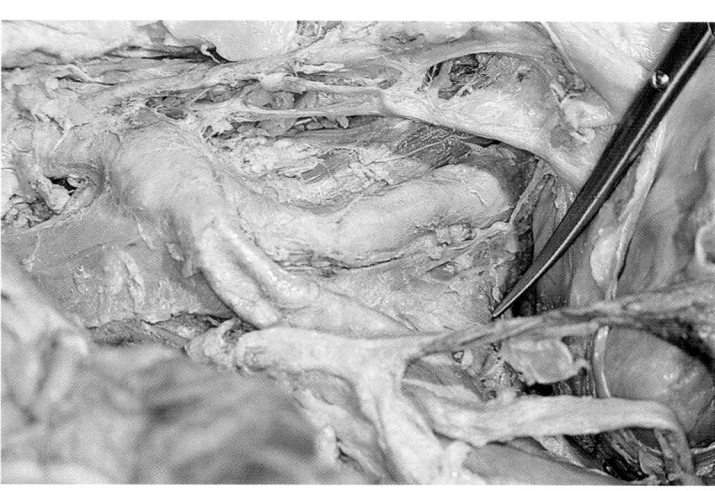

A

B

**FIGURE 38–5  A.** The scissors lie under the dissected left ureter (far lateral); the scissors tip points to the takeoff (origin) of the inferior mesenteric artery. The latter supplies the left and sigmoid colon. The right common iliac artery is seen in the foreground. **B.** The tip of the scissors points to the sacral promontory. The right ovarian vessels and the right ureter (below the vessels) cross the right iliac artery and descend into the pelvis at the right lateral margin of the presacral space.

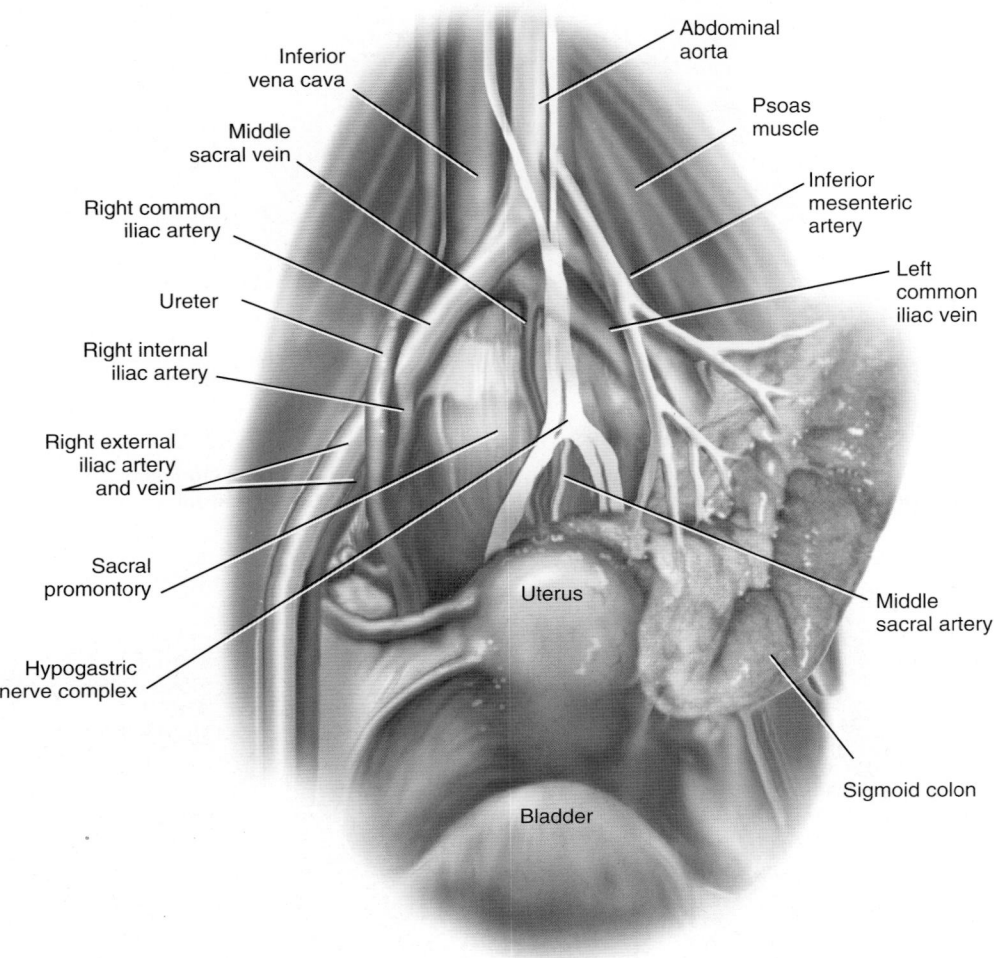

**FIGURE 38–6** The hypogastric nerve has been exposed by careful dissection. The important anatomic relationships must be recognized. Posterior to the nerve are the middle sacral vessels and the sacral bone. To the right are the common iliac vessels and the ureter. To the left and above are the left common iliac vein and the inferior mesenteric vessels.

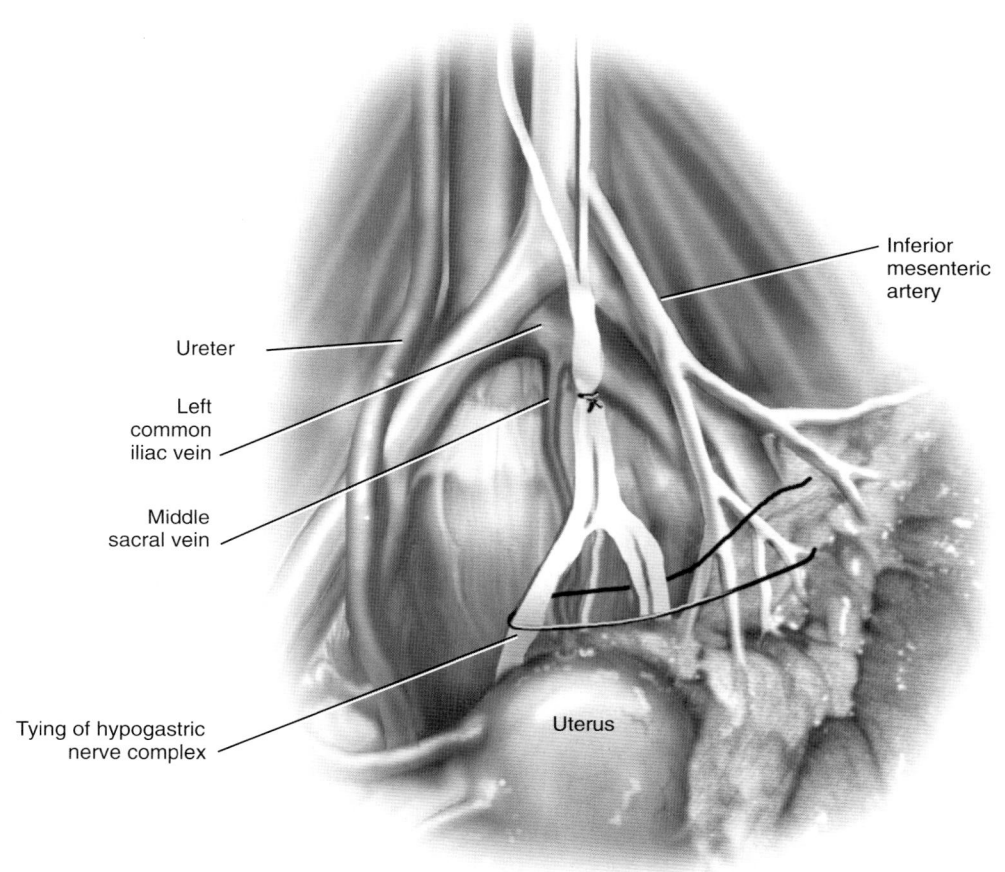

Inferior
mesenteric
artery

Ureter

Left
common
iliac vein

Middle
sacral vein

Tying of hypogastric
nerve complex

Uterus

**FIGURE 38–7** A 2-0 silk ligature is passed around the upper and lower margins of the nerve segment to be removed. The ligatures are tied tightly into place and cut.

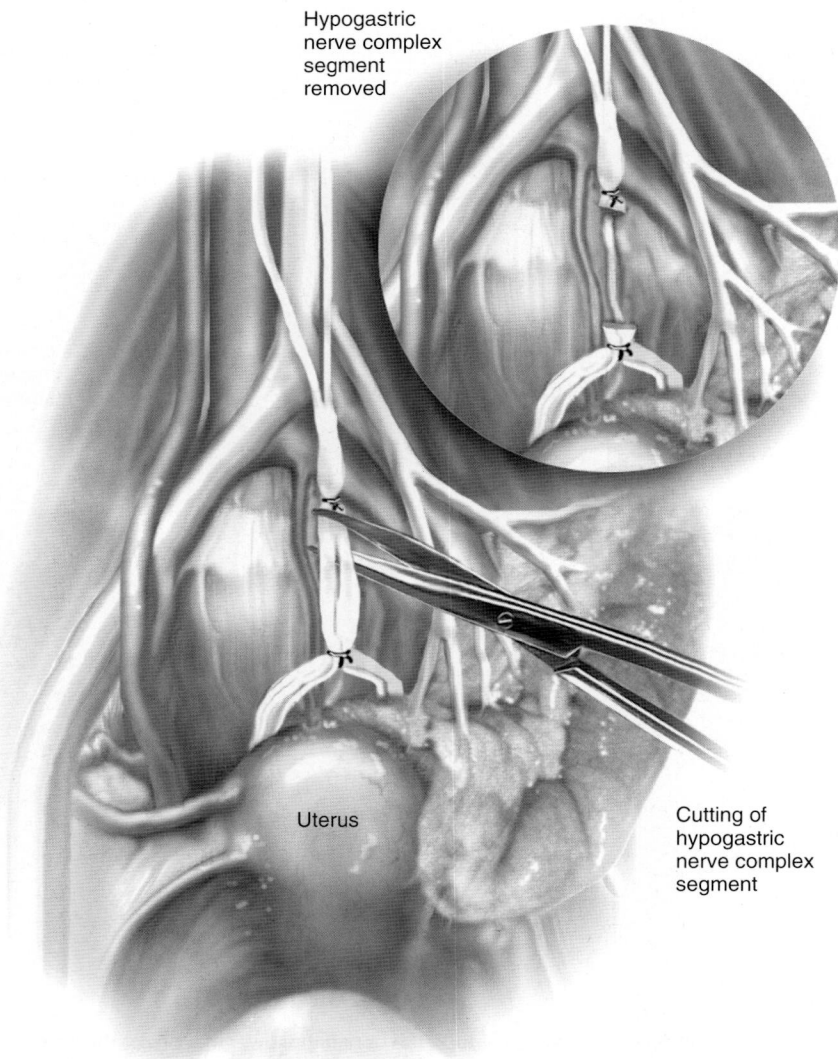

Hypogastric
nerve complex
segment
removed

Uterus

Cutting of
hypogastric
nerve complex
segment

**FIGURE 38–8** The segment of hypogastric nerve is cut out with the use of Metzenbaum scissors. The segment is placed in fixative and is sent to pathology. The field is irrigated with normal saline and is carefully examined for any bleeding.

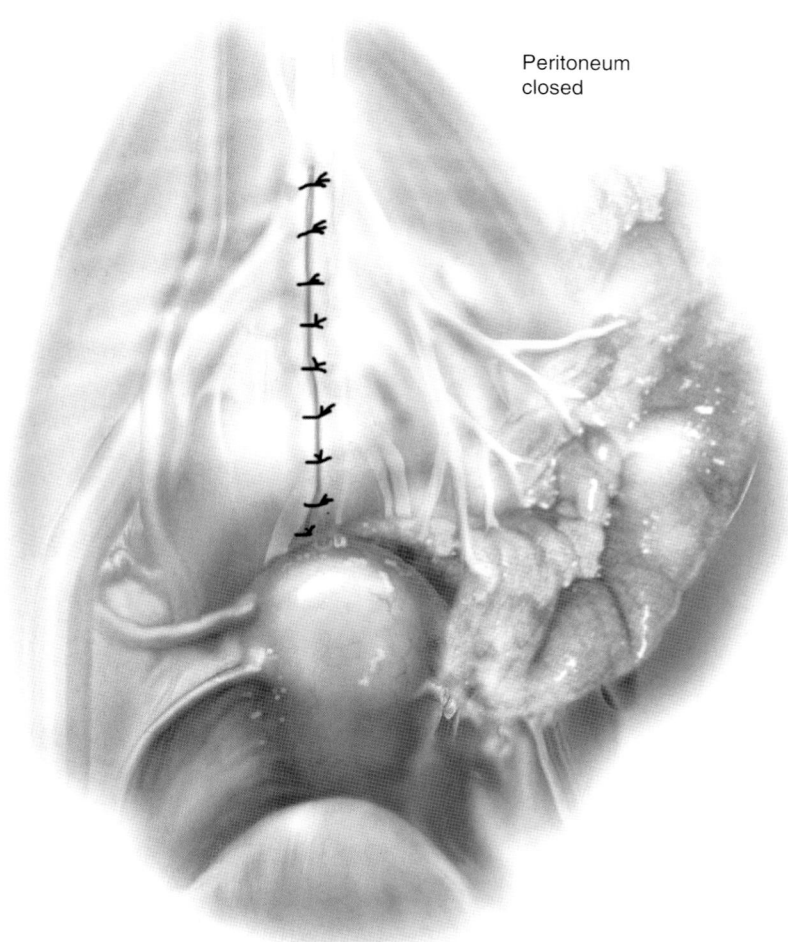

Peritoneum
closed

**FIGURE 38–9**  The peritoneum overlying the sacrum is closed with interrupted or running 3-0 Vicryl sutures. Care is taken to avoid encroaching on the right ureter or inferior mesenteric artery during closure.

# CHAPTER 39

# Uterosacral Nerve Transection

## *Michael S. Baggish*

Pain fibers emanating from the cervix and the lower portion of the uterine corpus traverse the uterosacral ligaments posteriorly to the sacrum and finally to the inferior hypogastric plexus (Fig. 39-1A, B). Section of these ligaments close to their origin at the junction of the upper vagina and the cervix has been advocated for the relief of dysmenorrhea. The operation does not relieve pain as completely as does presacral neurectomy. Nevertheless, uterosacral transection is a simpler operation to perform and usually is done via the laparoscopic approach.

The structures that must be identified to avoid injury are the right and left ureters and the uterine arteries. The latter are millimeters from the anterolateral aspect of the uterosacral ligaments. The former are within 1 to 2 cm of the ligaments (i.e., laterally located).

The uterosacral transection may be performed by laser ablation or by electrosurgical cutting. It is preferable to cut the ligament starting 1 to 2 mm from the lateral margin and to extend the cut medially toward the cul-de-sac (Fig. 39-2). The incision starts 4 to 5 mm distal from the locus where the ligament attaches to the uterus. The cut should be approximately 4 to 5 mm deep as well (Fig. 39-2, **Inset**). Some surgeons prefer to carry a 2-mm shallow incision across the posterior surface of the uterus, connecting the two severed uterosacral ligaments (Fig. 39-3).

Alternatively, the ligament can be doubly clamped and incised, and each end suture-ligated with permanent sutures. A 5- to 10-mm chunk of ligament thus is excised and is sent to pathology in fixative (Figs. 39-4 through 39-6).

At the terminus of the procedure, bleeding points are checked and secured. The ureters are again examined to ensure their integrity.

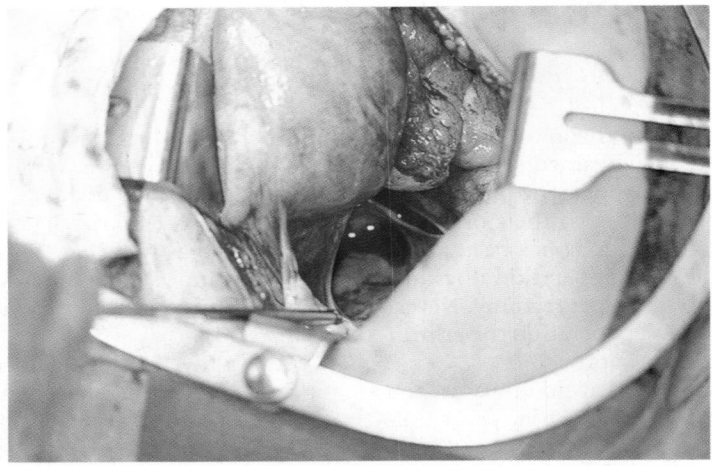

A

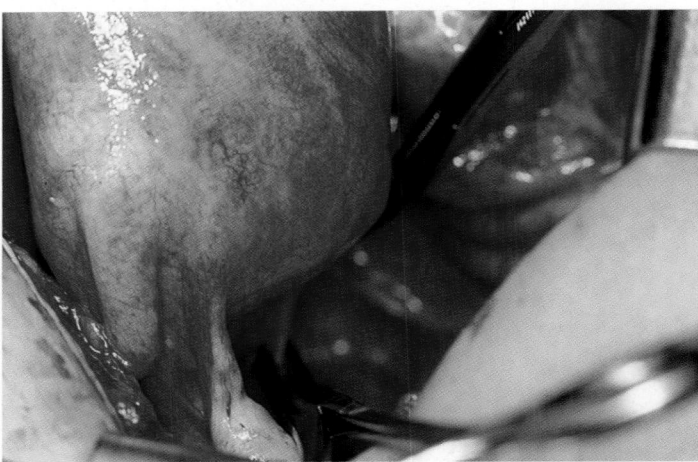

B

**FIGURE 39–1  A.** Normal uterus in situ. The left uterosacral ligament is grasped. **B.** Close-up of the same uterus as in Figure 39–1A. Pain fibers from the body of the uterus and the cervix are transmitted through the ligament, and pain is referred to the lower back via these fibers through the pelvic nerves and hypogastric plexus.

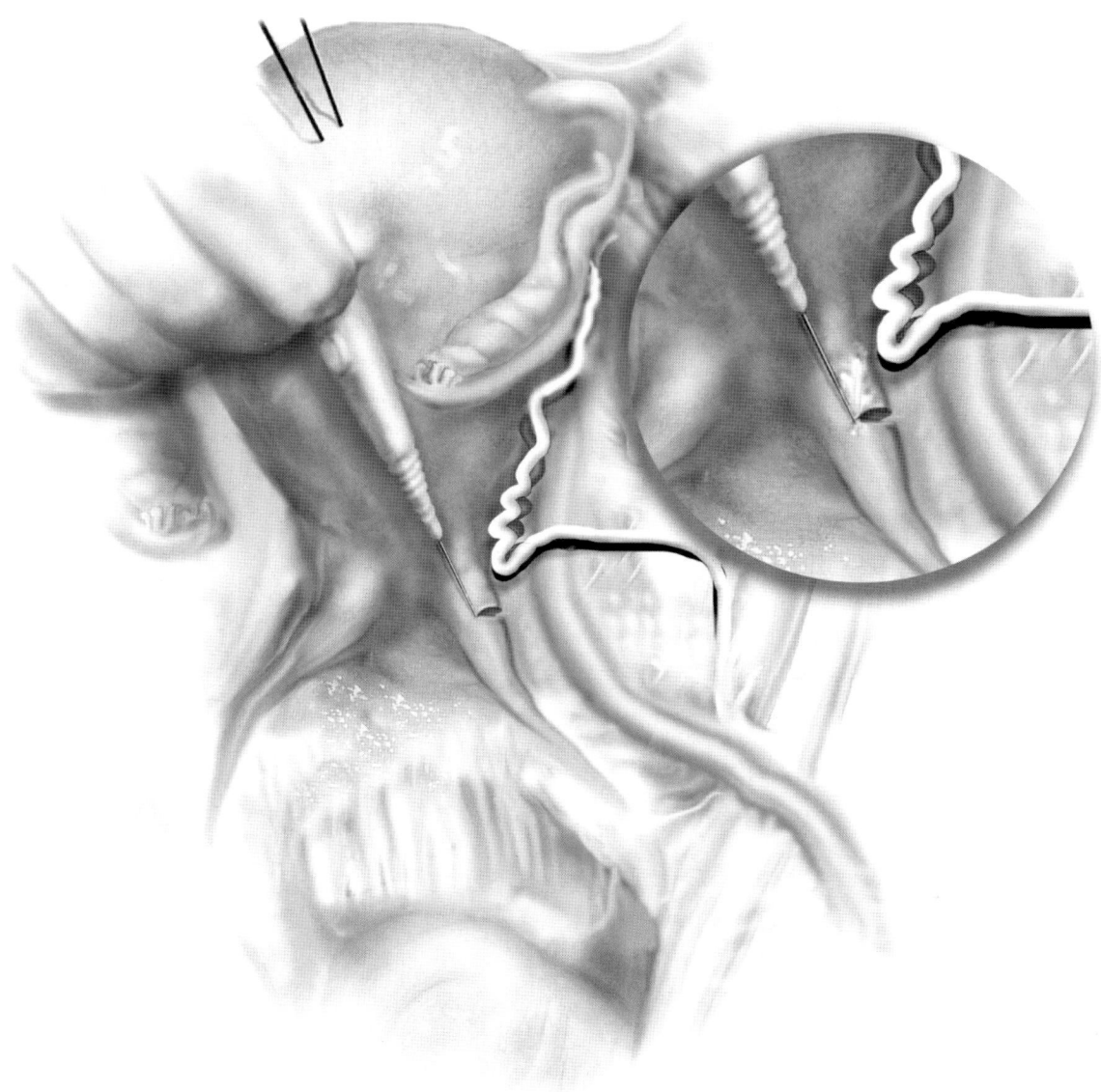

**FIGURE 39–2**  With an electrosurgical needle, the uterosacral ligament is transected. Note that the motion is from lateral to medial. The **inset** details the technique. Cutting current (blend one) at 30 to 40 W is applied at the lateral edge for short bursts to diminish conduction spread of thermal injury. Note that the ablation is initiated far enough posteriorly to avoid entry into the uterine artery. The sigmoid colon (medial) must be protected from conduction (electric current) injury.

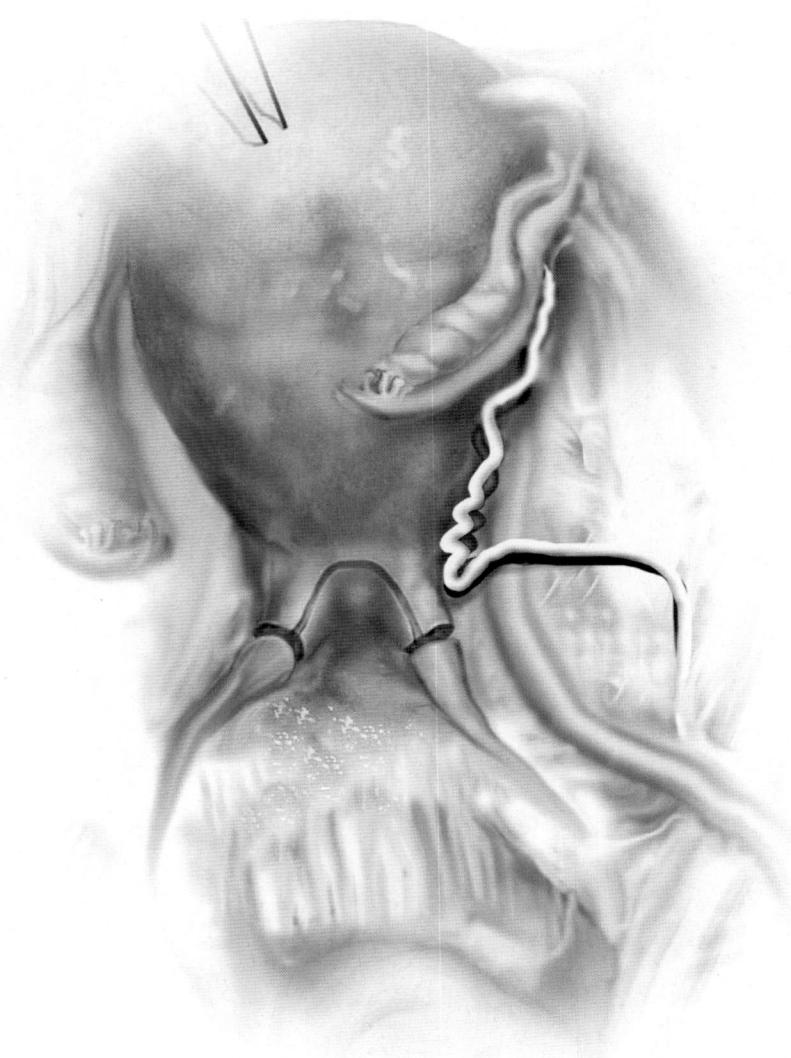

**FIGURE 39–3** The ablation is completed by continuing a 2- to 3-mm-deep extension across the back of the cervix (i.e., connecting the right and left uterosacral ablation lines).

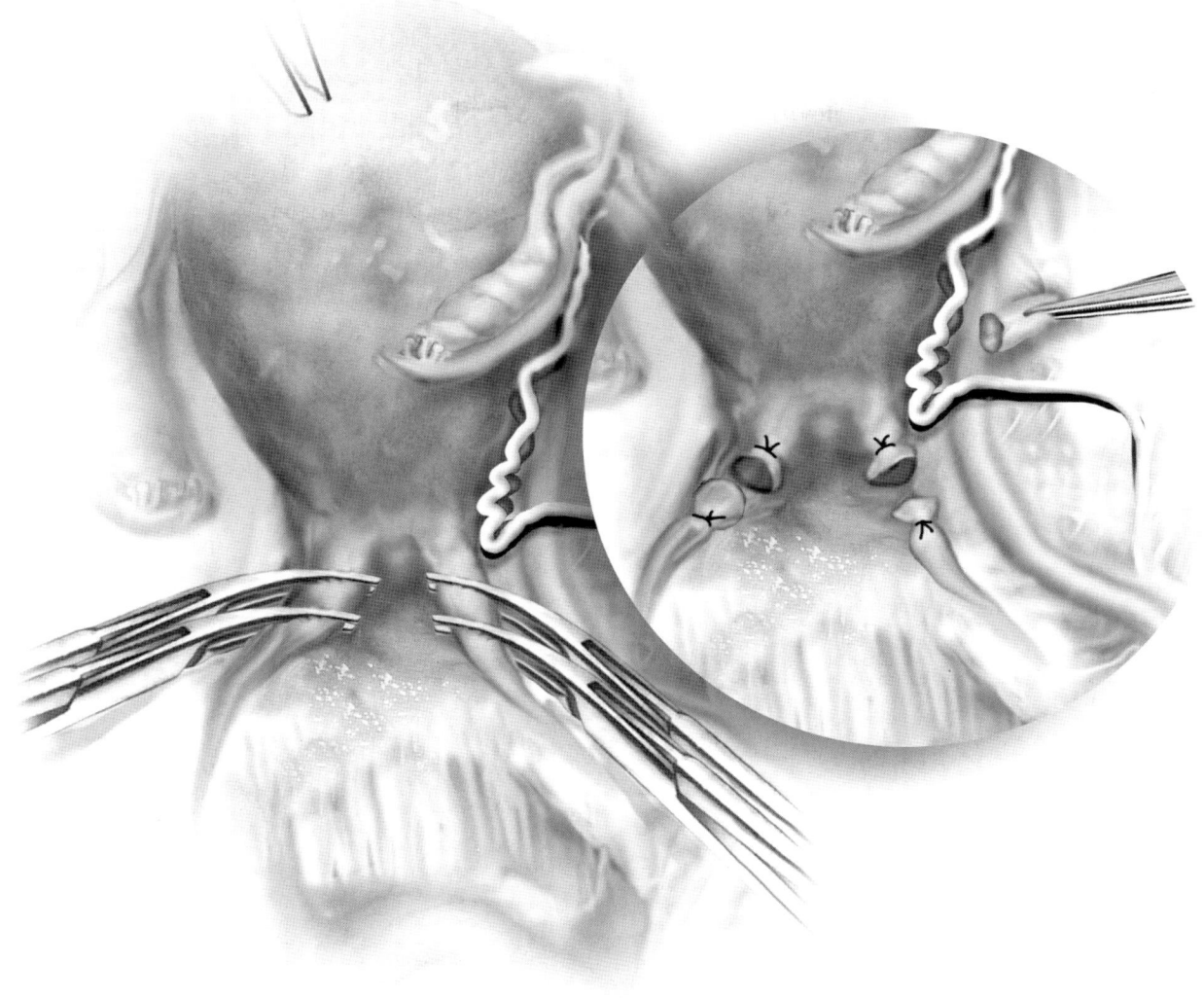

**FIGURE 39–4** Alternatively, the uterosacral ligaments may be clamped and cut. A segment of tissue (**inset**) may be sent to pathology to document excision and to determine whether any pathology exists within the ligament (e.g., endometriosis).

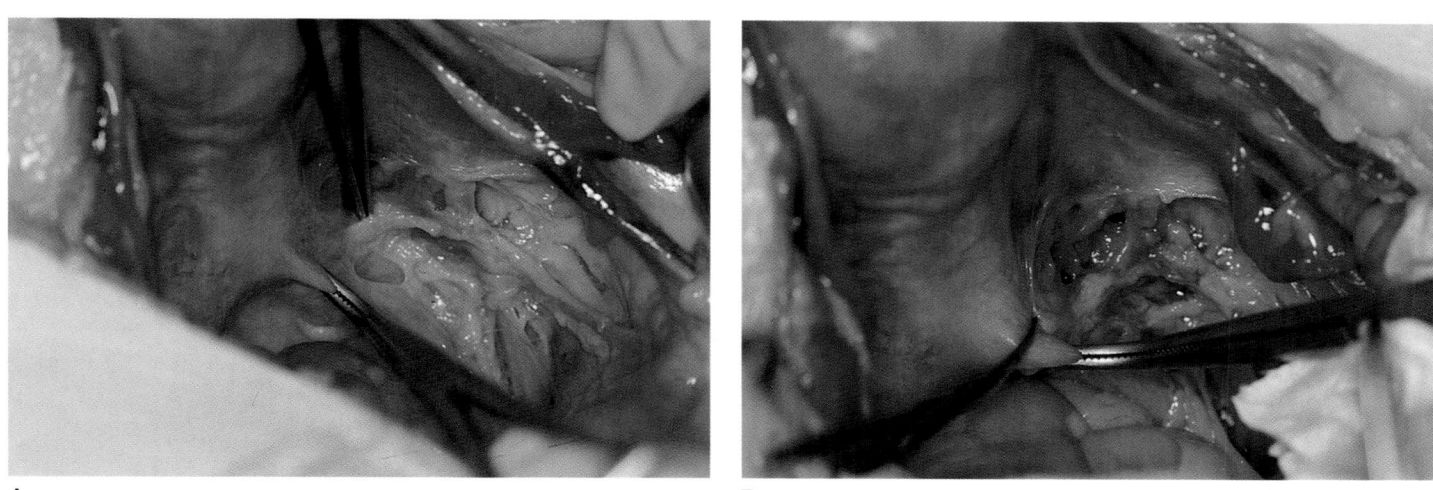

A

B

**FIGURE 39–5 A.** Actual application of the technique illustrated in Figure 34–4. **B.** The right uterosacral ligament is doubly clamped. The ureter has been identified lateral to the ligament.

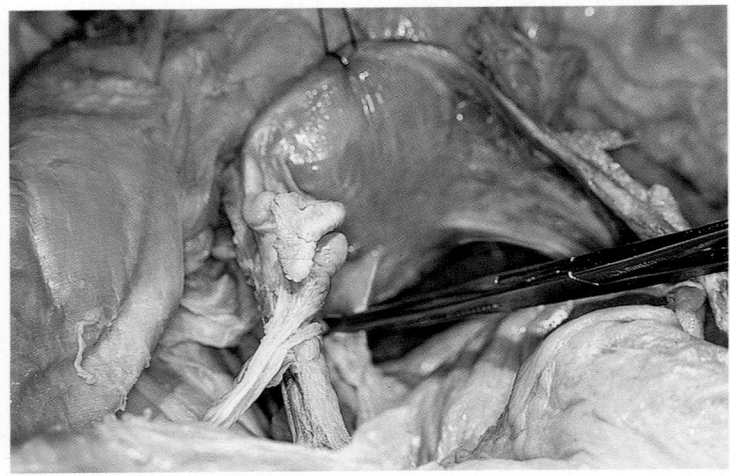

A

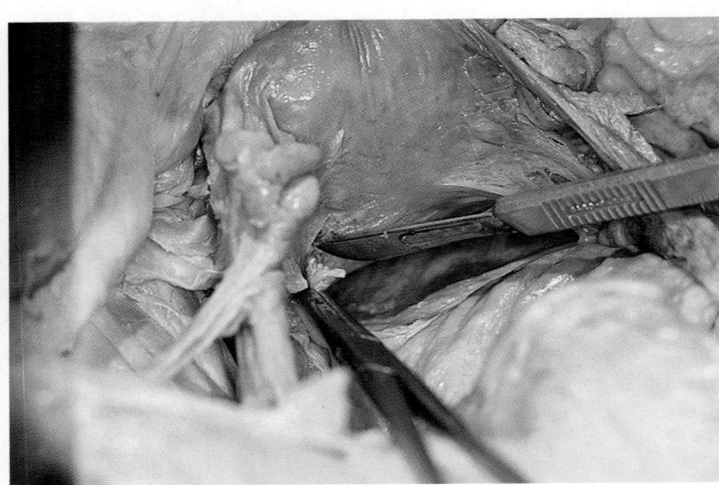

B

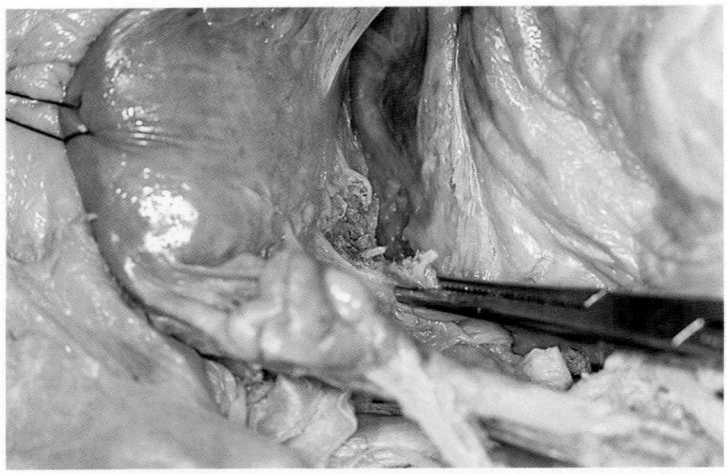

C

**FIGURE 39–6  A.** Fixed cadaveric uterus with left uterosacral ligament clamped. **B.** A scalpel divides the uterosacral ligament close to its uterine insertion. **C.** The ligament is completely divided. The key to accurate isolation and sectioning of the uterosacral ligaments is tension. The best demonstration of the ligaments can be produced only by pulling the uterus upward (cranially) and sharply dissecting in the anterior direction, as illustrated here.

# CHAPTER 40

# Lymph Node Sampling

*Michael S. Baggish*

In contrast to a complete lymphadenectomy (see Unit 1, Chapter 12), selective lymph node sampling is performed during simple hysterectomy for women who have been diagnosed with adenocarcinoma of the endometrium (see Unit 1, Chapter 13).

The lymph nodes typically sampled include the external iliac, internal iliac, common iliac, obturator, and periaortic nodes. These lymph nodes are closely associated with the large arteries and veins of the pelvis (Fig. 40–1).

The external iliac node sample is obtained by retracting the external iliac artery and removing some of the fatty tissue between the artery, the external iliac vein, and the lateral boundary formed by the psoas major muscle (Figs. 40–2A, 40–3 through 40–5).

The vein retractor is moved to the external iliac vein, which is gently elevated. Then with the use of ring pick-ups, some of the node-containing fatty tissue of the obturator fossa is teased away from around the obturator nerve (see Figs. 40–2B, 40–6 through 40–9).

Next, nodal tissue is excised from the hypogastric artery where it joins the external iliac artery to form the common iliac artery. Here the ureter must be identified and retracted medially to gain exposure (Figs. 40–2C and 40–10).

The tissue at the junction of the common iliac arteries and the aorta is sampled next (Figs. 40–2D and 40–11). Periaortic nodes are excised above the level of the takeoff of the inferior mesenteric artery (Figs. 40–12 and 40–13). The fat between the aorta and the inferior vena cava is carefully dissected and sampled (see Fig. 40–2E). When fatty tissue containing lymphatic tissue is cut, it typically bleeds. Therefore, when retroperitoneal lymph node sampling is performed, vascular clips should be applied to secure the small venules and arterioles (Fig. 40–14). Occasionally, it may be necessary to use a 3-0 or 4-0 Vicryl as a suture-ligature to achieve appropriate hemostasis (see Fig. 40–14).

Sampling should continue upward to the origin of the ovarian arteries from the aorta and of the ovarian veins from the vena cava and left renal vein areas (see Fig. 40–2F). For vulvar carcinoma, the lowest node in the external iliac chain is sampled. This can be done extraperitoneally by locating the inferior epigastric artery and tracing it to the iliac vessels at the point where the vessels cross under the inguinal ligament. The node is located just medial to the external iliac vein and lies in the femoral canal (Fig. 40–15A, B).

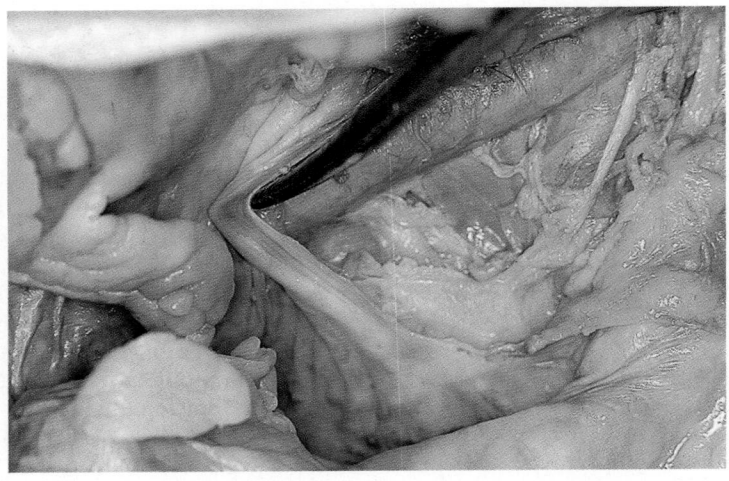

A

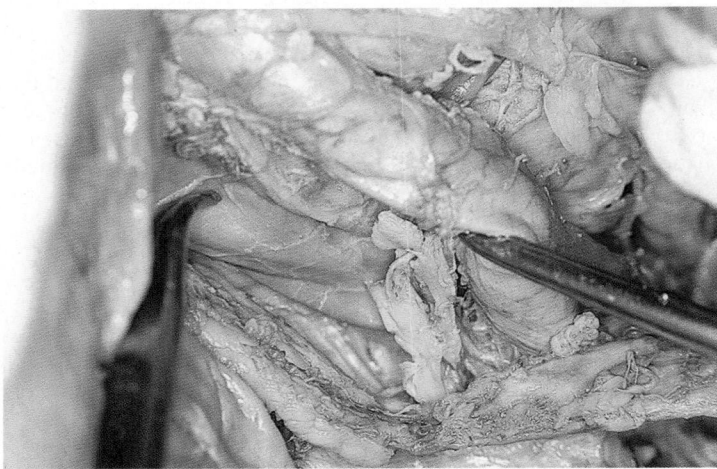

B

**FIGURE 40–1  A.** The peritoneum has been opened at the bifurcation of the right common iliac artery. The fat overlying the iliac arteries and veins contains lymphoid tissue. **B.** This clump of lymph nodes lies between the external iliac artery and vein. The scissor tip slightly elevates the external iliac artery; the clamp points to the external iliac vein. The ureter is in the foreground.

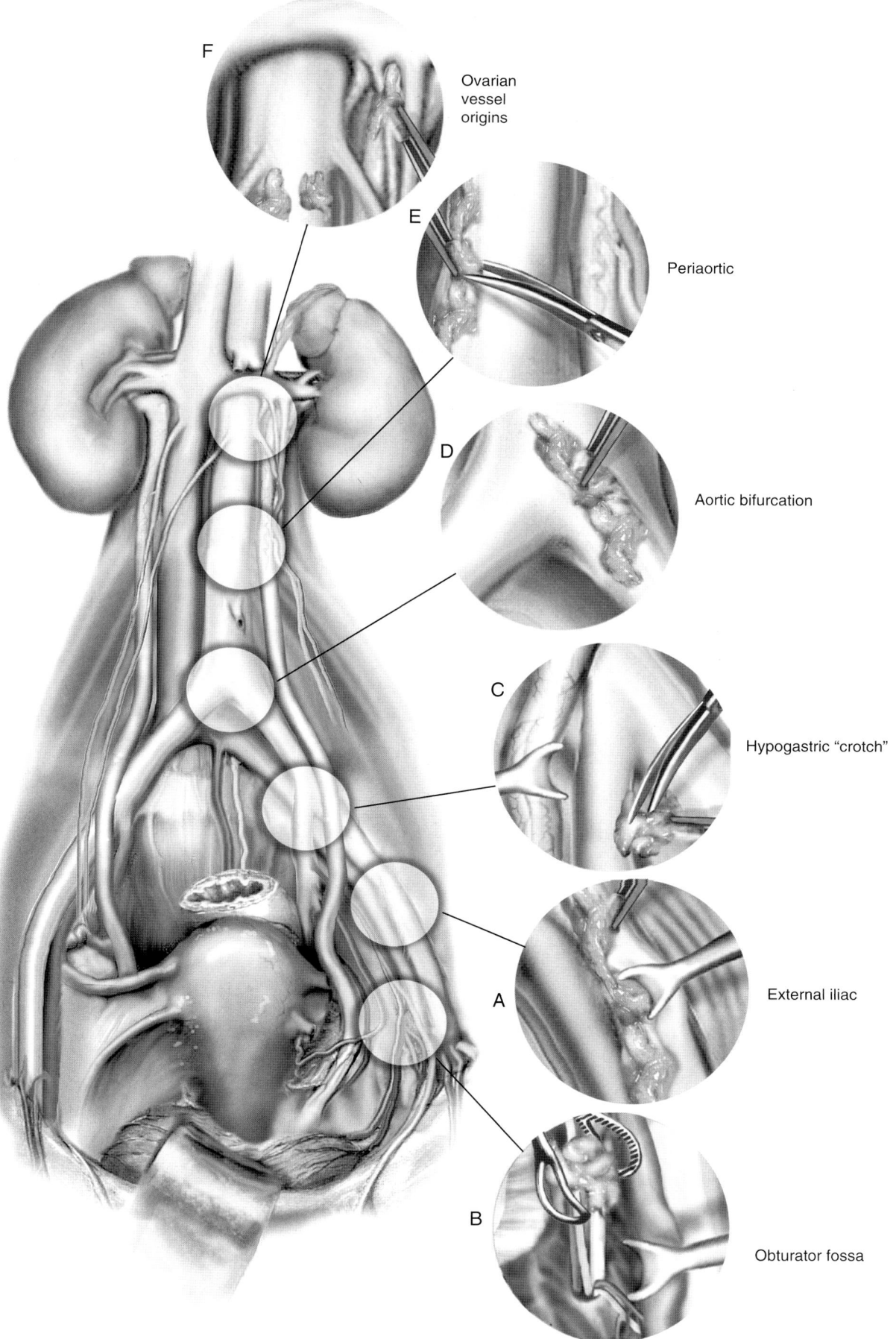

F  Ovarian
vessel
origins

E  Periaortic

D  Aortic bifurcation

C  Hypogastric "crotch"

A  External iliac

B  Obturator fossa

**FIGURE 40–2  A.** The external iliac artery is retracted with a vein retractor to allow the node-containing fat to be excised between the artery and the underlying external iliac vein. **B.** The obturator fossa is exposed by gently elevating the external iliac vein with a vein retractor. The fat is carefully teased out of the fossa with a ring forceps, and the obturator nerve and artery are exposed. **C.** The external iliac artery is followed cranially to reach its junction with the hypogastric artery. Fat is cleared from the crotch by sharp and blunt dissection. Care is taken to retract the ureter and to avoid injury to the underlying veins. **D.** The bifurcation of the aorta is located, and nodes are sampled between the aorta and vena cava and between the aortic bifurcation and the left common iliac vein. **E.** Periaortic nodes are sampled at and above the origin of the inferior mesenteric artery. The ureter lies close to the aorta on the left side and should be identified if the dissection carries over to the left side of the aorta. **F.** The ovarian arteries take origin from the aorta just below the renal arteries. Fat and nodes between these vessels typically are sampled at the upper limits of the dissection. Note that the left ovarian veins drain into the left renal vein and override the ureter.

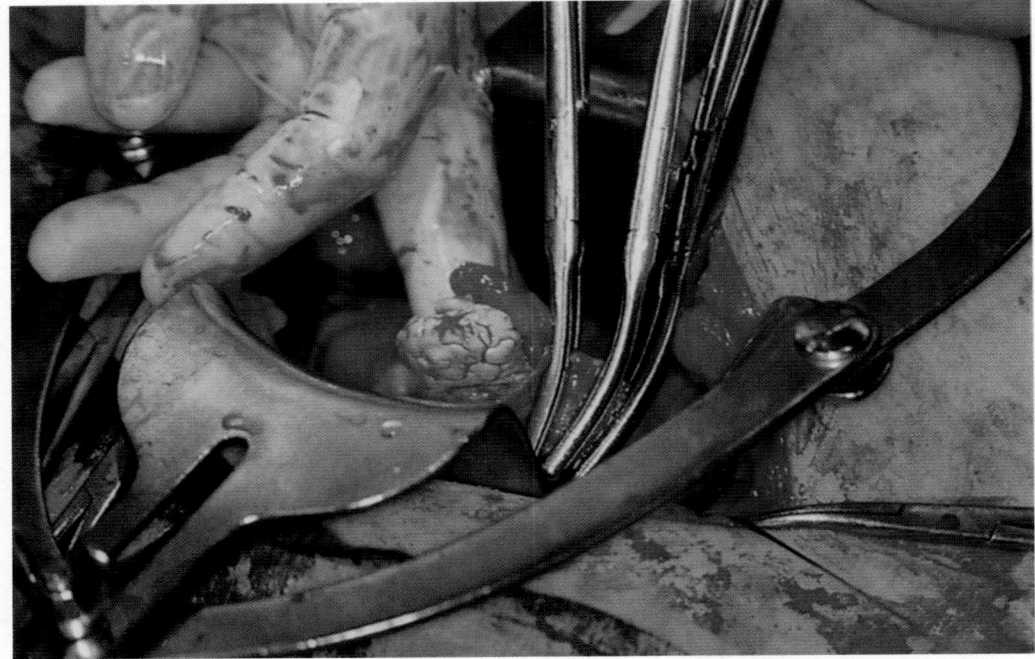

A

B

**FIGURE 40–3  A.** The infundibulopelvic ligament on the left side has been triply clamped. After the ligament is divided and the incision made following division of the round ligament is connected, the psoas muscle and the external iliac artery can be exposed easily. **B.** The lateral portions of the round ligament have been ligated and the infundibulopelvic ligament has been ligated for retraction (*arrows*). Fatty node-bearing tissue is dissected from the external iliac artery.

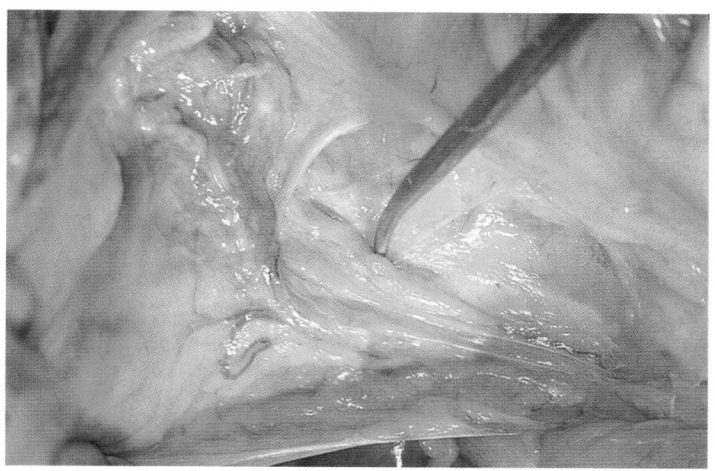

**FIGURE 40-4** The tonsil clamp is used to dissect fat and lymph nodes from the external iliac artery.

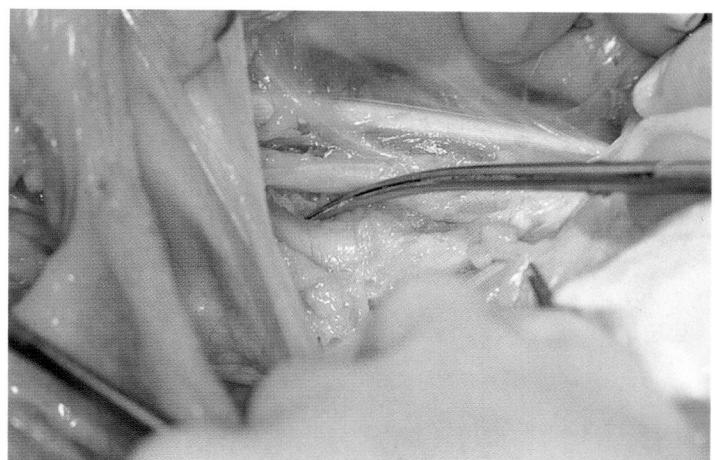

**FIGURE 40-5** Metzenbaum scissors dissect the lymphatic tissues between the external iliac artery and vein.

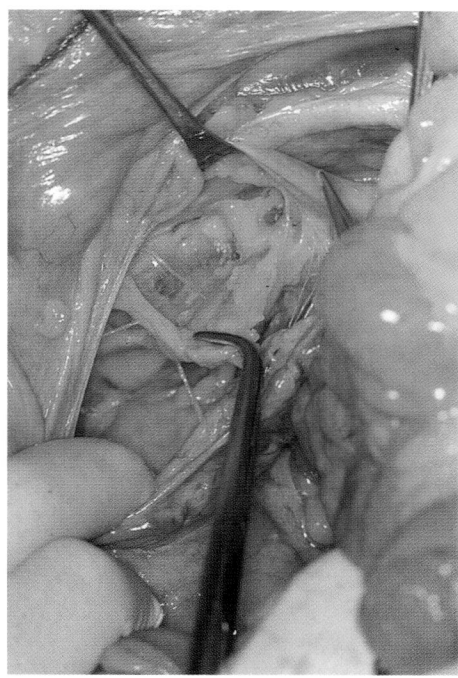

**FIGURE 40-6** A vein retractor exposes the obturator fossa by retracting the external iliac vein upward.

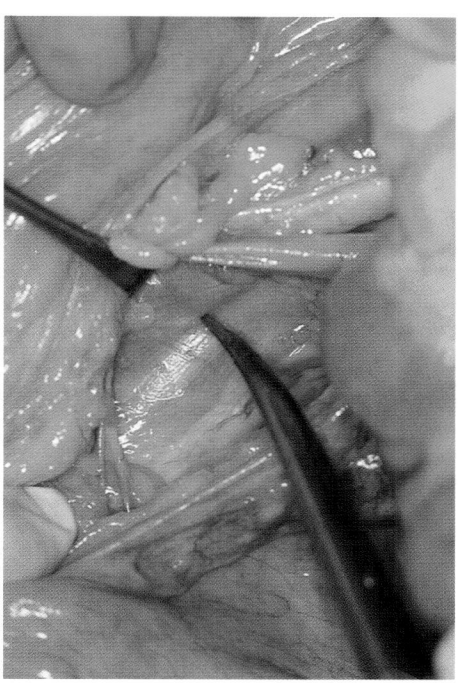

**FIGURE 40-7** The lateral border of the obturator fossa is made up of the obturator internus muscle.

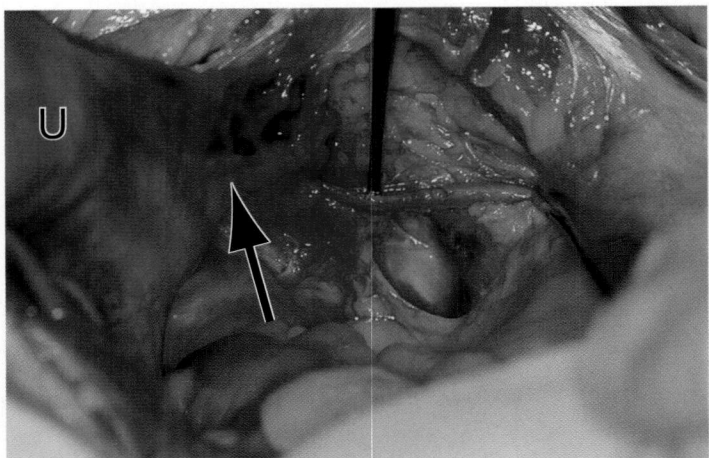

**FIGURE 40–8** The instrument is placed under the ureter to identify its position relative to the obturator fossa. The arrow points to the cardinal ligament. U, uterus.

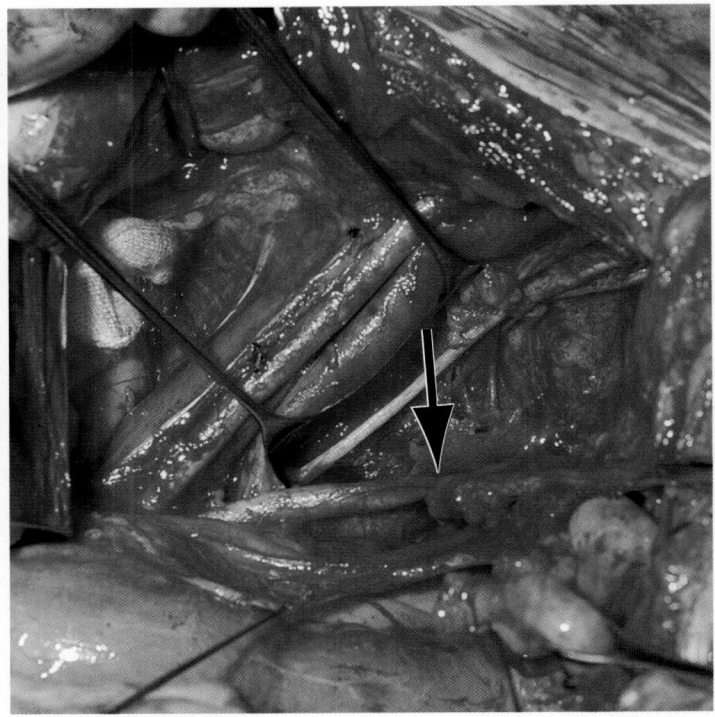

**FIGURE 40–9** The obturator fossa has been cleared of fat and nodes. The obturator nerve is clearly seen crossing the fossa. The arrow points to the hypogastric artery. The ureter is pulled medially by a suture placed at the peritoneal edge. (From Baggish et al: *In* Diagnostic and Operative Hysteroscopy, 2nd ed. Mosby, St. Louis, 1999, with permission.)

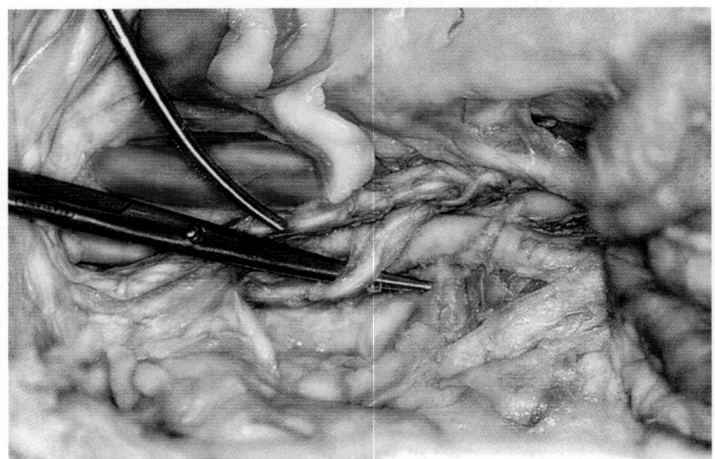

**FIGURE 40–10** The scissors lie beneath the ureter as it crosses the common iliac artery.

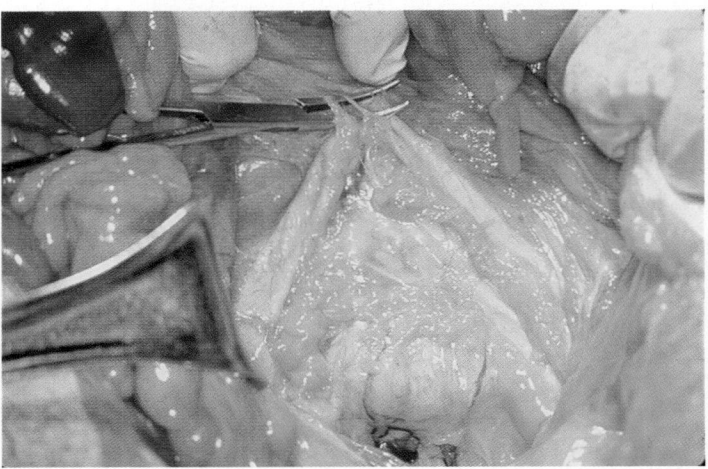

**FIGURE 40–11** The aortic bifurcation has been exposed. Fatty node-bearing tissue lies beneath the iliac arteries and the left common iliac vein.

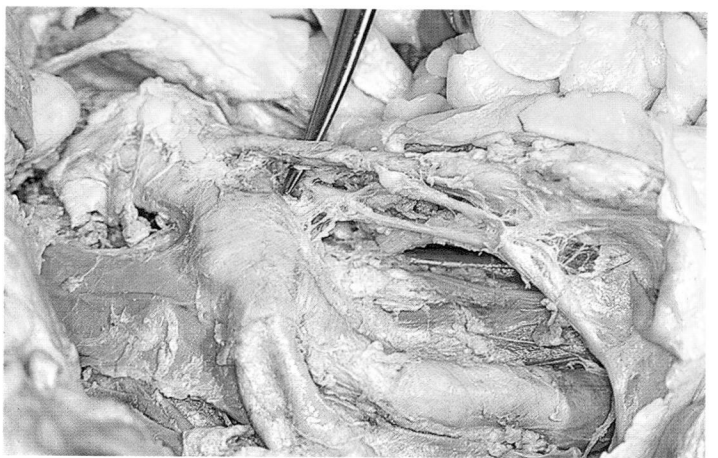

**FIGURE 40–12** The sigmoid colon has been pulled to the left. The peritoneum is opened and the fat is cleared to expose the aortic bifurcation and the inferior mesenteric artery.

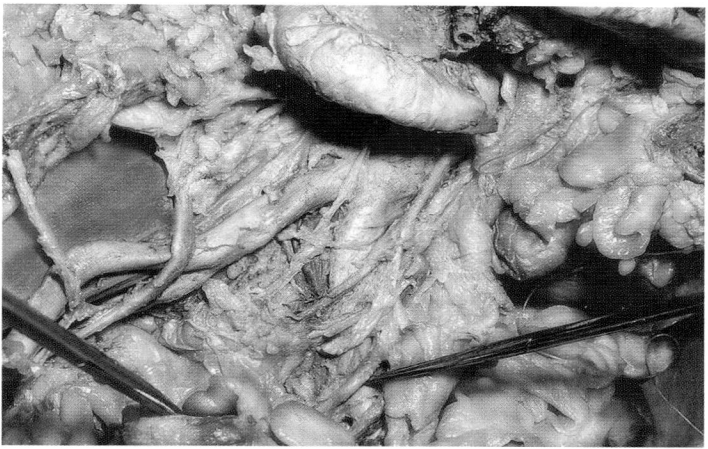

**FIGURE 40–13** The arrow points to the fully dissected inferior mesenteric artery.

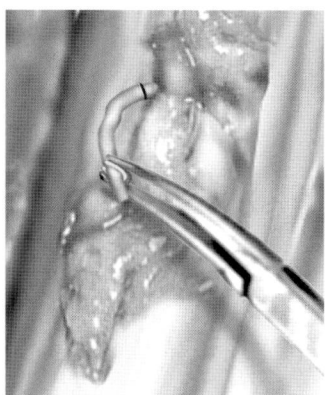

Vascular clip

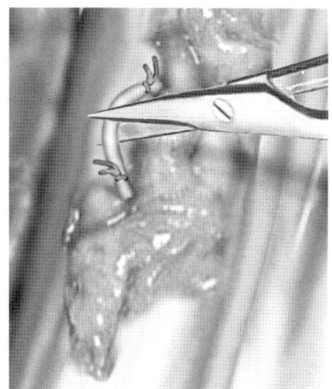

Suture ligature

**FIGURE 40–14** Small arteries and veins are typically encountered during lymphadenectomy. These may be clipped or, alternatively, clamped and ligated with 3-0 or 4-0 Vicryl.

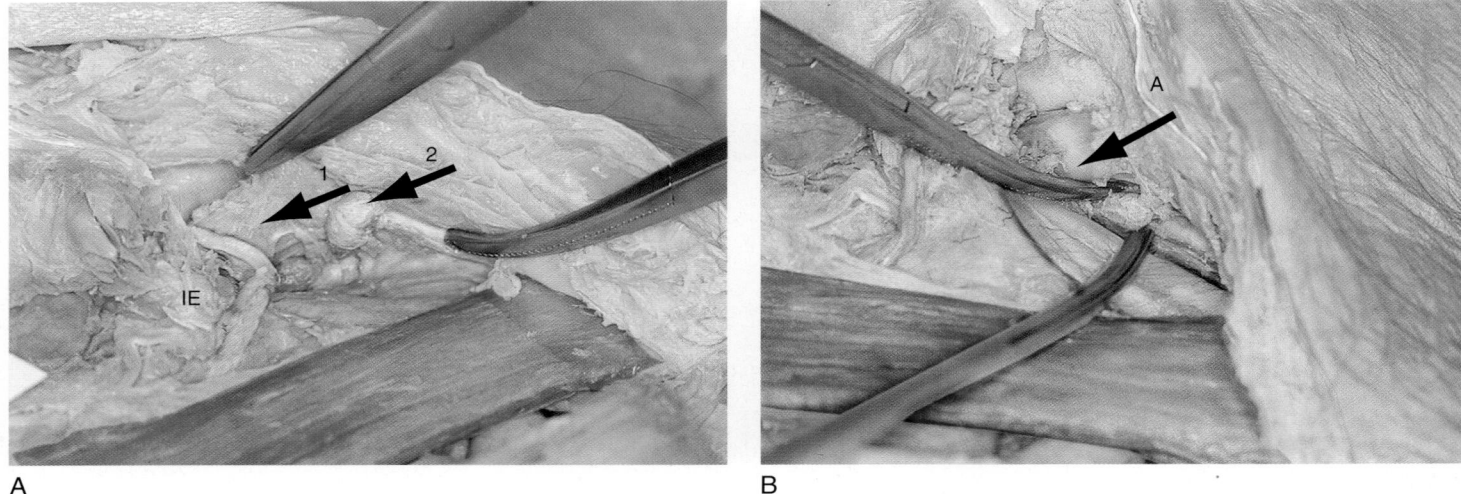

A                                                         B

**FIGURE 40–15** **A.** The left rectus abdominis muscle is seen in the foreground. The transversalis fascia covers the peritoneum and has a slate blue color. The inferior epigastric (*IE*) vessel can be seen originating from the external iliac artery. The scissors point to the iliac artery just before it passes beneath the inguinal ligament. Arrow 1 points to the external iliac vein. Arrow 2 points to Cloquet's node. The curved clamp rests on the inguinal ligament. **B.** Letter A is directly caudal to the external iliac artery. The *arrow* points to the external iliac vein. The lymph node is between the clamp and the scissors at the top of the femoral canal.

# SECTION G

# Abdominal Operations for Enterocele and Vault Prolapse

# CHAPTER 41

# Abdominal Enterocele Repair

*Mickey M. Karram*

Weakness in the support of the cervix or the vaginal vault can lead to uterovaginal prolapse or posthysterectomy vault prolapse. These defects are usually associated with an enterocele, a defect that results in attenuation or breakage of the rectovaginal or pubocervical fascia and thus allows the peritoneum to come into direct contact with the vaginal epithelium.

The posterior cul-de-sac (Fig. 41–1) should be addressed routinely when abdominal hysterectomy is performed, as well as in selected cases of retropubic urethropexy. At the time of abdominal hysterectomy, it is important to reconnect the vaginal vault to the cardinal uterosacral ligament complex (Fig. 41–2). Also, the continuity of the pelvic floor must be reinstated by approximating the fascia of the anterior vaginal wall (Figs. 41–3 and 41–4) to the fascia of the posterior vaginal wall (Fig. 41–5).

Three techniques of abdominal enterocele repair have been described: the Moschcowitz and Halban procedures and uterosacral ligament plication. The Moschcowitz procedure is performed by placing concentric purse string sutures around the cul-de-sac to include the posterior vaginal wall, the right pelvic sidewall, the serosa of the sigmoid, and the left pelvic sidewall (Figs. 41–6 and 41–7). The initial suture is placed at the base of the cul-de-sac. Usually three or four sutures completely obliter-

ate the cul-de-sac. The purse string sutures are tied so that no small defects remain that could entrap small bowel or lead to enterocele recurrence. Care should be taken not to include the ureter in the purse string sutures or to allow the ureter to be kinked medially when the sutures are tied.

Halban described his technique to obliterate the cul-de-sac by using sutures placed sagittally between the uterosacral ligaments. Four or five sutures are placed in a longitudinal fashion sequentially through the serosa of the sigmoid, into the deep peritoneum of the cul-de-sac, and up the posterior vaginal wall (Figs. 41–8 through 41–10). The sutures are tied, obliterating the cul-de-sac (Fig. 41–11).

Transverse plication of the uterosacral ligaments can be used also to obliterate the cul-de-sac (Fig. 41–12). Three to five sutures are placed into the medial portion of the uterosacral ligament, through the back of the vagina, and through the opposite uterosacral ligament. The lowest sutures incorporate the anterior rectal serosa to bring the rectum adjacent to the uterosacral ligaments and vagina (Figs. 41–13 and 41–14). Care must be taken to avoid injury or kinking of the ureter. Relaxing incisions can be made in the peritoneum lateral to the uterosacral ligaments to release the ureter if necessary.

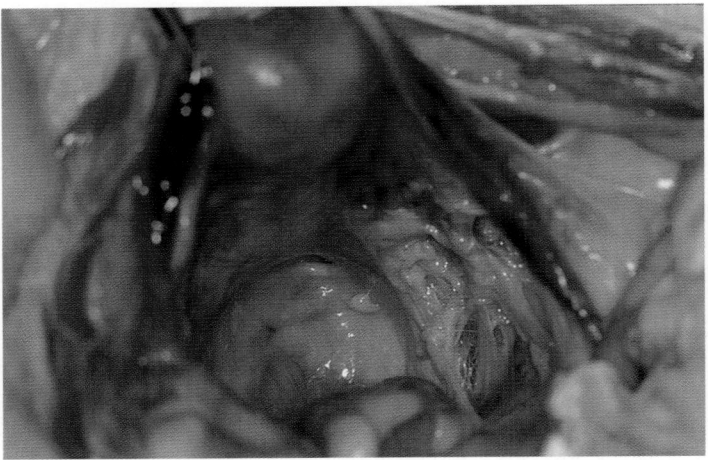

**FIGURE 41–1** Prominent cul-de-sac noted with uterus in place.

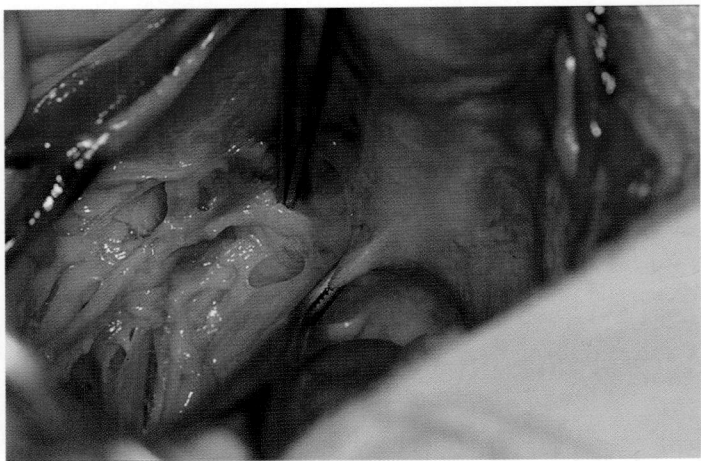

**FIGURE 41–2** Left uterosacral (clamped) and left cardinal ligaments. These structures are responsible for support of the cervix and the upper vagina.

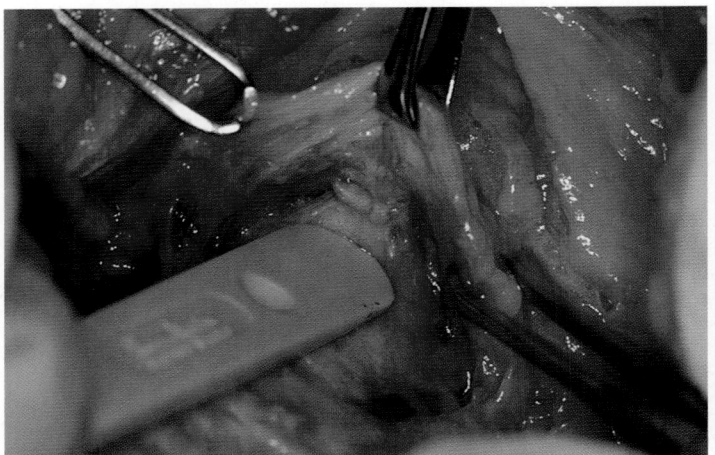

**FIGURE 41–3** The pubocervical fascia has been sharply dissected off the anterior cervix and vagina at the time of abdominal hysterectomy.

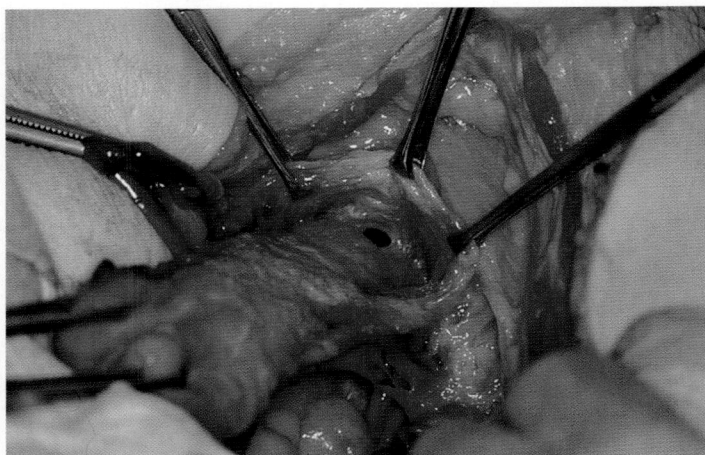

**FIGURE 41–4** The pubocervical fascia has been mobilized below the cervix. The anterior vaginal wall has been penetrated in preparation for removal of the uterus.

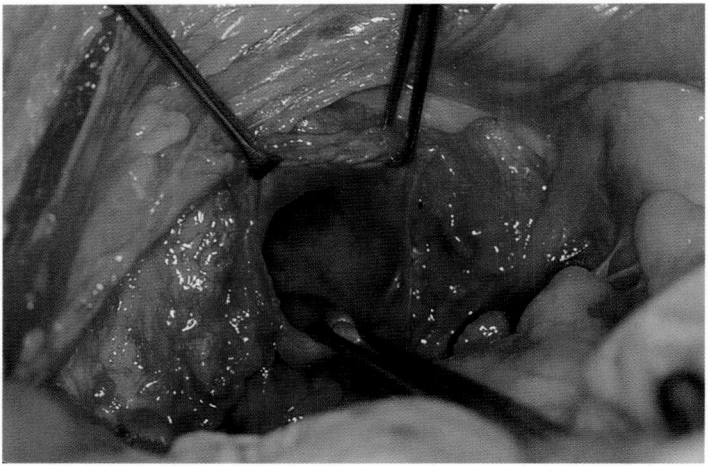

**FIGURE 41–5** The open vaginal cuff after removal of the uterus. Note the Allis clamps on the vaginal epithelium with the pubocervical fascia anteriorly and the vaginal epithelium with that rectovaginal fascia posteriorly. Closure of the cuff thus will restore fascial continuity between the anterior and posterior vaginal walls.

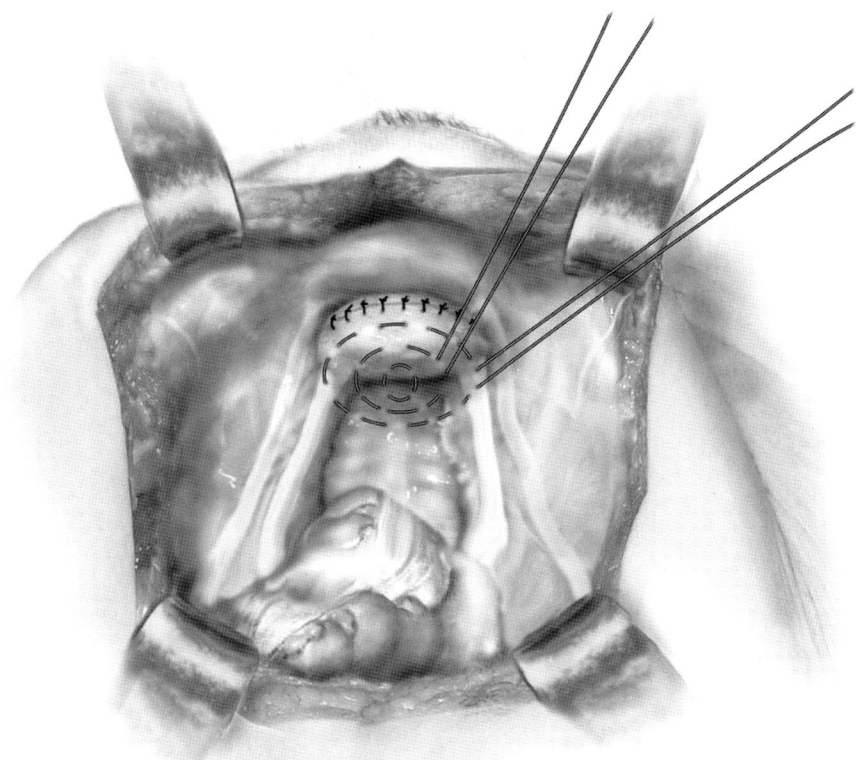

Moschcowitz procedure

**FIGURE 41–6** Moschcowitz procedure. Concentric purse string sutures are placed in the cul-de-sac. The suture should include the back of the vagina, the sidewall of the pelvis at the level of the distal uterosacral ligament, and the serosa of the sigmoid colon.

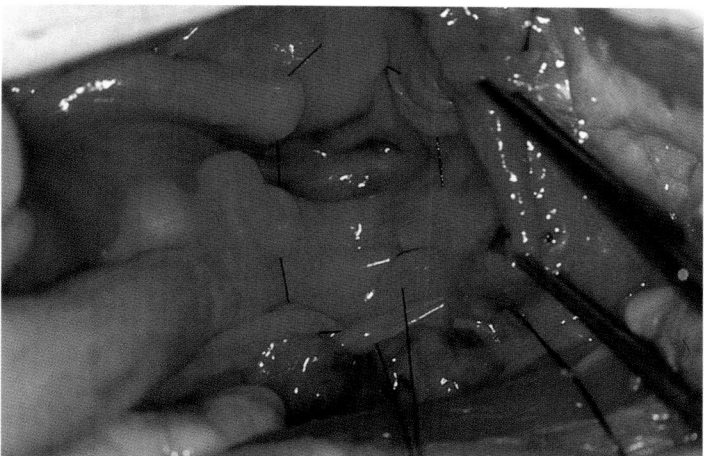

**FIGURE 41–7** Moschcowitz closure of the cul-de-sac. Initial purse string suture has been placed.

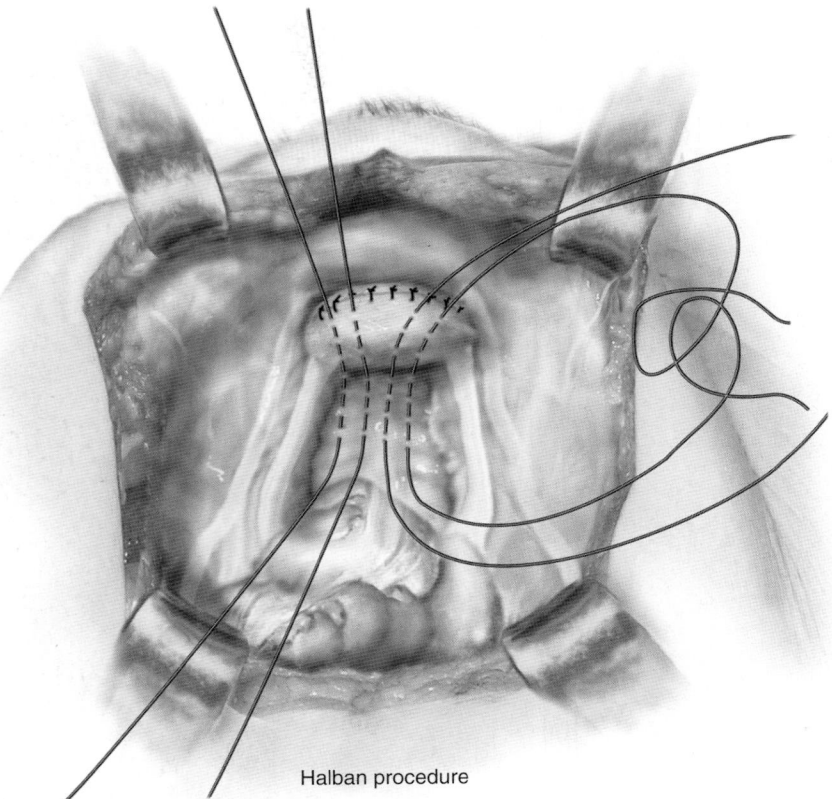

Halban procedure

**FIGURE 41–8** Halban closure of the cul-de-sac. Sutures are placed longitudinally through the serosa of the sigmoid, into the deep peritoneum of the cul-de-sac, and up the posterior vaginal wall.

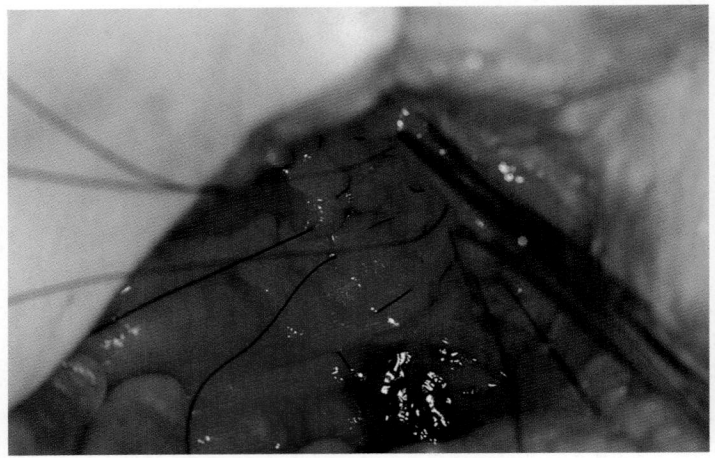

**FIGURE 41–9** Halban closure of the cul-de-sac showing suture placement. Clamps are placed on the vaginal vault for traction.

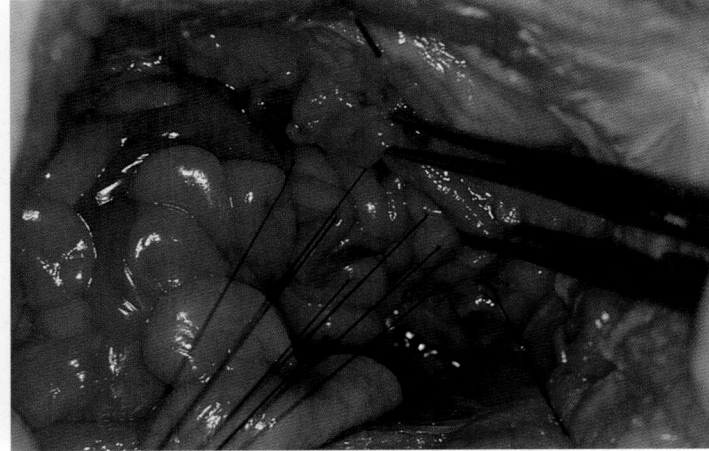

**FIGURE 41–10** Halban closure of the cul-de-sac. Pulling up of sutures brings the sigmoid into contact with the posterior vaginal wall.

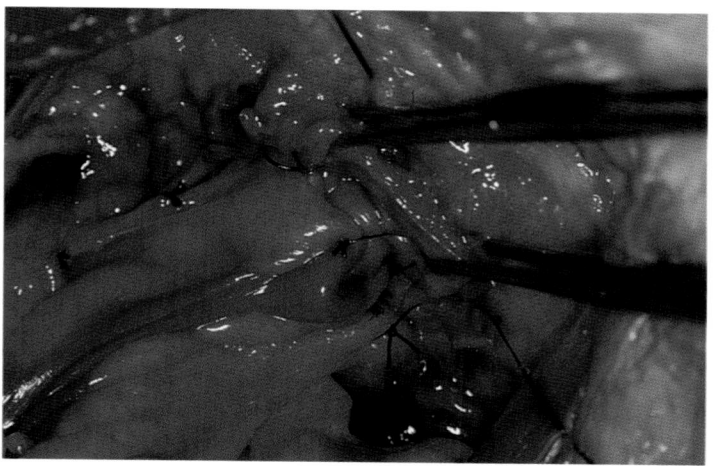

**FIGURE 41–11** Halban closure of the cul-de-sac. Tying of the sutures completely obliterates the cul-de-sac.

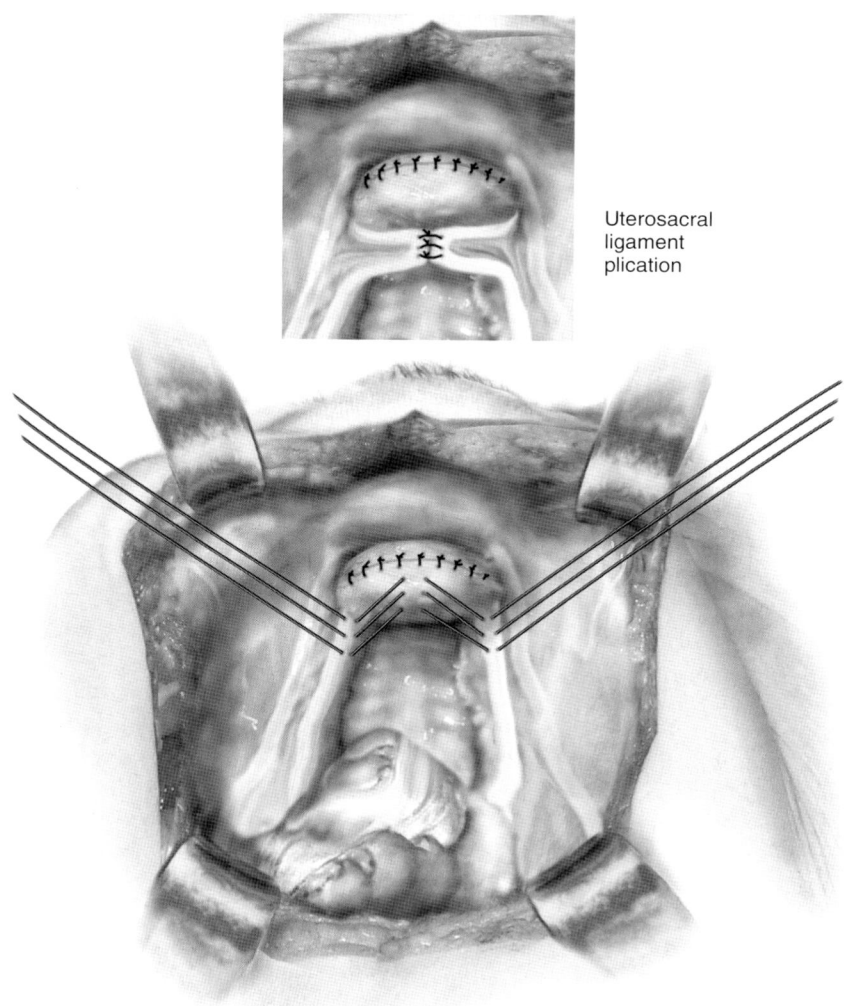

Uterosacral ligament plication

**FIGURE 41–12** Abdominal plication of the uterosacral ligament.

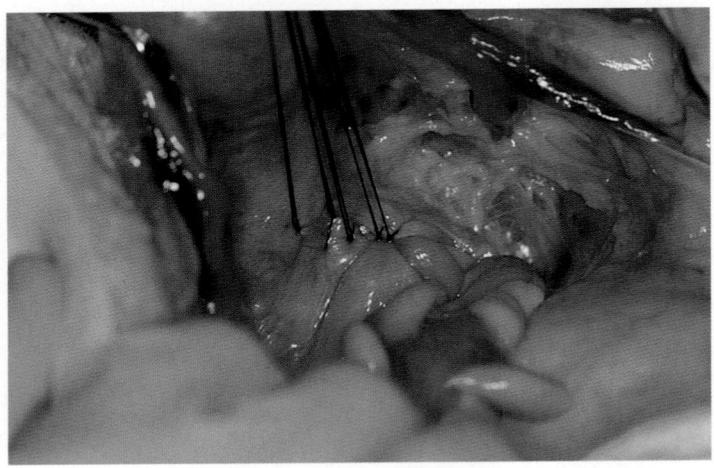

**FIGURE 41–13** A series of sutures have been placed to incorporate the uterosacral ligaments across the midline.

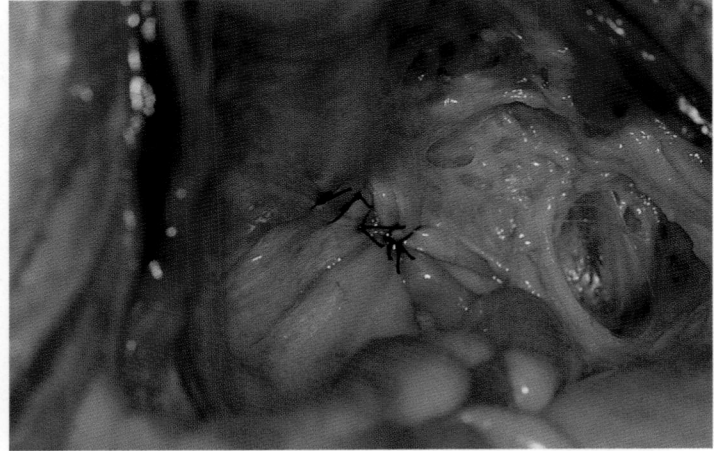

**FIGURE 41–14** Sutures have been cut. Note that the uterosacral ligaments have been plicated across midline, completely obliterating the cul-de-sac.

# CHAPTER 42

# High Uterosacral Ligament Suspension With Fascial Reconstruction: Abdominal Approach

*Mickey M. Karram*

This repair is based on the concept that the uterosacral ligaments do not attenuate in cases of uterovaginal prolapse or posthysterectomy vaginal vault prolapse but instead break at certain points. The remnants of the uterosacral ligaments or the most distal ends are identified and tagged. The remnants are usually found in the vicinity of the ischial spines on each side (Fig. 42–1).

The ureters are identified on each side, and the enterocele is addressed by excision of the sac or by abdominal obliteration of the cul-de-sac. Three or four permanent sutures then are placed to plicate the ends of the uterosacral ligaments across to the midline. This creates a durable ridge to which the vaginal vault can be attached (see Fig. 42–1). A sponge stick or an EEA (end-to-end anastomosis) sizer is usually placed in the vagina, and the peritoneum over the apex of the vagina is opened. The endopelvic fascia and the muscular component or fascia of the anterior and posterior vaginal walls are identified. Nonabsorbable sutures then are used to suspend the prolapsed vagina with its fascia to the uterosacral ligaments. This is usually accomplished by placing numerous longitudinal nonabsorbable sutures through the ridge of uterosacral ligaments down the cul-de-sac, through the upper edge of the rectovaginal fascia, into the vaginal vault, and finally through the edge of the pubocervical fascia (Fig. 42–2). Tying of the sutures (see Fig. 42–2, **inset**) elevates the apex of the vagina to the uterosacral ligaments and creates continuity between the pubocervical fascia and the rectovaginal fascia.

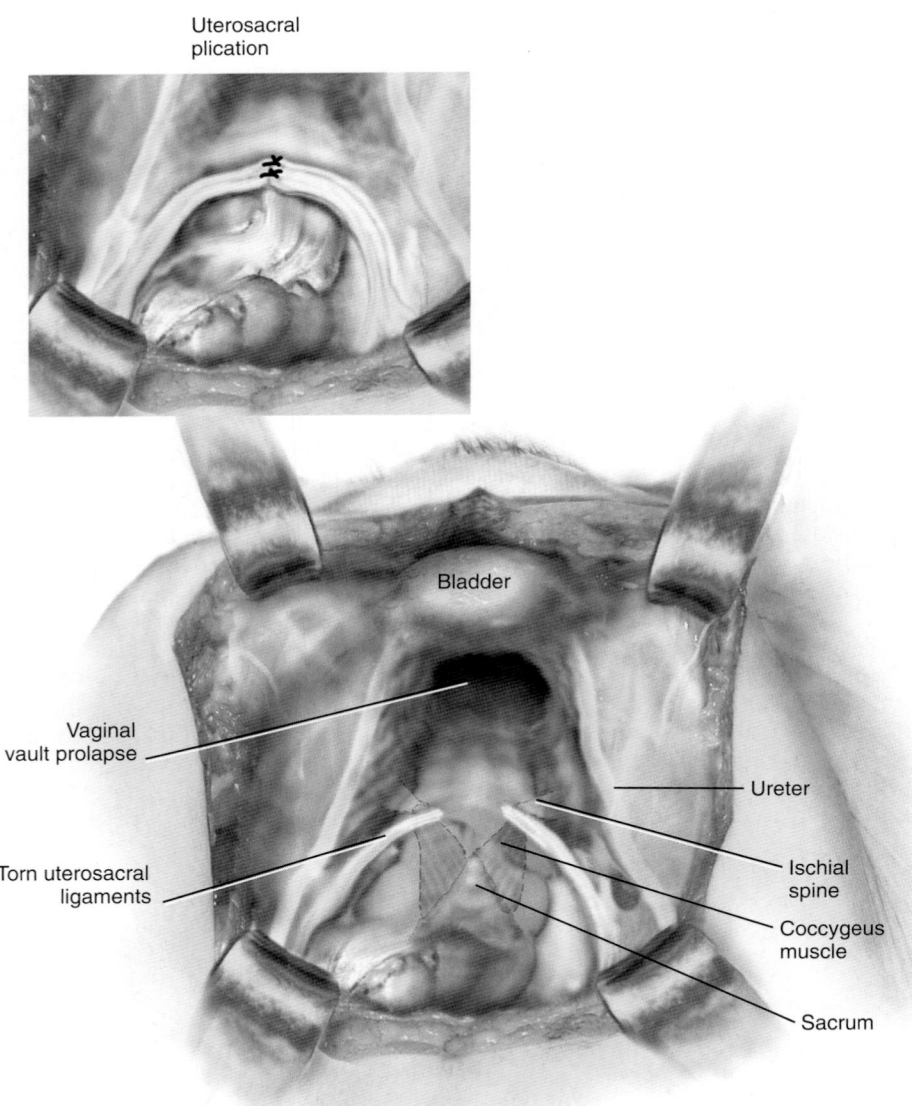

Uterosacral
plication

Bladder

Vaginal
vault prolapse

Torn uterosacral
ligaments

Ureter

Ischial
spine

Coccygeus
muscle

Sacrum

**FIGURE 42–1** Abdominal view of an enterocele and vaginal vault prolapse. Note the broken ends of the uterosacral ligaments at the level of the ischial spine. The **inset** demonstrates plication of ligaments, creating a firm durable ridge in the hollow of the sacrum to which the vaginal vault will be suspended.

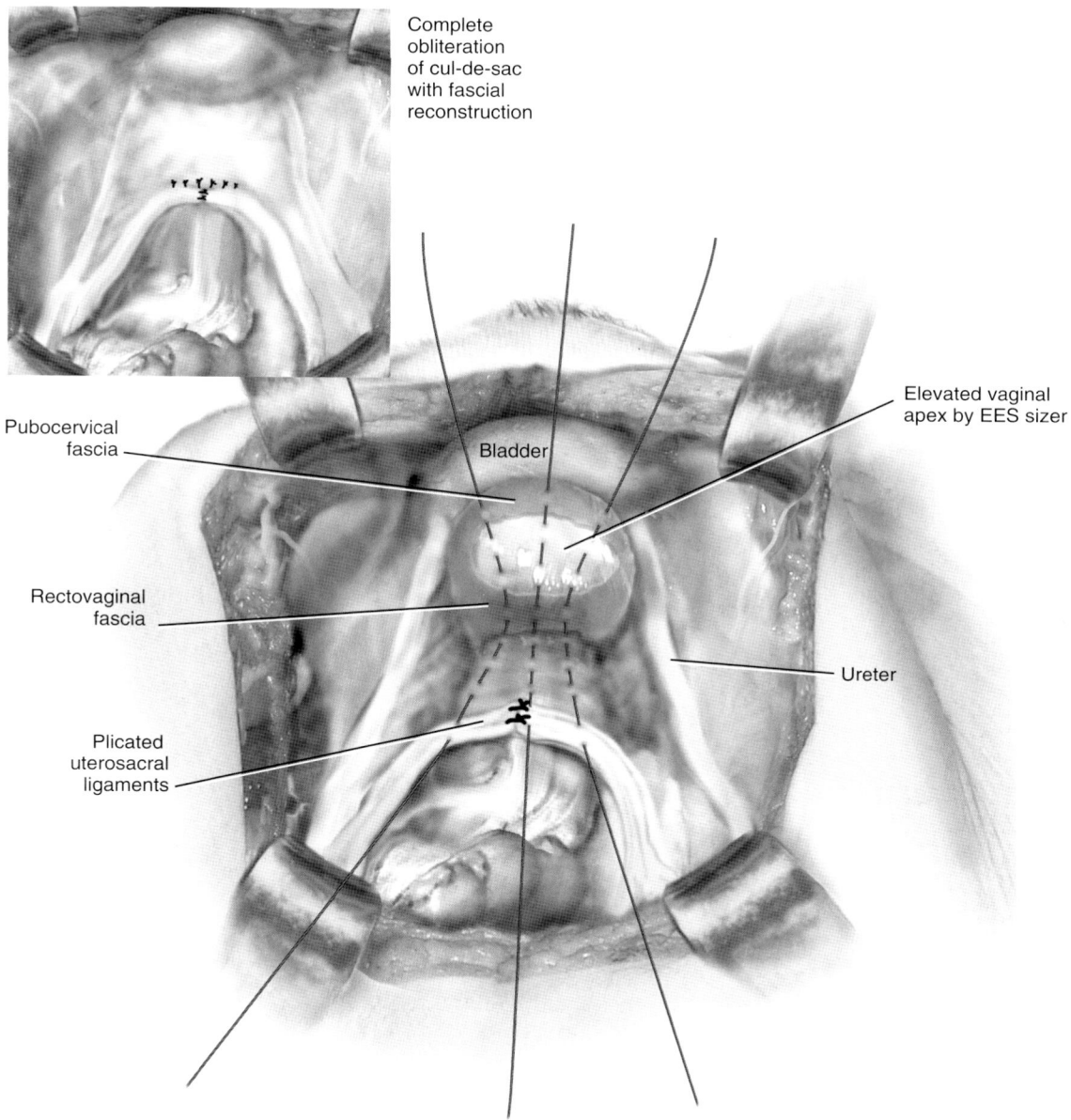

Complete
obliteration
of cul-de-sac
with fascial
reconstruction

Elevated vaginal
apex by EES sizer

Pubocervical
fascia

Bladder

Rectovaginal
fascia

Ureter

Plicated
uterosacral
ligaments

**FIGURE 42–2** Longitudinally placed nonabsorbable sutures are passed through the ridge of uterosacral ligaments, down the cul-de-sac to the edge of the rectovaginal fascia, into the vaginal vault, and finally through the edge of the pubocervical fascia. Tying of the sutures (inset) elevates the apex of the vagina to the uterosacral ligaments and reapproximates the pubocervical fascia with the rectovaginal fascia.

# CHAPTER 43

# Abdominal Sacral Colpopexy

*Mickey M. Karram*

Suspension of the vagina to the sacral promontory by means of an abdominal approach has been shown to be an effective treatment for uterovaginal prolapse and vaginal vault prolapse. Although the exact indications for abdominal sacral colpopexy are controversial, the author prefers it to a vaginal repair when there is obvious failure of the compensatory support mechanisms of the pelvis, especially in the very young patient (Fig. 43-1), or when the vagina has been foreshortened as a result of previous repairs (Fig. 43-2). Many different graft materials have been used for abdominal sacral colpopexy. Natural materials include fascia lata, rectus fascia, and dura mater. Synthetic materials have included polypropylene mesh, polyester fiber mesh, polytetrafluoroethylene mesh, Mersilene mesh, Silastic silicone rubber, and Marlex mesh. Although homologous tissue in the form of cadaveric fascia lata and other xenografts have also been utilized for this operation (Fig. 43-3), at the present time the material of choice is polypropylene. The technique for abdominal sacral colpopexy with graft placement is as follows:

1. The patient should be placed in Allen stirrups or in a frogleg position so that the surgeon has easy access to the vaginal area during the operation. A sponge stick or an EEA (end-to-end anastomosis) sizer (Fig. 43-4) can be placed in the vagina for manipulation of the apex if desired. A Foley catheter with a large (30-mL) balloon is placed in the bladder for drainage. Prophylactic perioperative antibiotics are generally used during this procedure.

2. A laparotomy is performed through a low transverse or midline incision, and the small bowel is packed into the upper abdomen. The sigmoid colon is packed, as much as possible, into the left pelvis. The ureters are identified bilaterally. If the uterus is present, a hysterectomy should be performed and the vaginal cuff closed. The depth of the cul-de-sac and the length of the vagina when completely elevated are estimated.

3. While the vagina is elevated cephalad using an EES sizer, the peritoneum over the vaginal apex is incised and the bladder dissected from the anterior vaginal wall (Figs. 43-5 and 43-6). The peritoneum over the posterior vaginal wall is incised into the cul-de-sac, longitudinally along the back of the vaginal wall (see Fig. 43-5). The vaginal apex then is elevated bilaterally with clamps or stay sutures.

4. As was previously mentioned, many different graft materials have been used, and many different techniques for fixation of the graft to the vagina have been described. The technique we use involves placement of a series of nonabsorbable sutures (usually 0) transversely in the posterior vaginal wall 1 to 2 cm apart (Fig. 43-7). All sutures are placed through the full fibromuscular thickness of the vagina but not in the vaginal epithelium. Biologic or synthetic grafts are prepared as in Figures 43-3 and 43-8. Sutures then are fed through the graft in pairs and tied (Fig. 43-9). The graft should extend at least halfway down the length of the posterior vaginal wall. The author prefers to attach a second piece of mesh or fascia to the upper part of the anterior vaginal wall (Fig. 43-10). This piece of fascia then is sewn to the posterior piece of fascia, which will be attached to the sacrum (see Fig. 43-10), or both pieces are taken back to the sacrum.

5. A longitudinal incision then is made over the peritoneum of the sacral promontory. The landmarks for this incision should be the right ureter and the medial edge of the sigmoid colon (Fig. 43-11). Very gentle dissection of the areolar tissue underneath the peritoneum is performed, usually in a blunt fashion, with a suction tip or a swab mounted on a curved forceps. The surgeon should be careful to palpate the aortic bifurcation and the common and internal iliac vessels and to mobilize the sigmoid colon to the left and the right ureter to the right, so that these structures can be avoided. The left common iliac vein is medial to the left common iliac artery

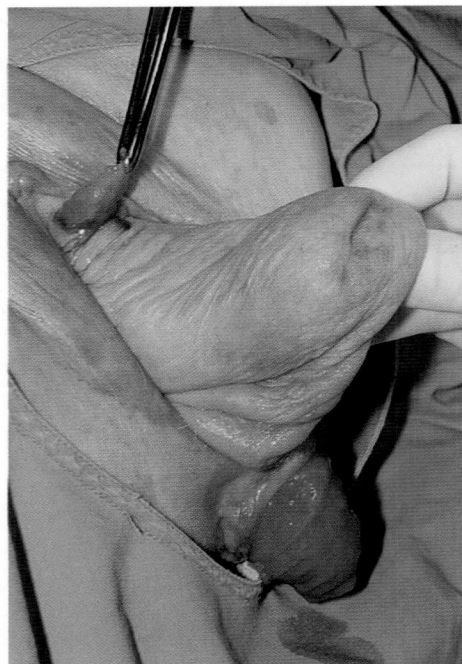

**FIGURE 43–1** This patient has very obvious weak pelvic connective tissue as indicated by urethral prolapse, uterine prolapse, and rectal prolapse. In the author's opinion, this patient would be an excellent candidate for abdominal sacral colpopexy.

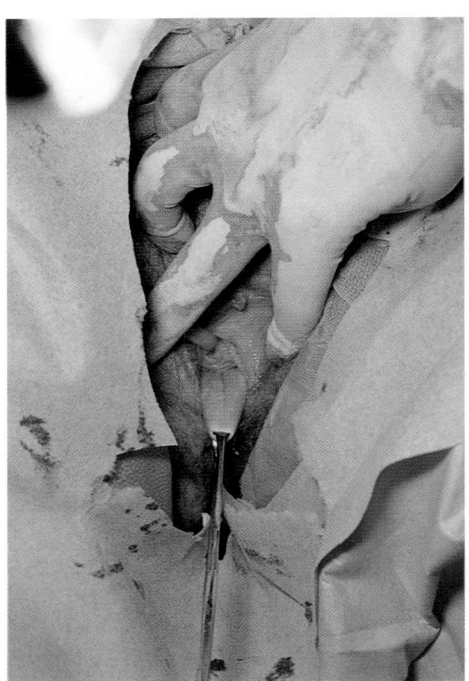

**FIGURE 43–2** This patient has had two previous anterior and posterior repairs. She now presents with a foreshortened vagina with an enterocele and vault prolapse. A properly performed abdominal sacral colpopexy will preserve her vaginal length and provide a durable repair.

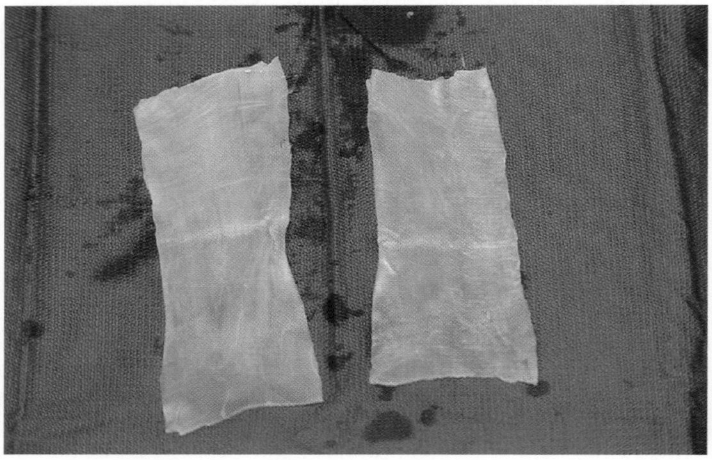

A

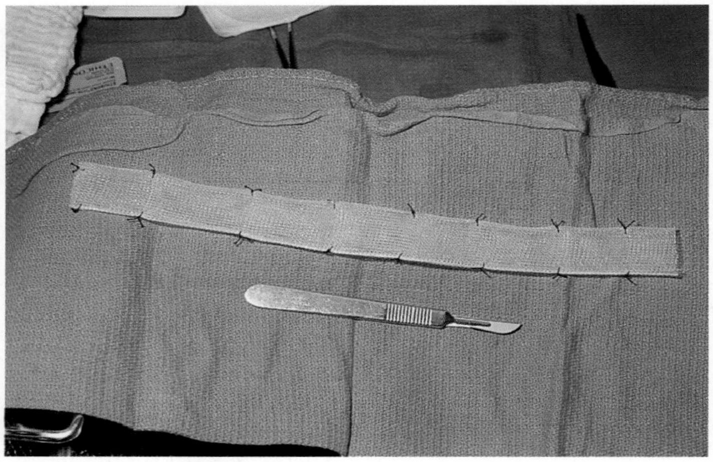

B

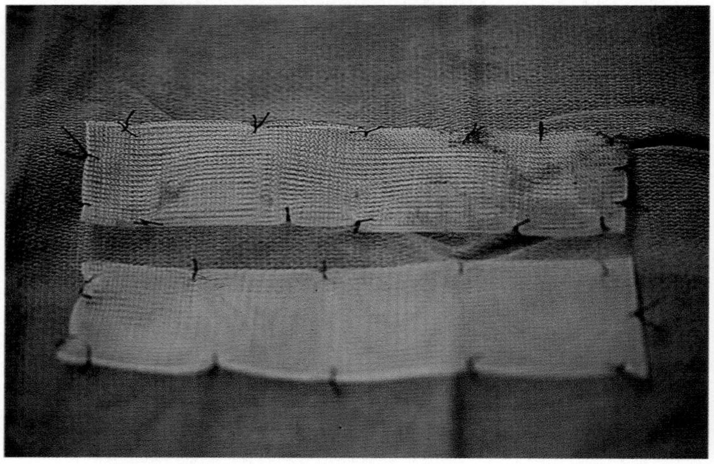

C

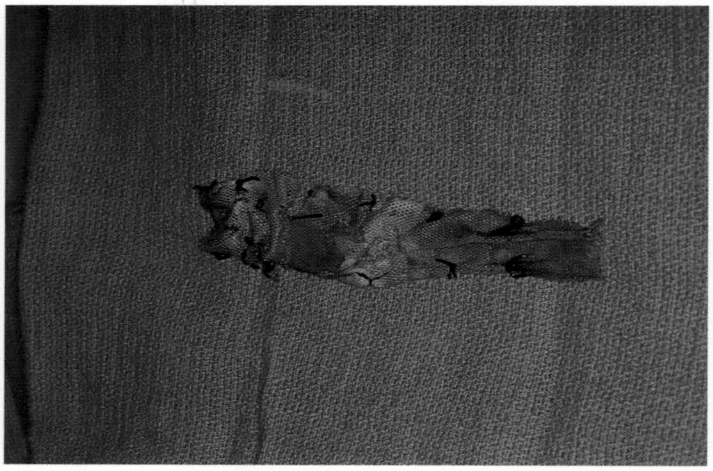

D

**FIGURE 43–3** Many different materials have been used for a graft to bridge the vagina to the sacrum. **A.** Fascia lata. **B.** Marlex mesh. **C.** Prolene mesh. **D.** Mersilene mesh, which has been removed transvaginally secondary to erosion.

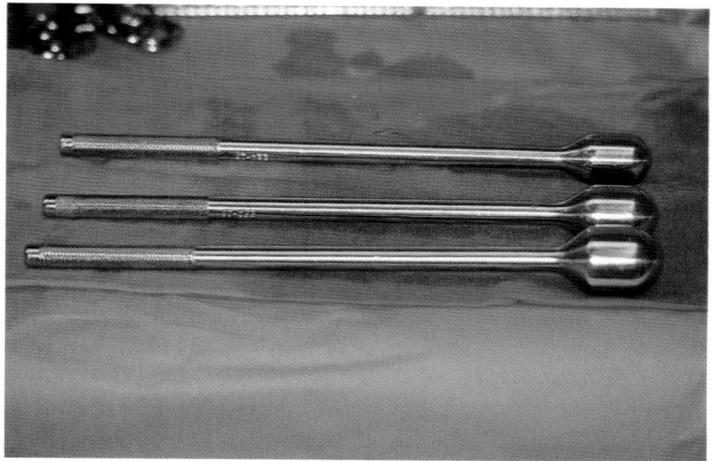

**FIGURE 43–4** EES sizers, used to elevate the vagina. They also can be placed in the rectum to assist in dissection of the vagina at the anterior rectal wall.

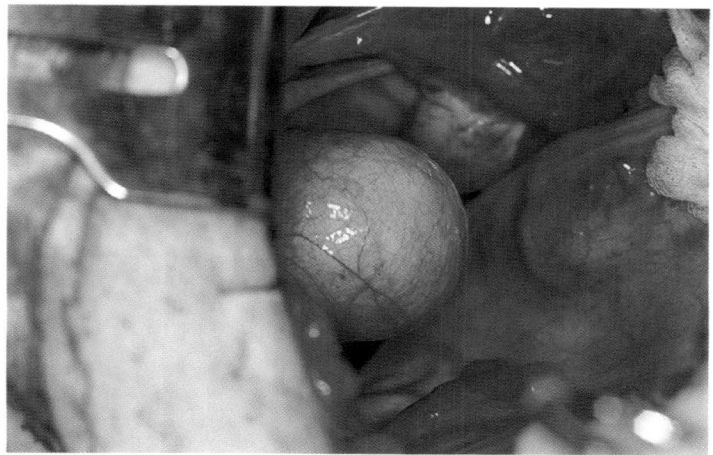

A

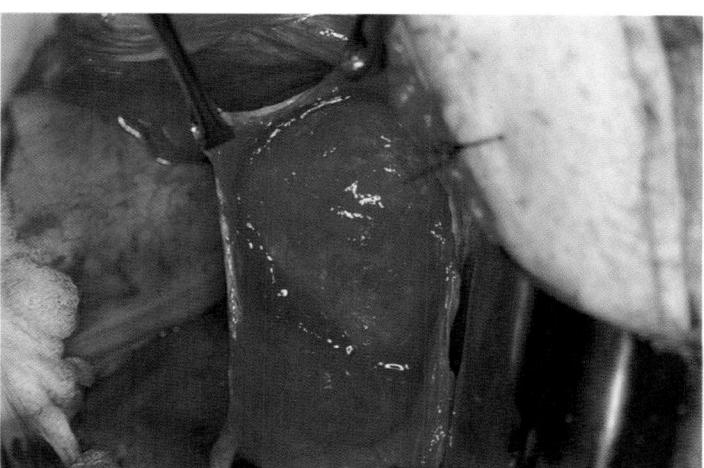

B

**FIGURE 43–5 A.** Elevated vagina, abdominal view. An EES sizer is used to elevate the vagina. **B.** The peritoneum over the vagina has been opened, exposing the vaginal cuff and anterior and posterior vaginal walls.

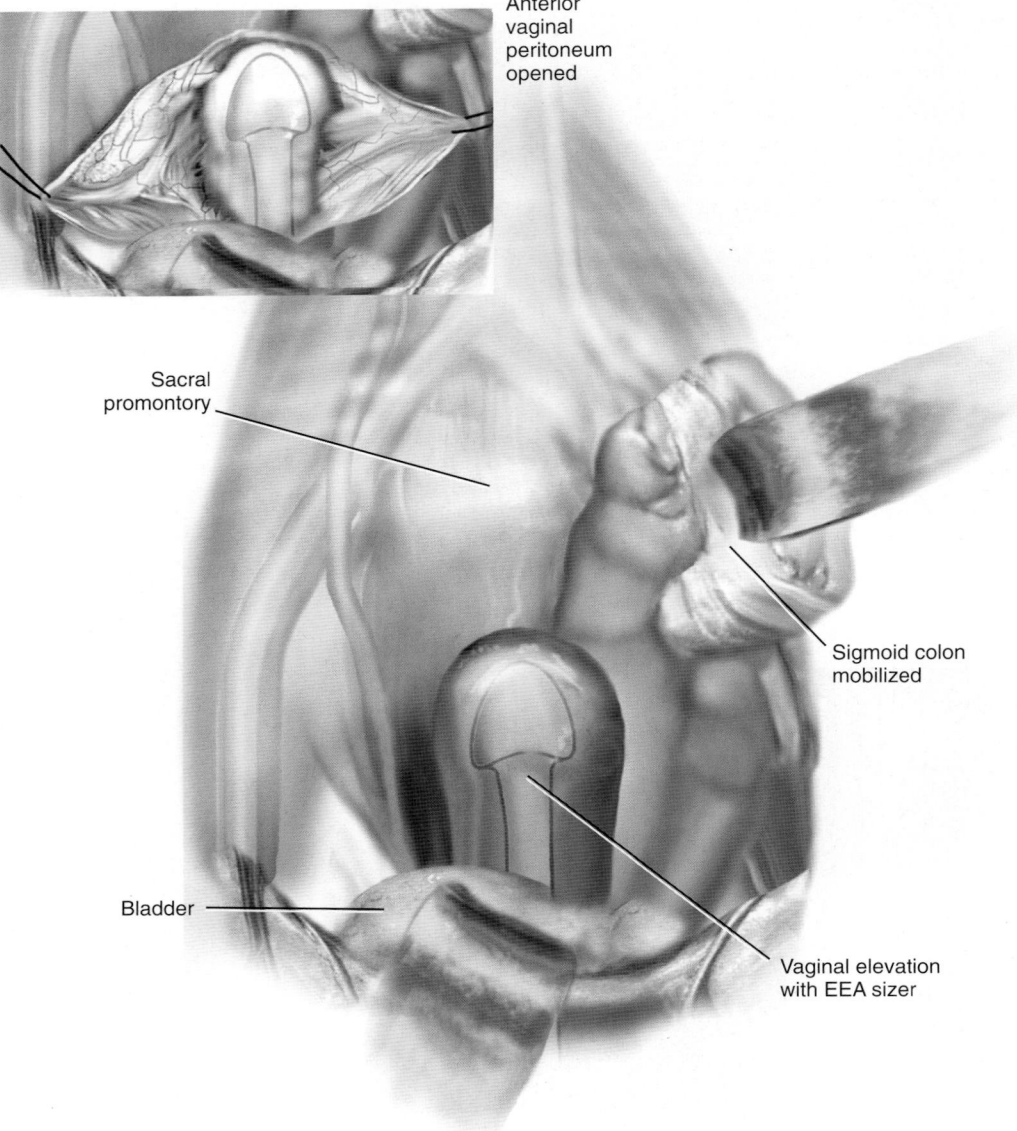

Anterior
vaginal
peritoneum
opened

Sacral
promontory

Sigmoid colon
mobilized

Bladder

Vaginal elevation
with EEA sizer

**FIGURE 43–6** The vagina is elevated with an EEA sizer. The peritoneum over the vagina is opened, exposing the muscular portion of the vaginal wall (**inset**).

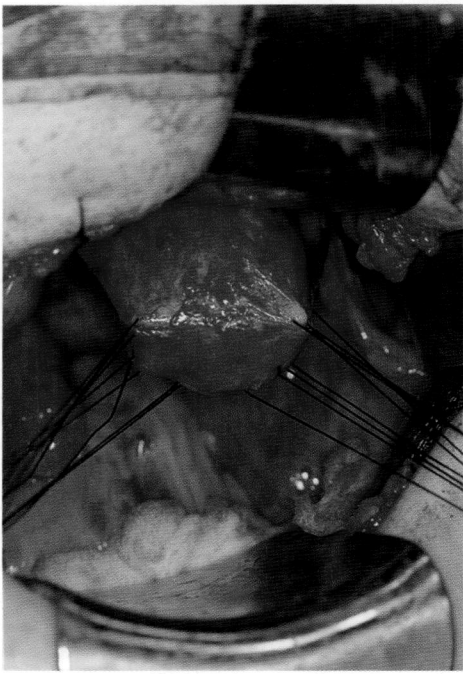

**FIGURE 43–7** A series of permanent sutures are taken through the full thickness of the posterior vaginal wall (excluding epithelium), starting at the apex.

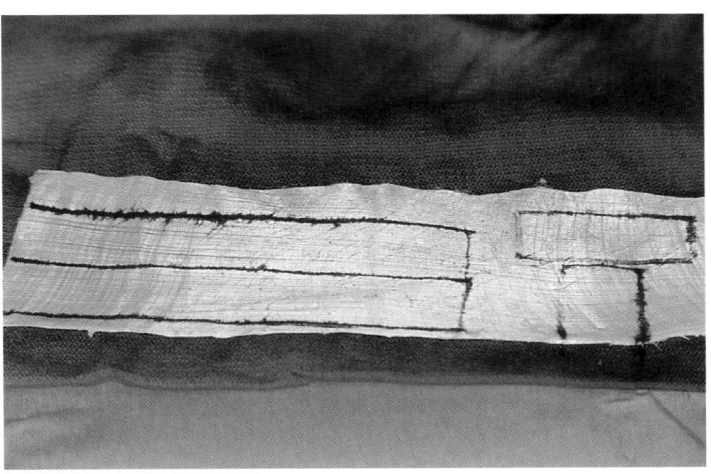

A

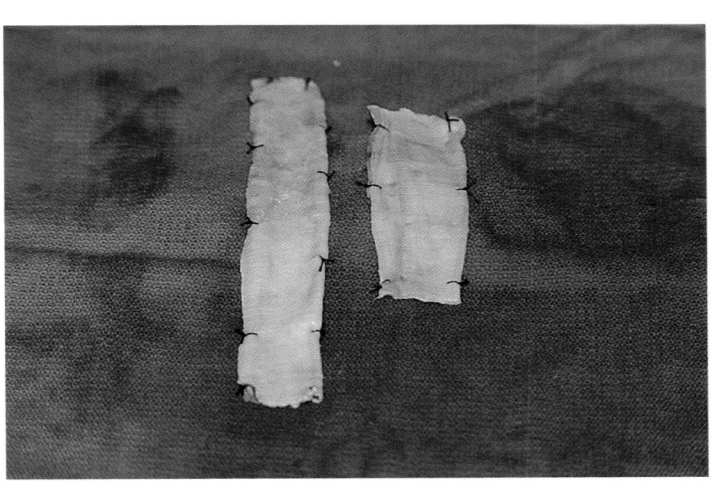

B

**FIGURE 43–8 A.** A large piece of cadaveric fascia lata. The marking pencil depicts how the fascia will be cut to prepare two pieces for colpopexy. **B.** The fascia has been cut and the pieces sutured to each other. A longer piece will extend from the posterior vaginal wall to the sacrum, and a shorter piece will attach to the anterior vaginal wall and the distal end of the longer piece.

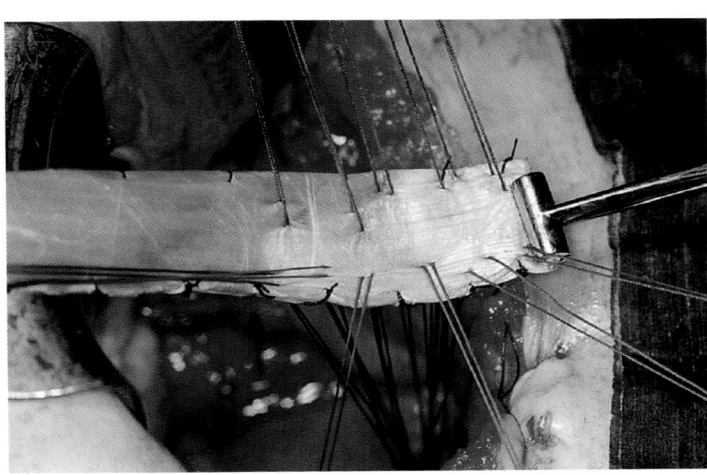

A

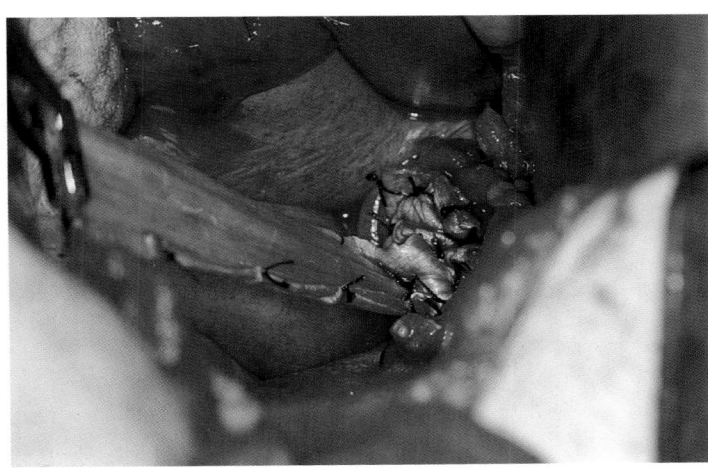

B

**FIGURE 43–9 A.** Passage of vaginal sutures through the cadaveric fascia lata. **B.** Sutures have been tied down, fixing the longer piece of fascia to the posterior vaginal wall.

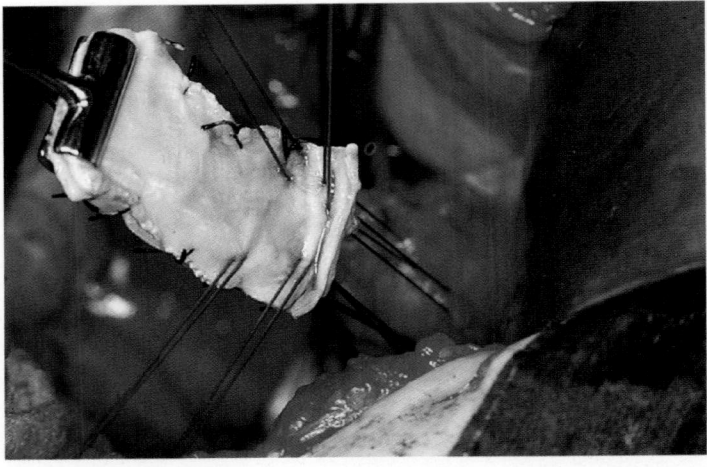

A

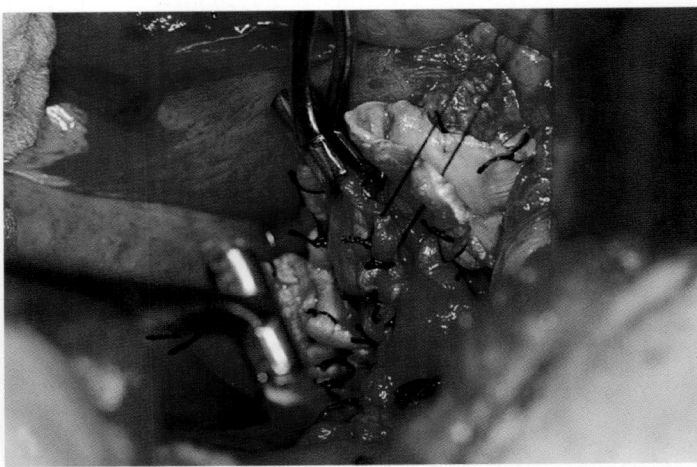

B

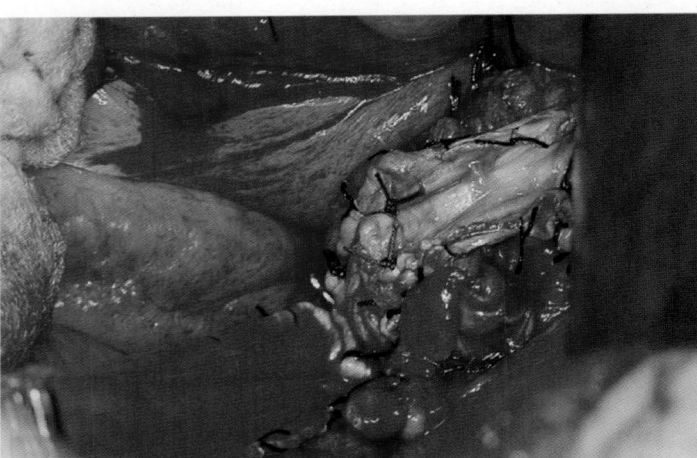

C

**FIGURE 43-10 A.** Sutures have been passed through the upper portion of the anterior vaginal wall and are brought up through the smaller piece of fascia. **B.** Sutures have been tied down and are being connected to the other piece of fascia. **C.** The two pieces of fascia lata have been attached to the upper part of the anterior vaginal wall and the posterior vaginal wall.

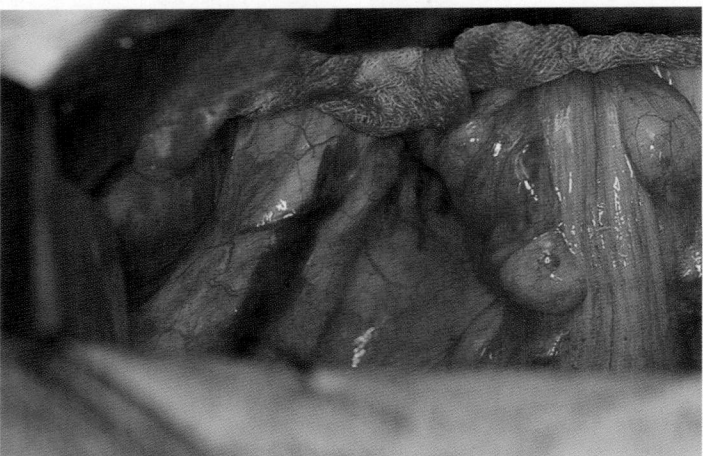

**FIGURE 43-11** An area of the sacral promontory is identified. The incision in the peritoneum should be well inside of the right ureter (*marked with purple marking pencil*) and the medial edge of the sigmoid colon.

and is particularly vulnerable to damage during this procedure. Very gentle dissection is performed down onto the sacral promontory to allow identification of the longitudinal ligament of the sacrum. The middle sacral vessels should also be easily visualized (Figs. 43–12 and 43–13). These vessels should be completely avoided. Ligation or cauterization should *never* be performed in the hope of preventing vascular injuries, as these vessels will retract into bone and create bleeding that is very difficult to control. If bleeding is encountered in this area, pressure should be applied on the bleeding vessels with a sponge stick. If this approach is unsuccessful, consideration can be given to the use of bone wax or the placement of sterile thumbtacks. The bony sacral promontory and the anterior longitudinal ligaments are directly visualized for approximately 4 cm with the use of blunt and sharp dissection through the subperitoneal fat. As dissection is carried caudad, special care should be taken to avoid the delicate plexus of presacral veins that is often present. With a stiff but small curved tapered needle, two to four 0 nonabsorbable sutures are placed through the anterior sacral longitudinal ligament over the sacral promontory (see Figs. 43–12 and 43–14). As few as one or two sutures can be placed, depending on the vasculature and exposure of the area. The graft should be trimmed to the appropriate length. The sutures then are fed through the graft and are paired and tied (Figs. 43–15 and 43–16). The appropriate amount of vaginal elevation should provide minimal tension and avoid undue traction on the vagina.

6. If necessary, a Moschcowitz or Halban procedure can be performed to obliterate the lower cul-de-sac, or the peritoneum over the cul-de-sac may be excised. Whatever technique is utilized, ultimately the graft must be extraperitonealized; thus the edges of the openings from the vagina to the sacrum are closed with a running delayed absorbable suture (Fig. 43–17).

7. When appropriate, retropubic urethropexy or paravaginal repair may be performed in conjunction with this procedure.

Also, posterior colporrhaphy and perineoplasty usually need to be performed to treat the remaining rectocele and perineal defect. A transvaginal midline repair of a cystocele may also be necessary.

Figure 43–18 reviews the entire procedure, utilizing synthetic mesh (Prolene mesh).

When these procedures fail and patients present with recurrent prolapse, most of the failures are due to inadequate attachment of the mesh to the vagina. For this reason, as was previously stated, it is very important to make sure that the mesh extends well down the posterior vaginal wall; we prefer to also attach a piece of mesh on the upper portion of the anterior vaginal wall. Figure 43–19 shows a patient who presented with recurrent vaginal vault prolapse after a previous abdominal sacral colpopexy performed with permanent mesh. On re-exploration, the previously placed mesh is found completely detached from the vagina (see Fig. 43–19). In this setting, the mesh was dissected away from the peritoneum and excised up to the level of the sacrum and then removed (Fig. 43–19B). The procedure was then repeated with a new synthetic mesh with a more aggressive fixation performed at the level of the vagina. Approximately 3% to 5% of patients who have undergone an abdominal sacral colpopexy with synthetic mesh will present with an erosion of the mesh into the vagina. Usually these patients will present with vaginal bleeding and a persistent malodorous vaginal discharge (Fig. 43–20). It has been our experience that most of these cases can be managed transvaginally by dissecting the mesh away from the vagina and utilizing aggressive downward traction on the mesh to assist in sharply dissecting it off the various tissues. The goal is to mobilize as much of the mesh as possible and then eventually cut the mesh as high up as possible. It is not necessary to remove the entire mesh. If a piece of mesh remains attached to the level of the sacrum and the distance between the distal end of that mesh and the closed vagina is sufficient, the potential for recurrent mesh erosion should be very low (Fig. 43–21).

UNIT 2 ■ SECTION G

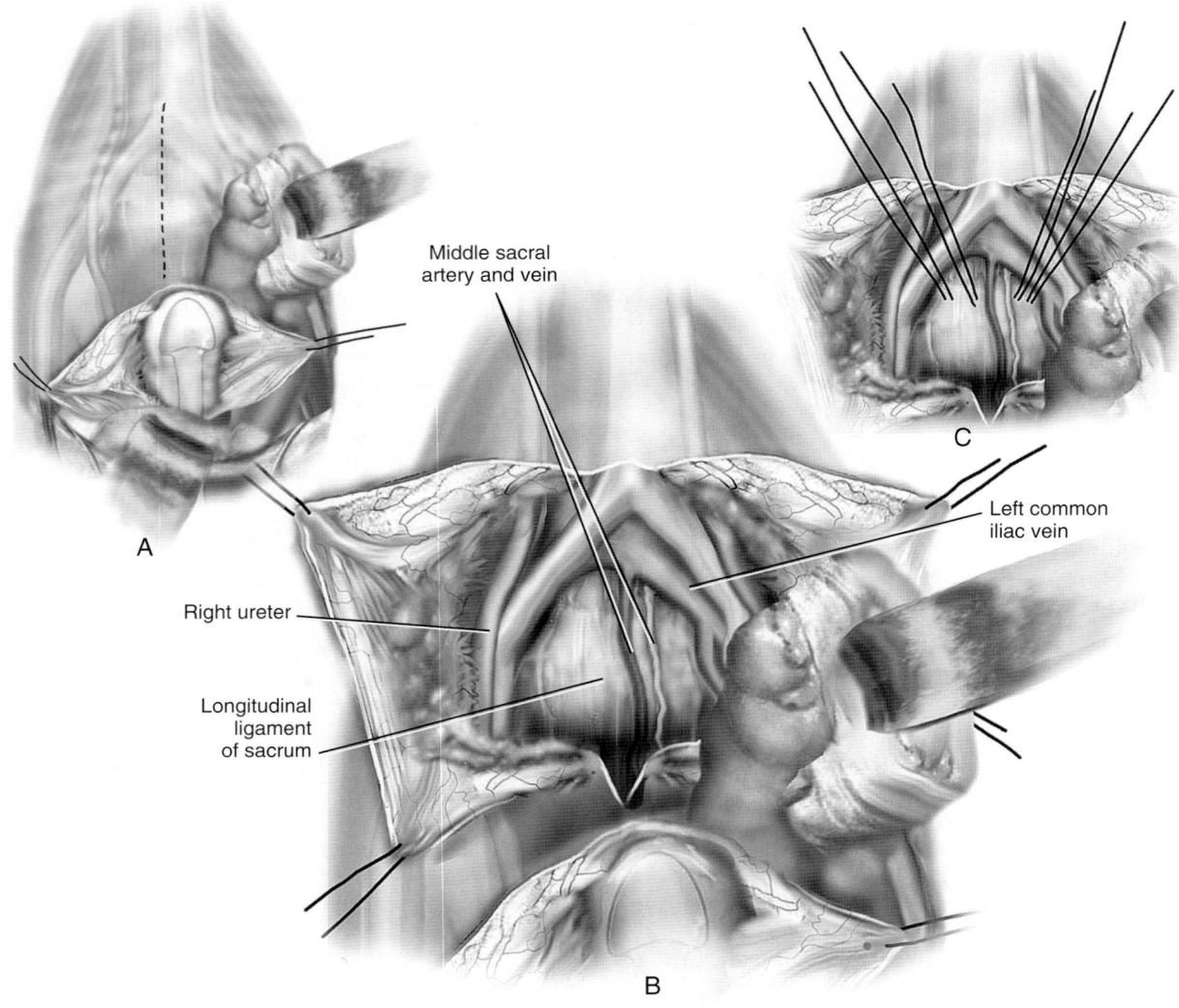

**FIGURE 43–12** Anatomy of the sacral promontory. **A.** Incision into the peritoneum. **B.** Dissection to the longitudinal ligament of the promontory. Note the vascularity of this area. **C.** Placement of permanent sutures through the longitudinal ligament of sacrum.

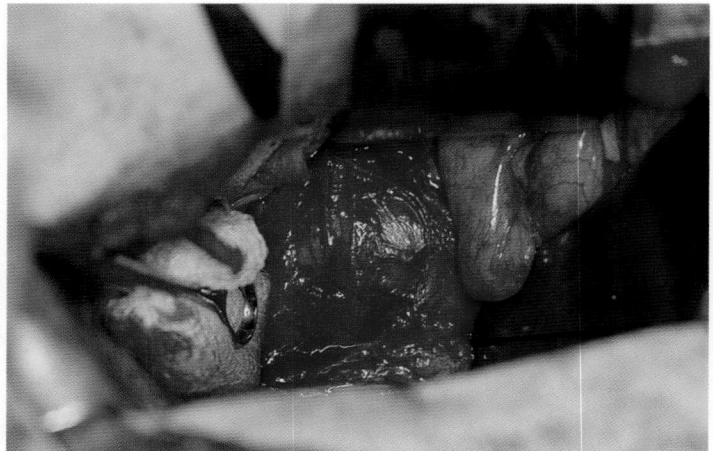

**FIGURE 43–13** Whitish-appearing periosteum of the sacral promontory.

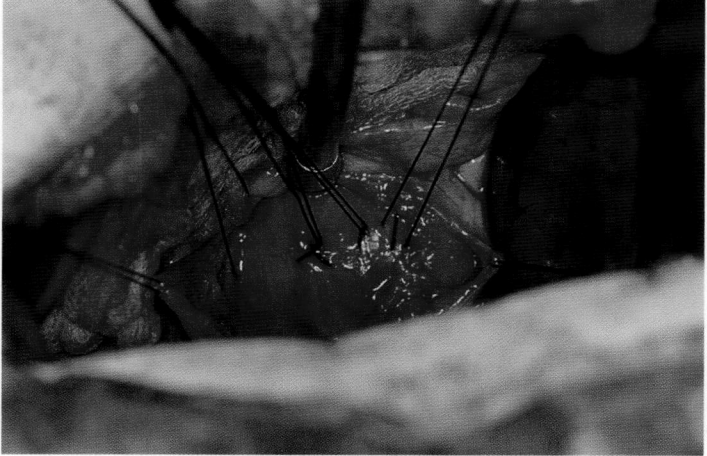

**FIGURE 43–14** Passage of permanent sutures through the longitudinal ligament of the sacrum.

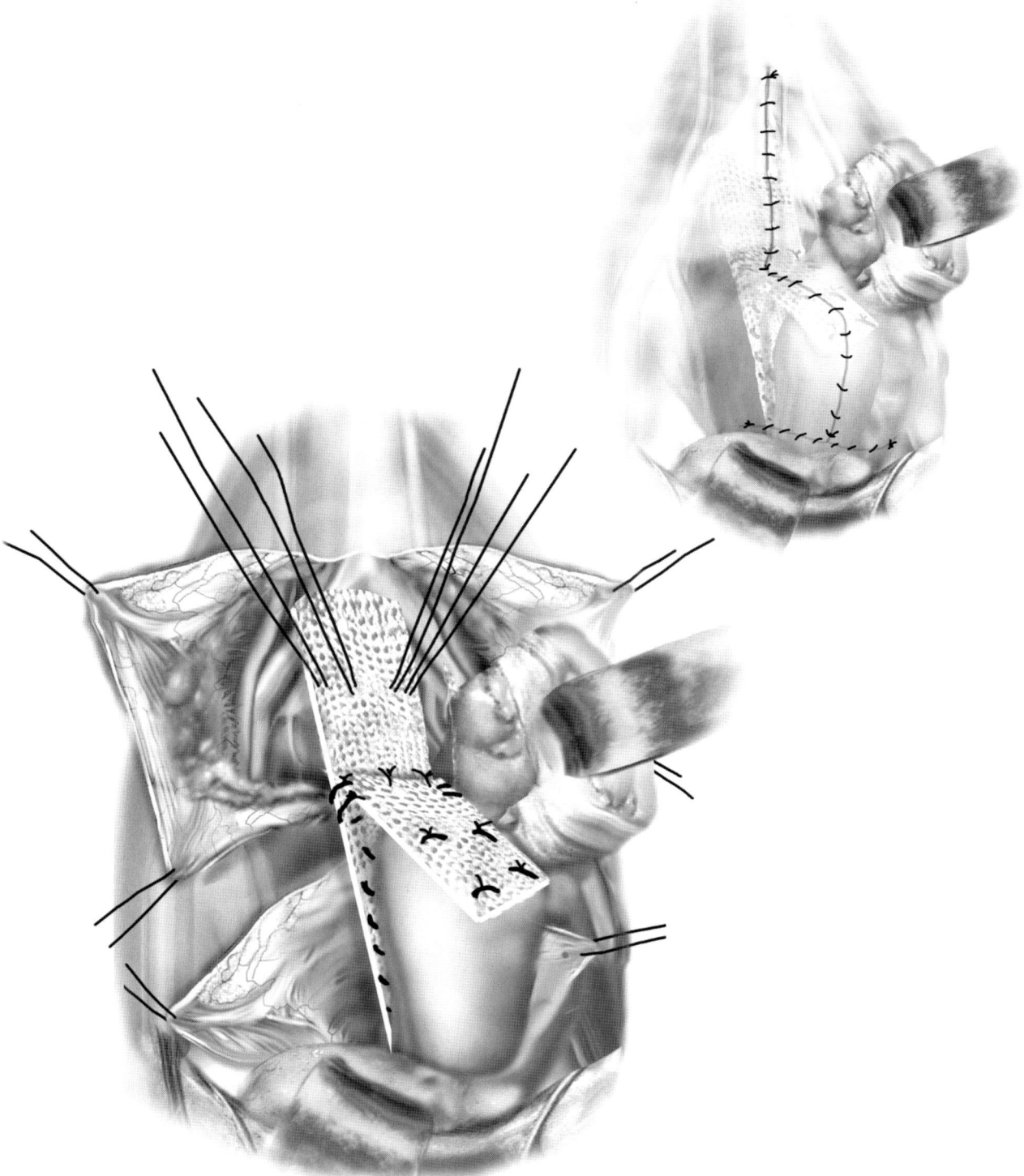

**FIGURE 43–15** Attachment of the mesh to the sacrum utilizing two pieces of mesh. Note that the anterior piece of mesh is fixed to the upper part of the anterior and extends much farther down the posterior vaginal wall. Both pieces are brought together and fixed to the sacral promontory. Closure of the peritoneum over the mesh is shown in the **inset**.

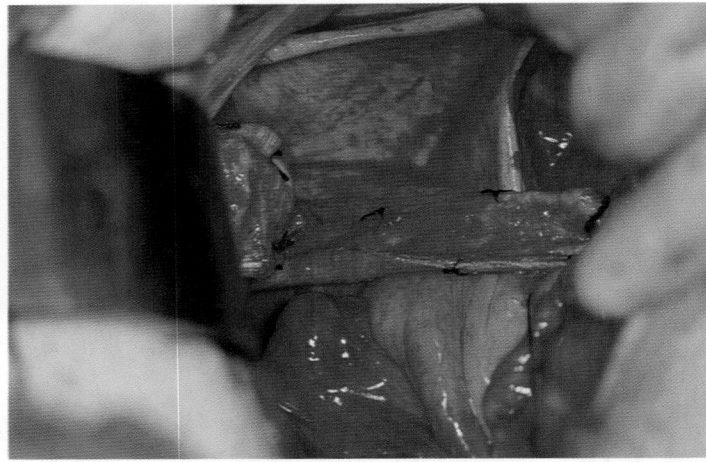

**FIGURE 43–16** Fascia lata has been attached to the sacrum. Note that the fascia should lay in the cul-de-sac under minimal tension.

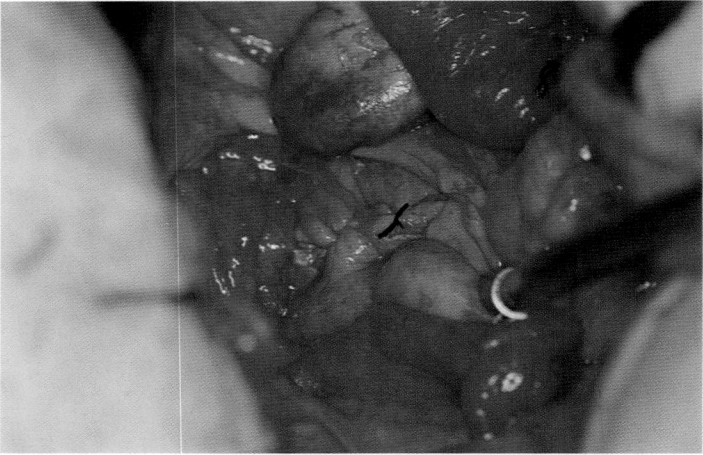

**FIGURE 43–17** The peritoneum has been closed over the mesh, thus placing the fascia retroperitoneally.

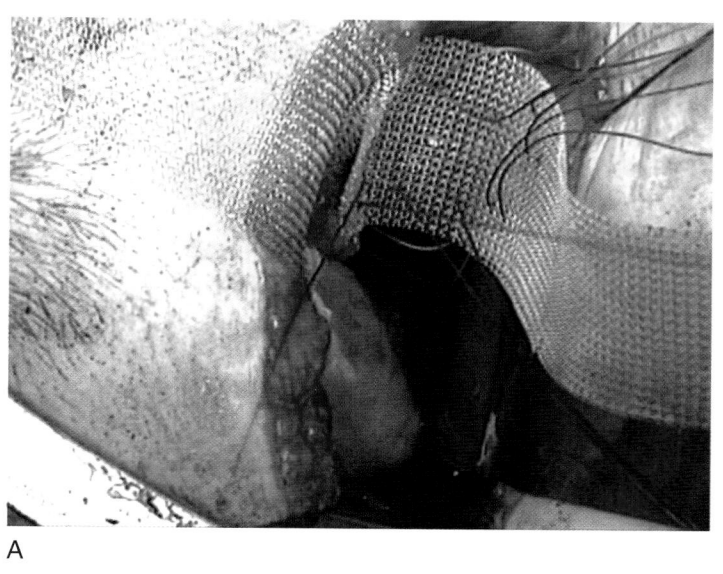

A

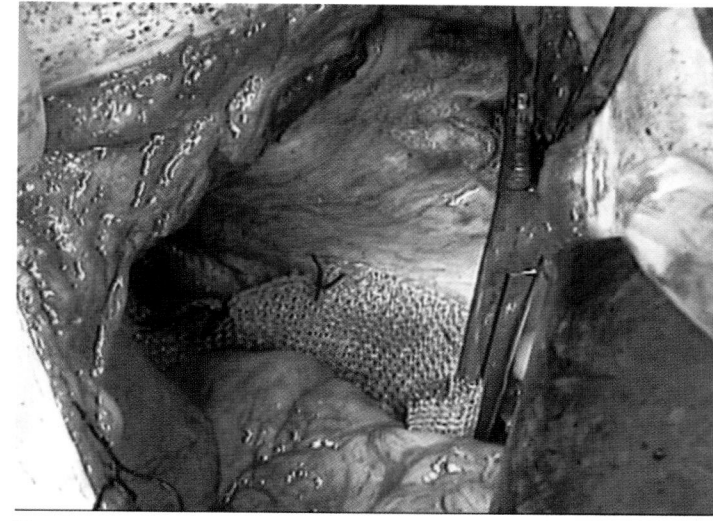

B

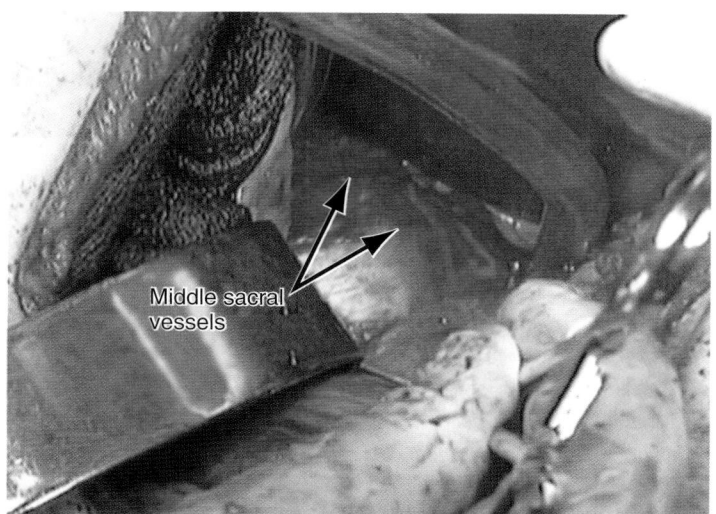

Middle sacral vessels

C

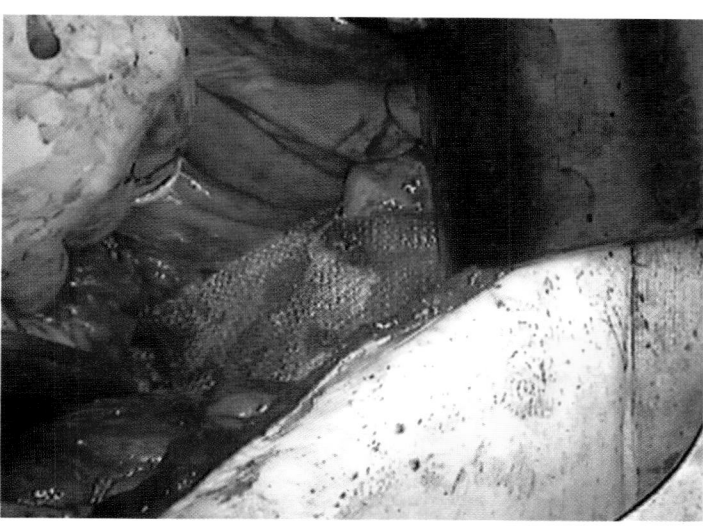

D

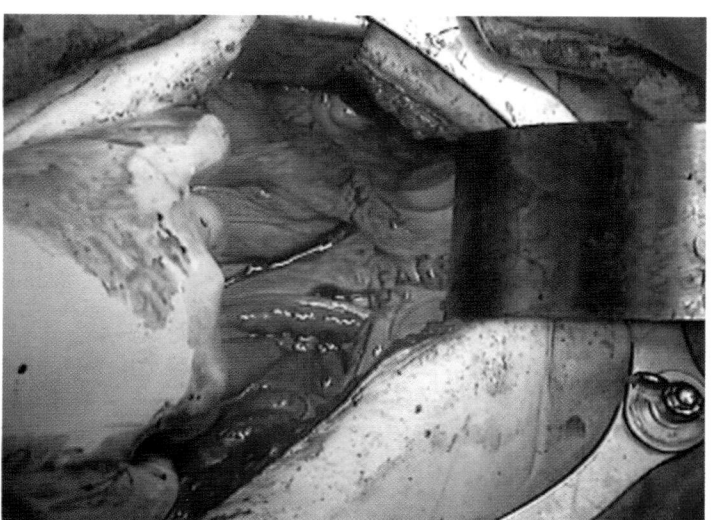

E

**FIGURE 43–18** Technique of abdominal sacral colpopexy performed with polypropylene mesh. **A.** A piece of polypropylene mesh is being attached with numerous permanent sutures to the anterior vaginal wall. **B.** A second piece of mesh has been attached down the posterior vaginal wall; the two meshes have been brought together in a Y fashion and will be attached to the sacral promontory. A Kelly clamp is used to determine the appropriate tension of the repair. In general, there should be little tension on the mesh, and it should sit very loosely in the cul-de-sac between the vagina and the sacral promontory. **C.** The area where the mesh will be attached at the level of the sacrum has been exposed. Again, this is at the level of the sacral promontory, and the sutures will be taken through the longitudinal ligament of the sacrum. Note that the middle sacral vessels are easily visualized at this level. **D.** The Prolene mesh has been attached at the level of the vagina and at the level of the sacrum. **E.** The peritoneum has been closed over the mesh, thus making the mesh an extraperitoneal structure. Note that with reperitonealization, most of the cul-de-sac is obliterated, as can be seen in this photograph.

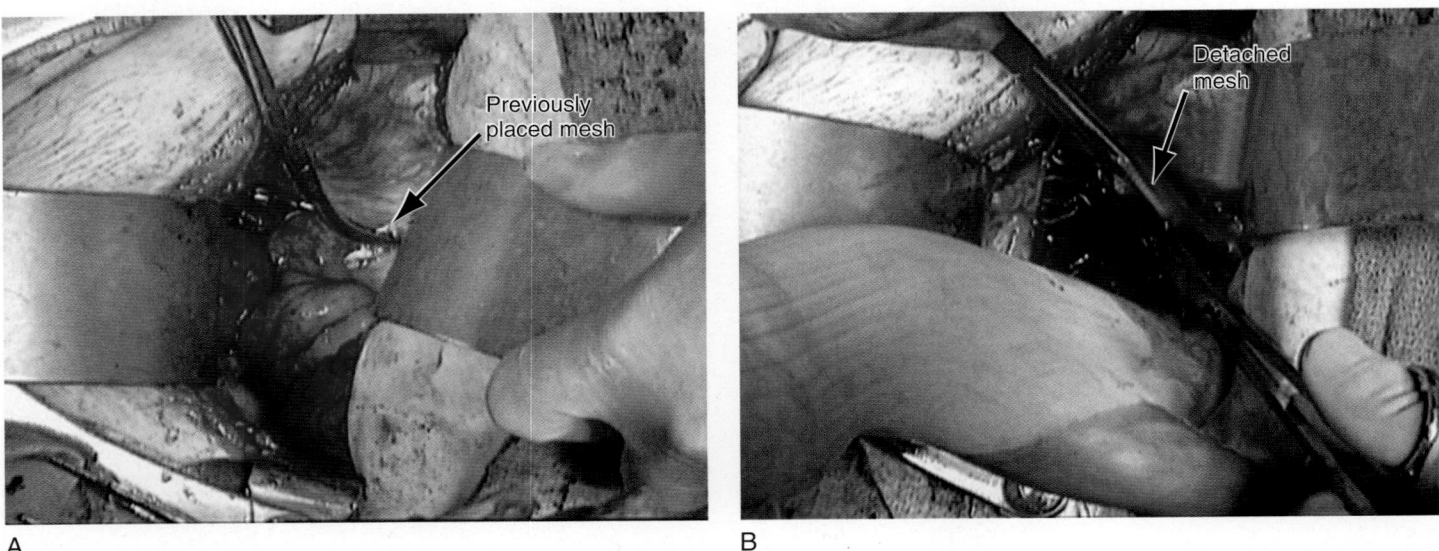

A                                    B

**FIGURE 43–19** A patient with recurrent prolapse who has previously undergone an abdominal sacral colpopexy. **A.** With re-exploration, the previously placed mesh is identified. As noted in this photograph, it is completely detached from the vagina. **B.** The detached mesh is dissected away from the tissue to be completely excised.

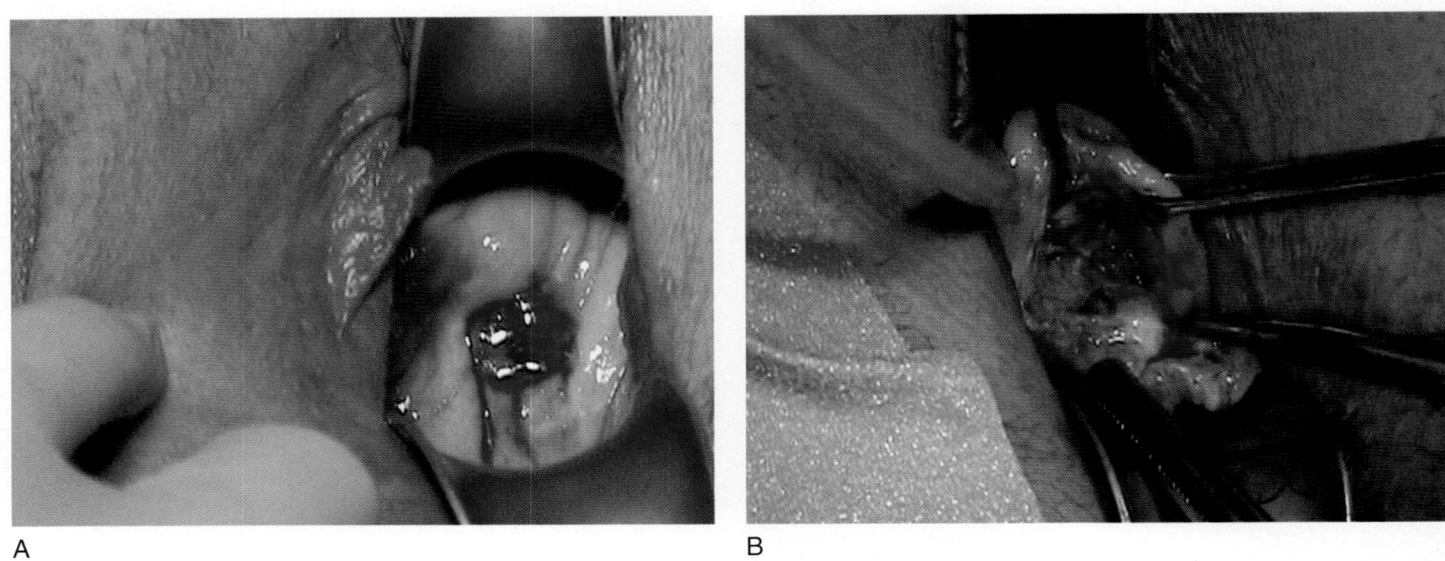

A                                    B

**FIGURE 43–20** A patient with an erosion of a synthetic mesh after a previous abdominal sacral colpopexy. **A.** Note that the mesh appears at the apex of the vagina. **B.** With sharp downward traction on the mesh, it is dissected away from the vaginal tissue, with the goal of completely dissecting the distal portion of the mesh and with aggressive downward traction excising it as high up as possible.

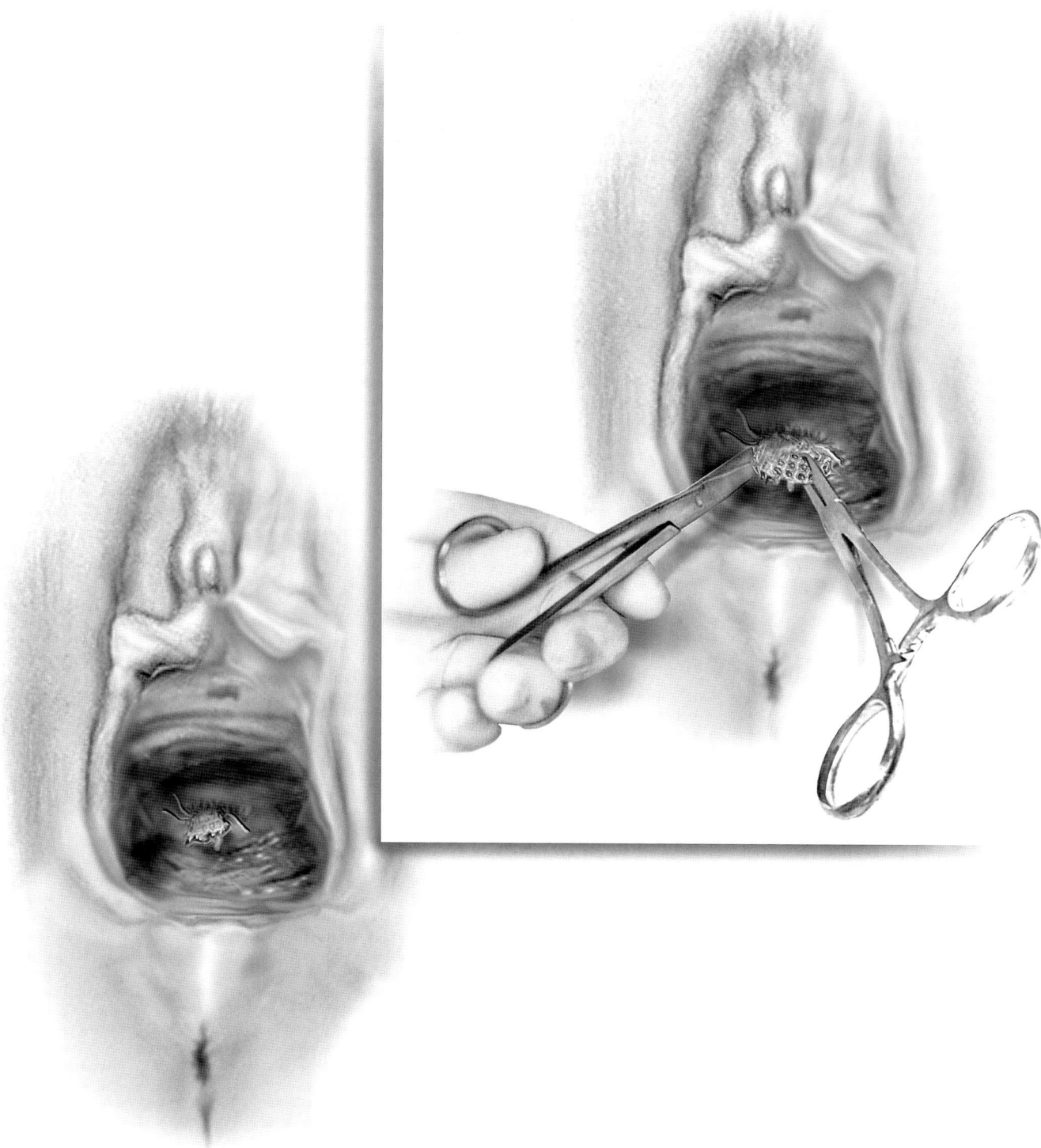

A

**FIGURE 43–21** The technique of vaginal removal of an eroded synthetic mesh after abdominal sacral colpopexy. **A.** Note that the mesh is identified and grasped (usually with Kocher-type clamps), with aggressive downward traction applied on the mesh.

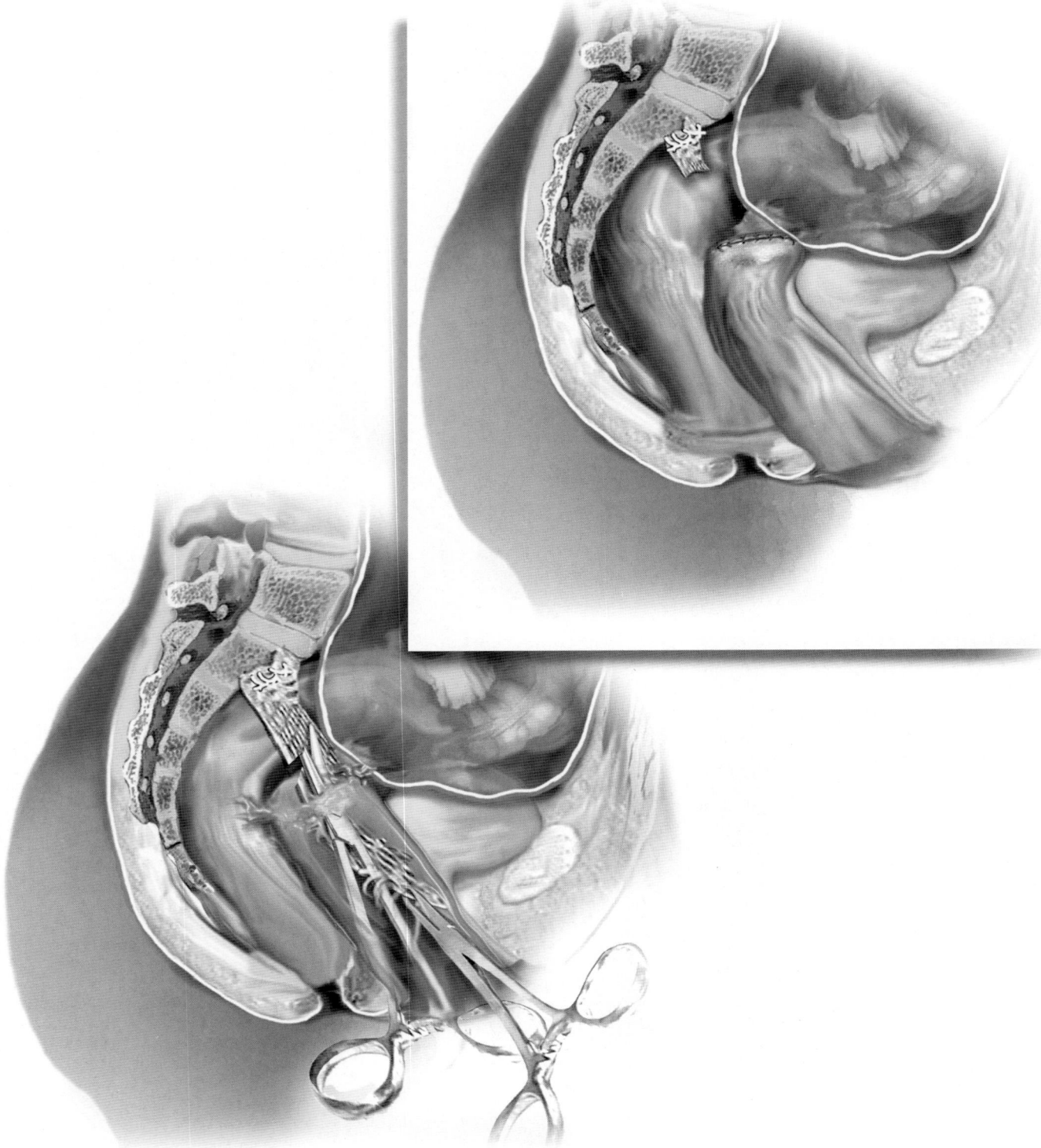

B

**FIGURE 43–21, cont'd  B.** The mesh is sharply dissected away from the vaginal tissue and any other tissue that it is adherent to, and, again with aggressive downward traction, it is excised as high up as possible. The goal is to create as much distance as possible between the closed vaginal cuff and the cut edge of the mesh (see **inset**).

# Cervical, Vaginal, Vulvar, and Perineal Surgery

# SECTION A

# Cervical Surgery

# CHAPTER 44

# Anatomy of the Cervix

*Michael S. Baggish*

The cervix uteri (cervix) is the lowest portion of the uterus (Fig. 44–1). The cervix consists of roughly equal supravaginal and vaginal portions. The part of the cervix that protrudes into and can be viewed from the vaginal aspect measures 2 cm (average) in length (Fig. 44–2). The supravaginal portion measures 1.5 cm (average) in length. Overall, the entire cervix in the nonpregnant, menstruating woman measures 3.5 cm in length and 2 cm in diameter. During the postmenopausal period or with prolapse, the relative length of the cervix may increase (Fig. 44–3A, B). Similarly, after cerclage, the relative length of the cervix may appear on ultrasound measurement to substantially increase (Fig. 44–4A, B). This apparent increase is undoubtedly due to the addition of a portion of the isthmus into the suture. As the cervix is viewed via an opened speculum, it is cylindrical in appearance with a central opening, the external os. The latter measures 3 to 5 mm in diameter (nulliparous) and up to 1 cm or more in a multiparous woman (Fig. 44–5). The reflection of the upper portion of the vagina (vault) around the protruding cervix forms recesses or fornices (anterior, posterior, right, and left lateral) (Fig. 44–6).

Most of the cervix is covered with multilayered squamous epithelium and has a pink appearance. The endocervical canal is lined by a single layer of glandular mucus-secreting epithelium and has a red coloration (Fig. 44–7). The endocervical canal is narrow (0.5 cm) and extends from the vaginal end (external os) to the point of entry into the lower portion of the uterine cavity (internal os) (Fig. 44–8A through C). The mucous epithelium is thrown into numerous folds and clefts that extend into the underlying stroma (collagen) for varying depths (Fig. 44–9). The purpose of the folds and clefts is to greatly increase the surface area of the endocervical canal without actually increasing its overall length (Fig. 44–10). Unfortunately, a popular misnomer has ingrained itself irreversibly in gynecologic literature and usage: "endocervical glands." These are not glands but rather an extension of the single-cell–layered endo-cervical canal. Several studies have shown that the endocervical mucosa projects 3 mm into the underlying stroma but may plunge as deep as 6 mm (Fig. 44–11A, B).

The cervix is endowed with a copious blood supply via the descending branch of the uterine artery and the vaginal artery. This accounts for its ability to miraculously heal and to survive the worst kind of iatrogenic insults.

During pregnancy, the cervix increases in length and even more so in diameter as a result of hyperplasia of both cellular and stromal elements. The greatly increased blood supply lends a dusky or bluish appearance to the tissue, as well as a mushy, soft feeling (Fig. 44–12). As a result of the high levels of estrogens, the endocervical mucosa everts onto the exposed surface of the cervix. In actuality, this is a process of metaplasia in which the reserve cells are programmed to form mucous cells rather than squamous cells.

The nerves supplying the cervix emanate from the vicinity of the sacral end of the uterosacral ligaments. This rather ill-defined combination of tissues constitutes the extra blood and vascular matter at the bottom of the pararectal space, which includes fat, lymphatics, nerves, and connective tissue. It is within this area that the otherwise well-defined uterosacral ligaments terminate.

The inferior hypogastric plexus supplies fibers to this plexus. In addition, fibers are supplied via the sacral roots, and sympathetic input occurs via the lumbar and sacral prevertebral chain (see Unit I, Section A, Chapters 1 and 2).

It is curious that the cervix and the vagina have few pain receptors compared with external skin surfaces or, for that matter, the mucosa of the oral cavity. However, the cervix is well endowed with pressure and temperature receptors. The paracervical plexus and ganglia (Frankenhaüser's ganglion) may be stimulated via the lateral vaginal fornices to elicit a pleasant sensation with light pressure or a very unpleasant pain elicited by greater pressure.

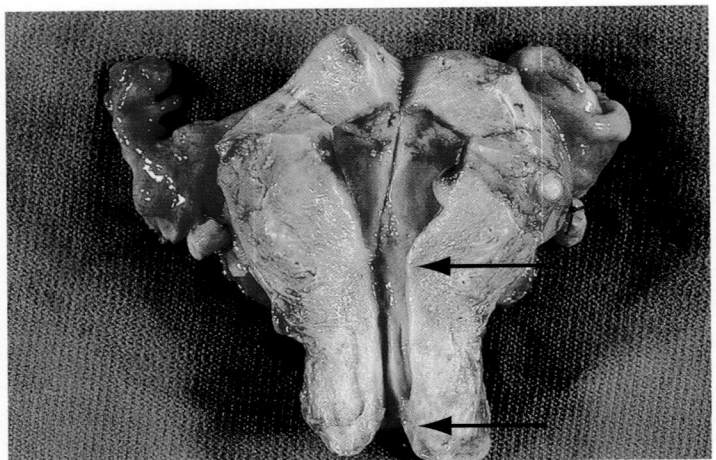

**FIGURE 44–1** The entire uterus is shown in an opened format. The two arrows indicate the entire cervical portion (length), including supravaginal and vaginal portions.

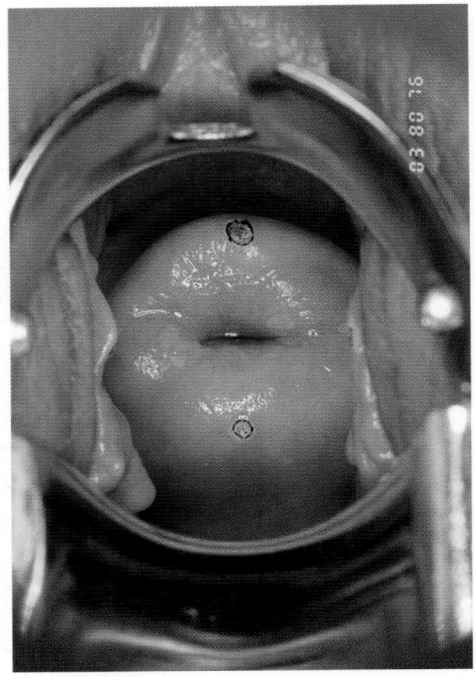

**FIGURE 44–2** The portio vaginalis of the cervix measures 2 cm in diameter and 2 to 2.5 cm in length. The cylindrical configuration is obvious. Imprints have been placed with a laser on the anterior and posterior lips of the cervix. The external os is midway between these points.

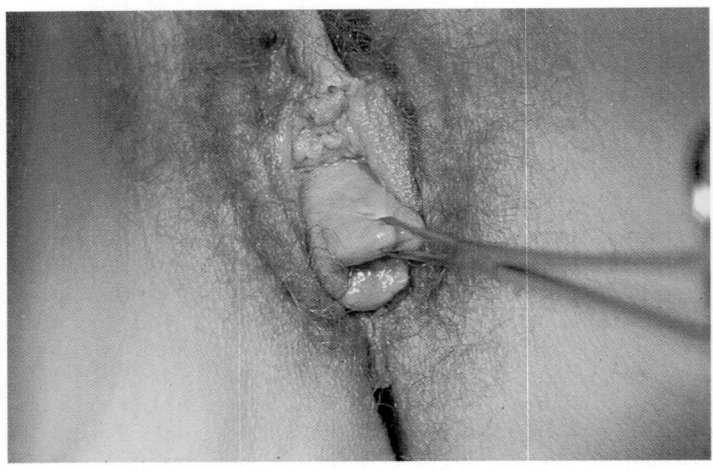

A

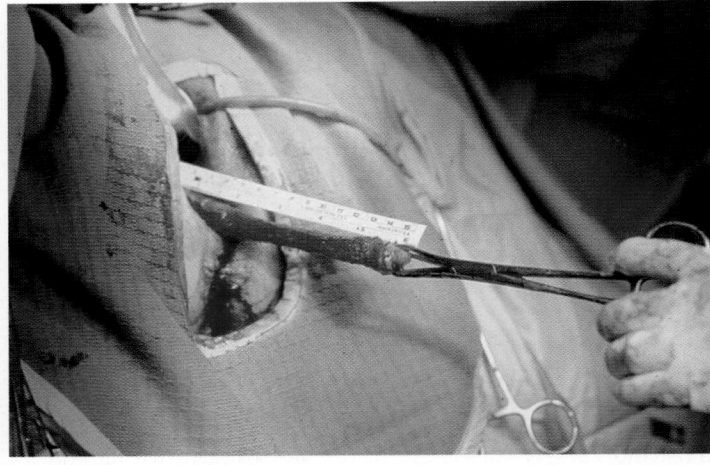

B

**FIGURE 44–3 A.** A greatly elongated cervix is not uncommon in elderly women with prolapse. **B.** At surgery, the actual length of this long cervix can be appreciated and quantified. Note that the yellowish skin color is due to the povidone-iodine prep.

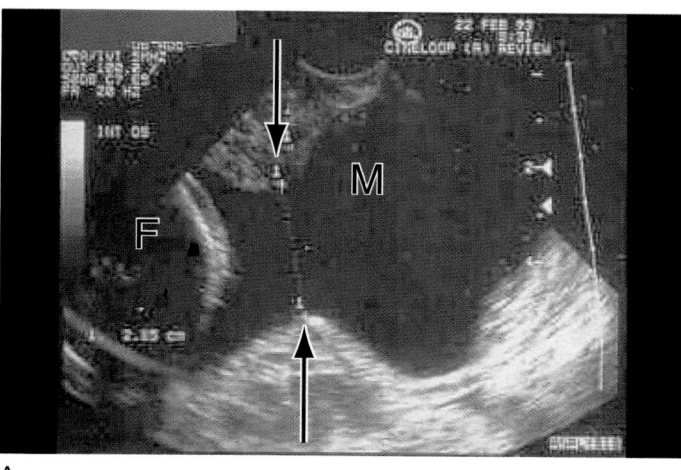 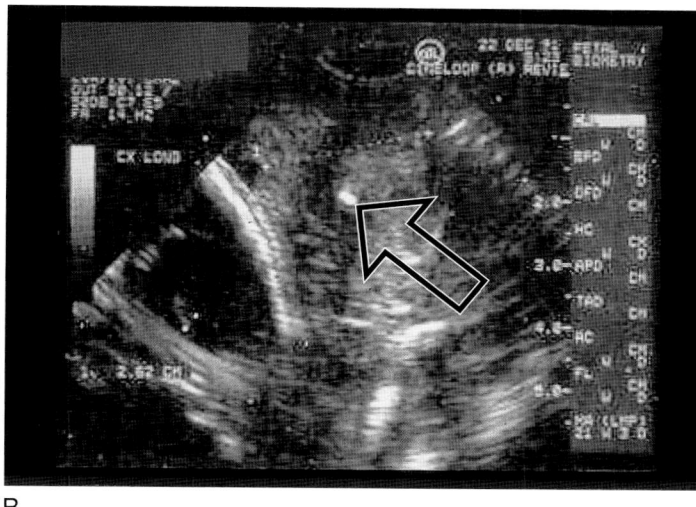

A                                 B

**FIGURE 44–4  A.** Ultrasonic view of a cervix detailing relative lengths before and after cervical suture placement. The cervix is less than 1 cm in length. The dilated os is at the arrows. Membranes (M) have prolapsed into the vagina. The fetal head is seen at F. **B.** The arrow points to the knot (*white density*) of the cervical stitch. Note that the length of the cervix has increased after placement of the suture.

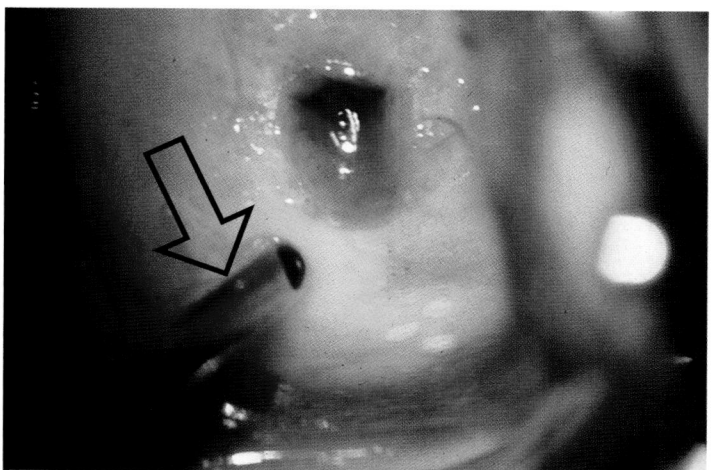

**FIGURE 44–5**  A contact hysteroscope measuring 6 mm in diameter (*arrow*) is positioned to enter the endocervical canal. Note that the canal is "more open" at the time of ovulation. The red tissue is mucous epithelium, which lines the endocervical canal.

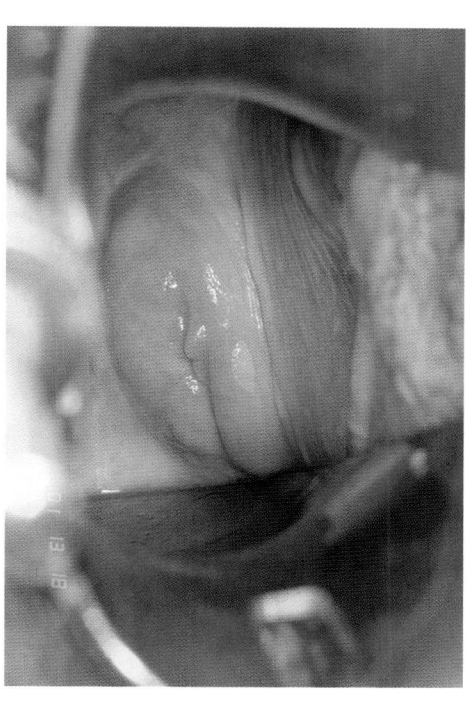

**FIGURE 44–6**  The vaginal fornices are created by the protrusion of the cervix through the vaginal vault. This picture clearly illustrates the anterior fornix and the left lateral fornix.

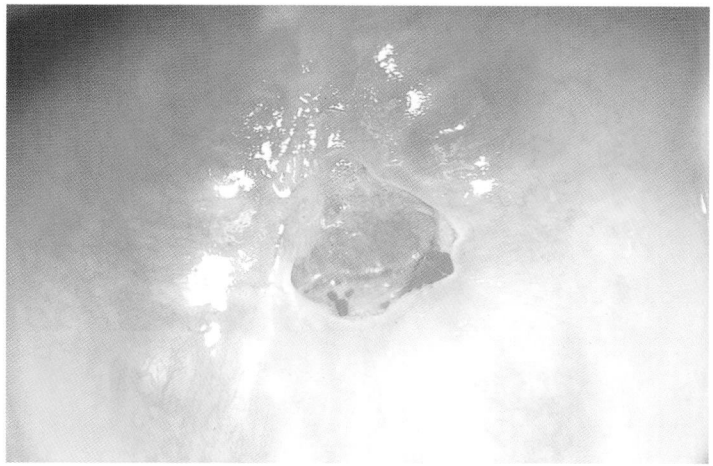

**FIGURE 44–7**  Close-up view of the cervix showing the squamocolumnar junction. The pink ectocervix sharply contrasts with the red endocervix. The color differences can be explained by the filtration of light between the surface mucosa and the underlying stromal blood vessels. The ectocervix consists of 20 to 40 layers of squamous cells versus the single layer of endocervical mucous epithelium.

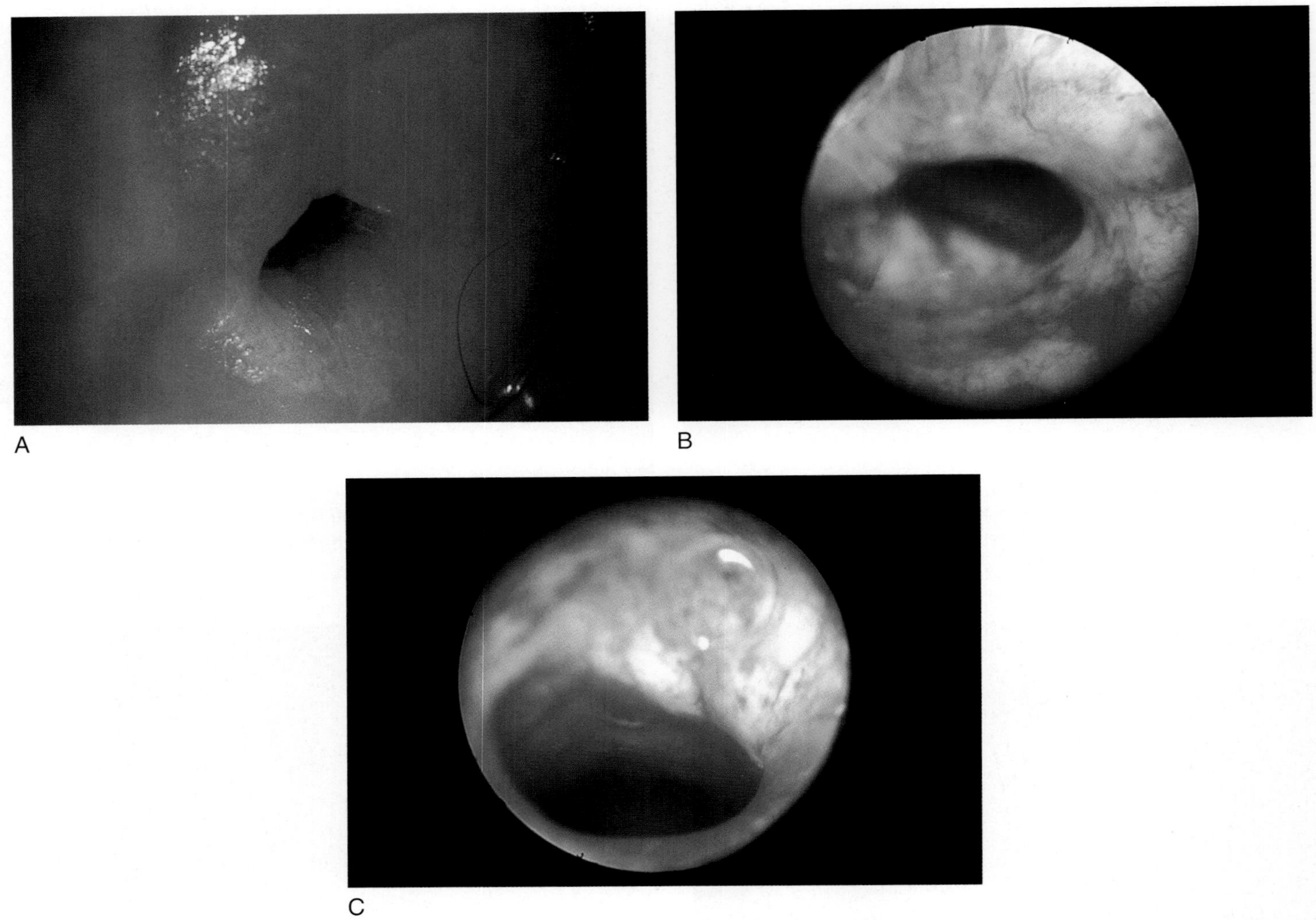

A

B

C

**FIGURE 44–8  A.** Close-up of the entry point to the cervical canal (external os). **B.** Hysteroscopic view within the endocervical canal looking upward at the internal os. **C.** Close-up view at the internal os looking into the lower portion of the uterine corpus (infundibular portion).

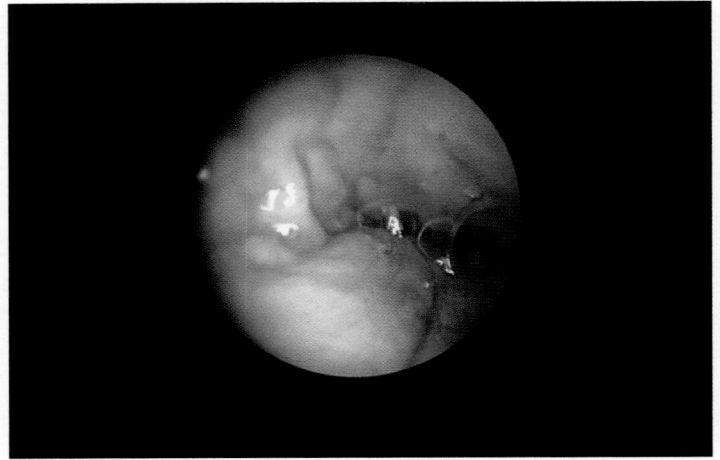

**FIGURE 44–9** Panoramic carbon dioxide ($CO_2$) hysteroscopic view of the endocervical canal. Note the numerous folds and clefts.

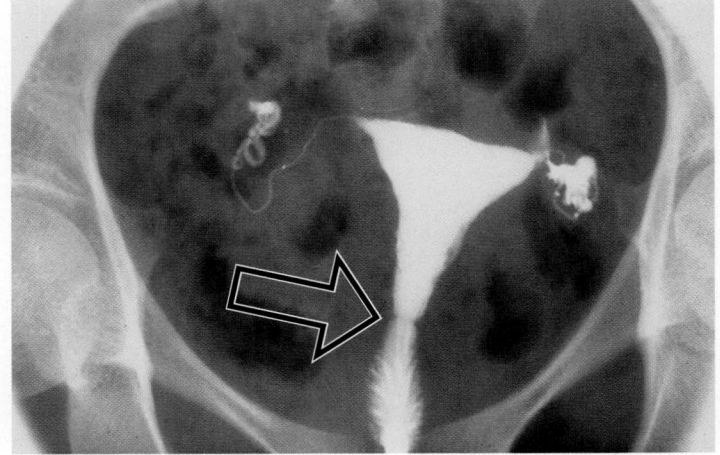

**FIGURE 44–10** Hysterosalpingographic detail of the cervix. The internal os is noted at the constriction points (*arrow*). The endocervical clefts create a feather-like pattern as a result of their extension into the underlying stroma.

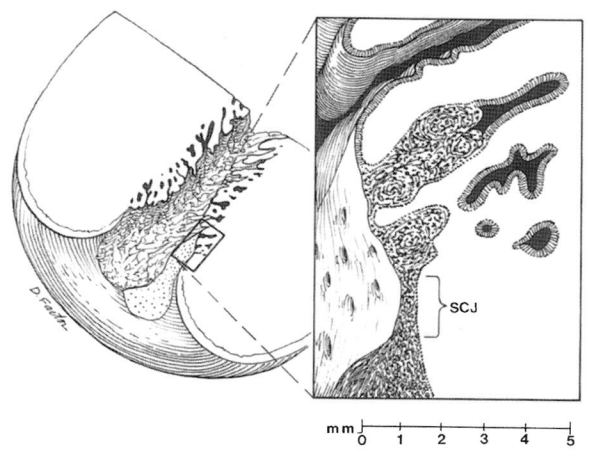

A

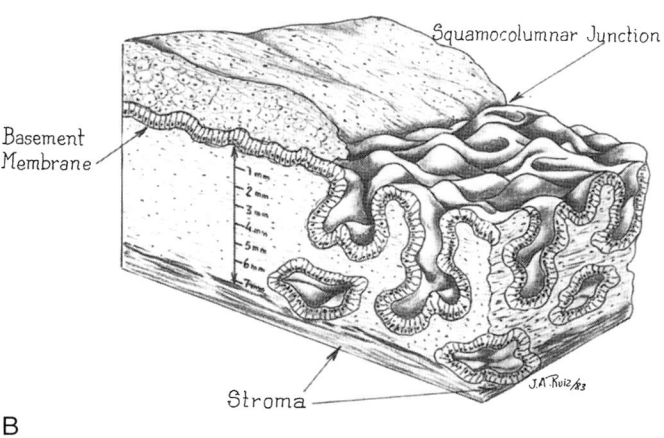

B

**FIGURE 44–11 A.** Schematic representation of the distribution and geography of the endocervical clefts. The **inset** shows a detail of the endocervical mucosal surface and the underlying stroma. Note the extent (millimeter rule) of the depth to which the endocervical clefts penetrate the collagenous stroma. **B.** This three-dimensional rendering further depicts the meandering endocervical canal. The deepest "gland" penetrates the stroma to a depth of 6 mm.

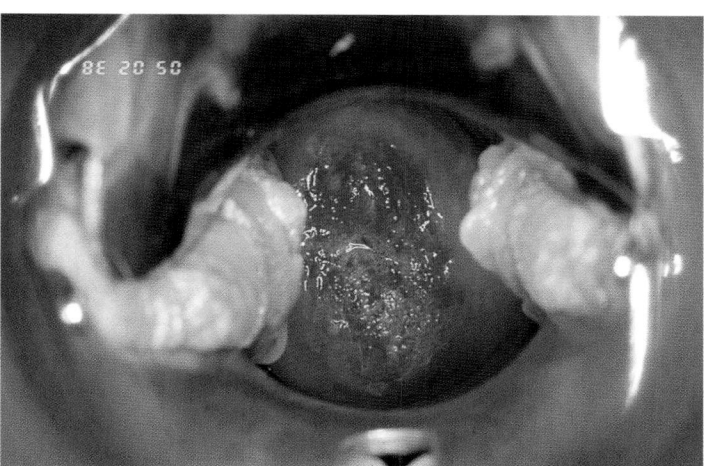

**FIGURE 44–12** The pregnant cervix is enlarged, bluish (cyanotic), soft, and everted. The hypervascularity must be considered and managed during any surgical procedure undertaken during the pregnant condition.

# CHAPTER 45

# Cervical Biopsy, Endocervical Curettage, and Cervical Biopsy During Pregnancy

*Michael S. Baggish*

## Cervical Biopsy

All cervical biopsies should be colposcopically directed. There is no reasonable excuse for not performing a directed biopsy in the 21st century. The abnormal transformation zone is identified by applying acetic acid 3% to 4% to the cervix with a cotton swab and then observing the whitish color that develops in the atypical area with or without vascular abnormalities (Fig. 45–1A, B). The areas selected for biopsy are based on the severity observed colposcopically. Analgesia usually is not required if the biopsy is performed in a timely fashion and if the biopsy forceps are suitably sharp. For patients anxious about the biopsy, 1% lidocaine may be injected directly into the cervix using a $1\frac{1}{2}$-inch 25- to 27-gauge needle. Most patients experience a pinching or light cramping sensation at the moment of biopsy.

The biopsy forceps are manipulated to the operative site by utilizing the magnification of the colposcope to guide it to the appropriate location (Fig. 45–2A, B). The large teeth of the forceps stabilize the cervix so that its rounded surface will not slip away from the clamp (Fig. 45–3). The jaws are closed, and with a click a piece of tissue is cut away from the cervix and is held within the jaws of the biopsy clamp (Fig. 45–4). The specimen is handed off, and a cotton-tipped applicator soaked with Monsel's solution (ferric subsulfate) is thrust into the crater at the biopsy site, held in place, and then slowly rolled to left and right until all bleeding stops (Fig. 45–5A, B).

If bleeding does not stop following the application of Monsel's solution, or if pulsatile bleeding is observed, a 3-0 Vicryl figure-of-8 suture should be placed while the magnification of the colposcope is used to accurately locate the stitch. A long, straight needle holder or a Haney needle holder should be used for this procedure (Fig. 45–6).

Alternatively, a biopsy may be performed with a large loop electrode (Fig. 45–7A, B).

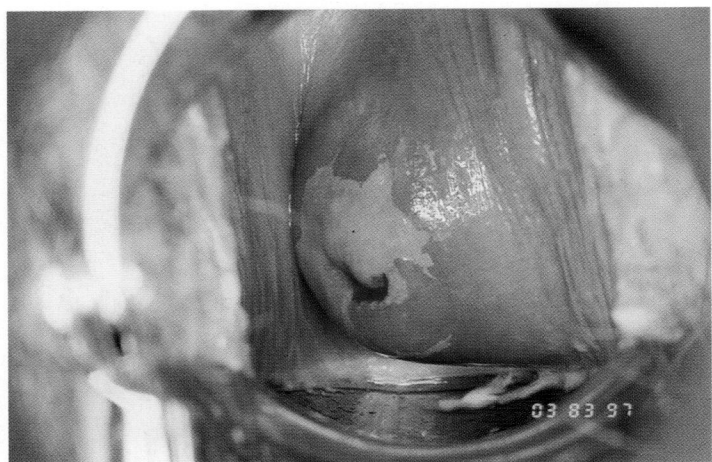

A

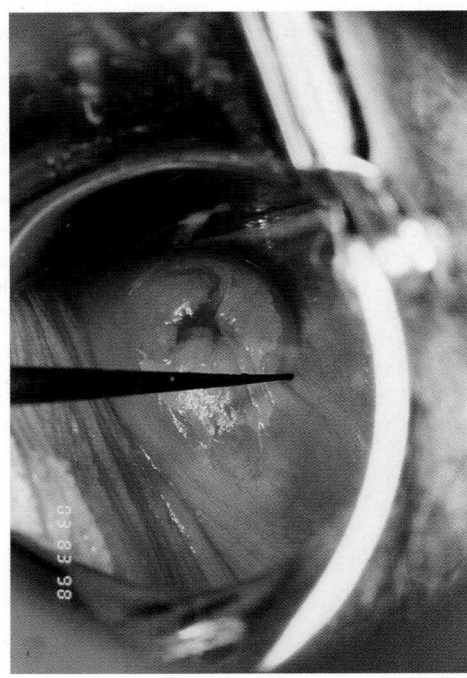

B

**FIGURE 45–1  A.** Colpophotograph of the cervix shows an atypical transformation zone involving predominantly the anterior lip of the cervix but also the posterior lip. **B.** A titanium hook is utilized to determine the ectocervical extent of the lesion.

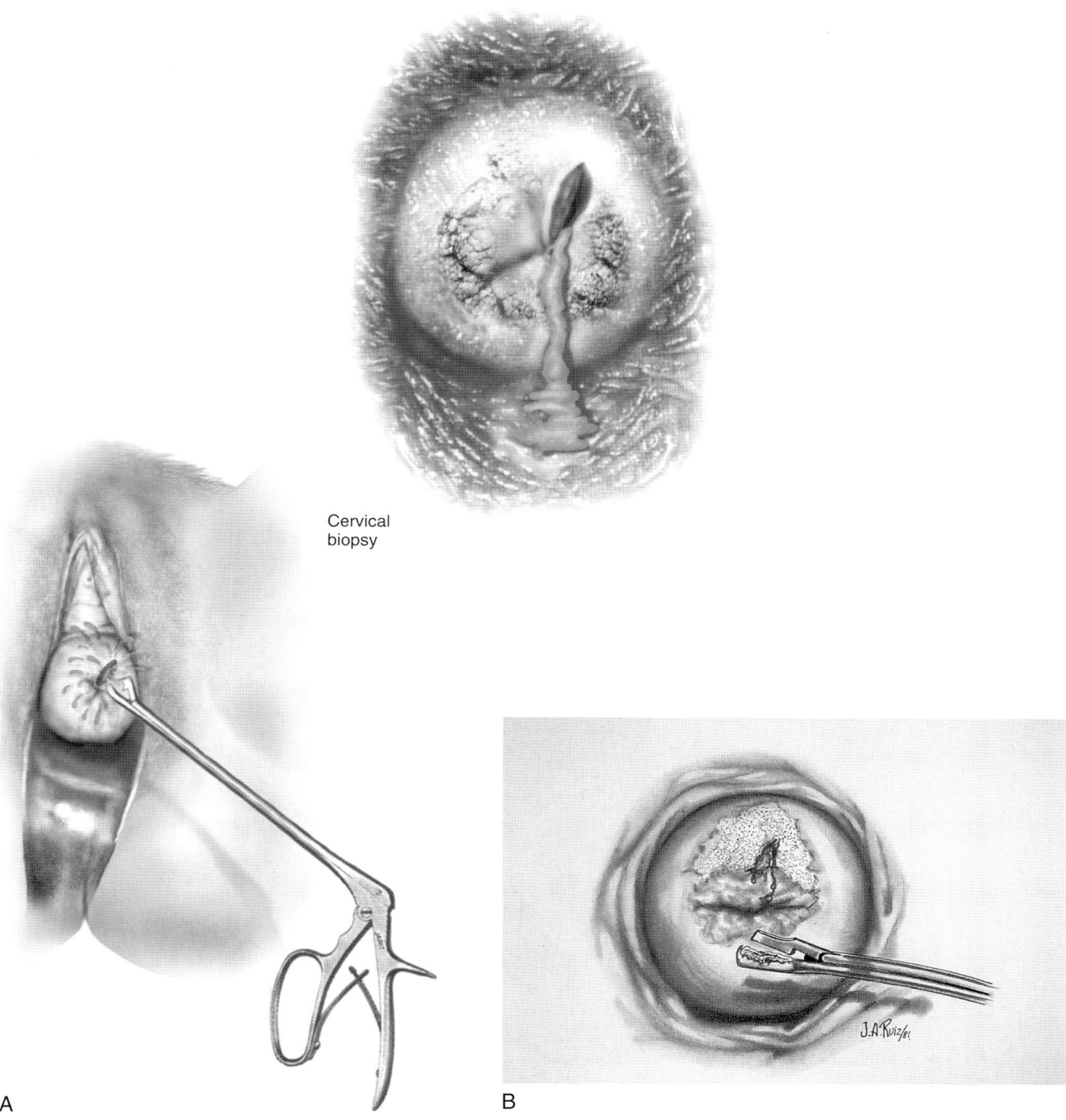

Cervical
biopsy

A

B

**FIGURE 45–2  A.** A directed biopsy of the cervix is performed. The **inset** demonstrates schematically the colposcopic view obtained.
**B.** An adequate sample will fill the cup of the biopsy forceps and will be sharply cut away from the surrounding cervical tissue.

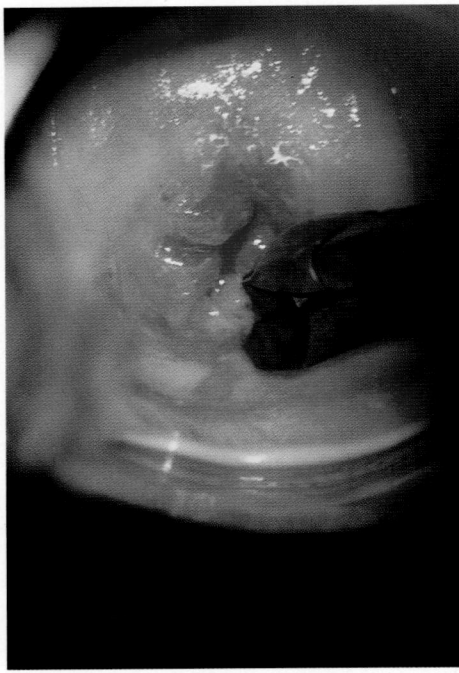

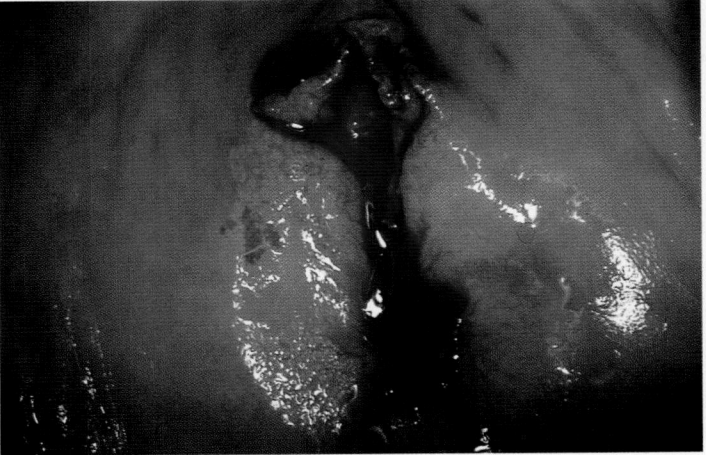

**FIGURE 45-4** This demonstrates an appropriately directed biopsy. Note that the borders of the specimen are sharp and that it extends completely through the atypical transformation zone. Further, this demonstrates that all biopsy specimens bleed.

**FIGURE 45-3** This view through the colposcope shows the biopsy forceps closing down on a piece of tissue at the squamocolumnar junction.

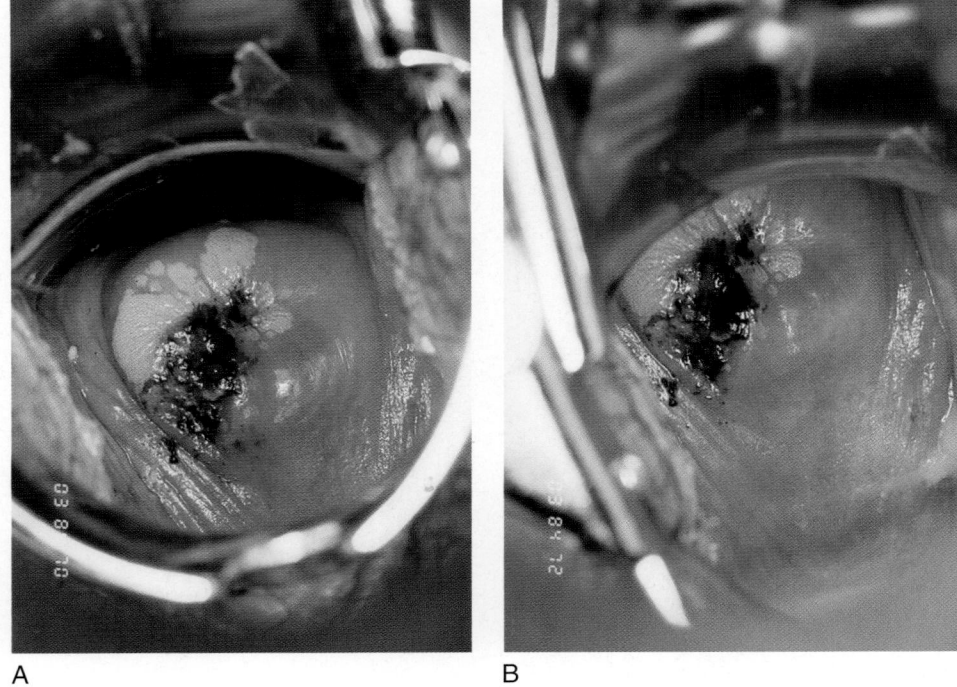

A                                        B

**FIGURE 45-5  A.** Monsel's solution (ferric subsulfate) has been applied to the biopsy site, creating a dark brown coloration to the tissue. **B.** Magnified view of the biopsy site after Monsel's solution has been applied. Note the excellent hemostasis.

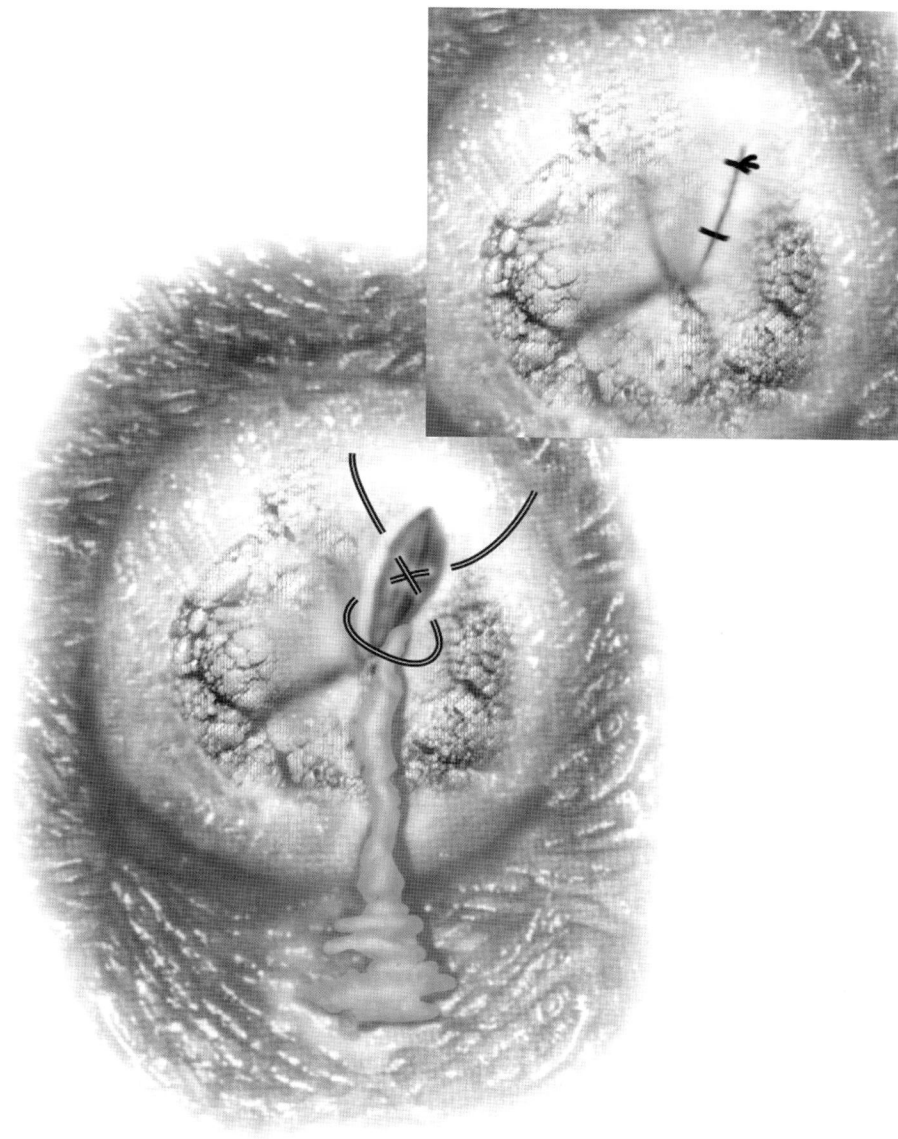

**FIGURE 45–6** If bleeding continues after Monsel's solution has been applied, the site must be sutured. This is performed by utilizing a long needle holder and closing the biopsy defect with a 3-0 Vicryl figure-of-8 suture.

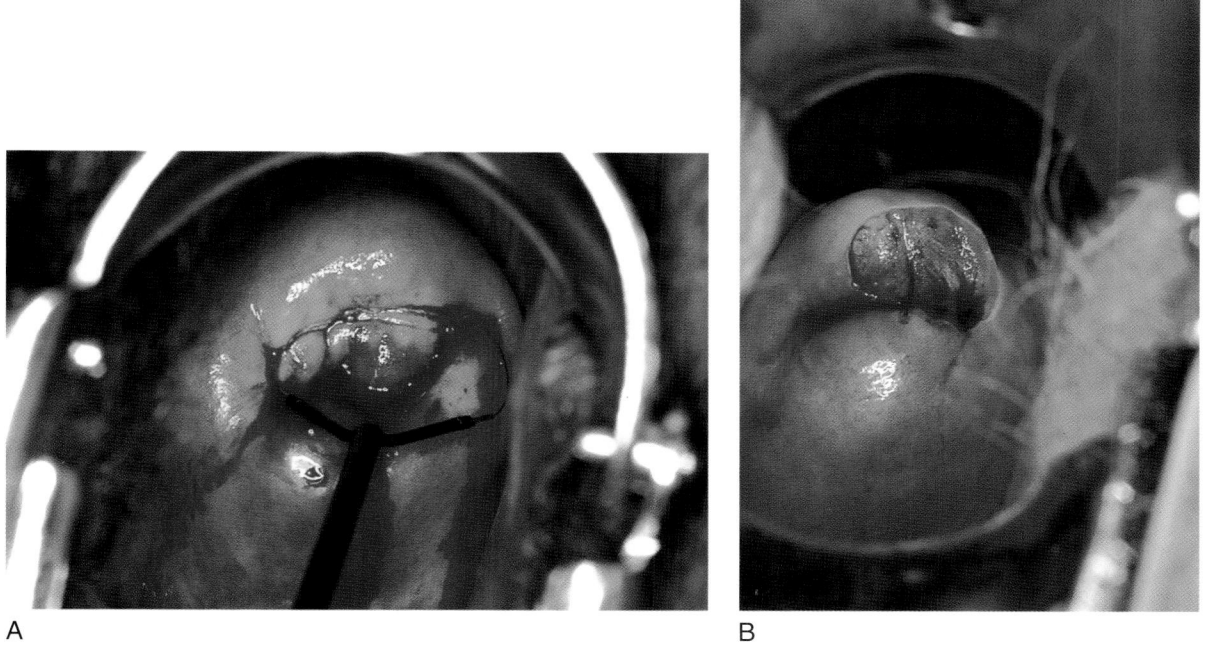

A

B

**FIGURE 45–7** **A.** A large loop electrode coupled to a monopolar cutting current is an alternative technique for obtaining a relatively "bloodless" biopsy specimen. **B.** The disclike sample is not deeply taken but is very easy for the pathologist to orient.

## Endocervical Curettage

To properly perform an endocervical curettage, the cervix must be stabilized. This is done by applying a single-tooth tenaculum to the anterior lip of the cervix. Next, a Telfa pad is placed below the posterior aspect of the cervix (i.e., into the posterior fornix of the vagina). A Kevorkian curette is engaged into the external os and is pushed along the axis of the cervical canal for a distance of 2.5 to 3 cm (Fig. 45–8). The sharp edge of the curette basket is aimed at the 12 o'clock position. The canal is vigorously curetted downward. Each subsequent stroke is rotated clockwise through 3, 6, and 9 o'clock positions until the device returns again to the 12 o'clock position (Fig. 45–9). Typically, the curettings are suspended in cervical mucus (Fig. 45–10). The specimen is retrieved from the Telfa pad by means of a long curved Kelly clamp, which twists the mucus sample as one would twist spaghetti on a fork. The specimen is deposited on a square of ordinary paper towel, and together these are placed immediately into a jar of fixative. Enhanced accuracy may be anticipated by directing the endocervical curettage to a targeted area for sampling. This is best accomplished by doing an endoscopic examination of the endocervix before curetting the canal (Fig. 45–11A through C).

## Cervical Biopsy During Pregnancy

Occasionally, a biopsy of the cervix during pregnancy is required to determine whether invasive cancer is present. It is inadvisable to perform an endocervical curettage during pregnancy. The pregnant cervix is blue because of its tremendous vascular supply. Obtaining even a small biopsy specimen can lead to significant blood loss (Fig. 45–12). Therefore, 3-0 Vicryl and appropriate long instruments should be at hand in the event that suture placement is needed. Following colposcopic examination and identification of the location at the biopsy site, the biopsy forceps are positioned on the cervix. The operator's free hand holds a cotton-tipped applicator to which Monsel's solution has been applied. As the jaws of the biopsy forceps close on the tissue, Monsel's swab is brought close to the cervix (i.e., just to the side of the forceps) (Fig. 45–13A). As the specimen is removed, Monsel's swab is stuffed into the wound crater and is gently rolled from one margin to the other while light pressure is maintained (Fig. 45–13B). The swab is kept in contact with the wound for a full 20 to 30 seconds, then is gently removed.

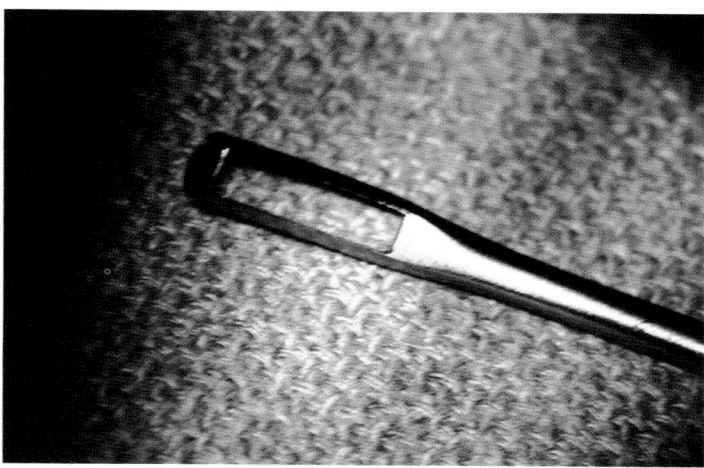

**FIGURE 45–8**  A Kevorkian curette is most suitable for endocervical curettage because of its narrow profile and sharp edges.

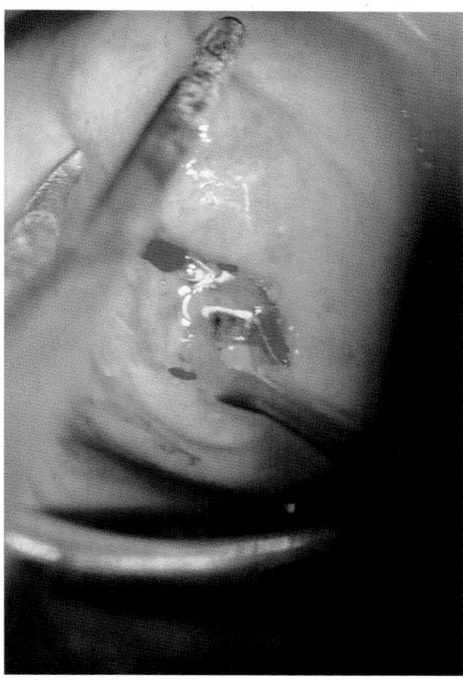

**FIGURE 45–9**  The cervix is grasped with a single-tooth tenaculum (12 o'clock position) for stability. The curette can be seen just before the cervical canal is entered.

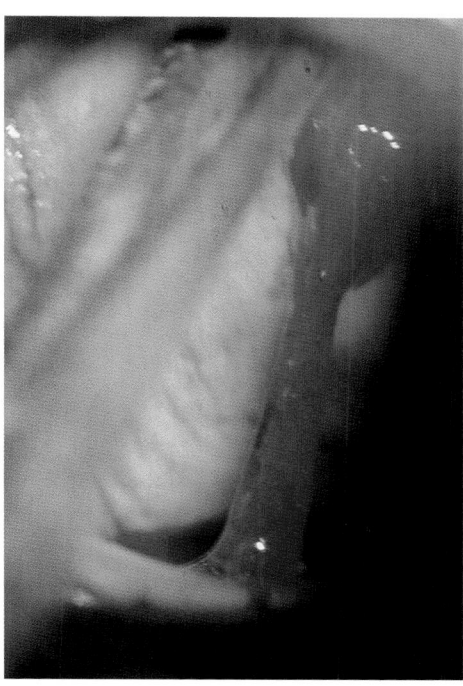

**FIGURE 45–10**  The curettage has been completed. Note the string of mucus containing fragments of endocervical mucosa.

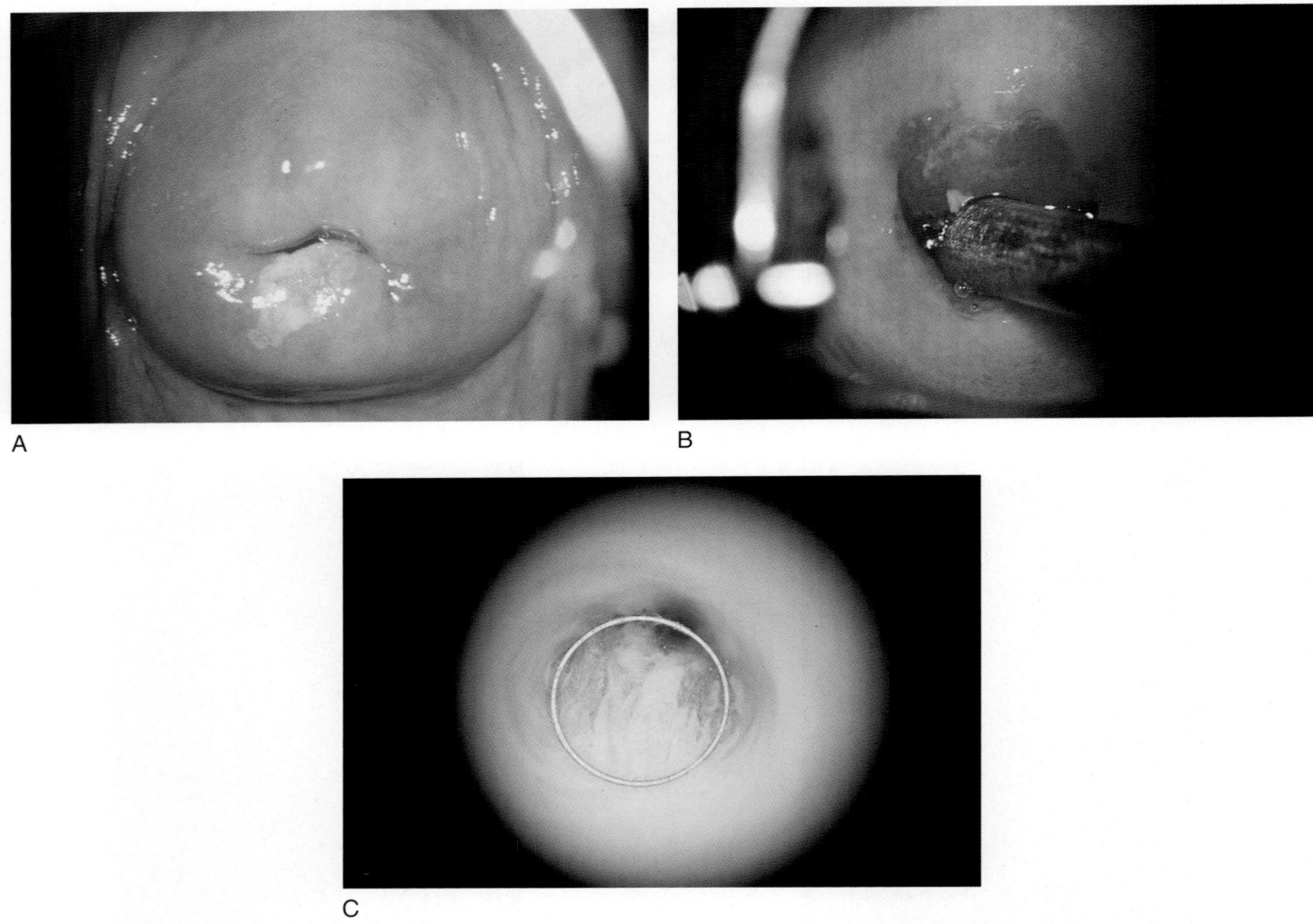

A

B

C

**FIGURE 45–11  A.** The abnormal transformation zone at 6 o'clock is extending into the endocervical canal. **B.** The barrel of the hysteroscope is engaged at the external os in preparation for an endoscopic examination of the cervical canal. **C.** Hysteroscopic view clearly shows how far and where in the canal the abnormal epithelium extends.

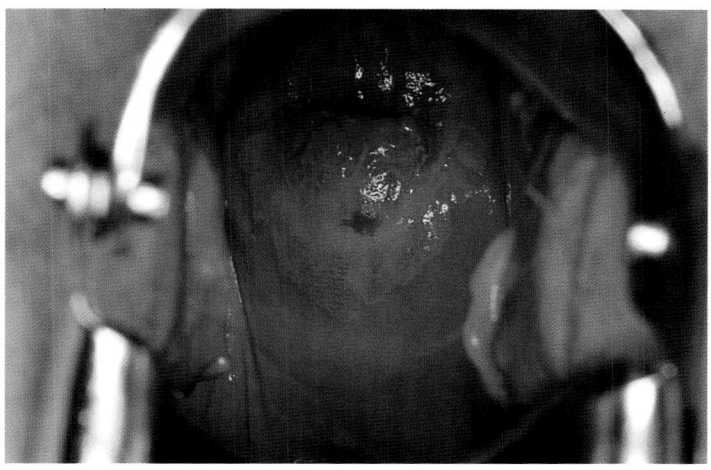

**FIGURE 45–12**  The pregnant cervix is cyanotic with extensive ectopy. An extensive abnormal transformation zone is visible in this colposcopic photograph.

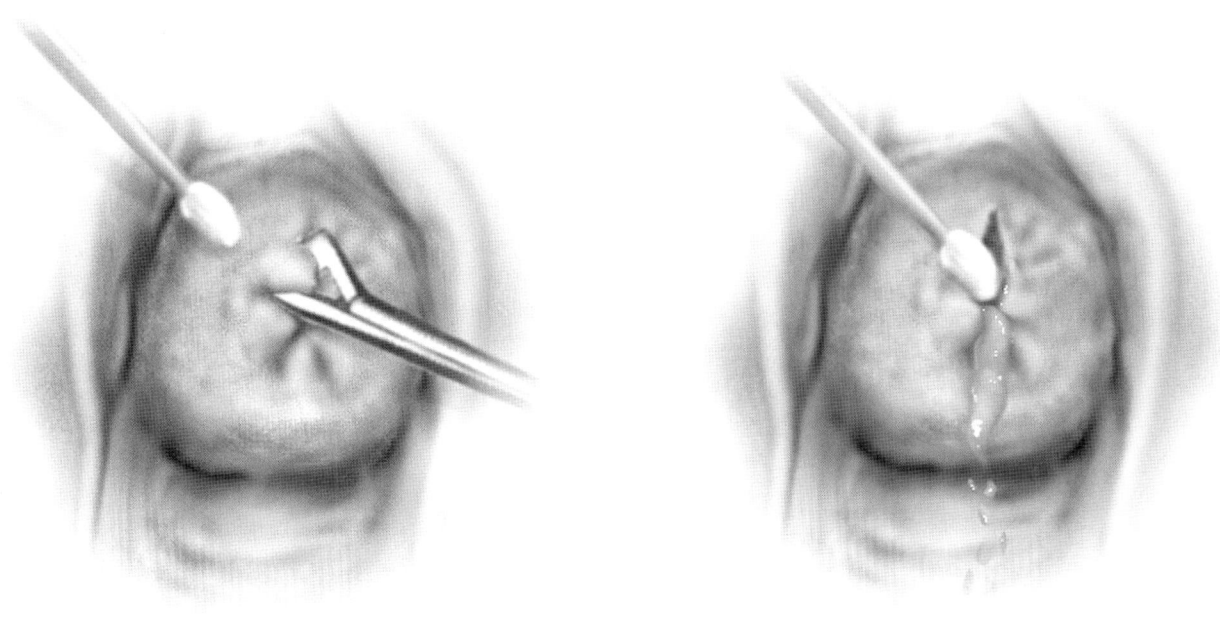

A                                                                                    B

**FIGURE 45–13  A.** The jaws of the biopsy clamp are closed on the tissue sample in this pregnant patient. Simultaneously, a cotton-tipped applicator soaked with Monsel's solution is positioned next to the biopsy forceps. **B.** As the biopsy forceps containing the tissue sample is removed, Monsel's swab is thrust into the defect and is gently rolled from side to side while light pressure is applied.

# CHAPTER 46

# Conization of the Cervix

*Michael S. Baggish*

The term *cone biopsy* has come to refer not only to biopsy of the geometric cone but also to cylinder and disc biopsies (loop excision of the T-zone). Over the past two decades, a great deal of research as well as discussion has focused on the specifications for conization of the cervix. Principally, the goal of the gynecologic surgeon is to obtain a clear (i.e., non-neoplastic) cell margin at the ectocervical, endocervical, lateral, and depth perimeters of the specimen. The strategy is to couple a diagnostic procedure to a therapeutic one. An additional goal of the operation should be maintenance of fertility because most patients who undergo this operation are within the reproductive age group. When performed in the pregnant patient, the procedure should not lead to pregnancy loss.

With the exception of adenocarcinoma in situ, which makes up a minority of premalignant neoplastic disorders of the cervix, neoplastic cells spread by direct continuity from the squamocolumnar junction by tracking a course into the endocervical canal or outward onto the portio. The former course is by far more common. Additionally, spread onto the ectocervix is visible by colposcopy, whereas movement into the canal is not. Squamous intraepithelial neoplasia (dysplasia, cervical intraepithelial neoplasia) rarely progresses more than 1 to 1.5 cm up into the endocervical canal. Similarly, when these lesions involve plunging into the endocervical clefts (glands), they penetrate the stroma to a depth of 3 to 3.5 mm and rarely to a depth of up to 6 mm. Thus, the height of the cone should be specified at no more than 15 mm and the peripheral margin around the canal 3 to 3.5 mm. This will encompass and cure 95% of high-grade lesions, including squamous intraepithelial neoplasia stages I (moderate dysplasia) and III (severe dysplasia, carcinoma in situ). An even more conservative approach should be adopted for low-grade squamous neoplasia (mild dysplasia, condylomatous atypia, cervical intraepithelial neoplasia stage I) because its propensity to spread into the canal is less than that of high-grade disorders. Low-grade disease should be excised to a maximal height of 8 to 10 mm with a 3-mm peripheral margin at the transformation zone.

On the basis of these facts, several methods can be used to perform a cone biopsy. This chapter does not describe ablative techniques because they do not provide a specimen for the pathologist (the only exception is a description of the unique combination cone).

## Cold-Knife Conization

As with other biopsy and therapeutic techniques, use of the colposcope throughout cold-knife conization provides great advantage because the surgeon's view of the field is magnified, permitting greater precision, the light is excellent and focused onto the field, and the instrument does not take up any space in the operative field.

Hemostasis is a key element in the performance of a knife conization. Stay sutures of 0 Vicryl are placed into the cervix at 9 o'clock or 3 o'clock to partially occlude the descending branch of the uterine artery and to provide stabilization of the cervix (Fig. 46–1A, B). The goal is better exposure of the operative field. Injection of vasoconstrictors into the cervical substance provides additional hemostasis (see Fig. 46–1A). The most potent vasoconstrictor is vasopressin, which must be diluted. Vasopressin is supplied as a powder; when mixed with sterile water, this agent contains 20 units per milliliter. An alternative preparation when mixed with sterile water contains 10 units of vasopressin per 0.5 mL (Fig. 46–2). For injection into the cervix, vasopressin should be diluted 1:100 (i.e., add 99 mL of diluent to 1 mL of reconstituted vasopressin solution such that each milliliter of the diluted solution will contain 0.2 unit). Typically, 10 mL of the solution is injected into the cervix. If 1% lidocaine without epinephrine is used to dilute the vasopressin, the resultant solution provides vasoconstriction and local anesthesia simultaneously when injected into the cervix (Fig. 46–3).

Before injection, however, a colposcopy should be performed, and the peripheral margins of the cone should be marked. Once the vasopressin is injected, the abnormal transformation zone (ATZ) will be difficult to see (Fig. 46–4).

The colposcope is set on scanning power. A circular knife cut is made 3 mm peripheral to the AZT. The knife is angled toward the endocervical canal and cuts deeper into the stroma to a height of 1.5 cm. The endocervical margin is cut (Fig. 46–5A through E). Hemostasis is carried out with a ball electrode utilizing spray or forced coagulation at a setting of 50 W. The stay sutures are cut close to the knot (intact), and the field is inspected for hemostasis. No sponges or packs are placed in the vagina or the crater. Performance of endocervical curettage is optional. If the surgeon wishes to curette the remaining endocervical canal, this should be done at the conclusion of the conization but before hemostatic coagulation occurs.

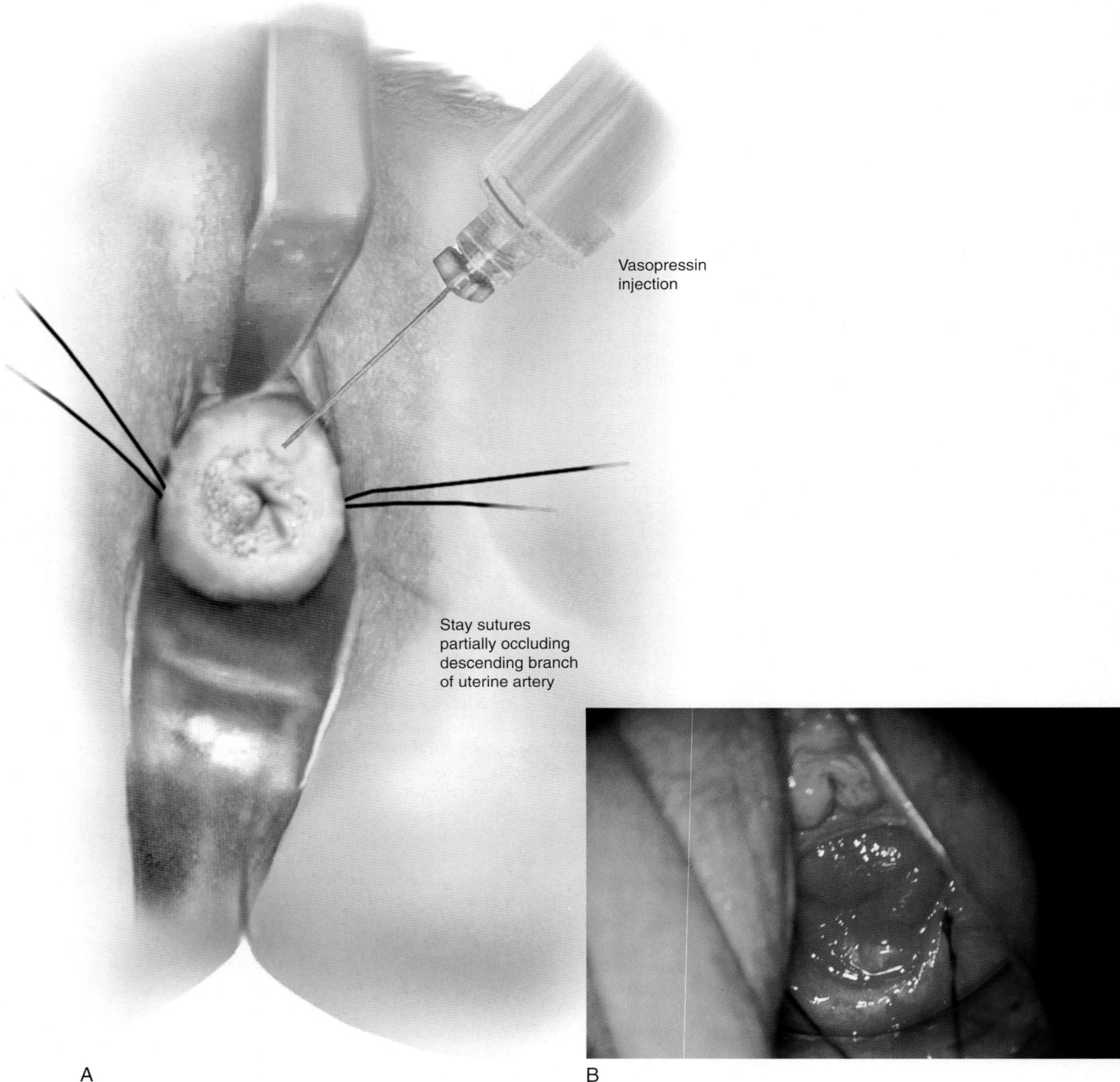

Vasopressin
injection

Stay sutures
partially occluding
descending branch
of uterine artery

A                                                                B

**FIGURE 46–1  A.** Two sutures of 0 Vicryl have been placed into the lateral aspect of the cervix at the 9 o'clock and 3 o'clock locations. These are placed to diminish bleeding and to stabilize the cervix during surgery. **B.** The stay sutures are pulled downward to better expose the cervix. Even with a deep retractor placed posteriorly, the vagina bulges beneath the posterior cervix.

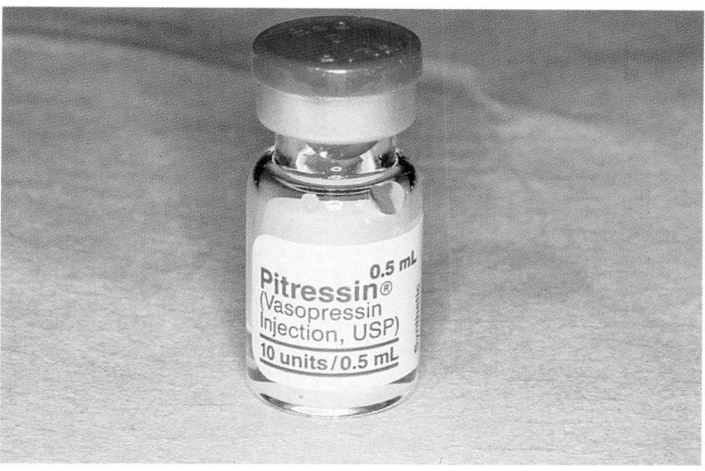

FIGURE 46–2  Vasopressin is diluted such that 1 mL (20 units) is diluted 100-fold. In the case illustrated, each 0.5 mL contains 10 units. Therefore, if 0.5 mL of this solution were mixed with 50 mL of sterile water, the resultant solution would be equivalent.

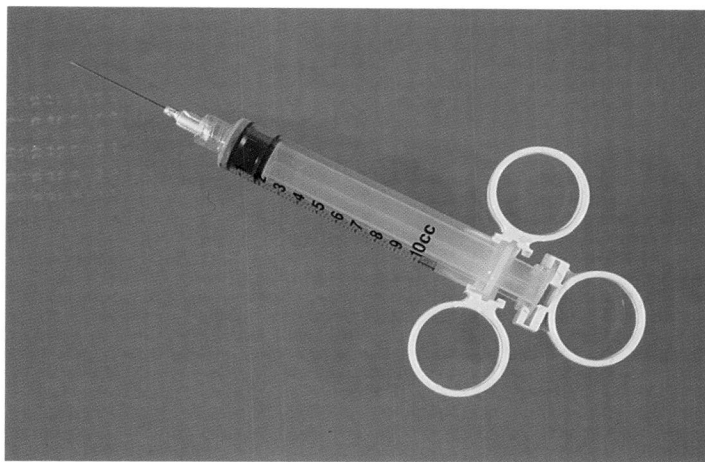

FIGURE 46–3  The vasopressin mixture is injected by using a 10-mL syringe with a 1½-inch, 25-gauge needle attached.

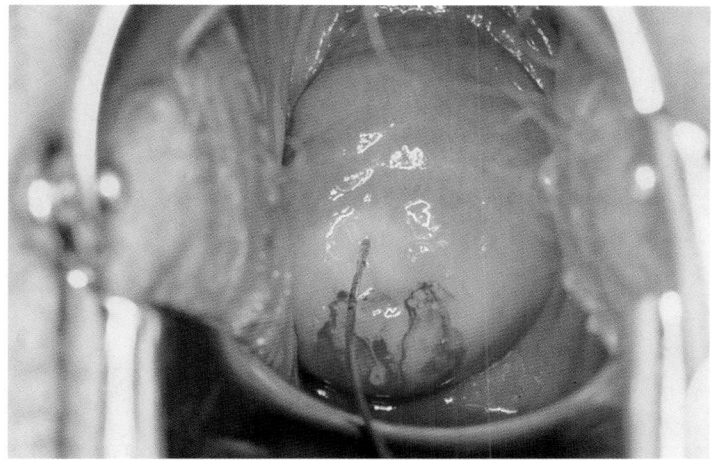

FIGURE 46–4  A very superficial needle stick is made into the cervix, and the vasopressin mixture is injected under pressure. As the vasopressin infiltrates, the tissue blanches.

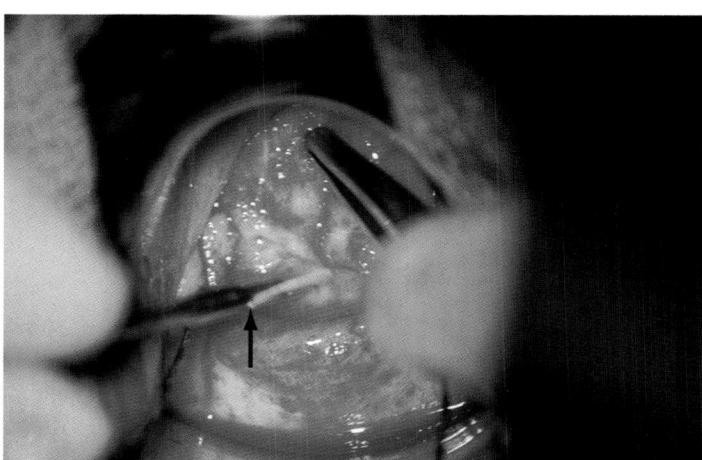

A

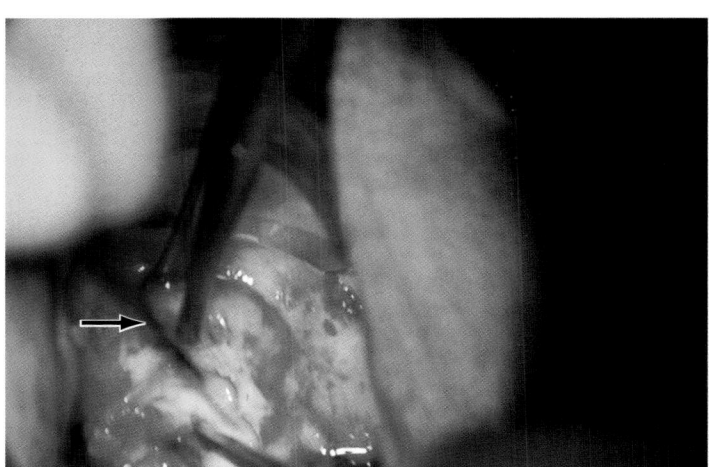

B

FIGURE 46–5  A. The knife cuts into the cervix at 6 o'clock with a margin 3 mm peripheral to the abnormal transformation zone (ATZ) (*arrow at knife*). B. The knife cut extends deep as traction is placed on the edge of the cut with an Allis clamp (*arrow at knife*).

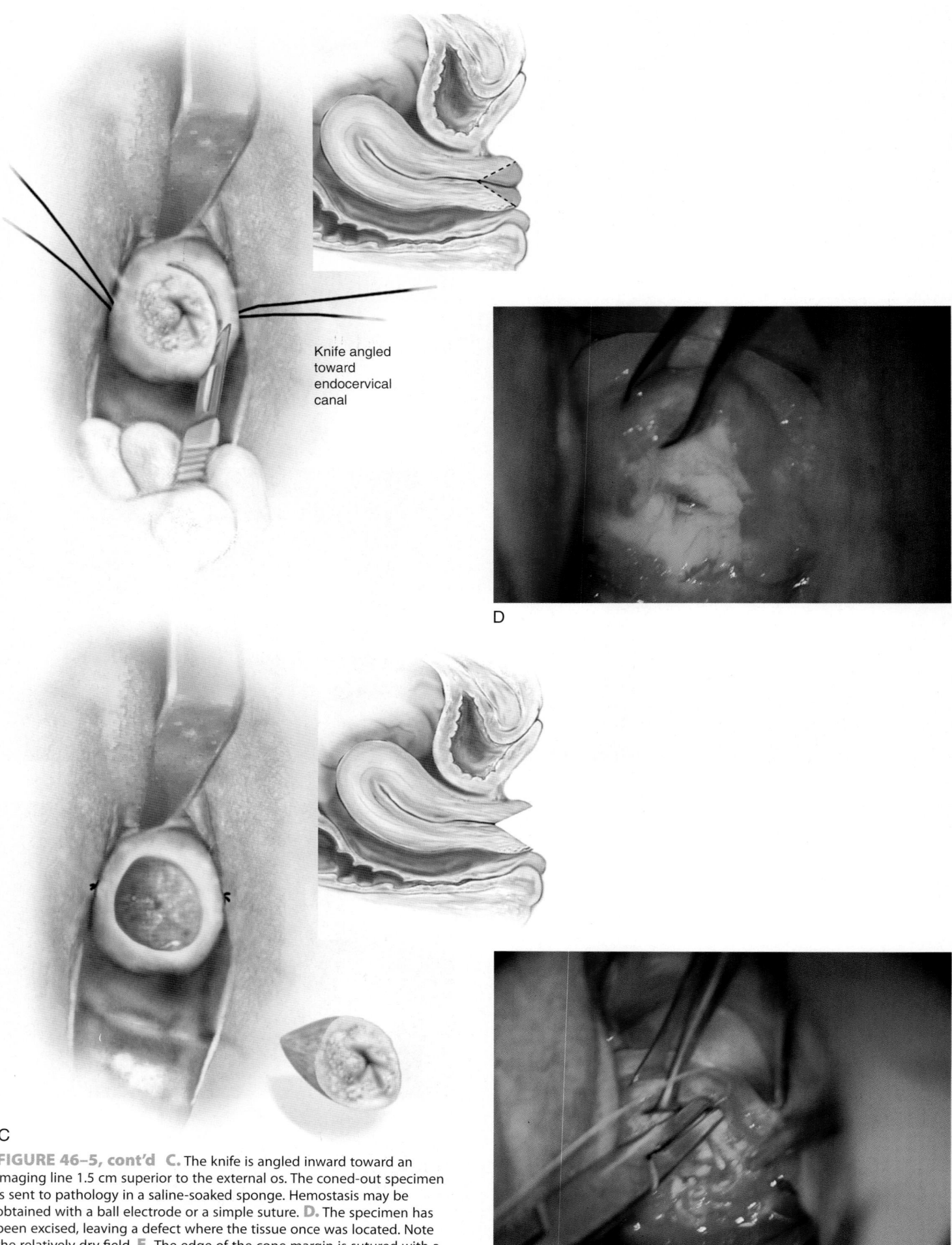

Knife angled toward endocervical canal

C

D

E

**FIGURE 46–5, cont'd** **C.** The knife is angled inward toward an imaging line 1.5 cm superior to the external os. The coned-out specimen is sent to pathology in a saline-soaked sponge. Hemostasis may be obtained with a ball electrode or a simple suture. **D.** The specimen has been excised, leaving a defect where the tissue once was located. Note the relatively dry field. **E.** The edge of the cone margin is sutured with a 0 Vicryl continuous suture.

## Laser Conization

This technique is similar to a knife conization with the exception that a superpulsed carbon dioxide ($CO_2$) laser beam is substituted for the scalpel (Fig. 46–6A through C). The advantage of the laser is that it is coupled to the microscope, thereby permitting a more precise cone (Fig. 46–7A through C). Additionally, the thermal action of the laser promotes better hemostasis. The disadvantages of the laser are that the procedure requires more time to finish and the laser may cause thermal injury (artifact) to the specimen (Fig. 46–8).

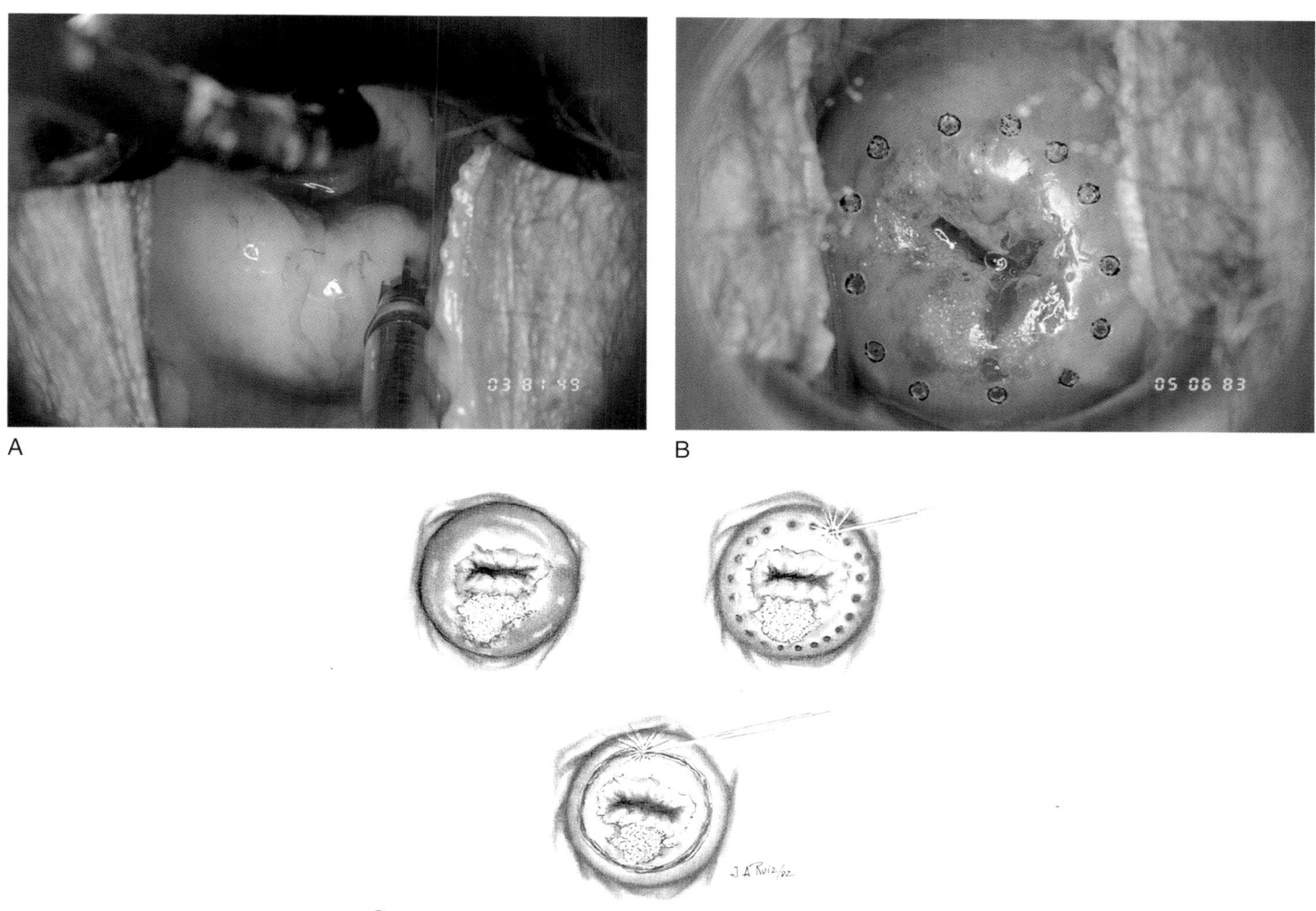

FIGURE 46–6 A. In the case of carbon dioxide ($CO_2$) laser conization, vasopressin is again injected into the cervix to create hemostasis. B. The laser beam traces a series of marking spots around the abnormal transformation zone (ATZ) to identify the outer margin(s) for excision. C. The laser beam diameter is reduced to a 1- to 1.5-mm spot. Power is set at 40 to 60 W. The dots are connected, and a peripheral crater is created.

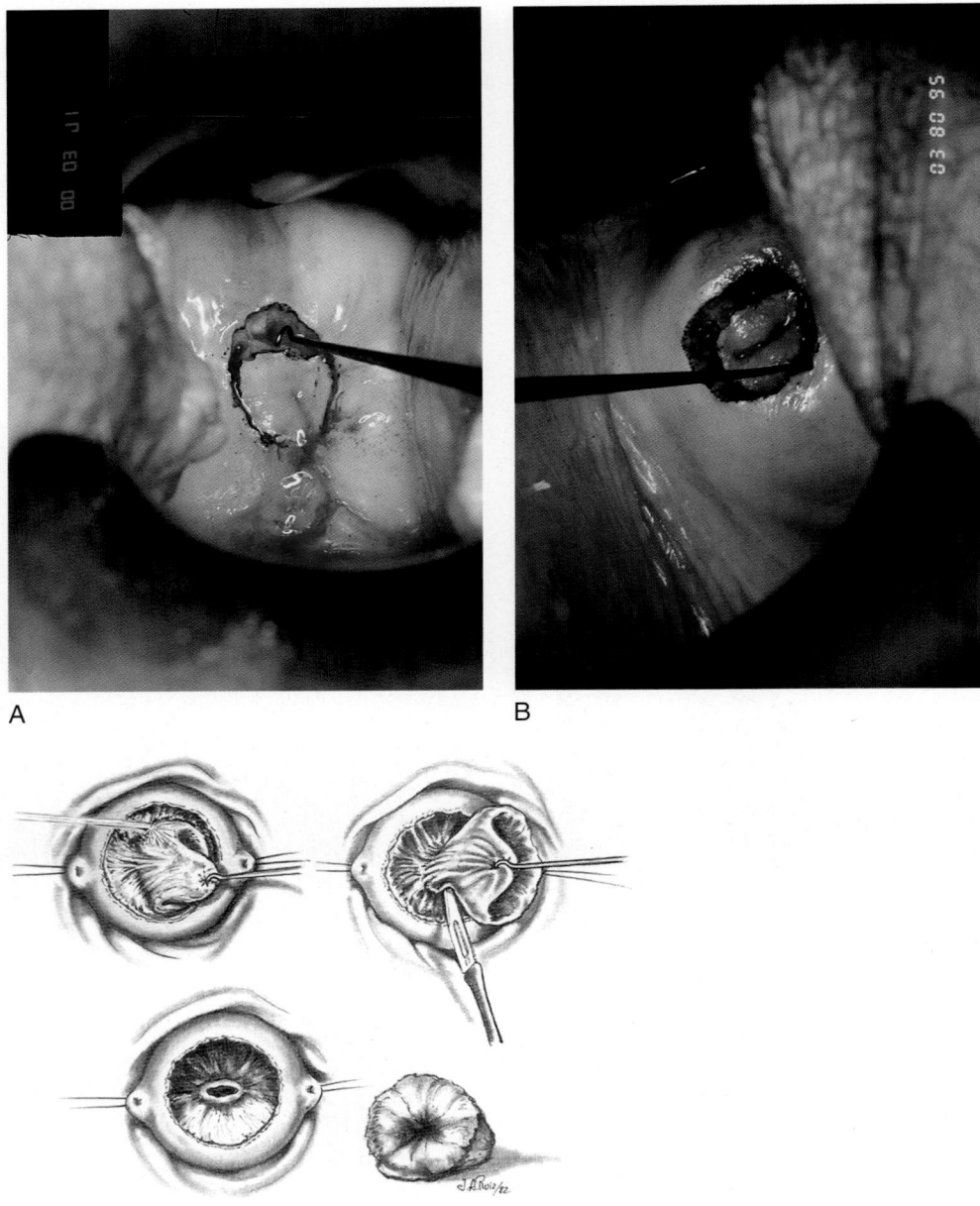

A    B

C

**FIGURE 46–7 A.** A laser titanium manipulating hook creates traction on the edge of the cervical incision, and the beam continues to cut deeper. **B.** The incision is focused inward to create the cone-shaped specimen. **C.** When the cervix has been cut to a sufficient height, the endocervical margin is cut and the specimen removed.

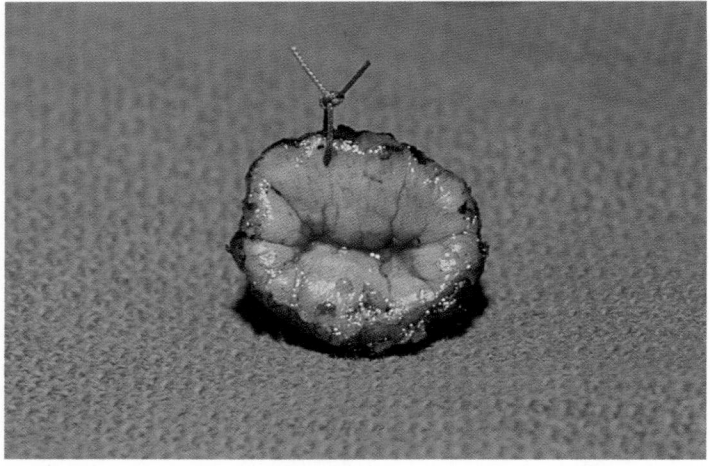

**FIGURE 46–8** The specimen is marked at 12 o'clock with a stitch and is sent to pathology for section.

## Conization During Pregnancy

As with punch biopsy, conization during pregnancy is associated with greater risk of bleeding. Therefore, the conization must be restricted to the lowest height possible while necessary information is secured to exclude or include the diagnosis of invasive cancer. A purse string or 0 Vicryl suture identical to that placed for the treatment of an incompetent cervix is placed (Fig. 46–9A). Next, with the use of a knife or energy device, the cone is taken. The purse string is tightened and tied (Fig. 46–9B).

## Loop Electrical Excision Conization

This technique is an office-based procedure. After the ATZ is marked, a 1:100 diluted vasopressin/lidocaine solution is injected into the cervix circumferentially (Fig. 46–10). Next, the loop electrode of proper size is selected. The electrosurgical unit is set to 50 to 60 W of cutting power. The electrode makes light contact with the cervix as power is applied (Fig. 46–11A, B). It sinks deep into the cervical matrix to a depth of 10 mm. The loop is swept across the entire T-zone by following a horizontal or a vertical pathway (Figs. 46–11C and 46–12). The loop is removed, and a large cotton swab is placed in the crater to absorb blood (Fig. 46–13A, B). The specimen is sent to pathology. The cutting loop electrode is removed from the handpiece, and a ball electrode is substituted for it. As the large swab is removed, the electrode is placed in the crater and is electrically activated to coagulate bleeding vessels and sinuses (Fig. 46–14). When hemostasis is complete, a small cotton-tipped applicator soaked with Monsel's solution may be utilized to stanch any persistent small vessel bleeding (Fig. 46–15).

## Loop Electrical Excision by Selective Double-Excision ("Top Hat") Technique

The selective double-excision technique is used for the treatment of high-grade lesions. Its goal is to conserve cervical stroma while removing an extra margin of cervical canal to provide clear margins and thus a high cure rate (Fig. 46–16A, B). Essentially, the first part of this operation is identical to the loop electrical excision conization described earlier (Fig. 46–17A, B). However, following specimen removal and the attainment of hemostasis, a small (4–5 mm) loop is placed into the handpiece and (by using 30–40 W of cutting current) a 5-mm endocervical sample is obtained. The sample then is marked and sent with the first specimen to pathology (Fig. 46–18A, B).

## Combination Conization

A young patient with extensive ectocervical intraepithelial neoplasia that additionally extends into the cervical canal beyond the view of the colposcope presents a dilemma for the gynecologist (Fig. 46–19). If adequate margins and depth were maintained, then the cervix would be more or less amputated by conventional cone techniques (Fig. 46–20A, B). The combination conization eliminates disease but preserves the stroma and volume of cervical tissue. This technique must be done with a superpulsed $CO_2$ laser for optimal results.

Two sets of trace spots are fired into the cervix: one set 3 mm beyond the ectocervical margin and a second set at the squamocolumnar junction. A narrow cylindrical excisional conization is performed to a height of 1.0 to 1.5 cm (Fig. 46–21A through C).

Next, a shallow 4- to 5-mm vaporization of the ectocervical disease is performed. (The lesion has been previously sampled, and its intraepithelial nature has been established via histopathologic diagnosis) (see Fig. 46–21D). The wound is copiously irrigated with saline.

The patient is seen at biweekly intervals for 4 to 6 weeks and returns 6 weeks later for a final check (Fig. 46–22).

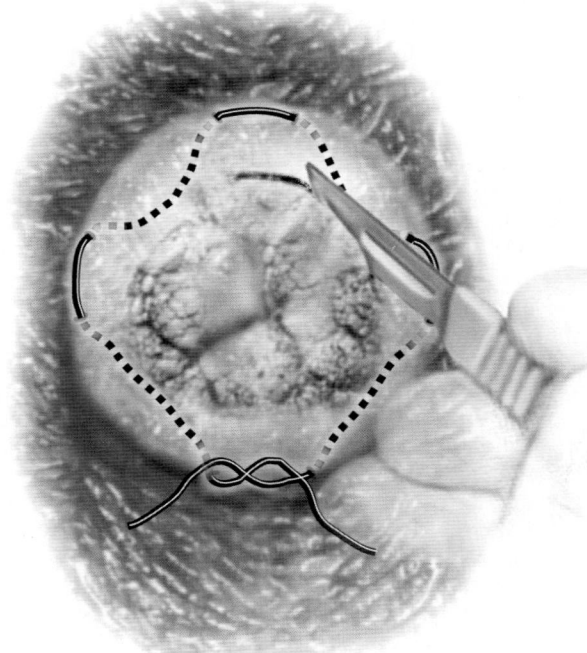

A

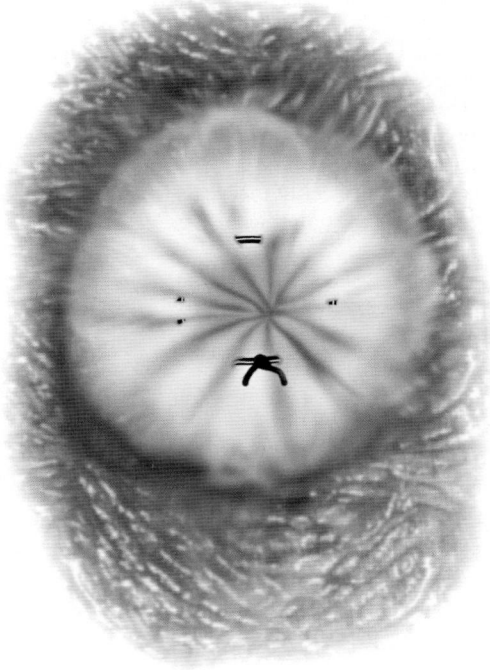

B

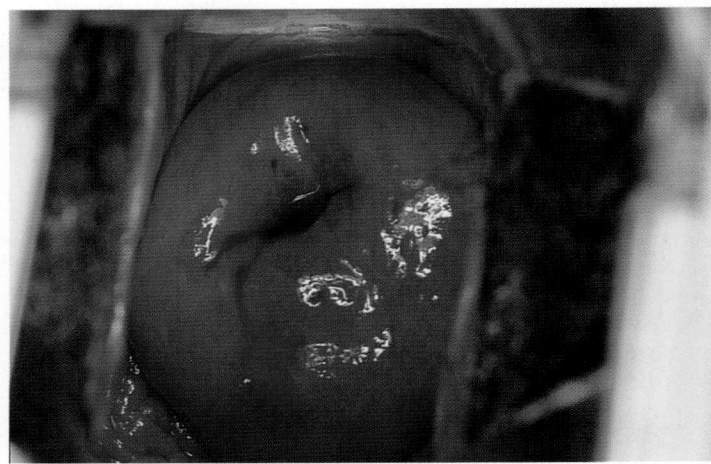

**FIGURE 46–10** The cervix has been injected with 1:100 vasopressin in preparation for loop excision. The injection was made deeper into the tissue, which accounts for the absence of blanching.

**FIGURE 46–9 A.** During pregnancy, a conization can be a very bloody procedure. To better control the bleeding, a purse string suture is placed high up on the cervix and is held with mosquito clamps. **B.** Immediately after completion of the operation, the stitch is snugged down and then tied. The constriction of the cervix will stop or significantly diminish bleeding secondary to conization.

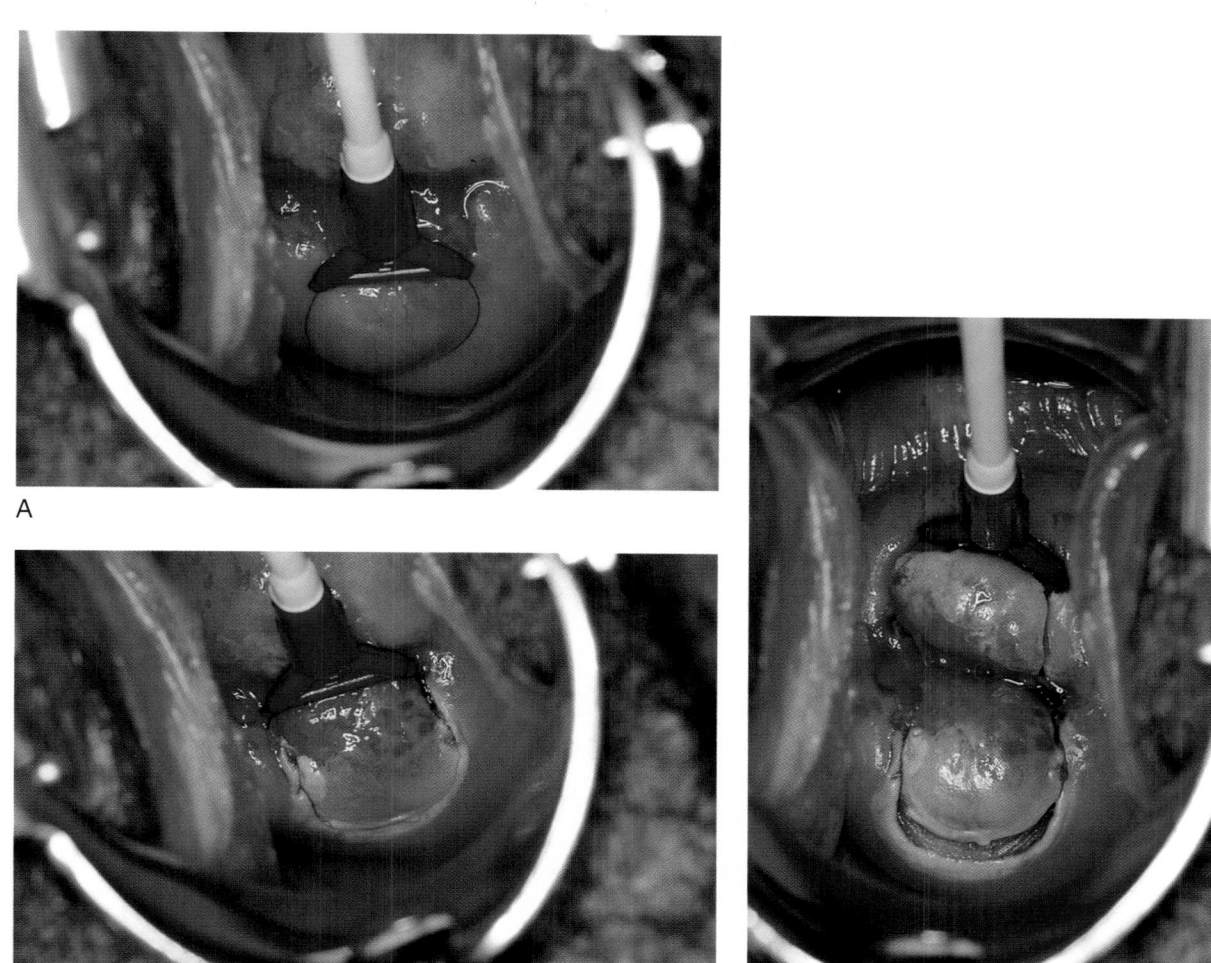

A

B

C

**FIGURE 46–11  A.** The loop electrode is placed at the 6 o'clock position (just before electrical activation). **B.** The electric current is activated, and the excision is initiated by moving the electrode vertically from 6 to 12 o'clock. **C.** In a single sweeping motion, the electrode has finished its excursion.

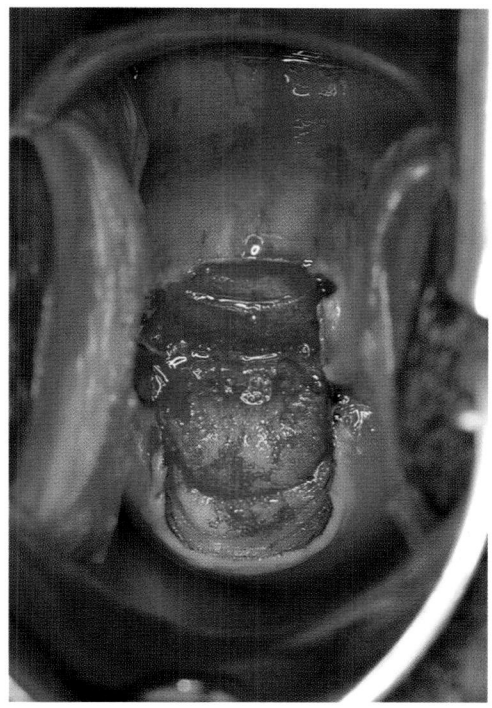

**FIGURE 46–12** The excision of the abnormal transformation zone (ATZ) is complete.

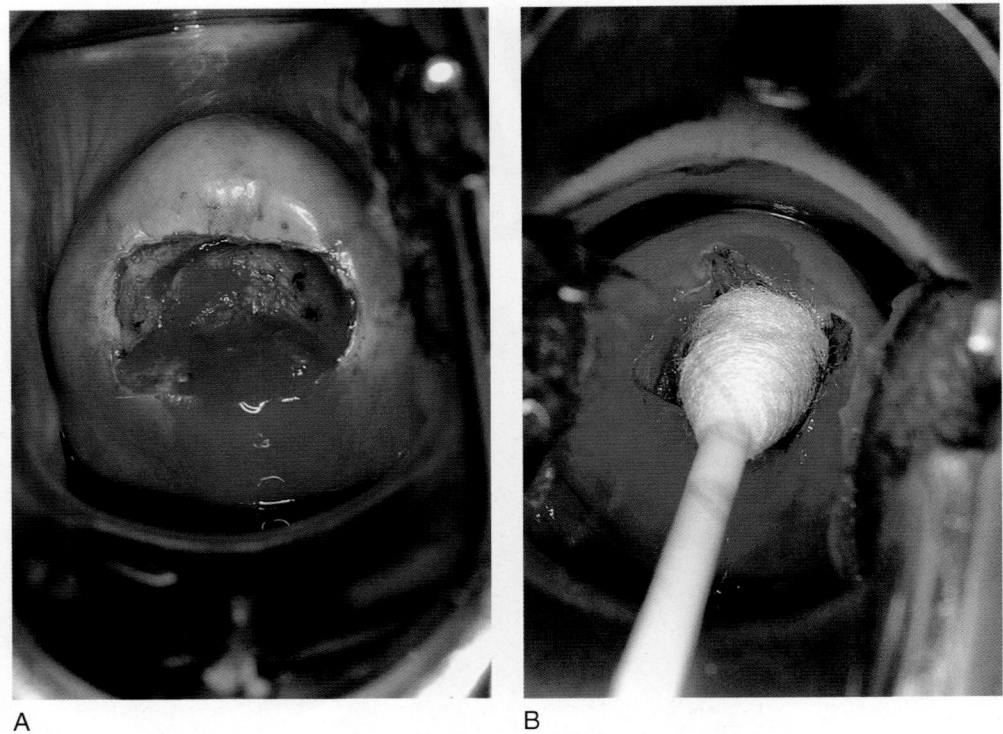

A                                                                 B

**FIGURE 46–13 A.** In this loop excision patient, bleeding was sufficient to warrant coagulation. **B.** A large cotton-tipped swab (proctoswab) tamponades the bleeding site while the loop electrode is changed to a ball electrode. The generator has already been set for coagulation mode.

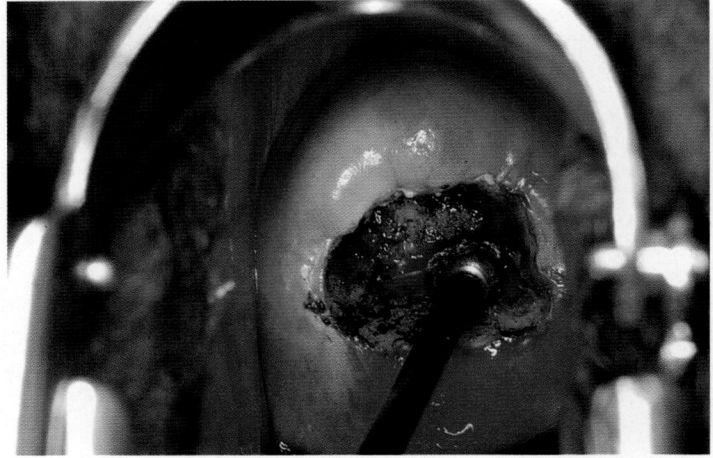

**FIGURE 46–14** The ball electrode coagulates the bleeding vessels by using forced or spray coagulation at 40 to 50 W of power.

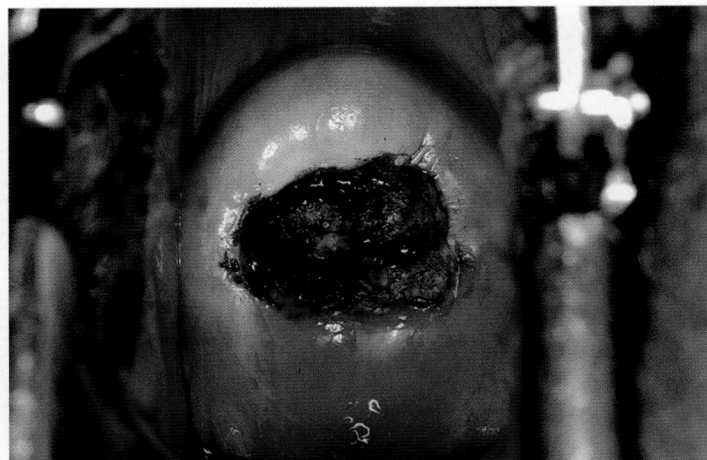

**FIGURE 46–15** The field is dry and the procedure is terminated. No packs are placed in the cervix. Any small additional bleeding may be staunched with a small cotton swab saturated with ferric subsulfate (Monsel's solution).

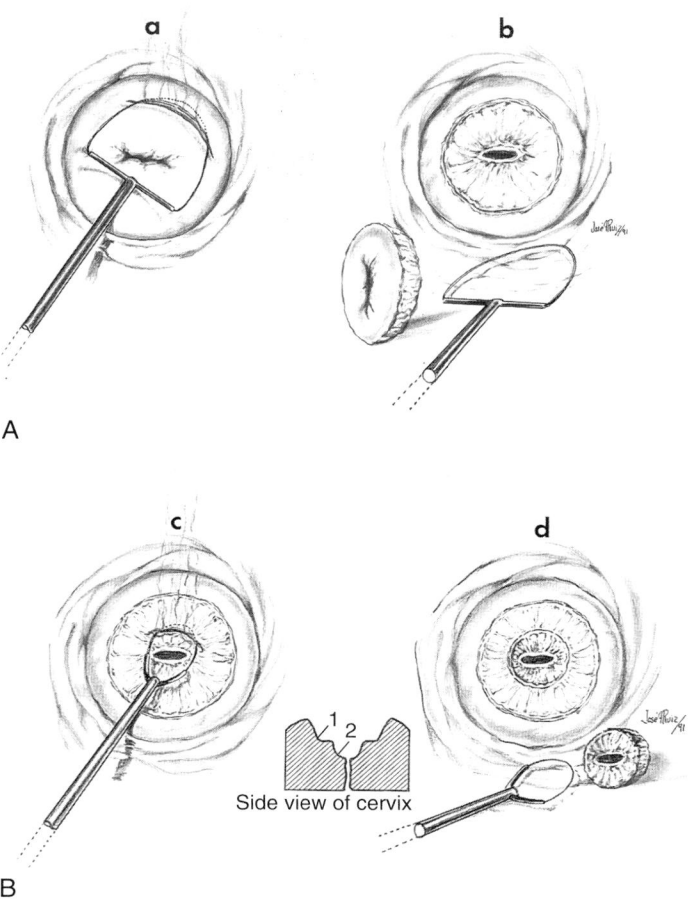

A

B

Side view of cervix

**FIGURE 46-16 A.** The technique of selective double excision is shown schematically. A loop excision of the T-zone is carried out to a depth not to exceed 10 mm (*a, b*). **B.** Next, a second smaller electrode is attached to the handpiece (control unit). This electrode measures 5 × 5 mm. A 5-mm excision of the endocervical canal is performed, and the specimen is submitted in a separate bottle to pathology. The defect produced resembles a cone.

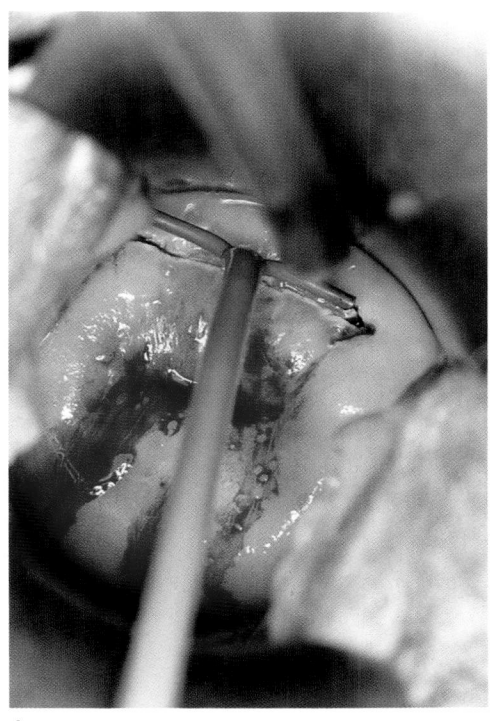

A

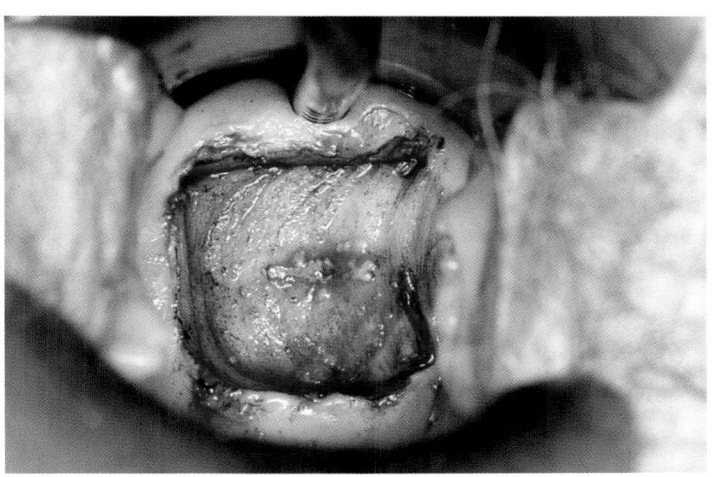

B

**FIGURE 46-17 A.** The loop electrode has been activated and cuts into the cervix at 12 o'clock. **B.** The T-zone has been excised to a 10-mm depth. Note the excellent hemostasis produced by injecting 12 to 15 mL of 1:100 vasopressin very superficially into the cervix before loop excision is performed.

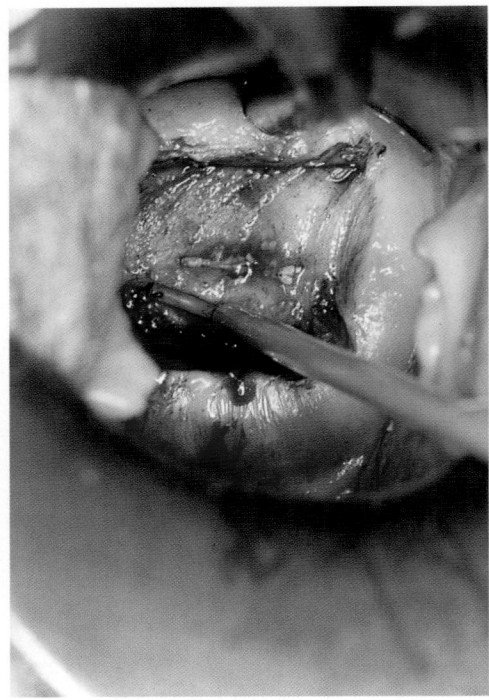

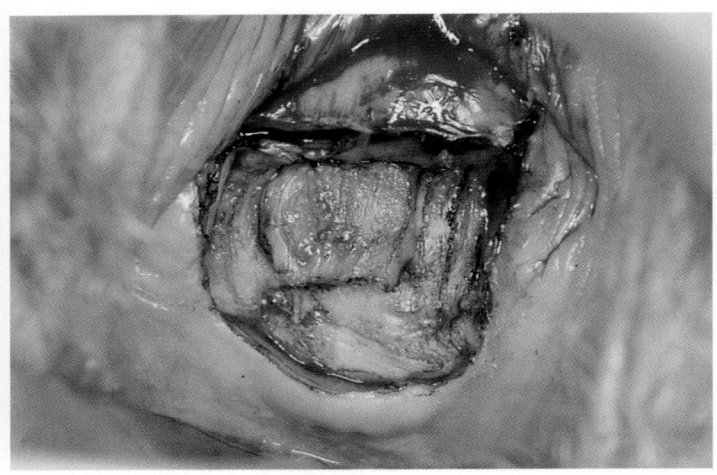

A                                                                    B

**FIGURE 46–18  A.** A 5-mm loop electrode is placed into the stroma just beneath the endocervical mucosa (6 o'clock). **B.** The second excision (5 mm) has been performed. The specimen is placed in a separate container of fixative. The defect has a top hat or a roughly conical shape and measures 15 mm in height.

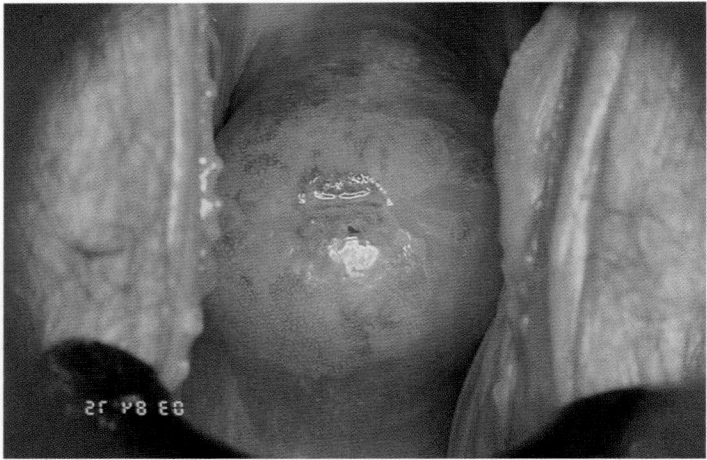

**FIGURE 46–19** This cervix shows a very extensive abnormal transformation zone (ATZ). The abnormal vessels are set in a white epithelial background and extend into the canal and out onto the portio, even to the vaginal fornices. Conventional conization performed by any means would eventuate in virtual amputation of the cervix.

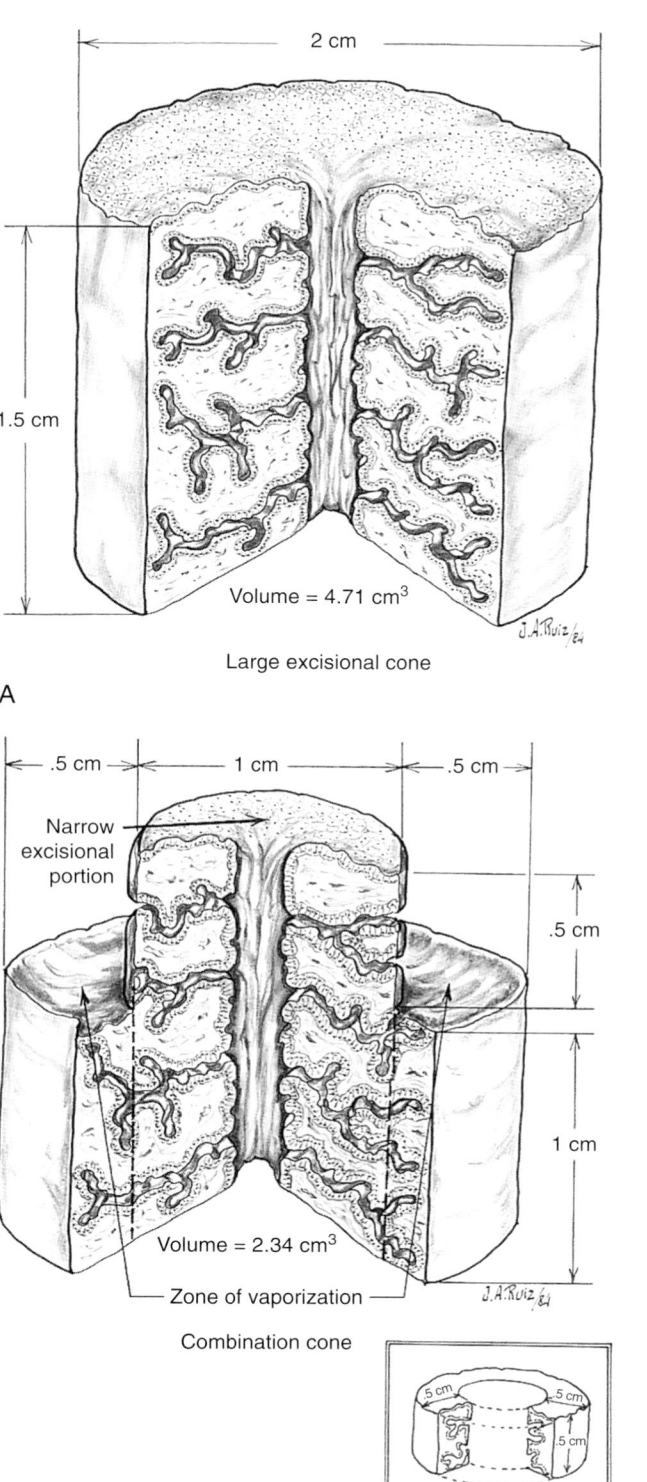

**FIGURE 46–20 A.** The situation described and shown in Figure 46–19 is quantified. A 1.5- × 2.0-cm cylinder conization results in tissue loss of 4.73 cm³. **B.** In contrast, a laser combination conization, which combines a narrow cylinder conization with superficial peripheral vaporization, calculates to a volume loss of cervix of 2.43 cm³. The combination of excision and vaporization thus preserves cervical integrity.

UNIT 3 ■ SECTION A

Combination laser excision and vaporization cylindration

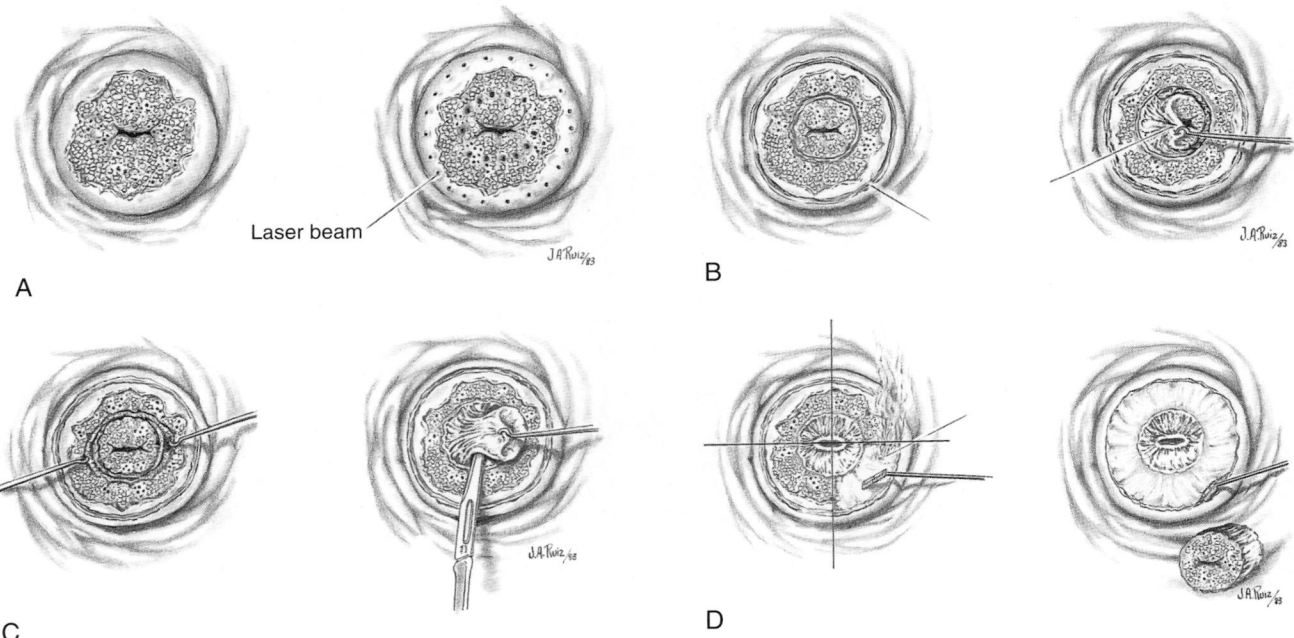

Laser beam

A

B

C

D

**FIGURE 46-21 A.** To perform a combination conization, a carbon dioxide ($CO_2$) laser is required. Two sets of laser trace spots are placed. The inner ring outlines the narrow excisional cone. The outer row is made peripheral to the ectocervical extension of the abnormal transformation zone (ATZ). **B.** The dots are connected by continuous firing of the laser beam, producing the inner and outer circular outlines. Excisional conization is performed by using the laser to cut the tissue (superpulsed and tightly focused beam), as described in Figures 46-4 through 46-8. **C.** The coned-out tissue (narrow cylinder) measures 1.5 cm in height. Its endocervical margin is cut with a scalpel, and the specimen is placed into fixative solution. **D.** The ectocervix is vaporized to a depth of 5 mm centrally, tapering to 2 mm peripherally. Vaporization eliminates the ectocervical disease. Note that the excised cylinder is pictured underlying the vaporized exocervix.

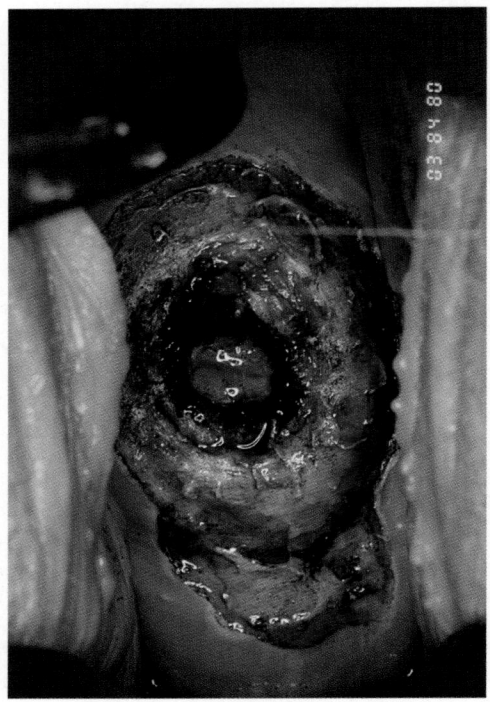

**FIGURE 46-22** A completed combination conization. Note the shallow but total ectocervical vaporization area and the deeper excised central cone (cylinder) cavity. Note also that peripheral vaporization of the abnormal transformation zone (ATZ) extends into the posterior fornix of the vagina.

# CHAPTER 47

# Cervical Polypectomy

*Michael S. Baggish*

Cervical polyps are usually benign but should always be removed and sent to pathology for microscopic examination. Polyps range greatly in size from small to large (Fig. 47–1). Large polyps may spill into the vagina (Fig. 47–2). In either circumstance, the presence of a polyp is commonly associated with contact bleeding and increased vaginal discharge. For small polyps, a Kelly clamp is placed across the pedicle and is twisted clockwise or counterclockwise until the polyp separates (Fig. 47–3). A swab soaked with Monsel's solution is placed onto the residual base pedicle for hemostasis.

Large polyps with thick, vascular pedicles must be clamped and suture-ligated or simply ligated then cut off (Fig. 47–4). If the base of the pedicle cannot be easily exposed, then the posterior wall of the cervix should be split to allow visualization. This is done by injecting 10 to 15 mL of 1:100 vasopressin into the posterior cervical lip. Then, by utilizing a carbon dioxide ($CO_2$) laser or a needle electrode, the cervix is cut vertically in the midline to a point 1 cm below the internal os (Fig. 47–5A, B). The cervix is closed with 3-0 Vicryl interrupted sutures (Figs. 47–6A through D and 47–7).

Alternatively, for a high polyp (i.e., attached at the level of the internal os), insertion of a hysteroscope and a needle electrode may provide the easiest access to the pedicle. In fact, a diagnostic hysteroscopy should be done for polyps attached by a high pedicle to differentiate a cervical polyp from a prolapsing endometrial polyp.

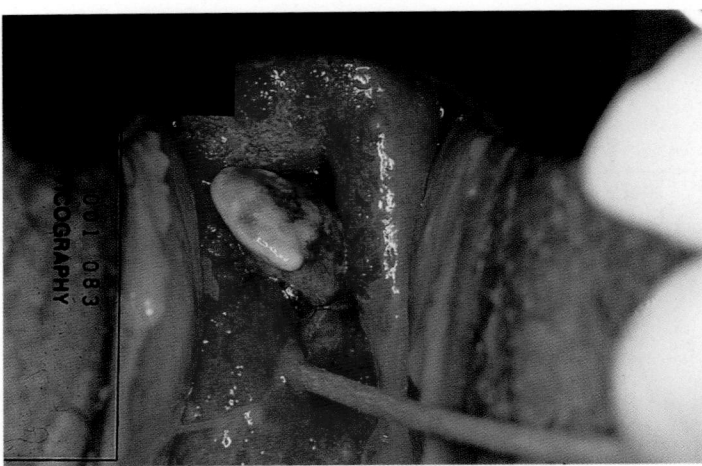

**FIGURE 47–1** A rather small endocervical polyp is exposed with the aid of a cotton-tipped applicator depressing the wall of the cervical canal.

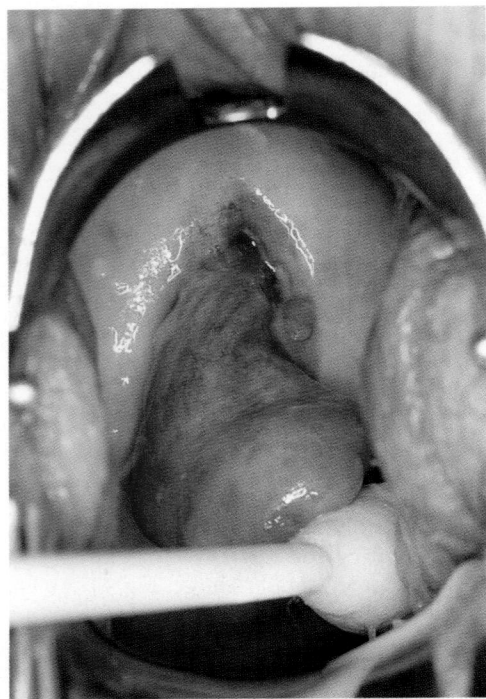

**FIGURE 47–2** A large cervical polyp protrudes into the vagina.

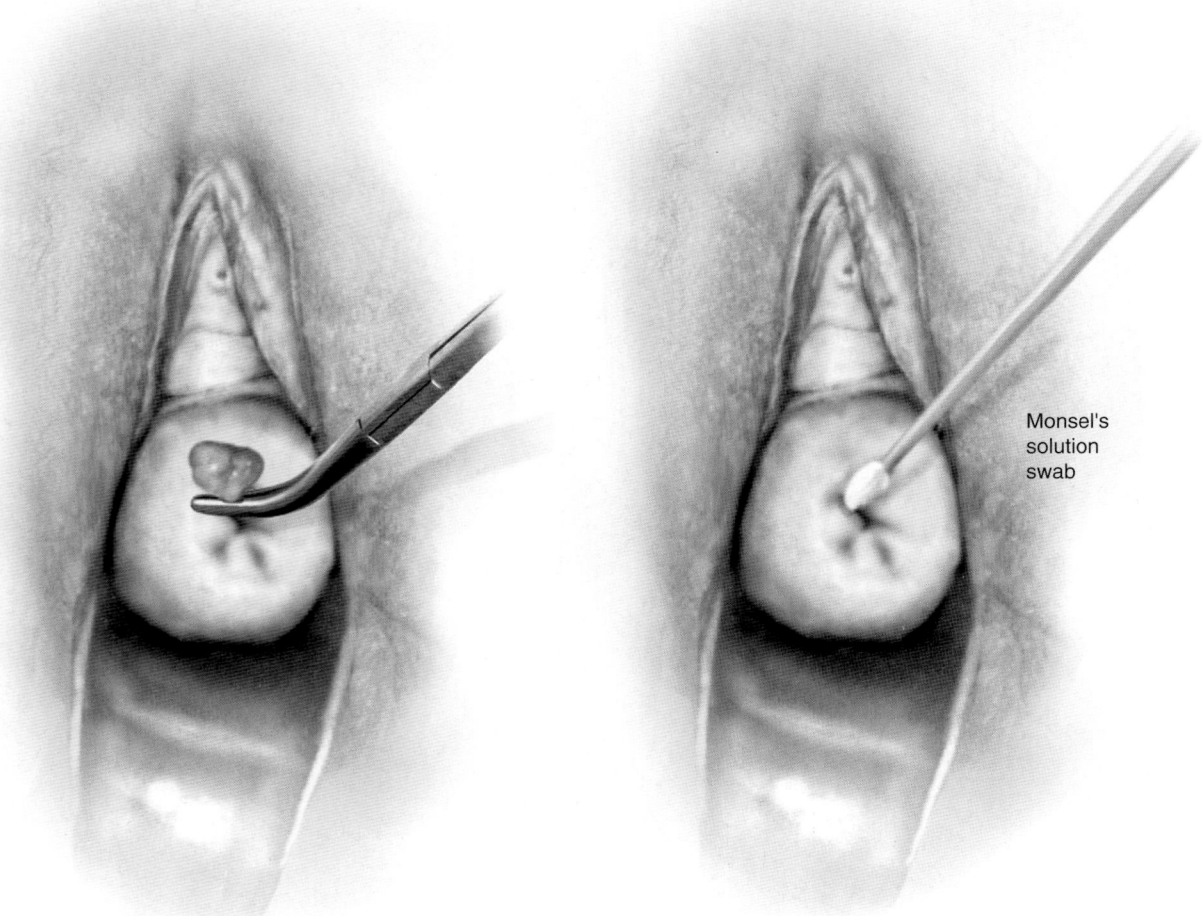

Monsel's solution swab

**FIGURE 47–3** A Kelly clamp is placed onto the pedicle of the polyp and twisted. The polyp separates from the endocervical canal and is sent to pathology. Monsel's solution is applied to the stump for hemostasis.

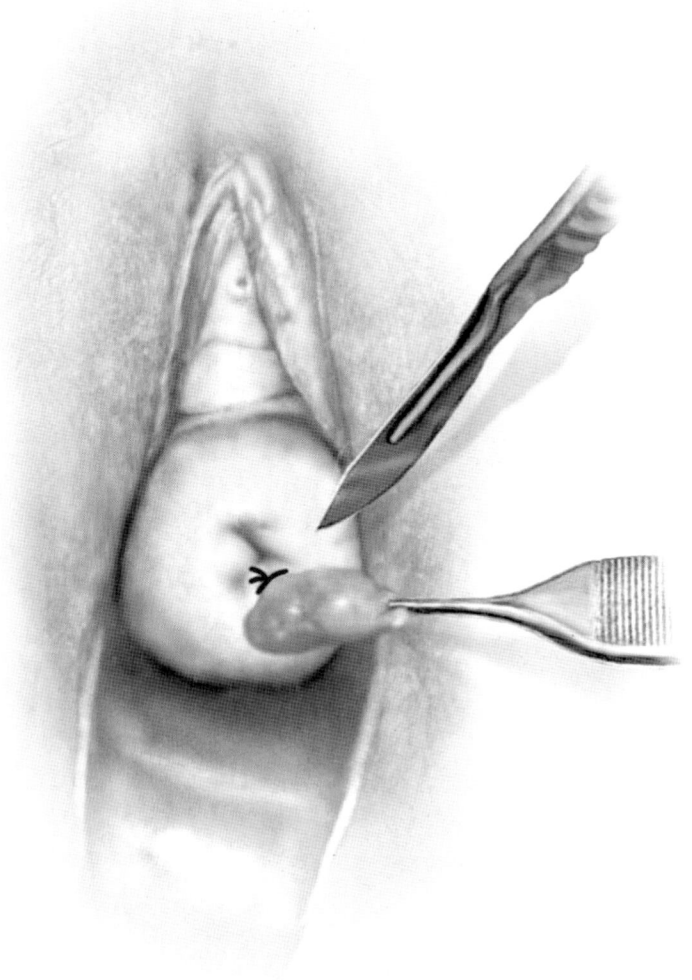

FIGURE 47–4 A larger polyp's pedicle is clamped and suture-ligated, then cut.

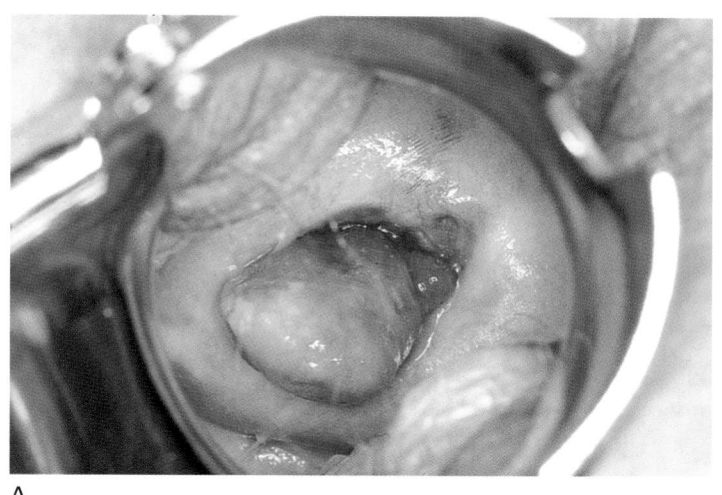

A

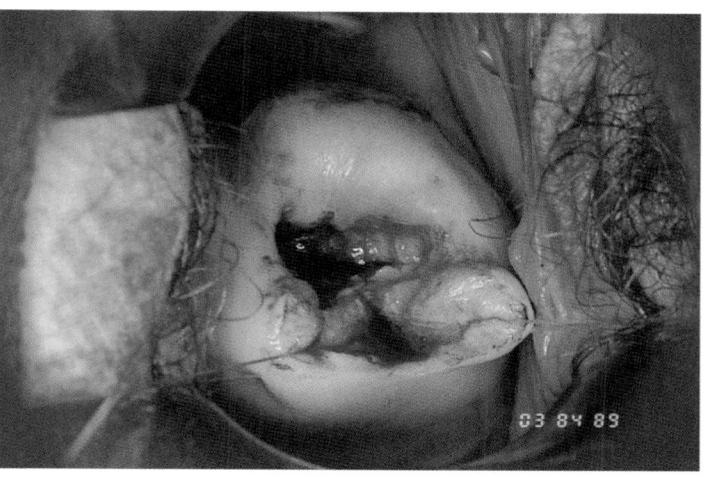

B

FIGURE 47–5 A. This large polyp's pedicle cannot be seen. B. An incision was made in the posterior lip of the cervix to expose the polyp's pedicle.

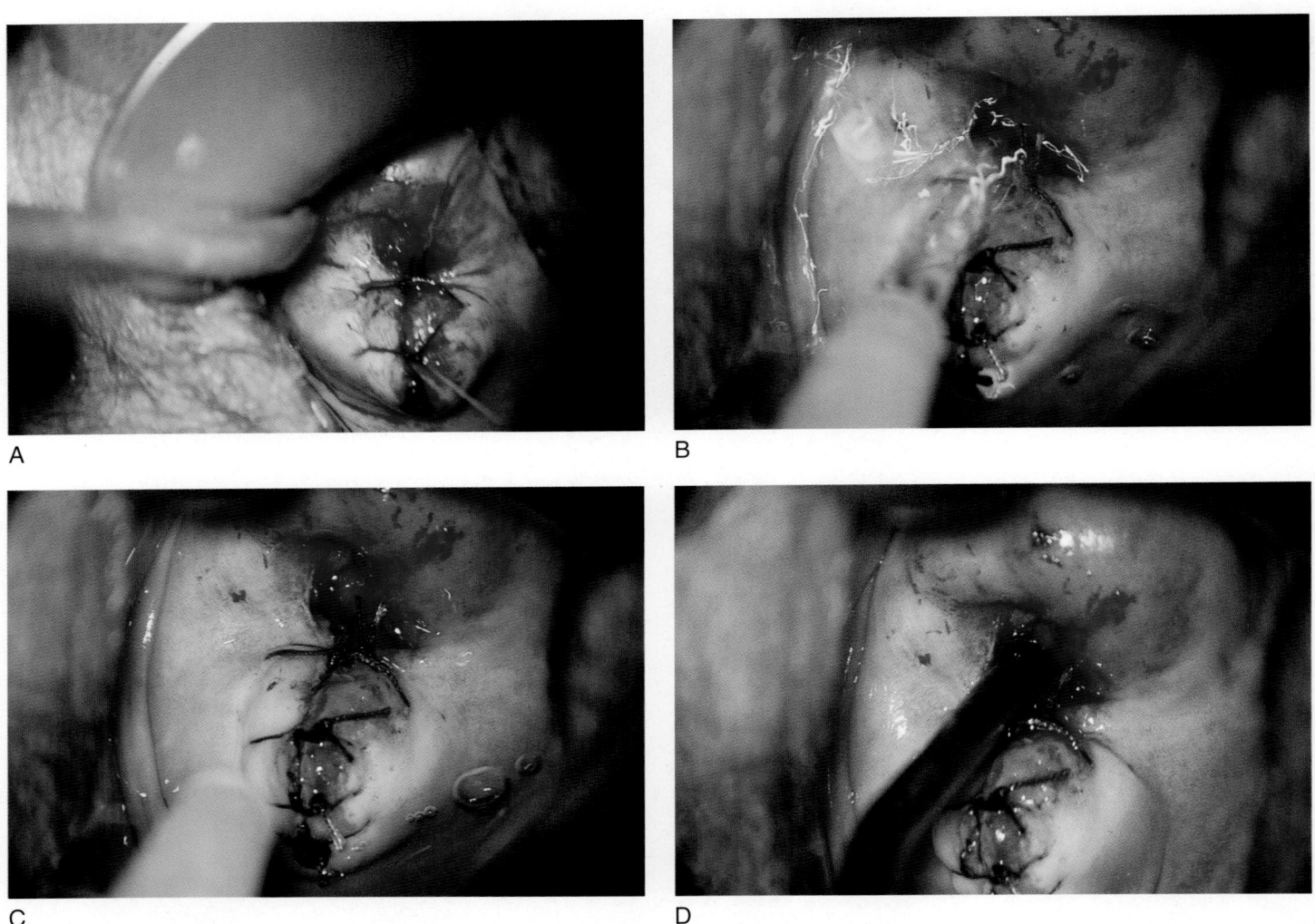

A

B

C

D

**FIGURE 47–6  A.** The ligature at the base of the polyp can be seen in the endocervical canal. Two stitches of 0 Vicryl have been placed into the previously opened posterior cervical lip. **B.** The wound is thoroughly irrigated with normal saline after the suture-ligature has been cut. **C.** A total of four sutures are placed into the posterior cervical lip. **D.** The cervical canal is sounded to ensure that no narrowing has occurred.

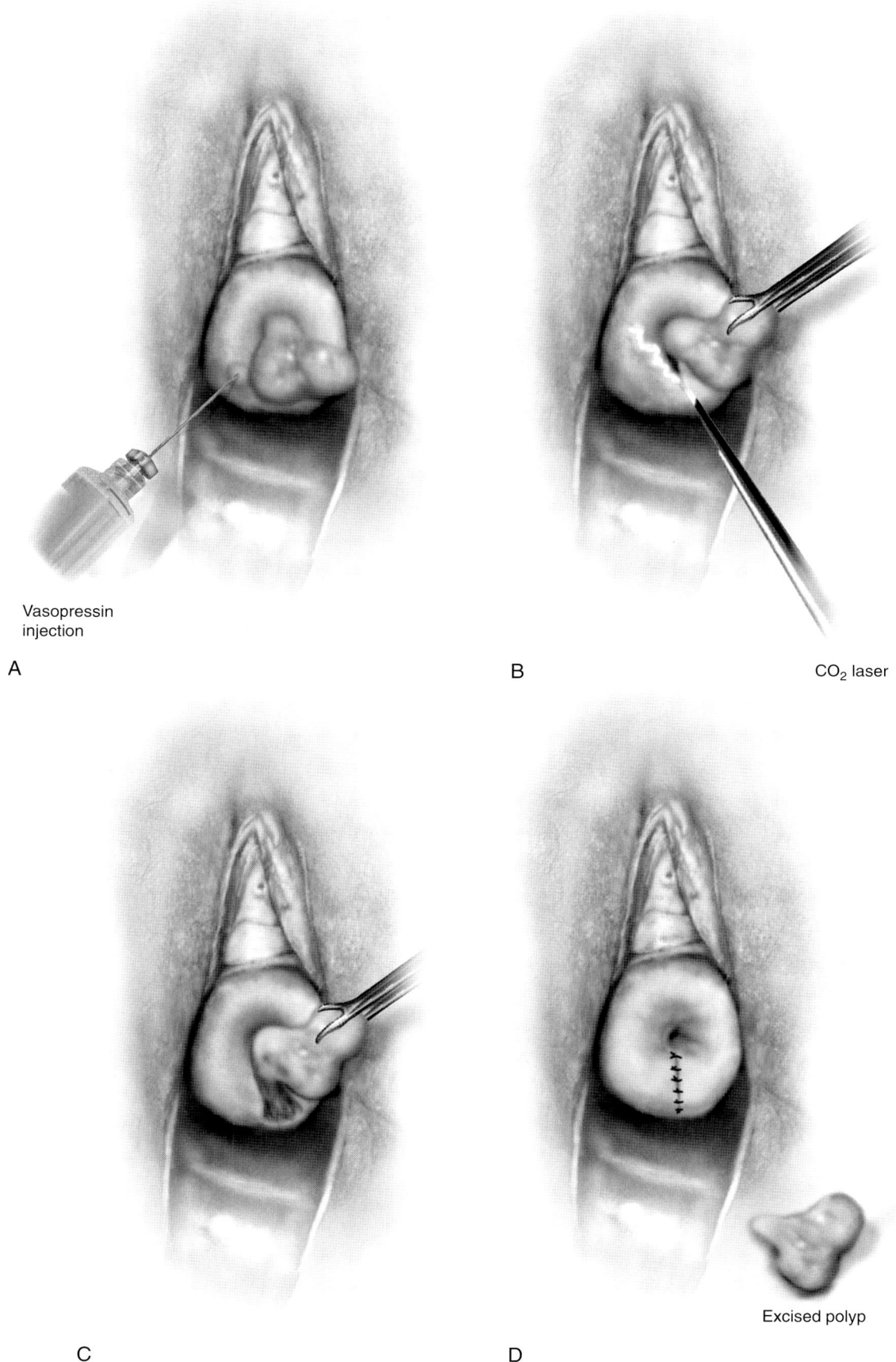

A

Vasopressin
injection

B

$CO_2$ laser

C

D

Excised polyp

**FIGURE 47–7 A.** Vasopressin is injected into the posterior portion of the cervix. **B.** The laser beam cuts the posterior lip of the cervix. **C.** The polyp base is ligated as the polyp is mobilized preparatory to cutting it off the cervix. **D.** The excised polyp and the repaired posterior cervical lip.

# CHAPTER 48

# Relief of Cervical Stenosis

*Michael S. Baggish*

Cervical stenosis is defined as a scarred endocervical canal measuring 1 mm or less in diameter. The stenosis ranges from mild at 2 mm to a pinhole opening of less than 0.5 mm (Fig. 48–1A through C). On occasion, the opening to the shrunken canal is marked only with a dimple. The cause of this problem is basically a quantitative reduction in cervical mucous glands secondary to obstetric trauma, sharp conization, electrosurgery, laser surgery, cryosurgery, or amputation. Dilatation and curettage, traumatic endocervical aspiration, and endocervical curettage more often lead to mild narrowing at the external os or adhesions rather than to true stenosis of the canal.

The diagnosis is made colposcopically and by the insertion of a small probe (Baby Hegar dilator) that measures 2 mm on one end and 1 mm on the other (Fig. 48–2). If required, a smaller lacrimal probe may be inserted into the canal with the intent to pass it along the canal's axis into the endometrial cavity.

The simplest therapeutic measure is directed at gently and gradually dilating the canal. It is advised to start with the Baby Hegar dilator and continue the dilatation with tapered Pratt dilators. This procedure should be repeated weekly in the office setting for 4 weeks. The patient should be checked and, if necessary, redilated monthly for 6 months. This method is useful for mild stenosis but is generally ineffective in more severe cases.

Severe stenosis can be relieved by removing the fibrotic tissue, finding viable glandular cells, exteriorizing them, and finally enlarging the canal. This technique requires a precision microsurgical procedure, which can and should be done by means of a superpulse-capable carbon dioxide ($CO_2$) laser coupled to the operating microscope via a micromanipulator. Small beam diameters (1 mm) must be used..

If a canal opening can be seen when the colposcope is used for magnification, a small probe can be inserted and gently advanced through the endocervical canal. Next, a 1:100 dilute vasopressin solution is injected into the cervix. The laser is set at 10 to 12 W ultrapulse, and trace spots are placed around the canal (Fig. 48–3A, B). The scar tissue around the canal is then vaporized layer by layer until orange-red endocervical mucosa is seen (Fig. 48–4). At this point, the endocervical canal is split by two radial cuts made from the center of the canal (probe) to its peripheral margin (Figs. 48–5A, B and 48–6A). A moist cotton-tipped applicator may be inserted through the canal and into the lower corpus of the uterus (Fig. 48–6B). Next, laser power is reduced to 5 to 10 W, and the beam is fired at the submucosal margin of the endocervical mucosa, thereby causing it to evert (see Fig. 48–6A). The field is irrigated with warm saline to expunge the carbonized, devitalized tissue.

Postoperatively, the patient is placed on the equivalent of 5 mg of conjugated estrogen (Premarin) per day for 30 days (Fig. 48–7).

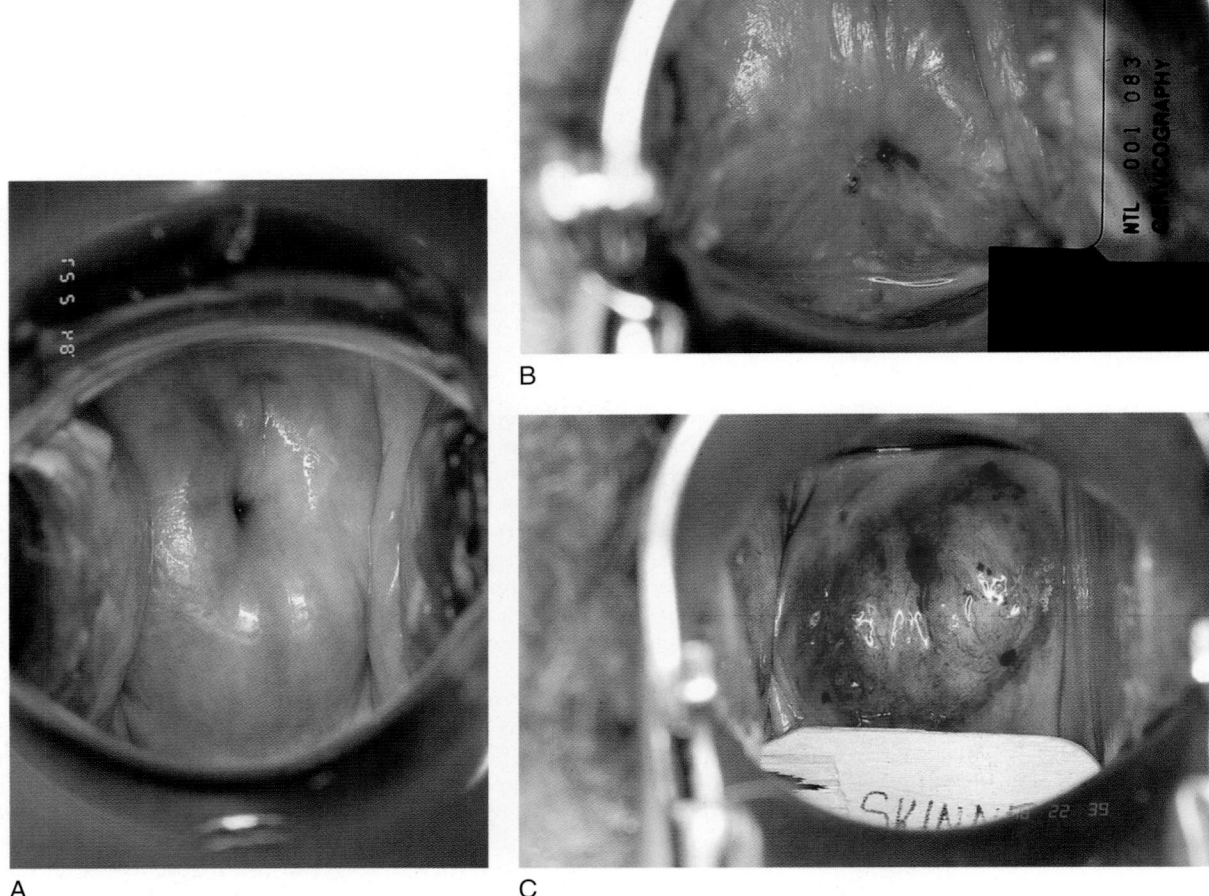

A

B

C

**FIGURE 48–1  A.** This cervix has been coned. The length has diminished by 30%, and the canal is moderately stenotic. **B.** Severe stenosis. The external os is located at the spot where a drop of blood is seen. **C.** Very severe stenosis. A pinhead opening is located centrally in this cervix.

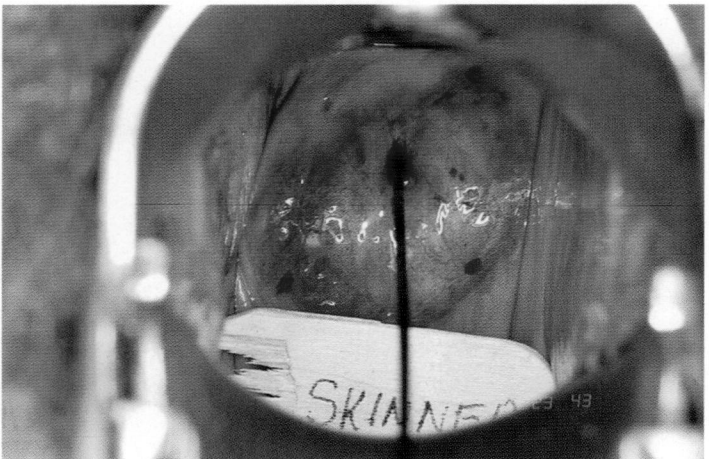

**FIGURE 48–2**  A Baby Hegar dilator is inserted in an attempt to enlarge the small opening in the cervical canal.

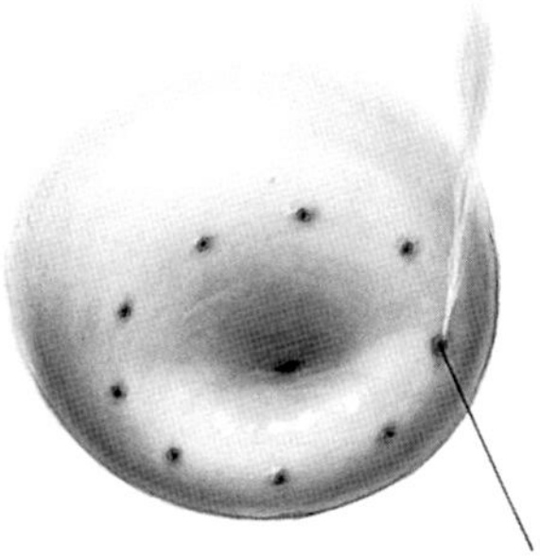

A

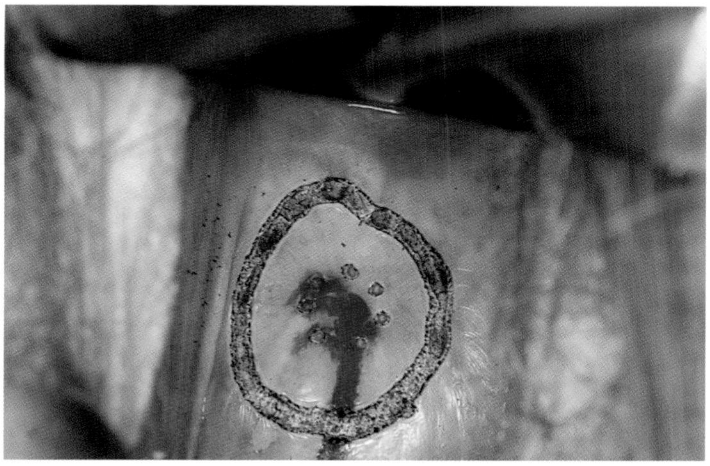

B

FIGURE 48–3 A. Following the injection of vasopressin, a superpulse laser is used to fire several trace spots into the cervix in preparation for reconstruction of the endocervical canal. B. The trace spots are connected 3 to 5 mm circumferential to the central stenotic opening of the cervical canal. The goal of this phase of the surgery is to vaporize the surrounding dense scar tissue to release the canal.

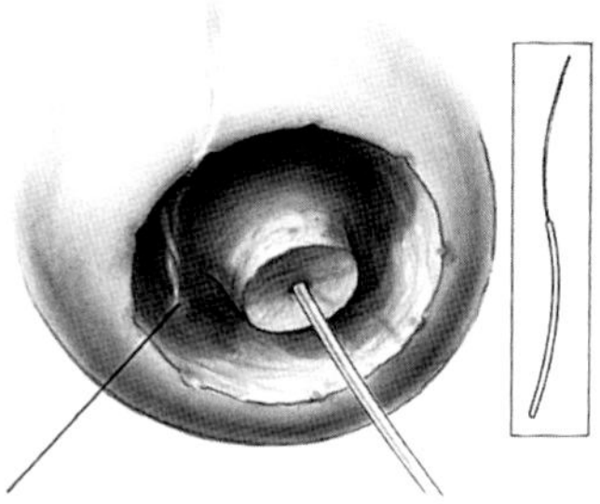

A

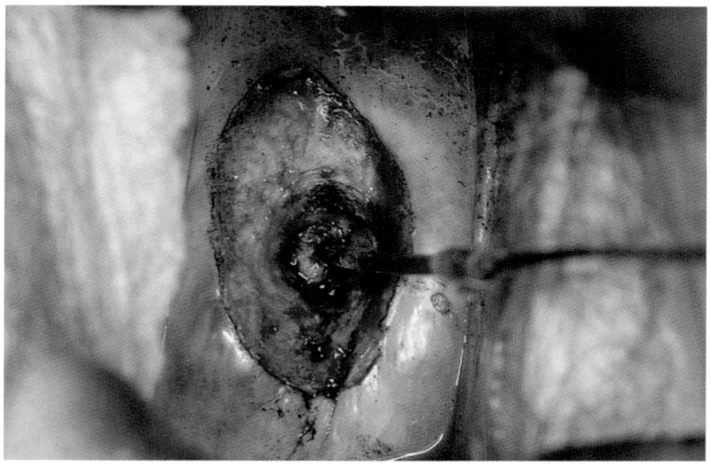

B

FIGURE 48–5 A. The Baby Hegar dilator is again inserted into the cervical canal. B. Once the canal has been released from the surrounding scar tissue, a greater degree of dilatation can be realized. Note that the 2-mm end of the dilator can now be accommodated.

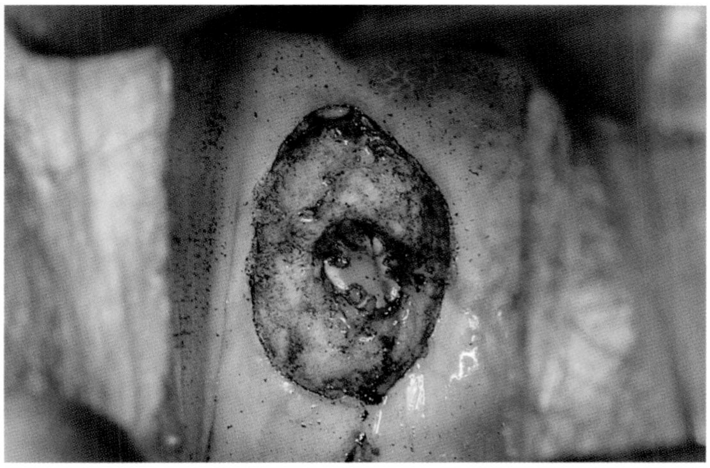

FIGURE 48–4 The peripheral scar tissue has been vaporized. Flexible tissue beneath the scar can be seen and palpated.

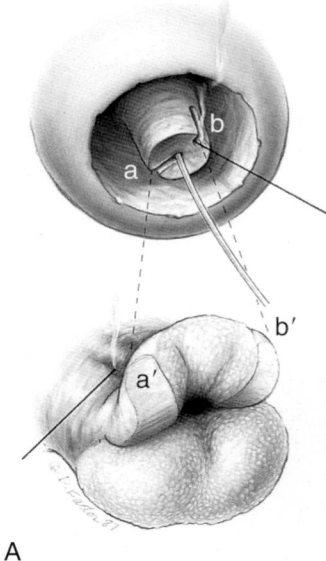

A

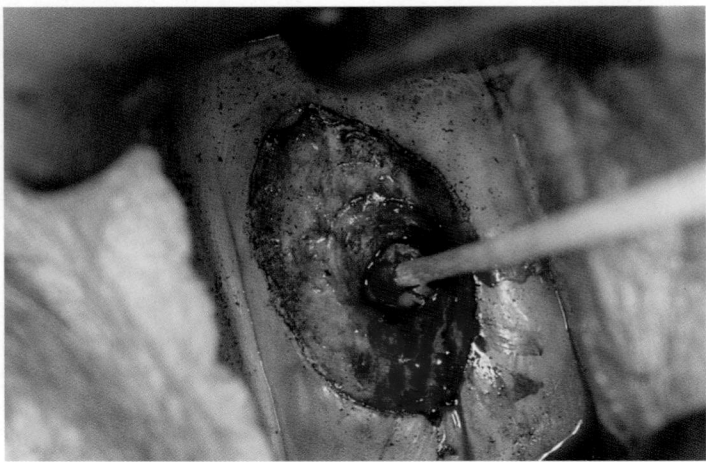

B

**FIGURE 48–6  A.** Red endocervical mucosa can now be recognized. The laser beam is tightly focused, and the canal is opened from the 1 o'clock position to 7 o'clock. The laser spot is then enlarged to 2 mm, and power is reduced to 5 to 10 W and is played directly behind the endocervical mucosa, resulting in eversion of the mucosa. **B.** A moist cotton-tipped applicator can be inserted through the now-enlarged canal.

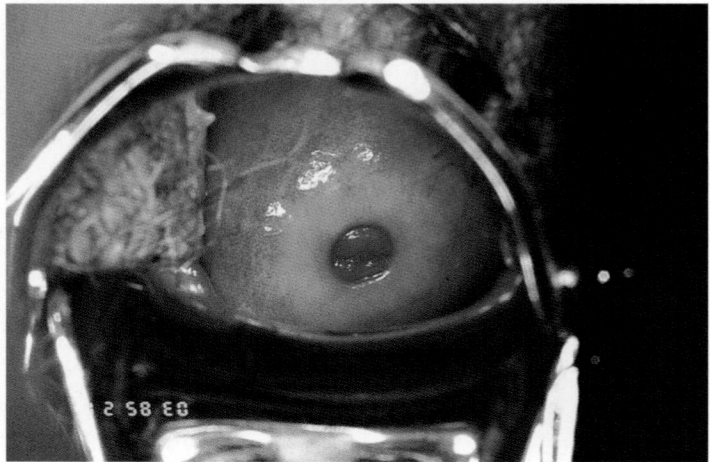

**FIGURE 48–7**  Six weeks postoperatively, a nonstenotic endocervical canal is visible.

# CHAPTER 49

# Cervical Cerclage

*Michael S. Baggish*

Cervical incompetence (cervical insufficiency) is a nebulous condition characterized by pain-free dilatation and shortening of the cervix in the second or early third trimester of pregnancy (Fig. 49-1). This is followed by prolapse of the membranes through the cervix and, ultimately, by expulsion of the fetus with or without membrane rupture (Fig. 49-2). The diagnosis of cervical insufficiency depends primarily on an obstetric history of one or more pregnancy losses associated with painless labor and dilatation.

Once the diagnosis has been at least presumptively made, a decision must be reached about whether to suture the cervix. Most cerclage operations are performed via the vaginal approach. The technique of abdominal cerclage is described and shown in Unit I.

The Shirodkar surgical procedure is aimed at restoring the cervix to a nondilated state as well as lengthening the cervical canal. Essentially, in this operation a nonresorbable suture is placed at or above the level of the internal os of the cervix. If lengthening is to be achieved, then a portion of the corporal isthmus should be incorporated into the encompassing suture. This will eliminate the funnel effect of the membranes at the top of the cervical canal and will add 1 to 2 cm of length to the canal. Care must be taken to dissect the vagina away from the cervix and to retract it superiorly and anteriorly to avoid injury to the terminal ureter (i.e., at the uterovesical junction). As is noted in Section F Unit II, the ureters cross the vagina at the anterior and anterolateral fornices to gain entry to the bladder base (trigone).

The cervix is exposed by placing a weighted retractor into the posterior fornix. Small Dever retractors are placed in the lateral vaginal fornices, and a finger (small Richardson) retractor is placed in the anterior fornix. Sutures of 0 Vicryl are placed into the cervix at the 3 and 9 o'clock positions in figure-of-8 fashion for traction (Fig. 49-3A). These sutures should not be placed too far back into the lateral fornix because they can occlude the ureter. The sutures must be placed in the cervix forward of the vaginal reflection.

Next, 10 to 20 mL of normal saline is injected into the anterior cervix at the point of the vaginal reflection to create a plane of dissection. A similar injection is made into the posterior aspect of the cervix. A 2-cm incision is made with a scalpel into the vaginal reflection. The vagina is easily separated and dissected from the cervix. A similar procedure is carried out posteriorly. Retractors can now be placed between the cervix and the vagina (Fig. 49-3B, C).

A Mersilene band on a double-armed needle is introduced into the anterior incision at or above the level of the internal os. The needle is slipped between the vagina and the cervix, respectively, on the right and left sides and is brought out at the posterior incision site (Fig. 49-3D). The suture is tied into place posteriorly taking care not to squeeze the cervix so much as to cause the band to cut into the substance of the cervix or, even worse, through the cervix. This can be prevented by inserting a metal catheter or a firm rubber catheter into the cervix and tightening over the catheter (Fig. 49-3E). A 3-0 Prolene stitch should be placed into the cervix and through the band both anteriorly and posteriorly to prevent the band from displacing. The mucosa is closed with simple interrupted 2-0 Vicryl sutures (Fig. 49-3F).

McDonald originally specified that a No. 4 braided silk suture should be placed into the cervix beginning anteriorly (12 o'clock) at the point where the rugose vagina is reflected onto the smooth mucosa of the cervix and is carried clockwise or counterclockwise, taking peripheral bites with the needle around the cervix through the 3, 6, and 9 o'clock positions until arriving back at the 12 o'clock position (Fig. 49-4A, B). At that point, the stitch is tightened over the assistant's index or little finger inserted into the patient's cervical canal and is secured with three or four throws of the knot (Fig. 49-4C). Although McDonald thought the cervicovaginal junction corresponded to the internal os, in reality it is below that location (Fig 49-4C, **inset**). Placing the suture at the internal os would mean suturing into the anterior vagina and possibly injuring the ureters or the urinary bladder. Currently, #2 Prolene and Mersilene are the suture materials most commonly used for this cerclage technique.

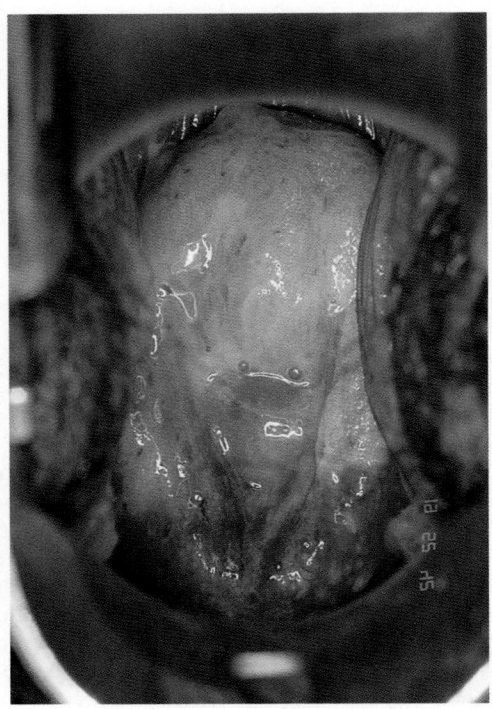

**FIGURE 49–1** This patient was referred for colposcopy and biopsy because of an abnormal Pap smear. The cervix is agape with the canal dilated and shortened. The blue-tinged membranes are clearly visible.

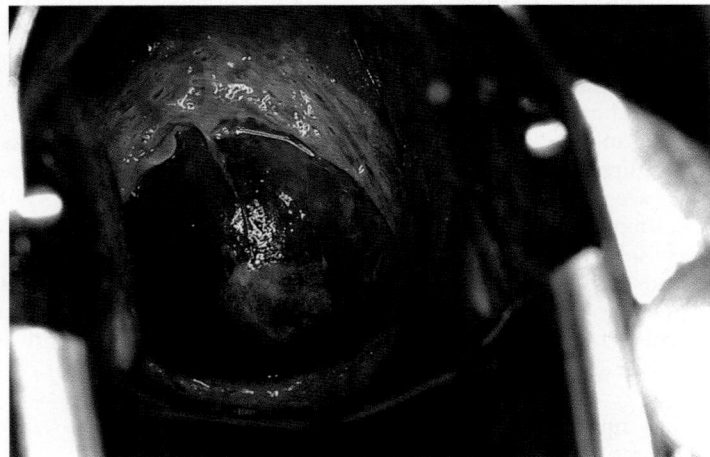

**FIGURE 49–2** This painless labor progressed rapidly. The cervix is 5 cm dilated and completely effaced, and the membranes are bulging into the vagina.

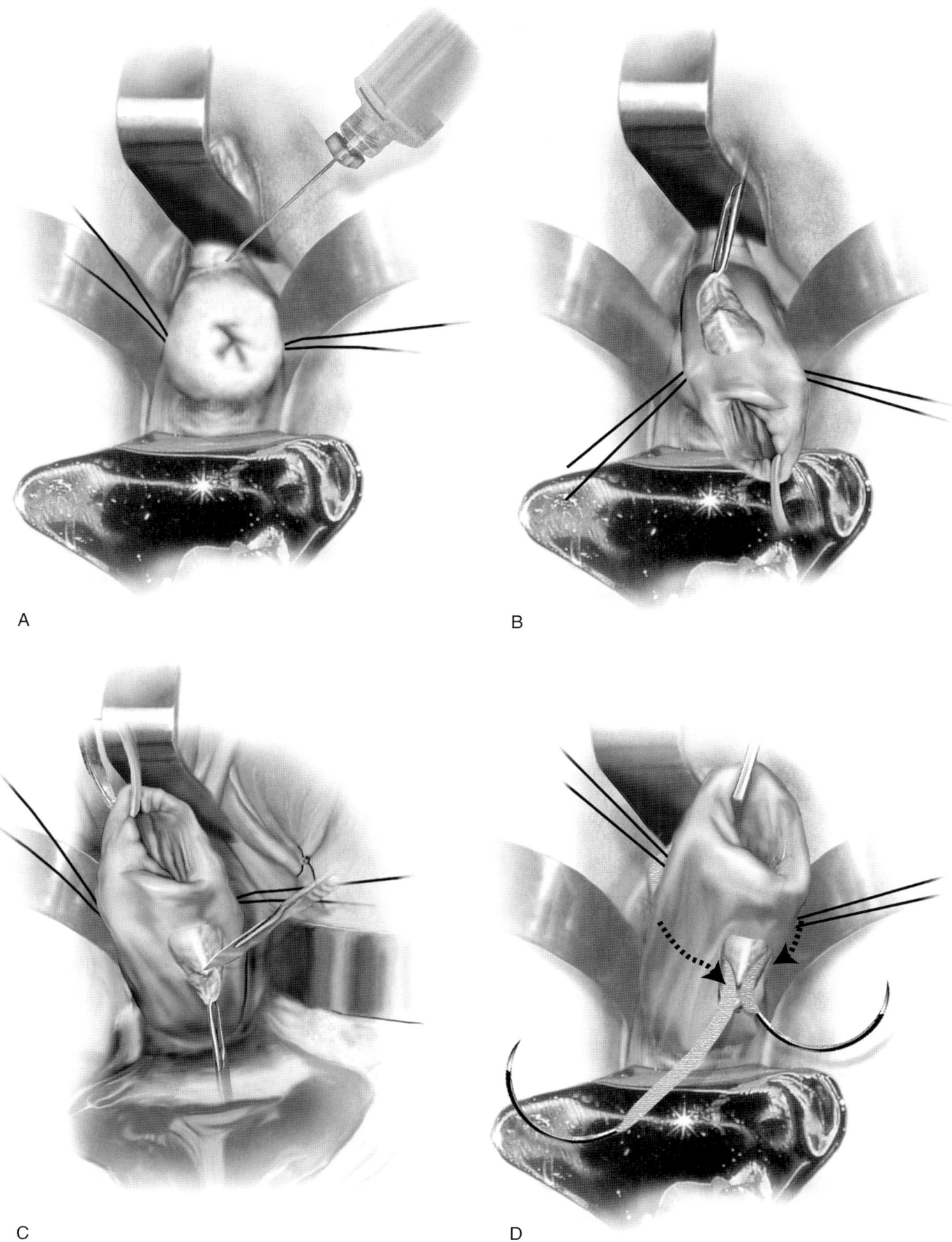

A

B

C

D

**FIGURE 49–3  A.** Shirodkar cerclage. The cervix is secured with two 0 Vicryl sutures placed at the 3 and 9 o'clock positions at the vaginal cervical reflections. An injection of 10 to 20 mL of normal saline is made just beneath the cervical mucosa to create a plane of dissection. **B.** A transverse 2-cm incision is made on the anterior aspect of the cervix at the 12 o'clock position and is carried down to the pubocervical fascia. The bladder is pushed cranially and is freed from the cervix (i.e., the bladder is advanced). **C.** A similar incision is made on the posterior surface of the cervix. In this case, the cul-de-sac is dissected away from the cervical tissue and is advanced. **D.** A Mersilene band swagged onto a large, curved needle enters via the anterior incision and exits via the posterior incision on the right and left. The cervix is now completely encircled by the band.

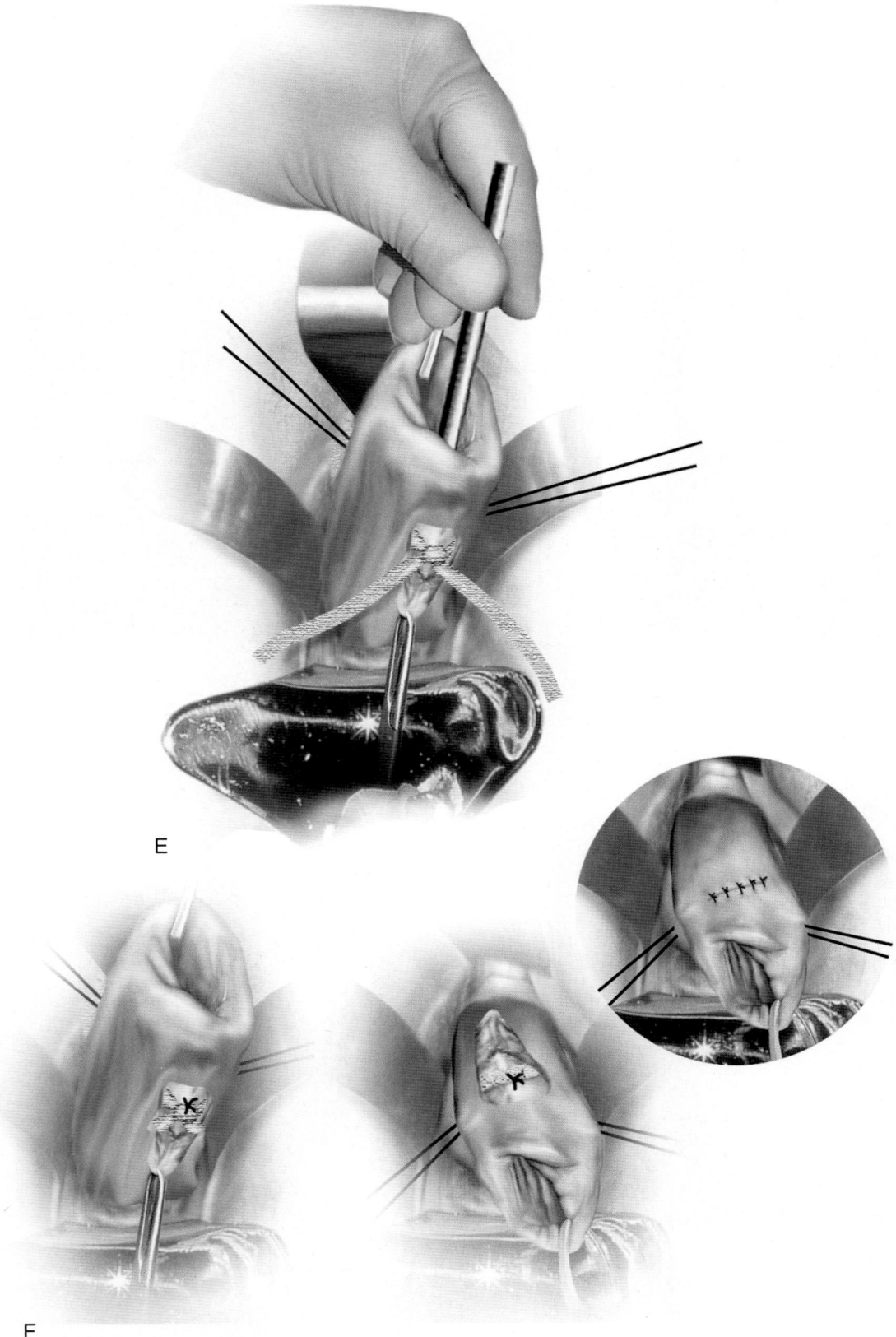

E

F

**FIGURE 49–3, cont'd  E.** The needles are cut off, and the band is tied at 6 o'clock over a rubber catheter.
**F.** Anteriorly and posteriorly, 3-0 nylon sutures are placed through the band and into the substance of the cervix to anchor the band and prevent migration. Finally, the incisions are closed with a 2-0 Vicryl running or interrupted suture.

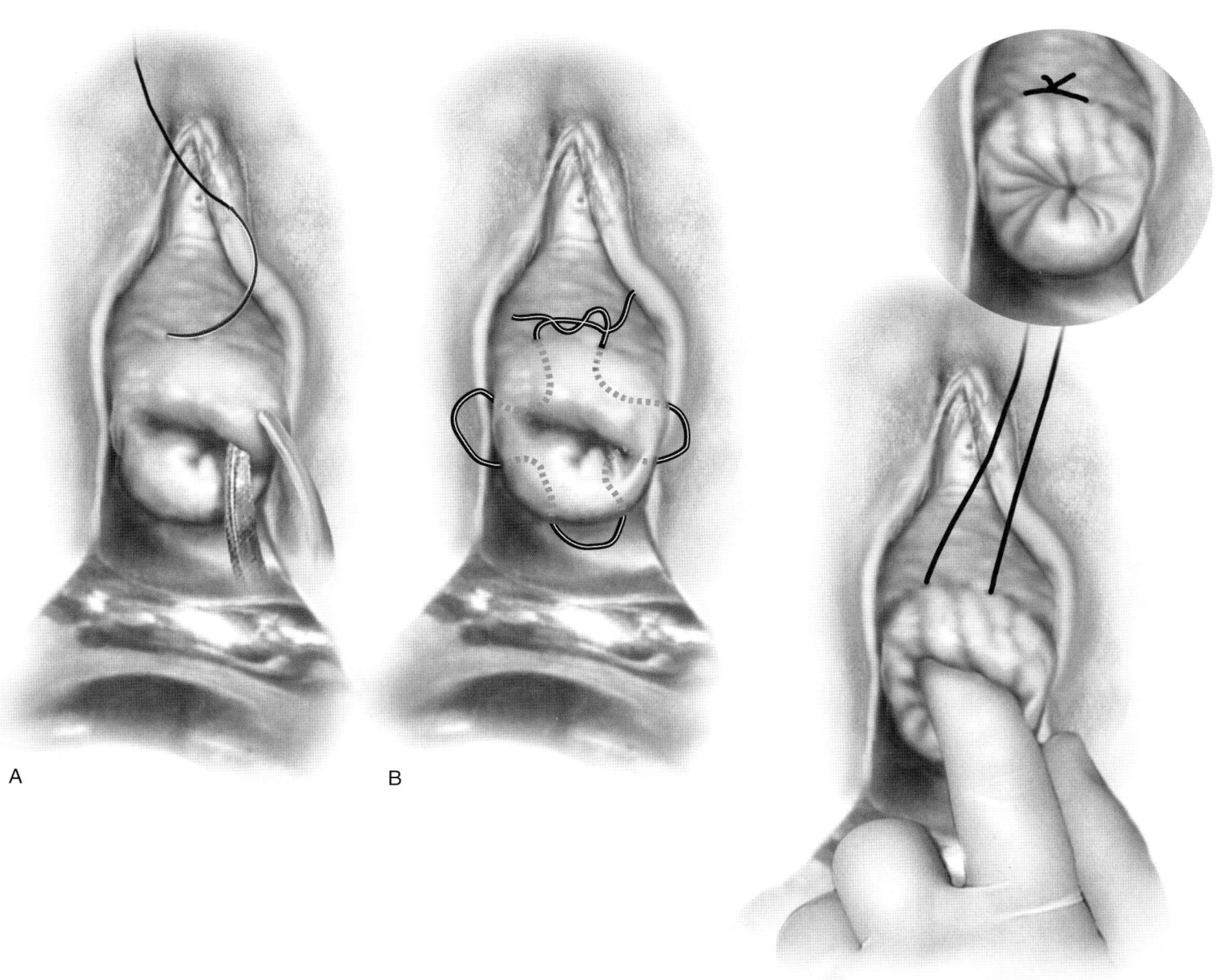

A                    B

C

**FIGURE 49–4  A.** McDonald cerclage. The anterior lip of the cervix is held with a tenaculum. A #2 Prolene suture is placed into the cervix beginning on the anterior surface below the junction of the cervical and vaginal mucosa. **B.** The suture is vectored counterclockwise around the cervix, while taking multiple, secure bites into the cervical mucosa and stroma throughout the circumnavigation of the cervix. **C.** The suture is squarely tied down over the finger of the assistant. This prevents excessive cinching down of the stitch and will reduce the chances of the suture cutting completely through the cervix. **Inset.** The final puckered appearance of the sutured cervix (purse string or tobacco pouch effect).

# CHAPTER 50

# Cervical Stump Excision (Trachelectomy)

*Mickey M. Karram* ■ *Michael S. Baggish*

A cervical stump is the remnant of the uterus that remains following a subtotal hysterectomy (Fig. 50–1). Historically, supracervical hysterectomy was performed under adverse circumstances whereby rapid termination of the operation was essential for the well-being of the patient (e.g., in the complicated pregnancy). However, more recently surgeons are electively performing laparoscopic or robotic subtotal hysterectomy. Subsequent removal of the stump, or trachelectomy, may be required for various reasons, including persistent bleeding, prolapse, pain, and abnormal cervical pathology.

The cervical stump is removed in an identical fashion to the initial steps of a vaginal hysterectomy. Although entering the peritoneal cavity is not mandatory, it is preferred to ensure complete removal of the cervix and to allow for obliteration of the cul-de-sac and suspension of the vagina in cases of prolapse. The stump is grasped with a single-toothed tenaculum and is pulled inferiorly. A 1:100 diluted vasopressin solution is injected beneath the cervical and vaginal mucosa with a 25-gauge needle and a triple-ring 10-mL syringe. The solution will help to develop a plane of dissection. The injections are performed circumferentially around the cervix (Fig. 50–2A). With a scalpel, an incision is made into the cervix and is circumscribed below the cervicovaginal junction (Fig. 50–2B). The bladder is dissected from the cervix anteriorly; the vagina, together with the ureters, is pushed upward (craniad) from the lateral aspect of the cervix (Figs. 50–2C and 50–3A). The cul-de-sac and the rectum are dissected free posteriorly (Fig. 50–3B). The lower portion of the cardinal ligaments is clamped with curved Zeppelin clamps (Figs. 50–2D and 50–4). The uterosacral ligaments are identified and clamped (Figs. 50–2E and 50–5). The clamped structures are cut and transfixed with 0 Vicryl sutures. The cervix is kept taut by downward traction of the tenaculum and is completely freed from the rectum posteriorly (i.e., the rectovaginal space is dissected free from the cervix) (Fig. 50–6). The bladder may be adherent to the stump; thus sharp dissection should always be utilized to mobilize the bladder off the cervix (Fig. 50–7). The Metzenbaum scissors are directed away from the bladder and toward the stump in a carefully executed spread-and-cut technique. The stump is cut free and removed (Figs. 50–2F, 50–8, and 50–9). The cardinal and uterosacral stumps are sutured into each vaginal angle, and the vagina is closed transversely with interrupted 0 Vicryl sutures. If prolapse is present, a culdoplasty or a vaginal vault suspension should be performed (see Chapters 53 and 55).

As a cautionary note, it should be understood that during the supracervical hysterectomy, the bladder peritoneum may be advanced over the top of the cervix and sutured down posteriorly as a means of covering and peritonizing the stump. Conversely, the peritoneum of the sigmoid colon may be advanced and sutured anteriorly for the same purpose.

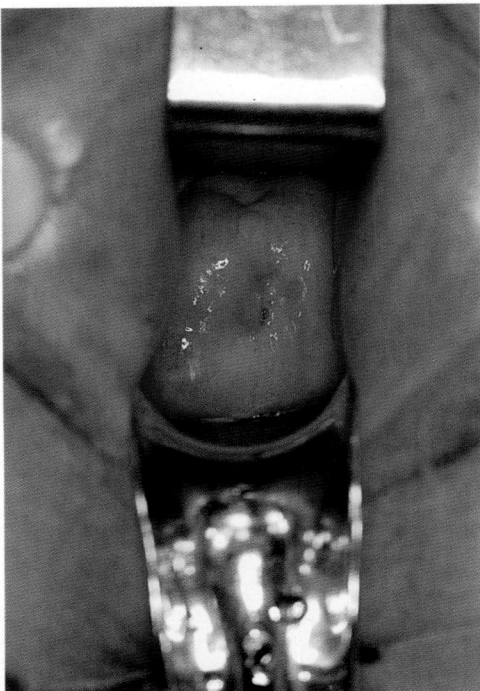

**FIGURE 50-1** This cervix remained in situ following a laparoscopic subtotal hysterectomy. The patient subsequently desired removal of the cervix because of a persistent foul discharge and postcoital bleeding.

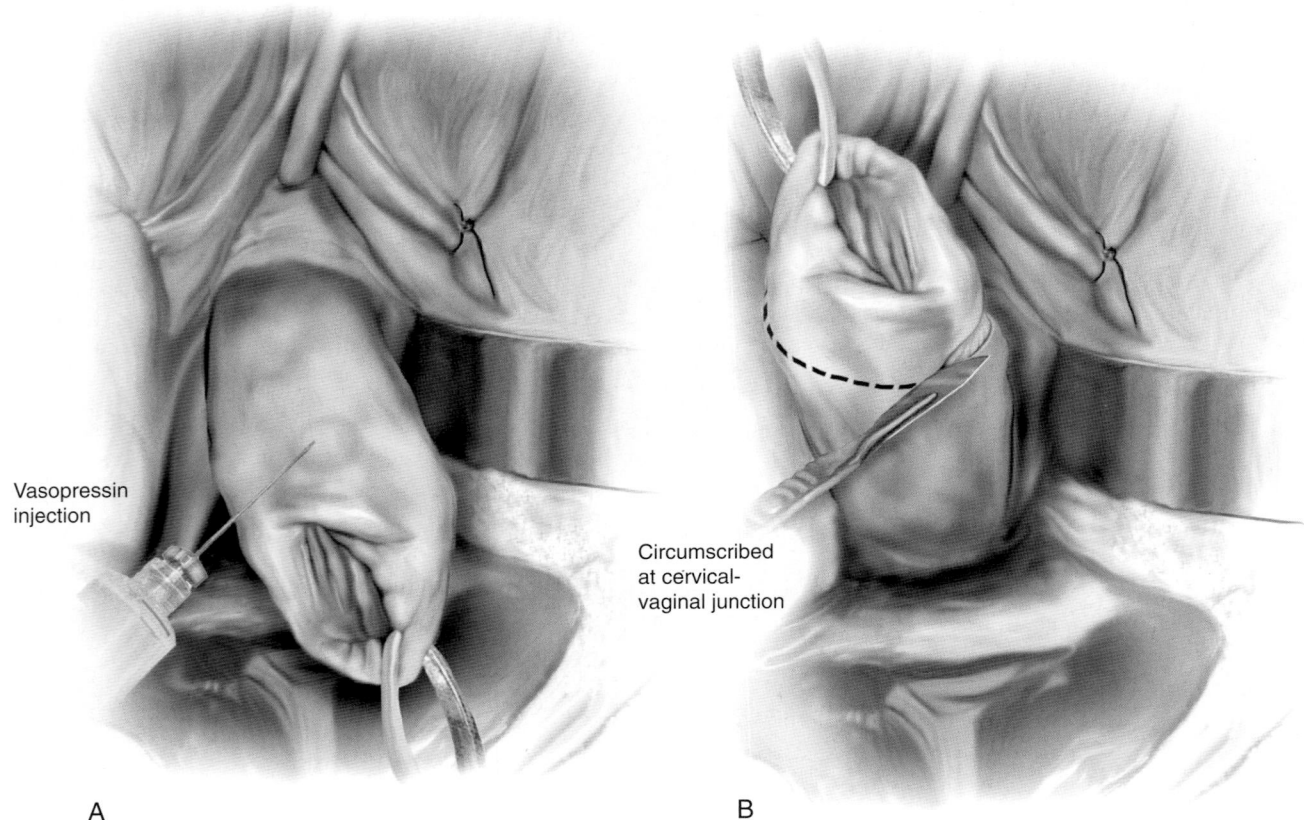

Vasopressin injection

Circumscribed at cervical-vaginal junction

A                                    B

**FIGURE 50-2 A.** The cervix is grasped with a tenaculum and is pulled downward. A fine needle is inserted submucosally, and a 1:100 vasopressin solution is injected at the 12 o'clock position and is continued circumferentially around the cervix. **B.** A scalpel is used to make a circumscribing incision into the cervix approximately 5 to 10 mm back from the external os.

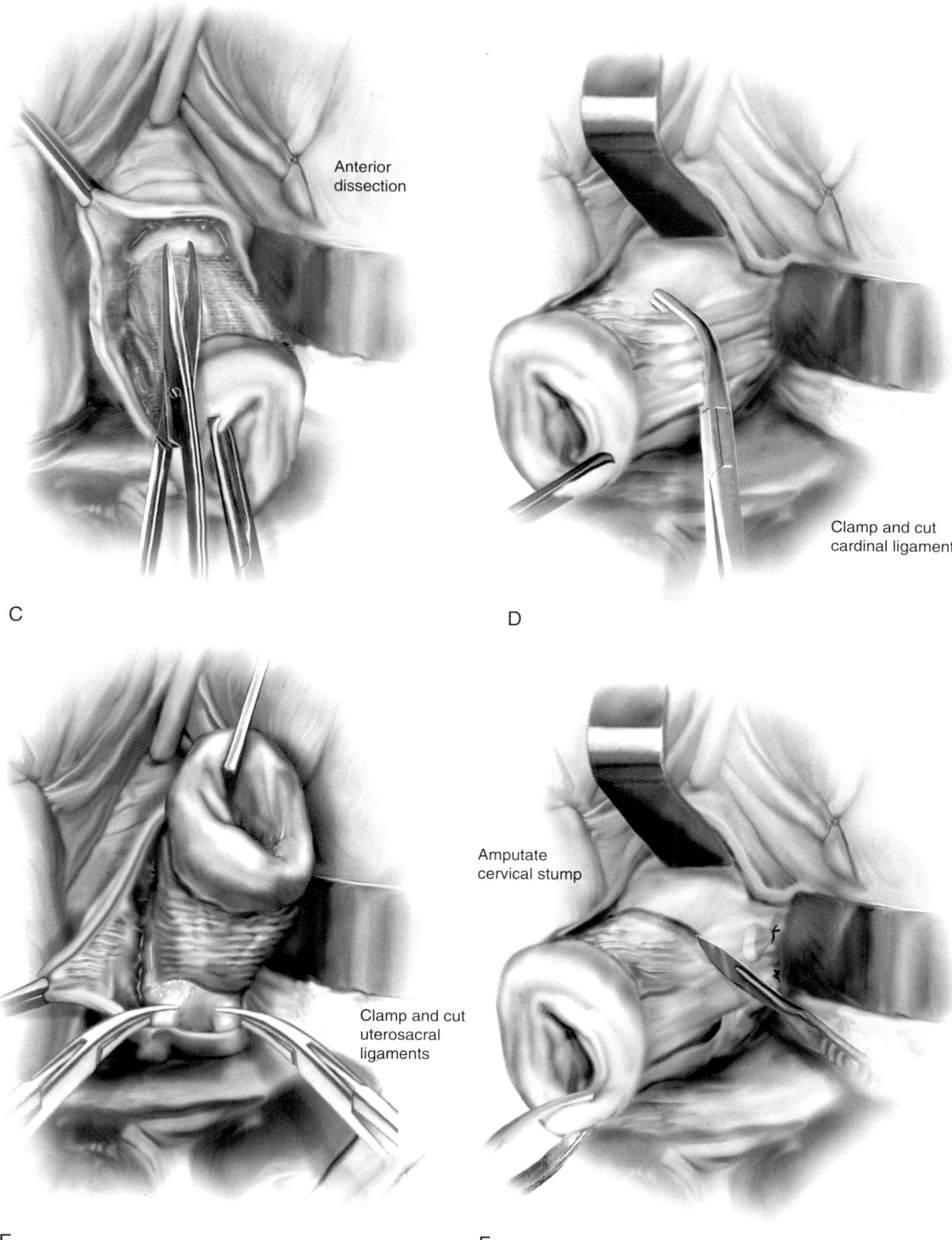

Anterior
dissection

C

Clamp and cut
cardinal ligament

D

Clamp and cut
uterosacral
ligaments

E

Amputate
cervical stump

F

**FIGURE 50–2, cont'd  C.** The bladder is sharply dissected from the cervix together with the anterior vagina; similarly, the posterior vagina and the cul-de-sac are dissected free of the cervix. **D.** The lower portion of the cardinal ligament is clamped. **E.** The uterosacral ligaments are similarly clamped, cut, and suture-ligated. **F.** The cervical stump, after having its ligamentous and vascular pedicles secured, is cut free by means of a sharp scalpel or scissors.

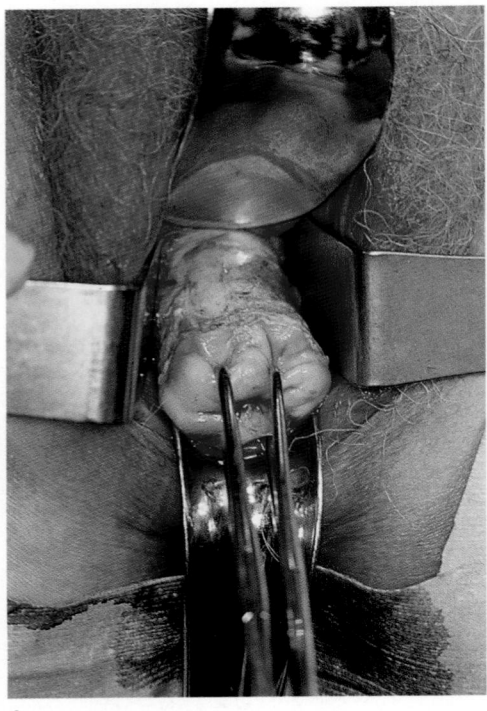
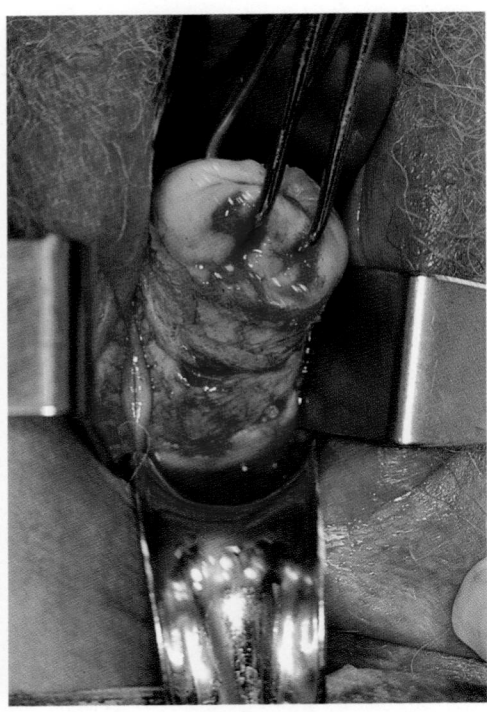

A                                                    B

**FIGURE 50–3  A.** The bladder has been dissected free from the anterior aspect of the cervix by means of Metzenbaum scissors. Note the downward tension on the cervix. **B.** The cul-de-sac and the rectum are freed from the posterior aspect of the cervix. Again, note the upward traction on the cervix, which facilitates the posterior dissection.

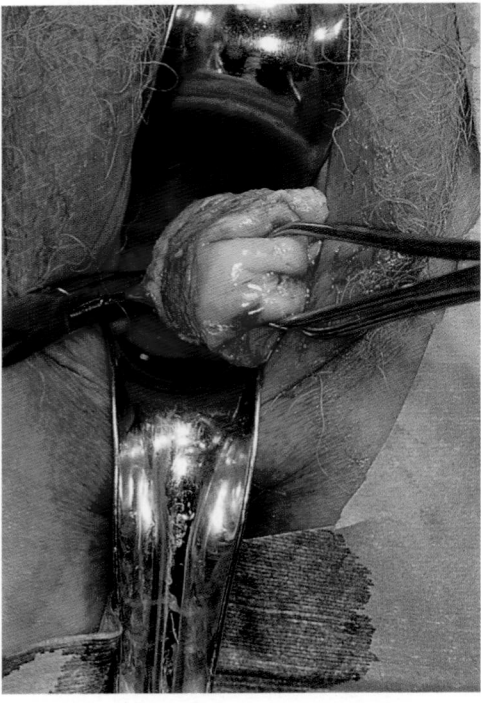

**FIGURE 50–4** The cardinal ligaments are clamped, cut, and suture-ligated with 0 Vicryl sutures.

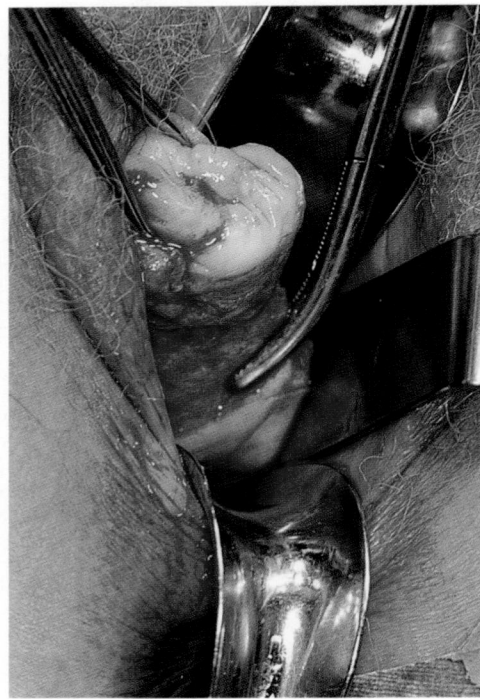

**FIGURE 50–5** The uterosacral ligaments are clamped, cut, and suture-ligated.

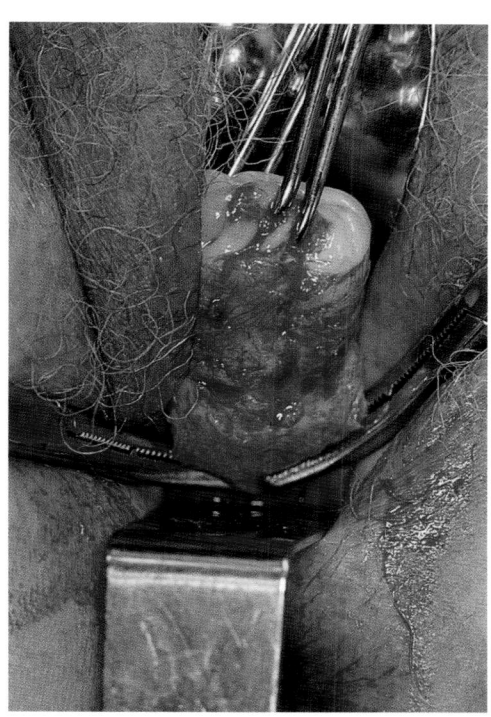

FIGURE 50–6 The top of the cervix is cross-clamped. Note that the rectum has been sufficiently mobilized off the posterior aspect of the cervix.

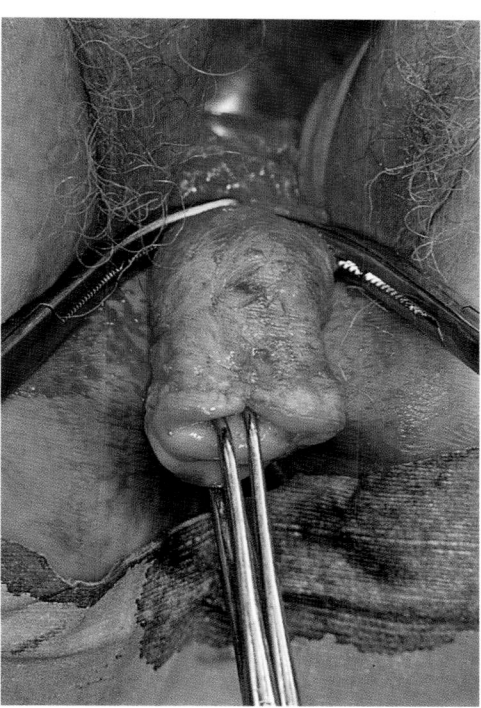

FIGURE 50–7 The bladder and ureters have been mobilized superiorly and out of the way of these clamps.

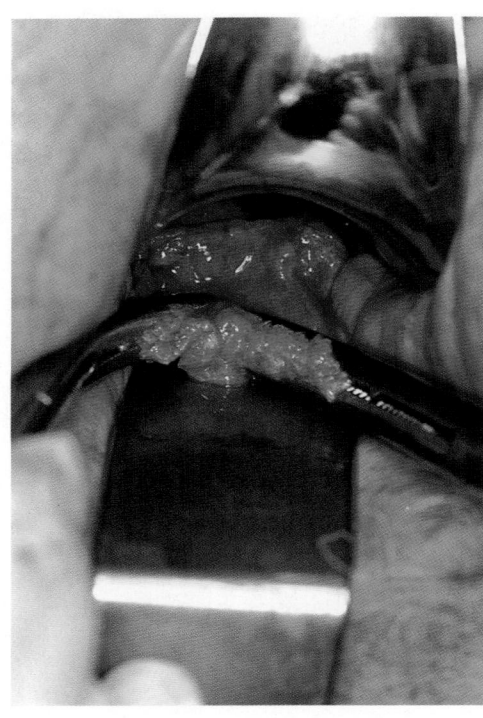

FIGURE 50–8 The stump has been excised over the clamps. The upper portions of the cardinal ligaments are suture-ligated with 0 Vicryl or polydioxanone (PDS).

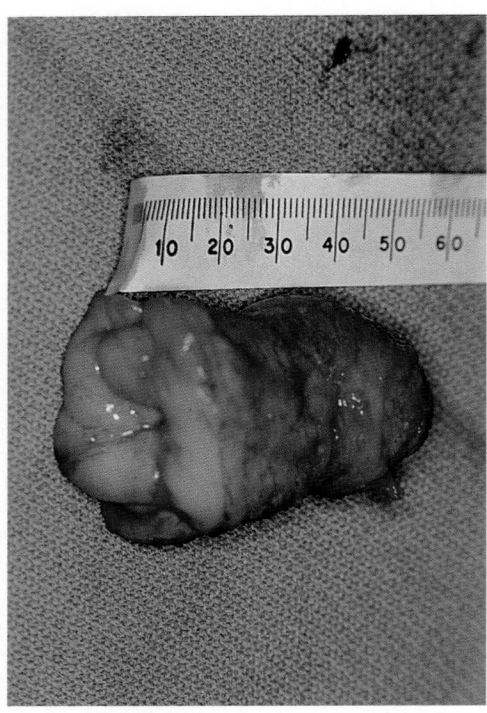

FIGURE 50–9 The 4-cm-long removed stump is sent to pathology for sampling. If intraepithelial neoplasia were present or suspected, the cervix would be cut up analogous to conization and serially sectioned.

# SECTION B

# Vaginal Surgery

# CHAPTER 51

# Anatomy of the Vagina

*Michael S. Baggish* ■ *Mickey M. Karram*

The vagina is a potential space that connects the lower portion of the uterus (cervix) to the outside environment. The vagina measures 8 to 8.5 cm from the hymenal ring to the top of the anterior fornix; 7 to 7.5 cm to the top of the lateral fornix; and 9 to 9.5 cm to the top of the posterior fornix. For the sake of organization, the vagina may be divided into thirds: upper, middle, and lower. The upper third of the vagina is closely related to the cervix uteri, to which it is attached (Fig. 51–1). Throughout its length, the vagina is intimately applied to the bladder and urethra anteriorly and is similarly applied to the rectum posteriorly. In its lower third, the vagina, rectum, and urethra share common walls. The lower third of the vagina also is closely related to the vulva, to which it is attached at the level of the vulvar vestibule (Fig. 51–2A). This particular transitional area can be considered the entry portal to or the exit portal from the vagina. In fact, in the lower third, one might consider the urethra, vagina, and anus–rectum as a single interdependent and interrelated structure rather than as independently functioning anatomic units (Fig. 51–2B, C). By sawing away the symphysis pubis and dissecting the bladder and urethra from the anterior vagina, important relationships can be seen and better understood (Fig. 51–2D through F).

The microscopic vagina consists of a mucosa that is made up of multilayered noncornified squamous epithelium. The underlying stroma consists of collagen admixed with elastic tissue. Beneath the stroma is smooth muscle interspersed with collagen. The epithelium measures 0.15 to 0.30 mm from top to bottom (surface to basement membrane). The entire vaginal wall thickness in a menstruating woman ranges from 2 to 3 mm.

## Lower Third

The hymenal ring forms the boundary between vagina and vestibule (Fig. 51–3A, B). Although the vagina contains no glandular elements under normal circumstances, several mucus-secreting structures are in close proximity: the paraurethral and vestibular glands (Fig. 51–4). The Bartholin glands (greater vestibular glands) are closely applied to the posterolateral wall of the vagina at a level 15 mm deep from the surface of the vestibule (Fig. 51–5A, B). At the 6-o'clock position, the rectum is 3 to 4 mm beneath the vagina, and at 12 o'clock, the urethra is 2 to 3 mm anterior to the vagina (Figs. 51–6A, B and 51–7A).

The vagina is highly vascularized, particularly on the anterolateral and lateral walls, from the level of the hymenal ring to the urethrovesical junction (Fig. 51–7B). Large venous sinuses and cavernous sinuses account for this vascularity, which is most plentiful at the level of the bulb of the vestibule. The bulb is encountered at a depth of 1.5 cm from the surface of the vestibule and lies in close proximity to the urethra and the anterolateral wall of the vagina. The urethra is covered on its anterior and lateral aspects with cavernous tissue emanating from the clitoris and the bulb (Fig. 51–8A through G). When one is dissecting in this area, consideration should be given to the pronounced vascularity along the lateral and anterolateral walls and the need for vasoconstrictive agents.

## Middle Third

The middle third begins just below the urethrovesical junction and crosses beneath the lower margin of the symphysis pubis (posterior-inferior margin) (2.5 to 3.5 cm from the hymenal ring). The levator ani muscle is applied to the lateral and posterior vaginal walls most prominently at the junction of the middle and lower thirds (see Fig. 51–7C). This portion, together with the cranial portion of the lower third, has the greatest degree of mobility compared with the rest of the vagina.

## Upper Third

The upper vagina is closely applied to the bladder but does not share the common wall encountered at the level of the urethra. A layer of loose areolar tissue permits the bladder to be easily dissected from the upper vagina (see Figs. 51–2D through F). Similarly, the rectum can be easily dissected from the upper vagina. However, as one dissects caudally, the wall shared among bladder, urethra, and vagina allows *no* easy plane of separation. The vagina terminates around the cervix, and the vaginal vault is divided into fornices by the protruding portio vaginalis of the cervix. The stroma of the vagina is actually inseparable from the cardinal and uterosacral ligaments (see Fig. 51–7D). Between the latter is a bloodless entry point between the posterior fornix of the vagina and the cul-de-sac (i.e., the entry into the peritoneal cavity). The relationships of the upper vagina to the bladder, urethra, and cervix require precise anatomic knowledge of the retroischial and retropubic (extraperitoneal) spaces. Many gynecologists refer to the lateral areas as paravaginal, but in reality these areas constitute the perivesical spaces in their entirety. The anterior boundary of the retropubic space is the symphysis pubis and the pubic bone. The posterior boundary is the main body of the urinary bladder. The perivesical spaces extend on either side of the bladder and end above at the pubic bone and the obturator internus muscle, and below at the obturator internus muscle and the ischial bone. The levator ani muscle originates from the lower margin of the inferior pubic ramus and the fascia of the obturator internus and funnels downward to the junction of the middle one third and the lower one third of

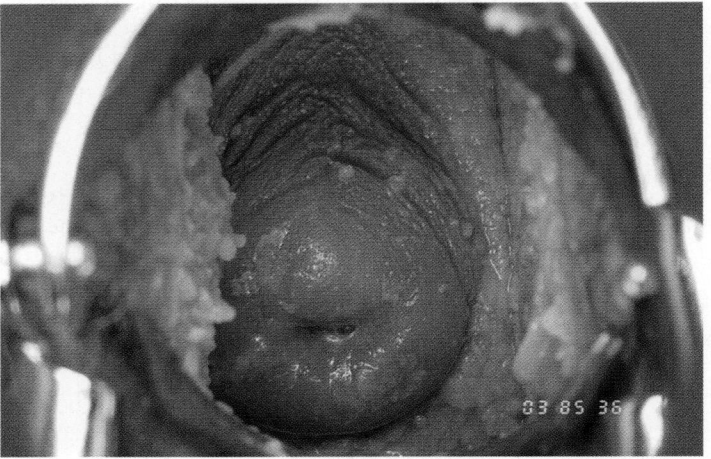

**FIGURE 51–1** The upper third of the vagina is closely related to the uterus, particularly the cervix uteri. The rugous vaginal mucosa can be seen to merge with the smooth cervical mucosa on the far periphery of the portio vaginalis of the cervix. The central cervix creates the vaginal fornices at the vault.

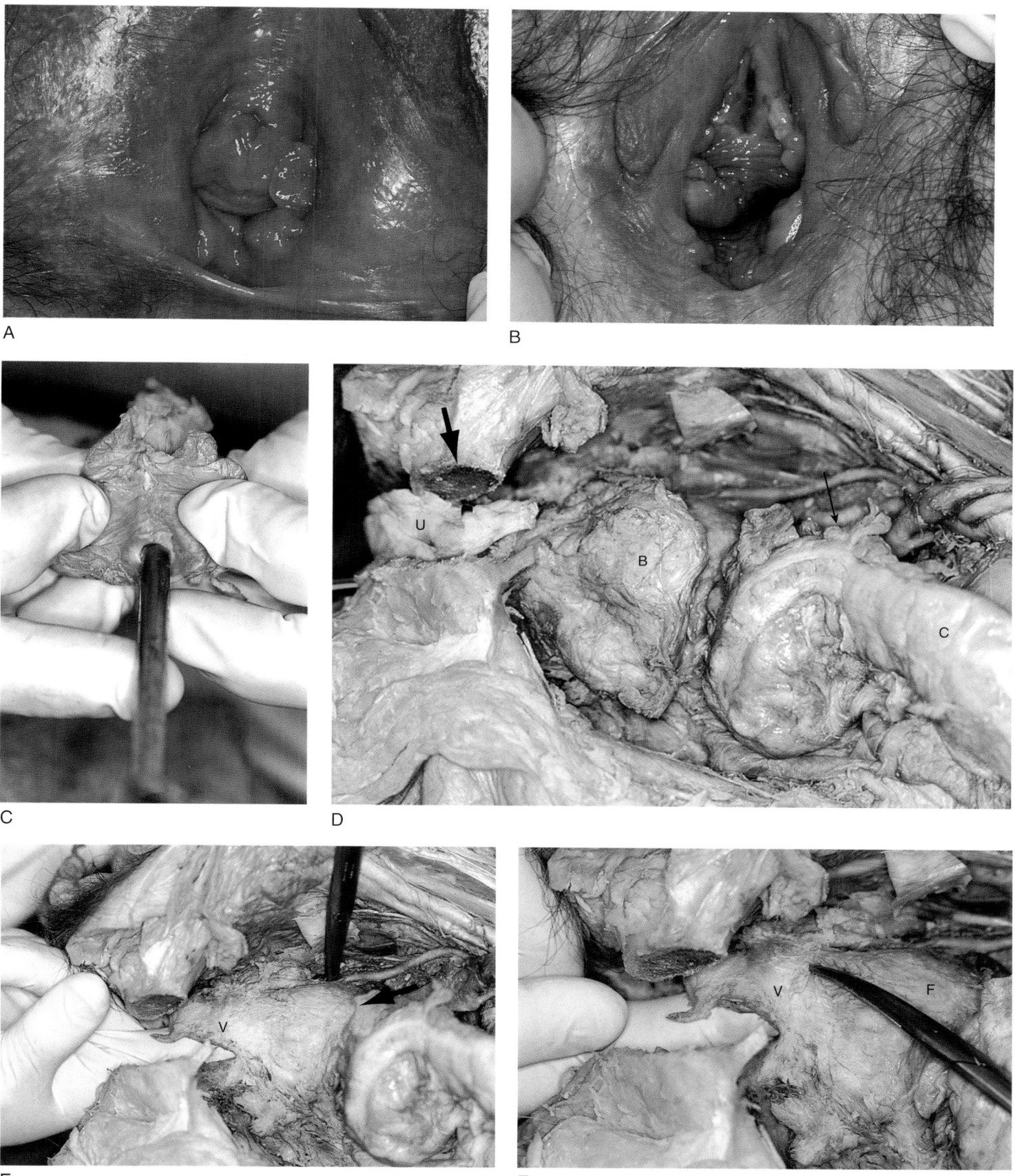

**FIGURE 51–2  A.** The lower third of the vagina forms a unit with the labia minora, vestibule, urethra, and rectum. The urethra is incorporated into the anterior vaginal wall. The anterior and posterior walls are in apposition. **B.** Compared with the lower vagina, seen in Figure 51–2A, this woman's vagina is agape with a definite space visible between the anterior and posterior walls. Note the size and shape of the enlarged external urethral meatus. **C.** The bladder, the urethra, and a portion of the vestibule have been dissected free of the anterior wall of the vagina and have been removed. A metal cannula traverses the urethra into the bladder. **D.** The pubic bone has been cut away with a saw (*large arrow*). The previously excised bladder (B) and urethra (U) (see Fig. 51–2C) have been replaced in the pelvis. The bladder covers the retroverted uterus, and the sigmoid colon (C) covers the uterus, which lies in the cul-de-sac. The small arrow points to the right ureter. **E.** The bladder-urethra complex has been removed, exposing the anterior (outside) wall of the vagina (V). The surgeon's finger is in the partially incised vagina and is located in the right lateral fornix (*arrow*). The scissors are directly lateral to the ureter. **F.** Detail of Figure 51–2E. The tip of the scissors is pointing to the pubocervical fascia of the vaginal wall. The blades of the scissors lie on that fascia and over the anterior vaginal fornix (F). Note the two sawed edges of the pubic bone overlying the surgeon's gloved hand.

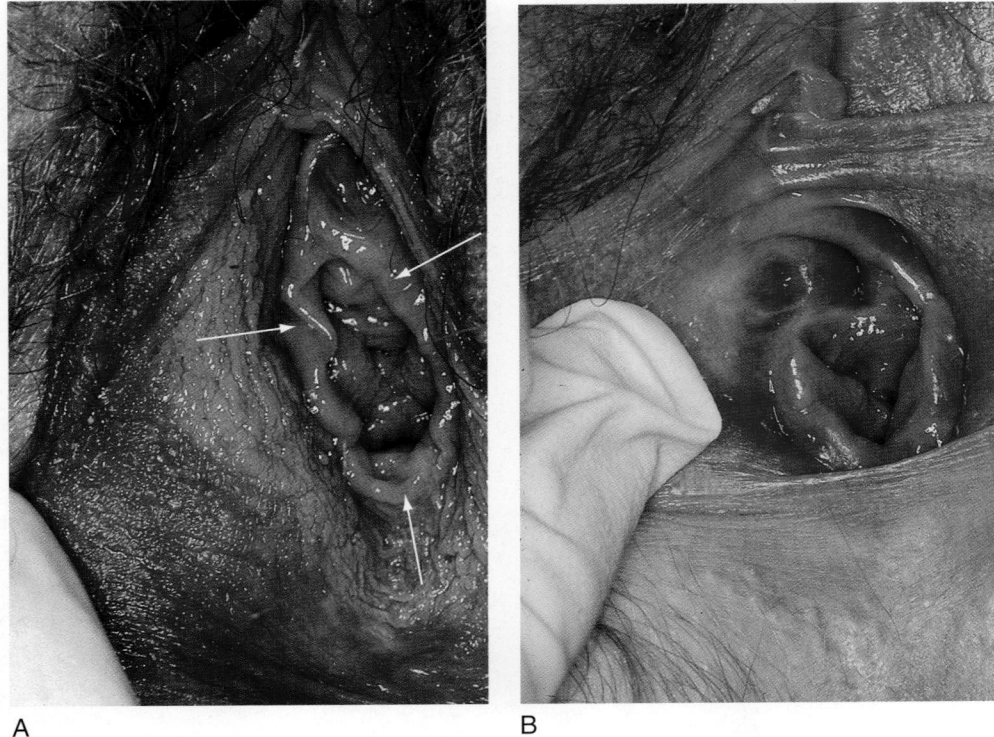

A          B

**FIGURE 51–3  A.** The hymenal ring (*arrows*) separates the vagina from the vestibule. **B.** In this case of vestibulitis, the boundary between the vagina and the vestibule is even more apparent.

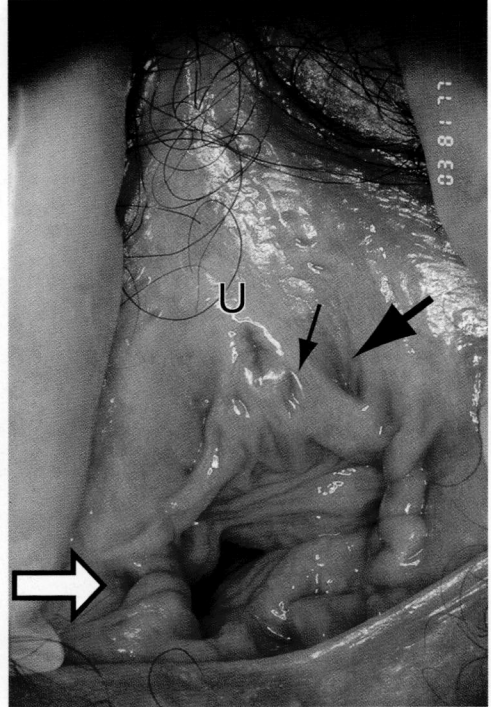

**FIGURE 51–4** The proximity of several mucous glands to the vagina is apparent. The Skene ducts (*small arrow*), paraurethral ducts (*large arrow*), and Bartholin ducts (*white arrow*) all are intimate with the outer wall of the vagina.

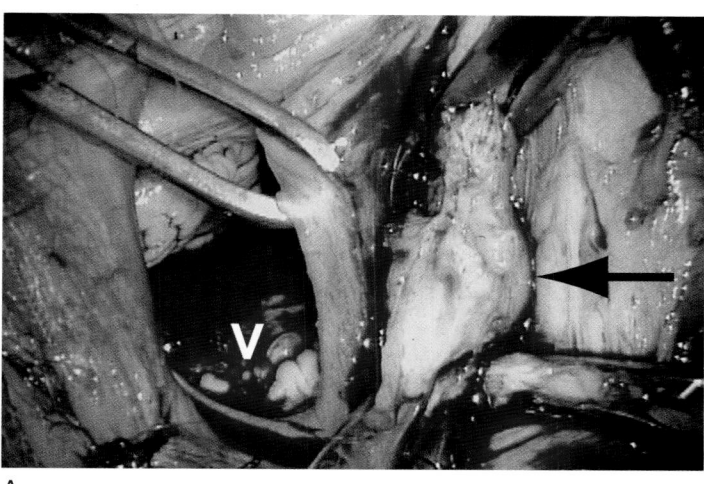
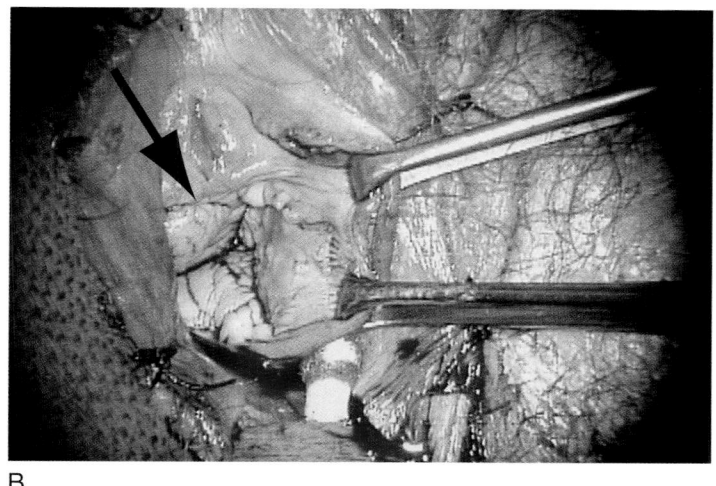

A                                                                                B

**FIGURE 51-5  A.** The relationship of the Bartholin gland to the posterolateral wall of the vagina (V) is shown here. The V overlies the bloody postvaginal mucosa. Clamps are placed across the upper and lower margins of the Bartholin gland (*arrow points to the gland*). The Allis clamp is attached to the lower vaginal lateral wall (introitus). **B.** The *arrow* points to the vagina. Allis clamps stretch the lateral wall of the vagina over the site where the Bartholin gland previously was located. A proctoscopic swab has been placed in the defect created by extirpation of the gland. The gland occupied a location 15 mm deep as measured from the outer edge of the introitus.

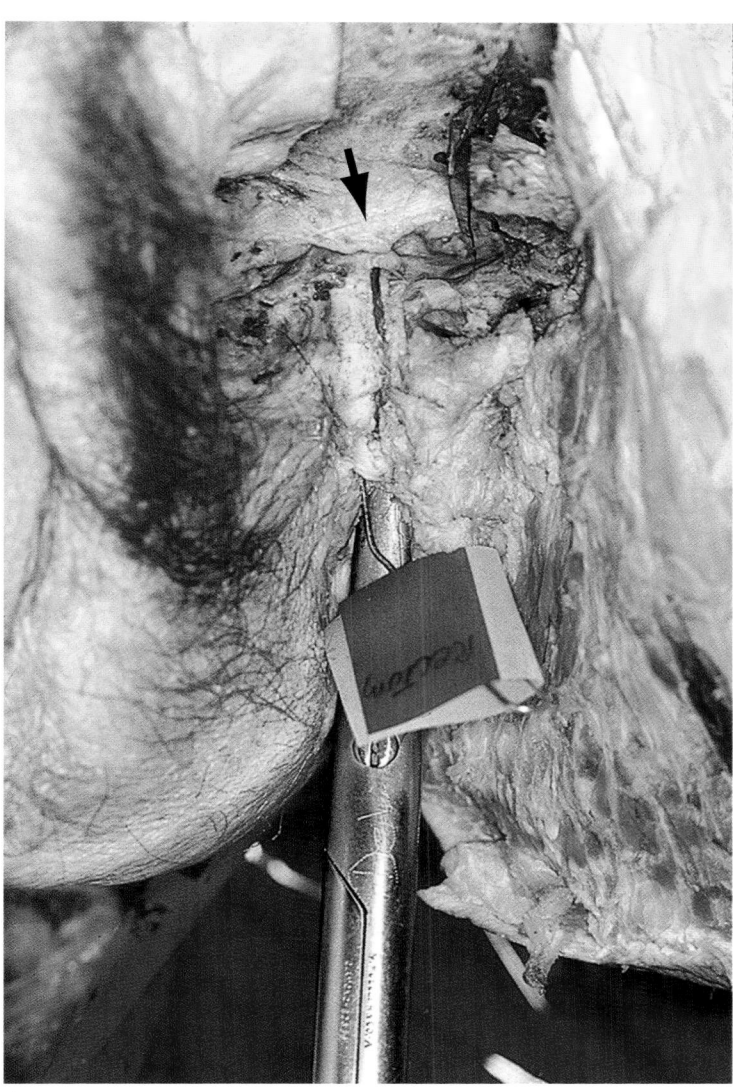
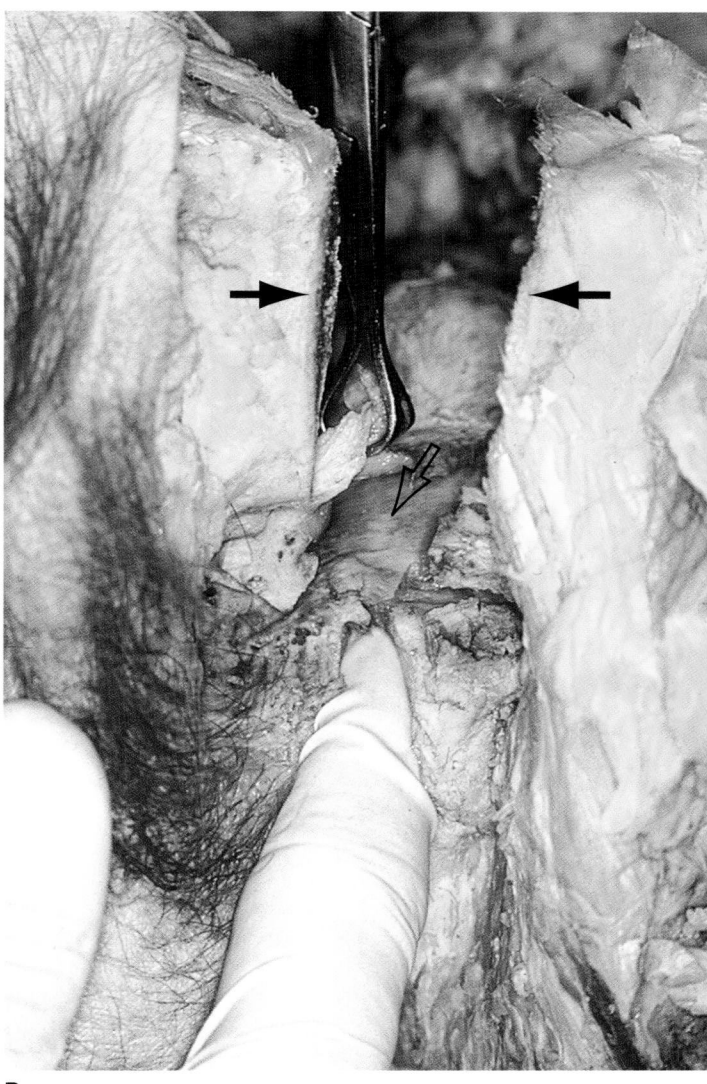

A                                                                                B

**FIGURE 51-6  A.** Scissors have been placed into the anus. Note the direction that the anus (scissors) takes to reach the posterior wall of the vagina. The bulge in the vagina is highlighted by the *arrow*. **B.** The anal sphincter and the perineal body have been cut, permitting a view of the direction of a finger placed in the anus relative to the posterior vagina. The Babcock clamp is attached to the incised anterior vaginal wall. The *open arrow* points to the posterior vaginal wall. The cut margins of the pubic bone are noted by *arrows*.

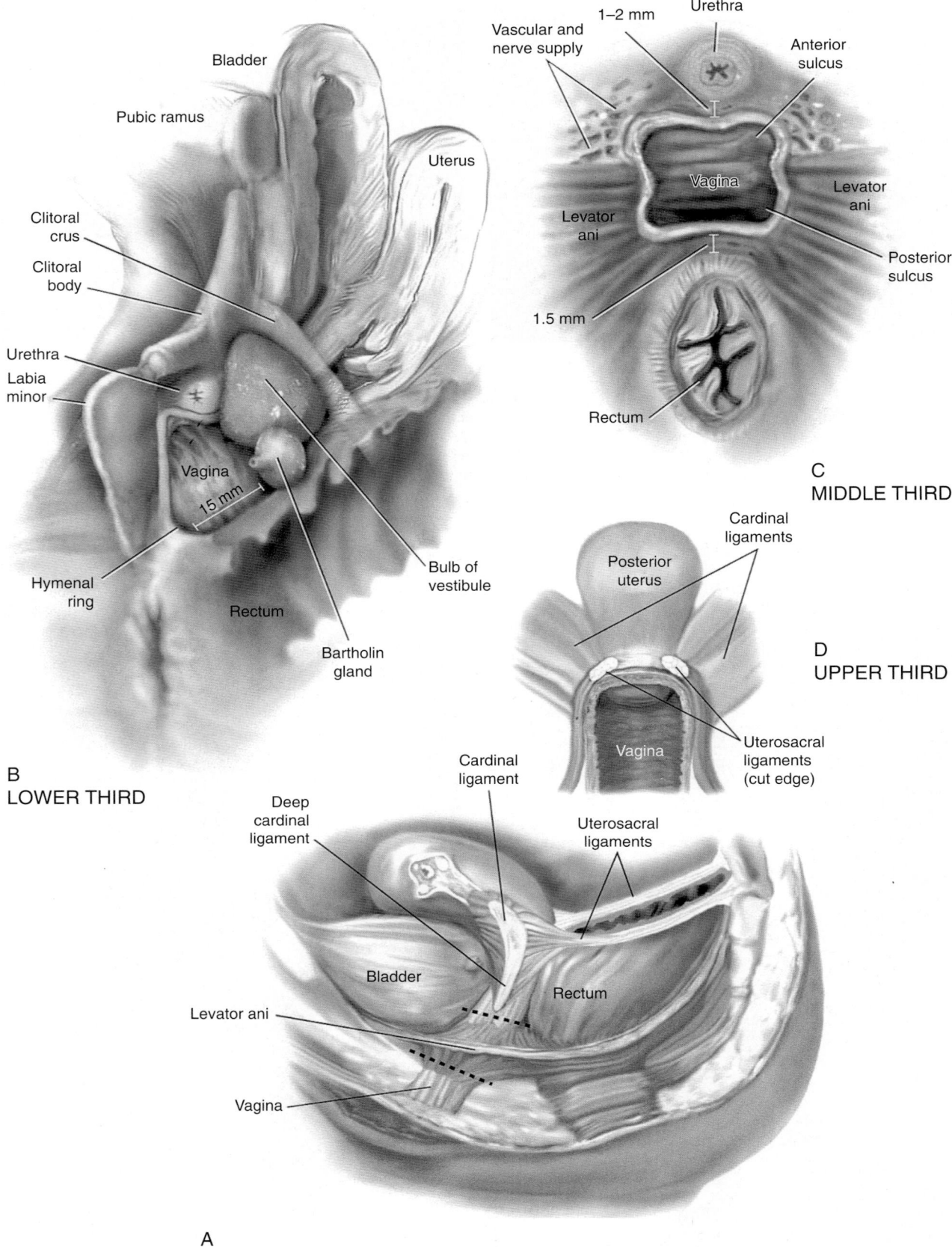

**FIGURE 51–7  A.** The vagina is divided into thirds of roughly equal length. The lower third is attached to the vestibule at the hymenal ring and is closely associated with vulvar vestibular structures. The middle third and upper lower third lateral walls are applied to the levator ani muscles. The upper third of the vagina is attached to the cervix. The cardinal and uterosacral ligaments likewise support the upper vagina as well as the uterus. Throughout its course, the vagina is intimately connected anteriorly to the bladder-urethra and posteriorly to the rectum. **B.** The lower portion of the left wall of the vagina has been removed. The lower right interior lateral wall of the vagina is seen. Approximately 15 mm deep from the surface of the vestibule is the left Bartholin gland and the left vestibular bulb. These are located at the lateral and posterolateral outer aspects of the left vaginal wall. Crossing above the vagina and urethra from the pubic ramus is the left clitoral crus (corpora cavernosum clitoris). **C.** A cross-section through the middle third of the vagina. Note the proximity of the rectum and the urethra. The levator ani inserts into the lateral vaginal walls. The anterior and lateral sulci are formed by the anterior and posterior walls, which are relatively relaxed compared with the fixed lateral walls. **D.** The posterior vaginal wall has been cut away at the level of the upper third of the vagina. Note the relationship of the uterosacral and lower cardinal ligaments to the vaginal vault.

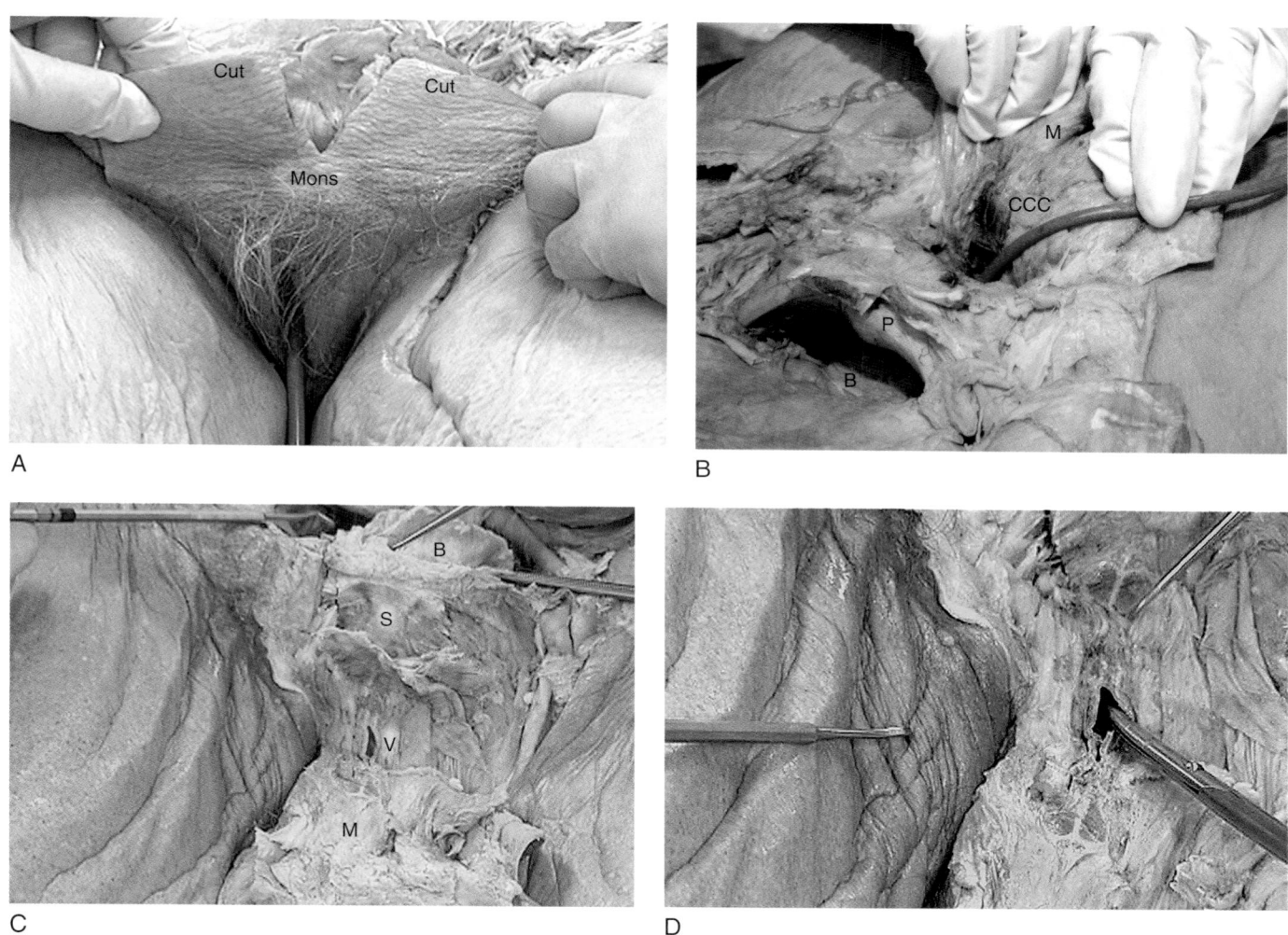

**FIGURE 51–8 A.** The incision line cut into the mons is shown. A catheter has been placed into the cadaver's urethra. **B.** The mons (M) has been cut and turned down. The distal portion of the corpora cavernosa clitoris (CCC) is seen in this view. The retropubic space has been opened and the relative positions of the pubic bone and symphysis (P) and the bladder (B) to the midvagina can be appreciated. **C.** This view is taken from the foot. The mons (M) is turned down. The midvagina (V) is seen as it passes beneath the symphysis (S) pubis. The bladder (B) is seen behind the pubic bone. **D.** Close-up of Figure 51–8C with the dissecting scissors placed into the midvagina. The upper hook marks the location of the corpora cavernosa clitoris.

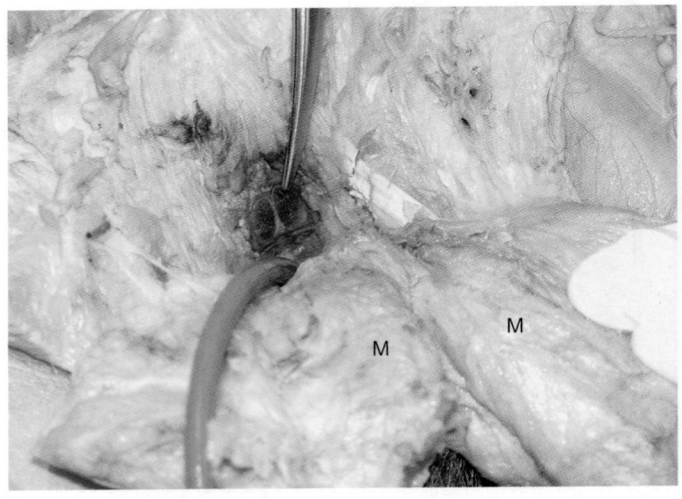

E

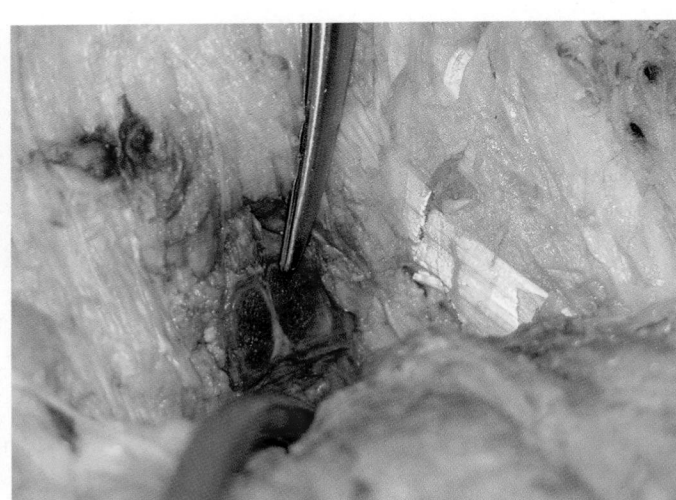

F

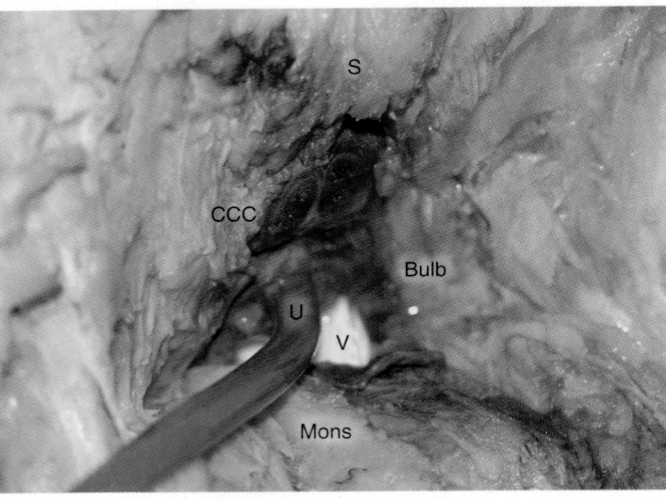

G

**FIGURE 51–8, cont'd** **E.** The catheter is in the urethra. The scissors point to the corpora of the clitoris located just above the midurethra. The mons (M) has been cut and reflected caudad. **F.** Close-up view showing the spongelike consistency of the cavernous tissue. **G.** The operator's gloved finger is in the vagina (V). The bulb of the vestibule surrounds the urethra (U) on three sides. The corpora cavernosa clitoris (CCC) lies immediately anterior to the urethra with bulb tissue interposed between the two structures.

the vagina and into the perineal and perianal areas. The anatomy can be demonstrated only by sawing away a portion of the pubic bone (Fig. 51–9A through D).

Much controversy has existed as to which structures support and maintain the position and integrity of not only the vagina but also its immediate neighbors: the bladder, the urethra, and the rectum. Specific anatomic sites of support to individual as well as paired structures can be identified (Fig. 51–10A through C). The ureters and the bladder base are closely related and applied to the area of the anterior upper vagina and the antero-lateral fornices (Fig. 51–11A, B). Common walls are shared by the urethra, bladder, and vagina anteriorly and with the rectum and vagina posteriorly. Figure 51–11C shows an overview of the urethra (urethrovaginal complex) and the bladder after the pubic bone was removed (Figs. 51–11C through G). The major support to the upper vagina consists of the cardinal ligaments as well as shared walls between bladder, rectum, and, to a lesser extent, uterosacral ligaments. The vaginal vault therefore is mainly supported (as is the cervix and bladder base) by the deep cardinal ligaments (Fig. 51–12A through C). Also, between the cervix, upper vagina, and bladder exists a well-defined fascial layer, silvery white in color. This layer is the pubovesicocervical fascia and could likewise be considered part of the paravaginal fascia (Fig. 51–13). The deep cardinal ligaments extend into the perivesical spaces to the pelvic side wall, that is, the obturator internus muscle, arcing posteriorly toward the ischial spine along the retroischial space (Figs. 51–14A through G, 51–15A through C).

The upper vagina is supplied via the pelvic plexus with input from the hypogastric plexus, prevertebral ganglia, and sacral nerves. The lower vagina is supplied by the pudendal nerve. Curiously, the vagina is relatively insensitive to biopsy forceps and to light touch (see Fig. 51–14A).

The blood supply emanates from the descending branch of the uterine artery, the vaginal artery, and the internal pudendal artery.

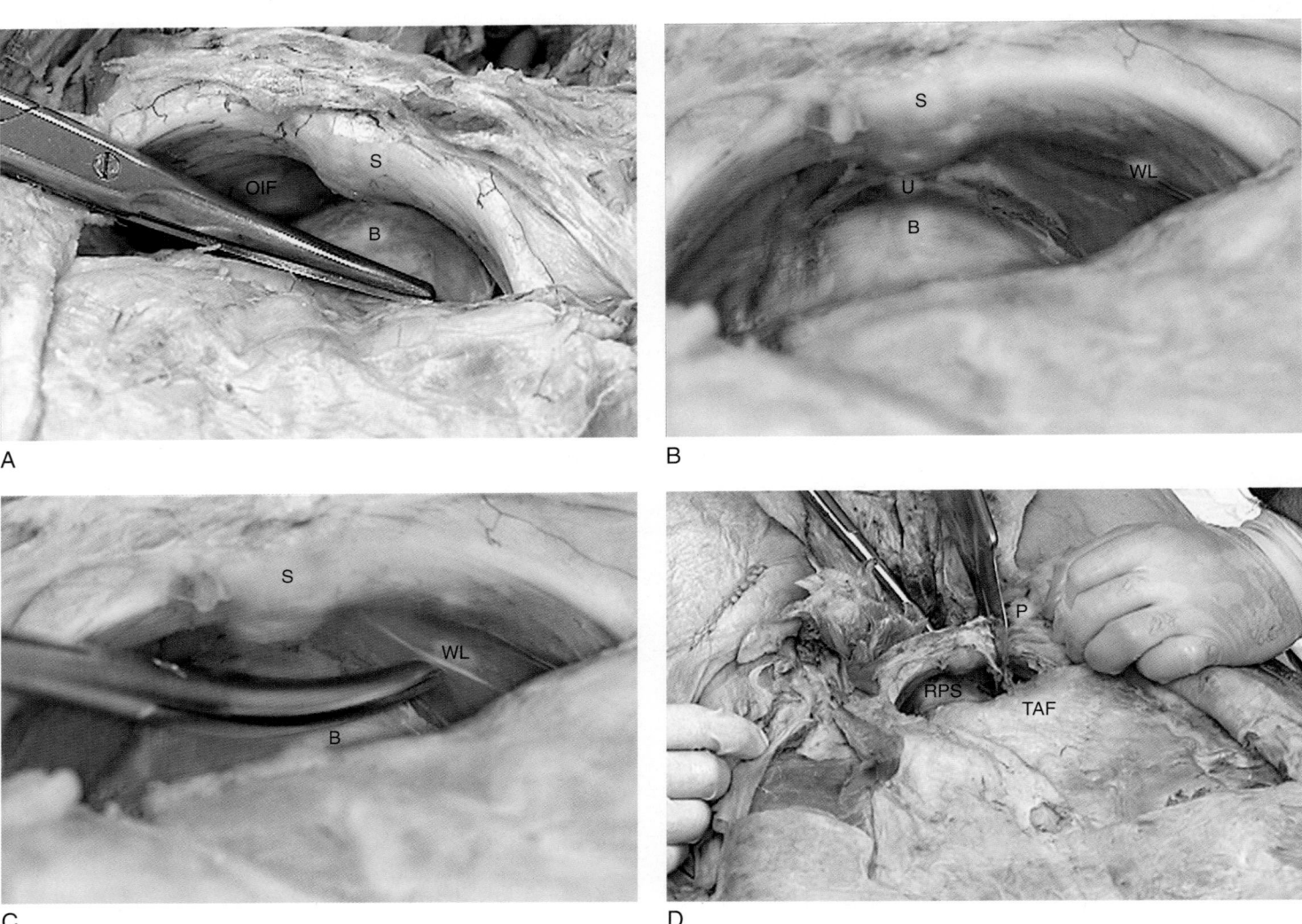

**FIGURE 51–9 A.** The relationships of the urethra, vagina, and bladder can be best understood by widely exposing the retropubic space. Important reference points include the symphysis pubis (S), the obturator internus muscle and its covering fascia (OIF), and the urinary bladder (B). **B.** This view of the retropubic space details the urethrovesical junction (U and B) at the lower margin of the caudal sloping symphysis pubis (S). A thickening in the obturator internus fascia creates a whitish appearance, i.e., a white line (WL). **C.** The scissors tip rests on the obturator internus fascia at the white line. **D.** The dissection into the retropubic space (RPS) is entirely extraperitoneal. Abdominal contents are contained under the transversus abdominis fascia (TAF), which is bound to the parietal peritoneum of the anterior abdominal wall. The relationships between the middle and upper vagina and the urethra and bladder base cannot be appreciated without removing a portion of the pubic bone (P) with a saw.

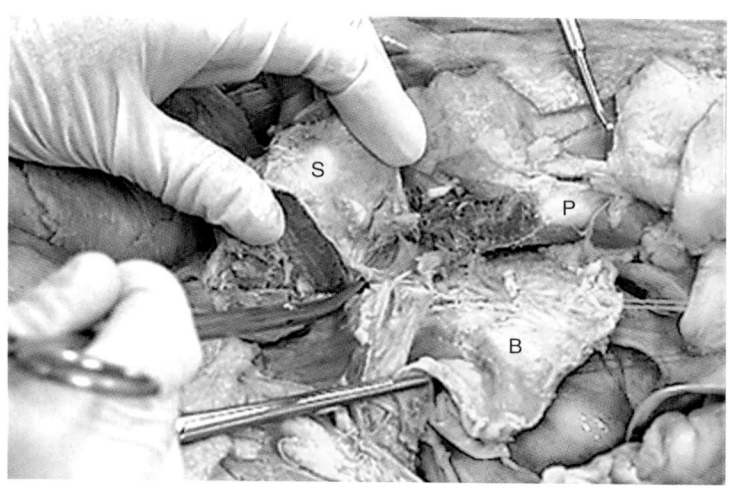

A

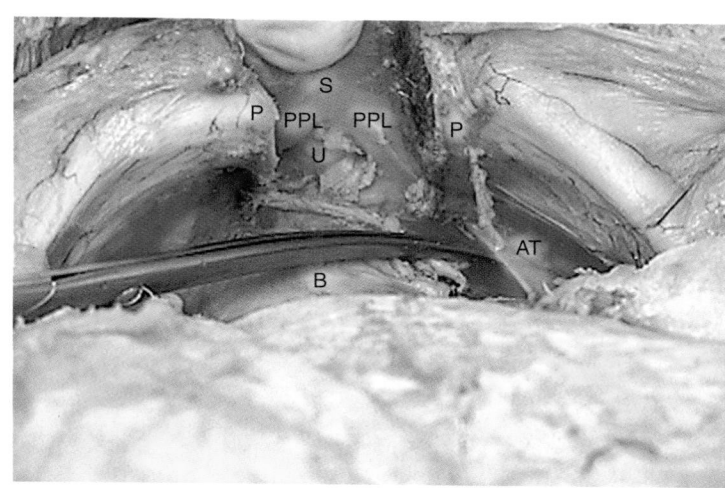

B

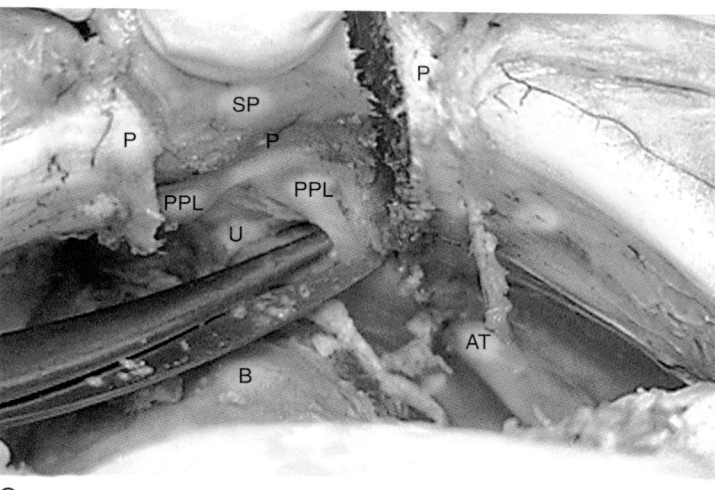

C

**FIGURE 51–10 A.** The symphysis pubis (S) has been sawed through. The cut edges of the pubic bone are clearly seen. The most prominent support of the urethra (U) as it passes beneath the symphysis (i.e., at its junction with the bladder [B]) is the posterior puboprostatic ligaments (pubourethral ligaments). The clamp points to the left ligament. **B.** The cut symphysis pubis (S) is pulled forward, exposing the urethra (U) at its junction with the bladder (B). Note the cut edges of the pubic bone (P). The right and left posterior puboprostatic ligaments (PPLs) are clearly seen at the lower margin of the symphysis. Note that the arcus tendineus (AT) terminates at the puboprostatic ligament on either side. **C.** The right puboprostatic ligament (PPL) is about to be cut to free the symphysis pubis (SP) from the urethra (U) and bladder (B). P, Cut edges of pubic bone; OIF, obturator internus fascia; AT, arcus tendineus.

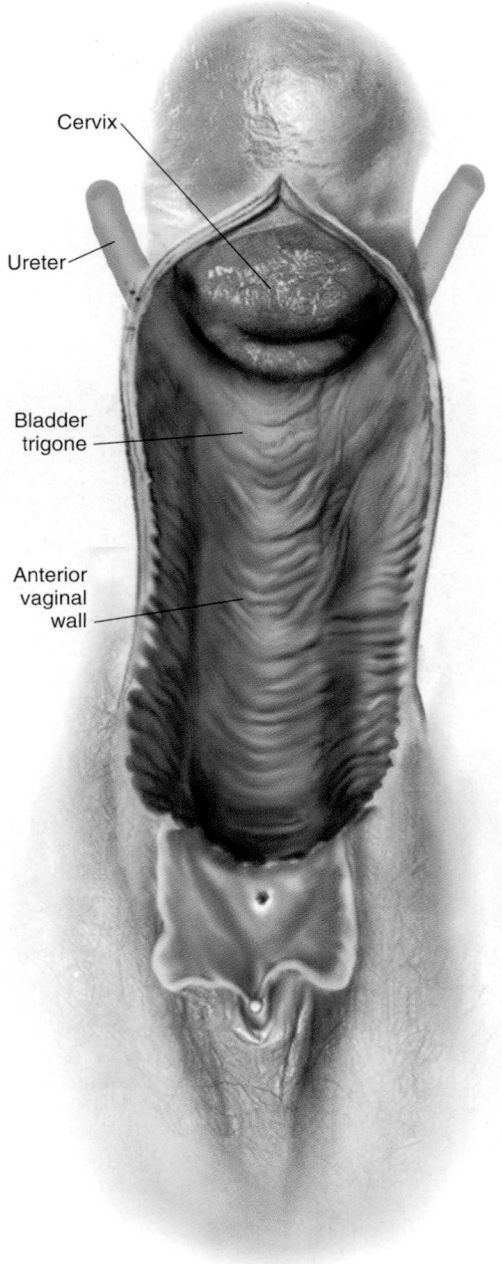

Cervix

Ureter

Bladder
trigone

Anterior
vaginal
wall

A

**FIGURE 51–11 A.** The rectum and the posterior wall of the vagina
have been excised. The relationship of the ureters and bladder base to
the anterior and anterolateral vagina is illustrated. Urinary tract structures
are pink. If the picture is inverted, the relationship of the urethra and the
vestibule to the anterior vagina can be better understood.

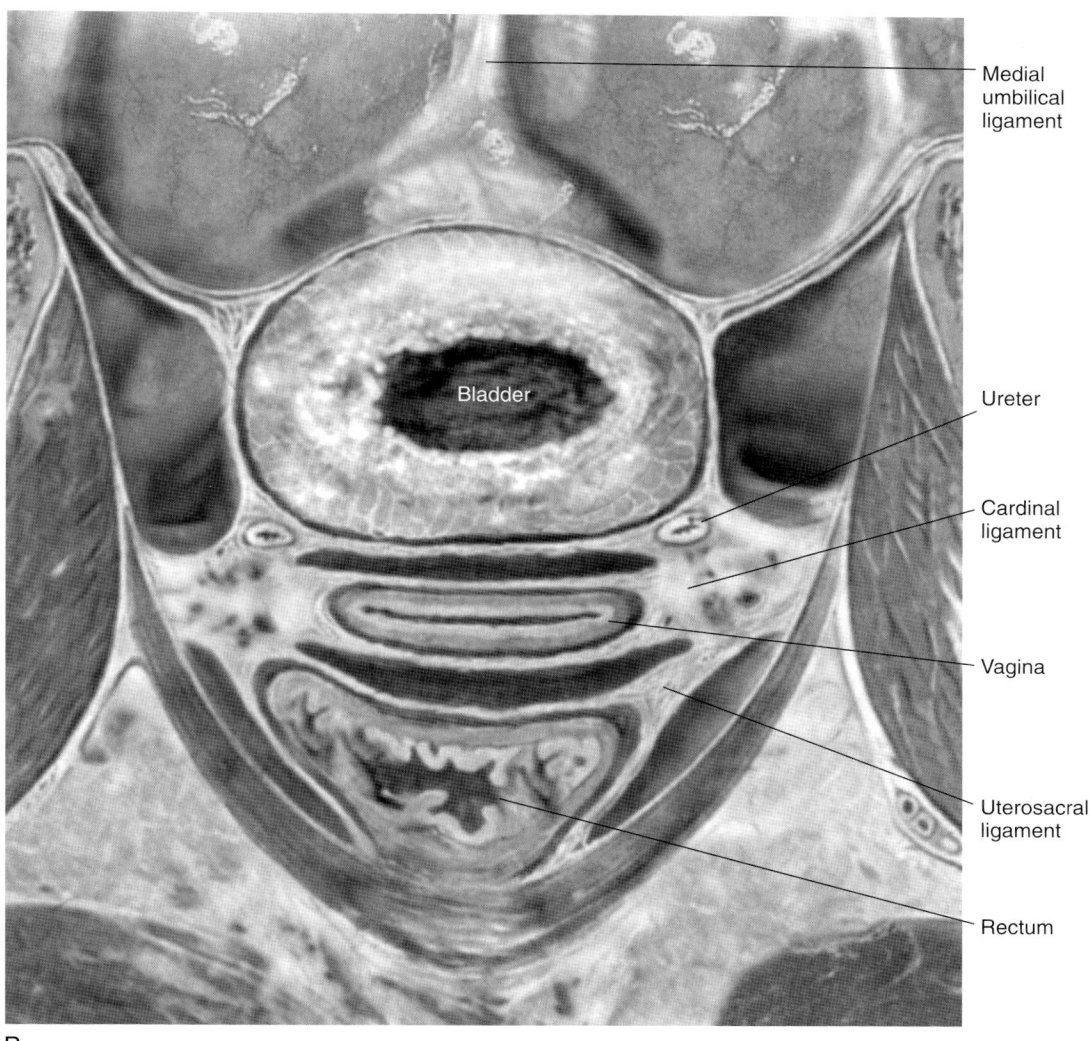

B

**FIGURE 51–11, cont'd   B.** Coronal section detailing the relationships of the upper vagina, ureters, cardinal ligaments, and vesicovaginal and rectovaginal spaces.

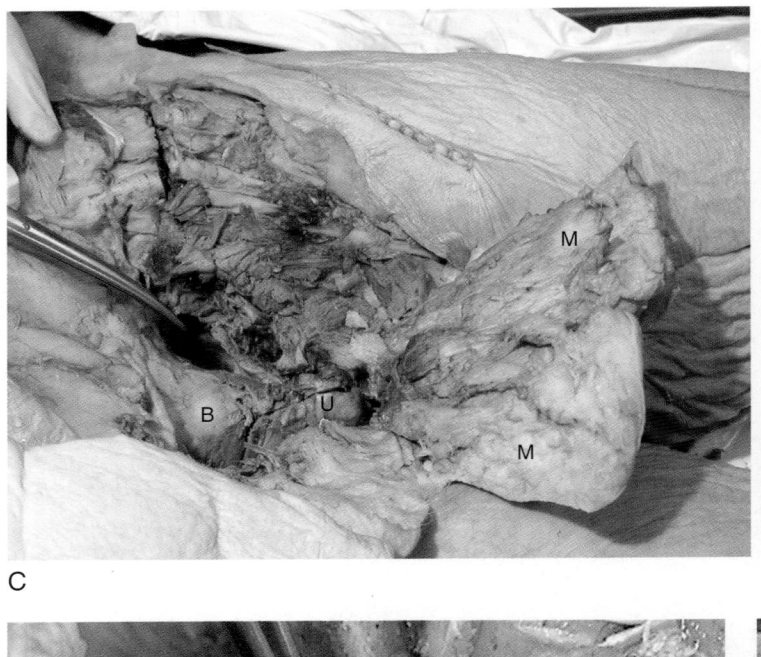

C

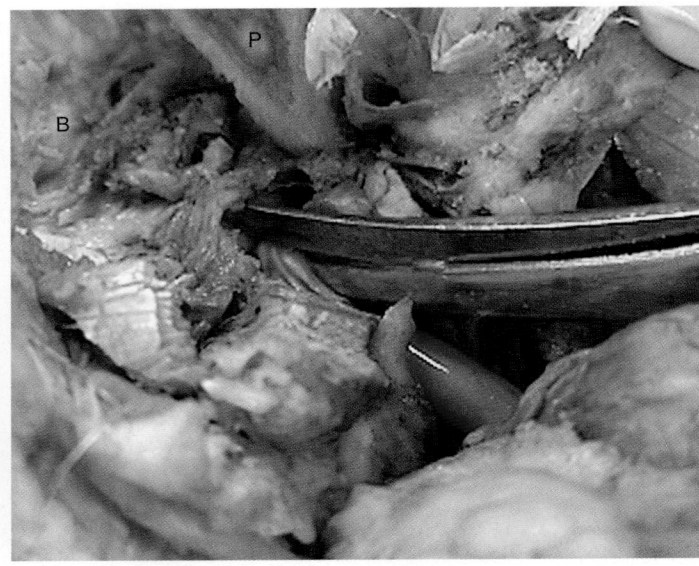

D

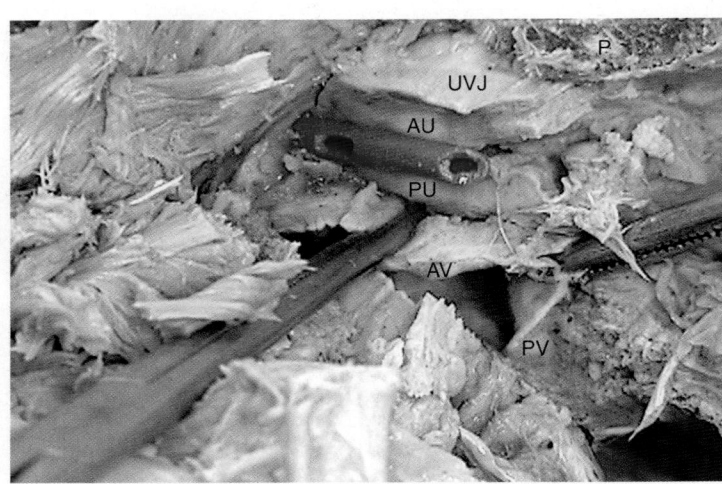

F

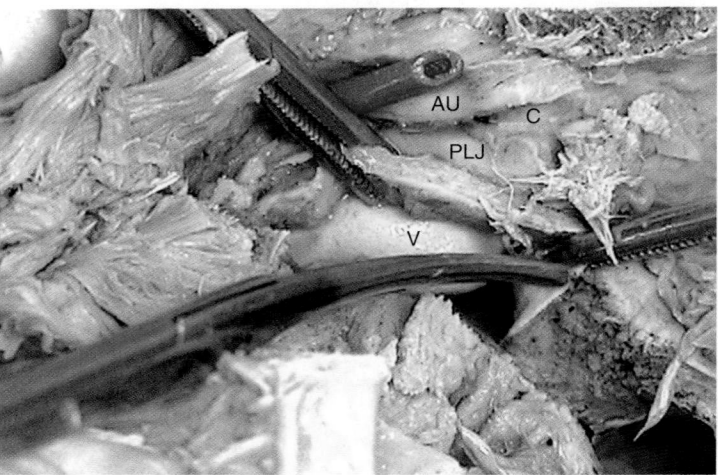

E

G

**FIGURE 51–11, cont'd** **C.** This panoramic view of the urethra (U), the bladder (B), and the perivesical space (scissors) can be seen only after the pubic bone is widely sawed away. **D.** The cut edge of the pubis allows dissection of the ureter beneath the area previously occupied by the symphysis pubis. The anterior wall of the urethra is being cut. **E.** The anterior wall of the urethra has been filleted open, as has the lower anterior bladder wall. **F.** The urethra and the vagina share a common wall. The catheter occupied the urethral canal before the urethra was cut open. A sagittal cut has been made through the urethrovesical junction (UVJ). The anterior (AU) and posterior (PU) urethral walls are seen. The scissors point to the common wall shared between the urethra and the vagina, specifically the anterior wall of the vagina (AV). The posterior wall of the vagina (PV) is also exposed. **G.** The relationship between the urethra (AU and PU) and the mid and upper vagina (V) is demonstrated by the surgeon's finger placement within the vagina.

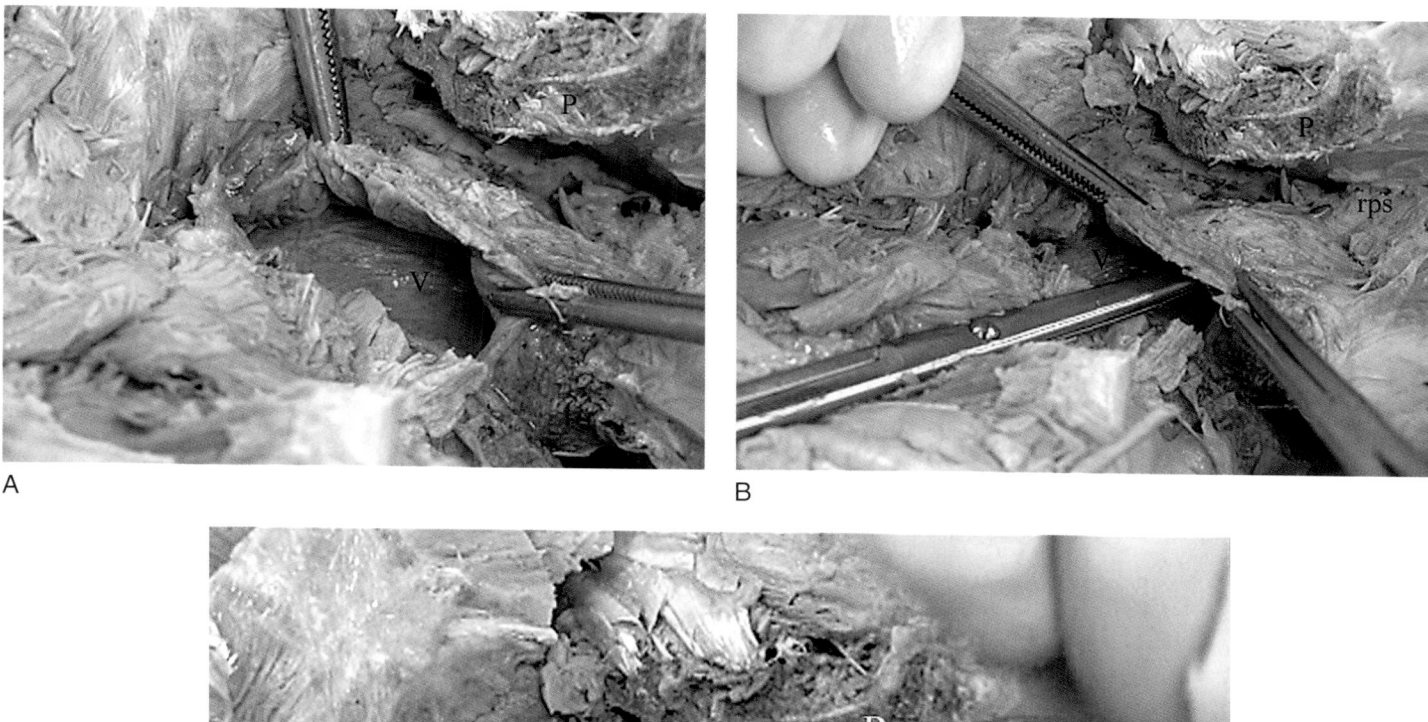

A

B

C

**FIGURE 51–12 A.** The junction of the upper one third and the middle one third of the vagina (V) beneath the symphysis (sawed away) is nicely demonstrated here. The cut and sloping edge of the pubic bone (P) is seen in the right upper corner. **B.** The scissors have been pushed through the right upper vaginal wall (V) into the retropubic space located behind (cranial) the cut pubic bone (P). **C.** The uterus (U) has been hemisected and is seen via sagittal view. The uterus is pulled upward via the blue fundal traction stitch. The Kocher clamp is located at the cervicovaginal junction. The cervix is also sagittally viewed. The vagina has been opened laterally, and the anterior and posterior vaginal (V) walls are in clear view. The scissors point to the obturator internus muscle (oim). P, Cut edge of the pubic bone.

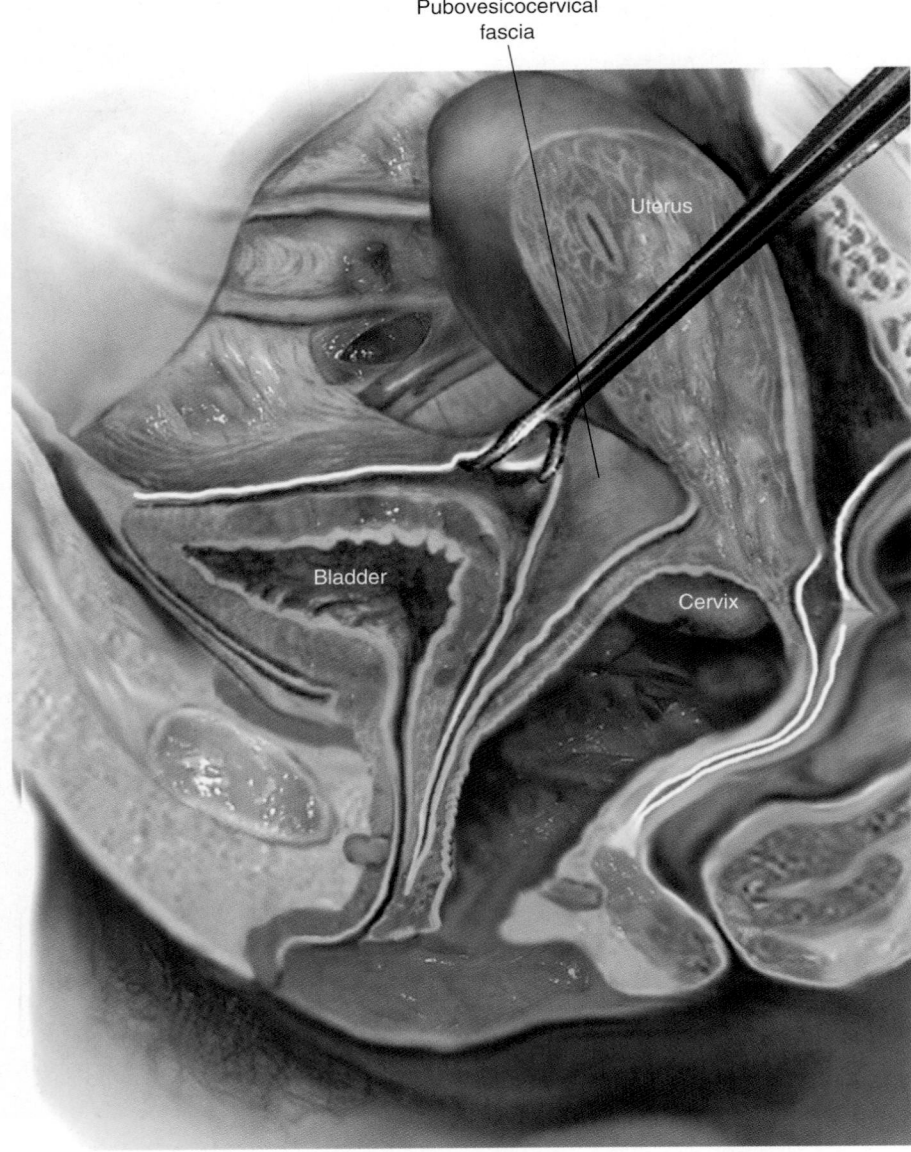

**FIGURE 51–13** The distribution of the pubovesicocervical fascia is shown here. The fascial space may be entered at the level of the cervix. As the space is developed, a nice plane of dissection permits identifiable separation of the vagina from the urinary bladder.

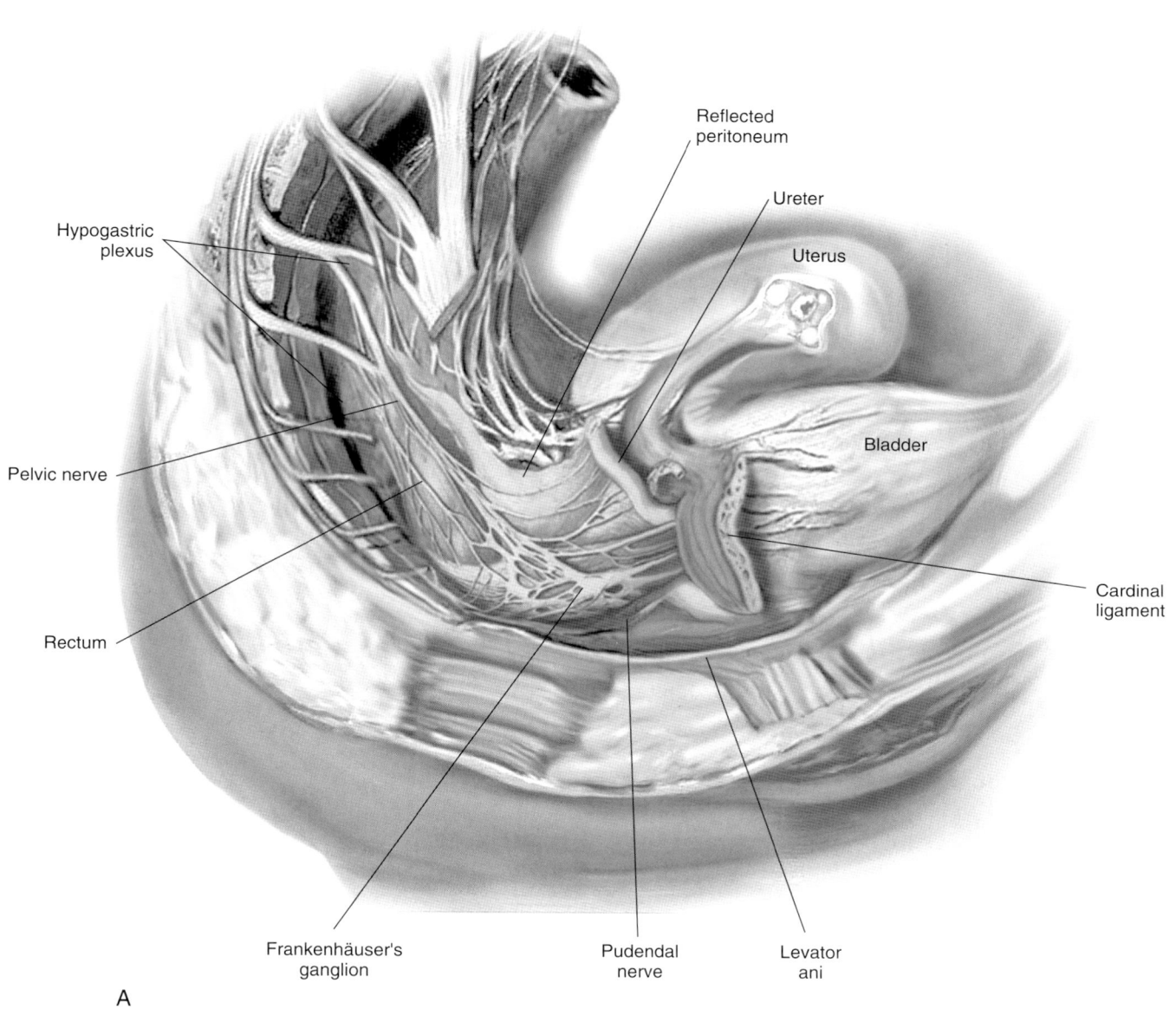

Reflected
peritoneum

Ureter

Uterus

Hypogastric
plexus

Bladder

Pelvic nerve

Cardinal
ligament

Rectum

Frankenhäuser's
ganglion

Pudendal
nerve

Levator
ani

A

**FIGURE 51–14  A.** The nerves supplying the cervix and the vagina are shown. The focal points of distribution are the pelvic nerves and the hypogastric plexus.

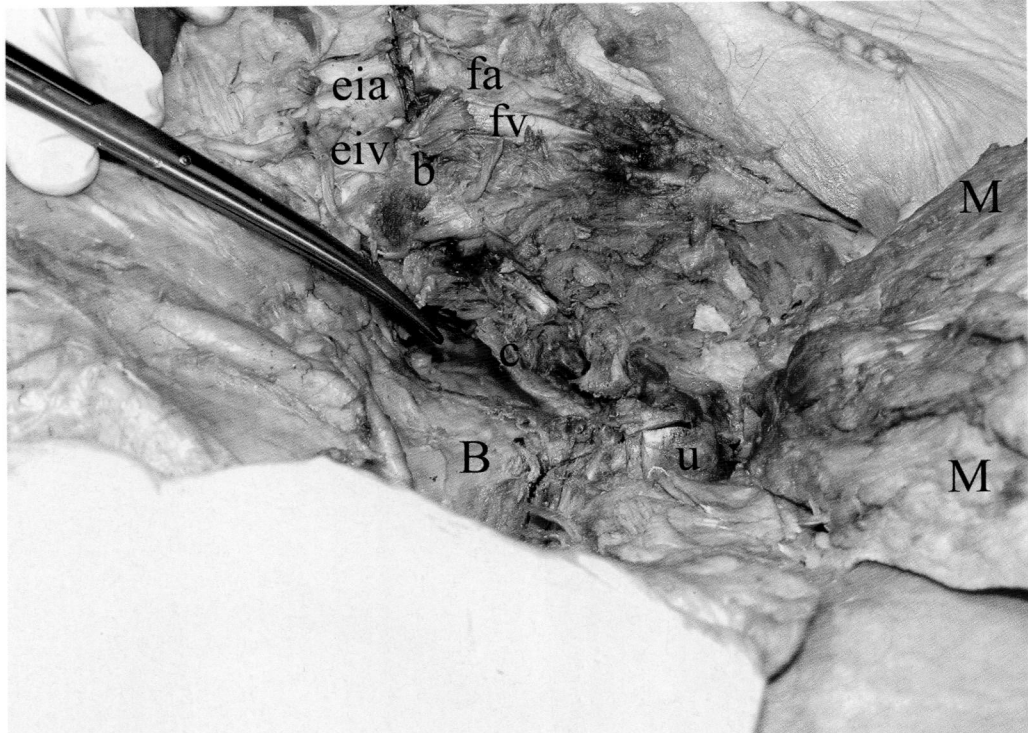

B

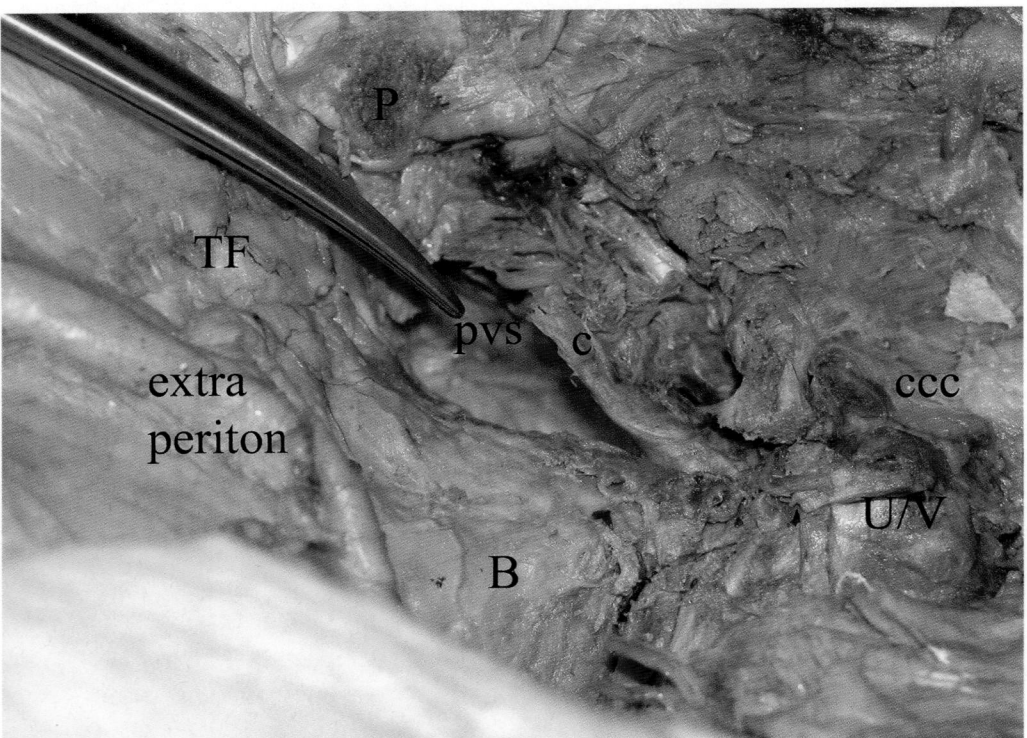

C

**FIGURE 51–14, cont'd   B.** The entire retropubic and subpubic areas have been exposed and are viewed from above. The external iliac artery and vein (eia, eiv) and the extension into the thigh as the femoral artery and vein (fa, fv) are seen crossing over the cut edge of the pelvic bone (b). The scissors point into the perivesical space to the left of the bladder (B). The urethra (u) has been cut along the anterior wall through most of its length. The deep cardinal ligament (c) attaches to the bladder base and upper vagina. The mons (M) has been cut and reflected caudally. **C.** This magnified view of part **B** shows details of the urethrovaginal complex (U/V), the bladder and the perivesical space (pvs), and the deep cardinal ligament (c). The left clitoral crus (ccc) can be seen to the left of the mid U/V complex. The widely cut edge of the pubic bone (P) is seen in the background. The transversus abdominis fascia (TF) covers the anterior intra-abdominal contents extraperiton, extraperitoneum.

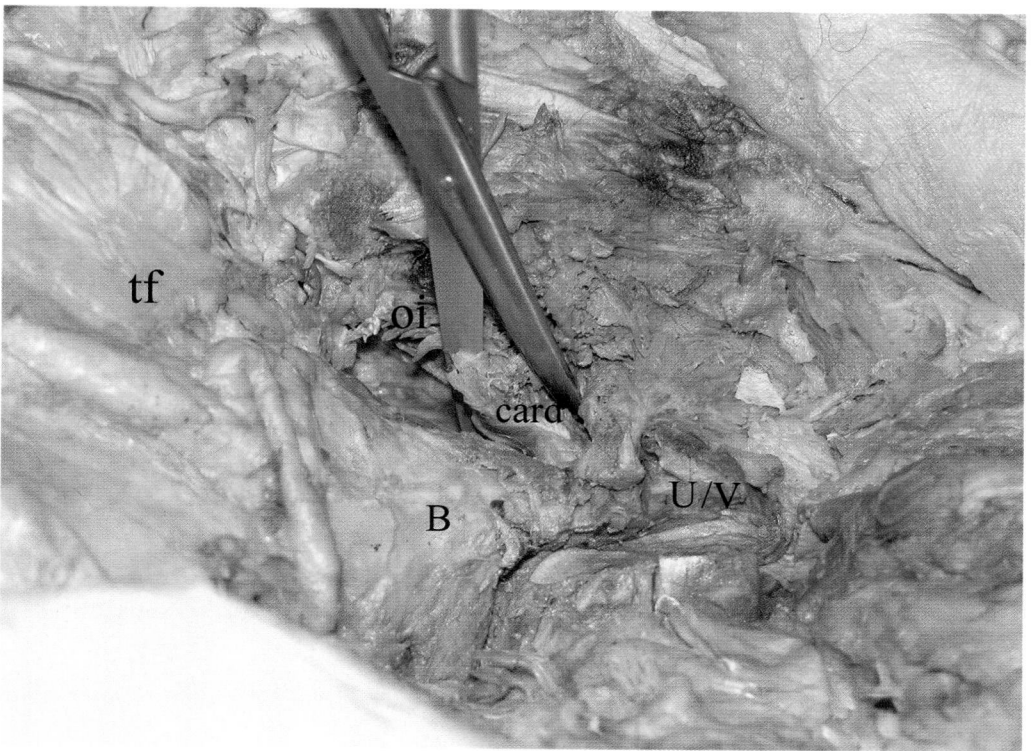

D

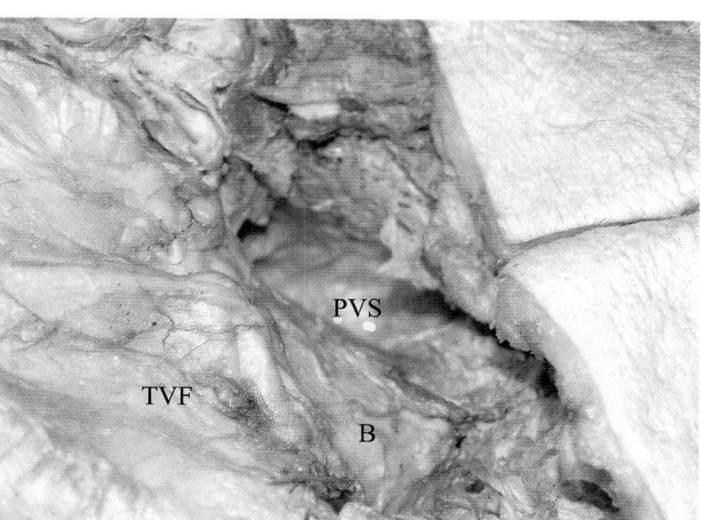

E

**FIGURE 51–14, cont'd   D.** The scissors are in place to cut the deep cardinal ligament (card).
**E.** The deep cardinal ligament has been severed, creating a large perivesical space (PVS), which extends posteriorly and caudally behind the ischial bone.

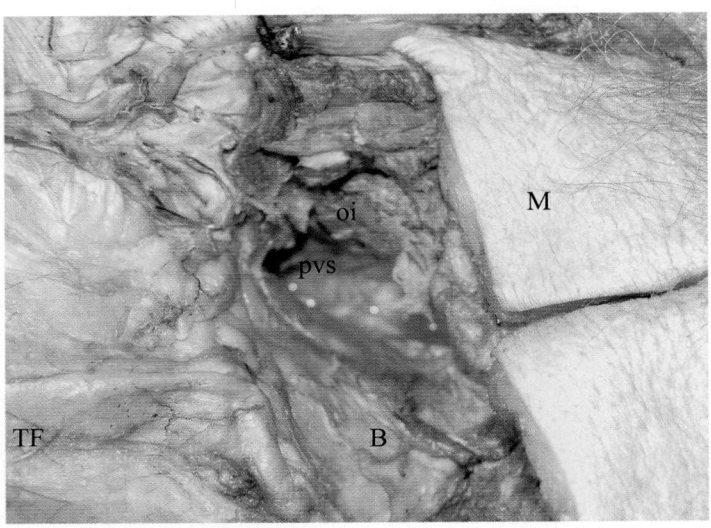

F

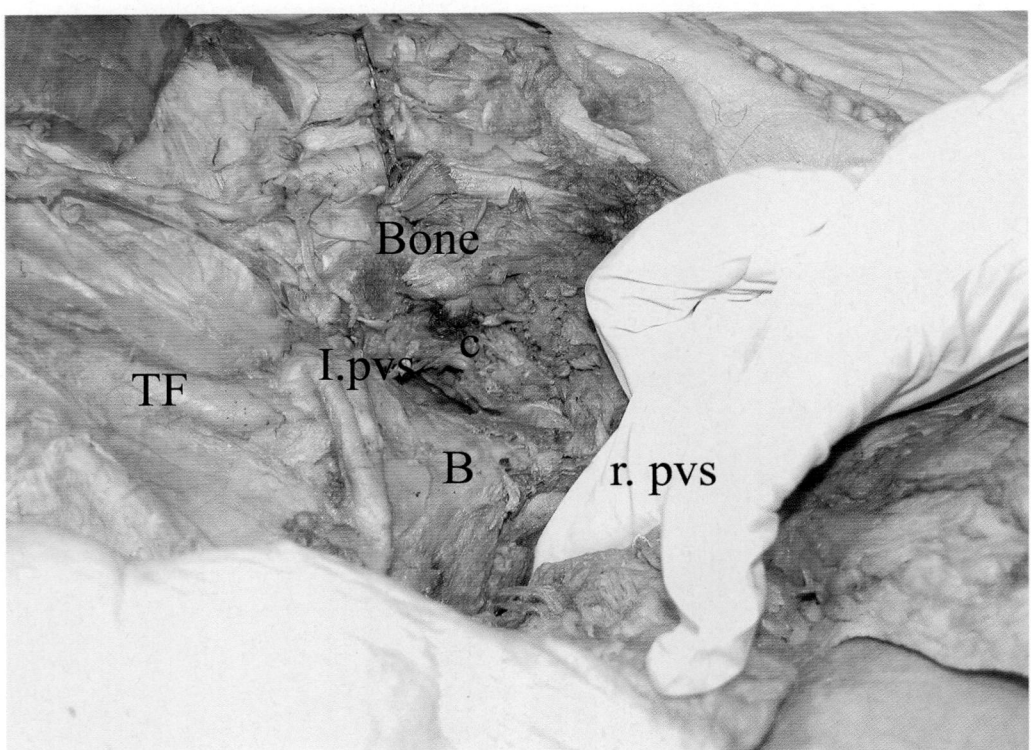

G

**FIGURE 51–14, cont'd   F.** This magnified view with the mons (M) replaced to its normal position shows the relationship of the obturator internus (oi) muscle to the deep perivesical space (pvs) after the cardinal ligament has been cut. **G.** This view shows the left deep cardinal ligament (c), the left perivesical space (l.pvs), and the bladder (B). The surgeon's finger has been placed into the right perivesical space (r.pvs).

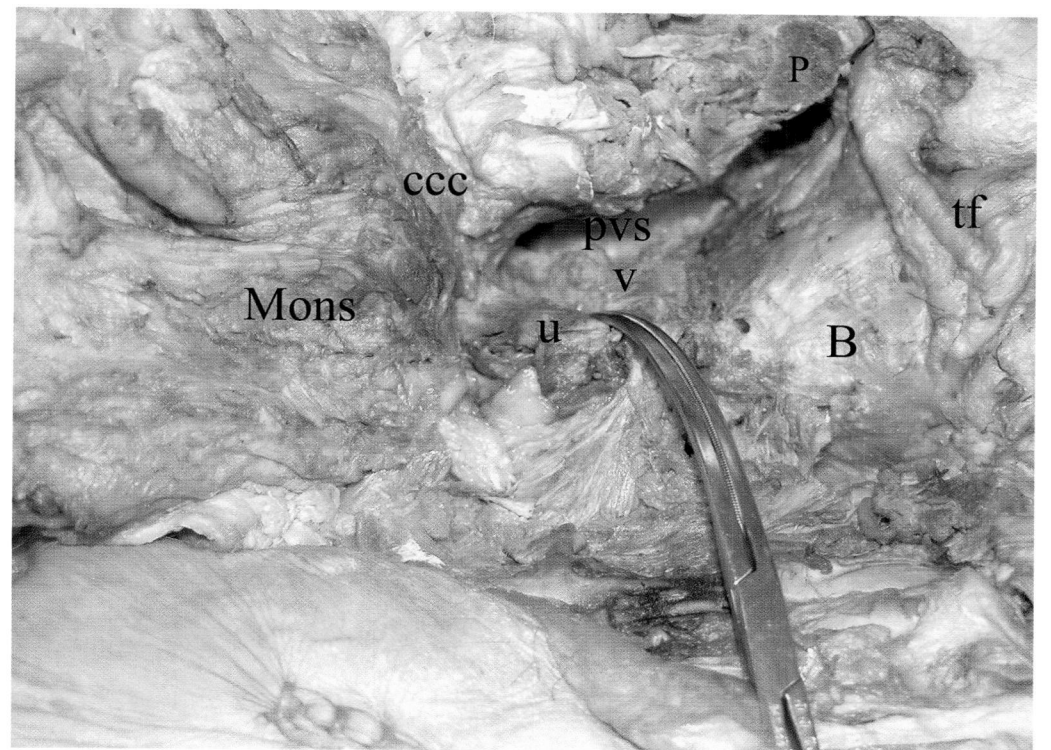

A

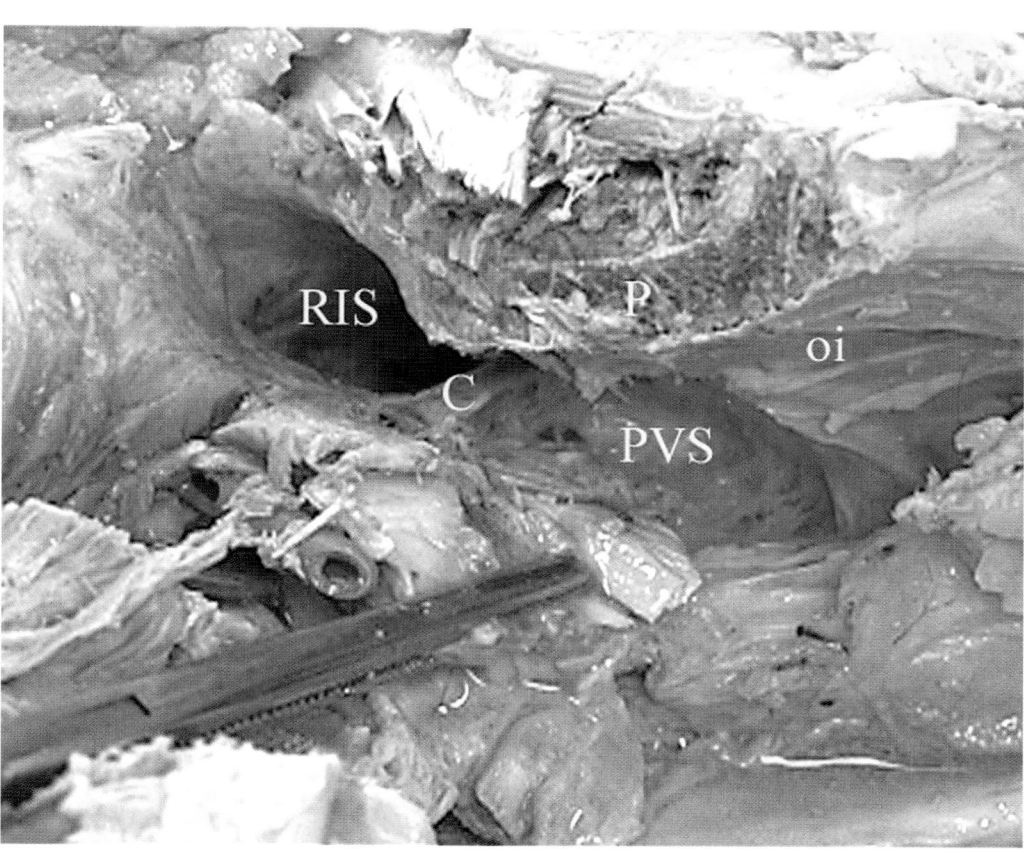

B

**FIGURE 51–15 A.** This picture is taken from the left side looking to the right. The mons again has been turned down. The pubic bone (P) has been sawed out. The operator's finger has been placed into the vagina (v), and the vagina has been pushed to the right of the urethra (u) at the junction of the urethra and the bladder (B). The clamp points to the bulging vagina. The right corpora cavernosa clitoris (ccc) is in front of where the symphysis pubis would have been located. The perivesical space (PVS) is lateral to the vagina. **B.** Detail of the right perivesical space (PVS) and retroischial space (RIS). Note that the deep cardinal (C) ligament curves and arcs posteriorly along the arcus tendineus and represents a much more substantive structure than the arcus formed by the obturator internus (oi) fascia.

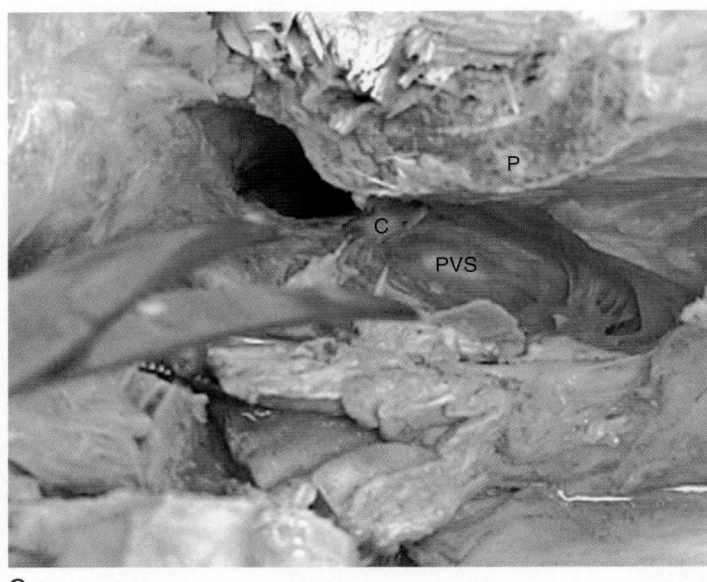

C

**FIGURE 51–15, cont'd   C.** The scissors are poised to cut the right cardinal ligament (C), which will connect the retroischial space with the perivesical (PVS) space. P, Cut edge of the pubic bone.

# CHAPTER 52

# Anatomy of the Support of the Anterior and Posterior Vaginal Walls

*Mickey M. Karram*

To safely perform procedures on the female pelvic floor, it is imperative that the surgeon has a good three-dimensional understanding of the anatomy in this area. This includes a full appreciation of where important blood vessels and nerves travel, as well as of the relationships between various structures used to support pelvic viscera. Figure 52–1 is a cross-sectional view of the pelvis, demonstrating the relationships of various blood vessels to the vagina, pelvic viscera, ureter, and coccygeus–sacrospinous ligament complex. Figure 52–2 demonstrates the support of the anterior vaginal wall viewed through the retropubic space. Note the white area labeled as the inside of the vaginal wall. In a woman with a well-supported anterior vaginal wall, it is attached to the arcus tendineus fascia pelvis (labeled as *white line*) laterally and the cervix or vaginal cuff proximally. Because many procedures for incontinence and prolapse involve the passing of needles and trocars through the inner thigh, a firm understanding of the anatomy of the structures in this area is necessary. Figure 52–3 reviews this anatomy as it relates to the retropubic space and vagina.

After the lower, middle, and upper thirds of the vagina are viewed, from the gross dissection it is helpful to consider what can be seen when the vagina is dissected for normal plastic operations. Initially, when the posterior vaginal wall is dissected from the anterior wall of the rectum, the vagina and the rectum are densely fused in the lower third of the vagina. This fusion is seen in operations such as perineorrhaphy and posterior colporrhaphy. As the operator attempts to separate the vaginal wall, no clear plane of dissection is evident from the anterior wall of the rectum. This is the case for approximately 3 to 4 cm from the posterior fourchette. Figure 52–4 shows a dissection of the posterior vaginal wall of a cadaver. Here one can see the upper edge of this dense, connective tissue. Above this edge, one enters the middle third of the vagina. At this point, a plane of cleavage is easily created between the vaginal and rectal walls. In Figure 52–4, this is the area marked *high rectocele*.

When the dissection is extended above the lower third of the vagina, a natural plane of cleavage is easily created and can be dissected bluntly without difficulty to the level of the cul-de-sac (see Fig. 52–4). The layers of the middle third of the vaginal wall, when viewed microscopically, reveal differences between this middle third of the vagina and the lower and upper thirds of the vagina.

The anterior wall of the vagina shows features similar to those of the posterior vaginal wall (Fig. 52–5). The vaginal wall is densely connected to the urethra in the distal third of the vagina. After extension approximately 3 to 4 cm into the vagina, a plane of cleavage or dissection easily allows the vaginal wall to be separated from the wall of the bladder (Fig. 52–6). Analogous to the posterior vaginal walls, the fibromuscular and adventitial layers of the vagina become thinner and less well defined as one moves toward the middle of the vagina and apically toward the cervix. Laterally a dense connection is seen between the adventitial and fibromuscular layers of the vagina and the arcus tendineus fascia pelvis (Fig. 52–7). In essence, the vagina is supported by the collagen and elastic fibers found in the adventitial and fibromuscular walls of the vagina. These connective tissues are attached laterally to the fascia overlying the levator ani muscles and apically to the uterosacral and cardinal ligament complexes. Disruption to the integrity of the levator ani muscles or of the elastin collagen network of fibers in the adventitial and fibromuscular walls of the vagina will predispose the patient to anatomic defects that may commonly result in functional derangements. Figure 52–8 demonstrates the lateral attachment of the vagina viewed from the retropubic space. Note that the tip of a pair of scissors has penetrated through the attachment of the muscular lining of the vagina to the arcus tendineus fascia pelvis. Figure 52–9 demonstrates complete detachment of the lateral support of the vagina when viewed vaginally. The lateral support of the vagina should extend to the level of the arcus, which inserts in the ischial spine. This creates the vaginal fornix on each side (Fig. 52–10). Grossly, the support of the anterior vaginal wall is best viewed as a trapezoid (Fig. 52–11) that consists of a lateral attachment to the arcus tendineus fascia pelvis, a transverse attachment to the vaginal apex or cervix, and durable midline tissue.

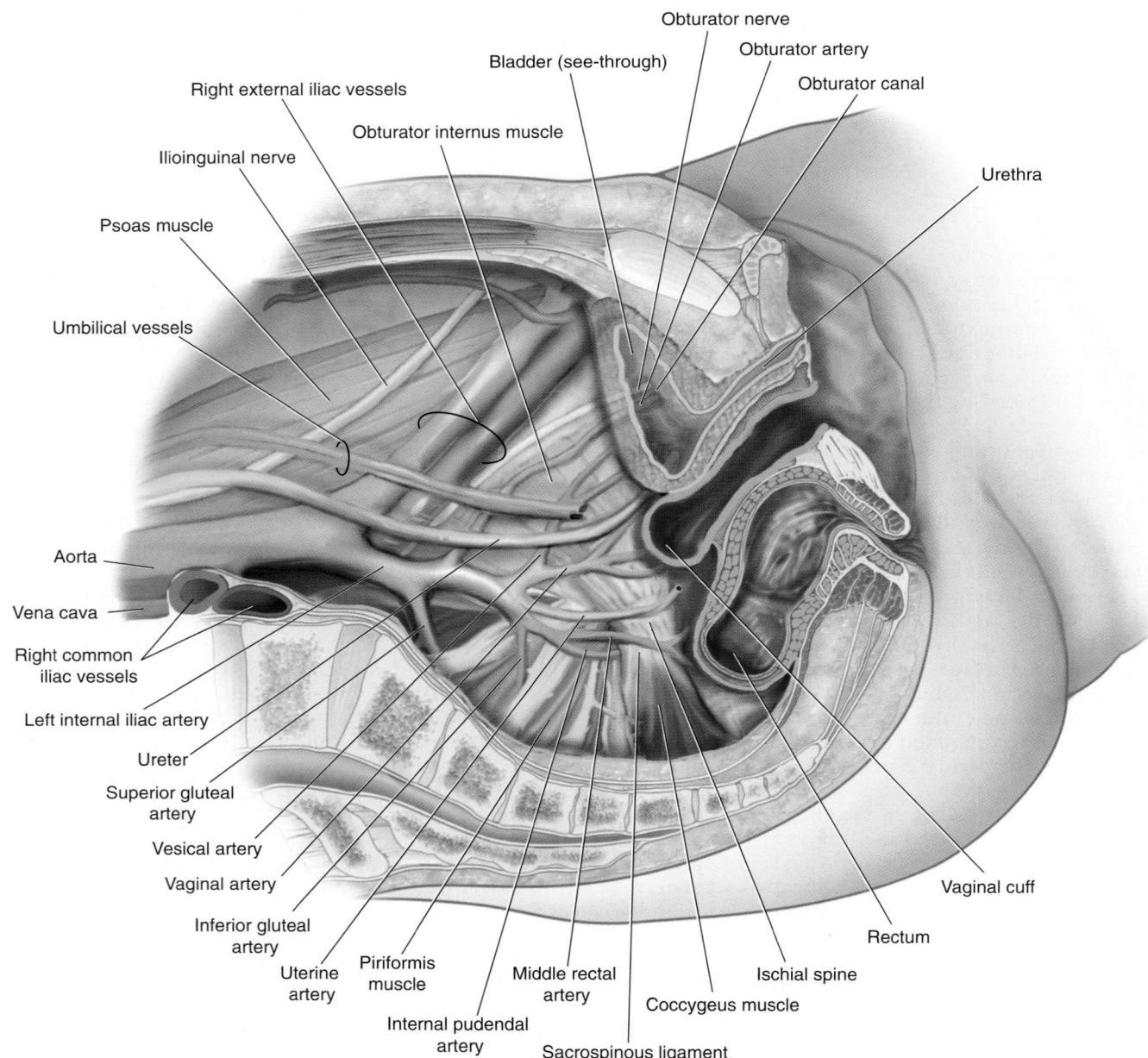

**FIGURE 52–1** Cross-sectional view of the pelvic structures. Note the relationships of vascular structures to the vagina, pelvic viscera, ureter, and coccygeus–sacrospinous ligament complex.

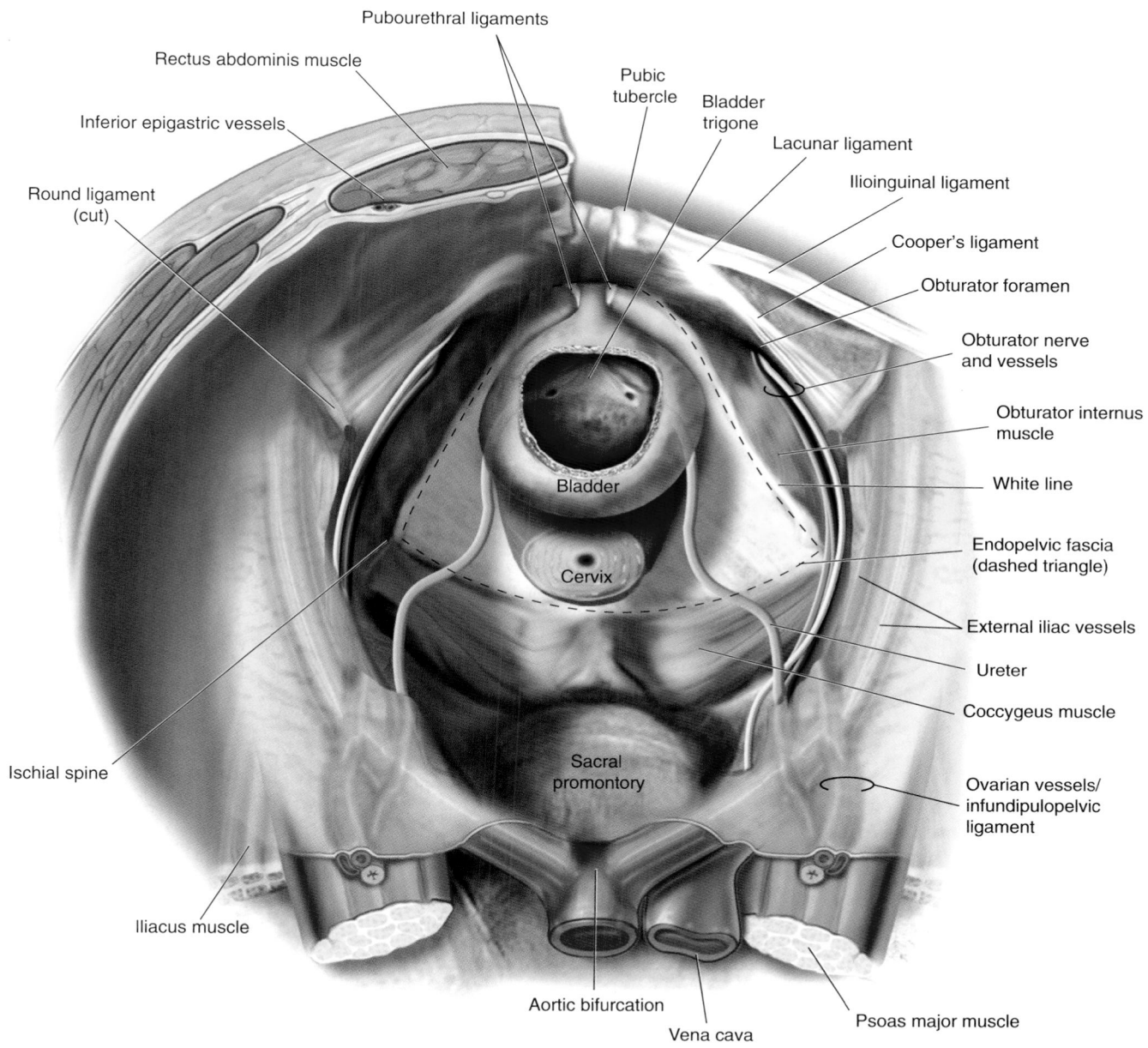

Pubourethral ligaments

Rectus abdominis muscle

Inferior epigastric vessels

Round ligament (cut)

Pubic tubercle

Bladder trigone

Lacunar ligament

Ilioinguinal ligament

Cooper's ligament

Obturator foramen

Obturator nerve and vessels

Obturator internus muscle

Bladder

White line

Cervix

Endopelvic fascia (dashed triangle)

External iliac vessels

Ureter

Coccygeus muscle

Ischial spine

Sacral promontory

Ovarian vessels/ infundipulopelvic ligament

Iliacus muscle

Aortic bifurcation

Vena cava

Psoas major muscle

Normal Antomy

**FIGURE 52–2** Support of the anterior vaginal wall as viewed through the retropubic space. The white area labeled as *endopelvic fascia* is actually the muscular lining of the inside of the vaginal wall. Note its normal attachment to the white line laterally and to the cervix or vaginal cuff proximally.

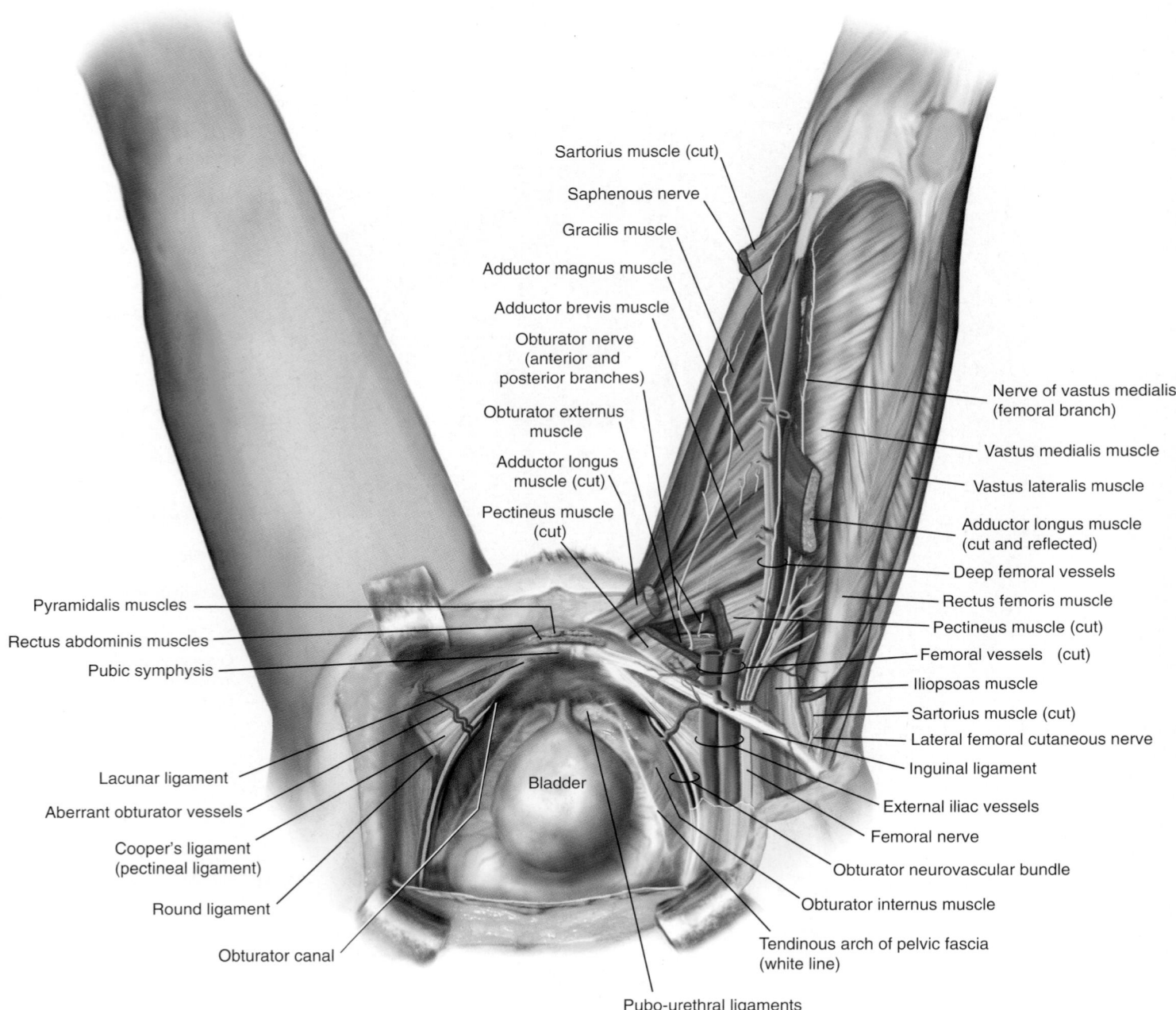

Sartorius muscle (cut)

Saphenous nerve

Gracilis muscle

Adductor magnus muscle

Adductor brevis muscle

Obturator nerve
(anterior and
posterior branches)

Obturator externus
muscle

Adductor longus
muscle (cut)

Pectineus muscle
(cut)

Pyramidalis muscles

Rectus abdominis muscles

Pubic symphysis

Lacunar ligament

Aberrant obturator vessels

Cooper's ligament
(pectineal ligament)

Round ligament

Obturator canal

Bladder

Pubo-urethral ligaments

Nerve of vastus medialis
(femoral branch)

Vastus medialis muscle

Vastus lateralis muscle

Adductor longus muscle
(cut and reflected)

Deep femoral vessels

Rectus femoris muscle

Pectineus muscle (cut)

Femoral vessels   (cut)

Iliopsoas muscle

Sartorius muscle (cut)

Lateral femoral cutaneous nerve

Inguinal ligament

External iliac vessels

Femoral nerve

Obturator neurovascular bundle

Obturator internus muscle

Tendinous arch of pelvic fascia
(white line)

**FIGURE 52–3** This drawing demonstrates the anatomy of the inner thigh and shows how these structures are related to the retropubic space and vagina.

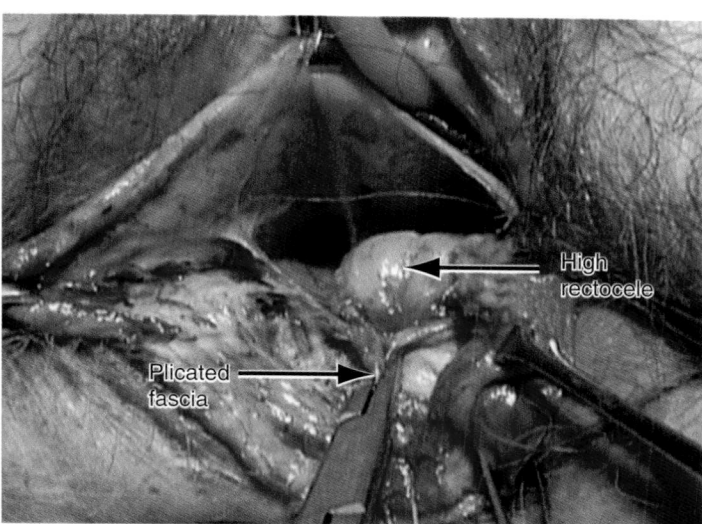

**FIGURE 52–4** Dissection of the posterior wall of the vagina on a cadaver. Note that the dense connective tissue is present only in the distal vagina. Note how the vagina and the anterior wall of the rectum are fused at this level. As the dissection extends proximally, a clear plane of dissection becomes apparent between the posterior vaginal wall and the anterior wall of the rectum that extends to the cul-de-sac. A finger in the rectum demonstrates a rectocele in the mid to upper vagina.

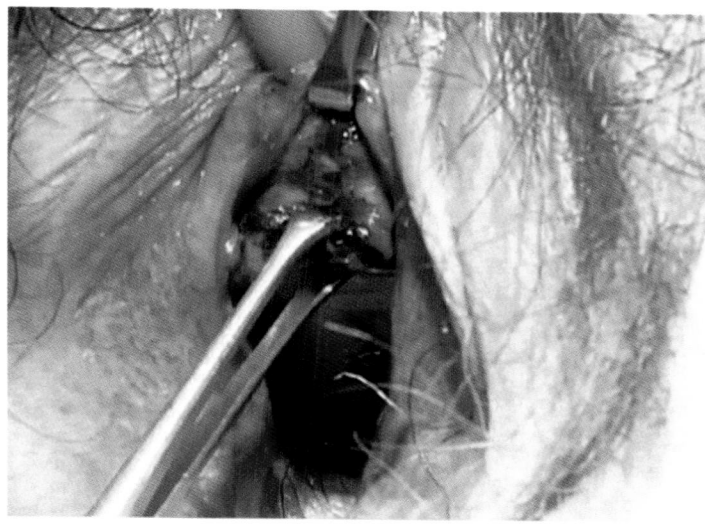

**FIGURE 52–5** The distal portion of the anterior vaginal wall of a cadaver. Note that the area of the vagina, at this anatomic location, is fused to the posterior urethra; this is very similar to what has been mentioned previously regarding the distal portion of the posterior vaginal wall.

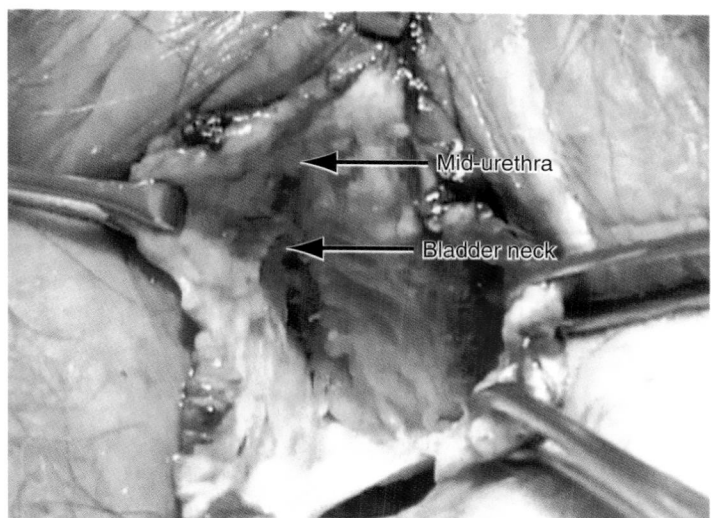

**FIGURE 52–6** The anterior vaginal wall of the same cadaver has now been opened from the external urethra meatus all the way back to the apex of the vagina. The levels of the midurethra and bladder neck are marked. No plane of dissection is seen at the level of the midurethra because in this area the vagina is fused to the posterior urethra. As the dissection extends proximally to the bladder neck, a very clear area of cleavage between the vagina and the bladder, which extends to the inferior pubic ramus, is demonstrated.

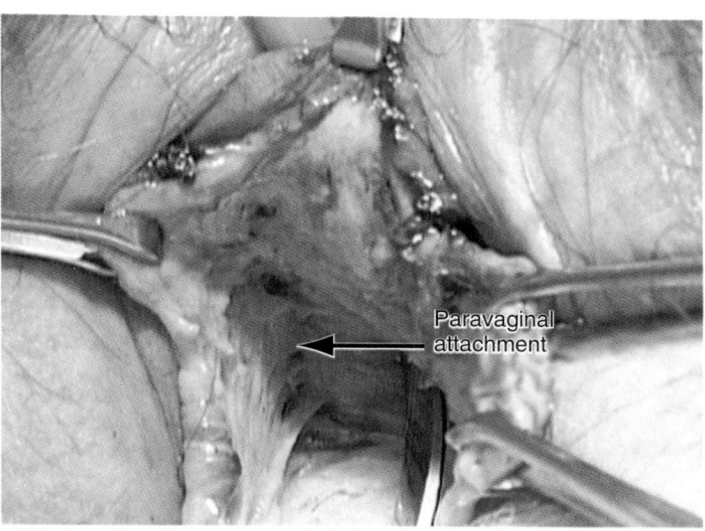

**FIGURE 52–7** This dissection has been extended farther laterally and proximally to demonstrate the normal paravaginal attachment of the anterior vaginal wall. The muscular lining of the vagina that supports the base of the bladder should extend laterally to the arcus tendineus fascia pelvis; this is the normal paravaginal attachment seen in a patient with a well-supported anterior vaginal wall.

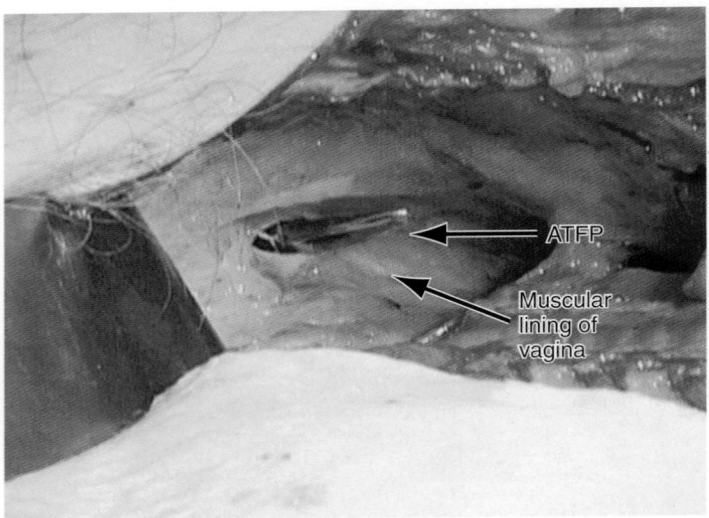

**FIGURE 52–8** A retropubic view of this anatomy is demonstrated. The muscular lining of the vagina that the base of the bladder sits on is shown, as is the arcus tendineus fascia pelvis on the right side. Note that the tip of the scissors has penetrated the urogenital diaphragm at the level of the proximal urethra or bladder neck.

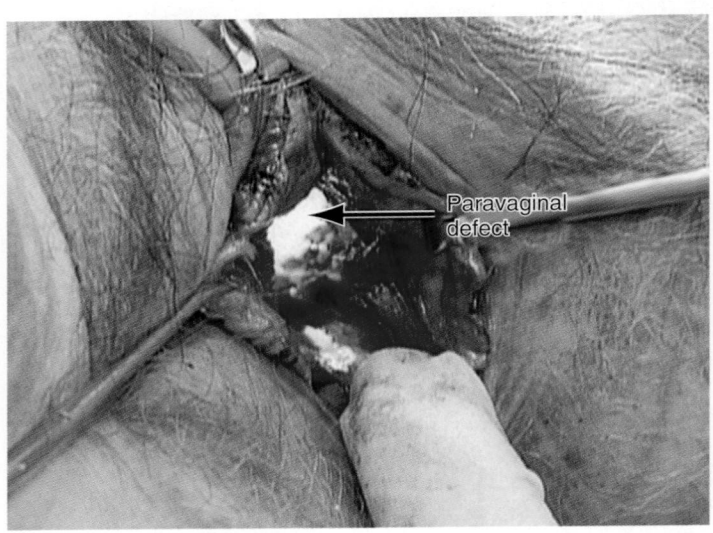

**FIGURE 52–9** Complete detachment of the normal attachment of the anterior vaginal wall on the right side of this cadaver.

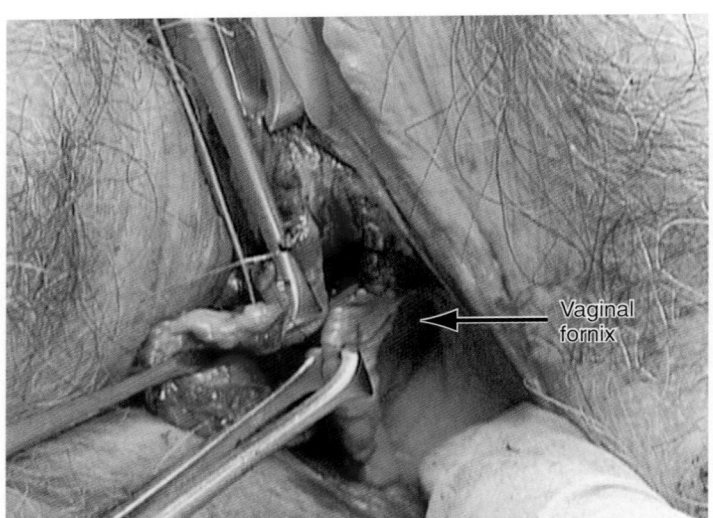

**FIGURE 52–10** Vaginal fornix of a well-supported anterior vaginal wall. The lateral attachment of the vagina proximally should attach to the arcus tendineus fascia pelvis as it inserts into the ischial spine. This normal anatomic attachment provides support and creates the lateral vaginal fornix of the anterior vaginal wall.

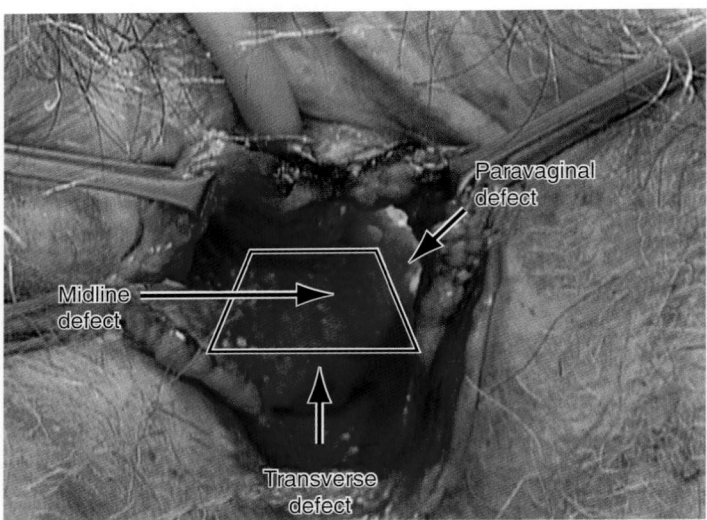

**FIGURE 52–11** The support of the anterior vaginal wall can be viewed as having the shape of a trapezoid, where the lateral aspects of the trapezoid represent normal paravaginal support, the transverse aspects represent the normal attachment of the muscular lining of the vagina to the apex of the vagina or the anterior portion of the cervix, and the midportion of the trapezoid represents durable tissue that should prevent the base of the bladder from descending in the midline.

# CHAPTER 53

# Vaginal Hysterectomy

*Mickey M. Karram*

## Simple Vaginal Hysterectomy

When hysterectomy is indicated, the most appropriate route of removal of the uterus must be chosen. Hysterectomy can be performed transvaginally, abdominally, laparoscopically, or with laparoscopic assistance. The decision to proceed with a vaginal hysterectomy depends on numerous factors. These include the surgeon's training and comfort level with the procedure, the size and mobility of the uterus, the presence of pelvic relaxation, and the benign or malignant nature of the condition. In general, vaginal hysterectomy is less morbid and results in a quicker recovery time than an abdominal or laparoscopy-assisted approach. In contrast to abdominal hysterectomy, vaginal hysterectomy is limited by the size and particularly the mobility of the uterus and by the capacity and elasticity of the vagina. Both are relative criteria because a large uterus can be morcellated, and a narrow vagina can be enlarged with an episiotomy.

Vaginal hysterectomy begins with appropriate positioning of the patient. Vaginal hysterectomy is performed with the patient in the dorsal lithotomy position with her feet in "candy-cane" stirrups. The patient's buttocks should extend slightly over the edge of the table so that a posterior retractor can be placed easily. The thighs are somewhat abducted and the hips flexed (Fig. 53-1). Excessive flexion and abduction of the thighs should be avoided, as this can lead to position-induced nerve injuries. The lateral aspects of the legs should be clear of the stirrups to avoid pressure on the peroneal nerve. The urinary bladder is then emptied with a catheter, and the vaginal area is prepped in a normal fashion. Examination under anesthesia is performed to confirm the degree of uterine descensus, the width of the vaginal outlet, and the presence or absence of pelvic pathology.

### Surgical Technique

1. With a speculum depressing the posterior vaginal wall, the anterior vaginal wall is lifted with a Dever or Haney retractor. The cervix is grasped with two single-toothed tenacula, and downward traction is placed on the cervix.

   Vasoconstrictors such as vasopressin (Pitressin), phenylephrine (Neo-Synephrine), or epinephrine may be injected into the paracervical tissue if no medical condition, such as hypertension or heart disease, contraindicates their use. We prefer to use a prepared solution of 1% or 2% lidocaine or 0.5% bupivacaine with 1:200,000 epinephrine. Use of these ready-made solutions negates the need for mixing in the operating suite and provides some preemptive analgesic at the surgical site. The surgeon should remember that the maximum amount of lidocaine with epinephrine used should not exceed 7 mg/kg or 500 mg total in the healthy adult, whereas the amount of bupivacaine with epinephrine generally should not exceed 225 mg. The total dosage for vaginal hysterectomy is usually 5 to 10 mL of injection. Should a medical contraindication to the use of vasopressors be present, injectable saline provides the benefits of hydrodistention without the cardiovascular risks.

   A knife or electrosurgical instrument is used to make the initial incision through the vaginal mucosa (Fig. 53-2). The position and depth of this incision are very important because they determine access to appropriate planes that will lead to the anterior and posterior cul-de-sacs. The appropriate location of the incision is at the site of the bladder reflection, which is indicated by a crease formed in the vaginal mucosa when the cervix is pushed slightly inward. If this location cannot be identified, one should make the incision low rather than high to avoid potential bladder injury. A circumferential cervical incision is accomplished (Fig. 53-3). Downward traction of the tenaculum and countertraction by the retractors help to determine the appropriate depth of the incision (Fig. 53-4). The incision should be continued down to the cervical stroma. Once the appropriate depth of the incision is reached, the vaginal tissue will fall away from the underlying cervical tissue because there is a distinct plane between these two tissues (Figs. 53-5 and 53-6).

2. The vagina is mobilized both anteriorly and posteriorly. Once the appropriate plane has been reached, blunt dissection of the posterior vaginal wall will lead to the posterior cul-de-sac, which can be entered sharply (Figs. 53-7 and 53-8). Once the peritoneum has been entered, the posterior cul-de-sac is explored for adhesive disease or any other potential abnormalities that may lead to difficulty in performing the hysterectomy. A Haney or weighted retractor is then placed in the posterior cul-de-sac.

3. The uterus is pulled outward and somewhat to the opposite side. Half of an open Haney or similar clamp is introduced into the posterior cul-de-sac, and the uterosacral ligament is clamped (Fig. 53-9). The tip of the clamp is advanced as far caudally to the cervix as possible so that the parametrium included in the clamp follows the line between the anterior and posterior incisions of the vagina (Fig. 53-10). The pedicle then is cut with heavy scissors or a scalpel. The author prefers to ligate the pedicle with an absorbable suture, usually 0 Dexon or Vicryl, with a strong needle attached to it (Fig. 53-11). At times, bleeding from the posterior vaginal cuff may be encountered. This usually can be controlled with cauterization or a running interlocking suture. The cut pedicle is suture-ligated with a transfixing-type suture in which the needle enters the upper part of the ligament pedicle just slightly beyond the end of the Haney clamp. It is withdrawn and then reintroduced into the pedicle at its midpoint. These sutures are usually tagged for later identification of the uterosacral ligaments. The author

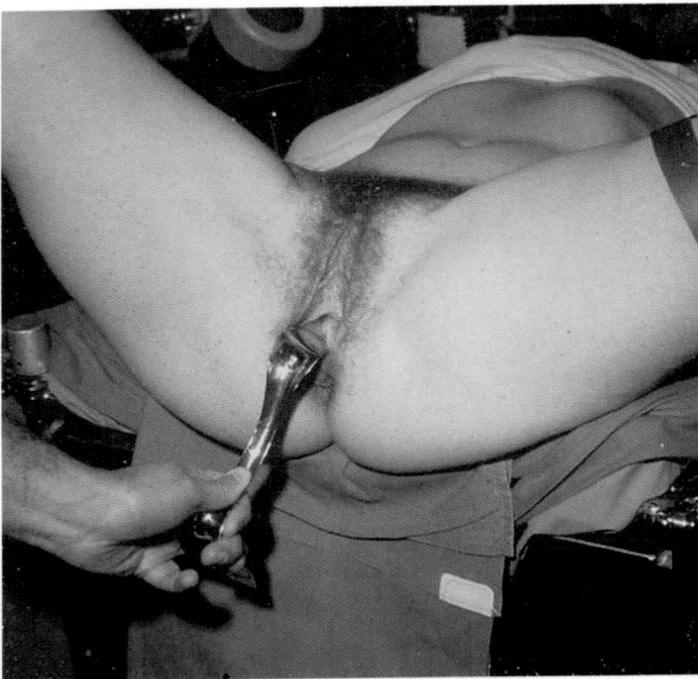

**FIGURE 53–1** Proper positioning of the patient in high "candy-cane" stirrups in preparation for vaginal hysterectomy.

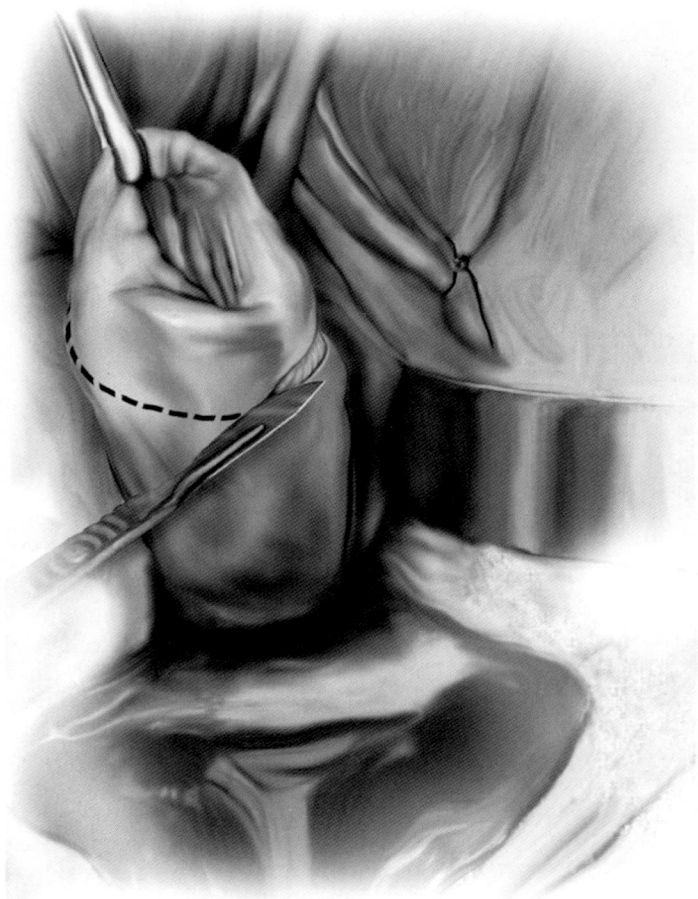

**FIGURE 53–2** The initial incision begins circumferentially at the reflection of the vaginal mucosa onto the cervix. A scalpel or electrosurgical instrument can be utilized.

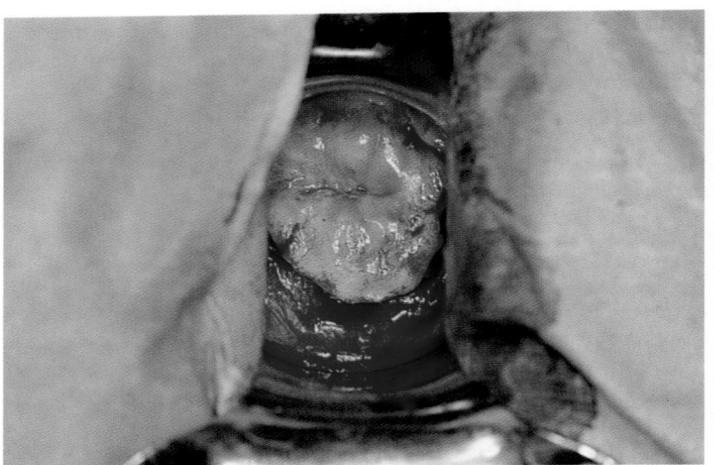

**FIGURE 53–3** The circumferential incision has been made around the cervix.

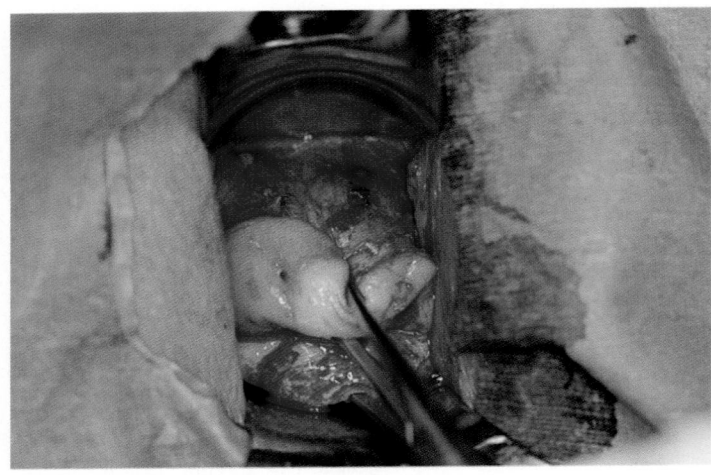

**FIGURE 53–4** The appropriate depth of the initial incision is demonstrated on the anterior cervix.

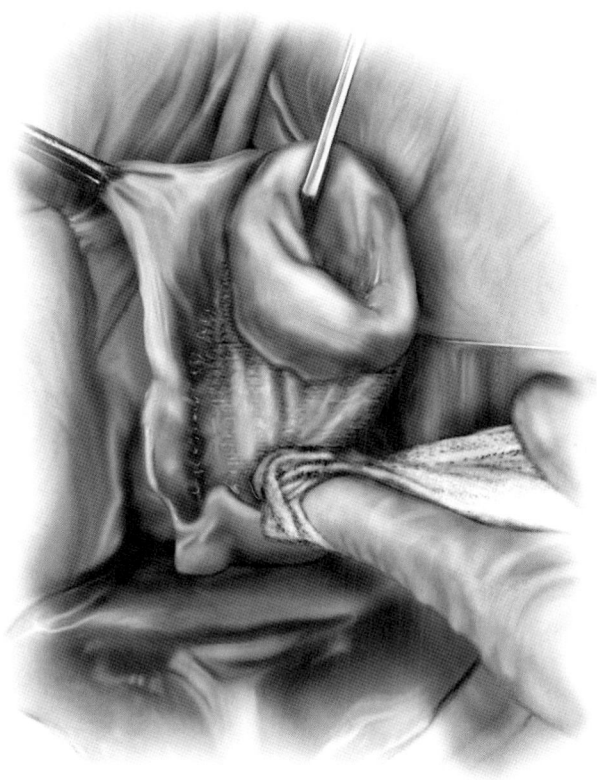

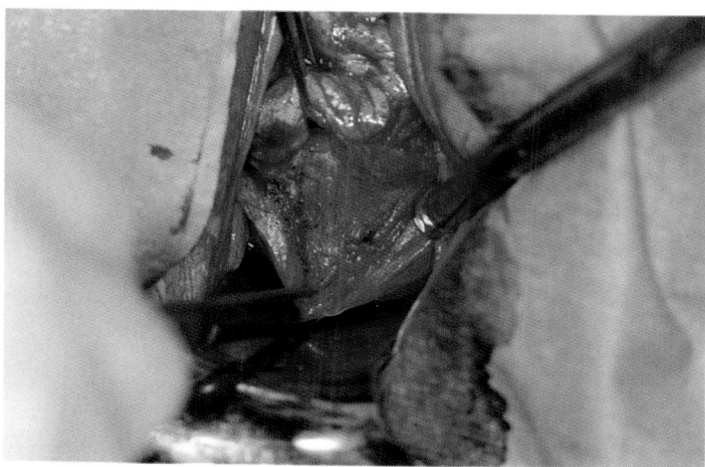

FIGURE 53–6 Dissection of the posterior vaginal wall off the back of the cervix.

FIGURE 53–5 Once the appropriate plane is reached, blunt dissection will usually lead to the posterior peritoneal reflection.

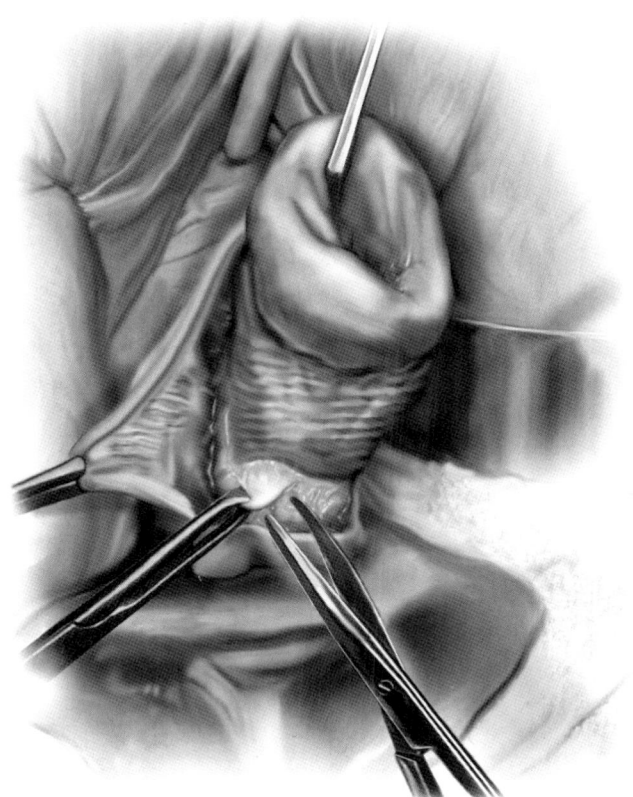

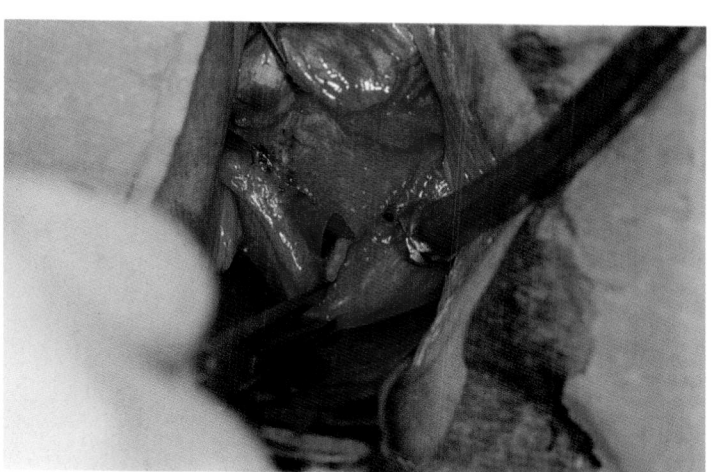

FIGURE 53–8 The posterior cul-de-sac has been entered.

FIGURE 53–7 Sharp entrance into the posterior cul-de-sac.

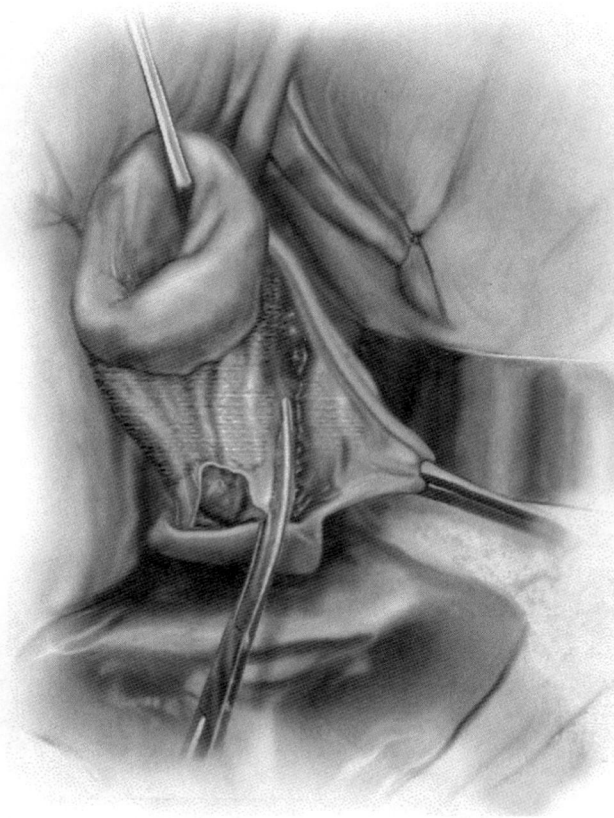

FIGURE 53–9  Clamping of the right uterosacral ligament.

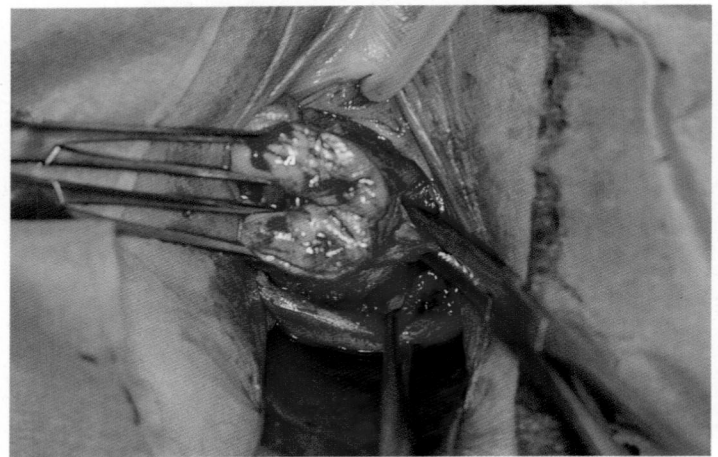

FIGURE 53–10  A Haney clamp is used to clamp the right uterosacral ligament.

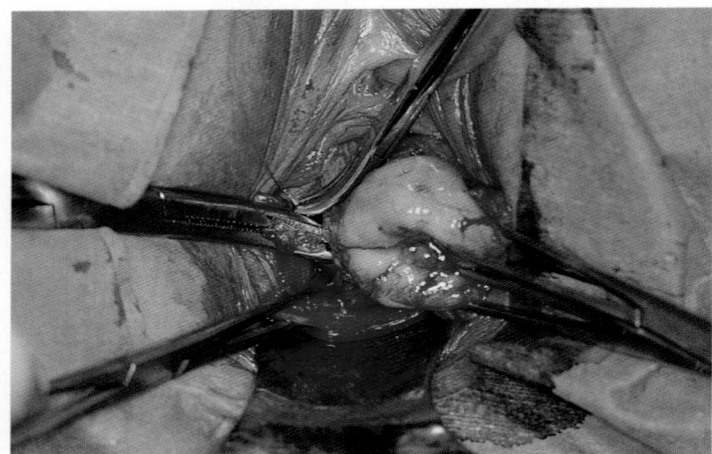

FIGURE 53–11  Passage of a 0 Vicryl suture through the tip of the Haney clamp after the left uterosacral ligament has been cut. Note that the clamp should be placed as perpendicular as possible to the cervix.

prefers to alternate clamping of pedicles on opposite sides instead of clamping up one side of the uterus and then the other. This will gradually improve uterine mobility and exposure. Sharp dissection is used to mobilize the bladder more anteriorly off the cervix (Figs. 53–12 and 53–13). There is never a benefit in rushing to enter the anterior cul-de-sac. This will only lead to inadvertent cystotomies. No attempt should be made to enter the anterior cul-de-sac until the vesicouterine space has been developed. Once the bladder has been mobilized (Fig. 53–14), the cardinal ligament is clamped on each side (Fig. 53–15). This pedicle, which should include peritoneal tissue posteriorly, is sutured in a similar fashion to the uterosacral ligaments. However, the second pass through the ligament is actually made through the previous pedicle, thus obliterating any dead space between the two pedicles to decrease the potential for bleeding or tearing of tissue.

4. After the cardinal ligaments have been incised, a retractor is placed in the vesicouterine space to elevate the bladder off the uterus (see Fig. 53–14). If the anterior cul-de-sac is easily accessible, it can be entered at this time (Figs. 53–16 through 53–18). The next clamp, which probably will include the uterine vessels, should incorporate the anterior and posterior peritoneal reflections if the anterior cul-de-sac has been entered (Fig. 53–19). These clamps should be placed perpendicular to the longitudinal access of the cervix, and the tips of the clamps should completely slide off the cervix to ensure no inadvertent lateral migration and to avoid excessive bleeding or ureteral injury (see Fig. 53–19). As was previously mentioned, suturing of all pedicles involves passage of the needle through the tissue at the tip of the clamp and then a second pass through the previous pedicle. This will obliterate any dead space and eliminate potential bleeding between pedicles (Fig. 53–20). Extra care should be taken to avoid passage of the needle through a vessel because this may lead to the development of a retroperitoneal hematoma.

5. The uterus is then delivered anteriorly or posteriorly into the vagina (Fig. 53–21). The fundus is grasped with the tenaculum and pulled into the vagina. The utero-ovarian ligament is supported by the index finger on the opposite side, and a clamp is placed close to the uterus. The last pedicle usually includes the fallopian tube and the round and ovarian ligaments. At times, these may be taken with one clamp, but usually a clamp placed from below is required, as well as a clamp placed from above (Fig. 53–22). A finger should be maintained behind this pedicle to ensure that the clamps overlap posteriorly, and that no other tissue has been included in the clamp (Figs. 53–22 through 53–24). Once the final pedicles have been cut, the uterus is handed off to be sent to pathology. These pedicles are then doubly ligated. If one clamp has been used, a free tie is initially placed, followed by a suture-ligature. If two clamps have been used, each pedicle is individually ligated, and then a figure-of-8 suture is placed through both pedicles. These sutures are tagged, and at this time all pedicles are inspected to ensure hemostasis (Fig. 53–25). Because all pedicles have been sutured into the previous pedicle, no tearing or dead space between the pedicles should be noted (see Fig. 53–25).

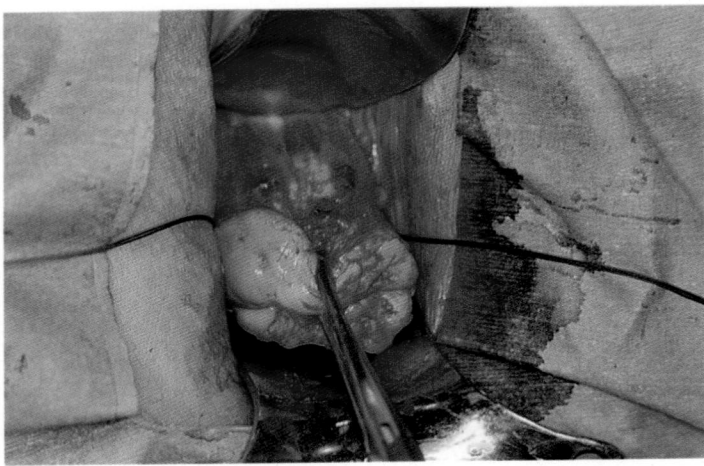

**FIGURE 53–12** The vagina has been mobilized off the anterior cervix.

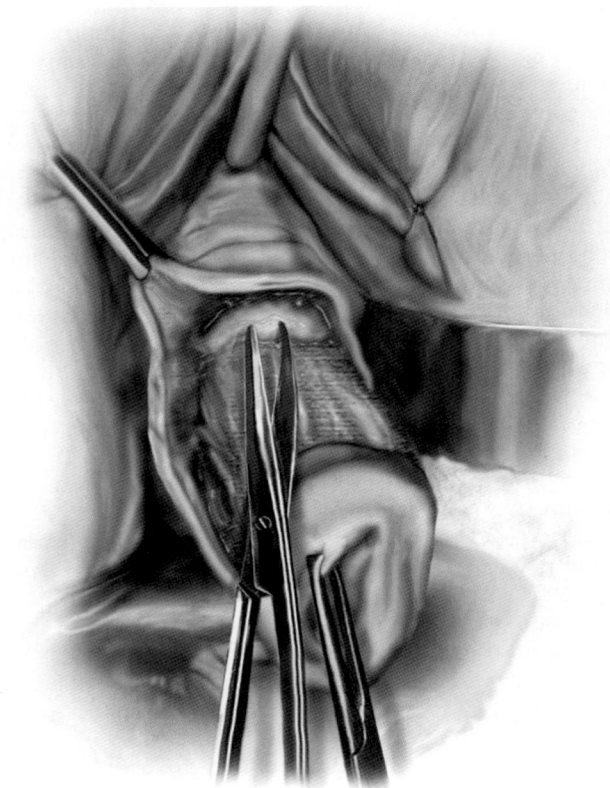

**FIGURE 53–13** Sharp dissection is then needed to incise the pubocervical fascia to enter the vesicouterine space before the anterior cul-de-sac is entered.

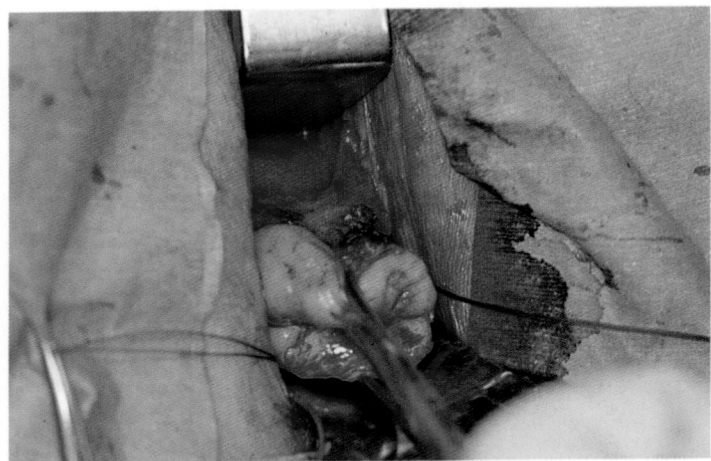

**FIGURE 53–14** The vesicouterine space has been entered. This allows placement of a retractor anteriorly, which mobilizes the bladder off the anterior cervix and exposes the peritoneal reflection of the anterior cul-de-sac.

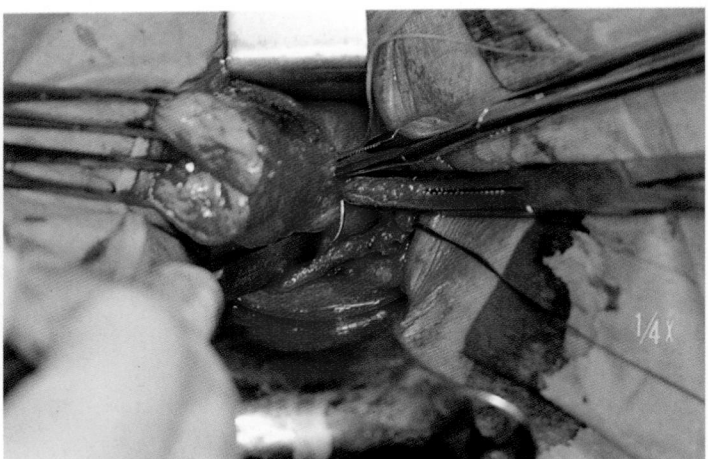

**FIGURE 53–15** The cardinal ligament has been clamped and cut and is being sutured. This suture will incorporate the pedicle into the previous uterosacral ligament pedicle.

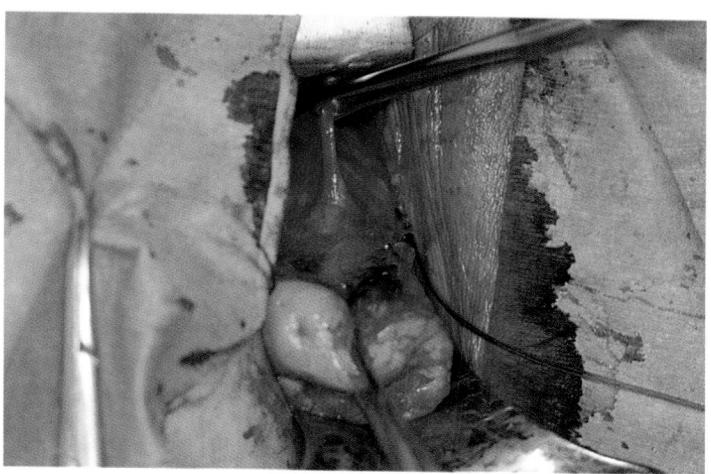

FIGURE 53–16  After the vesicouterine space has been entered, the anterior peritoneal reflection is usually easily accessible.

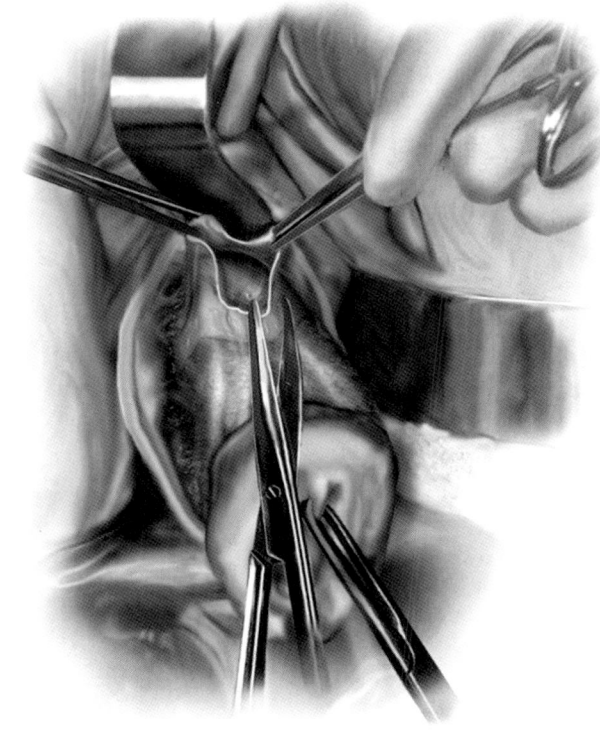

FIGURE 53–17  Sharp dissection into the anterior cul-de-sac.

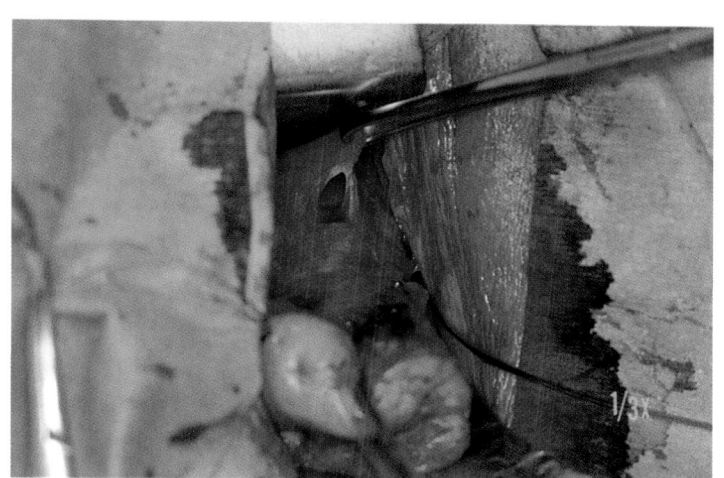

FIGURE 53–18  The anterior cul-de-sac has been entered.

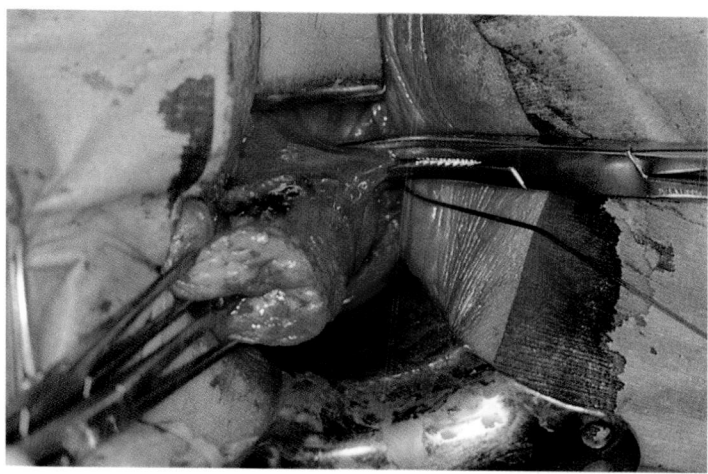

FIGURE 53–19  Clamping of the uterine vessels. The clamp incorporates the peritoneal reflections of the anterior and posterior cul-de-sac. Note the placement of the clamp at a right angle to the cervix.

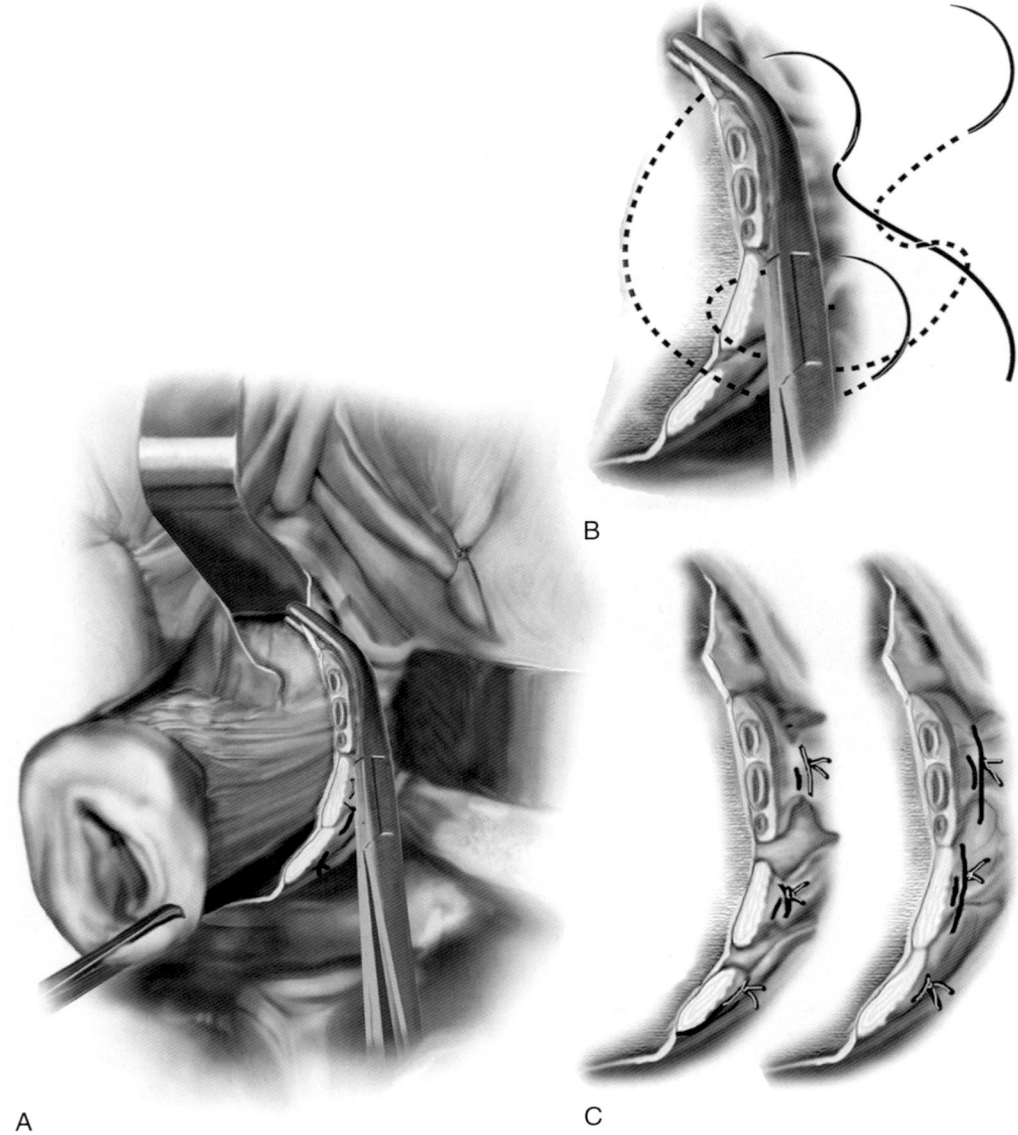

**FIGURE 53–20 A.** The proper technique for clamping of the uterine vessels. **B.** The pedicle is sutured to ligate the vessels, as well as to incorporate the pedicle into the previously ligated pedicle. A suture is initially passed through the tissue at the tip of the clamp, and then a second pass of the needle is made through the distal end of the previous pedicle. **C.** This technique of ligating pedicles completely obliterates the dead space between pedicles. This technique is contrasted with the technique of ligating each pedicle individually, which results in gaps between pedicles that may lead to tearing of tissue with bleeding between pedicles.

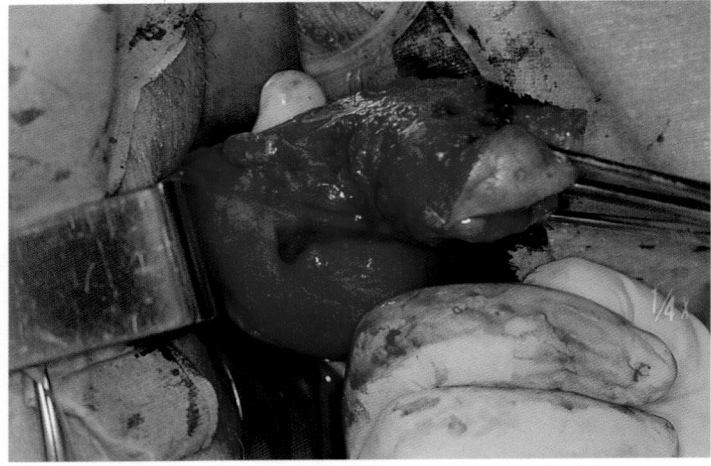

**FIGURE 53–21** The uterus is delivered through the posterior cul-de-sac.

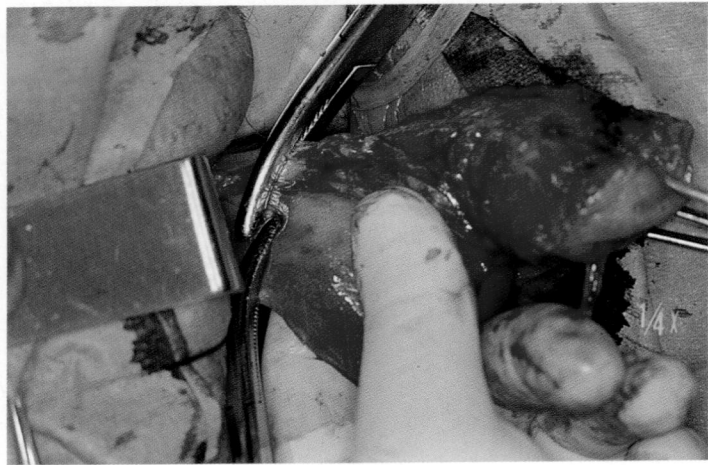

**FIGURE 53–22** Clamps have been placed close to the uterus. The pedicle includes the fallopian tube and the round and ovarian ligaments. Note that the tips of the clamps cross in the midline.

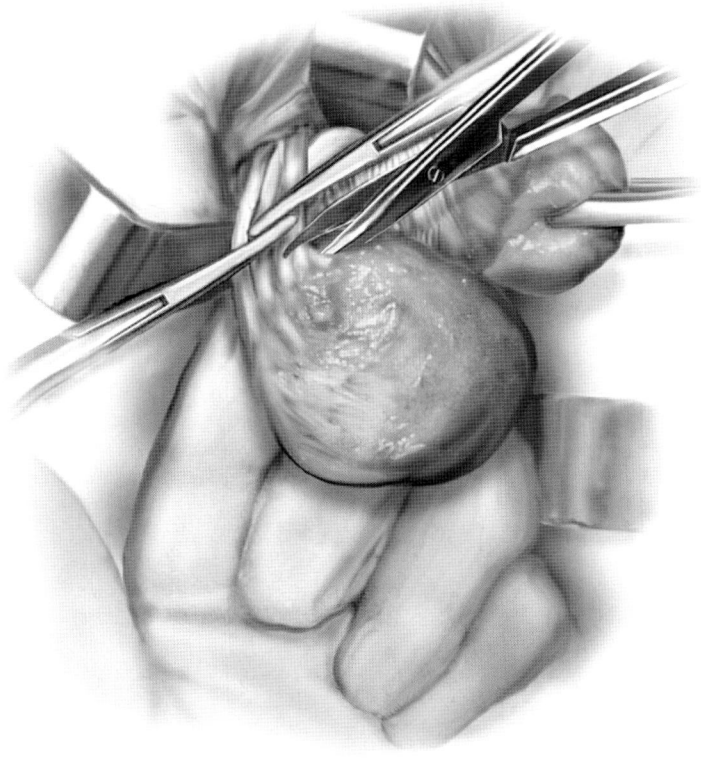

**FIGURE 53–23** The pedicle is cut with scissors or a knife. *Note:* A finger behind the pedicle prevents inadvertent cutting of other structures.

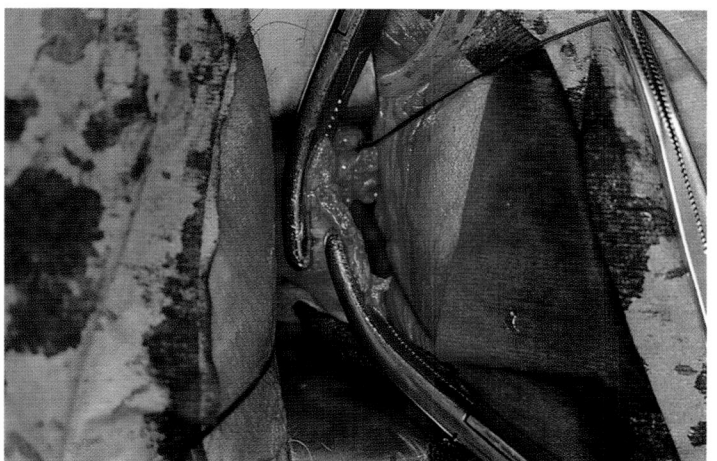

**FIGURE 53–24** The uterus has been removed and the adnexal pedicle is doubly ligated. Each clamp is individually ligated, and then a figure-of-8 suture is placed through both pedicles. This suture is usually tagged.

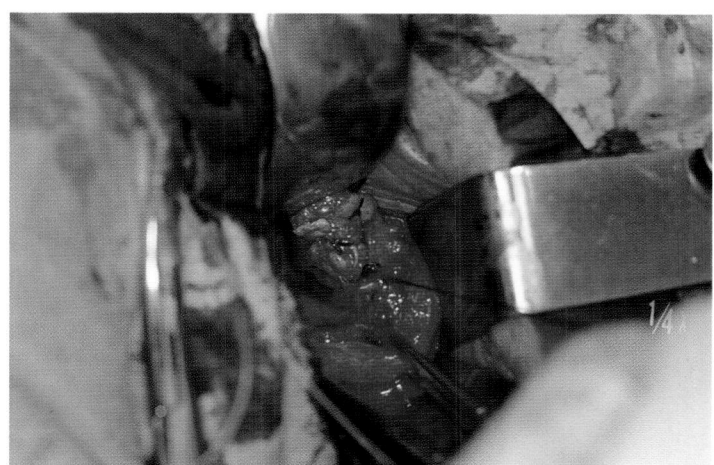

**FIGURE 53–25** The pedicles on the left side of the cuff are inspected, and hemostasis is ensured.

## Vaginal Salpingo-oophorectomy

Removal of the adnexa can be accomplished at the time of vaginal hysterectomy in at least 50% of patients and, according to some reports, in up to 90% of cases. The success of performing adnexectomy totally depends on the ability to expose the tube and ovary and to gain access to their pedicles. Utilization of suture tags to provide gentle traction on the round ligaments will aid in visualization of the tube and ovary. Most commonly it is best to grasp the adnexa with a Babcock clamp and pull them down as far as possible (Fig. 53–26). The round ligament, ovarian ligament, fallopian tube, and mesosalpinx are then clamped with a curved Haney clamp or, more ideally, a Statinsky vascular clamp. It is very important to place this clamp accurately and to ensure that the ovarian artery does not retract outside of the clamp. To avoid injuring the ureter, it is important to place the clamp as close to the ovary as possible. The tissue is then cut (Fig. 53–27) and the pedicle suture-ligated with a 2-0 delayed absorbable suture. An initial free tie is placed around the pedicle; this is followed by a transfixion suture-ligature distal to the first tie. If the ovary is inaccessible, this may be the result of a short, strong round ligament, which prevents the ligament from being pulled down and clamped. In this situation, the round ligament is separately clamped, and the adnexa is then mobilized, allowing direct clamping of the infundibulo-pelvic ligament.

## Evaluating the Posterior Cul-de-sac

The posterior cul-de-sac should be routinely assessed at the time of vaginal hysterectomy (Figs. 53–28 and 53–29). Many times, a potential or true enterocele is present. Also, in cases of uterovaginal prolapse, one has to decide whether a formal vaginal vault suspension needs to be performed, or whether simple obliteration of the cul-de-sac via a culdoplasty will result in adequate vaginal support and length.

The goal of a McCall-type culdoplasty is to obliterate the cul-de-sac by pulling the uterosacral ligaments across the midline. It also anchors and pulls the vagina inward, thus creating increased posterior vaginal wall length. The technique of a McCall culdoplasty usually involves the placement of one to three internal McCall sutures, which are permanent sutures that are placed to approximate the uterosacral ligaments and incorporate intervening peritoneum (Figs. 53–30 and 53–31). To place these stitches, the surgeon depresses the sigmoid colon down and to the right with the left index and middle fingers. A monofilament 0 suture is then placed deeply into the left uterosacral ligament. The suture is then continued across the top of the sigmoid colon and parietal peritoneum to reach the patient's right side, where it is placed deep into the right uterosacral ligament. This suture is then tagged, and a second (and even a third) suture is placed (see Figs. 53–30 and 53–31). The external McCall sutures are placed, beginning with passage of a delayed absorbable suture through the posterior vaginal wall and peritoneum. This suture is then incorporated into the left uterosacral ligament and is continued across the peritoneum over the sigmoid colon to the right uterosacral ligament; it then is brought back out through the vagina, where it is tagged (see Fig. 53–31). When the cul-de-sac is very shallow and redundancy in the posterior vaginal wall is minimal, a single external McCall suture may be sufficient (see Fig. 53–31). However, at times a second (and even a third) external McCall suture is placed, depending on the redundancy of the upper part of the posterior vaginal walls (Fig. 53–32). When the redundancy of the posterior vaginal wall and cul-de-sac is excessive, it is desirable to wedge out some vagina and actually excise the peritoneum up to the level of placement of the internal McCall sutures (Figs. 53–29 and 53–33).

The internal McCall sutures are tied, and the external McCall sutures are tagged but not tied until after closure of the vaginal cuff (Fig. 53–34). If an anterior colporrhaphy is to be performed, it is done at this time. If not, or after the anterior colporrhaphy is performed, the vaginal vault is closed with interrupted 2-0 delayed absorbable sutures approximating the anterior and posterior vaginal epithelia with their underlying fascia. The external McCall sutures are then tied (Figs. 53–35 through 53–38). These sutures anchor the posterior vaginal wall to the uterosacral ligaments, as well as obliterate the cul-de-sac and support the vaginal cuff. Cystoscopy to ensure ureteral patency should be considered routinely after McCall culdoplasty.

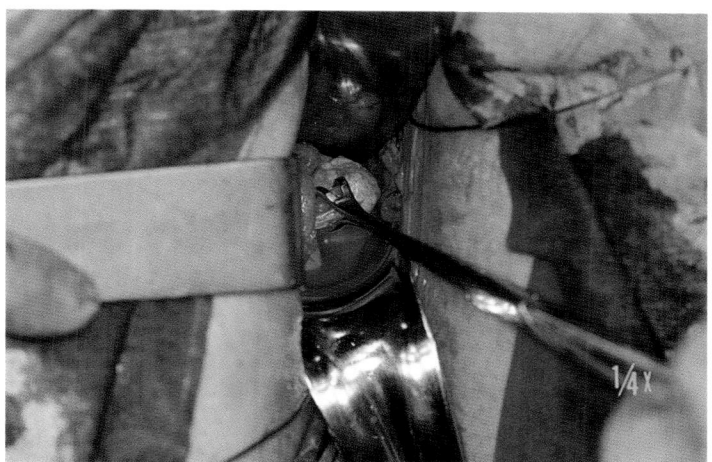

FIGURE 53–26  A Babcock clamp is used to grasp the ovary and pull it down into the vaginal field.

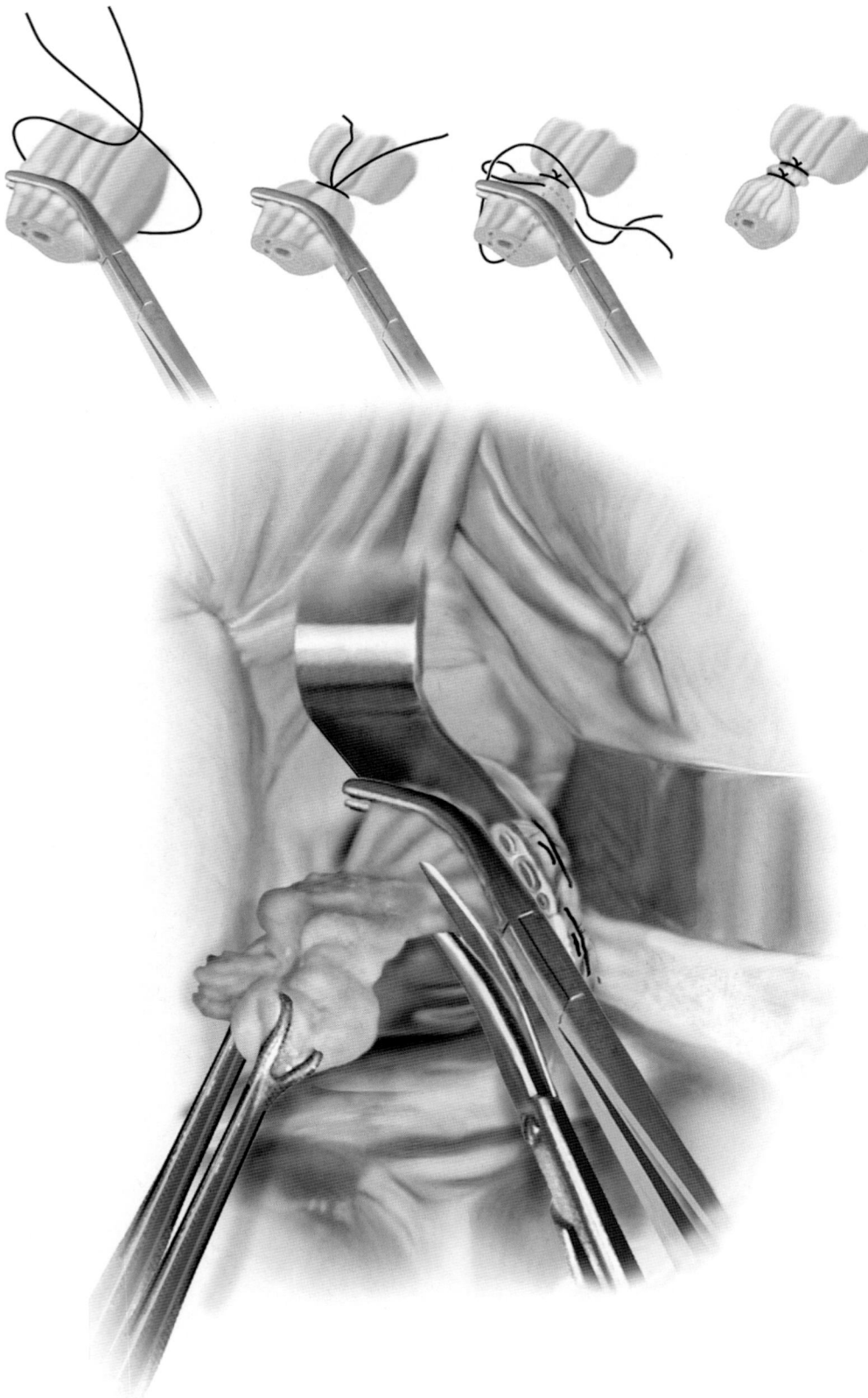

**FIGURE 53–27** A curved Haney or Statinsky vascular clamp is used to clamp across the adnexal pedicle. The adnexa is cut away with scissors, and the pedicle is doubly ligated (**inset**).

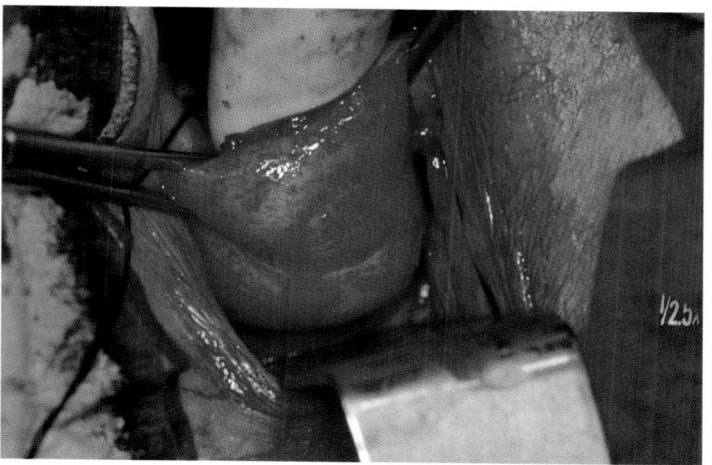

**FIGURE 53–28** Palpation of the posterior cul-de-sac after removal of the uterus. The index finger is placed in the cul-de-sac, and the peritoneum and upper posterior vaginal wall are mobilized distally.

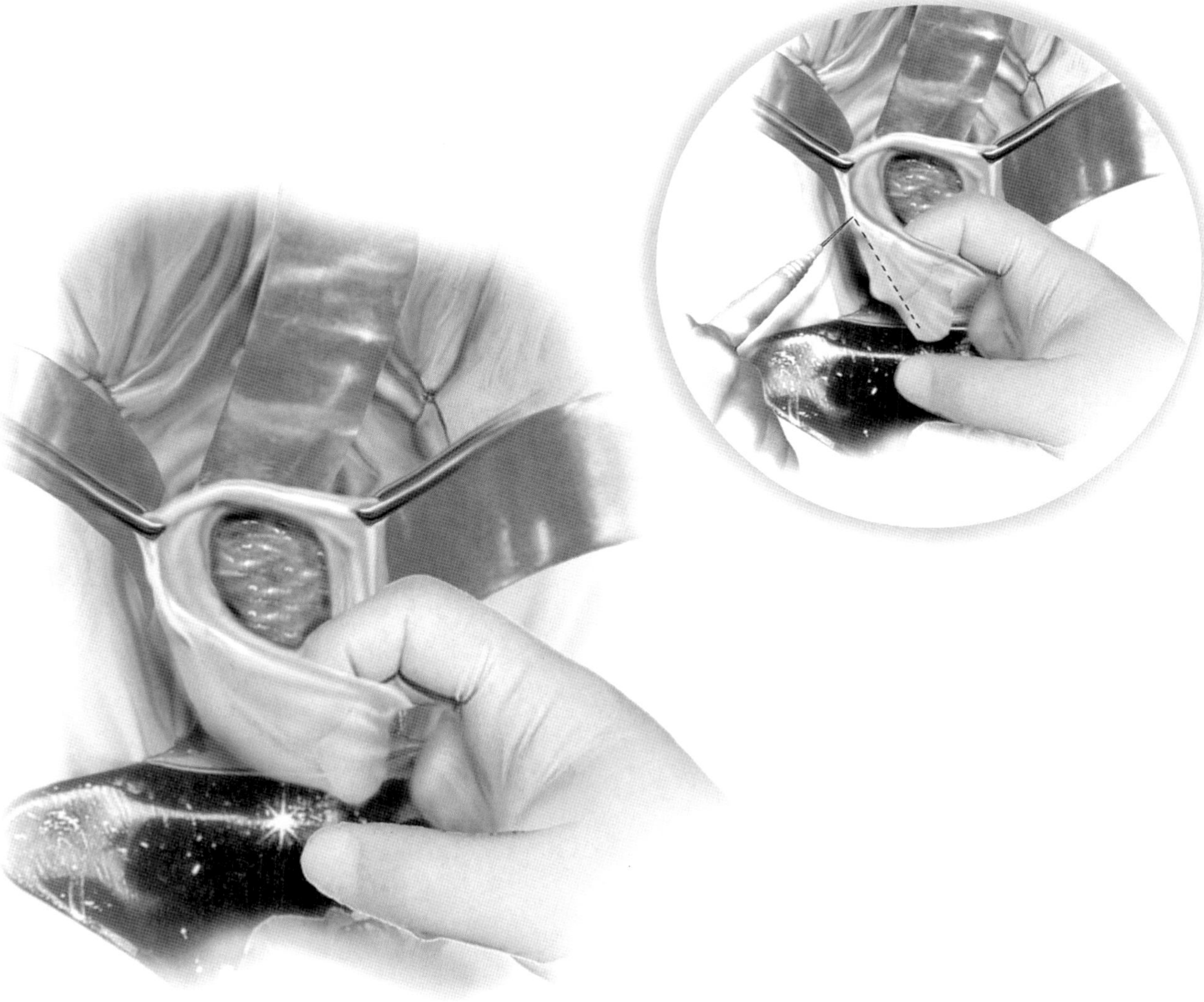

**FIGURE 53–29** Digital palpation of the posterior cul-de-sac and enterocele. **Inset.** The technique of removal of the redundant wedge of posterior vaginal wall and peritoneum.

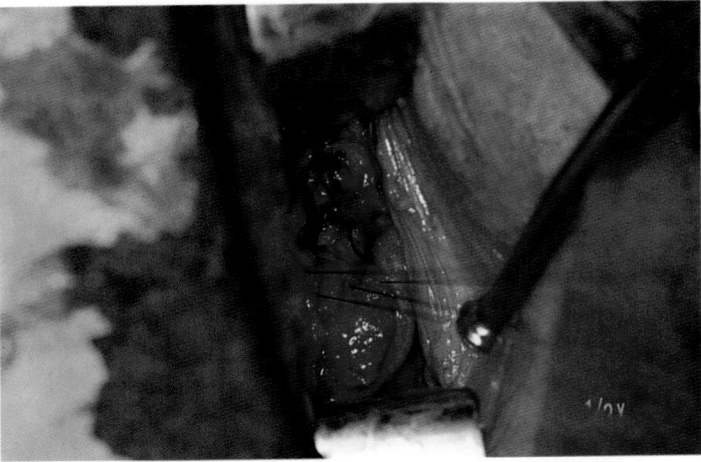

**FIGURE 53–30** Two internal McCall sutures have been placed; permanent sutures are passed through the uterosacral ligaments and intervening peritoneum of the cul-de-sac. Sutures are tagged to be tied after placement of the external McCall sutures.

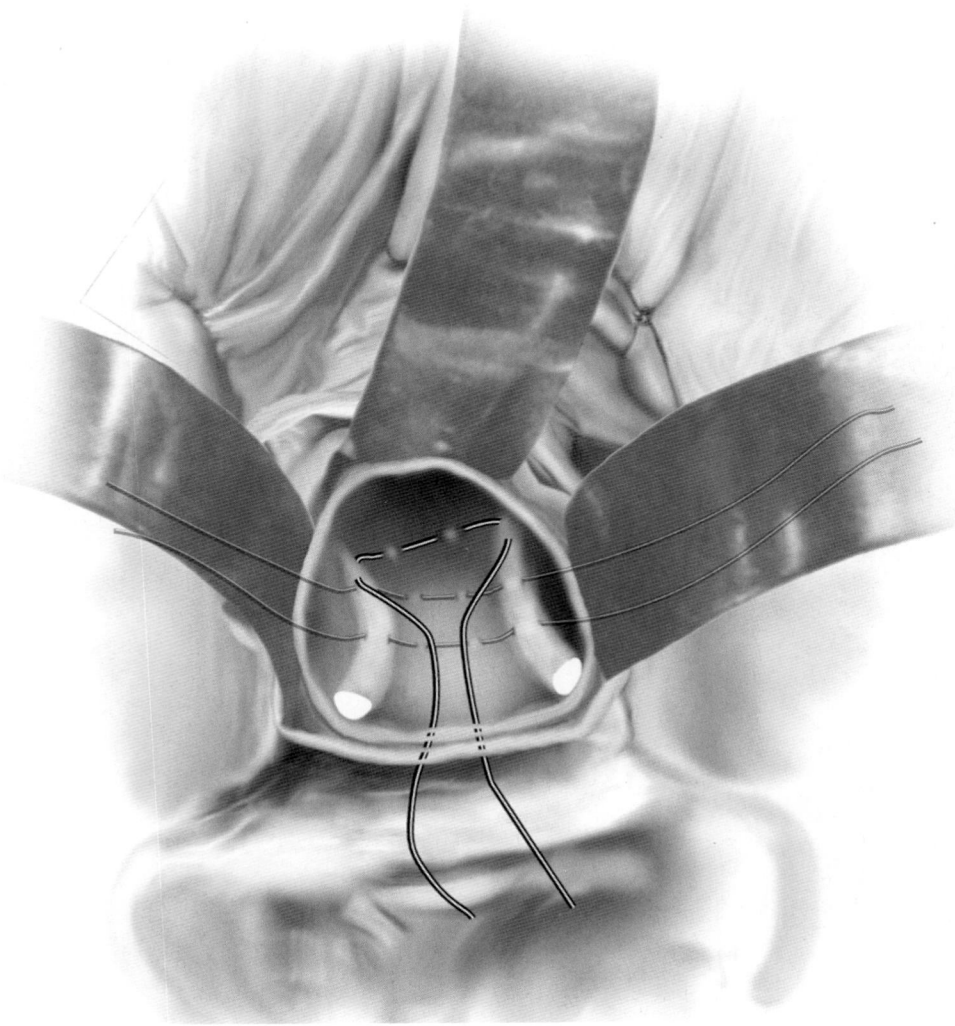

**FIGURE 53–31** McCall culdoplasty. Two internal sutures (permanent) and one external suture (delayed absorbable) have been placed.

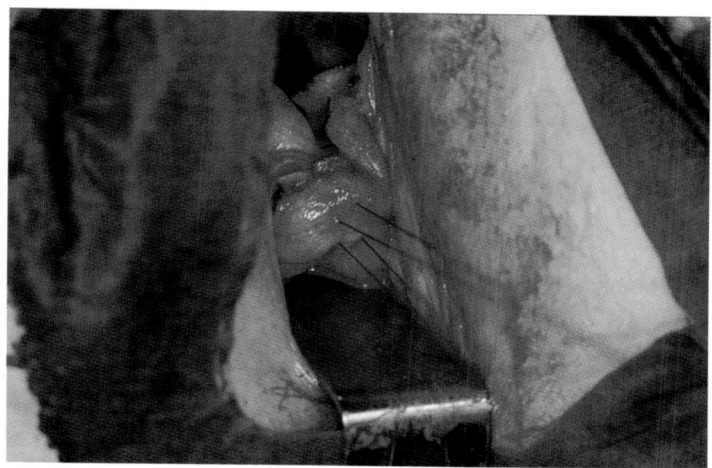

**FIGURE 53–32** Two external McCall sutures have been placed. These sutures will be tied after closure of the vaginal cuff.

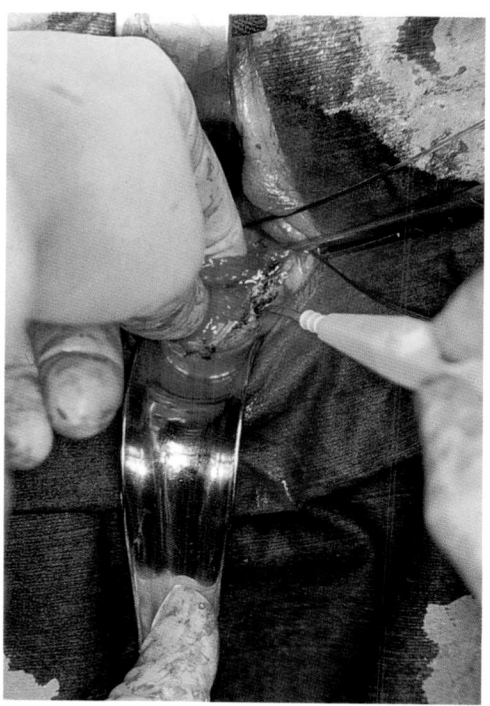

**FIGURE 53–33** A wedge of redundant posterior vaginal wall and peritoneum is being excised with Bovie cautery.

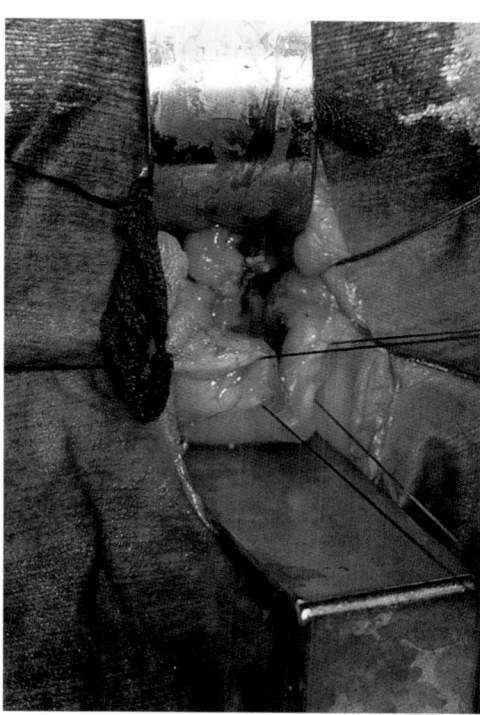

**FIGURE 53–34** Two tagged external McCall stitches, which have been placed after a wedge of posterior vaginal wall has been removed.

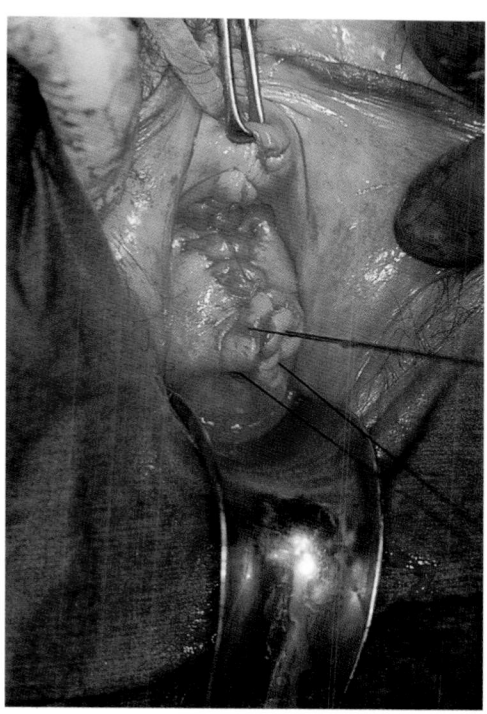

**FIGURE 53–35** Untied external McCall sutures after anterior colporrhaphy and closure of the vaginal cuff.

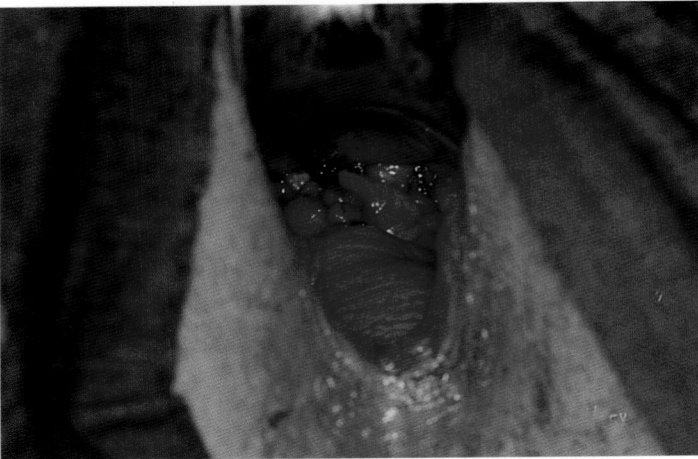

**FIGURE 53–36** The upper posterior vaginal wall after tying down of external McCall sutures.

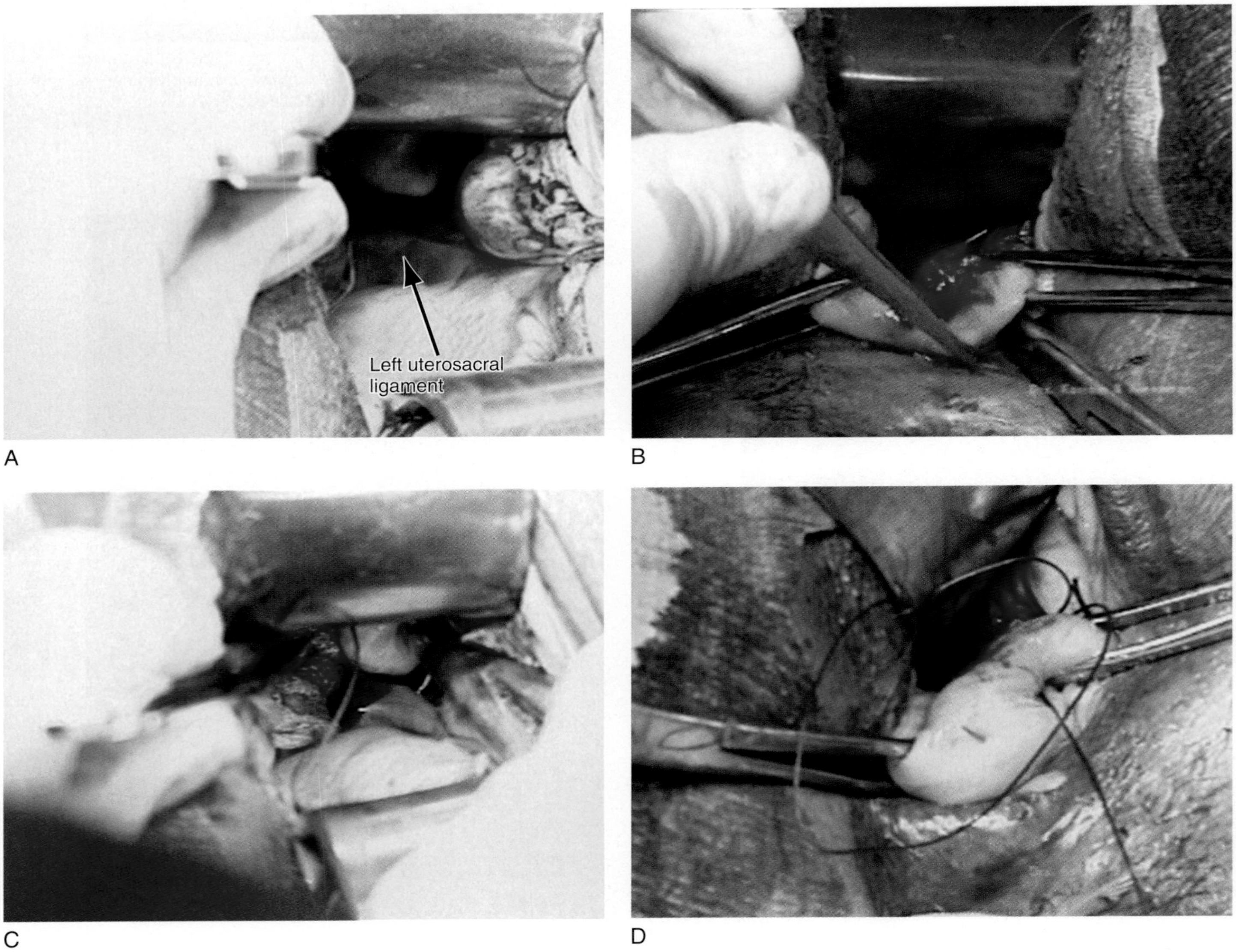

A

B

C

D

**FIGURE 53–37** Technique of McCall culdoplasty. **A.** The cul-de-sac has been exposed, and the left uterosacral ligament is visualized. **B.** The first external McCall suture is being passed from the inside of the vaginal lumen into the peritoneum of the cul-de-sac. **C.** The suture is then passed through the left uterosacral ligament. **D.** The suture has been passed across the intervening peritoneum through the right uterosacral ligament and is now being passed back out into the vaginal lumen through the posterior vaginal cuff.

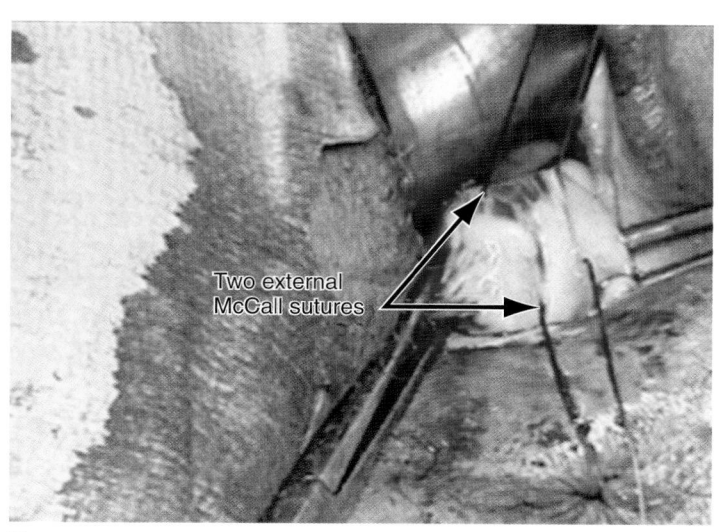

Two external
McCall sutures

E

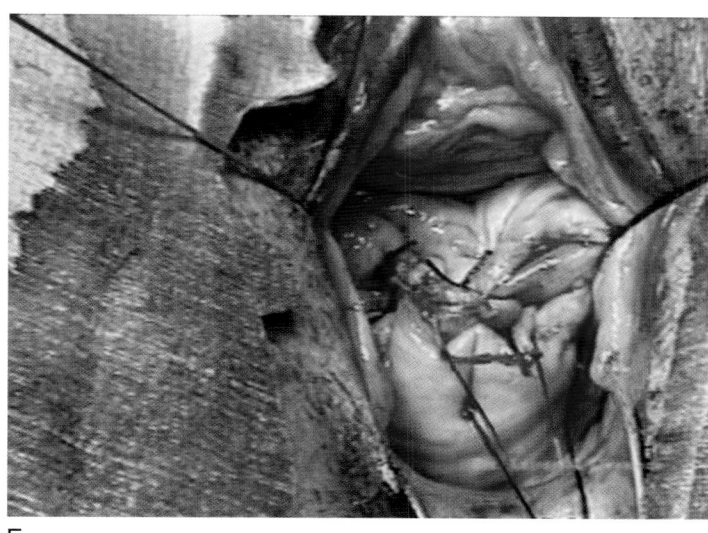

F

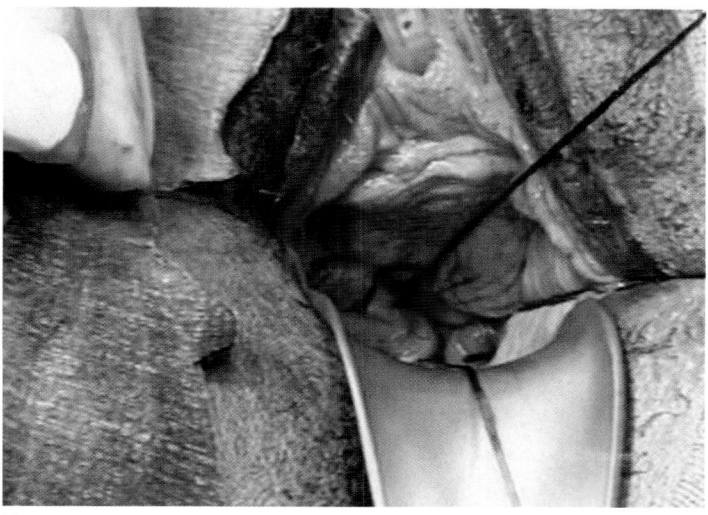

G

**FIGURE 53–37, cont'd  E.** A second McCall suture has been passed in an identical fashion more distal to the first. Demonstrated here are the two external McCall sutures before closure of the vaginal cuff and tying of the sutures. **F.** The vaginal cuff is closed with interrupted, delayed absorbable sutures. **G.** The McCall sutures are tied. Note the excellent elevation of the vagina into the hollow of the sacrum.

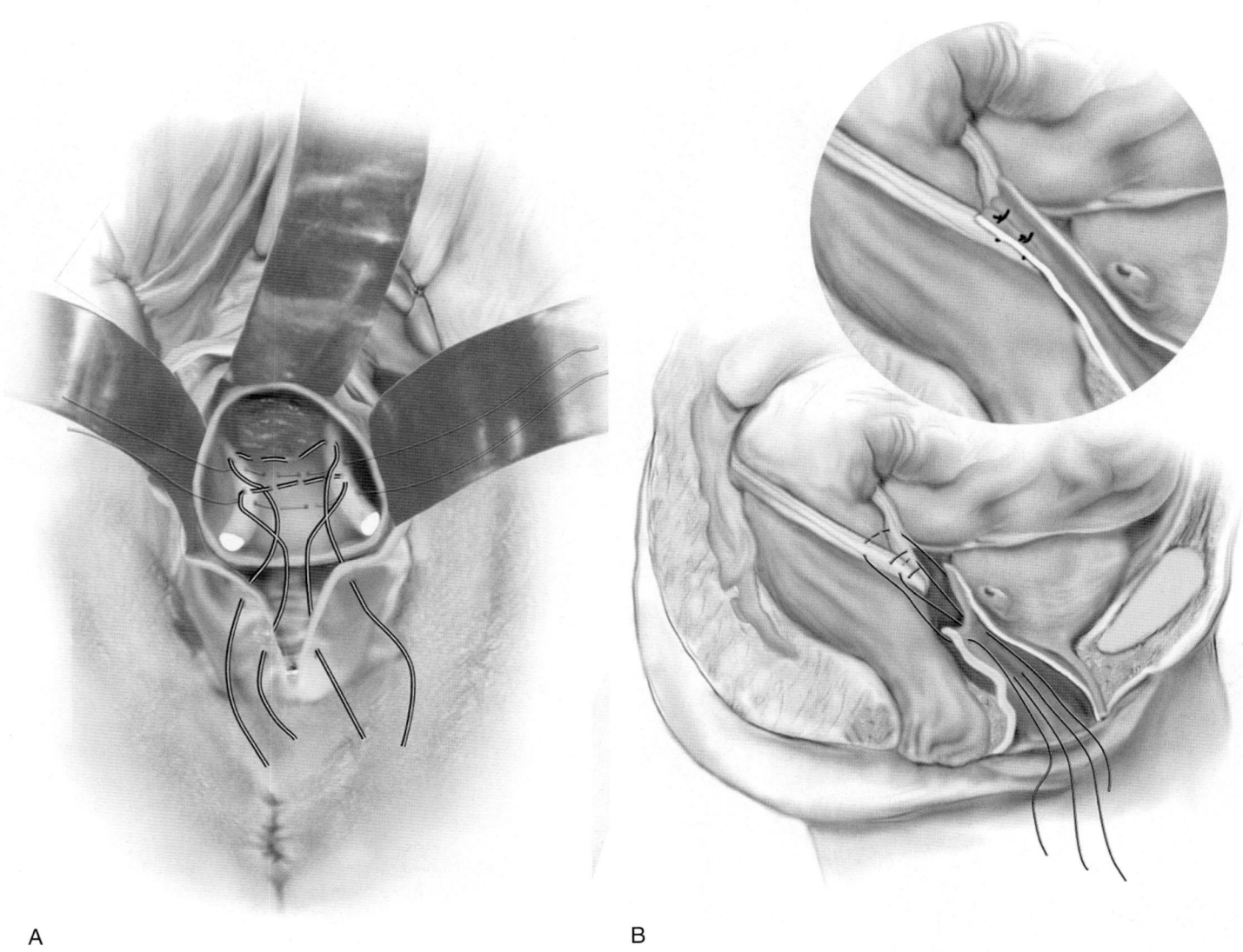

A                                                                                    B

**FIGURE 53–38  A.** Placement of internal and external McCall sutures after a wedge of posterior vaginal wall has been removed. **B.** Cross-section of the upper vagina and vaginal vault before and after tying of sutures.

## Difficult Vaginal Hysterectomy

The technical aspects of vaginal hysterectomy at times can be more challenging if abnormal pathology of the pelvis exists, resulting in adhesive disease or an enlarged uterus. Certain cases of significant uterovaginal prolapse may also be challenging.

### Complete Uterine Procidentia

In the preoperative assessment of complete uterine prolapse, it is important to determine whether this is true uterine procidentia, or whether it demonstrates a severely elongated cervix, and to assess in a site-specific fashion all other pelvic floor support defects. This should initially include palpation of the cervix (Fig. 53-39) to determine the extent of cervical elongation. The lateral fornices of the anterior and posterior vaginal walls should be evaluated (Fig. 53-40), and the extent of anterior (Fig. 53-41) and posterior vaginal wall eversion should be noted (Fig. 53-42). All of this information is very important in selection of the appropriate surgical procedure. The basic steps for vaginal hysterectomy in the patient with complete prolapse are identical to those for vaginal hysterectomy (Figs. 53-43 through 53-54). If the cervix is markedly elongated (Figs. 53-50 through 53-64), one must take numerous extraperitoneal bites in the paracervical tissue until the peritoneal reflection of the anterior and posterior cul-de-sac is reached (see Figs. 53-58 through 53-60). Severe descent of the uterus distorts the anatomy of the entire pelvis. It is important to keep in mind that the normal position of the ureter may be distorted as a result of long-standing traction commonly associated with advanced uterine prolapse and a large cystocele (Fig. 53-65).

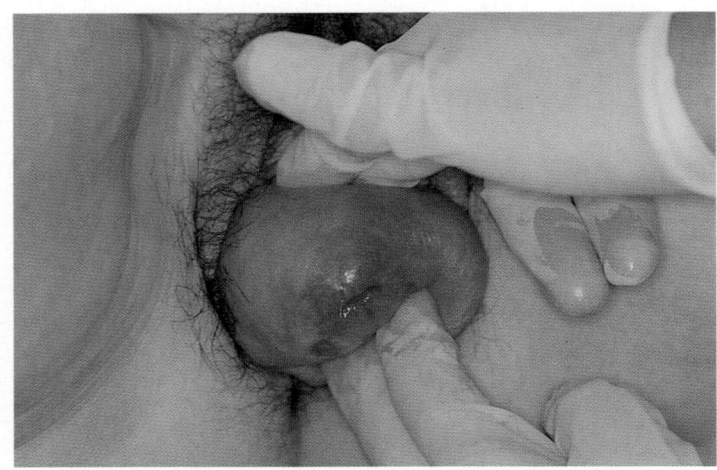

**FIGURE 53-39** Palpation of the cervix in a patient with complete prolapse to determine preoperatively whether the cervix is elongated.

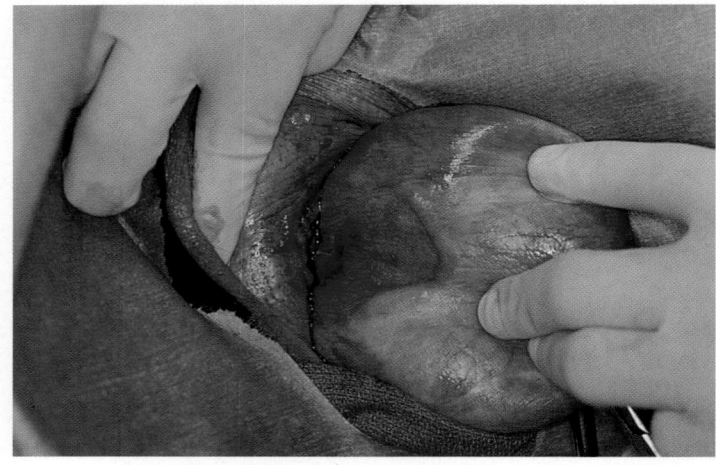

A

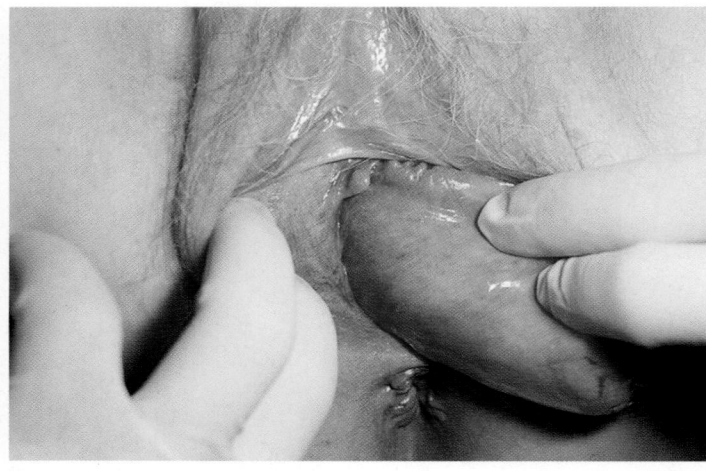

B

**FIGURE 53-40 A.** Lateral vaginal fornix. Note the large ulcer from long-standing prolapse. **B.** Complete eversion of the lateral aspect of the anterior vaginal wall.

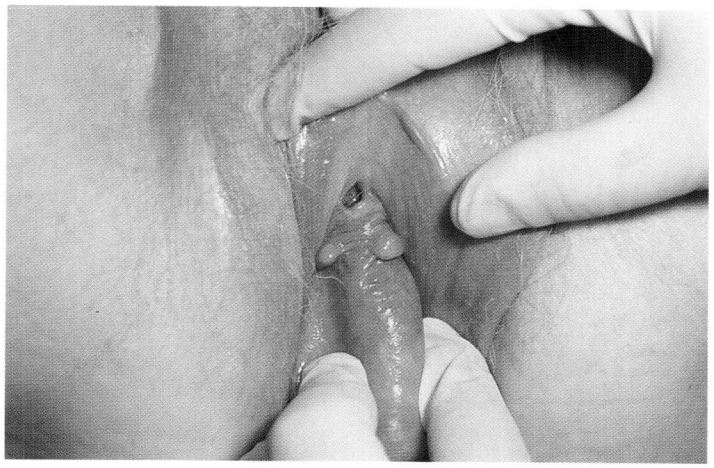

FIGURE 53–41 Complete eversion of the anterior vaginal wall.

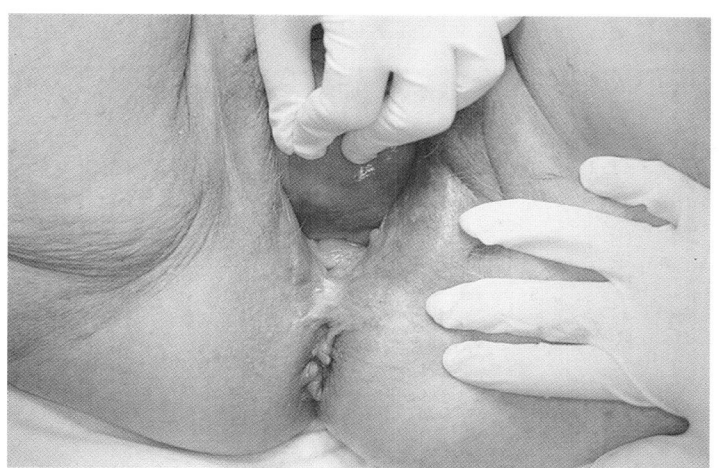

A

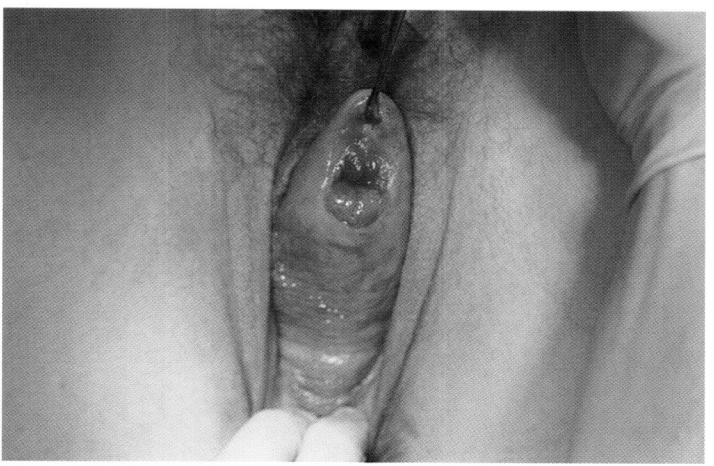

B

FIGURE 53–42 A. Approximately 75% of the posterior vaginal wall has been everted in this patient with uterine prolapse. B. Complete eversion of the posterior vaginal wall in a patient with an elongated cervix.

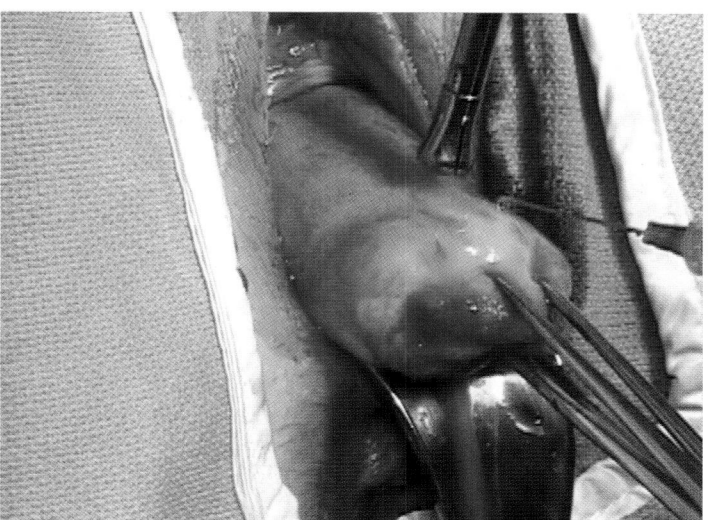

FIGURE 53–43 The level of the initial incision depends on the extent of cervical elongation. The so-called bladder sulcus often is not apparent. This incision is made in a relatively distal position because the cervix is not elongated.

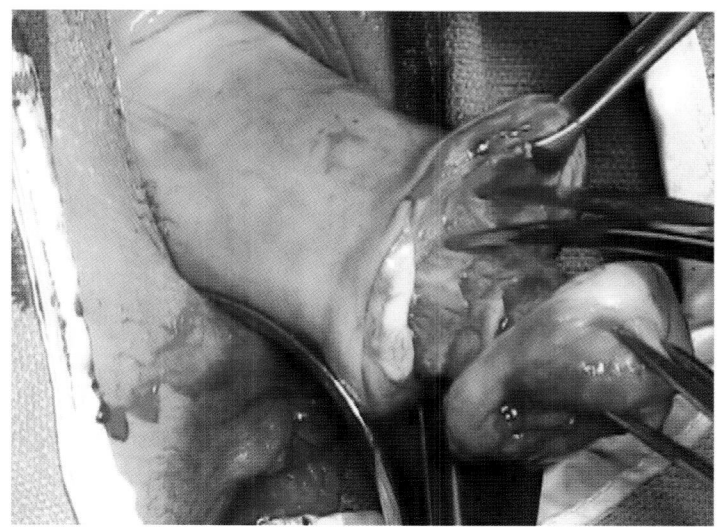

FIGURE 53–44 Sharp entrance into the posterior cul-de-sac.

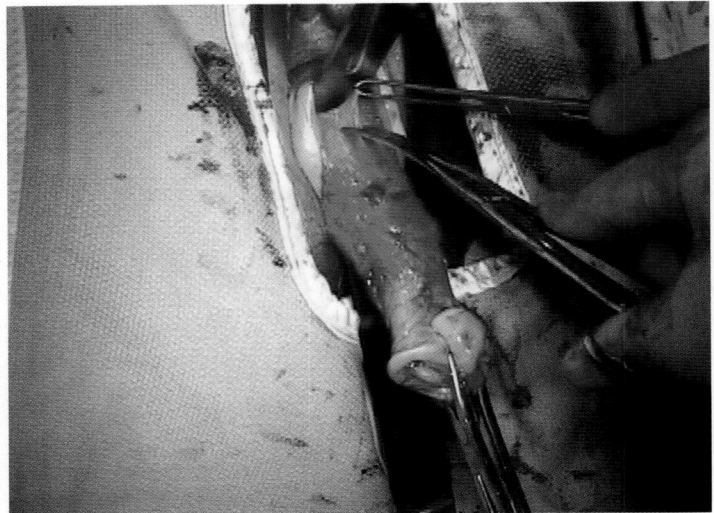

**FIGURE 53–45** A retractor has been placed in the posterior cul-de-sac. Note that the cervix is of normal length.

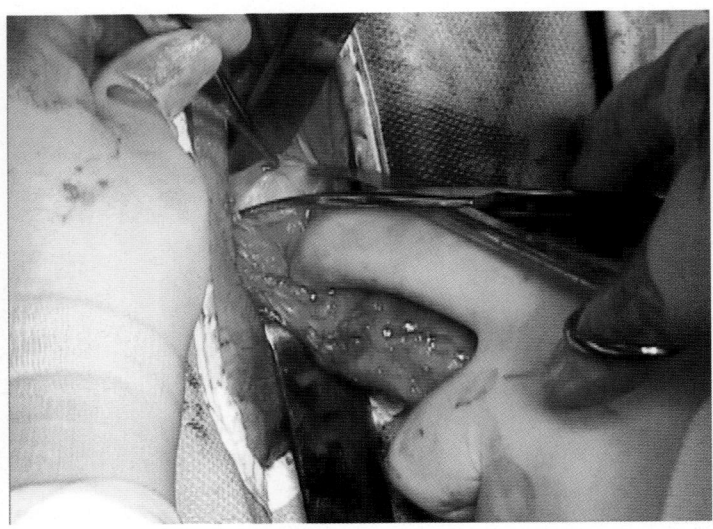

**FIGURE 53–46** Sharp dissection down to the pubocervical fascia, which is usually white and glistening.

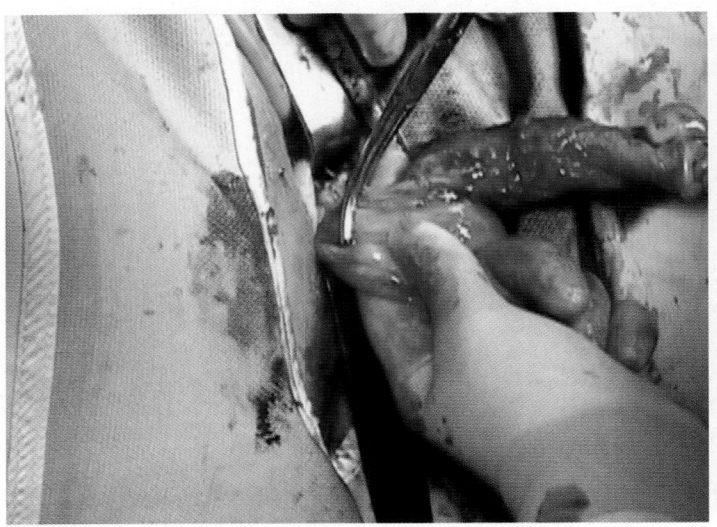

**FIGURE 53–47** A finger has been passed from posterior cul-de-sac up and around the uterus and is tenting up the peritoneum of the anterior cul-de-sac.

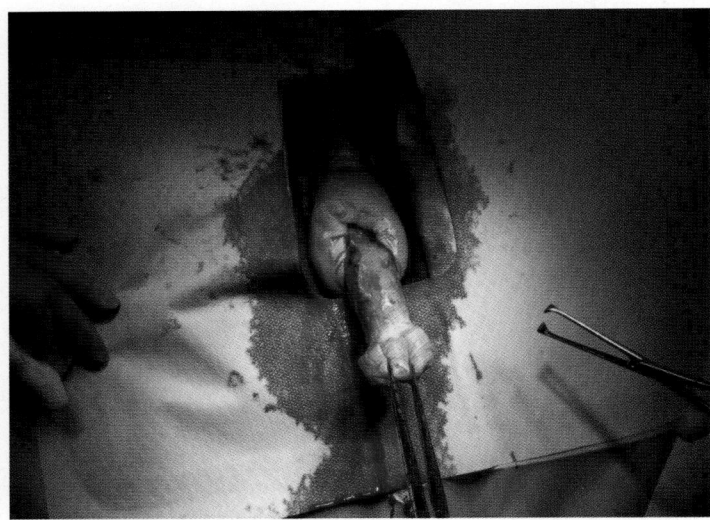

**FIGURE 53–48** The uterus has been delivered; posterior and adnexal structures have been clamped. *Note:* The clamps cross over each other in the midline.

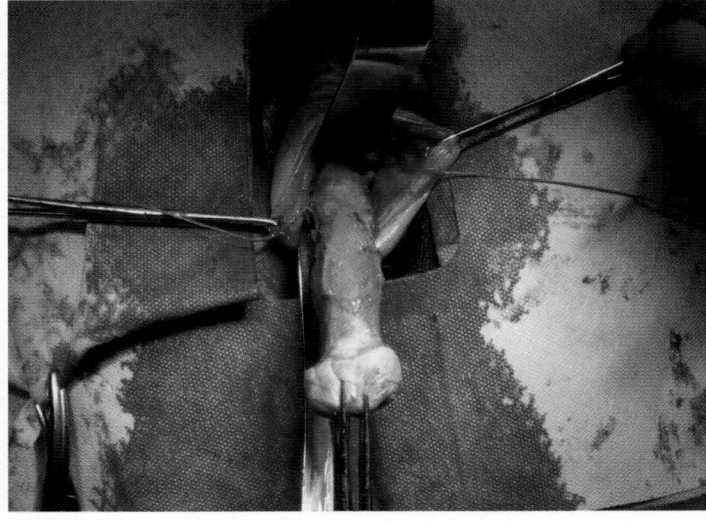

**FIGURE 53–49** Dissection and excision of the enterocele sac from the posterior vaginal wall.

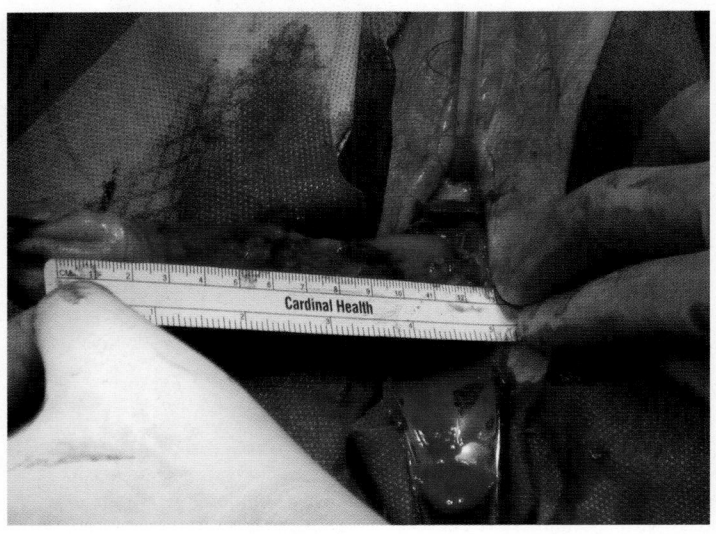

**FIGURE 53–50** Complete uterine procidentia with eversion of the anterior vaginal wall.

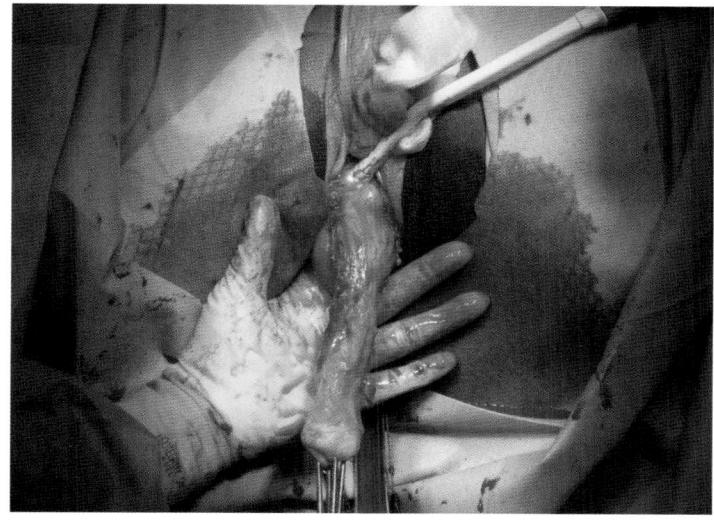

**FIGURE 53-51** Note a markedly elongated cervix. Sharp dissection of the bladder off the anterior cervical wall is demonstrated to the level of the vesicouterine space.

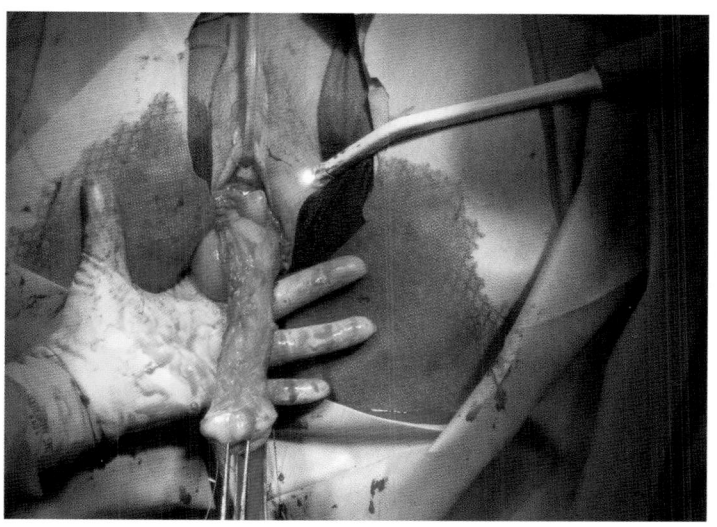

**FIGURE 53-52** The vesicouterine space has been identified.

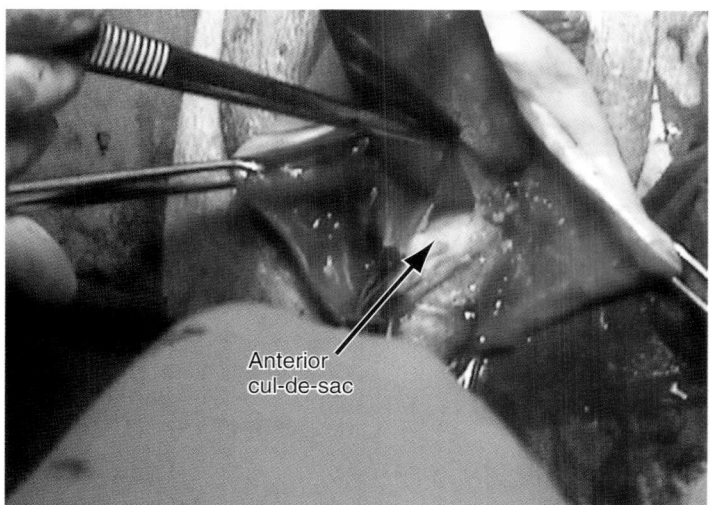

**FIGURE 53-53** Sharp dissection is used to enter the anterior cul-de-sac.

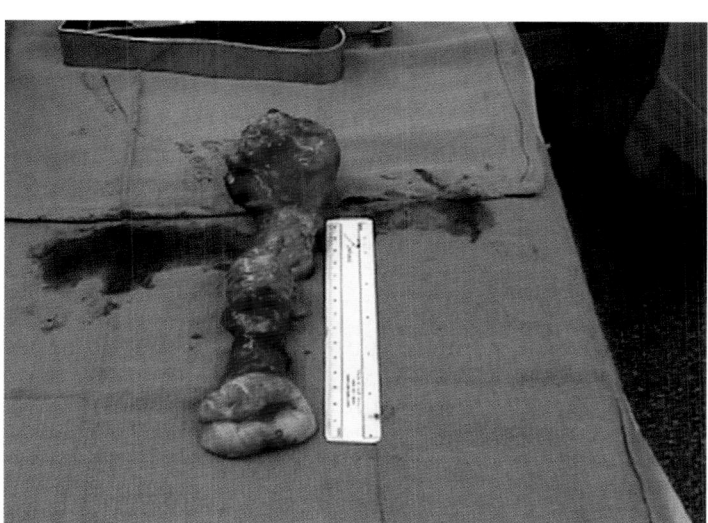

**FIGURE 53-54** A markedly elongated cervix in a patient with uterine procidentia.

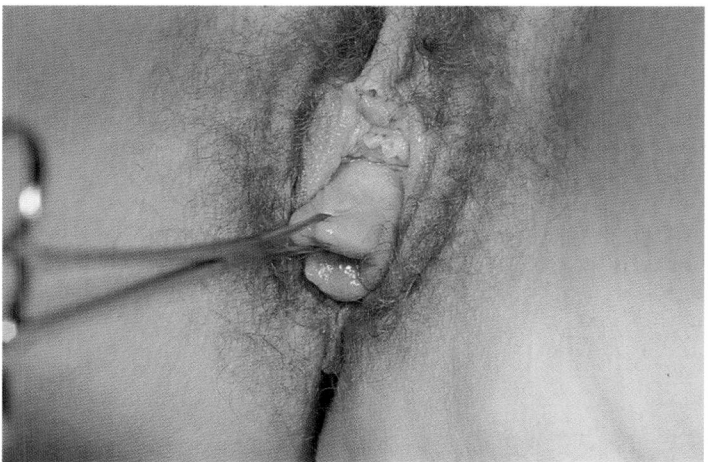

**FIGURE 53-55** Uterine prolapse with a markedly elongated cervix.

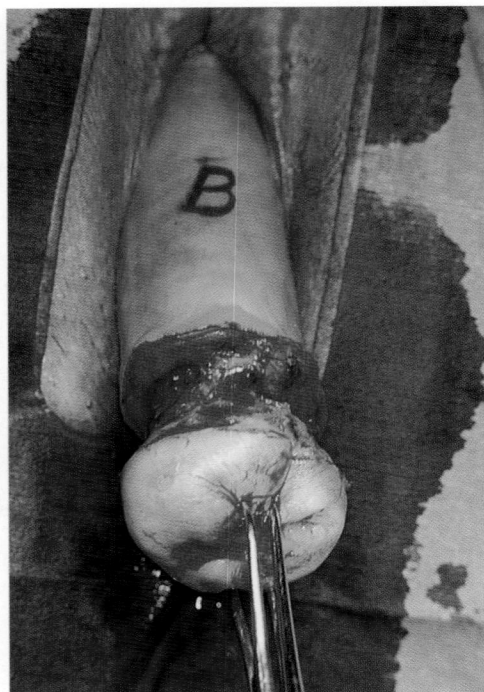

**FIGURE 53–56** The initial incision of the cervix. *B* indicates the approximate location of the bladder and anterior peritoneum.

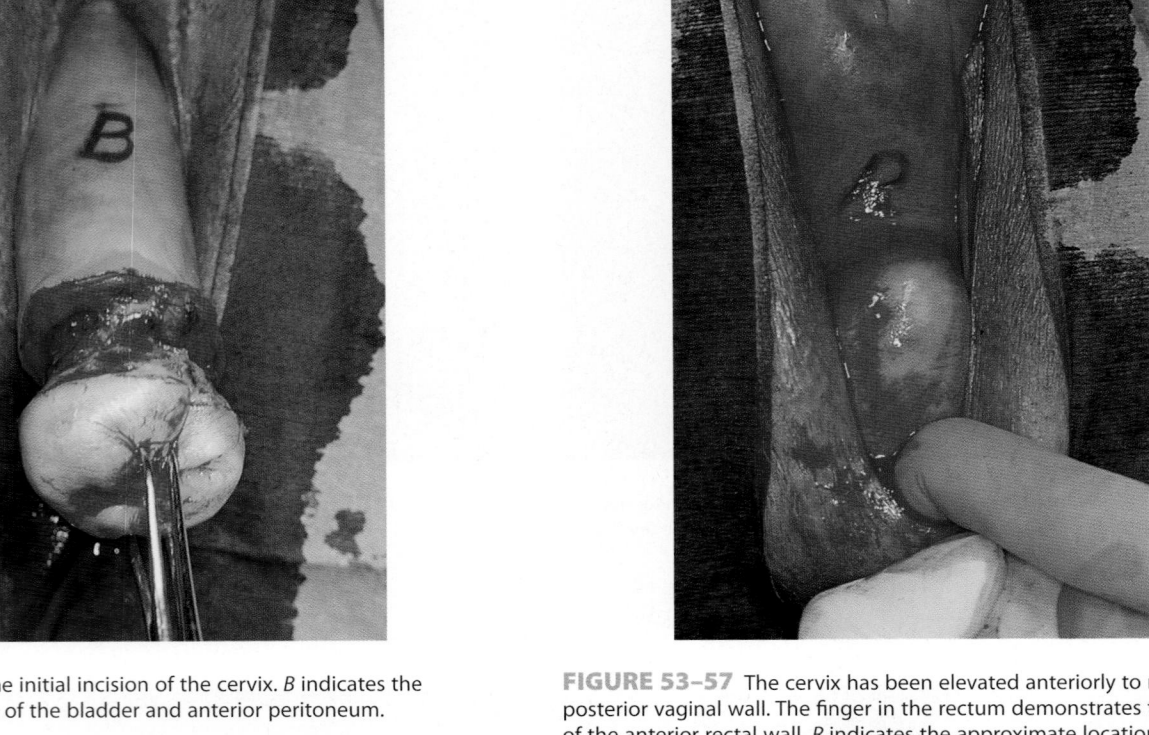

**FIGURE 53–57** The cervix has been elevated anteriorly to reveal the posterior vaginal wall. The finger in the rectum demonstrates the location of the anterior rectal wall. *R* indicates the approximate location of the posterior reflection of the peritoneum.

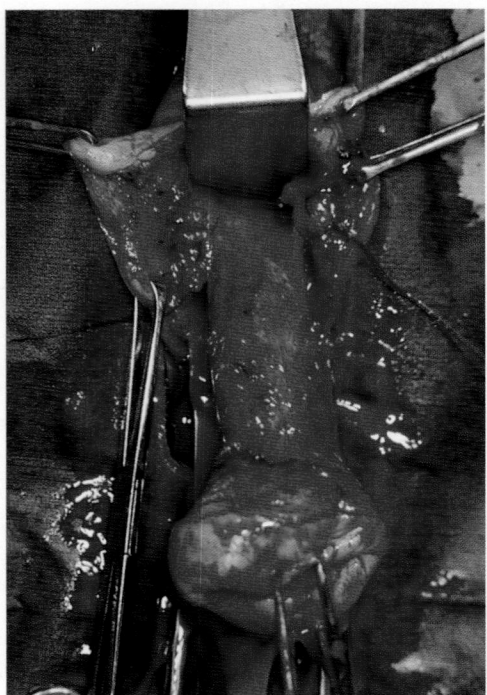

**FIGURE 53–58** Numerous extraperitoneal bites have been taken. High up on the anterior vaginal wall, the vesicouterine space has been reached.

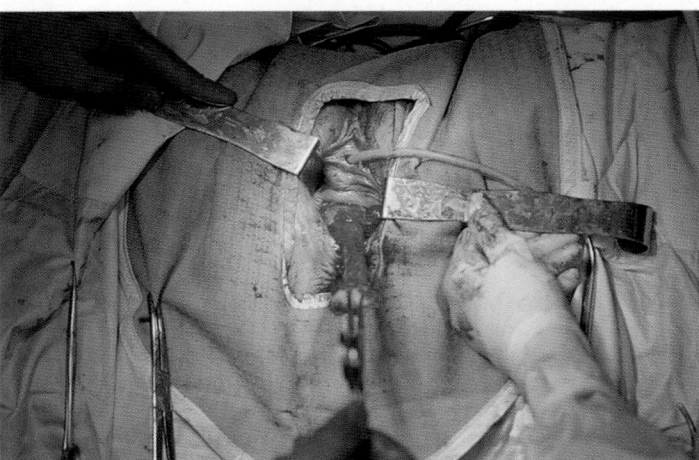

**FIGURE 53–59** Another photograph of an elongated cervix in which numerous extraperitoneal bites of tissue have been taken.

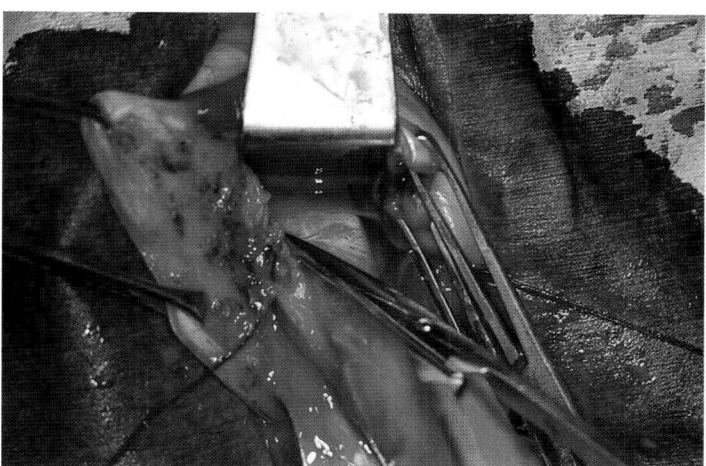

FIGURE 53–60 The anterior cul-de-sac is sharply entered high up at the top of an elongated cervix.

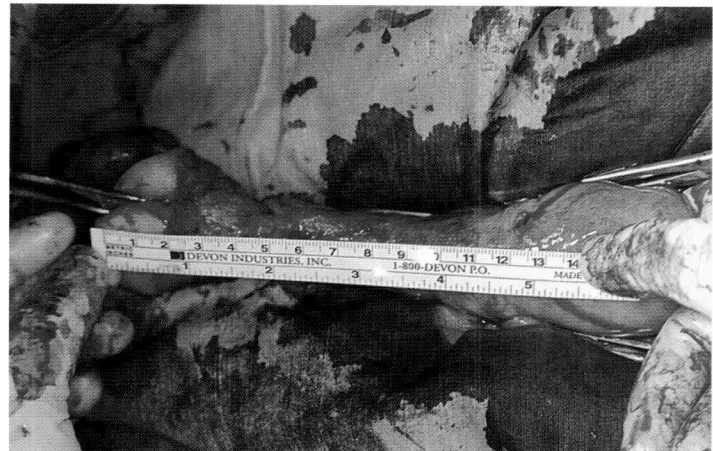

FIGURE 53–61 The tape measure documents a 12-cm cervix in this patient.

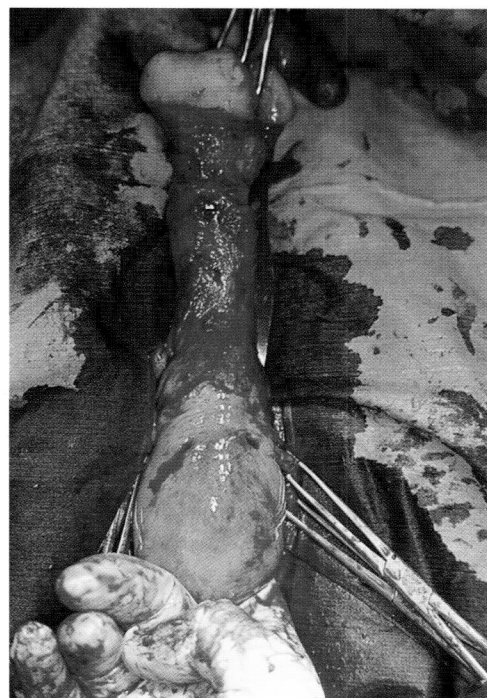

FIGURE 53–62 Once the posterior cul-de-sac has been entered, the uterus can usually be delivered.

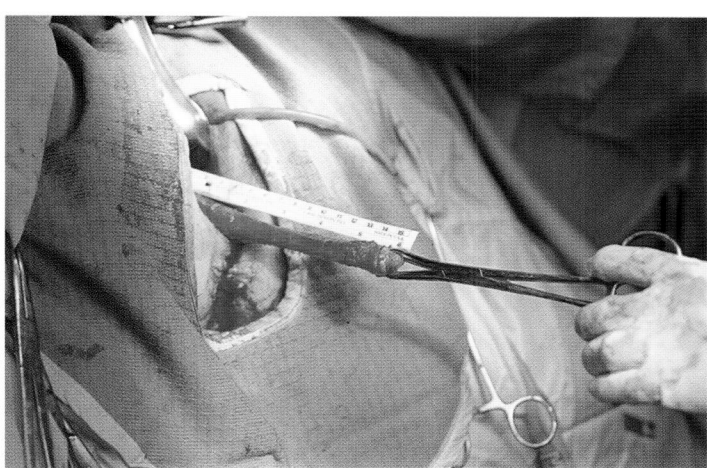

FIGURE 53–63 The tape measure documents a 15-cm cervix in this patient.

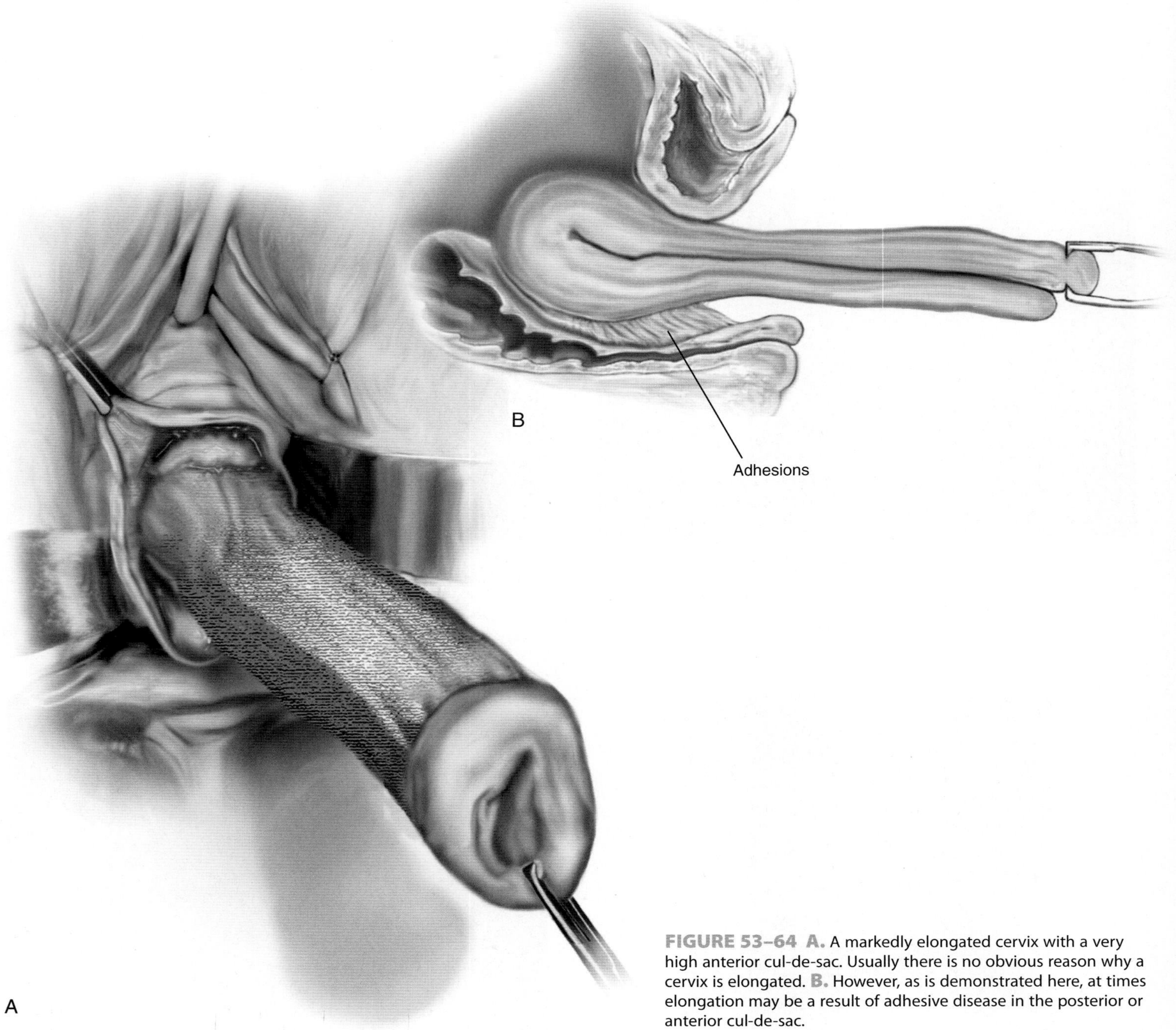

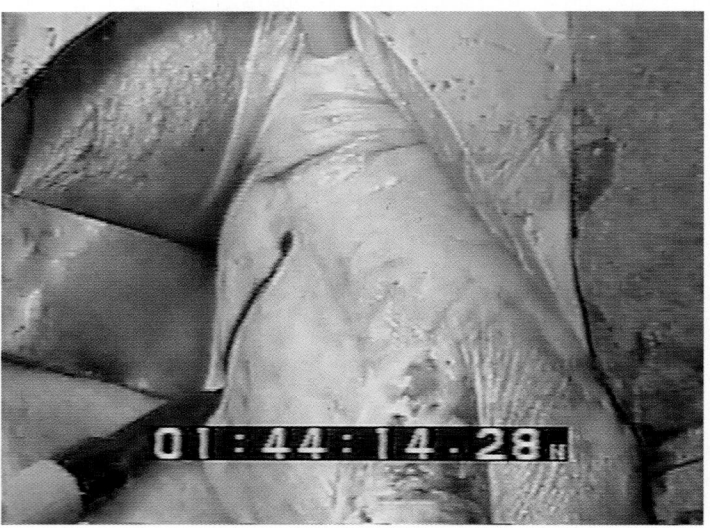

B

Adhesions

**FIGURE 53–64  A.** A markedly elongated cervix with a very high anterior cul-de-sac. Usually there is no obvious reason why a cervix is elongated. **B.** However, as is demonstrated here, at times elongation may be a result of adhesive disease in the posterior or anterior cul-de-sac.

A

**FIGURE 53–65** Marking on the anterior vaginal wall the approximate location of the right ureter in a patient with long-standing uterine procidentia and complete vaginal eversion.

## Obliteration of the Vesicouterine Fold

At times the peritoneal reflection of the anterior cul-de-sac cannot be found during vaginal hysterectomy because of previous inflammation or previous pelvic surgery, most commonly cesarean section. As was previously mentioned, the author routinely postpones entrance into the anterior cul-de-sac until the vesicouterine space is easily entered; this usually occurs after numerous clamps have been applied to the parametrium. It is very important in situations like this to use sharp dissection into this space because if aggressive blunt dissection is utilized, the chance of cystotomy is much greater (Figs. 53–66 and 53–67). Blunt dissection will ultimately result in passage of the finger into the plane of least resistance—many times this is directly into the bladder—if severe adhesive disease exists. If a cystotomy does occur at the time of vaginal hysterectomy, the cystotomy should be utilized to determine the appropriate plane through which the anterior cul-de-sac should be entered. The hysterectomy should then be completed and the cystotomy closed. Repair of a vaginal cystotomy should follow the guidelines for repair of any fistula. Cystoscopy initially should be performed to ensure that the ureteral orifices and trigone are not involved. The bladder wall is then mobilized to allow closure of the cystotomy under minimal tension. The cystotomy is usually closed in two layers with a 3-0 absorbable suture. After vaginal cystotomy, the bladder should be drained postoperatively for 7 to 10 days.

## Adhesions of the Posterior Cul-de-sac

Adhesions of the posterior cul-de-sac, although relatively rare, can occur, especially in cases of endometriosis. This should be highly suspected when some nodularity of the cul-de-sac is evident on examination, and certainly if the uterus is immobile. After the initial incision has been made and entry into the posterior cul-de-sac has been found to be impossible, it is probably best to proceed with anterior dissection and entry into the anterior cul-de-sac. If this cannot be accomplished, one should identify the anterior rectal wall by placing a finger in the rectum. Sharp dissection between the anterior rectal wall and the posterior cervix can be performed in the hope of safely reaching the posterior peritoneal reflection. If, however, the uterus is immobile and neither the anterior nor the posterior cul-de-sac can be comfortably entered, it is probably prudent to proceed with an abdominal or a laparoscopic approach to hysterectomy.

## Removal of the Large Uterus

At times the uterus will be enlarged and somewhat immobile, most commonly because of the presence of multiple leiomyomata.

Uterine morcellation, or removal of the uterus piecemeal, is a procedure most often used for the large myomatous uterus. The author prefers to do this by delivering as much of the uterus as possible into the posterior cul-de-sac and by morcellating the uterus via elliptical incisions. Elliptical incisions are taken through the posterior uterine wall. With each removal of tissue, the edges of the incision are brought together, thus decreasing the bulk of the uterus to the point where it ultimately can be completely delivered through the cul-de-sac (Figs. 53–68 through 53–70).

At times, amputating the cervix with a scalpel permits easier access to the uterus. From this point, the anterior uterine wall can be resected or bivalved (Figs. 53–71 and 53–72), assuming the anterior cul-de-sac has been entered, or submucosal myomata can be removed and a vaginal myomectomy performed to decrease the bulk of the uterus and assist in its delivery (Fig. 53–73).

Another technique for removal of a large uterus secondary to a uterine leiomyoma is intramyometrial coring. With strong downward traction, the cervix is circumscribed as high as possible, and a cylinder is developed parallel to the axis of the uterus with the scalpel (Fig. 53–74). The cylinder should be wide enough to include the endometrial cavity in the core specimen, but not so wide that the knife perforates the fundus. Downward traction delivers the cored specimen, eventually turning the uterus inside out.

Figure 53–75 demonstrates vaginal removal of a 17-week–size uterus in which a combination of morcellation and coring is utilized.

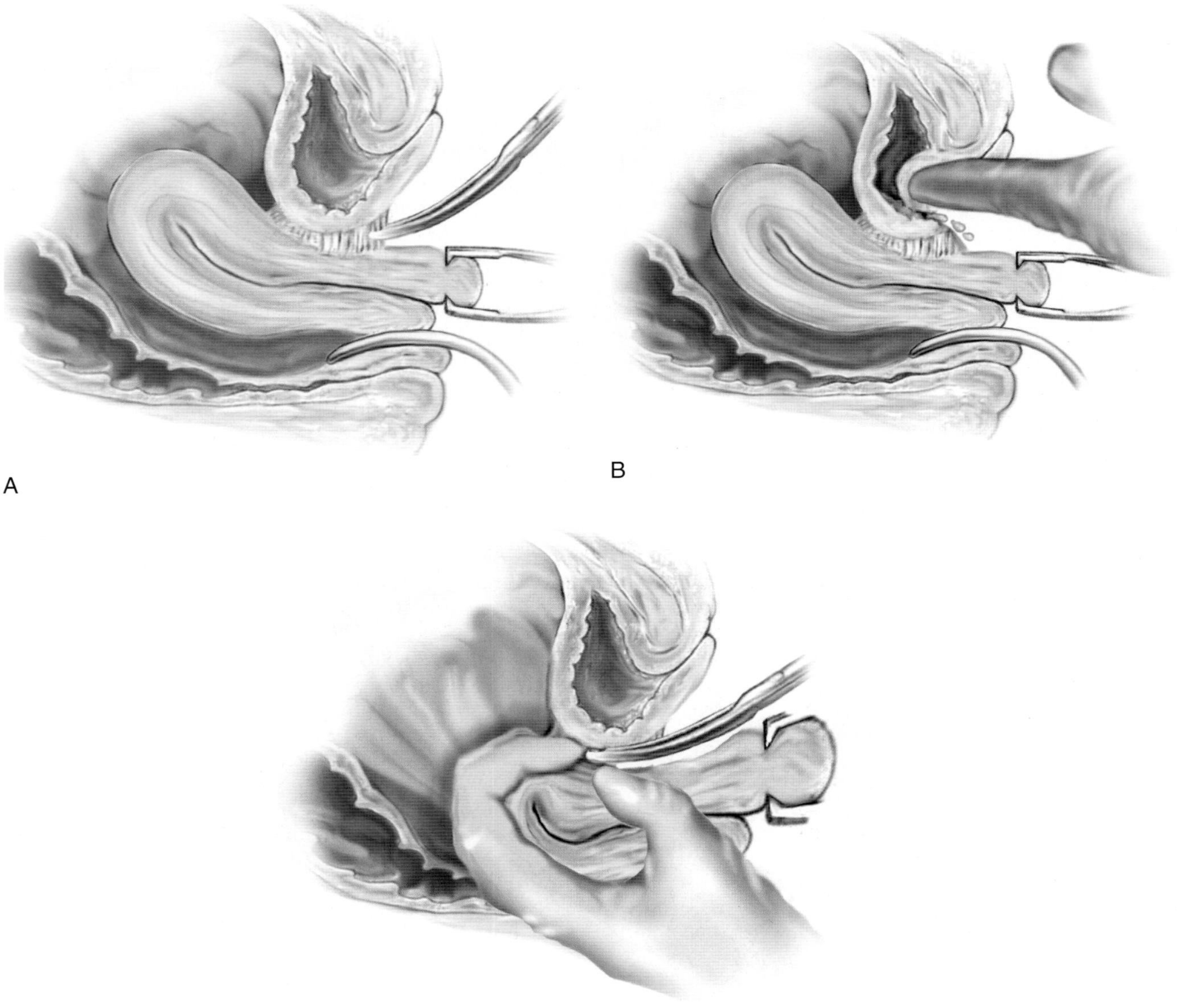

A

B

C

**FIGURE 53–66  A.** Dense adhesions noted between the base of the bladder and the anterior cervix. These are best taken down using sharp dissection. **B.** Blunt dissection in this situation may lead to inadvertent cystotomy, as the finger will pass into the area of least resistance. **C.** Passing a finger around the uterus, when possible, may help facilitate dissection in the appropriate plane.

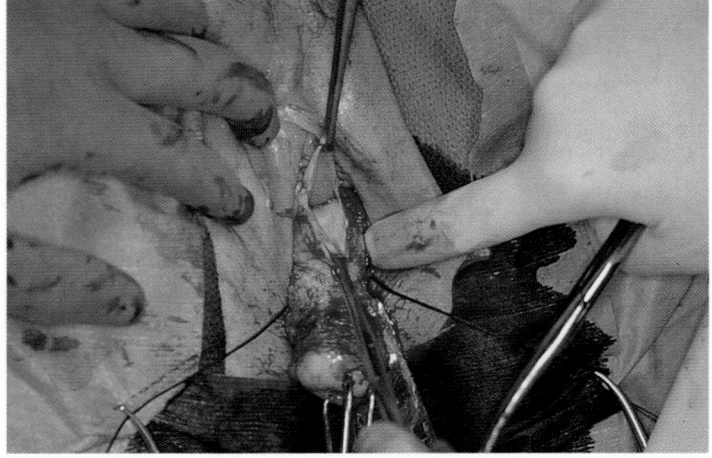

**FIGURE 53–67**  Sharp entrance into the anterior cul-de-sac has been performed in a patient who has anterior cul-de-sac adhesions secondary to a previous caesarean section.

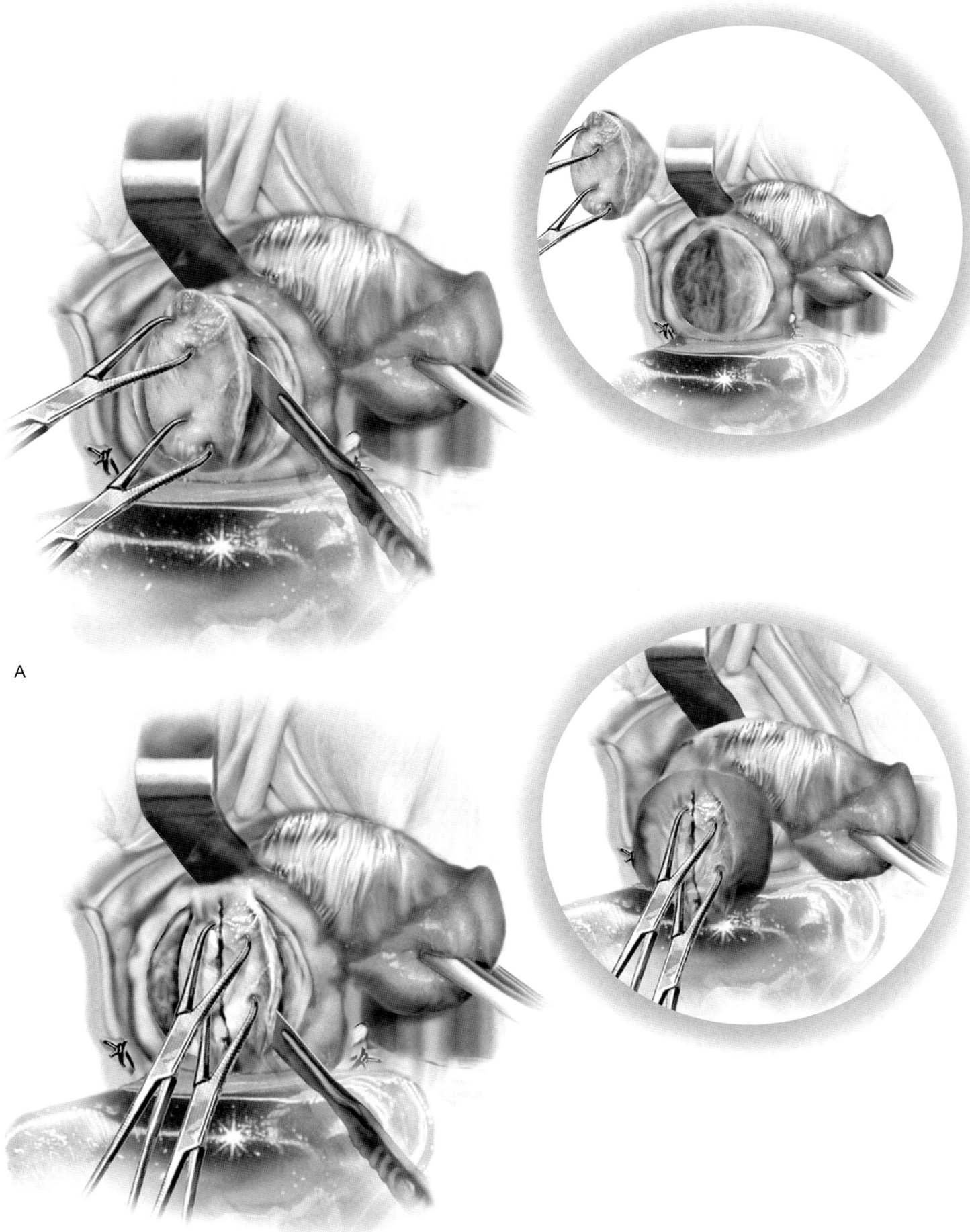

A

B

**FIGURE 53–68** Technique of uterine morcellation for vaginal removal of a large uterus. **A.** Elliptical wedge of tissue removed from the posterior uterus. **B.** Edges of the initial incision are brought together with two single-toothed tenacula, and another wedge of tissue is removed. This procedure is continued until the uterus can be completely delivered (**inset**).

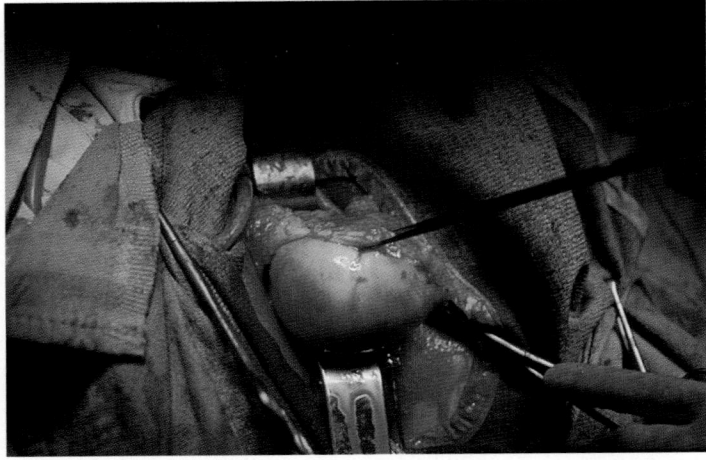

**FIGURE 53–69** Delivery of a large uterus after morcellation.

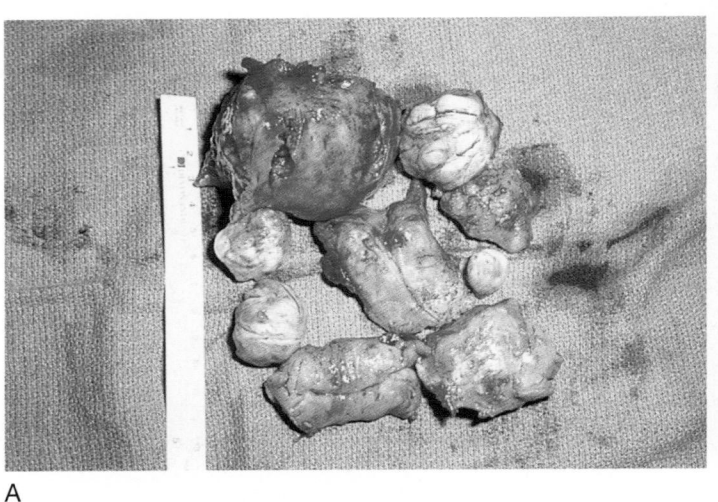

A

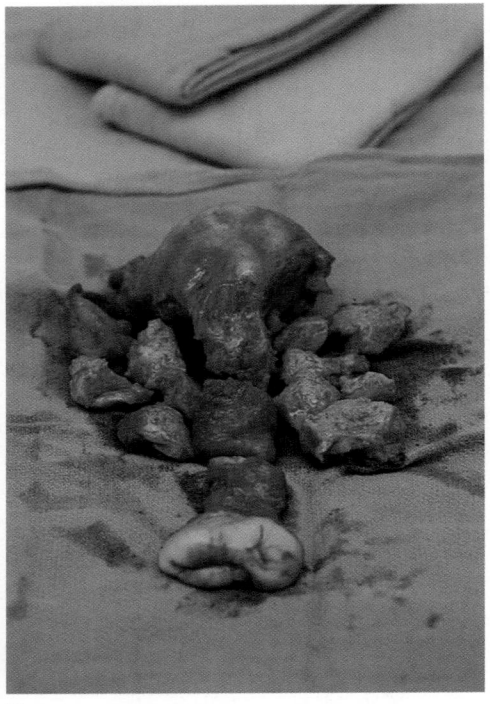

B

**FIGURE 53–70 A** and **B.** Two examples of morcellated uteri that have been removed transvaginally.

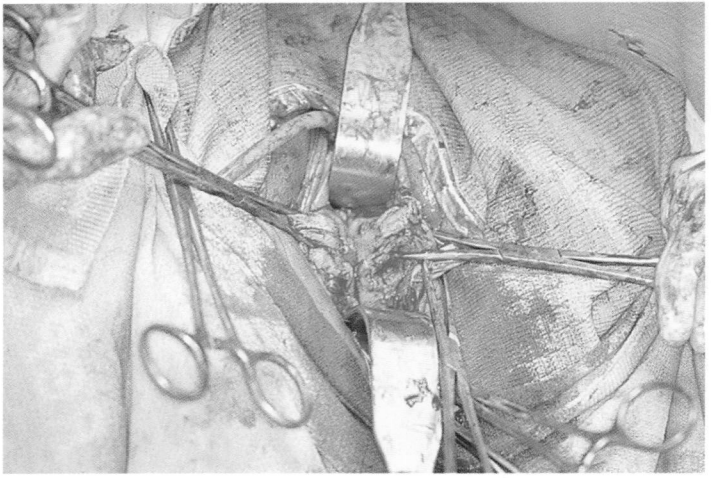

**FIGURE 53–71** The cervix has been amputated, and the uterus is being bivalved.

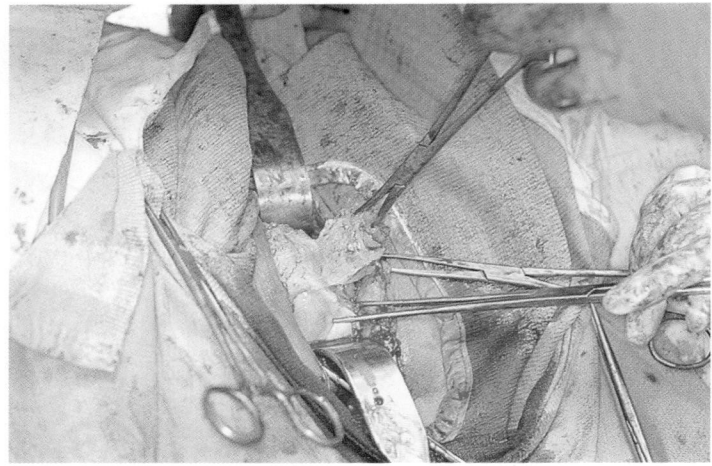

**FIGURE 53–72** Hemisection of the uterus after the cervix has been amputated. Note the multiple uterine leiomyomata.

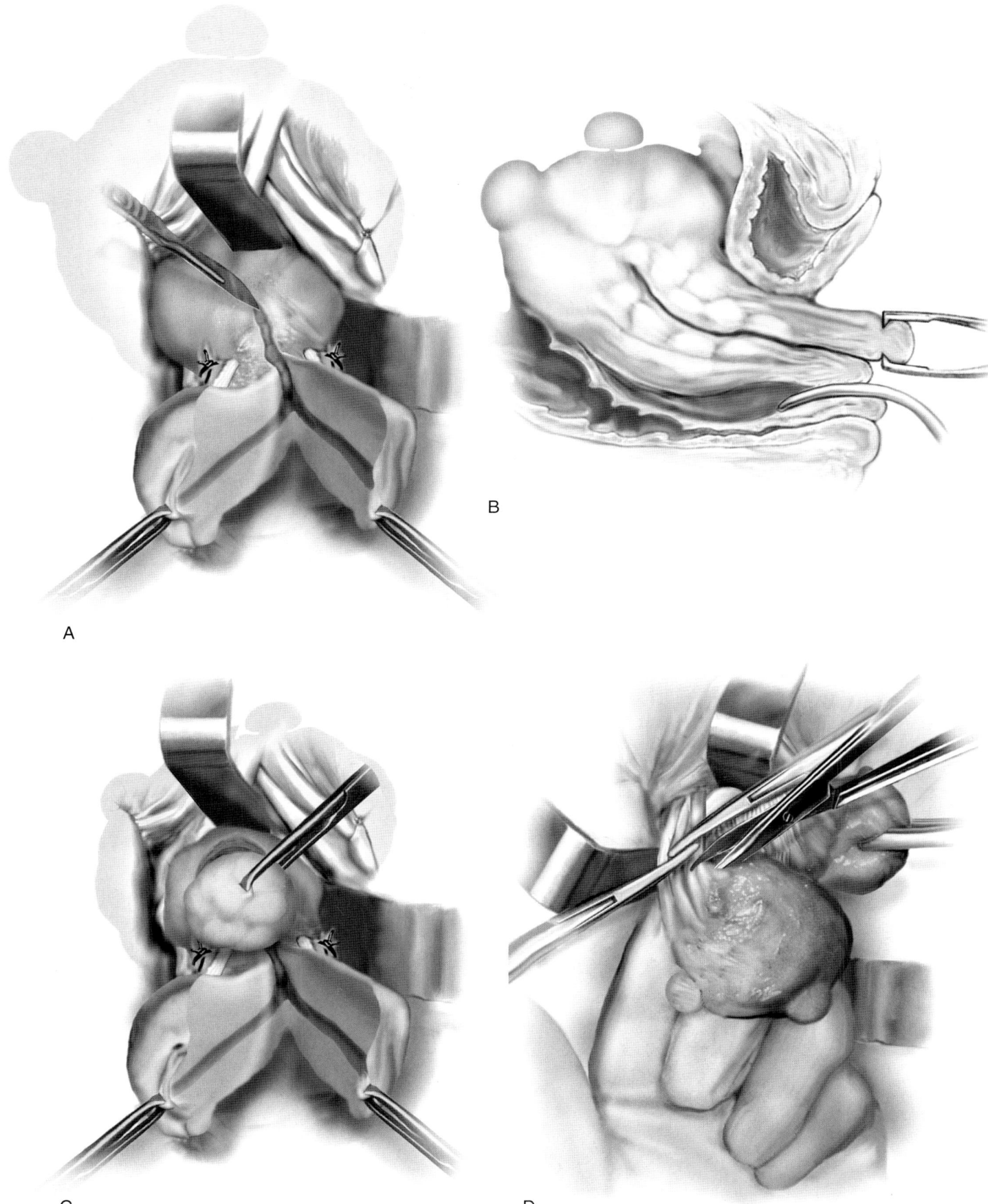

A

B

C

D

**FIGURE 53–73** Technique of hemisection of the uterus. **A.** The scalpel incises up the midportion of the uterus. **B.** The side view demonstrates multiple uterine leiomyomata. **C.** Vaginal myomectomy. **D.** Delivery of the uterus after its size has been reduced with clamping of adnexal pedicles.

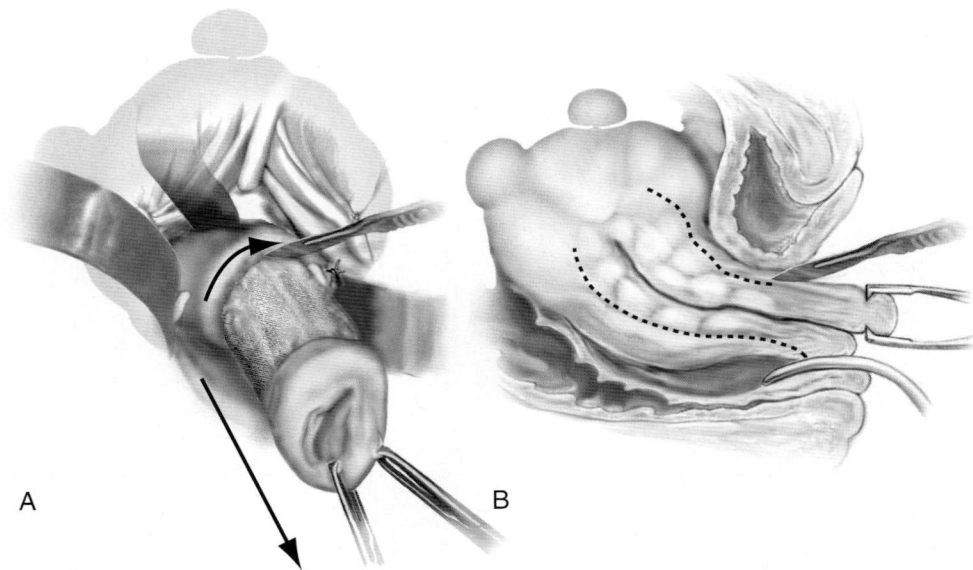

A                                                        B

**FIGURE 53–74** Technique of intramyometrial coring. **A.** The scalpel creates a cylinder of tissue, facilitated by strong downward traction on the cervix. **B.** Side view of the technique of intramyometrial coring. Downward traction delivers the cored specimen, eventually turning the uterus inside out.

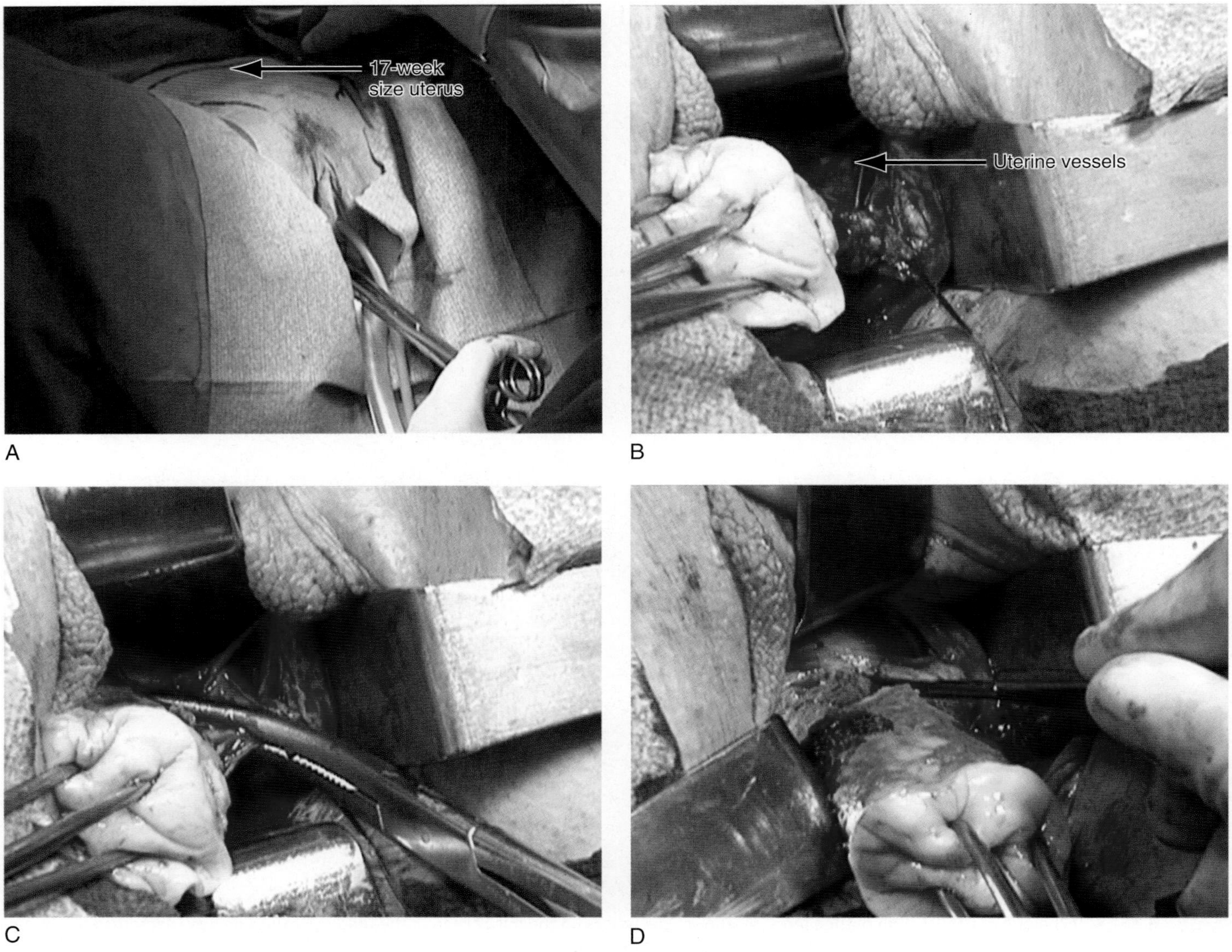

A                                                        B

C                                                        D

**FIGURE 53–75** Demonstrates vaginal removal of a 17-week–size uterus utilizing a combination of morcellation and intramyometrial coring. **A.** The uterus has been marked and is noted to be 17-week size. **B.** The vaginal hysterectomy has begun. It is important that before any morcellation or coring is done, the uterine vessels are clamped to ensure the blood supply of the uterus. **C.** The uterine vessels are clamped with a Haney clamp placed at right angles to the cervix. **D.** The cervix is being amputated to allow access to the enlarged body of the uterus.

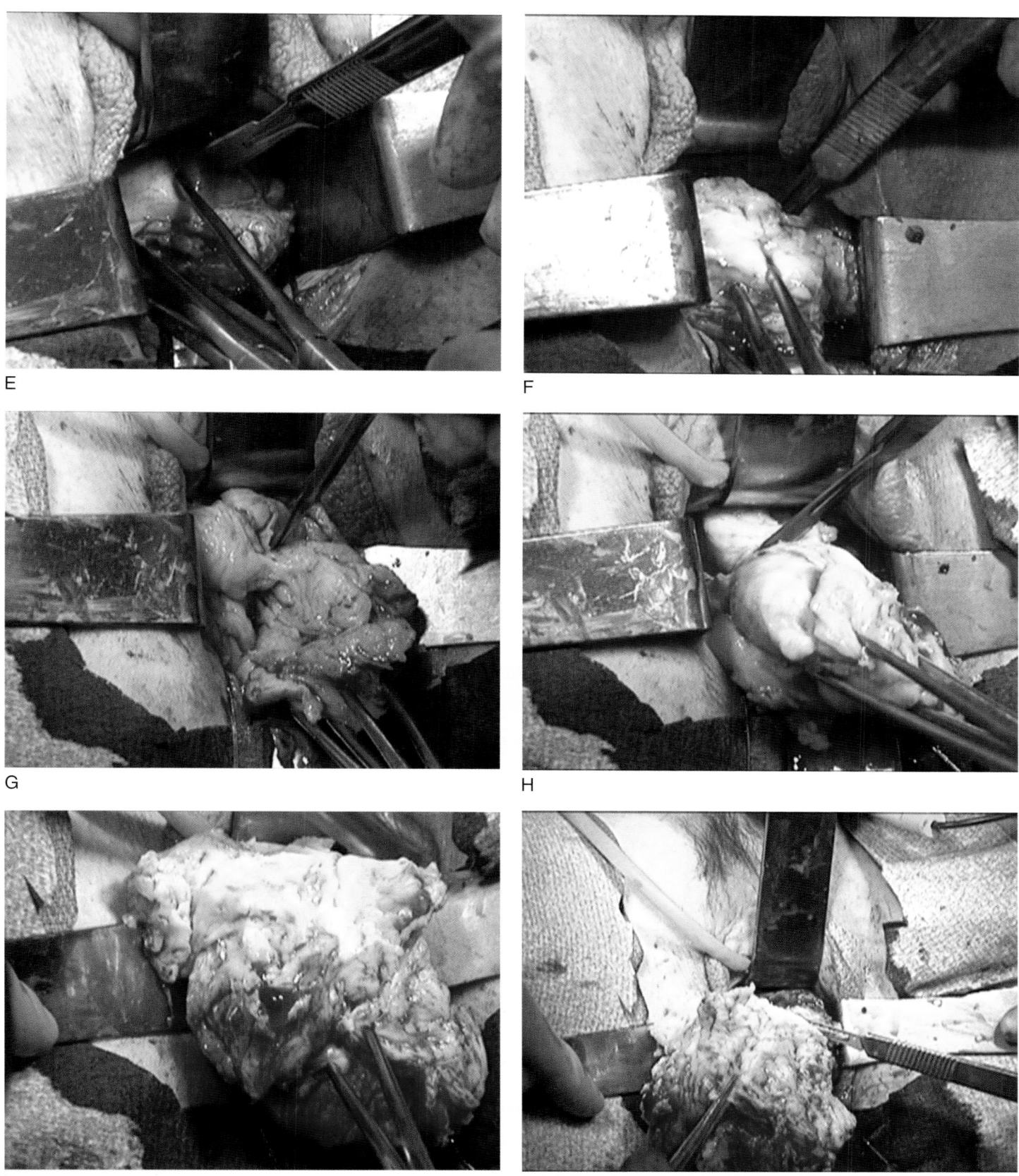

**FIGURE 53–75, cont'd  E.** The technique of intramyometrial coring is begun with a scalpel that is used to cut on the undersurface of the serosa of the anterior portion of the uterus. **F.** Downward traction with a single-toothed tenaculum allows removal of the uterus in pieces. **G.** The enlarged uterus is now morcellated and removed in pieces. **H.** Morcellation of the uterus is continued. **I.** The large fibroid has been delivered posteriorly. **J.** The large fibroid is being cut away from the remainder of the uterus.

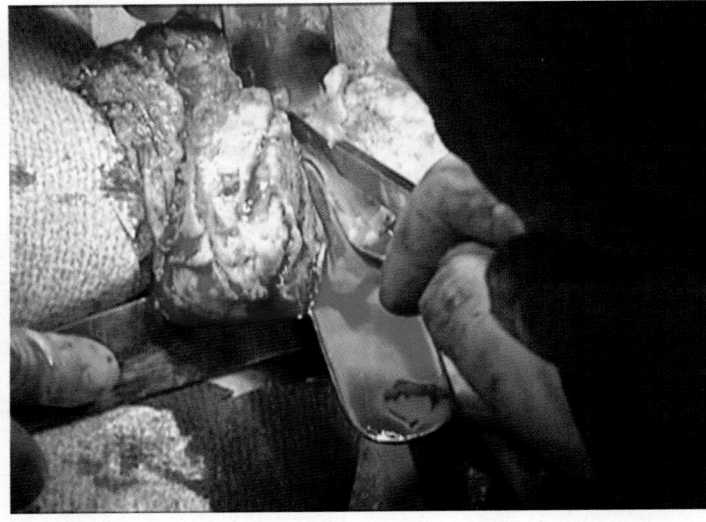

K

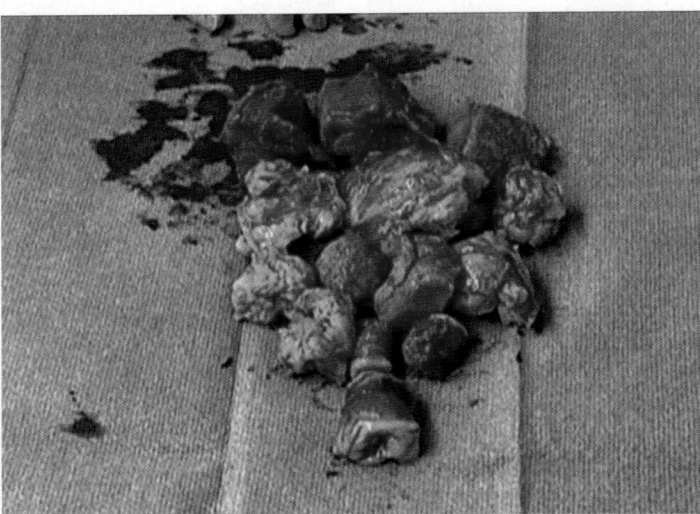

L

**FIGURE 53–75, cont'd   K.** The upper part of the uterus is being bivalved to allow facilitation of clamping of the adnexal pedicles. **L.** The 17-week–size morcellated uterus that has been removed vaginally is shown.

# CHAPTER 54

# Vaginal Repair of Cystocele, Rectocele, and Enterocele

*Mickey M. Karram*

## Anterior Vaginal Wall Prolapse

Anterior vaginal wall prolapse, or cystocele, is defined as pathologic descent of the anterior vaginal wall and overlying bladder base. The cause of anterior vaginal wall prolapse is not completely understood but is probably multifactorial, with different factors implicated in individual patients. Until recently, two types of anterior vaginal wall prolapse were described: distention and displacement cystocele. Distention cystocele was thought to result from overstretching and attenuation of the anterior vaginal wall, and displacement cystocele was attributed to pathologic detachment or elongation of the anterior lateral vaginal supports to the arcus tendineus fascia pelvis. More

recently, three distinct defects have been described that can result in anterior vaginal wall prolapse. The midline defect is what has been previously described as a distention-type cystocele; the paravaginal defect, which is a separation of the normal attachment of the connective tissue of the vagina at the arcus tendineus fascia pelvis (white line); and the transverse defect, which occurs when the pubocervical fascia separates from its insertion around the cervix or at the apex (Figs. 54–1 through 54–5). Anterior vaginal wall prolapse, especially in the posthysterectomy patient, may be commonly associated with an apical enterocele, or more rarely a true anterior enterocele (Fig. 54–6).

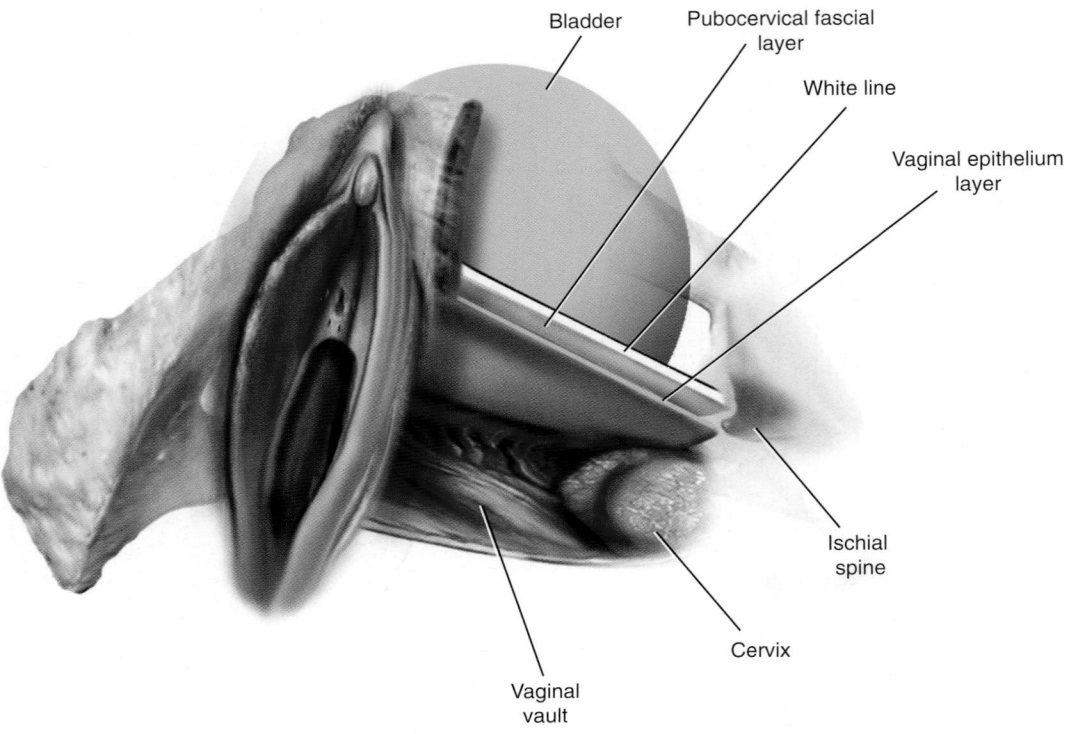

Bladder

Pubocervical fascial
layer

White line

Vaginal epithelium
layer

Ischial
spine

Cervix

Vaginal
vault

A                                    Normal support

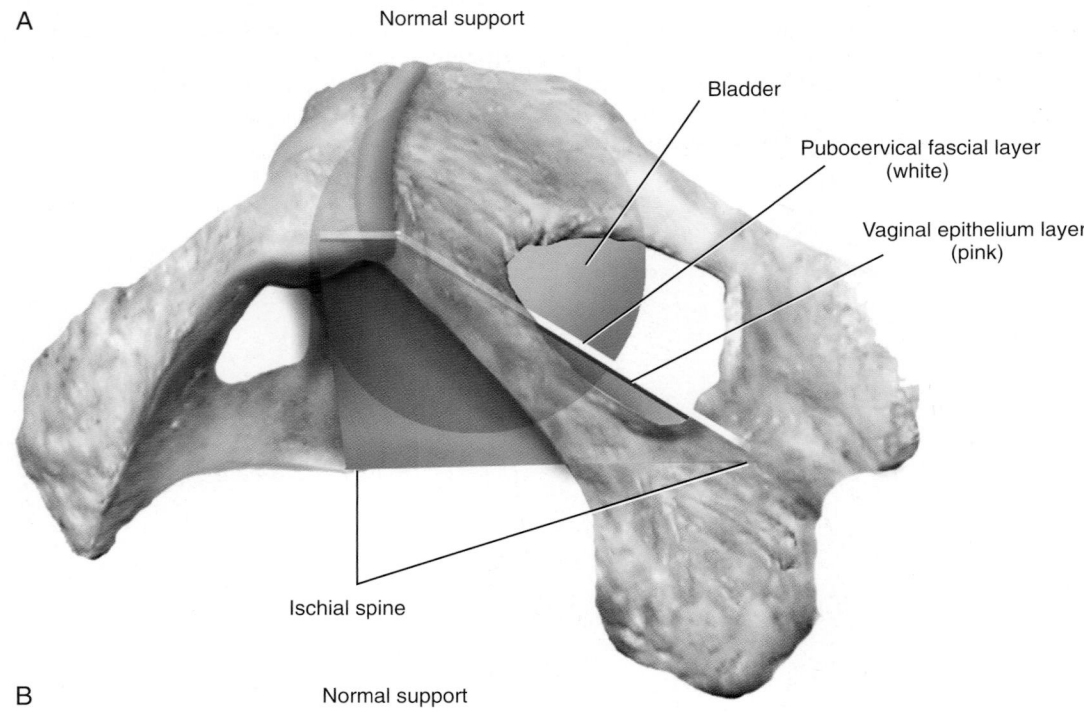

Bladder

Pubocervical fascial layer
(white)

Vaginal epithelium layer
(pink)

Ischial spine

B                                    Normal support

**FIGURE 54–1** Two views of normal and abnormal support of the anterior vaginal wall. **A.** Lateral view of normal anterior vaginal wall support with bladder support extending back to the level of the ischial spines. Note normal midline and lateral support. **B.** Trapezoid concept of the support of the anterior vaginal wall. Note that the trapezoid extends back to the ischial spine on each side, and the fascia or the muscular lining of the vagina extends from one side of the pelvic sidewall to the opposite side with good midline support and lateral and transverse attachments.

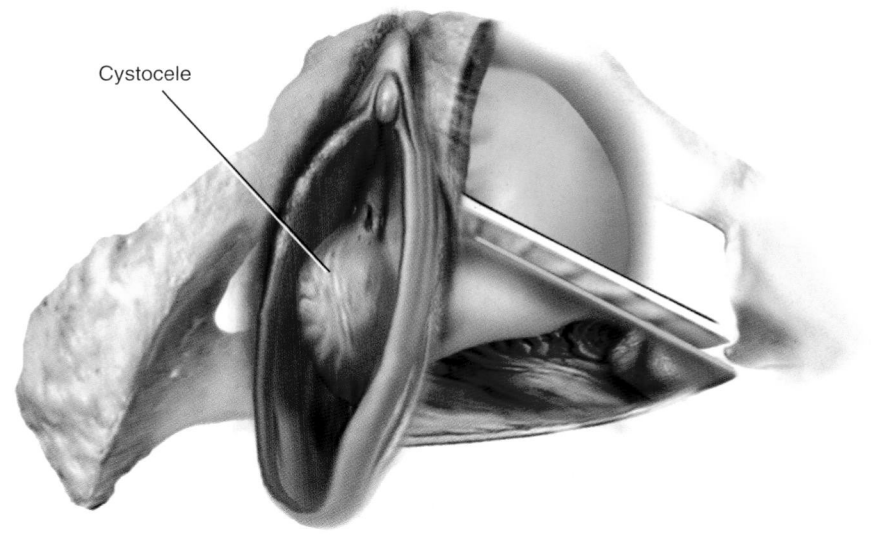

Cystocele

C                              Midline defect

Edges of midline
fascia defect
underneath
vaginal epithelium

Cystocele

D                              Midline defect

**FIGURE 54–1, cont'd  C.** Lateral view of a midline defect. Note the bulging of the bladder into the midportion of the vagina with maintenance of lateral support. Thus, the anterior vaginal fornix is maintained on each side. **D.** Midline defect demonstrates weakening in the midportion of the trapezoidal support of the anterior segment.

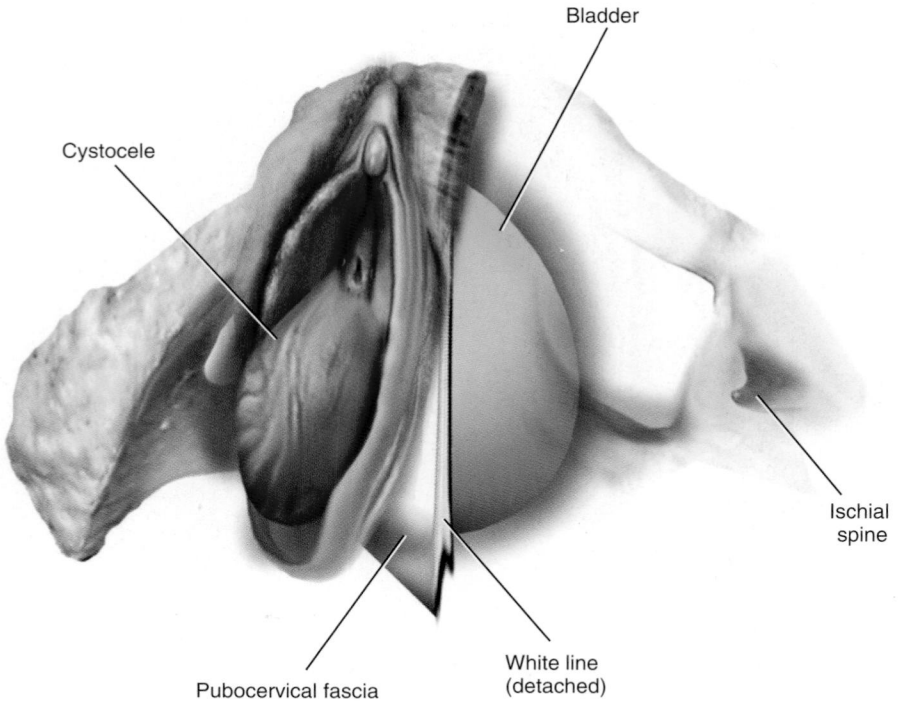

Bladder

Cystocele

Ischial
spine

Pubocervical fascia

White line
(detached)

E                          Bilateral paravaginal defects

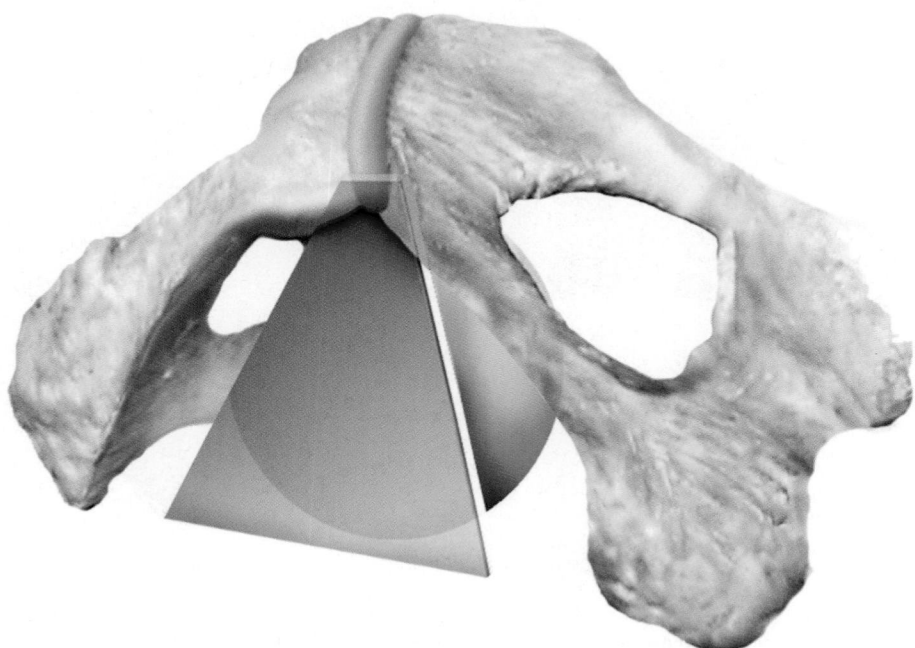

F                          Bilateral paravaginal defects

FIGURE 54–1, cont'd  E. Lateral view of bilateral paravaginal defects. Note the complete detachment of the white line from its normal attachment, resulting in complete loss of the anterolateral supports of the anterior segment. F. Bilateral paravaginal defects. Complete lateral detachment of the normal support is noted as the trapezoid rotates outwardly.

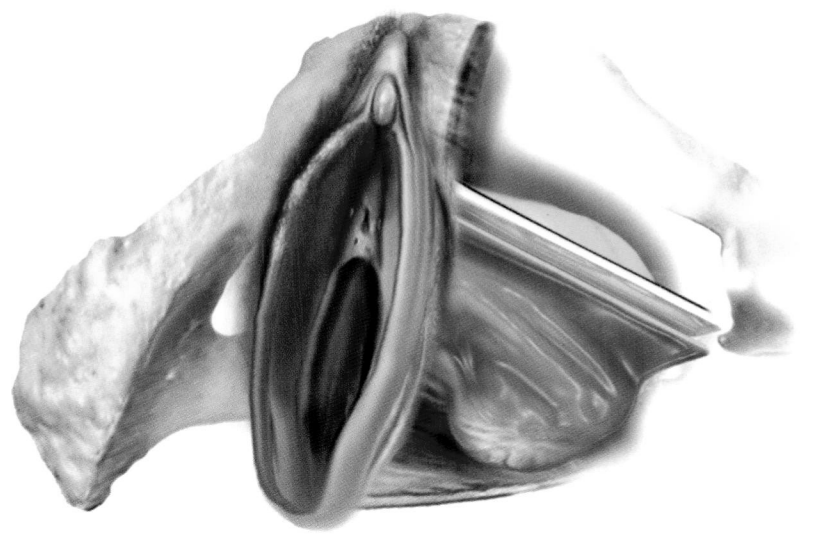

G                                    Transverse defect

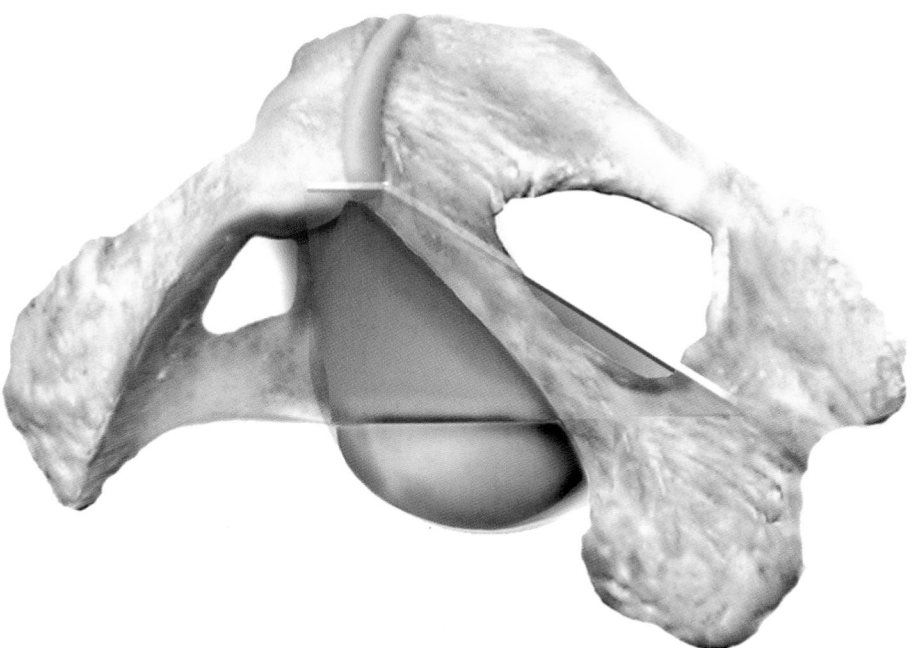

H                                    Transverse defect

**FIGURE 54–1, cont'd  G.** Lateral view of a transverse defect. Note that the bladder prolapse is between the normal upward attachment and the cervix or vaginal apex, usually resulting in what is termed a *high cystocele*. **H.** Note that the bladder descends around the normal upper attachment of the fascia or the muscular lining of the vagina.

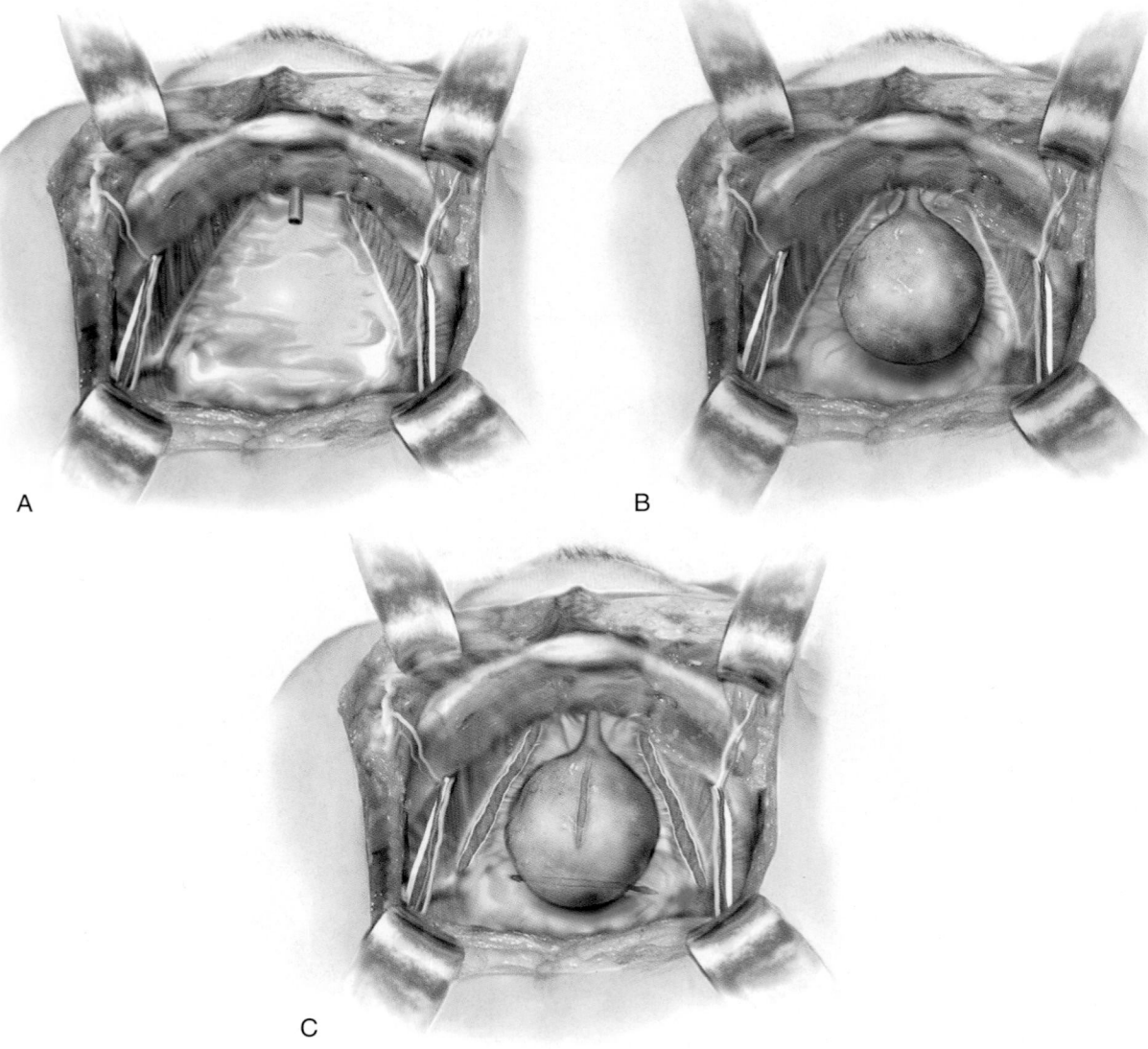

**FIGURE 54–2** Normal support of the anterior vaginal wall when viewed retropubically. **A.** *Note:* The bladder has been removed. The bluish area depicts the inside lining of the fascia or the muscular lining of the vagina. In a normally supported anterior segment, this is a trapezoid-shaped support that extends from the arcus tendineus fascia pelvis on one side all the way to the opposite side, with the support extending all the way back to the level of the ischial spine laterally and to the apex or the cervix transversely. **B.** The bladder has been placed back into the illustration to show its normal anatomic position. **C.** Different possible types of defects, noting paravaginal, midline, and transverse defects.

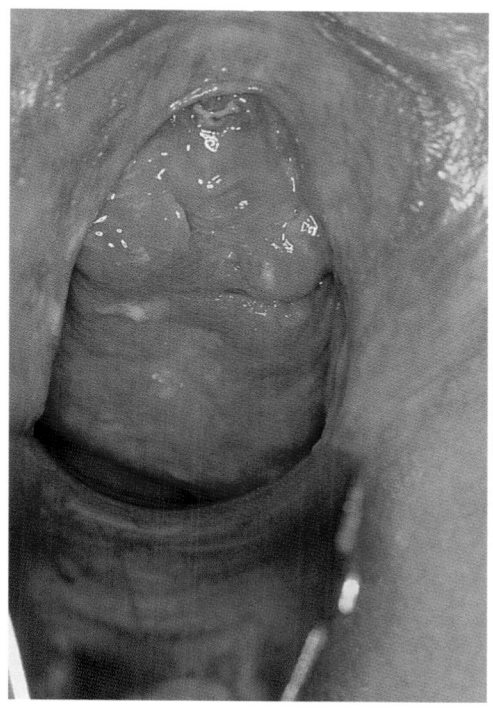

**FIGURE 54–3** The anterior vaginal wall showing the urethrovaginal crease. Note that the vagina over the bladder base shows minimal rugae, a situation that is more consistent with a midline defect.

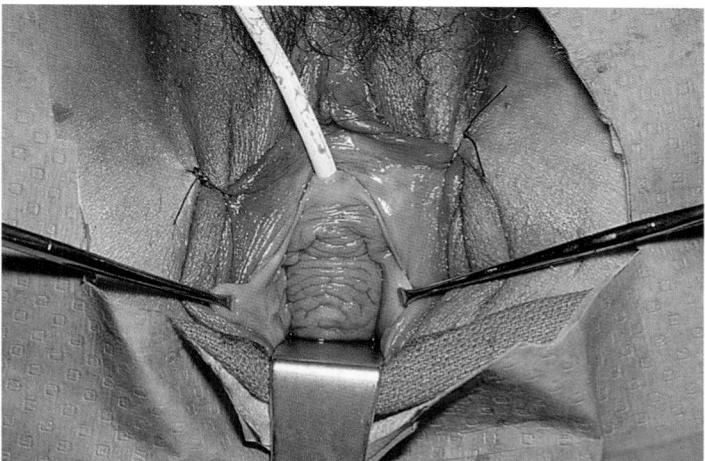

**FIGURE 54–4** The anterior vaginal wall with rugae, a situation that is more consistent with a paravaginal defect.

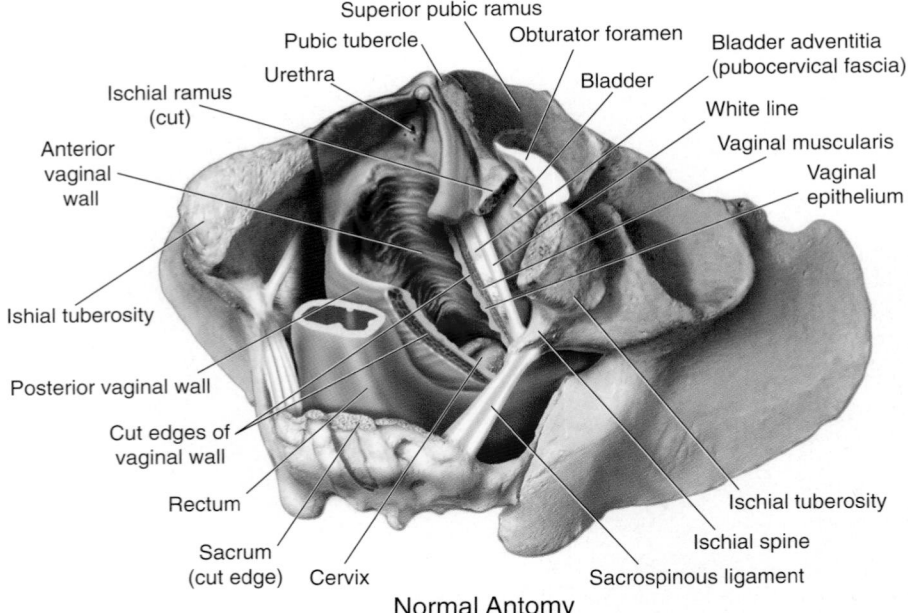

Normal Antomy

A

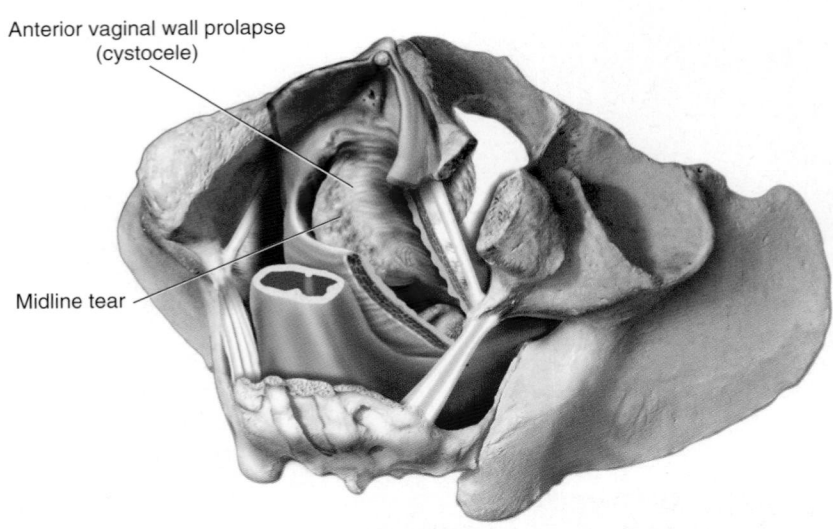

Midline Defect

B

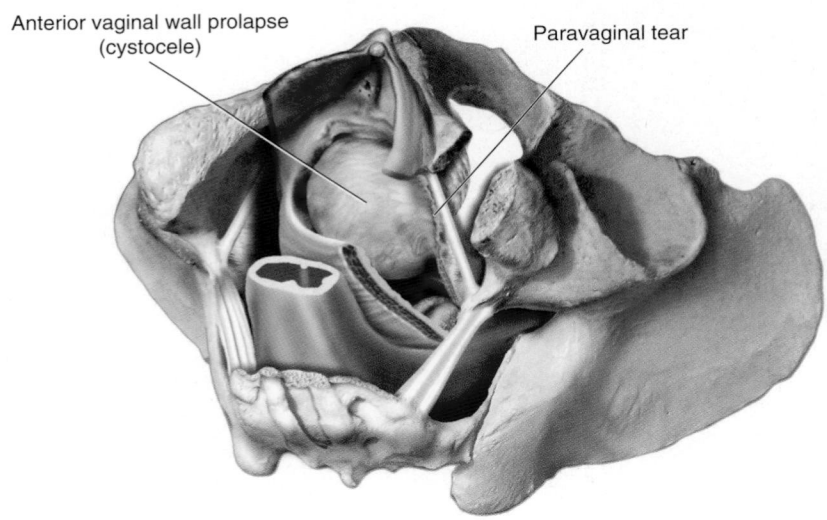

Paravaginal Defect

C

**FIGURE 54–5** Cross-sectional drawing of the pelvic floor to demonstrate (A) normal anatomy, (B) a midline defect of the anterior vaginal wall, and (C) a lateral or paravaginal defect of the anterior vaginal wall.

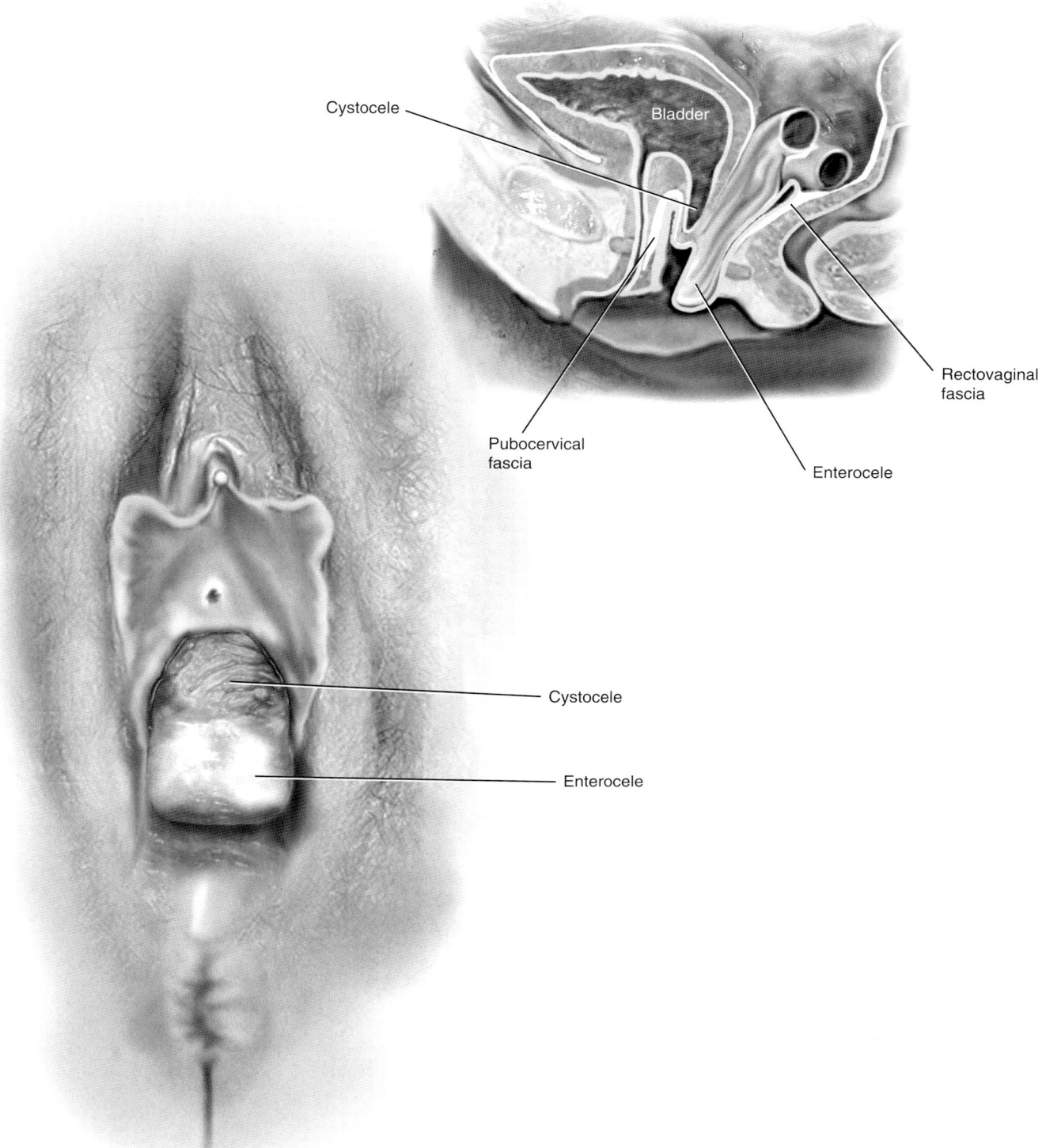

Cystocele

Bladder

Pubocervical fascia

Rectovaginal fascia

Enterocele

Cystocele

Enterocele

**FIGURE 54–6** Loss of anterior vaginal wall support. A cystocele that is coexistent with an apical or possibly an anterior enterocele in the posthysterectomy patient. Note that grossly the vaginal epithelium over an enterocele will appear to be much thinner than the vaginal epithelium over the prolapsed bladder.

## Midline Cystocele Repair

The objective of a midline anterior repair is to plicate the layers of the vaginal muscularis and adventitia overlying the bladder (*pubocervical fascia*). The operative procedure begins with the patient in the supine position and situated and prepped as for vaginal hysterectomy. A urethral Foley catheter is inserted for easy identification of the bladder neck. The anterior vaginal wall is then opened up via a midline incision (Fig. 54–7). If a vaginal hysterectomy has been performed, the incision is begun at the apex of the vagina by grasping this area with two Allis clamps (Fig. 54–8). Some prefer to inject a hemostatic solution before making any incisions. These various agents have been described in the chapter on vaginal hysterectomy. If there is only bladder base descensus and the bladder neck is well supported or has been previously supported via a retropubic suspension or sling procedure, then the incision need only extend to the level of the bladder neck. However, in most circumstances urethral hyper-mobility is present, and thus the anterior vaginal wall incision should extend to the level of the proximal urethra to allow for suburethral plication.

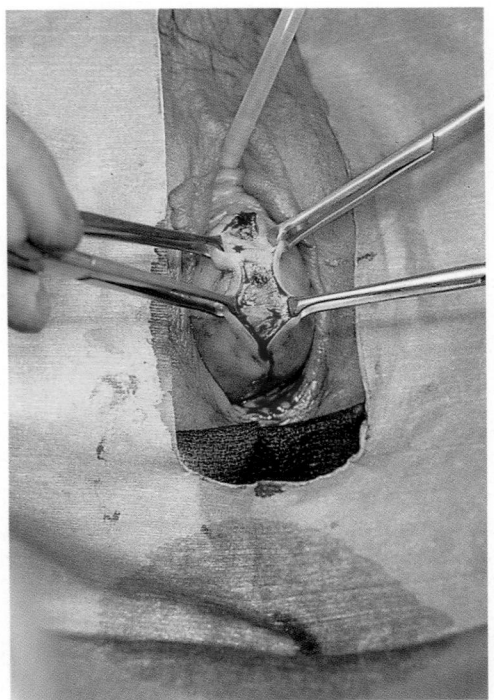

**FIGURE 54–7** Posthysterectomy cystocele showing the initial midline anterior vaginal wall incision.

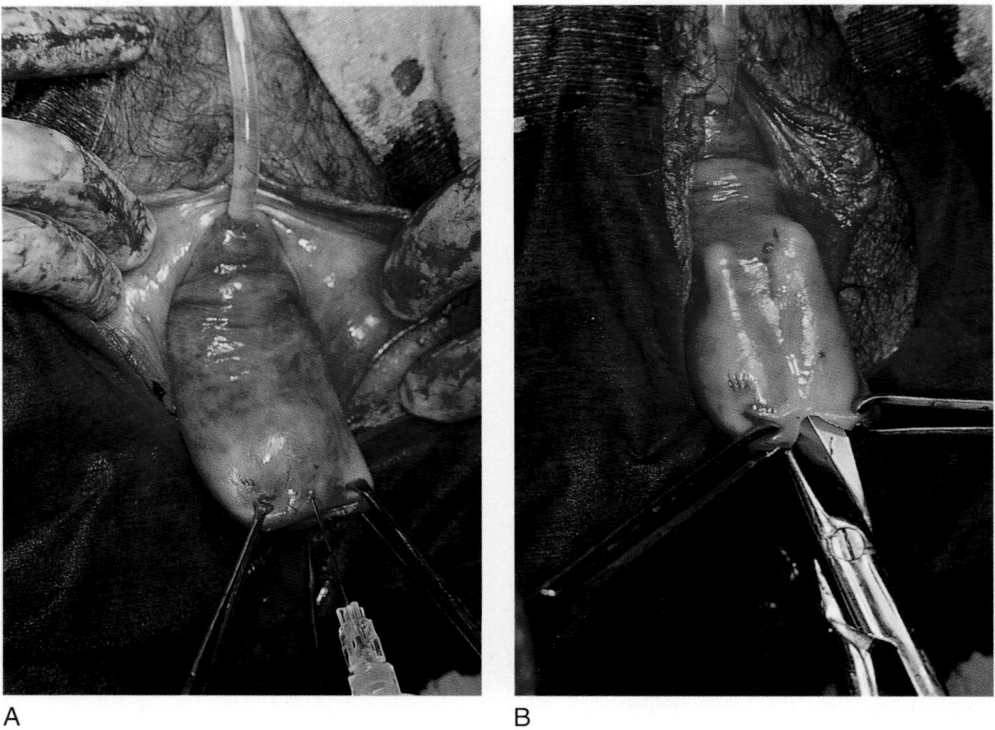

A                             B

**FIGURE 54–8 A.** Injection (hydrodistention) of the anterior vaginal wall. Note that Allis clamps grasp the anterior vaginal wall at the vaginal apex after completion of vaginal hysterectomy. **B.** The scissors are separated, creating an appropriate plane for midline anterior vaginal wall dissection.

After an initial incision is made, usually Mayo or Metzenbaum scissors are inserted between the vaginal epithelium and the vaginal muscularis or between the layers of the vaginal muscularis and are gently forced upward while they are partially opened and closed (Fig. 54–8B). The vagina is then incised, and the incision is continued to the desirable level, as was previously discussed. As the vagina is incised, the edges are usually grasped with Allis or T clamps and are drawn laterally for further mobilization. Dissection of the vaginal flap is then accomplished by turning the clamps back across the forefinger and incising the vaginal muscularis with scissors or a scalpel (Fig. 54–9). An assistant maintains constant traction medially on the bladder wall itself or on the remaining vaginal muscularis and underlying vesicovaginal adventitia. The dissection is extended bilaterally until the entire cystocele has been dissected off the vaginal wall (Figs. 54–10 to 54–13). Dissection should be continued until lateral assessment of vaginal support can be fully evaluated. This requires dissection to the inferior pubic ramus on each side. At this point the presence or absence of a paravaginal defect should be easily demonstrated (see Fig. 54–10). It is also important to sharply dissect the base of the bladder off the apex of the vagina in posthysterectomy cases (see Fig. 54–11). In most cases, regardless of whether the patient suffers from urinary incontinence, plicating sutures at the urethrovesical junction should be placed to augment the posterior urethral support in the hope of preventing de novo postoperative stress incontinence. To obtain durable tissue that can be plicated across the undersurface of the proximal urethra, it is important to extend the dissection all the way to the periurethral attachment at the level of the inferior pubic ramus (see Figs. 54–12 and 54–13). Usually a glistening white plane is present all the way to this area of attachment. Figures 54–14 and 54–15 demonstrate the technique of bladder neck plication in conjunction with midline cystocele repair. After stitches for the bladder neck plication have been placed and tied (see Fig. 54–14), attention is directed to the prolapsed bladder base. The goal of the midline cystocele repair is to reduce and provide support to the prolapsed bladder, as well as to provide preferential support to the bladder neck. The surgeon should try to avoid complete flattening of the posterior urethrovesical angle because this, in theory, may create incontinence (see Fig. 54–15). In the standard anterior colporrhaphy, 2-0 delayed absorbable sutures are placed in the muscularis and adventitia of the vaginal wall. Depending on the severity of the prolapse, one or two rows of plication sutures or a purse string suture followed by plication sutures is placed. The author prefers, if at all possible, to place two layers of sutures. For the initial layer, a 2-0 absorbable suture is used; this is followed by a second layer of 2-0 permanent suture (Figs. 54–16 and 54–17). The vaginal epithelium is then trimmed (Fig. 54–18), and the anterior vaginal wall is closed with a continuous 3-0 absorbable suture (Fig. 54–19). Figures 54–14 and 54–20 demonstrate, in succession, the steps of midline cystocele repair.

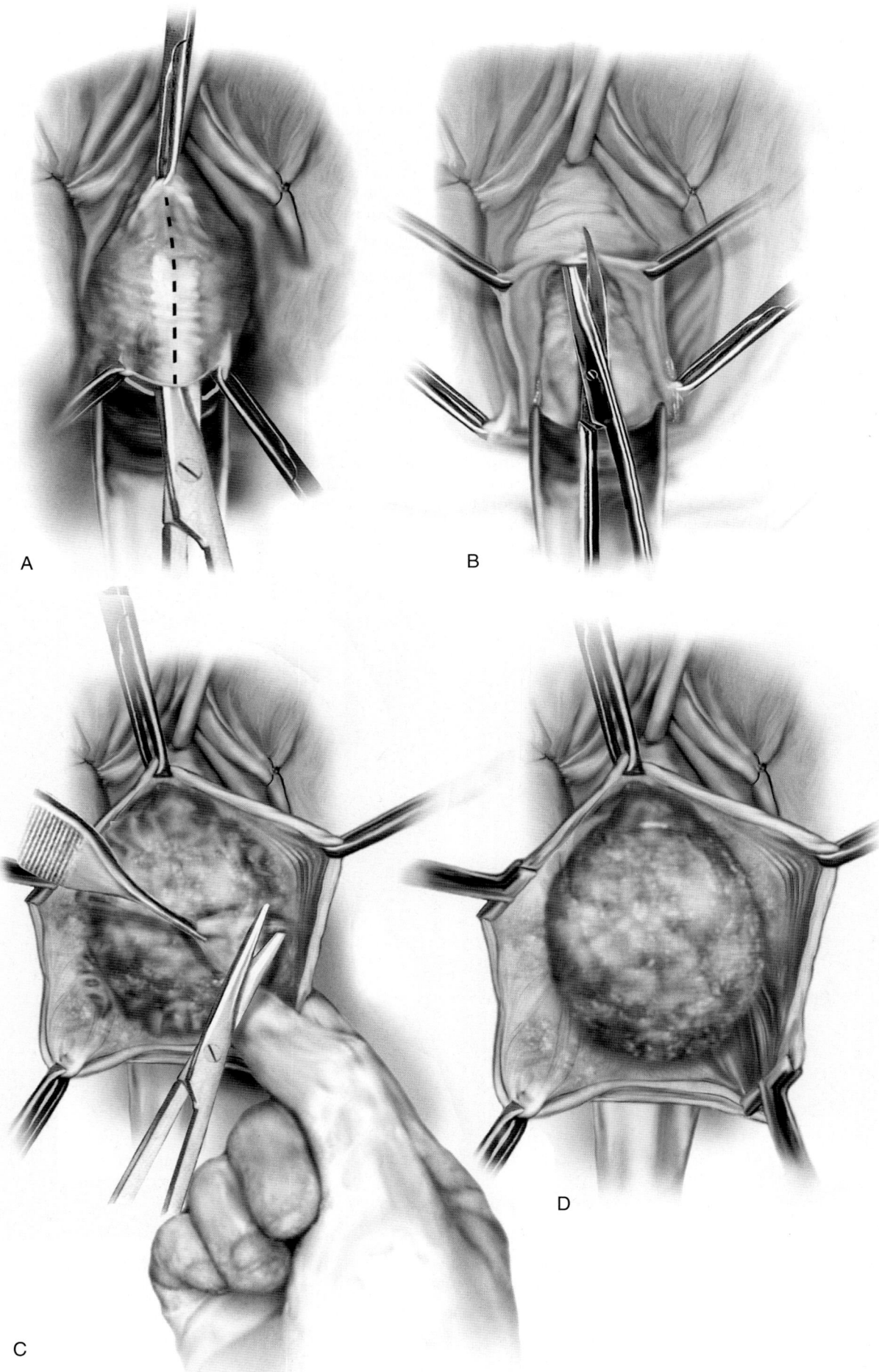

**FIGURE 54–9** **A.** Initial midline anterior vaginal wall incision. **B.** The incision is extended to the level of the proximal urethra. **C.** Sharp dissection and traction on the bladder facilitate dissection of the bladder off the vaginal wall. **D.** Mobilization of the cystocele off the vaginal wall is completed.

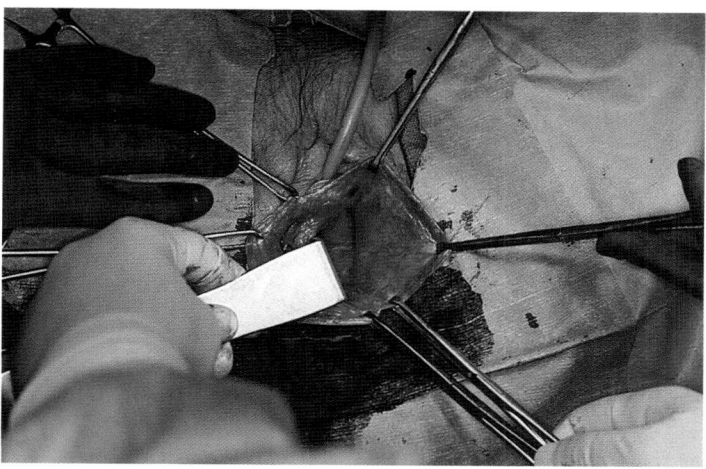

FIGURE 54–10 Dissection has been extended to the normal lateral attachment of the pubocervical fascia to the sidewall. Note that no paravaginal defect is present.

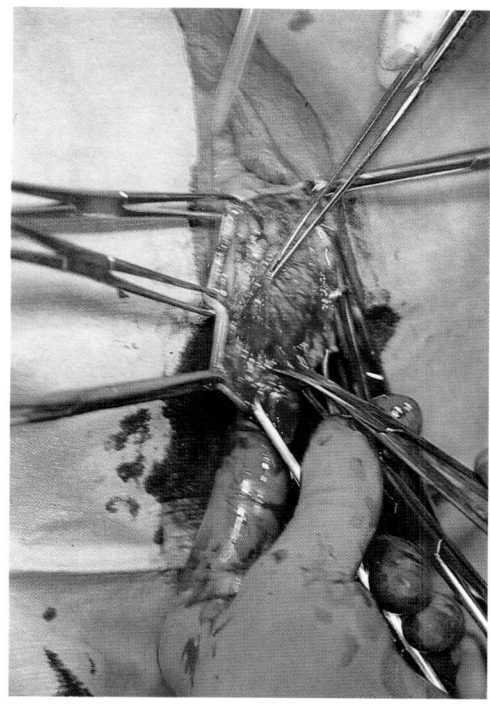

FIGURE 54–11 Dissection of the base of the bladder off the vaginal apex should be continued until the preperitoneal space is encountered.

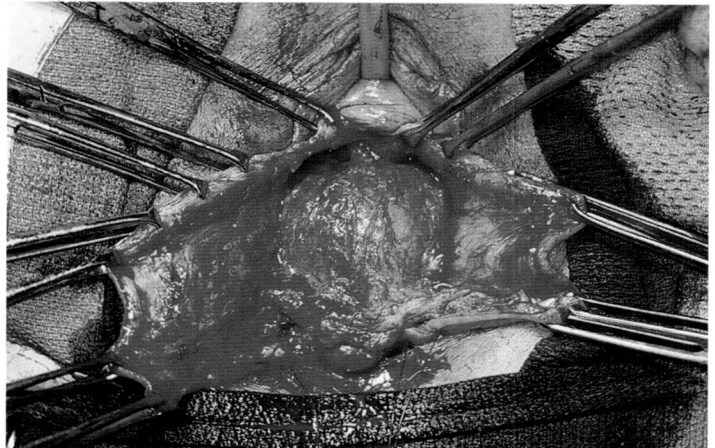

FIGURE 54–12 Lateral dissection of the cystocele off the vagina is complete. Note that the base of the bladder is still adherent to the apex of the vagina.

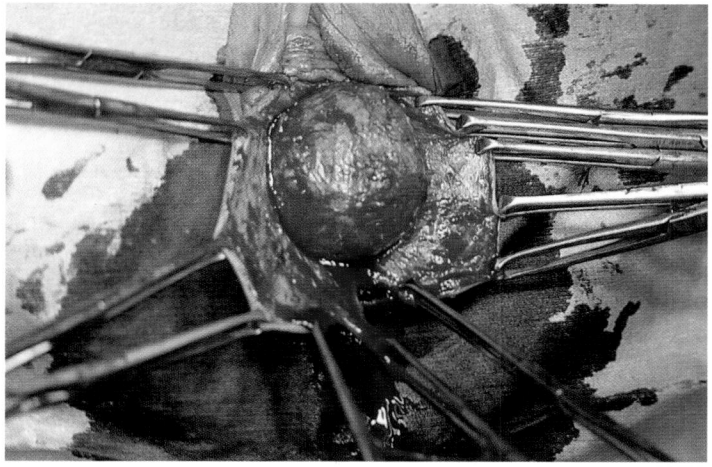

A

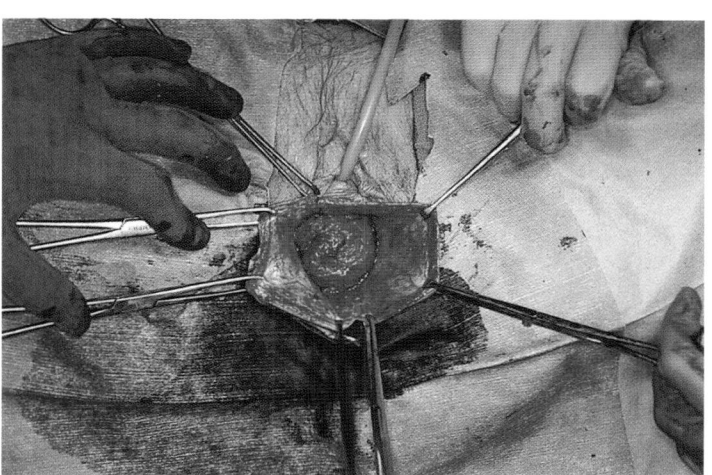

B

FIGURE 54–13 A and B. Two examples of cystoceles that have been completely mobilized off the vaginal epithelium.

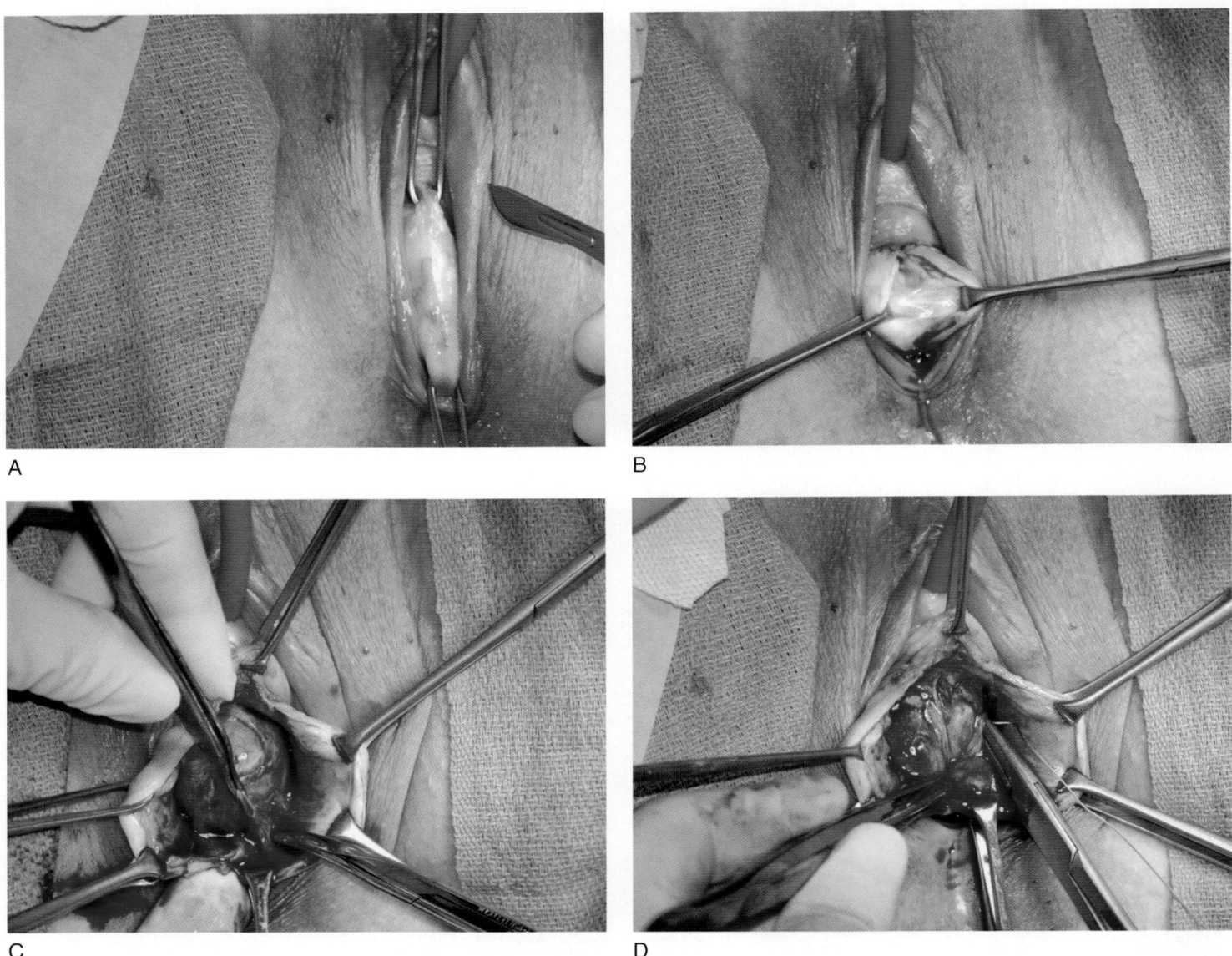

**FIGURE 54–14** Anterior colporrhaphy with Kelly plication in a patient with an isolated midline cystocele and bladder neck mobility. **A.** Midline anterior vaginal wall incision is made after hydrodissection. **B.** Appropriate plane of dissection is demonstrated. **C.** Dissection has occurred lateral to the level of the inferior pubic ramus; shown here is the sharp dissection of the base of bladder off the apex of the vagina. **D.** The first plication stitch is being placed at the level of the bladder neck.

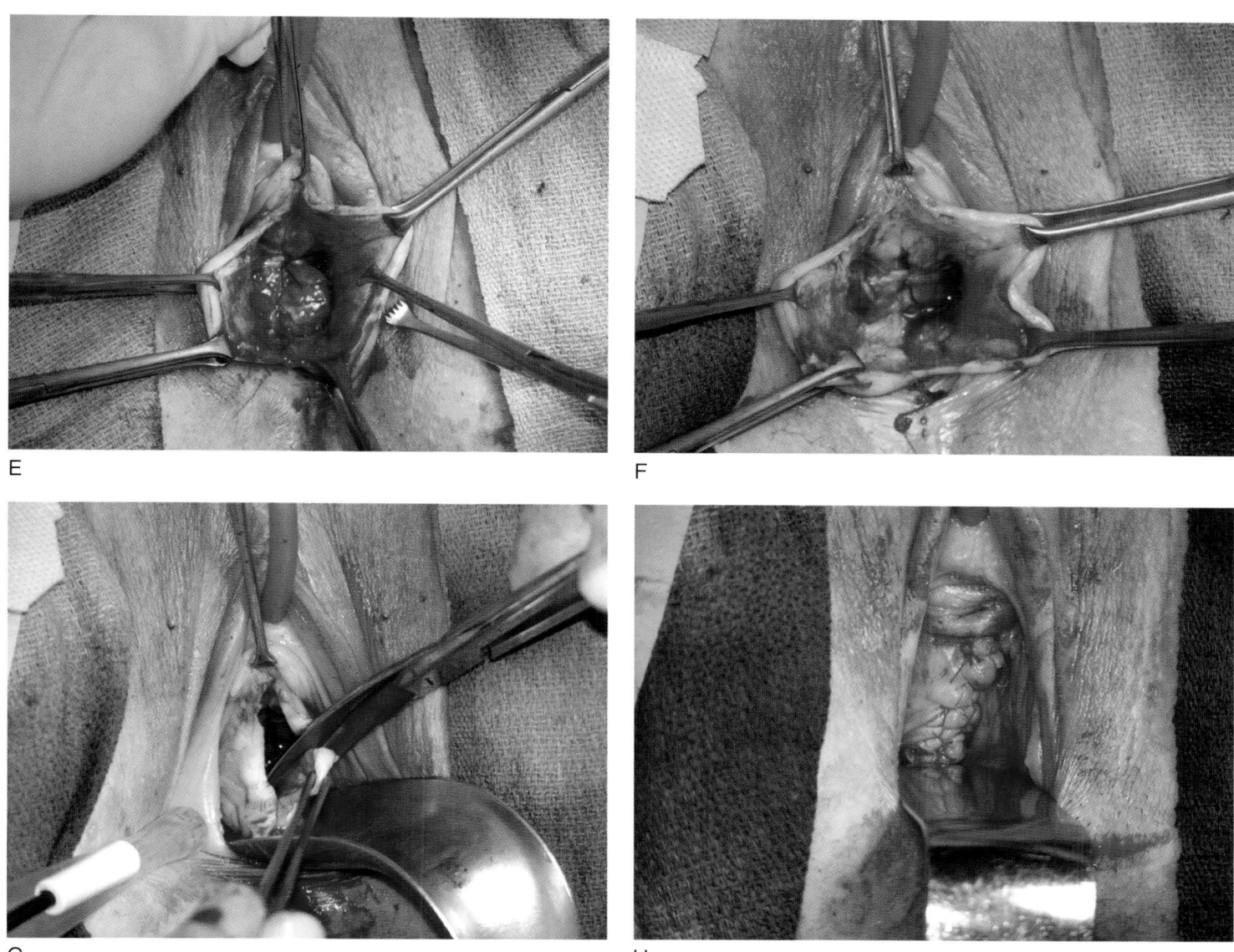

E

F

G

H

**FIGURE 54–14, cont'd   E.** The first stitch has been tied, providing preferential support to the proximal urethra and bladder neck (Kelly plication). **F.** Subsequent stitches have been placed, completing the anterior colporrhaphy. **G.** Excess mucosa is trimmed. **H.** The anterior vaginal wall is closed.

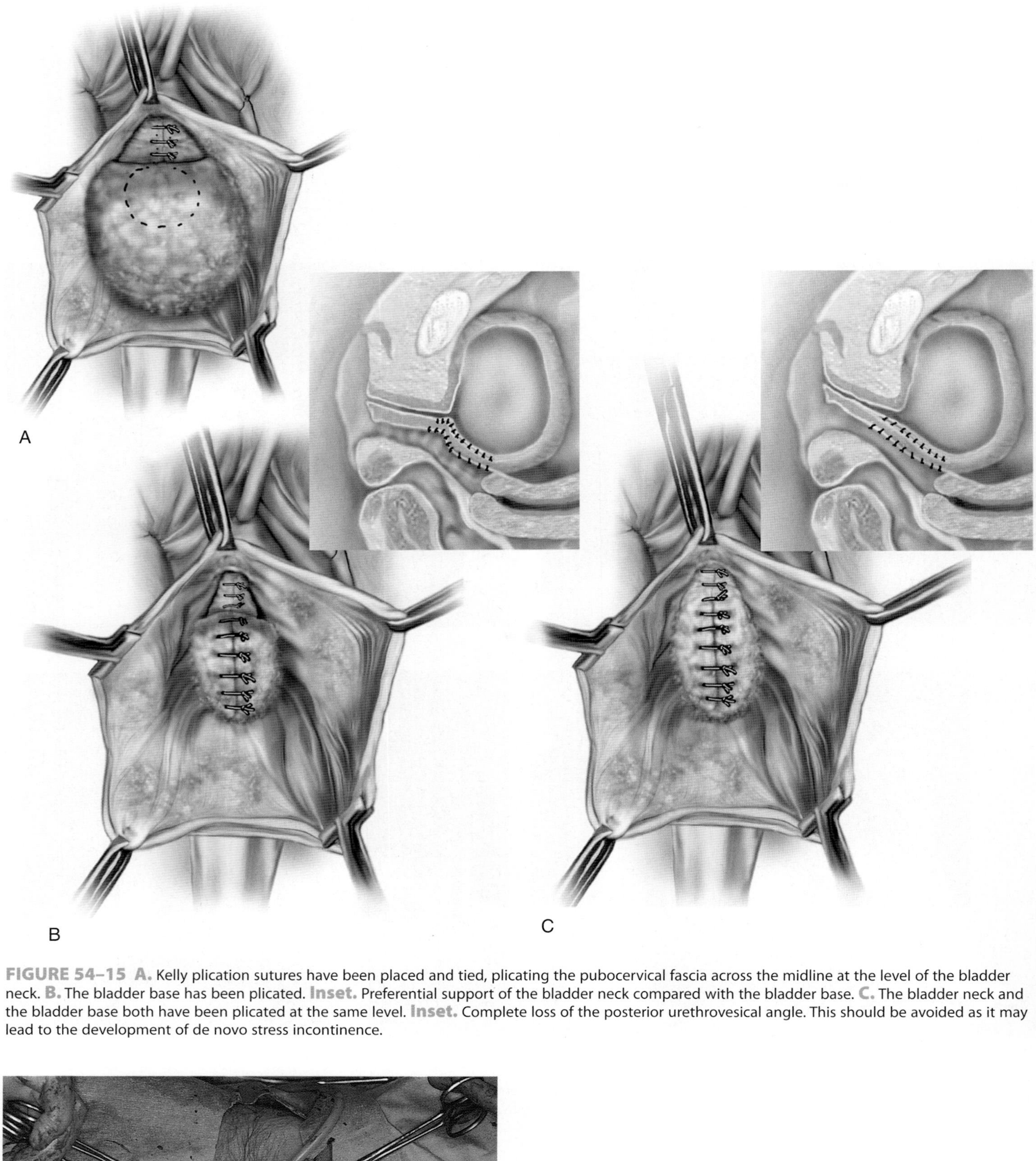

A

B

C

**FIGURE 54–15 A.** Kelly plication sutures have been placed and tied, plicating the pubocervical fascia across the midline at the level of the bladder neck. **B.** The bladder base has been plicated. **Inset.** Preferential support of the bladder neck compared with the bladder base. **C.** The bladder neck and the bladder base both have been plicated at the same level. **Inset.** Complete loss of the posterior urethrovesical angle. This should be avoided as it may lead to the development of de novo stress incontinence.

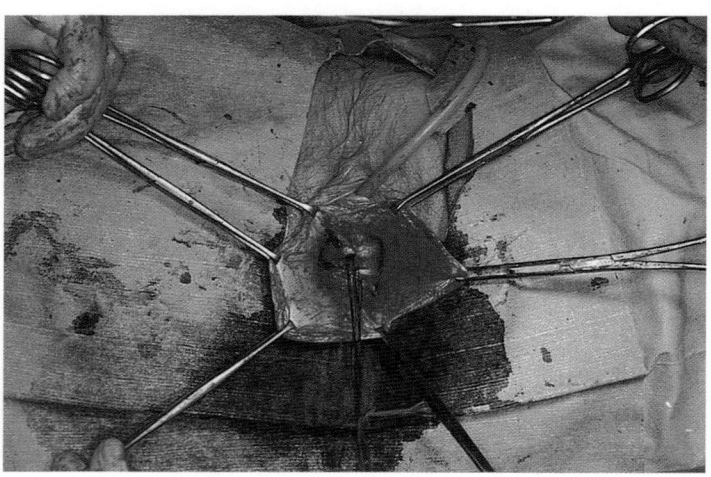

**FIGURE 54–16** Bladder base plication sutures have been placed and tied.

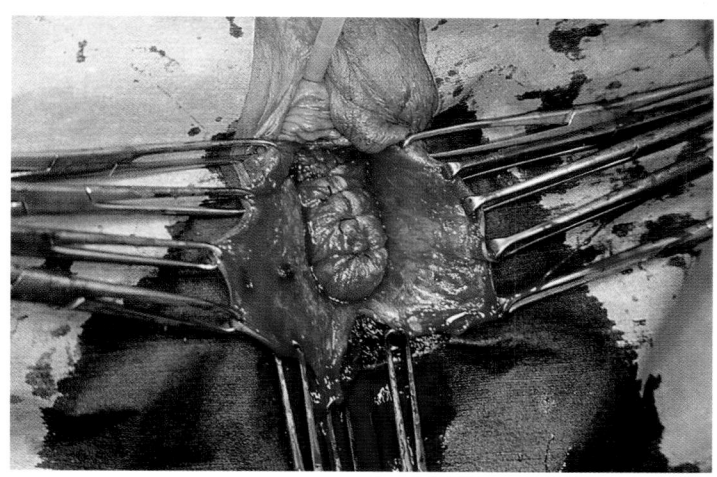

A

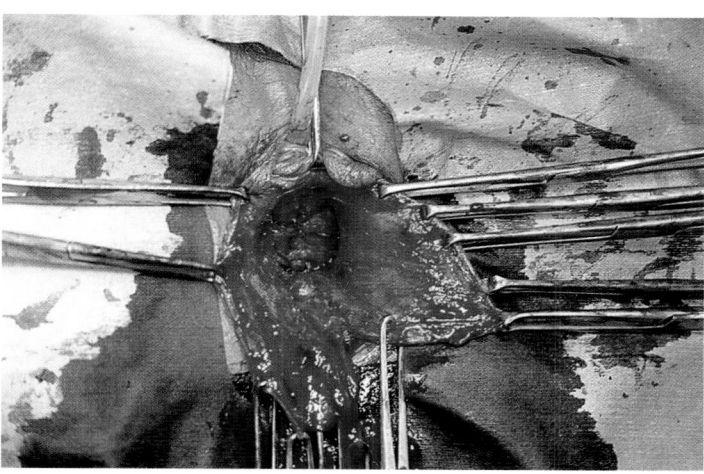

B

**FIGURE 54–17 A.** The initial layer of sutures has been placed, plicating the cystocele. **B.** The second layer of plication sutures completes the cystocele repair.

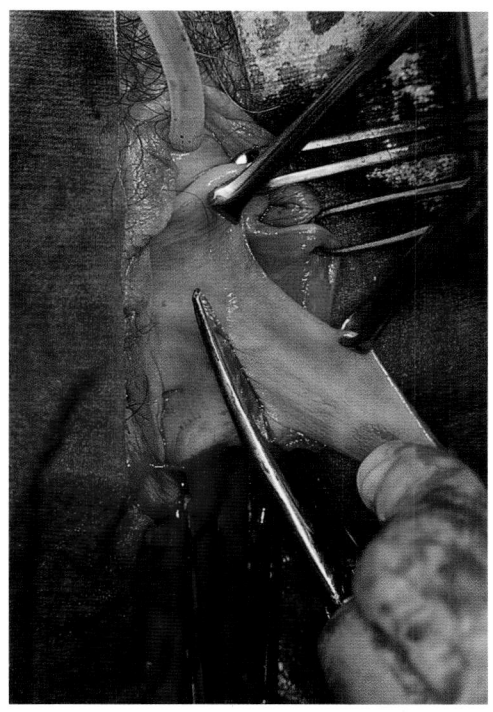

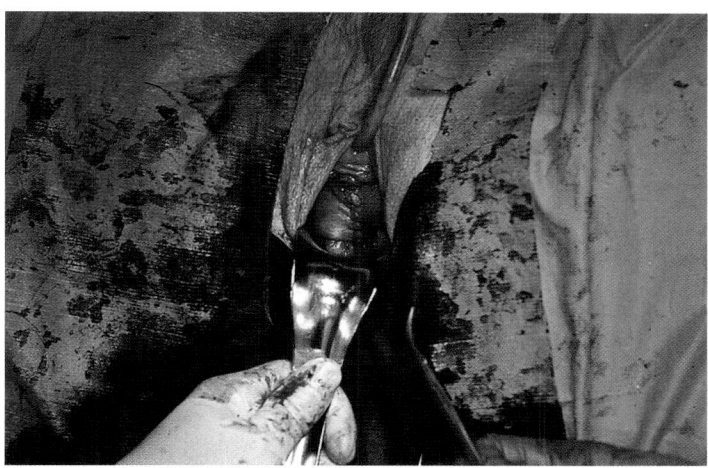

**FIGURE 54–19** The anterior vaginal wall is closed with continuous or interrupted 3-0 absorbable sutures.

**FIGURE 54–18** Excess anterior vaginal wall epithelium is excised.

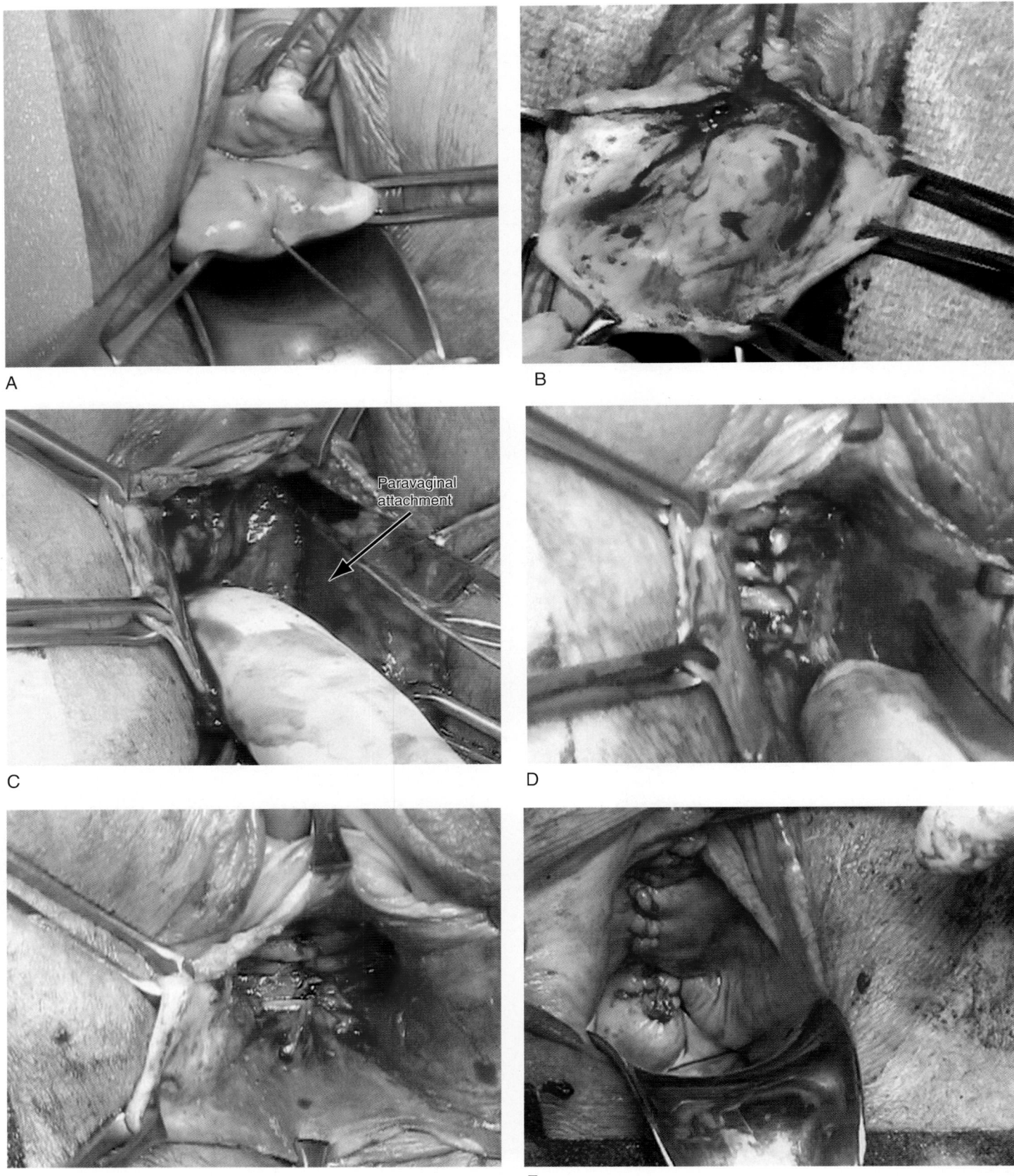

A

B

C

Paravaginal
attachment

D

E

F

**FIGURE 54–20** The technique of midline cystocele repair with Kelly plication. **A.** The anterior vaginal wall in this posthysterectomy patient is grasped with two Allis clamps, and a vasoconstrictive agent is injected to facilitate dissection in the appropriate plane. **B.** The anterior vaginal wall has been opened up, and dissection has been extended laterally on each side. Also, note that dissection must involve mobilizing the base of the bladder off the apex of the vagina. **C.** Dissection is extended to the inferior pubic ramus on each side. Note the good paravaginal attachment, ruling out any paravaginal defect in this patient. **D.** The midline cystocele has been initially plicated with delayed absorbable suture. *Note:* Plication sutures have been placed at the proximal urethral bladder neck to provide preferential support over those placed over the base of the bladder. **E.** Dissection has been extended farther laterally to facilitate the development of more fascia, and a second layer of permanent sutures is now used to complete the midline cystocele plication. **F.** After the anterior vaginal wall is trimmed, the anterior vaginal wall is closed with a 3-0 delayed absorbable suture. Note the excellent support of the anterior segment in the midline with maintenance of good lateral vaginal sulci on each side.

Some surgeons prefer to augment anterior vaginal wall repair with a free graft of tissue or mesh, which can be biologic or synthetic. The mesh or tissue is placed over the stitches and is anchored in place at the lateral limit of the previous dissection or at the inside of the anterior vaginal wall (Figs. 54–21 and 54–22). If bilateral paravaginal defects are present, the material can be attached to the arcus tendineus fascia pelvis on each side (Fig. 54–23). Materials that have been utilized have included rectus abdominis, fascia lata, and cadaveric fascia lata, as well as synthetic mesh such as Marlex, Mersilene, or Prolene. Indications for mesh-augmented prolapse repairs remain very controversial. Some surgeons believe that repairs should be augmented in recurrent cases and in women with a very poor or little muscular component to their vaginal skin, which is usually secondary to long-standing urogenital atrophy (Fig. 54–24).

At times a cystocele coexists with an enterocele (Fig. 54–25A). In this situation it is important to dissect out the individual defects, thus completely mobilizing the enterocele sac from the cystocele. Each defect is then individually repaired, and, if indicated, the vaginal vault is suspended (see Fig. 54–25).

## Vaginal Paravaginal Repair

The objective of a paravaginal defect repair for anterior vaginal wall prolapse is to reattach the detached lateral vagina to its normal place of attachment at the level of the arcus tendineus fascia pelvis (white line). This can be accomplished by using a vaginal or retropubic approach. Although at times a paravaginal defect can be accurately diagnosed preoperatively, many times it is an intraoperative diagnosis. To diagnose this defect via a transvaginal route, one must extend the plane of dissection between the vagina and the bladder all the way out to the inferior pubic ramus. When this lateral area is reached, the attachment must be assessed subjectively. At times complete detachment will be obvious, meaning that lateral dissection will lead directly into the retropubic space, and retropubic fat will be visualized. At times there will be an attachment, albeit a very weak one, and the decision must be made whether to completely detach the tissue, so it can be reattached in appropriate fashion. To perform a true vaginal paravaginal repair, there must be digital access into the retropubic space. The most important landmark is palpation of the ischial spine via the anterior segment. Once this is palpated, one can usually palpate the arcus tendineus fascia pelvis moving along the lateral pelvic sidewall toward the back of the symphysis.

Preparation for vaginal paravaginal repair begins as for an anterior colporrhaphy. Marking sutures are placed on the anterior vaginal wall or each side of the urethrovesical junction (identified by placing gentle traction on the catheter), and at the vaginal apex. If a culdoplasty is being performed, the sutures are placed but not tied until completion of the paravaginal repair and closure of the anterior vaginal wall. As for anterior colporrhaphy, vaginal flaps are developed by incising the vagina in the midline and dissecting the vaginal muscularis laterally. The dissection is performed bilaterally until the space is developed between vaginal wall and retropubic space. Blunt dissection with the surgeon's index finger is used to extend this space anteriorly along the pubic ramus, medially to the pubic symphysis, and laterally toward the ischial spine. If the defect is present and dissection is occurring in the appropriate place, one should easily enter the retropubic space, visualizing retropubic fat. The ischial spine then can be palpated on each side. The

arcus tendineus fascia pelvis coming off the spine can be followed to the back of the symphysis. After dissection is complete, midline plication of the vaginal muscularis can be performed at this point or after placement and tying of the paravaginal sutures. On the lateral pelvic sidewall, the obturator internus muscle and the arcus tendineus fascia pelvis are identified by palpation and then by visualization. Retraction of the bladder and the urethra medially is best accomplished with a Breisky-Navratil retractor, and posterior retraction is provided with a lighted suction device. With 0 nonabsorbable suture, the first stitch is placed through the white line just anterior to the ischial spine. If the white line is not visualized, is detached from the pelvic sidewall, or clinically is not thought to be durable, then the suture should be passed into the fascia overlying the obturator internus muscle. Placement of subsequent sutures is facilitated by placing tension on the first suture. A series of four to six sutures are placed and held, working anteriorly along the white line to the level of the urethrovesical junction. Starting with the most anterior suture, the surgeon picks up the edge of the periurethral tissue (vaginal muscularis or pubocervical fascia) at the level of the urethrovesical junction and then tissue from the undersurface of the vaginal flap at the previously marked site. Subsequent sutures move posteriorly until the last stitch closest to the ischial spine is attached to the undersurface of the vagina at the site of the marking sutures placed at the vaginal apex. Stitches in the vaginal wall must be carefully placed to allow adequate tissue for subsequent midline vaginal closure. After all stitches are placed on one side, the same procedure is carried out on the other side. The stitches are then tied in order from the urethra to the apex, alternating from one side to the other. This repair is a three-point closure between the vaginal epithelium, vaginal muscularis and endopelvic fascia (pubocervical fascia), and lateral pelvic sidewall at the level of the arcus tendineus fascia pelvis. Tissue-to-tissue approximation is necessary between these structures. Suture bridges must be avoided by careful planning of suture placement. Vaginal tissue should not be trimmed until all stitches are tied. As was previously stated, if not already performed, vaginal muscularis can then be plicated in the midline if necessary with several interrupted sutures. The vaginal flaps are then trimmed and closed with a running delayed absorbable suture. Figure 54–26 illustrates the entire procedure of a three-point vaginal paravaginal repair in a stepwise fashion. Other techniques can also be utilized to address a paravaginal defect. Some surgeons believe it is not necessary to include the inside of the vaginal wall in a vaginal paravaginal repair. This then becomes a two-point closure in which the detached fascia is sutured directly into the white line or the fascia over the obturator internus muscle (Figs. 54–27 and 54–28). If paravaginal support simply needs to be strengthened, or if the surgeon does not desire to fully enter the retropubic space to expose the arcus, a modified two-point closure in which the fascia is sutured to the upper part of the anterior vaginal wall can be performed (Fig. 54–29). This technique strengthens lateral support of the bladder but does not re-create the normal lateral vaginal sulcus because the fascia and the vagina are not reattached to the white line or the obturator internus fascia. Some surgeons routinely include the inside lining of the vaginal wall during traditional anterior colporrhaphy (Fig. 54–30). Although this will close off any paravaginal defect, it will commonly result in a scarred, foreshortened anterior segment.

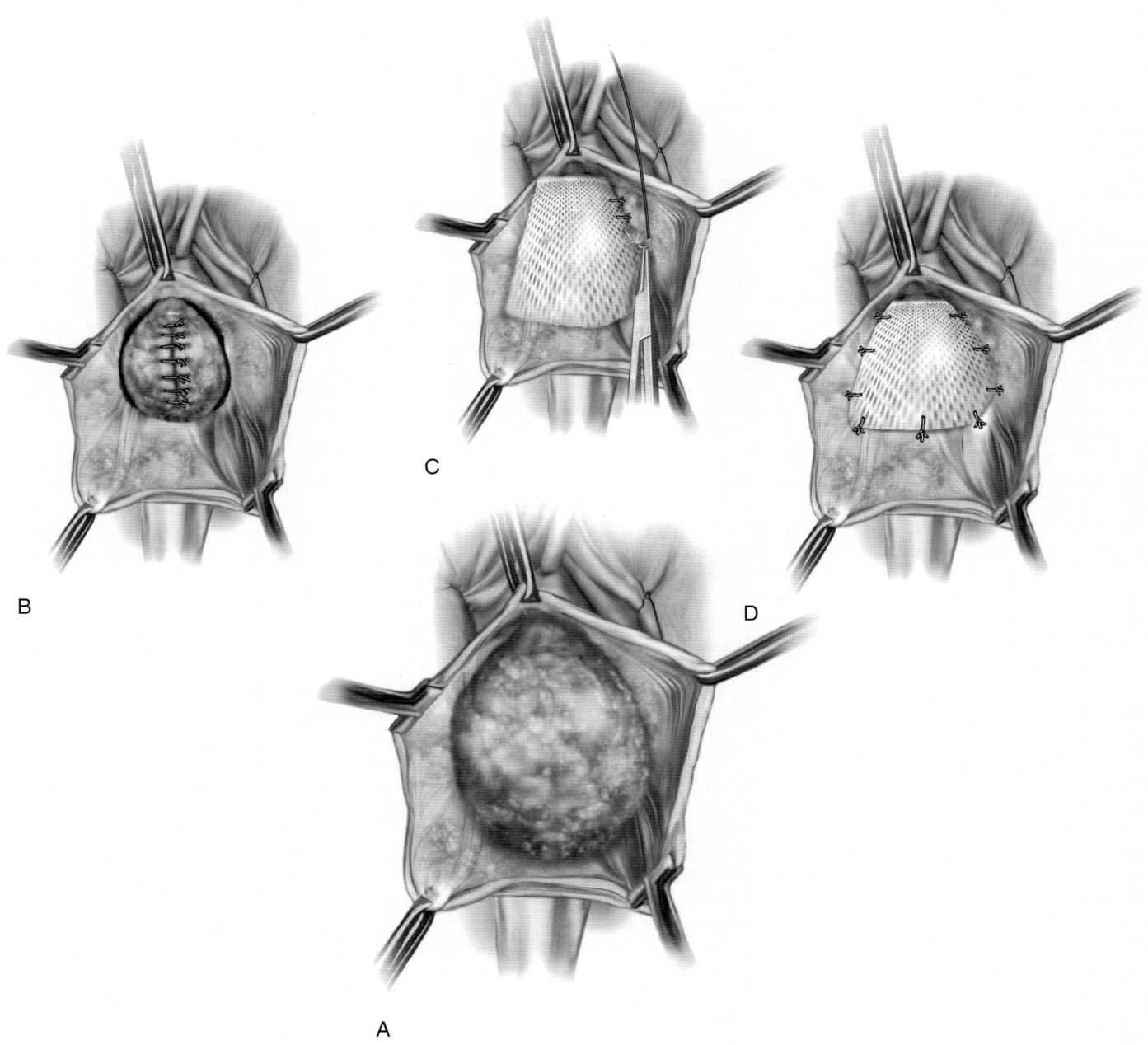

B

C

D

A

**FIGURE 54–21** Technique of placement of mesh in the anterior vaginal wall. **A.** The cystocele has been completely mobilized from the anterior vaginal wall. **B.** The cystocele has been plicated in the midline. **C.** The mesh is fixed to the upper portion of the anterior vaginal wall on the left. **D.** Fixation of the mesh is completed by fixing it to the opposite side, as well as to the inside lining of the vaginal wall at the level of the vaginal apex.

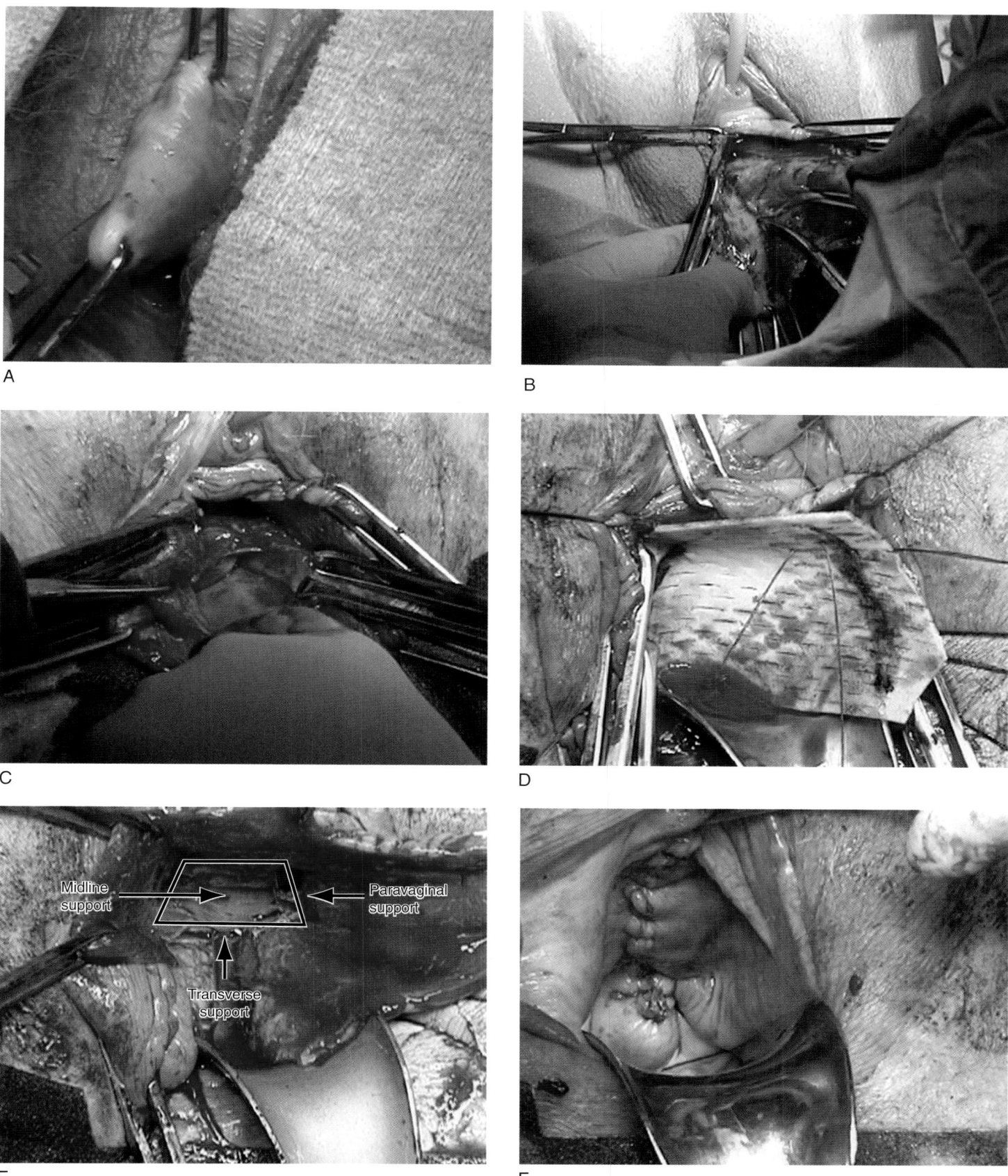

**FIGURE 54–22** Technique of a mesh-augmented anterior colporrhaphy in a patient with a recurrent cystocele and enterocele. **A.** The anterior vaginal wall is grasped with two Allis clamps and injected. **B.** Sharp dissection of the bladder from the anterior vaginal wall. **C.** An initial plication has been performed to reduce the cystocele. Note that the enterocele sac has been identified and entered. **D.** A trapezoid piece of Pelvisoft (Bard Urologic, Covington, Ga) is being fixed to the upper portion of the anterior vaginal wall on the left side. **E.** The mesh is fixed in place in the anterior segment; the trapezoid concept is demonstrated, showing how the mesh creates paravaginal, midline, and transverse support. **F.** The anterior vaginal wall has been trimmed and closed, and the vaginal vault has been suspended. Note the good support of the entire anterior segment.

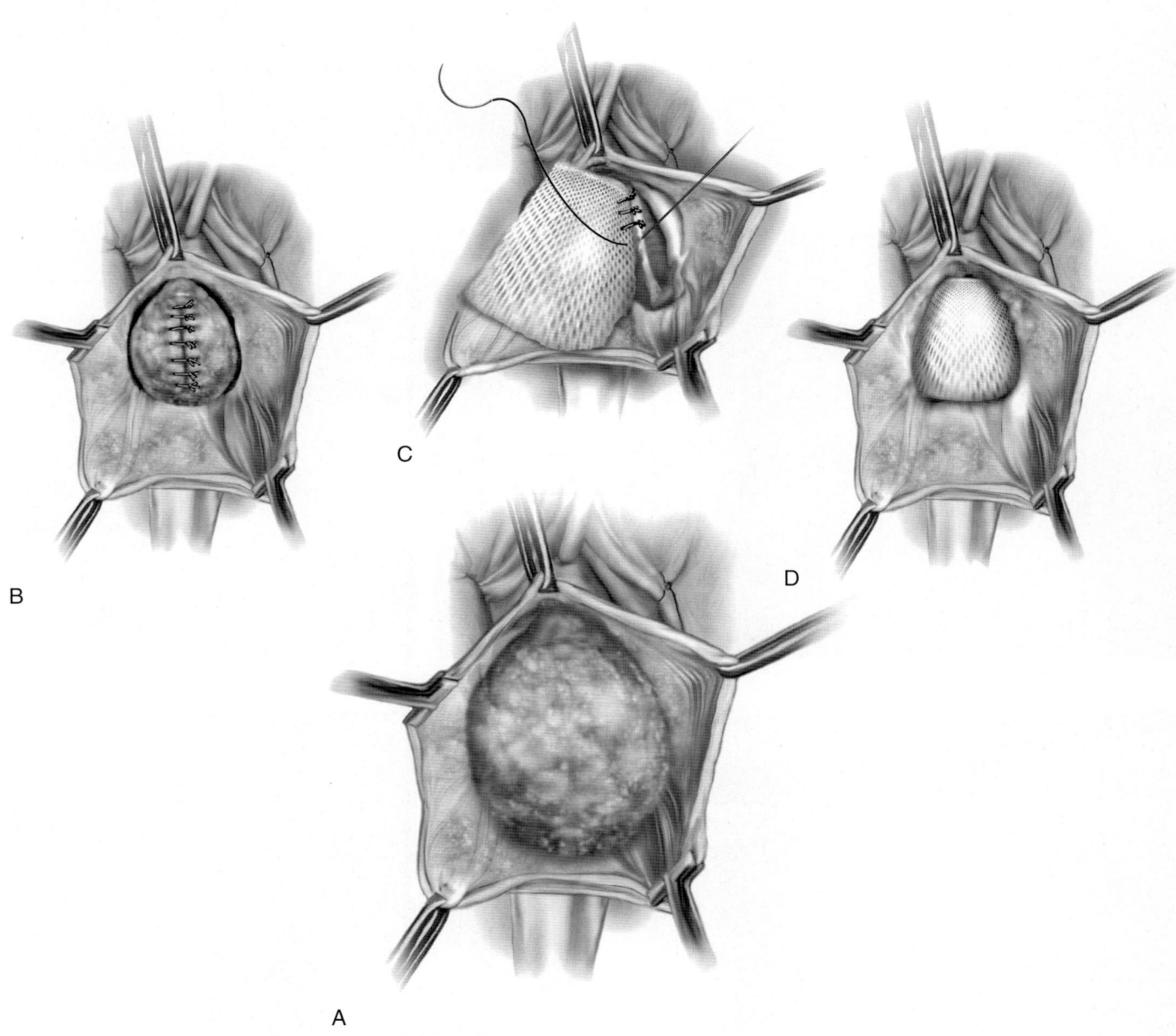

**FIGURE 54–23** Technique of utilizing a mesh to correct bilateral paravaginal defects. **A.** The cystocele has been dissected from the anterior vaginal wall. **B.** Midline plication has been created, and bilateral paravaginal defects are seen. **C.** The mesh is sutured directly to the arcus with interrupted sutures. **D.** The completed mesh repair shows the mesh fixed bilaterally to the arcus tendineus fascia pelvis.

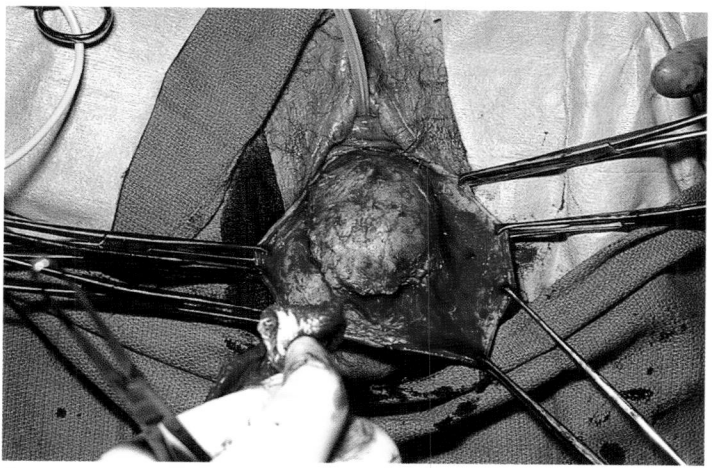

A

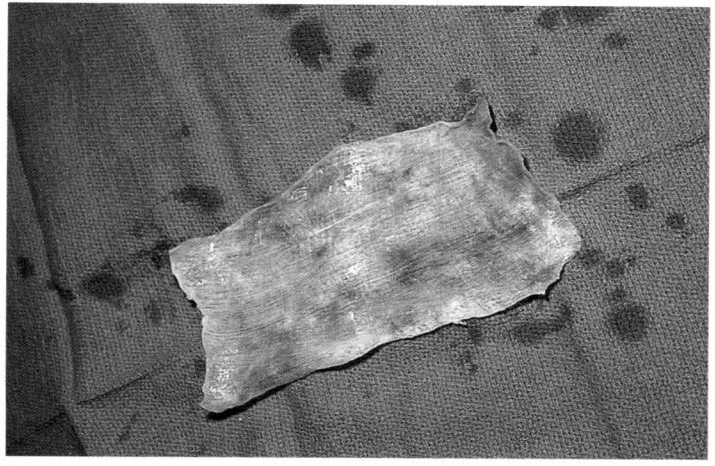

B

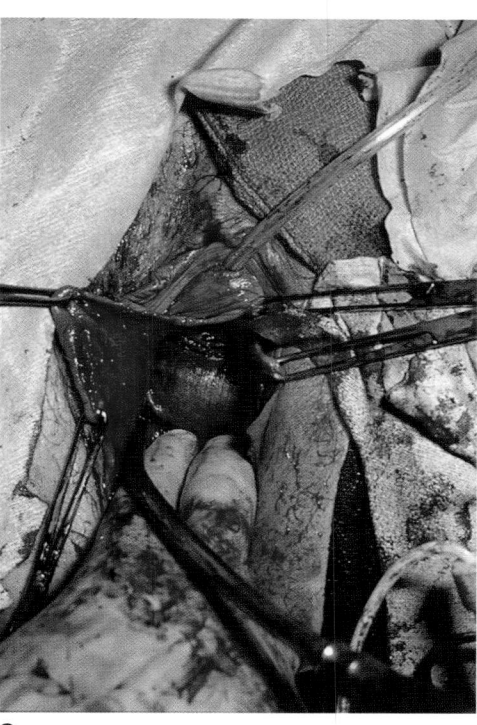

C

**FIGURE 54–24  A.** A large cystocele has been dissected off the vaginal epithelium. Note the minimal fascia present on the prolapsed bladder base. **B.** A piece of cadaveric fascia lata. **C.** The fascia has been attached to the inner aspect of the anterior vaginal wall, reducing the prolapsed bladder base.

UNIT 3 ■ SECTION B

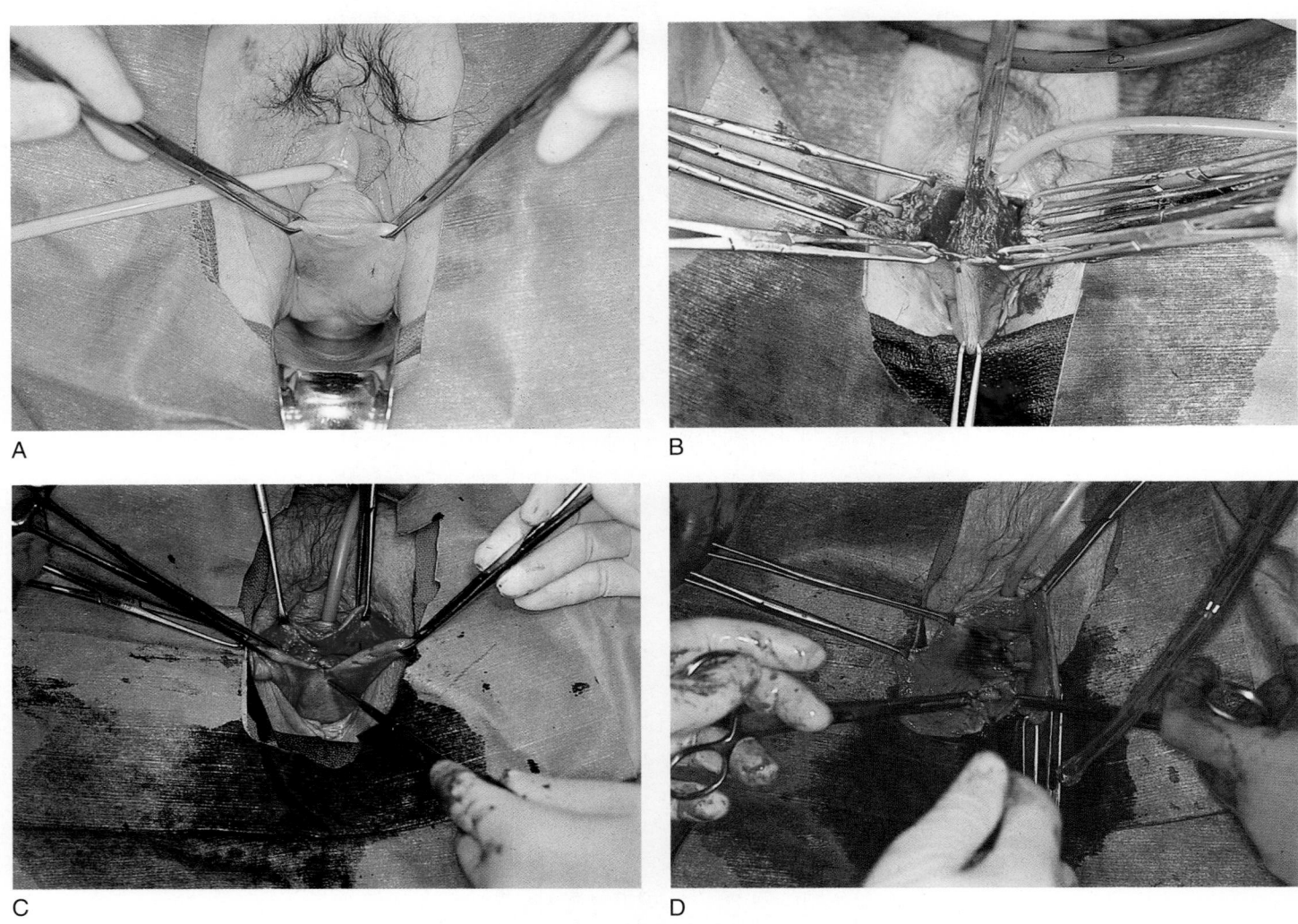

**FIGURE 54–25** Combined cystocele and enterocele repair **A.** Cystocele in conjunction with vaginal vault prolapse. **B.** An anterior vaginal wall incision has been made, and the anatomic location of the bladder base is noted. **C.** The vaginal incision is extended over the suspected enterocele. **D.** The bladder base prolapse has been plicated, the enterocele sac has been mobilized off the bladder base, and the peritoneal sac has been opened.

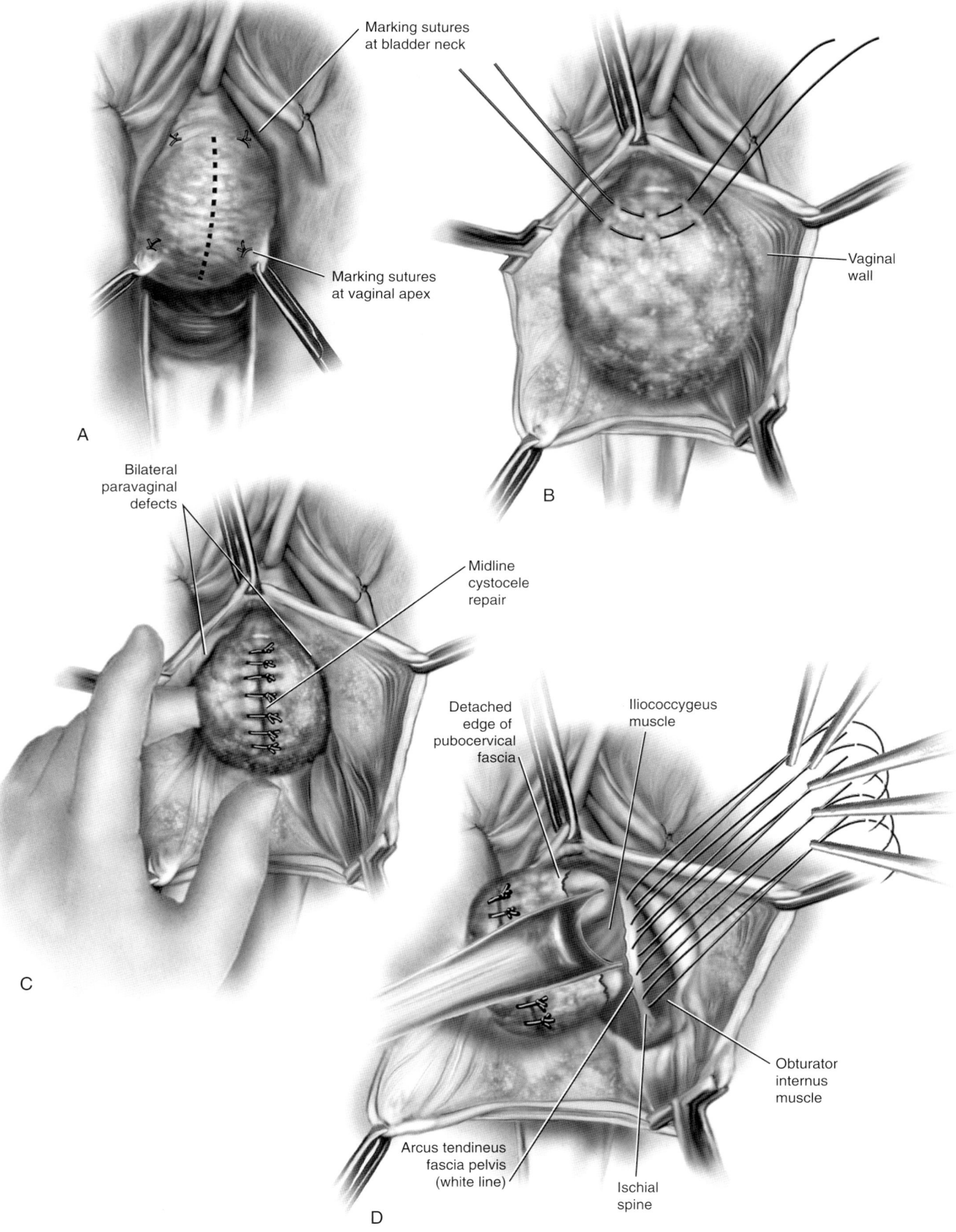

**FIGURE 54–26** Technique of vaginal paravaginal repair. **A.** Marking sutures are placed at the bladder neck and vaginal apex. A midline anterior vaginal wall incision is made. **B.** The bladder is dissected laterally and off the vaginal apex. Midline plication is performed. **C.** Midline plication is completed; obvious bilateral paravaginal defects are present. **D.** The bladder is retracted medially, and numerous sutures are passed through the arcus tendineus fascia pelvis (white line).

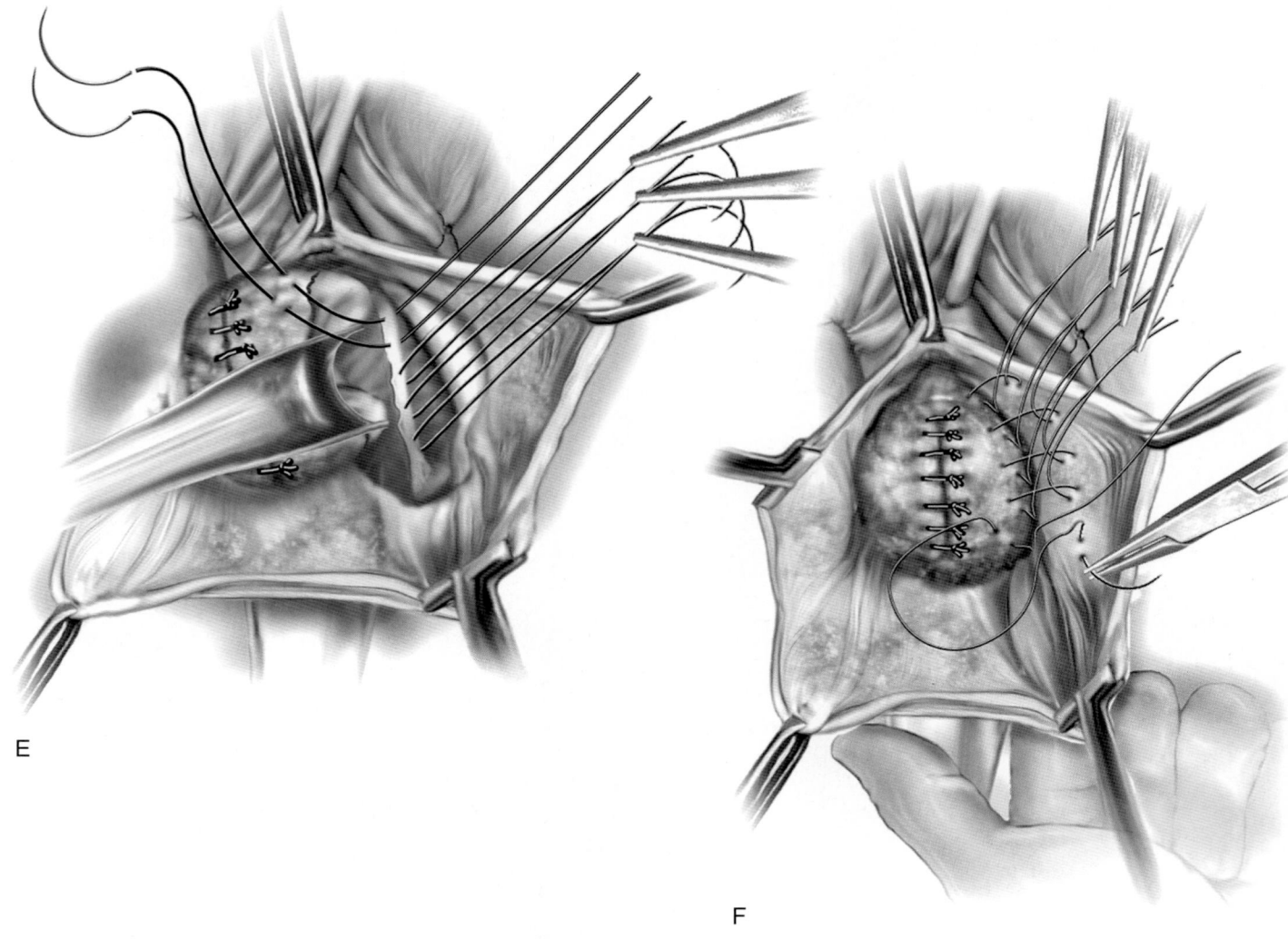

E

F

**FIGURE 54–26, cont'd   E.** Sutures are then passed through the detached pubocervical or endopelvic fascia. **F.** Sutures are passed through the inside of the vaginal wall, thus completing the three-point closure.

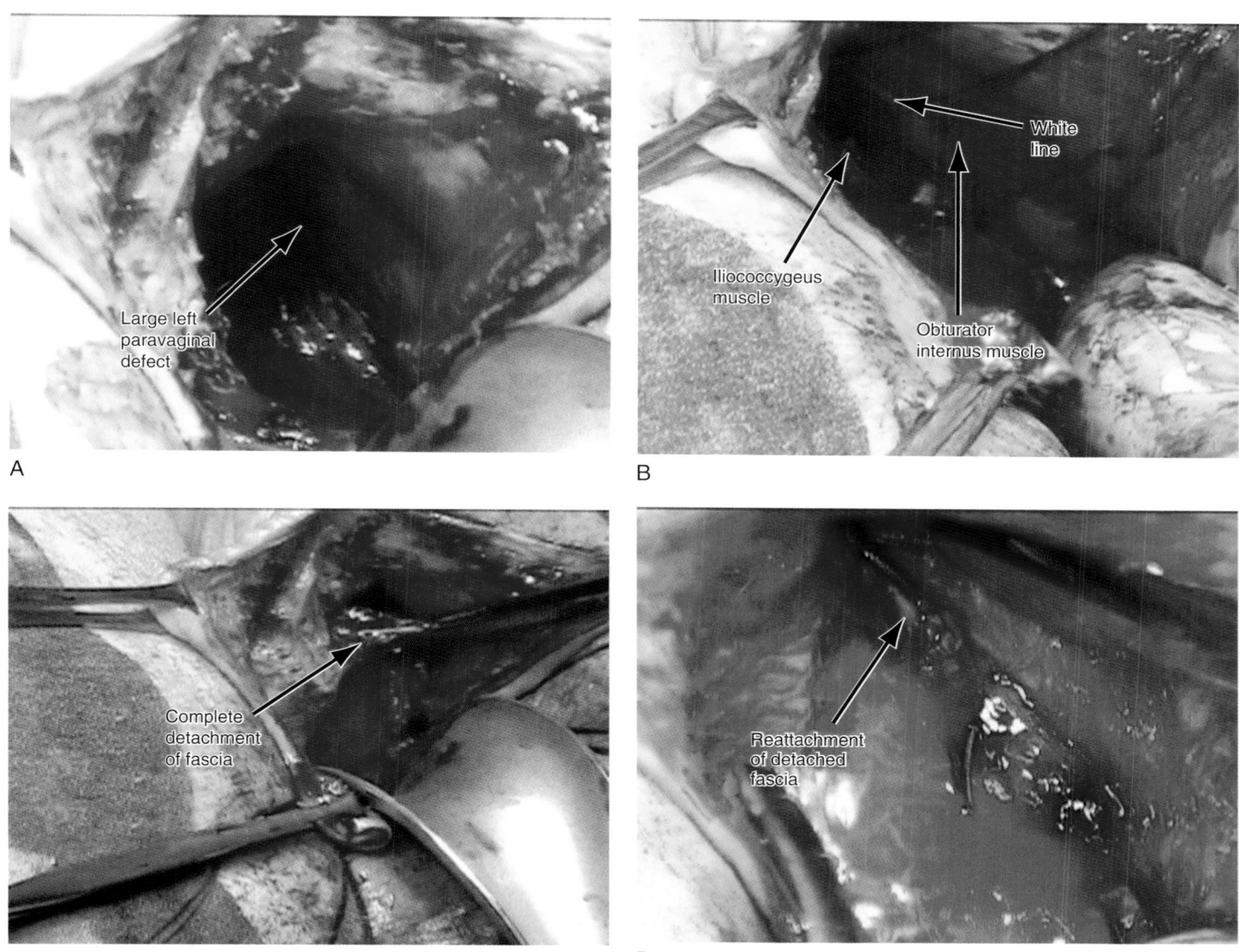

**FIGURE 54–27** Technique of two-point vaginal-paravaginal repair. **A.** Large paravaginal defect on the left side. **B.** Sutures have been passed through the arcus tendineus fascia pelvis on the left side. The obturator internus muscle and the iliococcygeus muscle, respectively, are seen above and below the white line. **C.** The detached fascia is noted. **D.** The detached fascia has been sutured into the arcus with numerous interrupted, permanent sutures.

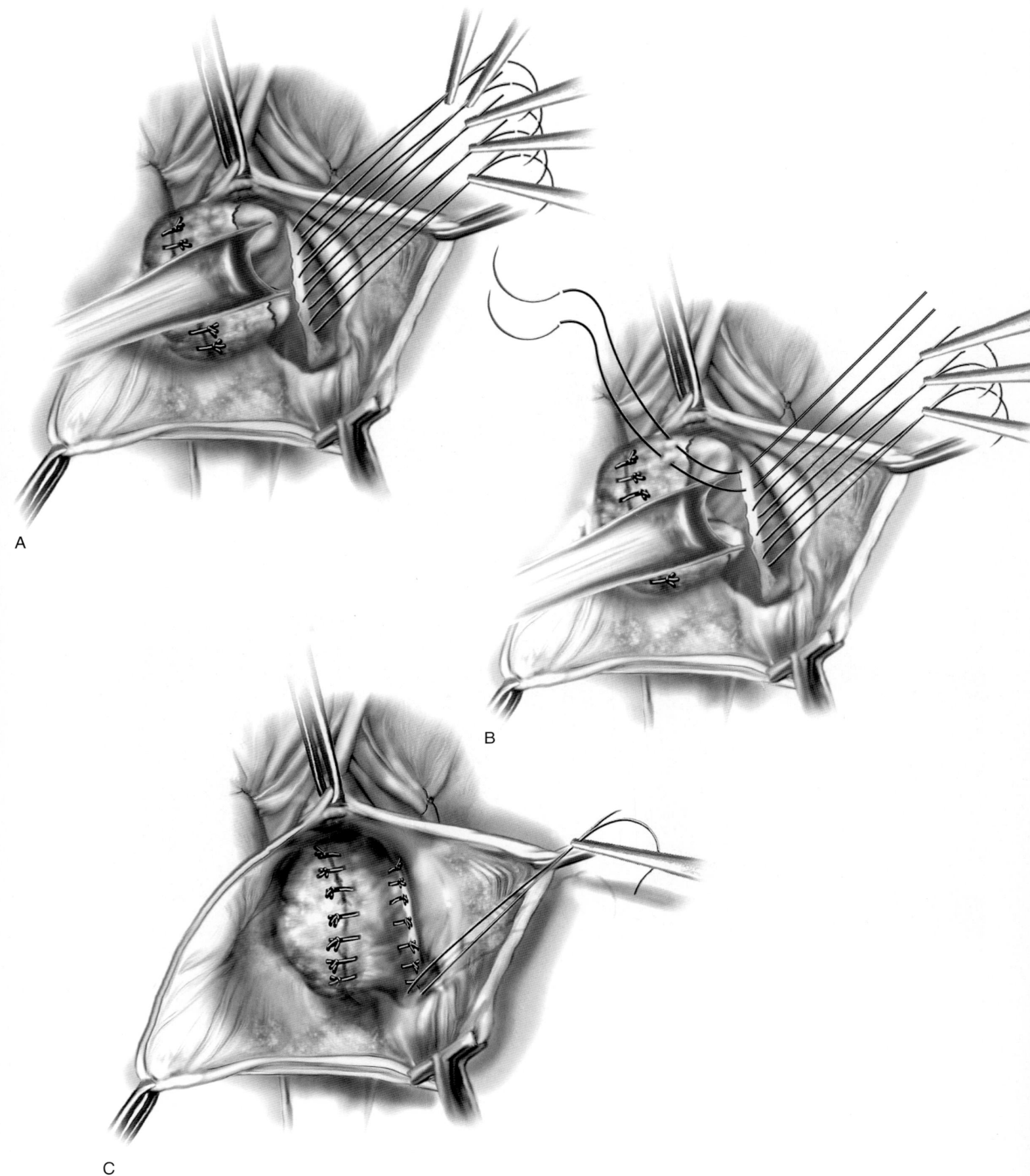

A

B

C

**FIGURE 54–28** Technique of two-point paravaginal defect repair, in which the detached fascia is sutured directly into the arcus tendineus fascia pelvis, or the white line. Note, in contrast to the three-point closure, the inside of the vaginal wall is not included in this repair.

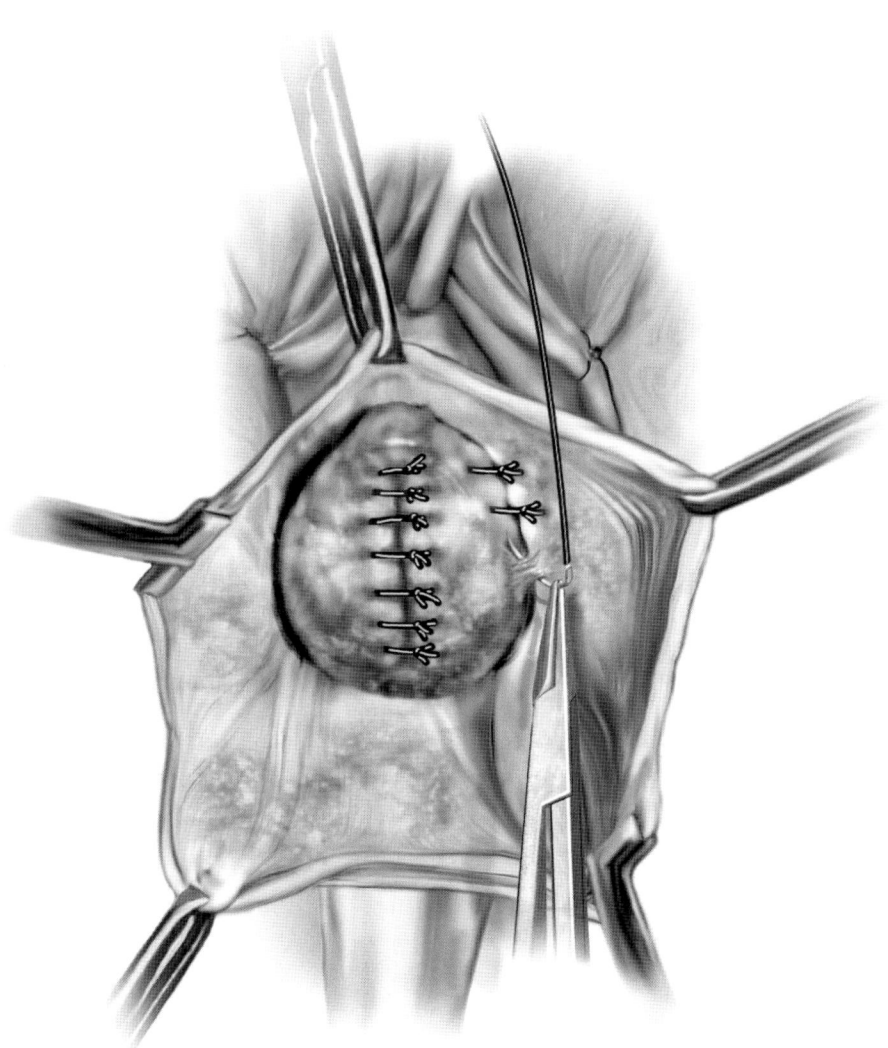

**FIGURE 54–29** Technique of two-point vaginal-paravaginal repair where the lateral edge of the detached fascia is sutured into the upper part of the anterior vaginal wall. Note that this technique does not require complete entrance into the retropubic space or visualization and identification of the obturator internus fascia and the arcus tendineus fascia pelvis.

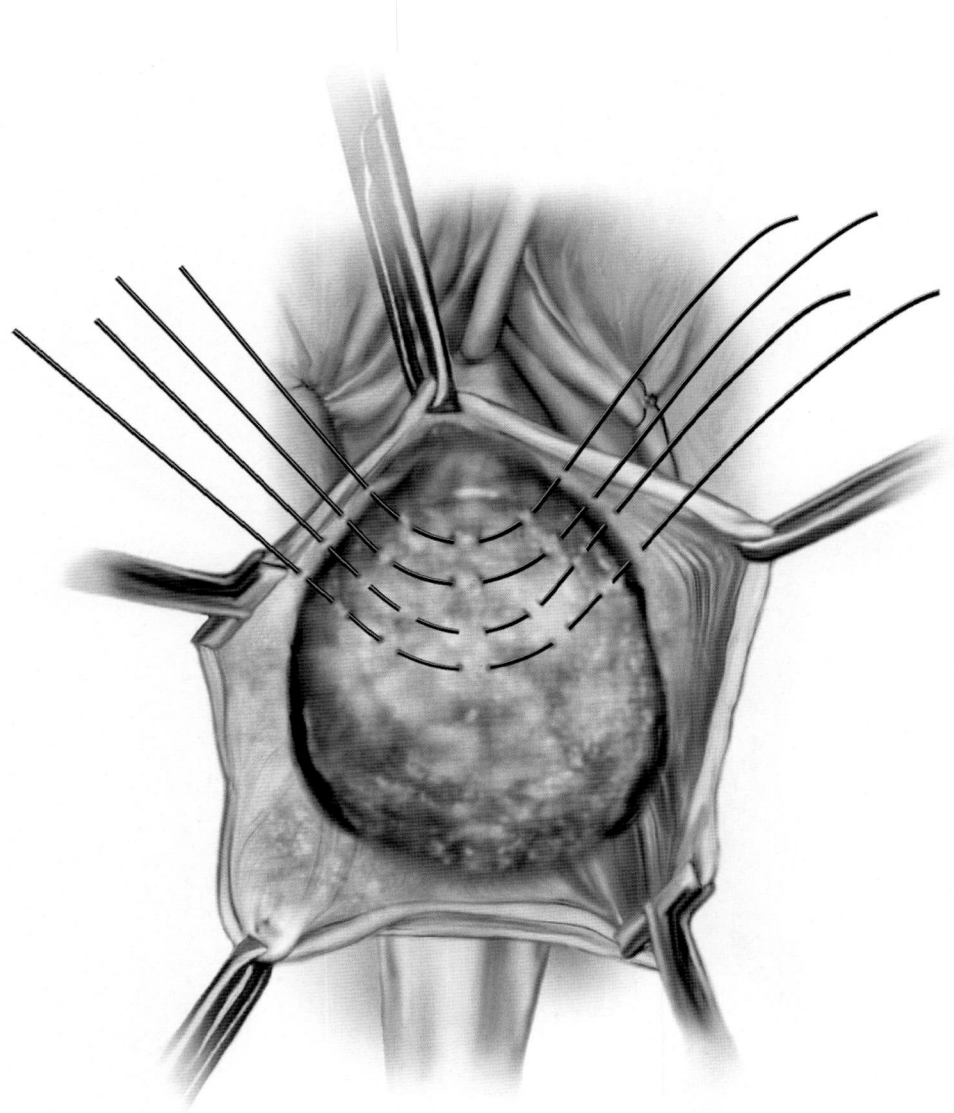

**FIGURE 54–30** Technique of simple anterior colporrhaphy in which the inside of the anterior vaginal wall is included in the plication stitches. Note that this technique will not restore any anterolateral vaginal sulcus and may result in a foreshortened and scarred anterior vaginal segment.

## Posterior Vaginal Wall Defects

Posterior vaginal wall defects can be due to an enterocele, a rectocele, or, very commonly, a combination of both. These defects are commonly associated with varying degrees of vaginal vault prolapsed, as well as anterior vaginal wall prolapse.

### Vaginal Enterocele Repair

Until recently, the anatomy of the cul-de-sac and its relationship to enterocele formation were poorly understood. After hysterectomy, the vaginal apex should be suspended or reattached to the cardinal and uterosacral ligaments. Enteroceles develop as the pubocervical and rectovaginal fasciae separate, allowing a peritoneal sac with its contents to protrude through the fascial defect (Fig. 54–31). Thus, by definition, an enterocele occurs when the peritoneum comes into direct contact with the vaginal epithelium with no intervening fascia. In a woman whose uterus is intact, enteroceles commonly occur posterior to the cervix and anterior to the rectum. Following hysterectomy, enteroceles may occur anterior to the vaginal apex, at the vaginal apex, or posterior to the vaginal apex. In apical enteroceles, the pubocervical fascia anteriorly and the rectovaginal fascia posteriorly separate at the apex. An anterior enterocele is a rare defect in the support of the transverse portion of the pubocervical fascia to the apex of the vagina and should not be confused with a cystocele. The peritoneal sac along with its intra-abdominal contents herniates anterior to the apex and posterior to the base of the bladder. A posterior enterocele is a defect at the superior or transverse portion of the rectovaginal fascia in which the peritoneal sac, with its intra-abdominal contents, herniates anterior to the rectum but posterior to the vaginal apex.

Because an enterocele is a true hernia, it is best repaired by identification of the fascial defect, dissection and excision of the peritoneal sac, reduction of intra-abdominal contents, and closure of the defect. The technique of vaginal enterocele repair involves placing the patient in the dorsal lithotomy position. The bladder should be drained before the first incision. The vagina over the enterocele is grasped with Allis clamps, and the boundaries of the defect are visualized (Figs. 54–32 and 54–33A). A midline incision is made through the vaginal epithelium over the enterocele (see Fig. 54–33A). The vaginal epithelium is dissected sharply away from the enterocele sac, and the sac is completely mobilized all the way up to its neck (Figs. 54–33 through 54–36). This may involve mobilization of the hernia off the urinary bladder (Fig. 54–37), as well as mobilization of the peritoneal sac off the anterior rectal wall (Figs. 54–36 and 54–38). When an enterocele sac is difficult to distinguish from the rectum, differentiation is aided by a rectal examination with simultaneous dissection of the enterocele sac off the anterior rectal wall (see Figs. 54–36A and 54–38B). At times, distinguishing the enterocele sac from a large cystocele may prove difficult (see Fig. 54–40). In this situation, placement of a probe into the bladder or transillumination with a cystoscope may prove helpful. After the enterocele sac has been dissected from the vagina and the rectum, traction is placed on it with two Allis clamps, and the sac is sharply entered (see Figs. 54–36B, 54–37C, 54–38C, 54–39C). The enterocele sac is explored digitally to ensure that no small bowel or omental adhesions are present. The method of closure of the defect depends on whether a vaginal vault suspension procedure is indicated and, if so, what type is to be performed. If adequate vaginal length exists and no suspension procedure is necessary, purse string sutures incorporating the distal portions of the uterosacral ligaments can be used to close the defect (see Fig. 54–34). Fascial reconstruction is accomplished by reapproximating the vagina

with its underlying fascia. However, if a vaginal vault suspension is needed, then the defect is closed as part of the suspension procedure. If a sacrospinous or ileococcygeus suspension is to be performed, the enterocele is closed with a purse string suture, and the pararectal space is entered lateral to the enterocele sac to allow access to these sutures (see Chapter 55, Vaginal Repair of Vaginal Vault Prolapse).

### Rectocele Repair

Repair of a relaxed perineum and repair of a rectocele are two distinct operative procedures, although they are usually performed together. Before beginning the repair, the surgeon should estimate the severity of the rectocele and the perineal defect, as well as the desired postoperative caliber of the vagina and introitus (Fig. 54–40). The ultimate size of the vaginal orifice is determined by placing an Allis clamp on the inner aspect of the labia minora bilaterally and approximating them in the midline. The final vaginal opening should admit two or three fingers, but the surgeon must take into account that the levator ani and perineal muscles are completely relaxed from the anesthesia, and the vagina may further constrict postoperatively.

To begin the repair, a triangular incision is made in the perineal skin (see Fig. 54–40). Sharp dissection is used to detach the posterior vaginal wall off the underlying anterior rectal wall (see Fig. 54–40). The dissection is extended to the apex of the vagina and bilaterally to the rectovaginal space. Many times a strip of vaginal epithelium in the midline is removed, leaving enough vagina to repair the rectocele and leave appropriate vaginal caliber. Historically, posterior colporrhaphy has involved a levatorplasty in which the dissection is extended laterally as far as possible to mobilize perirectal fascia and expose the medial margins of the puborectalis muscle (Fig. 54–41). The terminal ends of the bulbocavernosus and transverse perineal muscles are also freed from the epithelium adherent to the lower vagina. The author prefers to avoid levatorplasty during posterior colporrhaphy except in cases of massive prolapsed, when a levatorplasty is the only mechanism available to decrease the size of the vaginal introitus. Routine use of levatorplasty at the time of posterior colporrhaphy may create vaginal distortion, constriction, postoperative pain, and dyspareunia. The author prefers a site-specific defect approach to rectocele repair. This is best performed by identifying rectovaginal fascial defects with a finger in the rectum elevated toward the vagina (Figs. 54–42 and 54–43). Various possible defects are transverse, longitudinal, or oblique (see Figs. 54–42 and 54–43). The edges of the defects are identified and approximated with interrupted 2-0 absorbable sutures (see Fig. 54–43). Whereas rectocele repair is accomplished by identification of fascial defects and reapproximation of connective tissue, evaluation of the levator hiatus is an entirely different issue. As was previously mentioned in women with an enlarged levator hiatus, it may be appropriate to place another set of interrupted sutures horizontally to narrow the levator hiatus (see Fig. 54–41). This portion of the operation is not necessary in all patients and is independent of the rectocele.

Perineorrhaphy is the third part of the posterior segment reconstruction. The perineal body consists of the anal sphincter, superficial and deep transverse perineal muscles, the bulbocavernosus muscles, and the junction of the rectovaginal fascia to the anal sphincter. Perineorrhaphy involves identification and reconstruction of these components and is discussed separately under the section on perineal surgery.

Figure 54–44 demonstrates repair of a low rectocele with various defects; note the mobilization and approximation of the fascial edges.

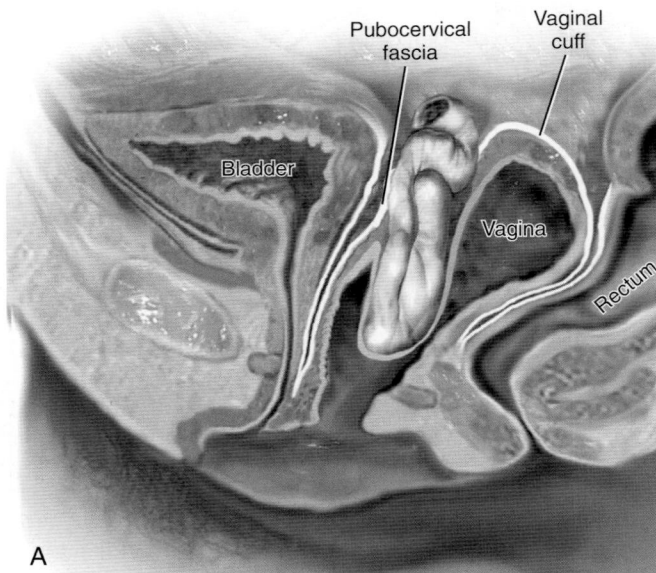

A

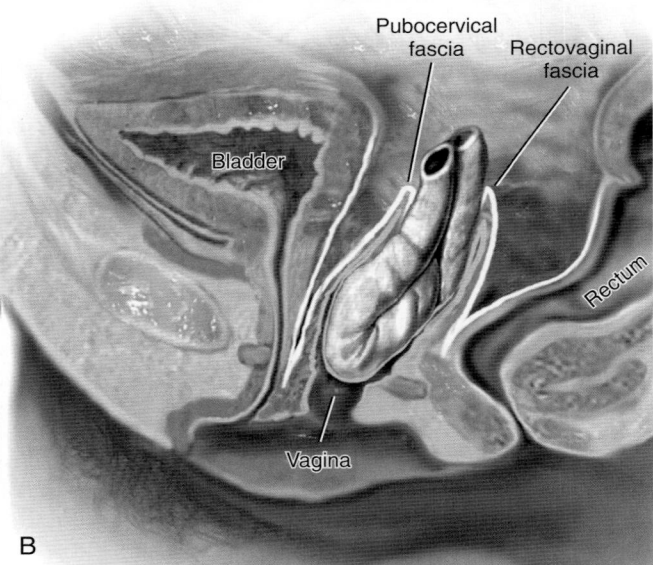

B

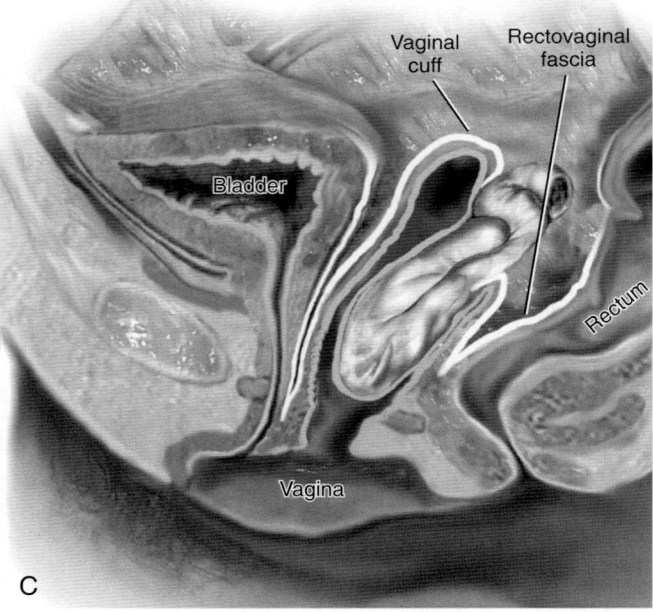

C

**FIGURE 54–31** Cross-section of the pelvic floor showing various anatomic locations of enteroceles. **A.** Anterior enterocele defect in the pubocervical fascia near its attachment to the vaginal apex. The peritoneal sac with its contents protrudes into the vaginal opening. **B.** Apical enterocele defect at the vaginal apex; the peritoneal sac protrudes between the pubocervical fascia anterior and the rectovaginal fascia posterior. **C.** Posterior enterocele defect posterior to the vaginal cuff. The peritoneal sac protrudes through the defect into the rectovaginal fascia.

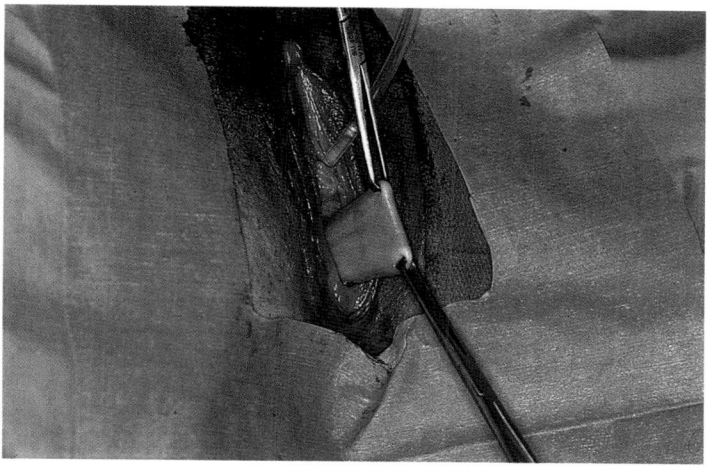

**FIGURE 54–32** High posterior enterocele. Allis clamps apply traction to the most dependent portion of the enterocele. In this patient, the vaginal apex, anterior vaginal wall, and distal posterior vaginal wall are all well supported. This thus represents an isolated high posterior enterocele.

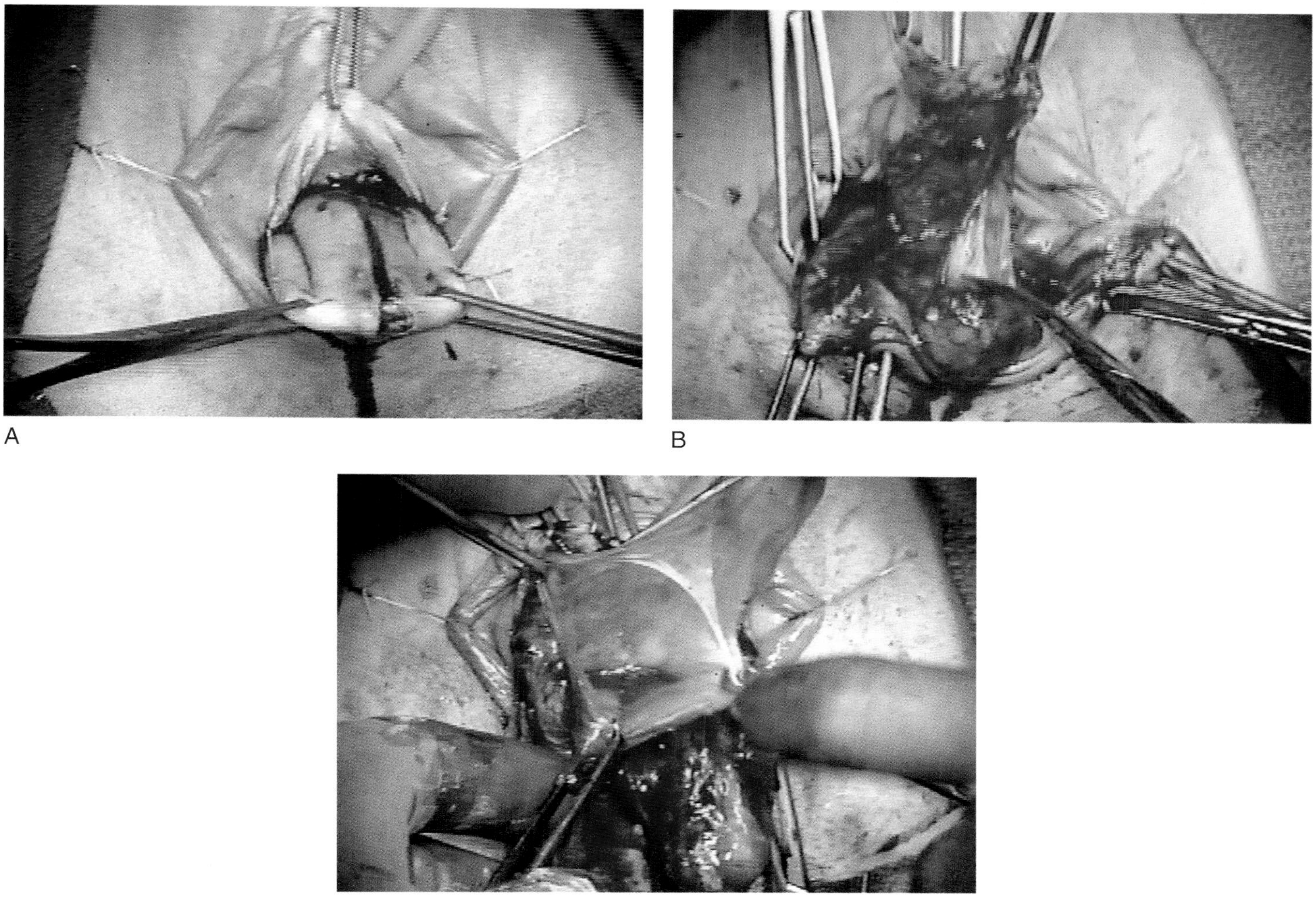

A

B

C

**FIGURE 54–33** Large enterocele associated with vaginal vault prolapse. **A.** The midline posterior vaginal wall incision extends from the proximal edge of the pubocervical fascia to the proximal edge of the rectovaginal fascia. **B.** Sharp dissection is used to separate the enterocele sac from the anterior rectal wall. **C.** The enterocele sac has been excised to its neck.

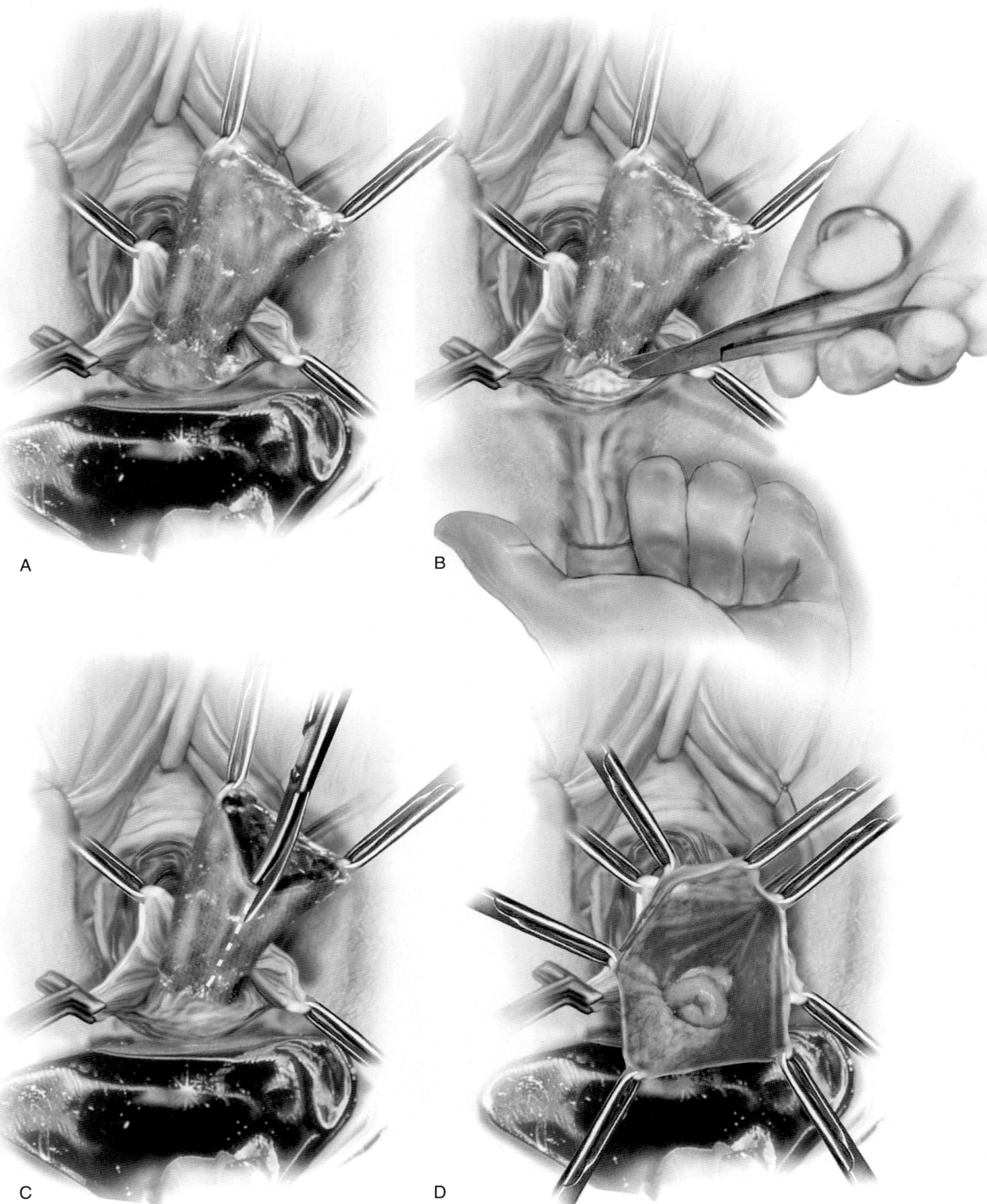

A

B

C

D

**FIGURE 54–34** Dissection and vaginal repair of enterocele. **A.** The enterocele sac has been completely mobilized off the vaginal epithelium. **B.** A finger in the rectum facilitates sharp dissection of the enterocele sac off the anterior wall of the rectum. **C.** The enterocele sac is sharply entered. **D.** The peritoneum has been excised, and the cul-de-sac is exposed.

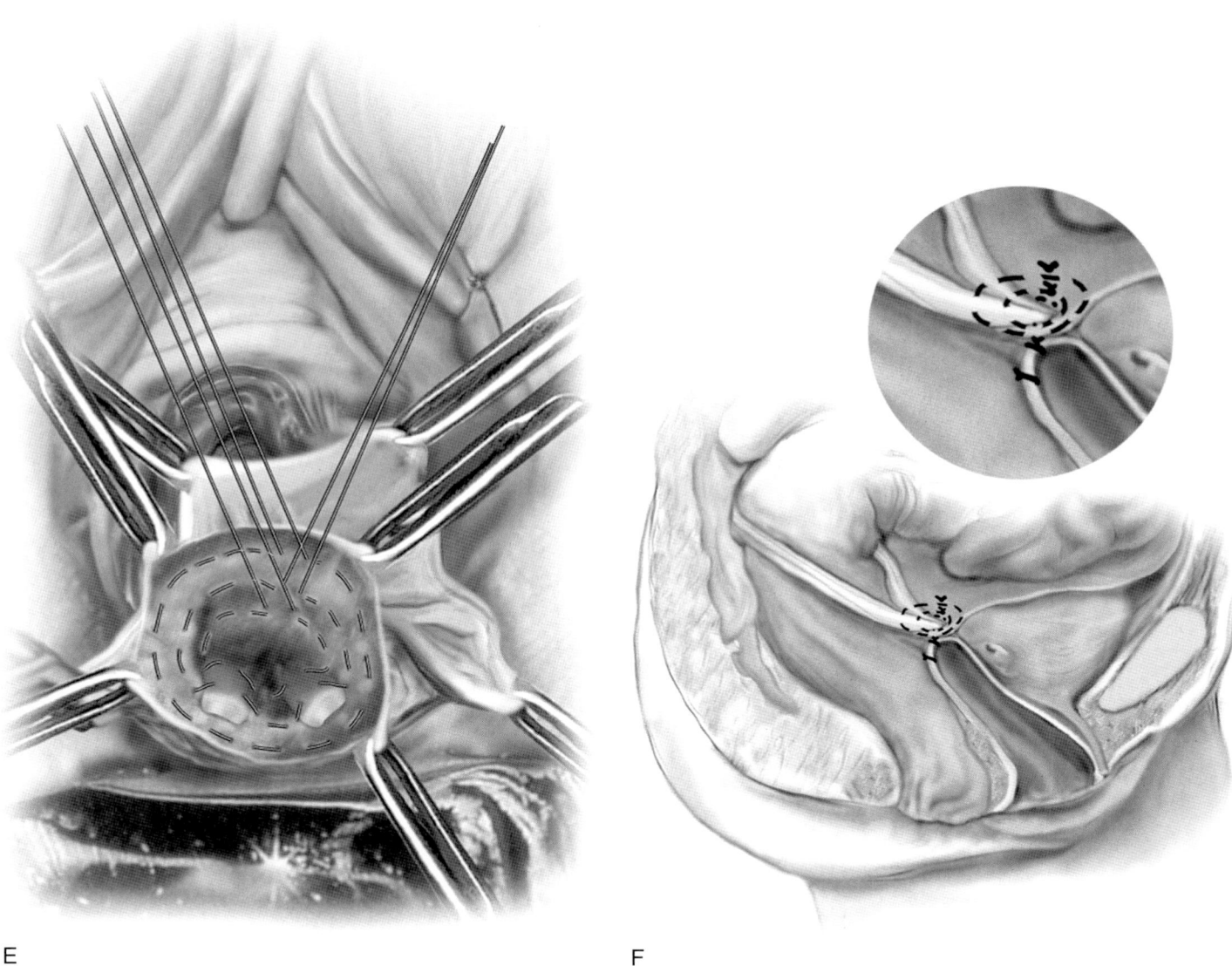

E

F

**FIGURE 54–34, cont'd  E.** A series of purse string sutures incorporating the distal ends of the uterosacral ligaments are placed to close the defect at its neck. **F.** The vaginal apex is attached to the plicated uterosacral ligaments.

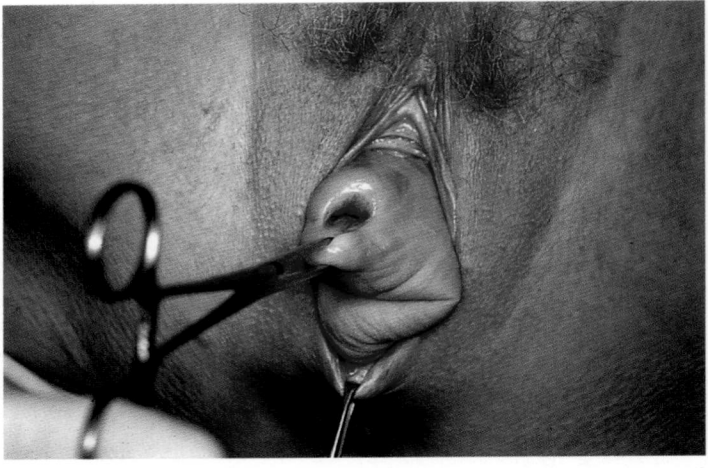

A

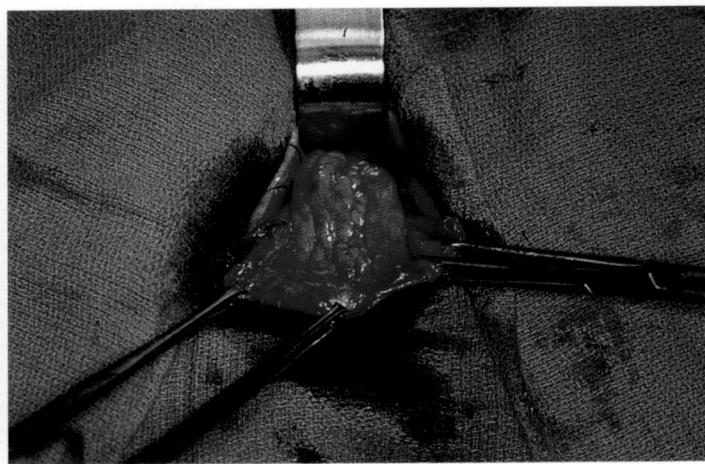

B

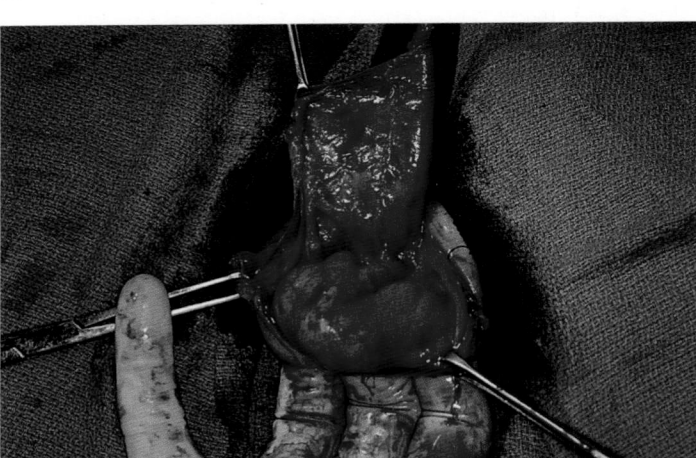

C

**FIGURE 54–35  A.** Complete uterine prolapse with a large enterocele. **B.** The uterus has been removed; note the complete prolapse of the vaginal vault with a large enterocele. **C.** The enterocele sac is sharply dissected off the posterior vaginal wall up to the level of the neck of the hernia.

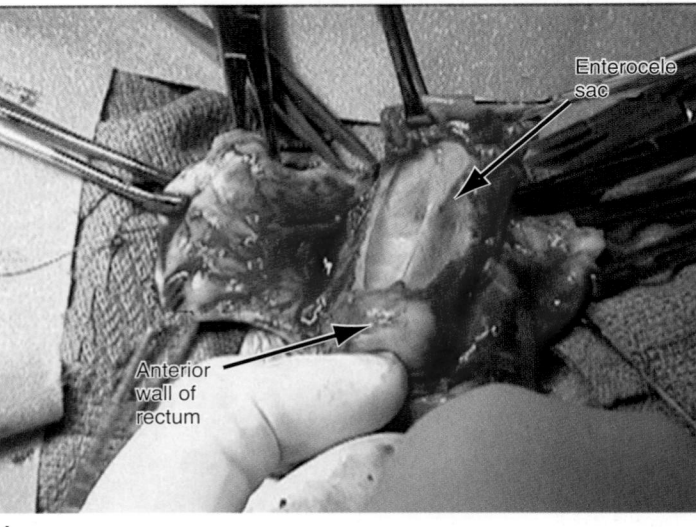

Enterocele sac

Anterior wall of rectum

A

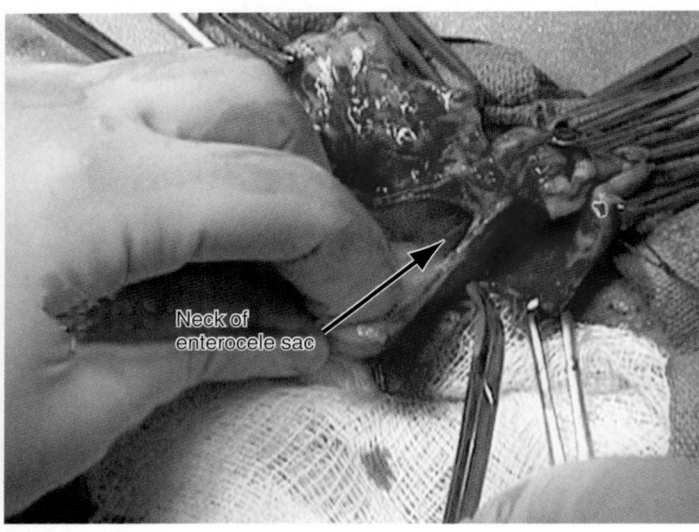

Neck of enterocele sac

B

**FIGURE 54–36  A.** Note that the posterior enterocele is identified with a finger in the rectum, and the enterocele sac has been mobilized off the anterior wall of the rectum. **B.** The enterocele sac has been sharply entered, and the neck of the enterocele is identified.

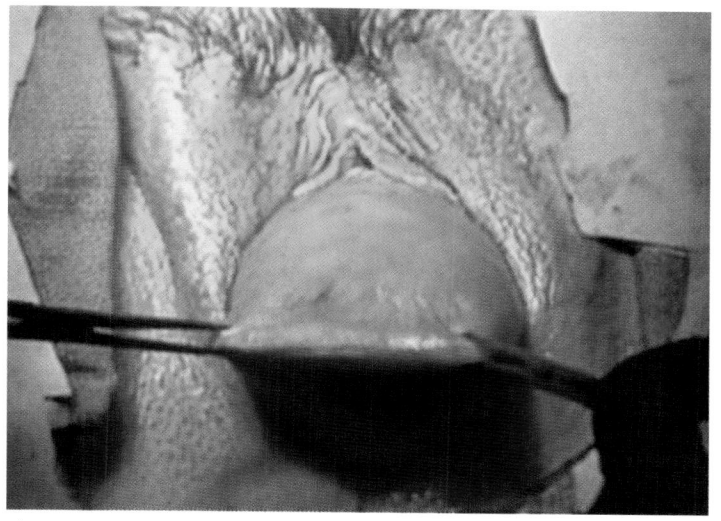

A

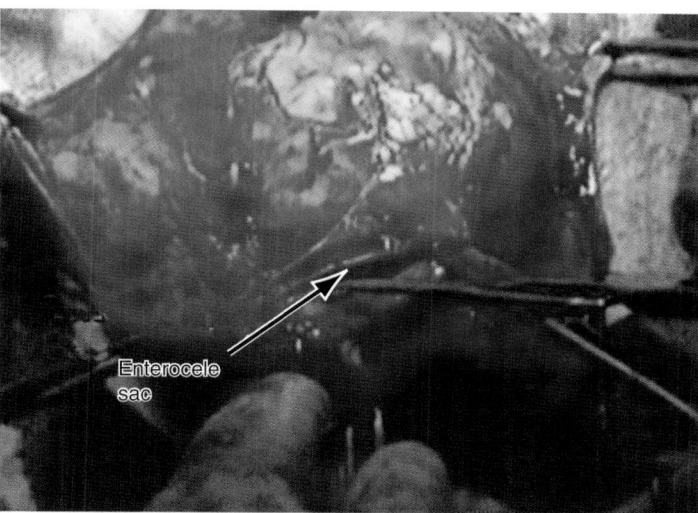

B

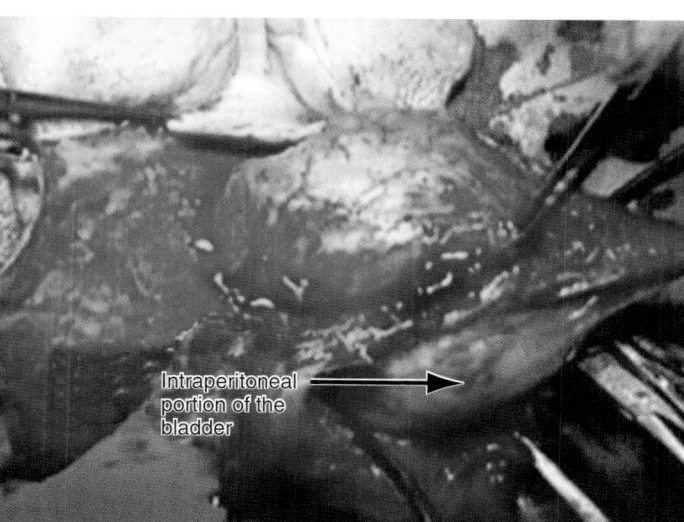

C

**FIGURE 54–37  A.** Note complete vaginal vault eversion secondary to a large enterocele and cystocele. **B.** The Allis clamps are grasped at the apex of the vagina. **C.** The anterior vaginal wall has been dissected off the underlying cystocele. At the base of the cystocele or the apex of the vagina, the enterocele sac is identified and sharply entered. The large intraperitoneal portion of the cystocele is identified.

UNIT 3  ■  SECTION B

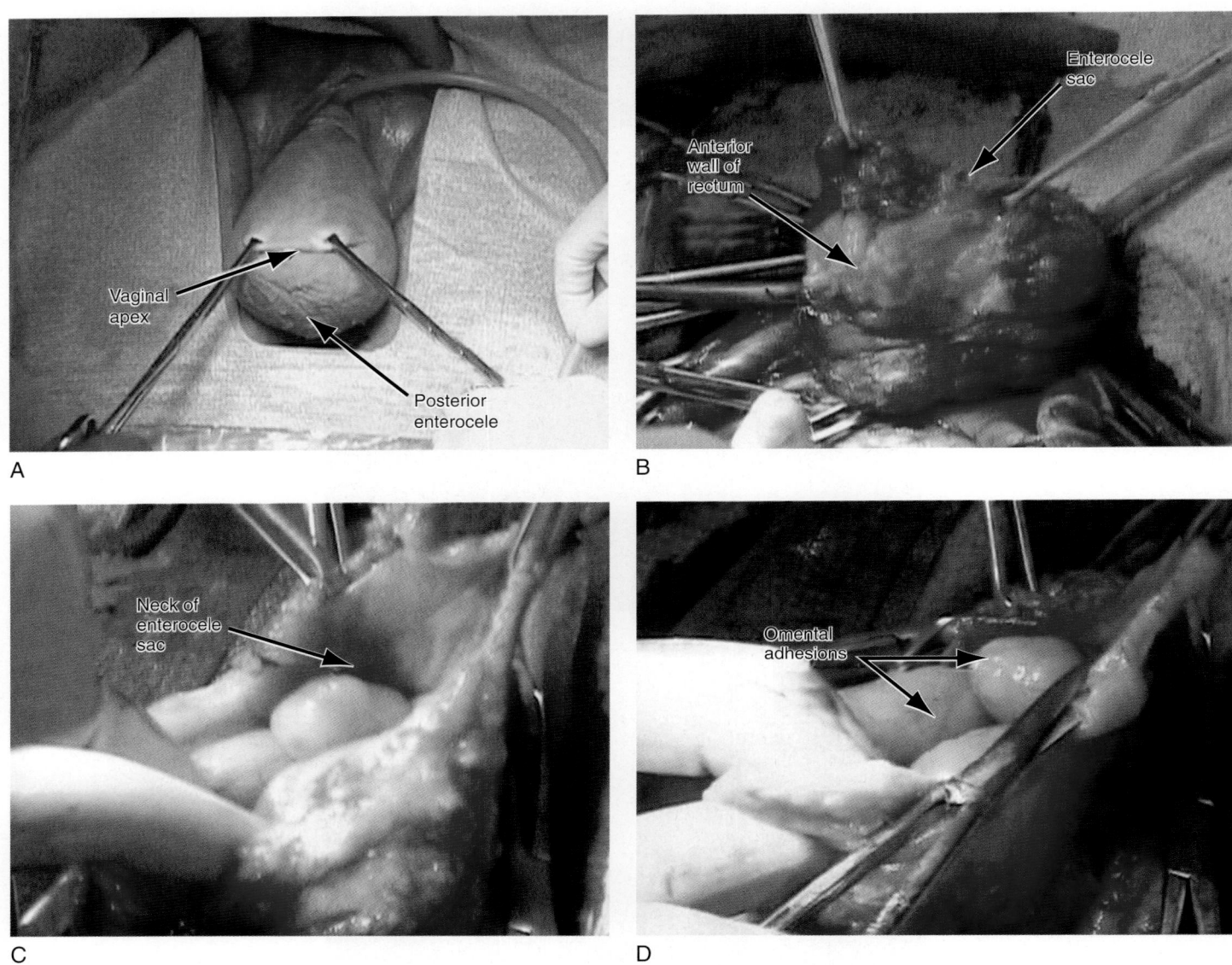

**FIGURE 54–38** Large vaginal prolapse. **A.** The apex of the vagina is grasped with two Allis clamps, and posterior to this a large enterocele is identified. **B.** Sharp dissection with a finger in the rectum facilitates dissection of the enterocele sac away from the anterior wall of the rectum. **C.** The enterocele sac has been sharply identified, and the neck of the enterocele is noted. **D.** Note extensive omental adhesions in the cul-de-sac.

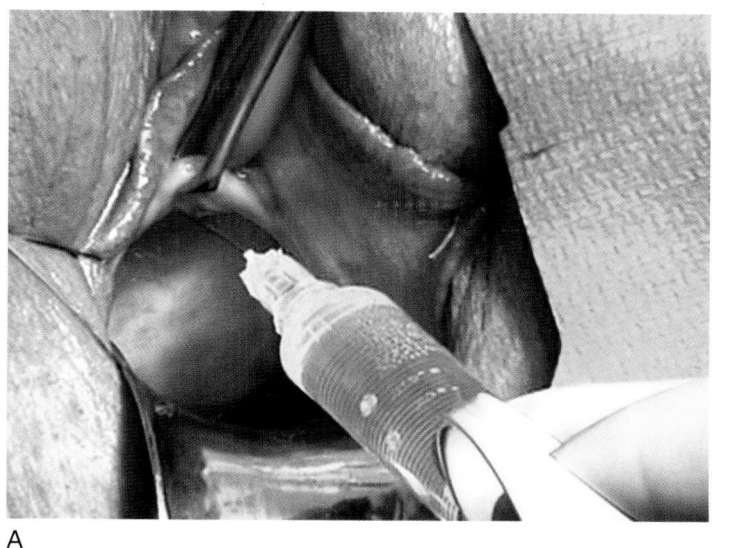

A

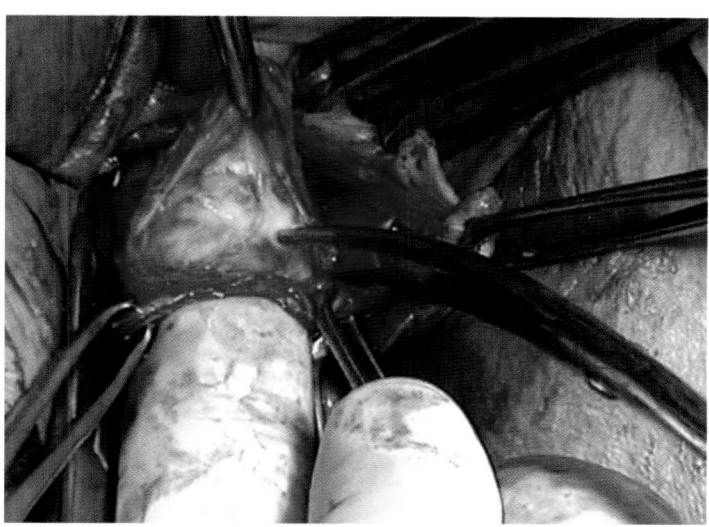

B

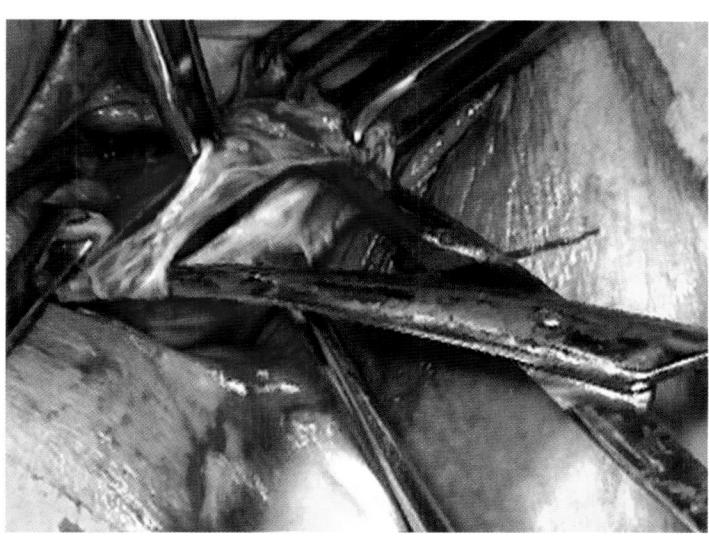

C

**FIGURE 54–39** Anterior enterocele. **A.** The prolapse is identified; note that the prolapse is anterior to the apex of the vagina, denoting that this is a high cystocele or an anterior enterocele. **B.** The vaginal wall has been opened, and dissection of the prolapse off the apex of the vagina is being performed. **C.** The enterocele sac is identified and sharply entered.

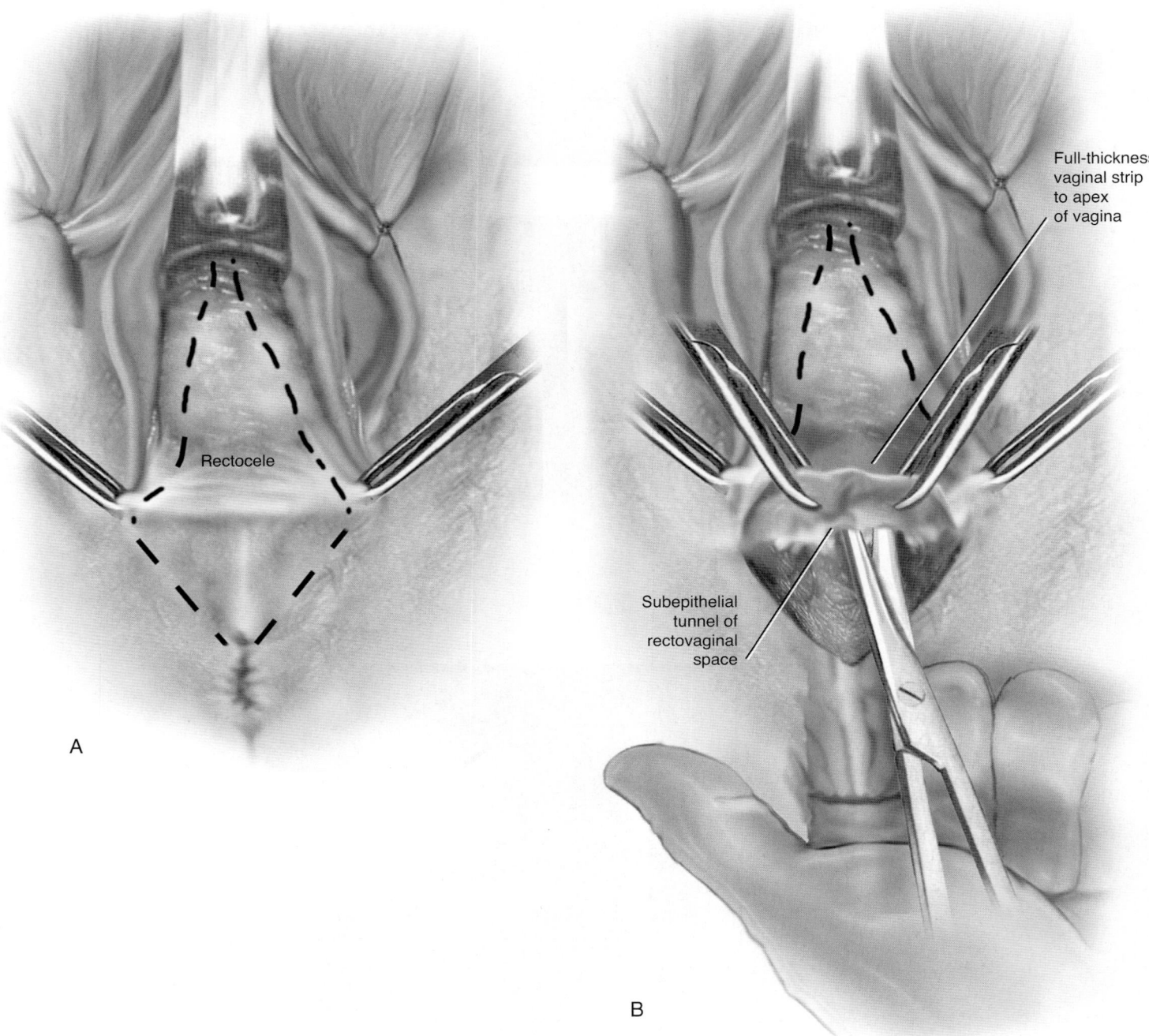

Rectocele

A

Full-thickness
vaginal strip
to apex
of vagina

Subepithelial
tunnel of
rectovaginal
space

B

**FIGURE 54–40  A.** The dashed line indicates the area of perineal skin and posterior vaginal wall to be excised. **B.** Sharp dissection of the posterior vaginal wall from the anterior rectal wall; dissection is aided with a finger in the rectum.

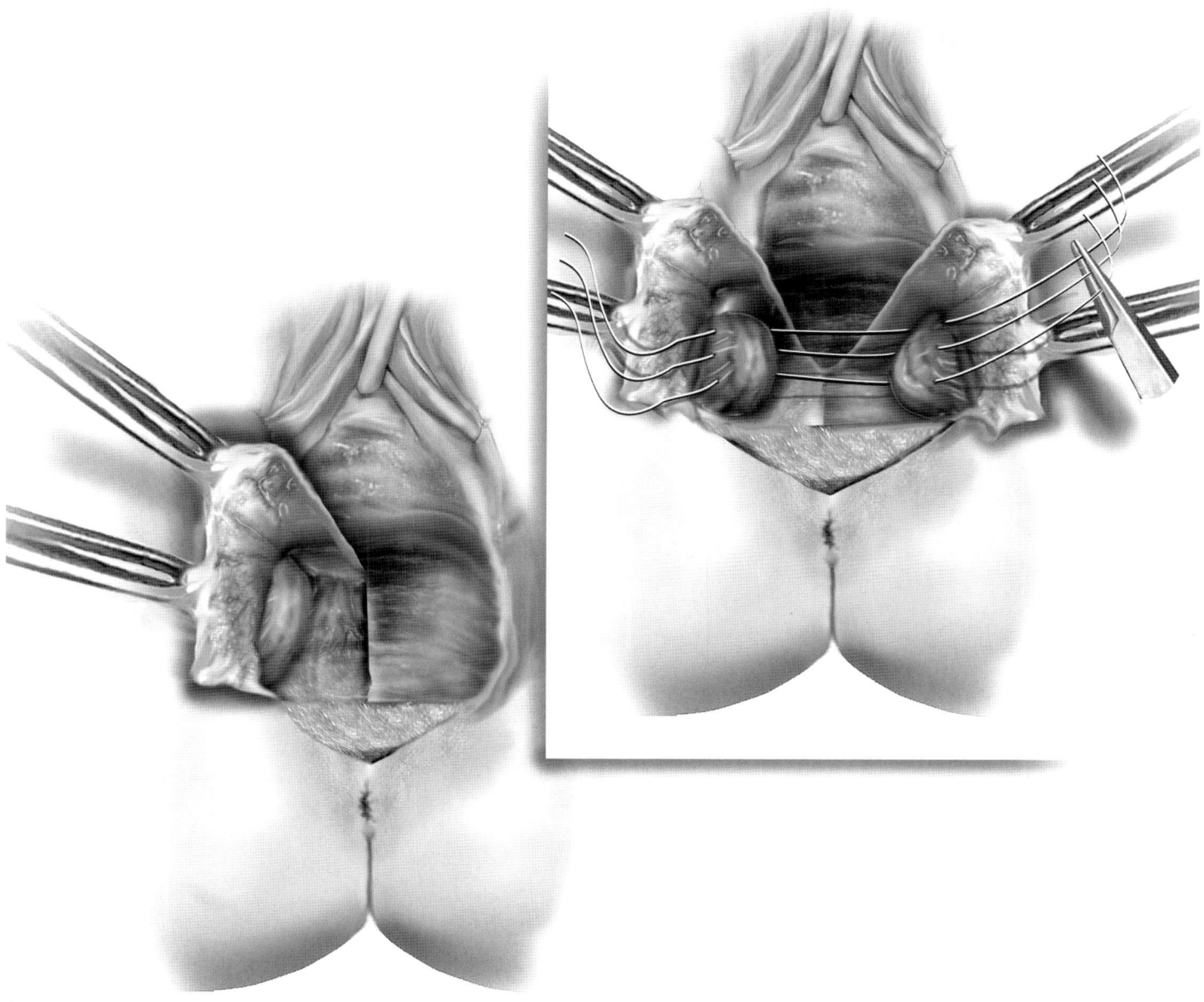

A

**FIGURE 54–41** Technique of levatorplasty. **A.** The posterior vaginal wall has been opened up, and the levator muscles are identified laterally. Absorbable sutures are taken through the levator muscles on each side. Note that the fascia over the anterior wall of the rectum is totally ignored, and the support that occurs is based on the levator muscles' being tied across the midline.

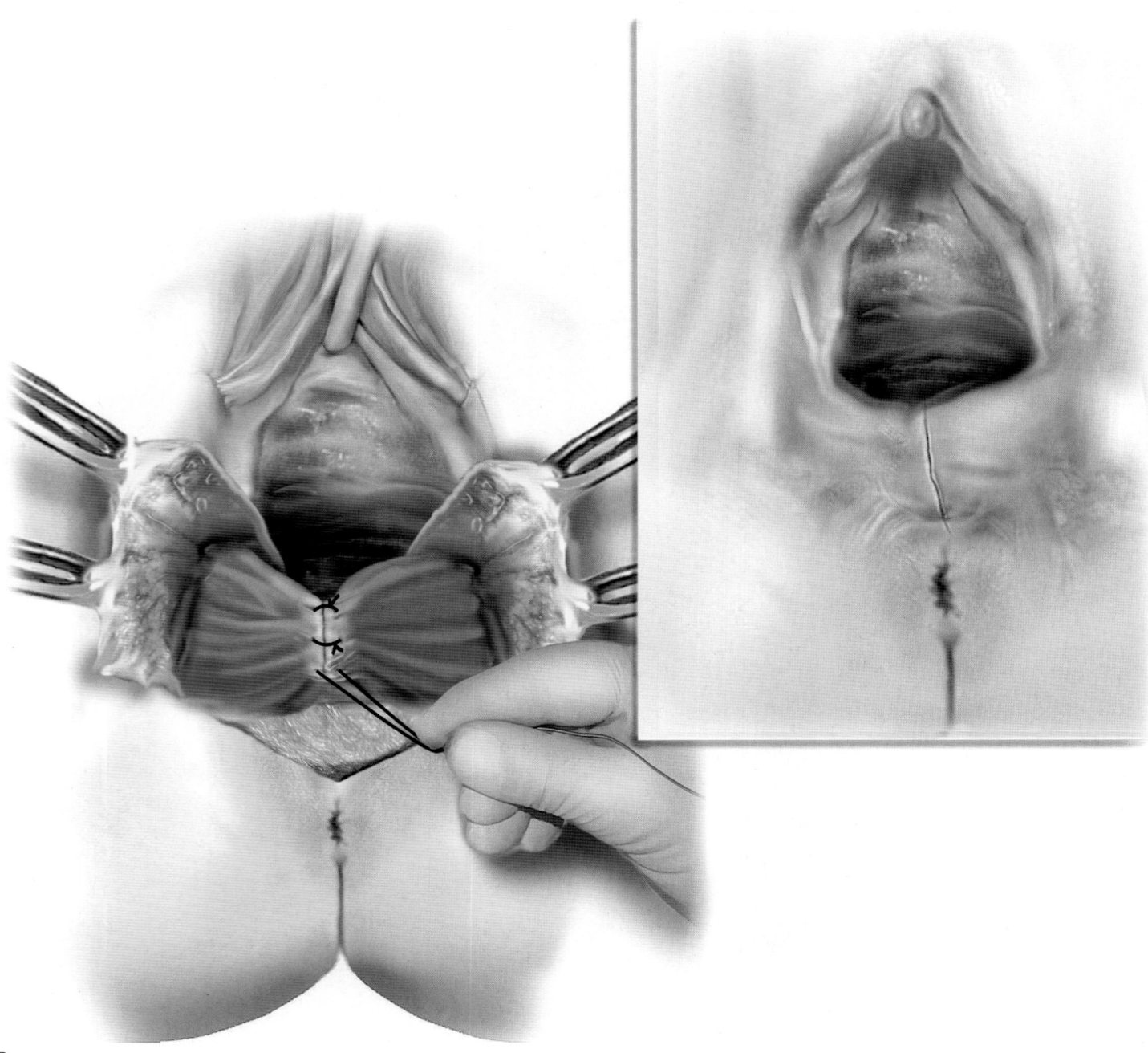

B

**FIGURE 54–41, cont'd B.** The levators have been tied, and a posterior vaginal ridge is created that is intended to support the posterior vaginal wall.

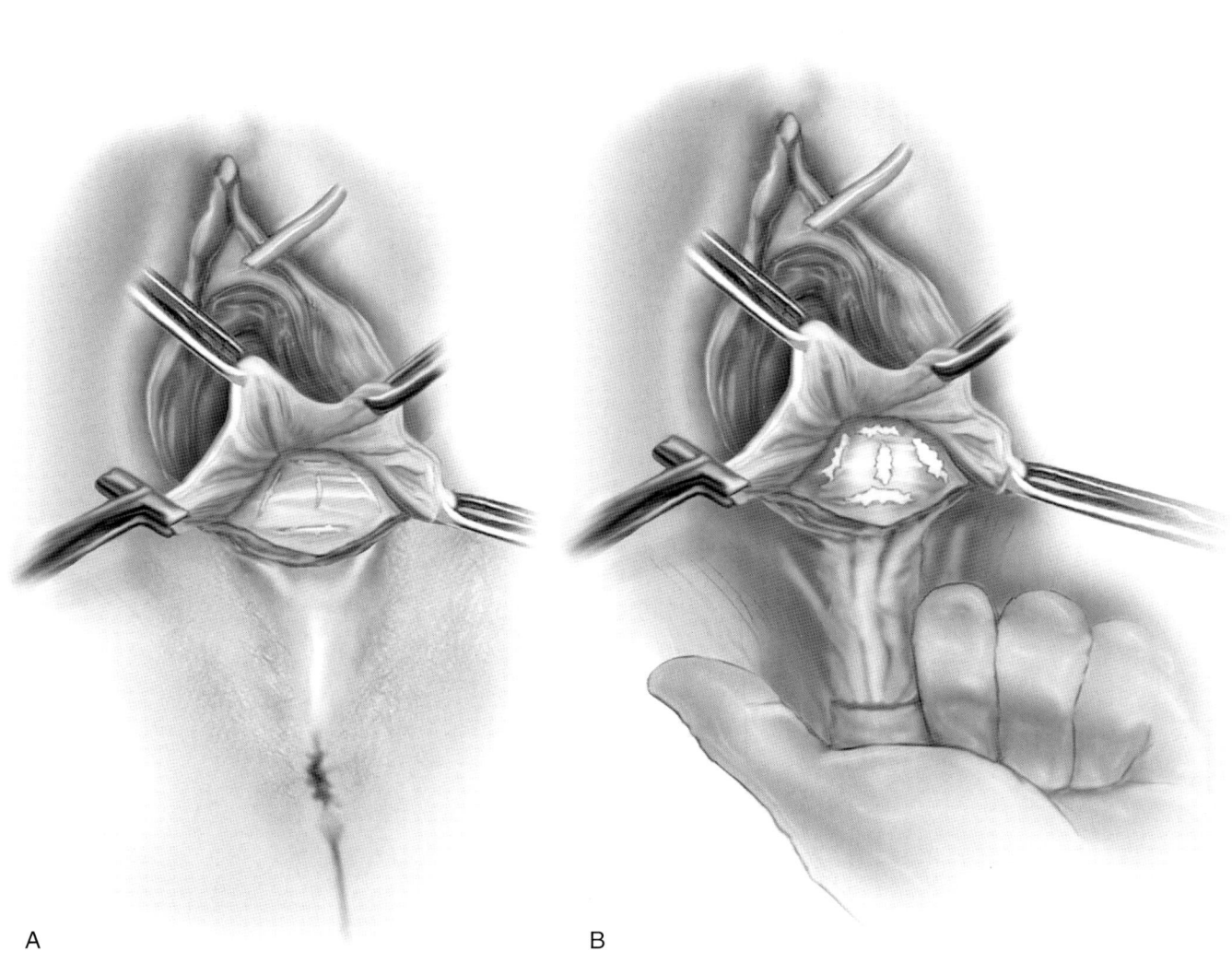

A

B

**FIGURE 54–42 A.** Various potential defects that may be encountered at the time of rectocele repair. **B.** Placing a finger in the rectum and elevating the anterior rectal wall help to further delineate fascial tears.

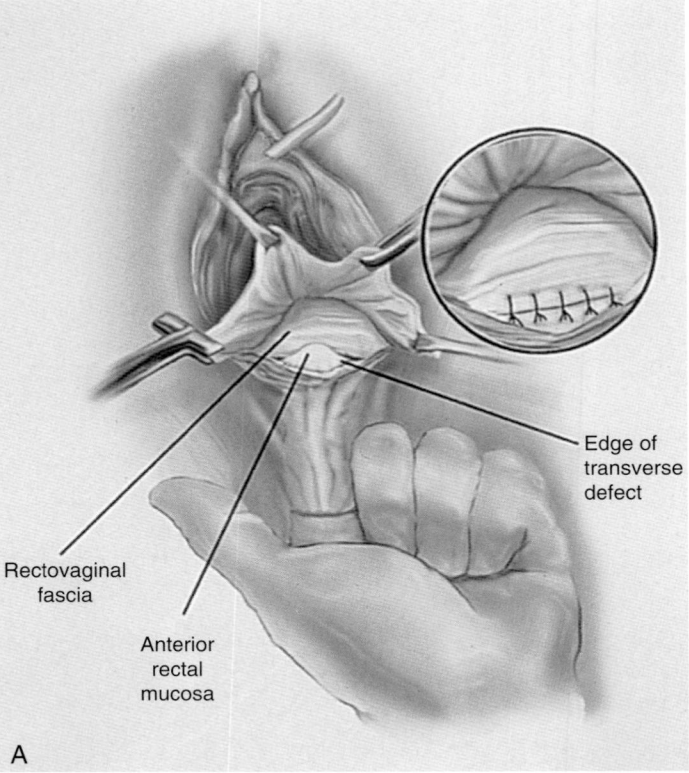

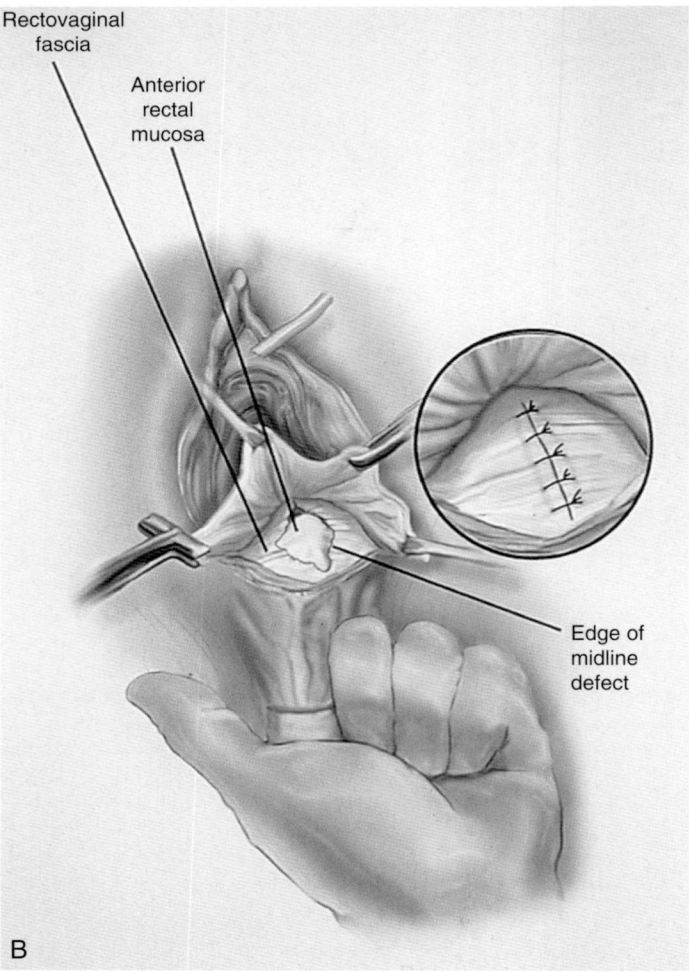

**FIGURE 54–43  A.** A low transverse defect between the perineum and the distal edge of the rectovaginal fistula. **Inset.** Defect-specific closure with interrupted sutures. **B.** A midline longitudinal defect. **Inset.** Defect-specific closure with interrupted sutures.

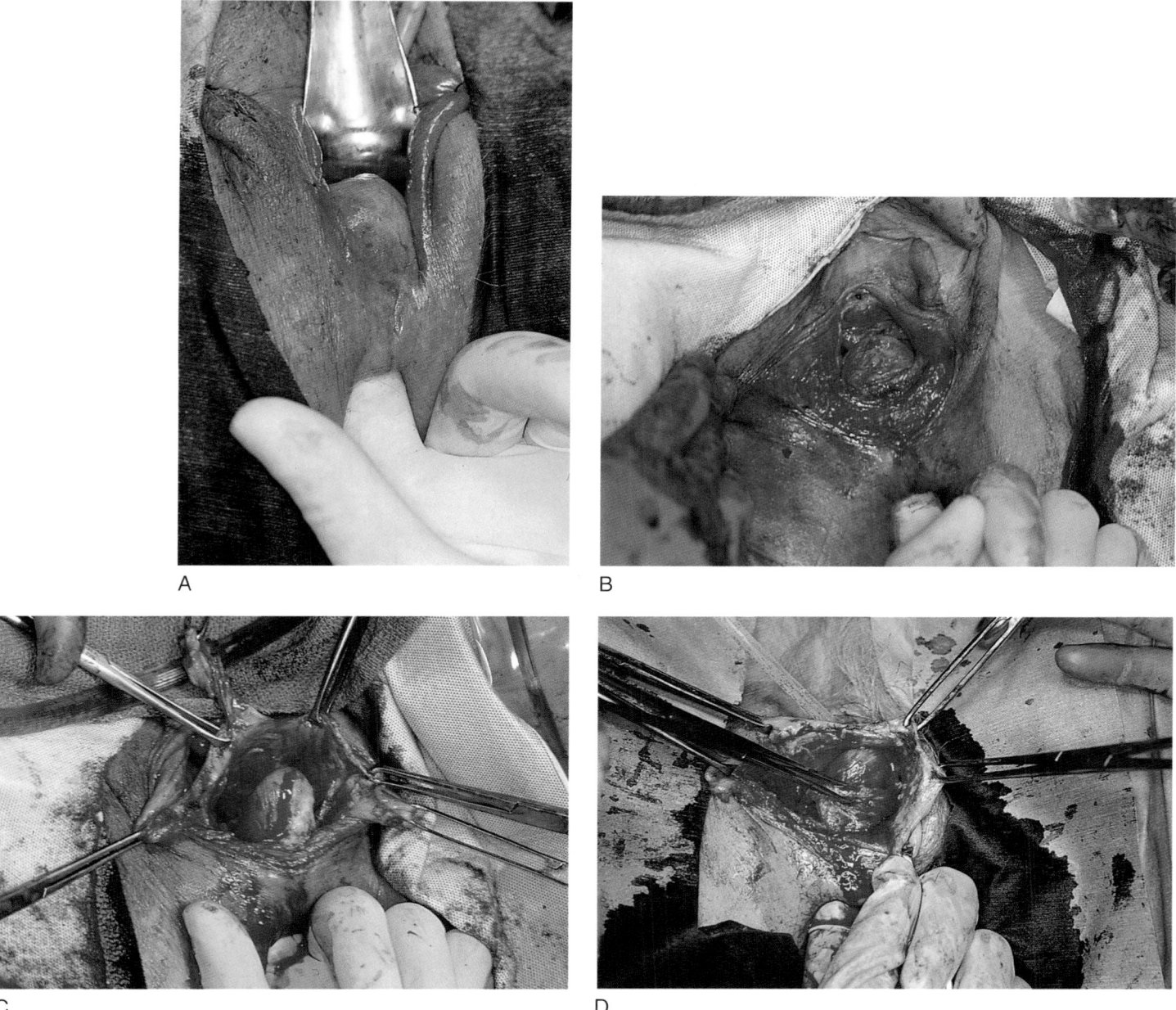

A

B

C

D

**FIGURE 54–44 A.** A distal rectocele with attenuated perineum. **B.** The initial wedge of perineal skin has been removed. This incision should be tailored to the desired size of the introitus. This can be estimated by placing two Allis clamps on the edges of the incision and approximating them across the midline. **C.** Sharp dissection has been utilized to completely mobilize the posterior vaginal wall from the anterior rectal wall. Note that a narrow piece of vagina has been dissected in the midline. The width of this segment of vagina is determined by estimating the amount of vagina that will need to be trimmed. **D.** Identification of fascia to be utilized for plication over the anterior rectal wall.

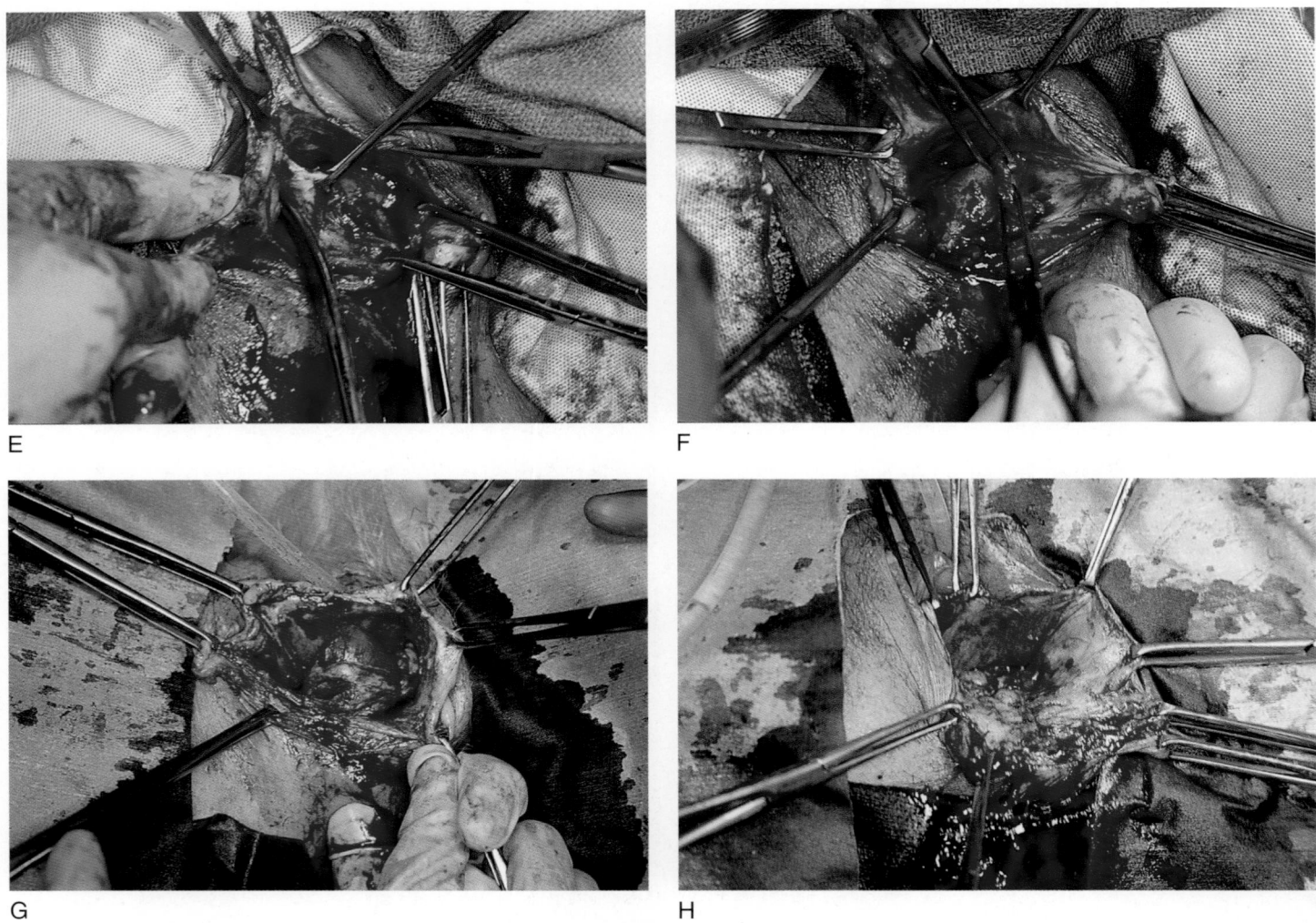

E

F

G

H

**FIGURE 54–44, cont'd   E.** Mobilization of the fascia off the posterior vaginal wall. **F.** The fascia has been completely mobilized off the right vaginal wall. Note that the midline wedge of vaginal skin has no underlying fascia, confirming a midline defect. **G.** A high transverse defect is demonstrated. Note that the fascia is present over the distal anterior rectal wall. **H.** Completed fascial defect repair. Note that durable fascia has been plicated over the entire anterior wall.

High rectoceles are very commonly associated with an enterocele. On examination the vagina over an enterocele will usually have a thin, smooth appearance in comparison with the thicker-appearing mucosa over the rectocele (Fig. 54–45). In cases of high posterior vaginal wall defects, it is important to dissect up to the vaginal apex in search of an enterocele sac. Figure 54–46 demonstrates the technique of rectocele repair in conjunction with vaginal suspension and perineal reconstruction. Figure 54–47 shows how suspending the full thickness of the posterior vaginal wall overlying an enterocele can contribute to the overall support of the entire posterior vaginal wall (see section on high uterosacral ligament suspension in Chapter 55). At times, posterior colporrhaphy with perineoplasty is done in conjunction with external anal sphincter repair (Fig. 54–48).

Some surgeons have advocated augmenting posterior colporrhaphy with an intervening mesh. At present, the indications and preferred material for such a repair remain controversial. Figures 54–49 and 54–50 demonstrate the technique of utilization of a mesh to augment posterior vaginal wall repair.

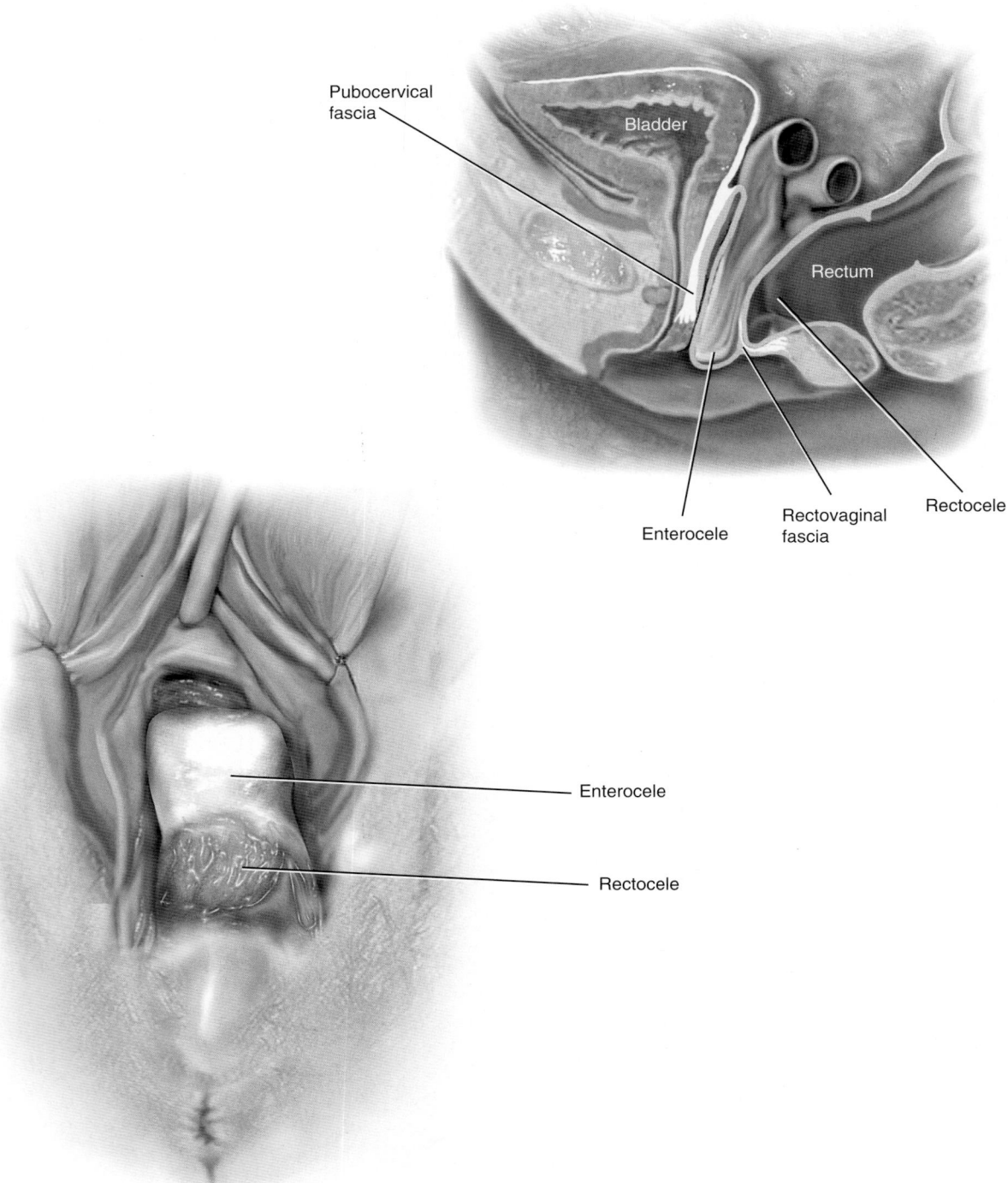

**FIGURE 54–45** High posterior vaginal wall defect secondary to a posterior enterocele in conjunction with a rectocele. On examination, the vagina over the enterocele wall appears smoother and thinner.

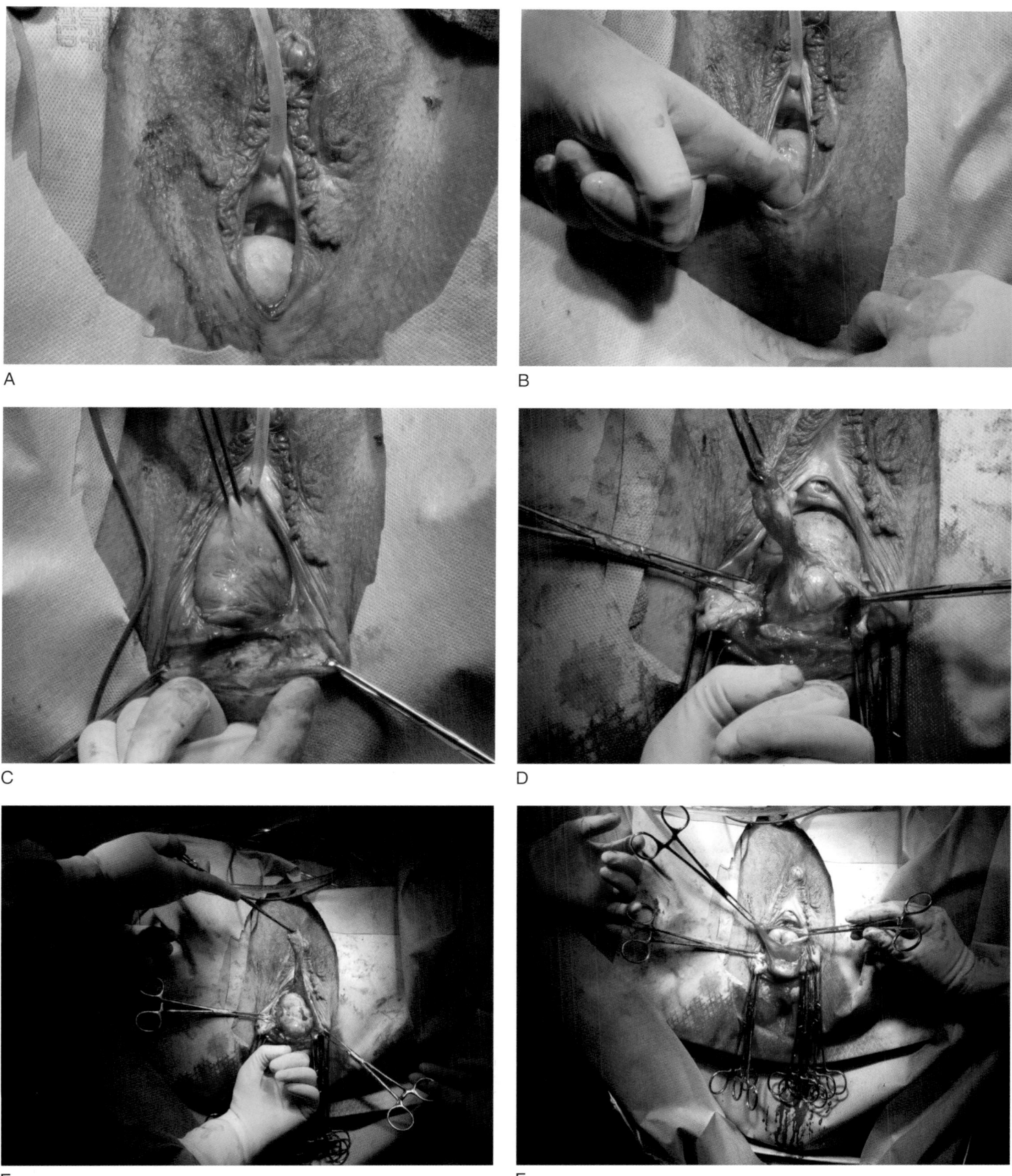

**FIGURE 54–46** Patient with recurrent prolapse secondary to a rectocele and enterocele. **A.** Large posterior vaginal wall defect with a somewhat foreshortened vagina. **B.** Note the previous inappropriate buildup of perineal skin. **C.** The perineal skin has been cut longitudinally down to the level of the posterior fourchette. **D.** With a finger in the rectum, sharp dissection is used to mobilize the posterior vaginal wall off the anterior wall of the rectum. **E.** The dissection is extended cephalad; note the excessive amount of pararectal, preperitoneal fat encountered. **F.** The enterocele sac is sharply entered.

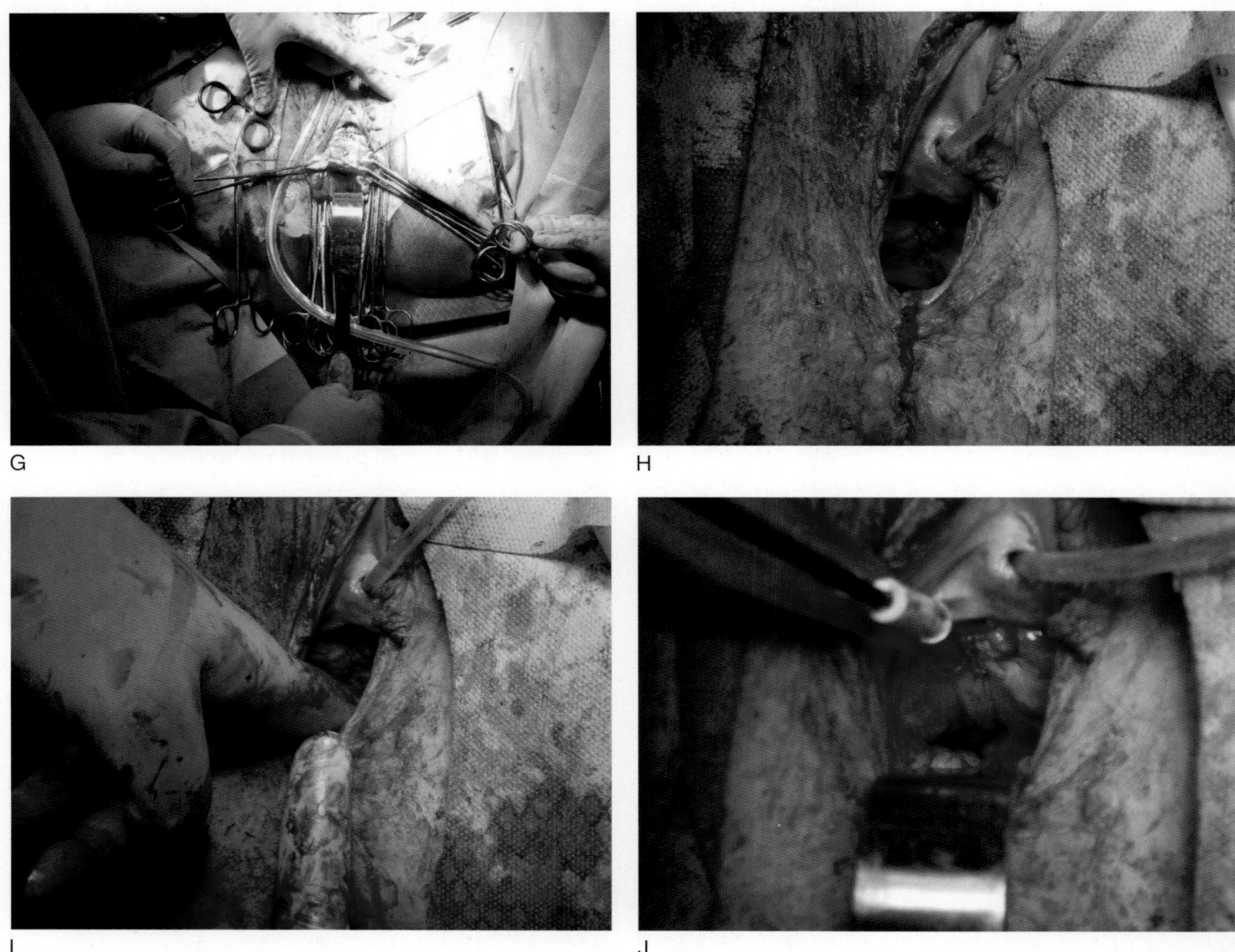

**FIGURE 54–46, cont'd** **G.** High intraperitoneal uterosacral sutures have been placed (see Chapter 55) and passed through the vaginal apex to suspend the vaginal vault. **H.** The vaginal vault stitches have been tied, the rectocele plicated, and the perineum reconstructed. **I.** Note the perpendicular relationship between the perineum and the posterior vaginal wall. **J.** Note the good vaginal depth with no deviation of the vaginal axis.

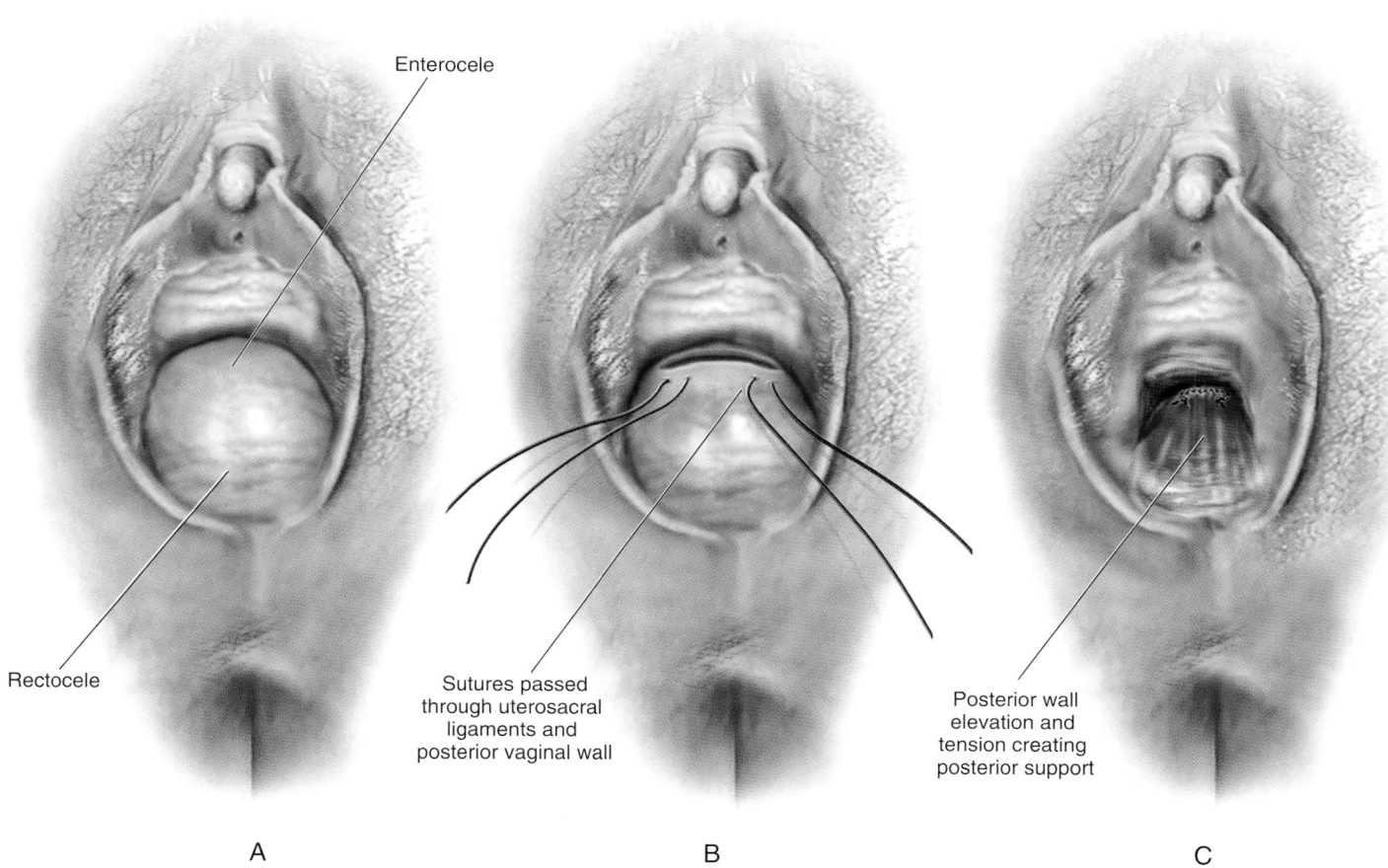

Enterocele

Rectocele

Sutures passed
through uterosacral
ligaments and
posterior vaginal wall

Posterior wall
elevation and
tension creating
posterior support

A                                          B                                          C

**FIGURE 54–47  A.** Posterior vaginal wall defect secondary to an enterocele and rectocele. **B.** After entry into the enterocele sac, intraperitoneal suspension sutures are brought out through the full thickness of the vaginal wall at the level of the apex. **C.** Tying of these sutures after closure of the vaginal incision at the apex not only will result in an increase in vaginal length but also will contribute to the overall support of the entire posterior vaginal wall.

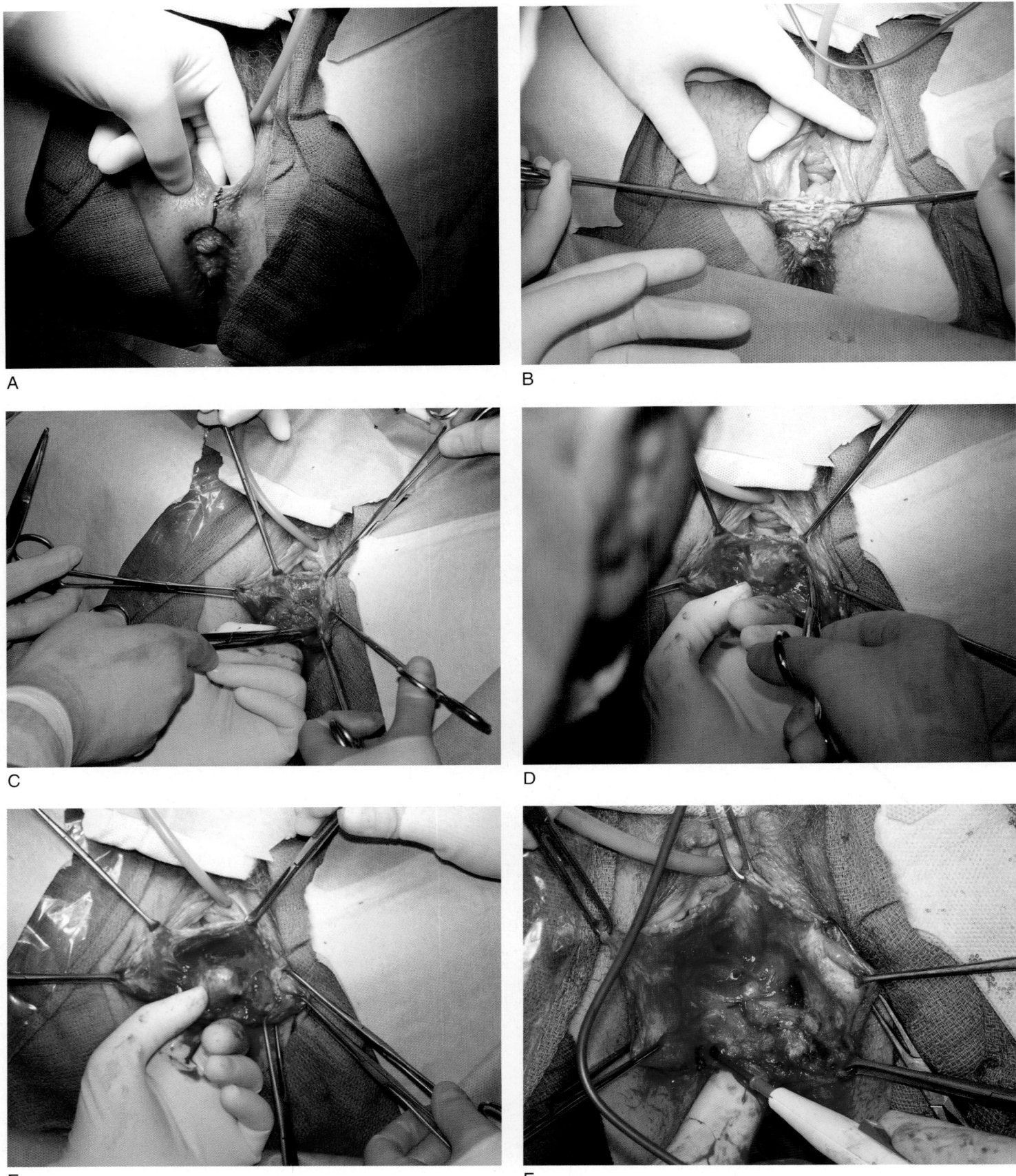

**FIGURE 54–48** Patient with a symptomatic rectocele and fecal incontinence secondary to a sphincter defect. **A.** Perineal incision to be made is marked. **B.** After hydrodissection, a perineal incision is made. **C.** Sharp dissection, with a finger in the rectum, is utilized to mobilize the perineal skin and the posterior vaginal wall. **D.** Sharp dissection is extended cephalad toward the vaginal apex. **E.** The rectocele is isolated. **F.** A defect-specific rectocele repair has been performed and monopolar cautery is being used to identify viable external anal sphincter.

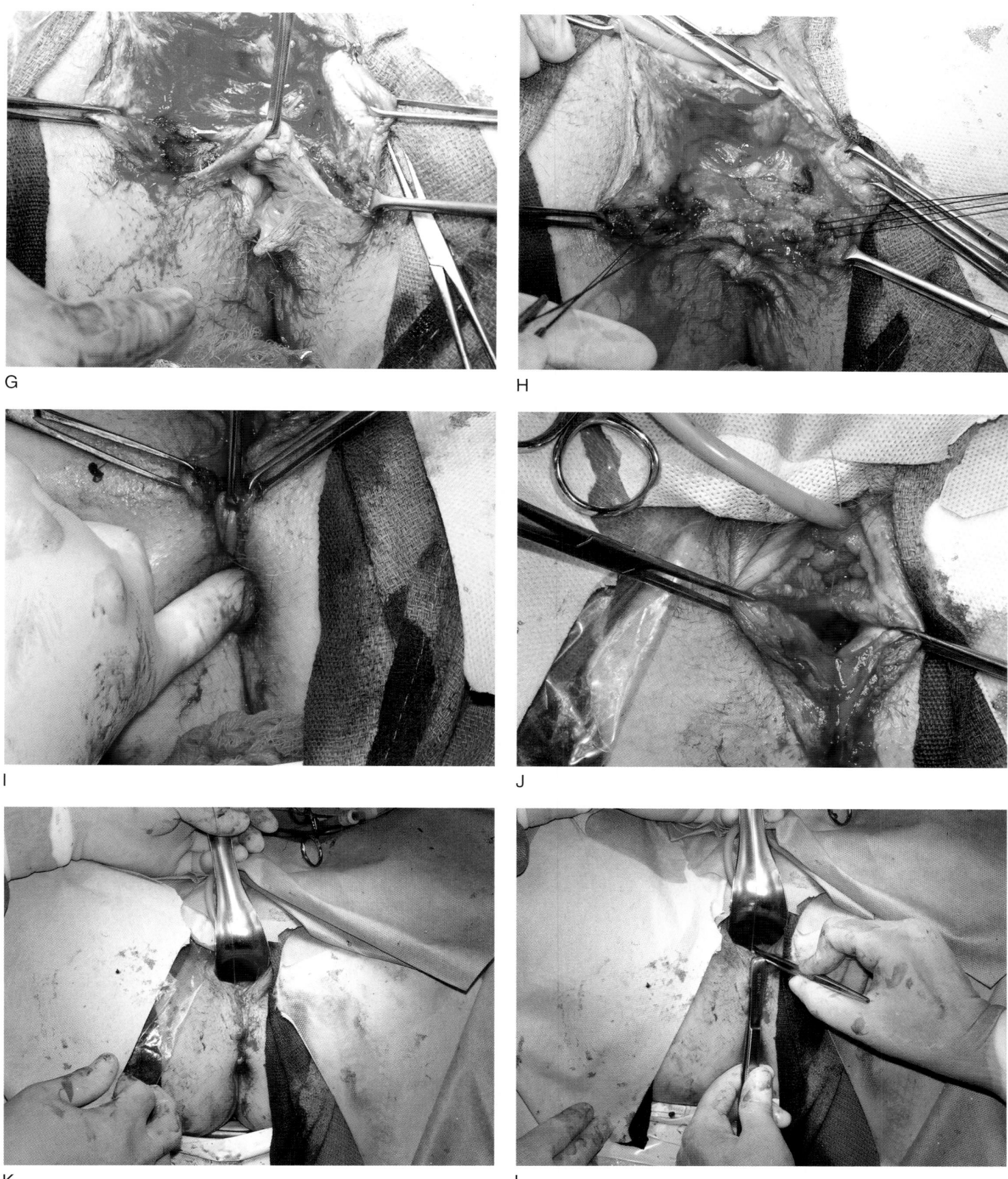

**FIGURE 54–48, cont'd  G.** Note the widened caliber of the anal opening before sphincter repair. **H.** Sutures have been passed through the retracted ends of the external anal sphincter. **I.** After the sphincteroplasty has been performed, note the significant decrease in caliber of the opening of the anus. **J.** The upper portion of the vaginal incision is closed with a fine continuous absorbable suture. **K.** The repair is completed. Note the significant building up of the perineal body. **L.** The appropriate perpendicular relationship between the perineum and the posterior vaginal wall is demonstrated.

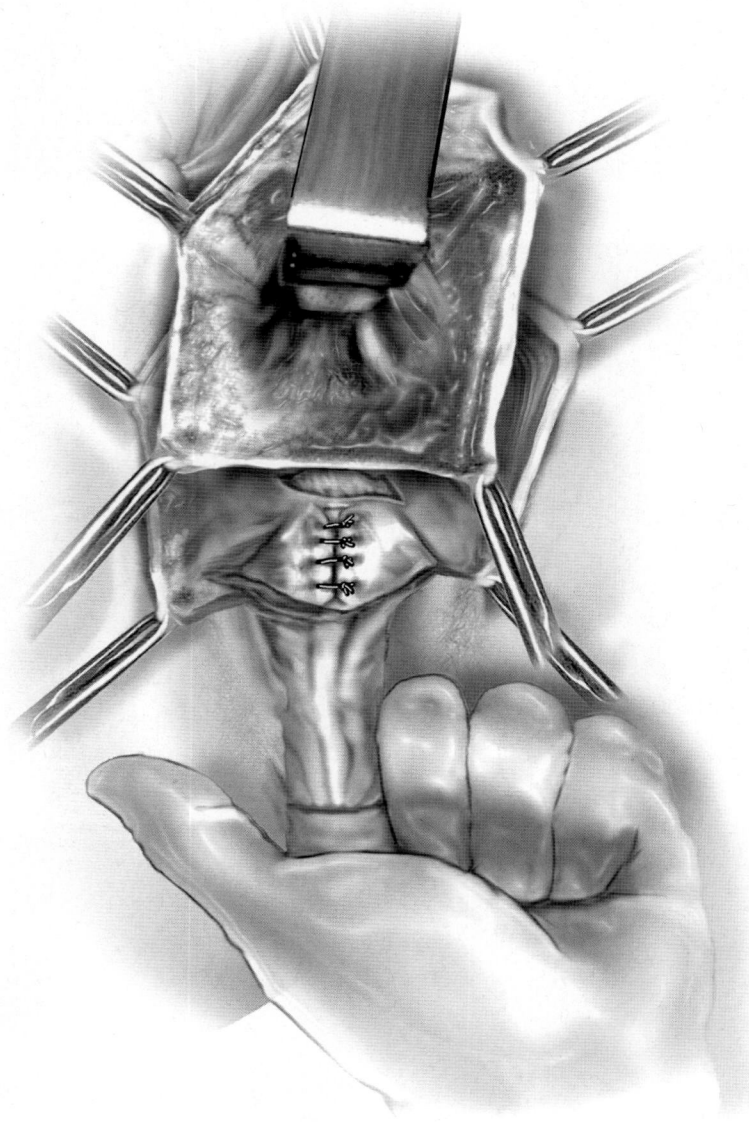

A

**FIGURE 54–49** Posterior vaginal wall defect. **A.** Note that the rectocele has been plicated in the middle and distal vagina. A high rectocele remains, and the enterocele sac has been opened.

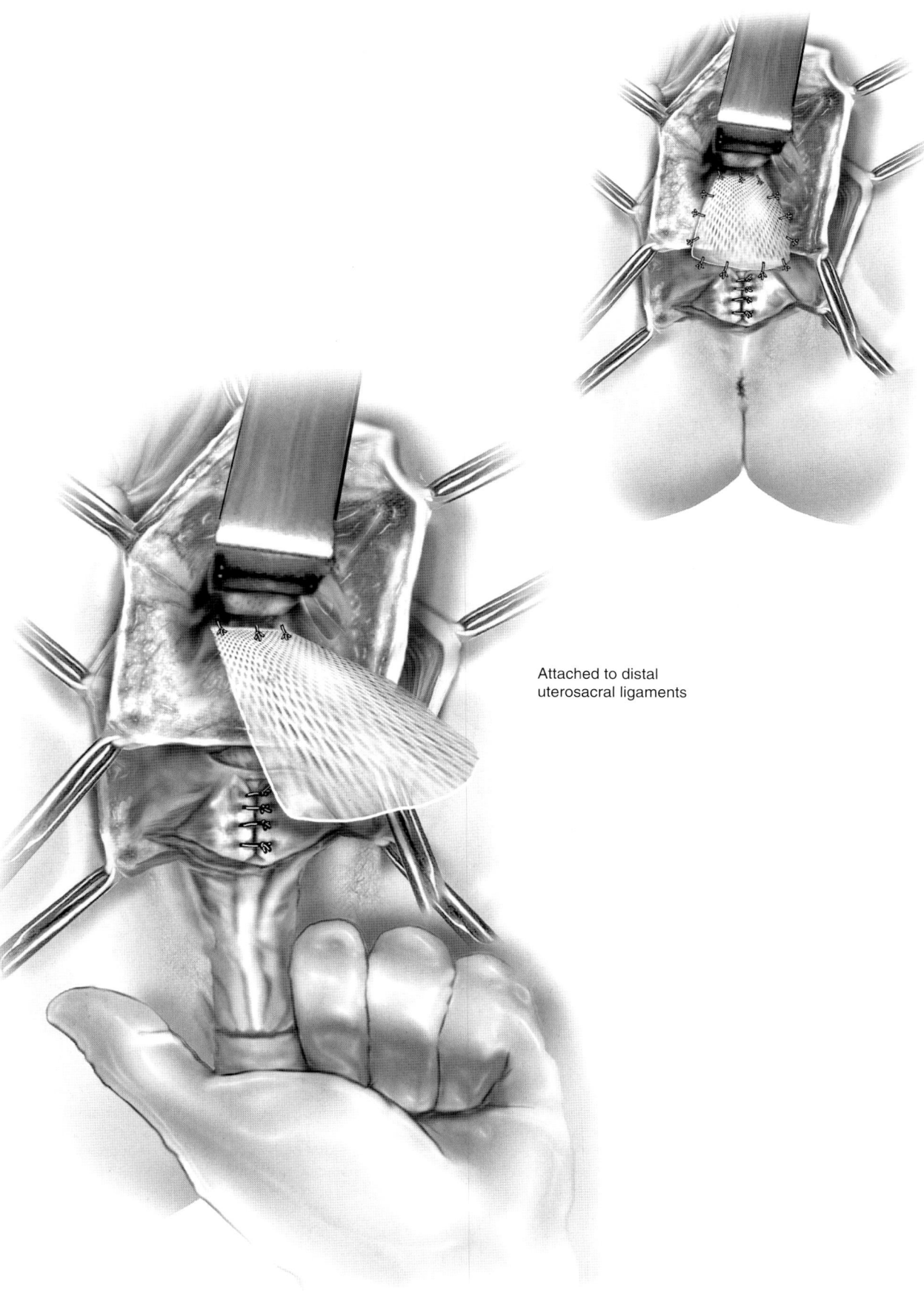

Attached to distal
uterosacral ligaments

B

**FIGURE 54–49, cont'd   B.** In such a situation, mesh can be attached proximally to the distal portions of the uterosacral ligaments intraperitoneally and distally to the upper margin of the plicated rectovaginal fascia, thus supporting the high rectocele.

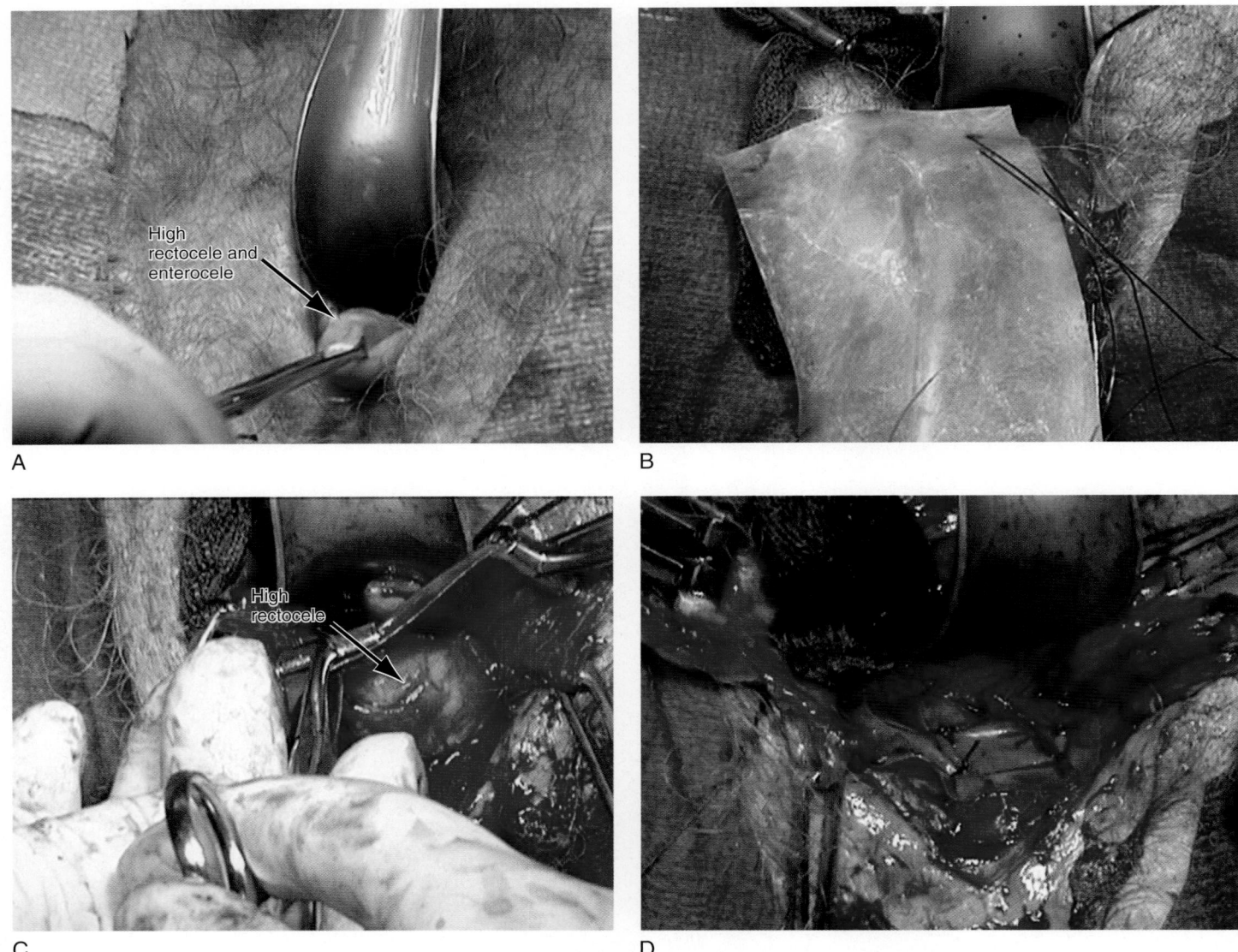

A

B

C

D

**FIGURE 54–50** Patient with a somewhat tightened vaginal introitus who has a recurrent prolapse of the upper portion of the posterior vaginal wall, secondary to a high rectocele and an enterocele. **A.** An Allis clamp is used to identify the prolapsed portion of the posterior vaginal wall. **B.** The vagina has been opened in the midline. A piece of biologic mesh is being attached proximally to the distal portions of the uterosacral ligaments intraperitoneally. **C.** The mesh has been attached proximally to the uterosacral ligaments, and the high rectocele is noted. A finger in the rectum identifies the defect, and the mesh will be placed over this defect and sutured to the proximal margins of the rectovaginal fascia. **D.** The mesh has been attached proximally and distally, as well as laterally, to the levator muscles. Note that the mesh nicely supports the previously noted high rectocele.

# CHAPTER 55

# Vaginal Repair of Vaginal Vault Prolapse

*Mickey M. Karram* ■ *Christine Vaccaro*

The true incidence and prevalence of vaginal vault prolapse are unknown. Eversion of the vagina probably occurs in about 0.5% of patients who have undergone vaginal or abdominal hysterectomy. Prophylactic measures performed at the time of hysterectomy probably decrease the incidence of vaginal vault prolapse. These measures include routine reattachment of the vaginal vault to the cardinal-uterosacral ligament complex, routine use of culdoplasty sutures, and cul-de-sac obliteration or enterocele excision after removal of the uterus. When isolated uterovaginal prolapse or posthysterectomy vaginal vault prolapse is mild (i.e., the presenting part of the prolapse descends to the midportion of the vagina), vaginal hysterectomy with culdoplasty or a vaginal enterocele repair will usually be sufficient to relieve the patient's symptoms and to restore normal vaginal function and vaginal length. However, when descent of the vault of the vagina or the uterus is significant, formal suspension of the apex of the vagina is necessary to preserve vaginal function. The vaginal procedures used to suspend the apex of the vagina discussed in this section include sacrospinous ligament suspension, iliococcygeus fascia suspension, and high uterosacral ligament suspension.

## Sacrospinous Ligament Suspension

To perform this procedure correctly and safely, the surgeon must be familiar with pararectal anatomy, as well as the anatomy of the sacrospinous ligament and its surrounding structures. This area at times is difficult to expose, and when vascular complications are encountered, life-threatening hemorrhage can occur. The sacrospinous ligaments extend from the ischial spine on each side to the lower portion of the sacrum and coccyx (Fig. 55–1). The ligament itself is a cordlike structure lying within the substance of the coccygeus muscle. However, the fibromuscular coccygeus muscle and the sacrospinous ligament are basically the same structure and are best referred to as the coccygeus-sacrospinous ligament complex (CSSL). The coccygeus muscle has a large fibrous component that is present throughout the body of the muscle and on its anterior surface, where it appears as white ridges. The CSSL is best identified by palpating the ischial spine and tracing the flat, triangular thickening posterior to the sacrum. The coccygeus muscle and the sacrospinous ligament are directly attached to the underlying sacrotuberous ligament.

It is extremely important to appreciate the close proximity of the many vascular structures and nerves to the CSSL (Fig. 55–2). Posterior to the complex are the gluteus maximus muscle and the ischial rectal fossa. The pudendal nerves and vessels lie directly posterior to the ischial spine. The sciatic nerve lies superior and lateral. Also superiorly lies an abundant vascular supply that includes the inferior gluteal vessels and the hypogastric venous plexus (see Fig. 55–2). The CSSL complex can be exposed via posterior perirectal dissection, as well as by anterior paravaginal dissection. The ability to safely identify and palpate this structure is mandatory when a mesh prolapse kit is used (see Chapter 57). The complex also can be palpated easily transperitoneally (see Figs. 55–3 and 55–15).

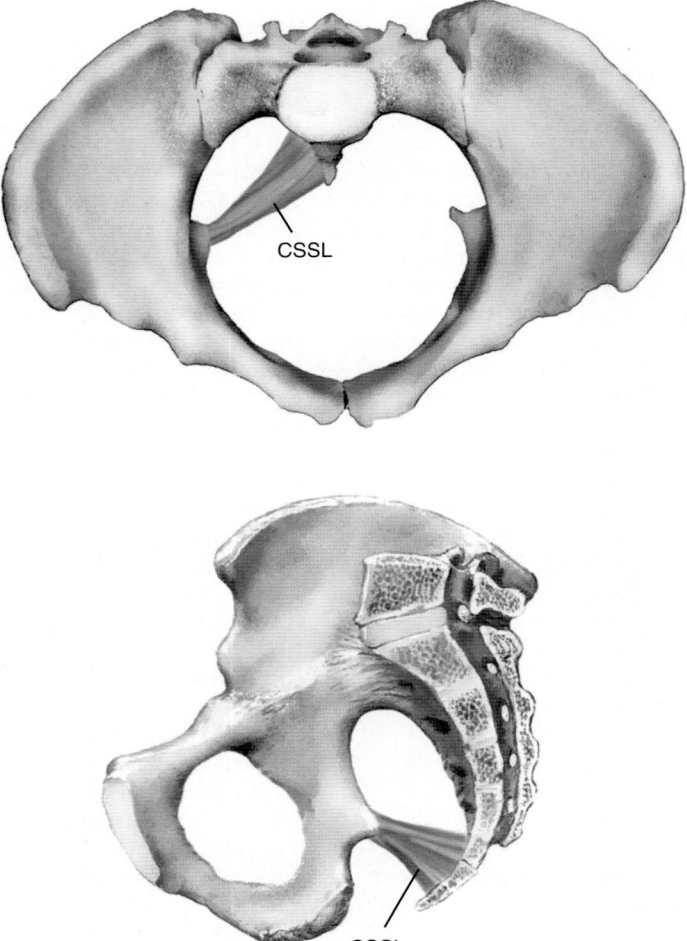

**FIGURE 55–1** Coccygeus–sacrospinous ligament complex. Note that the sacrospinous ligament lies within the coccygeus muscle.

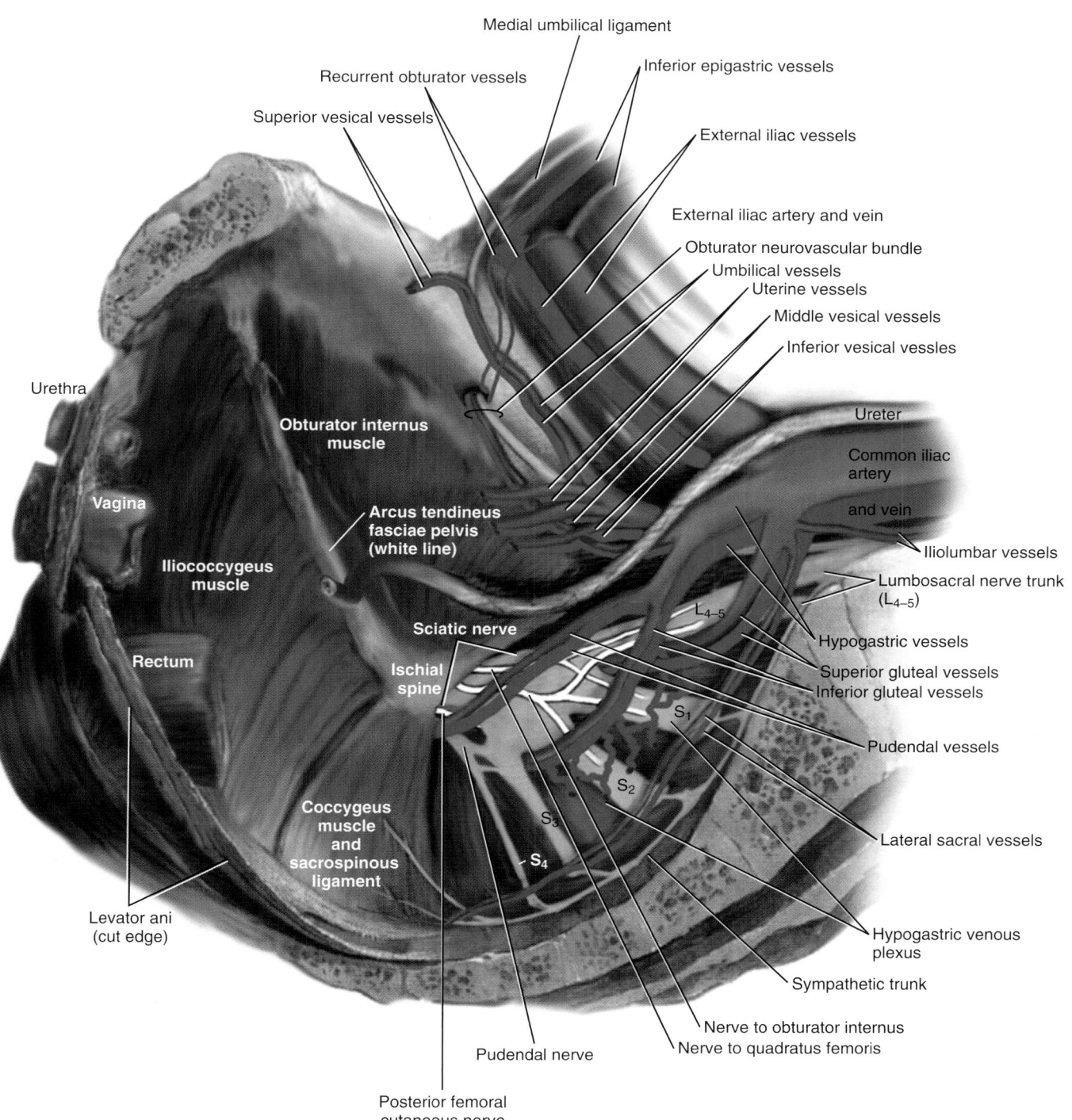

Medial umbilical ligament

Recurrent obturator vessels

Superior vesical vessels

Inferior epigastric vessels

External iliac vessels

External iliac artery and vein

Obturator neurovascular bundle

Umbilical vessels

Uterine vessels

Middle vesical vessels

Inferior vesical vessles

Urethra

Obturator internus muscle

Ureter

Common iliac artery

and vein

Vagina

Arcus tendineus fasciae pelvis (white line)

Iliolumbar vessels

Iliococcygeus muscle

Lumbosacral nerve trunk $(L_{4-5})$

$L_{4-5}$

Sciatic nerve

Hypogastric vessels

Rectum

Ischial spine

$S_1$

Superior gluteal vessels

Inferior gluteal vessels

$S_2$

Pudendal vessels

Coccygeus muscle and sacrospinous ligament

$S_3$

$S_4$

Lateral sacral vessels

Levator ani (cut edge)

Hypogastric venous plexus

Sympathetic trunk

Nerve to obturator internus

Nerve to quadratus femoris

Pudendal nerve

Posterior femoral cutaneous nerve

**FIGURE 55–2** Anatomy surrounding the coccygeus–sacrospinous ligament complex (CSSL).

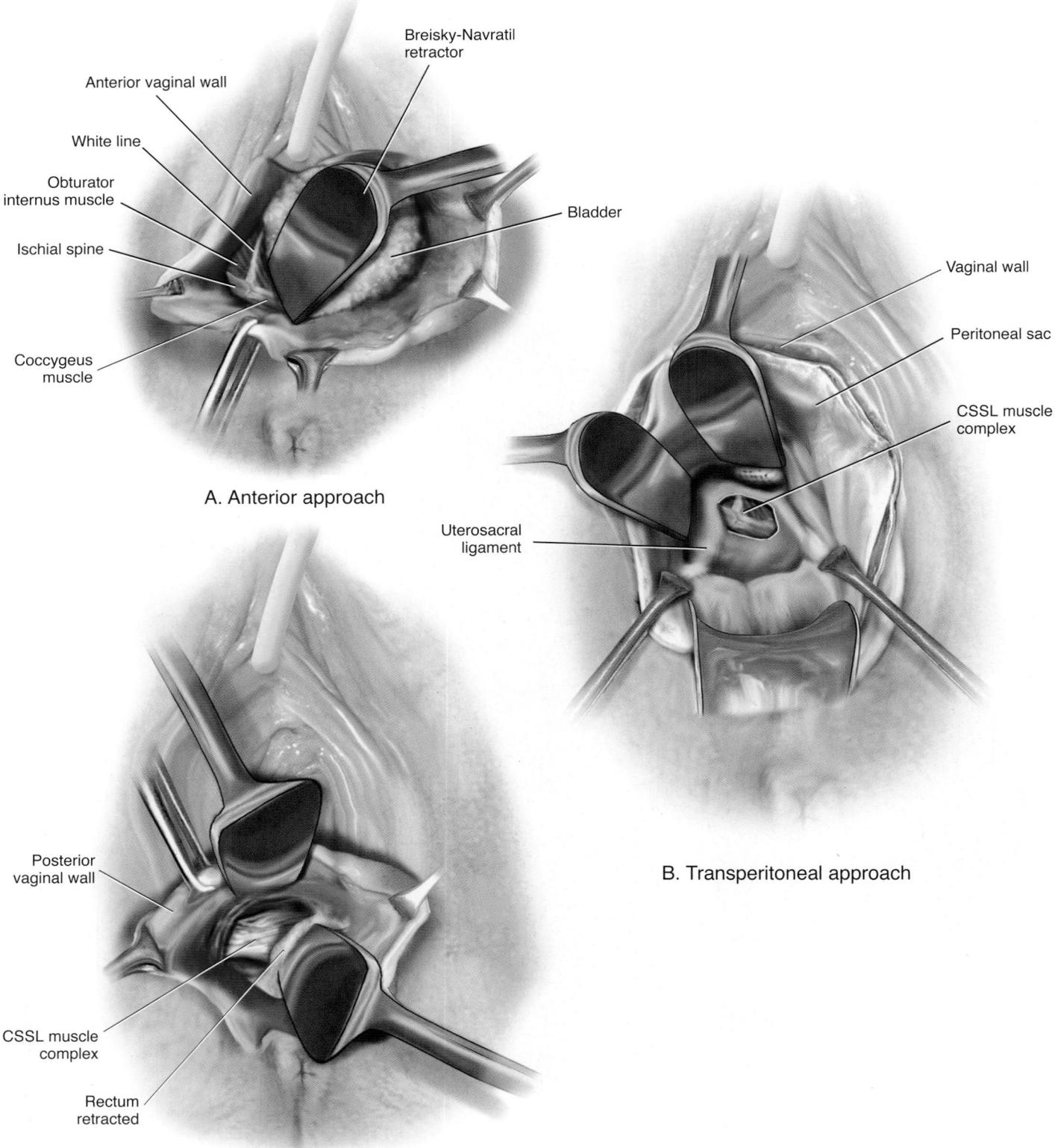

A. Anterior approach

B. Transperitoneal approach

C. Posterior approach

**FIGURE 55–3** The sacrospinous ligament can be palpated and or exposed via the (**A**) anterior paravaginal approach, (**B**) transperitoneal approach, or (**C**) posterior pararectal approach.

Although unilateral and bilateral sacrospinous ligament suspensions have been described, the author prefers unilateral suspension via perirectal or posterior dissection. Before beginning the operation, the surgeon should recognize the ischial spine and palpate the CSSL on pelvic examination. Performance of this operation almost always requires simultaneous correction of an enterocele and the anterior and posterior vaginal walls. Preoperatively elevating the prolapsed vaginal apex to the ligament that is to be utilized for the suspension at times assists the surgeon in determining whether an anterior and posterior colporrhaphy will also be necessary. If, when the patient is asked to perform a Valsalva maneuver, the anterior and posterior vaginal segments descend, then repairs most likely will be necessary. Patient consent should be routinely sought for these repairs because it is often difficult to discern the extent of various defects preoperatively in an office setting. The technique of unilateral sacrospinous ligament fixation is performed as follows:

1. With the patient in the dorsal lithotomy position, the vaginal area is prepped and draped, and prophylactic perioperative antibiotics are given on call to the operating room.
2. The apex of the vagina is grasped with two Allis clamps, and downward traction is used to determine the extent of the vaginal prolapse and associated pelvic support defects. The vaginal apex is then reduced to the sacrospinous ligament intended to be used. If bilateral sacrospinous fixation is to be performed, then each side of the vaginal apex should be reduced to the respective ligament on that side. At times, the true apex of the vagina is foreshortened and will not reach the intended area of fixation. This is commonly associated with a shortened anterior vaginal wall and a very prominent enterocele. In this setting, the apex should be moved to a portion of the vaginal wall over the enterocele, thus allowing sufficient vaginal length for suspension to the sacrospinous ligament. The intended apex is tagged with sutures for later identification. If the patient has complete eversion of the vagina that requires anterior vaginal wall repair or bladder neck suspension, the author prefers to do this portion of the operation first. During this procedure, one can separate the bladder base away from the vaginal apex, thus lowering the risk of cystotomy.
3. The upper part of the posterior vaginal wall is then incised, usually at least halfway down the length of the posterior vaginal wall. The enterocele sac is mobilized off the vaginal apex and is entered and excised. If the patient has undergone a vaginal hysterectomy, the peritoneum over the posterior vaginal wall is removed to the level of the neck of the enterocele, and the enterocele is closed as previously described.
4. The next step is entering the perirectal space. The right rectal pillar separates the rectovaginal space from the right perirectal space. The rectal pillar is nothing more than areolar tissue that extends from the rectum to the arcus tendineus fascia pelvis and overlies the levator muscle. It may contain a few small fibers and blood vessels. In most cases, entry into the perirectal space is best achieved by breaking through this fibroareolar tissue just lateral to the enterocele sac at the level of the ischial spine. This maneuver can usually be accomplished by gently mobilizing the rectum medially. At times, however, the use of gauze on the index finger or a tonsil clamp is necessary to break through into the space.
5. Once the perirectal space has been entered, the ischial spine is identified by palpation. With dorsal and medial movement of the fingers, the coccygeus sacrospinous ligament is palpated and its superior edge is identified.
6. Blunt dissection is used to further remove tissue from this area. The surgeon should take care to ensure that the rectum is adequately retracted medially. It is recommended that a rectal examination be performed at this time to ensure that

no inadvertent rectal injury has occurred. Breisky-Navratil retractors are used to expose the complex (Fig. 55–4).

7. Two techniques have been popularized for the actual passage of sutures through the ligament. The first involves use of a long-handled Deschamps ligature carrier and nerve hook (Fig. 55–5A). Long straight retractors are used to expose the coccygeus muscle, ideally Breisky-Navratil retractors (Fig. 55–5B). One must take great care that the assistant does not let the tip of the retractor be pushed across the anterior surface of the sacrum, which would risk potential damage to the vessels and nerves. If the right sacrospinous ligament is to be used, the middle and index fingers of the left hand (in a right-handed surgeon) are placed on the medial surface of the ischial spine, and under direct vision, the CSSL is penetrated by the tip of the ligature carrier at a point two fingerbreadths medial to the ischial spine. When the ligature carrier is pushed through the body of the ligament, considerable resistance should be encountered. This must be overcome by forceful, yet controlled rotation of the handle of the ligature carrier. If visualization of the CSSL is difficult, the muscle and the ligament can be grasped in the tip of a long Babcock or Allis clamp, which helps to isolate the tissue to be sutured from underlying vessels and nerves. After the suture has been passed, the fingers of the left hand are withdrawn, the retractor is suitably repositioned, and the tip of the ligature carrier is visualized. The suture is then grabbed with a nerve hook. A second suture is placed similarly 1 cm medial to the first. To avoid a second passage of the ligature carrier, the original long suture can be cut in the center and each end of the cut loop paired with its respective free suture. This obtains two sutures through the ligament with only one penetration of the ligature carrier. To ensure that an appropriate bite of tissue has been obtained, one should be able to gently move the patient on the table with traction of the sutures.

A second technique popularized for passing the sutures through the CSSL is the Miyazaki technique (Fig. 55–6). The proposed advantages of this technique are that it is safer and easier because the ligature carrier enters the CSSL under direct palpation of distinct landmarks and is then pulled down into the safe perirectal space below. To perform this modification, the tip of the right middle finger is placed on the CSSL just below its superior margin, approximately two fingerbreadths medial to the ischial spine. The Miya hook in the left hand in a closed position is slid along the palmar surface of the right hand. The hook point should come to rest just beneath the previously positioned tip of the right middle finger. The handles are then opened and lowered to a near horizontal position. This points the hook into the CSSL at about a 45° angle. If a high perineum prevents lowering of the handle, an episiotomy should be performed. With the tip of the middle finger, the hook point is placed two fingerbreadths medial to the ischial spine approximately 0.5 cm below the superior edge (see Fig. 55–4). With experience, the hook point can be passed along the superior edge. With the middle and index fingers, firm pressure is applied downward just behind the hook hump so that the hook point penetrates the CSSL. Downward pressure with two fingers on the tip plus traction with the back of the thumb on the back handle produces enough force to penetrate the ligament. The handle of the Miya hook is closed and elevated, and tissues from the hook point are pushed downward with the index and middle fingers so as to make the suture clearly visible. If too much tissue is in the hook, the hook is simply backed out a little, and a smaller bite taken. An assistant should hold the elevated handles in the closed position. A long retractor is then placed to mobilize the rectum medially, and a notched speculum is inserted by palpation under the hook point. A nerve hook is then used to retrieve the suture (see Fig. 55–4).

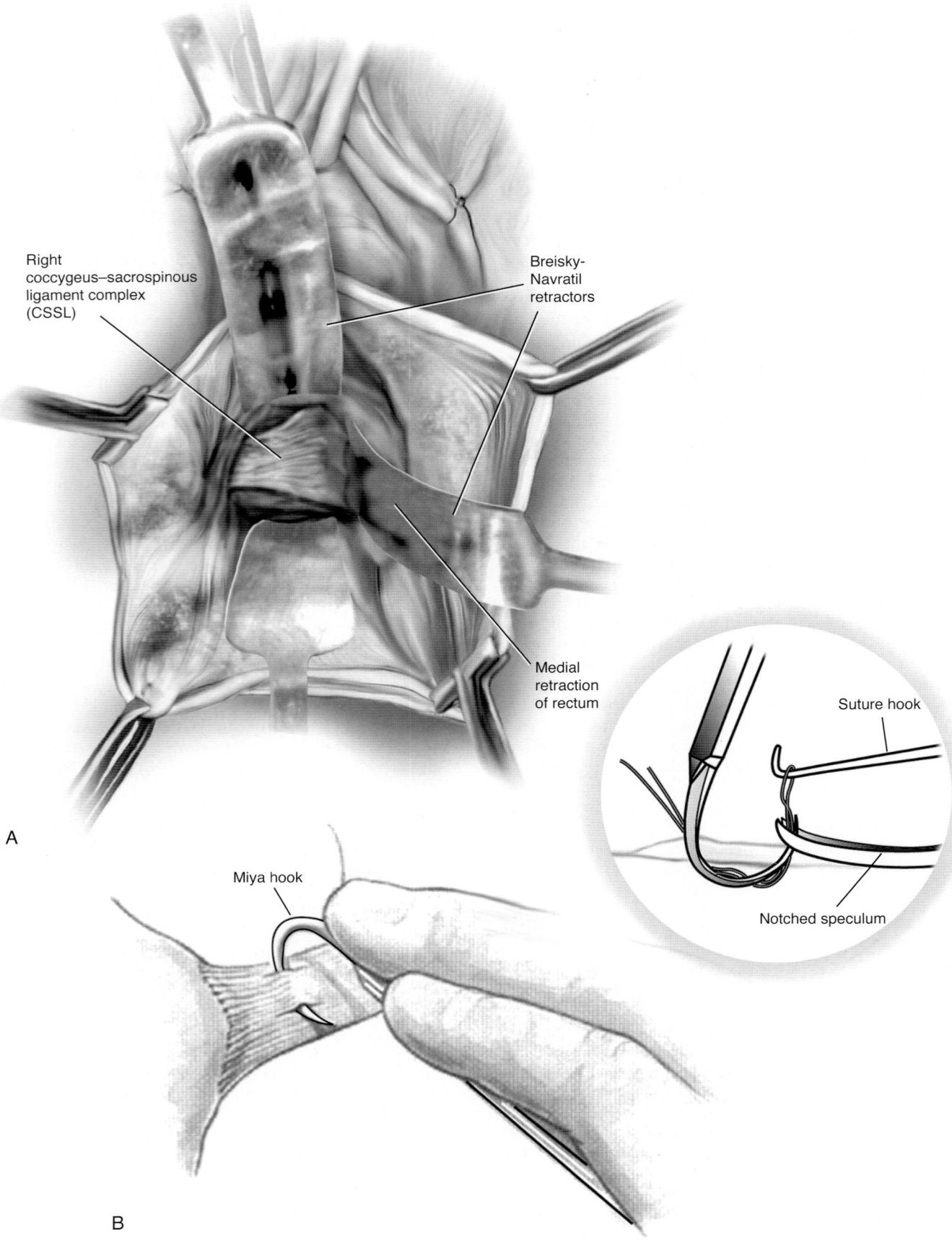

Right
coccygeus–sacrospinous
ligament complex
(CSSL)

Breisky-
Navratil
retractors

Medial
retraction
of rectum

Suture hook

Notched speculum

Miya hook

A

B

**FIGURE 55–4 A.** Breisky-Navratil retractors are used to retract the rectum medially and the bladder superiorly. **B.** Technique of passage of a Miya hook through the ligament. **Inset.** Technique of retrieval of the suture.

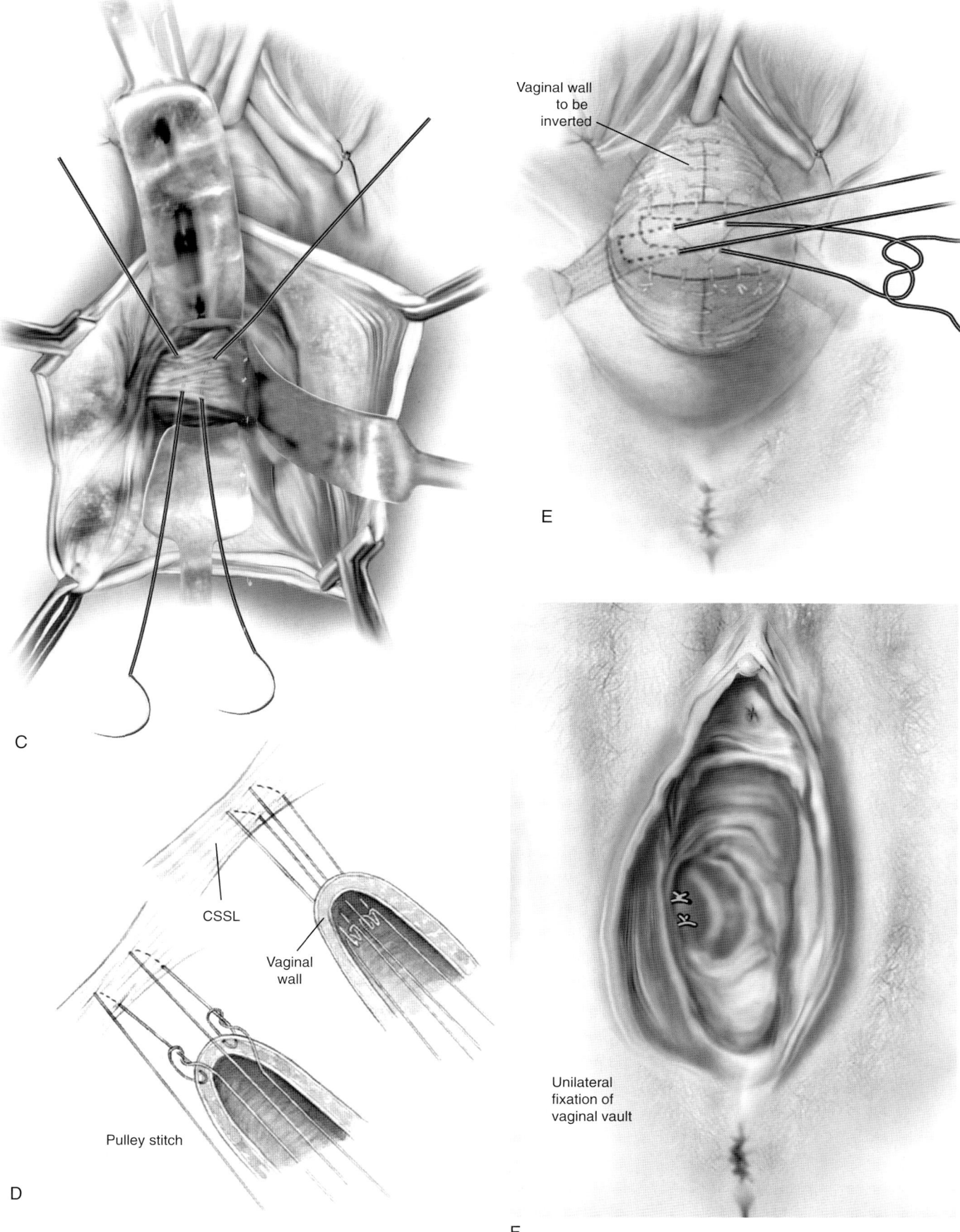

**C**

**D**

CSSL

Vaginal
wall

Pulley stitch

**E**

Vaginal wall
to be
inverted

**F**

Unilateral
fixation of
vaginal vault

**FIGURE 55–4, cont'd** **C.** Two sutures have been passed through the complex. **D.** Technique of fixing the vaginal apex to the coccygeus-sacrospinous ligament complex (CSSL). If a pulley stitch is performed, then permanent sutures should be used. If the sutures are passed through the vaginal epithelium and tied in the vaginal lumen, then delayed absorbable sutures should be used. **E.** The vagina is closed before the suspension sutures are tied. **F.** Tied sacrospinous sutures.

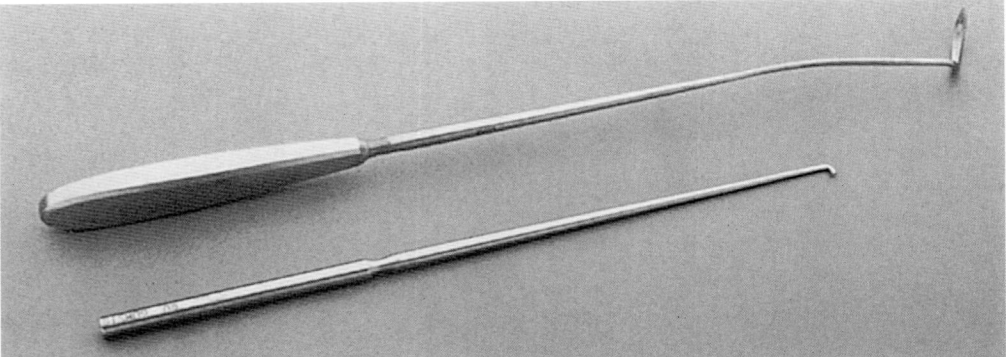

A

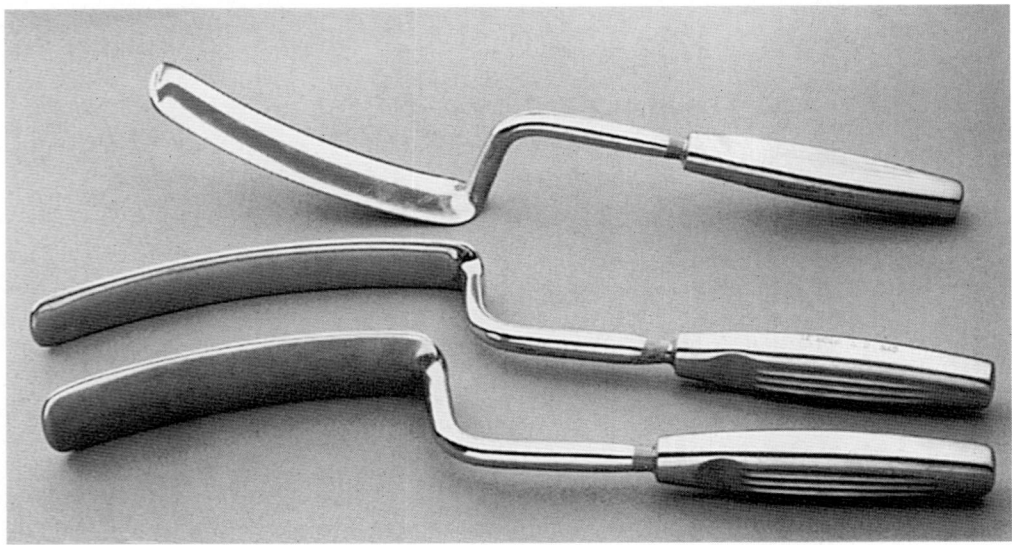

B

**FIGURE 55–5 A.** Long-handled Deschamps ligature carrier and nerve hook. Note the slight bend near the tip to facilitate suture placement into the coccygeus–sacrospinous ligament complex (CSSL). **B.** Breisky-Navratil retractors, various sizes. (From Walters MD, Karram MM: *In* Urogynecology and Reconstructive Pelvic Surgery, 2nd ed. CV Mosby, St. Louis, 1999, with permission.)

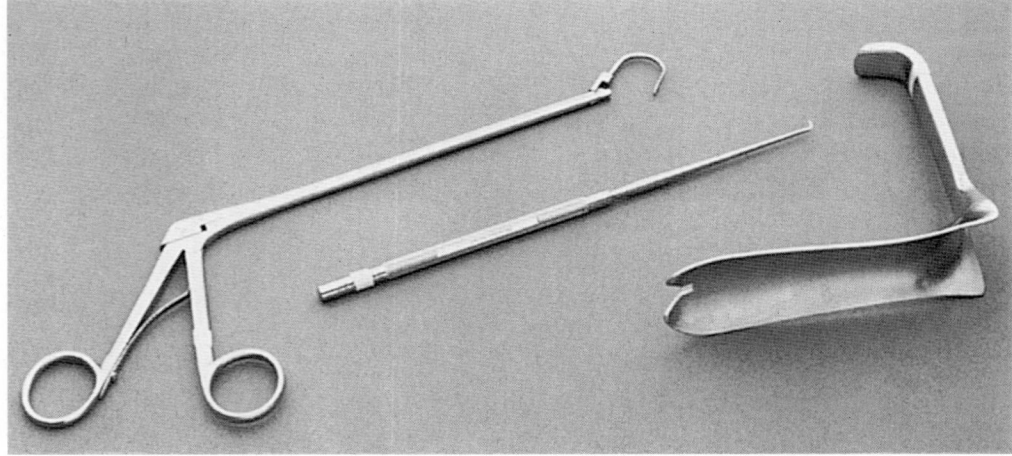

**FIGURE 55–6** Left to right: Miya hook, notched speculum, and suture hook for use during sacrospinous ligament fixation. (From Walters MD, Karram MM: *In* Urogynecology and Reconstructive Pelvic Surgery, 2nd ed. CV Mosby, St. Louis, 1999, with permission.)

Two other instruments that are commonly utilized to facilitate passage of a suture through the ligament are the Capio needle driver (Microvasive-Boston Scientific Corp, Watertown, Mass) and the Nichols-Veronikis ligature carrier (BEI Medical Systems, Chatsworth, Calif) (Fig. 55–7).

8. Now the surgeon is ready to bring stitches out to the apex of the vagina. Two techniques are commonly performed for this maneuver. The first involves bringing the vaginal apex to the surface of the CSSL with the use of a pulley stitch (see Fig. 55–4). After the stitch has been placed in the ligament, one end of the suture is rethreaded on a free needle, sewn into the full thickness of the fibromuscular layer of the undersurface of the vaginal apex, and tied by a single half-stitch, while the free end of the suture is held long. Traction of the free end of the suture pulls the vagina directly into the muscle and ligament. A square knot then fixes it in place. With this type of fixation, a permanent suture should be used because the suture is not exposed through the epithelium of the vagina.

Some surgeons prefer a second technique (see Fig. 55–4), especially if the vaginal wall is thin or if greater vaginal length is desired. With this method, both ends of the sutures are passed through the vaginal epithelium. When this method is used, a delayed absorbable suture should be used because the knot remains in the vagina. We recommend a #2 delayed absorbable suture. After the sutures have been brought out through the vagina, the vagina is trimmed if necessary, and the upper portion of the vaginal wall is closed with an interrupted or continuous suture. The vaginal vault suspension sutures are then tied, thus elevating the apex of the vagina to the CSSL (Figs. 55–8 through 55–10). It is important that the vagina comes into contact with the coccygeus muscle and that no suture bridge exists, especially if delayed absorbable sutures are being used. While these sutures are being tied, it may be useful to perform a rectal examination to detect any suture bridge.

9. After these sutures are tied, the posterior colpoperineorrhaphy is completed as needed, and the vagina is packed with moist gauze for 24 hours.

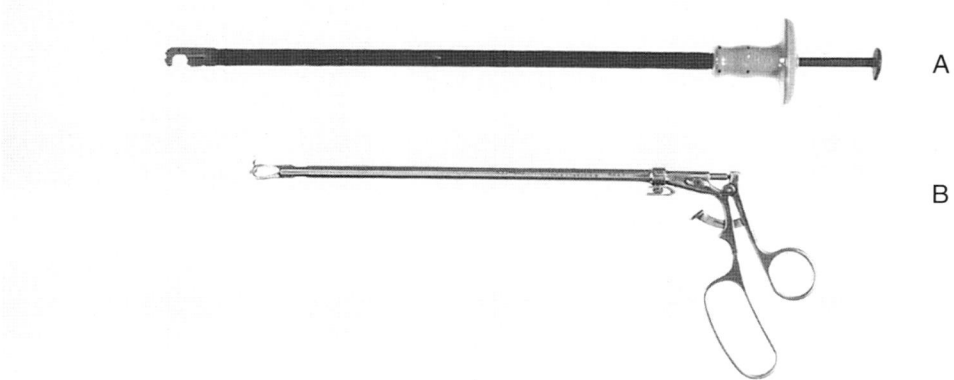

A

B

FIGURE 55–7 Two specially designed instruments to facilitate passage of sutures through the sacrospinous ligament. A. Capio needle driver (Microvasive-Boston Scientific Corp, Watertown, Mass). B. Nichols-Veronikis ligature carrier (BEI Medical Systems, Chatsworth, Calif). (From Walters MD, Karram MM: *In* Urogynecology and Reconstructive Pelvic Surgery, 2nd ed. CV Mosby, St. Louis, 1999, with permission.)

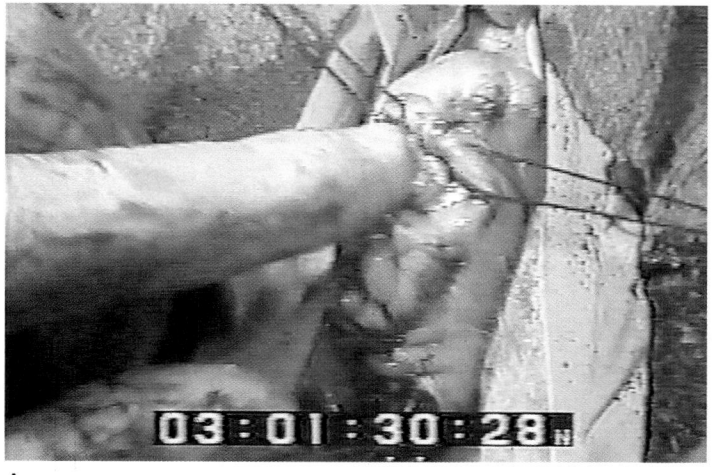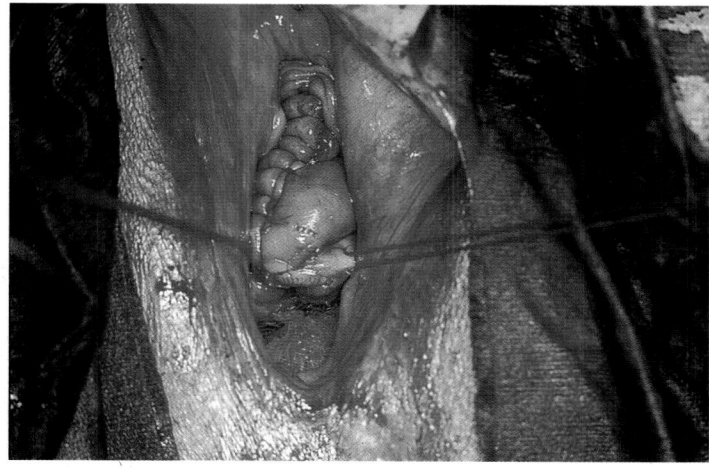

A                                                              B

FIGURE 55–8 A and B. Two examples of cases in which sacrospinous ligament fixation has been performed. The anterior vaginal wall and the vaginal cuff have been closed. Sacrospinous suspension sutures have been brought out through the vaginal apex.

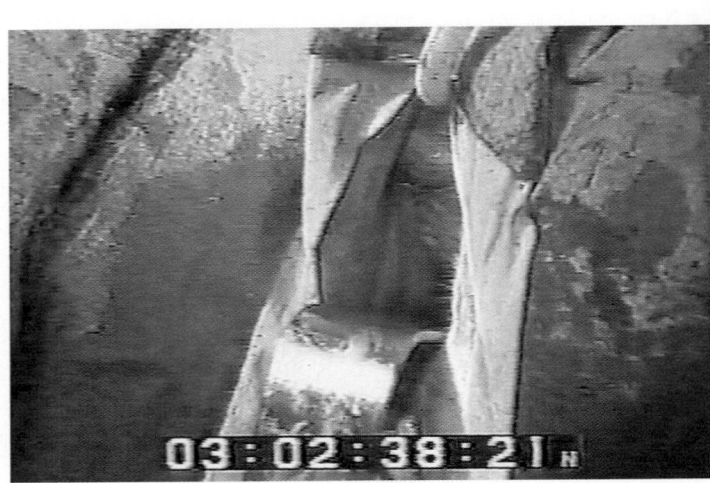

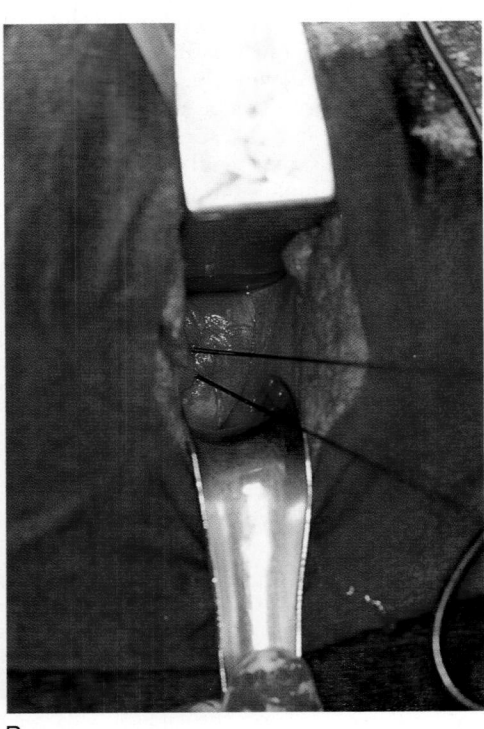

A

B

**FIGURE 55–9  A** and **B.** Two examples of cases in which sacrospinous ligament fixation has been performed. Sutures are being tied, approximating the apex of the vagina to the coccygeus–sacrospinous ligament complex (CSSL). Note that the vagina is distorted posteriorly and to the right.

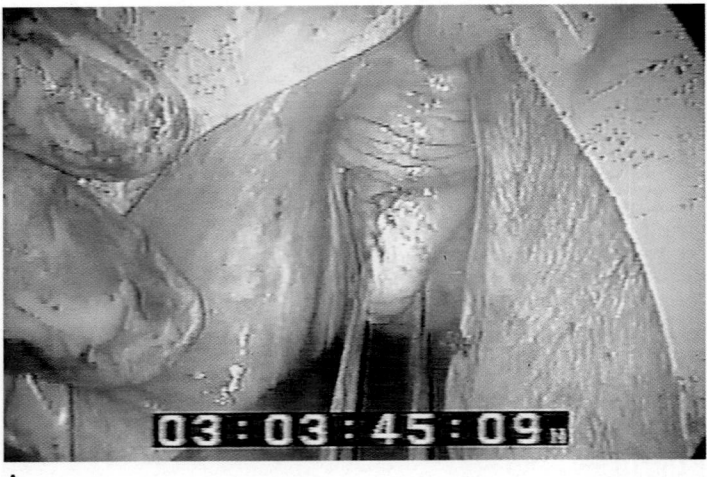

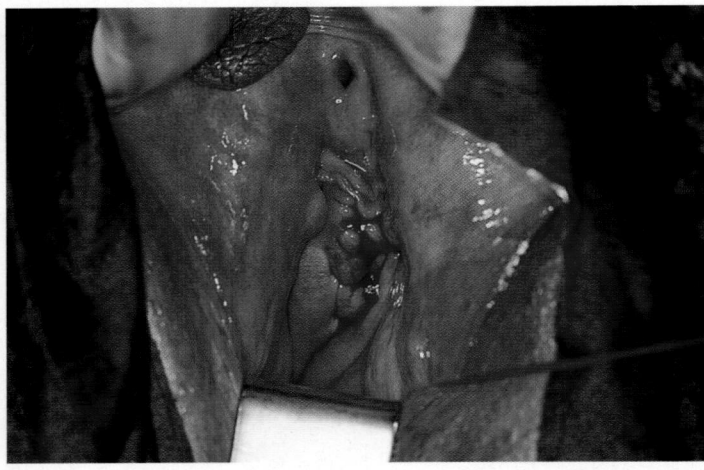

A

B

**FIGURE 55–10** The anterior vaginal wall after tying of the sacrospinous sutures. **A.** An Allis clamp has been placed on the anterior vaginal wall, which is the segment of the prolapse most likely to recur. **B.** Note the posterior distortion of the anterior segment after tying of the sacrospinous sutures.

## Iliococcygeus Fascia Suspension

In 1963, Inmon described bilateral fixation of the everted vaginal apex to the iliococcygeal fascia just below the ischial spine. The technique for this repair is as follows:

1. The posterior vaginal wall is opened in the midline as for posterior colporrhaphy, and the rectovaginal spaces are dissected widely to the levator muscles bilaterally.
2. The dissection is extended bluntly toward the ischial spine.
3. With the surgeon's nondominant hand pressing the rectum downward and medially, an area 1 to 2 cm caudad and posterior to the ischial spine in the iliococcygeus muscle and fascia is exposed (Fig. 55–11). A single, 0 delayed absorbable suture is placed deeply into the levator muscle and fascia. Both ends of the suture are then passed through the ipsilateral posterior vaginal apex and are held with a hemostat. This is repeated on the opposite side.
4. The posterior colporrhaphy is completed, and the vagina is closed. Both sutures are tied, while the posterior vaginal apices are elevated (see Fig. 55–11). This repair is often done in conjunction with a culdoplasty or uterosacral suspension.

## High Uterosacral Ligament Suspension

Another popular approach to the management of enterocele and vault prolapse is based on the anatomic observation that connective tissue of the vaginal tube does not stretch or attenuate but rather breaks at specific definable points. This concept has been discussed briefly in the section on posterior vaginal wall defects (see Chapter 54).

A uterosacral ligament suspension requires entrance into the peritoneum as it is an intraperitoneal suspension. This is currently the author's preferred procedure for vaginal vault prolapse because it can be utilized for all degrees of prolapse. Since it does not significantly distort the vaginal axis, it does not predispose the patient to recurrent anterior or posterior vaginal wall prolapse. The procedure can be easily tailored for a particular prolapse, depending on the extent of the vault prolapse and whether coexistent anterior and posterior vaginal wall defects are present. Figure 55–12 demonstrates three degrees of vaginal vault prolapse. The goal of any vault suspension should be to re-create a well-supported, functional vagina of appropriate length. A suspension to the level of the ischial spines usually results in a vagina that is at least 9 cm in length. The complexity of such a repair is based on how much coexistent anterior and posterior vaginal wall eversion is present. Figure 55–12A illustrates an isolated vaginal vault prolapse secondary to an apical enterocele with well-supported anterior and posterior vaginal walls. In such a situation, all that is required is excision of the enterocele sac and closure of the defect at the level of the neck of the enterocele. In contrast, Figure 55–12C demonstrates complete vault prolapse in conjunction with complete eversion of the anterior and posterior vaginal walls. Such a situation

requires a much more complex repair to reconstruct a functional, well-supported vagina of appropriate length. Over the years, intraperitoneal procedures utilized to support or suspend the vaginal apex as well as address apical or posterior enteroceles have evolved. A McCall culdoplasty (see Chapter 53), originally described in 1957, remains a very good procedure that can be utilized at the time of a vaginal hysterectomy because it suspends the vagina to the plicated distal portions of the uterosacral ligaments. A traditional high uterosacral suspension attempts to pass sutures bilaterally through the uterosacral ligament at the level of the ischial spine. More recently, we have modified our technique to pass the sutures higher and more medially. Figure 55–13 illustrates the anatomy of the uterosacral ligament and surrounding structures. Figures 55–14 through 55–17 illustrate placement of sutures for McCall culdoplasty, traditional uterosacral suspension, and a modified high uterosacral suspension. Note the modified technique attempts to pass sutures that incorporate a portion of the CSSL muscle complex or the presacral fascia (see Figs. 55–14 and 55–15). Figure 55–18 is an intraperitoneal photograph of the uppermost portion of the uterosacral ligament as it inserts into the CSSL complex. This modified high uterosacral suspension has led to the creation of a deeper vagina and has significantly reduced the rate of ureteral compromise (Figs. 55–19 and 55–20). The technique of high uterosacral vaginal vault suspension (Fig. 55–21) is as follows:

1. The vaginal apex is grasped with two Allis clamps and incised with a scalpel. The vaginal epithelium is dissected off the enterocele sac up to the neck of the hernia. The enterocele is opened, exposing intraperitoneal structures.
2. Numerous moist tail sponges are placed in the posterior cul-de-sac. A wide retractor is used to elevate the sponges and the intestines out of the pelvis, thus exposing the uppermost portion of the uterosacral ligament on each side (see Fig. 55–18).
3. Allis clamps are placed at approximately 5 o'clock and 7 o'clock, incorporating the peritoneum and the full thickness of the posterior vaginal wall. Downward traction on the Allis clamp allows palpation of the uterosacral ligament on each side. The ischial spines are palpated transperitoneally, and the ureter can usually be palpated along the pelvic sidewall anywhere from 1 to 5 cm ventral and lateral to the ischial spine.
4. Two to three delayed absorbable sutures are passed through the uppermost portion of the uterosacral ligament on each side. Each of these sutures is individually tagged.
5. The delayed absorbable sutures that previously had been passed through the uterosacral ligament are individually brought out through the full thickness of the posterior vaginal wall.
6. If indicated, an anterior colporrhaphy is performed at this time.
7. After appropriate trimming, the vagina is closed and the vault sutures are tied, elevating the vaginal apex high up to the uterosacral ligaments on each side.

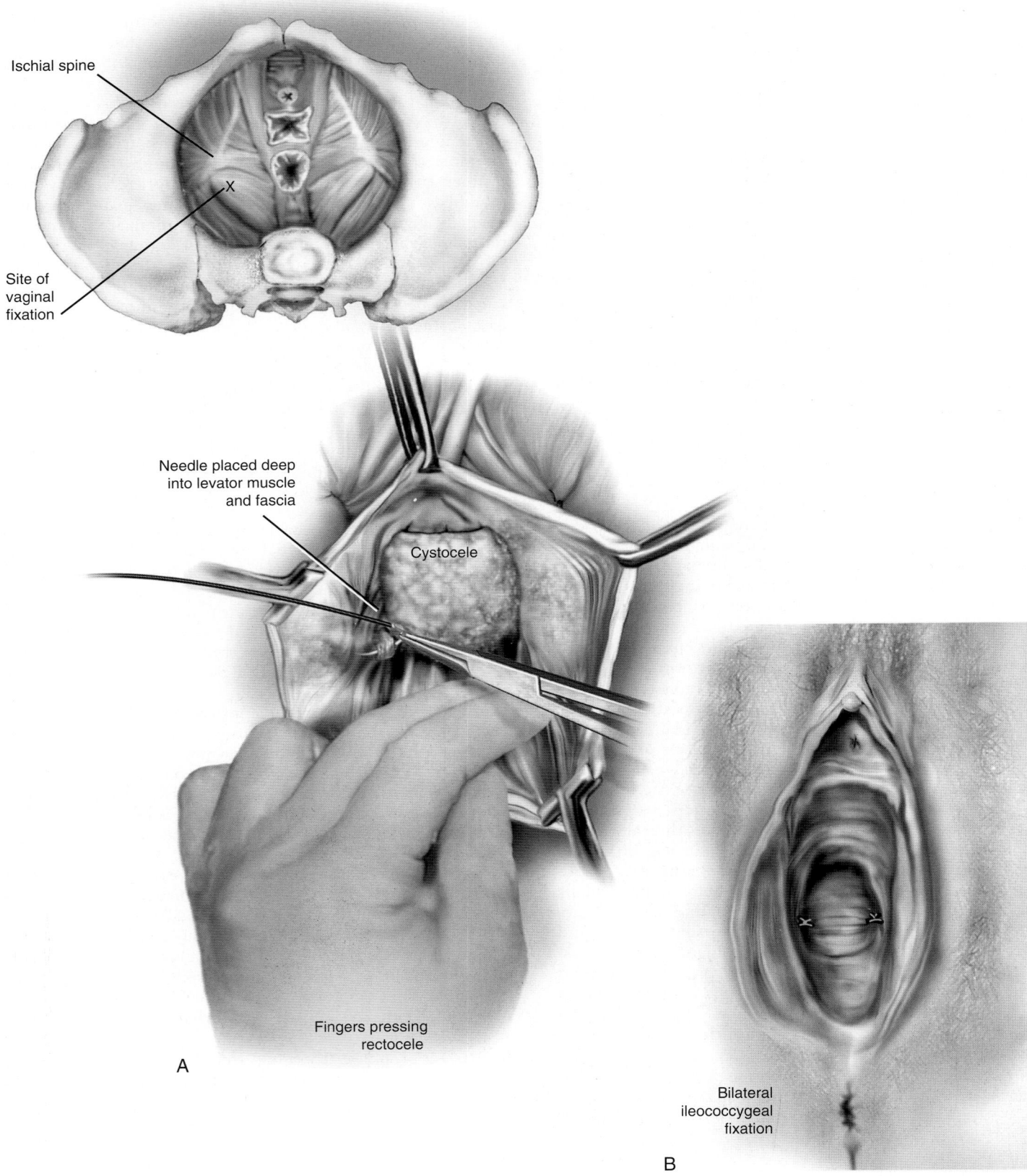

Ischial spine

Site of
vaginal
fixation

X

Needle placed deep
into levator muscle
and fascia

Cystocele

Fingers pressing
rectocele

A

Bilateral
ileococcygeal
fixation

B

**FIGURE 55–11** Ileococcygeus fascia suspension. **A.** With the surgeon's finger pressing the rectum downward, the right ileococcygeus fascia suture is placed. **Inset.** Approximate location of the ileococcygeus fascia sutures. **B.** Bilateral ileococcygeus fascia suspension.

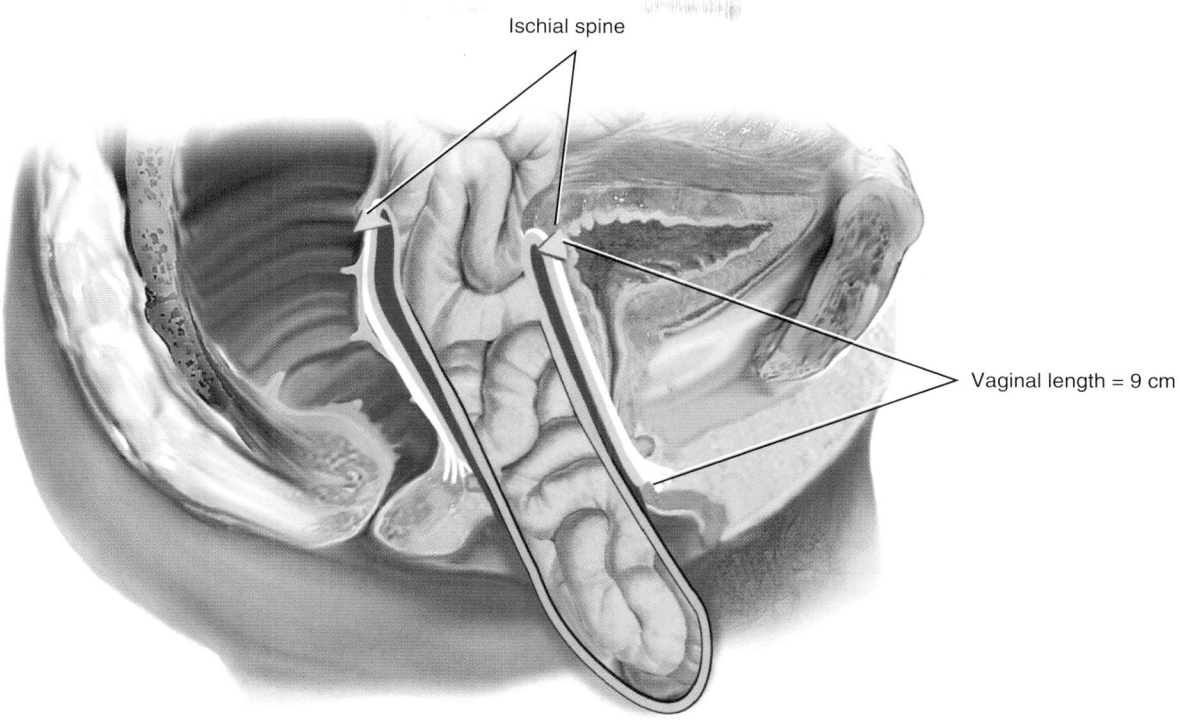

Ischial spine

Vaginal length = 9 cm

A

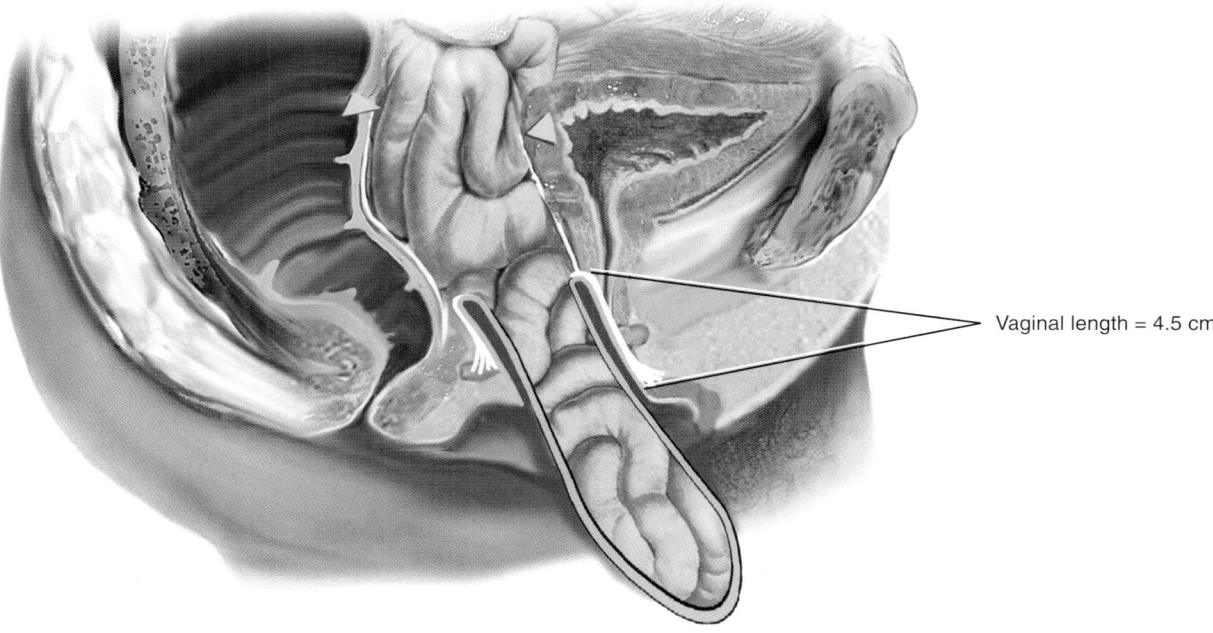

Vaginal length = 4.5 cm

B

**FIGURE 55-12  A.** Vaginal vault prolapse in isolation. Note the good support of the anterior and posterior vaginal walls. Such a situation simply requires excision of the enterocele sac and closure of the defect at the level of the neck. This will support the apex of the vagina, maintaining adequate vaginal length. **B.** Fifty percent of the length of the anterior and posterior vaginal walls is everted. Such a situation would require suspension of the apex to the level of the ischial spine, in conjunction with restoration of support of the upper portion of the anterior and posterior vaginal walls.

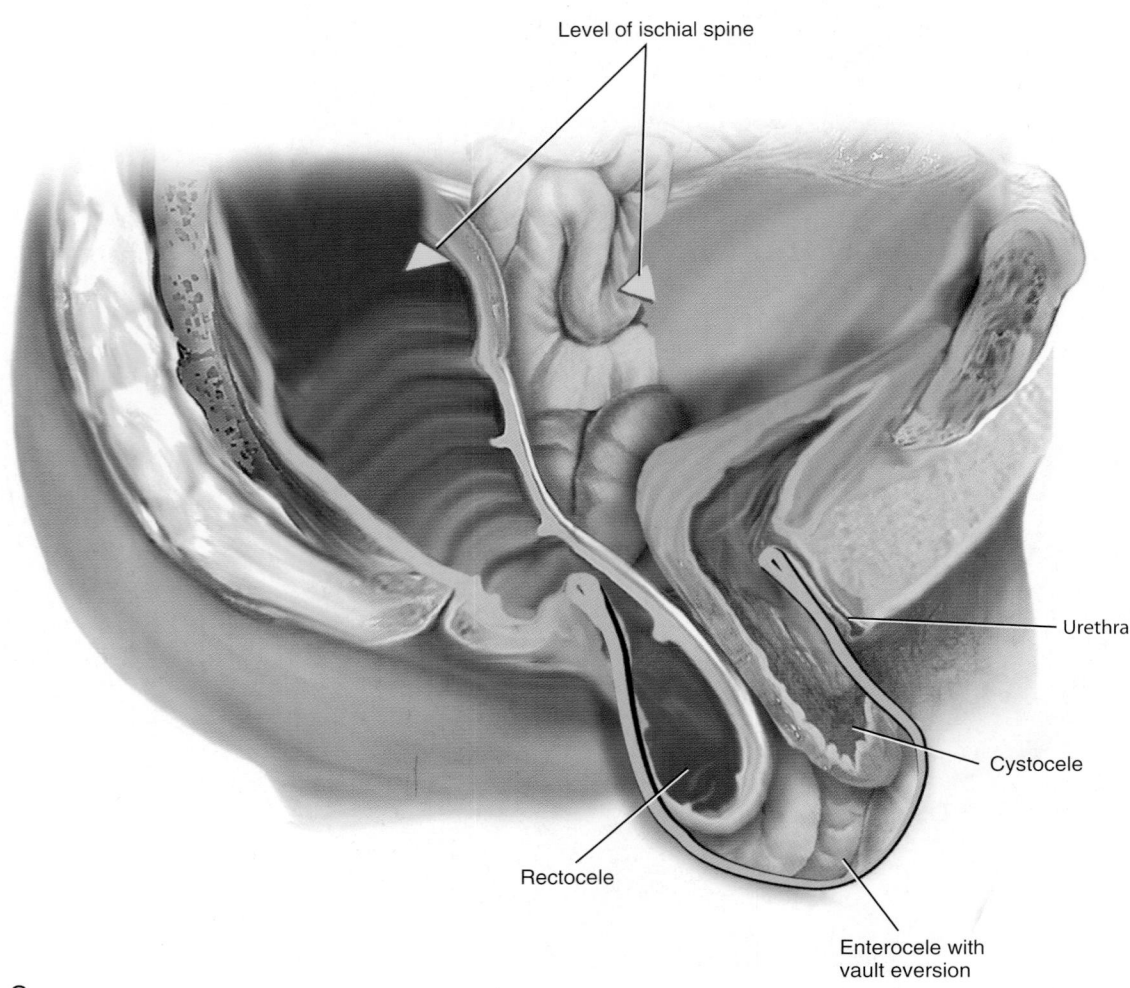

Level of ischial spine

Urethra

Cystocele

Rectocele

Enterocele with
vault eversion

C

**FIGURE 55–12, cont'd    C.** Complete vaginal vault prolapse with complete eversion of the anterior and posterior vaginal walls. Such a situation requires a much more complex repair, in that the prolapsed vaginal vault now needs to be suspended high up into the pelvic cavity to the level of the ischial spines. This must be done in conjunction with other procedures that would need to be performed to provide durable support to the anterior and posterior vaginal walls.

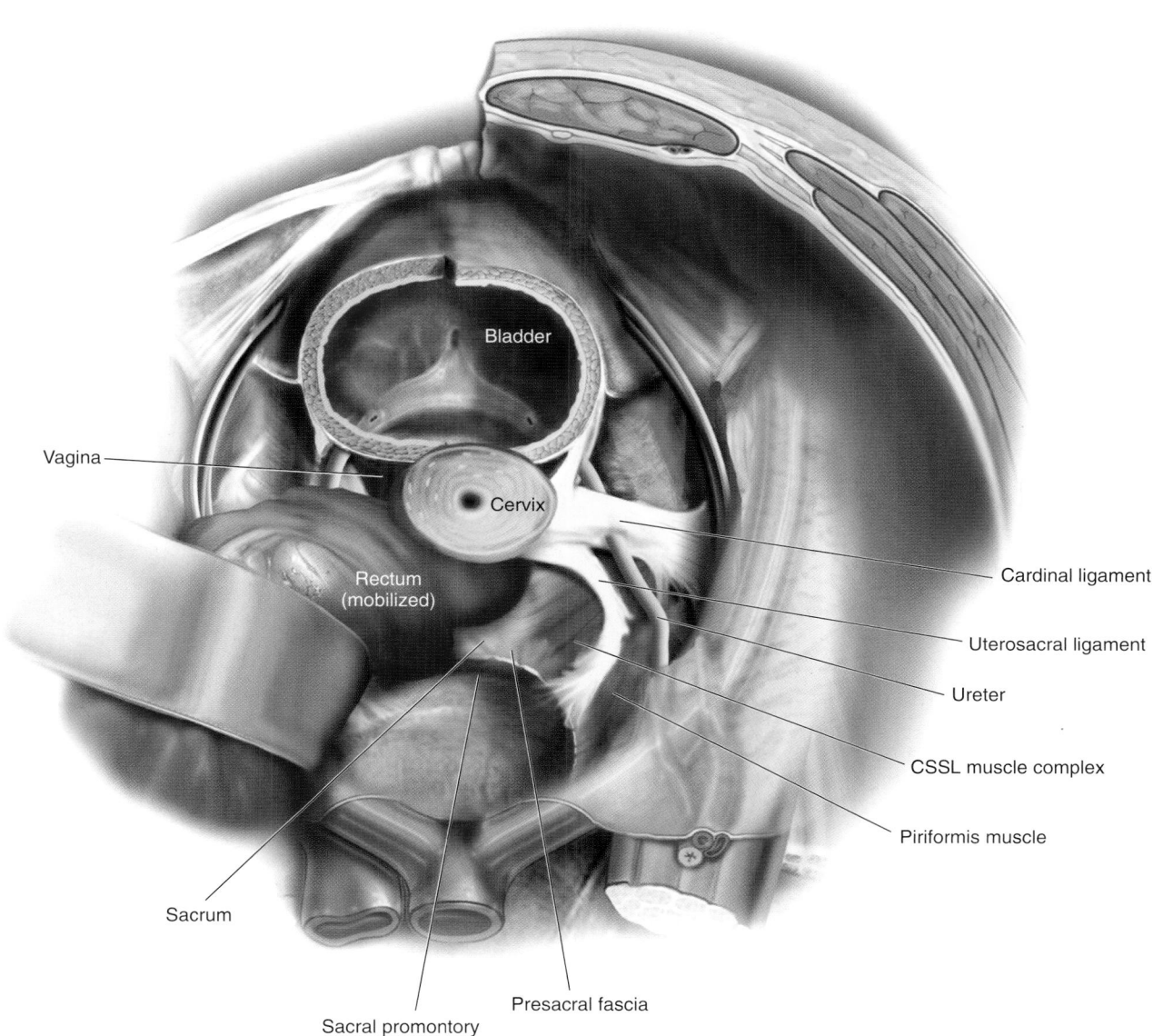

**FIGURE 55–13** Demonstrates the anatomy of the support of the uterus and upper vagina. Note the relationship between the uterosacral ligament, the ureter, the CSSL muscle complex, and the presacral fascia.

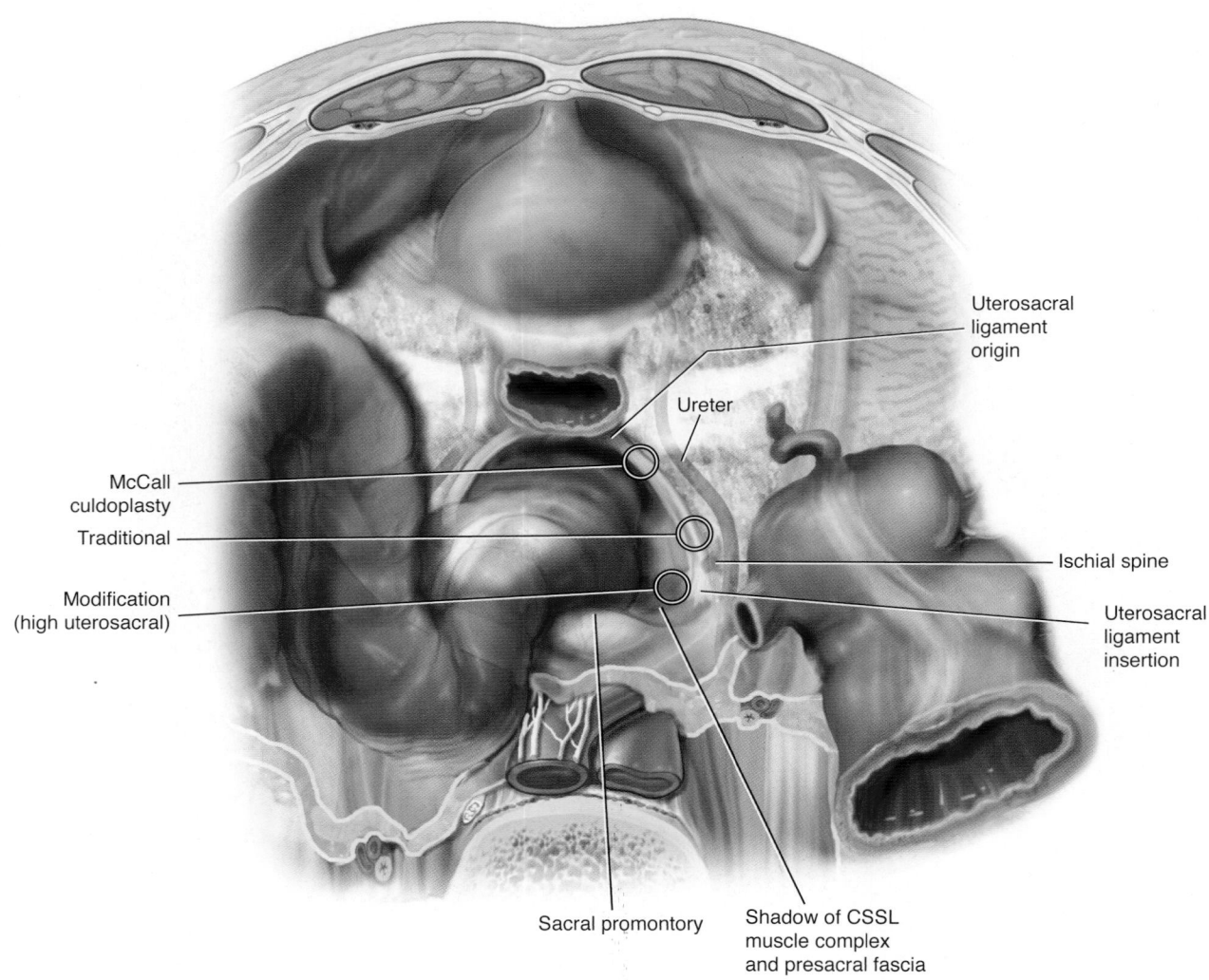

**FIGURE 55–14** Intraperitoneal view of the uterosacral ligament with circles demonstrating suture placement for McCall culdoplasty, traditional uterosacral suspension, and modified high uterosacral suspension. Note the close proximity of the ureter to the uterosacral ligament.

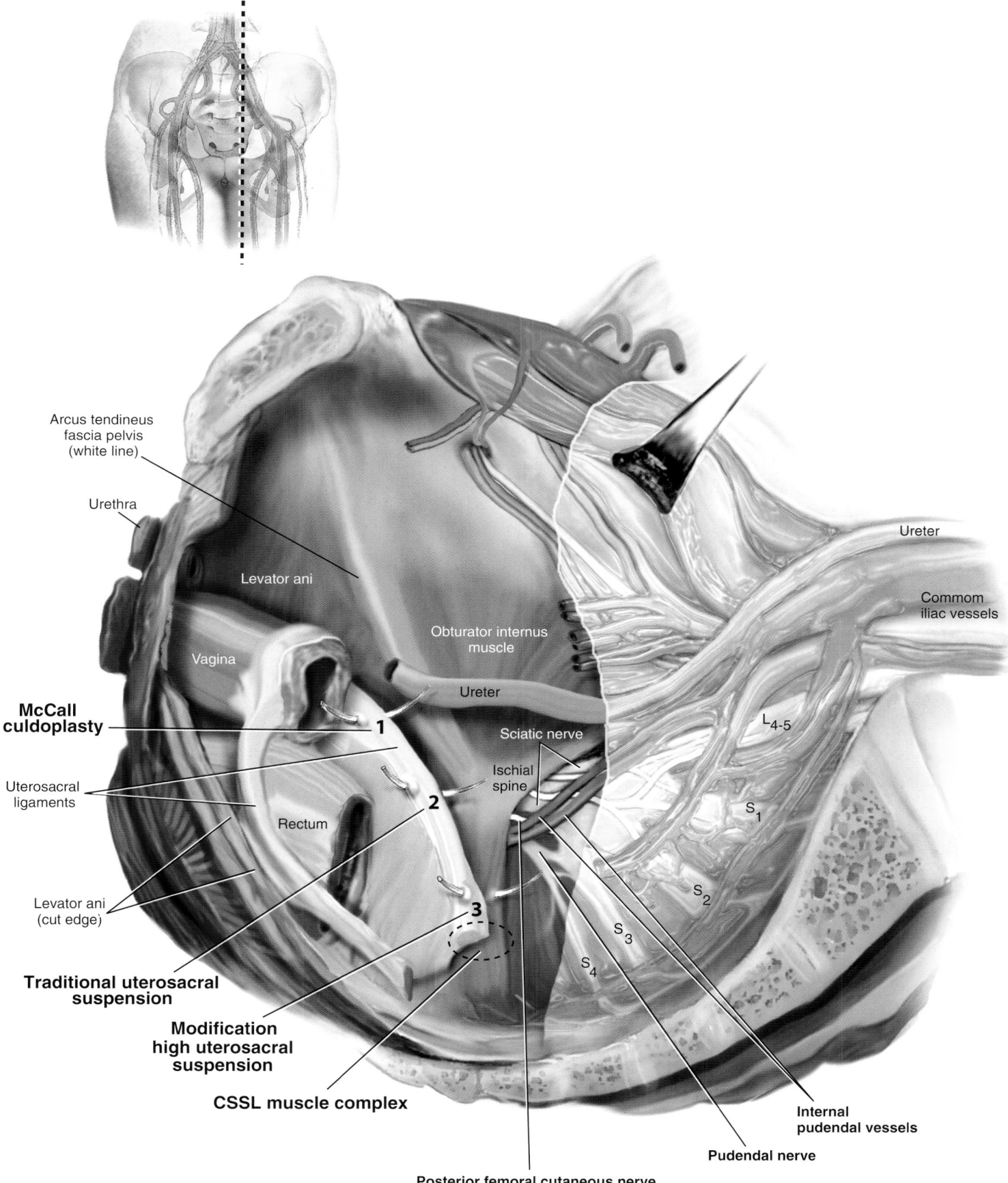

**FIGURE 55–15** Cross-section of the pelvic floor demonstrating intraperitoneal placement of sutures for (1) McCall culdoplasty, (2) traditional uterosacral suspension, and (3) modified high uterosacral suspension. Note that high uterosacral suspension may involve passage of the suture through the CSSL muscle complex, as a portion of the uterosacral ligament inserts into this structure.

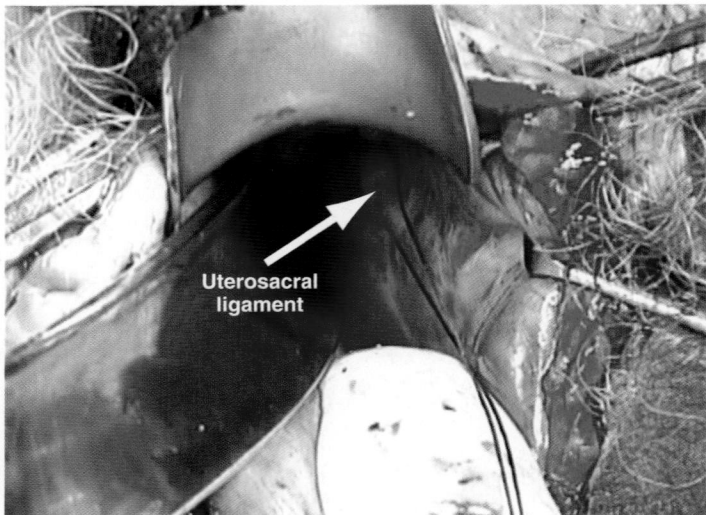

**FIGURE 55–16** Suture placement for traditional uterosacral suspension. Note that the suture is passed through the upper portion of the uterosacral ligament just below the level of the ischial spine.

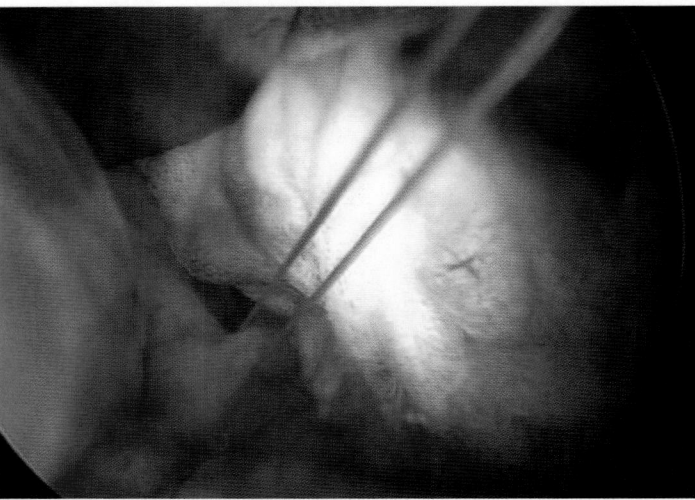

**FIGURE 55–17** Suture placement for modified high uterosacral suspension. Note that the suture is passed above and medial to the ischial spine, incorporating the coccygeus–sacrospinous ligament complex (CSSL) or the presacral fascia.

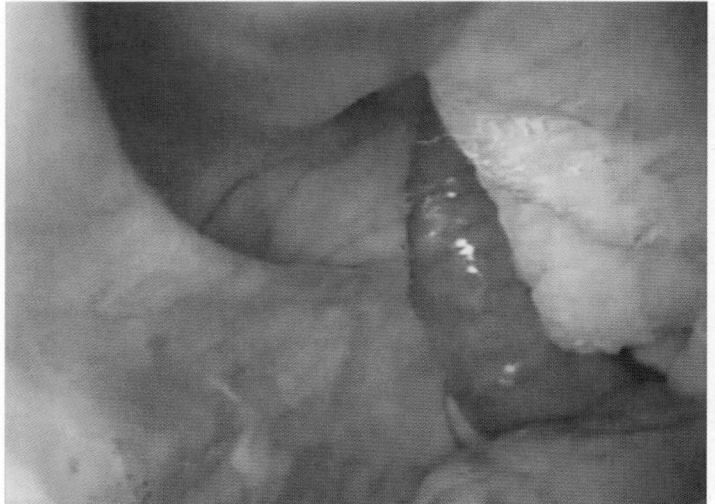

**FIGURE 55–18** An intraperitoneal photograph of the uppermost portion of the right uterosacral ligament. Note that a portion of this structure inserts directly into the coccygeus–sacrospinous ligament complex (CSSL).

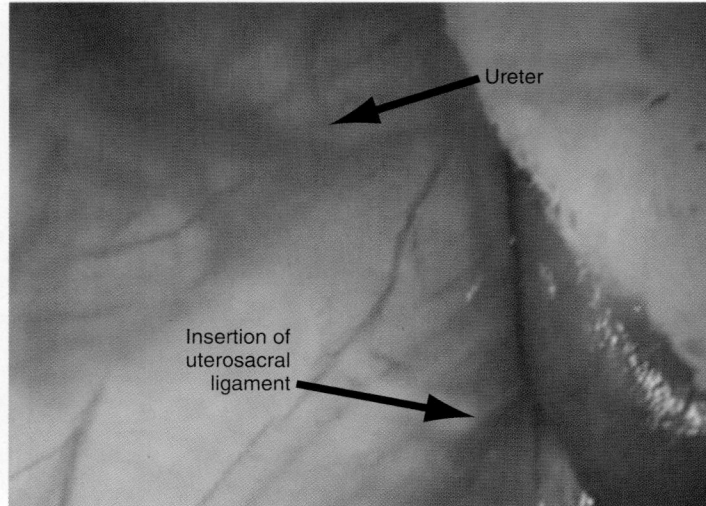

**FIGURE 55–19** An intraperitoneal photograph shows the relationship between the right ureter and the uppermost portion of the right uterosacral ligament.

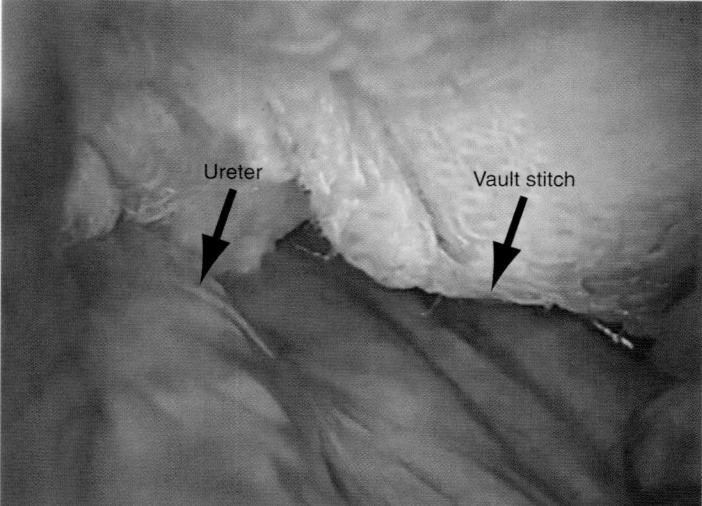

**FIGURE 55–20** Intraperitoneal photograph illustrating the location of the suture for modified high uterosacral suspension. Note that the suture is placed at least 2 cm medial to the ureter.

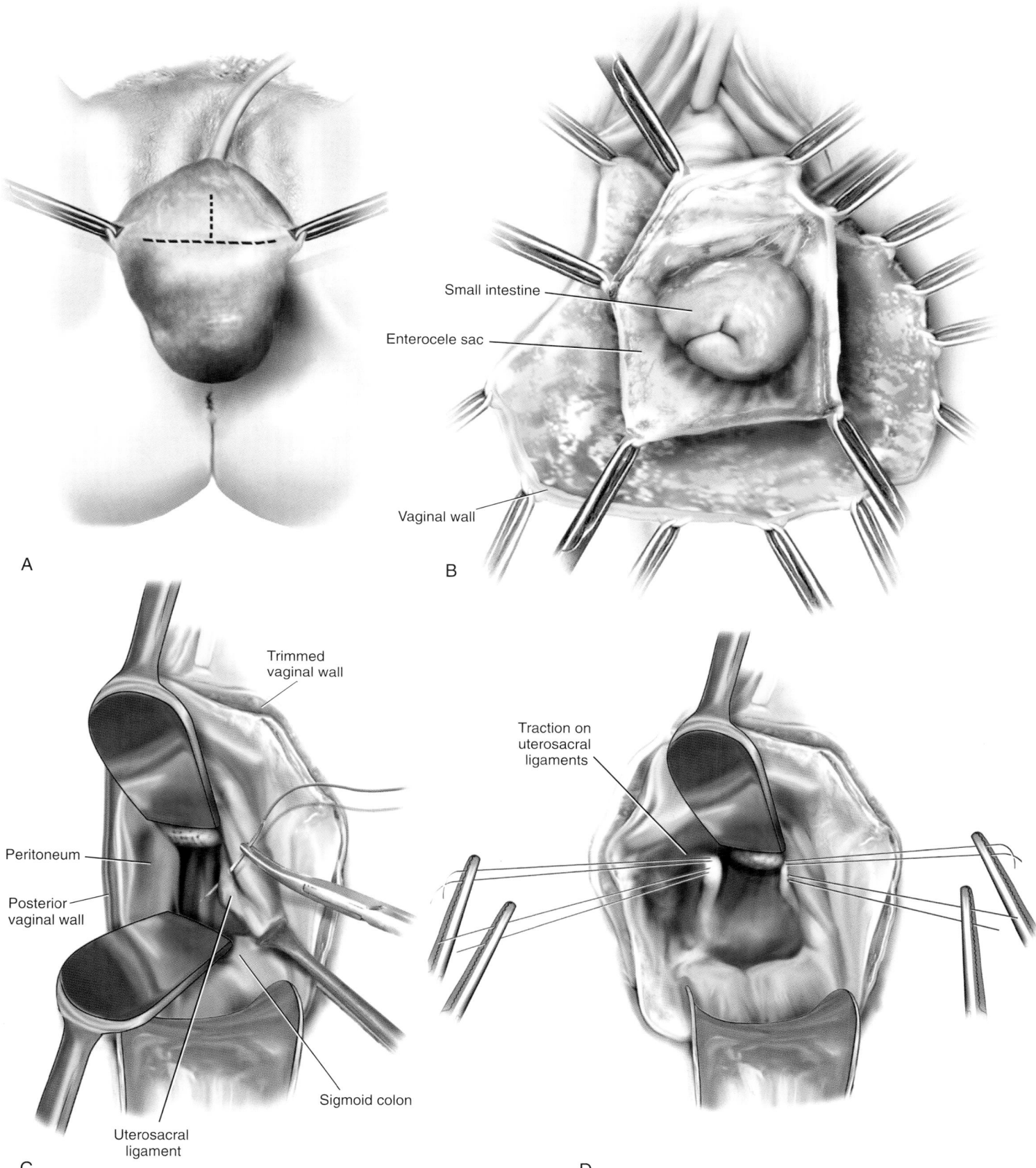

A

B

Small intestine

Enterocele sac

Vaginal wall

Trimmed
vaginal wall

Peritoneum

Posterior
vaginal wall

Sigmoid colon

Uterosacral
ligament

C

Traction on
uterosacral
ligaments

D

**FIGURE 55–21** Technique for high uterosacral vaginal vault suspension. **A.** The most prominent portion of the prolapsed vaginal vault is grasped with two Allis clamps. **B.** The vaginal wall is opened up, and the enterocele sac is identified and entered. **C.** The bowel is packed high up into the pelvis using large laparotomy sponges. The retractor lifts the sponges up out of the lower pelvis, thus completely exposing the cul-de-sac. When appropriate traction is placed downward on the uterosacral ligaments with an Allis clamp, the uterosacral ligaments are easily palpated bilaterally. **D.** Delayed absorbable sutures have been passed through the uppermost portion of the uterosacral ligaments on each side and have been individually tagged.

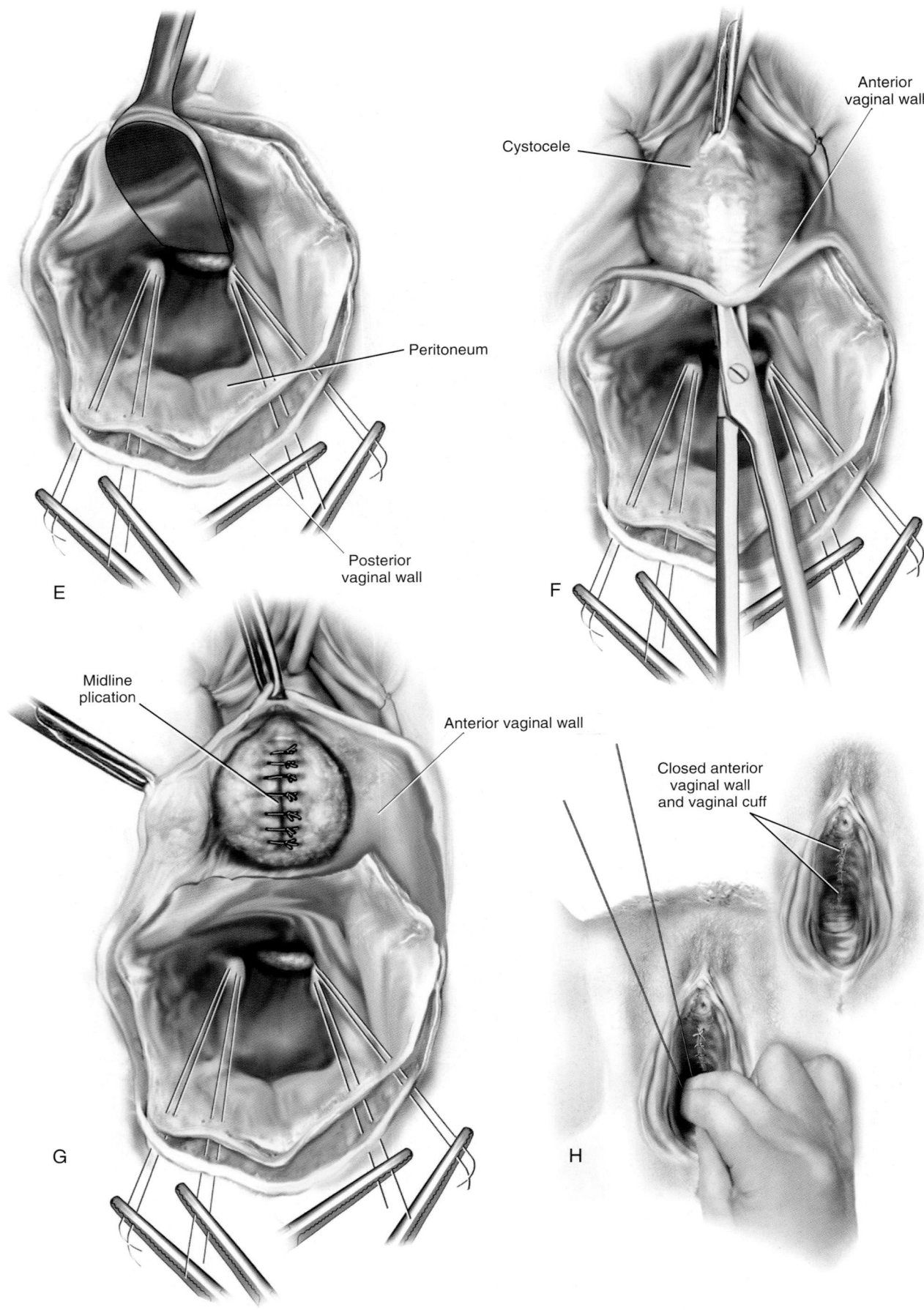

**FIGURE 55–21, cont'd  E.** Each end of the previously passed sutures is brought out through the posterior peritoneum and the posterior vaginal wall. (A free needle is used to pass both ends of these delayed absorbable sutures through the full thickness of the vaginal wall.) **F.** The anterior colporrhaphy is begun by initiating a dissection between the prolapsed bladder and the anterior vaginal wall. **G.** The anterior colporrhaphy has been completed. **H.** The vagina has been appropriately trimmed and closed with interrupted or continuous delayed absorbable sutures. After closure of the vagina, the delayed absorbable sutures that were previously brought out through the full thickness of the posterior vaginal wall are tied, thereby elevating the prolapsed vaginal vault high up into the hollow of the sacrum.

Figures 55–22 and 55–23 illustrate important anatomic relationships between the uterosacral ligaments and surrounding structures. Figures 55–24 and 55–25 show two examples of cases in which a traditional uterosacral suspension is performed. Figure 55–26 demonstrates the increased vaginal length that can be obtained when a modified high uterosacral suspension is performed. Figure 55–27 illustrates the high suspension of the vaginal apex with the creation of a normal vaginal axis. Figure 55–28 compares vaginal shape and configuration after traditional uterosacral suspension and modified high uterosacral suspension.

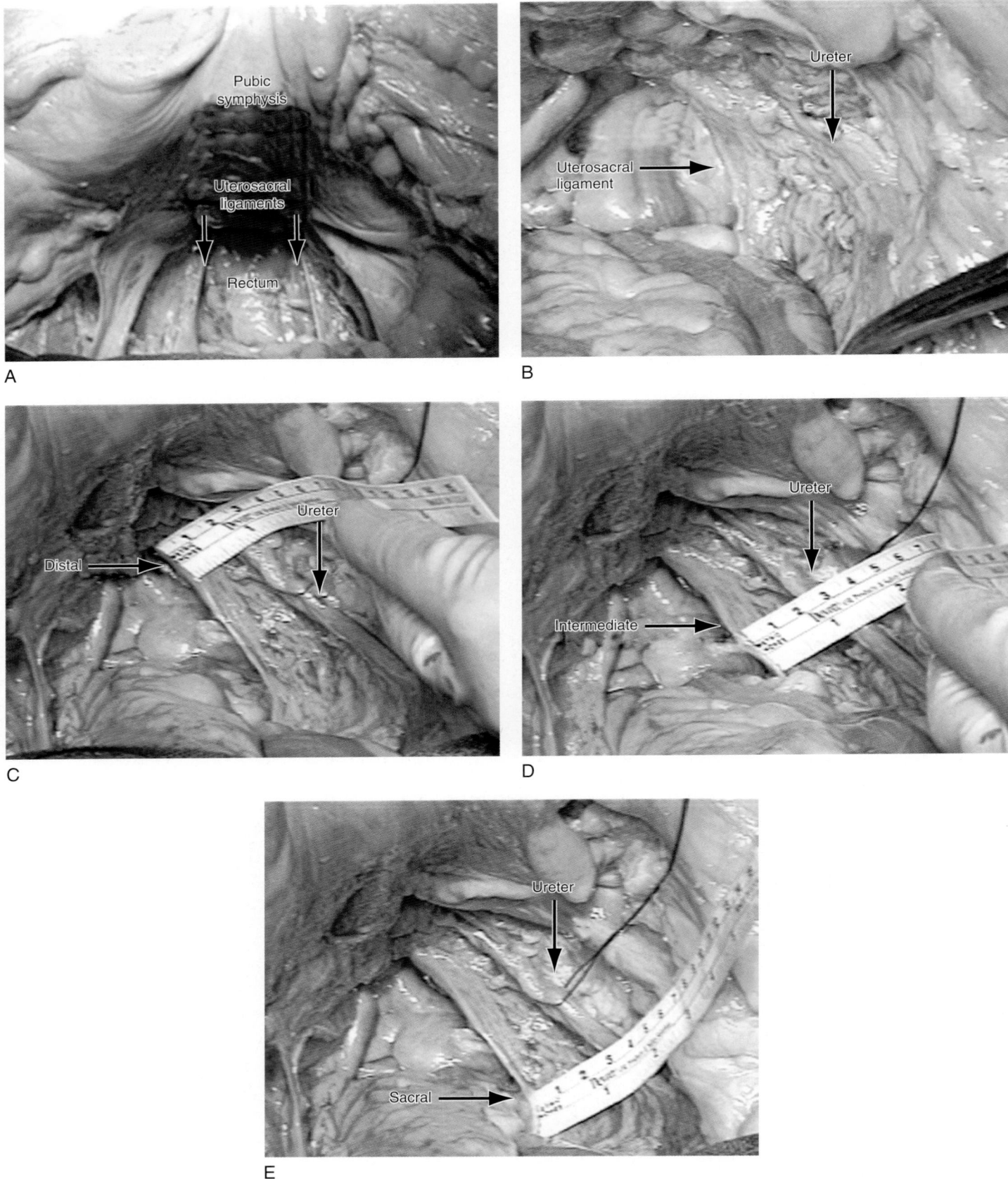

A

B

C

D

E

**FIGURE 55–22** Important anatomic relationships between the uterosacral ligament and surrounding structures with cadaveric dissection. **A.** An abdominal view of the uterosacral ligaments as they relate to the rectum. **B.** Abdominal view of the uterosacral ligaments and their relationship to the ureter. **C.** The distal uterosacral ligament is noted to be 2.5 cm medial to the ureter in this specific cadaveric dissection. **D.** The relationship between the intermediate portion of the uterosacral ligament and the ureter. Again, the ureter is 2.5 to 3 cm lateral to this portion of the uterosacral ligament. **E.** The relationship between the ureter and the uppermost portion or the most proximal portion of the uterosacral ligament. The ureter is approximately 3.5 cm lateral to this portion of the uterosacral ligament. (Compliments of The Cleveland Clinic Foundation.)

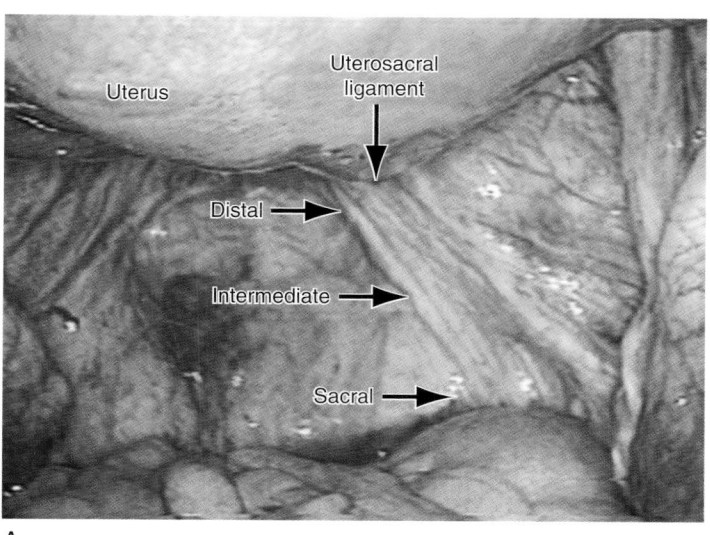
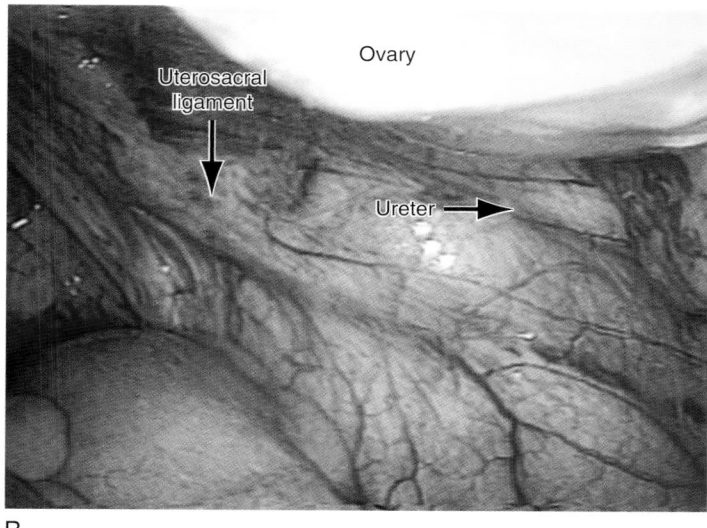

A                  B

**FIGURE 55–23** Laparoscopic view of the relationship between the uterosacral ligament and the other pelvic organs. **A.** Note that the distal, intermediate, and sacral portions of the uterosacral ligament are demonstrated on the patient's right side. **B.** Note the relationship of the uterosacral ligament to the right ureter viewed laparoscopically. (Compliments of The Cleveland Clinic Foundation.)

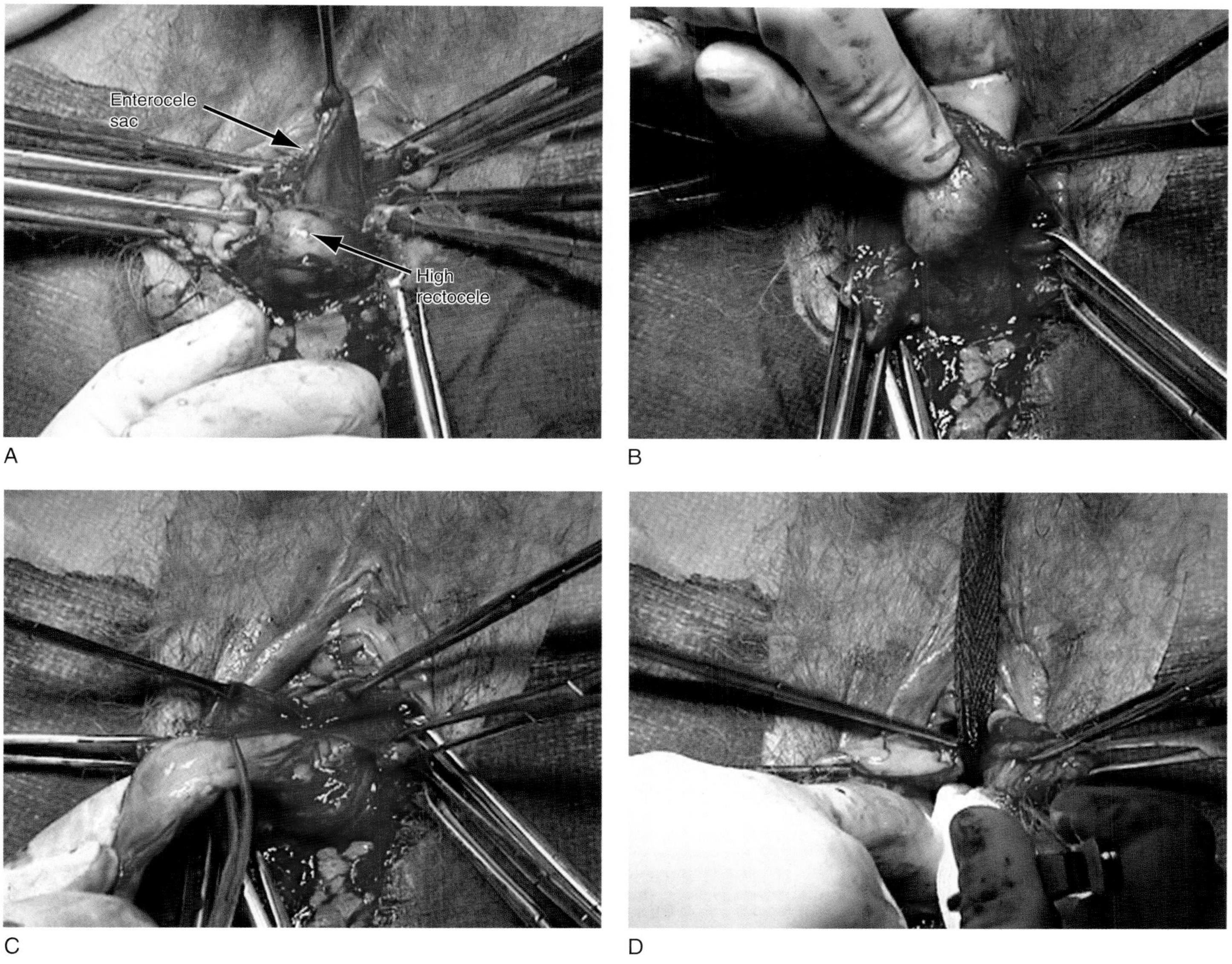

A                  B

C                  D

**FIGURE 55–24** Technique for traditional uterosacral suspension. **A.** The patient has a large posterior vaginal wall defect. A high rectocele and the enterocele sac have been identified. **B.** The enterocele sac has been entered, and the cul-de-sac is being palpated in preparation for excising the peritoneal sac. **C.** The peritoneal sac is being excised. **D.** The intraperitoneal contents have been packed with large laparotomy tail sponges to facilitate exposure of the posterior cul-de-sac.

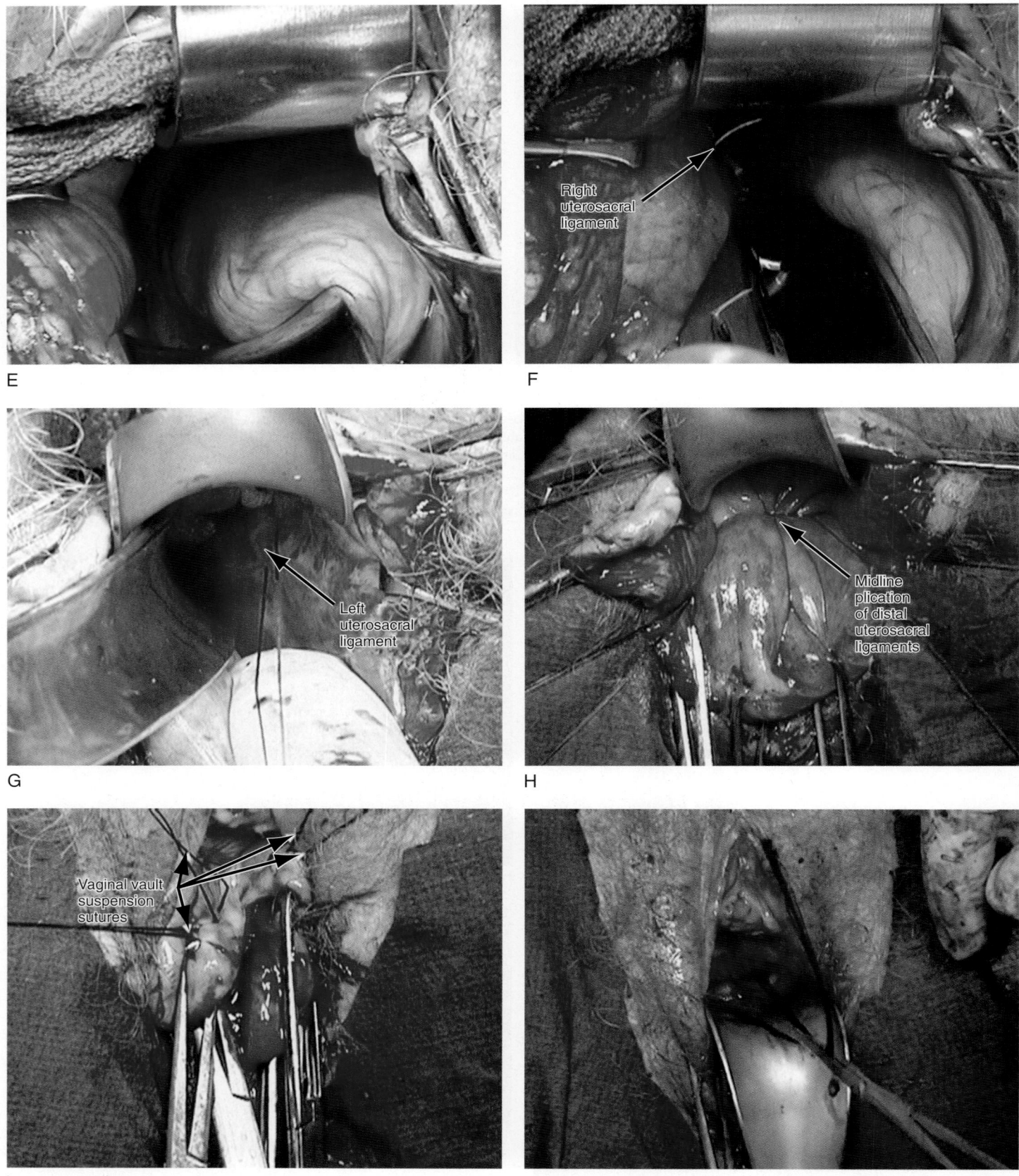

**FIGURE 55–24, cont'd** **E.** A large retractor has been placed intraperitoneally, and the lap sponges have been elevated high up into the abdomen, thus nicely exposing the entire cul-de-sac. **F.** The right uterosacral ligament has been identified, and a delayed absorbable suture has been passed through the right uterosacral ligament at the level of the ischial spine. **G.** The left uterosacral ligament has been identified, and a delayed absorbable suture has been passed through the ligament at the level of the ischial spine. **H.** The distal portion of the cul-de-sac has been plicated across the midline with permanent sutures. **I.** The sutures previously passed through the uterosacral ligament on each side have now been passed through the full thickness of the vaginal wall at the level of the apex of the vagina. The vagina has been closed, and the vaginal vault stitches have been tied. **J.** Note the excellent elevation of the apex of the vagina high up into the hollow of the sacrum, without any significant distortion of the vaginal axis.

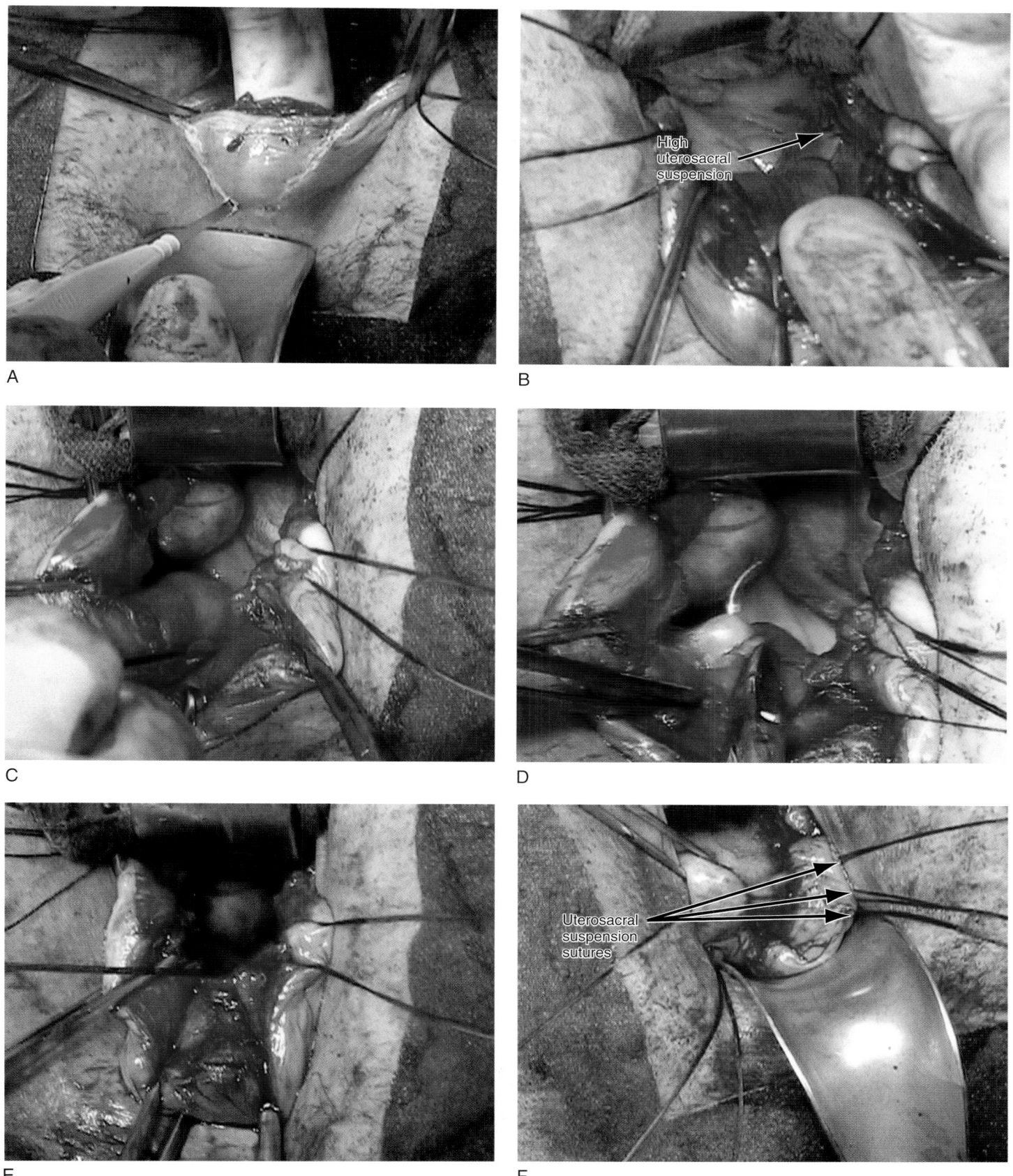

A

B

High
uterosacral
suspension

C

D

E

F

Uterosacral
suspension
sutures

**FIGURE 55–25** Technique of a high uterosacral vaginal vault suspension in a patient who has undergone a vaginal hysterectomy. **A.** Note that the cul-de-sac is being palpated and excess posterior vaginal skin and peritoneum are being excised. **B.** Uterosacral suspension sutures have been passed on the patient's left side. These again are delayed absorbable sutures that are individually tagged. **C.** The distal portion of the cul-de-sac is visualized in preparation for midline plication. **D.** A permanent suture is being passed across the cul-de-sac to plicate the distal portions of the uterosacral ligaments. **E.** The permanent sutures that were previously passed to plicate the distal portions of the uterosacral ligaments are now tied in the midline, creating midline support of the cul-de-sac. **F.** The sutures that were previously passed through the upper portion of the uterosacral ligament are now individually taken out through the posterolateral aspects of the vaginal vault.

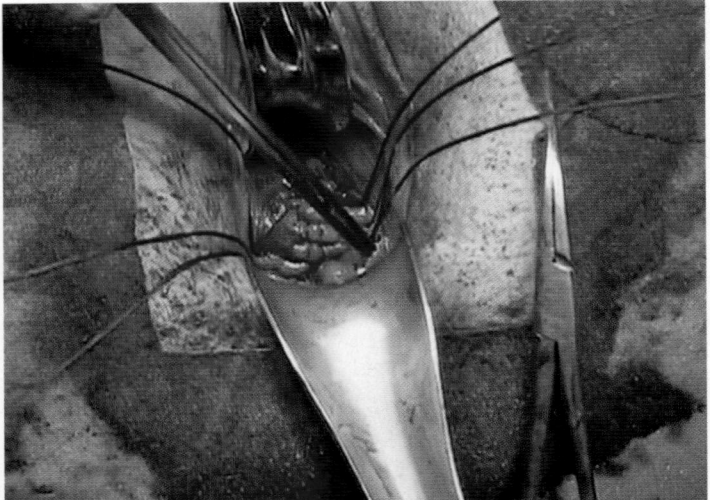

G

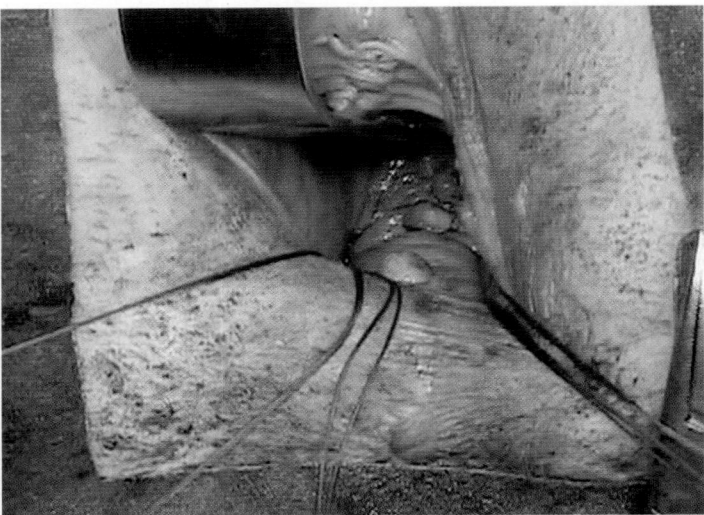

H

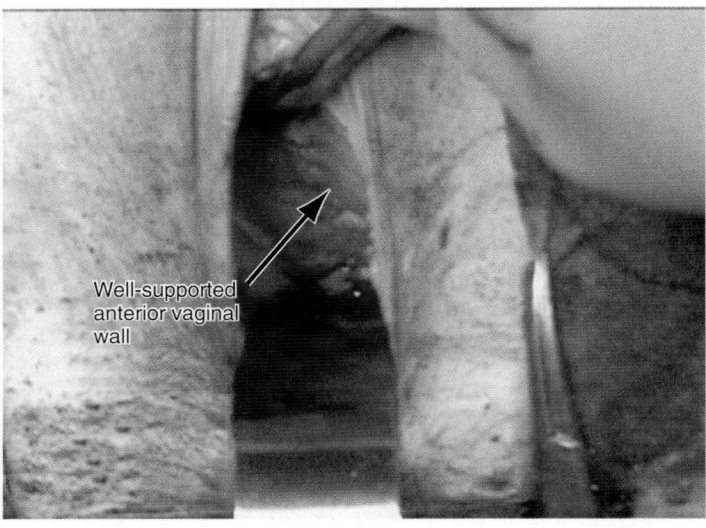

Well-supported
anterior vaginal
wall

I

**FIGURE 55–25, cont'd  G.** The vagina has been closed. **H.** The vaginal vault sutures have been tied. Note the excellent elevation of the apex of the vagina into the hollow of the sacrum without any significant distortion of the vaginal apex. **I.** Note the normal support of the anterior vaginal wall after the apical sutures have been tied.

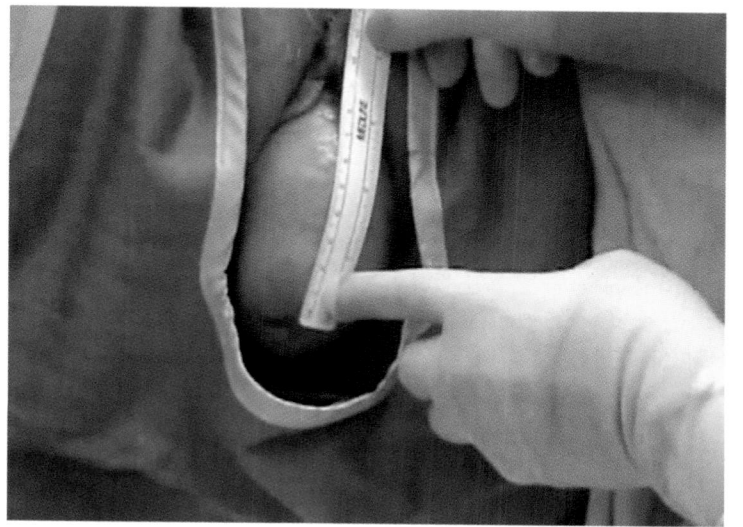

A

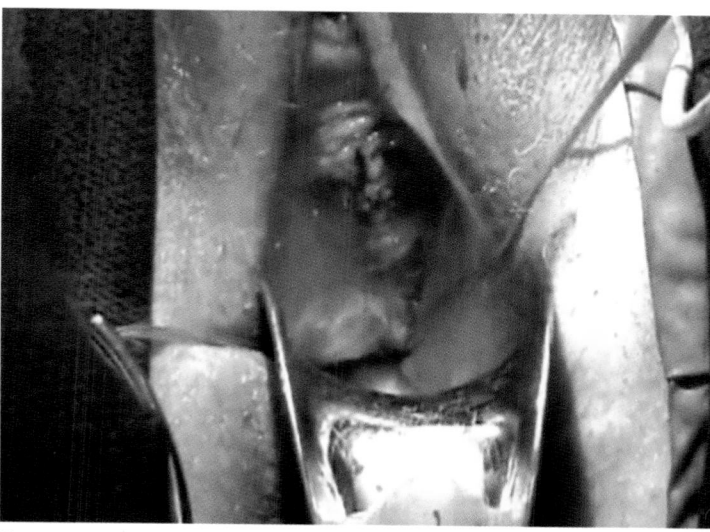

B

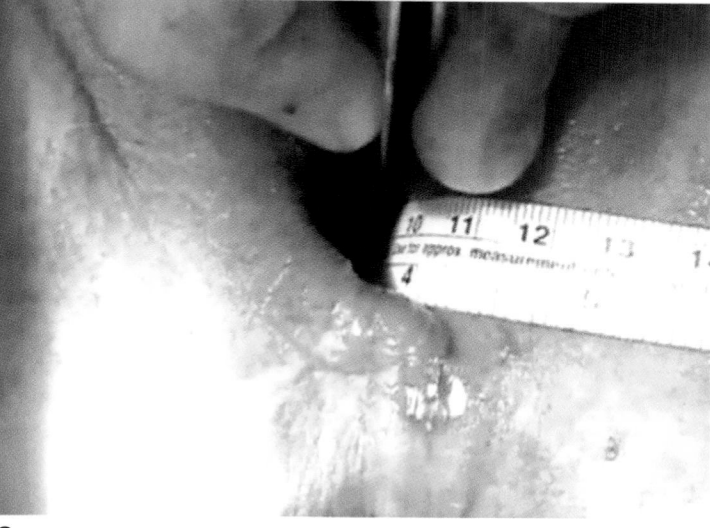

C

**FIGURE 55–26 A.** Patient with complete uterine procidentia and vaginal eversion extending 11 cm beyond the introitus. **B.** View of the suspended vaginal vault after vaginal hysterectomy with repairs and modified high uterosacral vaginal vault suspension. **C.** Note that the vagina is 11 cm in length after completion of the repair.

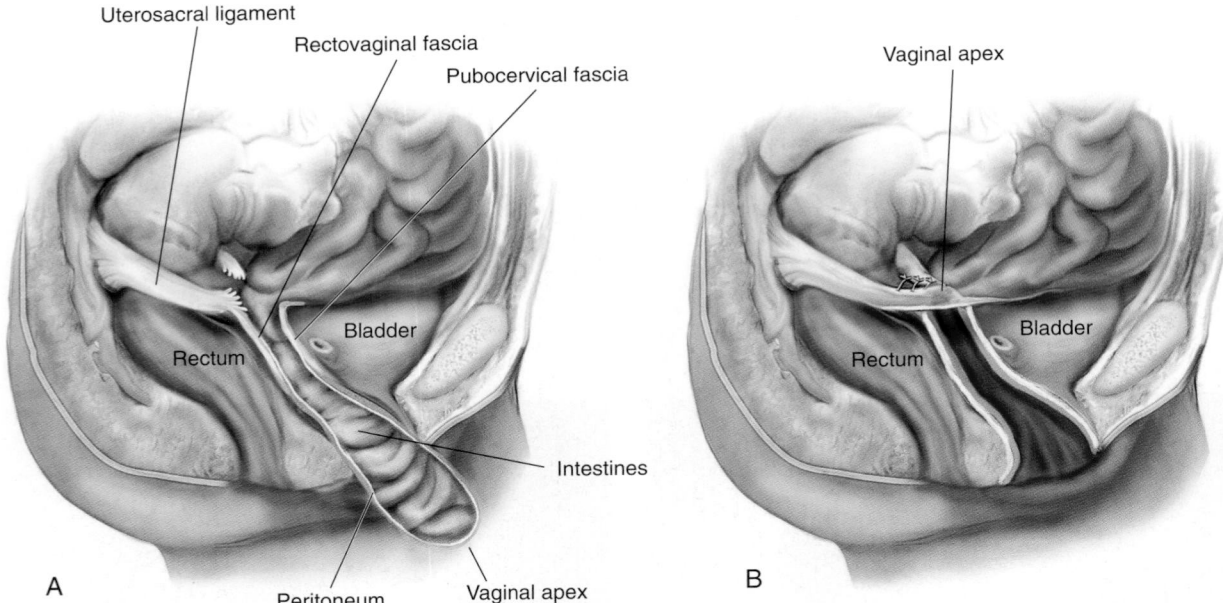

**FIGURE 55–27  A.** Cross-section of pelvis demonstrating enterocele and vaginal vault prolapse. **B.** Cross-section of the pelvis after excision of the enterocele sac and suspension of the vaginal apex to the uppermost portions of the uterosacral ligaments.

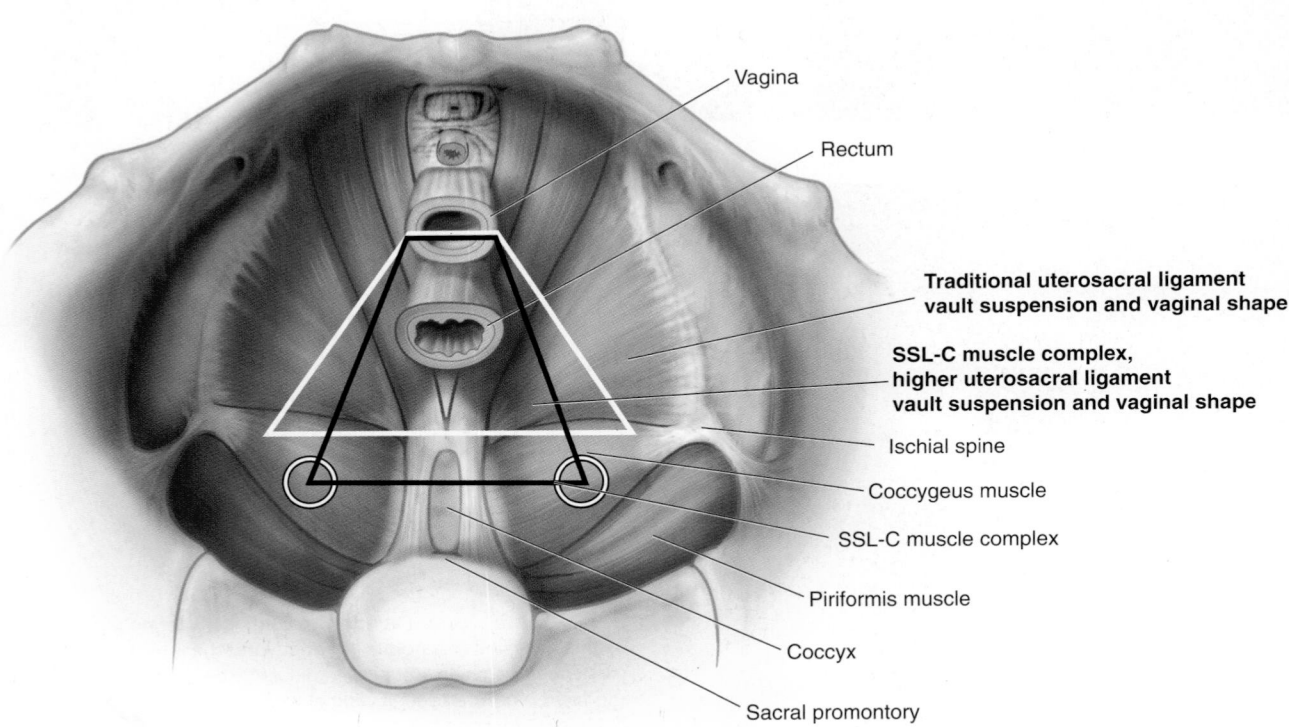

**FIGURE 55–28** Vaginal shape and configuration after bilateral traditional uterosacral suspension (*white trapezoid*) versus high modified uterosacral suspension (*black trapezoid*).

# CHAPTER 56

# Obliterative Procedure for the Correction of Pelvic Organ Prolapse

*Mickey M. Karram*

## Obliterative Procedure

### LeFort Partial Colpocleisis

In elderly, fragile, or medically compromised patients with advanced prolapse, the best management option is sometimes an obliterative procedure. The advantages of these procedures are that they can be performed quickly with minimal morbidity, often with the patient under a local anesthetic. When a uterus is present, a LeFort partial colpocleisis (Fig. 56–1) is performed as follows:

1. Traction is placed on the cervix to evert the vagina completely, and a 0.5% solution of lidocaine or bupivacaine (marcaine) with epinephrine is used to inject the vaginal tissue below the epithelium. A pudendal nerve block can be used if the procedure is being performed with the patient under local anesthetic. A Foley catheter with a 30-mL balloon is placed for easy identification of the bladder neck.
2. A dilatation and curettage should be performed if it was not performed preoperatively to ensure that no premalignant or malignant process is present in the uterus.
3. Areas to be denuded anteriorly and posteriorly are marked out with a scalpel or a marking pencil, as indicated in Figure 56–2. The rectangular piece of anterior vaginal wall should extend from 2 cm proximal to the tip of the cervix to approximately 5 cm below the external urethral meatus (see Fig. 56–2).
4. Sharp and blunt dissection is used to remove the vaginal epithelium. These flaps should be thin, leaving the maximum amount of fascia on the bladder and rectum. Sufficient vagina should be left bilaterally to form canals for draining cervical secretions or blood. We almost routinely perform a plication of the bladder neck (see Fig. 56–1). Posteriorly, the cul-de-sac peritoneum may be encountered when the vaginal mucosa is excised, but it does not have to be entered. Bleed-

ing is controlled with fulguration. Absolute hemostasis is necessary to avoid a postoperative hematoma in the vaginal canal.

5. The cut edge of the anterior vaginal wall is sewn to the cut edge of the posterior vaginal wall with interrupted delayed absorbable sutures (Figs. 56–3 and 56–4). This is achieved in such a way that the knot is turned into and remains in the epithelium-lined tunnels that are created bilaterally (Fig. 56–5). Suturing in this way gradually pushes the uterus and the vaginal apex inward. When the entire vagina has been inverted, the superior and inferior margins over the rectangle can be sutured horizontally (Fig. 56–6).
6. Perineorrhaphy and distal levatorplasty is usually performed to increase posterior pelvic muscle support and narrow the introitus. Postoperatively, the patient is mobilized early; however, heavy lifting is avoided for at least 2 months to prevent recurrence of the prolapse secondary to breakdown of the repair. Figure 56–7 reviews the technique of LeFort partial colpocleisis with perineorrhaphy.

### Colpectomy and Colpocleisis

In cases of posthysterectomy vaginal vault prolapse in which obliteration of the vagina is chosen as the procedure of choice, it is best to proceed with a colpectomy and complete colpocleisis. This operation is performed in cases of vault prolapse when operating time is best kept at a minimum and future vaginal intercourse is not anticipated. This procedure can also be performed with the patient under local anesthetic. The operation is performed by completely excising the vaginal mucosa from the underlying vaginal or endopelvic fascia. It is not necessary to enter the peritoneum. A series of purse string delayed absorbable sutures are placed, slowly inverting the vaginal muscularis and fascia (Figs. 56–8 through 56–20). Similar to the LeFort procedure, bladder neck plication and perineorrhaphy with levatorplasty are often performed with a colpectomy.

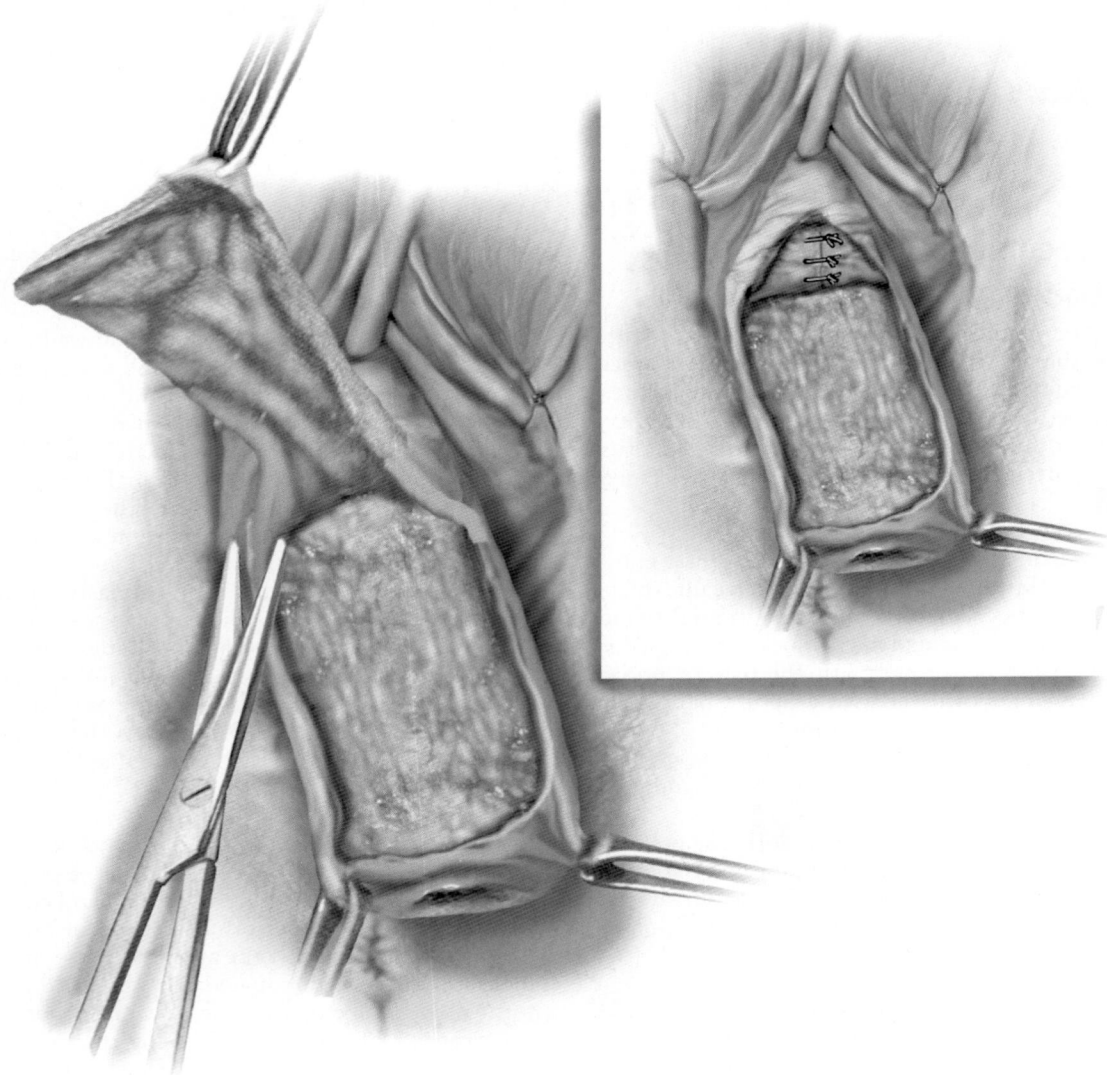

A

**FIGURE 56–1** LeFort partial colpocleisis. **A.** A rectangular piece of anterior vaginal wall has been removed. Note in the **inset** that the dissection has been extended laterally at the level of the proximal urethra to perform a Kelly-Kennedy plication in the hope of providing preferential support to the bladder neck and thus preventing any occult or potential stress incontinence.

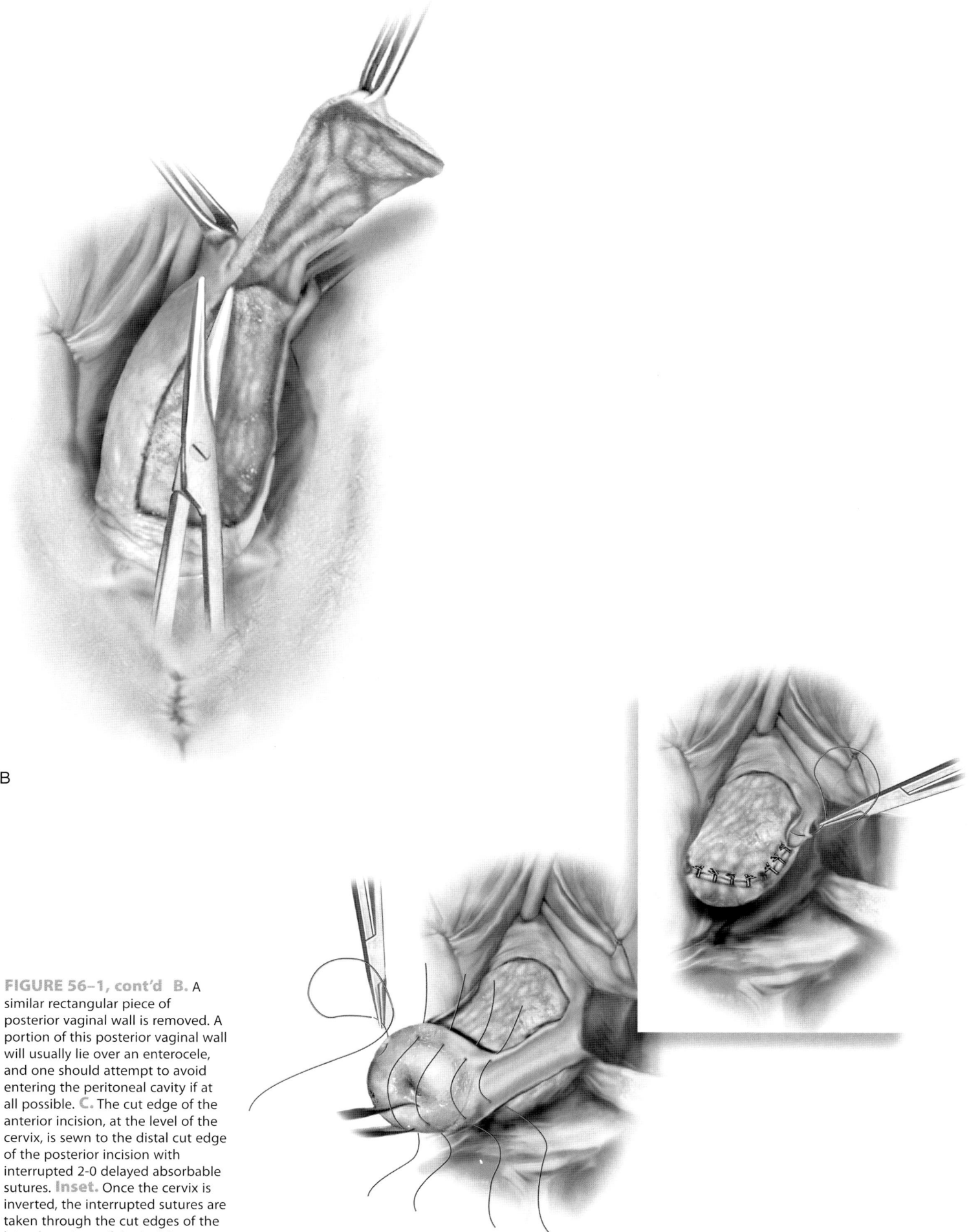

B

C

FIGURE 56–1, cont'd  B. A similar rectangular piece of posterior vaginal wall is removed. A portion of this posterior vaginal wall will usually lie over an enterocele, and one should attempt to avoid entering the peritoneal cavity if at all possible. C. The cut edge of the anterior incision, at the level of the cervix, is sewn to the distal cut edge of the posterior incision with interrupted 2-0 delayed absorbable sutures. Inset. Once the cervix is inverted, the interrupted sutures are taken through the cut edges of the lateral portions of the incision on each side.

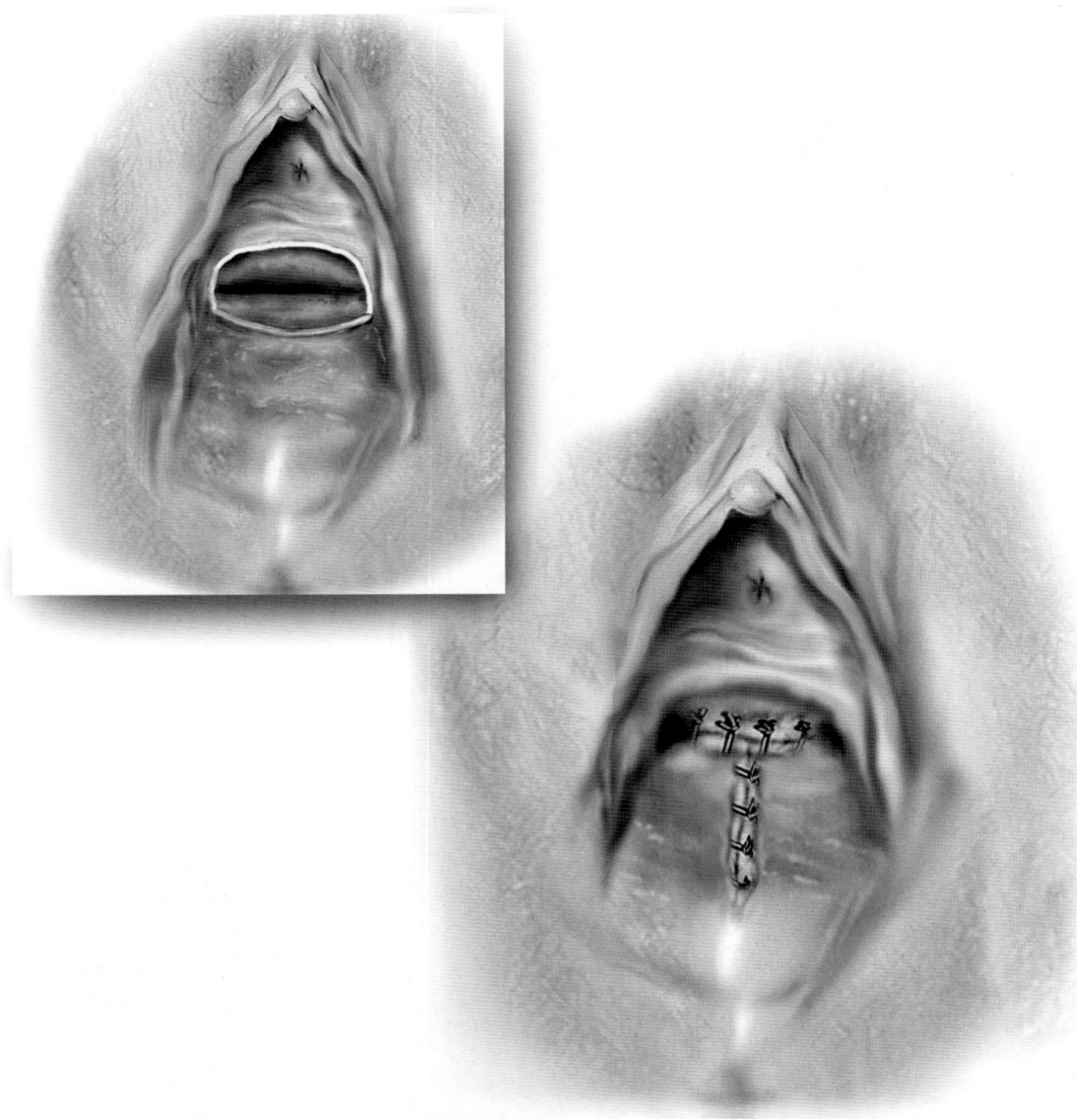

D

**FIGURE 56–1, cont'd  D.** Once the entire vagina has been inverted, the superior and inferior margins over the rectangle can be sutured horizontally, thus completely obliterating the midportion of the vagina. *Note:* Draining channels are left in the lateral portions of the vagina to facilitate drainage of any cervical discharge. A levatorplasty is commonly performed to increase posterior pelvic muscle support and to narrow the introitus.

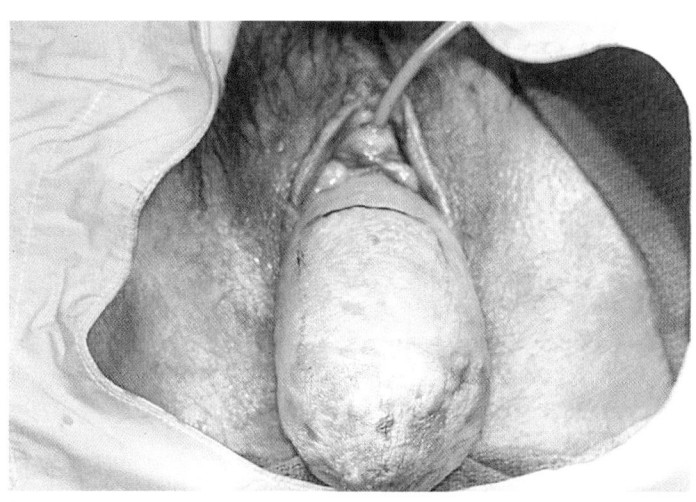
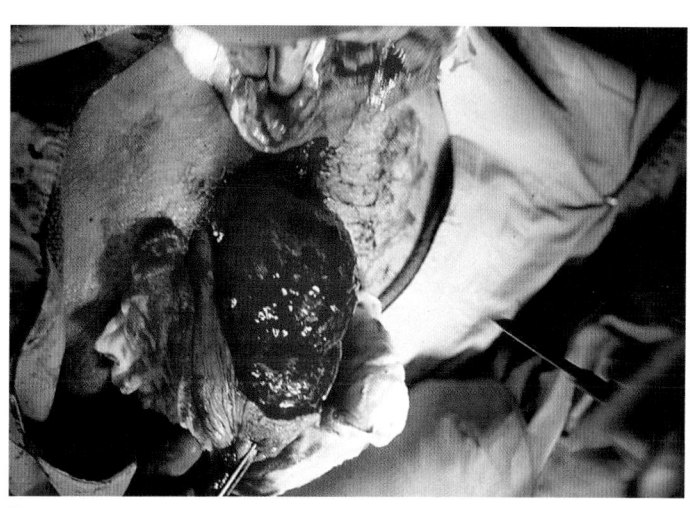

A
B

FIGURE 56–2 A. Complete procidentia. B. A rectangular piece of anterior vaginal wall has been excised.

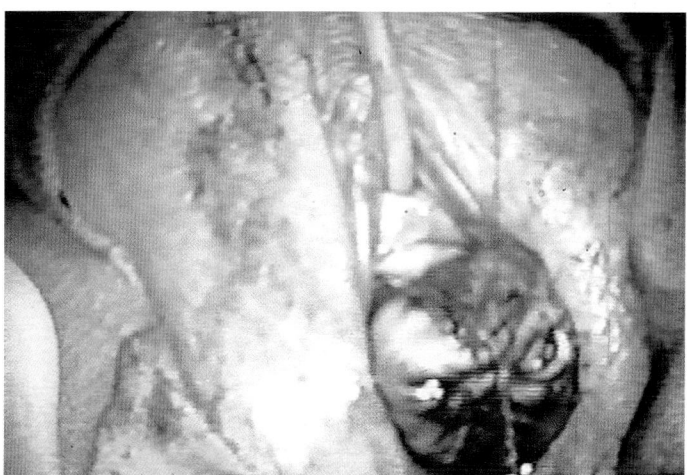
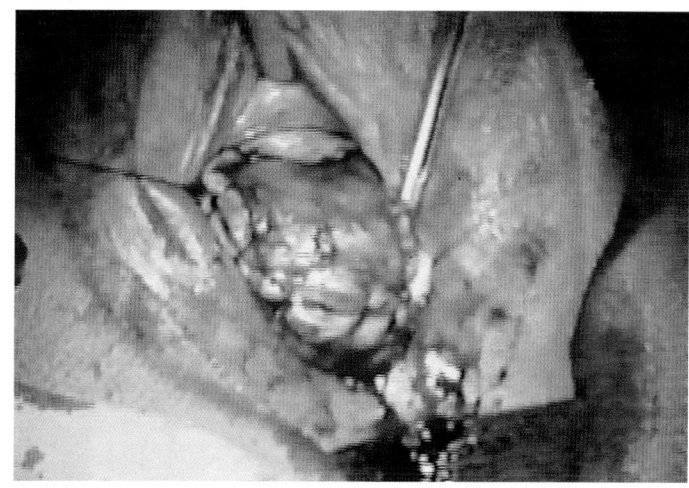

FIGURE 56–3 Interrupted 2-0 absorbable sutures are placed initially, approximating the lower transverse edge of the anterior vaginal wall incision to the upper transverse edge of the posterior vaginal wall. This row of sutures reduces or buries the cervix.

FIGURE 56–4 Sutures are placed all the way to the distal incisions on the anterior and posterior vaginal walls.

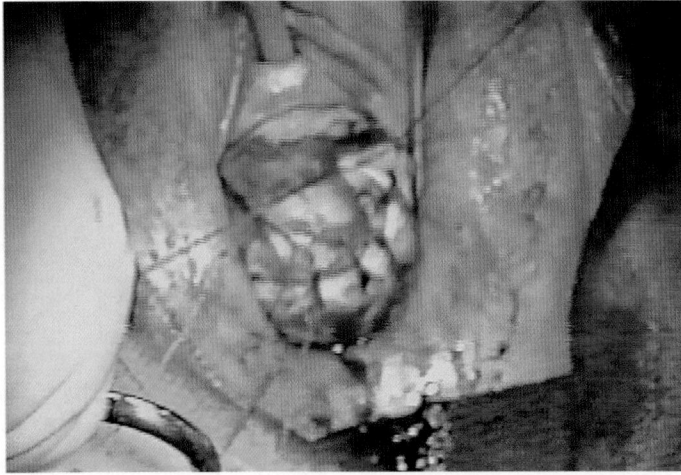

**FIGURE 56–5** As the uterus is reduced, draining channels are created on each side.

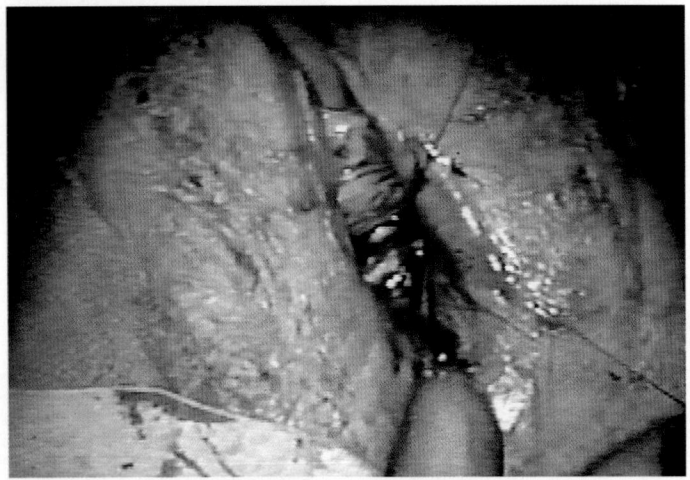

A

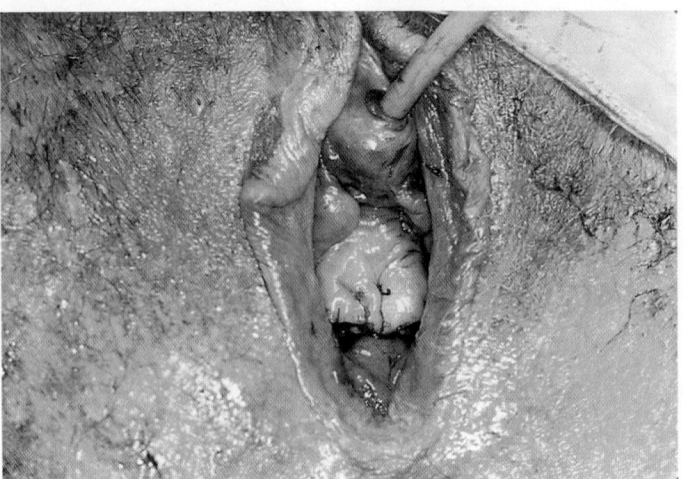

B

**FIGURE 56–6  A.** Once the uterus is reduced, the distal transverse incision on the anterior vaginal wall is sewn to the distal transverse incision on the posterior vaginal wall. **B.** Note the closed vagina with lateral draining channels.

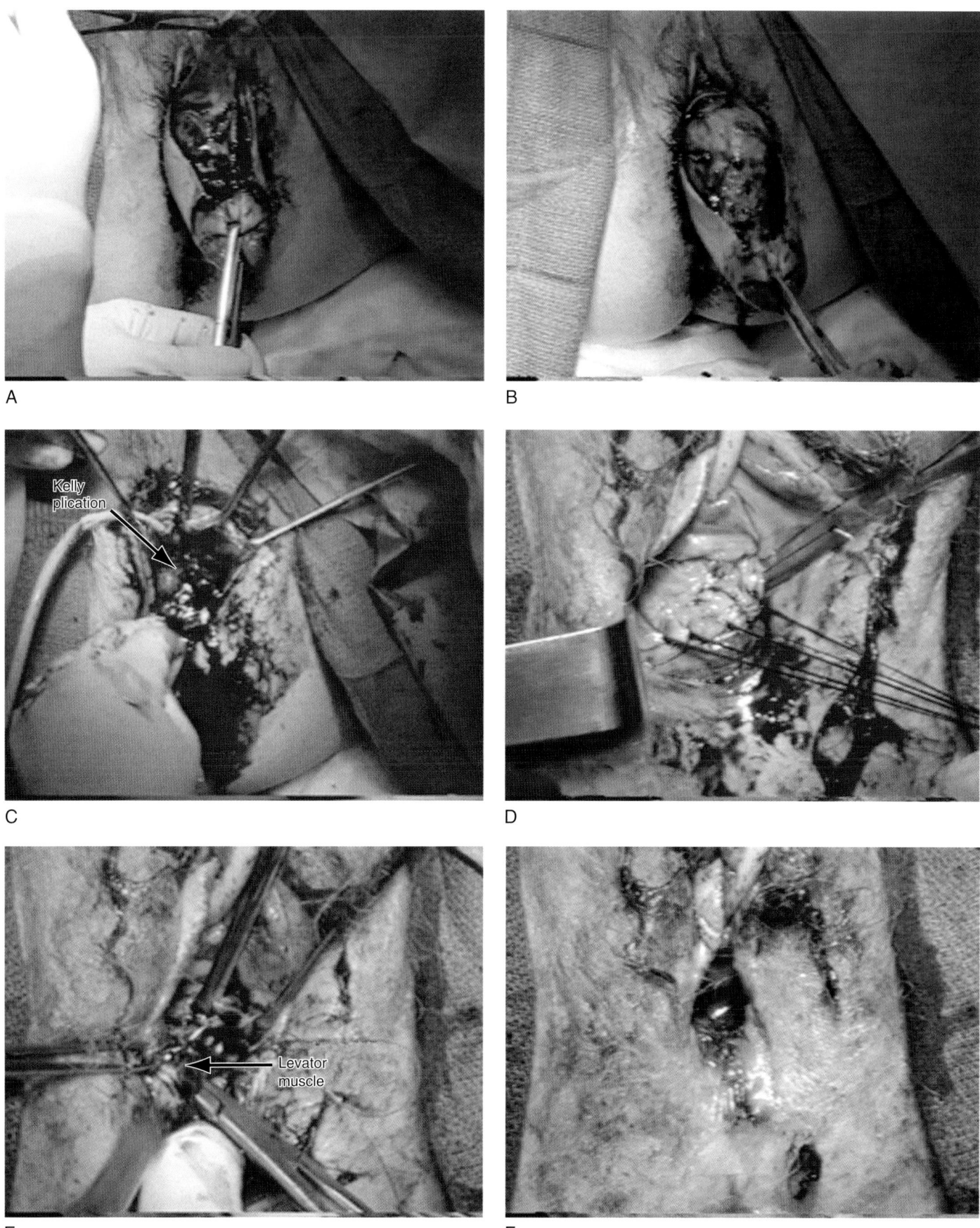

**FIGURE 56–7** Technique of a LeFort partial colpocleisis in conjunction with a perineorrhaphy. **A.** A rectangular piece of anterior vaginal wall is being excised. **B.** The entire anterior dissection has been completed. Note that the rectangular piece of vagina has been removed to the level of the bladder neck to facilitate the performance of a Kelly-Kennedy plication. **C.** The dissection has been extended laterally at the level of the bladder neck, and the Kelly-Kennedy plication stitch has been placed. **D.** The cut edges of the anterior and posterior vaginal wall incisions have been sewn together as previously described. The completed LeFort is shown here. Note that the horizontal superior and inferior edges have been sewn in the midline and the Kelly clamp is placed in the left lateral draining channel. **E.** An incision has been made at the level of the perineum to identify the levator muscle. **F.** A levatorplasty has been performed by plicating the distal portions of the levator muscle across the midline to facilitate posterior vaginal wall support.

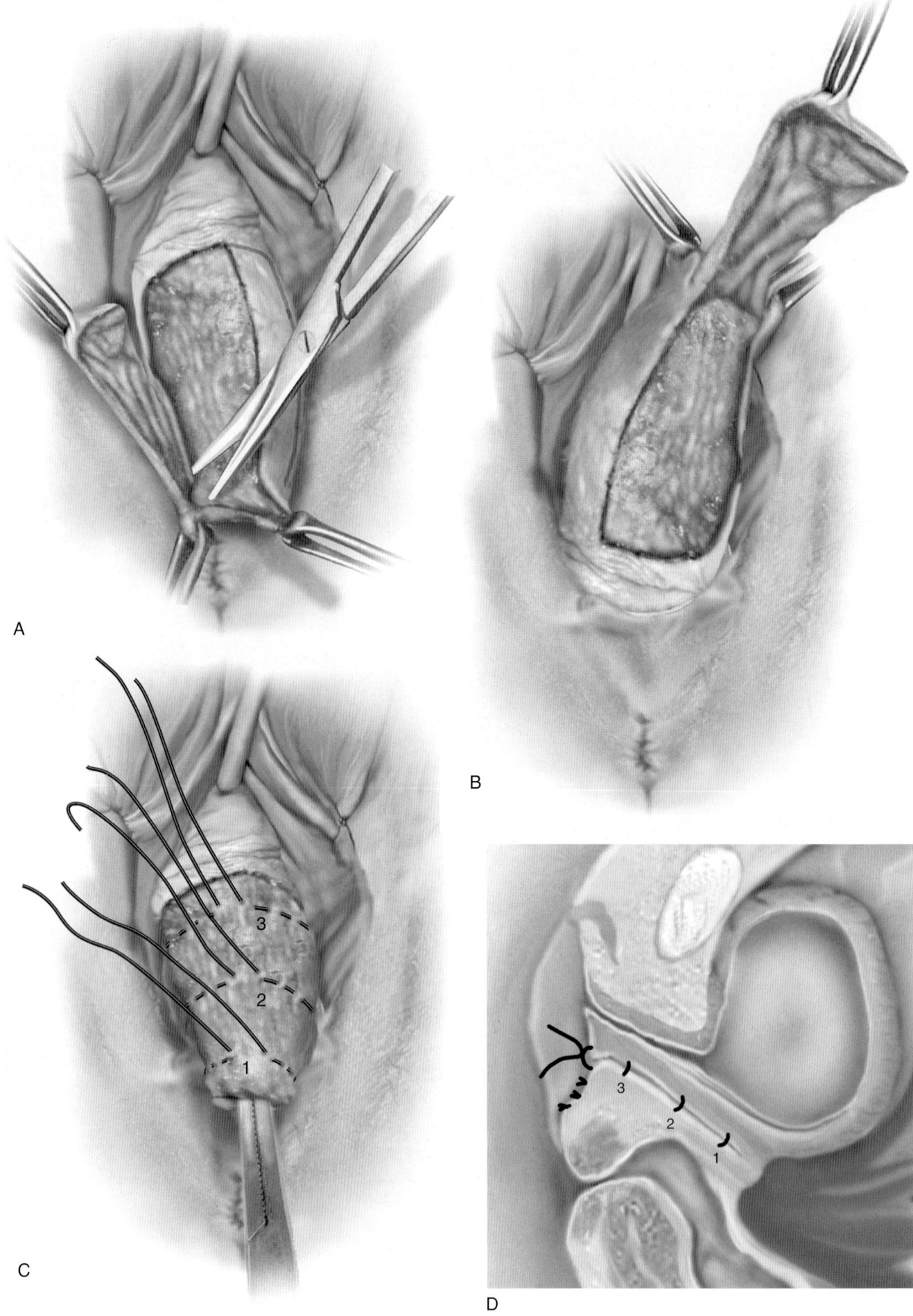

A

B

C

D

**FIGURE 56-8** Colpectomy and complete colpocleisis. **A** and **B.** After subcutaneous infiltration with lidocaine or bupivacaine in 1:200,000 epinephrine solution, the vagina is circumscribed by an incision at the site of the hymen and is marked into quadrants. Each quadrant is removed by sharp dissection. **C.** Purse string delayed absorbable sutures are placed. The leading edge of the soft tissue is inverted by the tip of a forceps. Purse string sutures are tied 1 before 2 and 2 before 3, with progressive inversion of the soft tissue before the tying of each suture. **D.** The final relationship is shown in cross-section. A perineorrhaphy is also usually performed.

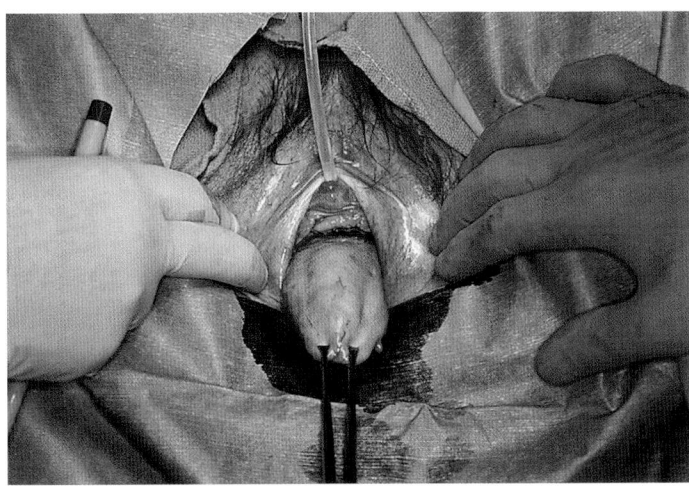

FIGURE 56–9  The base of the prolapse has been marked with a marking pencil.

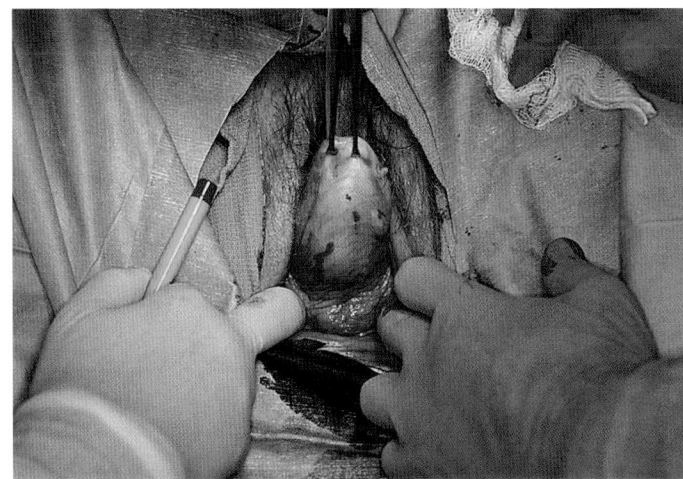

FIGURE 56–10  The level of the posterior aspect of the incision is demonstrated.

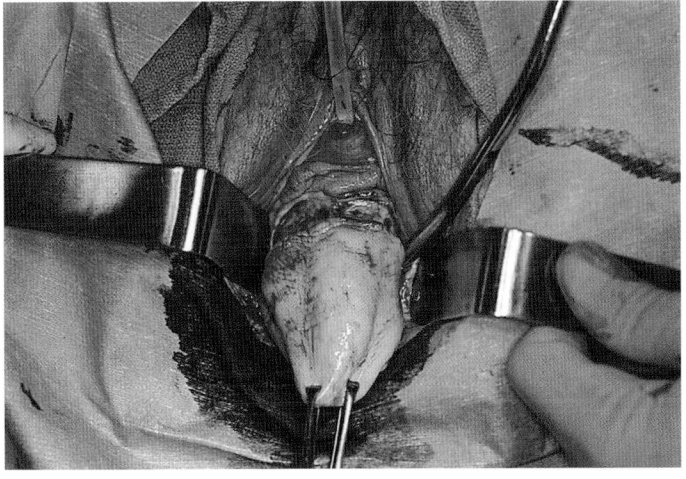

FIGURE 56–11  An incision has been made at the base of the prolapse very near the hymenal ring.

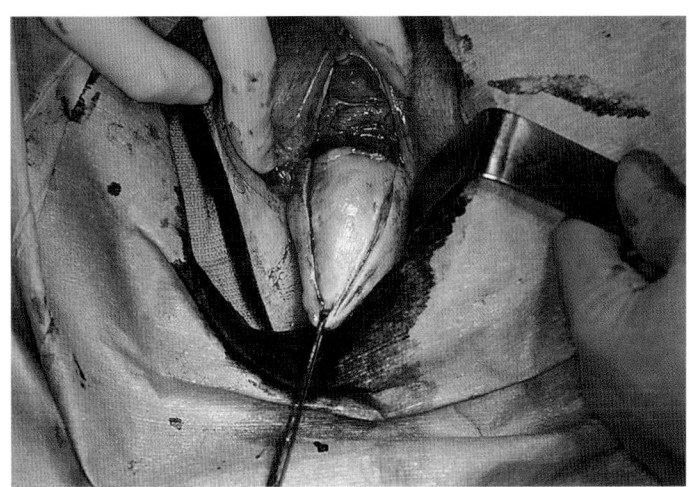

FIGURE 56–12  An incision is made through the vaginal mucosa in preparation for removal of the first quadrant of the vagina.

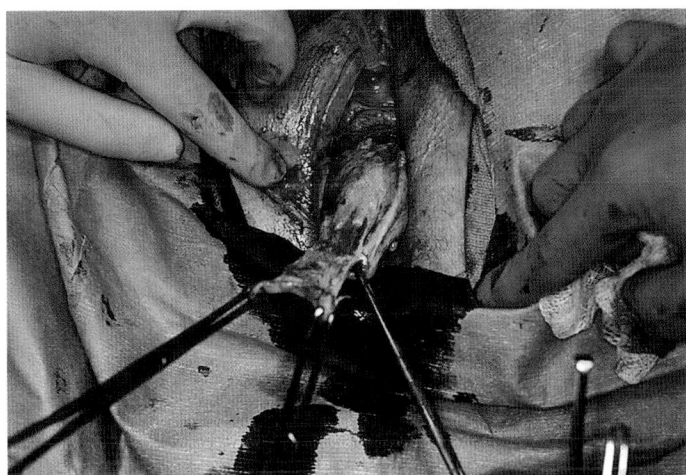

FIGURE 56–13  The first quadrant of the vagina over the prolapse is sharply removed from the underlying tissue.

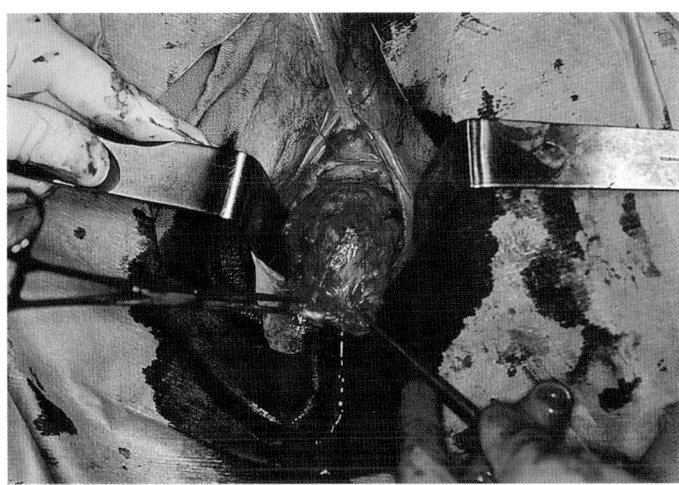

FIGURE 56–14  The remainder of the vaginal epithelium has been removed.

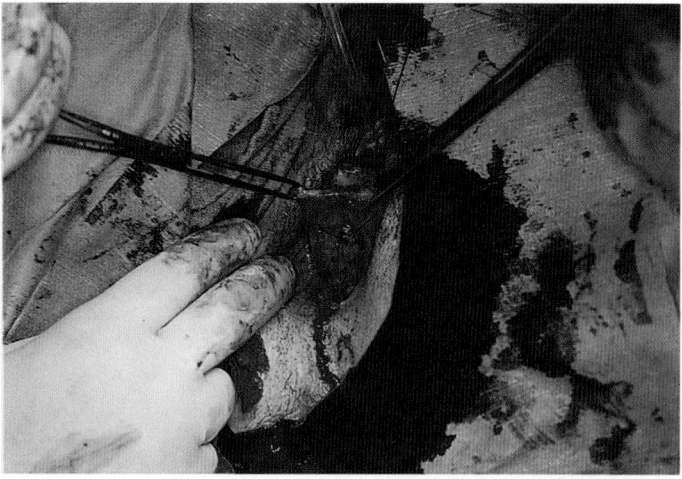

**FIGURE 56-15** The initial purse string 2-0 absorbable suture has been placed.

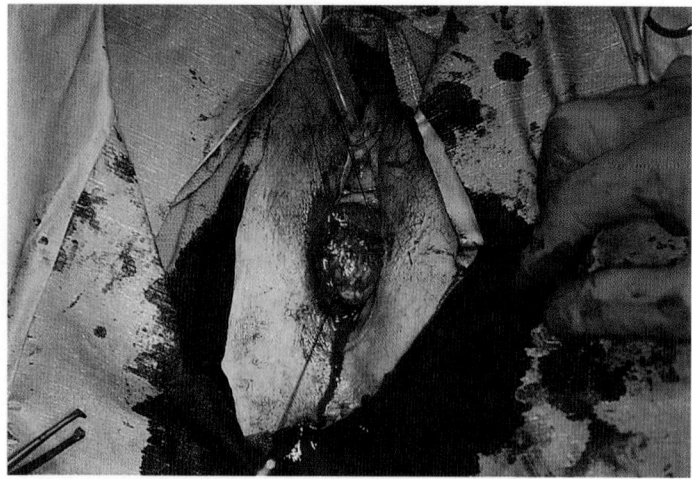

**FIGURE 56-16** The first purse string suture has been tied, and the second purse string suture has been placed.

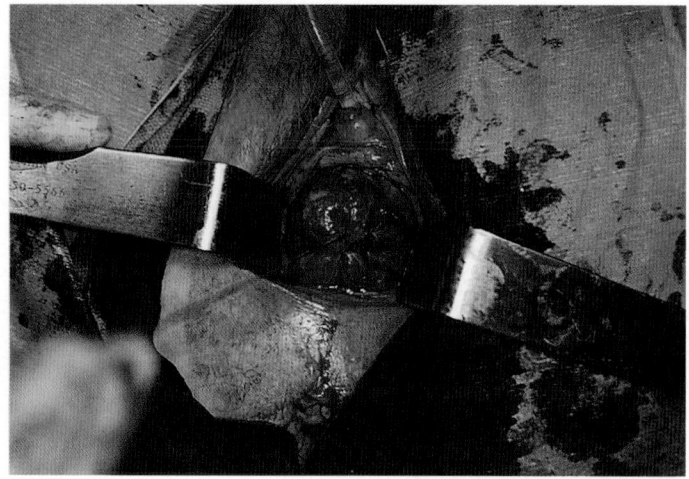

**FIGURE 56-17** The second purse string suture has been tied.

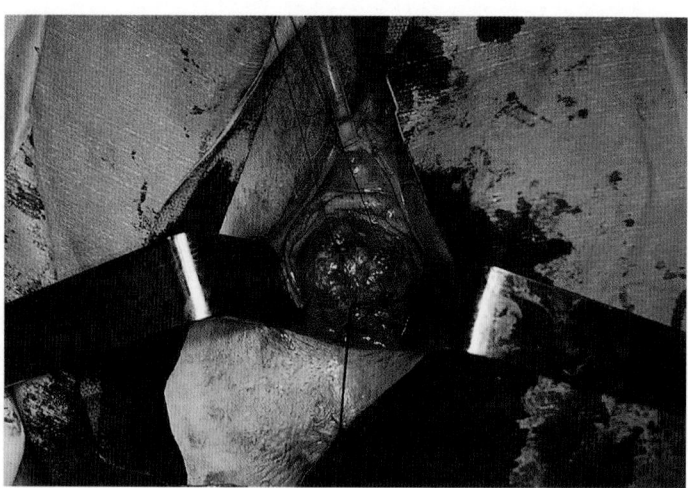

**FIGURE 56-18** The third purse string suture has been placed.

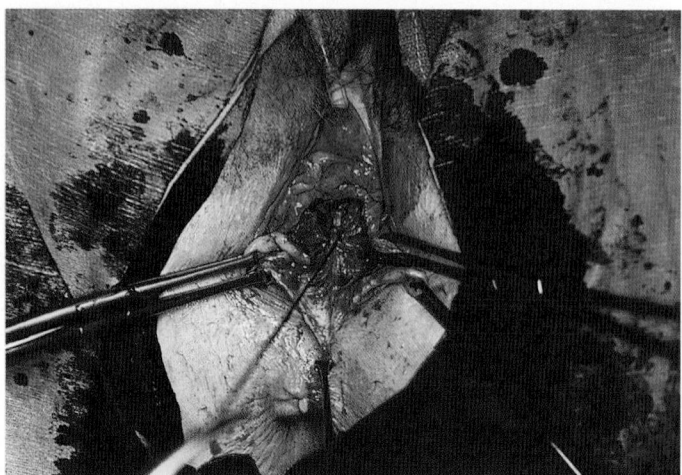

**FIGURE 56-19** The third purse string suture has been tied.

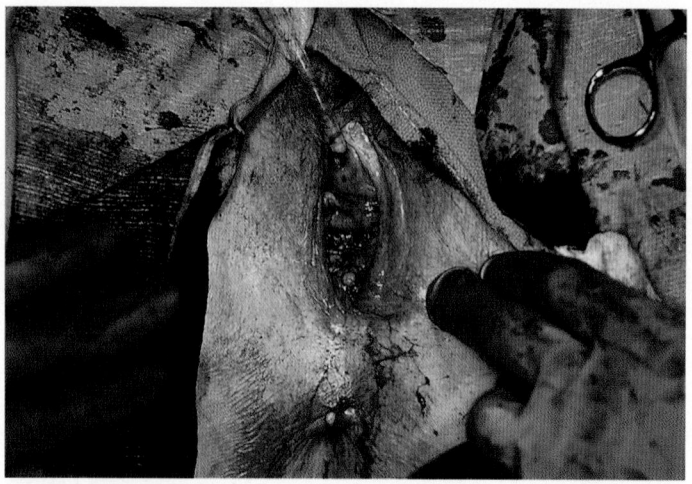

**FIGURE 56-20** The vaginal epithelium is closed, completing the repair.

# CHAPTER 57

# Trocar-Based Synthetic Mesh Kits Used to Correct Pelvic Organ Prolapse

*Vincent Lucente* ■ *Patrick Culligan*

Some surgeons believe that for many patients, native connective tissues are inadequate for successful long-term results in reconstructive pelvic surgery. Recently, meshes have been developed with the hope of meeting the unique requirements for use in the vagina. Innovative tension-free approaches to the placement of these meshes have been described in the hope of facilitating successful surgical outcomes while maintaining a minimally invasive surgical approach.

The most commonly utilized mesh kits for prolapse are the Prolift system marketed by Ethicon Women's Health and Urology (Fig. 57–1), the Apogee and Perigee Systems marketed by American Medical Systems (Fig. 57–2), and the Avaulta System marketed by Bard. These kits make use of an optimal mesh material (polypropylene) and an innovative trocar-based delivery system designed to facilitate tension-free placement. This chapter describes techniques used by the authors for placement of these systems.

Patients undergoing pelvic reconstructive surgery via a transvaginal mesh system require appropriate and standard preoperative medical clearance, especially those patients at increased risk for operative adverse events, such as those resulting from fluid shifts, blood loss, susceptibility to infection, or impaired wound healing. Additional unique considerations must be carefully reviewed before a transvaginal mesh procedure is performed.

Perhaps most important, as for many surgeries, is the provision of a very clear and understandable informed consent process. As with all evolving newer technologies and surgical procedures, one must have even a higher level of commitment to reviewing with the patient where in the development of evidence-based medicine (as well as your own surgical expertise) the surgical technology currently exists. At our centers, we have developed dedicated consent forms specifically designed to clearly communicate to patients the nuances of undergoing these relatively new approaches to pelvic reconstructive surgery. We go to great lengths to explain definitions of the term *experimental* versus *standard of care*. We discuss that the surgery has indeed gone through the review process of the FDA and has stood the test of earlier observational and comparative trials and has developed a growing body of literature supporting the benefits, as well as defining the associated risks. We candidly discuss our own success rates, as well as complication rates, especially those related to exposure or erosion and de novo dyspareunia. We also stress with our patients that we have found relative risks such as younger age, a history of undergoing a prior reconstructive procedure utilizing any permanent material or suture, and the presence of chronic pain disorder (especially pelvic pain) to be associated with the possibility of developing new-onset pelvic pain or, more specifically, dyspareunia. Last, each patient is given the option of a more traditional suture repair of endogenous tissue, as well as the alternative of an open or laparoscopic abdominal sacral colpopexy.

All of our patients receive appropriate thromboembolic precautions, a rectal prep, including an enema the night before and the morning of surgery, preoperative antibiotic prophylaxis utilizing a second-generation cephalosporin, and careful operative prep of the vaginal canal and surgical site. We recommend that patients receive preoperative topical transvaginal estrogen and encourage patients to continue to use transvaginal topical estrogen for an extensive period of time postoperatively. It is important that patients realize that to optimize sexual function and comfort, the vaginal lining itself should be kept as healthy as possible with the support of topical estrogen.

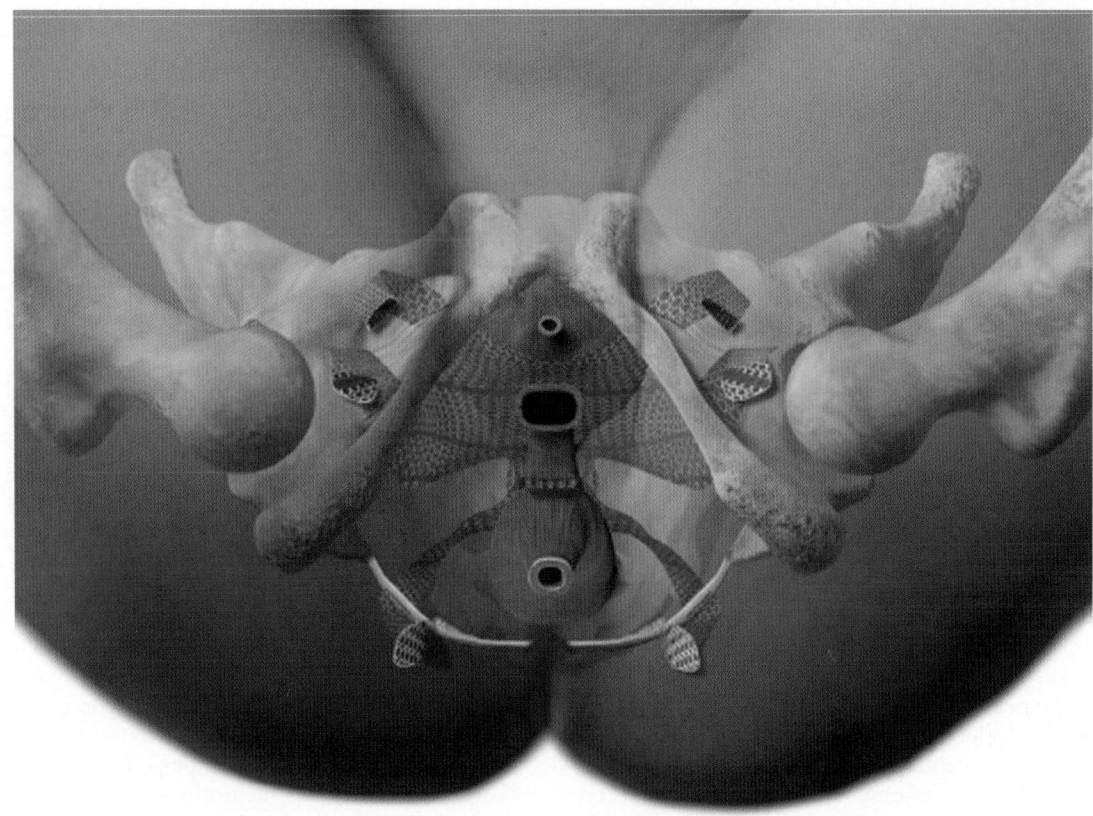

**FIGURE 57–1**  The Prolift system (Ethicon Women's Health & Urology).

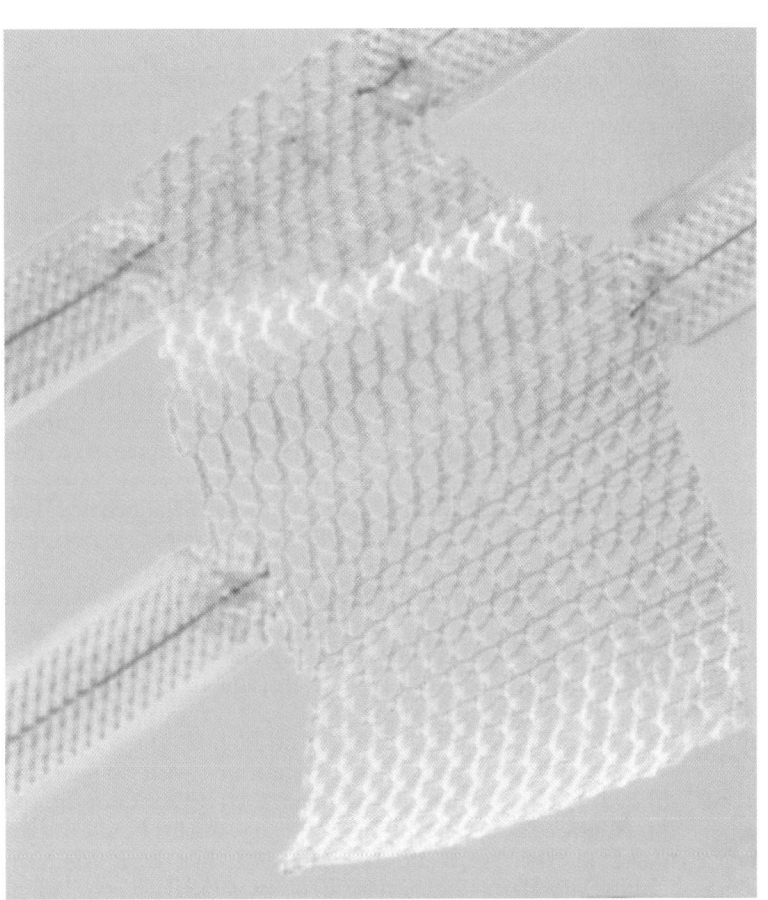

A

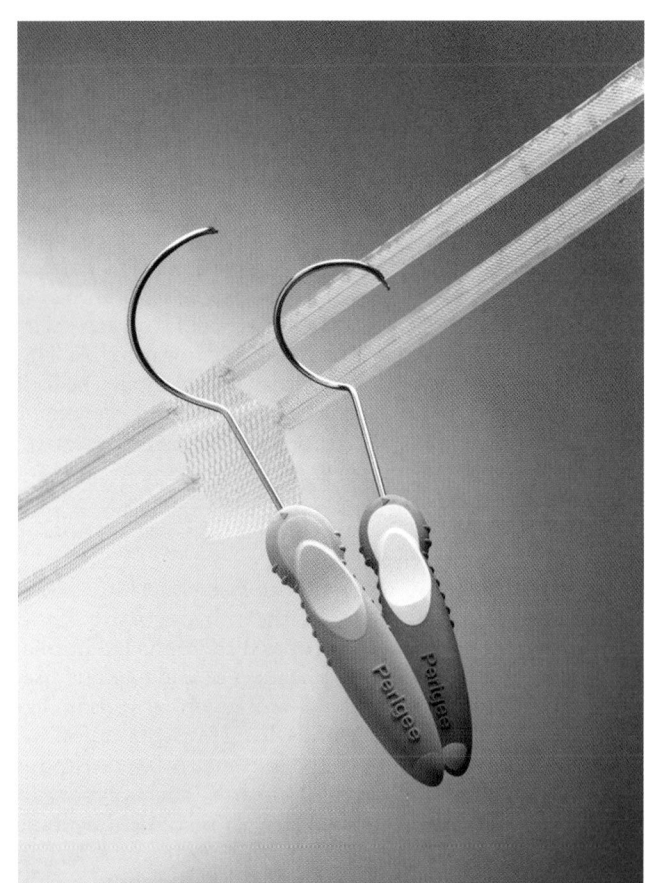

B

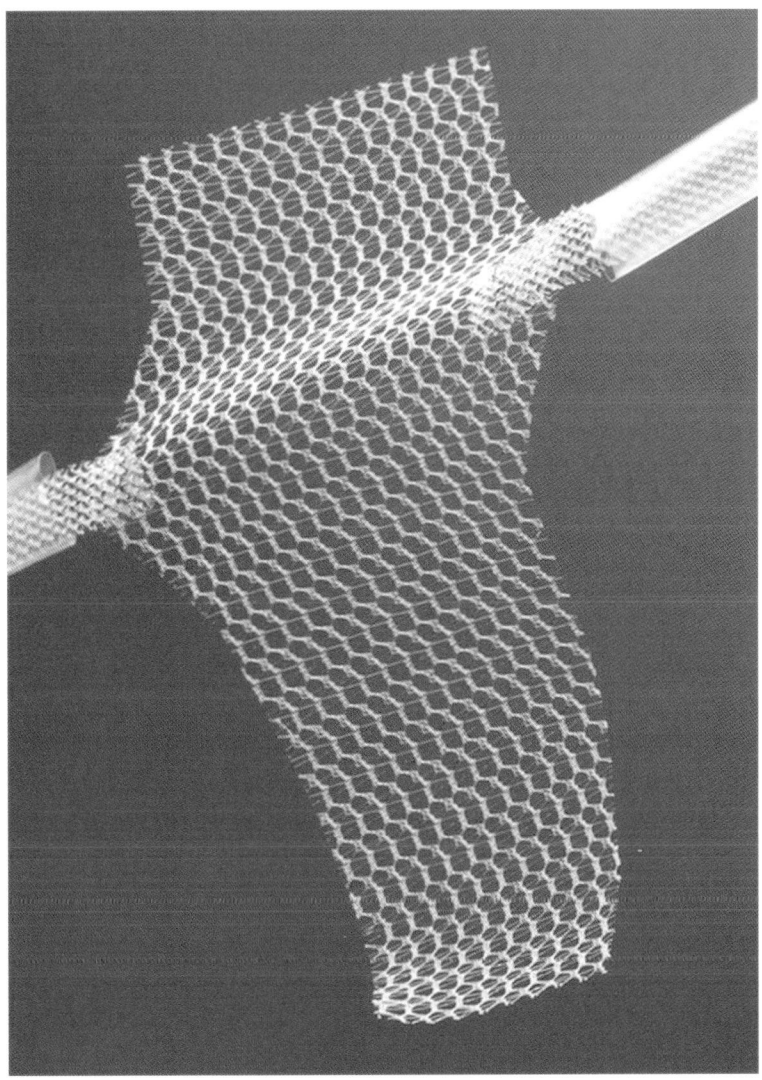

C

**FIGURE 57–2** The Apogee and Perigee Systems. (Courtesy American Medical System, Inc., Minnetonka, Minnesota. www. AmericanMedicalSystems.com.)

We believe it is our responsibility to position the lower extremities carefully in adjustable Allen-type stirrups. From the lateral perspective, hip flexion should be no greater than 90°, and the leg should be abducted such that the knee is not in line with the foot and the contralateral shoulder (Fig. 57–3). Even with careful positioning, some patients will experience muscle strain and discomfort caused by hip flexion. Therefore, we often recommend that our patients perform specific stretching exercises for several weeks before undergoing surgery. Patients are instructed to perform these exercises while lying in bed in the morning or evening. Patients are instructed to grasp their knee or behind the knee, then while flexing toward their chest as much as they physically can, they can gently rotate the leg laterally and hold that position for a count of 10 seconds. Since embracing this exercise as part of our routine preoperative care, we have anecdotally seen a significant decrease in patient complaints of hip, back, and leg pain associated with the exaggerated dorsal lithotomy position required for transvaginal mesh surgery.

In the authors' opinion, the most technically challenging aspect of placement of any of the transvaginal trocar-based mesh kits is performing the proper dissection. Traditional dissection involved with suture plication of endogenous tissue of the anterior or posterior vaginal wall involves "splitting" of the vaginal epithelium from the underlying muscularis, followed by various forms of plication of the muscularis layer, trimming of the redundant epithelium, and closure. This splitting dissection, if utilized with transvaginal mesh placement, will inevitably result in a significantly high mesh exposure rate. To emulate and achieve the same low exposure rate experienced with transabdominal placement of the pelvic mesh, the transvaginal approach must enter the same pelvic spaces, placing the mesh deep to all of the histologic layers and compromising the vaginal wall. The surgeon must be skilled at entering the true vesicovaginal space anteriorly, as well as the rectovaginal space posteriorly, and placing the mesh into these spaces, as opposed to within the vaginal wall (Figs. 57–4 through 57–6). This specific full-thickness dissection is accomplished by utilizing first a very precise hydrodissection, then careful sharp dissection, and is finally completed with blunt dissection into the paravesical and pararectal spaces. Anteriorly, surgical entrance into the vesicovaginal space can be difficult because the lumen of the space is extremely small. Given the minimal amount of fat that exists in this potential space, it is best viewed as a balloon with little to no air within the lumen, which must be carefully entered. Recently, we adopted the use of an 18-gauge Tuohy needle, which provides increased tactile and visual feedback for precise bevel placement, allowing proper fluid dissection and distention of the vesicovaginal space (Fig. 57–7).

Our approach to entering this space involves the placement of two Allis clamps on the anterior vaginal wall approximately 3 to 4 cm apart, in the area corresponding with the most pronounced portion of the anterior prolapse. Very commonly, the inferior margin of the bladder can be easily palpated through the vaginal wall. With a gentle pinch, the bladder can be pushed cephalad, potentiating the space between the bladder and the full-thickness vaginal wall. A Tuohy needle is then utilized to enter the vesicovaginal space, while a point closer to the inferior Allis clamp is chosen and the needle is held perpendicular to the plane of the vaginal wall edge. The needle offers 5-mm colored segments to provide the surgeon with a measured visual reference, which aids in accurate placement. The needle is carefully advanced through the full thickness of the vaginal wall, which most often is approximately 5 to 7 mm. Commonly, a popping sensation is distinctly palpable as the rounded tip of the needle enters the true vesicovaginal space. With the needle bevel-faced ventral in a 12-o'clock position, fluid can be infused easily into the space, creating hydrodissection. We prefer a dilute solution of 0.25% marcaine with epinephrine diluted 1:1 with injectable saline. A 20-mL aliquot of the fluid is placed along the midline. Next, a standard needle is used to reenter the 20-mL fluid pocket and then is directed off midline laterally, while the needle is kept parallel with the lateral aspects of the anterior vaginal wall. A vigorous push of the syringe will help force fluid laterally, physically separating the underlying detrusor muscle from the overlying full-thickness vaginal wall.

Next, the anterior vaginal wall is incised with a scalpel or with the use of electrocautery to enhance hemostasis. Extreme care must be utilized to ensure that the surgeon has penetrated through *all* of the histologic layers of the vagina and has surgically entered the previously established fluid pocket. Often, this fluid pocket appears as a silver-gray jelly-like space that often contains yellow wisps of adipose tissue, which are easily visible without magnification. The incision is extended for a total length of approximately 4 cm (Fig. 57–8).

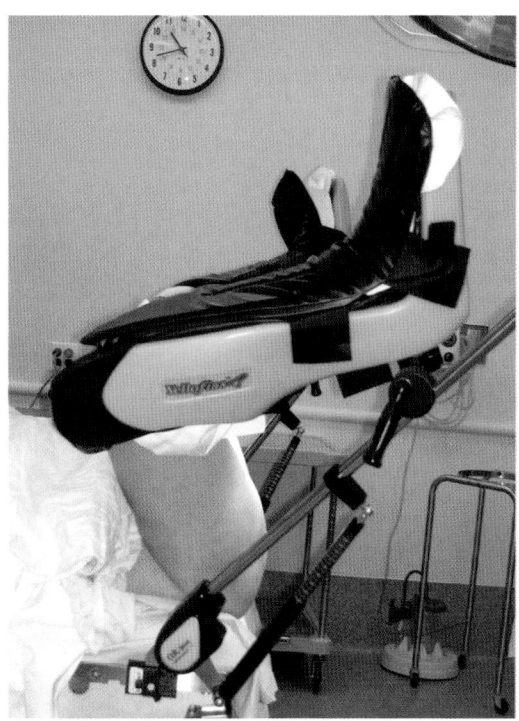

**FIGURE 57-3** Patient positioning on the operating room table with hip flexion not greater than 90°.

UNDERSTANDING THE HISTOLOGY

Nonkeratinized squamous epithelium ——

Thin lamina propria

Concentric layers of smooth muscle

Vesicovaginal/ rectovaginal space ——

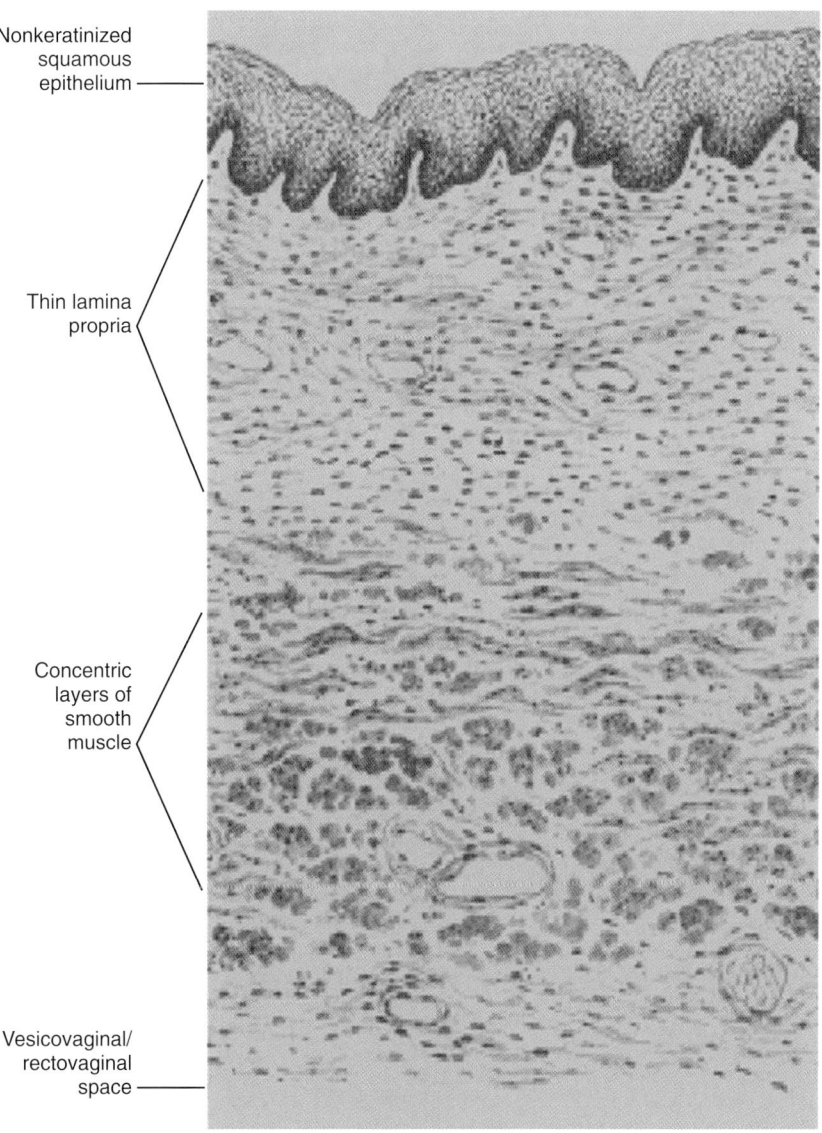

**FIGURE 57-4** Histologic layers making up the vaginal wall.

VAGINAL WALL ANATOMY
*Surgical placement of mesh*

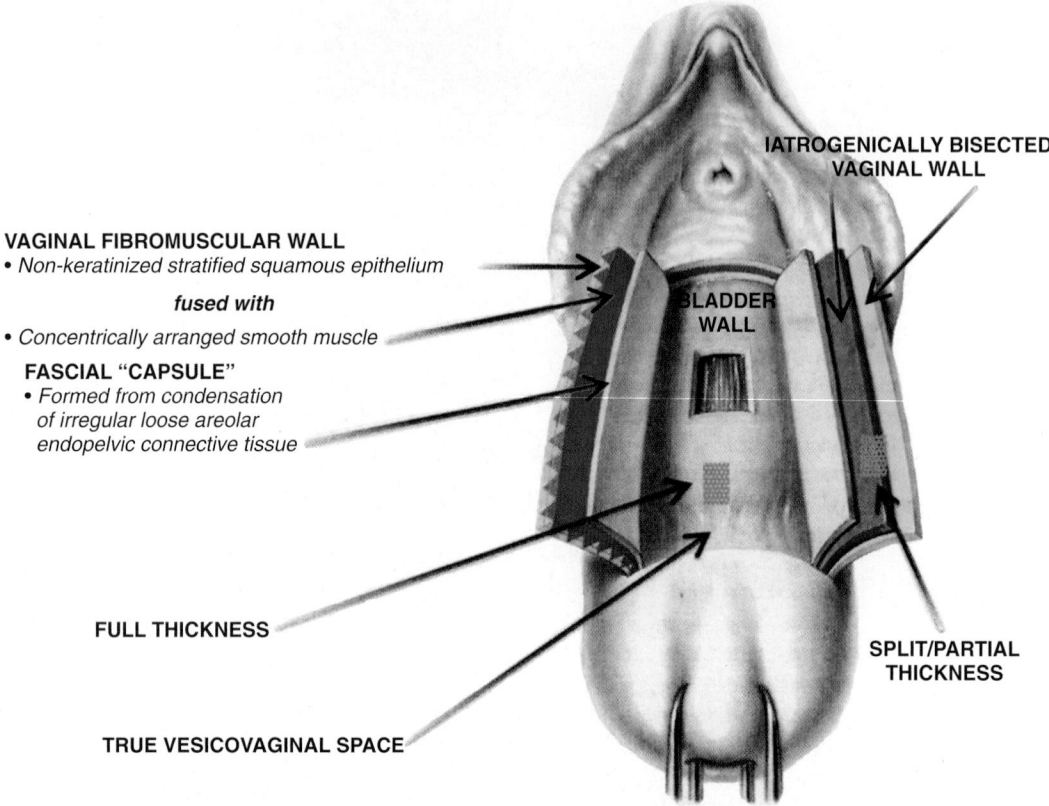

**IATROGENICALLY BISECTED VAGINAL WALL**

**VAGINAL FIBROMUSCULAR WALL**
• *Non-keratinized stratified squamous epithelium*

**fused with**

• *Concentrically arranged smooth muscle*

**BLADDER WALL**

**FASCIAL "CAPSULE"**
• *Formed from condensation of irregular loose areolar endopelvic connective tissue*

**FULL THICKNESS**

**SPLIT/PARTIAL THICKNESS**

**TRUE VESICOVAGINAL SPACE**

**FIGURE 57–5** Diagrammatic representation of different layers of the vaginal wall for optimal placement of mesh.

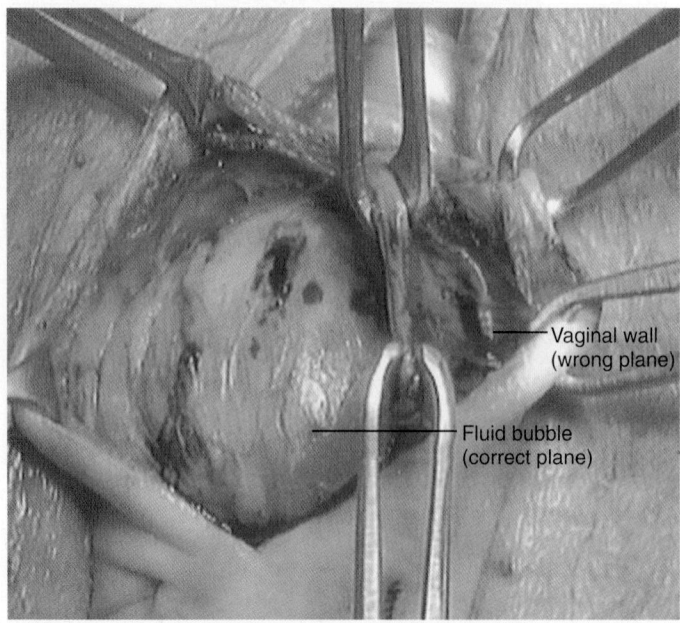

Vaginal wall (wrong plane)

Fluid bubble (correct plane)

**FIGURE 57–6** Tissue layer grasped between middle Allis clamps represents the inner aspects of the vaginal wall, inadvertently split or separated (wrong plane) from the full thickness of the wall.

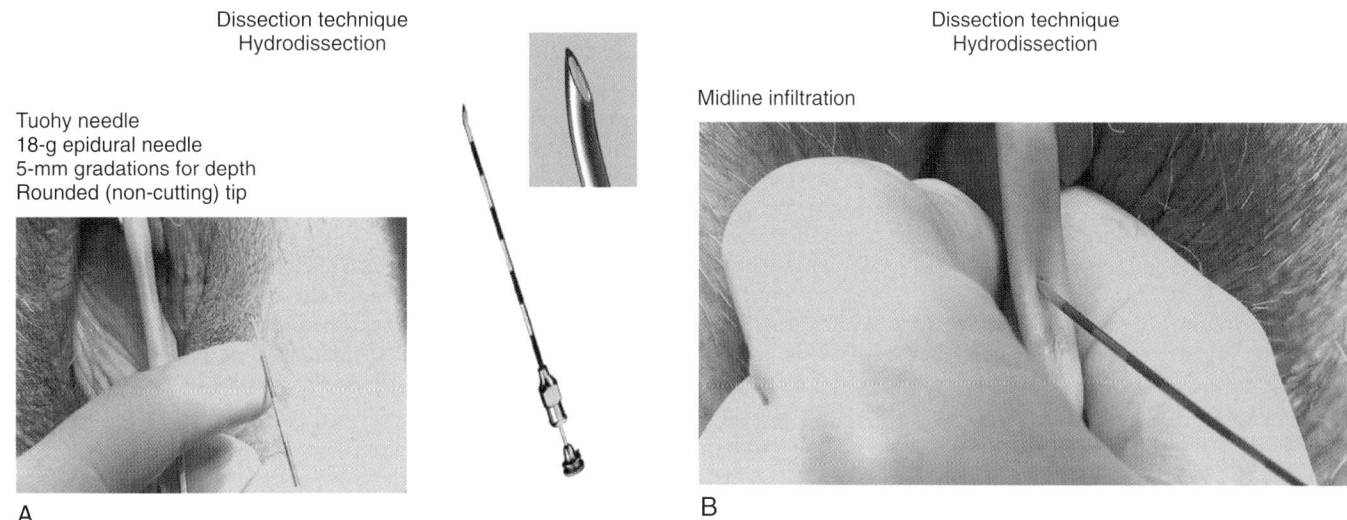

Dissection technique
Hydrodissection

Tuohy needle
18-g epidural needle
5-mm gradations for depth
Rounded (non-cutting) tip

Dissection technique
Hydrodissection

Midline infiltration

A

B

**FIGURE 57–7  A.** Dissection technique with a Tuohy needle for precise distention of the vesicovaginal space. **B.** Midline infiltration with a Tuohy needle.

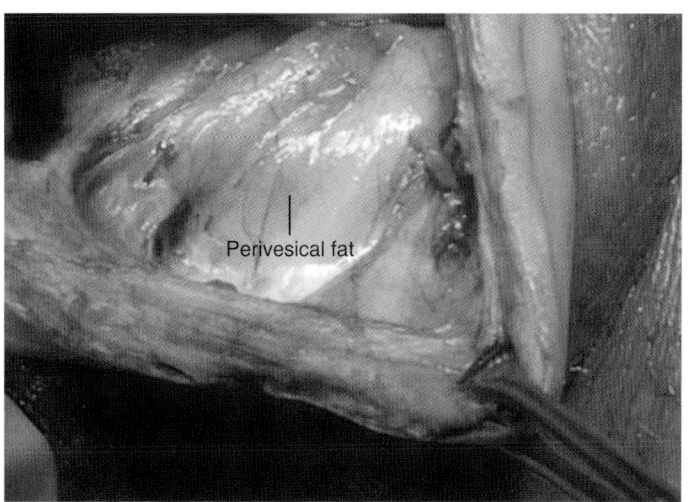

Perivesical fat

**FIGURE 57–8** True vesicovaginal space identified by gross visualization of perivesical fat.

Sharp dissection with Metzenbaum scissors is then used by dissecting the overlying vaginal wall from the underlying detrusor muscle. The natural tendency to avoid the bladder can result in the adverse outcome of dissecting into the vaginal wall. Surgical entrance into the vaginal wall can be identified by excessive bleeding, as well as by surgical resistance when an attempt is made to advance the dissection plane laterally. It is helpful to keep the shaft of the scissors parallel with the plane of the vaginal wall and to allow the natural curve of the scissors to create gentle pressure on the underside of the anterior vaginal wall, while avoiding digging or burrowing into the vaginal wall.

Blunt dissection completes development of the surgical spaces. It is preferable to switch from sharp to blunt dissection once safe visualization of scissor placement is no longer feasible because of lateral advancement and deviation of the dissection. The tip of the surgeon's index finger is used to sweep the loose areolar tissue, with pressure directed laterally toward the medial aspect of the obturator internus muscle. This allows the development of a surgical space, enabling direct palpation of pelvic sidewall structures, including the ischial spine, the iliococcygeus fascia, and the arcus tendineus fascia pelvis. Patients who have had prior dissection in this area, such as those who have undergone a prior paravaginal defect repair with suture attachment, can pose great technical difficulty for developing this space. We have found it helpful to utilize cystoscopic guidance to avoid inadvertent blunt dissection or injury into the bladder wall for patients who may have adhesive disease in the paravesical space.

Trocar or needle placement for the anterior Prolift utilizes the obturator foramen, with the needle traversing the obturator membrane at the superior medial edge of the inferior ramus and superior ramus, as well as at the inferior medial aspect of the foramen along the inferior ramus (for the posterior [or kindly referred to as] "deep pass"). A marking pen is utilized to demarcate the incisions, beginning with the superior medial notch, which is often palpable, and a pinch technique is used to internally feel the notch with the surgeon's index finger and with the thumb externally pinching to identify the exact location of the notch, given the various pelvic shapes and bone thicknesses that are seen in diverse populations. Once the superior medial notch has been palpated and marked on the skin, measurement 1 cm lateral and 2 cm inferior from the first mark is used to establish the location of the incision for the deep anterior pass. Both skin sites are then infiltrated with approximately 10 mL of dilute 0.25% marcaine epinephrine to promote hemostasis and provide perioperative anesthetic. A vertical 4-mm skin incision is made. We have preferred to place the deep anterior trocar first. The key to optimal needle placement is to appreciate the three-dimensional aspects of the pelvis (Fig. 57-9) to encourage alignment of the needle and proper trajectory of the needle to reach the level of the ischial spine and slightly ventral to it. This can be accomplished only with rotation of the needle such that the curve of the needle becomes concentric with the curve of the pelvis as downward pressure is maintained on the needle handle, encouraging the tip of the needle to maintain intermittent contact with the medial aspect of the ischium until the tip of the needle reaches the ischial spine (Fig. 57-10). Because of the inward or medial curvature of the ischium, which actually creates the ischial spine itself, the needle must take an "arced" approach rather than a "straight" approach to the ischial spine to drop the needle down onto the anterior aspect of the ischial spine, providing optimal vaginal lengthening or apical support (Fig. 57-11). Unfortunately, a common error that occurs when an anterior Prolift is performed is that the surgeon fails to properly utilize the design and curvature of the needle, often placing the needle and cannula only within 2 cm of the ischial spine, resulting in suboptimal apical support or vaginal foreshortening.

Once the tip of the deep anterior trocar has truly reached the level of the ischial spine, the handle is elevated slightly, allowing the tip to point; additional advancement of the needle creates a small hole through the condensation of the arcus tendineus and iliococcygeal fascia, allowing the needle to enter the dissected space, and the needle is advanced for a distance of approximately 1 to 2 cm. It is critical to carefully remove any surrounding areolar tissue so that the deployed cannula can be controlled and the forthcoming retrieval suture easily passed down the cannula and advanced outwardly through the dissected space.

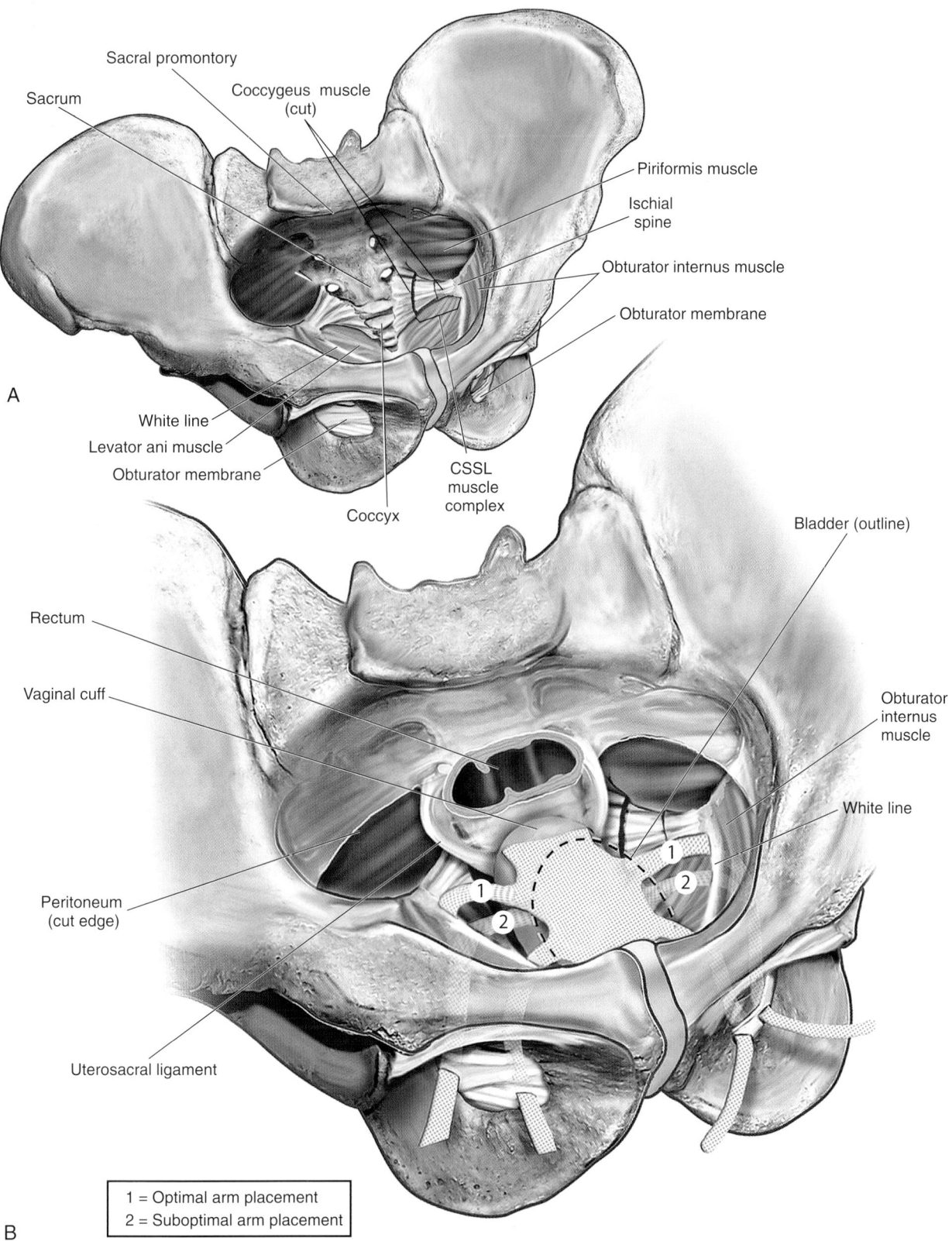

1 = Optimal arm placement
2 = Suboptimal arm placement

**FIGURE 57–9** Three-dimensional view of the pelvis. **A.** Bony anatomy and ligaments; insertions of muscles. **B.** Placement of anterior mesh kits.

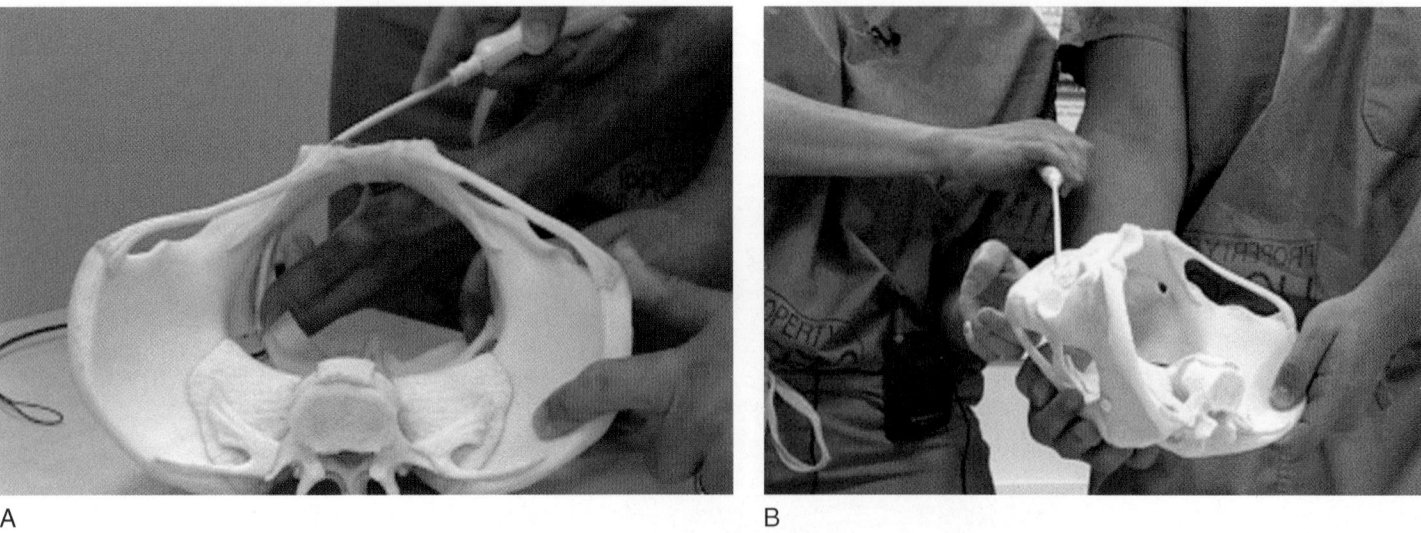

A                                                                                    B

**FIGURE 57–10** Concentric alignment of the needle curve and pelvic curve achieved with trocar rotation. **A.** View from above, aligning the needle curve with the pelvic curve. **B.** Lateral view of the alignment of the needle with the pelvic curve.

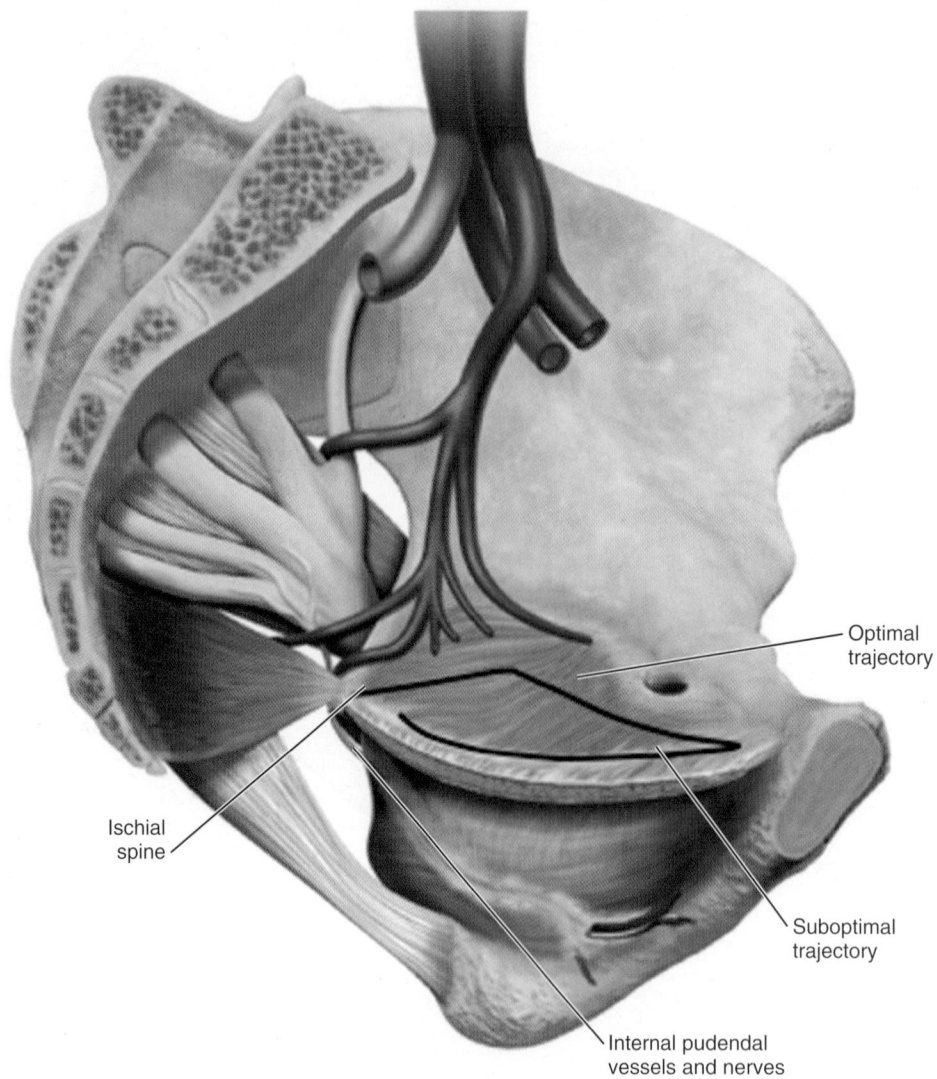

Optimal trajectory

Ischial spine

Suboptimal trajectory

Internal pudendal vessels and nerves

**FIGURE 57–11** Trajectory of the needle with respect to pelvic anatomy, aiming to provide optimal support. (Trocar Placement With Respect To Pelvic Anatomy © Ethicon, Inc, Women's Health and Urology Division, Somerville, NJ. Reproduced with Permission.)

Attention is then directed toward the superior medial cannula, which is easily placed with direct palpation guidance by placing the index finger at the superior medial notch, bringing the trocar to the index finger, piercing the obturator internus muscle, and then deploying the cannula and removing the needle. Given the short distance of this trajectory, it is often feasible to bring the cannula completely out, allowing easier retrieval suture placement. Once both cannulas have been placed, it is critical to perform an assessment of the curved linear distance between the two cannulas. This distance should be 5 cm or greater, thereby representing the appropriate origin and insertion of the arcus tendineus fascia pelvis.

Once all four cannulas of the anterior Prolift have been placed with the corresponding retrieval suture, proper mesh sizing and securement of the mesh must be achieved. The surgeon should appropriately size the mesh based on the distance between the urethrovesical junction and the vaginal cuff or apex or the anterior aspect of the cervix for patients who have not had a prior hysterectomy. Suture securement of the mesh, which primarily serves to prevent the mesh from folding, shifting, or bunching, is simple tacking of the mesh along the midline, both distal and proximal. At the level of the urethrovesical junction, a 2-0 delayed absorbable polydioxanone (PDS) suture is utilized. Proximally, suture selection is dependent on the presence or absence of the cervix. For those patients who have a cervix, we prefer to use a permanent 2-0 polypropylene suture by placing at least two or three sutures through the cervical stroma and then securing the sutures to the mesh itself. For those patients who have had a prior hysterectomy, we favor a 2-0 PDS suture.

The dissection techniques and incisions used for the Prolift and Avaulta procedures are identical. Because the area of the Avaulta mesh body is quite a bit smaller than that of the Prolift system, we believe that an anterior colporrhaphy is a helpful first step for this operation. However, because of the deep dissection required to get into the true vesicovaginal space, little to no connective tissue is left for plication. Therefore, extreme care must be taken to avoid intravesical suture placement or ureteral compromise when an anterior colporrhaphy is performed as the first step in this procedure.

As is the case with the anterior Prolift, the anterior Avaulta arms are delivered through two distinct aspects of the obturator foramen, and the same trocar is used for both deep and superficial passes. With any needle pass through the obturator foramen (deep or superficial), the surgeon should always be aware of the exact location of the needle tip immediately after placement and through the level of resistance. If the needle is inadvertently placed too far as it goes through a level of resistance (i.e., overshoot), the surgeon might not be able to feel the needle tip easily. In these instances, the best course of action is to remove the needle and start over, rather than "finding" the needle by moving it about within the patient because this may result in vascular or visceral damage.

Vigorous irrigation of the surgical site is then performed. This facilitates debridement of the area and provides obvious dilution of any possible bacterial inoculants. Once vigorous irrigation is completed, the incision is closed with a running lock delayed absorbable suture (2-0 Vicryl or Monocryl). After the incision has been closed, one of the most critical steps of the procedure is deployment of the mesh. Setting of the mesh is accomplished with the vagina completely closed then displaced inwardly, replicating or reproducing inward vaginal displacement such that occurs with coital function. Because transvaginal meshes are not in line with the axis of the vagina, they can create resistance to inward displacement during sexual intercourse. The arrangement of mesh used for an abdominal sacral colpopexy has the advantage of not providing such resistance; therefore, mesh is placed very loosely to avoid excessive tightness, which may cause a pulling sensation when

the patient stands erect. For transvaginal meshes, if the mesh is set too loose, symptoms of relaxation may result; alternatively, if the mesh is set too tight, deep penetrating dyspareunia can occur.

After the cannulas have been removed, thereby deploying or setting the mesh, the vagina is immediately packed with gauze in the upper vaginal and midvaginal areas before any additional surgery, such as a sling procedure, or even posterior colporrhaphy, is performed. Patients then undergo final packing of the vagina upon completion of any concomitant surgeries. An indwelling Foley is placed until the following day. Most patients have both the packing and the Foley removed and next-day discharge with minimal analgesic use. For those patients who may pose a risk for avulsion of the vagina off the mesh before adequate fibrin adherence or tissue ingrowth (morbid obesity, chronic coughing, etc), packing remains in place until postoperative day number 3.

## Placement of Posterior Mesh System

Dissection for a posterior Prolift again must require a full-thickness incision and dissection of the posterior vaginal wall. Unlike the true vesicovaginal space, the rectovaginal space is easier to enter because the space is distended with pararectal fat. Most surgeons are more comfortable and have a higher degree of accuracy when correctly entering and dissecting within the true rectovaginal space. This dissection continues cephalad toward the apex of the vagina, again with care taken to make the length of the incision as minimal as possible to still execute the surgery. Therefore, tunneling below the posterior vaginal wall to the posterior cervix or cuff as much as possible is preferred. Once the rectovaginal space has been properly developed, the pararectal spaces are entered with sharp and blunt dissection through the right and left rectal pillars. Once the pararectal space has been entered, surgical landmarks are identified with palpation of the ischial spine, iliococcygeus muscle, and coccygeus muscle and the sacrospinous ligament (running within the lower third of the coccygeus). Less dissection is needed than for a traditional sacrospinous ligament fixation because a posterior mesh placement does not require direct visualization, as is often required when other instrumentation is used to secure the sacrospinous ligament for vaginal vault suspension.

Once dissection is completed, attention is directed toward needle placement. With the mid anal skin verge used as an anatomic reference point, two skin marks are made 3 cm lateral and 3 cm posterior to the mid anal verge. Once again, dilute local anesthetic solution is infiltrated, with the needle directed approximately 15° to 20° degrees off the midline to allow safe and ample spacing away from the rectum residing in the midline. Two small 4-mm skin incisions are then made. For the Prolift device, a trocar needle and overriding cannula are guided via palpation through the gluteal muscle, with a curved approach to the sacrospinous ligament at a point two fingerbreadths medial to the ischial spine. Gentle upward movement of the needle can often identify the tip as it ascends under the iliococcygeus muscle toward the coccygeus and accompanying sacrospinous ligament. Care must be taken to avoid the rectum at all times. This is best accomplished again by using a slight 15° to 20° angle away from the midline during the beginning journey or trajectory of the needle, and then drifting the needle back toward the midline as it approaches the sacrospinous ligament preidentified spot. This again allows safe passage without jeopardizing or encroaching the pudendal neurovascular bundle residing within Alcock's canal. Many surgeons have the tendency to repeatedly check the location of the ischial spine as a reference point during passage of the trocar. This, unfortunately, will result in inadvertent directing of the needle toward the ischial spine itself, rather than at the desired location of two fingerbreadths medial to the ischial spine along the lower one third of the coccygeus muscle. It is much better to repeatedly rub or push down on the coccygeus to facilitate spatial reference as opposed to retouching or reaching toward the ischial spine. Once the trocar tip has approximated the appropriate location under the muscle ligament complex, it is directed upward through the sacrospinous ligament complex. The areolar tissue is then easily swept away with an index finger, allowing the cannula to be deployed and the introducing trocar removed. As with the anterior Prolift, the retrieval suture is placed down the cannula and delivered through the dissected field, exiting the vaginal introitus.

Although it is possible to place the posterior Avaulta needle directly through the sacrospinous ligament, it is not specifically designed for this. Instead, the posterior Avaulta needle is initially placed in exactly the same way as the posterior Prolift needle, but the endpoint of deep posterior needle placement is the iliococcygeus muscle, about 1 cm medial and inferior to the ischial spine. Once the needle has pierced this aspect of the muscle, the surgeon should deploy the snare, as is done for the anterior mesh arm placement previously described. The two deep passes of the posterior Avaulta should be performed first. If tacking sutures are desired near the apex along the body of the mesh, they should be placed at this point. A rectal exam should be performed after each step of posterior mesh placement. We are less inclined to perform a posterior colporrhaphy when placing posterior Avaulta than we are to perform an anterior colporrhaphy at the time of anterior Avaulta placement. Our decision regarding the posterior colporrhaphy step is based on the caliber of the distal rectum. If the rectum has become significantly wider than the body of the mesh, we will perform a traditional plication colporrhaphy before setting the tension of the mesh.

Another major difference between the posterior Prolift and the posterior Avaulta is the presence of distal arms on the Avaulta mesh. These arms are deployed with the same needle used for the deep pass of the device. The same buttock incisions are used as well. The needle is placed through the buttock incision, with care taken to avoid snagging of the proximal arm. The needle is placed through the subcutaneous tissue lateral to the anal sphincter. The endpoint for distal needle placement is the junction of the bulbocavernosus and transverse perineal muscles. Particular care must be taken to avoid vessels and nerves in the region such as the inferior rectal artery and nerve.

As with the anterior Prolift, the mesh itself must be properly sized to the patient's vaginal and pelvic dimensions. It is advised that the mesh should be cut approximately to correspond with the upper two-thirds length of the posterior vaginal wall. We have found that bringing the mesh distally all the way to the perineum across the perineal body will result in a higher exposure rate at the level of the perineal body. We, therefore, do not bring mesh beyond a point 3 cm above the posterior fourchette. We have also found that it is beneficial to narrow the distal aspect of the posterior mesh to avoid rolling or folding of the mesh in the lower region. Once again, as with the anterior Prolift, if a cervix is indeed in place, two to three permanent 2-0

Prolene sutures are used to permanently fixate the cervix to the mesh itself. A cervical notch is cut in the apical aspect of the Prolift mesh, approximating the size of the cervix. In the absence of a cervix, 2-0 PDS is utilized, and the tail of the Prolift is removed if indeed there is no enterocele. For those patients who have an enterocele, depending on size, the sac itself may be opened, removed, then closed or inverted with an extraperitoneal purse string suture, or it may simply be inverted with the mesh placed over the enterocele. It is important to realize that keeping the tail of the mesh intact to cover the apex to prevent or treat the enterocele requires double tacking of the mesh. The proximal edge of the mesh bridge or tail must be secured with sutures to the apical aspect of the anterior pubocervical fascia. A second tacking suture must be placed at the cephalad aspect of the posterior vaginal wall. Once the mesh has been sized and secured, the arms or straps of the mesh are retrieved by using the retrieval sutures previously placed.

Once the mesh has been retrieved through the cannula, vigorous irrigation is carried out for the purposes previously described. The posterior vaginal wall is again closed with a running lock 2-0 Vicryl suture. For those patients who have a significant rectocele and a dilated ampule with defecatory dysfunction more often requiring digital splinting to facilitate bowel movements, rectal plication of the outer layer of the rectal muscularis is carried out with a delayed absorbable suture under digital guidance of an index finger placed within the rectal cavity itself. Before complete closure, the distal aspect of the mesh is secured to the cephalad aspect of the perineal body with the use of interrupted 2-0 Monocryl sutures. It is best to place these sutures after the mesh has been deployed, as it is nearly impossible to predict how far the mesh will pull up once the arms of the mesh have been retrieved. Final adjustment is again achieved by creating a certain amount of slack into the mesh setting by placing the exam finger into the rectum and then displacing the anterior rectal wall ventrally to simulate a large bolus of stool, so that the mesh will not restrict rectal distention necessary for the passage of large-caliber stool. It is also imperative that the surgeon ensure that the rectal wall has not been involved with the mesh system, and that it is clearly separated from any mesh material. A bimanual exam with an index finger within the rectum and a second index finger in the pararectal space following the mesh material downward easily ensures that the rectum has not been involved during mesh placement. We follow the same steps postoperatively as for the anterior Prolift. Figures 57–12 and 57–13 illustrate placement of a total mesh kit.

Our utilization of trocar-based transvaginal mesh systems has evolved over the past 5 years. We began with selective cases on older patients who were not sexually active and had undergone prior surgery, which had failed. Recently, with our expertise in proper dissection and confidence in optimizing needle placement and mesh deployment, and with the latest developments in lower-weight hybrid mesh construction, we routinely began to offer mesh kit placement to most women with advanced pelvic organ prolapse. Although recent interest has been expressed in nontrocar delivery systems, at the present time experience and published data are insufficient to allow objective commentary on these procedures.

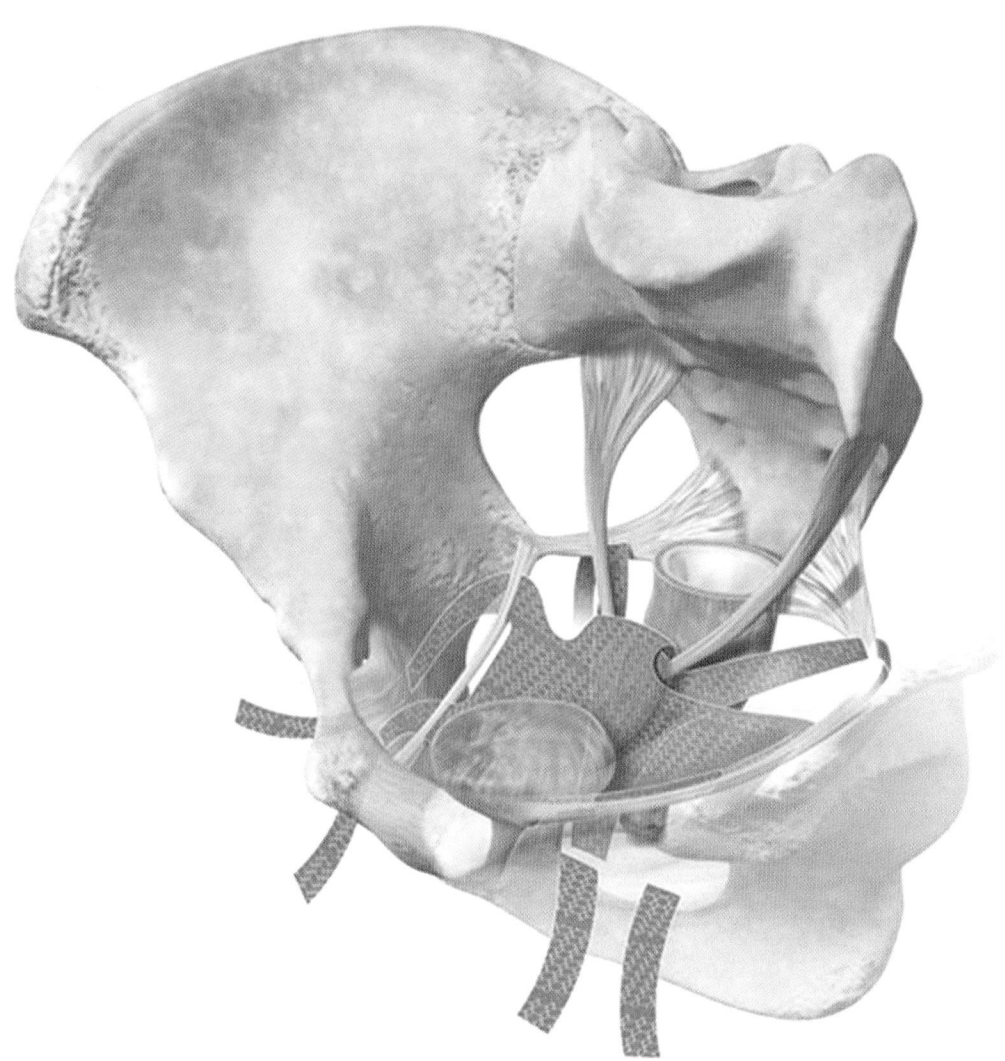

**FIGURE 57–12** Total mesh placement as it is related to the bony pelvis. (Placement of GYNECARE PROLIFT Pelvic Floor Repair System © Ethicon, Inc, Women's Health and Urology Division, Somerville, NJ. Reproduced with Permission.)

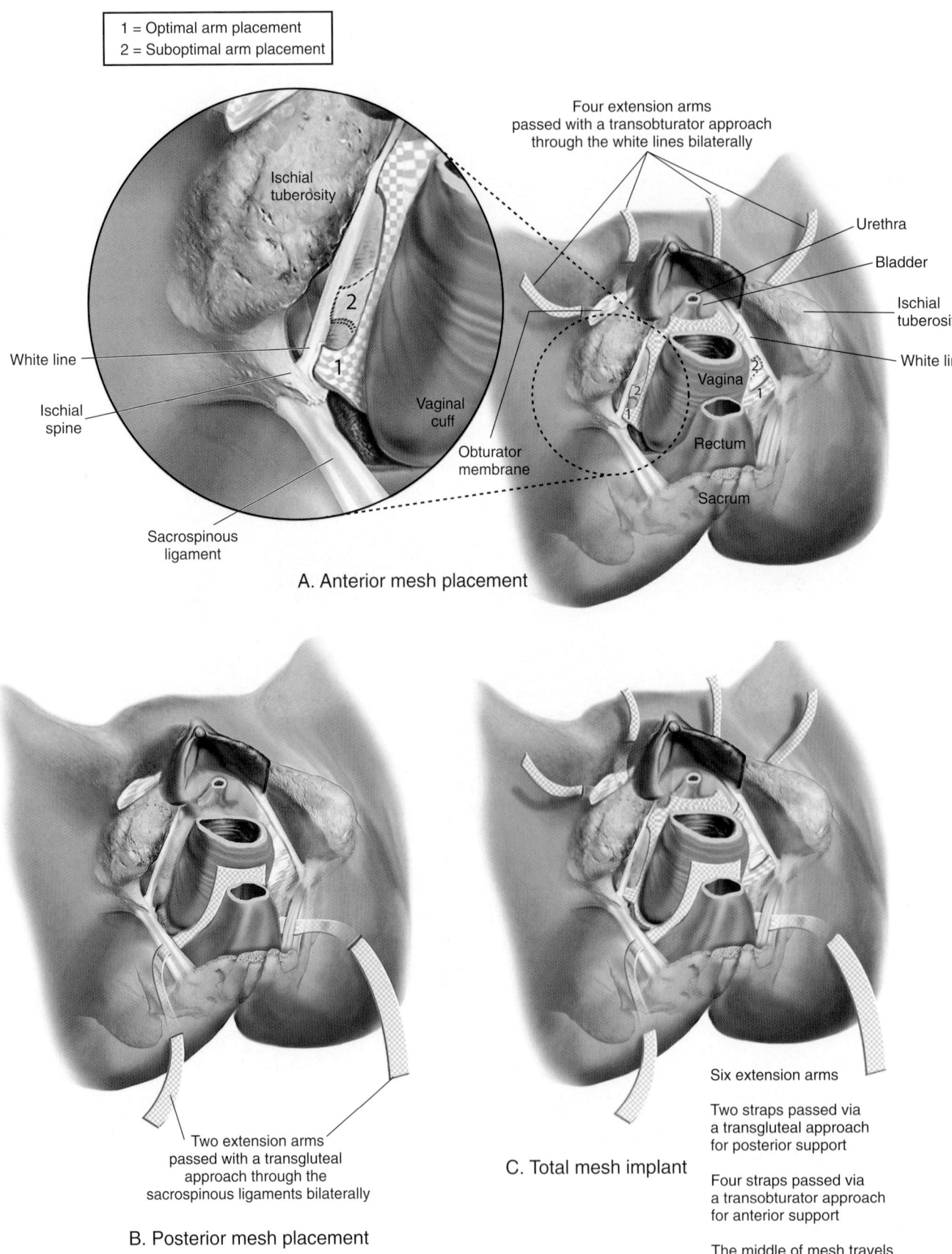

1 = Optimal arm placement
2 = Suboptimal arm placement

Ischial
tuberosity

White line

Ischial
spine

Sacrospinous
ligament

Vaginal
cuff

Obturator
membrane

Four extension arms
passed with a transobturator approach
through the white lines bilaterally

Urethra

Bladder

Ischial
tuberosity

White line

Vagina

Rectum

Sacrum

**A. Anterior mesh placement**

Two extension arms
passed with a transgluteal
approach through the
sacrospinous ligaments bilaterally

**B. Posterior mesh placement**

**C. Total mesh implant**

Six extension arms

Two straps passed via
a transgluteal approach
for posterior support

Four straps passed via
a transobturator approach
for anterior support

The middle of mesh travels
behind the vaginal cuff

**FIGURE 57–13 A.** Completed anterior mesh placement. **B.** Completed posterior mesh placement. **C.** Total mesh implant.

# CHAPTER 58

# Synthetic Midurethral Slings for the Correction of Stress Incontinence

*Mickey M. Karram* ■ *Apurva B. Pancholy*

In 1996, Ulmsten et al introduced the first synthetic midurethral sling, which they named the tension-free vaginal tape (TVT) procedure. This procedure introduced the concept of placing a synthetic material (polypropylene) under the midportion of the urethra in a tension-free fashion. The technique quickly gained popularity because it involved minimal vaginal dissection, was easy to learn, and could be performed with the patient under local anesthesia on an outpatient basis. To date several studies have compared the TVT procedure with more traditional retropubic procedures such as the Burch colposuspension and have shown equal to superior cure rates with less morbidity. The success of the original TVT midurethral sling has led to the development of other midurethral slings in an effort to decrease morbidity while maintaining efficacy. In 2001, Delorme described the first transobturator synthetic midurethral sling. The motivation behind the development of this approach was to reduce the risk of bladder perforation and eliminate the risk of bowel or major blood vessel injury, which had been reported with the TVT procedure. Subsequent studies have shown that a transobturator midurethral sling is as efficacious as a retropubic synthetic midurethral sling, if the patient does not have intrinsic sphincter deficiency. More recently, single-incision midurethral slings have been described. The newest version of a polypropylene sling requires only one incision in the vagina because the sling has no exit points. This chapter discusses anatomy and currently recommended techniques for the placement of these various synthetic midurethral slings.

## Retropubic Synthetic Midurethral Slings

The tension-free vaginal tape procedure was the first retropubic synthetic midurethral sling. This ambulatory procedure aims to restore the pubourethral ligament and suburethral vaginal hammock by using specially designed needles attached to a synthetic sling material (Fig. 58-1). The synthetic sling material is made of polypropylene and is approximately 1 cm wide × 40 cm in length. This sling material is attached to two stainless steel needles, which are passed on each side of the urethra blindly through the retropubic space. The needles exit through a previously created stab wound in the suprapubic area. Because this type of sling requires blind passage of a needle through the retropubic space, it is imperative that the surgeon have a clear understanding of the important anatomic structures of the retropubic space, to avoid potential complications (Figs. 58-2 through 58-5). Besides the potential for damaging the urethra or the bladder, there is also potential for injuring important vascular structures, including the obturator neurovascular

bundle and the external iliac vessels as they exit the pelvis (see Figs. 58-2 through 58-5).

The technique for placement of a retropubic synthetic midurethral sling is as follows:

1. The procedure can be performed with the patient under local, regional, or general anesthesia. If local anesthesia is used, a combination of an anesthetic and a vasoconstrictive agent is usually injected into the abdominal skin just above the pubic symphysis and downward along the back of the pubic bone into the space of Retzius. A small suprapubic incision is made on each side medial to the pubic tubercle at the superior pubic ramus of the pubic bone (Fig. 58-6).

2. Even if the procedure is performed with the patient under general or regional anesthesia, the anterior vaginal wall is always hydrodissected with an anesthetic solution before the incision is made. A midline anterior vaginal wall incision is made at the level of the mid to distal urethra. It should be noted that this area of the vagina is fused to the posterior urethra. This vaginal wall must be sharply separated from the underlying urethra (Fig. 58-7).

3. With Metzenbaum or Mayo scissors, two tunnels are created through the tissue to the level of the inferior pubic ramus on each side. The direction of the tips of the scissors should be toward the ipsilateral shoulder. The tunnel needs to be only large enough to admit the 5-mm TVT needle (see Fig 58-7).

4. The needle is then brought into the field and is attached to a nondisposable handle. The tip of the needle is placed in the tunnel so it is pointing toward the ipsilateral shoulder. The dominant hand holds the handle, and the index finger of the nondominant hand is placed in the anterior vaginal wall with the thumb placed on the back of the disposable needle (Fig. 58-8). In this way, the appropriate tension required to penetrate the urogenital diaphragm with the needle is best appreciated. Once the tip of the needle has penetrated the urogenital diaphragm, the handle should be dropped in an inferior direction, and the tip of the needle moved medially and superiorly so that it hugs the back of the pubic bone (Fig. 58-9). The needle is then advanced to the posterior aspect of the rectus muscle and penetrates up through the anterior abdominal fascia to exit from the previously created suprapubic stab wound.

5. With the needle in place, cystoscopy is performed with a 70° cystoscope to ensure that no inadvertent penetration of the needle through the bladder occurs. During cystoscopy, it is important to aggressively distend the bladder so that any subtle indentations or penetrations from the needle will be

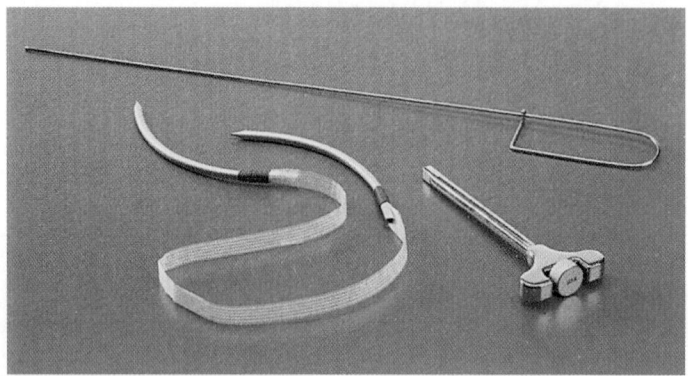

A

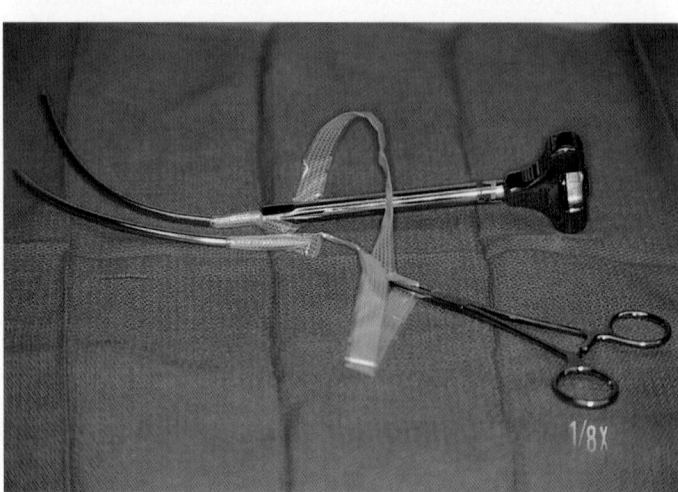

B

**FIGURE 58–1** **A.** Tension-free vaginal tape (TVT) instrumentation, including (clockwise from top) a Foley catheter guide, a needle introducer/handle, and specially designed needles attached to a synthetic suburethral sling tape. **B.** Needles have been attached to the handle. A hemostat has been placed on the overlapping plastic sheath.

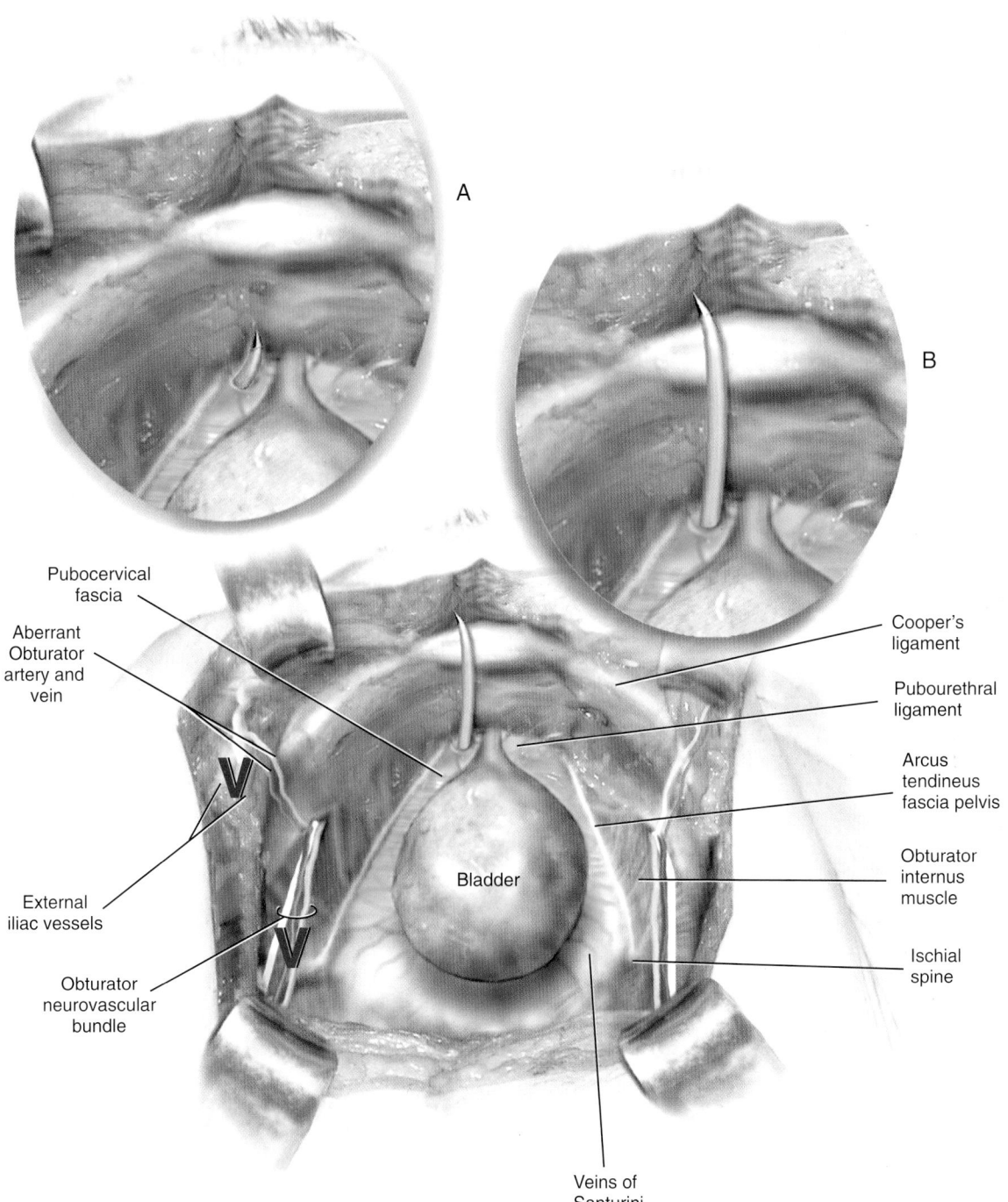

Pubocervical
fascia

Aberrant
Obturator
artery and
vein

External
iliac vessels

Obturator
neurovascular
bundle

Cooper's
ligament

Pubourethral
ligament

Arcus
tendineus
fascia pelvis

Obturator
internus
muscle

Ischial
spine

Bladder

Veins of
Santurini

**FIGURE 58–2** The retropubic space is visualized. The urethra and the bladder sit on the muscular lining of the vagina (*green*). **A.** The needle should penetrate the urogenital diaphragm and enter the retropubic space just medial to the arcus tendineus fascia pelvis and lateral to the urethra. **B.** It should then maintain direct contact with the back of the pubic bone as it passes toward the anterior abdominal stab wound. Marked with a red "V" are the obturator neurovascular bundle and the external iliac vessels, which should be well away from the tip of the tension-free vaginal tape (TVT) needle.

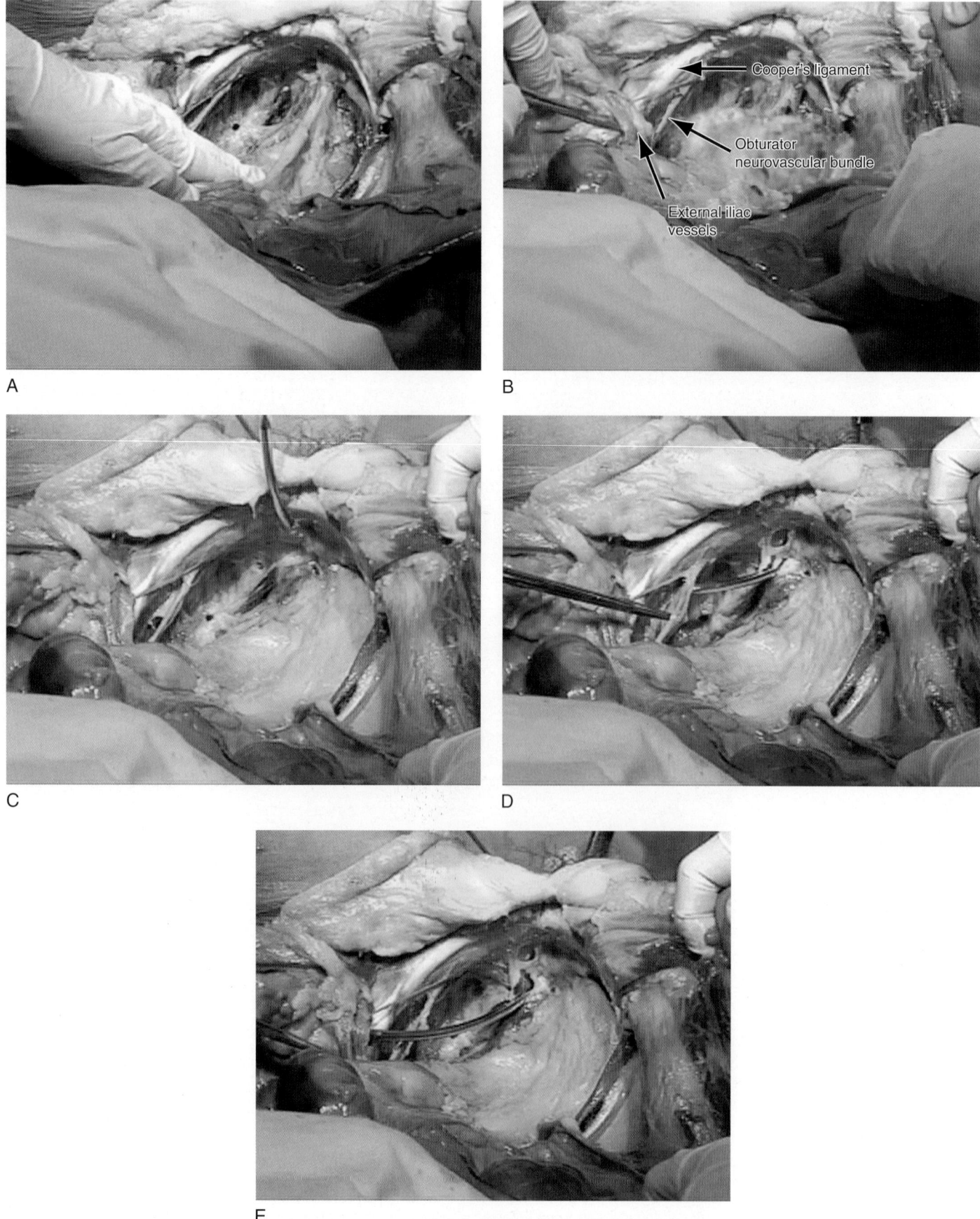

**FIGURE 58–3  A.** View of the retropubic space of a fresh cadaver. **B.** Cooper's ligament, the obturator neurovascular bundle as it exits the pelvis through the obturator foramen, and the external iliac vessels as they exit the pelvis under the inguinal ligament are marked. **C.** A tension-free vaginal tape (TVT) needle has been passed in an appropriate fashion on the left side of this cadaver. **D.** The TVT needle is intentionally continued in a cephalad-lateral direction, and one can see how it can easily come into contact with the obturator neurovascular bundle in the retropubic space. **E.** The TVT needle is intentionally continued in this direction, and one can see how it could potentially come in contact with the external iliac vessels.

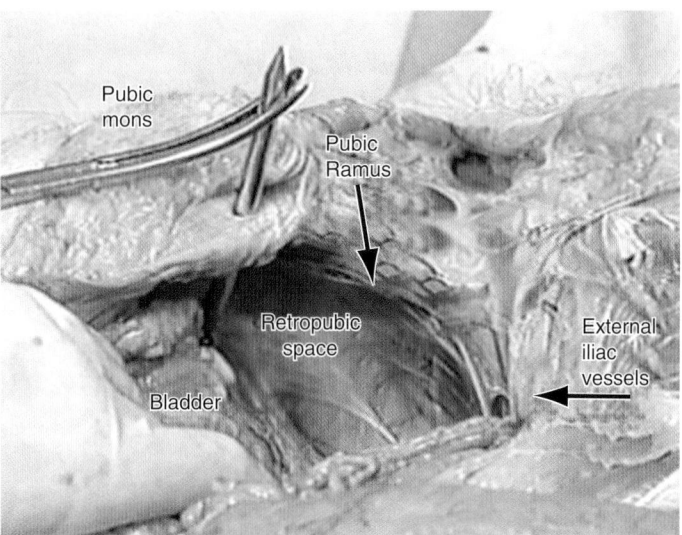

**FIGURE 58-4** Retropubic view of an embalmed cadaver. Note the appropriate passage of the tension-free vaginal tape (TVT) needle on the right side and the normal anatomy of other structures in the retropubic space.

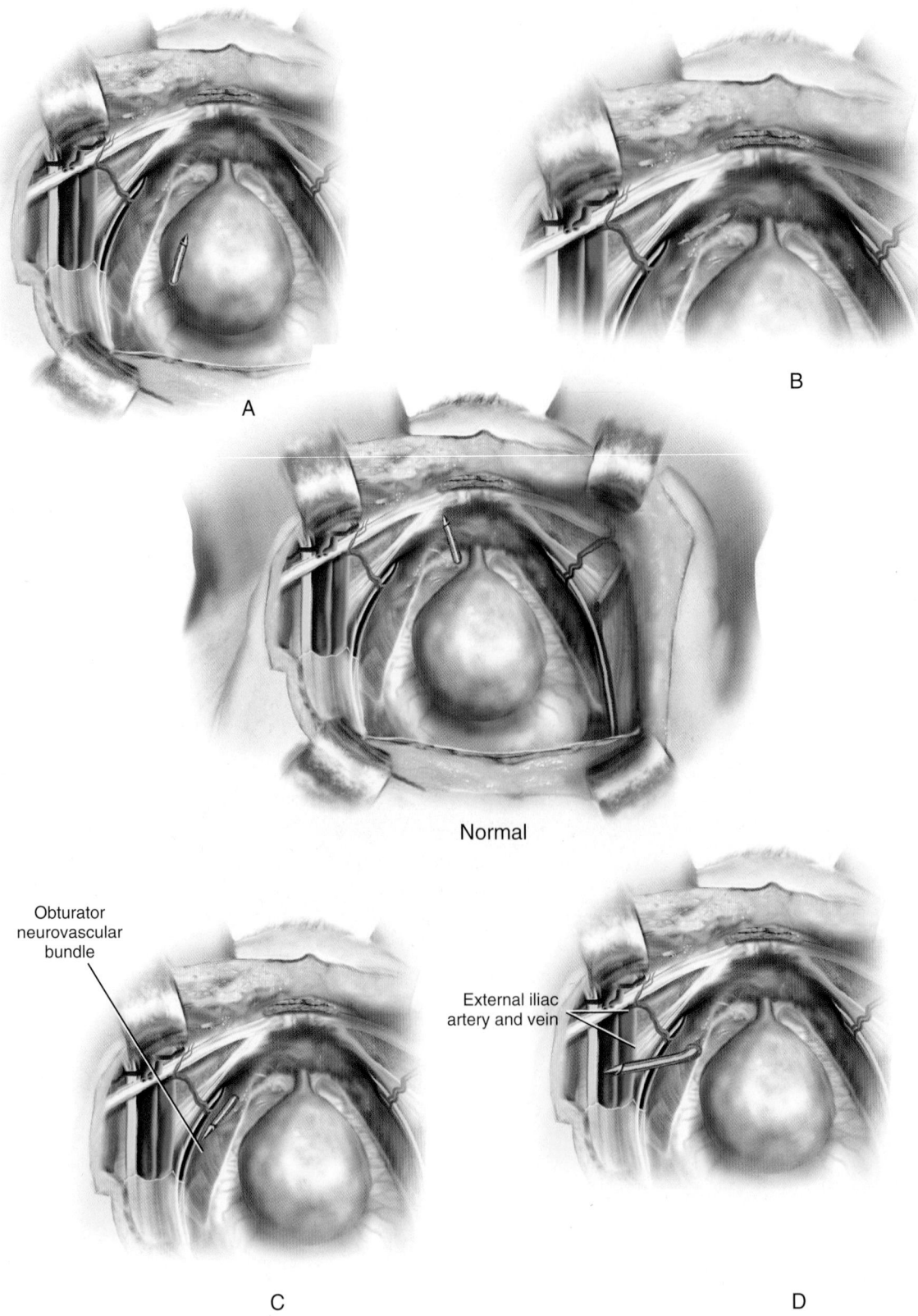

**FIGURE 58–5** Retropubic view of appropriate safe passage of a retropubic tension-free vaginal tape (TVT) needle (*middle illustration*). **A.** Cephalad migration of the needle away from the back of the pubic bone is the most common cause of bladder perforation. **B.** External rotation of the handle will initially result in penetration of the obturator internus muscle by the needle tip, with the potential to injure aberrant vessels along the lateral pelvic sidewall. **C.** Continued external rotation of the handle with cephalad migration of the needle may result in injury to the obturator neurovascular bundle or (**D**) the external iliac vessels.

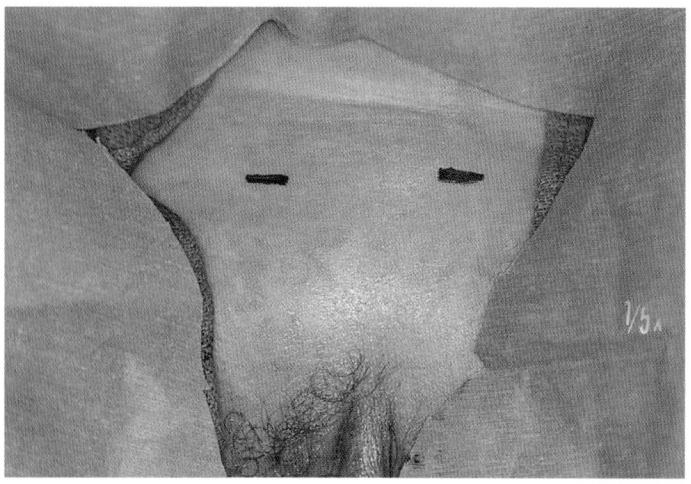

**FIGURE 58–6** Site of suprapubic incisions for the tension-free vaginal tape (TVT) procedure.

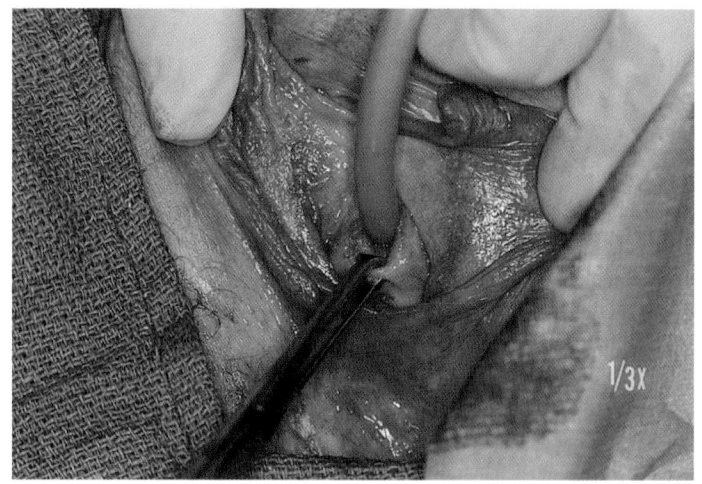

A

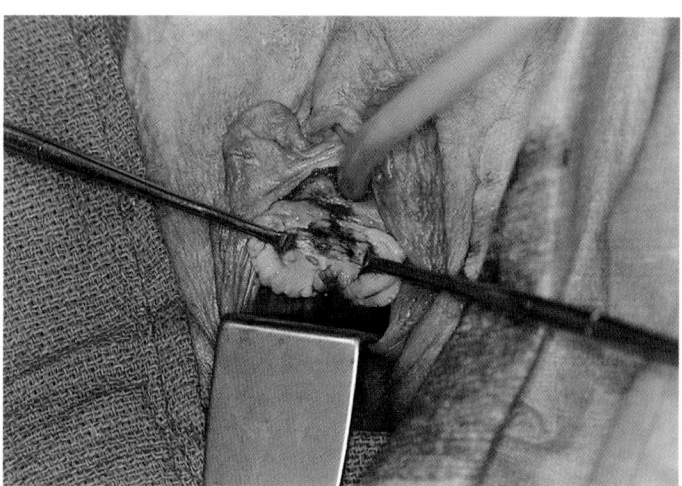

B

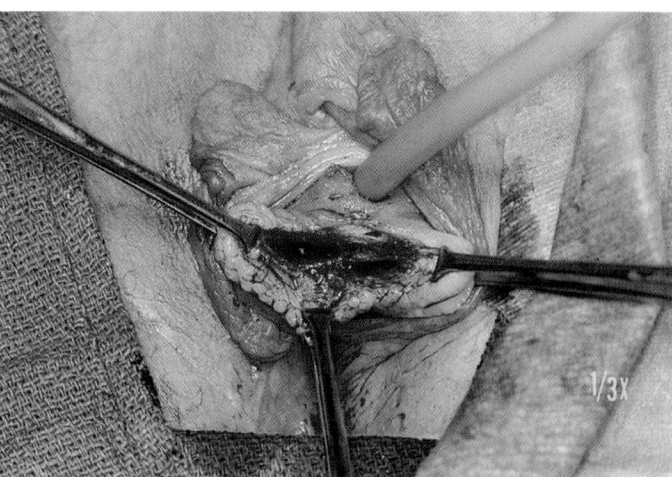

C

**FIGURE 58–7 A.** The external urethral meatus is grasped with an Allis clamp at 6 o'clock. **B.** A small midline incision is made at the level of the midurethra. **C.** Mayo or Metzenbaum scissors are utilized to create a tunnel to the inferior pubic ramus. The urogenital diaphragm is not penetrated.

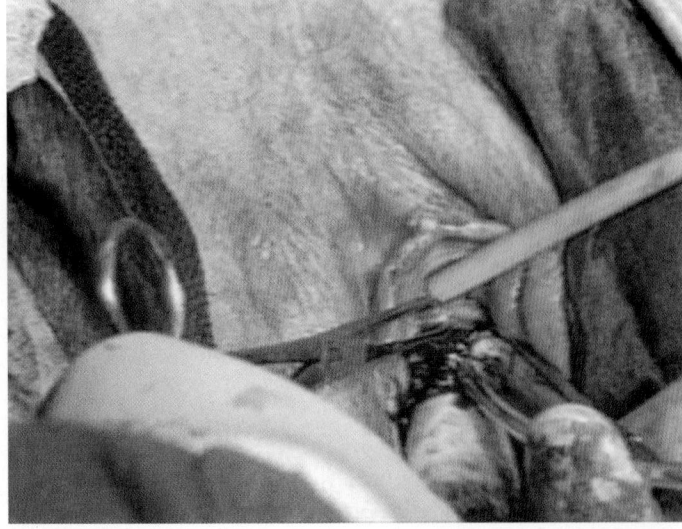

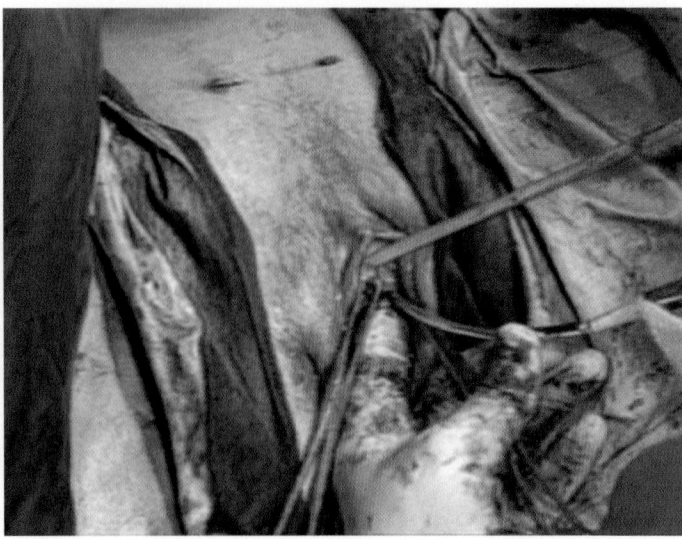

A

B

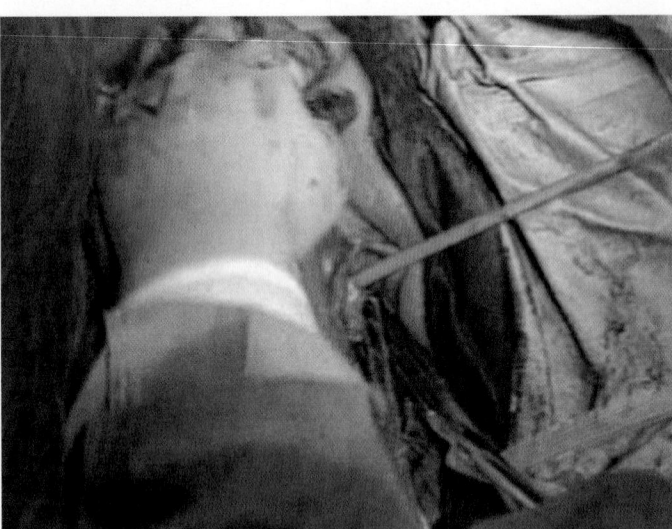

C

**FIGURE 58–8** Proper technique for passing a tension-free vaginal tape (TVT) needle. **A.** The tip of the needle is placed in the small tunnel that has been created and should come into direct contact with the inferior pubic ramus, pointing toward the ipsilateral shoulder. **B.** With the index finger of the nondominant hand in the vagina and the thumb on the shaft of the needle, the tip is pushed through the urogenital diaphragm. **C.** Once the resistance of the urogenital diaphragm is overcome, the handle is dropped and the needle is moved in a medial and superior direction, while direct contact with the back of the pubic bone is maintained. Cephalad migration must be avoided. The tip of the needle is then palpated suprapubically and is guided to exit through the previously created stab incision.

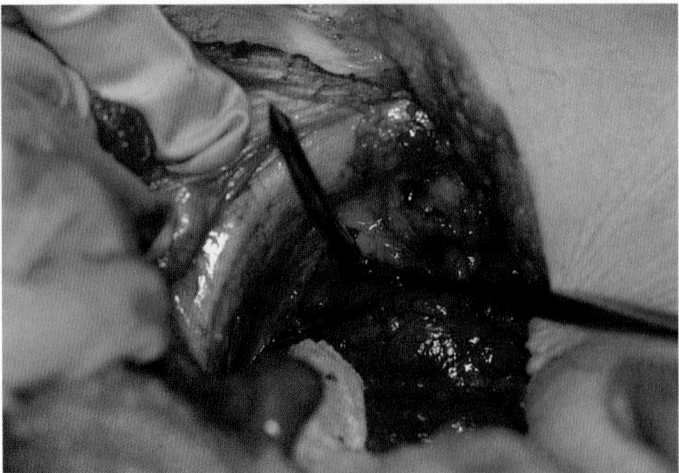

**FIGURE 58–9** The direction of the needle along the back of the pubic bone is demonstrated in a cadaver.

visualized (Fig. 58-10). The needle is then withdrawn through the stab incision, and the same procedure is repeated exactly on the opposite side. In this way, the Prolene tape covered by a plastic sheath is placed in a U shape around the urethra (Figs. 58-11 and 58-12). The technique utilized to determine the appropriate tension of the TVT sling is done at the discretion of the surgeon. If local anesthesia is used, a cough stress test can be attempted to create the sign of stress incontinence (see Fig. 58-11). If general anesthesia is used, suprapubic pressure can be used to create urinary leakage. The sling material is adjusted until only a slight amount of leakage is visualized with these provocative maneuvers. The plastic sheath is then removed while the tape is stabilized with a right-angle clamp or Metzenbaum scissors (Figs. 58-13 and 58-14). The tape can be further adjusted after the plastic sheath is removed by stretching with a right-angle clamp. Ultimately, in most patients, the tape should sit very loosely at the level of the midurethra, easily allowing placement of an instrument between the tape and the urethra (Fig. 58-15). The sling material is not fixed or sutured to the endopelvic fascia or the rectus fascia, but is simply cut on each side at the level of the skin. The vaginal and abdominal incisions are closed.

More recently, a suprapubic approach to synthetic retropubic midurethral slings has been described. The needle is passed from the suprapubic stab wound along the back of the symphysis to exit into the vaginal incision. The needle should maintain direct contact with the posterior aspect of the pubic bone as it passes through the retropubic space. To ensure that the needle exits in the midurethra, not at the level of the bladder neck, it should be laid down flat on the abdomen as it transcends through the retropubic space (Figs. 58-16 and 58-17).

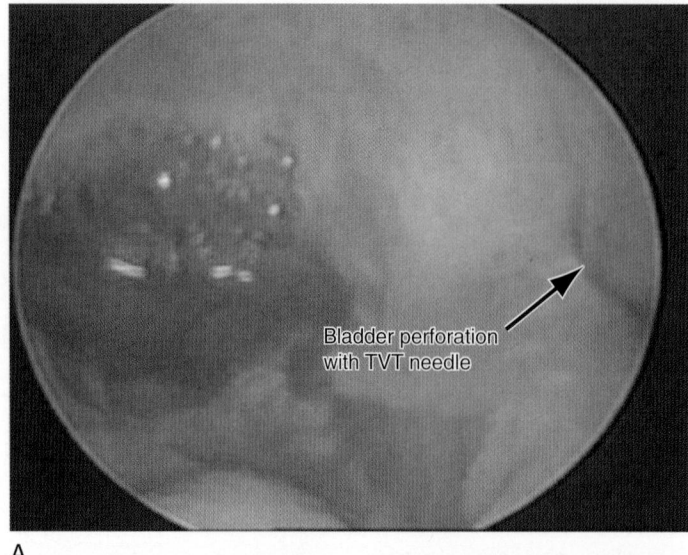

A

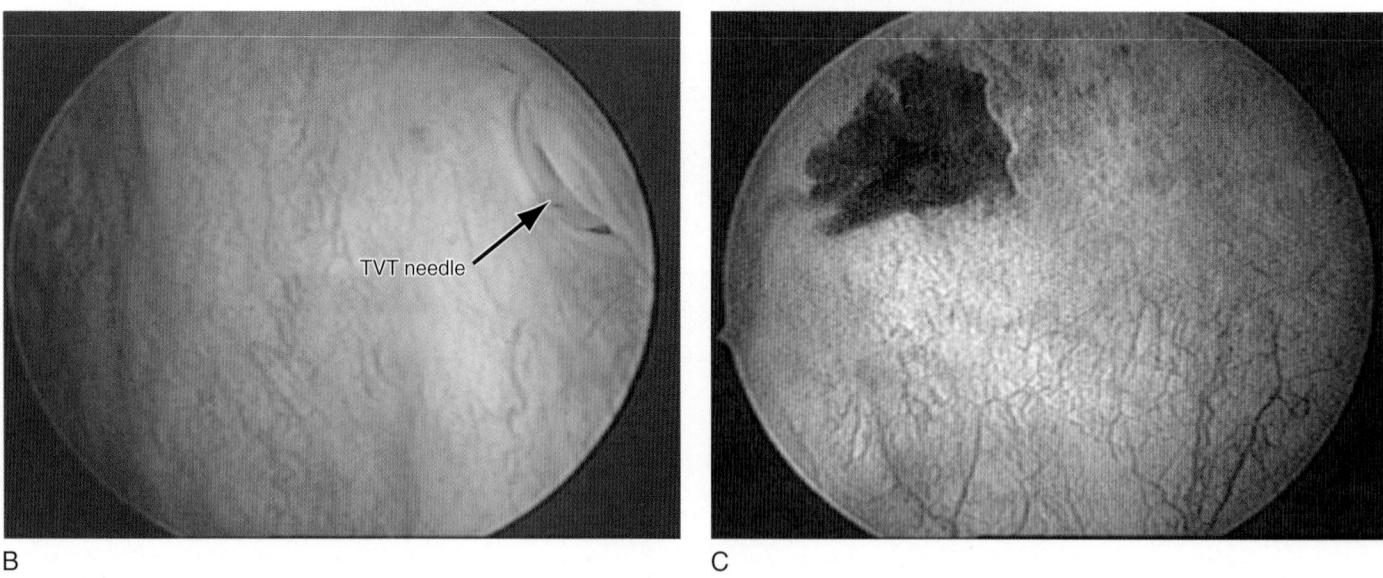

B                                                         C

**FIGURE 58–10  A.** Bladder perforation with a tension-free vaginal tape (TVT) on the patient's left side. **B.** The shaft of the needle is now visible as it is withdrawn back into the vagina. **C.** The defect that is left in the bladder.

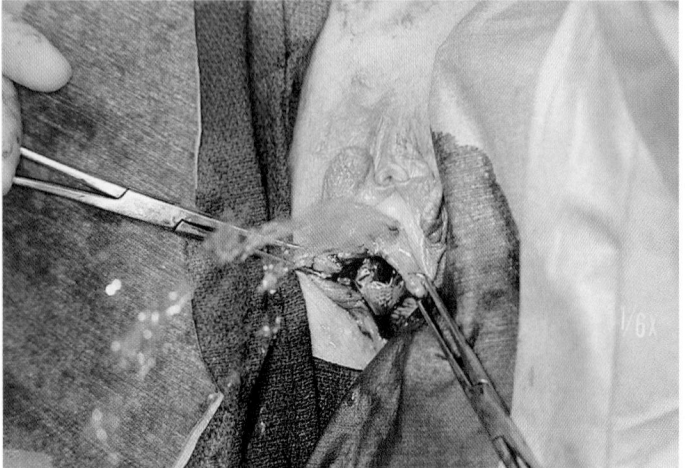

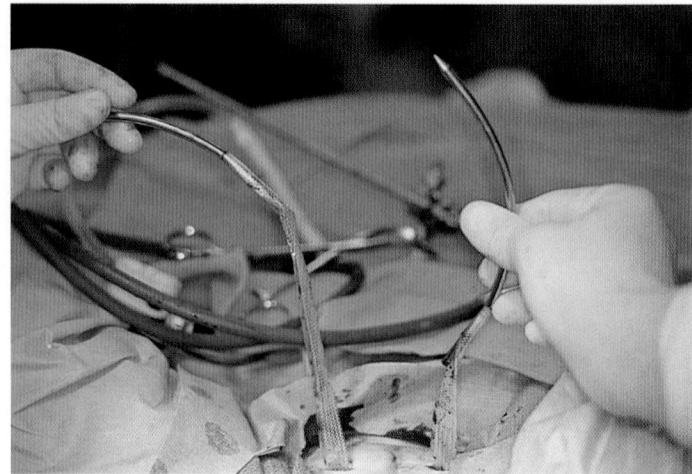

**FIGURE 58–11**  The tape has been passed suprapubically on both sides. Leakage of urine during a coughing stress test indicates the need for adjustment of the sling material.

**FIGURE 58–12**  Tension-free vaginal tape (TVT) needles and a plastic sheath containing Prolene tape have been passed up through suprapubic stab wounds.

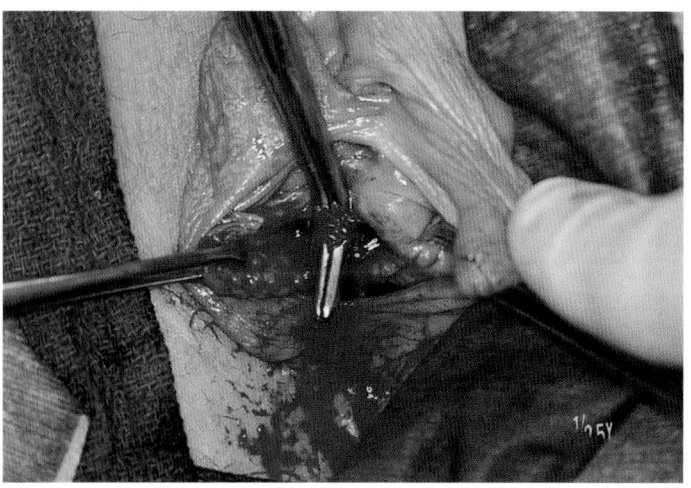

**FIGURE 58–13** A right-angle clamp stabilizes the Prolene while the plastic sheath is being withdrawn suprapubically.

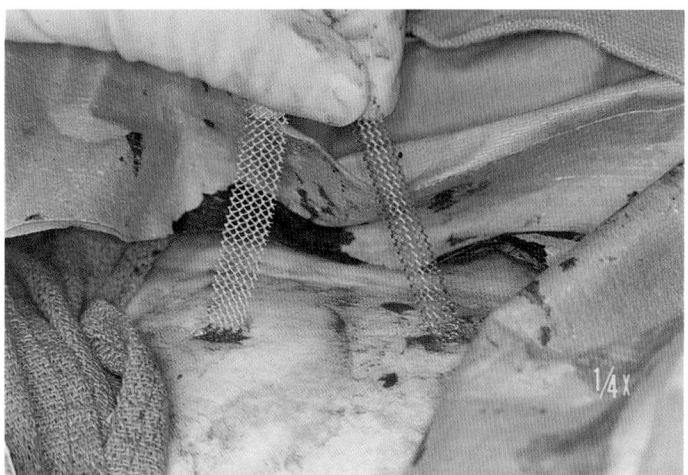

**FIGURE 58–14** Prolene tape after the plastic sheath has been removed.

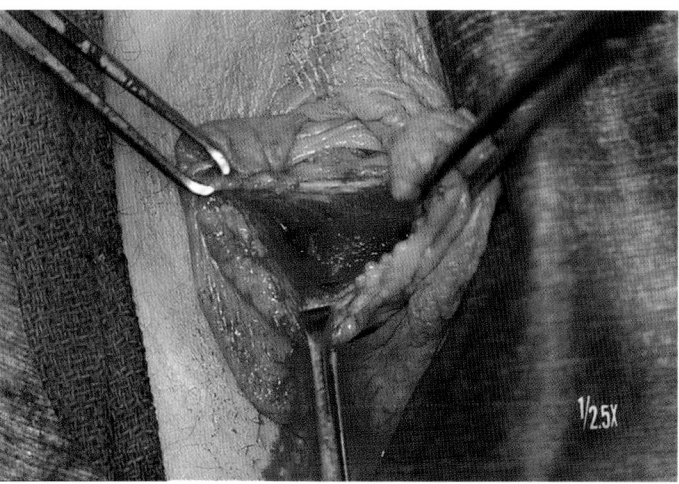

**FIGURE 58–15** Tension-free Prolene tape at the level of the midurethra.

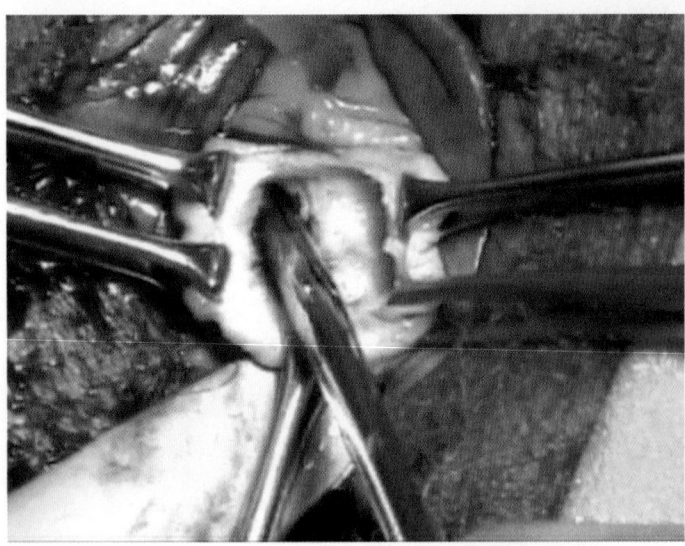
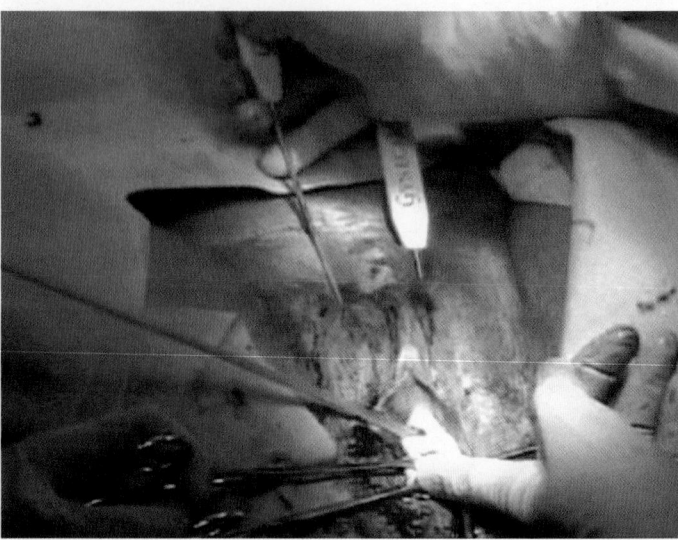

A                                                                                          B

**FIGURE 58–16  A.** Dissection for an abdominal guide procedure (Gynecare, Somerville, NJ). *Note:* The vaginal incision is larger to allow the tip of the finger to palpate the inferior pubic ramus and pick up the needle as it passes through the urogenital diaphragm. **B.** Needles being passed suprapubically into the vagina.

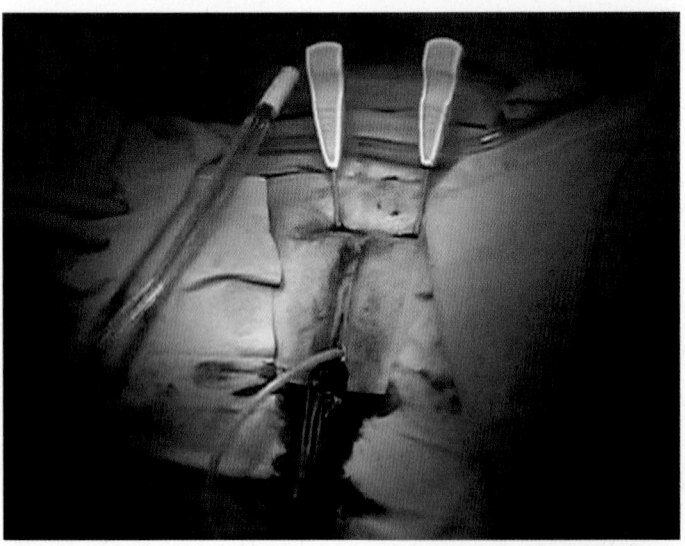
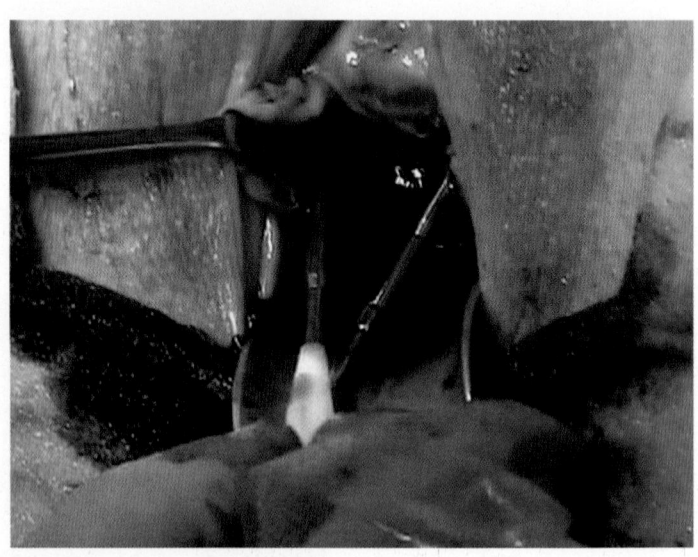

A                                                                                          B

**FIGURE 58–17  A.** The SPARC procedure (American Medical Systems, Minneapolis, Minn), which is a suprapubic approach to a retropubic synthetic midurethral sling. **B.** The connector utilized with the SPARC procedure allows transfer of the sling into the suprapubic area.

## Transobturator Synthetic Midurethral Slings

DeLorme described the first transobturator synthetic midurethral sling. The theoretical advantages of a transobturator sling include less bladder injury, because the device largely avoids the space of Retzius, and reduced potential for vascular and bowel injury. These slings are passed through a group of inner thigh muscles, specifically, the gracilis tendon, the adductor brevis, and the obturator externus. Figure 58-18 illustrates the origins and insertions of these muscles, as well as other medial thigh muscles. Currently, two techniques are available for placing a transobturator sling. Both techniques involve specially designed needles that are passed from the obturator region into the vagina or from the vagina into the obturator region. Figures 58-19 through 58-26 demonstrate the anatomy of the region via extensive cadaveric dissection. When passed from outside-in, the sling is directed from a small incision lateral to the clitoris at the inferior edge of the adductor longus tendon, through the obturator foramen, around the ischiopubic ramus, and into the anterior vagina at the level of the midurethra. It passes in order through the following structures: gracilis, adductor brevis muscle, obturator externus muscle, obturator membrane, and beneath or through the obturator internus muscle and periurethral endopelvic connective tissue; it finally exits into the opened vagina. In the technique utilized for the inside-out approach, the same structures are passed through in the opposite direction. Figures 58-27 and 58-28 demonstrate the technique for placement of a transobturator sling via an outside-in approach and an inside-out approach.

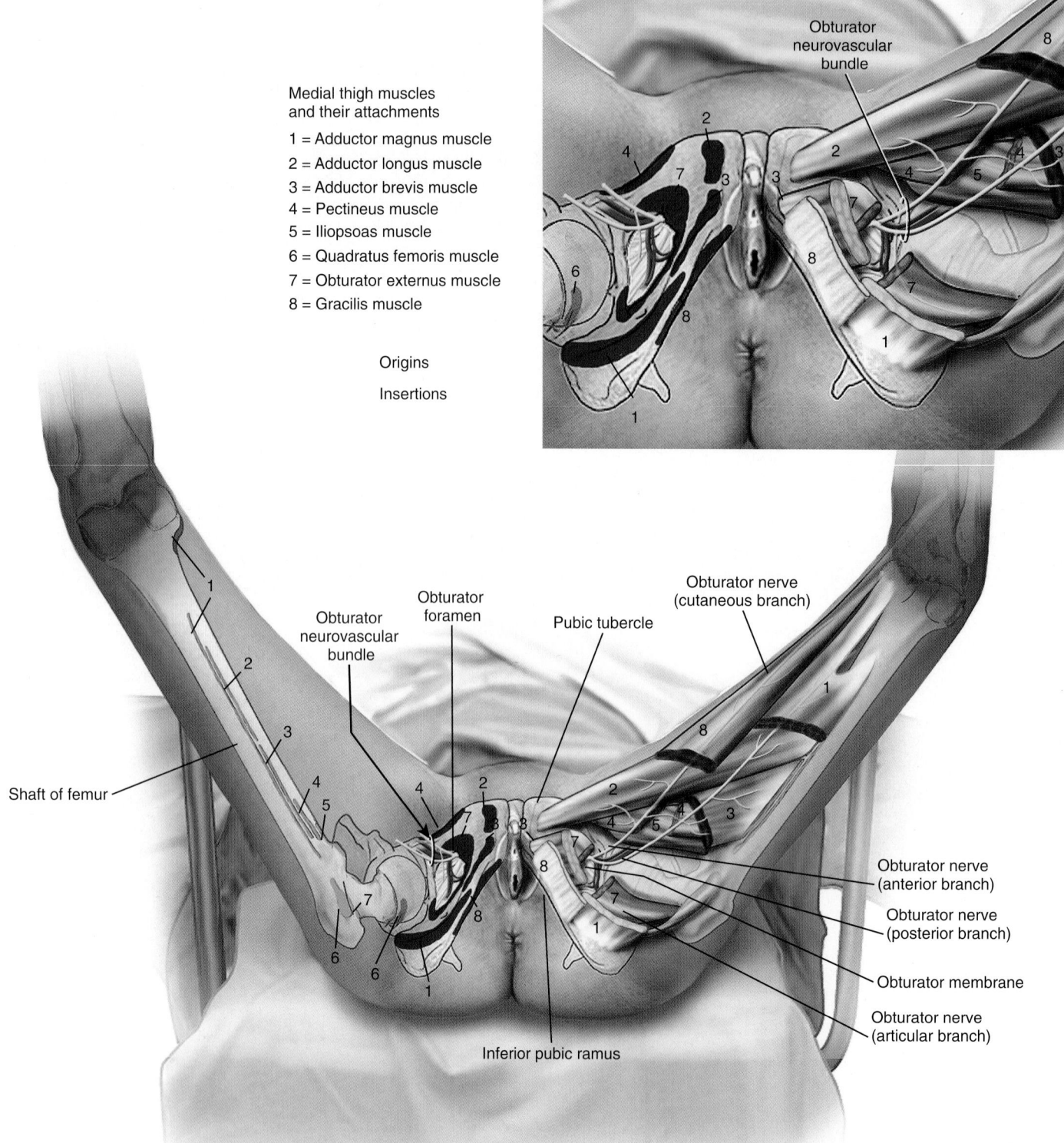

Medial thigh muscles
and their attachments

1 = Adductor magnus muscle
2 = Adductor longus muscle
3 = Adductor brevis muscle
4 = Pectineus muscle
5 = Iliopsoas muscle
6 = Quadratus femoris muscle
7 = Obturator externus muscle
8 = Gracilis muscle

Origins

Insertions

Obturator
neurovascular
bundle

Obturator nerve
(cutaneous branch)

Obturator
foramen

Pubic tubercle

Obturator
neurovascular
bundle

Shaft of femur

Obturator nerve
(anterior branch)

Obturator nerve
(posterior branch)

Obturator membrane

Obturator nerve
(articular branch)

Inferior pubic ramus

**FIGURE 58–18** Illustration of the anatomy of the inner thigh. Note the origins and insertion of medial thigh muscles.

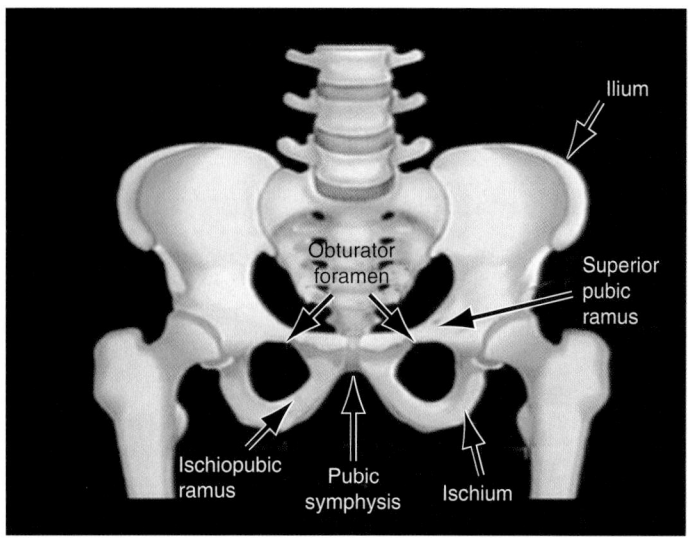

**FIGURE 58–19** The bony pelvis. Note the superior pubic ramus and the obturator foramen.

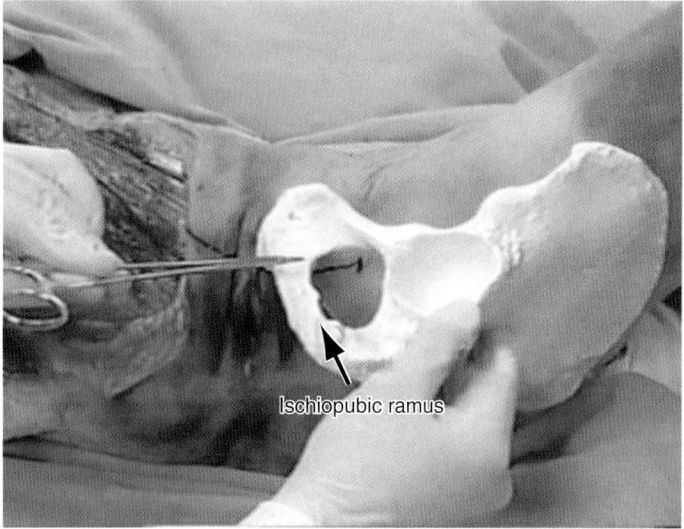

**FIGURE 58–20** The bony pelvis held in front of a cadaver to demonstrate the anatomic location of the ischiopubic ramus and the obturator foramen.

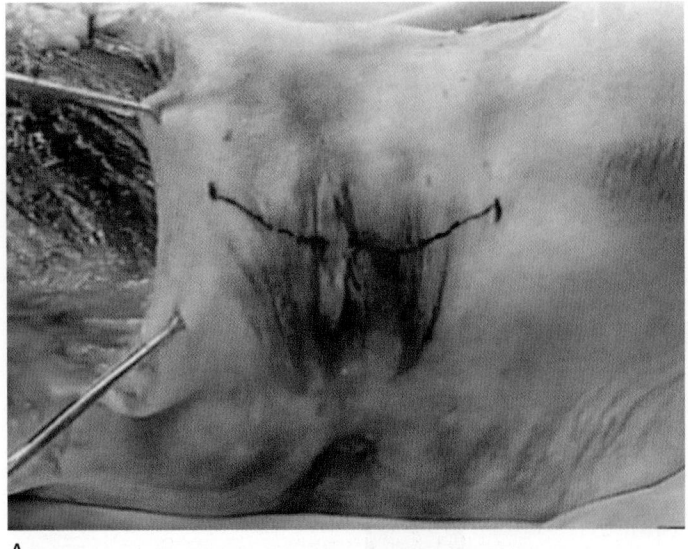

A

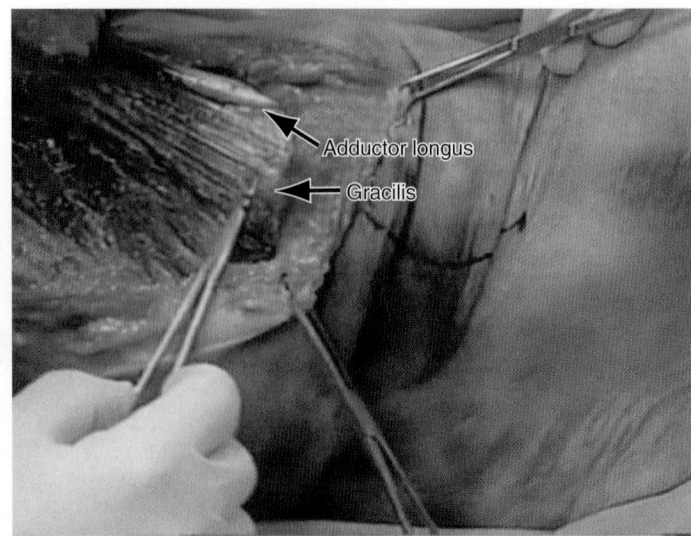

B

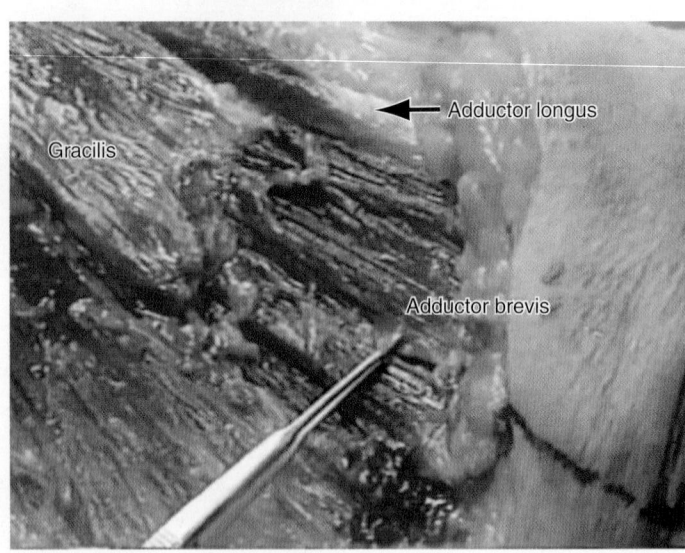

D

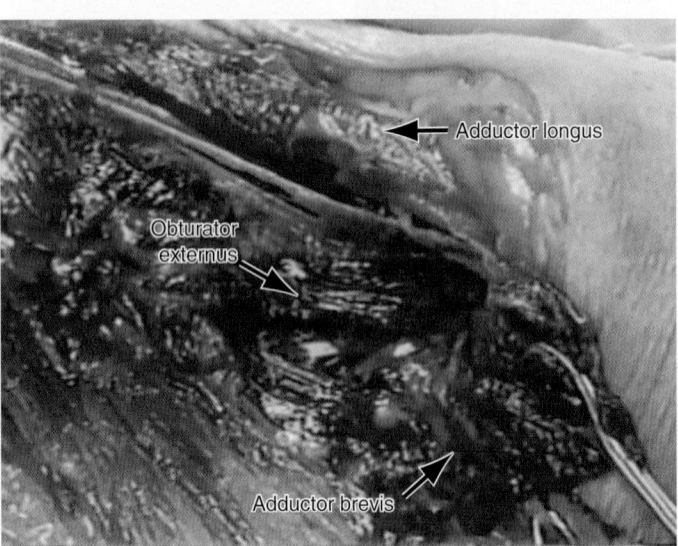

E

**FIGURE 58–21  A.** The anatomic location of a transobturator suburethral sling is drawn on the cadaver. **B.** The obturator region on the cadaver's left side is open to demonstrate the anatomic site of the gracilis and adductor longus muscles. **C.** Muscles of the inner thigh. **D.** The gracilis muscle has been cut to expose the adductor brevis muscle. **E.** The adductor brevis muscle is displaced to demonstrate the location of the obturator externus muscle, the site of which lies directly on the obturator membrane.

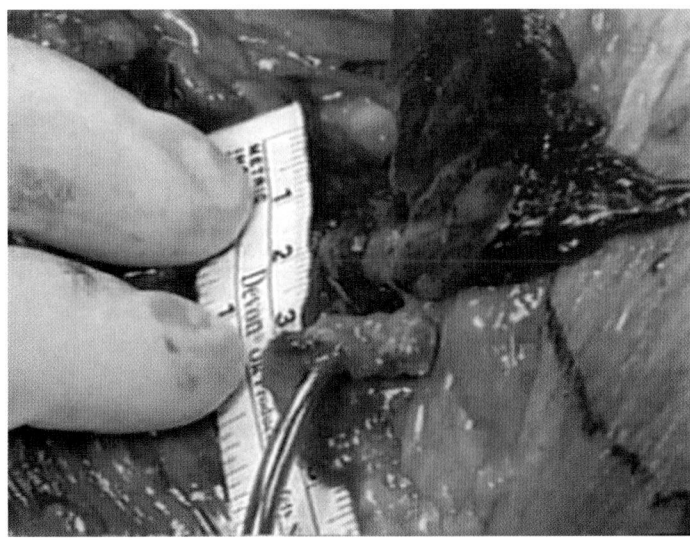

FIGURE 58–22 Distance from the entrance point of the transobturator needle to the obturator neurovascular bundle as it exits the obturator canal.

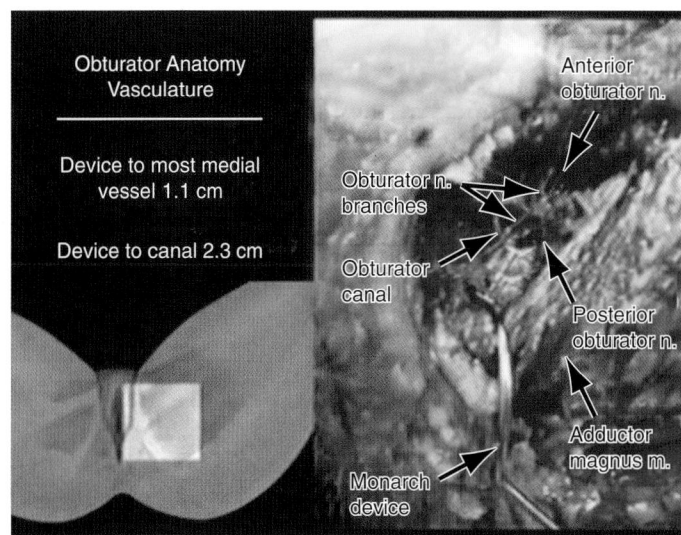

FIGURE 58–23 Anatomy of the obturator region. Average distance from the Monarch device to the obturator vessels in six fresh-frozen cadavers.

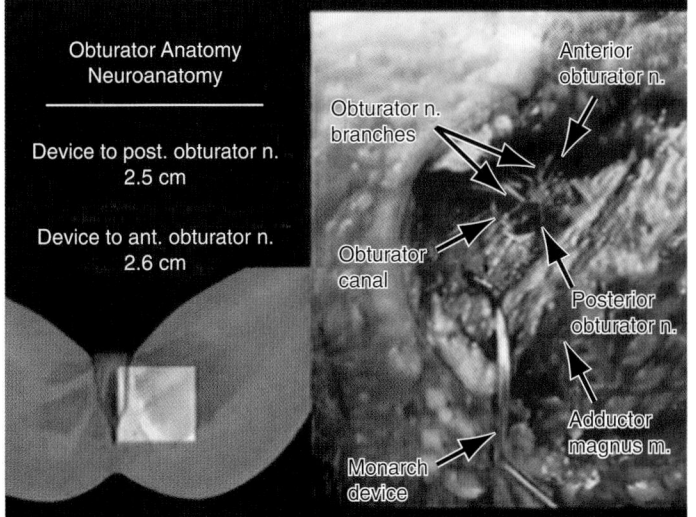

FIGURE 58–24 Anatomy of the obturator region. Average distance from Monarch device to obturator nerves in six fresh-frozen cadavers.

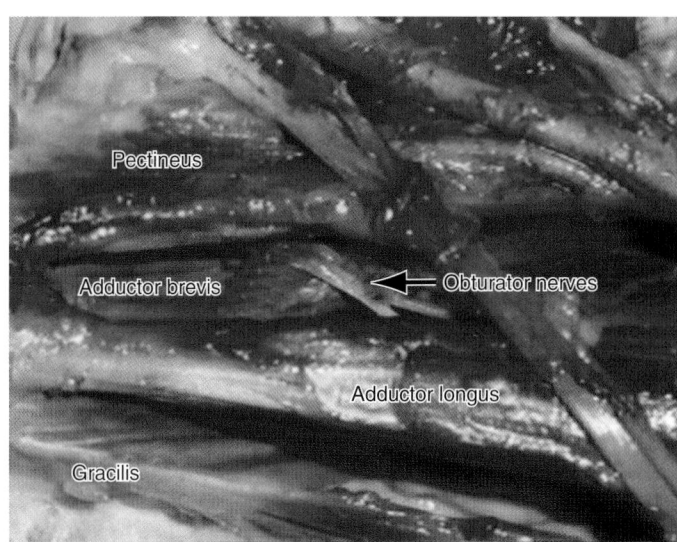

FIGURE 58–25 Relationship of the obturator nerves to the muscles of the obturator region.

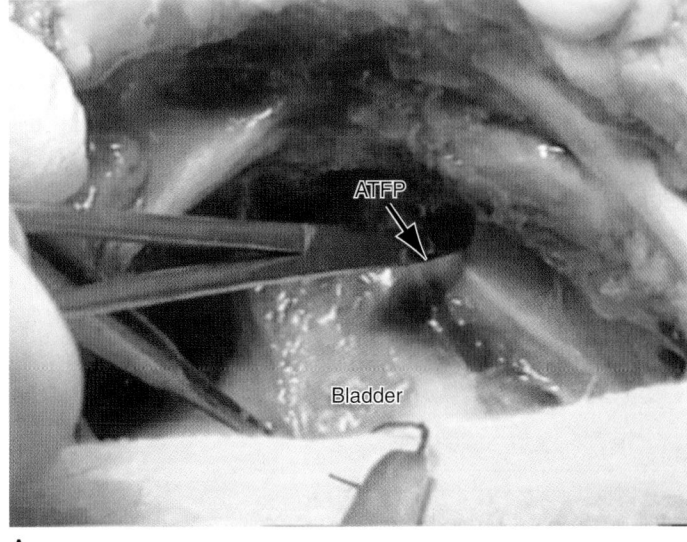

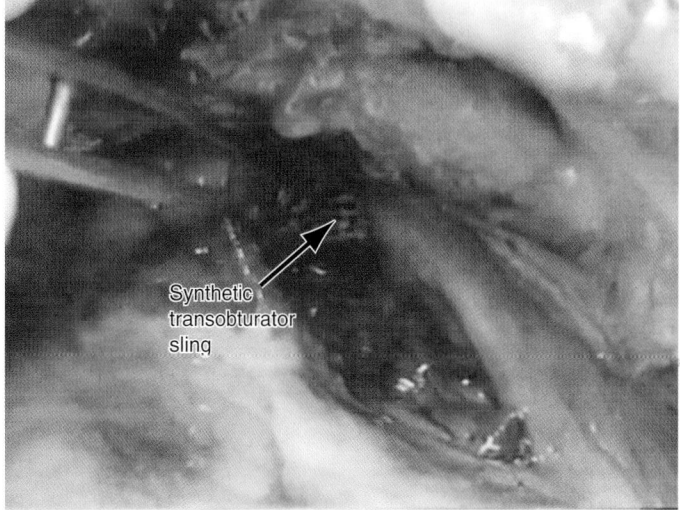

A  B

FIGURE 58–26 A. View of the retropubic space of a cadaver. The clamp is pointing to the arcus tendineus fascia pelvis and the obturator internus muscle. B. This area has been opened up to demonstrate the normal anatomic location of a transobturator sling. Note: The sling should not enter the retropubic space. It should remain deep to the arcus tendineus fascia pelvis and the obturator internus muscle.

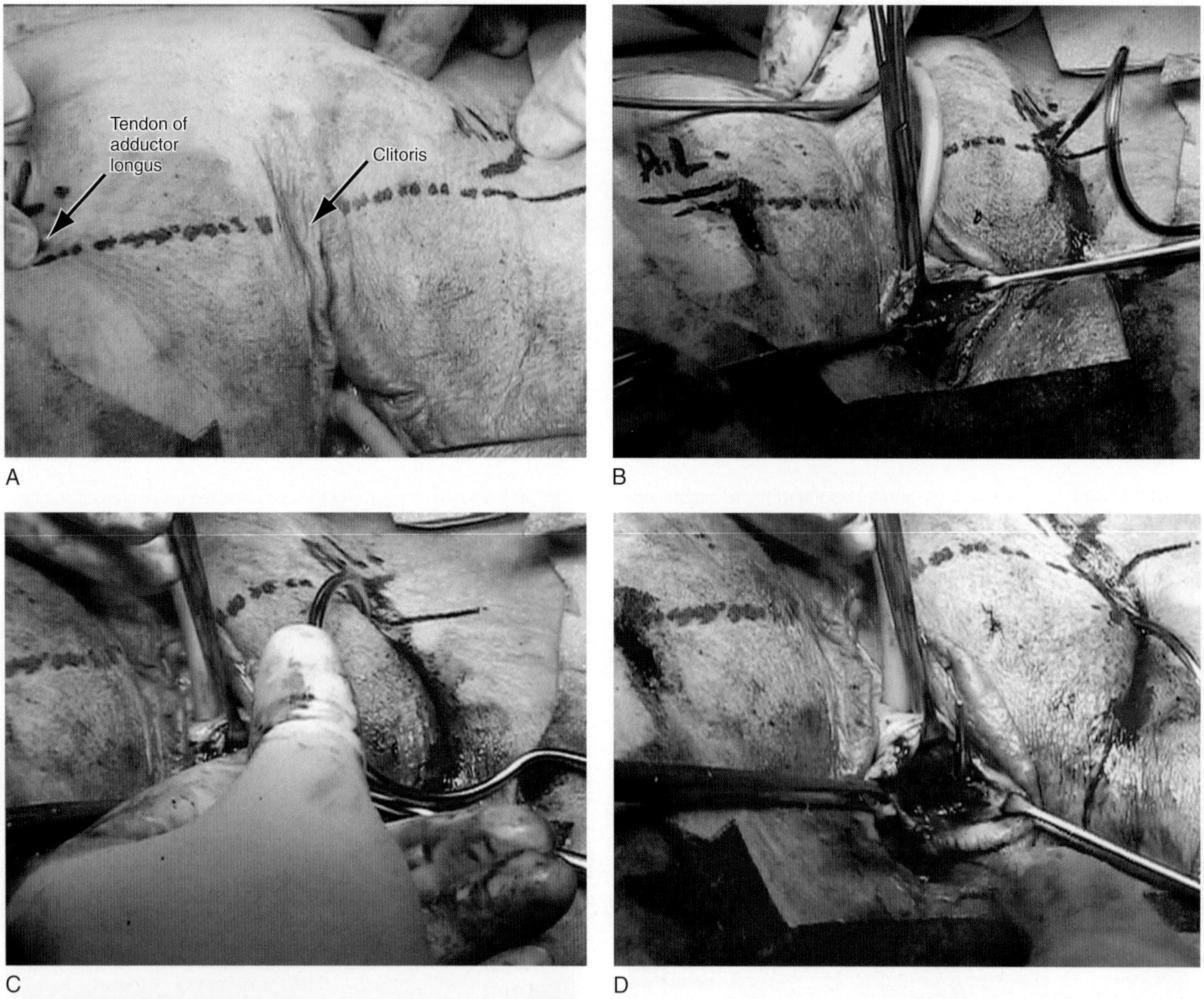

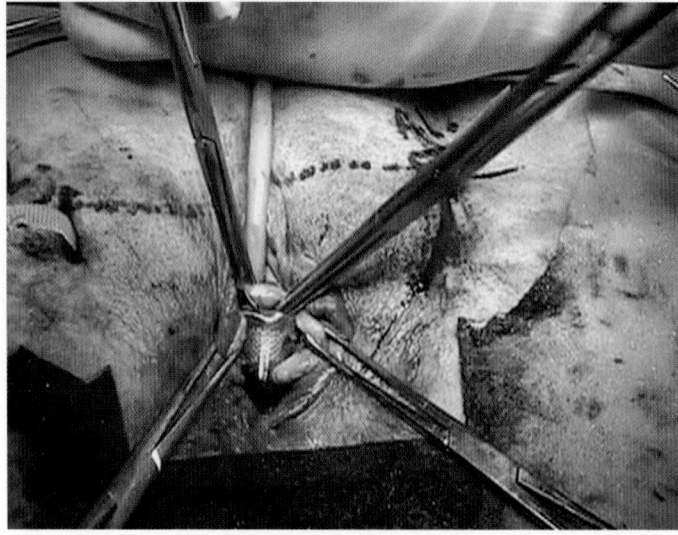

A

B

C

D

E

**FIGURE 58–27 A.** Anatomic location of the clitoris and tendon of the adductor longus. These are important landmarks when a transobturator sling procedure is performed. **B.** Monarch needle being passed into the obturator region. **C.** Appropriate positioning of the nondependent hand on the curvature of the needle so that downward pressure can be applied to facilitate penetration of the needle through the obturator membrane. **D.** The needle has been passed through the obturator membrane around the ischiopubic ramus and is shown exiting into the lateral part of the vaginal incision. **E.** The sling has been placed, and a right-angle clamp is used to stabilize the sling while the plastic sheath is removed.

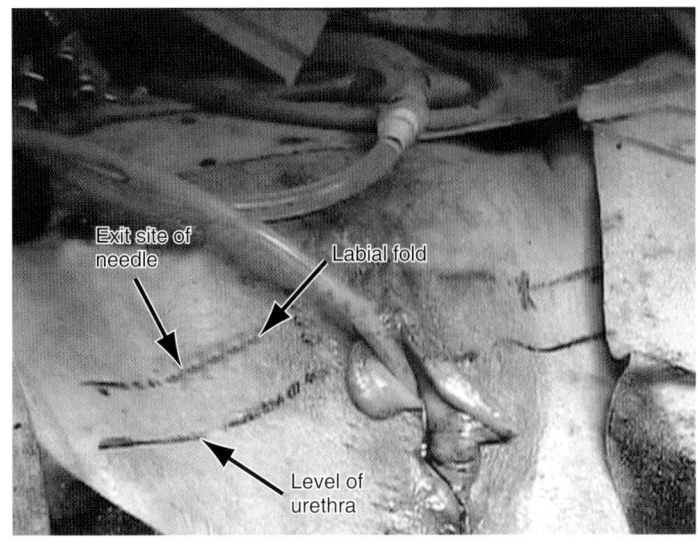

A

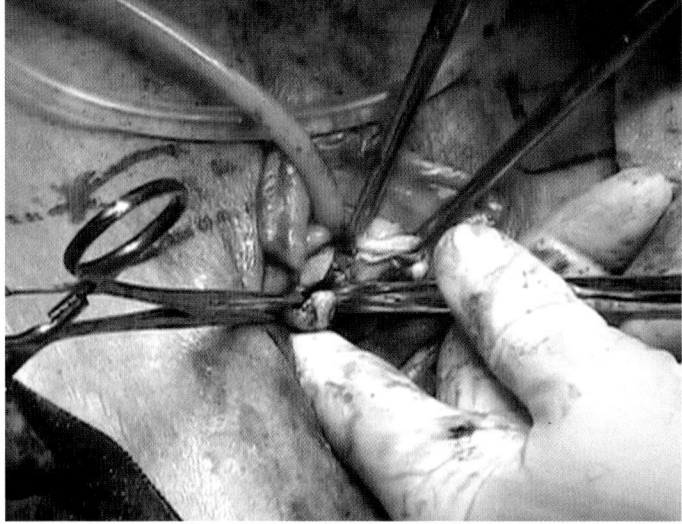

B

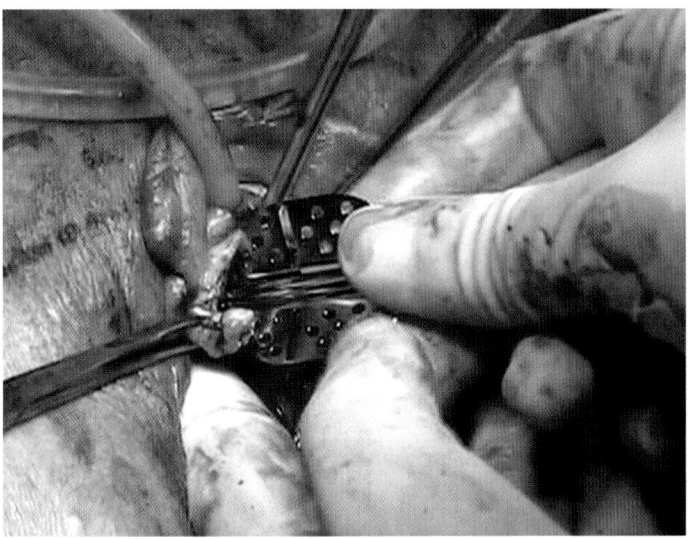

C

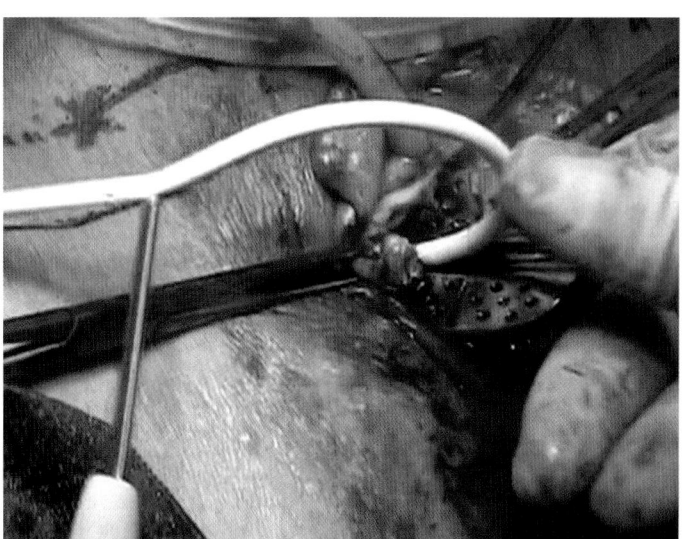

D

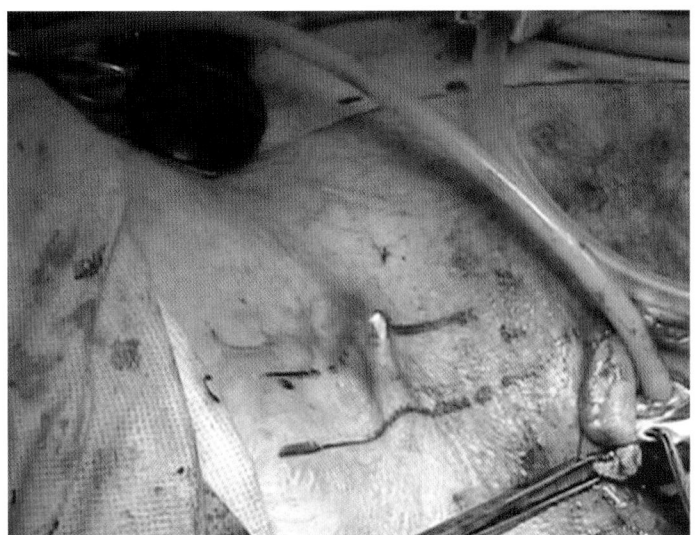

E

FIGURE 58–28 Technique for the tension-free vaginal tape (TVT)-O procedure (GyneCare, Somerville, NJ). This procedure utilizes specially designed needles that are passed from a vaginal incision into the obturator region. A. The exit site of the needle is marked. It should be 2 cm above the level of the urethra and 2 cm lateral to the labial fold. B. After a midline anterior vaginal wall incision is made, Metzenbaum scissors directed at a 45° angle are used to tunnel under the inferior pubic ramus toward the obturator region. The tips of the scissors should penetrate the obturator membrane. When this occurs, distinct resistance is overcome. C. A guide is then placed in the tunnel that is created by the scissors. D. A specially designed needle is passed, with the help of the guide, through the obturator membrane. E. The guide is then removed and the needle is passed into the obturator region, exiting at the previously marked exit site.

## Synthetic Single-Incision Midurethral Slings

Single-incision midurethral slings are approximately 10 cm in length, if one assumes that they are symmetrically and appropriately placed at the midline; the various anatomic structures that the sling can penetrate include the periurethral attachment to the pubic bone, or what is sometimes termed the *urogenital diaphragm* or *obturator internus muscle*. When a single-incision sling is performed, the anatomic objective is for the sling to be placed in durable tissue. If the sling is placed in a more lateral direction, it would penetrate directly into the obturator internus muscle with the possibility of duplicating a transobturator-type sling. The length of the sling does not allow the sling to pass through the obturator membrane; thus the inner thigh muscles, nerves, and blood vessels could not be damaged. If the sling is placed in a more medial fashion, stimulating the original retropubic synthetic sling, it will penetrate the urogenital diaphragm or the paraurethral attachment to the inferior pubic ramus and enter the lowest portion of the retropubic space. Structures at risk include the urethra, the bladder, and the aberrant retropubic blood vessels that drape down the lateral pelvic sidewall, as well as the large veins of the anterior vaginal wall. Of note, the sling, if placed appropriately, is not long enough to reach the obturator neurovascular bundle as it exits the pelvis through the obturator canal. Figure 58-29 illustrates a variety of potential placements of a single-incision sling based on the technique and device that are utilized.

At the present time, indications for these procedures are very controversial because of the lack of a standard technique for placement and minimal outcome data. The perceived advantages of the mini-slings are that they are less invasive, quicker to place, and safer.

The procedure can be performed with the patient under general, regional, or local anesthesia. The bladder is drained with a catheter, and a 2- to 3-cm incision is made in the mid to distal portion of the anterior vaginal wall (Fig. 58-30). Hydrodistention facilitates dissection of the anterior vaginal wall epithelium off the urethra. This may minimize bleeding during dissection. The dissection is taken laterally to the inferior pubic ramus, with assurance that the lateral portion of the urethra is dissected away from the anterior vaginal wall (Figs. 58-31 and 58-32). The sling is then inserted with an inserter or a sling carrier device. The other end of the sling is inserted in a similar manner. Appropriate tensioning of these slings remains the most challenging aspect of the procedure. In our experience, these slings need to be tensioned much more tightly than retropubic or transobturator synthetic slings (Fig. 58-33). The single-incision sling should be left in direct contact with the posterior urethra. This is in direct contradiction to what has been taught with previous synthetic slings, which should be placed very loosely. Once the appropriate position of the sling is reached, the surgeon must go to great lengths to avoid inadvertently loosening the sling while removing the needle attachment. Patients under monitored anesthesia care (MAC) or local anesthesia can undergo a cough test to aid in tensioning. Once the mesh is in place, cystourethroscopy is performed to ensure that no inadvertent injury to the urethra or bladder occurs.

Currently available synthetic midurethral slings include the TVT Secur System (Ethicon Women's Health & Urology, Sommerville, NJ), which was the first commercially available sling; it utilizes an 8 × 1.1-cm laser-cut Prolene mesh. At the ends of the Prolene mesh are absorbable fixation tips made of Vicryl and polydioxanone (PDS) suture material. The sling is attached to a steel inserter with a spade needle tip (Fig. 58-34). The mesh can be placed in a "hammock" or U shape. The urethra is deflected in the opposite direction with the use of a catheter guide in the Foley catheter when the U-shaped sling is placed. The inserter is used to deliver the mesh and allow adjustment until the wire is released. Figures 58-35 through 58-39 demonstrate appropriate techniques for placement of a TVT Secur device. The second single-incision sling that came to market was the MiniArc (American Medical Systems, Minnetonka, Minn) sling. This 2.3-mm-diameter blunt needle requires a lesser insertion force as compared with the TVT Secur (4.5 lb vs. 2.5 lb). The sling is an 8.5 × 1.1-cm polypropylene mesh with a midline mark. The MiniArc uses a blunt-tip needle to deliver the sling's self-fixating tip. The needle has a redocking feature that provides the ability to reconnect to the mesh and allow for additional tensioning. Compared with the TVT Secur, the MiniArc sling has a smaller needle diameter (8.1 mm vs. 2.3 mm) (Figs. 58-40 and 58-41). Another slim needle design sling is the Solyx SIS System (Boston Scientific, Natick, Mass). This sling features a different delivery and tensioning system. The sling is a polypropylene mesh that measures 9 cm in length. The mesh itself snap-fits to the delivery device, which prevents premature release of the mesh off the device. The delivery device has a deployment mechanism that allows appropriate tensioning without premature release of the mesh. The mesh has "De-Tanged" edges in the middle portion of the sling measuring 4 cm. After appropriate tensioning, the mesh is set in place by grasping the deployment mechanism and pulling the delivery device handle back (Figs. 58-42 and 58-43). Both MiniArc and Solyx single-incision slings are intended to be passed directly into the obturator internus muscle.

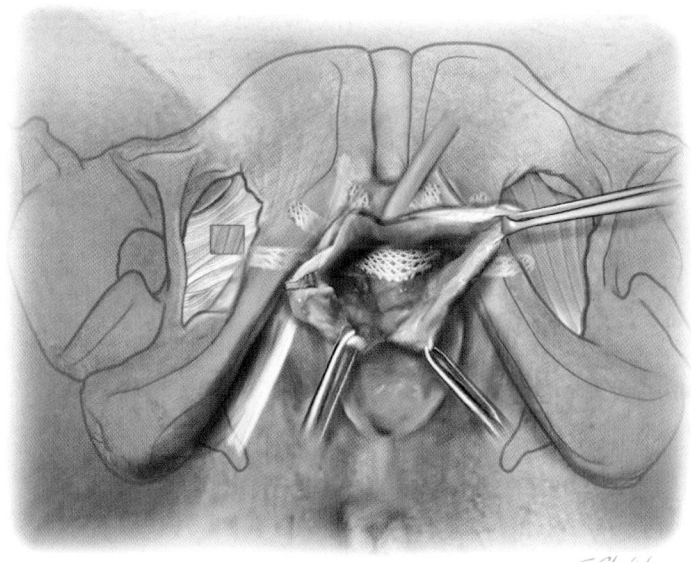

**FIGURE 58–29** Illustration demonstrating a variety of potential placements of a single-incision sling based on the technique and the device that are utilized.

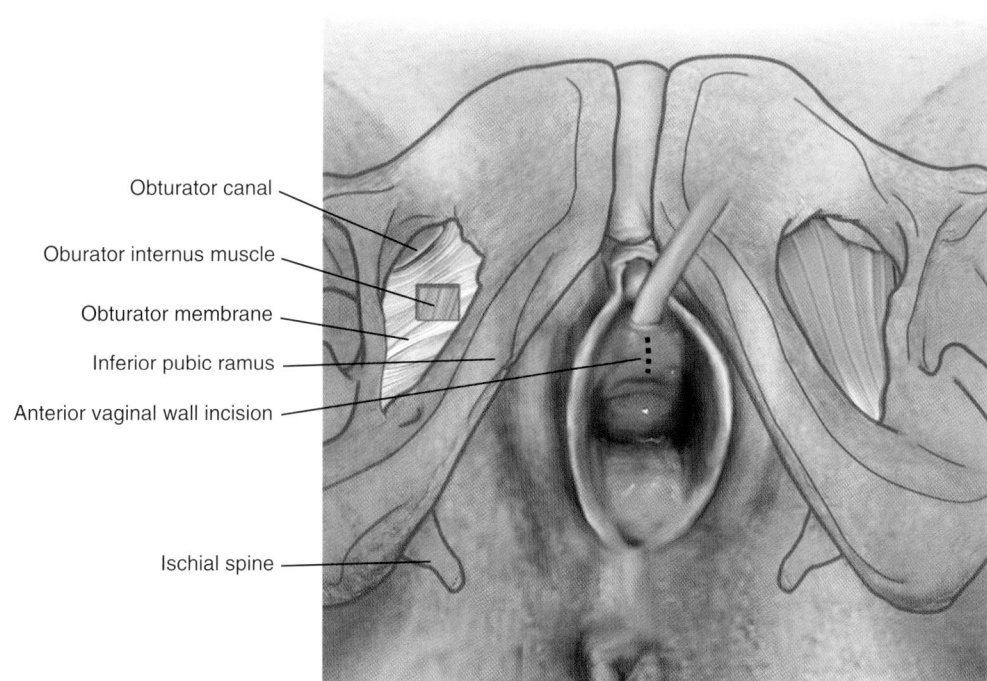

Obturator canal

Oburator internus muscle

Obturator membrane

Inferior pubic ramus

Anterior vaginal wall incision

Ischial spine

B

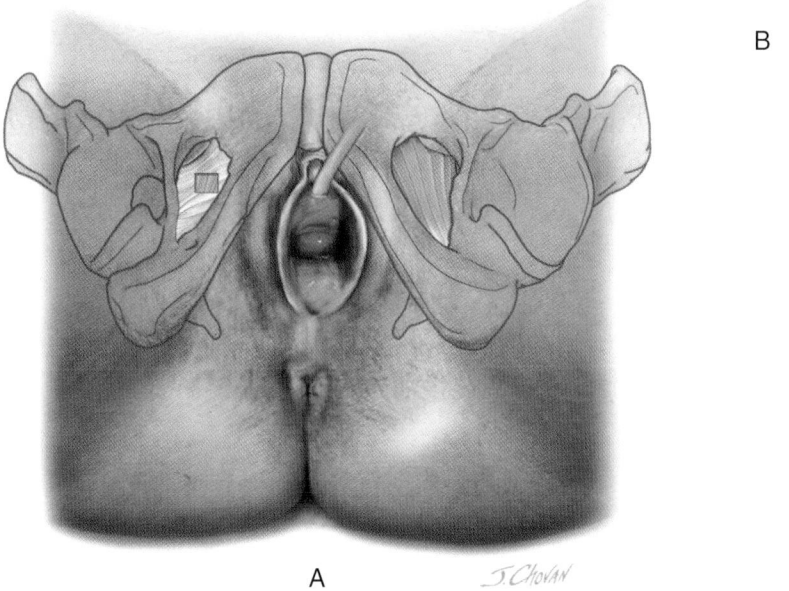

A

**FIGURE 58–30 A.** View of the anterior vaginal wall as it relates to the obturator membrane and the obturator internus muscle. **B.** Level of anterior vaginal wall incision is marked.

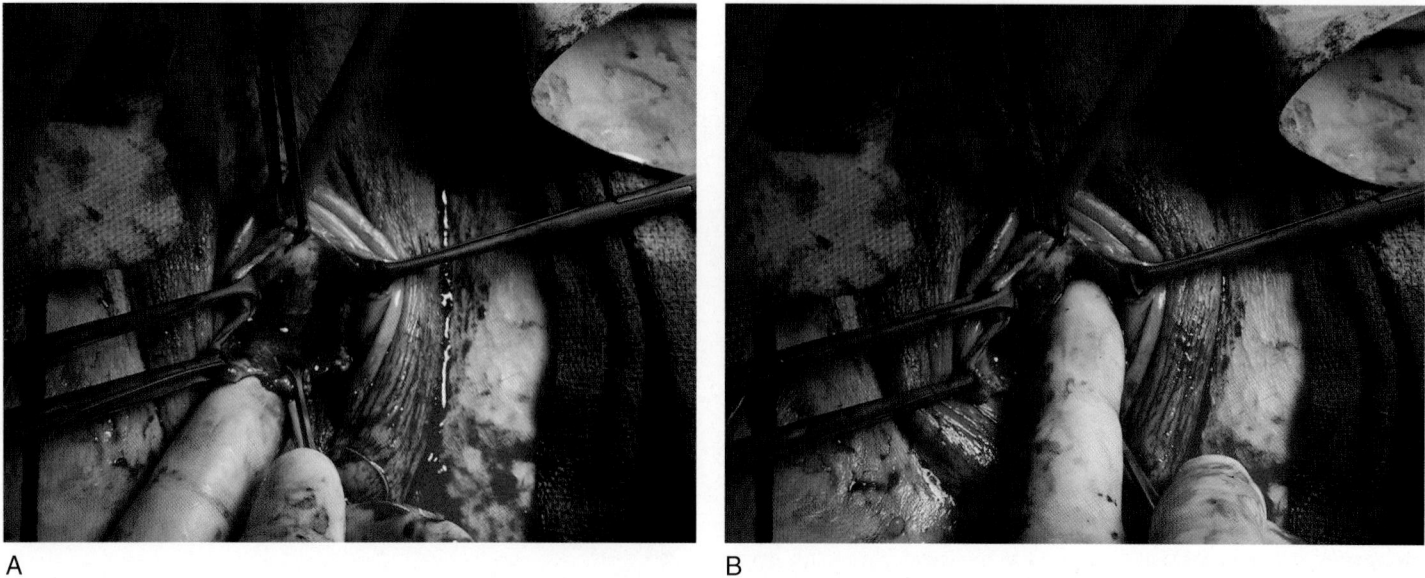

A    B

**FIGURE 58-31 A.** Anterior vaginal wall incision for a single-incision sling should completely mobilize the distal anterior vaginal wall off the posterior urethra. **B.** The incision should be large enough for placement of the surgeon's index finger.

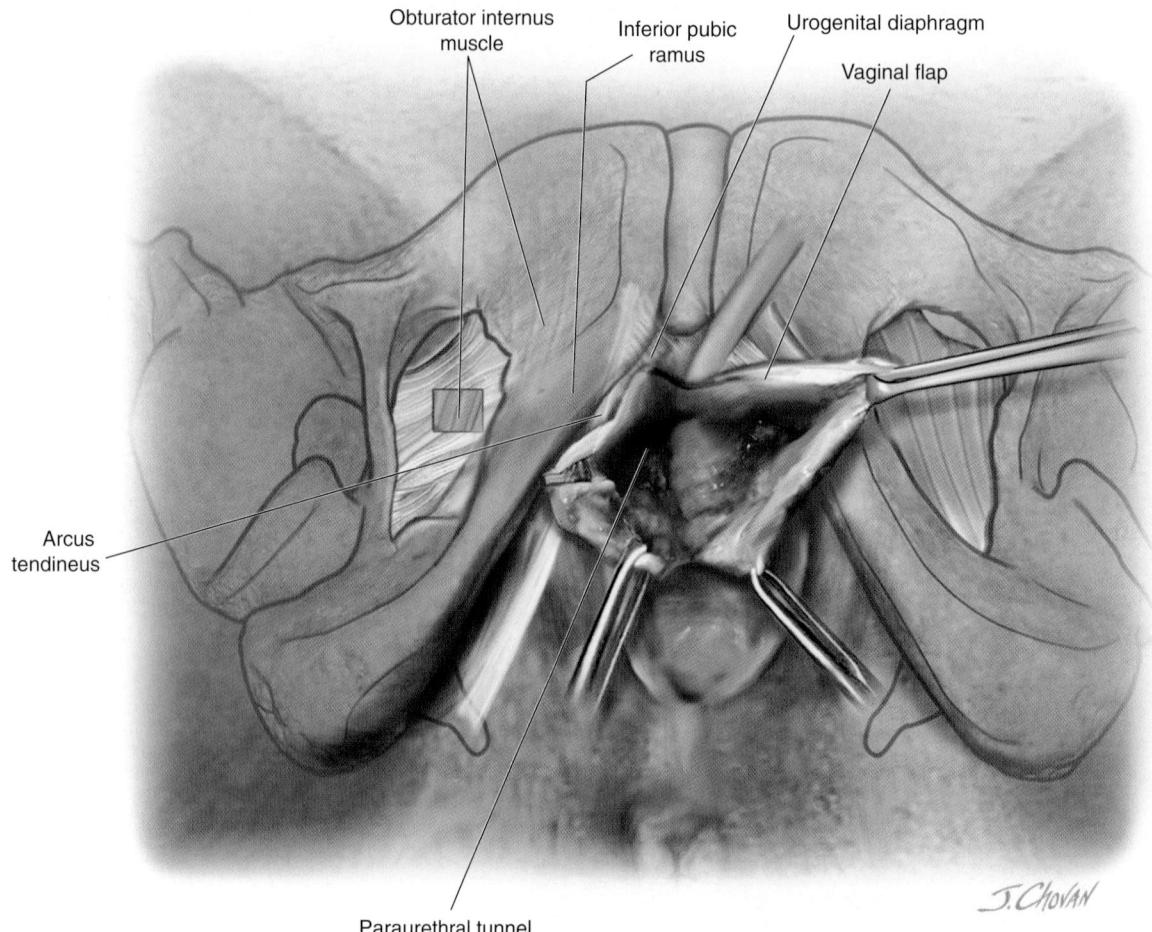

**FIGURE 58-32** Illustration of appropriate anterior vaginal incision made for a single-incision sling. Note that dissection extends paraurethrally to the inferior pubic ramus.

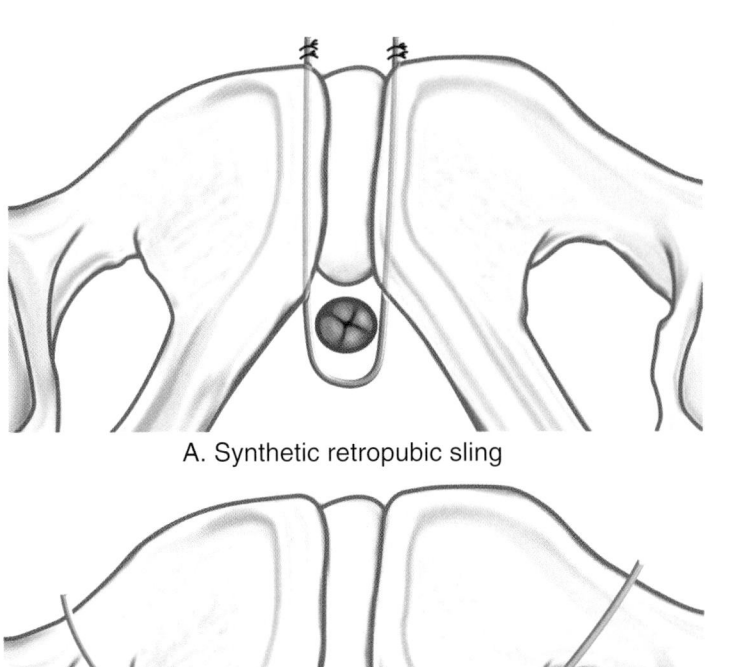

A. Synthetic retropubic sling

B. Synthetic transobturator sling

C. Synthetic single-incision slings

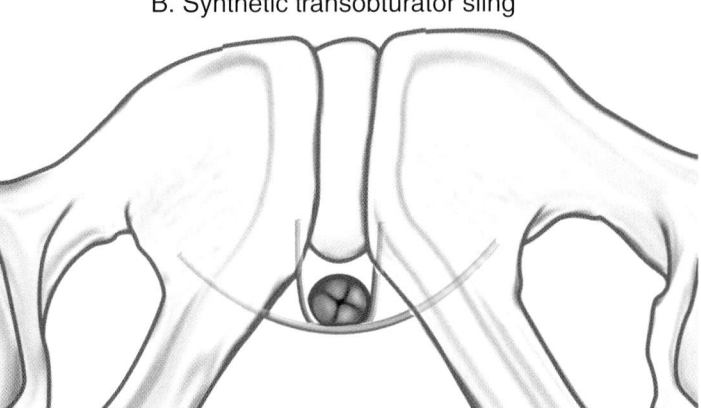

**FIGURE 58-33** Tensioning of synthetic midurethral slings.
**A.** Synthetic retropubic slings are usually left very loose, easily allowing an instrument to be passed between the sling and the posterior urethra. **B.** Transobturator synthetic midurethral slings are usually tensioned slightly tighter than retropubic slings. **C.** Single-incision slings are tensioned so that they come in direct contact with the posterior urethra, making it very difficult to pass an instrument between the sling and the posterior urethra.

**FIGURE 58-34** The tension-free vaginal tape (TVT) Secur sling (Ethicon Women's Health & Urology).

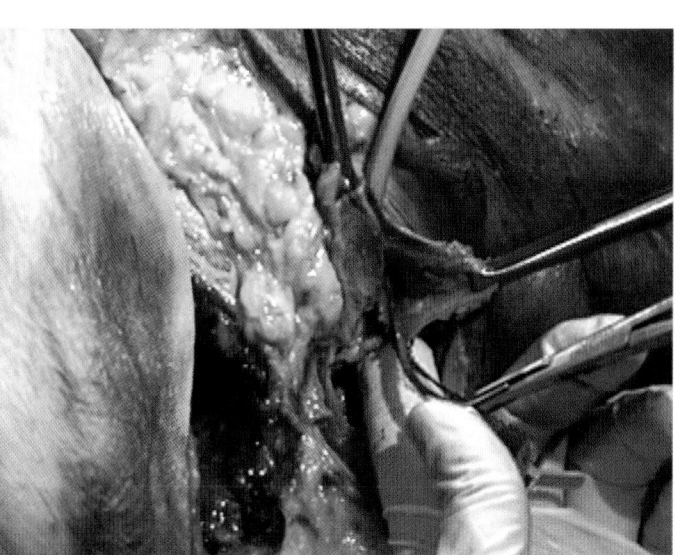

**FIGURE 58-35** Techniques utilized for passage of a tension-free vaginal tape (TVT) Secur device. Note that the vaginal incision should be large enough to allow the tip of the needle to come in direct contact with the inferior pubic ramus. The index finger of the nondominant hand is placed in the anterior vaginal fornix, and the thumb of the nondominant hand is used to advance the tip into the tissue. A needle holder is used as the handle for the device.

UNIT 3 ■ SECTION B

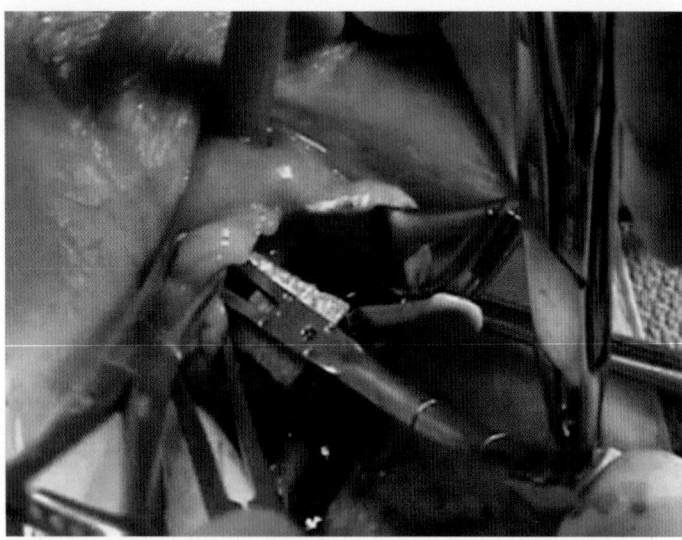

**FIGURE 58-36** Patient undergoing tension-free vaginal tape (TVT) Secur procedure with U-shaped placement. Note that the needle tip should penetrate the urogenital diaphragm just lateral to the urethra. A catheter guide should always be utilized when a U placement procedure is performed.

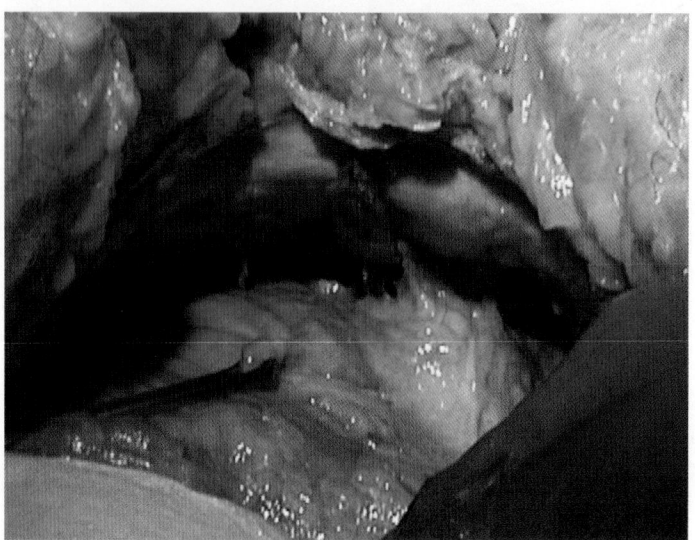

**FIGURE 58-37** Retropubic view of a cadaver in which a tension-free vaginal tape (TVT) Secur needle has been passed via the U-shape technique. Note that the needle tip should be in direct contact with the back of the pubic bone.

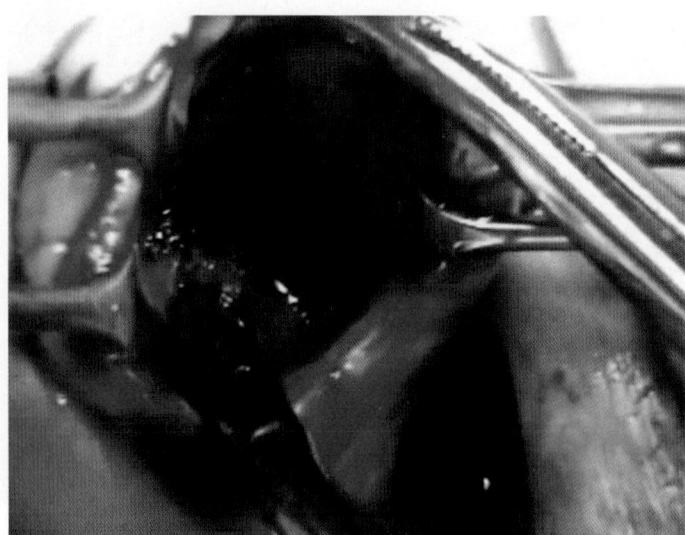

**FIGURE 58-38** U-placed tension-free vaginal tape (TVT) Secur sling after removal of the inserter. Note that the sling should be tensioned so that it is in direct contact with the posterior urethra.

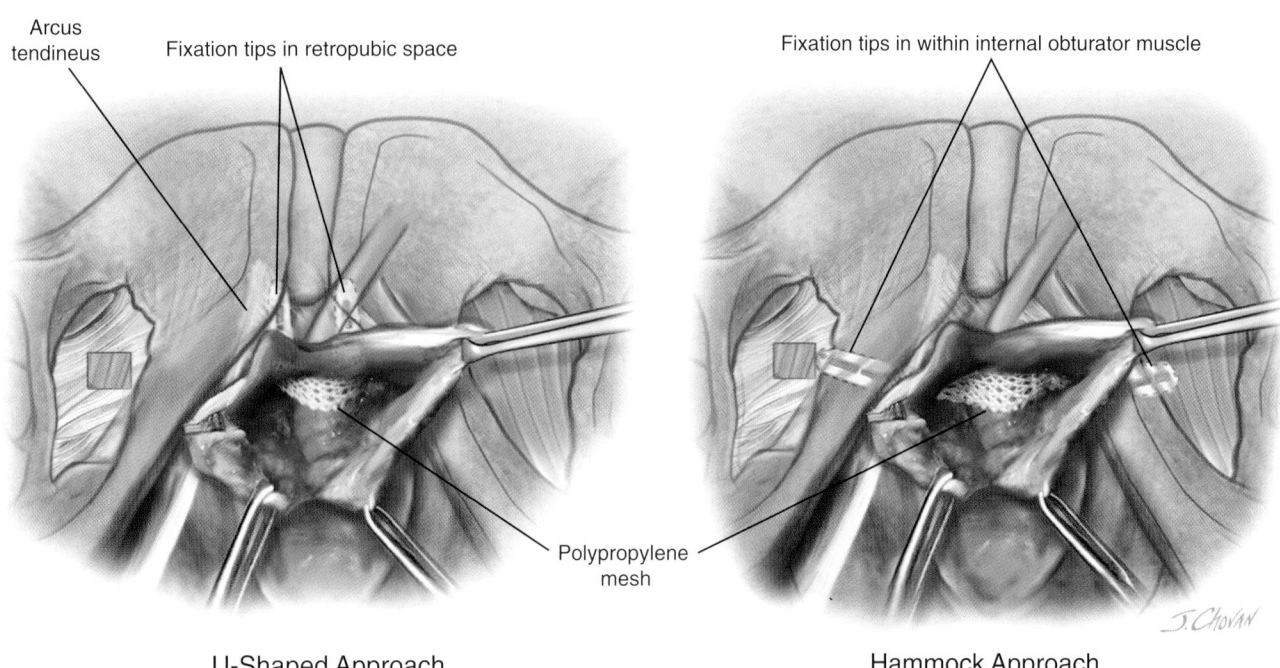

U-Shaped Approach             Hammock Approach

**FIGURE 58–39** Placement of tension-free vaginal tape (TVT) Secur single-incision sling, illustrating U-shaped placement where the needle penetrates the urogenital diaphragm, and hammock placement where the needle is passed directly into the obturator internus muscle.

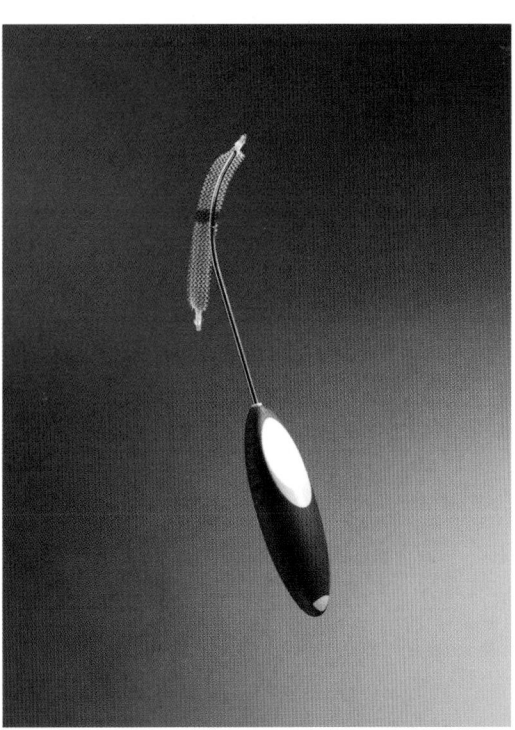

**FIGURE 58–40** The MiniArc sling. (Courtesy American Medical Systems, Inc., Minnetonka, Minnesota. www.AmericanMedicalSystems.com)

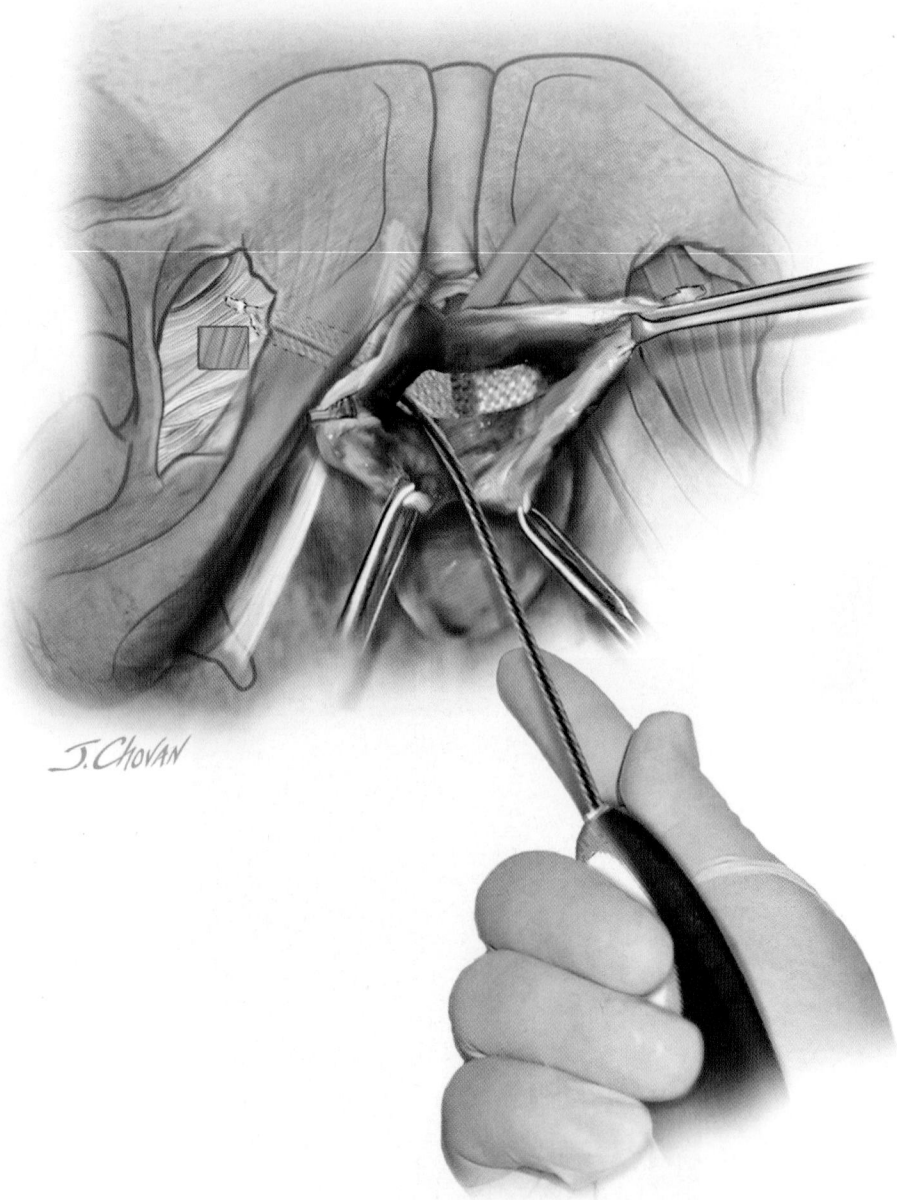

**FIGURE 58–41** Technique for placement of the MiniArc single-incision sling (American Medical Systems). Note that the sling is placed directly into the obturator internus muscle.

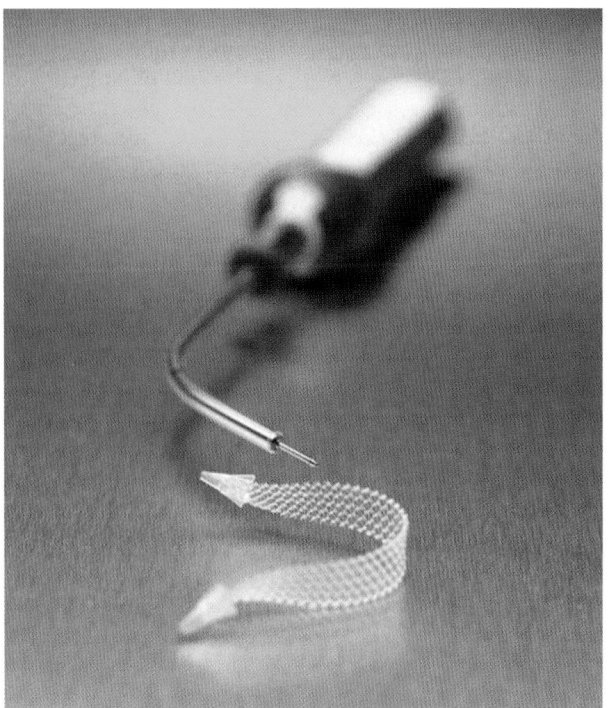

FIGURE 58–42  The Solyx sling (Boston Scientific, Natick, MA). (Photos courtesy Boston Scientific Corporation.)

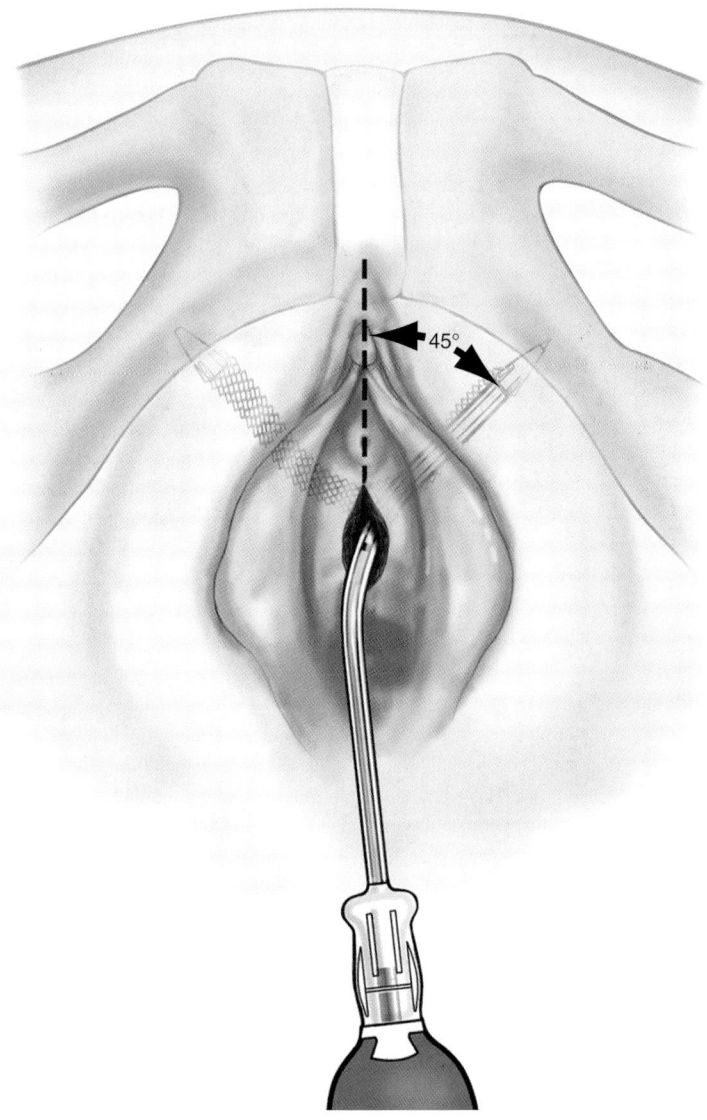

FIGURE 58–43  Illustration demonstrating placement of the Solyx sling (Boston Scientific, Natick, MA). (Photos courtesy Boston Scientific Corporation.)

## Techniques Used to Cut or Remove Sling Material

A certain percentage of women undergoing a suburethral sling procedure will require the sling to be cut or removed secondary to urethral obstruction or voiding dysfunction, at times because of erosion or excursion of the sling into the vagina, urethra, or bladder, or rarely, because of severe infection or allergic reaction. Urethral obstruction or voiding dysfunction can occur with any anti-incontinence procedure and usually results from a sling being tied or placed too tightly. It also may relate to the fact that the sling material is irritating and may cause symptoms of urgency and frequency, which can occur de novo anywhere from 5% to 20% of the time after sling procedures are performed. When this occurs, the sling must be adjusted, cut, or taken down. The technique used to perform this procedure depends on the sling material and how it interacts with the patient's tissue. For example, certain autologous or allograft slings may aggressively incorporate with the surrounding tissue, making it impossible to differentiate the sling material from the patient's tissue. In contrast, certain other materials, whether synthetic or biologic, may be easily identifiable and easily dissected away from the patient's tissue. Whether the patient redevelops stress incontinence or maintains her continence is based on the degree of scarification, how aggressive the takedown is, and what sling material was utilized. Figure 58–44 demonstrates the technique of isolating and cutting a cadaveric fascial sling with subsequent interposition of another piece of cadaveric fascia. Figure 58–45 demonstrates the technique of cutting a synthetic midurethral sling. Very rarely, synthetic midurethral slings may be placed inappropriately in the wall of the urethra or may erode into the urethra. Figure 58–46 demonstrates the technique of isolating, mobilizing, and cutting the suburethral portion of the sling and then fixing the defect within the urethra. The urethral defect should be repaired as one would repair a urethrovaginal fistula. Figures 58–47 through 58–50 provide examples of vaginal excursions and permanent sling material in the bladder.

At times patients who have undergone bladder neck suspension or a suburethral sling procedure for stress incontinence may develop severe voiding dysfunction or even retention, requiring a vaginal urethrolysis.

The technique of vaginal urethrolysis (Fig. 58–51) involves placement of a transurethral Foley catheter with a 30-mL balloon within the bladder. Initial traction on the catheter with simultaneous vaginal palpation of the bladder neck subjectively assesses the degree and extent of scarring, elevation, and fixation of the urethrovesical junction. The goal of a vaginal urethrolysis is to create some mobility at the proximal urethra and bladder neck. This may at times require removal or loosening of the sling material.

An inverted-U incision (see Fig. 58–51A) or a midline anterior vaginal wall incision is made. Urethral mobility is created by dissecting toward the inferior pubic ramus on each side (see Fig. 58–51B). This may involve perforating the urogenital diaphragm. Urethral mobility is subjectively assessed via traction on the Foley catheter. Some also advocate the placement of a labial fat pad around the urethra to prevent rescarification. The author would discourage any attempts at resuspension.

Figure 58–52 reviews a technique of removal of a synthetic sling that had created significant voiding dysfunction.

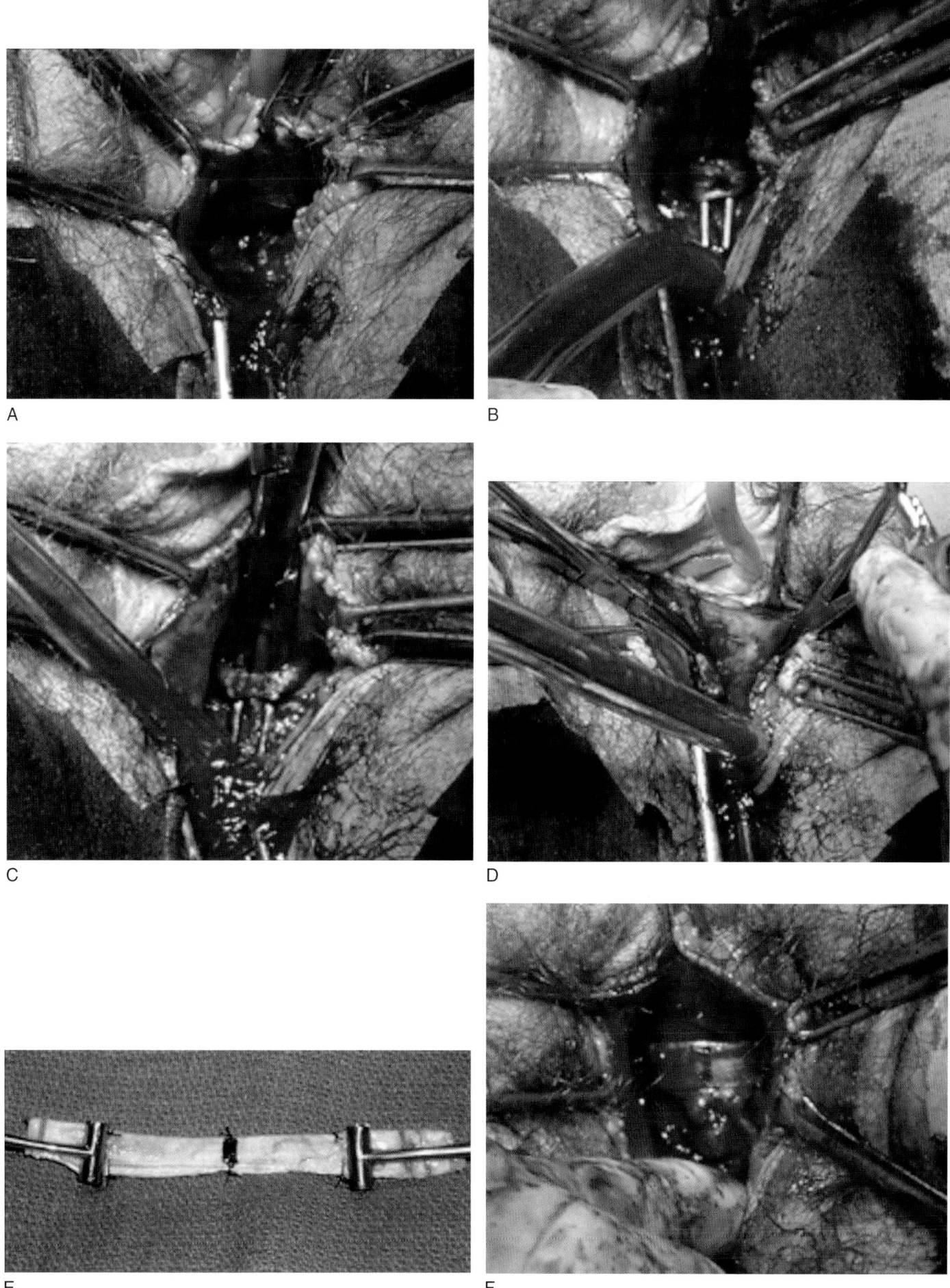

A

B

C

D

E

F

**FIGURE 58–44** **A.** Cadaveric fascia lata sling causing urethral obstruction. **B.** Right-angle clamp has been passed between the sling and the urethra. **C.** Sling is being cut. **D.** Sling has been cut, and retracted ends are held in clamps. **E.** Cadaveric fascia to be interposed between the two cut ends. **F.** Piece of cadaveric fascia has been interposed. Note appropriate placement of tension of the sling.

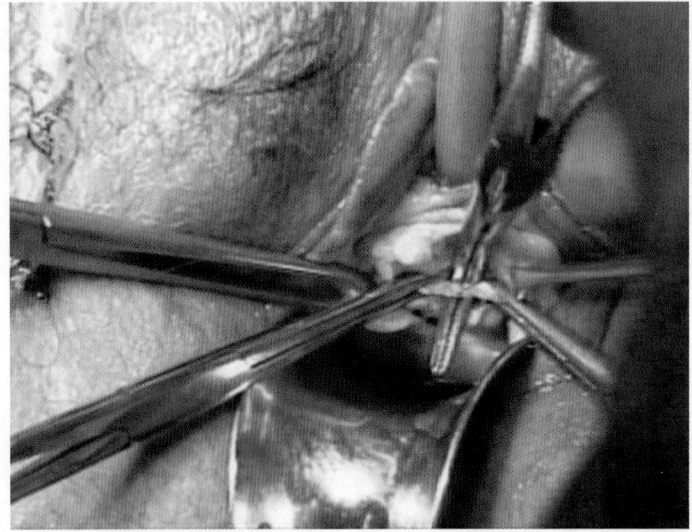

A

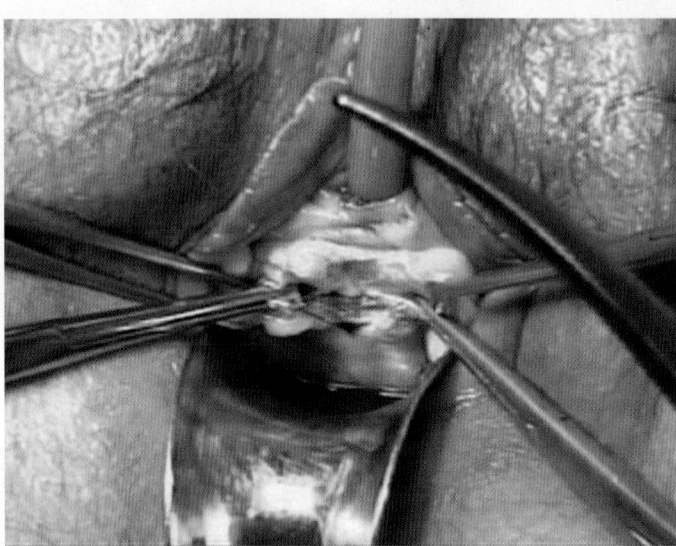

B

**FIGURE 58–45  A.** Technique for takedown of a synthetic midurethral sling. Note that the sling is identified, and a right-angle clamp is passed between the sling and the urethra. The edges of the sling are grasped with clamps, and the sling is cut at the midline. Of note, it is important to completely dissect the sling away from the urethra to ensure that the voiding dysfunction will be resolved. **B.** The sling has been cut, and the edges of the sling remain on the vaginal side of the urogenital diaphragm.

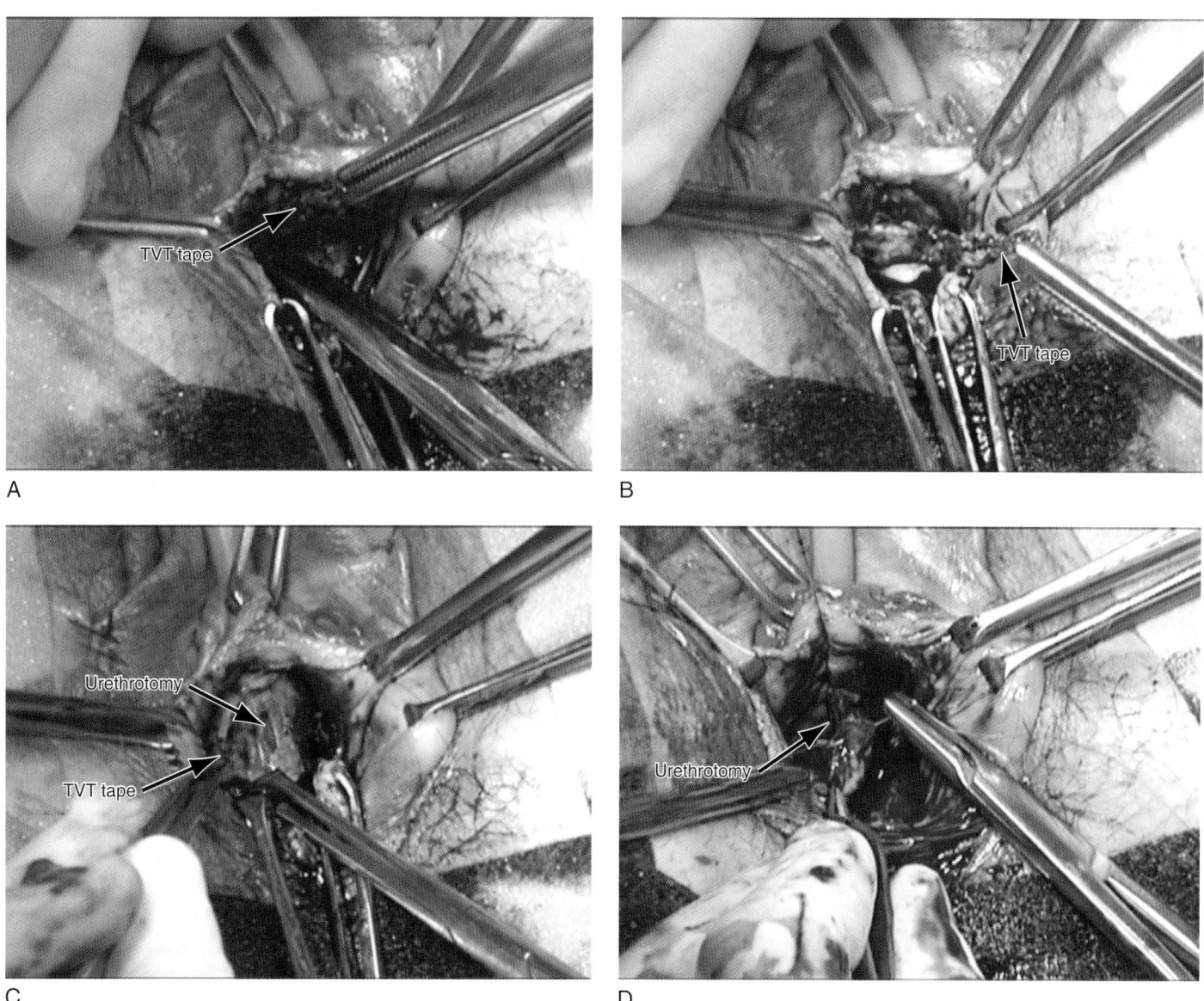

**FIGURE 58–46** Synthetic midurethral sling eroded or placed in the wall of the urethra. **A.** Tape present in the wall of the urethra. **B.** Tape has been dissected away from the urethral wall. **C.** Resultant urethral defect is seen. **D.** Repair of the urethral defect should be done with interrupted 4-0 delayed absorbable sutures.

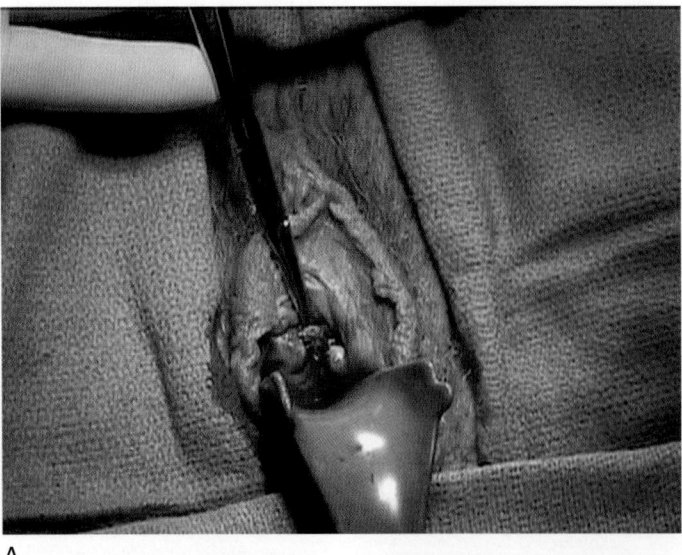

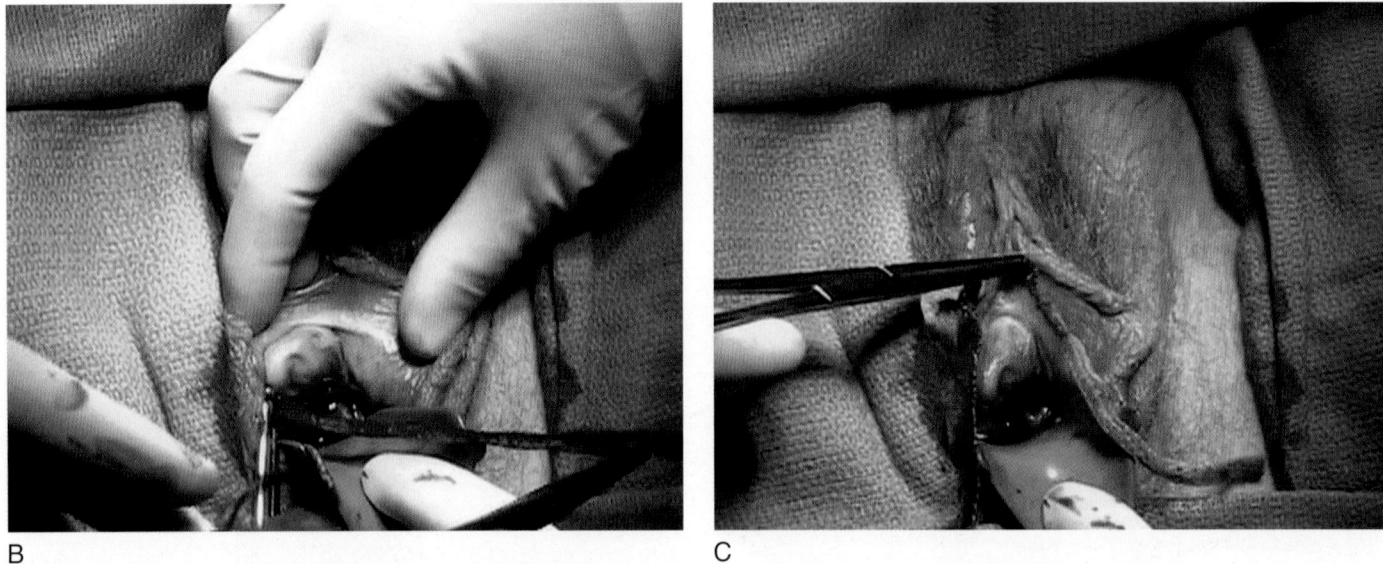

**FIGURE 58–47 A.** Excursion of an OB-Tape procedure (Mentor, Santa Barbara, CA). **B.** The tape is removed from one side. **C.** The entire tape is removed intact 4 weeks after the procedure.

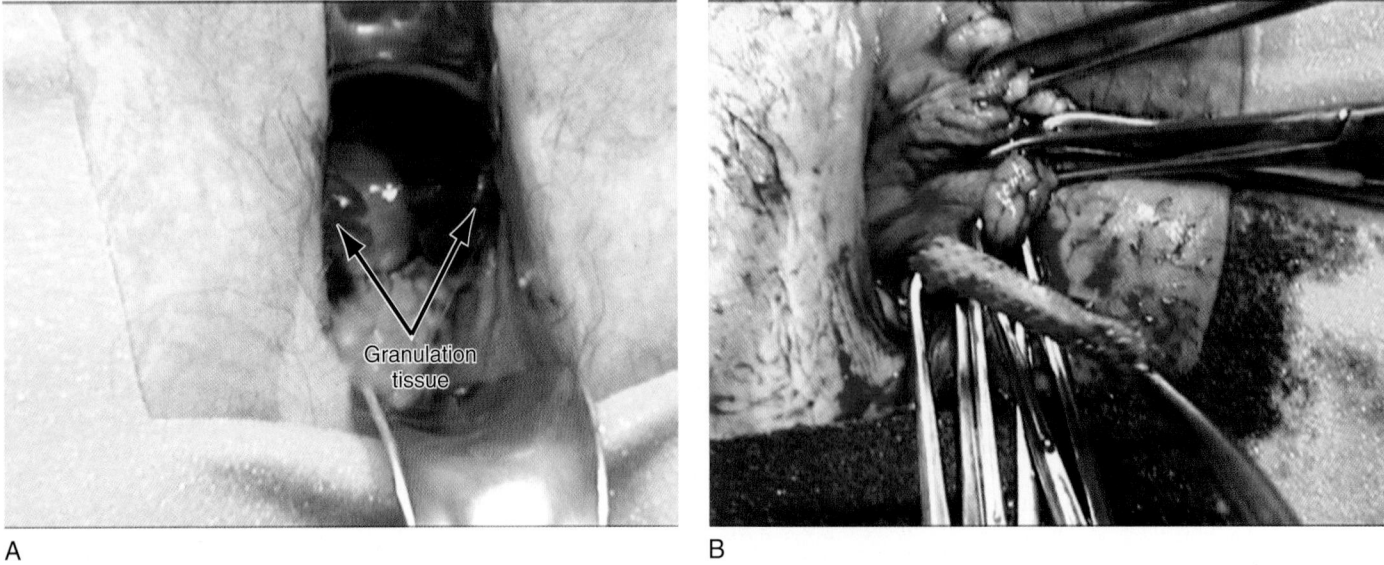

**FIGURE 58–48 A.** Large areas of granulation tissue secondary to excursion or erosion of an OB-Tape (Mentor, Santa Barbara, CA). **B.** The OB-Tape is removed intact 6 months after it was placed.

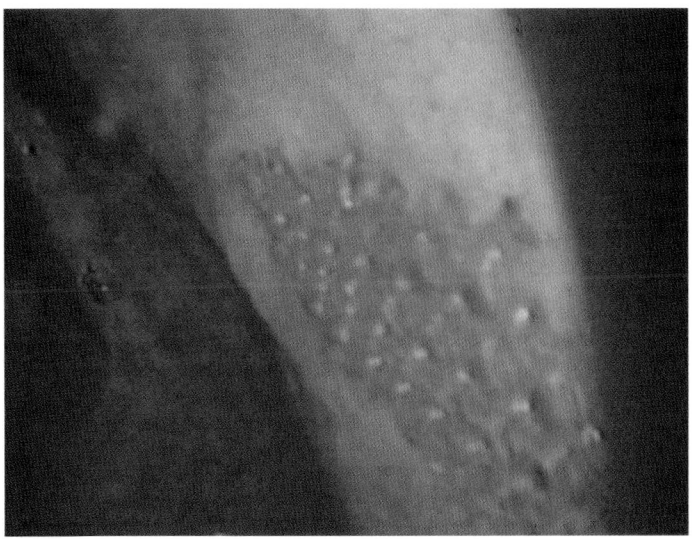

**FIGURE 58–49** Synthetic sling material in the bladder 3 months after a synthetic midurethral sling procedure.

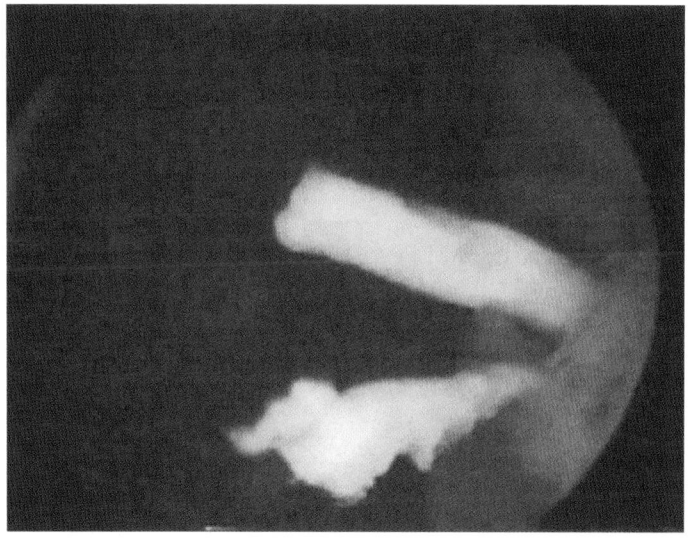

**FIGURE 58–50** Permanent suture in the bladder a year after a bone anchor sling.

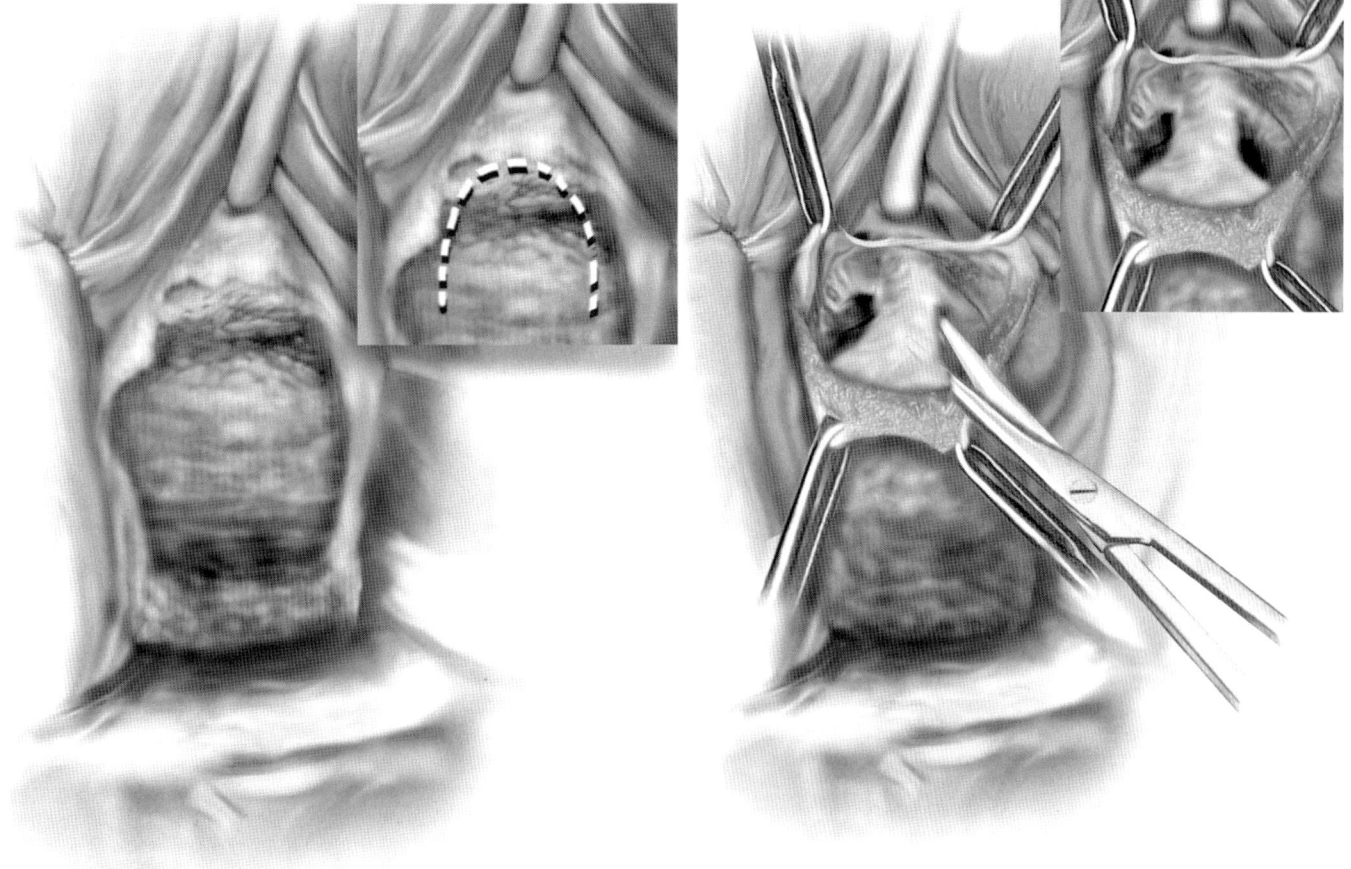

A

B

**FIGURE 58–51** Technique of vaginal urethrolysis. **A.** An inverted-U incision is made on the vagina. **B.** Sharp dissection lateral to the bladder neck with sharp penetration of the urogenital diaphragm allows entry into the retropubic space with the possibility of creating some urethral mobility.

UNIT 3 ■ SECTION B

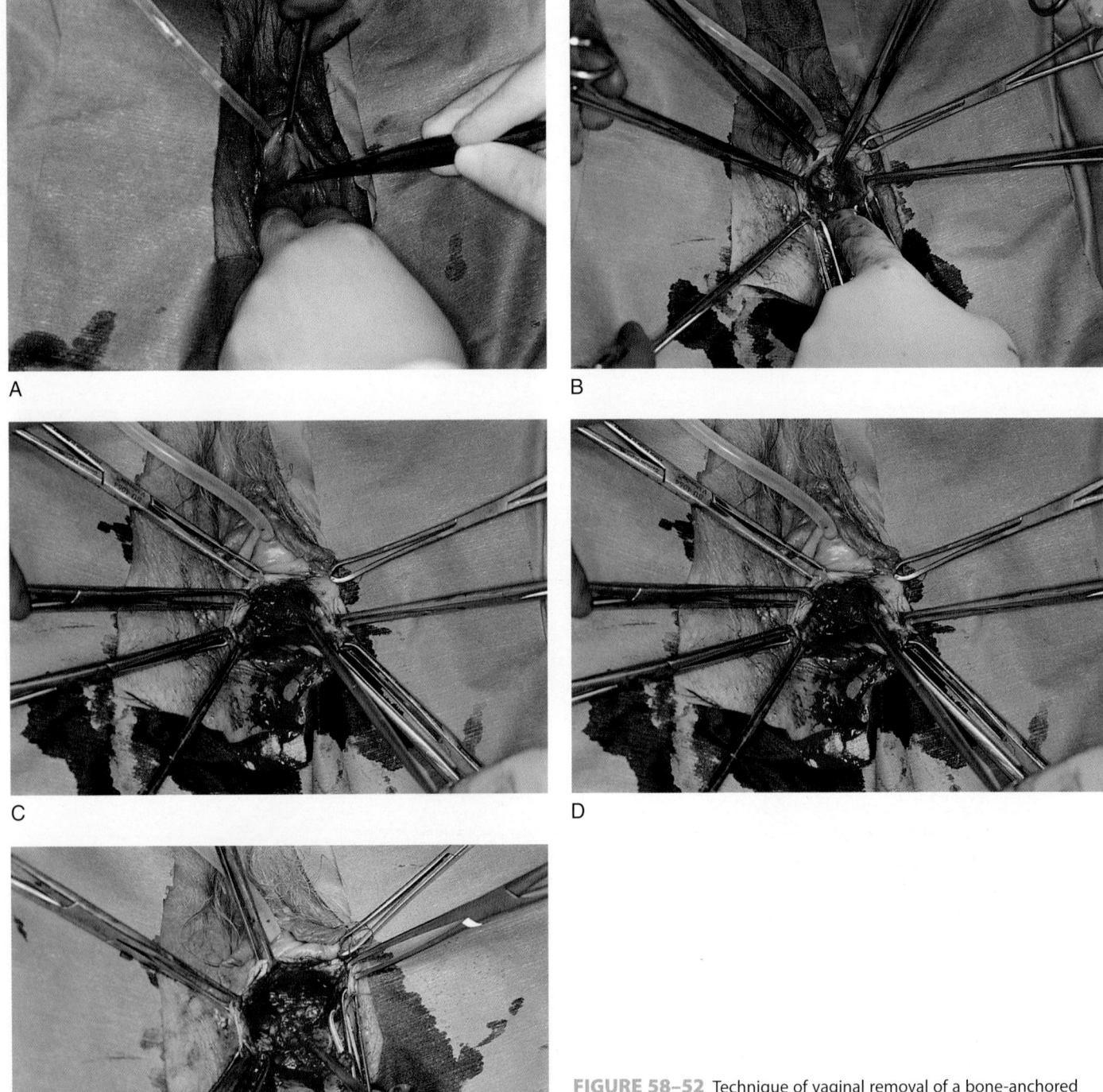

**FIGURE 58–52** Technique of vaginal removal of a bone-anchored Protogen suburethral sling. **A.** Anatomic location of the level of the sling. **B.** Identification of the Protogen sling (Boston Scientific, Natick, MA). **C.** Dissection of sling material off the urethra. **D.** Retrieval of sutures that had been anchored in bone on the left side. **E.** Removal of sling material and suture from the right side. Note that after complete removal of the sling material, the obstruction at the level of the proximal urethra has been relieved.

# CHAPTER 59

# Pubovaginal Slings for the Correction of Stress Incontinence

*Mickey M. Karram* ▪ *Mark D. Walters*

Pubovaginal slings are well-accepted procedures utilized for the correction of stress incontinence. Materials utilized for pubovaginal slings are always biologic and are placed at the proximal urethra and bladder neck. Currently used biologic materials are divided into autologous tissue, which is harvested from the patient who is undergoing the sling; allograft material, which is most commonly cadaveric fascia lata; and xenografts, which are harvested from various animal sources. Technically, bladder neck slings are called *pubovaginal slings* when the arms of the material used are connected to the anterior rectus fascia on each side. Various modifications of a traditional pubovaginal sling have been described and involve various patch-type slings in which the sling materials are placed vaginally at the level of the proximal urethra and then are attached to sutures that are passed suprapubically. Proximal suburethral slings work best when bladder neck mobility and vaginal pliability are present. Although plenty of data are available to support the use of pubovaginal slings as a primary operation, these procedures are usually reserved for patients who have failed synthetic midurethral slings, or who have a contraindication for the use of a synthetic material.

If the surgeon decides to utilize autologous tissue, this will most commonly be fascia lata or rectus fascia. Harvesting of these tissues usually will occur before any vaginal dissection is performed. The technique used to harvest fascia lata is determined by whether the surgeon prefers to do a complete pubovaginal sling, in which the fascia will need to extend from the anterior abdominal fascia to below the proximal urethra and back to the anterior abdominal fascia on the opposite side, or if the surgeon prefers to place a patch-type sling. If a patch-type

sling is used, a patch of rectus fascia or fascia lata is harvested. To harvest a patch of fascia lata, a 3- to 4-cm transverse skin incision is made about 8 cm above the midpatella lateral to the knee and the lower thigh. Blunt dissection exposes the underlying fascia lata. A 4 × 6-cm piece of fascia lata is removed and will serve as the patch for the sling procedure (Figs. 59-1 and 59-2). Subcutaneous tissue is reapproximated, the skin is closed, and a pressure bandage is placed. If a full pubovaginal sling is to be utilized, then a long piece of fascia lata can be obtained by using a Wilson or Crawford fascial stripper. The technique used to obtain a full strip of fascia involves a similar incision as described with the patch technique; however, fat is bluntly dissected away from the fascia lata, all the way up the lateral side of the leg toward the greater trochanter. A 1-cm-wide piece of fascia is then removed with the fascial stripper. This usually will produce a 20-cm-long piece of fascia. A second piece of fascia lata of similar length can be obtained by repeating the same procedure. A 1-cm-wide bridge of fascia lata should remain between the two areas where the stripper has removed the tissue (Fig. 59-3). These two pieces of fascia can then be sutured to each other, thus providing a 30- to 35-cm-long piece of fascia for use in providing the pubovaginal sling. If the rectus fascia is used for a pubovaginal sling, a transverse abdominal incision is made, usually 4 cm above the pubic symphysis. Blunt dissection is performed until the underlying rectus fascia is identified. Via a transverse incision in the fascia, a 1- to 2-cm-wide strip of fascia is sharply dissected away. If the goal is to have the arms extend to the anterior abdominal wall, then a 20-cm-long piece of fascia is harvested (Fig. 59-4). If a patch sling is to be placed, then a 2 × 8 piece of fascia is harvested.

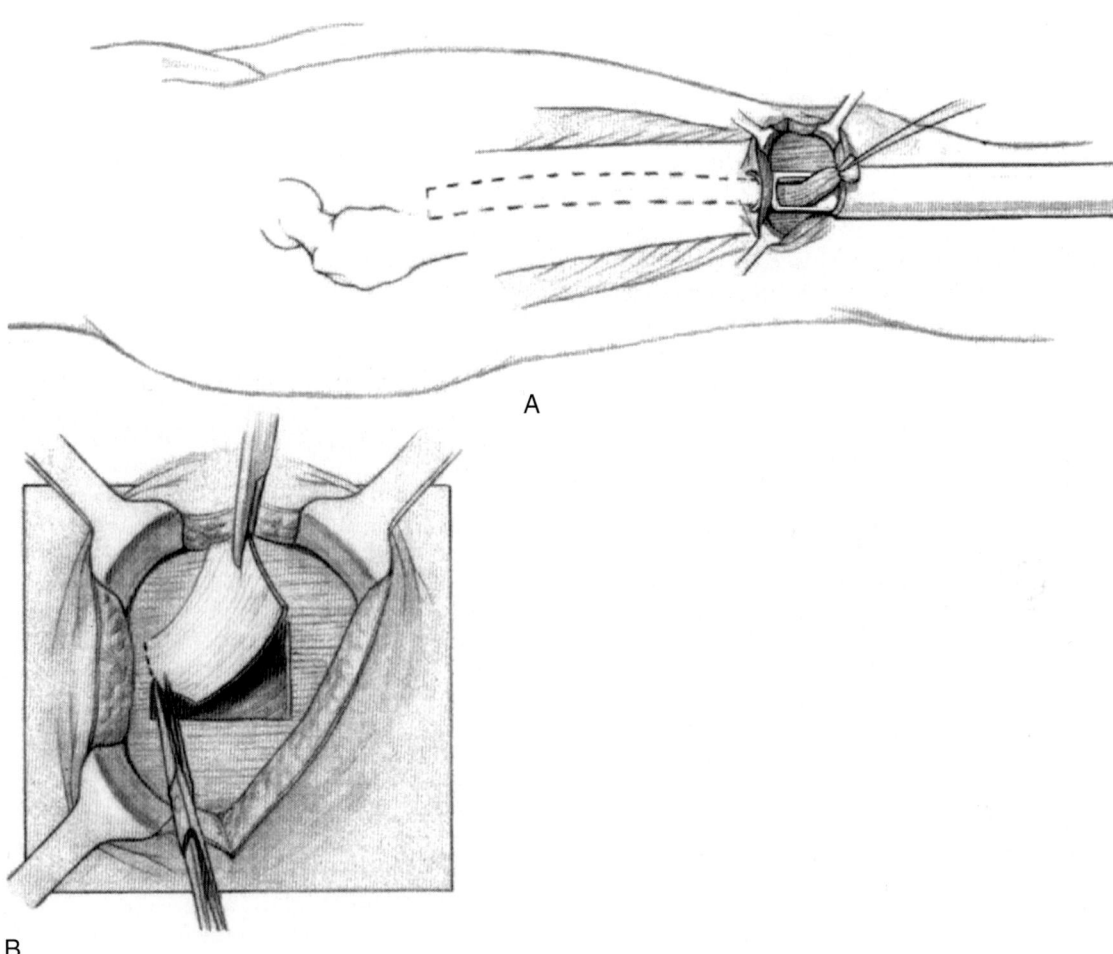

A

B

**FIGURE 59–1  A.** Technique for obtaining a strip of fascia lata using a vein stripper. **B.** Technique for obtaining a patch of fascia lata. Fascia lata patch has been excised.

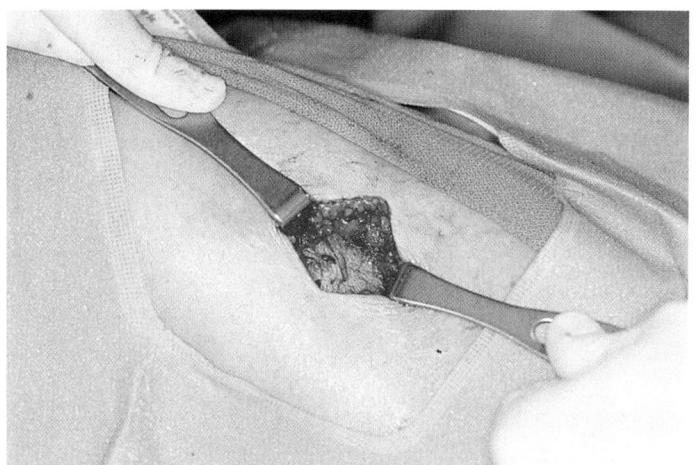

A

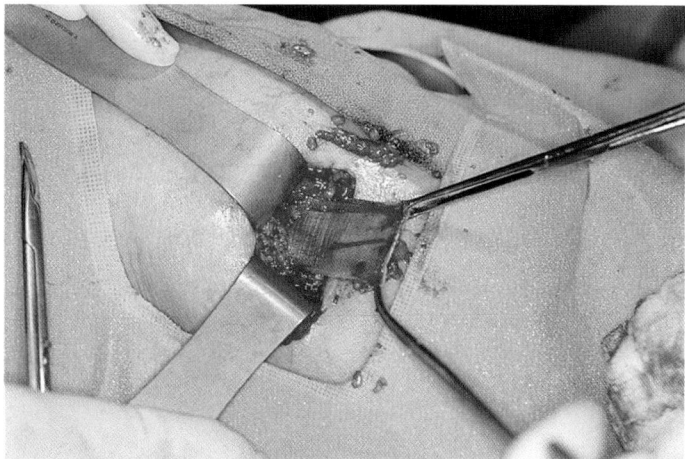

B

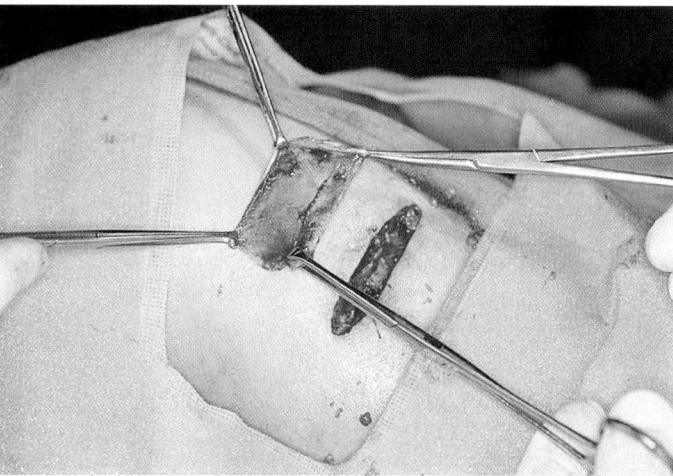

C

**FIGURE 59–2  A.** An incision on the lower leg is made about 8 cm above the midpatella lateral to the knee, exposing fascia lata. **B.** A patch of fascia is being excised. **C.** A fascia lata patch has been excised.

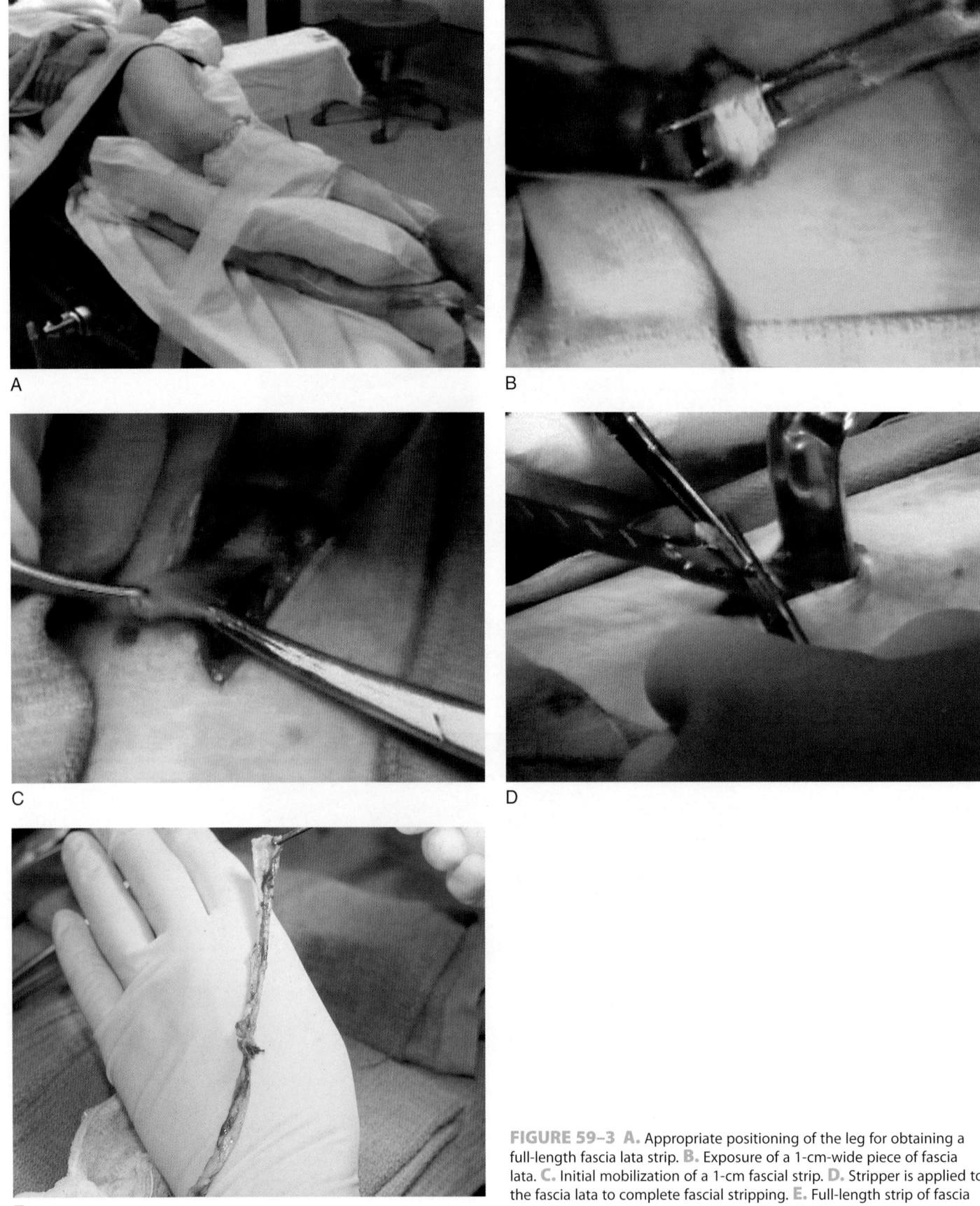

FIGURE 59–3  A. Appropriate positioning of the leg for obtaining a full-length fascia lata strip. B. Exposure of a 1-cm-wide piece of fascia lata. C. Initial mobilization of a 1-cm fascial strip. D. Stripper is applied to the fascia lata to complete fascial stripping. E. Full-length strip of fascia lata. (Photographs A–D compliments of Dr Alfred Bent.)

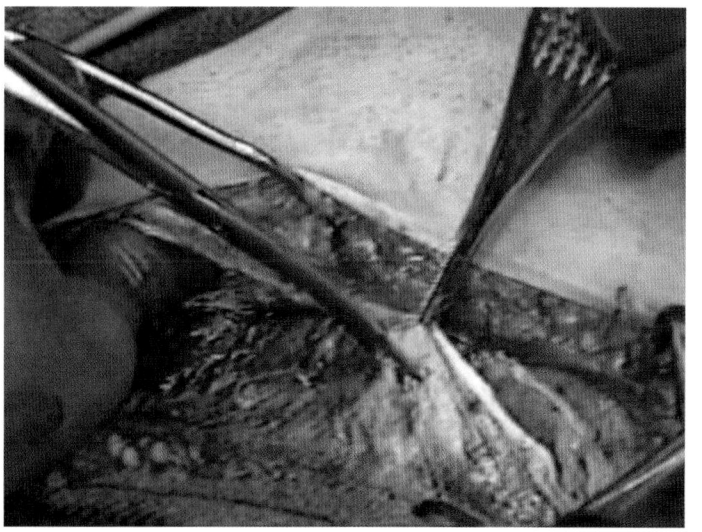

A

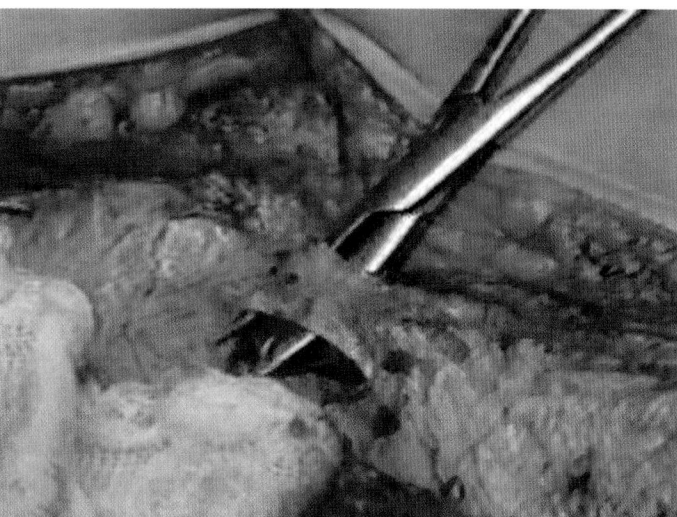

B

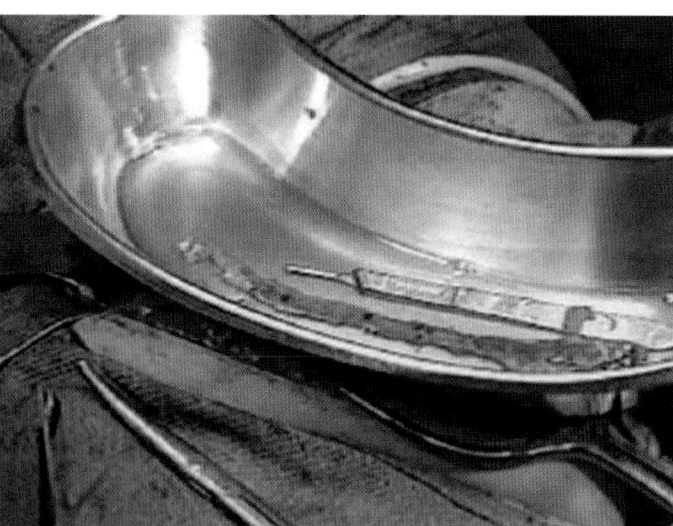

C

**FIGURE 59–4 A.** Rectus fascia has been exposed via a low transverse skin incision. **B.** A 1-cm-wide piece of fascia lata is exposed at the midline. **C.** Full-length piece of rectus fascia has been completely excised. (Photographs compliments of Dr Jerry Blaivas.)

## Operative Details

1. The patient is placed in high stirrups in the dorsal lithotomy position, and the vagina and lower abdomen are appropriately prepped and draped. Preoperative antibiotics are usually given on call to the operating room.

2. Hydrodissection of the anterior vaginal wall is usually utilized by injecting beneath the epithelium of the anterior vaginal wall at the level of the bladder neck (Fig. 59–5A). This facilitates dissection of the appropriate plane and also may have a hemostatic effect.

3. A midline vaginal incision or an inverted-U vaginal incision is made at the level of the proximal urethra or bladder neck (Fig. 59–5B). This is easily determined by palpation of the anterior vaginal wall with a Foley catheter in place. The vaginal epithelium is carefully dissected off the underlying periurethral and perivesical fascia with the use of blunt and sharp dissection. This dissection is extended bilaterally to the inferior lateral aspect of the pubic rami (Fig. 59–5C).

4. The retropubic space is then entered via blunt or sharp dissection (Fig. 59–5D, E). Once the periurethral attachment of the urethra has been penetrated on each side, one should be able to pass a finger along the back side of the pubic bone all the way to the inferior aspect of the rectus muscle.

5. If a traditional pubovaginal sling procedure is to be performed, an abdominal incision is made. This is usually made approximately two fingerbreadths, or 4 cm, above the level of the pubic symphysis and is a transverse incision usually no longer than 8 cm. The incision is extended down to the rectus fascia.

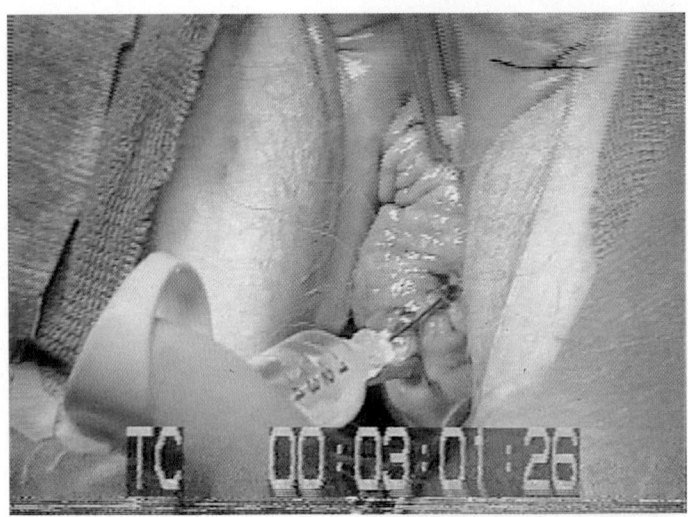

A

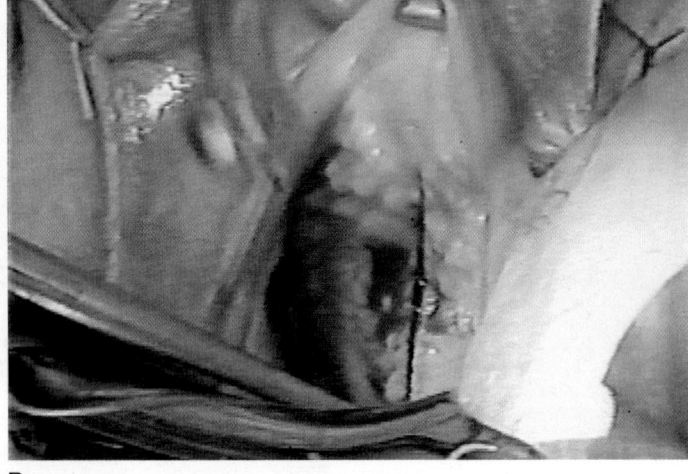

B

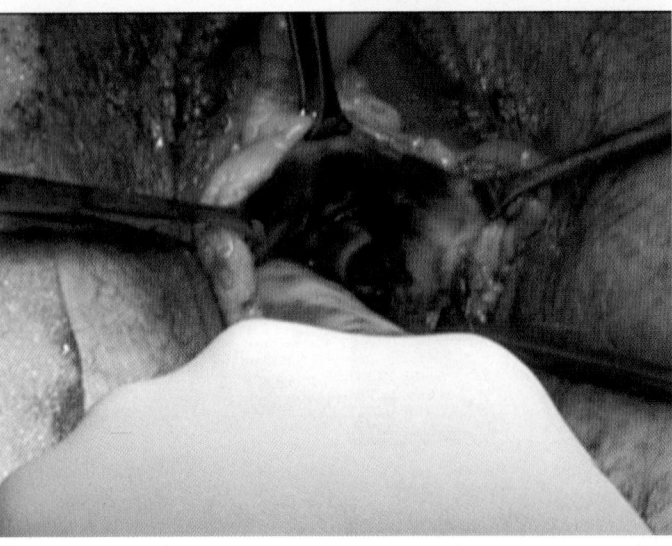

C

**FIGURE 59–5  A.** Hydrodissection of the anterior vaginal wall to facilitate dissection in the appropriate plane. **B.** A midline anterior vaginal wall incision is made that extends from the level of the proximal urethra to the level of the bladder base. **C.** The anterior vaginal wall has been opened up, and the dissection has been extended on the left side to the inferior pubic ramus.

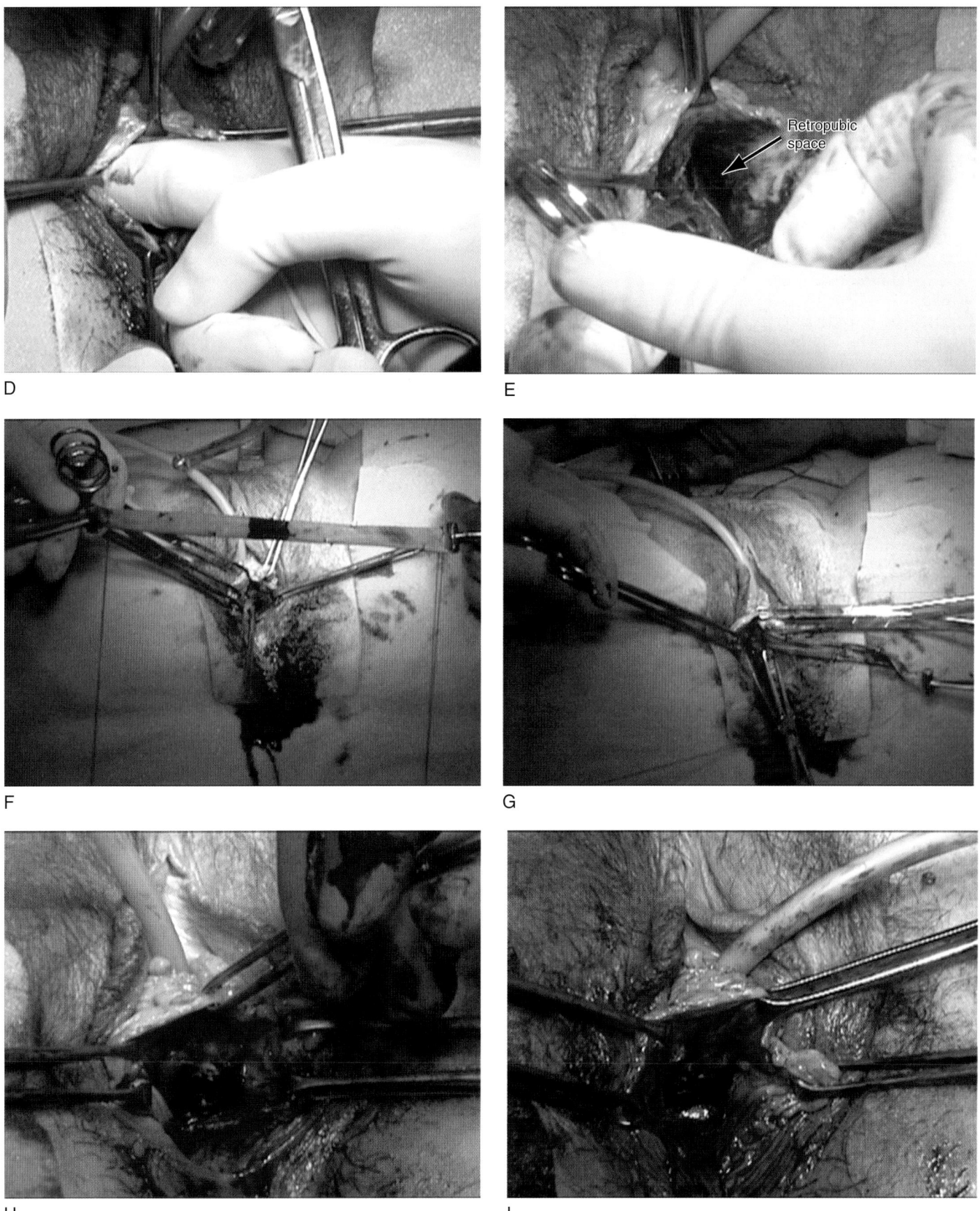

**FIGURE 59–5, cont'd  D.** The index finger is now placed in the plane of dissection, and blunt dissection is utilized to penetrate the urogenital diaphragm and enter the retropubic space. **E.** The retropubic space has been entered sharply on the patient's left side with the use of Mayo scissors. The scissors are directed toward the ipsilateral shoulder and are maintained in direct contact with the inferior pubic ramus. Once the urogenital diaphragm has been penetrated, the scissors are spread to complete the dissection. **F.** The sling material is brought into the field. It has been attached to a suture on each side, which will facilitate passage of it into the suprapubic incision. The area has been darkened at the midportion of the sling because this area sits under the proximal urethra. **G.** One arm of the sling has been passed into the suprapubic incision, and a Pereyra needle ligature carrier has been passed on the right side; the sutures from the other end of the sling have been passed through the eye of the ligature carrier. **H.** The sling is in place at the level of the proximal urethra and bladder neck. **I.** The arms of slings have been tied suprapubically, and the sling is resting loosely at the level of the proximal urethra and bladder.

6. The sling is then brought into the field and is transferred from the vaginal incision to above the anterior abdominal fascia (Fig. 59–5F). Each arm is transferred with the use of a dressing forceps or some type of needle ligature carrier (Fig. 59–5G). Small incisions in the fascia allow each arm to come up through the fascia. Transfer of each arm of the sling is done under direct finger guidance with the use of a dressing forceps or a Stamey or Pereyra needle (Fig. 59–6A through C). A full-length pubovaginal sling should sit loosely at the level of the proximal urethra (Fig. 59–7).

7. If a patch-type sling is utilized, the length of the patch is determined, and the longitudinal edges of the patch are usually attached to permanent sutures, which are passed into the anterior abdominal incision (Figs. 59–8 and 59–9). With some bone fixation techniques, sutures, or the sling itself, are directly anchored into bone. When the sling is directly anchored into bone, this can be done entirely via a vaginal incision, so an abdominal incision is not required. For patch slings, some surgeons do not enter the retropubic space and thus transfer the sutures after blind passage of the ligature carrier through the retropubic space.

8. Cystourethroscopy is performed to ensure no inadvertent injury or passage of any material through the bladder. Also, visualization of the proximal urethra and bladder neck documents that the sling is in the appropriate position. Elevation of the arms of the sling or the sutures should elevate or compress the proximal urethra. If no mobility occurs at this area, then the sling may be placed in the wrong anatomic position, or further periurethral dissection may need to be performed to create urethral mobility (Figs. 59–10 and 59–11).

9. The final step in proximal suburethral sling placement involves appropriate tensioning of the sling. Unfortunately, no standardized method can be utilized on all patients. One must individualize the surgery on the basis of the severity of the patient's incontinence and the state of her pelvic tissue. In general, the sling should be placed loosely at the level of the proximal urethra and should act as a backboard to prevent descent of the proximal urethra during increases in intra-abdominal pressure. Thus, after tying of the sling, downward traction on a Foley catheter should document that this area has been appropriately supported with the previously mentioned backboard mechanism. The author routinely places a right-angle clamp between the urethra and the sling material during tying, with the goal of maintaining zero tension at rest (Fig. 59–12). Ideally, a compressive mechanism initiated only during increases in abdominal pressure creates continence.

10. After the sutures are tied, the anterior vaginal wall is closed, and a transurethral or suprapubic catheter is left in place. A vaginal packing is also commonly utilized.

Figures 59–13 through 59–18 show a similar technique in which a piece of rectus fascia is used as the sling material.

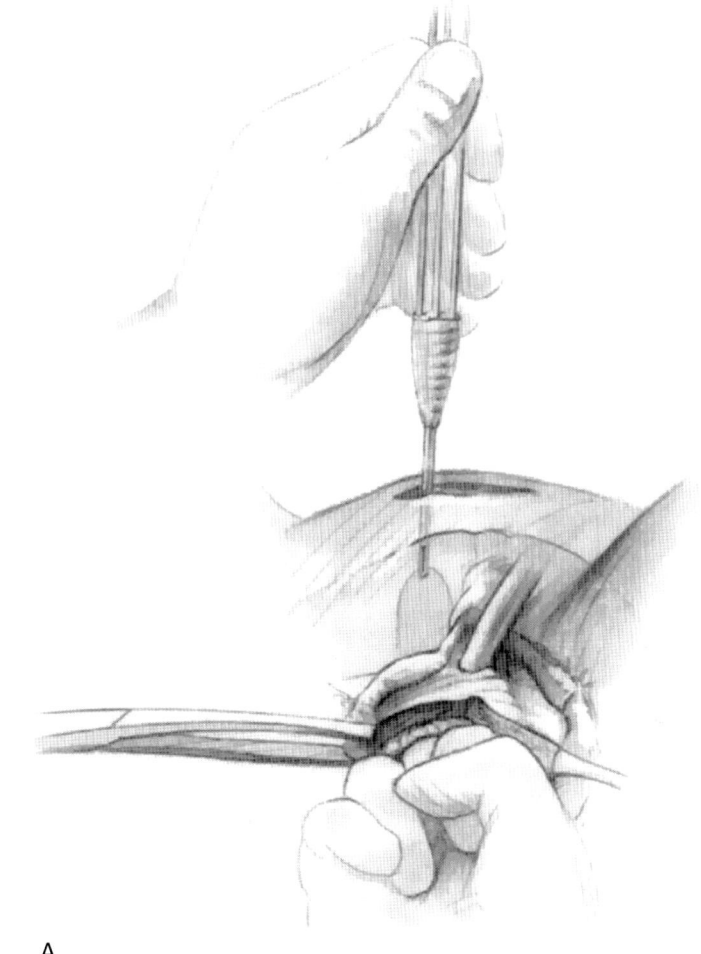

A

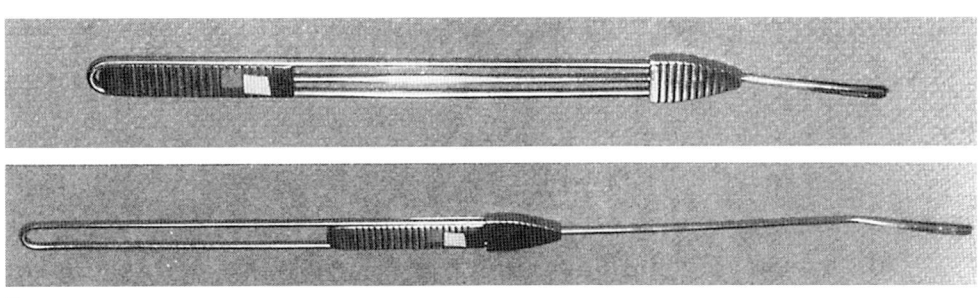

B

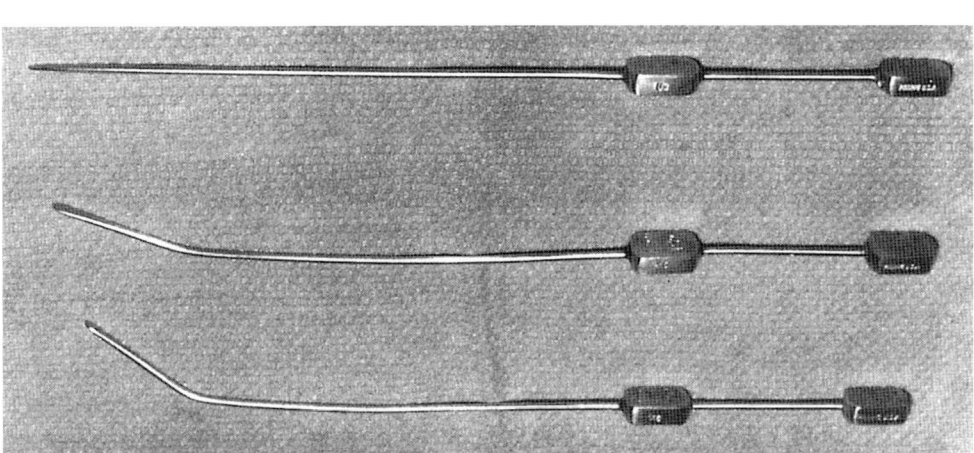

C

**FIGURE 59–6 A.** The needle is passed under direct finger guidance. A finger in the vagina is inserted to the posterior aspect of the rectus muscle. (From Hurt WG: *In* Urogynecologic Surgery, 2nd ed. Lippincott, Williams & Wilkins, Philadelphia, 2000, with permission.) **B.** Pereyra ligature carrier. (Courtesy El Ney Industries, Inc., Upland, Calif.) **C.** Series of Stamey needles: straight needle (*top*), 15° angled needle (*middle*), and 30° angled needle (*bottom*). (Courtesy Pilling Company, Fort Washington, Pa.)

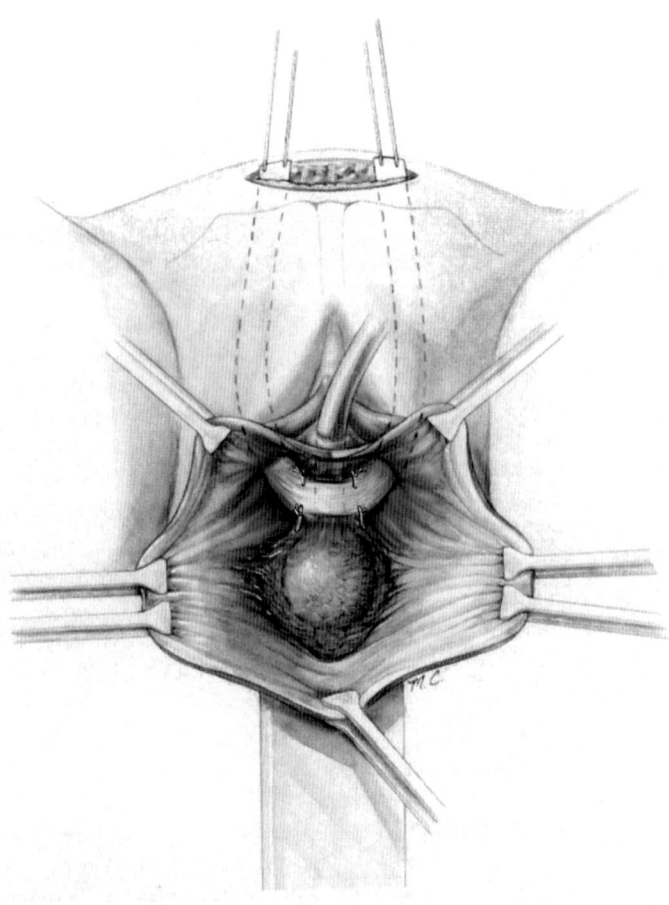

**FIGURE 59–7** Full-length suburethral sling in which the sling material is passed and tied above the anterior rectus fascia.

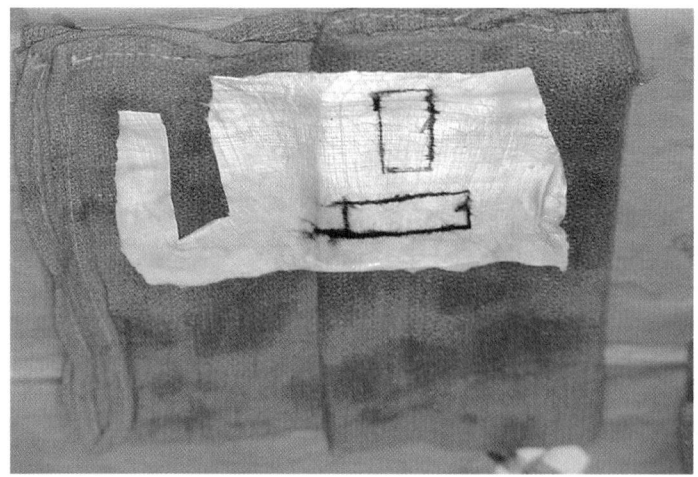

A

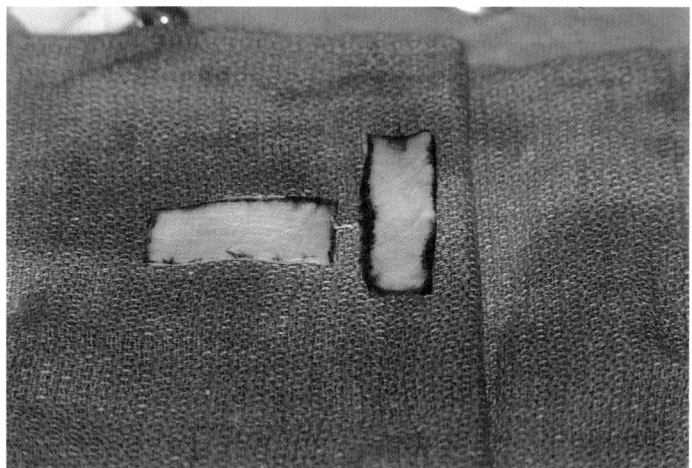

B

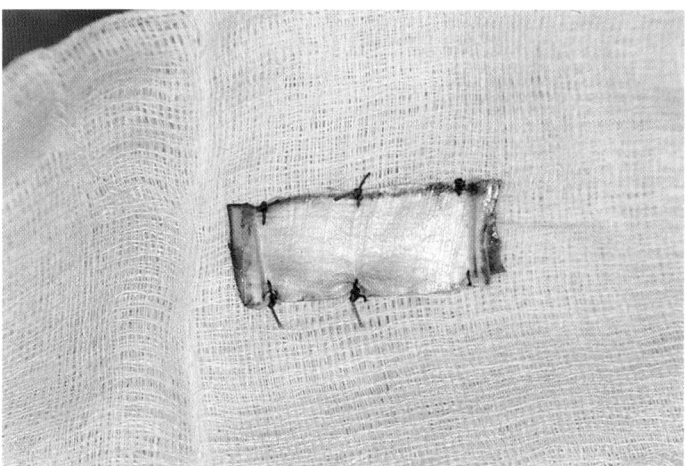

C

**FIGURE 59–8 A** through **C.** Cadaveric fascia lata. Two pieces with the fibers running in opposite directions have been attached to each other.

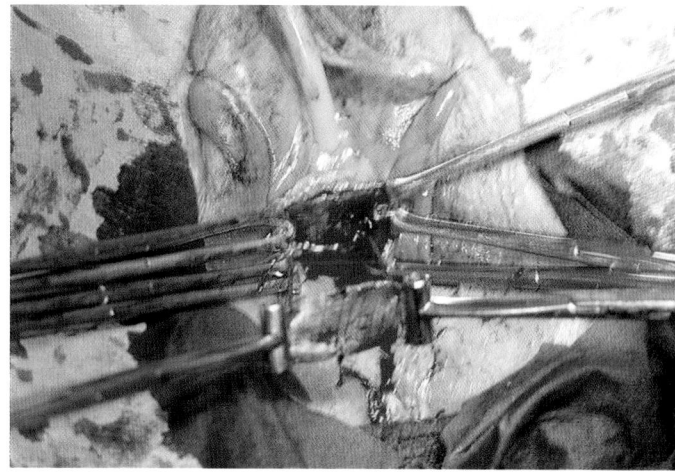

**FIGURE 59–9** A patch sling has been attached to sutures that have been passed via a long needle to the suprapubic area. The sling material is being held away from the urethra with T-clamps.

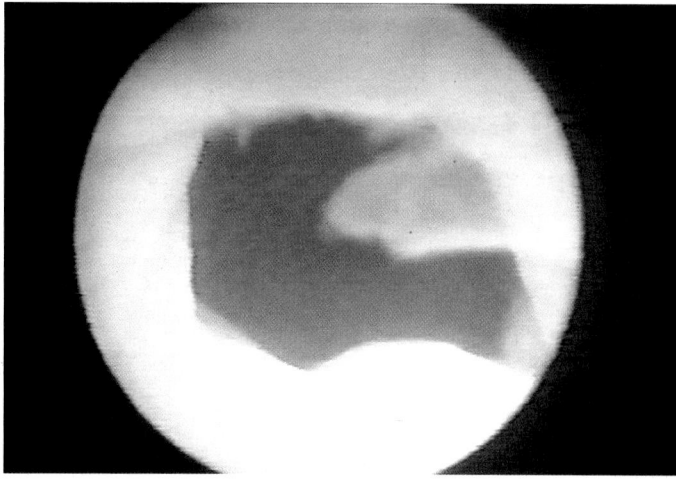

A

B

**FIGURE 59–10** Urethroscopic view of the proximal urethra to confirm proper placement of the suburethral sling. **A.** Proximal urethra and bladder neck before elevation of sling. **B.** Elevation of the sling closes the bladder neck. This maneuver ensures proper placement of the sling under the proximal urethra.

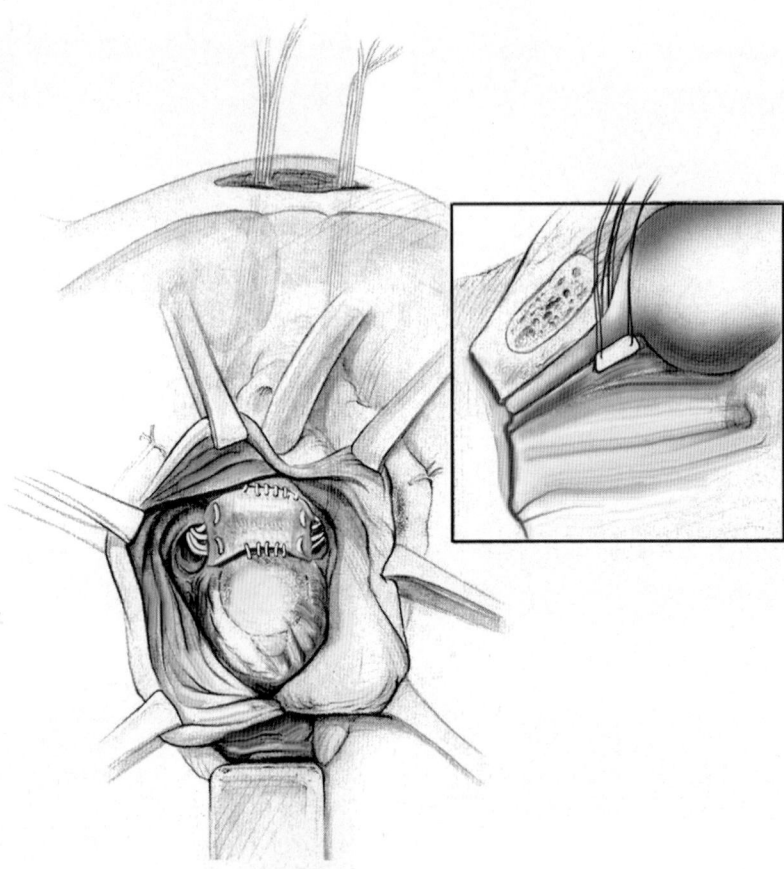

**FIGURE 59–11** A patch sling in which a suburethral patch of fascia or synthetic material is suspended to the anterior rectus fascia with permanent sutures.

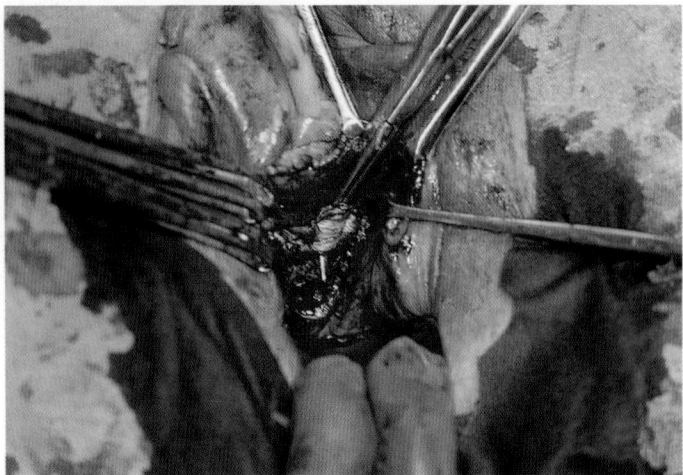

**FIGURE 59–12** A right-angle clamp is placed between the patch and the urethra to prevent excess tension as sutures are being tied suprapubically.

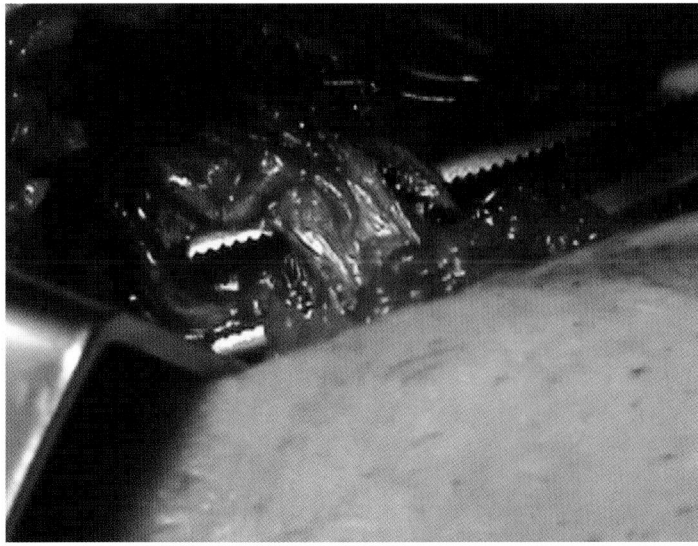

A

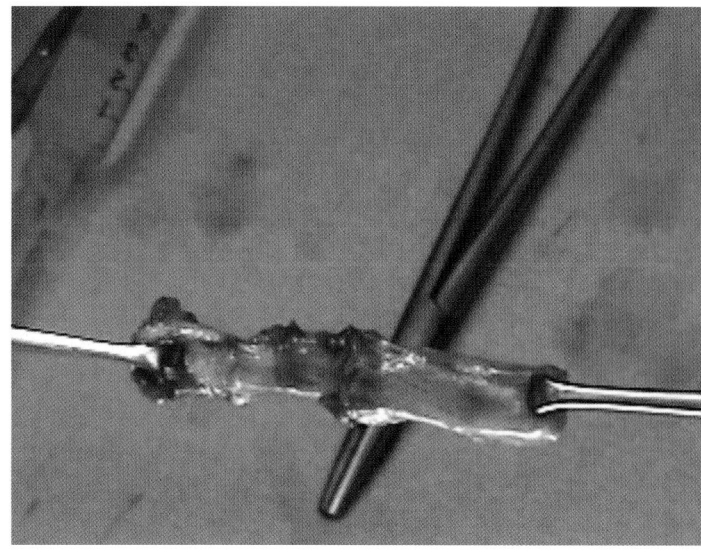

B

**FIGURE 59–13 A.** A 1.5- to 2.0-cm-wide piece of rectus fascia is isolated and mobilized off the underlying rectus muscle. **B.** The mobilization is then extended laterally, resulting in an 8- to 10-cm-long piece of rectus fascia that will be used for the sling material.

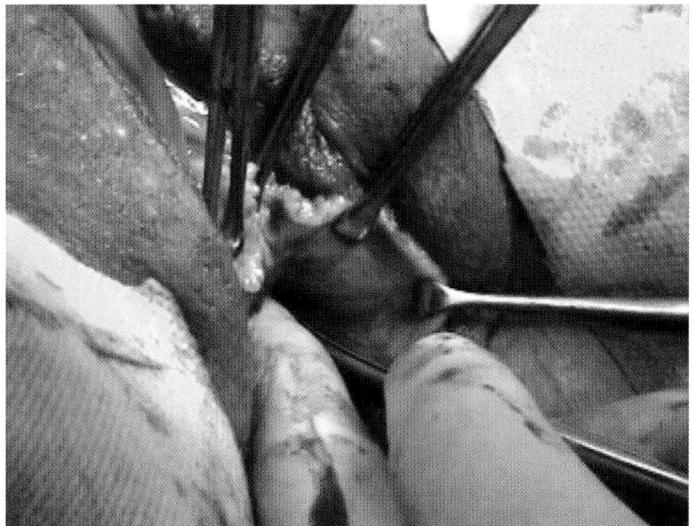

**FIGURE 59–14** After an anterior vaginal wall incision is made, the inferior pubic ramus is dissected on each side of the urogenital diaphragm sharply (*shown on this figure*) or bluntly to enter the retropubic space.

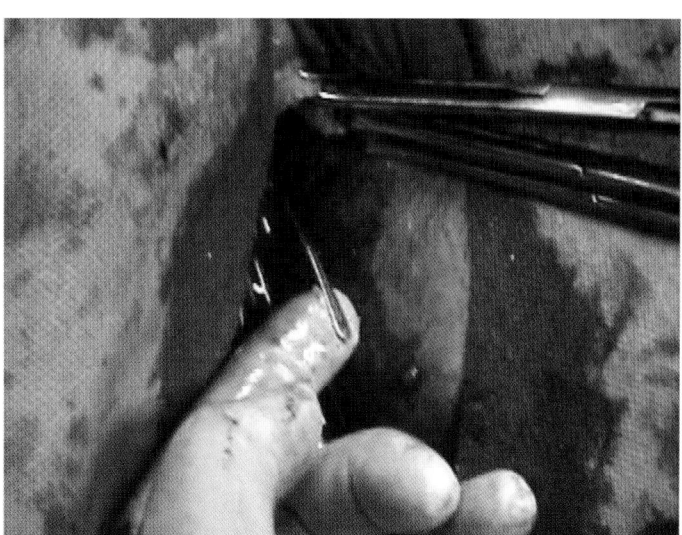

**FIGURE 59–15** A Stamey needle is then passed from the suprapubic incision under direct finger guidance into the vaginal incision. This needle will be used to transfer a permanent suture that is attached to the lateral aspects of the sling into the suprapubic incision.

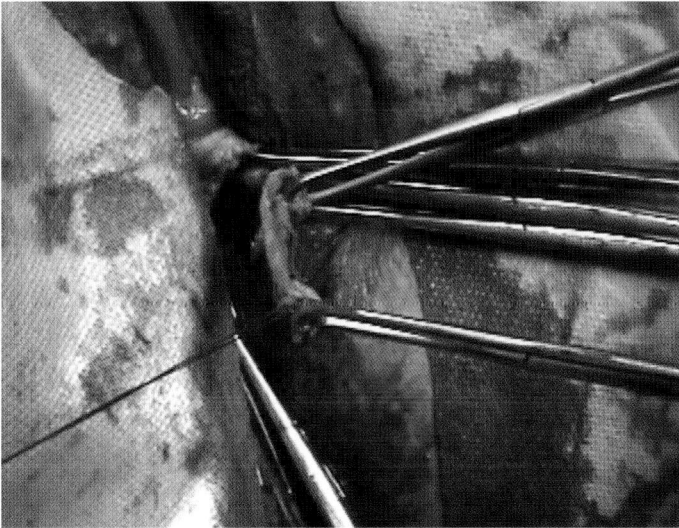

**FIGURE 59–16** A permanent suture has been attached to the lateral edge of the rectus fascia sling.

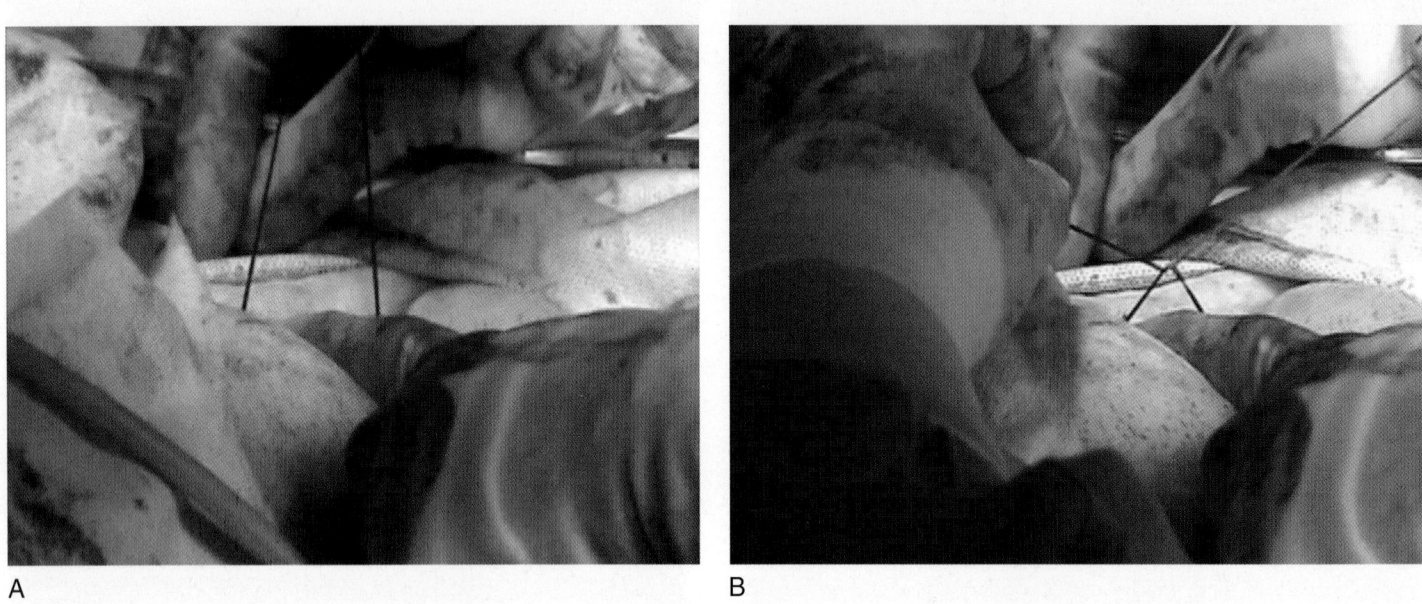

A                                                                      B

**FIGURE 59–17  A.** Both sutures have been transferred into the suprapubic incision and (**B**) are loosely tied across the midline to each other.

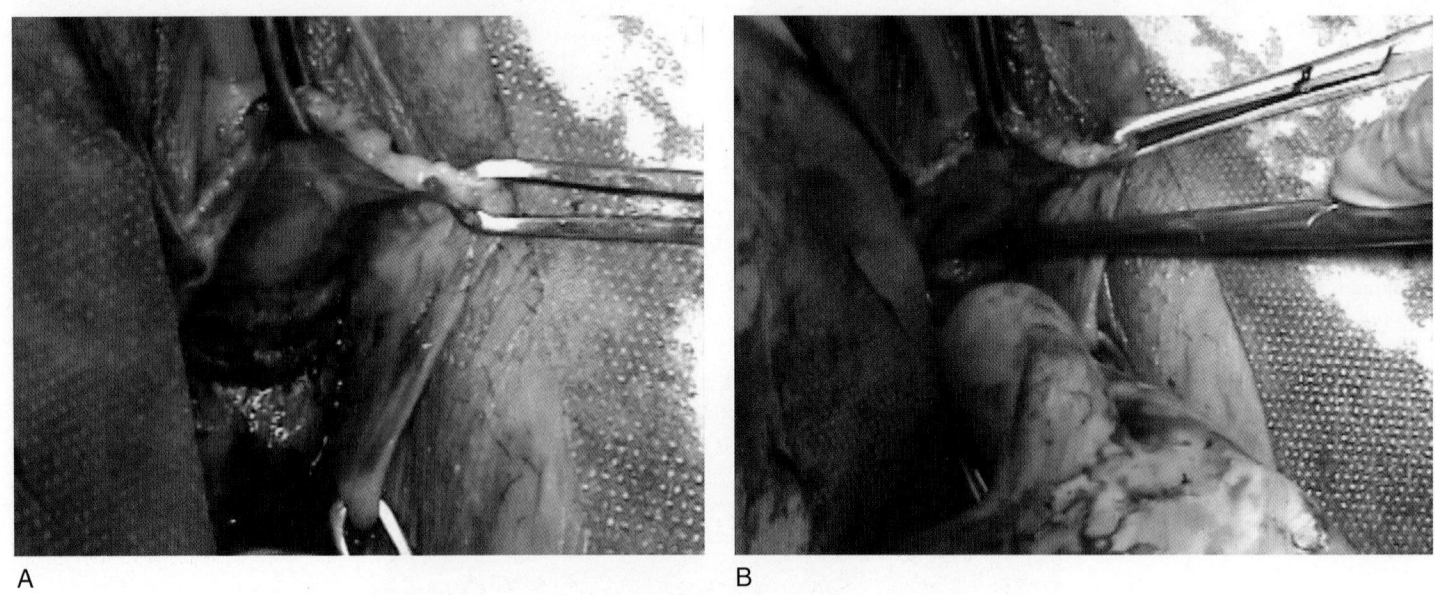

A                                                                      B

**FIGURE 59–18  A.** The rectus fascia sling is shown supporting the proximal urethra. **B.** To ensure that the sling is not placed too tightly, a right-angle clamp can be passed easily between the sling material and the posterior urethra.

# CHAPTER 60

# Benign Lesions of the Vaginal Wall

## Michael S. Baggish

Under normal circumstances, the vagina does not contain any glands. However, when the condition of adenosis exists (i.e., occurs spontaneously or as the result of antenatal diethylstilbestrol [DES] exposure), mucosal and submucosal mucus-secreting glands may be identified (Fig. 60–1A, B). These lesions appear as granulation-like tissue, clefts, holes, or cysts (Fig. 60–2A, B). Whenever adenosis is suspected, the lesion should be biopsied to ensure that adenocarcinoma does not exist within or around it. Additionally, the risk of squamous intraepithelial neoplasia is increased because of the multiple squamocolumnar junctions exposed to environmental factors associated with coitus.

## Biopsies

Vaginal biopsies are performed in a manner similar to that used for cervical disease (i.e., with a long-shanked biopsy forceps) (Fig. 60–3). Exposure can be a problem for vaginal lesions, and the use of a manipulating hook allows the examiner to properly display the lesion to colposcopic vision (Fig. 60–4A, B).

## Cysts

Cysts 2 cm or larger should be excised in the operating room with the patient under local or general anesthesia. Clearly, these lesions may run the gamut from mucous inclusions (adenosis), to squamous inclusions, to Gartner duct cysts (mesonephric remnants). Viewing a cyst from the vagina provides little insight as to its origin or potential risk(s). An unusual condition that produces small cysts—some up to 1 to 1.5 cm—is **vaginitis emphysematosa.** This condition is associated with multiple gas-filled spaces (Fig. 60–5A through D).

**The Gartner duct (mesonephric)** is found deep in the lateral wall of the vagina; although it may wander anteriorly or posteriorly, a cyst duct may extend cranially through the entire length of the vagina and via the cervix into the broad ligament (Fig. 60–6A through E). Before embarking on an operation to remove the cyst, it is important for the gynecologist to obtain as much preoperative information about the cyst and its neighboring structures as possible (Fig. 60–6F through H). The technique of excising any vaginal cyst is similar. The relationship of the cyst to the bladder and the ureter must be known (Fig. 60–6I). If necessary, the ureter should be catheterized.

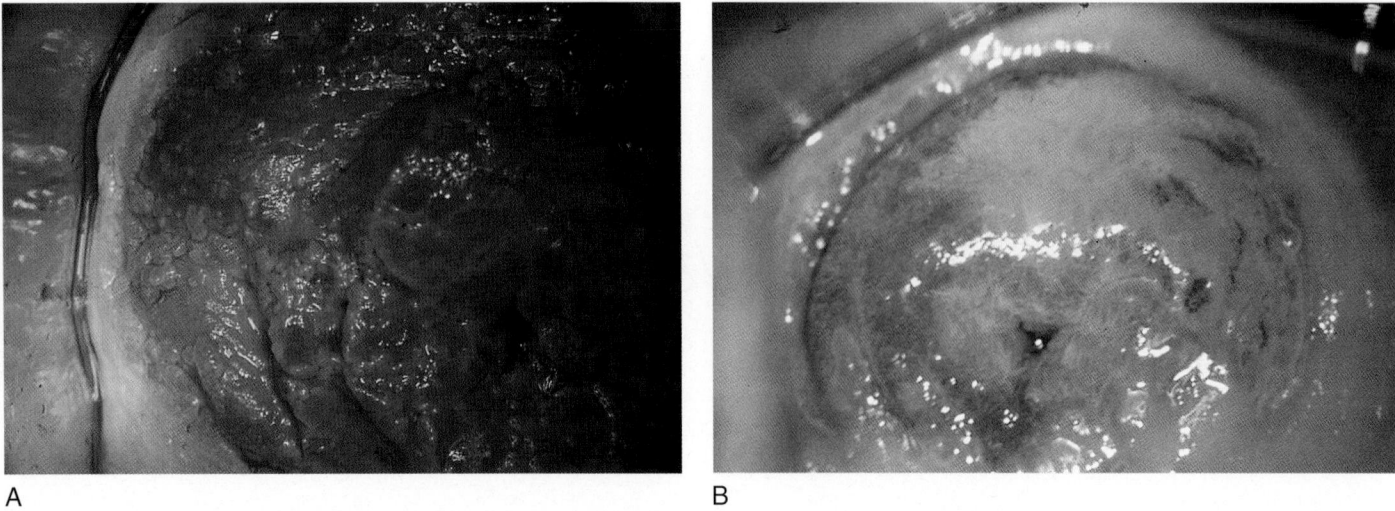

A          B

**FIGURE 60–1  A.** The cervix and the vagina of this diethylstilbestrol (DES)-exposed woman reveal total absence of a squamous epithelial covering of the ectocervix. The vaginal fornices likewise contain only glandular tissue. **B.** Another DES-exposed woman's cervix and vagina show extensive squamous metaplasia (*pink*) interspersed with glandular tissue (*red*).

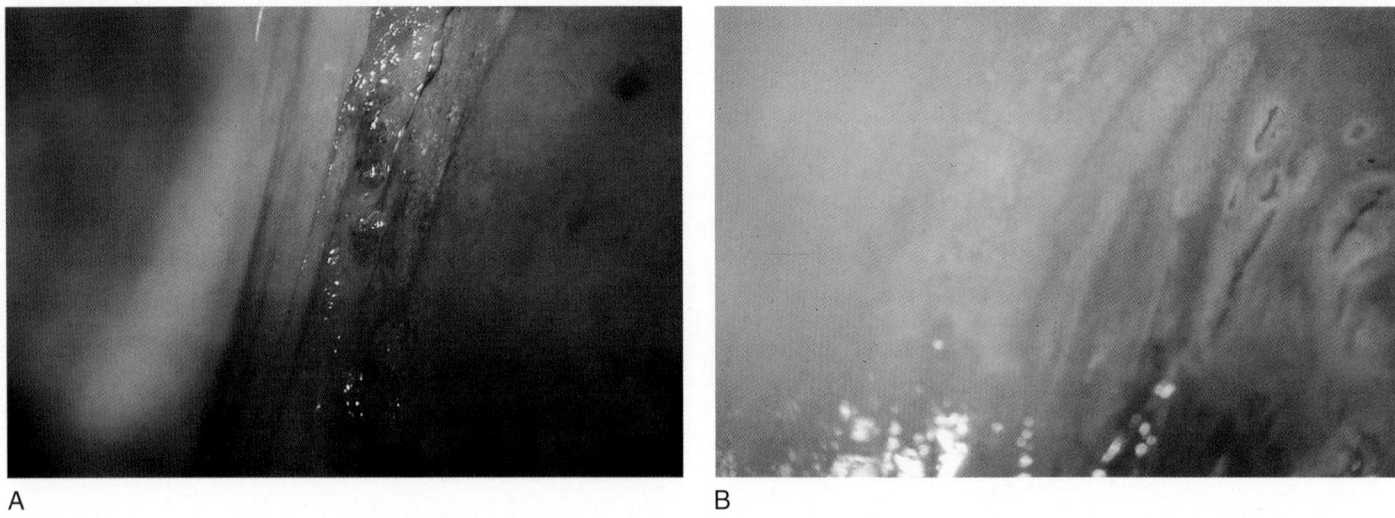

A          B

**FIGURE 60–2  A.** Granulation-like glandular tissue located in the lateral vaginal fornix is diagnostic of adenosis. **B.** Clefts and gland openings are apparent in this patient's vagina. A biopsy into this area will reveal mucous glands beneath the surface squamous metaplastic epithelium.

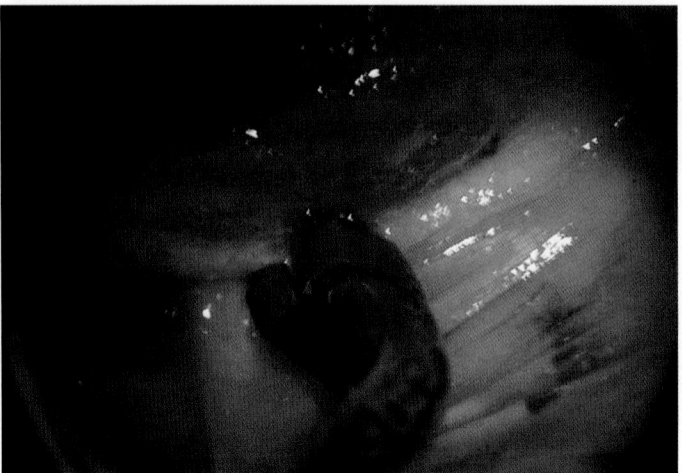

**FIGURE 60–3**  A directed vaginal biopsy is performed under colposcopic guidance. Patients feel little, if any, discomfort if the biopsy is performed in a timely manner with a sharp biopsy clamp.

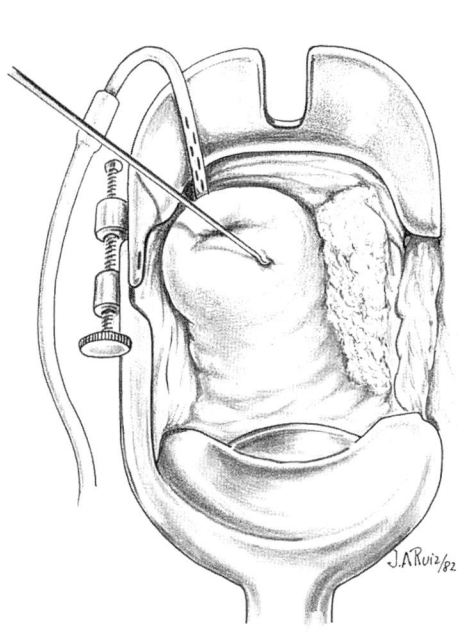

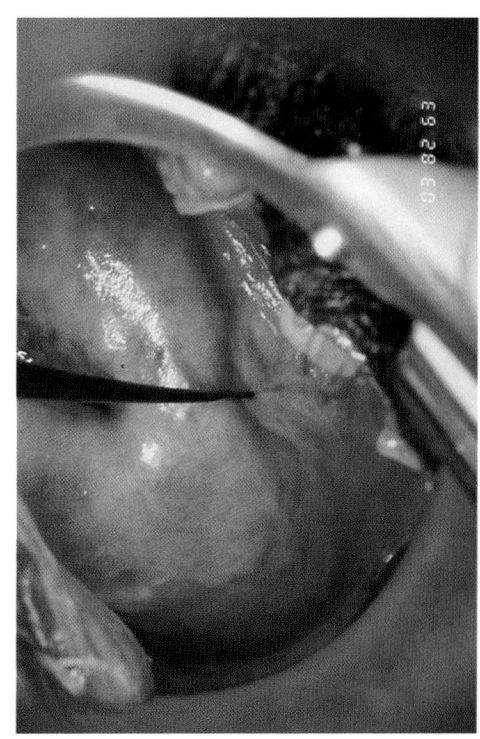

**FIGURE 60-4 A.** To expose the vaginal fornices to facilitate a directed biopsy, a long-handled titanium hook pulls the cervix out of the way. **B.** Without the benefit of the hook, it would be exceedingly difficult to obtain an adequate colposcopic view of the lateral fornices.

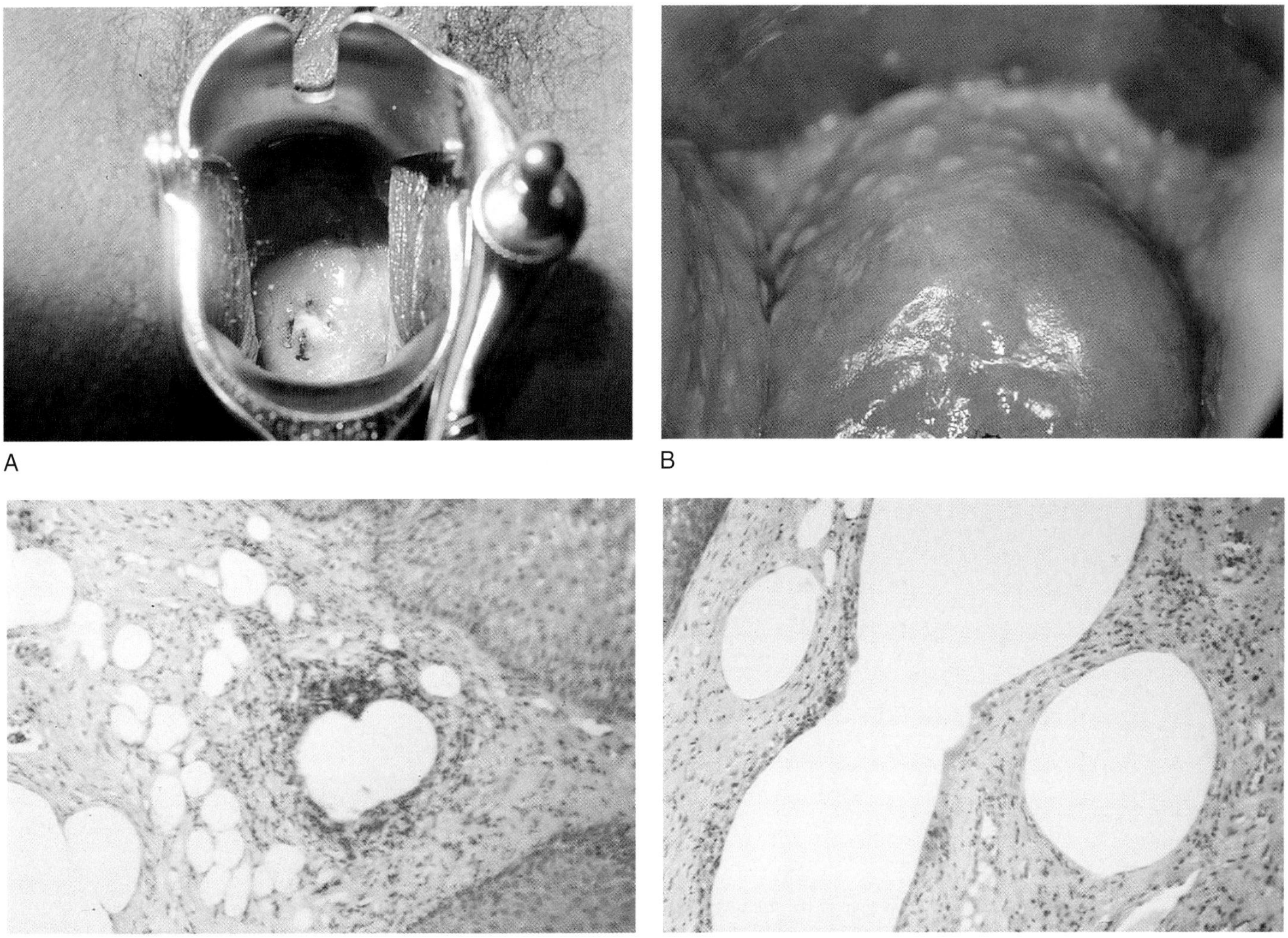

A

B

A

B

C

D

**FIGURE 60-5 A.** Numerous small cysts are seen in the anterior vaginal fornix. These cysts are filled with gas. **B.** A magnified view of part **A** reveals the appearance of vaginitis emphysematosa. **C.** Microscopic section through the vaginal wall (part **A**) showing air spaces beneath the epithelial pegs. **D.** Vaginitis emphysematosa is characterized by gas-filled spaces surrounded by multinucleated giant cells.

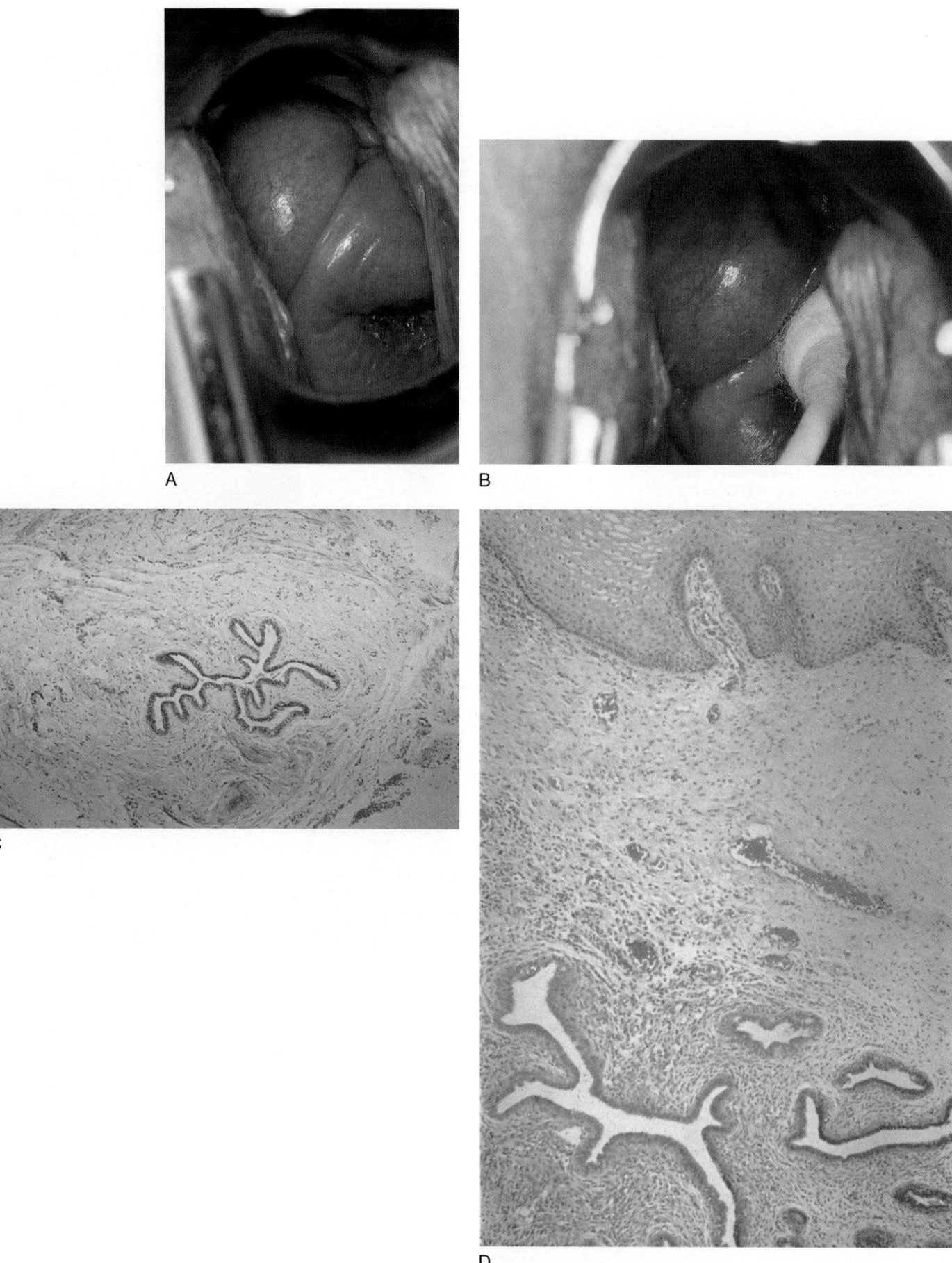

A

B

C

D

**FIGURE 60–6 A.** A large Gartner duct cyst is seen in the right anterolateral wall of the vagina. The cervix is displaced downward and to the left. Preoperatively, the cyst should be injected with radiopaque dye and fluoroscopically studied. An intravenous pyelogram and cystoscopy should be performed to determine the exact location of the bladder and ureter relative to the cyst. Ureteral catheterization is recommended if the cyst will be excised. **B.** A large cotton swab displaces the cervix posteriorly to better delineate the relationship of the Gartner duct cyst to the urinary bladder. **C.** Microscopic section through mesonephric duct remnant in the lateral wall of a normal vagina. Obstruction of this duct leads to a Gartner duct cyst. **D.** Above is the stratified squamous epithelium of the vagina. The glandular structures lying (below) in the vaginal stroma (wall) are remnants of the mesonephric duct and tubules.

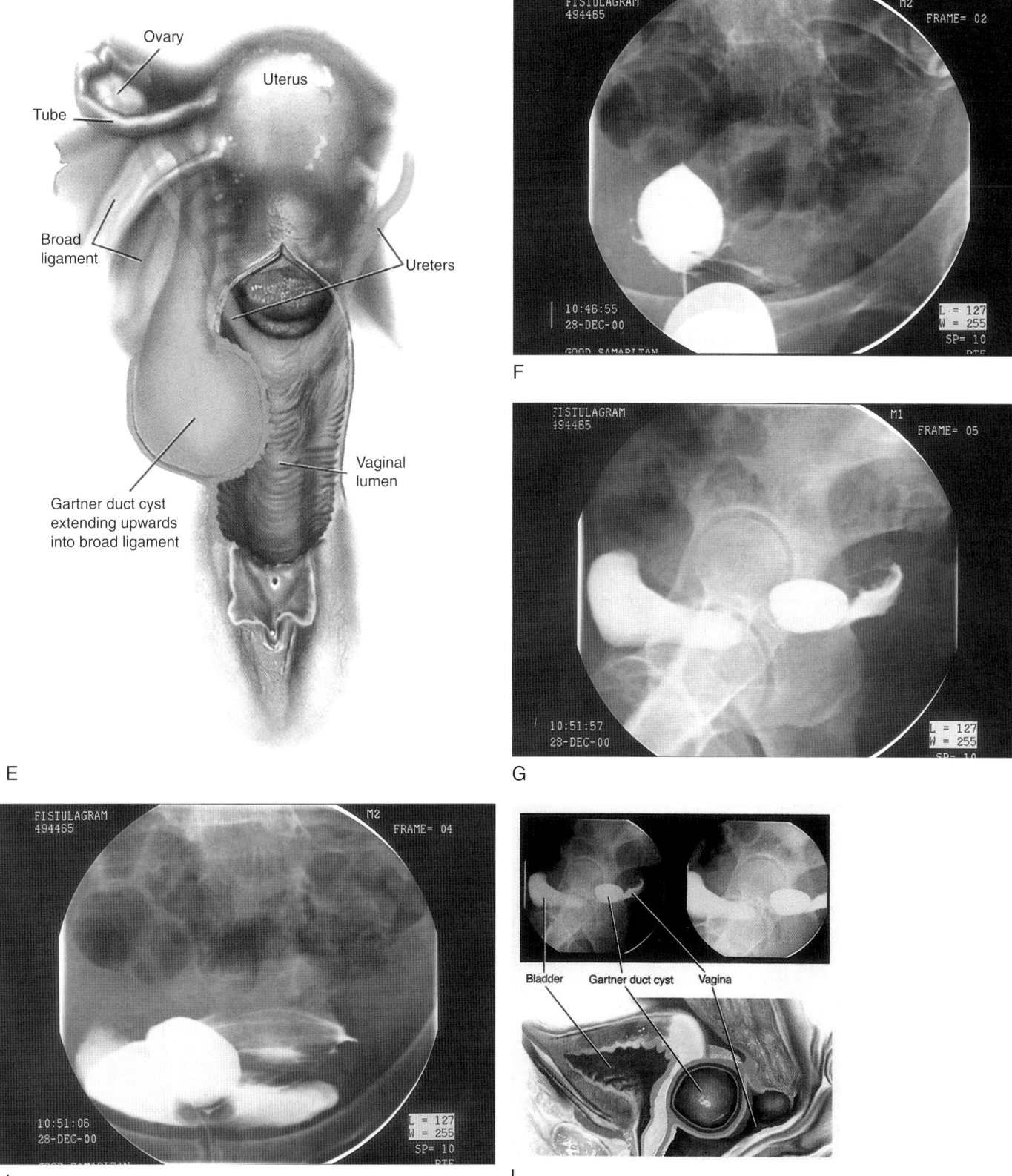

**FIGURE 60–6, cont'd E.** Gartner duct cysts may become quite large, as is illustrated in part **A.** The relationship of the cyst to the bladder and ureters must be clearly defined. This drawing illustrates several key issues. The mesonephric duct and hence any Gartner duct may extend craniad from the vagina into the broad ligament of the uterus. The ureters and the bladder base have been superimposed onto the anterior wall of the vagina. The Gartner cyst in this case illustrated impinges on both the right ureter and the right side of the bladder. **F.** To better define the critical relationships between the cyst and surrounding structures, a water-soluble contrast medium is injected into the cyst and fluoroscopic examination is carried out. **G.** Dye is also instilled into the bladder to determine the proximity of the Gartner cyst (*to the right*) to the bladder (*to the left*). **H.** Anterior-posterior view of the cyst relative to the bladder. **I.** This picture shows the relationships of the drawn-in cyst and the radiographic images.

A Gartner duct cyst extending down to the lower vagina should be radiologically investigated to determine the upward extent of the cyst. Figures 60-7 through 60-10 show a cyst of the left anterior-lateral vaginal wall and its relationship to the urinary bladder.

An easy reliable technique for dealing with this type of cyst is described below.

The cyst is injected with a $1:100$ diluted vasopressin solution (Fig. 60-11). Next, carbon dioxide ($CO_2$) laser trace spots outline the area of the cyst that will be excised (Fig. 60-12). The excision essentially uncaps the cystic mass (Fig. 60-13). The interior of the cyst can now be viewed (Fig. 60-14). The $CO_2$ laser beam diameter is enlarged to 2.3 mm (spot), and the interior of the cyst is systematically vaporized (Fig. 60-15). The vaporization completely denudes the thin epithelial lining of the cyst (Fig. 60-16). The opposing collapsed walls will effi-ciently agglutinate to one another. The fenestration site is reefed with a running lock suture of 3-0 Vicryl (Fig. 60-17). Six to 8 weeks postoperatively, the mass and the opening are gone (Fig. 60-18). The excised cyst wall is sent to pathology for confirmation.

On occasion, a Gartner duct cyst may reach a large size (i.e., greater than 5 to 10 cm) and may extend upward into the lateral aspect of the cervix. Figure 60-19 illustrates a large posterior vaginal wall Gartner duct cyst that ended up in the right lateral fornix of the vagina. In such instances, it may be advantageous to resect a significant portion or all of the cyst (Figs. 60-20 through 60-25). If a portion of the cyst remains unresected, then the interior should be vaporized to diminish the chances for recurrence (Figs. 60-26 through 60-28). At the completion of the procedure, the vaginal wall is carefully reapproximated to avoid scar formation.

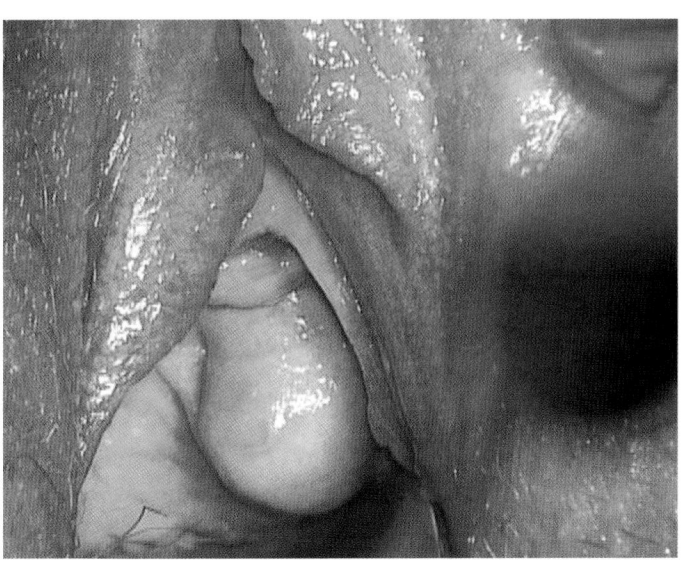

**FIGURE 60–7** Moderate-sized cyst attached firmly to the left anterolateral vaginal wall.

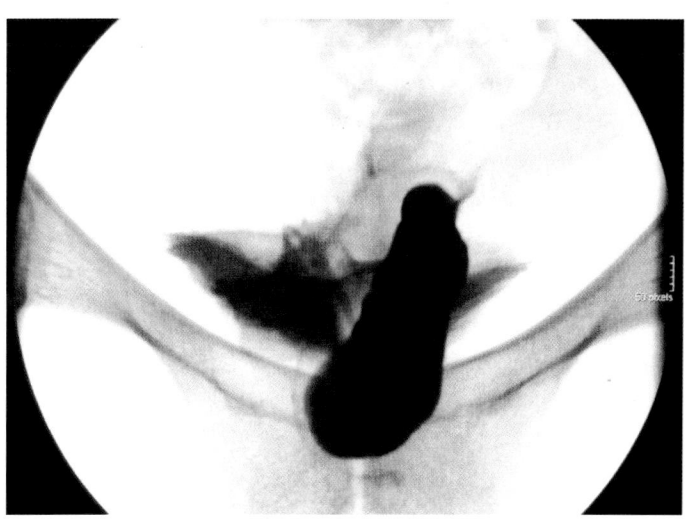

**FIGURE 60–8** The cyst has been injected with radio-opaque medium. The cyst extends for 3 to 4 cm cranially.

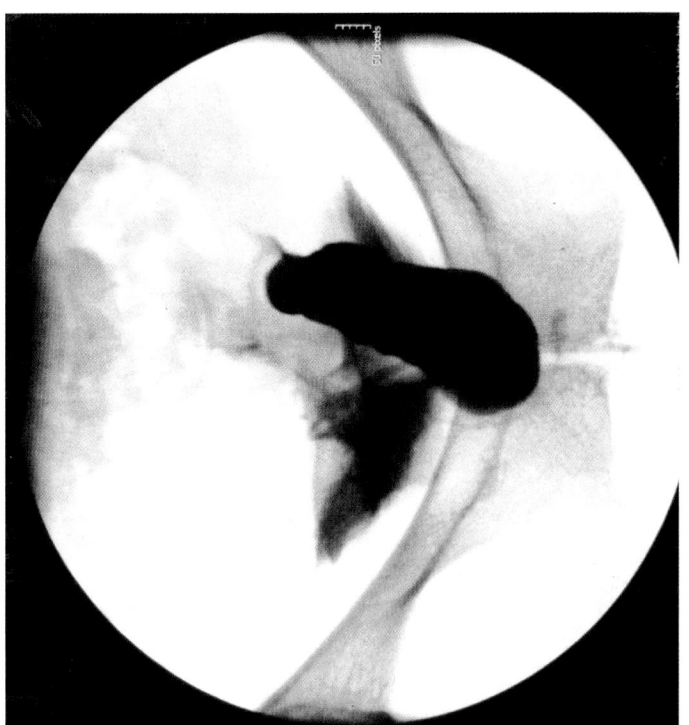

**FIGURE 60–9** The bladder has been filled with dye to determine its relationship to the cyst wall.

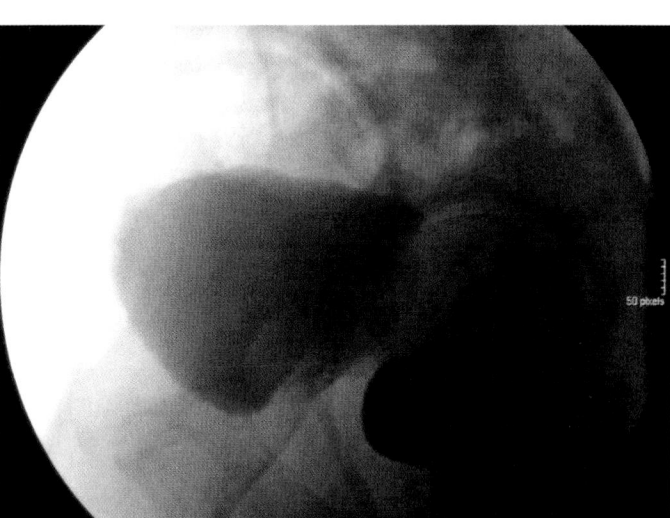

**FIGURE 60–10** This view shows that the posterior bladder wall is safely away from the cyst wall.

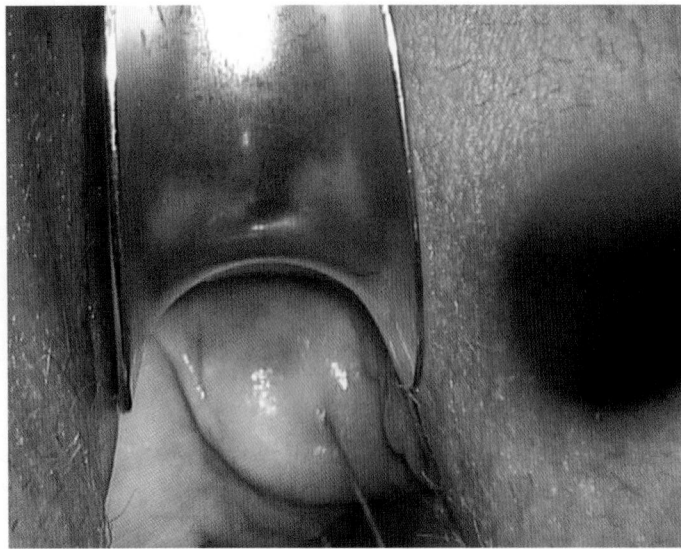

**FIGURE 60–11** Vasopressin, 1:100 dilution, is injected into the cyst wall for hemostasis.

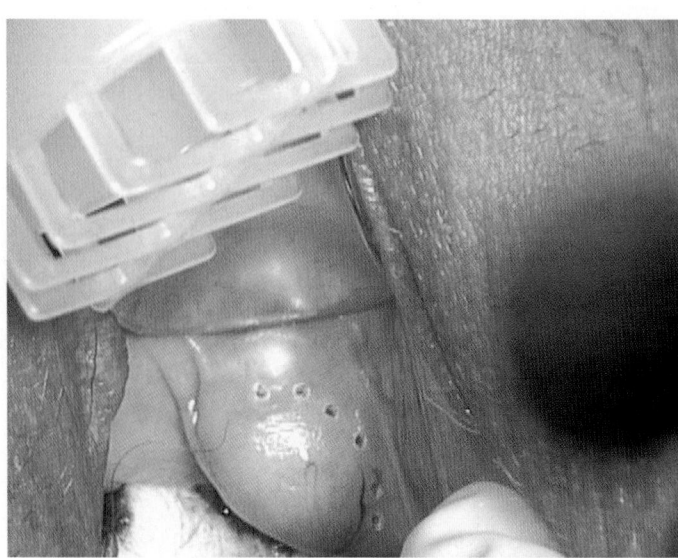

**FIGURE 60–12** Carbon dioxide ($CO_2$) laser trace spots are placed into the cyst.

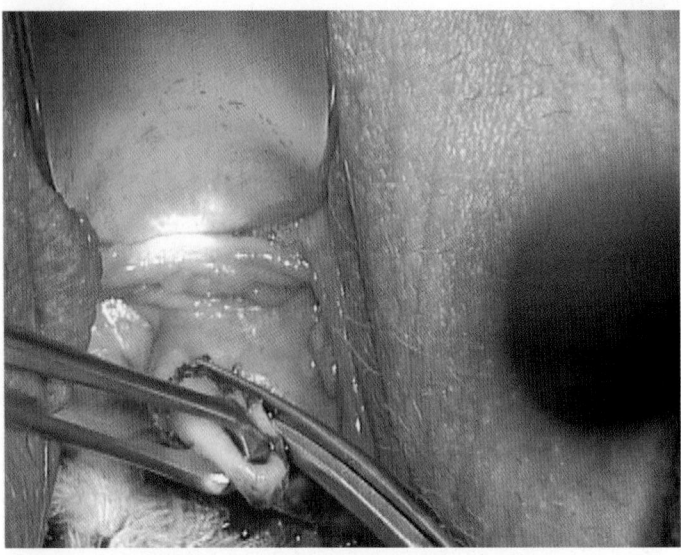

**FIGURE 60–13** The cyst is uncapped by means of carbon dioxide ($CO_2$) laser cutting or by means of scissors.

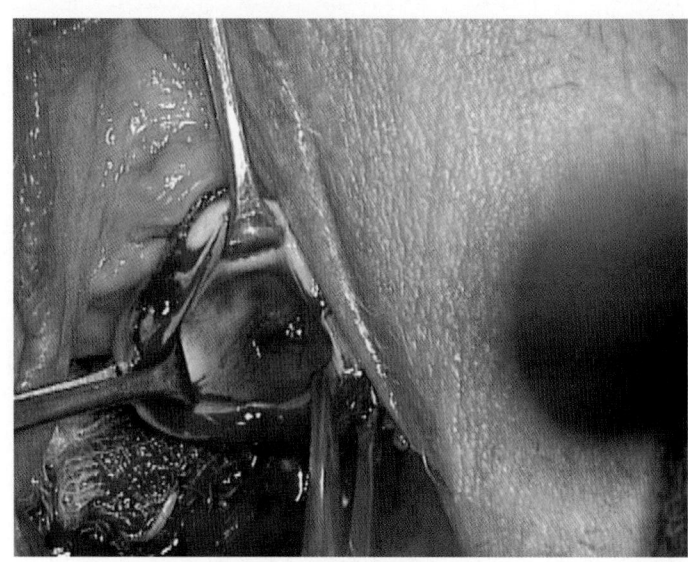

**FIGURE 60–14** The interior of the cyst is now visible.

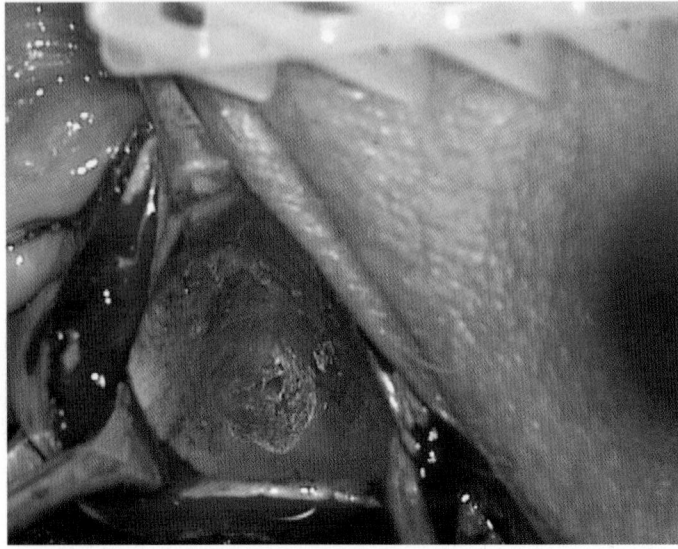

**FIGURE 60–15** The laser spot size is increased to 2 to 3 mm, and vaporization of the cyst lining commences.

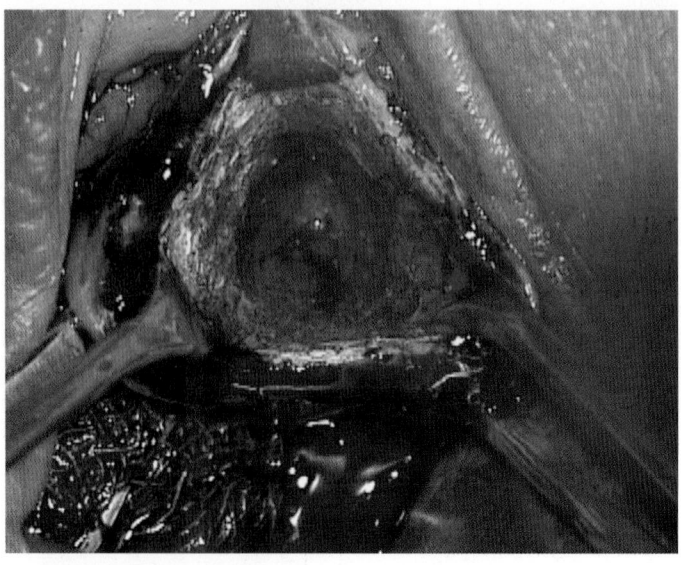

**FIGURE 60–16** The epithelium of the cyst has been completely vaporized.

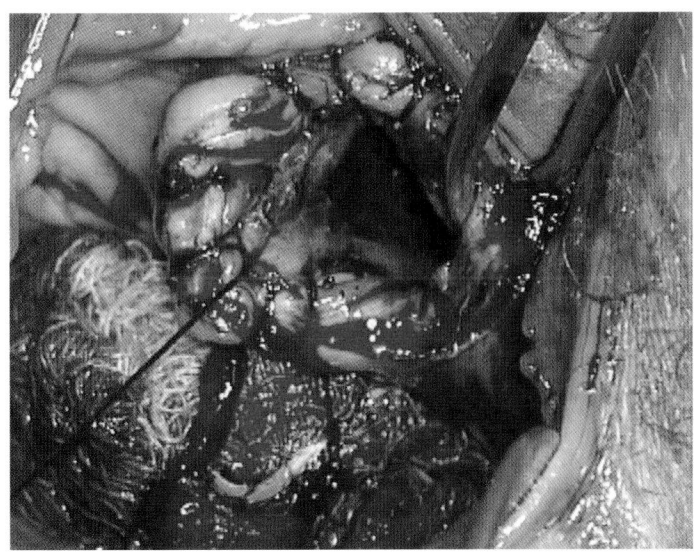

FIGURE 60–17 The margins of the uncapped portion of the cyst are closed with a 3-0 Vicryl reefing stitch.

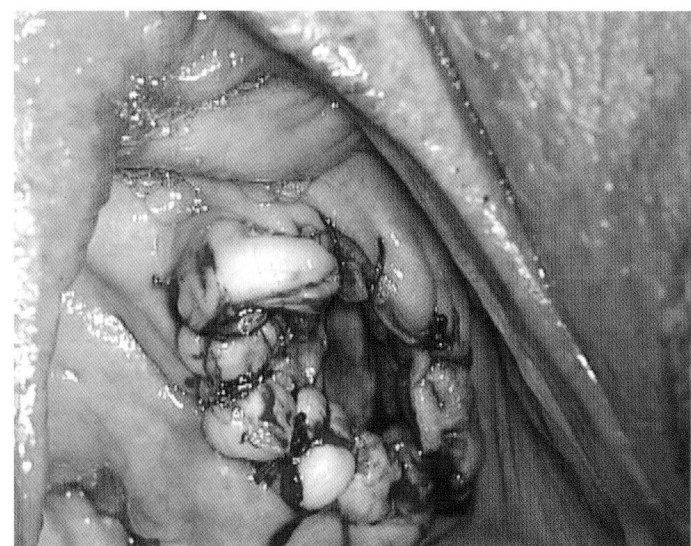

FIGURE 60–18 The operation is completed and the field is homeostatic.

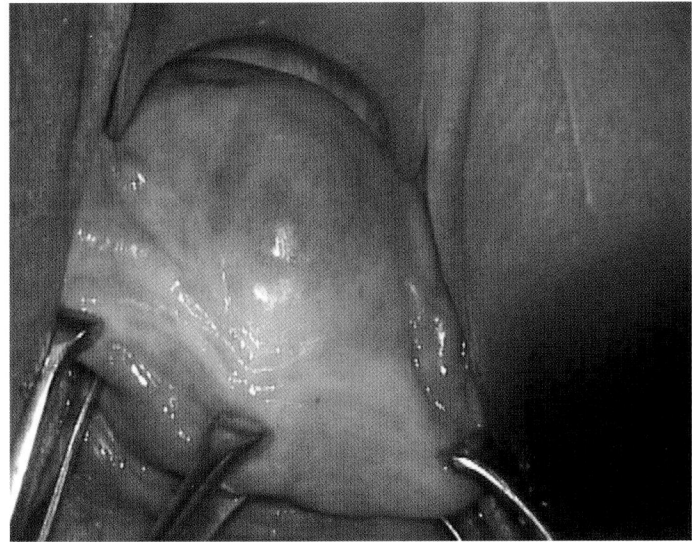

FIGURE 60–19 A large Gartner duct cyst involving the posterior vaginal wall and extending up the vagina to the level of the cervix. The cyst gradually shifted to the right and occupied the right lateral vaginal fornix.

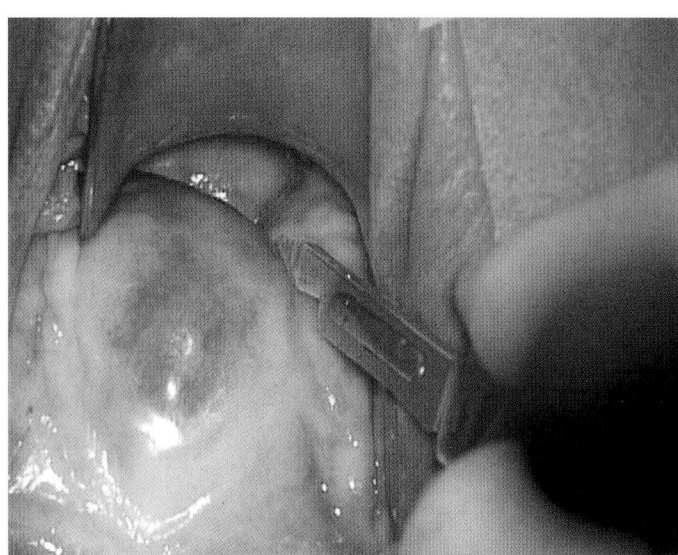

FIGURE 60–20 After injection of a 1:100 diluted vasopressin solution, a knife cut is made into the left posterior vaginal wall.

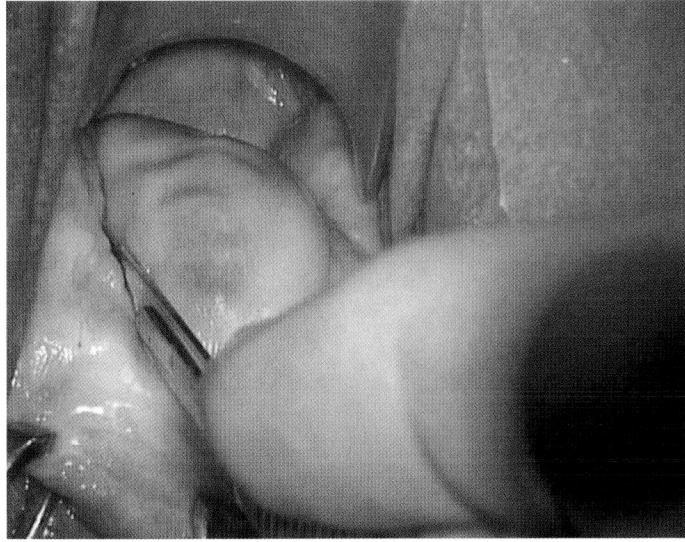

FIGURE 60–21 A similar incision is made on the right posterior vagina.

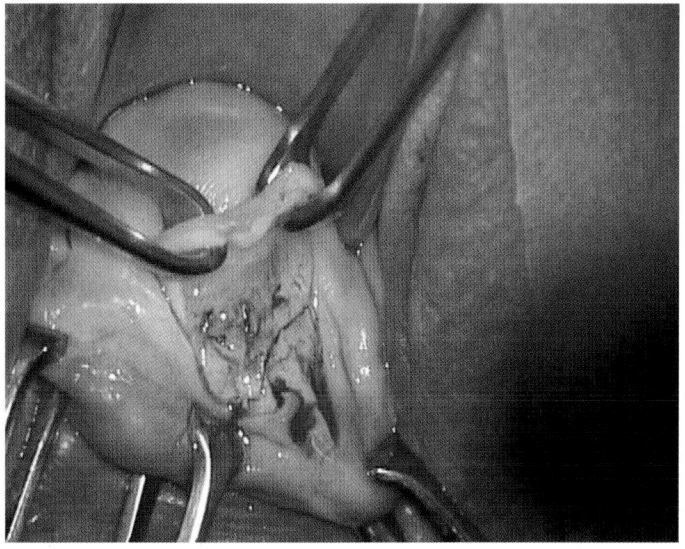

FIGURE 60–22 The cyst wall is dissected and removed, together with the adherent posterior vagina.

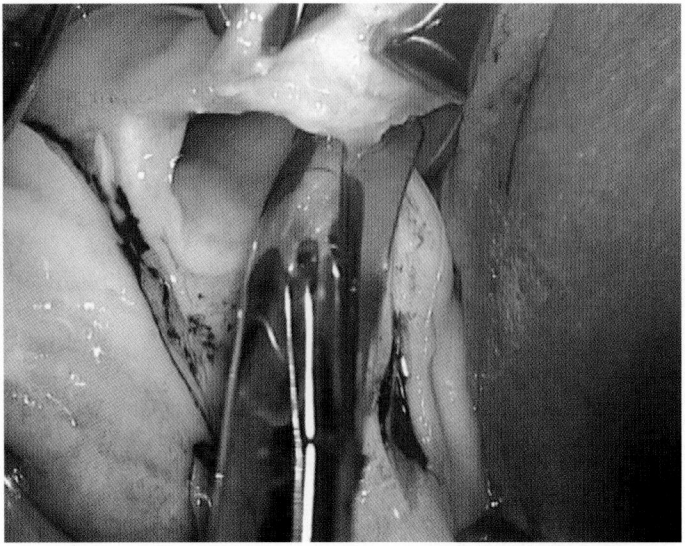

FIGURE 60–23  The cyst is entered and then is widely opened.

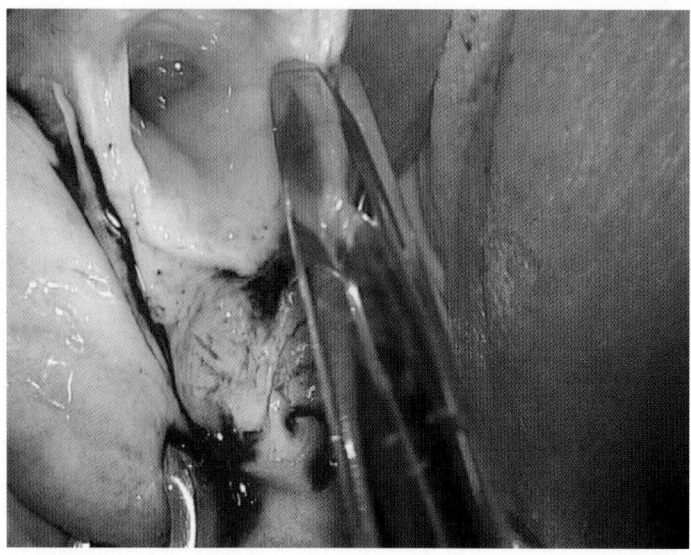

FIGURE 60–24  The interior of the cyst can be viewed, and the depth of its upward extension can be determined.

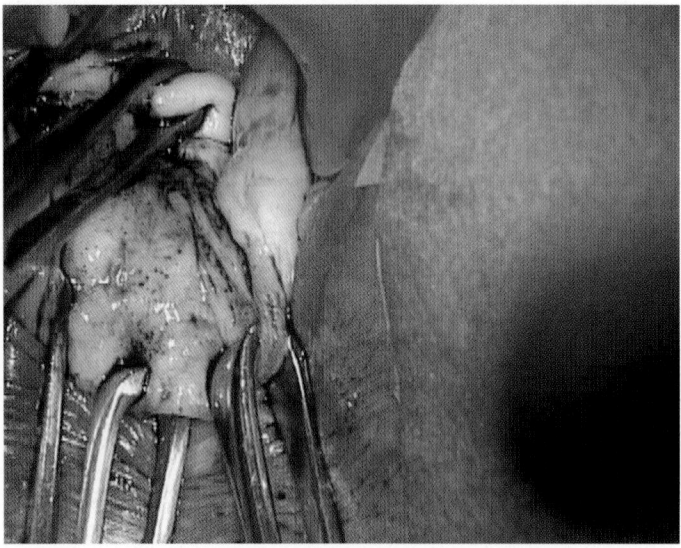

FIGURE 60–25  The posterior wall of the cyst remains. Traction is placed with the three (lower) Allis clamps. The upper two Allis clamps are attached to the remaining margin of the posterior vagina.

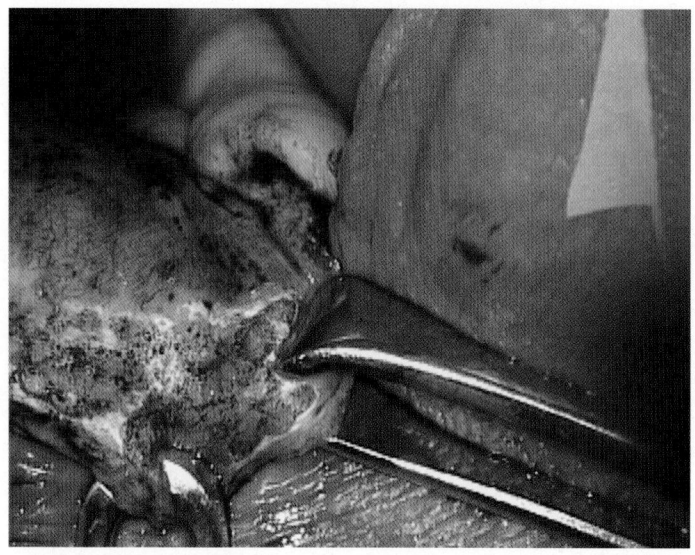

FIGURE 60–26  Laser vaporization of the posterior cyst lining the epithelium is initiated.

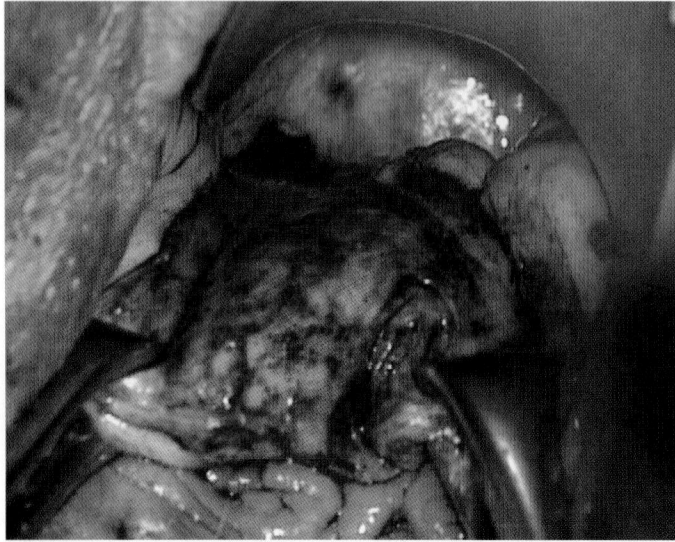

FIGURE 60–27  The entire posterior cyst wall has vanished (i.e., the vaporization has been completed).

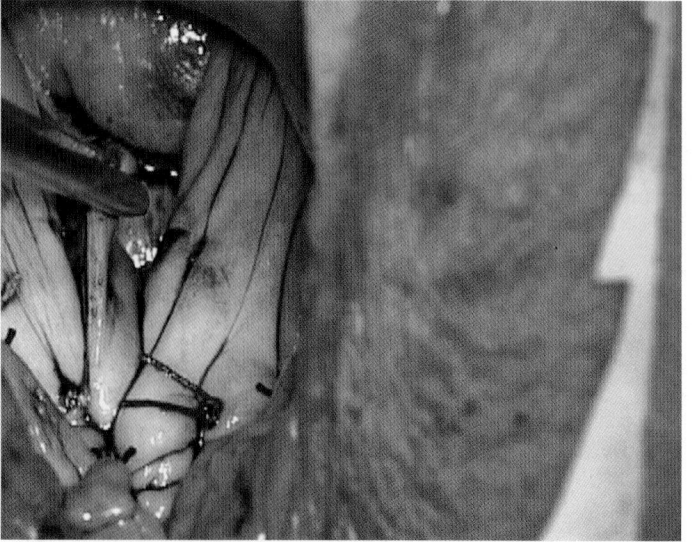

FIGURE 60–28  The posterior vaginal wall is vertically closed with 3-0 Vicryl interrupted sutures. Note that the forceps grasps the open vaginal edge as the incision swings into the right vaginal fornix. Note the cervix just cranial to the end of the forceps.

## Ulcers

Ulceration may be created in the vagina through the application of toxic chemicals, tampon injury, surgery, and trauma. The ulcer is typically infected via vaginal bacteria and may expand or perpetuate as a result of the infection (Fig. 60-29A through C). The initial treatment is to perform a biopsy of the ulcer to exclude a neoplastic process; simultaneously, the ulcer should be cultured for bacteria, as well as fungi and viruses. The vagina should be irrigated two or three times daily, and a topical antibiotic (clindamycin cream) applied several times per day (Fig. 60-30A through G). Systemic antibiotics, antifungals, or antivirals are administered according to the sensitivity of the specific organism identified. If, because of a poor vascular supply, the ulcer does not regress, it should be excised. The margins should be demarcated, and the periphery injected with a 1:100 vasopressin solution. If the ulcer is large, a graft should be taken preoperatively. If the lesion measures less than 2 cm, it usually can be closed without constricting the vagina (Fig. 60-31A through C).

## Solid Masses

Solid masses may present in the vagina, particularly in the fornices or the vesicovaginal or rectovaginal spaces. These lesions cause pain and must be excised. Frequently, they represent infiltration of endometriosis. This type of surgery is performed by utilizing the microscope and a combination of instruments, including the $CO_2$ laser and long tenotomy scissors. Tissue planes between the endometriosis and the normal tissue in these circumstances may be difficult to identify. Wide excision of the subepithelial mass therefore is required. Attention must be focused on neighboring structures (ureter, bladder, rectum) to avoid injuring them (Fig. 60-32A through D).

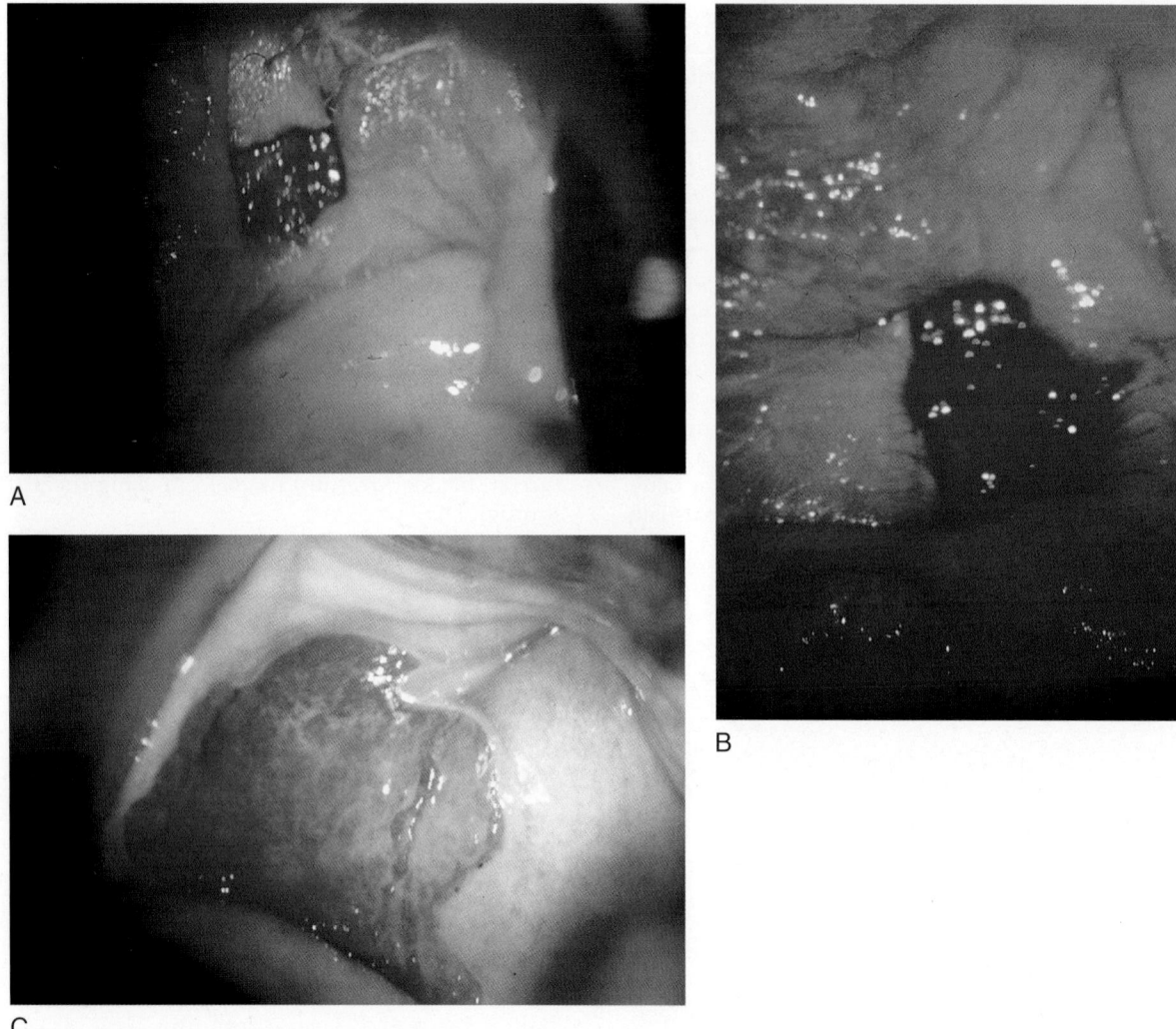

**FIGURE 60–29 A.** This patient complained of an uncomfortable sticking-like pain during coitus. Note the ulcer on the anterior wall of the vagina. **B.** The ulcer most probably was caused by a tampon. Initial treatment for this lesion is a topical antibiotic. **C.** This large ulcer resulted after laser vaporization of vaginal intraepithelial neoplasia. It represents devitalized tissue and should be excised.

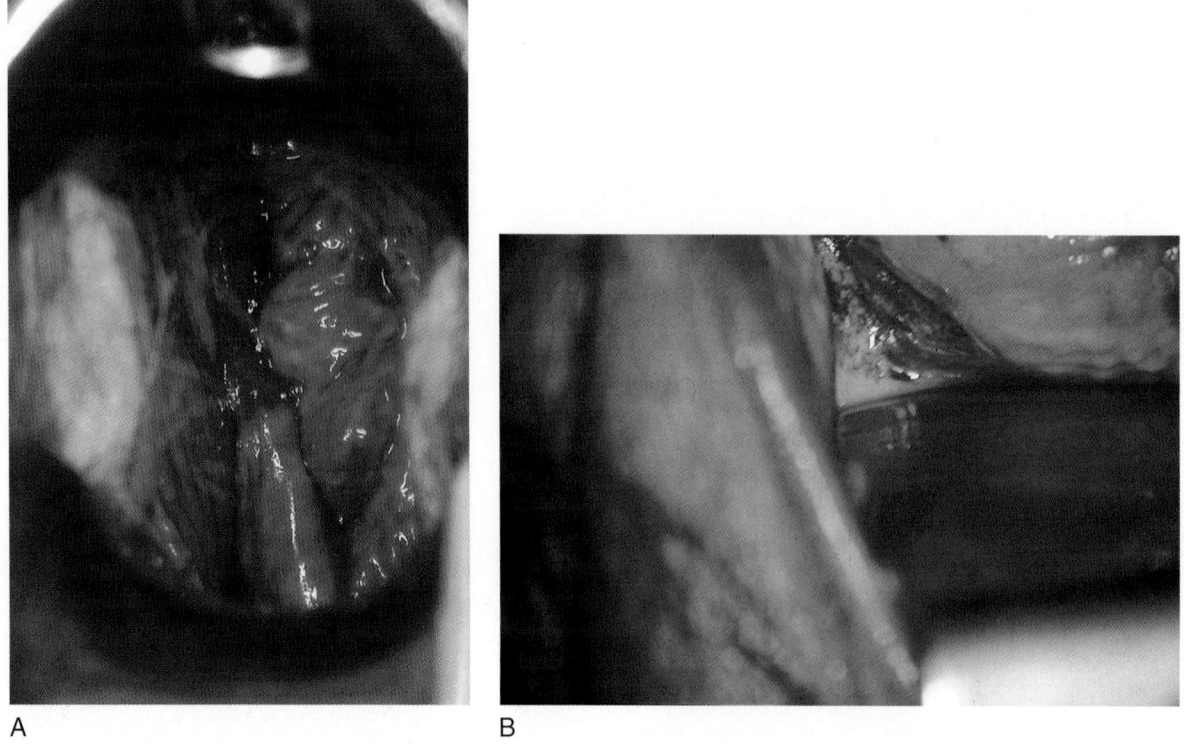

**FIGURE 60–30 A.** This young woman presented with a large ulcer of the right lateral vaginal wall and right fornix. This photo was taken during an office examination. **B.** The ulcer is fully exposed at surgery. A 1:100 vasopressin solution is injected with a 1½-inch, 25-gauge needle. Note the blanching beneath the ulcer. Traction sutures have been placed at the periphery of the ulcer.

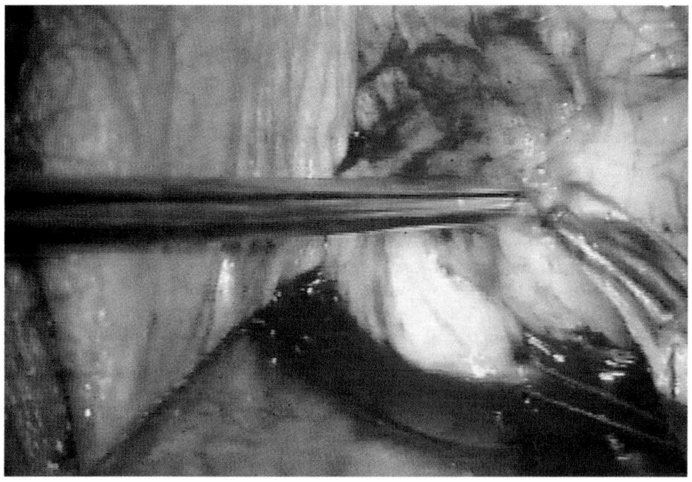

C

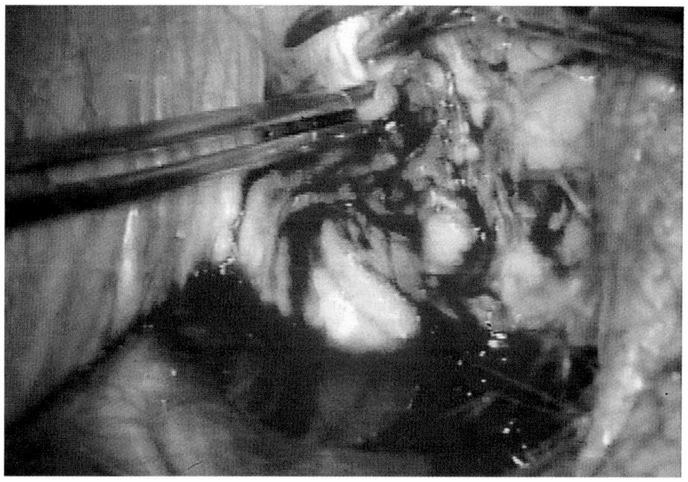

D

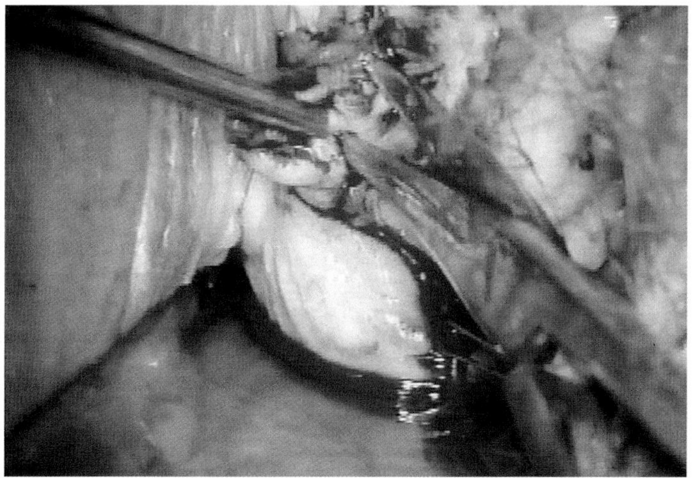

E

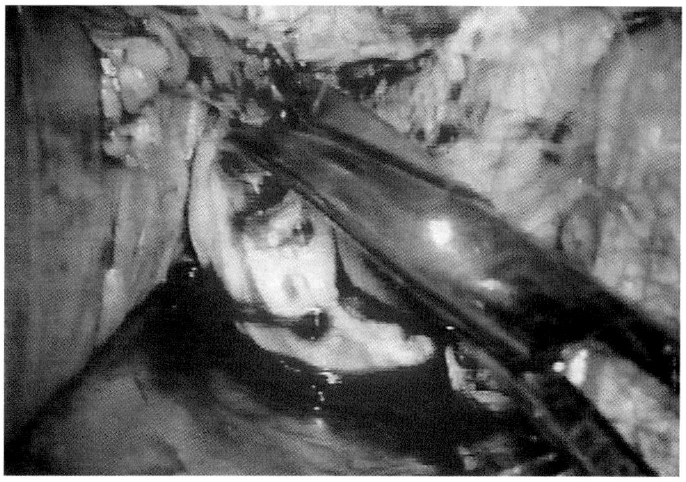

F

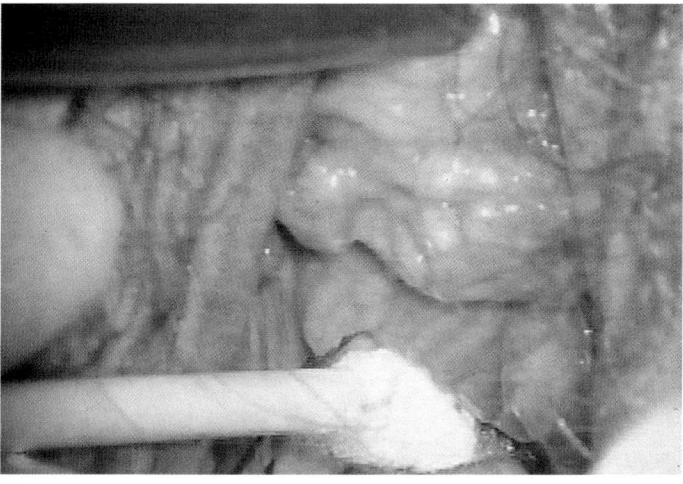

G

**FIGURE 60–30, cont'd** **C.** Dissection of the ulcer is initiated with Stevens scissors at the left lateral margin of the ulcer. The lesion itself occupies the right anterolateral fornix of the vagina. **D.** The dissection is carried above the ulcer (right anterolateral fornix) just beneath the bladder. A plane has been established, and one blade of the scissors is within the dissection plane. **E.** The bulk of the ulcer is held within the teeth of the forceps as the Stevens scissors separates it from the vaginal stroma. **F.** The ulcer is cut free from the right lateral margin of the ulcer. **G.** A catheter has been placed into the bladder and methylene blue dye injected. A proctoswab is placed on the ulcer bed to check for transvesical leakage of dye (bladder base disruption).

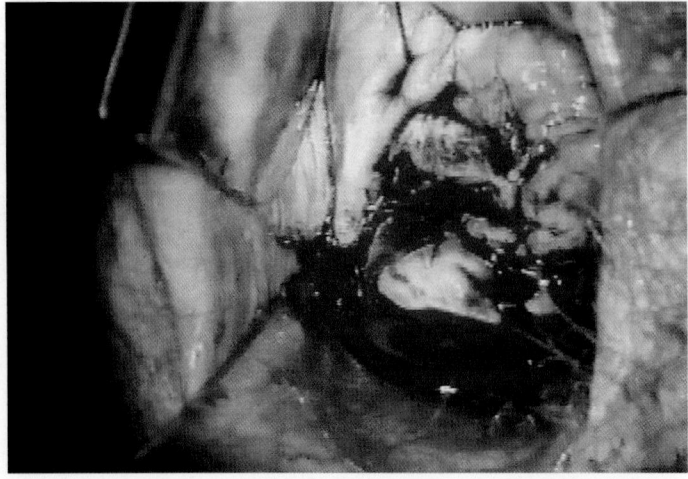

A

B

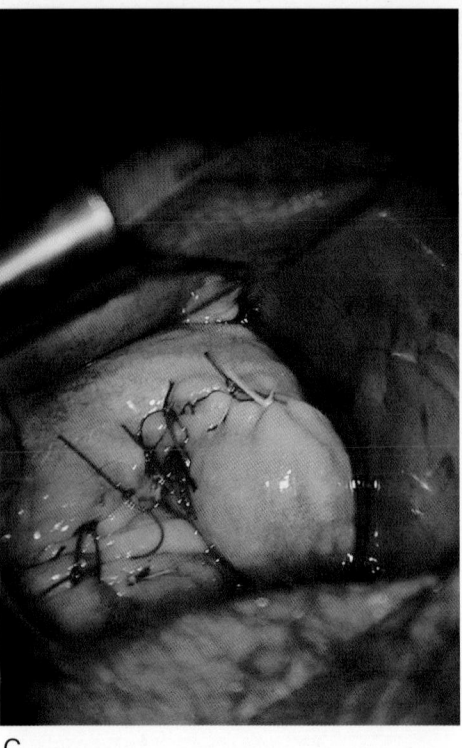

C

**FIGURE 60–31  A.** The dissected bed of the excised ulcer (Fig. 60–13A through G) is exposed in the right anterolateral vaginal fornix. **B.** The undermined walls of the vagina are closed over the operative site with interrupted 3-0 Vicryl sutures. **C.** The vaginal fornix is completely closed by primary suture. The wound is then irrigated with normal saline.

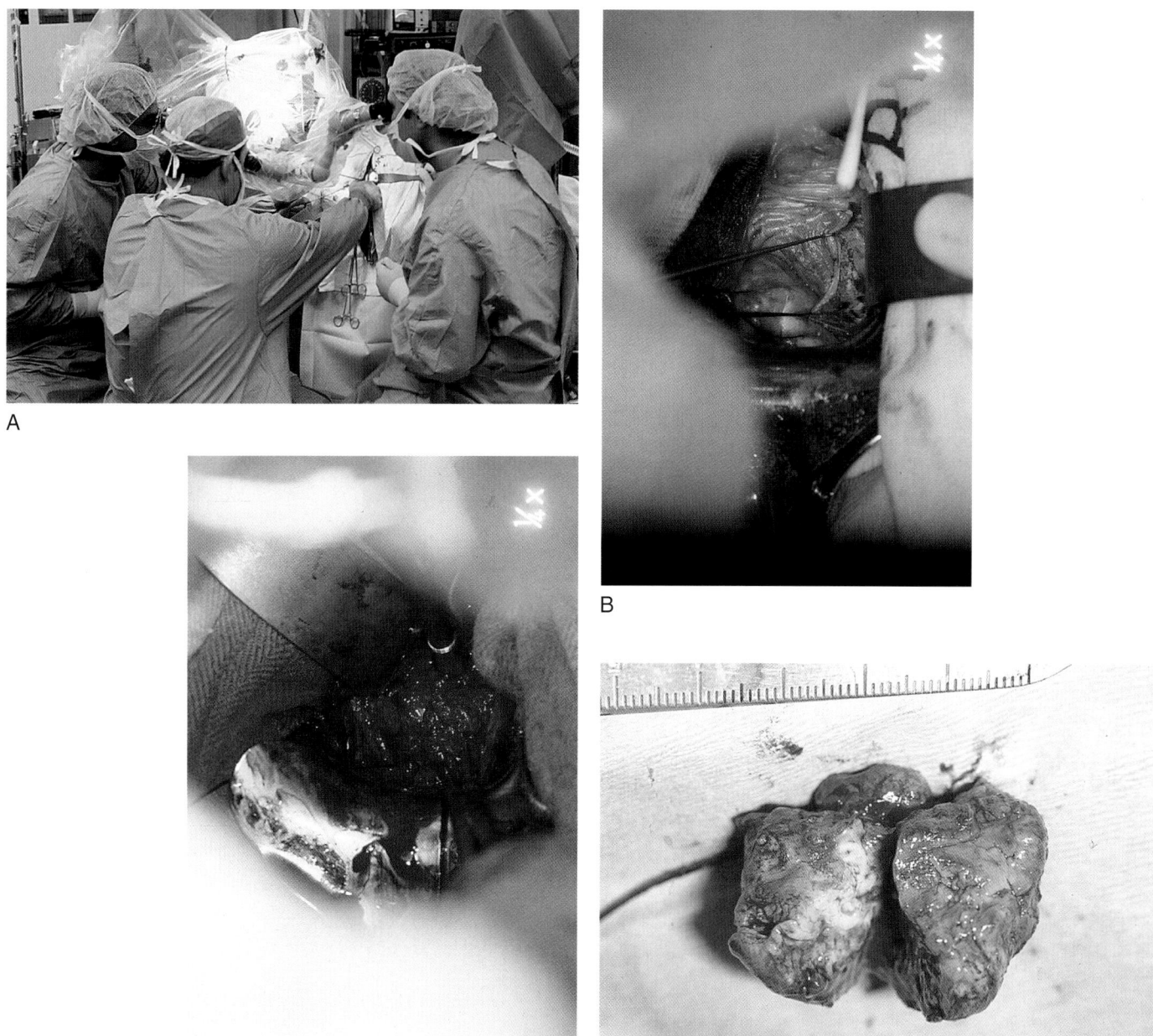

A

B

C

D

FIGURE 60–32 A. Solid masses in the vagina must be surgically removed in all cases. The dissecting microscope is the best tool for this difficult dissection. B. An incision is made into the left anterolateral fornix of the vagina over a rock-hard 3-cm painful mass. The red aiming beam of a carbon dioxide ($CO_2$) laser is located at the lower margin of the incision. The vaginal manipulating hooks are at the upper and middle margins of the incision. C. The mass has been reached and is being dissected from the bladder base. A ureteral catheter has been placed into the left ureter. D. The excised mass has been cut to reveal endometriosis of the vaginal wall. Note the brownish siderophagic coloration of the tissue and the hemosiderin-laden fluid matter.

# CHAPTER 61

# Congenital Vaginal Abnormalities

*John B. Gebhart* ■ *Lesley L. Breech* ■ *Bradley S. Hurst* ■ *John A. Rock*

## Imperforate Hymen

A child or adolescent with an imperforate hymen presents with pain and a thin, translucent membrane distended by blood or mucus. An imperforate hymen is often treated in the operating suite with sedation or general anesthesia.

First, an incision is made in the center of the membrane, and the blood and mucus are evacuated. The incision is extended transversely to the lateral margins of the obstructing membrane (Fig. 61-1A, B). Next, the membrane is divided anteriorly, then posteriorly, to complete a cruciate incision. Finally, the redundant avascular tissue is excised (Fig. 61-1C).

Bleeding should be minimal following resection of the hymenal membrane. Pressure applied with a damp sponge will control most bleeding sites. If the resection has been carried out too far, and the bleeding cannot be controlled with a sparing application of Monsel's solution (ferric subsulfate) or light pressure, then simple interrupted sutures of 3-0 polyglycolic acid should be placed. A continuous running simple suture should be avoided because this may cause constriction of the hymenal ring. The appropriate result is a capacious introitus that functionally permits comfortable coitus (Fig. 61–2A).

Other developmental abnormalities of the hymen, including cribriform and septated hymens (Fig. 61–2B), may require surgical intervention. As with the aforementioned, the goal of the surgery is to create a nonconstricting, functional vaginal introitus.

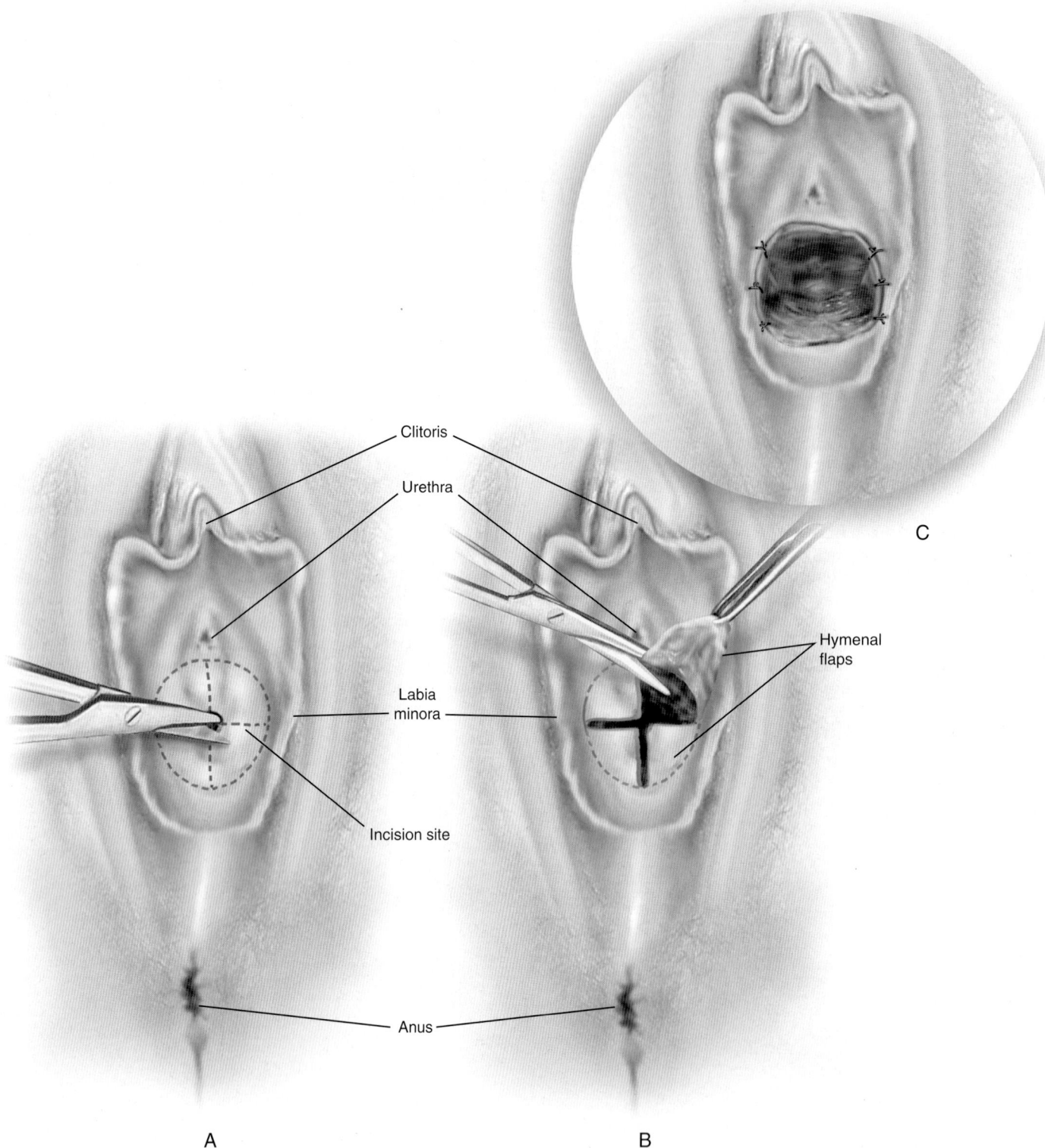

Clitoris

Urethra

Labia
minora

Incision site

Anus

Hymenal
flaps

A

B

C

**FIGURE 61–1 A.** The incision is extended laterally into the hymenal membrane from 3 to 9 o'clock, then along the midline from 12 to 6 o'clock. **B.** Resection of the hymenal membrane is completed as the avascular quadrants are excised. **C.** The hymenal flaps have been resected, and the areas between 1 and 5 o'clock and between 11 and 7 o'clock have been sutured to the vestibular margin with interrupted 3-0 Vicryl sutures.

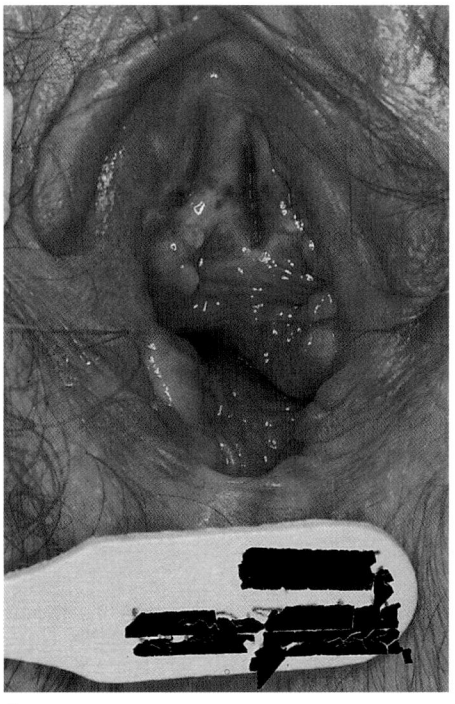

A

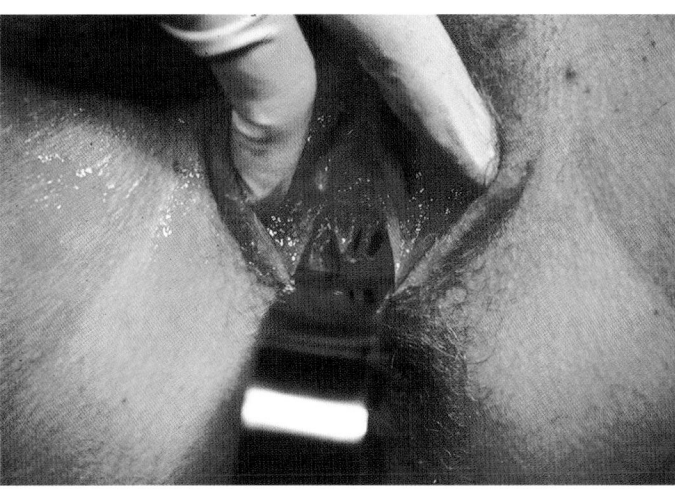

B

**FIGURE 61–2  A.** Eight weeks after resection of the hymen. The introitus is widely open. The patient has been inserting a large vaginal form for 4 weeks. **B.** This young woman has a cribriform hymen. It is excised in a manner similar to the imperforate hymen (see Fig. 61–1A through C).

## Vaginal Agenesis

Müllerian agenesis occurs once in approximately 4000 to 5000 female births. Typical findings of Rokitansky-Kuster-Hauser syndrome include a small vaginal pouch and a normal perineum (Fig. 61–3A). Vaginal agenesis may also occur in a male pseudohermaphrodite. Genital appearance varies depending on the underlying causes. Occasionally, a "flat" perineum is found (Fig. 61–3B).

Vaginal dilation using the Ingram method is the primary approach used to prepare the vagina for intercourse when a vaginal pouch is present. A series of progressively wider and longer dilators are used (Fig. 61–3C). The patient is instructed to position the dilator against the perineum, and to apply her weight gradually onto a bicycle seat that is affixed to a stool. In a motivated patient, the vagina can be prepared for intercourse after a few weeks of dilation. More than 90% of women who comply with this regimen achieve anatomic and functional success.

The McIndoe vaginoplasty is the primary surgical approach for vaginal agenesis when dilation is unsuccessful or is not possible. The patient must be physically and emotionally prepared for the surgery and must anticipate intercourse in the not too distant future.

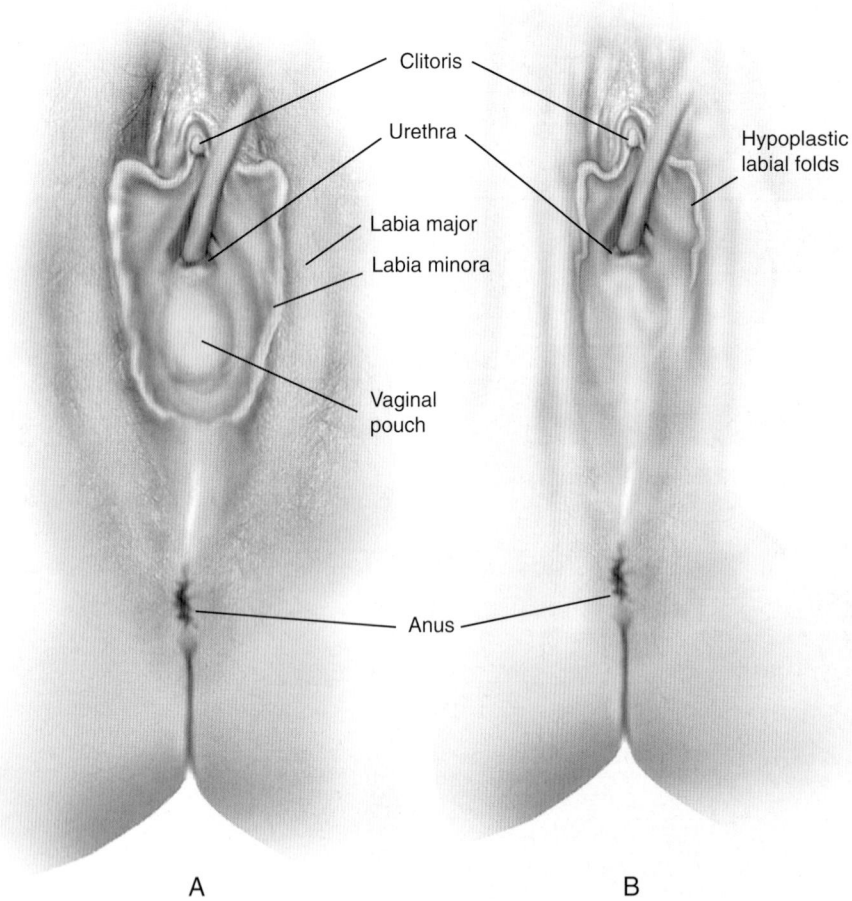

A                                        B

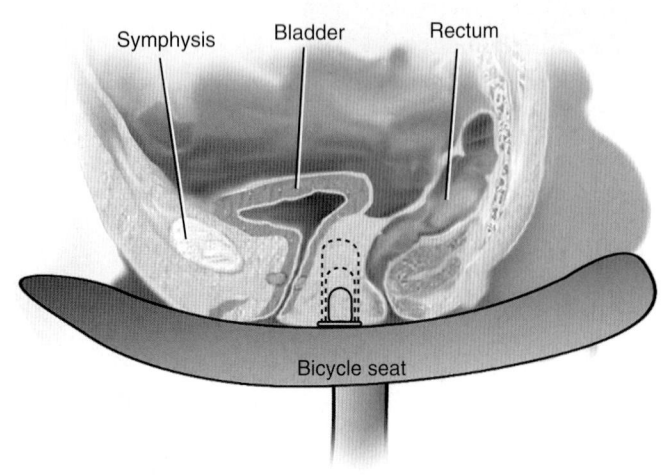

C

**FIGURE 61–3  A.** Müllerian agenesis. The perineum is normal. A small vaginal pouch is evident. **B.** A flat perineum, which may be found in a male pseudohermaphrodite. No vaginal pouch is present. Labial folds, if present, terminate near the urethral meatus. **C.** Vaginal dilation with graduated dilators. Using a bicycle seat, the patient slowly sits on the dilator. Pressure on the dilator from the body's weight allows complete dilation within a few weeks.

First, a transverse incision is made at the apex of the vaginal pouch in the patient with müllerian agenesis (Fig. 61–3D). If the perineum is flat, a 3- to 4-cm incision is made in the posterior fourchette, anterior to the anal sphincter (Fig. 61–3E). The neovaginal space is bluntly dissected laterally, then toward the midline. One finger is placed in the rectum for guidance (Fig. 61–3F).

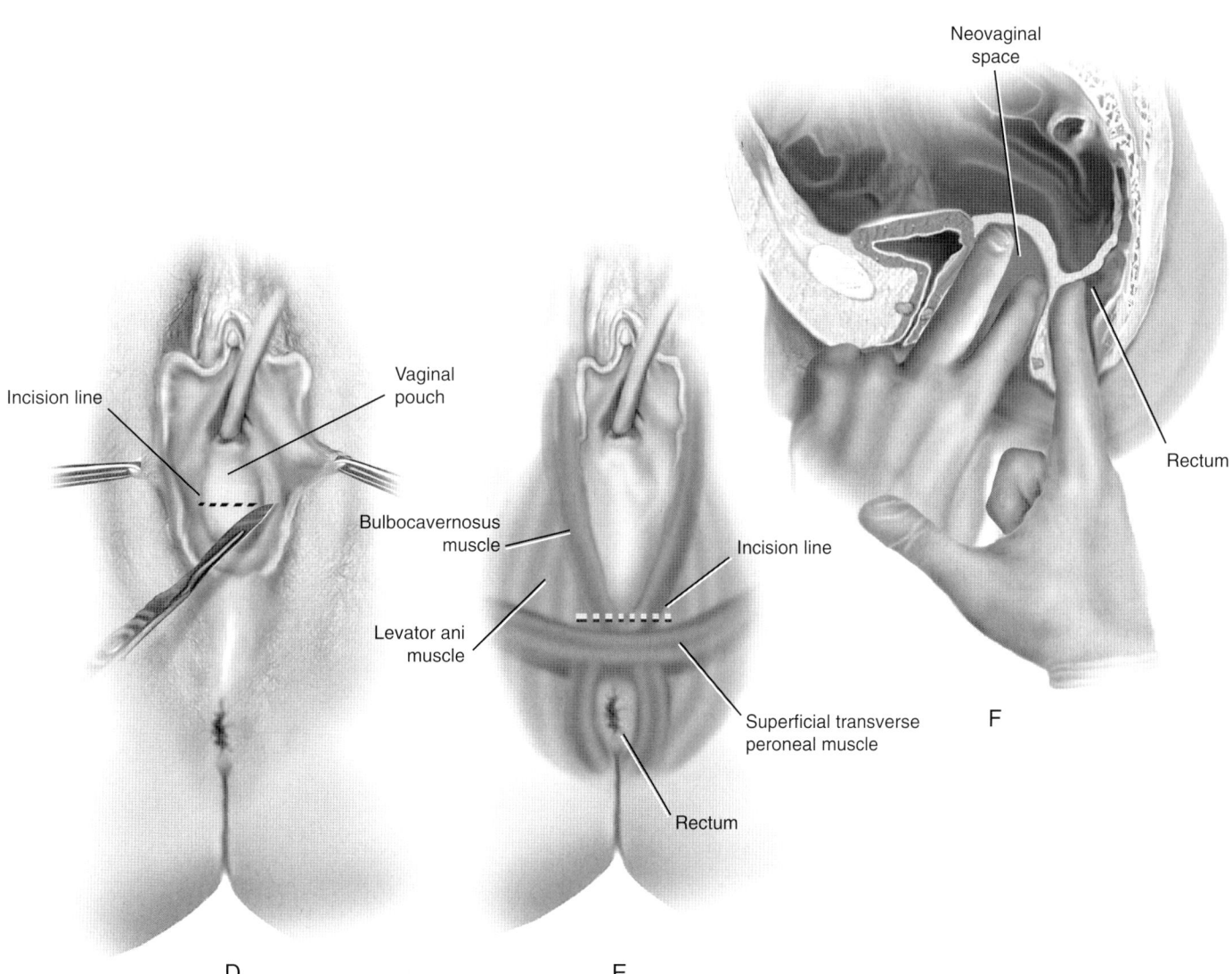

D                                    E

**FIGURE 61–3, cont'd   D.** Initial transverse incision into the apex of the vaginal pouch in a woman with vaginal agenesis. The initial incision should be at least 3 to 4 cm. **E.** Initial transverse incision is made immediately anterior to the superficial transverse peroneal muscle in the patient with a flat perineum. Relationships among the urethra, labia, rectum, and underlying musculature are shown. **F.** Blunt dissection into the neovaginal space. Dissection is performed laterally, then medially. If the patient is 46XY, sharp resection of the prostate may be necessary to avoid damage to the rectal mucosa. Care is taken not to dissect too large an area near the peritoneum because herniation may occur.

Sharp dissection is necessary in the male pseudohermaphrodite if the prostate remnant is adherent to the rectum. A thick band of connective tissue between the bladder and rectum—the median raphe—is sharply divided near the neovaginal fornix (Fig. 61–3G). The space should easily accommodate the surgeon's index and middle fingers. If necessary, the levator muscles can be divided lateral to the incision to provide more space. Meticulous hemostasis is obtained.

Next, sterile 10 × 10 × 20-cm foam rubber form is shaped with scissors (Fig. 61–3H). The form is placed inside a sterile condom and compressed (Fig. 61–3I). The compressed form is inserted completely into the neovaginal space (Fig. 61–3J). The form is then allowed to expand for 1 to 2 minutes. The external end of the condom is tied with a silk suture and the form removed. A second condom is placed over the form, and the free end is tied with a silk suture.

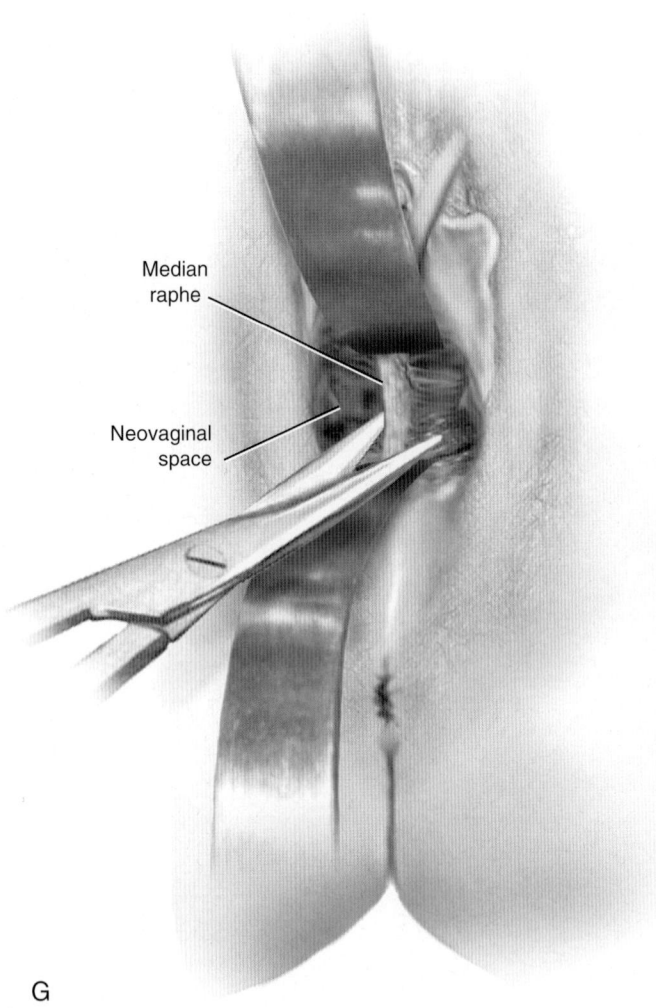

G

**FIGURE 61–3, cont'd  G.** Retractors are placed into the neovaginal space. The median raphe, a thick band of connective tissue, is divided sharply.

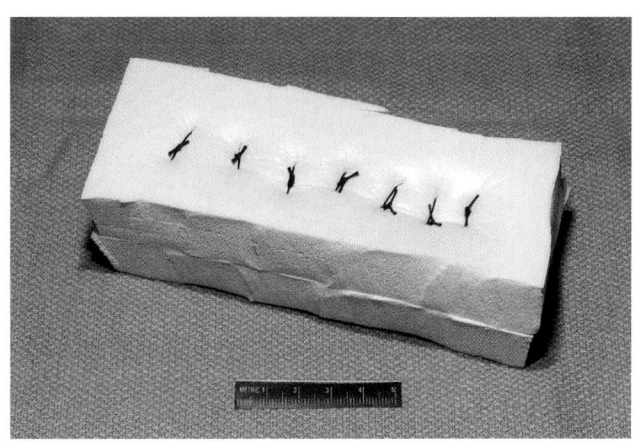

H¹

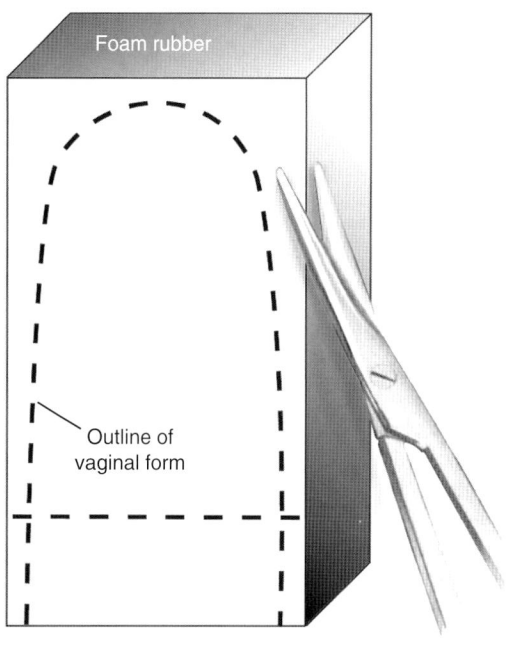

Foam rubber

Outline of
vaginal form

H²

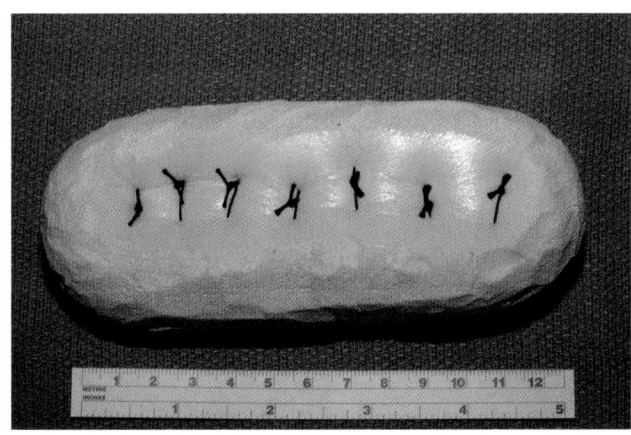

H³

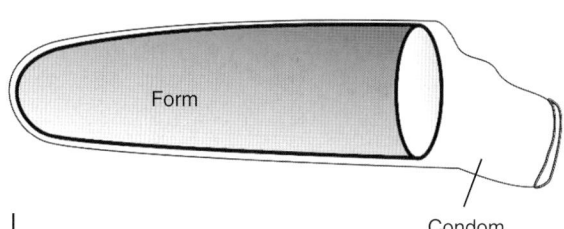

Form

I

Condom

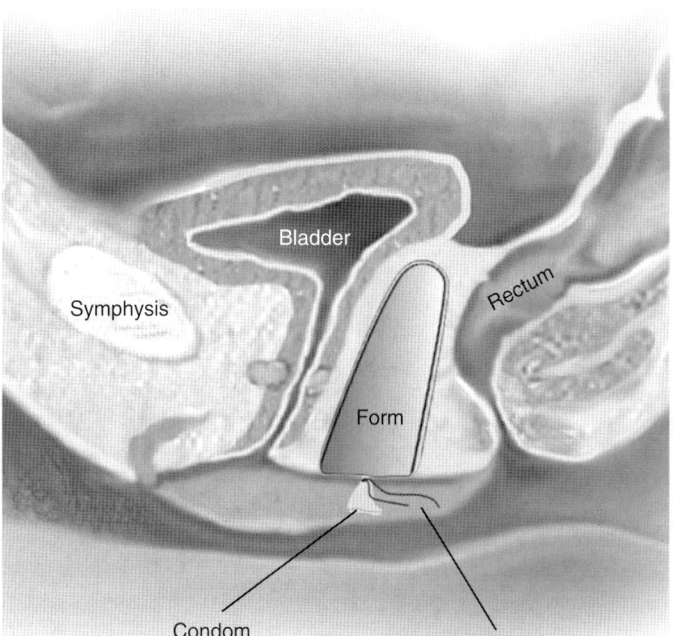

Bladder

Symphysis

Rectum

Form

Condom

Silk tie

J

**FIGURE 61–3, cont'd** **H.** A 10 × 10 × 20-cm sterile block of soft foam rubber is shaped according to the outline. The base is cut to accommodate the vaginal depth. The cut end is saved and later is used to protect the neovagina. **I.** A sterile condom is placed over the shaped vaginal form. **J.** After the form and the condom have been compressed, they are placed into the neovaginal space and allowed to expand for approximately 1 minute. A 2-0 silk tie is then secured at the base of the condom, and the form is removed. A second condom is placed over the first condom, and the base tied with 2-0 silk.

Next, a split-thickness skin graft is harvested. The patient is repositioned into a lateral position. After the harvest site is cleaned, sterile mineral oil is applied to the buttock. A 10-cm Padgett electrodermatome blade, set at 0.017 inch (0.45 mm), is used to obtain a 15- to 18-cm graft from the buttock inside the bikini (tan) line if possible (Fig. 61–3K). The graft site is covered with a sterile plastic adhesive sheet. The patient is then placed back in the lithotomy position.

Interrupted 5-0 absorbable nonreactive sutures are used to sew the graft over the vaginal form with the skin surface touching the form (Fig. 61–3L). During preparation of the graft, a suprapubic catheter is placed in the urinary bladder. The suprapubic catheter prevents pressure necrosis on the graft, which may occur with a urethral Foley catheter.

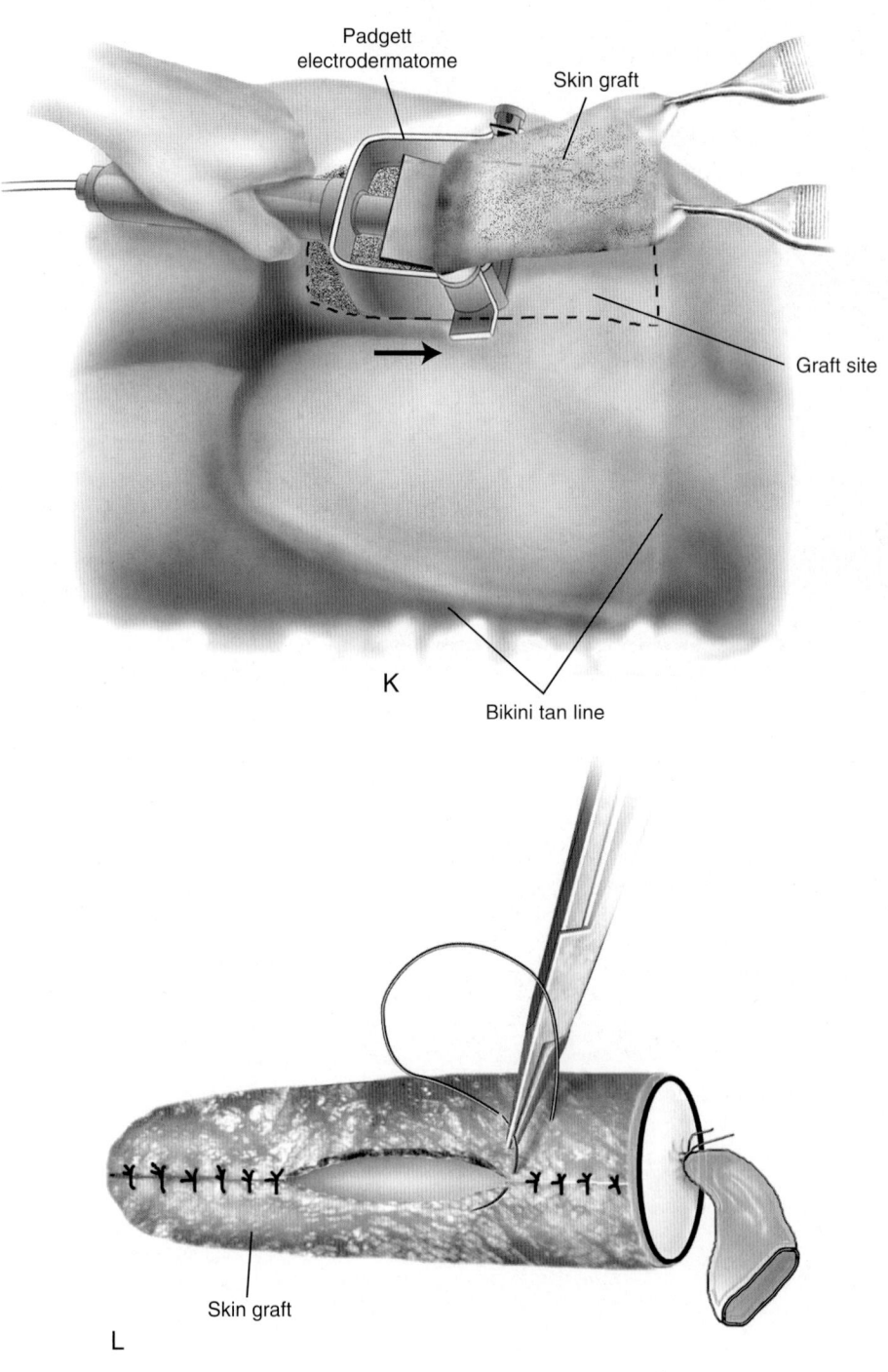

**FIGURE 61–3, cont'd  K.** The patient is placed in a lateral position. The buttock is prepped and draped, then is coated with sterile mineral oil. A Padgett electrodermatome with a 10-cm-wide blade is used to harvest a 0.45-mm-thick graft 15 to 18 cm long inside the bikini (tan) line if possible. **L.** The edges of the graft are approximated around the form with interrupted vertical mattress sutures of 5-0 polyglycolic acid. The skin surface touches the form.

After the edges are sutured, the graft and form are placed in the neovaginal space. The graft edges are sutured to the skin edges with 5-0 polyglycolic acid, allowing approximately 1 cm between suture sites to provide drainage of blood or serous fluid (Fig. 61–3M). A supporting foam pad is placed over the perineum and is anchored into place with labial sutures (Fig. 61–3N).

Postoperatively, the patient is kept on strict bedrest for 1 week. A constipating regimen of diphenoxylate-atropine (Lomotil) or codeine is prescribed, along with a low-residue diet. The patient is allowed to log roll but should be moved as a single unit to prevent "shearing" of the graft from the neovaginal walls. Pneumatic compression stockings are worn during the entire postoperative interval. Patient-controlled analgesia, administered by an epidural catheter placed preoperatively, provides for additional comfort and may improve compliance with bedrest.

After 1 week, the patient is brought back to the operating room. The vaginal form is removed and the vagina irrigated. The suprapubic catheter is removed. The graft is carefully inspected to assess viability. Small nonviable areas can be excised and allowed to heal by granulation. However, repeat skin grafting is necessary with large necrotic areas or total failure of the graft.

Postoperative compliance with dilation is essential. The form is removed daily to allow a warm-water douche. It is worn continuously for 2 to 4 weeks, then is used nightly. After healing is complete, rigid dilation may be necessary until the patient initiates sexual activity. Intercourse may be possible 4 to 8 weeks after surgery. Approximately 80% of women report long-term satisfaction after McIndoe vaginoplasty. Ninety percent are sexually active, and 75% are able to achieve orgasm.

Several alternatives to skin grafting have been proposed, including barrier products to prevent adhesions (Interceed), artificial dermis, autologous buccal mucosa, and simply allowing the neovaginal space to heal by secondary intention. The adhesion barrier is used to cover the vaginal form after creation of the neovaginal space, and skin grafting is avoided. However, we have seen severe contracture and scarring of the neovagina in a patient referred after this approach, and these alternatives cannot be recommended.

The Vecchietti procedure is a surgical alternative to passive dilation and the McIndoe vaginoplasty and is the preferred approach in some European centers. The Vecchietti procedure is performed by placing progressive tension on abdominal sutures that are attached to an olive-shaped device at the perineum. This method was originally performed during laparotomy, but a laparoscopic approach provides comparable outcomes and a faster recovery.

Like the McIndoe vaginoplasty, the Vecchietti procedure should be performed only when passive dilation is unsuccessful, and when the patient is physically and emotionally prepared for the surgery and anticipates intercourse in the not too distant future. However, it may be considered a primary approach if laparoscopy or laparotomy is required for other indications such as pelvic pain.

Special instruments required for the Vecchietti procedure include a 2.2 × 1.9-cm acrylic "olive," an abdominal traction device, and a long perineum suture passer (Fig. 61–3O). An alligator-jaw needle passer is also helpful. The laparoscope is placed through the umbilicus. An additional port is placed approximately 2 to 3 cm above the symphysis. A #2 polyglycolic acid suture is passed through the olive, and both free ends of the suture are placed in a long needle passer (Fig. 61–3P). Concurrent cystoscopy is performed, and one finger is placed in the rectum to ensure that the bladder and the bowel are not punctured during the procedure. The long needle is inserted through the perineum and the vesicorectal space into the peritoneal cavity under direct laparoscopic visualization (Fig. 61–3Q). The free ends of the suture are removed from the needle with graspers placed through the suprapubic port, and the needle is removed from the perineum.

The Vecchietti traction device is placed 2 to 3 cm above the symphysis, and a marking pen is used to identify the sites in the right and left lower quadrants where the sutures will be passed through the abdominal wall (see Fig. 61–3Q). The traction device is removed temporarily, and a needle passer is placed through the marked skin into the abdomen. One end of the suture is grasped with the needle passer, and the suture is pulled through the skin (see Fig 61–3Q). This procedure is repeated through the left lower quadrant, so that both ends of the suture are removed through the abdomen.

The sutures are attached to the Vecchietti traction device (Fig 61–3R). Traction is applied to allow downward movement of the olive of 1 cm with countertraction. Tension should be equal on both sides of the device. Excessive traction may cause tissue necrosis, and inadequate traction will not accomplish vaginal lengthening.

Patients are hospitalized for 2 to 3 days, then are seen every day or every other day after discharge until adequate depth has been attained. Tension on the traction sutures is adjusted every 24 to 48 hours, at a maximal daily rate of 1.0 to 1.5 cm. Using constant pressure allows creation of a 7- to 10-cm vagina within 7 to 9 days in most cases. Early ambulation is believed to accelerate vaginal dilation by increasing traction on the olive with contraction of the rectus muscles.

All patients require analgesics for perineal pain as suture tension is increased. A serosanguineous discharge related to tension on the olive is normal during this stage.

The sutures are removed during heavy sedation or general anesthesia after vaginal dilation of at least 7 cm is achieved. Postoperatively, a soft latex 1.5-cm-diameter, 10-cm dilator is used continuously for approximately 8 to 10 hours daily during the first month. The patient gradually advances to larger dilators, first 2.0 cm followed by 2.5 cm. Intercourse may be allowed beginning 20 days after the olive is removed. Long-term sexual satisfaction is greater than 80% with this approach, which is comparable with passive dilation and the McIndoe vaginoplasty.

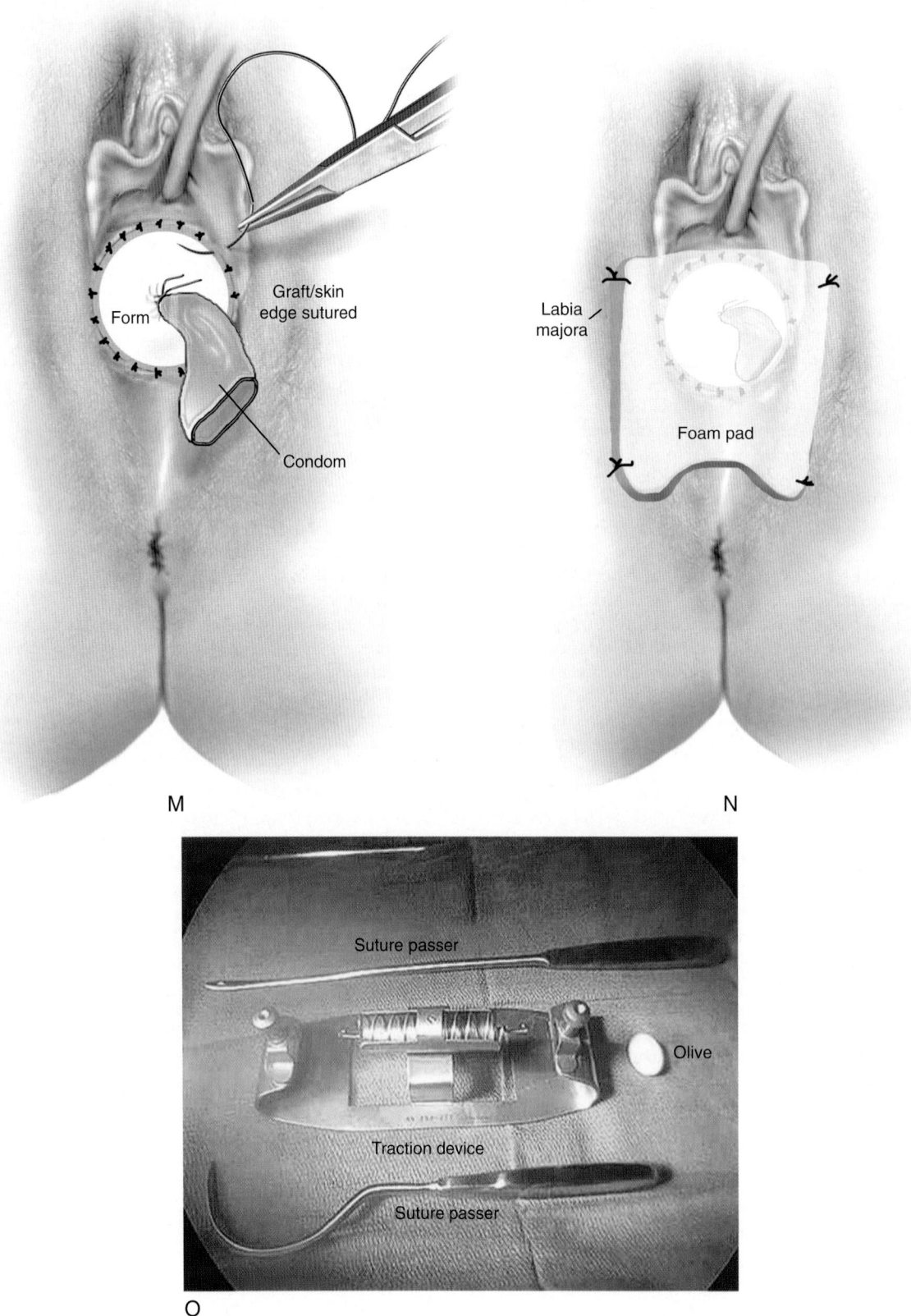

**FIGURE 61–3, cont'd   M.** The form and the covering graft are placed into the neovaginal space. The edges of the graft are sutured to the perineal skin with interrupted absorbable suture material, approximately 1 cm apart, to allow drainage. **N.** A foam pad is placed over the perineum and is secured into the labia minora with 0 silk suture. A gap is cut near the anus to avoid contamination of the pad during a bowel movement. **O.** Instruments required for the Vecchietti vaginoplasty include a 2.2 × 1.9-cm acrylic "olive," an abdominal traction device, a long perineum suture passer, and an alligator-jaw needle passer.

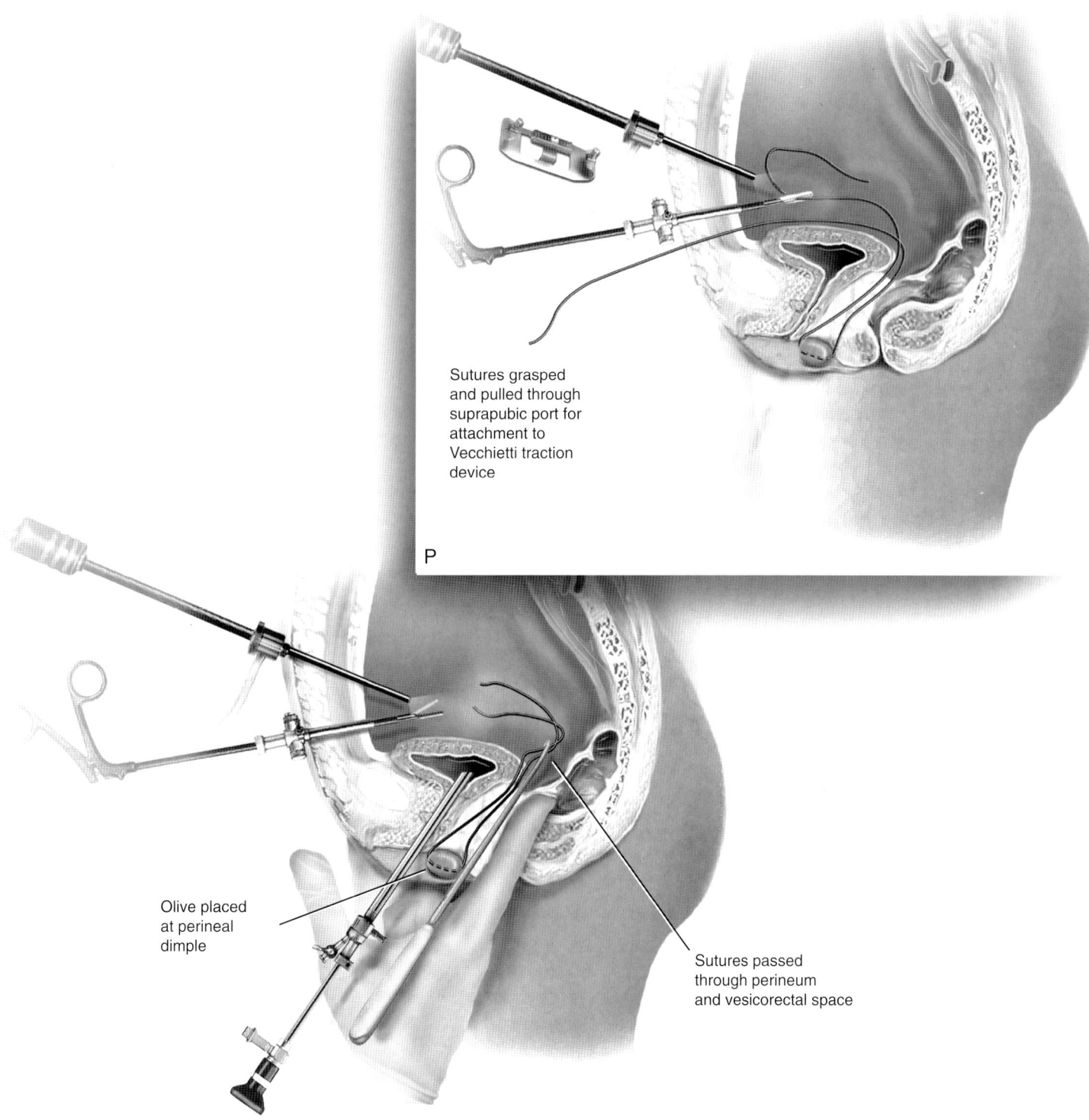

Sutures grasped
and pulled through
suprapubic port for
attachment to
Vecchietti traction
device

P

Olive placed
at perineal
dimple

Sutures passed
through perineum
and vesicorectal space

Q

**FIGURE 61–3, cont'd** **P.** A #2 polyglycolic acid suture is passed through the olive, and both free ends of the suture are placed in a long needle passer. **Q.** A laparoscope is placed through the umbilicus, and a secondary port is inserted above the symphysis. Concurrent cystoscopy is performed, and one finger is placed into the rectum to identify puncture of the bladder or bowel. The long needle passer is inserted from the perineum into the peritoneal cavity under direct laparoscopic visualization. A suture passer is placed through the skin into the abdomen in the right lower quadrant, approximately 2 to 3 cm above the symphysis. One end of the suture is grasped and pulled through the skin. This procedure is repeated through the left lower quadrant, so that both ends of the suture are removed through the abdomen.

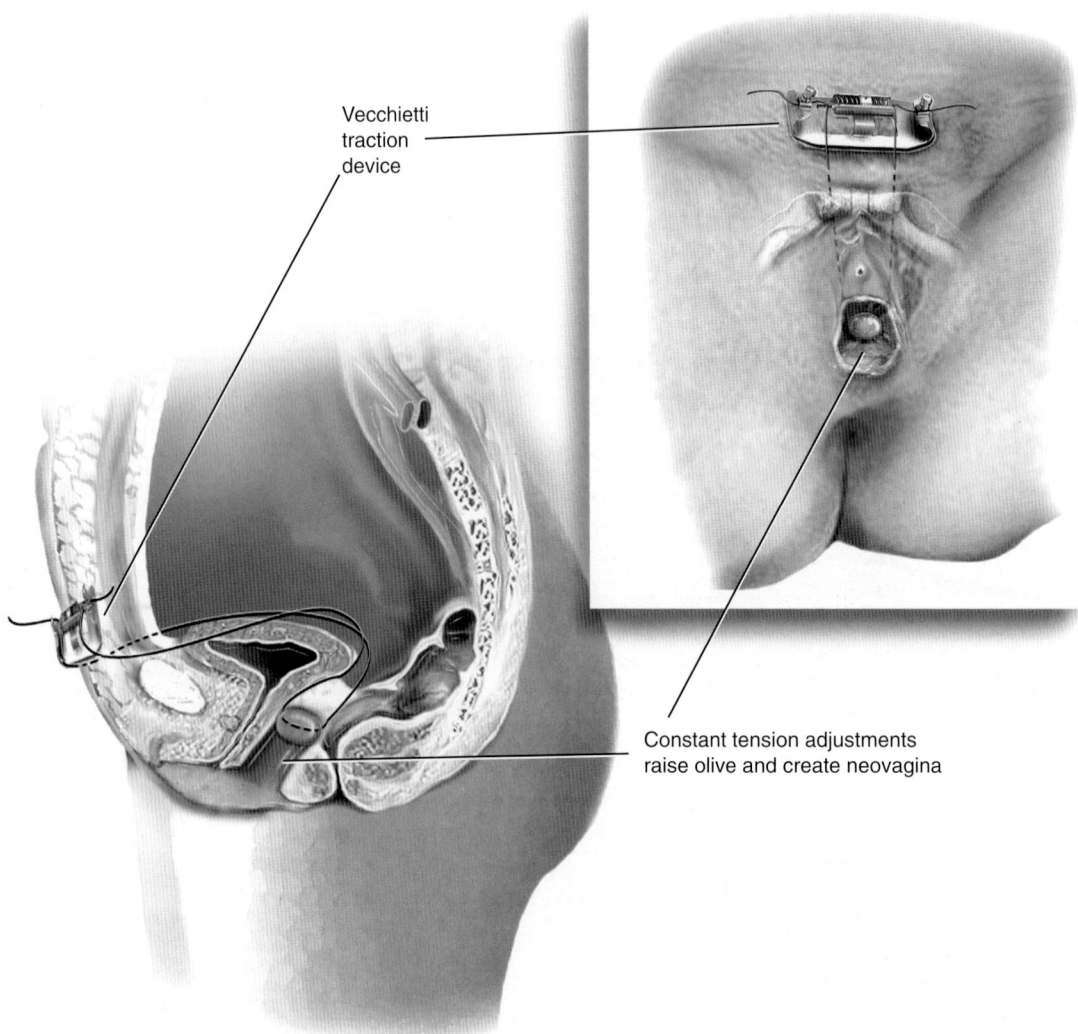

Vecchietti
traction
device

Constant tension adjustments
raise olive and create neovagina

R

**FIGURE 61–3, cont'd  R.** The sutures are attached to the Vecchietti device, and traction is applied to allow downward movement of the olive of 1 cm with countertraction. Tension should be equal on both sides of the device. Within 7 to 9 days, a 10- to 12-cm vagina is created.

## Transverse Vaginal Septum

The patient with a transverse vaginal septum typically presents with progressive pain and amenorrhea at the time of expected menses. Examination reveals a normal perineum, a blind vaginal pouch, and a palpable mass (the hematocolpos) during rectal examination.

Magnetic resonance imaging (MRI) should be done before surgery to determine the extent of the transverse vaginal septum, to confirm the presence of the cervix, and to evaluate the uterus (Fig. 61–4). Surgical resection of the septum is usually necessary soon after the diagnosis is established.

Temporizing measures to relieve pain and reduce the hematocolpos may be beneficial if MRI confirms a high transverse vaginal septum. The hematocolpos can be evacuated in the operating room under abdominal ultrasonographic guidance. After prophylactic antibiotics have been administered, a large-bore (12- to 14-gauge) needle is placed into the hematocolpos under abdominal ultrasonographic visualization (Fig. 61–5). The fluid is extremely viscous, and saline irrigation may be required repeatedly to evacuate the blood (Fig. 61–6). With persistence, the clot can be broken up and the fluid eventually completely evacuated. After this, a regimen to reduce uterine bleeding is initiated, such as Depo-Provera, continuous oral contraceptives, or gonadotropin-releasing hormone analogues. Emergent decompression allows for vaginal dilation. Dilation of the lower vagina improves the chances for a direct anastomosis of the upper and lower vaginal mucosa.

Surgical resection of a transverse vaginal septum may present an unexpected challenge to an inexperienced surgeon. First, a cruciate incision is made at the vaginal opening and the connective tissue is bluntly dissected toward the hematocolpos. Occasionally, it may be difficult to locate the upper vagina. If this is a problem, abdominal ultrasonography can be performed to identify the hematocolpos (Fig. 61–7). Once the upper vagina is visualized with ultrasound, a needle is passed into the upper vagina (Fig. 61–8A). If small, the hematocolpos can be distended to enlarge the upper vagina. An incision is made along the needle tract into the upper vagina.

Laparotomy may be necessary if the upper vagina still cannot be visualized. A probe is placed through the uterine fundus, through the cervix, and into the upper vagina (Fig. 61–8B). With this probe used as a guide, the upper vagina can be readily identified and opened without risk of injury to the bowel or bladder.

Once open, the septum is progressively dilated with cervical dilators. A transverse incision is made to increase the width of the vagina. Next, the upper and lower vaginal mucosa is reanastomosed transversely with interrupted 3-0 nonreactive absorbable sutures (Fig. 61–8C). If needed, the upper and lower vaginal mucosal edges are undermined and mobilized to bring down the tissues.

A Z-plasty repair may be beneficial if there is a wide gap between the lower and upper vagina (Fig. 61–8D). This approach allows anastomosis with minimal shortening of the vagina. The upper vagina must be identified, as discussed previously (see Figs. 61–7, 61–8). After the initial incision connects the lower and upper vagina, a balloon catheter is placed into the upper vagina to provide traction and orientation. An X-shaped incision is made at the apex of the lower vagina. The shape of the incision avoids extension of the incision into the bladder or rectum. The edges of the flaps are tagged with 3-0 nonreactive absorbable sutures. The lower vaginal flaps are mobilized by dissecting the connective tissue from the mucosa. Next, the connective tissue between the lower and upper vaginal tubes is resected laterally. The upper vaginal mucosa is mobilized and opened with an X-shaped incision. The edges of the upper vaginal flaps are tagged with suture. The Z-plasty is completed by suturing the tagged edge of the lower flaps to the base of the upper flaps, then suturing the edge of the upper flaps to the base of the lower flaps. The remaining vaginal mucosa is approximated with interrupted absorbable sutures.

When the gap between the upper and lower vagina is too large to accommodate these closures, skin grafting from the buttock may be necessary. The graft is prepared as described for the McIndoe vaginoplasty, but the length is limited to the size needed to approximate the upper and lower vaginal edges. The graft is then sutured to the upper vagina with simple interrupted sutures of 4-0 polyglycolic acid, then to the lower vagina. The redundant tissue is excised.

Alternatively, when a small gap between the upper and lower vagina cannot be approximated, a Neoprene dilator with a hollow center to allow cervical drainage may be placed in the vagina. Eventually, stratified squamous epithelium covers the denuded area.

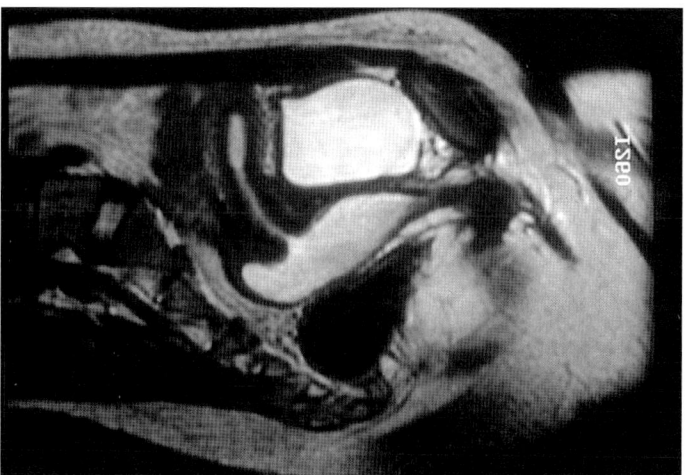

FIGURE 61–4 Magnetic resonance image of a patient with a large transverse vaginal septum. The hematocolpos is white. The vagina communicates with the uterus, and a hematometrium is evident.

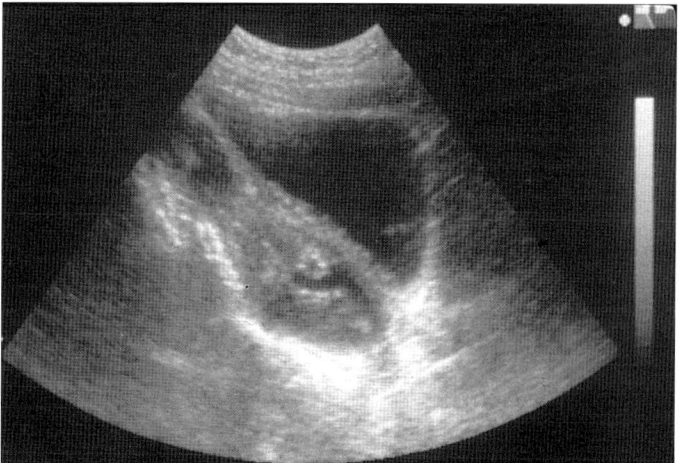

FIGURE 61–5 Hematocolpos caused by a transverse vaginal septum is seen with abdominal ultrasound (midline sagittal). Ultrasound-directed placement of a large-bore needle from the lower vagina, followed by persistent flushing and drainage, will eventually decompress the hematocolpos. This approach may increase the risk of upper genital tract infection and is appropriate only when a large transverse vaginal septum is present, and when the patient will benefit from dilation of the lower vagina before resection of the septum and anastomosis.

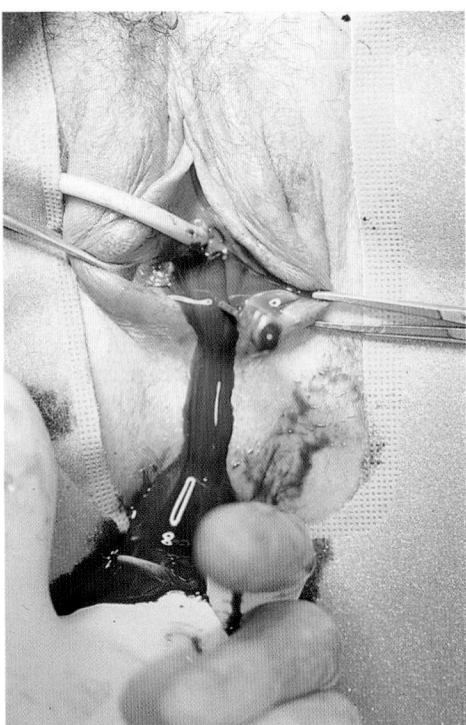

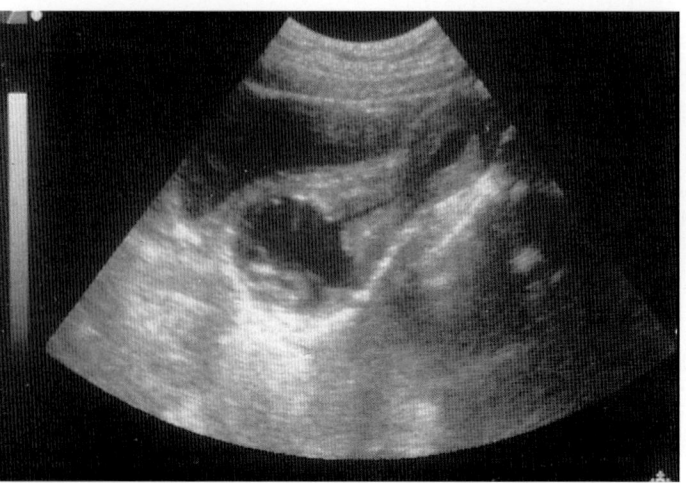

**FIGURE 61–7** Abdominal ultrasound (midline sagittal) is used to identify the upper vagina after the bladder is filled with saline. Here, a complex hematocolpos is identified inferior to the cervix and uterus.

**FIGURE 61–6** The septum has been incised, and the pent-up viscous blood and mucus drains from the vagina. The operator's left finger has been inserted into the rectum. The guide, a 16-gauge needle, is noted just to the patient's left (of the flowing dark blood).

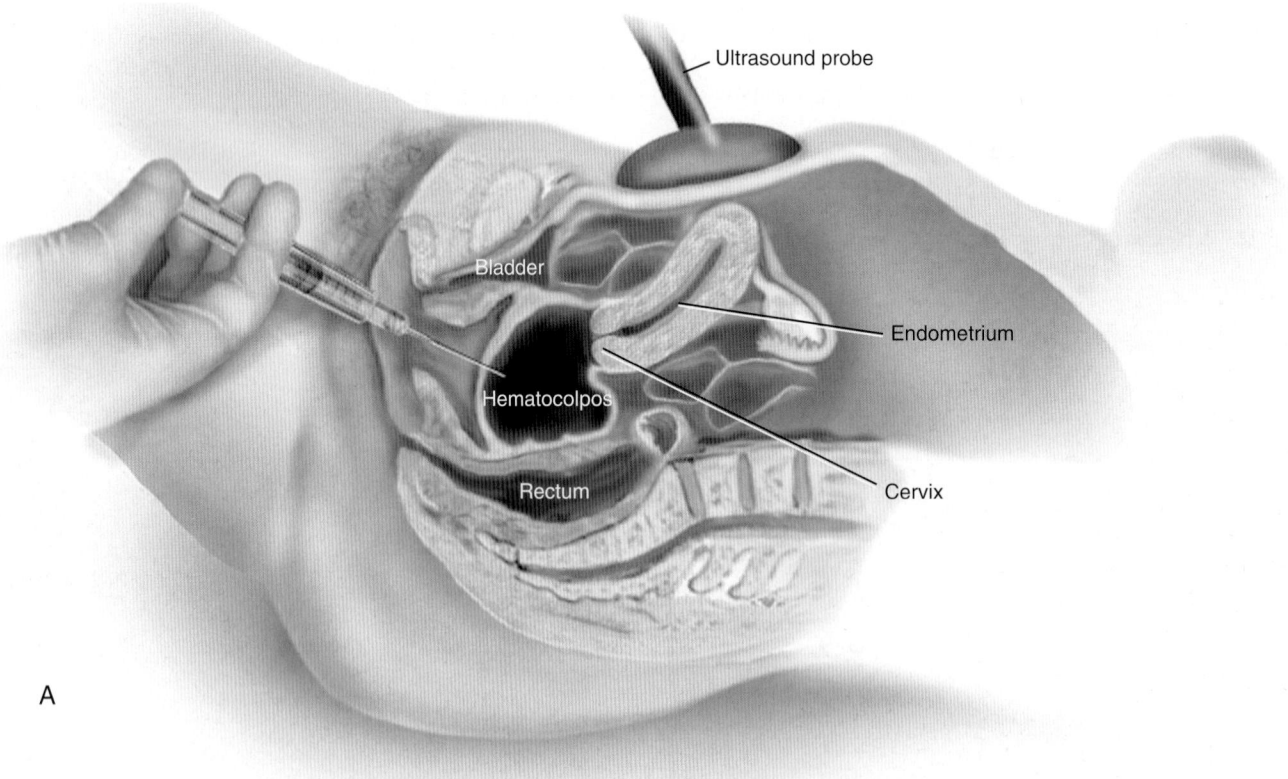

A

**FIGURE 61–8 A.** A needle is passed from the lower vagina into the hematocolpos under abdominal ultrasound guidance when the upper vagina cannot be identified after dissection.

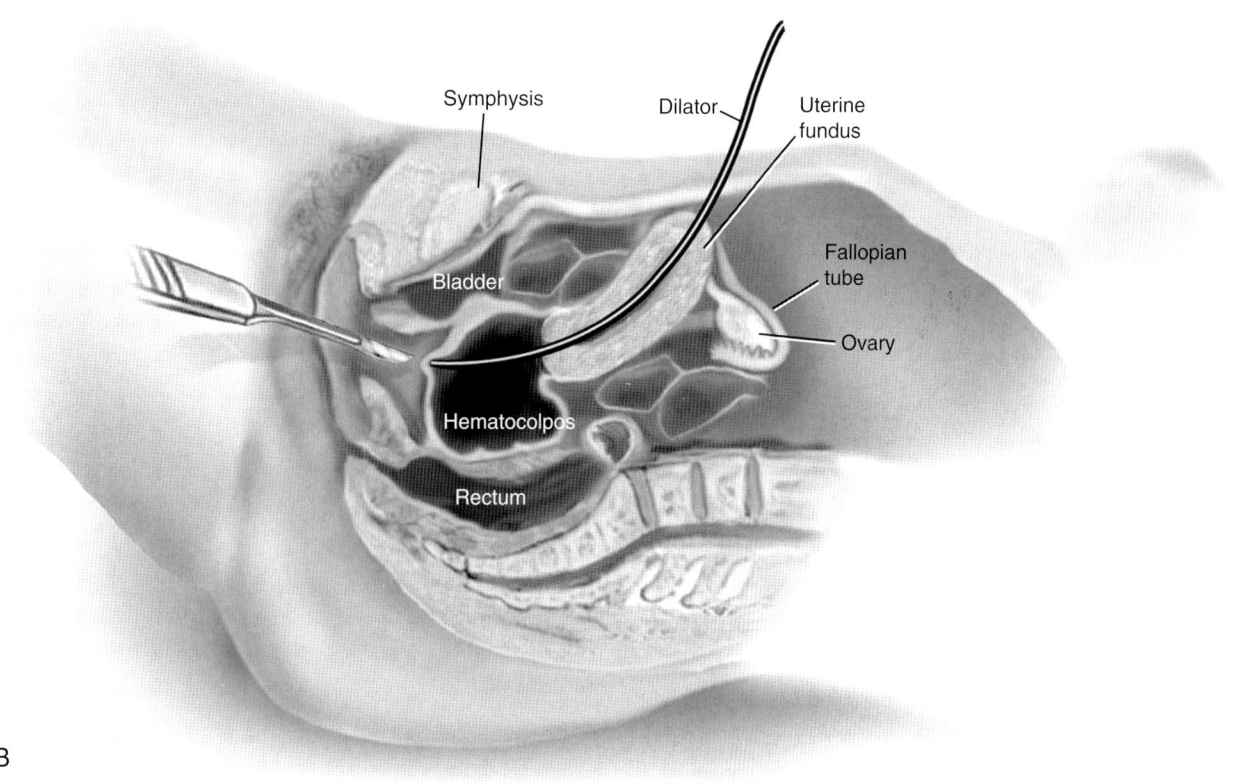

B

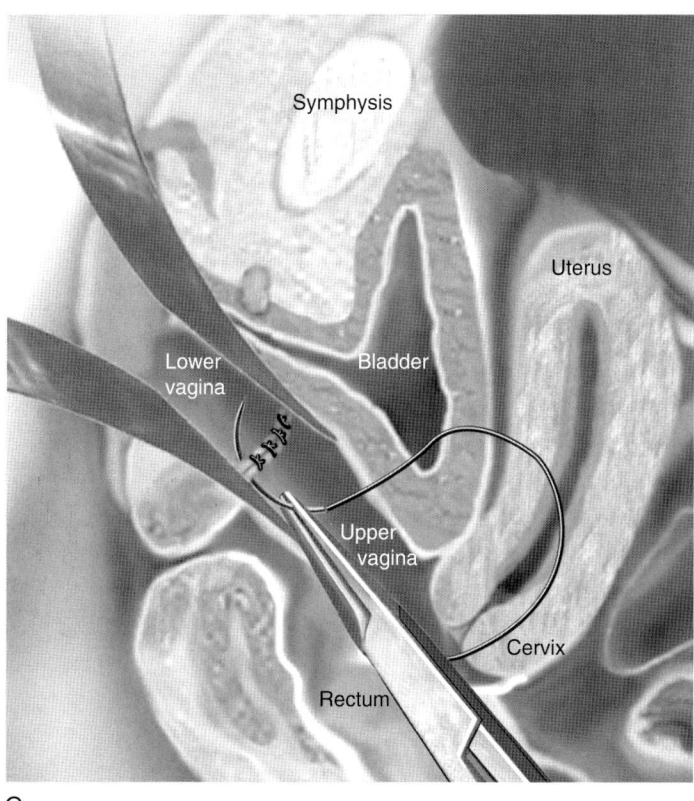

C

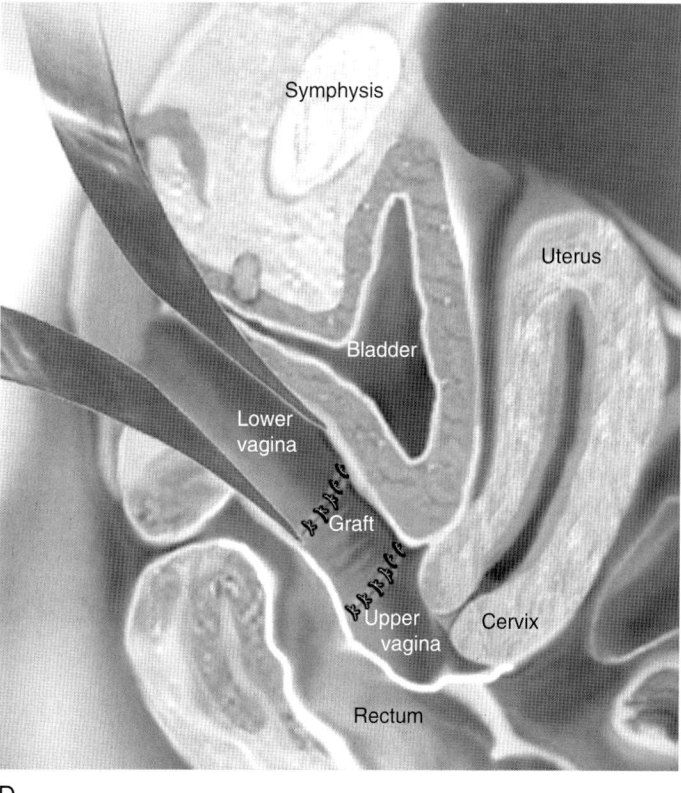

D

**FIGURE 61–8, cont'd B.** Laparotomy is necessary when the upper vagina cannot be identified after surgical exploration or with the use of abdominal ultrasound. After the abdomen has been opened, a long cervical dilator or uterine sound is passed through the fundus into the uterine cavity and cervix. Pressure is placed against the upper vagina. The rigid dilator is identified vaginally. The upper vaginal mucosa is sharply entered. **C.** The upper and lower vaginal mucosal edges are approximated with interrupted 3-0 nonreactive, delayed absorbable sutures. **D.** A split-thickness skin graft may be used when the upper and lower vaginal edges cannot be approximated. An appropriately sized graft is harvested from the buttock and is sutured into place. A foam pad covered with a sterile condom can be placed into the vagina, as described for a McIndoe vaginoplasty, to provide maximal contact of the graft with the paravaginal connective tissue.

UNIT 3 ■ SECTION B

## Longitudinal Vaginal Septum

A longitudinal vaginal septum is usually asymptomatic, although some women may complain of dyspareunia or leakage when using tampons, and a septum may tear during vaginal birth. A longitudinal vaginal septum is caused by failure of distal vaginal cannulation; it is usually accompanied by cervical duplication. Repair is not required in asymptomatic patients. However, some women may request resection of the septum to enable the use of tampons and to prevent rupture during delivery.

The septum is exposed for surgery by placing two fingers or two narrow retractors in each side of the vaginal septum and retracting posteriorly (Fig. 61–9). A Haney or Kelly clamp is placed across the septum near the anterior and posterior vaginal walls. Bladder injury is avoided by leaving a small segment of the septum on the anterior wall. If the septum is narrow, the central aspect is cut, and each wall is sutured with absorbable suture. If the septum is wide, excess tissue may be excised. The dissection continues until the upper vagina near the cervix has been divided. However, complete excision of the upper vaginal septum is often unnecessary.

## Obstructed Hemivagina

An adolescent with a double uterus and cervix typically presents with severe pain caused by an obstructed hemivagina. The obstruction is caused by canalization failure and failure to absorb the vaginal septum. A high incidence of renal anomalies has been noted on the side of the obstructed hemivagina. A hematocolpos forms in the obstructed hemivagina with menarche, and each episode of bleeding from the ipsilateral hemiuterus causes additional distention and pain (Fig. 61–10). A pelvic mass is identified during pelvic and rectal examination. On speculum examination, the nonobstructed cervix may not be visible, especially if the vagina is greatly distorted from a large hematocolpos from the contralateral obstruction. Findings on vaginal ultrasonography may be confusing because the obstructed hematocolpos is found inferior to the nonobstructed cervix. The diagnosis can be made with abdominal ultrasonography and confirmed with MRI if needed.

The initial incision is most important for safe resection of the obstructed hemivagina. A deep lateral incision made in the distended hemivagina should be followed by an immediate release of dark blood from the hematocolpos. Although the mass should be easily identified by palpation of the distended cystic mass and the bulge into the vagina, abdominal ultrasonography may be used to ensure that the initial incision is made into the hematocolpos. After release of the hematocolpos, the vagina is irrigated. The vaginal septum superior to the initial incision site is then resected as described for the longitudinal vaginal septum. The entire inferior margin of the vaginal septum is resected to avoid formation of a vaginal pocket. A residual pocket may trap menstrual blood and cervical secretions and cause bothersome intermenstrual bleeding or discharge.

## Bladder Exstrophy

A variant of the exstrophy-epispadias complex, bladder exstrophy is a rare defect that occurs in 1:30,000 to 1:50,000 live births. Bladder exstrophy is characterized by (1) absence of the lower anterior abdominal wall in the midline, (2) an absent anterior bladder wall, such that the posterior bladder wall and ureters open directly into the abdominal wall defect, (3) wide separation of the rectus muscles, (4) absence of the symphysis pubis and wide separation of the pubic rami connected by a bridge of fibrous tissues(s), (5) separation of the clitoris into two bodies and division of the pubic hair and mons, (6) a poorly defined bladder neck and a short patulous urethra, and (7) an anteriorly displaced vagina and anus with a short perineum and deficient pelvic floor musculature. These defects are thought to be due to overdevelopment of the cloacal membrane, which does not permit migration of the anterior abdominal wall mesoderm. The cloacal membrane is left unsupported and subsequently ruptures, leading to lack of lower abdominal wall development. The condition necessitates multiple reconstructive surgeries throughout childhood to preserve bladder function and continence. Numerous procedures have been used in the past to facilitate urinary diversion, with ureterosigmoidostomy probably being the most common (Fig. 61–11A). However, primary bladder closure, with or without osteotomy, later followed by bladder neck reconstruction and bilateral ureteroneocystostomy, is currently the most common sequence of urologic operations performed. A significant number of these women develop a significant pelvic organ prolapse, especially those who have experienced childbirth. Figure 61–11B through D demonstrates a posthysterectomy vault prolapse in a woman with bladder exstrophy. Previously mentioned vaginal abnormalities are seen.

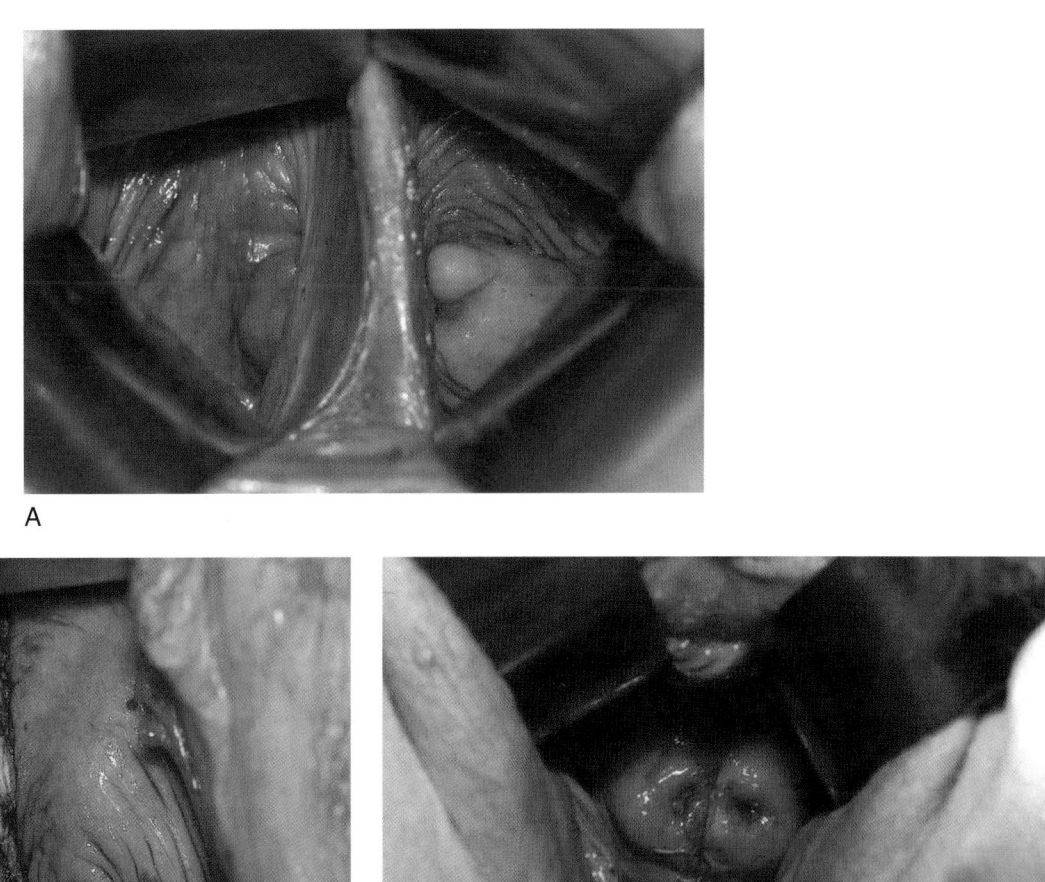

A

B

C

**FIGURE 61-9 A.** Two narrow, curved retractors are placed on each side of the vaginal septum and retracted posteriorly. A curved Kelly clamp is placed across the septum on the anterior and posterior walls. **B.** The septum is cut, and each wall is sutured with absorbable suture. If the septum is wide, excess tissue may be excised. **C.** The dissection continues until the upper vagina near the cervix has been divided. However, complete excision of the upper vaginal septum is not necessary.

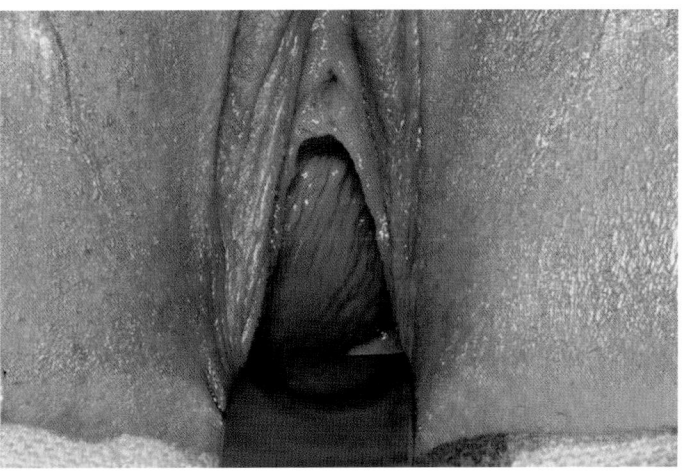

**FIGURE 61-10** This patient had uterine didelphys with a right-sided vaginal mass, which represents an obstructed right hemivagina. She presented with vaginal and abdominal pain in the setting of regular menses (occurring from the patent left hemivagina and uterus). Preoperative evaluation revealed an absent right kidney.

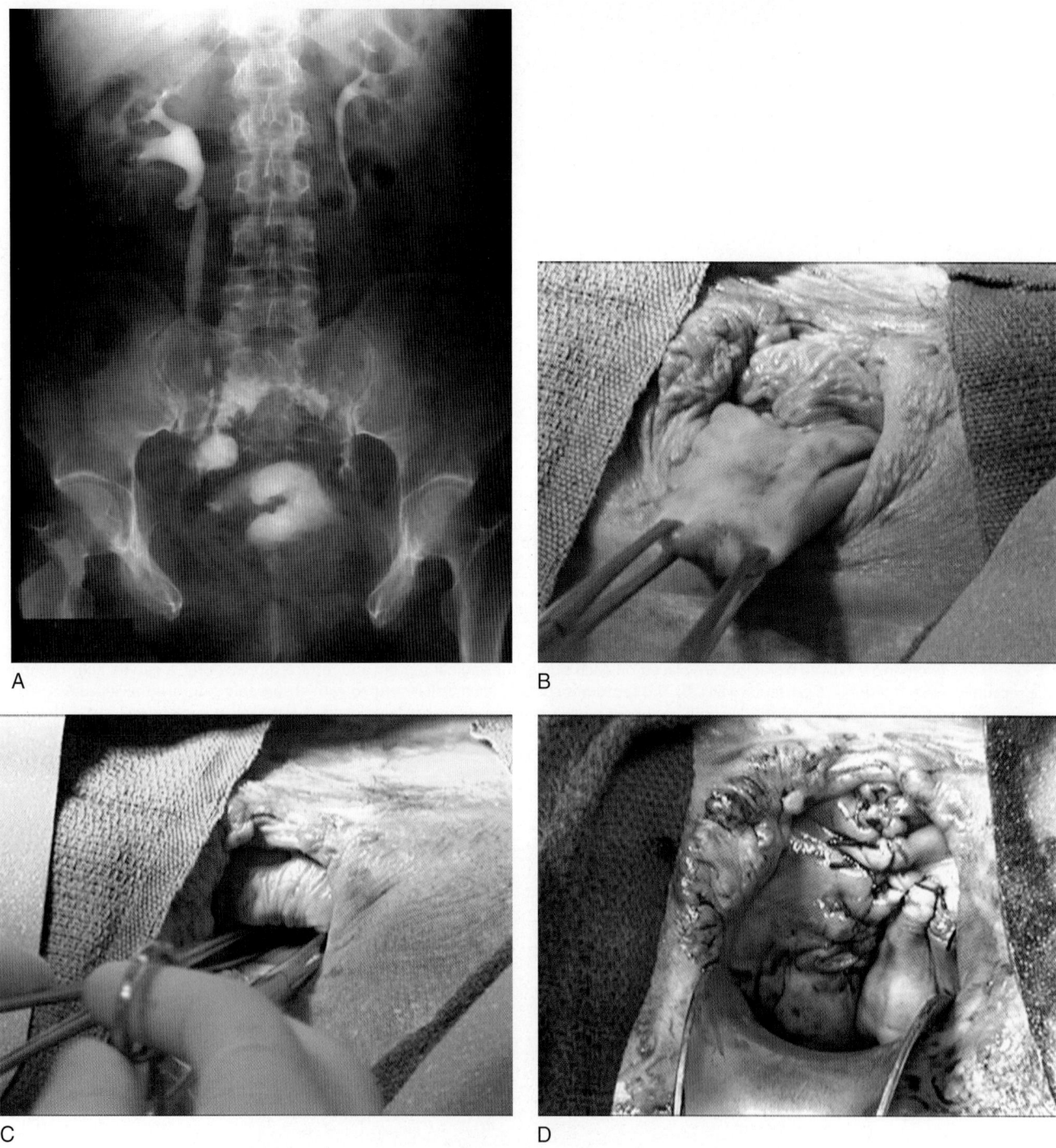

**FIGURE 61–11  A.** Intravenous pyelogram in a patient with bladder exstrophy who underwent bilateral ureterosigmoidostomy. **B.** Complete posthysterectomy vault prolapse in a patient with bladder exstrophy. **C.** The prolapse has been reduced in the posterior direction with two Allis clamps. **D.** The prolapse has been surgically corrected.

# CHAPTER 62

# Iatrogenic Vaginal Constriction

*John B. Gebhart* ■ *Mickey M. Karram*

## Introduction

Vaginal stricture may occur secondary to inflammatory conditions of the vagina, vaginal surgery, episiotomy repair, or radiotherapy. The surgical approach to the stenosis depends on its anatomic location, underlying cause, and severity. For introital or vaginal stenosis, the procedure can treat both upper and lower vaginal strictures or can correct lower vaginal strictures specifically. Operations that correct upper and lower vaginal strictures include incision of the vaginal constriction ring or ridge, vaginal advancement, Z-plasty, free skin graft, perineal flaps, and abdominal flaps. Restenosis risk is high after these interventions; therefore, postoperative care must include rigid dilation that is initiated immediately in the postoperative period.

## Incisions

The simplest approach to a vaginal constriction is a midline incision of the contracting scar or ridge. The midline incision is made, and the vaginal mucosa is mobilized from the underlying scar (Fig. 62–1). Excessive scar tissue may be excised completely to increase the vaginal or introital diameter. When hemostasis is achieved, the wound may be left to heal by secondary intention, or the vaginal tissue may be undermined and advanced and the incision closed transversely in a tension-free manner (Fig. 62–2). When a single midline incision with transverse closure is inadequate, numerous vertical incisions may be made (Fig. 62–3). Separate vertical incisions are closed transversely—after mobilization of surrounding vaginal tissues—to obtain sufficient introital or vaginal diameter (Fig. 62–4).

Figure 62–5A shows a midvaginal constriction ring after an overzealous anterior and posterior colporrhaphy. The stenotic site was initially enlarged with the use of Hegar dilators passed from the lower vaginal segment into the upper segment. When the vagina was dilated to at least 10 mm, bilateral longitudinal incisions were made in the lateral aspect of the stenotic site and were taken along the vaginal axis (Fig. 62–5B). The tight fibrous band was completely excised, and the dissection continued until loose connective tissue was encountered in the ischiorectal space (Fig. 62–5C). Some surgeons prefer to leave the space open; others prefer to close it transversely and perpendicular to the original incision, using interrupted, 3-0 absorbable sutures.

## Z-Plasty

The Z-plasty technique involves transplantation of two interdigitating triangular flaps. The orientation of the Z may be vertical or transverse, depending on the stricture. The degree of stenosis determines the incision length of the flap arms and the flap angles. Typically, the flaps are 2 cm long and at 60° angles. Additional diameter is gained by increasing the angle. The midpoint, or the site of the most severe contracture, is identified, and a transverse incision is made (this incision becomes the common limb of the Z-plasty). The upper arm of the Z is extended into the vagina; the lower arm is extended toward the perineum (Fig. 62–6). Scar tissue, if present, may be excised, and the transposed flaps are reapproximated with interrupted, 3-0 or 4-0 absorbable sutures (Fig. 62–7).

Introital stricture may be amenable to a transverse Z-plasty. This technique results in the absence of a midline suture line. Duplication of the flaps at the 4- and 8-o'clock positions of the introitus results in an increase in introital diameter (Fig. 62–8). Care must be taken to approximate the apices of the incisions and thereby to gain maximum transverse diameter. "Dog ears" should be trimmed and absorbable sutures used to produce a smooth approximation of tissues (Fig. 62–9).

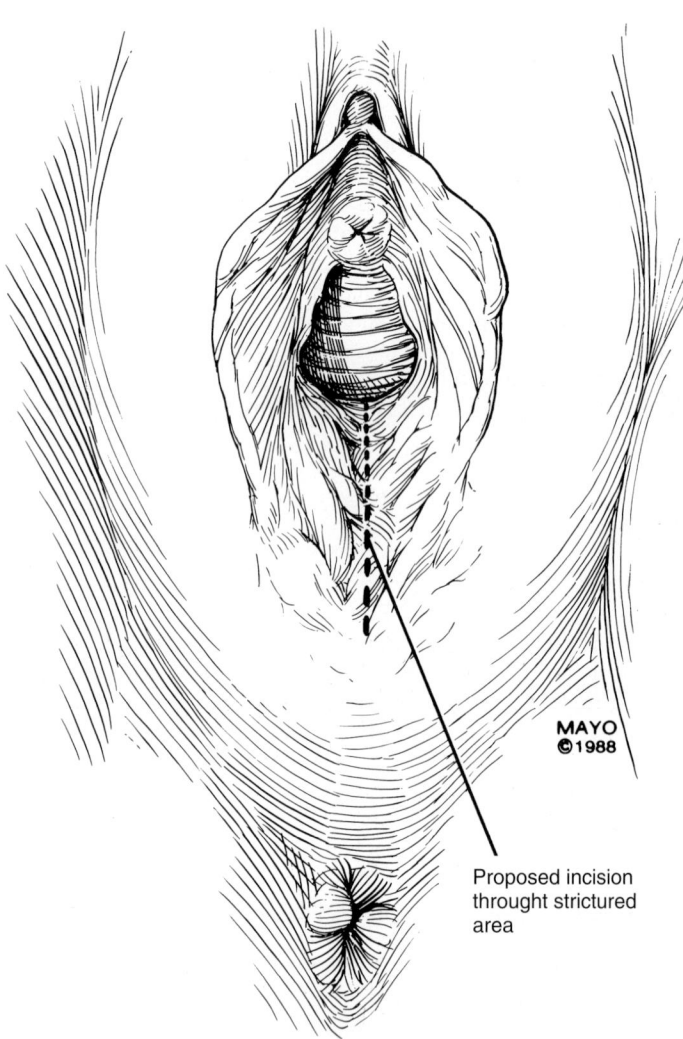

MAYO
©1988

Proposed incision
throught strictured
area

**FIGURE 62–1** A midline incision is made and the vaginal mucosa
is widely mobilized, excising the underlying scar tissue as needed.
(Adapted from Lee RA: Atlas of Gynecologic Surgery. Philadelphia,
WB Saunders, ©1992. Used with permission of Mayo Foundation for
Medical Education and Research.)

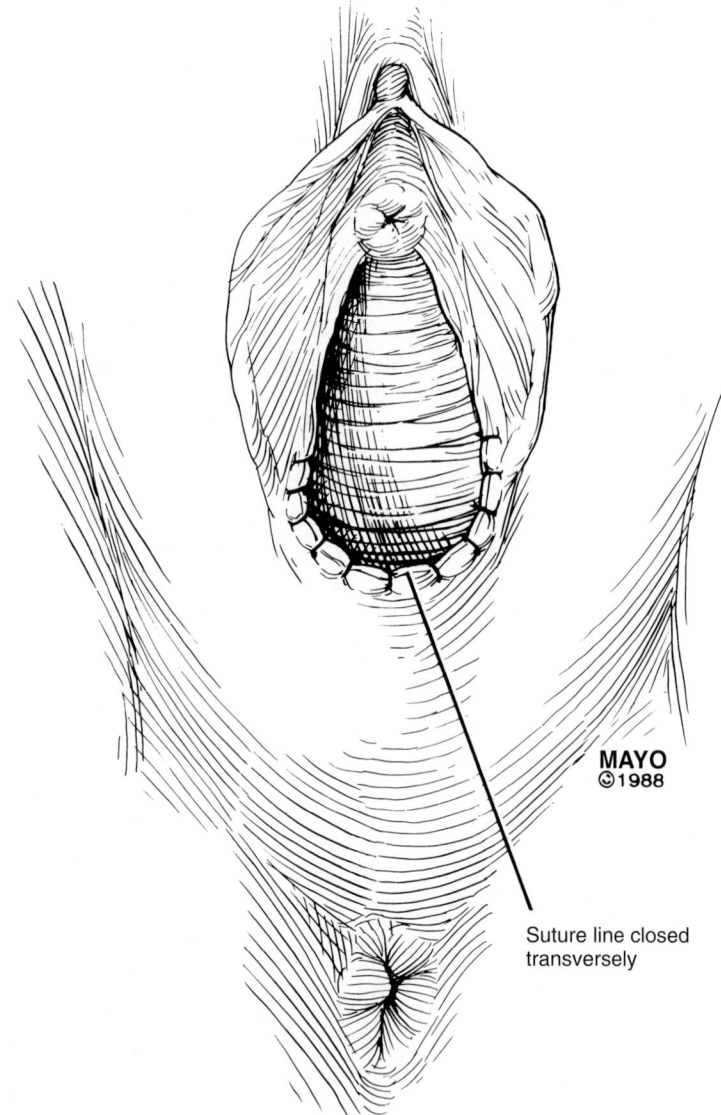

MAYO
©1988

Suture line closed
transversely

**FIGURE 62–2** To increase vaginal diameter, the initial vertical incision
is closed in a transverse manner. (Adapted from Lee RA: Atlas of
Gynecologic Surgery. Philadelphia, WB Saunders, ©1992. Used with
permission of Mayo Foundation for Medical Education and Research.)

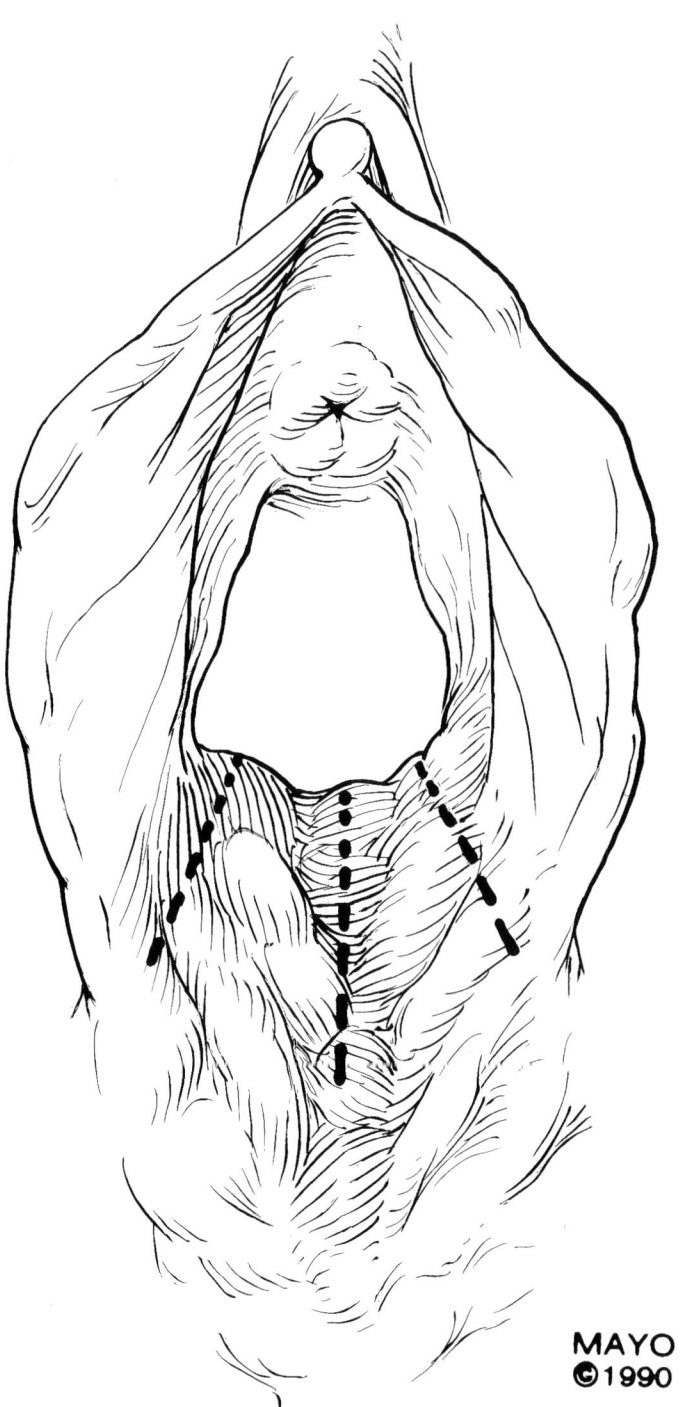

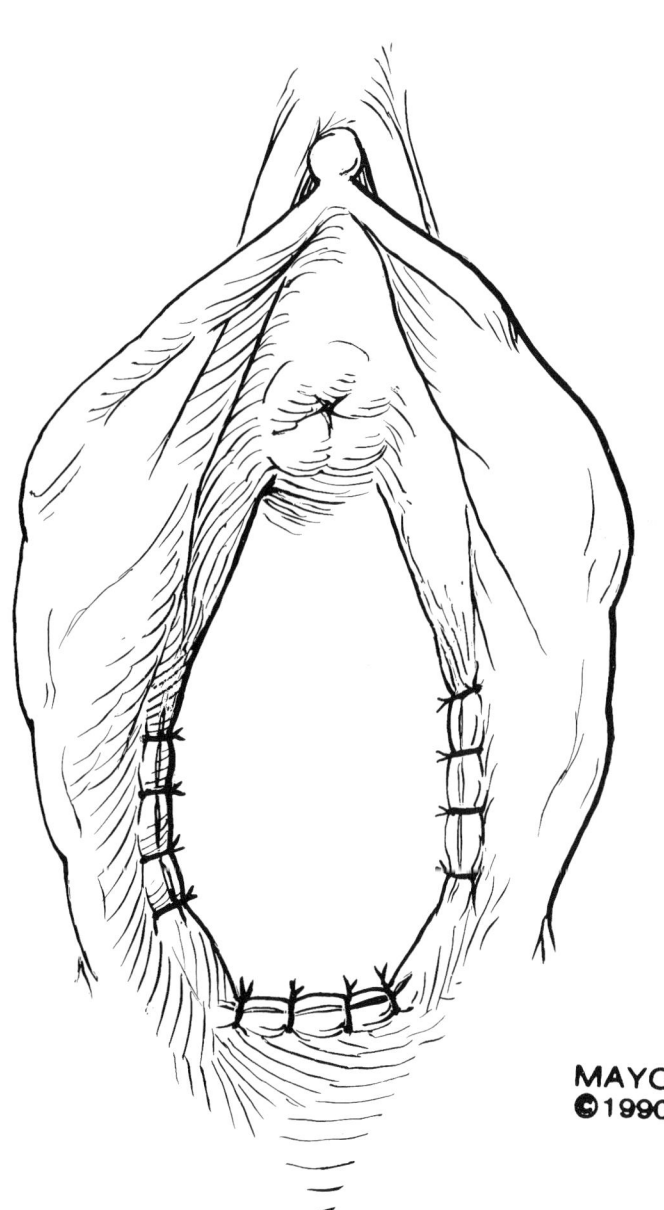

**FIGURE 62–3** In cases of broader areas of scarring and stenosis, numerous vertical incisions may be used. The surrounding tissues are mobilized, and excessive scar tissue is excised. (Adapted from Lee RA: Atlas of Gynecologic Surgery. Philadelphia, WB Saunders, ©1992. Used with permission of Mayo Foundation for Medical Education and Research.)

**FIGURE 62–4** Numerous vertical incisions may be converted to multiple transverse closures, thereby increasing the diameter at the area of stricture. (Adapted from Lee RA: Atlas of Gynecologic Surgery. Philadelphia, WB Saunders, ©1992. Used with permission of Mayo Foundation for Medical Education and Research.)

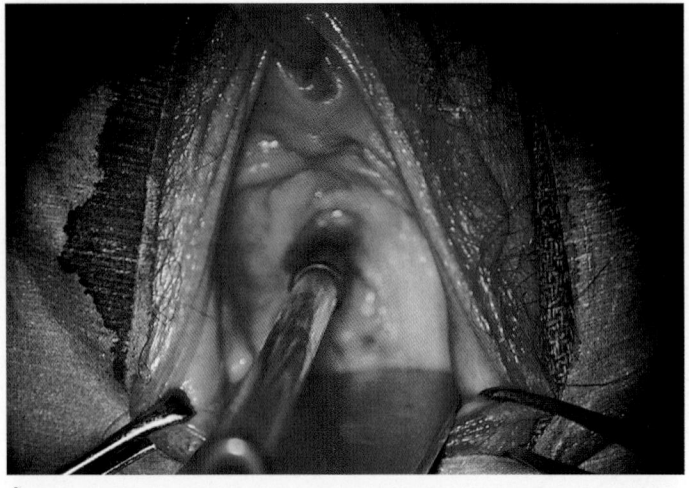

A

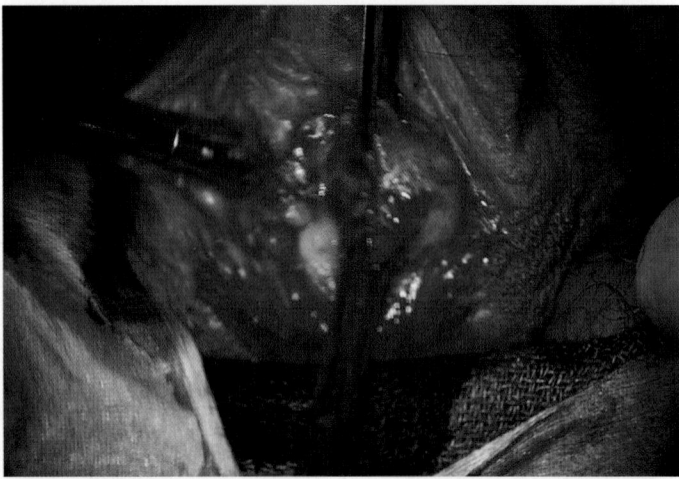

B

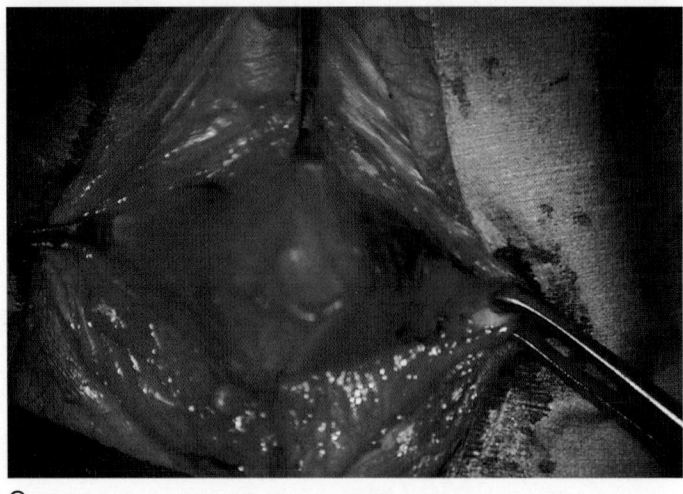

C

**FIGURE 62–5 A.** Midvaginal constriction ring that occurred after an overzealous anterior and posterior repair. The image shows the Hegar dilator in the small opening. **B.** Because the vagina was sufficient above this ring, bilateral relaxing incisions were performed to reopen the vagina. Allis clamps were used to grasp the ring in preparation for the incision. An incision was made at both 4 and 7 o'clock. **C.** The incisions were continued until the band was completely incised and loose areolar tissue was encountered. The incision was left open to heal by secondary intention.

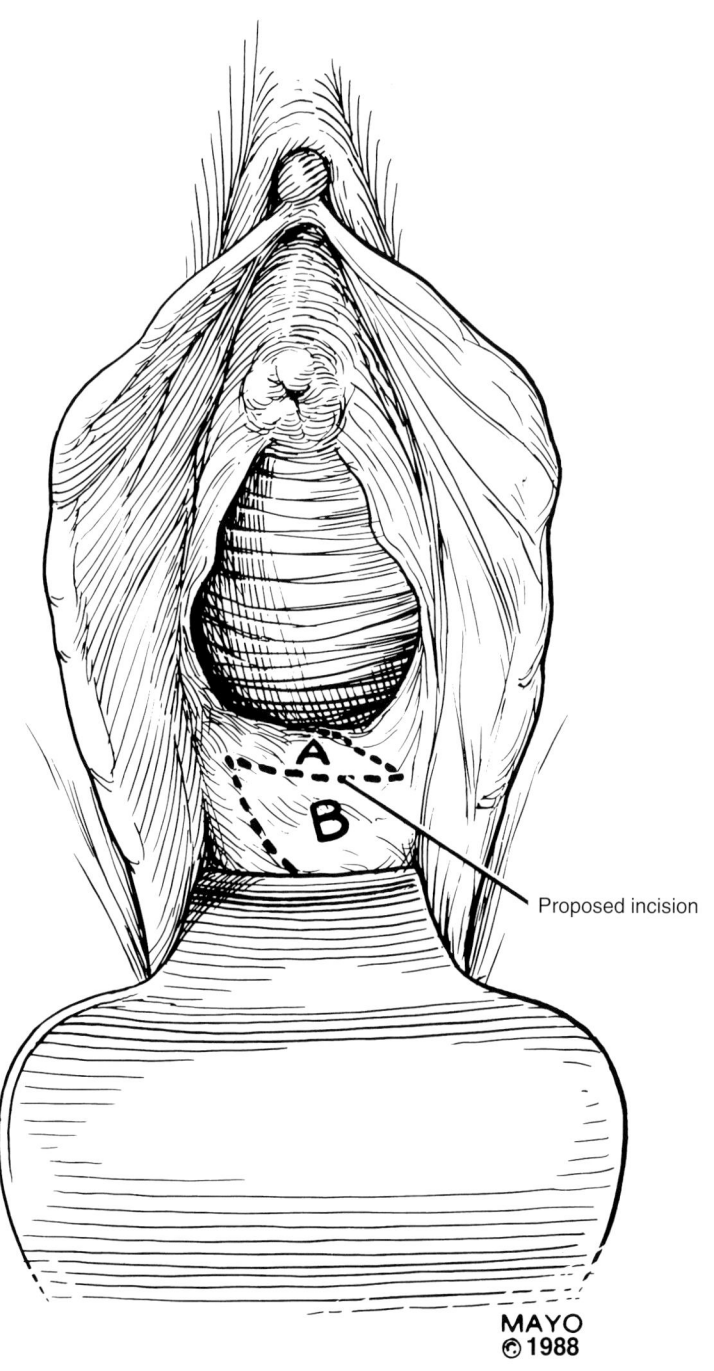

Proposed incision

MAYO
© 1988

**FIGURE 62–6** The midpoint of the scar is identified, and a transverse incision made. This incision site becomes the common arm of the Z-plasty. The upper arm of the Z is extended into the upper vagina; the lower arm of the Z is extended toward the perineum. The area of stricture determines the length and angle of the incisions. (Adapted from Lee RA: Atlas of Gynecologic Surgery. Philadelphia, WB Saunders, ©1992. Used with permission of Mayo Foundation for Medical Education and Research.)

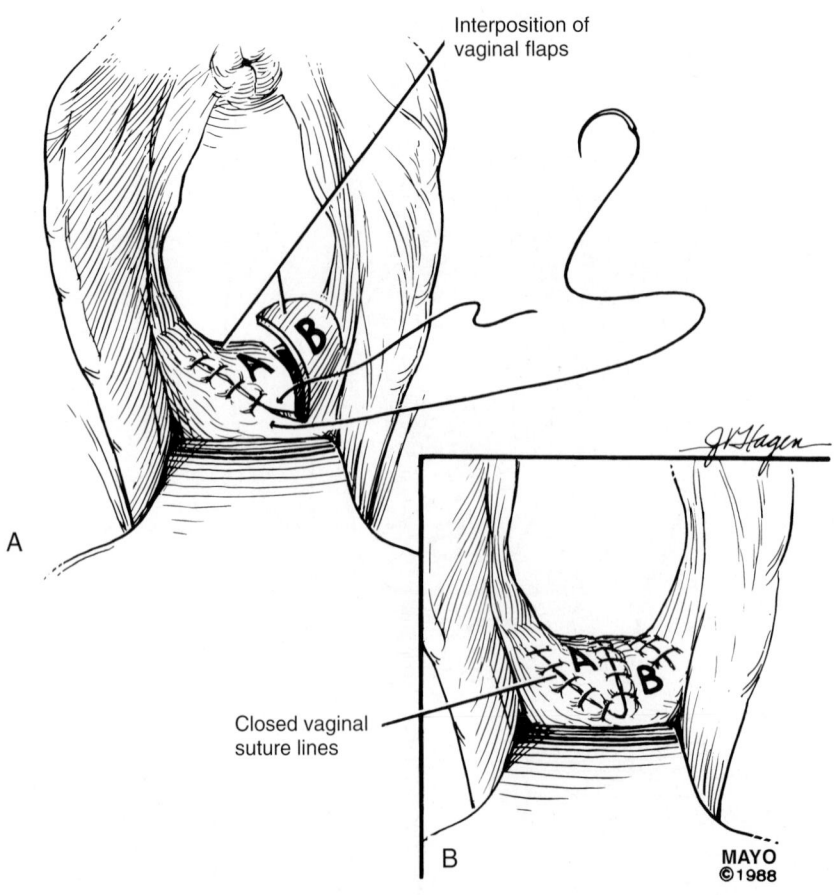

Interposition of
vaginal flaps

Closed vaginal
suture lines

A

B

MAYO
©1988

**FIGURE 62–7  A.** After mobilization, the scar tissue is excised and the flaps interposed. **B.** The transposed flaps are reapproximated in a tension-free manner with interrupted sutures. (Adapted from Lee RA: Atlas of Gynecologic Surgery. Philadelphia, WB Saunders, ©1992. Used with permission of Mayo Foundation for Medical Education and Research.)

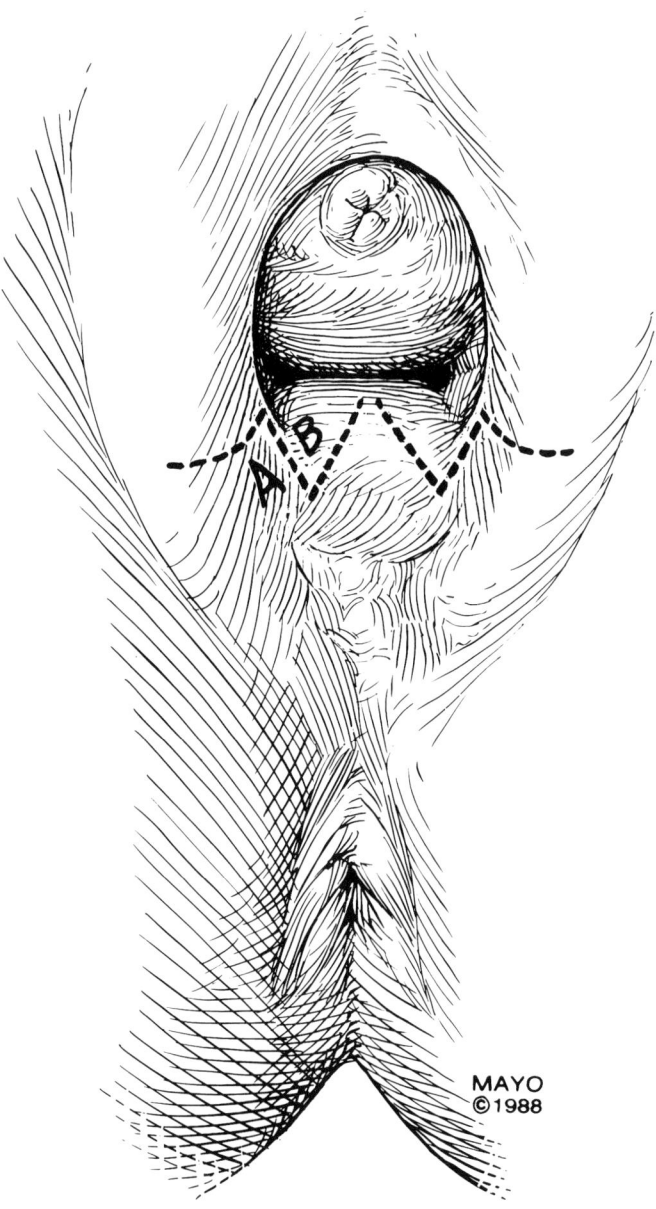

**FIGURE 62–8** The Z-plasty may be made on either side of the introital opening, which results in a lateral incision closure and the absence of an incision in the midline. (Adapted from Lee RA: Atlas of Gynecologic Surgery. Philadelphia, WB Saunders, ©1992. Used with permission of Mayo Foundation for Medical Education and Research.)

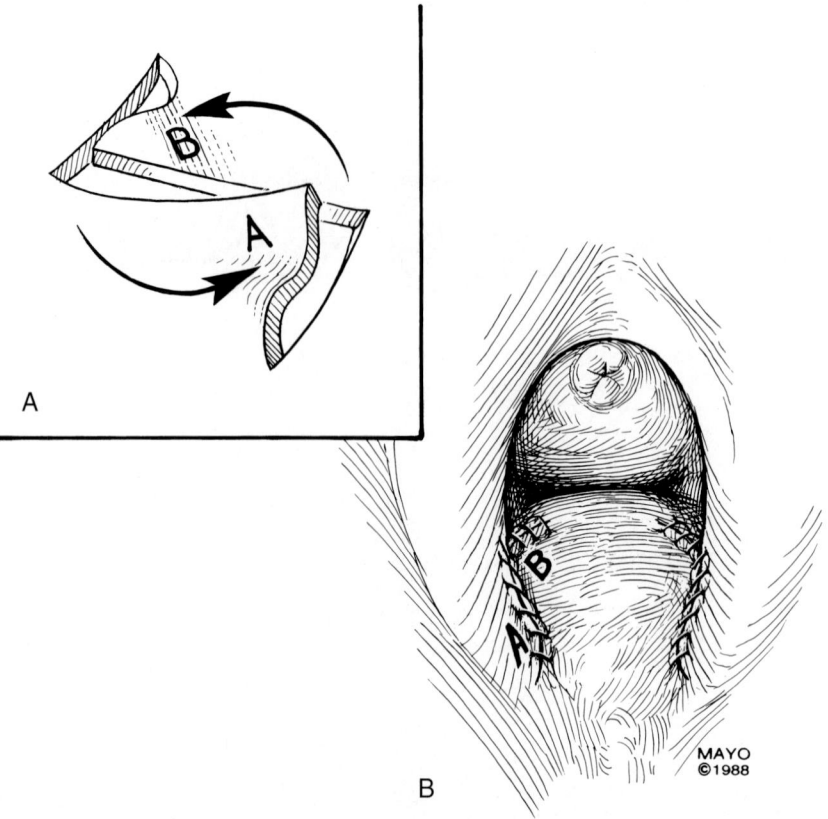

**FIGURE 62–9  A.** After the incisions are made and the tissues mobilized, the subcutaneous tissues are separately approximated. **B.** The overlying mucosa is closed with interrupted, 4-0 delayed absorbable suture. (Adapted from Lee RA: Atlas of Gynecologic Surgery. Philadelphia, WB Saunders, ©1992. Used with permission of Mayo Foundation for Medical Education and Research.)

## Free Skin Grafts

Full-thickness skin grafts may be used for repair of vaginal stenosis or vaginal shortening. These grafts, in contrast to split-thickness grafts, are used because they cause less postoperative contracture. A full-thickness graft composed of dermis and epidermis (with all fat removed) can be harvested from any site on the body. Relaxing incisions can be made in the vagina through the area of stenosis, and the graft is sewn into place with fine absorbable sutures. The vagina should be packed with moistened gauze for at least 24 hours after the procedure.

### Xenografts

Xenografts are acellular extracts of collagen—with or without additional extracellular matrix components—that are harvested from nonhuman sources. They differ in the source species (bovine or porcine), in the site of harvest (pericardium, dermis, or small intestine submucosa), and by whether chemical cross-linking is used in processing the material.

Xenograft materials include Surgisis (Cook Biotech Inc, West Lafayette, Indiana), an extracellular matrix material derived from the submucosa of the porcine small intestine. It contains structural and functional proteins arranged in a tissue-specific orientation for direct healing and tissue remodeling. Surgisis has been used as an alternative to split-thickness skin grafting in human patients with full-thickness chronic leg ulcers and granulating open dermal wounds. It is available in various sizes and thicknesses.

We have used four-layer Surgisis successfully to bridge gaps in vaginal epithelium or perineal skin in cases where approximating the tissue would cause narrowing or foreshortening. In this use, the surrounding vaginal epithelium is undermined, and the graft is laid flat beneath the epithelium and is secured in place with sutures (Fig. 62-10). The graft is generally well accepted by the body and remodels to become nearly indistinguishable from surrounding tissue. It is essentially used in lieu of a skin graft. Porcine small intestine submucosa is recommended over porcine dermis when used to replace or bridge epithelial defects.

## Perineal Flaps

Lateral strictures near the introitus or farther up the vaginal canal may result in dyspareunia or in a functionally shortened vagina. In addition, inflammatory conditions (e.g., lichen planus, Behçet disease) may cause vaginal obliteration. Perineal flaps provide a potentially large and vascular tissue source to aid in management of various strictures and obliterative conditions.

An incision is made throughout the entire longitudinal extent of the introital and vaginal scar (Fig. 62-11). The area is undermined to open the contracture completely. After measurements are taken to calculate the desired flap length, a hinged perineal flap is created immediately lateral to the labium majus on the side of the contracture (Fig. 62-12). The blood supply (in the flap base) generally supports a flap length several times the width of the flap base. A portion of subcutaneous fat is preserved on the flap to maintain a blood supply and results in a soft pad at the previous contracture site. The flap is rotated into the vaginal space and is secured in place with fine, absorbable, interrupted sutures after hemostasis is obtained. A suction catheter may be placed beneath the flap and generally is removed in 24 to 48 hours (Fig. 62-13).

Occasionally, bilateral flaps (Fig. 62-14) are required to adequately address a large stricture or a complete vaginal obliteration. The resultant vagina and introitus should have adequate diameter and depth and should be completely free of any contracting bands or scars (Fig. 62-15).

Figure 62-16 shows an example of vaginal obliteration from Behçet disease. Several prior attempts at repair were unsuccessful. After meticulous vaginal dissection and the placement of relaxing incisions at 4 and 8 o'clock, measurements were taken, and the left perineal flap was mobilized (Fig. 62-16A) and rotated into the dissected area (Fig. 62-16B). Interrupted sutures secured the flap in place after placement of a drain. Measurements were taken on the right side, and the right perineal flap was mobilized (Fig. 62-16C). Again, interrupted sutures were used to secure the flap after placement of a drain beneath the mobilized flap (Fig. 62-16D). Deaver and right-angle Heaney retractors were used to gain exposure to the vaginal apex and secure the proximal interrupted sutures (Fig. 62-16E). The skin surrounding the groin harvest sites was undermined to aid in a tension-free closure. (Bringing the patient's legs down from the lithotomy position may be helpful for this part of the procedure.) The groin incisions were then closed in two layers: an interrupted subcutaneous layer to ease tension on the skin, and a subcuticular layer to close the skin (Fig. 62-16F). An ice pack was applied to help limit swelling, and a Foley catheter was left in place for several days to assist in bladder drainage.

## Abdominal Flaps

When other, more traditional options have failed or circumstances dictate that a new tissue source must be used, abdominal flaps provide an alternative. Abdominal flaps are often used in other surgical procedures, such as breast reconstruction, and they may be applicable in gynecologic reconstruction as well. Vertical rectus abdominis myocutaneous flaps and transverse rectus abdominis myocutaneous flaps may be used for vaginal reconstruction in patients with vaginal stricture who have had previously unsuccessful procedures, and for vaginal reconstruction in patients with gynecologic malignancy.

Figure 62-17 illustrates the use of a vertical rectus abdominis myocutaneous flap in a patient who underwent radical resection of a rhabdomyosarcoma of the perineum at a very young age. Several subsequent operations failed to create a functional vagina. Figure 62-17A shows a multioperated perineum with a sigmoid neovagina, in which stricture developed over time (bilateral labial flaps and bilateral Singapore flaps had previously failed). In the planning of surgical incisions, preoperative markings were made (Fig. 62-17B). The sigmoid neovagina was isolated and mobilized from above (Fig. 62-17C). The mobilized sigmoid neovagina was everted (Fig. 62-17D) and excised at the perineum (Fig. 62-17E). The left rectus abdominis muscle, overlying skin, and adipose tissue (i.e., the vertical rectus abdominis myocutaneous flap) were isolated (Fig. 62-17F), sacrificing the superior blood supply while preserving the inferior blood supply (i.e., the inferior epigastric artery). The flap was then configured in a helical manner with interrupted and continuous, delayed absorbable sutures (Fig. 62-17G) and was rotated into the pelvis, where it was secured to the perineum (Fig. 62-17H) with interrupted, delayed absorbable sutures. (The bulk of the neovagina may make this step a challenging part of the reconstruction.) The fascial defect was then approximated directly or with the use of a graft, and the overlying skin was closed primarily (Fig. 62-17I).

The advantages of abdominal flaps for vaginal reconstruction include the availability of a large, well-vascularized, and generally undisturbed tissue source that usually does not require dilation postoperatively. Disadvantages include the potential for partial graft skin slough, which may require further surgical intervention and grafting. In addition, these tissue flaps are often bulky (depending on the patient's body habitus) and may be difficult to interpose between the bladder and the rectum and to attach to the perineum.

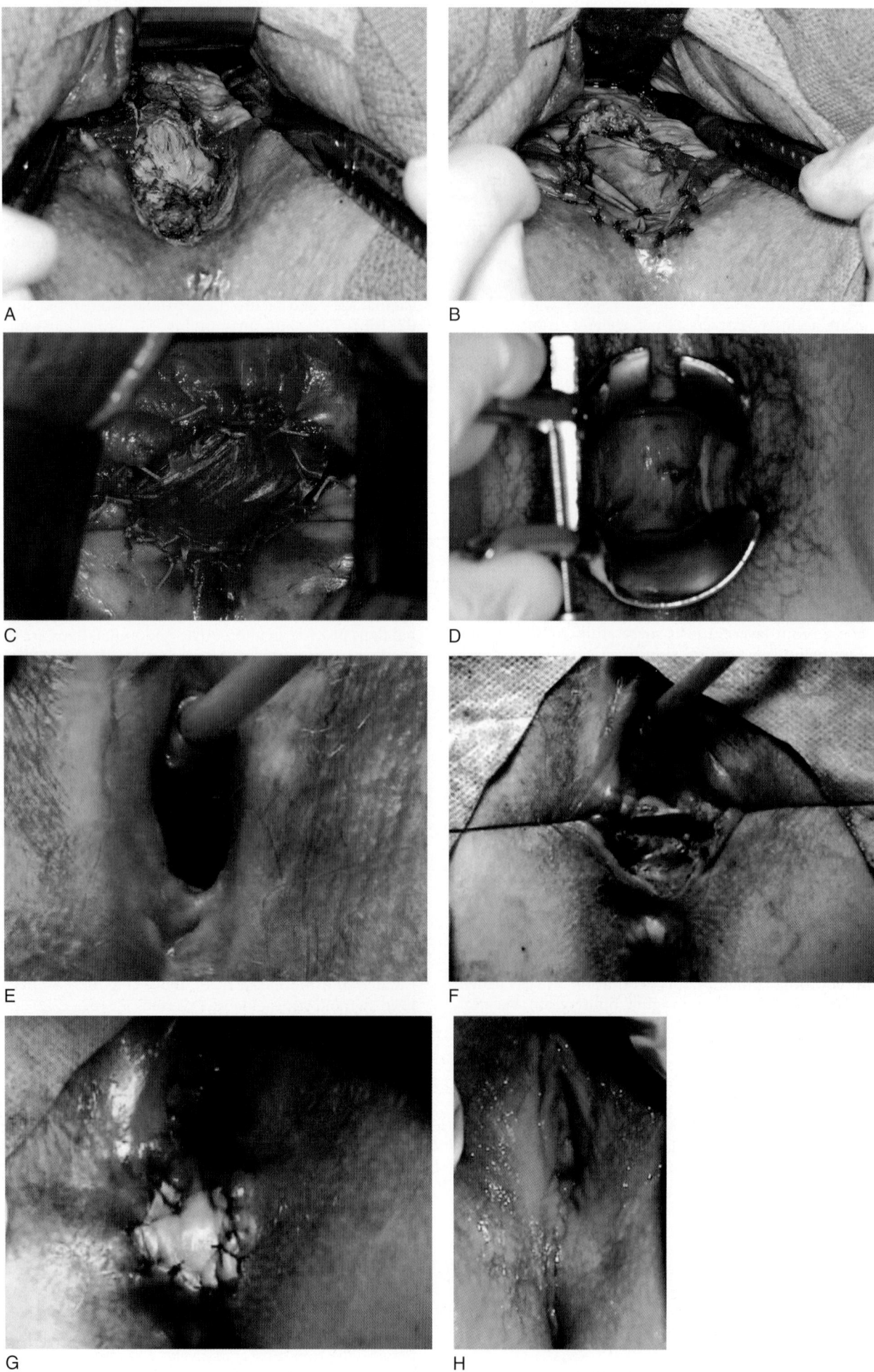

**FIGURE 62–10** Operative photos show the use of four-layer extracellular matrix material (Surgisis; Cook Biotech Inc, West Lafayette, Indiana) in replacing epithelium after vaginal and perineal reconstruction. **A.** A large defect along the distal posterior vaginal wall and perineal body after excision of vaginal mesh secondary to dyspareunia. Closing the wound primarily would cause introital narrowing. **B.** The graft sutured into place. **C.** A painful vertical scar at the vaginal apex excised and the defect bridged with the graft. **D.** The vaginal apex 6 weeks later. **E.** Perineal scarring after an episiotomy, causing dyspareunia. **F.** Large perineal defect after excision of the scarred tissue. **G.** Graft sutured into place to bridge the defect. **H.** The perineum 6 weeks after surgery.

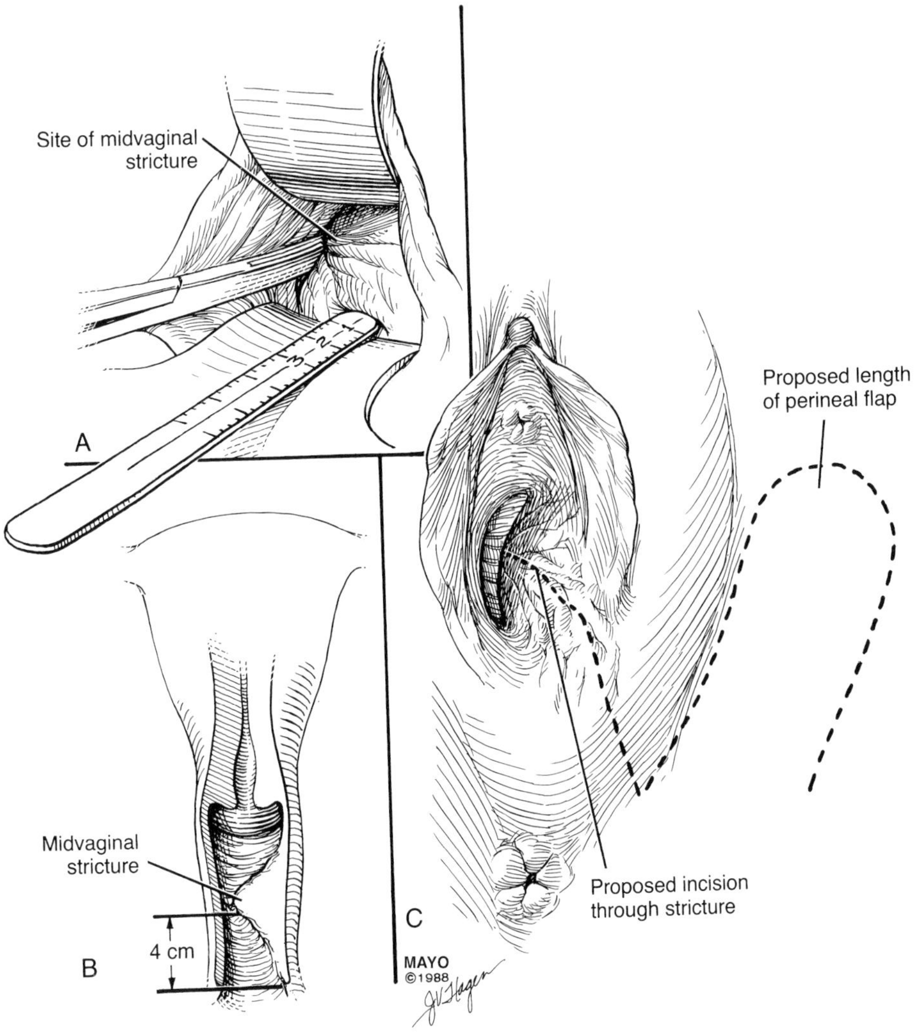

**FIGURE 62–11 A.** A ruler and curved tissue forceps used to define the area of stricture and to plan the size of graft needed for harvest. **B.** A narrowed midvaginal contracture in a longitudinal view, emphasizing a thick scar with a narrow passage connecting the upper and lower vagina. **C.** The proposed incision and perineal flap. An incision is made in the introitus and is extended through the constriction. The scar is incised and completely excised, and the surrounding tissues are adequately mobilized in preparation for a perineal flap. The region and extent of contracture determine the size of the perineal graft. (Adapted from Lee RA: Atlas of Gynecologic Surgery. Philadelphia, WB Saunders, ©1992. Used with permission of Mayo Foundation for Medical Education and Research.)

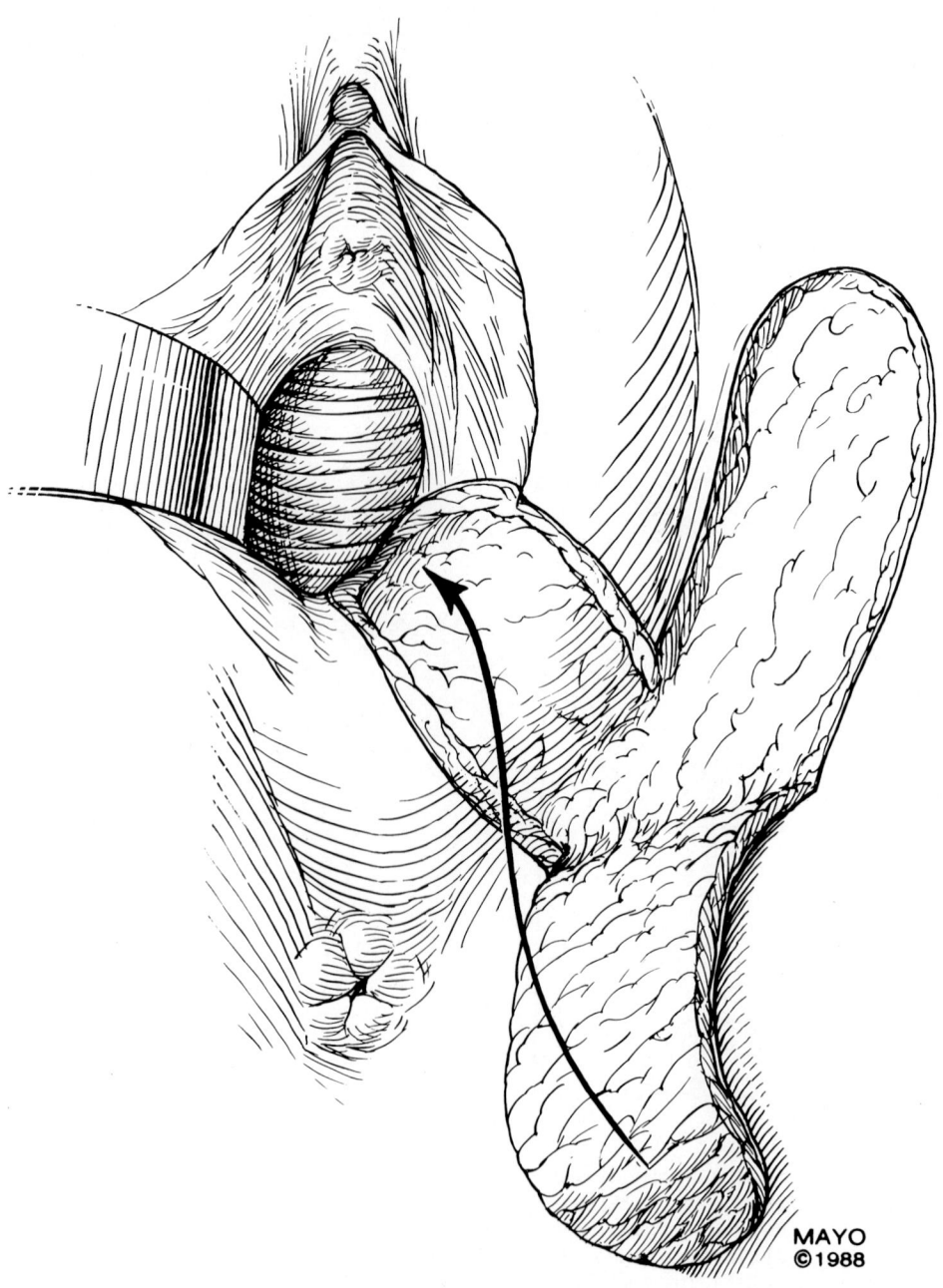

**FIGURE 62–12** After the contracture has been excised and the surrounding tissues mobilized, measurements are taken to determine the size of graft required. A hinged perineal graft is then created immediately lateral to the labium majus on the side of the contracture. The blood supply in the hinge region must be preserved. Making the distal end of the flap round rather than pointed is advised, to reduce the risk of slough of the distal aspect of the graft. (Adapted from Lee RA: Atlas of Gynecologic Surgery. Philadelphia, WB Saunders, ©1992. Used with permission of Mayo Foundation for Medical Education and Research.)

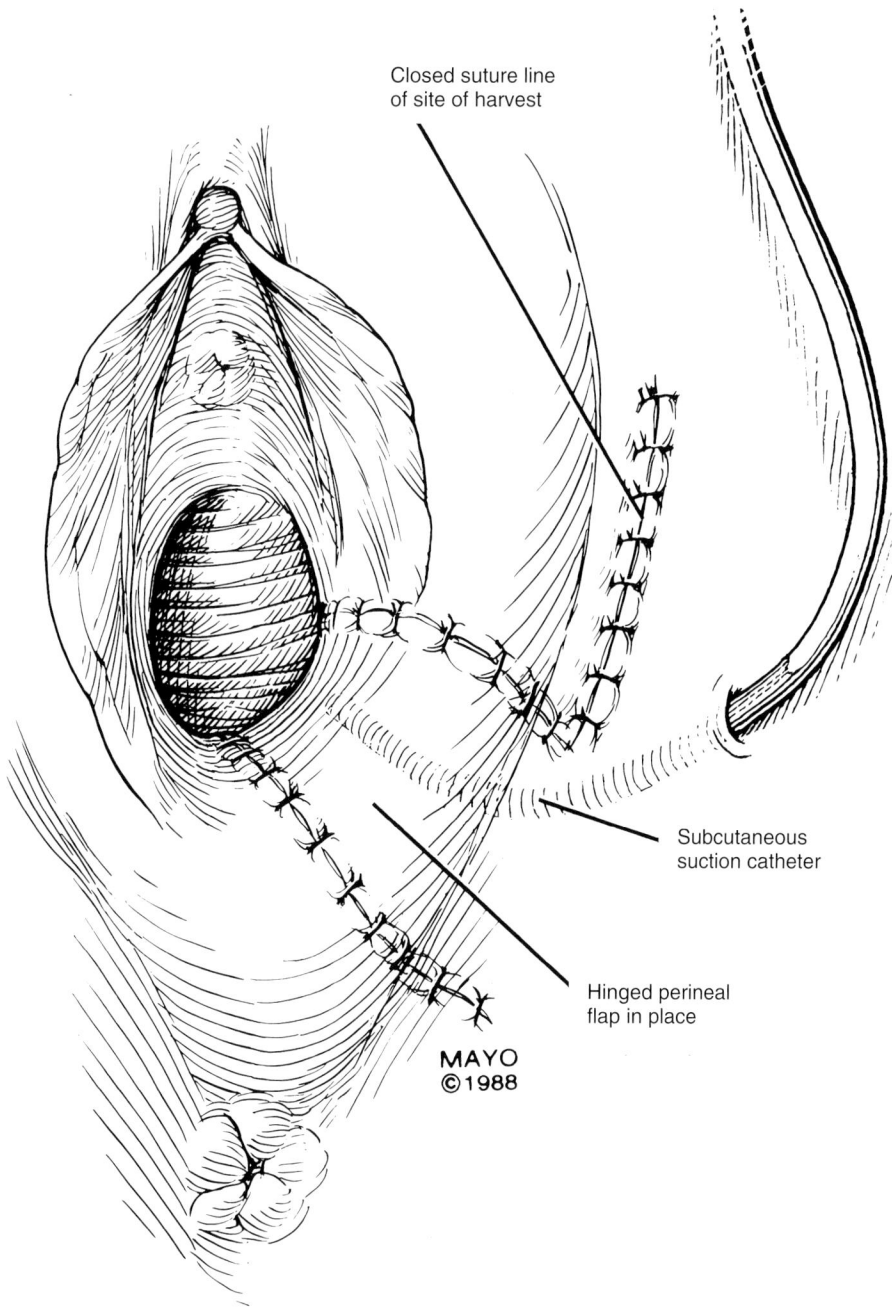

Closed suture line
of site of harvest

Subcutaneous
suction catheter

Hinged perineal
flap in place

MAYO
©1988

**FIGURE 62–13**  A suction catheter is placed in the wound bed and is extended laterally. The flap is rotated into the defect and is secured to the adjoining tissue with interrupted sutures. The initial sutures secure the flap near the vaginal apex; subsequent sutures are placed toward the introitus, with care taken to avoid asymmetry. The tissue lateral to the labium majus is circumferentially mobilized to allow the incision to be closed in a tension-free manner. (Adapted from Lee RA: Atlas of Gynecologic Surgery. Philadelphia, WB Saunders, ©1992. Used with permission of Mayo Foundation for Medical Education and Research.)

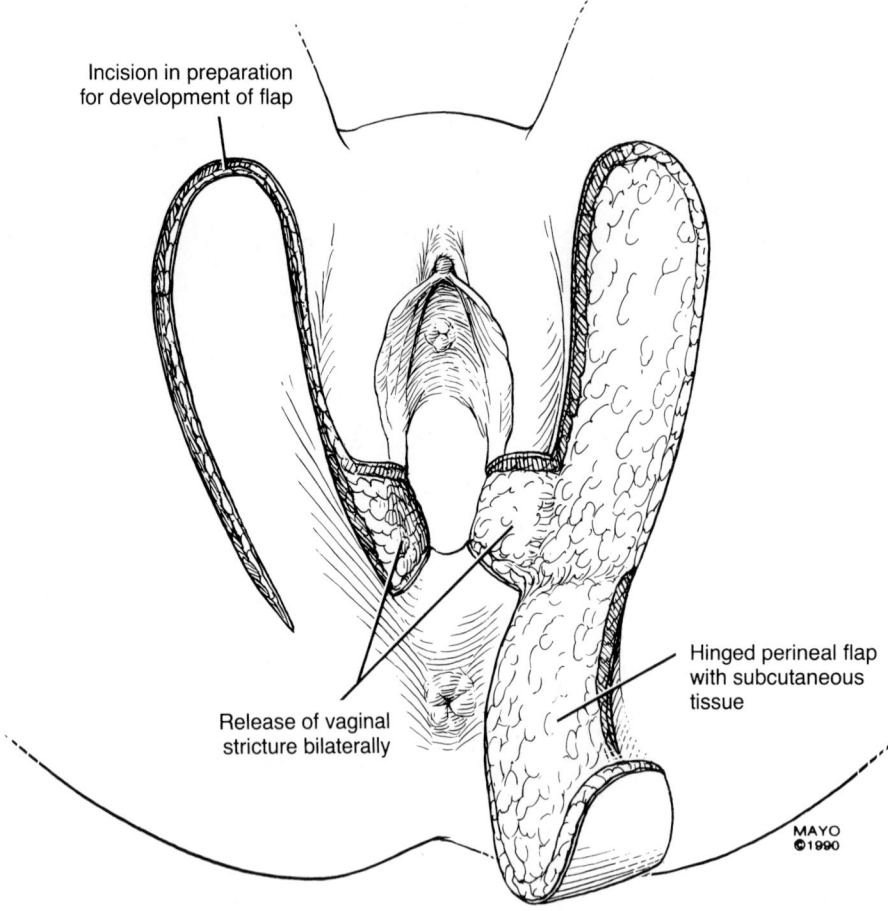

Incision in preparation
for development of flap

Release of vaginal
stricture bilaterally

Hinged perineal flap
with subcutaneous
tissue

MAYO
©1990

**FIGURE 62–14** When a circumferential constriction or vaginal obliteration is encountered, bilateral perineal flaps may be required. The principles described in Figures 59–10 through 59–12 apply to this type of repair as well. (Adapted from Lee RA: Atlas of Gynecologic Surgery. Philadelphia, WB Saunders, ©1992. Used with permission of Mayo Foundation for Medical Education and Research.)

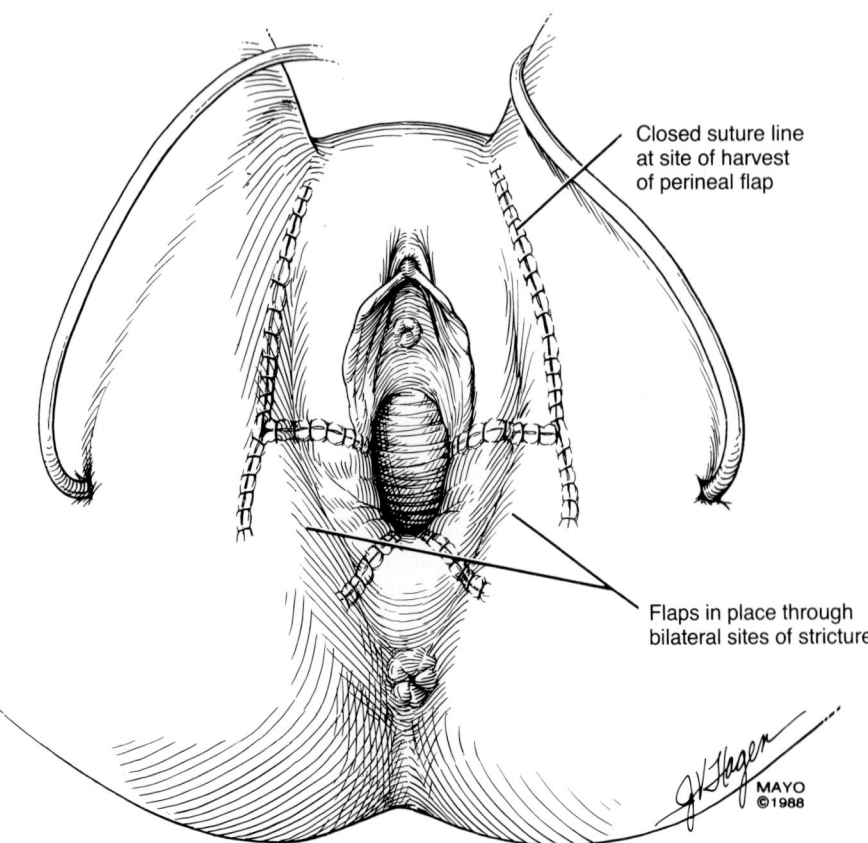

Closed suture line
at site of harvest
of perineal flap

Flaps in place through
bilateral sites of stricture

MAYO
©1988

**FIGURE 62–15** Bilateral perineal flaps should yield a functional vagina. Meticulous hemostasis is required. Harvesting a graft that is approximately 1 cm longer than the vaginal incision is advised, to ensure adequate graft length and a tension-free closure. (Adapted from Lee RA: Atlas of Gynecologic Surgery. Philadelphia, WB Saunders, ©1992. Used with permission of Mayo Foundation for Medical Education and Research.)

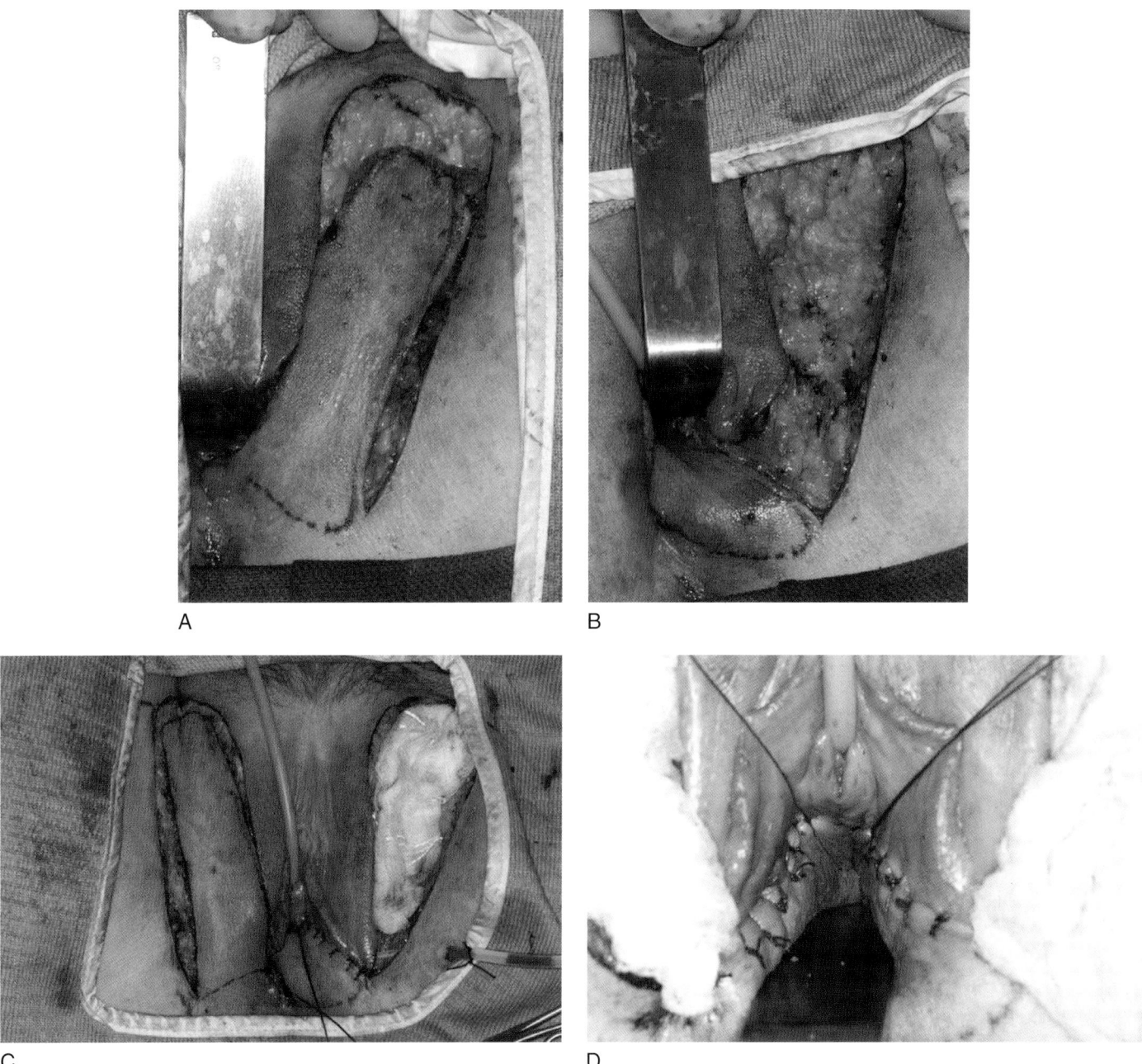

A

B

C

D

**FIGURE 62–16** Bilateral perineal flaps in a patient with vaginal obliteration from Behçet disease. The patient previously underwent two vaginal dissections that quickly resulted in restenosis of the vagina. Adequate control of her underlying disease process, the desire for a functional vagina, and the failure of previous vaginal dissections led to the advice to use bilateral perineal flaps for reconstruction. **A.** The vaginal dissection has been completed, and measurements have been taken to determine the size of graft needed. The left perineal flap was thus mobilized. A broad base at the hinge preserved the blood supply, and rounding of the distal tip was performed. **B.** The left perineal flap was rotated into the defect and was secured to surrounding tissue with interrupted sutures. **C.** When the left perineal flap was secured, vaginal dissection was repeated on the right side, measurements were taken, and the right perineal flap was mobilized. **D.** Interrupted sutures, starting at the apex and working toward the introitus, were placed to secure the grafts in a symmetrical and tension-free manner.

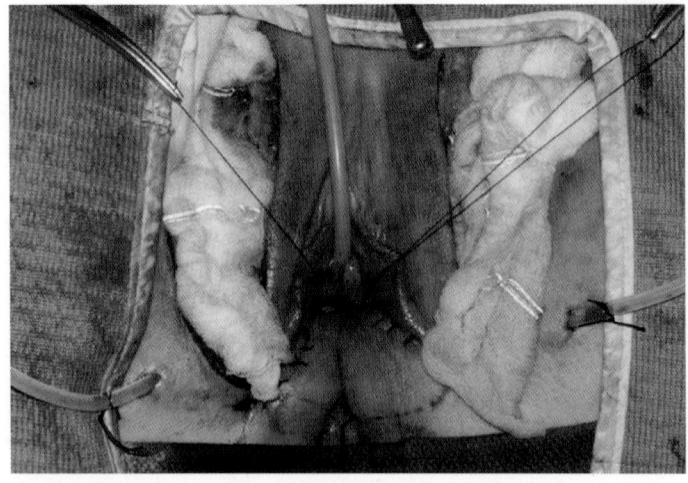

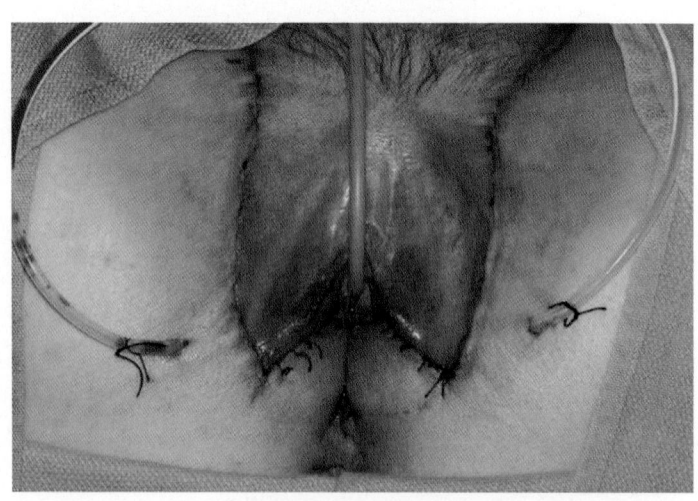

E

F

**FIGURE 62–16, cont'd  E.** After the flaps were secured in place, the tissue surrounding the incisions lateral to the labia majora was mobilized. Often, the lateral aspect of the incision can be mobilized to a greater degree than the medial aspect, to avoid a tethering effect on the remaining labial and periclitoral tissues. **F.** An initial layer of interrupted sutures was placed to reapproximate the subcutaneous tissues in the lateral incisions. This placement reduced tension on the overlying skin closure. The skin was then reapproximated with a running subcuticular, delayed absorbable suture. A Foley catheter was left in place to drain the bladder, and an ice pack was applied to limit edema. Tissue edema in the perineal flaps was not uncommon, and the grafts were monitored for evidence of vascular compromise.

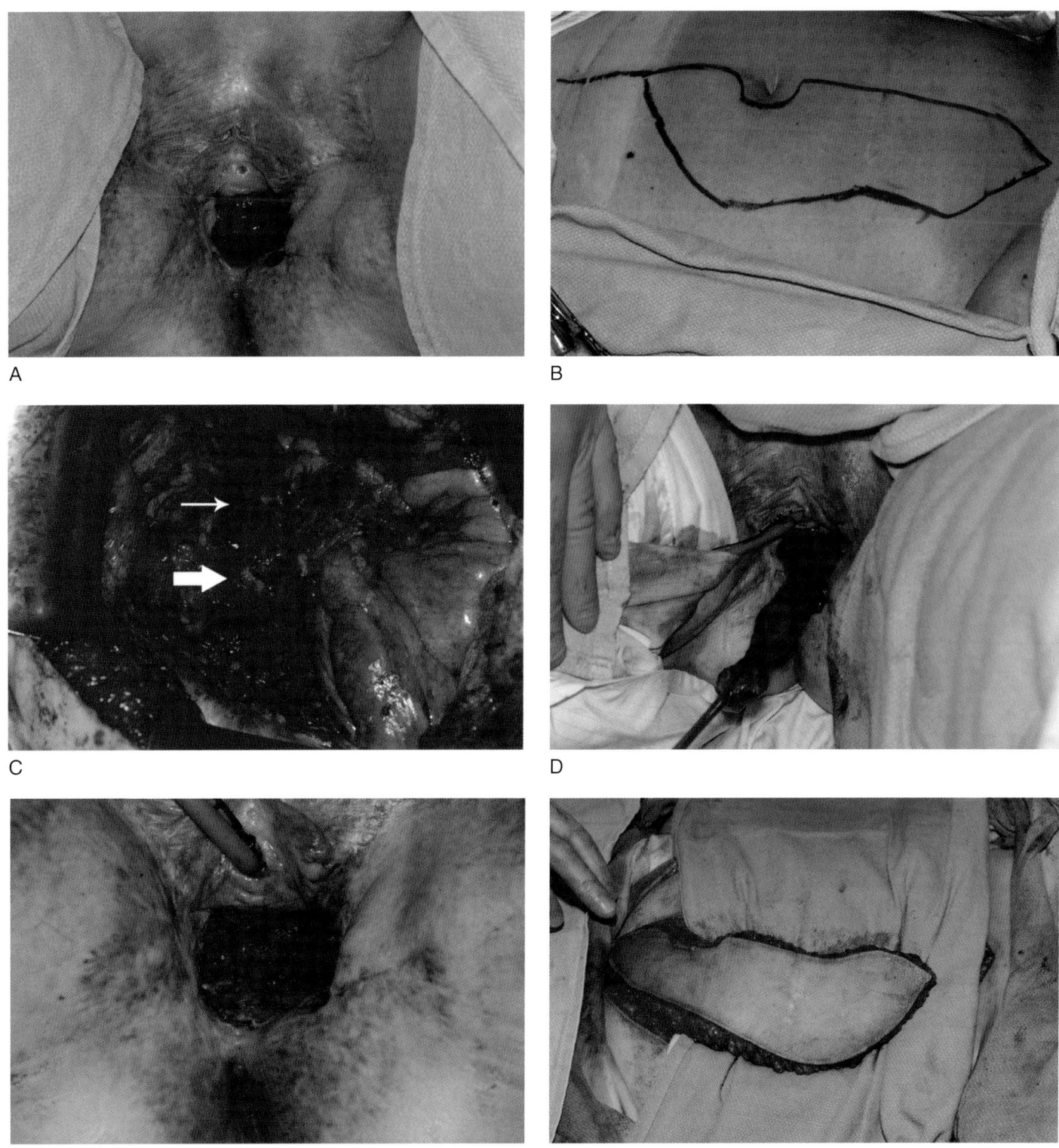

**FIGURE 62–17** Use of a vertical rectus abdominis myocutaneous (VRAM) flap for vaginal reconstruction in a patient who at a very young age underwent radical resection of a rhabdomyosarcoma of the perineum, followed by pelvic irradiation. Vaginal stricture and hematocolpos developed. She eventually underwent hysterectomy, bilateral perineal flap, bilateral Singapore flap construction, and, finally, construction of a sigmoid neovagina, in which stenosis ultimately developed. **A.** The perineal area showed extensive scarring from previous operations and pelvic irradiation. The mucosa of the sigmoid neovagina had erythema from chronic irritation. **B.** The left rectus abdominis muscle was marked for future harvest. **C.** The sigmoid neovagina with a Lucite dilator in place (*thick arrow*) underwent stenosis and was mobilized from the left pelvic sidewall and adjacent rectum (*thin arrow*). **D.** After mobilization abdominally, the sigmoid neovagina was everted through the vagina and excised. **E.** With sharp dissection and cautery, the sigmoid neovagina was dissected free from the overlying bladder and urethra and underlying rectum. A preoperative left external ureteral stent was placed to aid the identification and dissection of the left ureter. **F.** The left VRAM flap was isolated, sacrificing the superior blood supply.

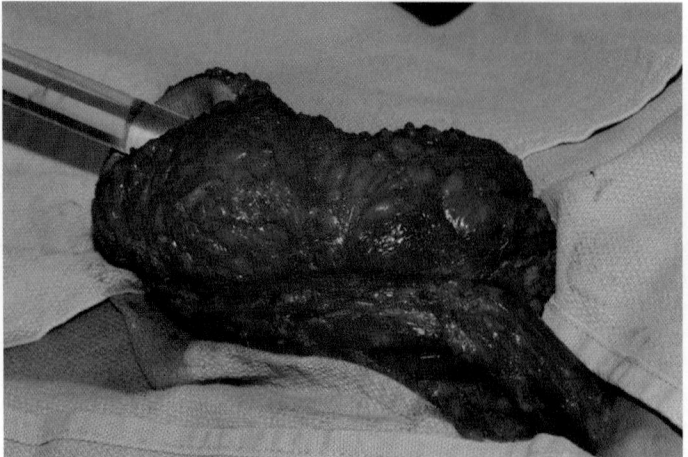

G

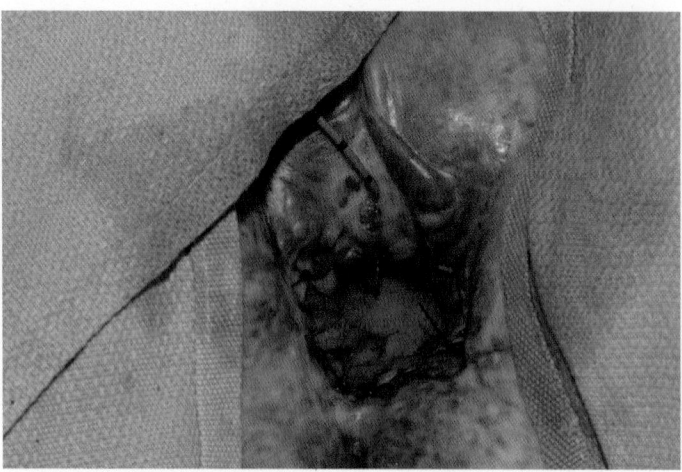

H

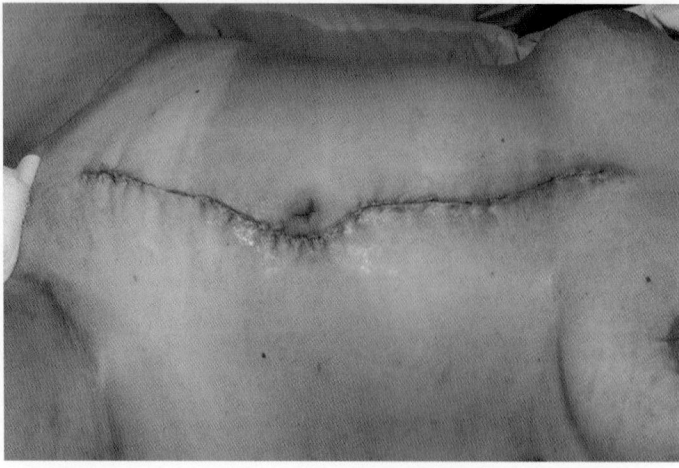

I

**FIGURE 62–17, cont'd**  **G.** The VRAM flap was rolled in a helical fashion to create a neovagina, and the skin edges were secured with interrupted and continuous delayed absorbable sutures. **H.** The VRAM-flap neovagina was then rotated into the pelvis and secured to the perineum with interrupted sutures. **I.** After the fascial edges were reapproximated, the skin was closed, leaving a long, vertical midline scar.

# CHAPTER 63

# Vaginectomy

## Michael S. Baggish

Partial or total excision of the vagina is performed most often because of vaginal neoplasia. The diagnosis is suspected following an atypical cytology report. Vaginal intraepithelial neoplasia (VAIN) may follow or exist concurrently with cervical intraepithelial neoplasia (CIN) or vulvar intraepithelial neoplasia (VIN), or may occur de novo. A de facto vaginectomy may be performed as a result of treatment for extensive condyloma acuminata. The goal of vaginectomy is twofold: (1) to remove the pathology, and (2) to retain a functioning structure. The latter translates into maintaining the vagina as a supple, nonconstricted, and suitably lengthy structure. The factor most often responsible for vaginal deformity and accompanying dyspareunia is scar formation. As was noted in Chapter 50, neighboring organs are exceedingly close (2 to 4 mm) to the vaginal mucosa. The vagina itself is a rather simple structure—essentially a potential space with its anterior and posterior walls in light contact in vivo. The vagina is attached at its lower margin to the vulva and at its upper margin to the uterus, together with the uterine supports. The vagina is attached laterally to the levator ani and a mass of surrounding connective tissue (endopelvic fascia). The loose peripheral attachments allow movement as well as flexibility between the points of relative fixation. Anteriorly, the vaginal wall and the bladder and urethral walls are in apposition. Similarly, an identical set of circumstances exists between the rectal and vaginal walls posteriorly. When reduced to its lowest common denominator, the vagina is a pleated, lightly muscled, highly vascularized skin tube.

Intraepithelial neoplasia in the absence of glands occupies less than 1 mm of a vaginal wall cross-section. Treating the vagina more deeply to eradicate the disease adds nothing to the cure but may adversely influence the functional outcome. Unfortunately, VAIN is multifocal; therefore, to diminish the chances of persistence or recurrence, very wide excisional margins around visible lesions must be undertaken. This translates into dividing the vagina into thirds and removing a minimum of one third to a maximum of three thirds.

## Excision

Because the vagina is highly vascular, particularly beneath the urethra and at the bulb of the vestibule, brisk bleeding should be anticipated when it is cut. The sources of much of the bleeding are sinusoidal and cavernous structures. These sites are better sutured as they are encountered rather than clamped. If substantial areas of the vagina are going to be excised, a split-thickness skin graft should be obtained before the vaginal part of the operation is begun (Fig. 63–1). The colposcope will be used throughout the intravaginal operation. Initially, the extent of the lesion is mapped (Fig. 63–2A, B).

A 1:100 vasopressin solution is injected subepithelially into the vaginal stroma (Fig. 63–3A). This provides some hemostasis and a convenient dissection plane (Fig. 63–3B). An axis-oriented incision is made into the anterior or posterior wall, and flaps are created to the right and left of the midline cut as a submucosal plane is created (Fig. 63–4). The dissecting microscope (colposcope) has the great advantage of providing good, bright light as well as variable magnification. Stevens (tenotomy) scissors are ideal for this type of dissection (Fig. 63–5). The lateral wall is divided into two recesses, or sulci, which create an H appearance to the vagina as viewed head on. These are located anterolaterally and posterolaterally on the right and left walls. Between the sulci lies the insertion of the levator ani muscle on the right and left sides, respectively. Above and below the insertion on the muscle is fat, through which course blood vessels, lymphatics, and nerves. The vagina is dissected across the point of levator attachment but superficial to that attachment (i.e., remaining well within the immediate submucosal plane) (Fig. 63–6). Anterior and posterior dissections meet in the anterolateral and posterolateral sulci, and the specimen is removed (Figs. 63–7 and 63–8). Care must be taken at the vaginal fornices to not damage the ureter, which is quite close to the anterior and anterolateral fornices.

Depending on the size of the removed tissue, the vagina may be closed edge to cut edge or grafted. Generally the latter approach is selected because any substantial excision will lead to constriction, should the vagina be reconstituted by primary closure, particularly if the suture lines are closed under tension.

For split-thickness closure, a graft is taken from the buttock or thigh. Upon completion of the vaginectomy, the defect is measured and the graft is cut to fit the defect. The graft is removed from its saline-soaked sponge roll, remoistened with normal saline, and carefully placed to cover the wound (Fig. 63–9). It is sutured into place with multiple 4-0 Vicryl sutures and is covered with fine-mesh gauze (Fig. 63–10A, B). The donor site is covered with a urethane dressing. Although it is obvious, the point must be made that absolute hemostasis must be accomplished before any graft is placed over a surgical bed. This location is preferable to avoid electrosurgical coagulation, which devitalizes tissue and increases the risk of infection. Instead, bleeding areas should be irrigated and suture-ligated with fine absorbable sutures (e.g., 3-0 or 4-0 Vicryl) (Fig. 63–11).

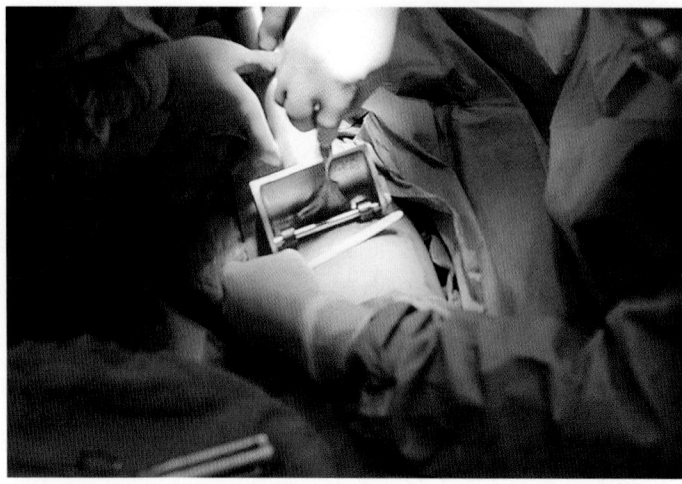

**FIGURE 63–1** In preparation for a large vaginal excision (partial vaginectomy) involving the upper and middle thirds of the vagina, a split-thickness skin graft is obtained from the thigh.

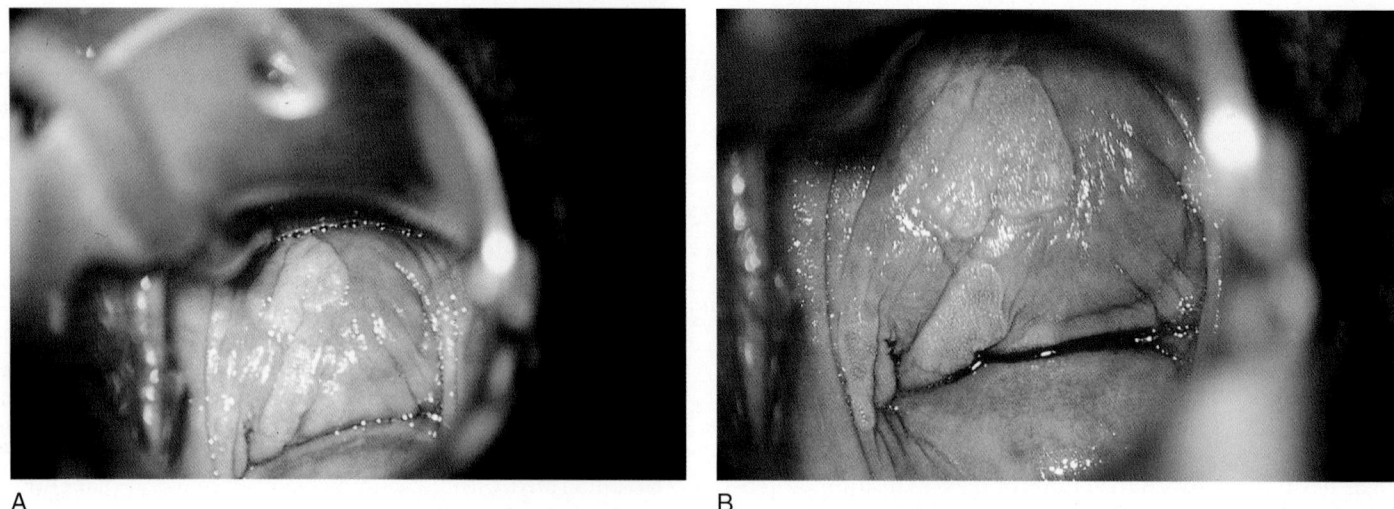

A

B

**FIGURE 63–2 A.** An extensive area of vaginal intraepithelial neoplasia (VAIN) is seen on the anterior and lateral walls of the vagina. **B.** Close-up view of Figure 63–2A documents the flat, warty pattern of VAIN.

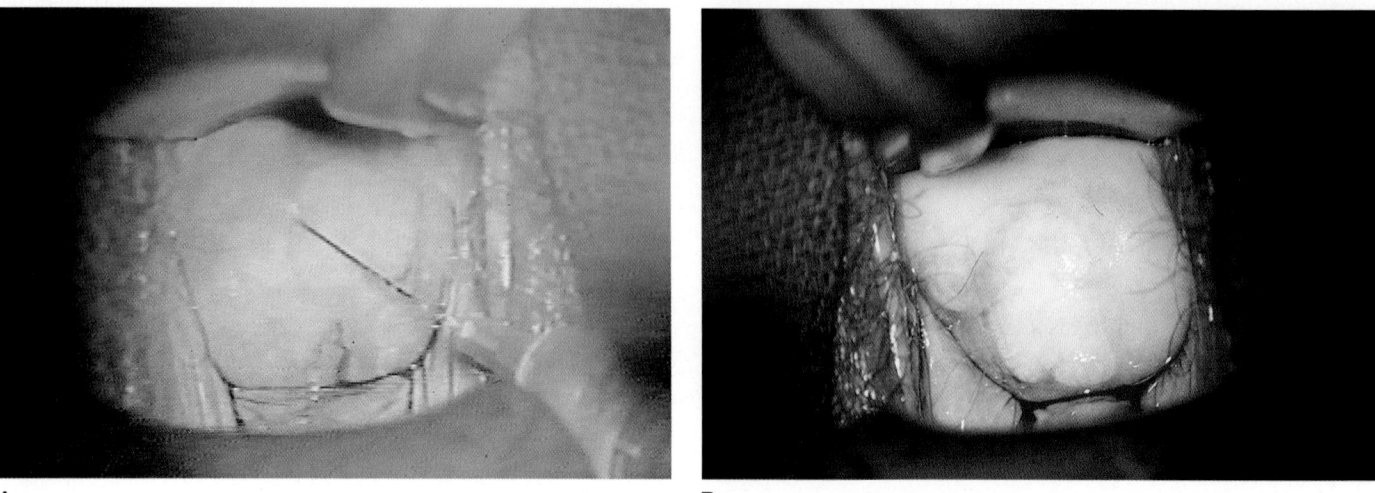

A

B

**FIGURE 63–3 A.** An injection of 1:100 vasopressin solution is made into the vagina in preparation for surgery. The vasopressin provides hemostasis, and the solution helps to identify a plane for the vaginectomy. **B.** Note the extreme blanching produced by the injection of vasopressin. Actually, it is advisable to map the lesion and identify the margins before injection.

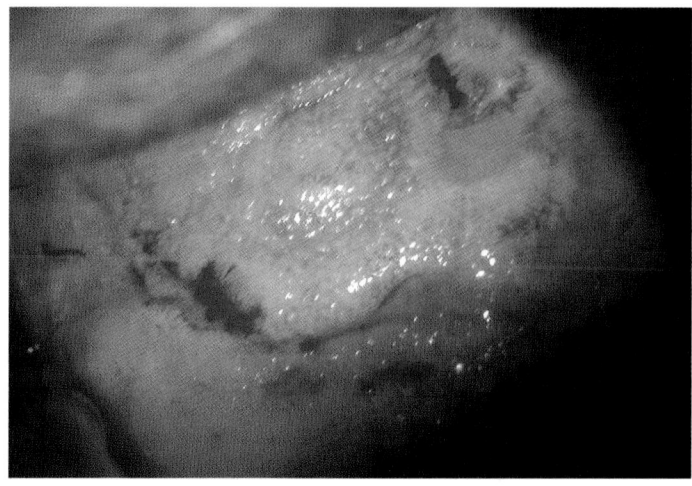

FIGURE 63–4 A trace incision is made into the vagina with a 3-mm margin around the visible neoplasia.

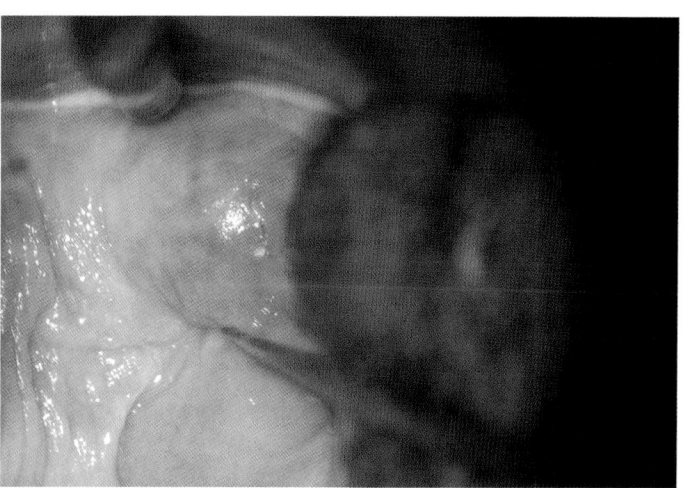

FIGURE 63–5 The excision is begun at the distal margin with the use of Stevens tenotomy scissors and with the optical advantage of the dissecting microscope.

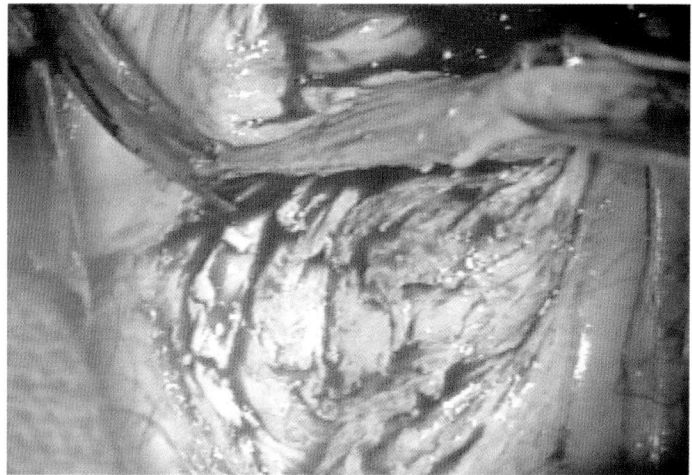

FIGURE 63–6 The full thickness of the vaginal epithelium is dissected from the underlying vaginal stroma. In actuality, a bit of stroma is also excised because the epithelial pegs extend down into the underlying stroma.

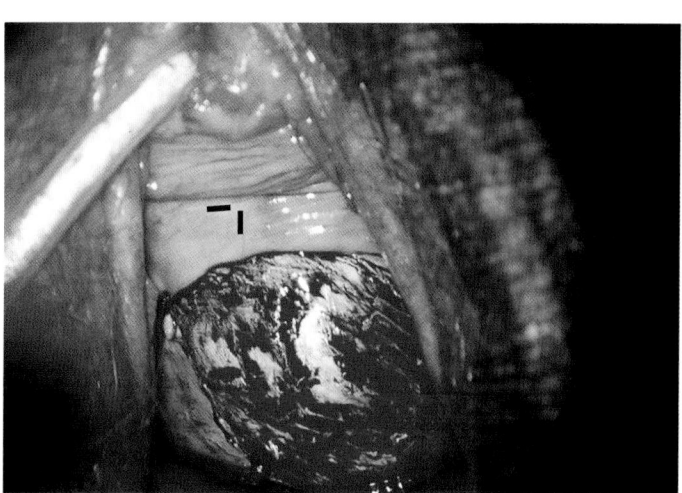

FIGURE 63–7 A large portion of the anterior vaginal wall has been excised. The black markers are beneath the area of the bladder neck (urethrovesical junction).

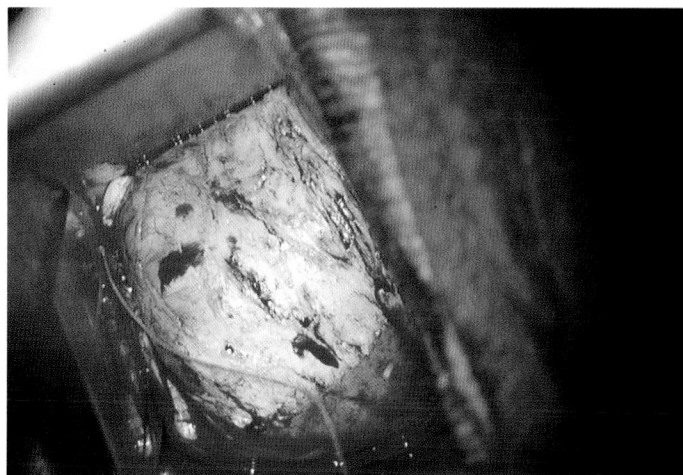

FIGURE 63–8 The lateral vaginal wall has been primarily sutured, closing the excisional defect. The anterior wall cannot be primarily closed without constricting the vagina.

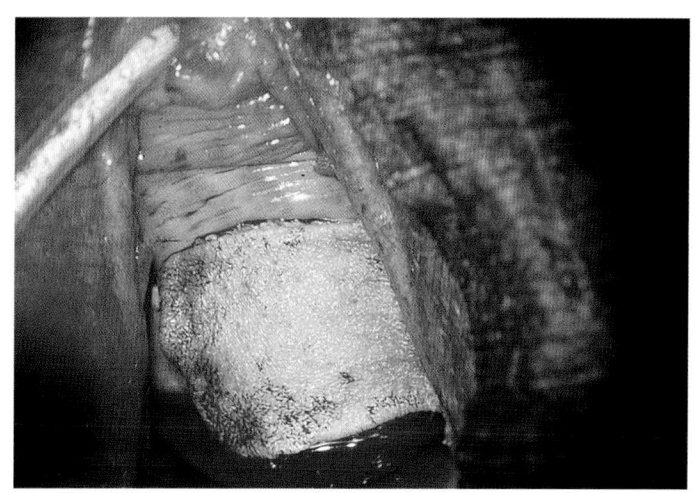

FIGURE 63–9 A split-thickness graft is placed over the defect extending from just cranial to the urethrovesical junction to the anterior vaginal fornix.

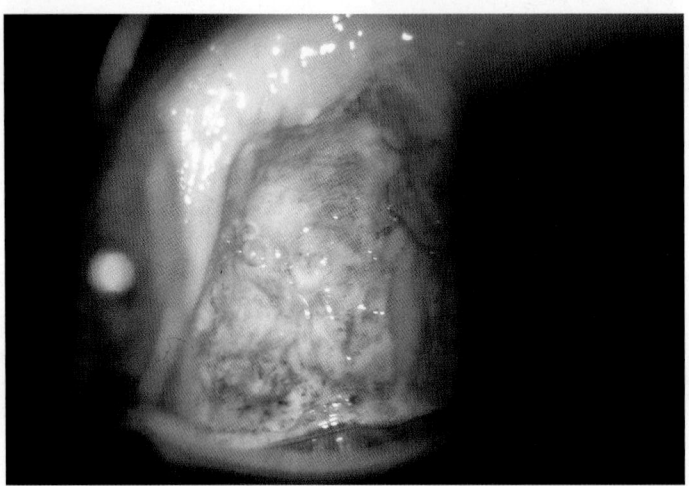

**FIGURE 63–10** No electrosurgical devices are used for hemostasis. Instead, bleeding points are suture-ligated with 4-0 Vicryl.

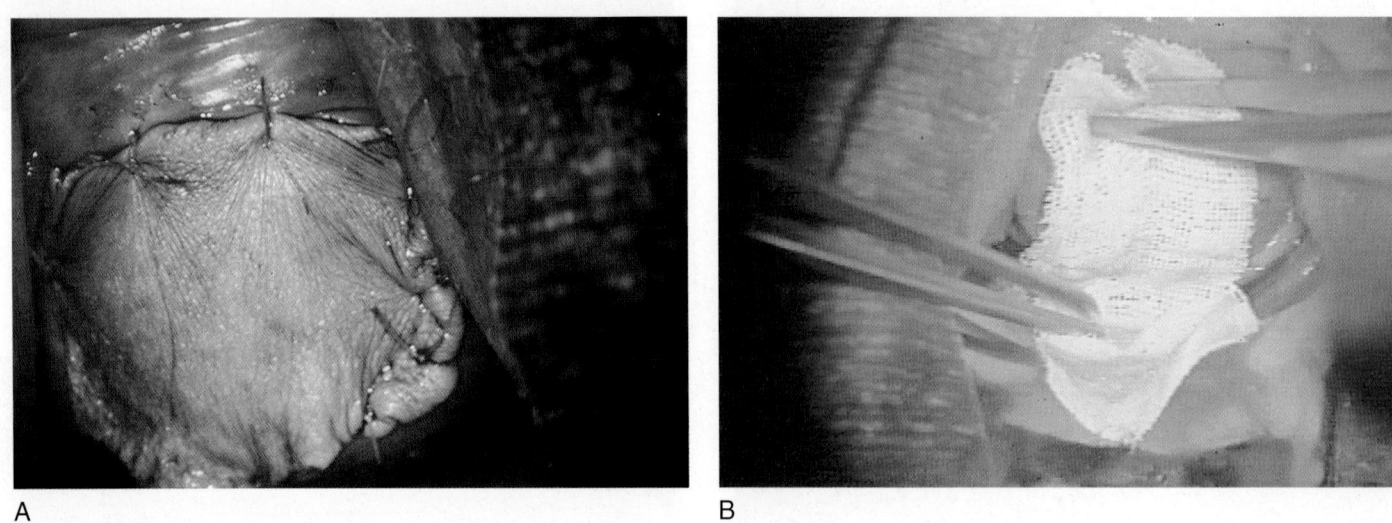

A

B

**FIGURE 63–11 A.** The slightly stretched graft is sutured into place over a *dry* vaginal bed. **B.** Fine-mesh gauze is placed over the graft.

## Carbon Dioxide Laser

The only practical laser to use in the vagina is the carbon dioxide laser ($CO_2$ laser) delivered via microscope and micromanipulator. The technique for ablation depends on a suitably large laser spot size to avoid deep penetration, and the use of superpulsing to avoid excessive heat conduction. Power should be adjusted so the beam (spot) penetrates no farther than 1 mm.

Typically, VAIN appears as white, flat, warty lesions (Fig. 63–12). Neoplastic areas are separated by normal tissue (i.e., multicentricity is the rule for VAIN) (Fig. 63–13). Before treatment, multiple biopsies performed on the lesions have confirmed them to be intraepithelial neoplasia (i.e., the disease has been mapped). For ablative operations, vasopressin is not injected. The margins of the area to be vaporized are outlined by the laser on the basis of prior colposcopically directed mapping (Fig. 63–14). The dots are connected, thereby clearly outlining the area to be vaporized and permitting a ready reference for orientation (Fig. 63–15). Next, the laser spot size is increased to 2.5 mm, and the area within the outlined margins is vaporized (Fig. 63–16). Power settings depend on the surgeons' skill and experience with laser technology and range from 15 to 40 W. The goal is to vaporize the tissue to a depth not to exceed 1 mm. All char is washed away with 4% acetic acid (Fig. 63–17). When the fornices are to be vaporized, a titanium hook is utilized to manipulate the cervix so as to expose completely the vaginal recesses (Fig. 63–18A through C).

For women who have undergone hysterectomy and who have upper-third VAIN, the vaginal vault must be vaporized to effectively treat the disease. This in fact constitutes a high-risk group for invasive disease. Therefore, in the pretreatment and intraoperative phases, particular attention to detail is a requisite. The vault and tunnels must be multiply sampled and mapped. During the treatment phase, the vault recesses (tunnels) must be drawn out by means of a titanium hook and completely exposed and vaporized (Fig. 63–19A, B). Postoperatively, the vaginal walls can agglutinate and must be separated by application of a vaginal cream daily or twice daily. A sulfa-based vaginal cream or clindamycin (Cleocin) cream is suitable.

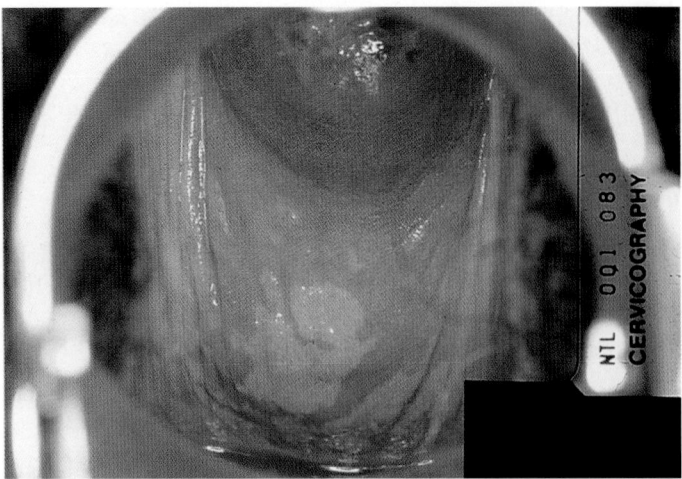

**FIGURE 63–12** Extensive, white condylomatous lesions characteristic of VAIN are seen on the posterior wall of the vagina.

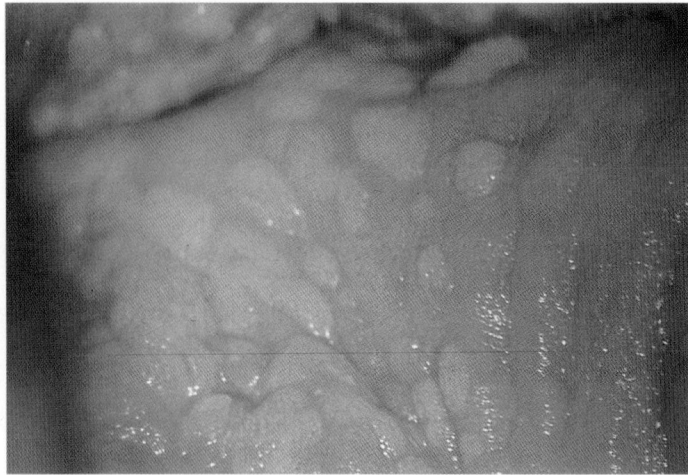

**FIGURE 63–13** Magnified detail of VAIN illustrates the multifocal nature of the disease.

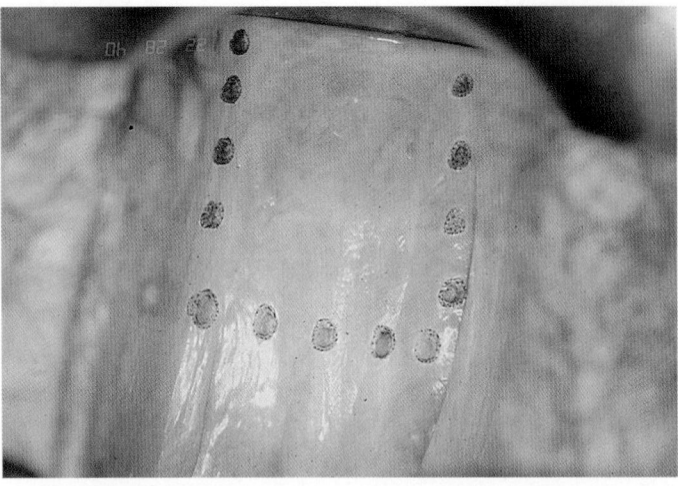

**FIGURE 63–14** Initially, the power density of the carbon dioxide ($CO_2$) laser (coupled to the operating microscope) is reduced to map the area to be vaporized by means of multiple trace spots.

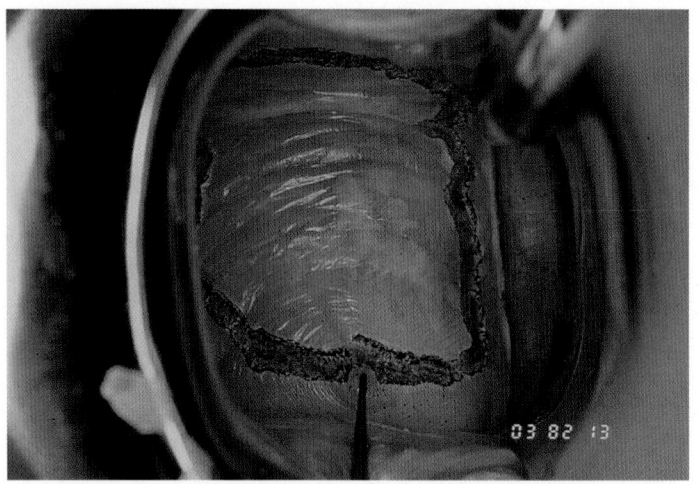

**FIGURE 63–15** The dots are connected by a superficial incision.

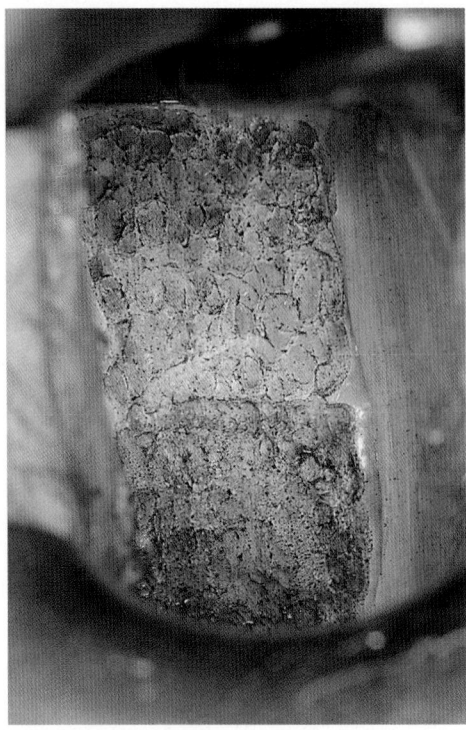

**FIGURE 63–16** The entire posterior wall of the vagina is vaporized to a depth of no more than 1 mm.

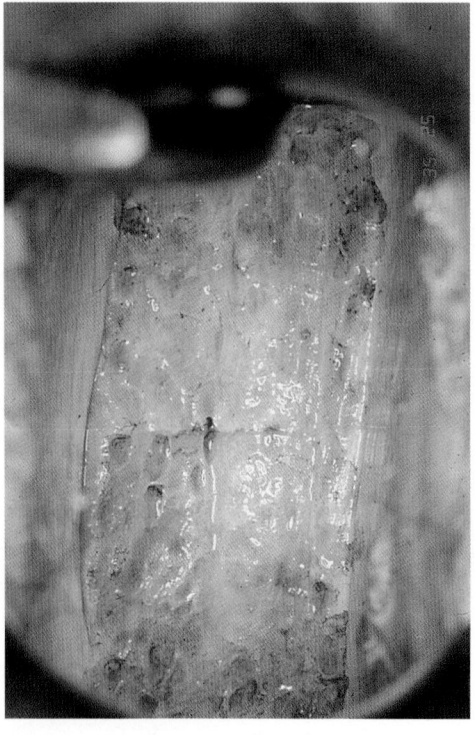

**FIGURE 63–17** The superpulsed laser creates minimal char formation. The laser wound is swabbed clean of all debris with the use of sodium chloride solution.

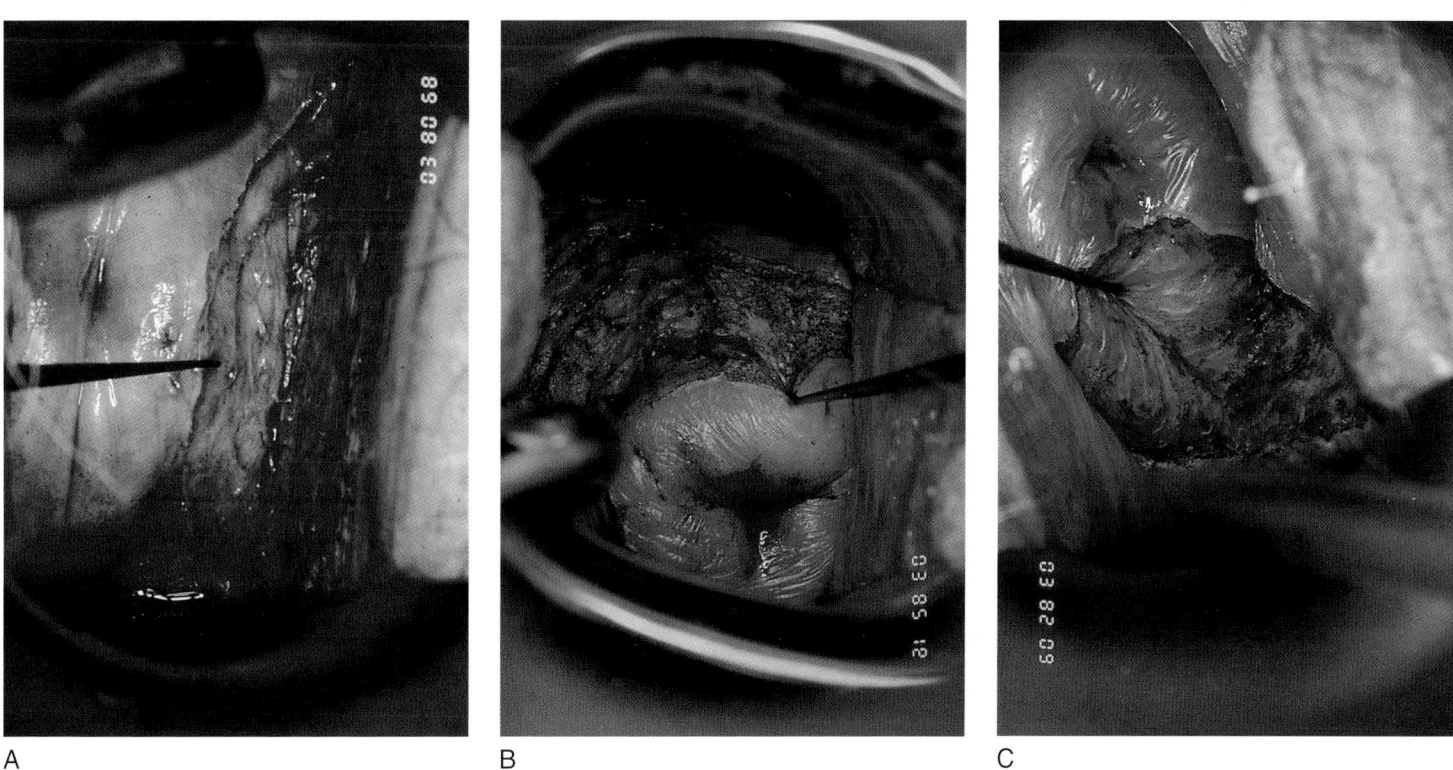

A          B          C

FIGURE 63–18 A. The cervix is placed on traction with a titanium hook to expose the lateral fornix. The lateral fornix is vaporized. B. Next, the cervix is pulled downward and posteriorly by manipulating hook to expose the anterior fornix. This is also vaporized. C. The posterior fornix is exposed by pulling the cervix downward and anteriorly. The posterior fornix is vaporized.

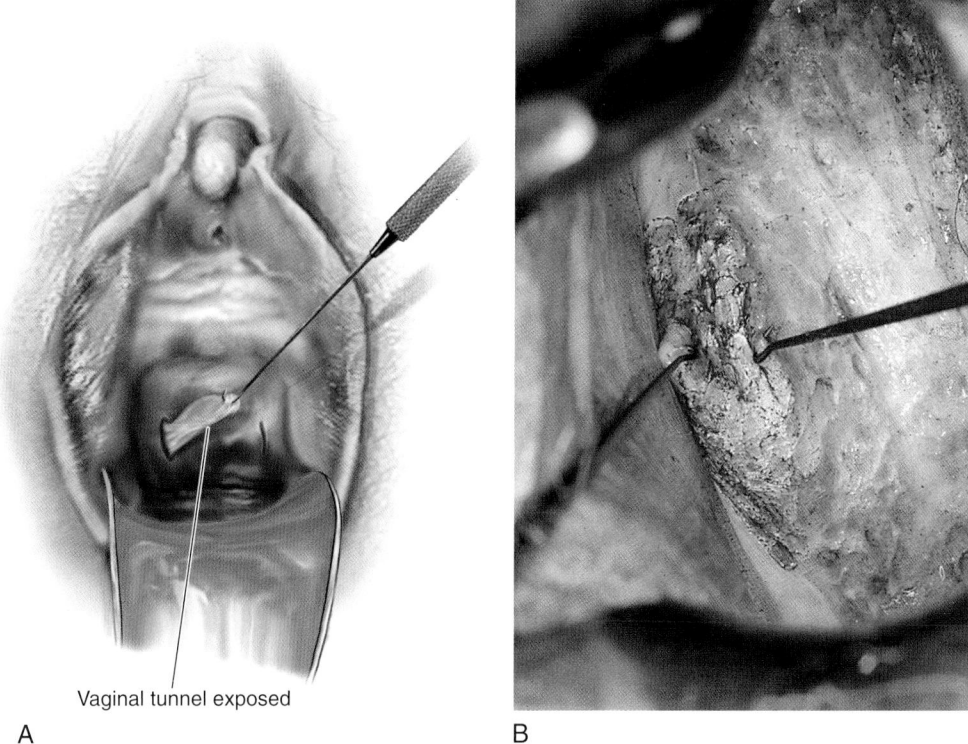

Vaginal tunnel exposed

A          B

FIGURE 63–19 A. The exposure and vaporization of vaginal tunnels created as the result of hysterectomy are vitally important when VAIN is treated. B. This vaginal tunnel has been exposed with the use of two titanium hooks. Note that the epithelium has been completely destroyed by laser vaporization.

# Vulvar and Perineal Surgery

# Vulvar and Perineal Anatomy

*Michael S. Baggish*

The external genitalia in the female are homologues to structures in the male. The former are unfused, the latter are fused.

The labia majora are homologous to the scrotum; the labia minora, to the median raphe of the penis and scrotum. The glans clitoris, clitoral body, and corpora cavernosa clitoris are direct homologues to equivalent penile structures in the male. The hood of the clitoris and the penile foreskin are likewise of similar origin.

The labia majora consist of skin and appendages, including hair follicles, sebaceous glands, and sweat glands, and create two prominent swellings on either side of the vulva. Subdermal fat deposits produce these bulges (Figs. 64–1A, B and 64–2). The prominence diminishes with age as the fat atrophies. Superficial branches of the pudendal artery supply the labia, and branches of the pudendal, ilioinguinal, genital femoral, and femoral cutaneous nerves supply the neural components (Fig. 64–3A through E).

The labia minora contribute to the structure of the clitoral frenulum and sheath (Fig. 64–4A, B). These structures contain no hair follicles but are copiously supplied with sebaceous glands and sweat glands. The labia are sites for specially adapted large sweat glands, the apocrine glands. These are also present in the perineum and perianal skin.

The area bounded anteriorly by the clitoral frenula, laterally by the medial aspects of the labia minora, and posteriorly by the fossa navicularis and posterior commissure constitutes the vulvar vestibule (see Figs. 64–1B and 64–5A). The external urethral meatus opens into the vestibule, as does the vaginal introitus. The hymenal ring frames the vaginal opening and is considered to be a portion of the vestibule (Fig. 64–5B). Additionally, several mucous glands open into the vestibule [Bartholin (major vestibular), minor vestibular, Skene ducts, paraurethral] (see Figs. 64–1B and 64–5C, D).

Below (caudad to) the external genitalia lies a flattened area extending between the anus and the lower portions of the labia majora and posterior commissure (Fig. 64–6). This region is referred to as the *perineum*, although the term also may encompass the whole area from the mons to the anus to the medial aspects of the buttocks and junction with the thighs. The perianal skin and anus constitute a part of the perineum and have much in common with the rest of the vulva (Fig. 64–7).

A flap may be cut to expose the underlying anatomy by incising from the top of the mons through the right or left interlabial sulcus to the perineum above the perianal skin. The flap is then cut from medial to lateral and is reflected laterally (Fig. 64–8). Ninety-five percent of the tissue beneath the skin of the labia majora is fat, through which course superficial vessels and nerves (branches of internal pudendal and pudendal) (Fig. 64–9). A membranous condensation of fat is located superficial to the thin muscles of the urogenital diaphragm. This is Colles'

fascia, which may easily be dissected with the fingers upward over the symphysis and above the inguinal ligament to Scarpa's fascia of the anterior abdominal wall. Just lateral and juxtapositioned to the hymenal ring beneath the vestibular skin is the bulbocavernosus muscle (Fig. 64–10A, B). During actual dissection, the muscle is thinner than depicted in the schematic illustrations shown in most anatomic texts (Fig. 64–11A through C). The same can equally be said for superficial transverse perineal muscle, which extends anterolaterally from its junction with the bulbocavernosus to the ischial tuberosity (Fig. 64–12A, B). Inferior to the latter muscle is the septated and fat-filled ischiorectal fossa. The fossa borders the anus and rectum medially (Fig. 64–13A through F). The levator ani descends through the ischiorectal fossa peripheral to the external sphincter and rectum (Fig. 64–14A through C). The ischiocavernosus muscle lies directly along the superior ischial ramus partly overlying the corpora cavernosa clitoris (crus). In relative size, the crus dwarfs the muscle (Fig. 64–15). A tough membrane encompasses the clitoral crus, the bulb of the vestibule, and the body of the clitoris. The membrane is tightly adherent to the cavernous vascular structures, which constitute the bulb, clitoris, and corpora (Fig. 64–16). The deep perineum is in fact revealed to be a vascular lake, and the most impressive structures in the deep perineum are these cavernous vascular structures. The cavernous structures impart a bluish hue because of the venous blood held within the vascular sinuses (Fig. 64–17A, B). The bulb is closely applied to the lateral aspect of the vaginal wall, which is also honeycombed with large cavernous and venous sinuses. Between the lateral margin of the bulb, the pubic, and the ischial rami is the fascia-muscle complex of the levator ani (Fig. 64–18). Similarly, the urethra is covered by an umbrella-like mass of cavernous tissue emanating from the bulb of the vestibule (Fig. 64–19A, B). The urethra, vagina, and cavernous structures are intimately applied to one another immediately below and at the urethrovesical junction (Fig. 64–20).

The anal opening is below the perineum. The course of the anus/rectum is upward (cephalad), deep to the broad anal sphincter and perineum, to situate itself 3 to 4 mm beneath the fossa navicularis and the lower vagina. The rectum is located in the posterior midline directly beneath the perineum (see Fig. 64–20). The space between the perineal and vestibular skin surfaces and the rectum depends to a great extent on the development, mass, and integrity of the perineal body and the anterior sphincter ani muscle (Fig. 64–21). At the point where the rectum reaches within a few millimeters of the posterior vagina, it parallels the vagina and follows a posterior and cephalad course (Fig. 64–22). The vagina may be freed from the rectum by careful incision and dissection of the rectovaginal septum from below upward, or by entry into the rectouterine space from above.

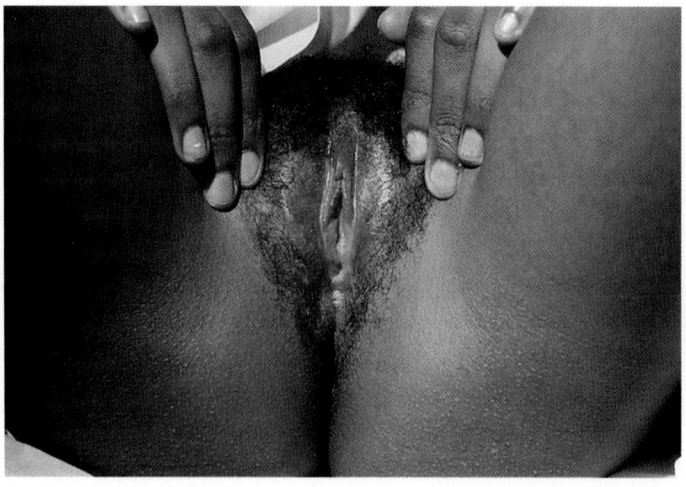

A

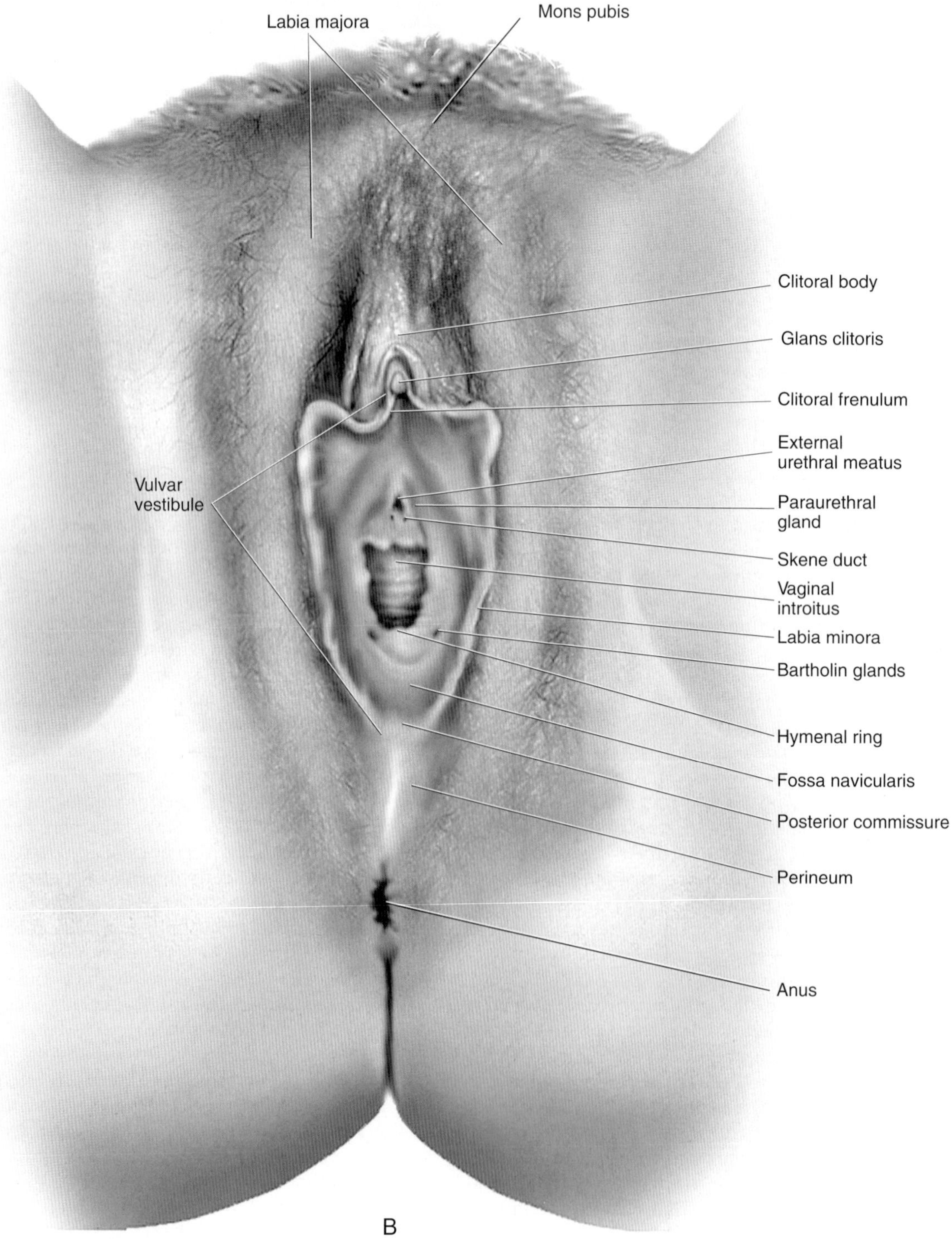

Labia majora          Mons pubis

Clitoral body

Glans clitoris

Clitoral frenulum

External
urethral meatus

Paraurethral
gland

Skene duct

Vaginal
introitus

Labia minora

Bartholin glands

Vulvar
vestibule

Hymenal ring

Fossa navicularis

Posterior commissure

Perineum

Anus

B

**FIGURE 64–1  A.** The labia majora form two prominent swellings that are produced by fat deposits lying between the dermis and Colles' fascia. These hair-bearing areas are rich in sebaceous glands, hair follicles, and sweat glands. **B.** This panoramic view of the vulva details the outermost areas, consisting of the mons (anteriorly), the labia majora (laterally), and the perineum (posteriorly). The innermost portions consist of the labia minora, the vestibule, the hymenal ring, the clitoral hood, and the glans clitoris. The clitoral body lies deep to the glans clitoris and is suspended from the pubic symphysis by a ligament.

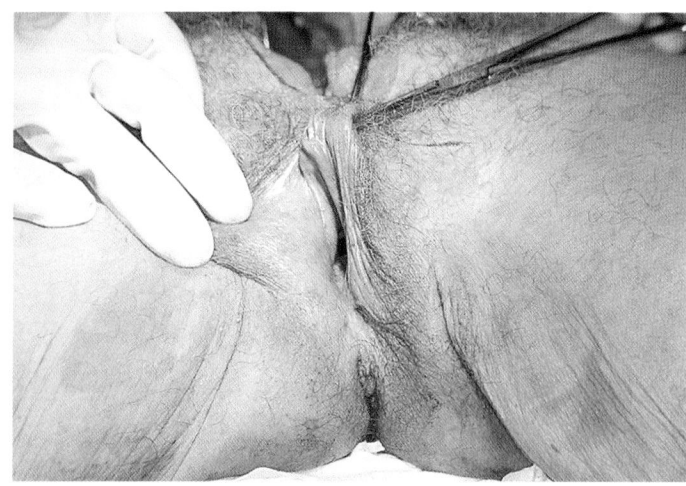

**FIGURE 64–2** The fresh cadaver specimen illustrates labial atrophy secondary to fat mobilization and deterioration following menopause.

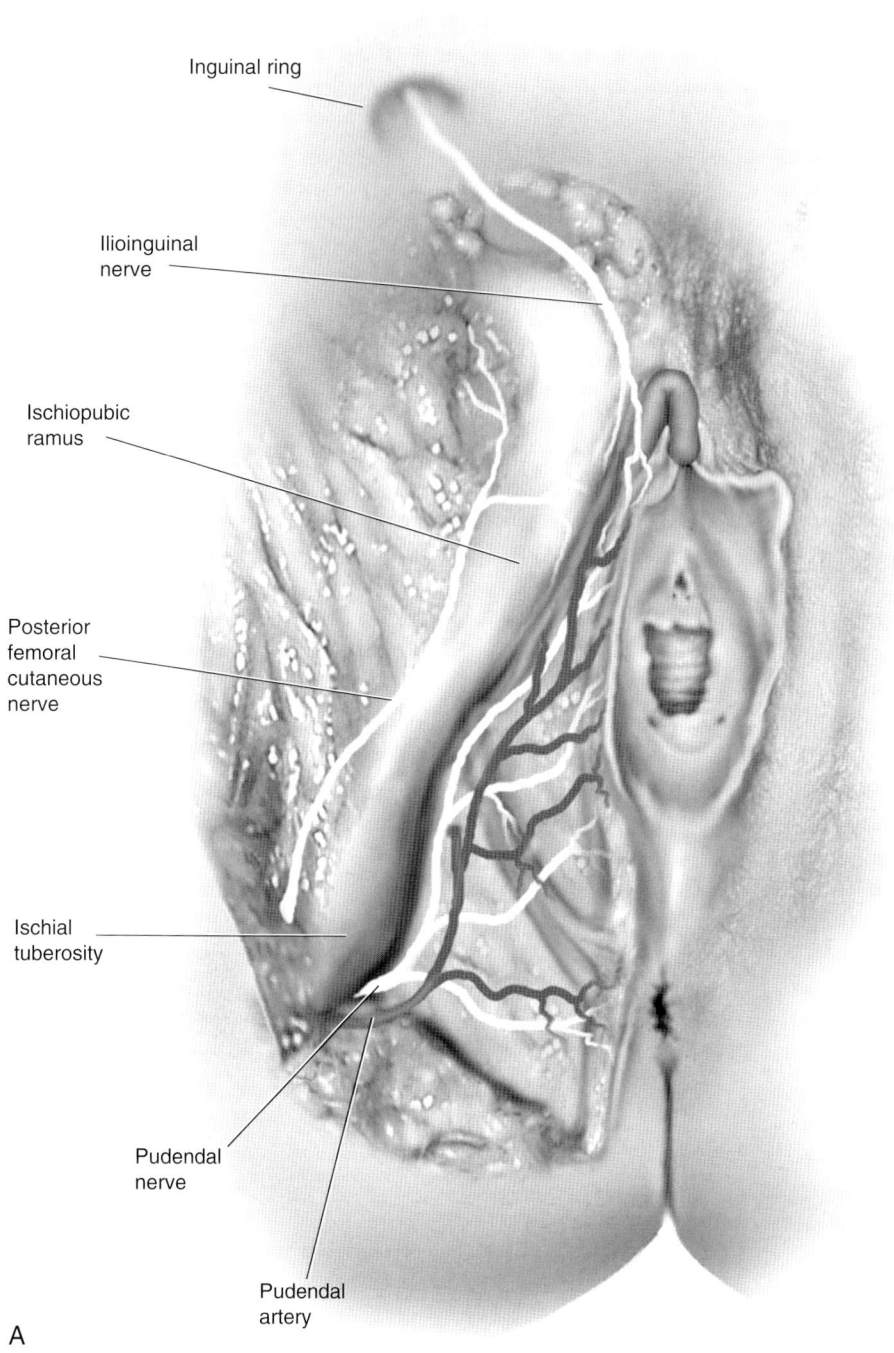

Inguinal ring

Ilioinguinal
nerve

Ischiopubic
ramus

Posterior
femoral
cutaneous
nerve

Ischial
tuberosity

Pudendal
nerve

Pudendal
artery

**FIGURE 64–3 A.** The vascular and neural supply to the vulva emanates from the internal pudendal artery (perineal branches) and from the pudendal nerve as they emerge from Alcock's canal and from beneath the ischial tuberosity. The posterior femoral cutaneous, ilioinguinal, and genital femoral nerves also supply portions of the vulva.

A

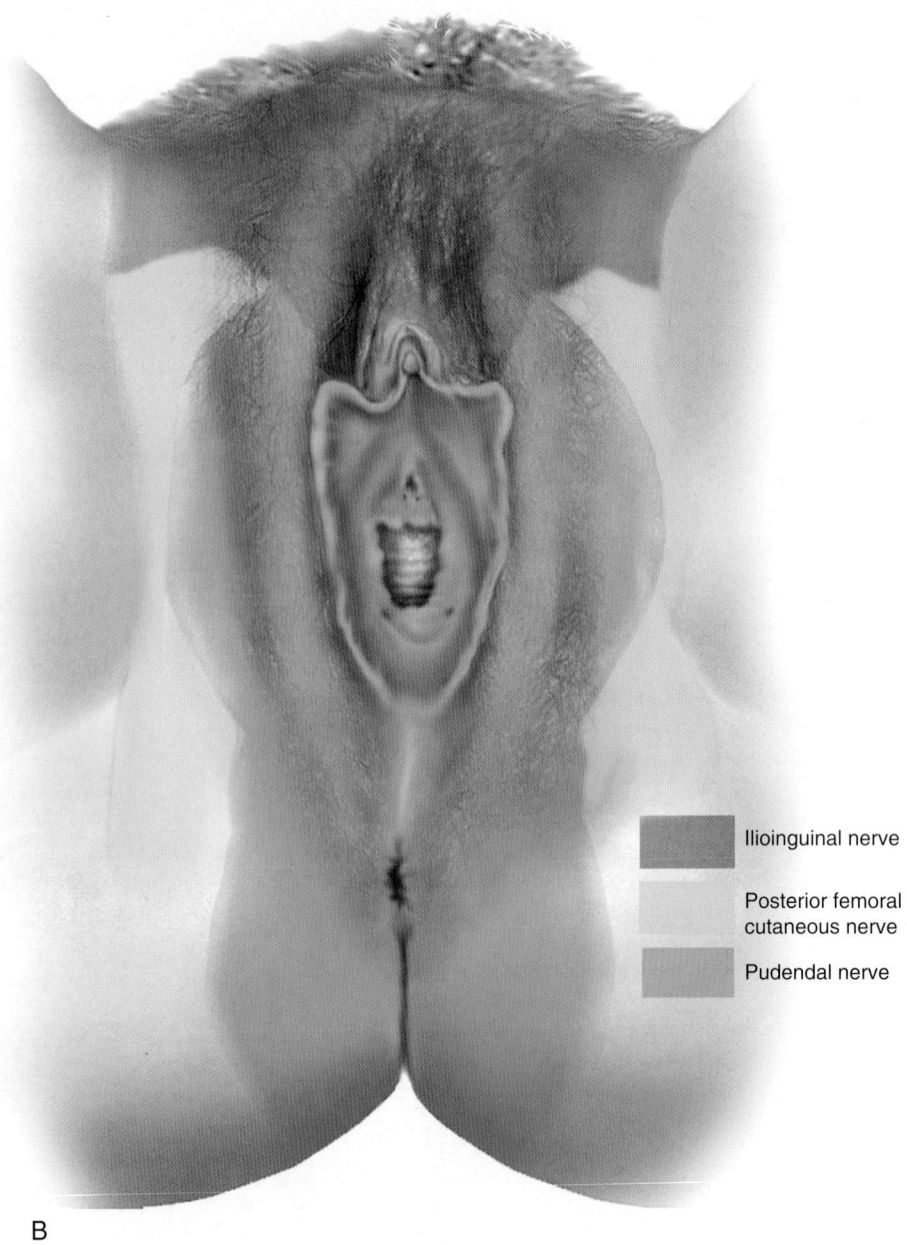

Ilioinguinal nerve

Posterior femoral
cutaneous nerve

Pudendal nerve

B

**FIGURE 64–3, cont'd  B.** The pink areas (mons, upper labia majora) are supplied by the ilioinguinal and genital femoral nerves. The yellow crural areas are supplied by the posterior femoral cutaneous nerves. The remainder of the vulva and the perianal skin are supplied by the pudendal nerves.

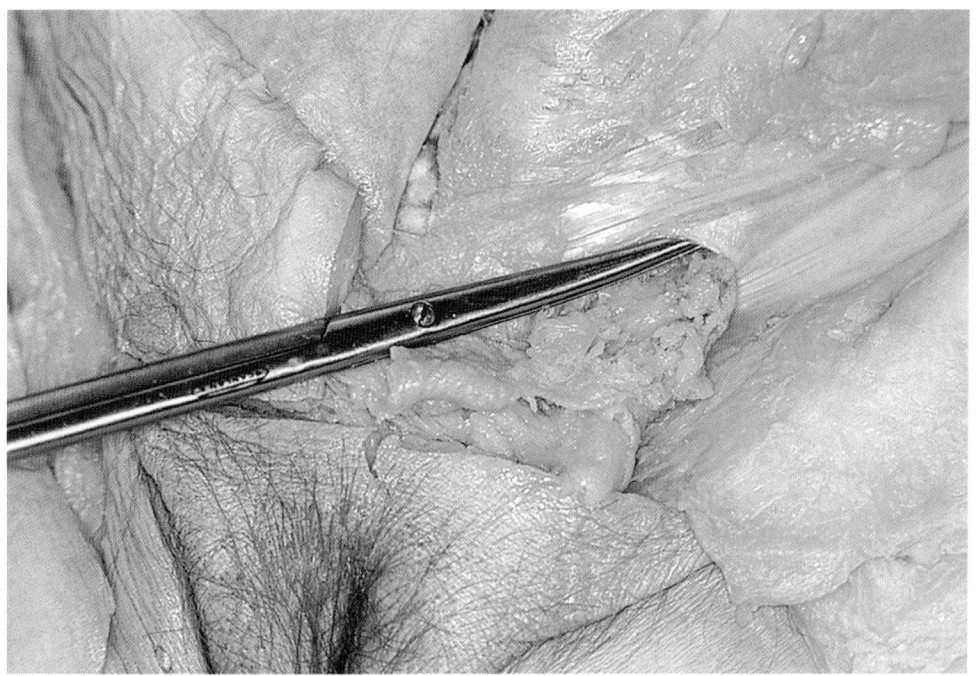

C

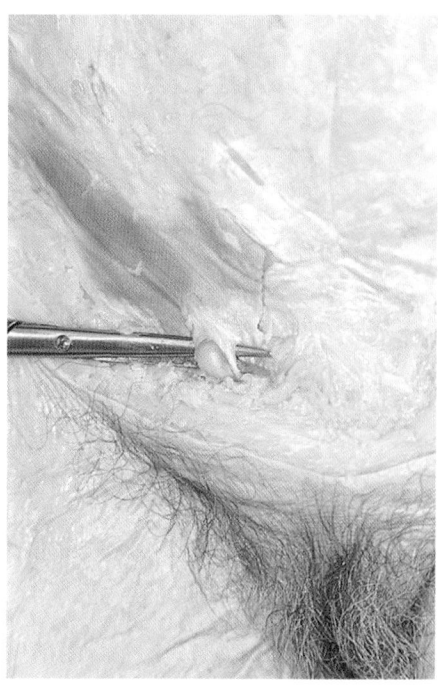

D

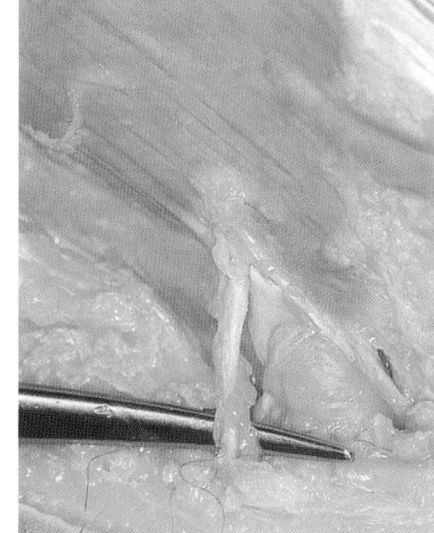

E

FIGURE 64–3, cont'd **C.** The tip of the scissors points to the external inguinal ring. The genital femoral (genital branch) and ilioinguinal nerves emerge in the fat, accompanied by the round ligament, which itself extends to the labium majus. The external inguinal ring illustrated in this photo is prominent because of the herniated fat emerging from it. **D.** The scissors are spread beneath the round ligament. The round ligament traverses the mons fat to terminate within the fat of the labium majus. **E.** The ilioinguinal nerve has been dissected free from the round ligament and surrounding fatty tissue. The branches of the nerve supply the mons skin and the upper aspects of the labia majora.

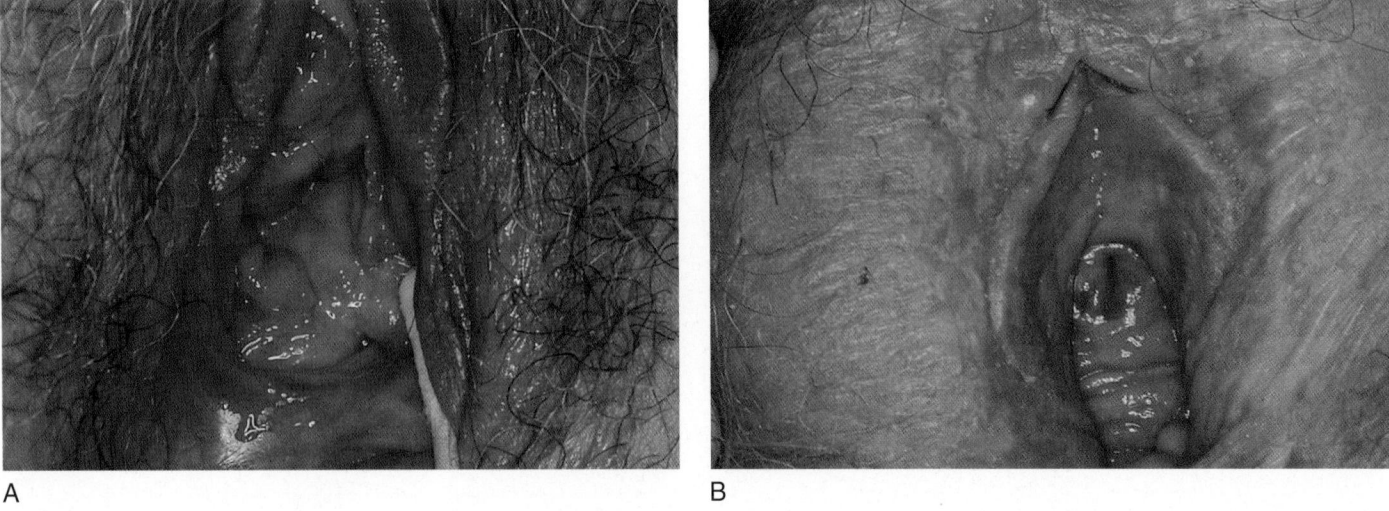

**FIGURE 64–4  A.** The labia minora are finely sculpted, hairless folds of skin that enclose the vestibule. The labia minora receive a rich neural and vascular supply and are more sensitive to touch than are the labia majora. **B.** This photograph illustrates the contribution of the labium minus to the clitoral frenulum and hood. As the labia come together beneath (posterior to) the clitoral glans, they form the upper limits of the vestibule. Note the external urethral meatus opening into the vestibule.

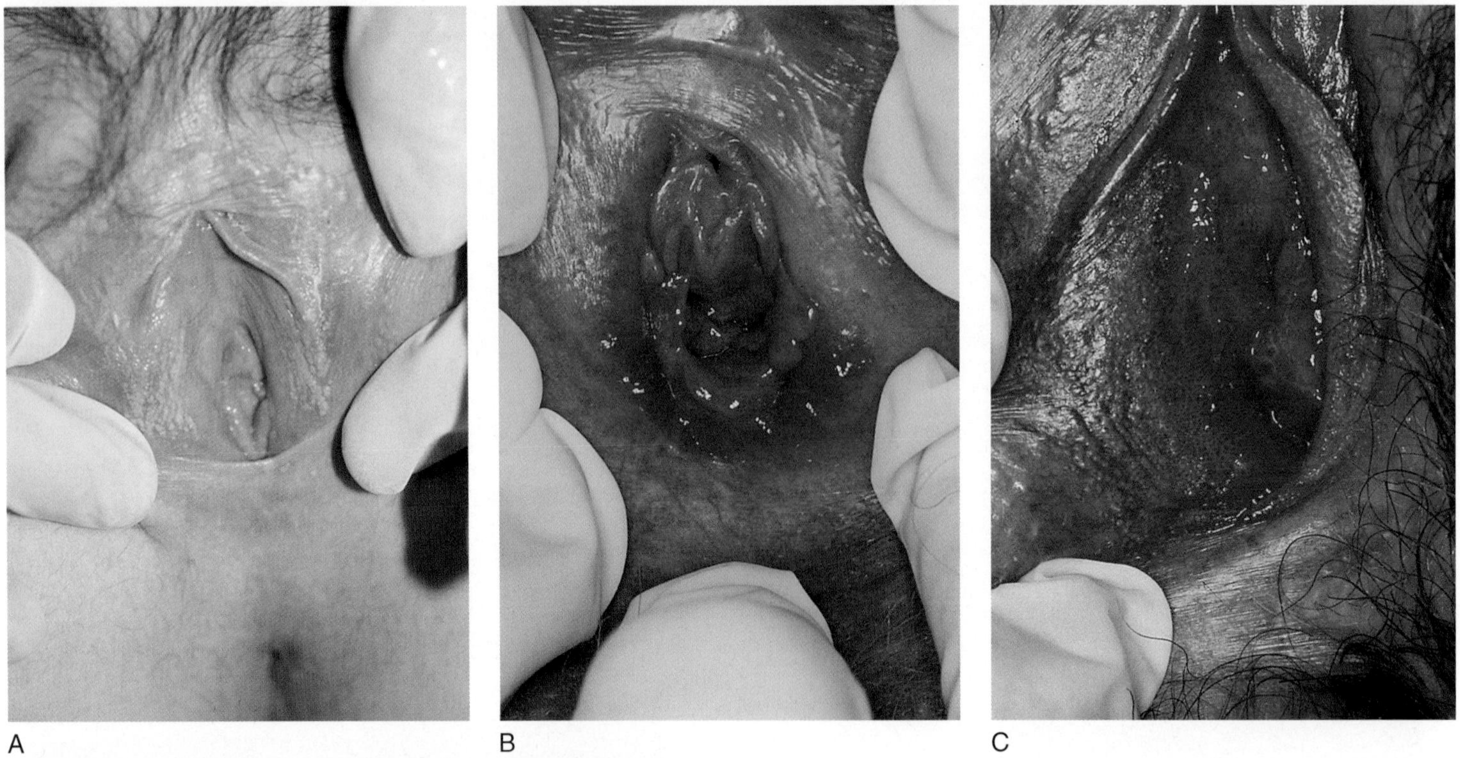

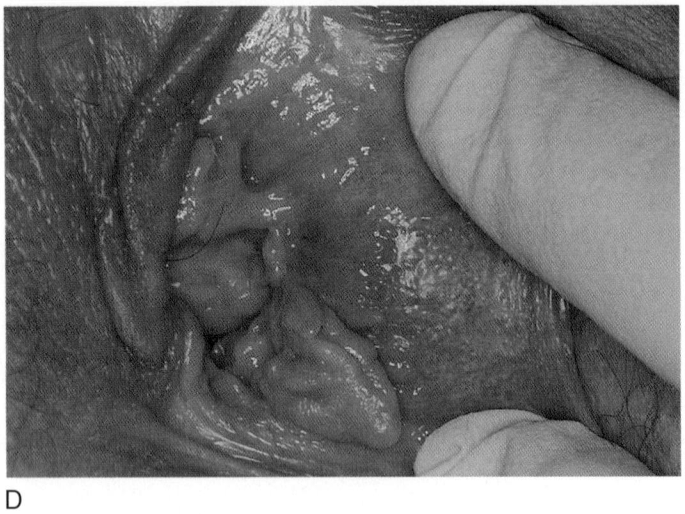

**FIGURE 64–5  A.** The vestibule is bounded anteriorly by the fused labia minora and the clitoral frenula. Laterally, the vestibular margins coincide with the medial surfaces of the labia minora. The posterior boundary of the vestibule is constituted by the fossa navicularis and the posterior commissure (see also Fig. 64–1B). **B.** The hymenal ring extends from the lower paraurethral area to the upper margin of the fossa navicularis. It frames the boundary between the vestibule and the entrance to the vagina. **C.** Paraurethral gland ducts are prominent and are located on either side of the urethral meatus (see also Fig. 64–1B). **D.** The opening of the left Bartholin gland duct is seen adjacent to the lower lateral aspect of the hymen. The gland is located 12 mm deep to the surface and slightly posterior and lateral to the duct opening.

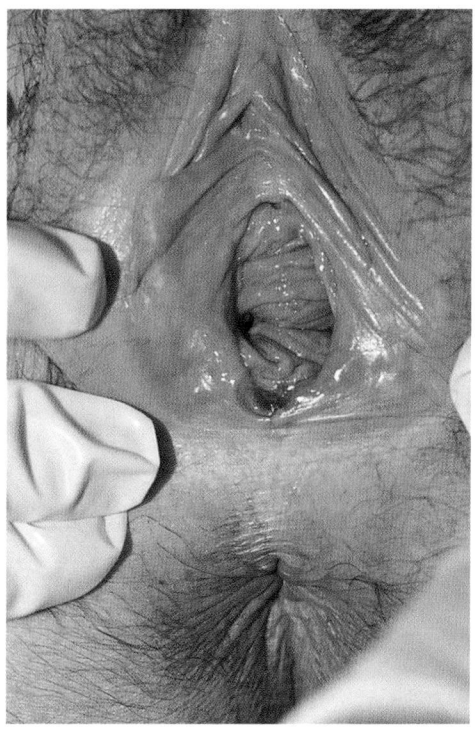

FIGURE 64–6 The perineum constitutes part of the vulva. It lies between the posterior commissure and the perianal skin. Deep to the skin are the "perineal body" and the external sphincter ani.

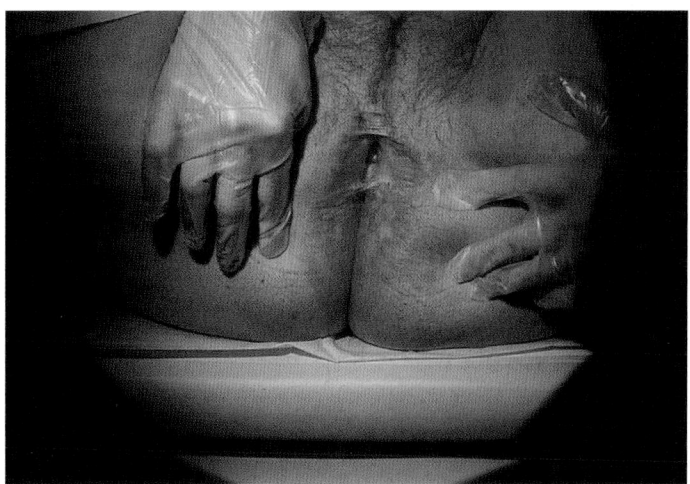

FIGURE 64–7 The perianal skin lies in the immediate vicinity of the anus and is subject to fecal contamination and inflammation if it is not kept clean and relatively dry. The skin in this area is usually more pigmented than the skin peripheral to it.

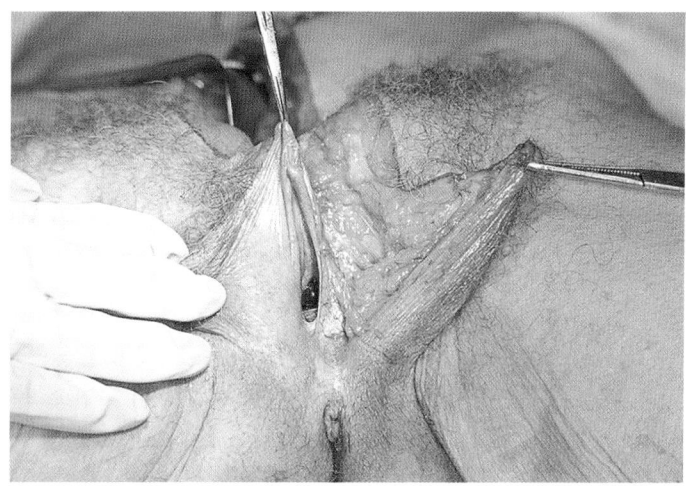

FIGURE 64–8 A flap has been cut in the skin of the left labium majus. Ninety-five percent of the subdermal content is fat. The glistening white membrane at the bottom of the incision is Colles' fascia.

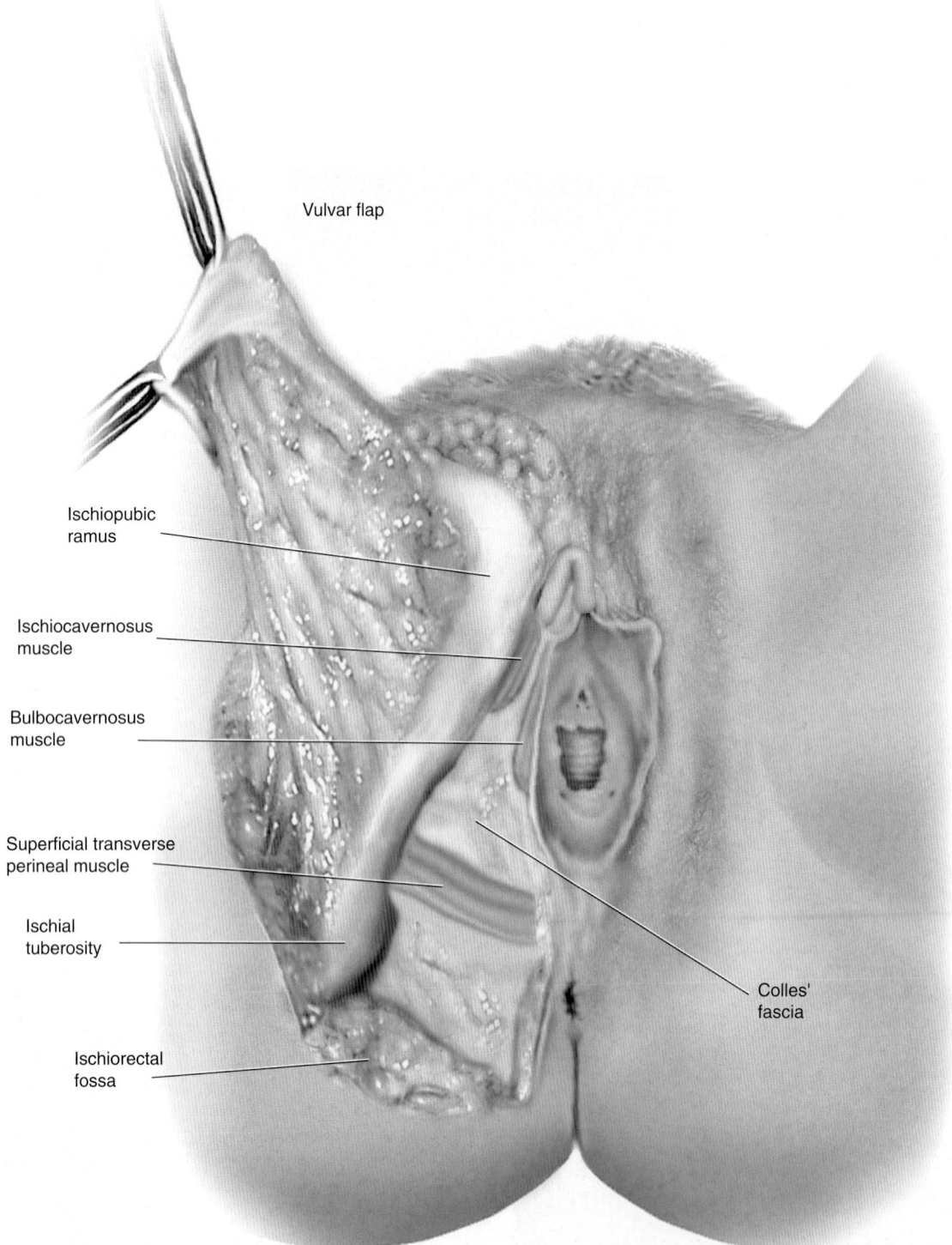

Vulvar flap

Ischiopubic
ramus

Ischiocavernosus
muscle

Bulbocavernosus
muscle

Superficial transverse
perineal muscle

Ischial
tuberosity

Colles'
fascia

Ischiorectal
fossa

**FIGURE 64–9** The fascia has been dissected away from the three superficial perineal muscles. These muscles are very thin structures and are represented in the drawing as they are seen during cadaver dissection. Between and covering the muscles is the tough Colles' fascia. Although others have described another fascial layer below Colles' fascia, the author has not found this layer to be a separate entity.

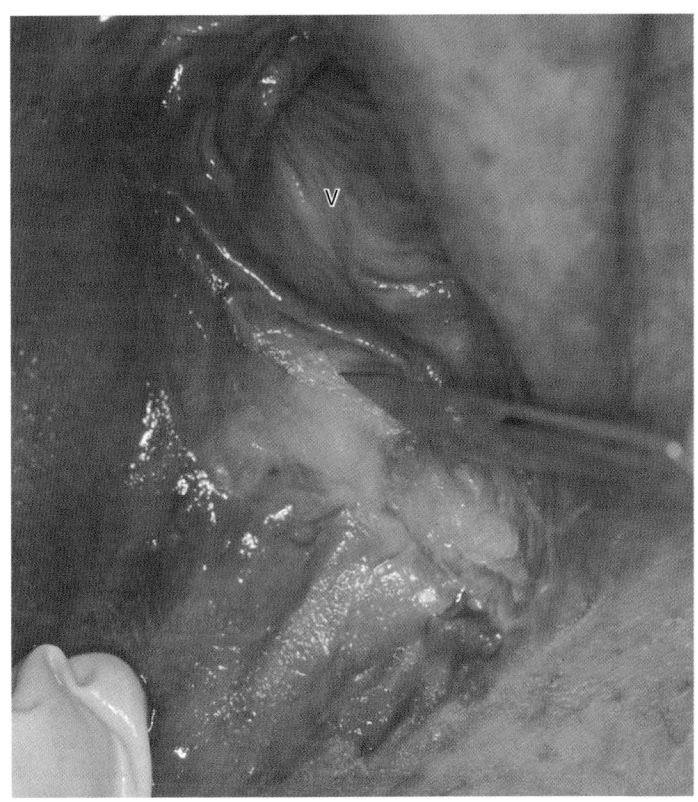

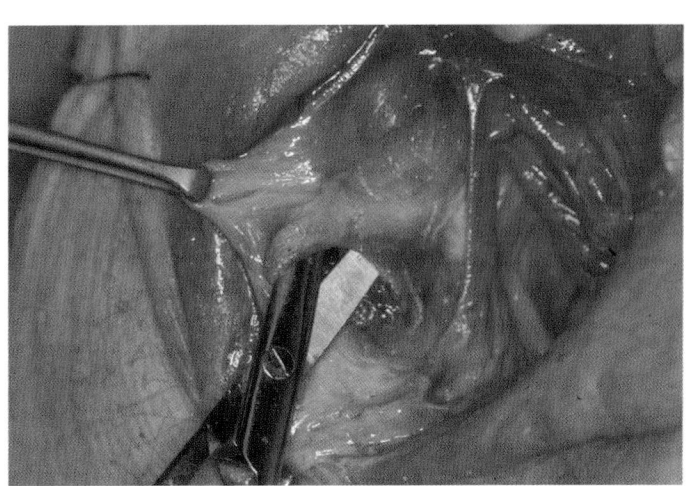

A

B

**FIGURE 64–10 A.** An incision is made immediately lateral to the hymenal ring. The white membrane is Colles' fascia. The vagina (V) is seen medial to the incision. **B.** Colles' fascia has been incised, and the bulbocavernosus muscle is dissected.

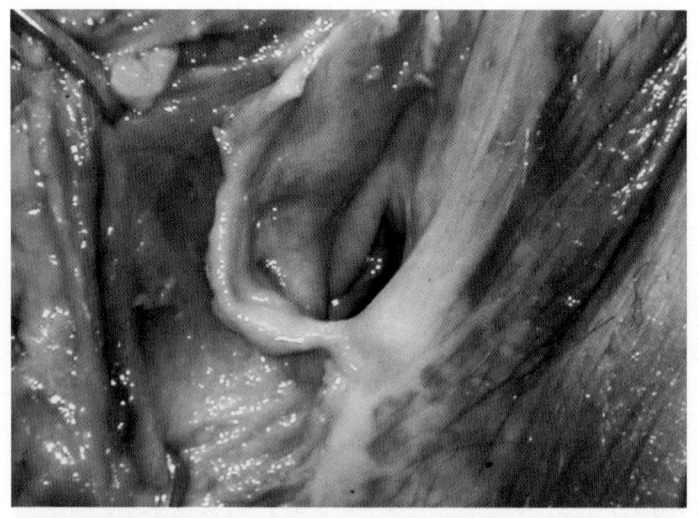

A

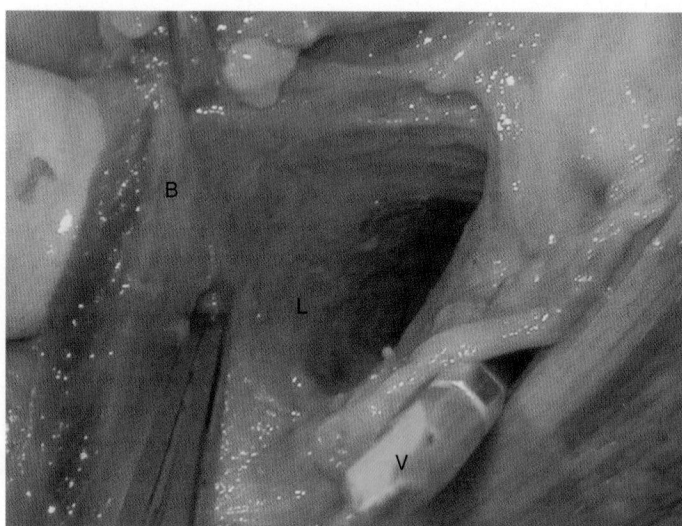

B

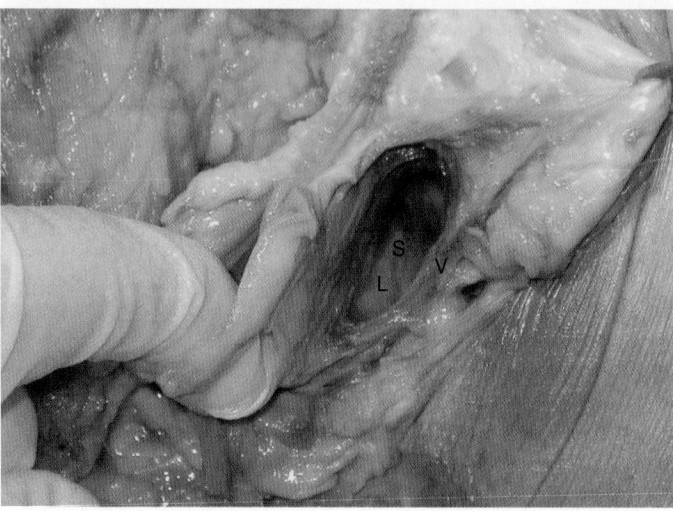

C

**FIGURE 64–11 A.** The bulbocavernosus muscle is held on edge with two Allis clamps. **B.** The green scalpel handle has been placed into the vagina (V). The scissors point to the junction of the bulbocavernosus (B) with the deeper lying levator ani muscle (L). The surgeon's gloved finger is behind and lateral to the bulbocavernosus muscle. **C.** The surgeon's finger is lateral to the right bulbocavernosus muscle. The space (S) dissected along the right inner vaginal wall (V) exposes the levator ani muscle (L).

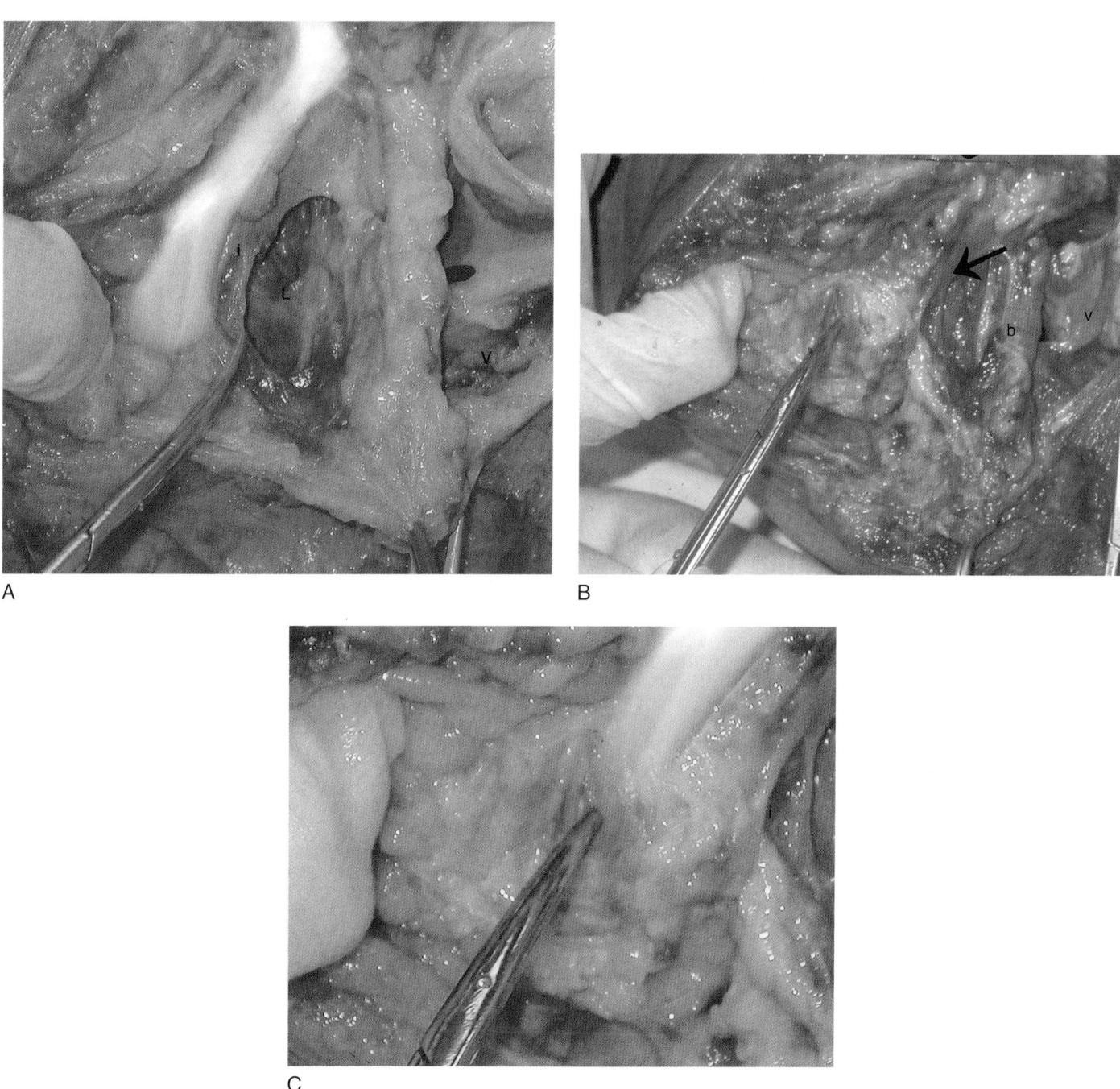

A

B

C

**FIGURE 64–12 A.** The scissors point to the superficial transverse perineal muscle. The ischiocavernosus muscle (i) lies along the pubic and ischial ramus. The perineal membrane has been removed to expose the underlying levator ani muscle (L). The vagina (V) has been dissected anteriorly, producing the hole in the anterior wall. **B.** The scissors point to the ischial tuberosity. The arrow points to the ischiocavernosus muscle. The bulbocavernosus (b) muscle is to the right of the vagina (V). **C.** Same photo as part **B**, but the ischial ramus has been added. The ischiocavernosus muscle (i) lies along the ramus.

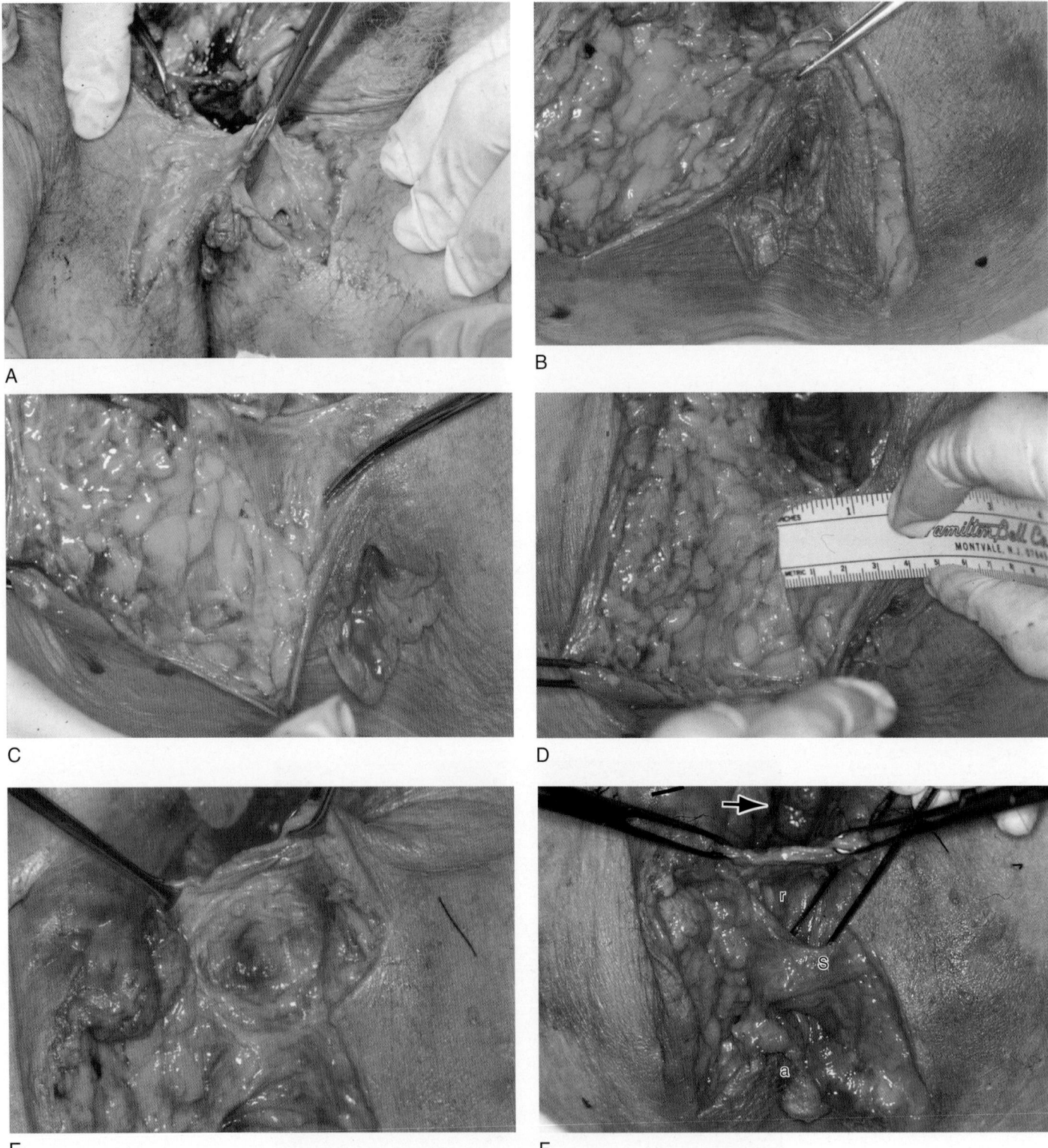

**FIGURE 64–13** **A.** An inverted-U incision has been made in the perineum and perianal skin, exposing the fat in the ischiorectal fossa. **B.** Magnified view of part **A.** The anal sphincter lies within the fat peripherally around the anus. It measures approximately 1 inch in width. **C.** The forceps point to the right lateral margin of the pink external anal sphincter. **D.** The ruler documents the width of the right portion of the external anal sphincter. **E.** The posterior vaginal wall, which measures 4 mm thick, has been dissected free from the rectum. **F.** The arrow points to the vagina. The Allis forceps hold the dissected posterior vaginal wall. The outer wall of the rectum (r) constitutes the inner sphincter mechanism. The external sphincter (S) has been partially separated from the rectum (r). The anal opening (a) is seen at the lower margin of the photo.

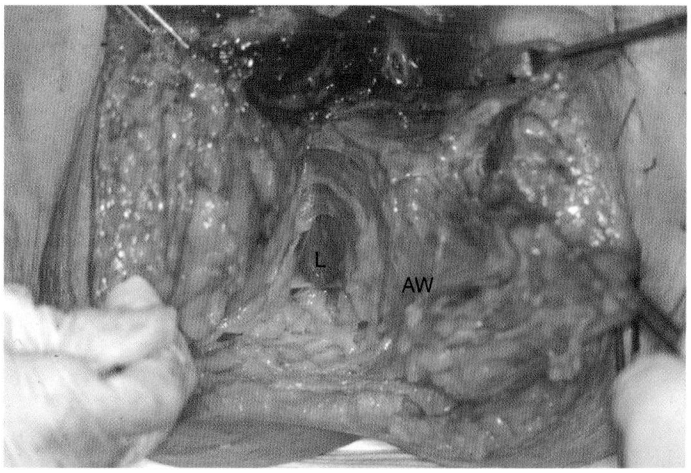

A

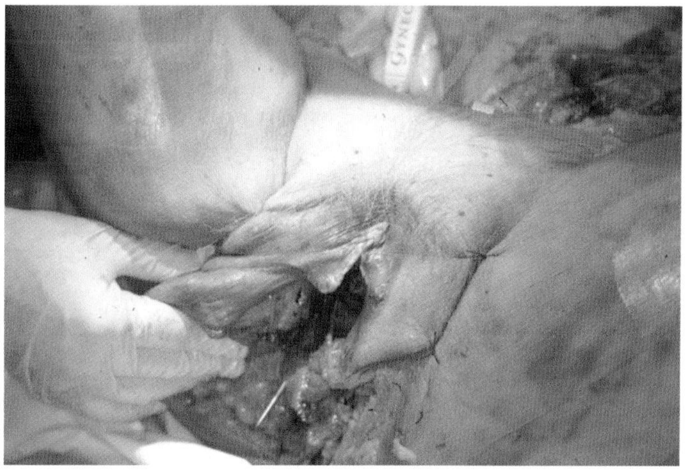

B

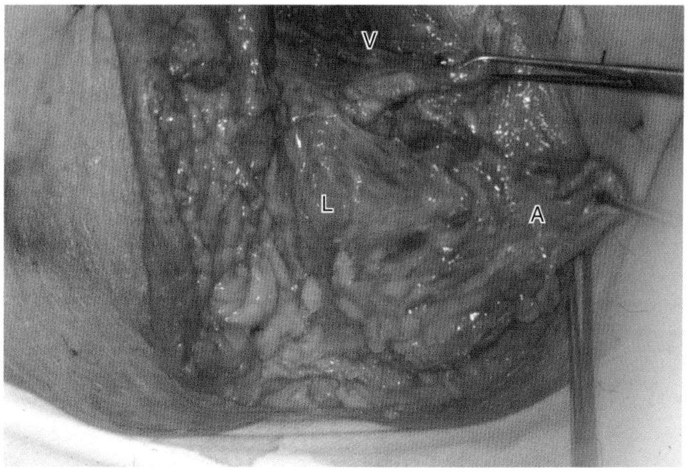

C

**FIGURE 64-14 A.** The levator ani (L) is seen adjacent to the anal sphincter and the anorectal inner wall (AW). **B.** A needle has been placed to mark the location of the levator ani muscle. The handle of the needle is seen above the mons in the retropubic space. The needle tip emerges in the dependent portion of the levator ani lateral to the anorectal wall, where it interdigitates with the external sphincter ani. **C.** Close-up of the right levator ani muscle (L). The upper Allis forceps hold the edge of the posterior vagina (V). The lower Allis forceps hold the edge of the anus (A).

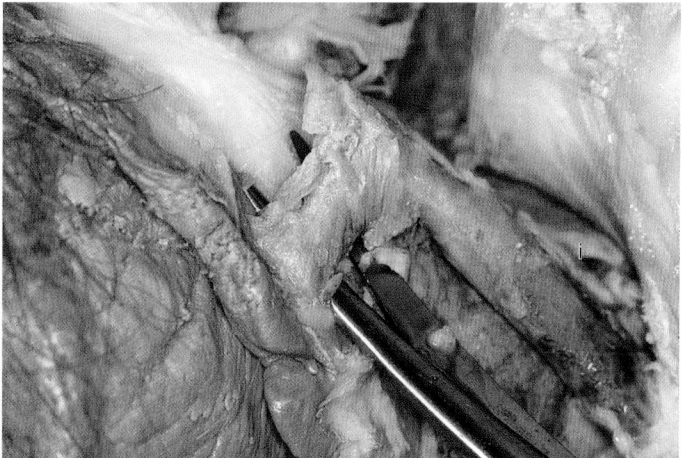

**FIGURE 64-15** The scissors are spread beneath the body of the clitoris. The large left corpora of the clitoris lies along the pubic ramus and is more prominent than is the ischiocavernosus muscle (i).

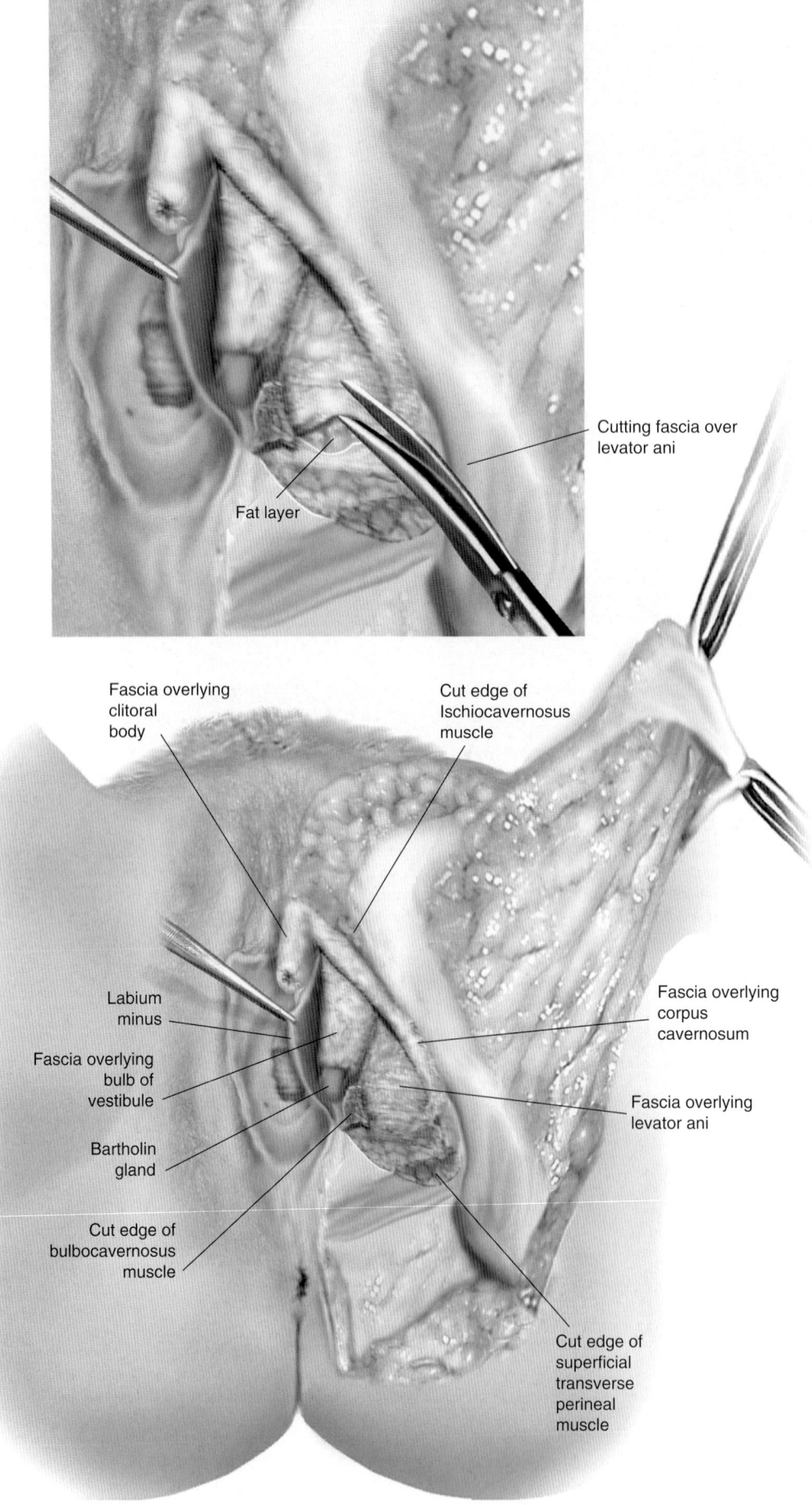

**FIGURE 64–16** The tissues situated deep to the superficial perineal muscles and Colles' fascia constitute a "blood lake" and are composed of a tightly applied tough connective tissue membrane overlying cavernous vascular spaces. These constitute the clitoral crura, the vestibular bulbs, and the body of the clitoris. The bulb of the vestibule shares a common wall with the urethra (anterior and lateral). Situated deep to and exposed between the bulb and the clitoral crus is the fascia covering the levator ani muscle. Between the fascia and the muscle is a thin layer of fat.

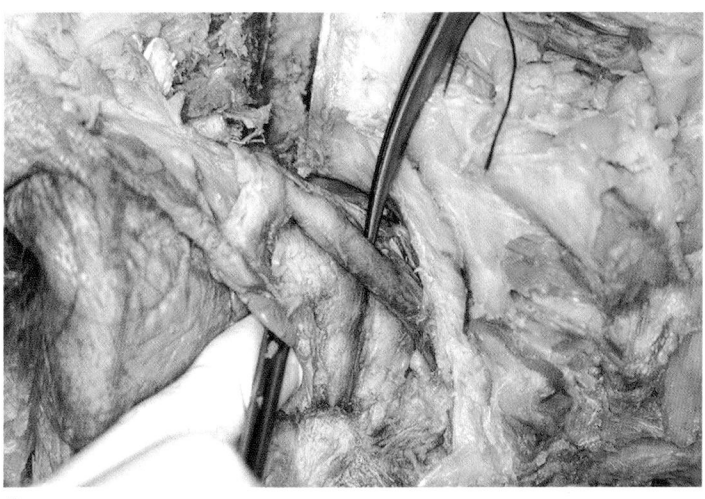
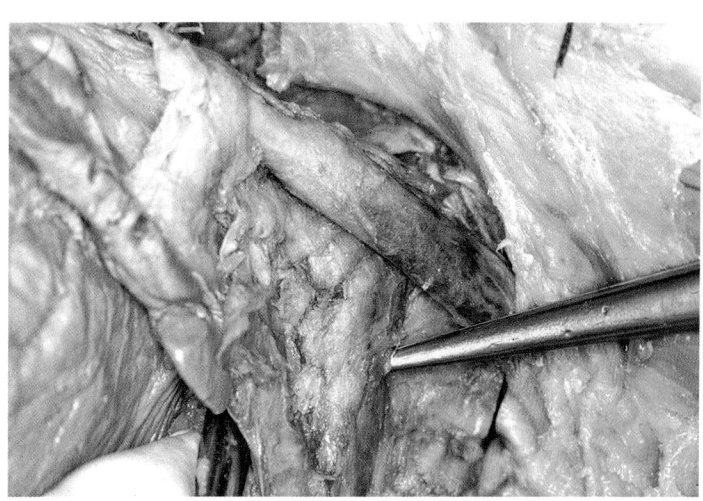

A

B

FIGURE 64–17 A. A portion of the fascia has been stripped from the left clitoral crus (corpora), revealing the deep blue coloration produced by the engorged cavernous spaces. B. The scissors point to the bulb of the vestibule.

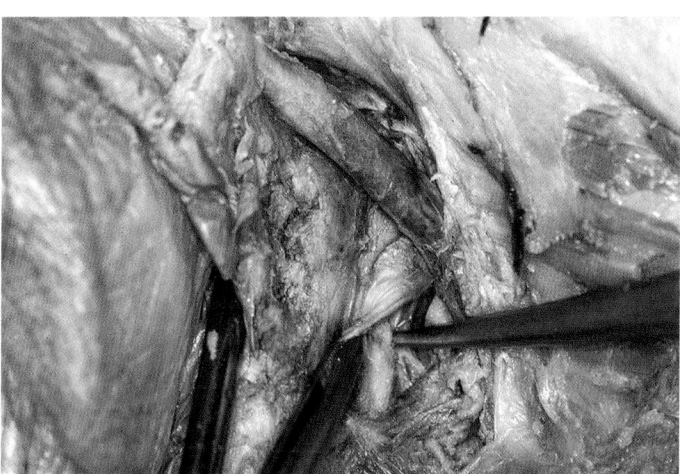

FIGURE 64–18 The tip of the scissors lifts the fascia of the levator ani muscle. If one were to push the scissors upward, the tip of the scissors would be seen to emerge in the retropubic space.

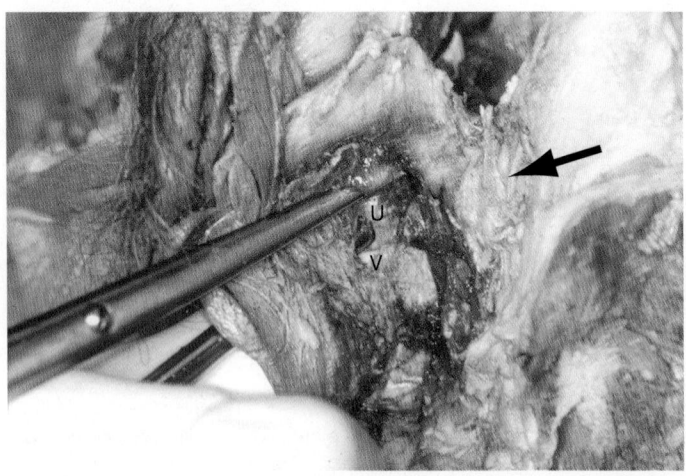

A

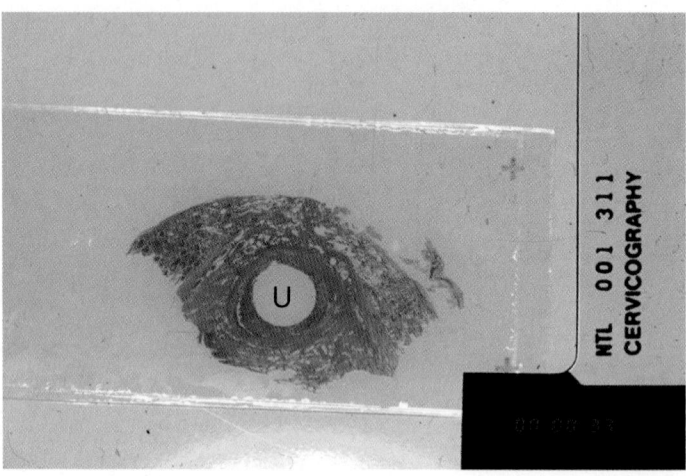

B

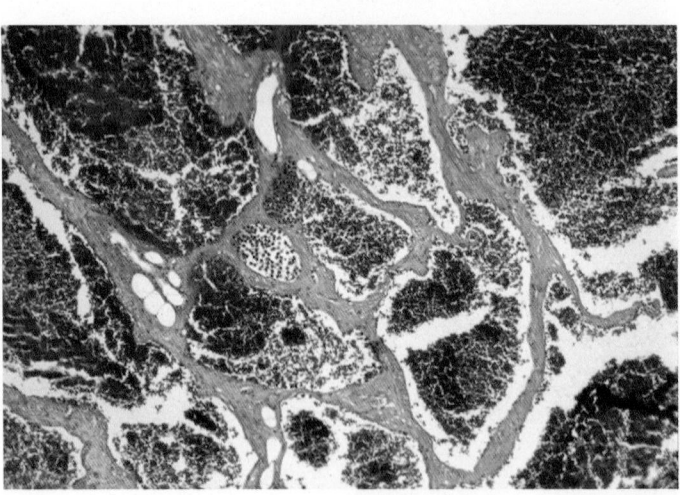

C

**FIGURE 64–19  A.** The surgeon's gloved finger has been inserted into the vagina of the cadaver. The metal tube has been placed into the urethra. The scissors have dissected through the bulb of the vestibule and have opened through the lateral urethral wall (U). A small bit of the white gloved finger (V) can be seen beneath the metal urethral cannula. The arrow points to the left corpora and pubic ramus. **B.** Microscopic section shows the urethra covered in umbrella-like fashion by the cavernous and blood-filled spaces of the bulb of the vestibule (Verhoeff–van Gieson stain). The urethral lumen is labeled (U). **C.** High-powered view of part B (hematoxylin and eosin stain).

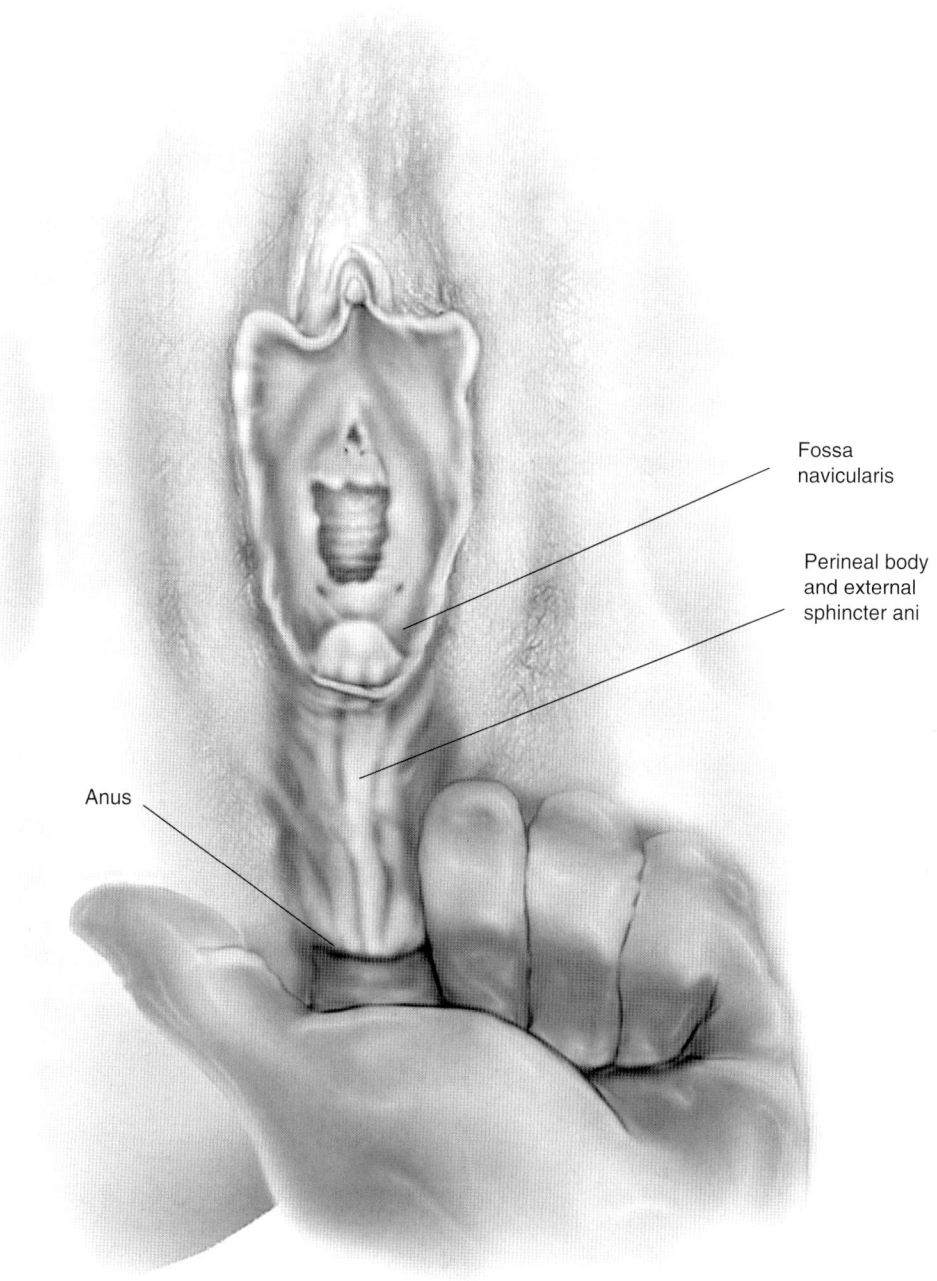

Fossa
navicularis

Perineal body
and external
sphincter ani

Anus

**FIGURE 64–20** The anus passes along the axis of the vagina after initial anterior vectoring. The mass of tissue between the perineum and the anorectal wall is the anterior sphincter ani muscle.

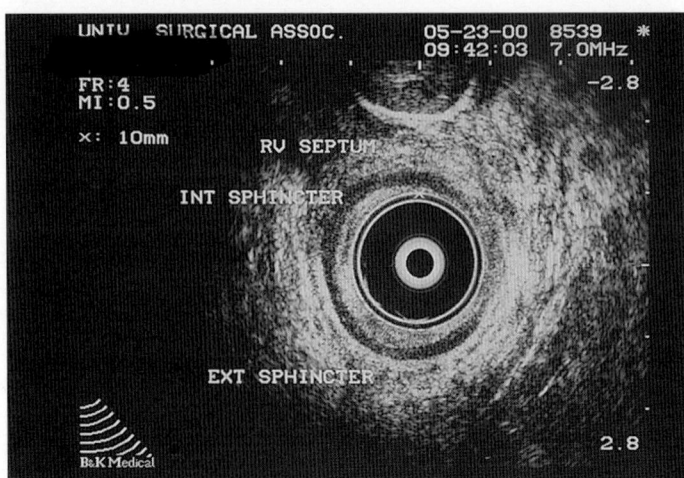

**FIGURE 64–21** Anal ultrasound image showing the relationship of the anus to its sphincter and the posterior wall of the vagina.

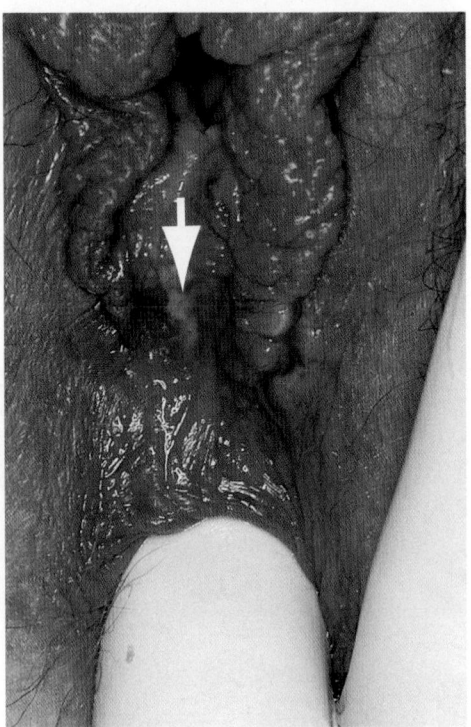

**FIGURE 64–22** This patient has an anovaginal sinus tract. Note the direction of the anal canal. The whitish discharge (*arrow*) emits from the lower, posterior wall of the vagina.

The microanatomy of the vulva is essentially that of specialized skin. The epithelium is composed of stratified and cornified squamous cells. Where the epithelium abuts the underlying stroma, it is characterized by finger-like downward-plunging pegs and upward-extending projections of the dermis known as the *dermal papillae*. Within the connective tissue stroma lie the sebaceous glands, ordinary sweat glands, and the large modified sweat (scent) glands, that is, the apocrine glands. In close proximity to the sebaceous glands are hair shafts and follicles. The follicles may extend deeply (3 to 4 mm) into the underlying fat. The dermis itself is divided into a small zone of papillary dermis and a larger zone of recticular dermis (Fig. 64-23).

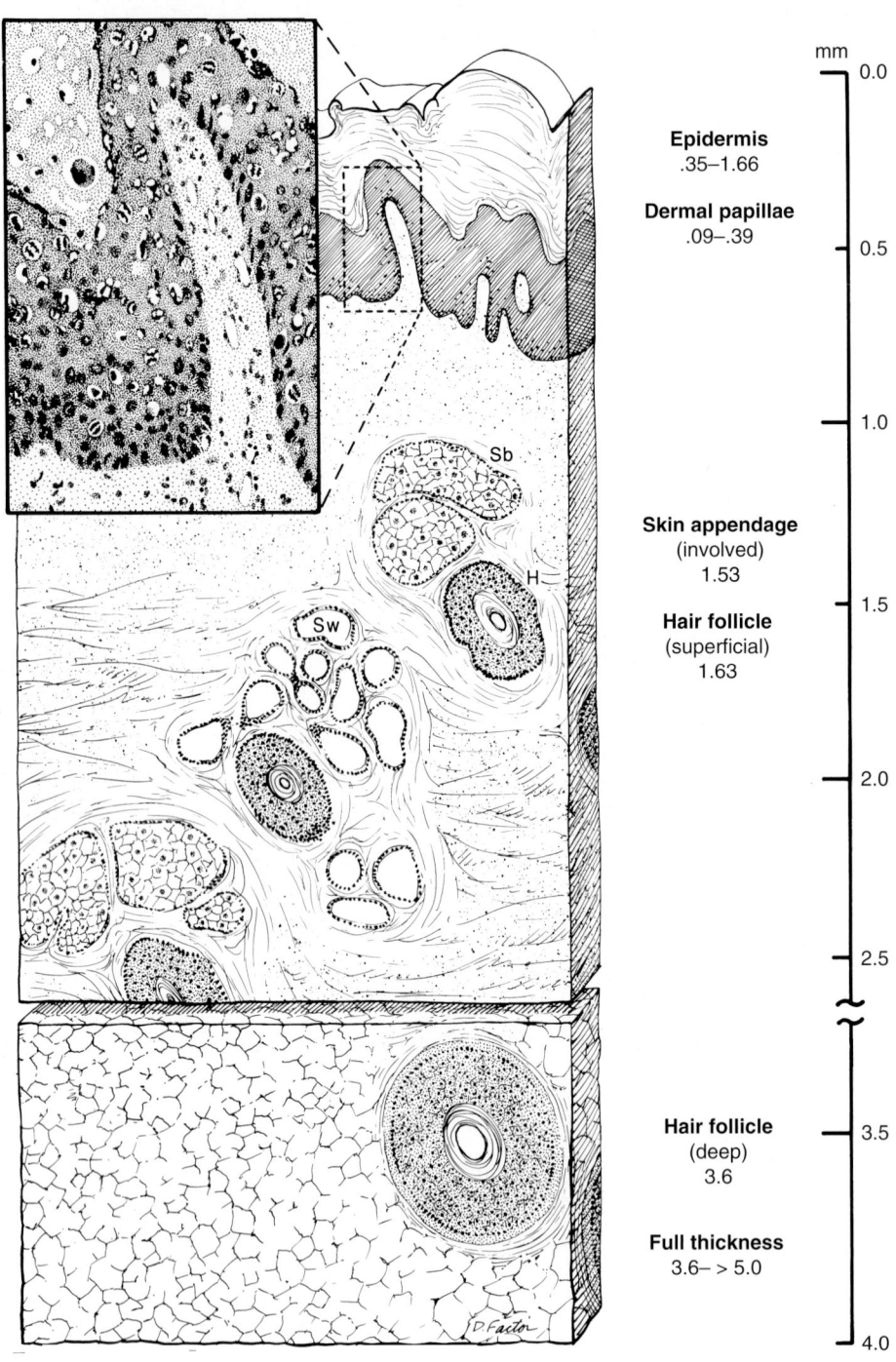

**FIGURE 64–23** Schematic microanatomic cross-section of vulvar skin based on micrometer measurements of actual histologic material. The papillary dermis is located directly beneath the epithelial pegs. The reticular dermis extends down to the subcutaneous tissue. H, hair follicle/shaft; Sb, sebaceous glands; Sw, sweat glands.

# CHAPTER 65

# Vulvar Biopsy

## Michael S. Baggish

A number of techniques have been reported that use vulvar biopsy. Regardless of the technique selected, the vulvar skin, unlike the cervix, has many pain receptors, and biopsy specimens cannot be taken without the aid of local anesthesia. Injection of 1% lidocaine with a 27-gauge needle will create sufficient anesthesia to permit the biopsy to be done painlessly. The injection discomfort itself may be significantly diminished by having the patient apply EMLA cream 30 minutes before the anticipated injection.

Dermatologists prefer to use a dermal punch and scissors for biopsies. The major advantage of the punch relates to the fact that it creates a flat disc sample that is easy for the pathologist to orient. This type of sample therefore is unlikely to result in a tangential tissue section.

After the creation of adequate anesthesia (objectively tested by squeezing the site with toothed forceps), the skin is flattened with one hand, and the sharp punch is applied and twisted back and forth two or three times until a full-thickness cut has been made through the skin (Fig. 65–1A, B). Next, with a fine forceps, the skin disc is elevated and its base cut away from surrounding fat and connective tissue (Fig. 65–2A through C). The sample is placed into fixative and transported to the pathol-ogy laboratory. The biopsy site is compressed with a sterile sponge and then is closed with two or three interrupted Vicryl sutures.

The dermal punch may be omitted by elevating the piece of skin to be biopsied and then simply cutting it off at the base with scissors or a knife (Fig. 65–3). As with the dermal punch technique, this requires the placement of sutures for hemostasis.

The least complex method for sampling vulvar skin is the punch biopsy technique. The same biopsy instrument used for the cervix and vagina is applied to the vulva. After the specimen is obtained, the biopsy skin defect is touched with Monsel's solution (ferric subsulfate) to stop bleeding (Fig. 65–4A through E).

The use of electrosurgical devices (e.g., loop electrodes) to perform a skin biopsy is decried because thermal injury devitalizes the skin and slows healing; it also increases the risk of infection. The same argument may be made when the use of Monsel's solution is discussed. Here, the amount of caustic Monsel's solution is a critical factor in that a large glob of the solution will retard healing and devitalize tissue, whereas a sparing application will not have significant detrimental actions.

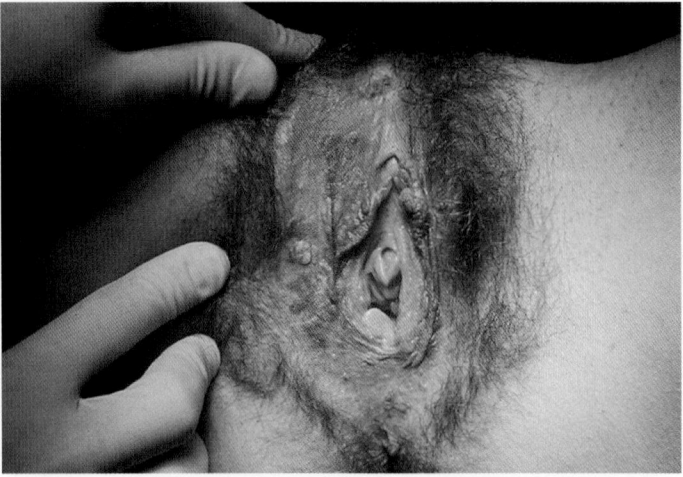

A

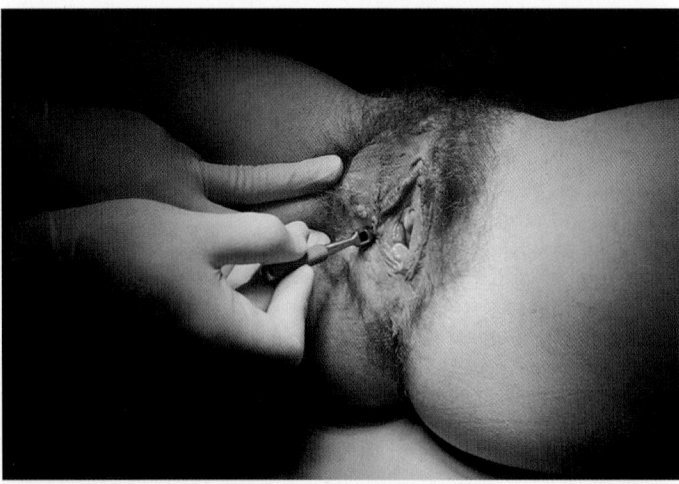

B

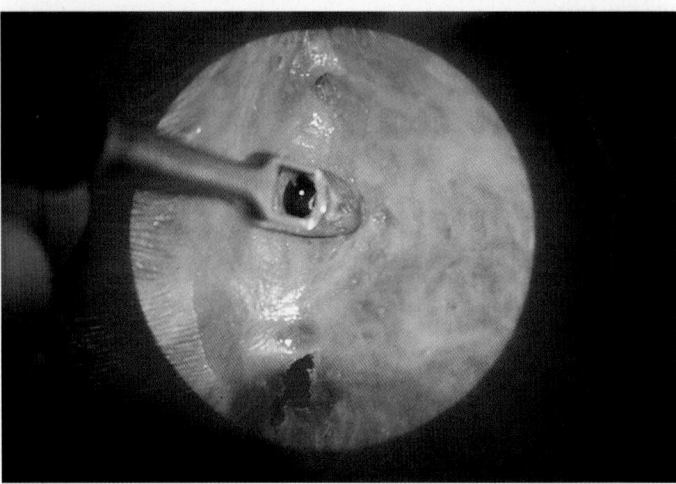

C

**FIGURE 65–1 A.** The vulva pictured here shows several areas suggestive of carcinoma in situ. These include flat warts and pigmented warty areas. **B.** The vulvar skin is anesthetized with a local anesthetic. The skin is flattened. The dermal punch is applied over the area of skin that will be subsequently sampled. **C.** The punch is rotated back and forth two or three times.

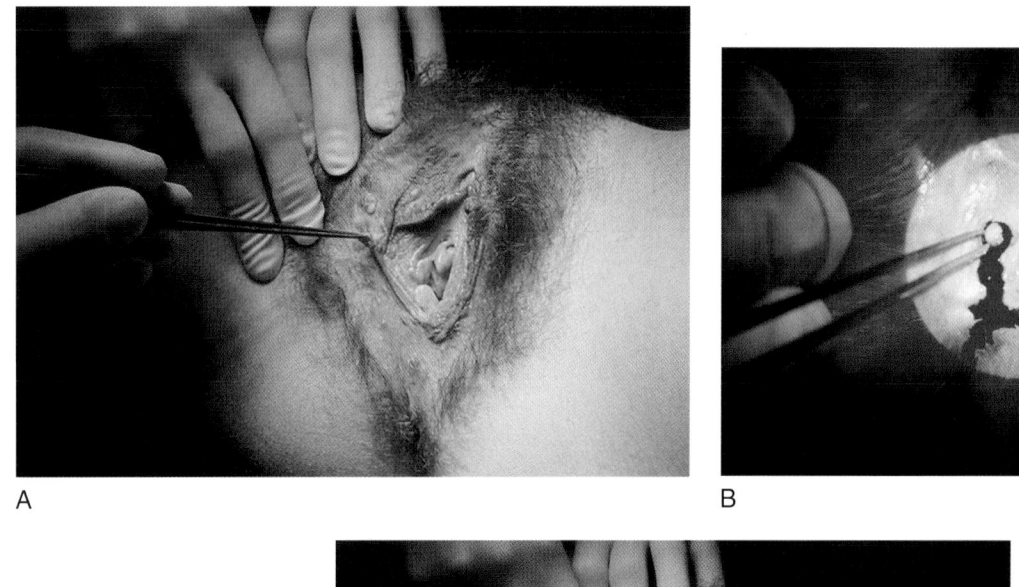

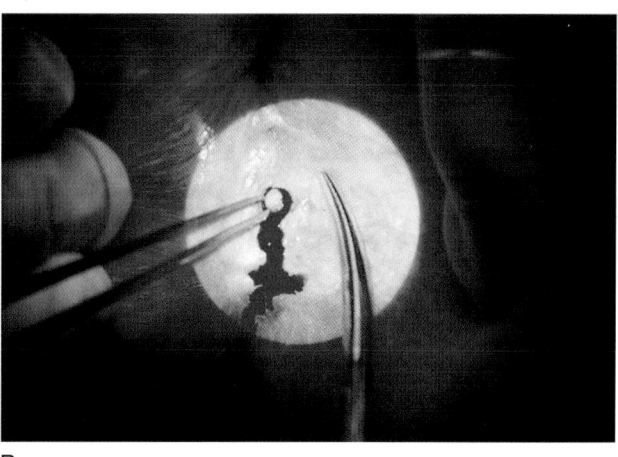

A

B

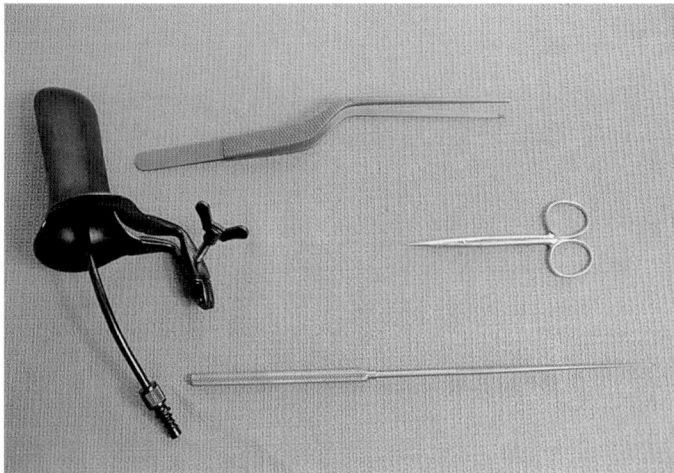

C

**FIGURE 65–2  A.** The disc of skin that has been cut by the sharp edge of the punch is now elevated with forceps. **B.** The disc is cut free from its base with fine, sharp scissors. **C.** After the specimen is separated from the surrounding skin, it is placed in fixative. If necessary, one or two 3-0 Vicryl sutures are placed for hemostasis.

**FIGURE 65–3** Another technique for biopsy utilizes a forceps or hook and a fine scissors. The skin to be sampled is elevated by a hook or forceps. The scissors snip across the base of the elevated skin, and the specimen is removed. As with the dermal punch technique, one or two stitches may be required for hemostasis.

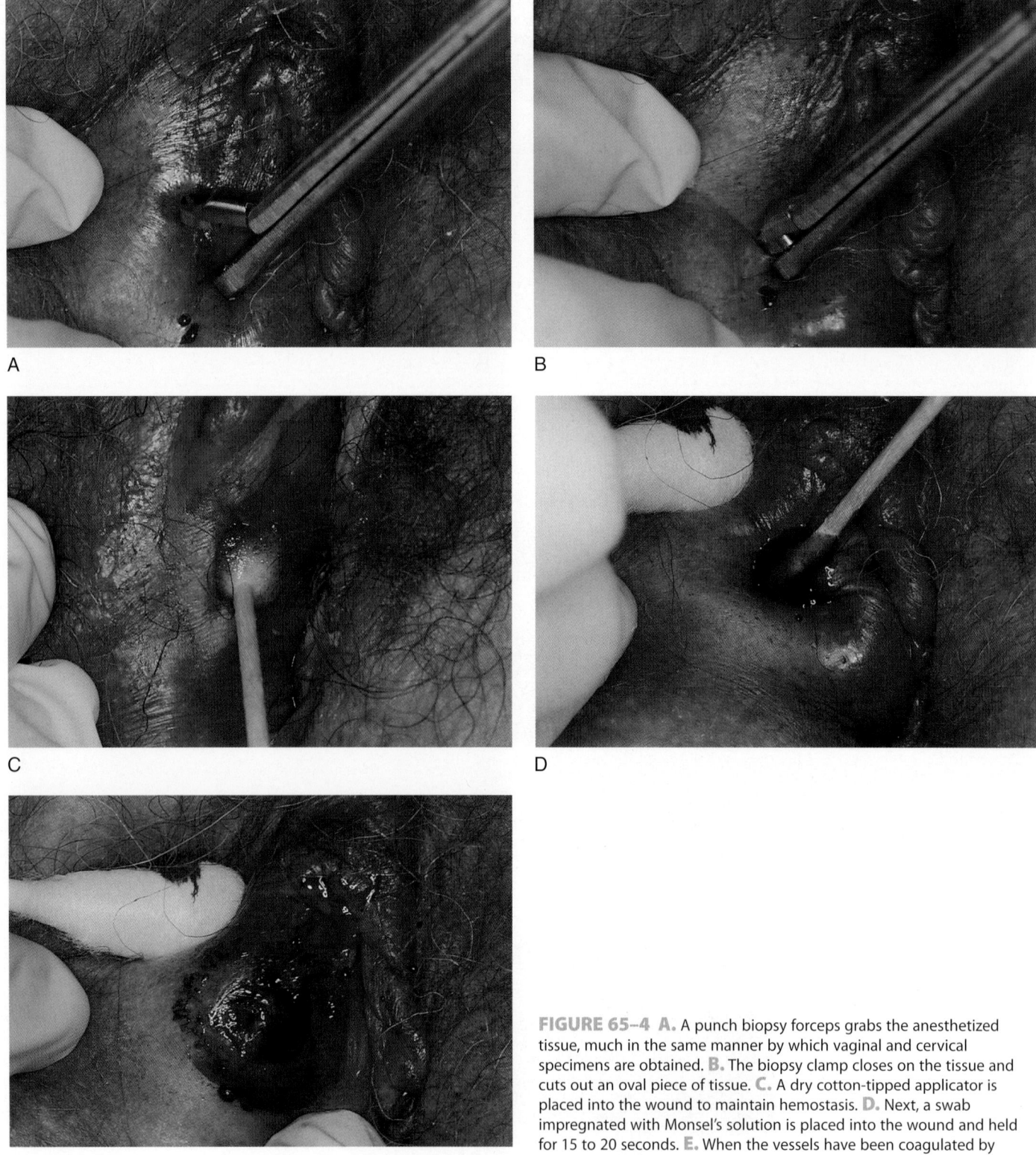

**FIGURE 65–4  A.** A punch biopsy forceps grabs the anesthetized tissue, much in the same manner by which vaginal and cervical specimens are obtained. **B.** The biopsy clamp closes on the tissue and cuts out an oval piece of tissue. **C.** A dry cotton-tipped applicator is placed into the wound to maintain hemostasis. **D.** Next, a swab impregnated with Monsel's solution is placed into the wound and held for 15 to 20 seconds. **E.** When the vessels have been coagulated by Monsel's solution, the swab is removed. The wound is dry.

# CHAPTER 66

# Bartholin Duct Cyst and Abscess

*Michael S. Baggish*

Frequently, gynecologists refer to obstruction of the Bartholin duct as a Bartholin gland cyst. The obstruction usually occurs at the surface (vestibule), and secretion of mucus by the gland leads to progressive dilation of the closed-off duct. As a consequence, the ballooned duct produces a swelling in the vestibule adjacent to the posterolateral margin of the hymenal ring (Fig. 66–1A). Pressure causes the swelling to be sensitive and even painful to touch (Fig. 66–1B). If the duct is colonized via vaginal or rectal flora, then the mucous cyst may become septic, producing a Bartholin duct abscess. This disorder is associated with cellulitis, erythema, and fever.

Treatment for a Bartholin cyst or abscess is drainage. A large opening should always be made in the cyst and its walls prevented from coapting and closing for 1 to 2 weeks. This may be accomplished by a variety of techniques, including marsupialization of residual margins of the open duct, insertion of a drain, and insertion of a Word catheter. The simplest technique is usually the best treatment regimen (Fig. 66–2A through C).

The patient may be anesthetized with general, regional, or local anesthesia. Two or three 0 Vicryl sutures are placed into the labia on the affected side and into the crural fold for retraction. The cystic swelling is incised vertically, and the draining interior fluid is cultured. Next, the skin and cyst wall are cut away, thereby greatly enlarging the opening (Fig. 66–3A through E). The cut edges are closed by a running lock stitch of 3-0 polydioxanone (PDS) or Vicryl. A small drain is sutured into the cavity with 3-0 chromic or plain catgut (Fig. 66–4). The patient is instructed to soak for 10 to 15 minutes in a tub bath to which 2 cups of salt (e.g., Instant Ocean sea salt) has been added twice per day for 1 to 2 weeks. She should rinse with fresh water after the soaking. The genital area may be blown dry with a hair dryer on the nonheat cycle or gently towel-dried.

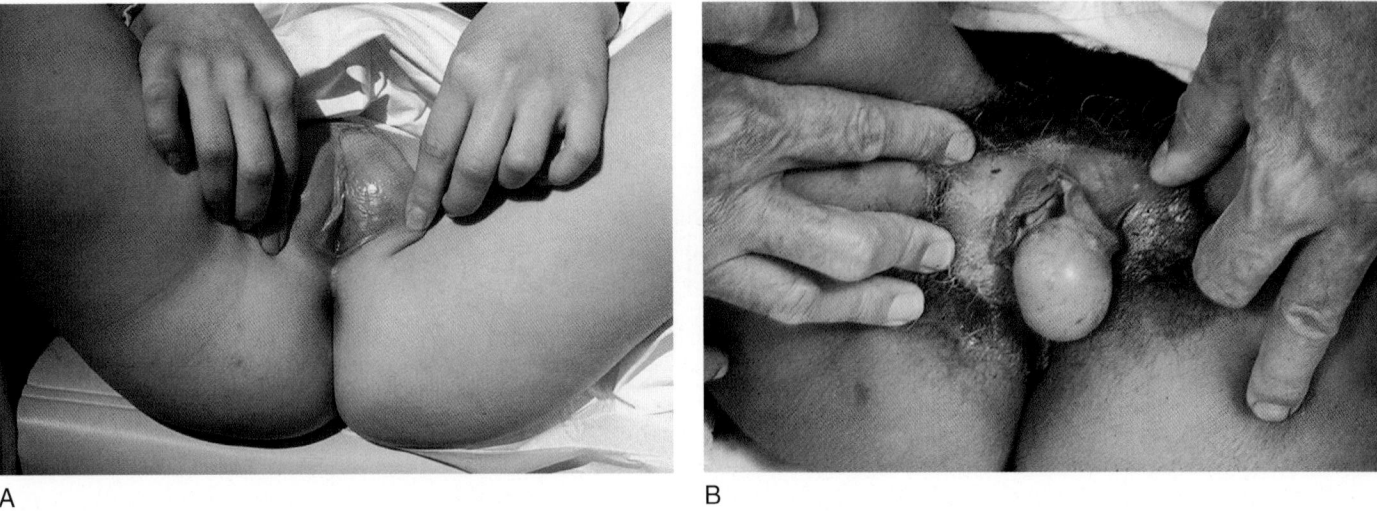

A

B

**FIGURE 66–1 A.** The obstructed duct of the Bartholin gland produces swelling in the vestibule. This will produce discomfort for the patient. In this case, no evidence of infection is noted. **B.** This cystic lesion is secondary to an obstructed Skene duct.

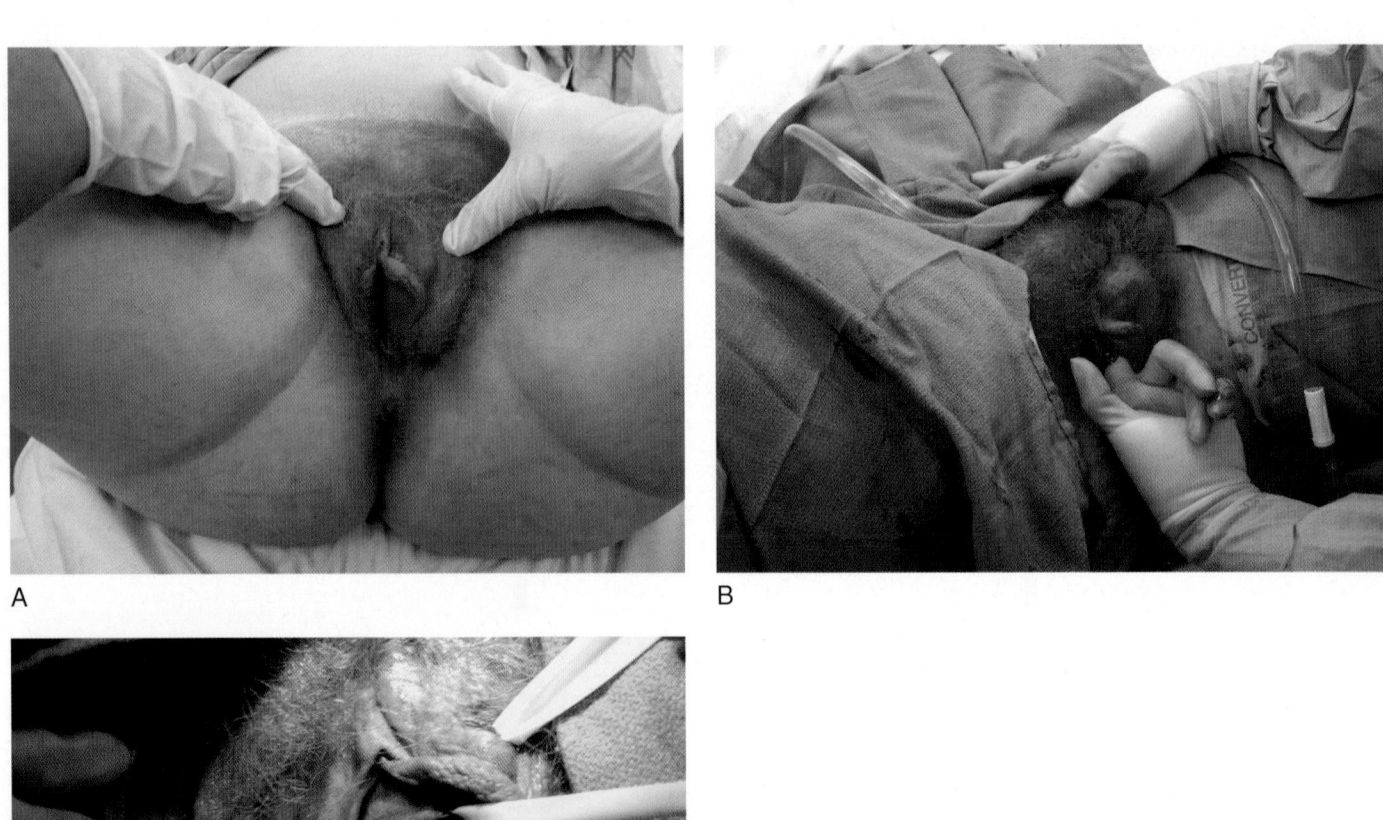

A

B

C

**FIGURE 66–2 A.** This woman was hospitalized with a painful vulvar mass, which failed to respond to administration of oral antibiotics. She had a past history of recurrent Bartholin duct cysts. This photo shows tremendous swelling of the left vulva and cellulitis extending into the mons. **B.** Drainage was accomplished by an incision into the mass at its most dependent, medial (vestibular) site. The operator's finger is inserted into the abscess cavity to break up all septa to ensure complete drainage. *Note:* The finger is extended into the lower portion of the mons. **C.** A circular piece of skin has been excised (2-cm diameter), and the perimeter of the opening has been sutured via a running 0 Vicryl stitch. A through-and-through ¾-inch Penrose drain has been placed.

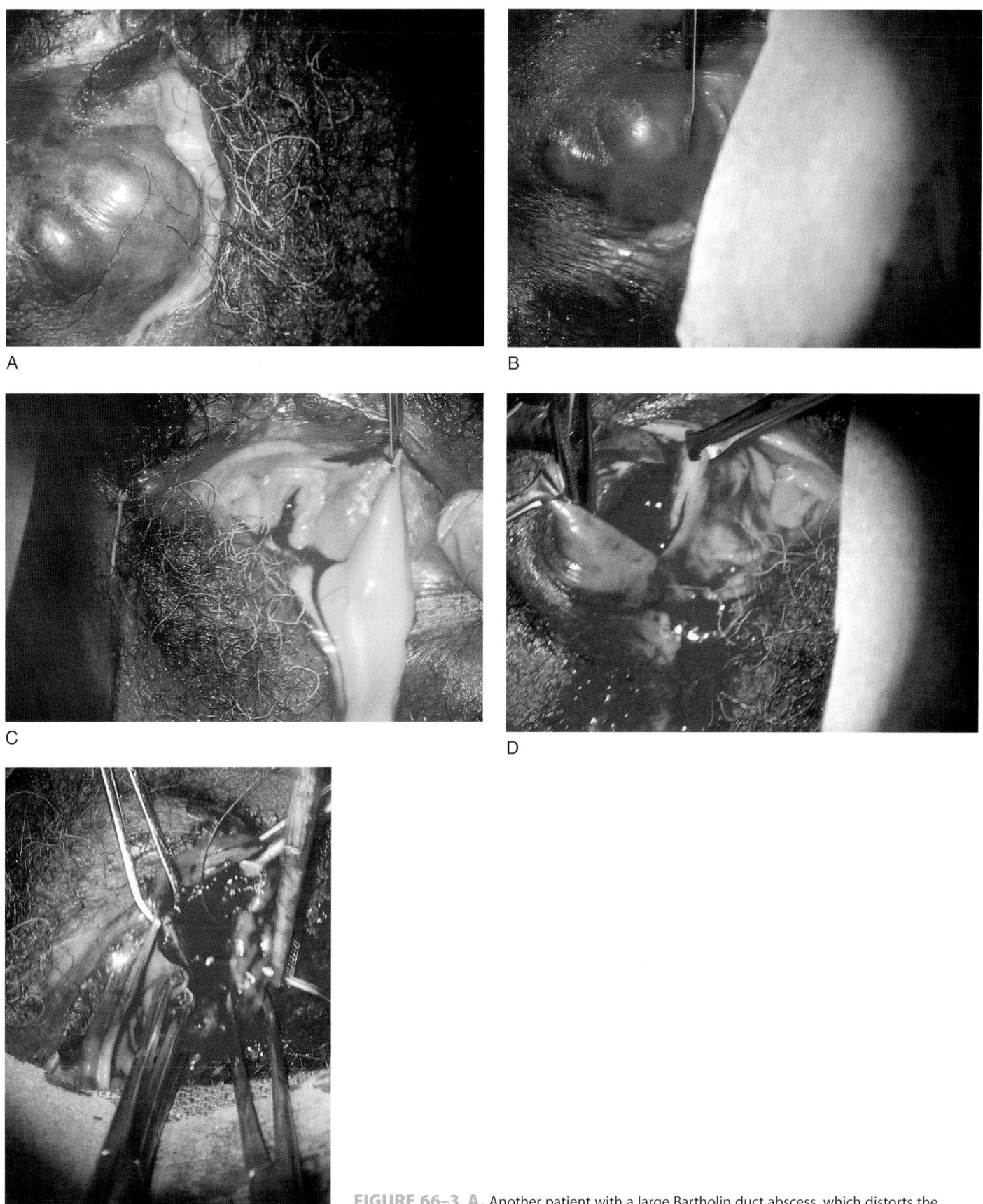

**FIGURE 66–3 A.** Another patient with a large Bartholin duct abscess, which distorts the vulva. **B.** The knife blade is prepared to cut the skin and penetrate the abscess cavity medially and dependently. **C.** Pus pours from the drainage site. **D.** A scissors is placed into the crater and spread open to break up any septa. **E.** The perimeter of the large opening (into the abscess cavity) is closed with a running 0 Vicryl suture.

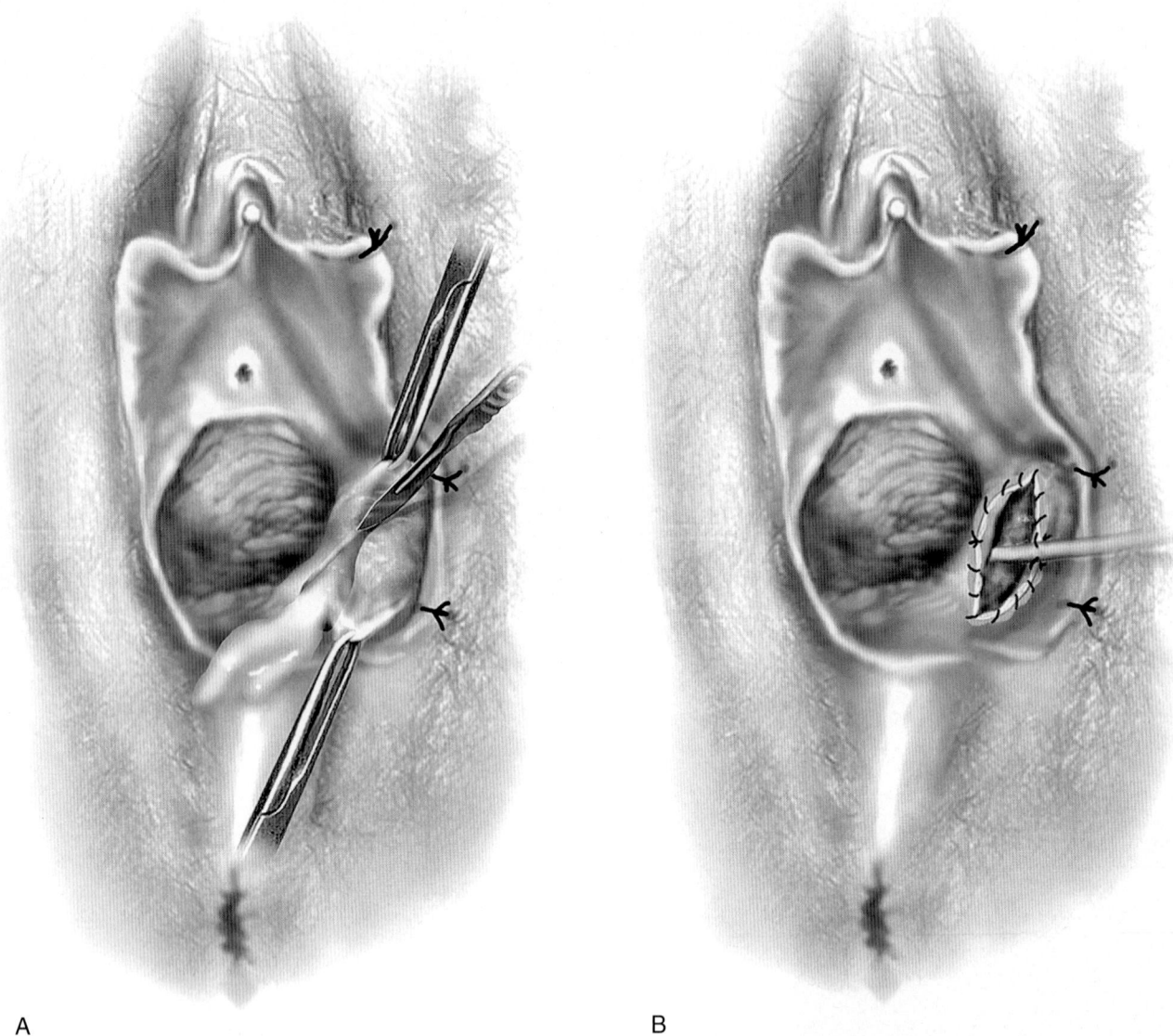

A

B

**FIGURE 66–4  A. and B.** The labia on the affected side are sutured back with 0 Vicryl to provide exposure. A vertical incision is made into the cyst. The edges of the incision are grasped with forceps and Allis clamps. The skin, together with a portion of the cyst lining, is widely cut away with a scalpel or Stevens scissors. The edges of the cut are sutured circumferentially with 3-0 Vicryl or polydioxanone (PDS). A drain is placed into the wound and secured with 3-0 chromic catgut. The cyst thus has been "marsupialized."

# CHAPTER 67

# Surgery for Vulvar Vestibulitis Syndrome (Vulvodynia)

*Michael S. Baggish*

Vulvar vestibulitis syndrome is a disorder of unknown cause that produces erythema, hyperesthesia, and extreme discomfort to light pressure, principally around the Bartholin duct and the underlying Bartholin gland. Although other vulvar mucous glands (i.e., the paraurethral and minor vestibular glands) may be sensitive to touch, major signs and symptoms are related mainly to Bartholin glands (Fig. 67–1A through C). Afflicted women complain of a burning raw feeling during and after sexual intercourse to such a degree that apareunia eventuates. All patients in whom this diagnosis is made should undergo a conservative regimen over a period of 2 to 4 months. If conservative treatment does not lead to substantial amelioration of symptoms and an objective decrease in erythema and light touch–induced pain, then the patient should be offered the surgical option (Fig. 67–2).

Surgery for the treatment of vestibulitis presents two options. The first and simpler procedure is vestibulectomy with or without excision of the paraurethral duct(s) and vaginal advancement. This operation excises the inflamed tissue(s) to include depth into Colles' fascia and margins to Hart's line, as well as removal of a centimeter of the lower vagina. The advantage of this operation is shortened operative time (1.5 hours or less) and less morbidity in the form of postoperative pudendal neuralgia (Fig. 67–3A through E).

The alternative operation includes radical excision of the Bartholin glands, vestibulectomy, and vaginal advancement. This operation requires 2.5 hours to perform and is associated with a 15% to 20% risk of postoperative pudendal neuralgia. It is currently recommended for severe cases of vestibulitis; for cyst formation post simple vestibulectomy; and for failure of the simple vestibulectomy operation.

Success rates for the above procedures vis-à-vis elimination of entry pain associated with intercourse is greater than 90%. Additionally, the vestibular pain is unlikely to return. Both operations are performed with the patient in the low to medium lithotomy position. The operating microscope is recommended to perform this surgery most effectively.

## Simple Vestibulectomy

The initial part of this surgery is identical with the technique used for Bartholin gland excision.

Stay sutures of 0 Vicryl retract the labia to expose the vestibule, and a 1:100 solution of vasopressin is injected via a 25-gauge needle into the subdermis of the vestibule (Fig. 67–4A, B).

A carbon dioxide ($CO_2$) laser is coupled to a microscope via a micromanipulator. The laser control is adjusted to deliver a 1- to 1.5-mm spot at a focal distance of 300 mm. The format is set for a superpulsed beam at 12 W power. The laser beam traces the dimensions of the incision, and the trace spots are then connected by incising the vestibular skin (Fig. 67–5A, B). The initial incision is U-shaped.

Next, with a Stevens tenotomy, the vestibule with attached Colles' fascia is sharply excised (Fig. 67–6). Additionally, a 0.5- to 1-cm margin of the lower vagina (which includes the hymenal ring) is removed. Hemostasis and wound approximation are obtained by placing a series of pleating fascial stitches of 3-0 Vicryl (Fig. 67–7A). Next, the skin is closed with interrupted 3-0 Vicryl stitches. Cosmetically, the operative result is quite good. At the same time, the vaginal inlet has been reshaped and widened to permit two fingerwidths (2.5 to 4 cm) for easy coital entry (Fig. 67–7B).

## Vestibulectomy With Radical Bartholin Gland Excision

This operation is more complex. It begins with the same trace incision described for simple vestibulectomy (Fig. 67–8A, B). A mosquito clamp is then inserted parallel to and along the outer wall of the vagina to develop a space 2 cm deep from the introital surface (Fig. 67–8C).

Next, the mosquito clamp is moved 1 to 1.5 cm laterally to develop a similar space into the fat of the ischiorectal fossa (Fig. 67–8D). The two spaces differ significantly. The medical space is dominated above (superiorly) by the vestibular bulb and the vaginal wall sinuses. The lateral space contains a few small arteries and veins, but principally fatty tissue. At this point, the bulbocavernosus muscle is identified (Fig. 67–9). Immediately below the muscle is the Bartholin gland (Fig. 67–10). Under magnification, the lobules and the texture of the gland can be identified as distinct from surrounding muscle, fat, and connective tissue (Fig. 67–10B, C). The gland is isolated anteriorly and posteriorly by the application of mosquito clamps (Fig. 67–11). The gland is excised and all pedicle sutures ligated with 4-0 Vicryl. All vessels are suture-ligated, and the field is secured from bleeding and irrigated (Fig. 67–12A, B). The fossa previously occupied by the gland measures approximately 1 to 1.5 cm from the surface of the vestibule. The dead space is closed with interrupted 3-0 Vicryl sutures. A doubly gloved finger is placed in the anus to verify its location relative to the operative field, as well as its integrity. Next, the vestibular skin is cut away (Fig. 67–13A through C). The vagina is advanced to cover the defect and is closed transversely to the surrounding perineal skin (Fig. 67–14). The overall effect is to actually enlarge the vaginal opening.

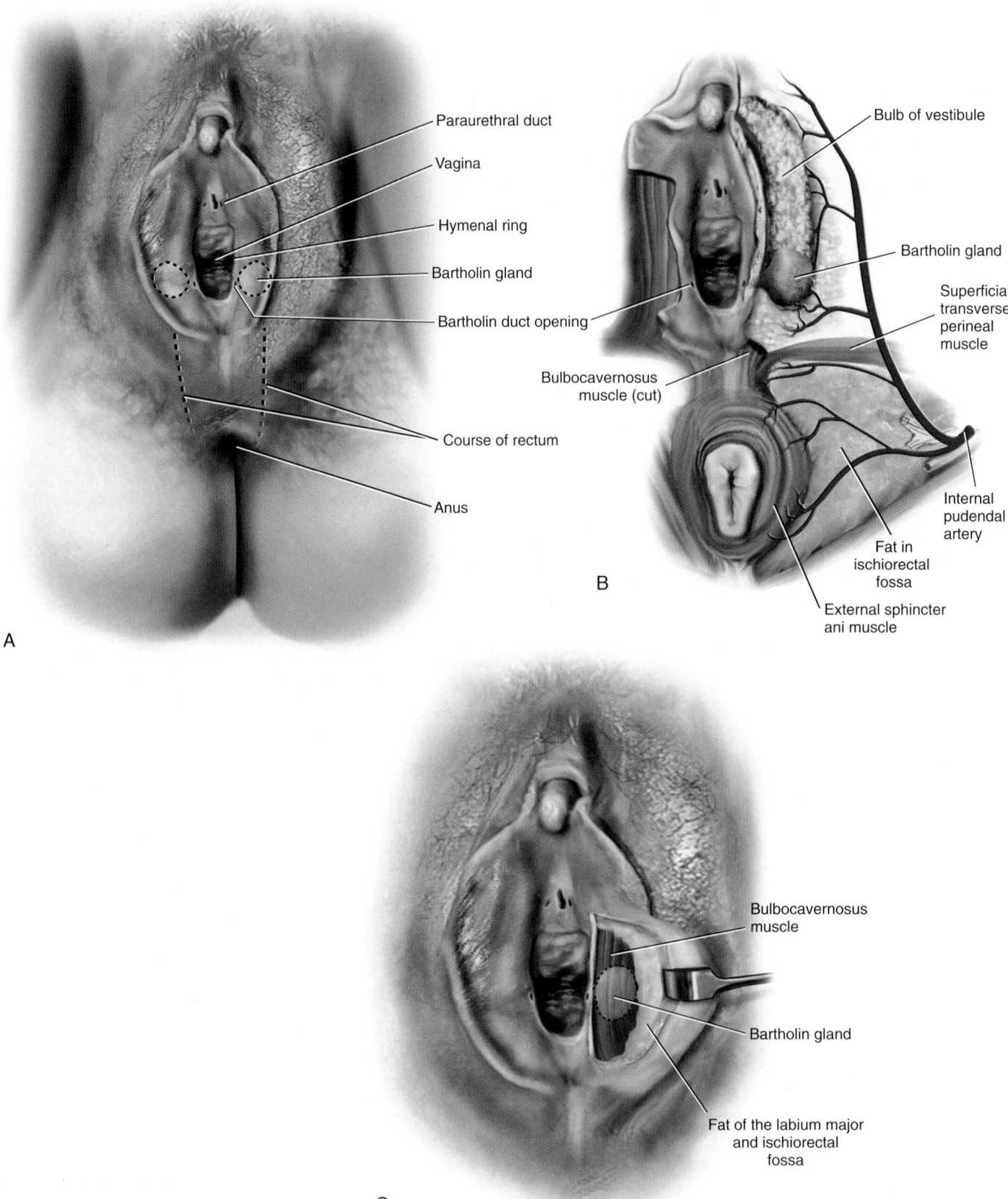

**FIGURE 67–1  A.** This drawing illustrates the topographic anatomy of the vestibule and Bartholin glands/ducts. It also shows the relationship of the paraurethral ducts to the ureter. Noteworthy is the relationship of the anus to the posterior aspect of the vestibule and lower vagina. **B.** A deep dissection of the vestibule (*left*) and a superficial dissection (*right*) are shown here. The bulbocavernosus muscle has been removed on the left side. The arterial blood supply emanates from the internal pudendal artery. The vessel enters the perineum with the pudendal artery. The vessel enters the perineum with the pudendal nerve medial to the ischial tuberosity (i.e., from a posterolateral direction). **C.** The bulbocavernosus muscle overlies the Bartholin gland; lateral to the gland is the fat of the labium majus and ischiorectal fossa.

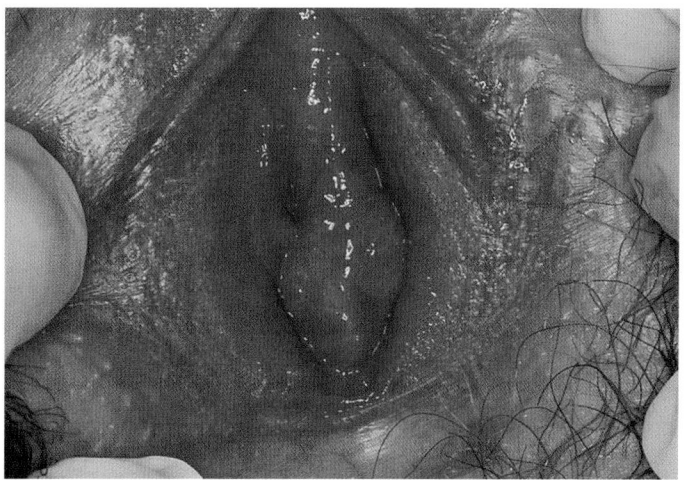

FIGURE 67–2  Preoperative view of the vestibule in a woman afflicted with vulvar vestibulitis syndrome. Note the erythema around the Bartholin ducts, as well as the vascular ectasia (punctation).

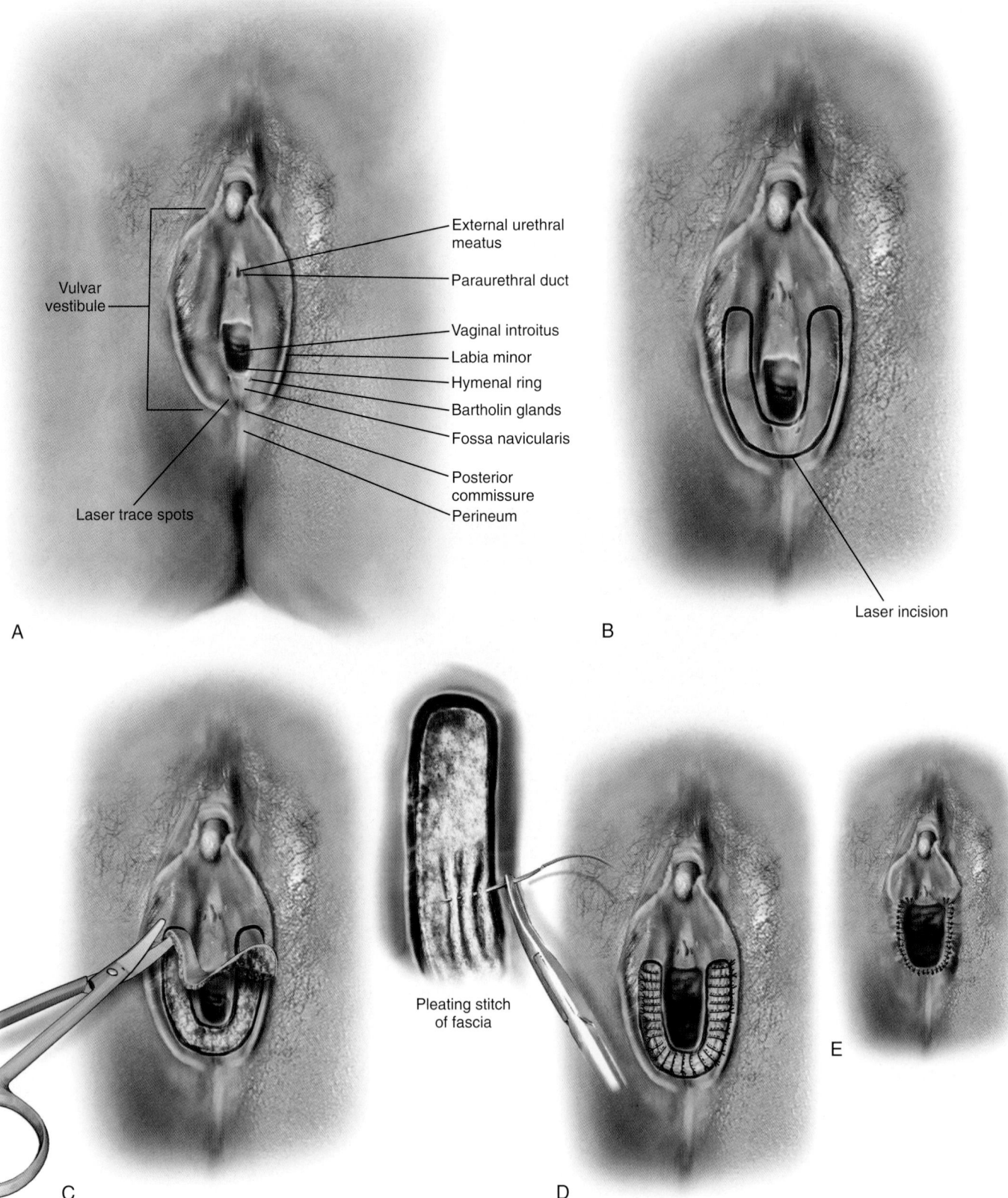

**FIGURE 67–3  A through E.** The technique of simple vestibulectomy is illustrated here. **A.** Initially, carbon dioxide ($CO_2$) laser spots trace the boundaries of the U-shaped incision. **B.** Via a tightly focused laser beam, the dots are connected and a deeper incision is completed **(C)** with Stevens scissors. The skin and a thickness of Colles' fascia are removed, and the specimen sent to pathology. **D.** Hemostasis and wound apposition are accomplished with fascial pleating stitches. **E.** Finally, the skin is closed with interrupted sutures. The vagina has been advanced, and the introitus has been widened.

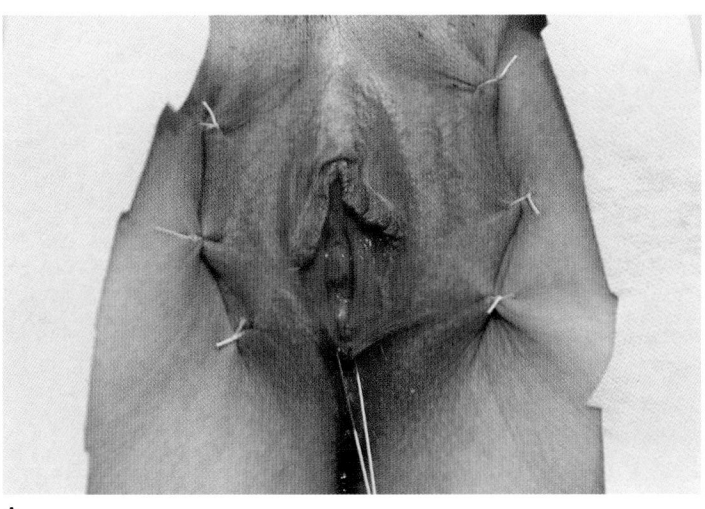
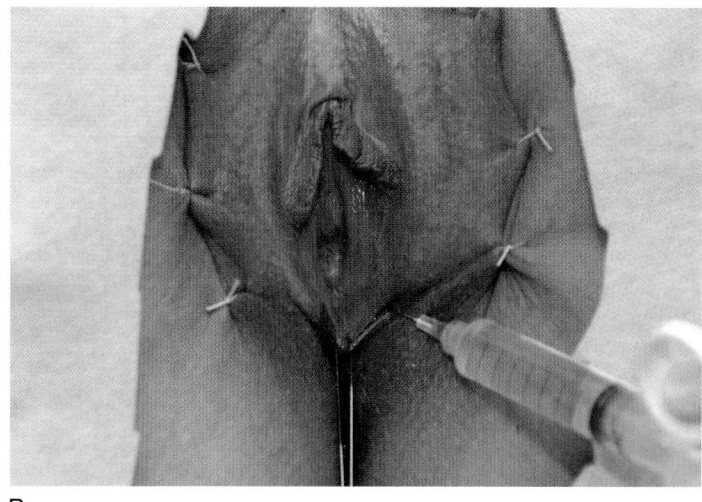

A                                           B

**FIGURE 67-4** **A.** Exposure to the vestibule is provided by suturing back the labia majora. The suture at the fossa navicularis is not tied but is pulled caudad for traction. **B.** A 1:100 dilution of vasopressin is injected subdermally to provide hemostasis, as well as a heat sink to absorb the carbon dioxide ($CO_2$) laser beam.

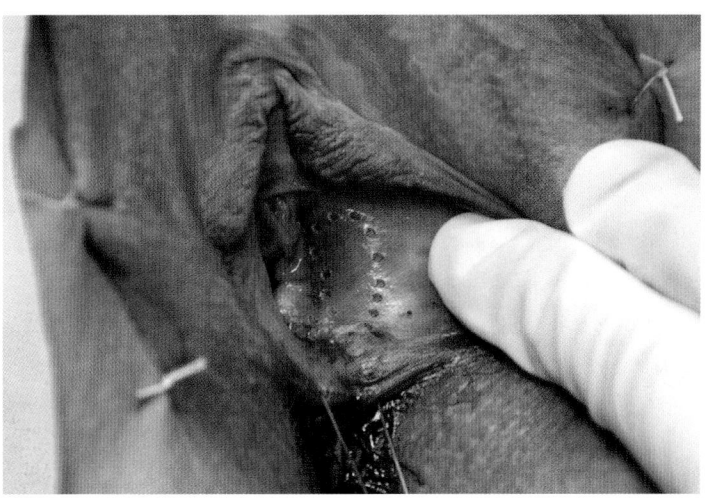
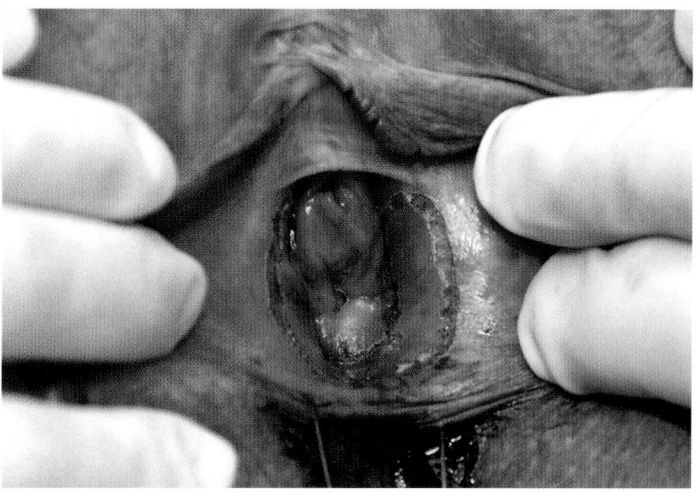

A                                           B

**FIGURE 67-5** **A.** Trace spots are placed via the attached carbon dioxide ($CO_2$) laser into the vestibule. This outlines where the incision will be placed. **B.** The trace spots are connected via a deeper incision. Note that the completed incision is U-shaped.

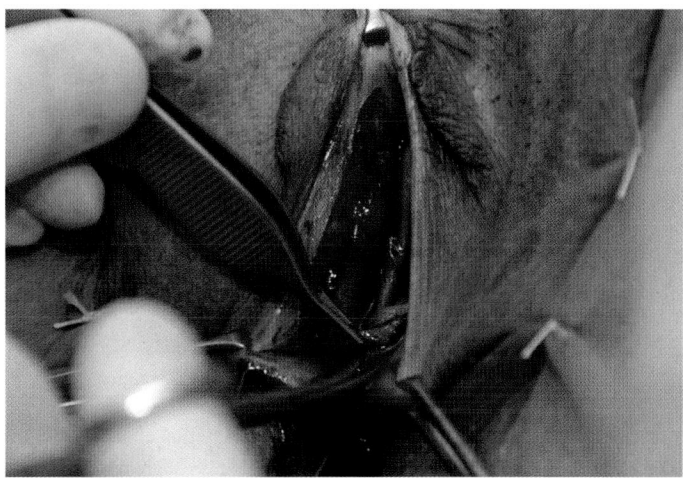

**FIGURE 67-6** The vestibule and a 3-mm margin of Colles' fascia are cut away.

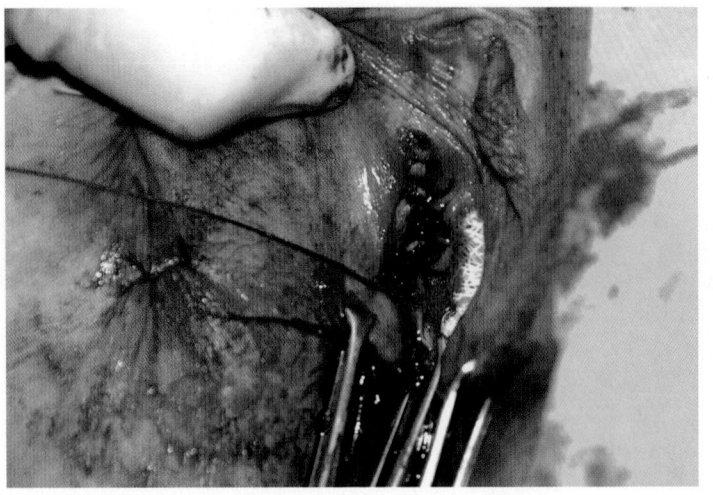

A

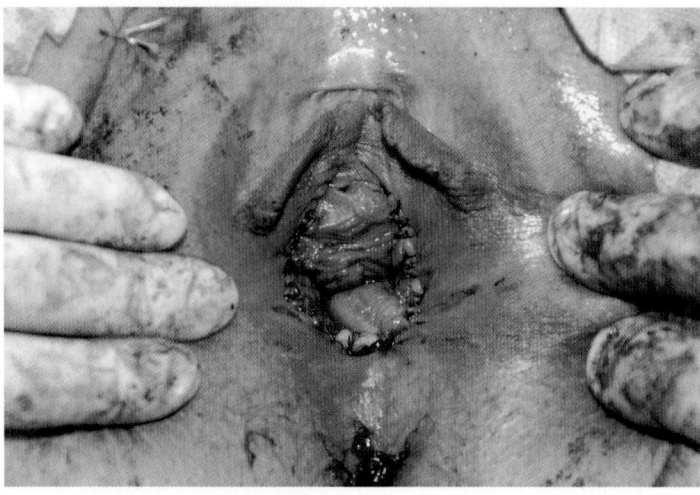

B

**FIGURE 67–7  A.** Pleating sutures are placed in Colles' fascia. This technique pulls the vagina outward toward the distal margin of the incision. **B.** The skin is closed, advancing the vagina and widening the introitus.

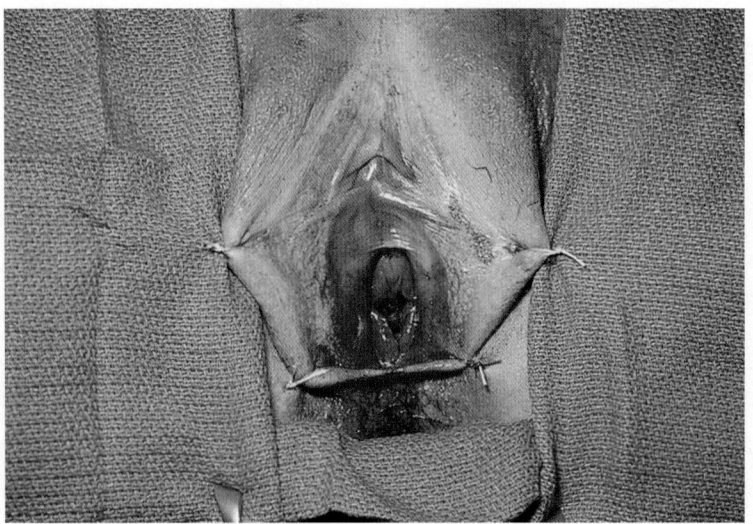

A

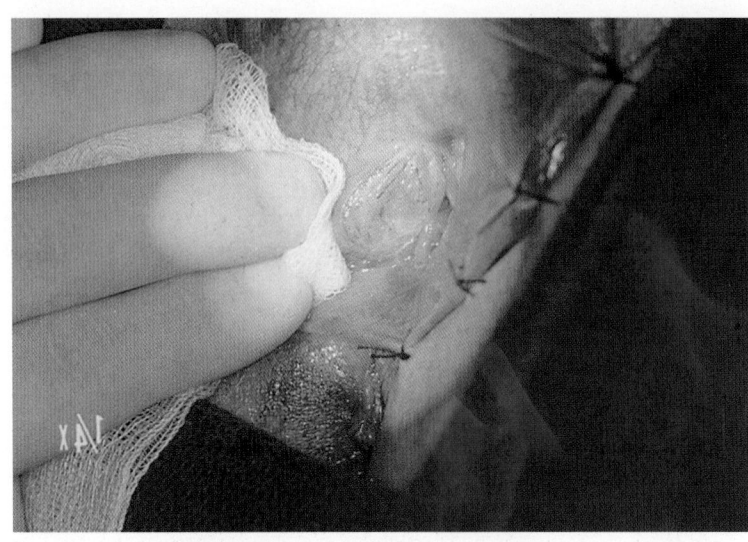

B

**FIGURE 67–8  A.** The labia are sutured back for retraction and continuous exposure of the vestibule. **B.** A 2-cm bloodless incision is made immediately lateral to and above and below the right Bartholin duct opening.

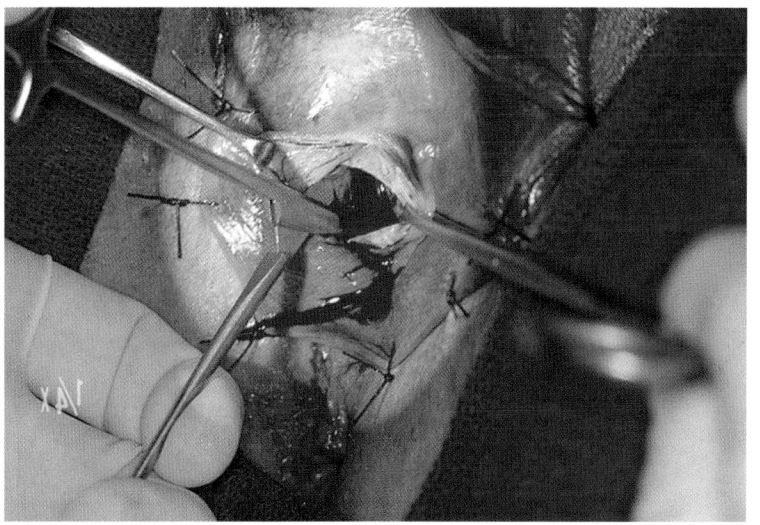

C

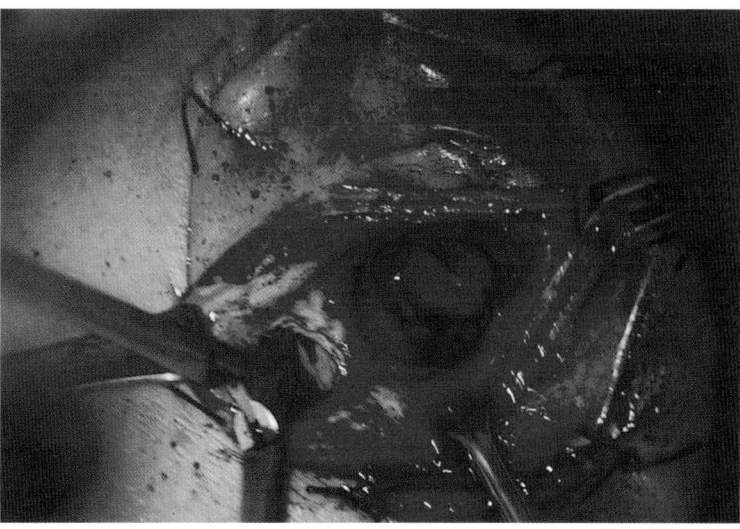

D

**FIGURE 67–8, cont'd  C.** A mosquito clamp dissects the space between the bulb, the Bartholin gland, and the inner wall of the vagina. Invariably, some bleeding will occur from the bulb. **D.** A second space is dissected lateral to the gland and the bulb. This space is dissected into the fat of the labium majus and the ischiorectal fossa.

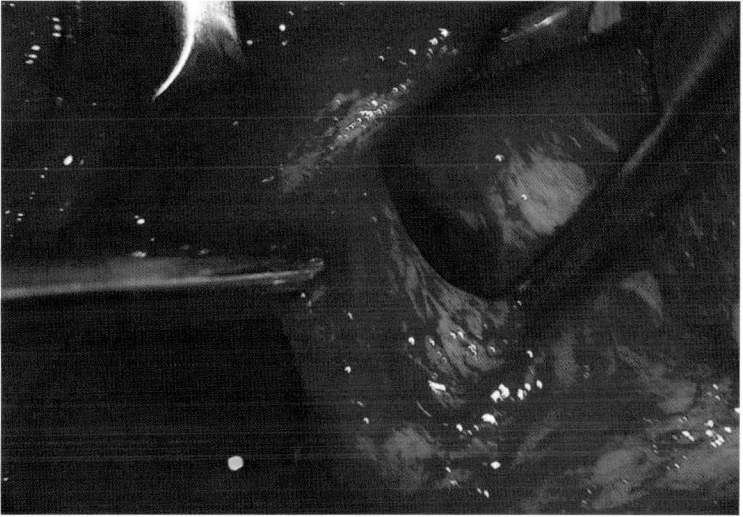

**FIGURE 67–9** The edge of the bulbocavernosus muscle is held in the clamps overlying the Bartholin gland.

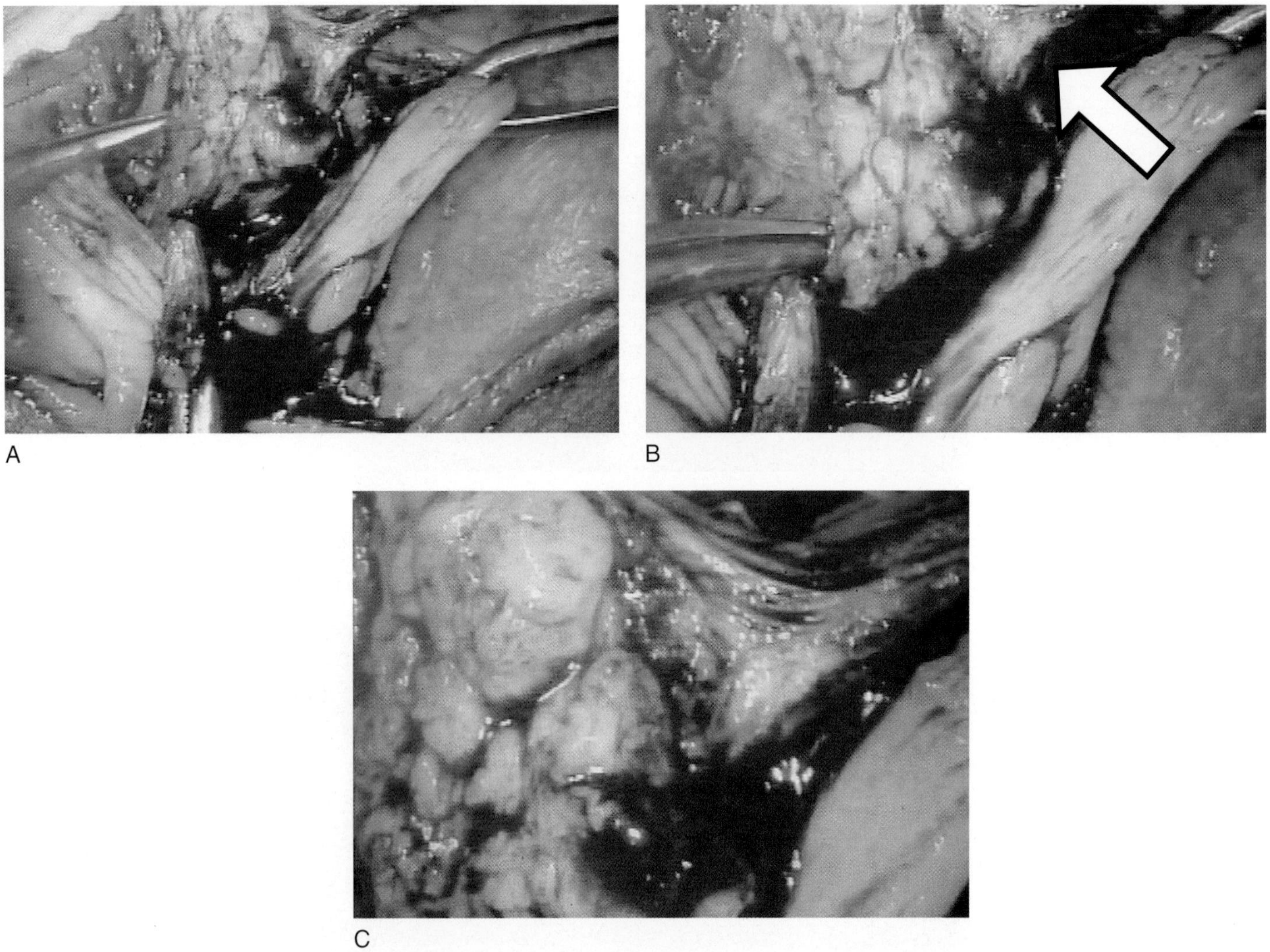

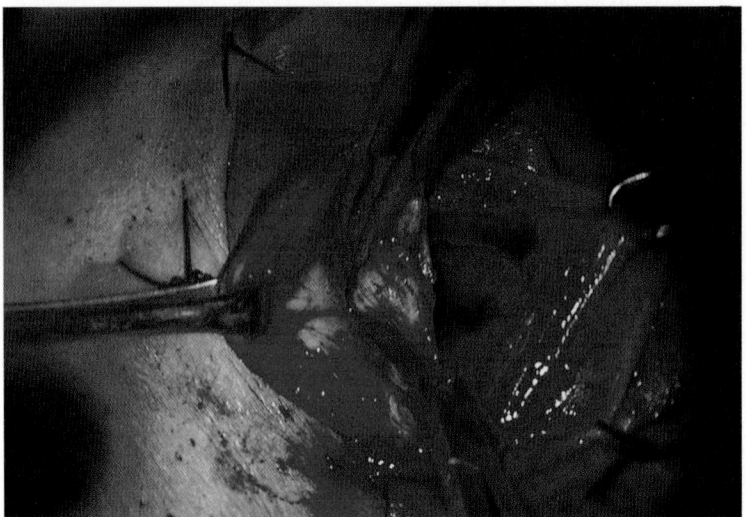

**FIGURE 67–10** **A.** The lobed Bartholin gland clings to the bulbocavernosus muscle. The scissors point to the gland. **B.** Higher magnification of part **A.** The arrow points to the bulbocavernosus muscle. The scissors point to the gland. **C.** Further magnification of part **B.** This shows the distinct lobed pattern of the Bartholin gland.

**FIGURE 67–11** The gland is isolated between the upper and lower clamps. The lateral edge of the incision is pulled with an Allis clamp to provide exposure. Medially, the vagina is retracted with an Allis clamp.

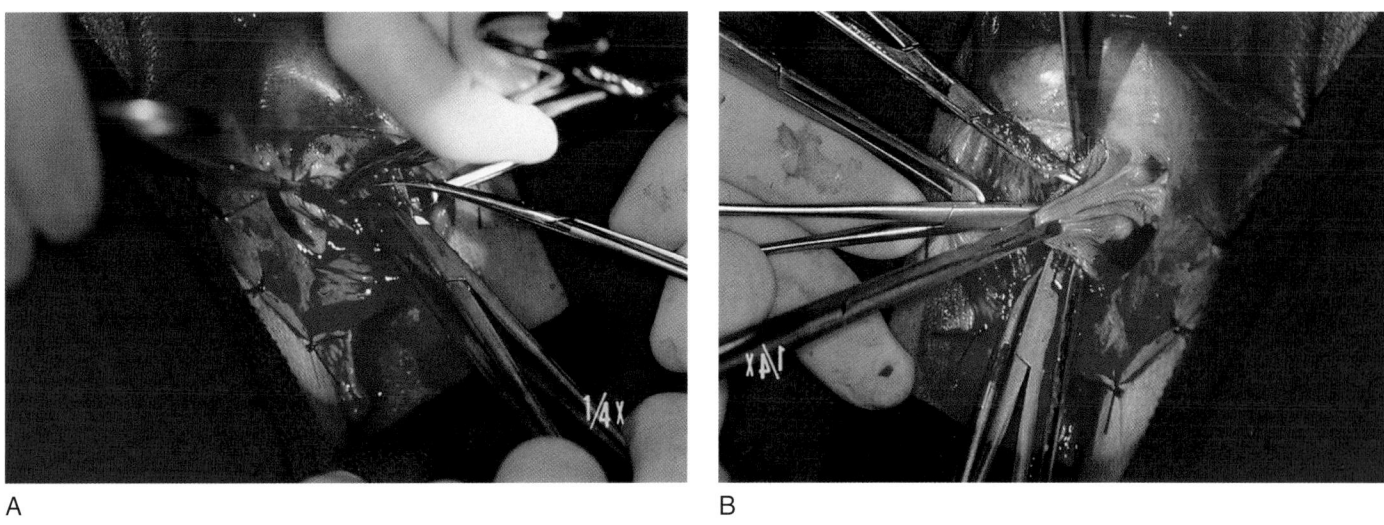

A                                                                    B

FIGURE 67–12 A. The Bartholin gland is cut free from the surrounding tissue with Stevens scissors. B. The gland has been excised on the right side. The pedicles will be suture-ligated with 4-0 Vicryl sutures. The right wall of the vagina is pulled caudally with an Allis clamp.

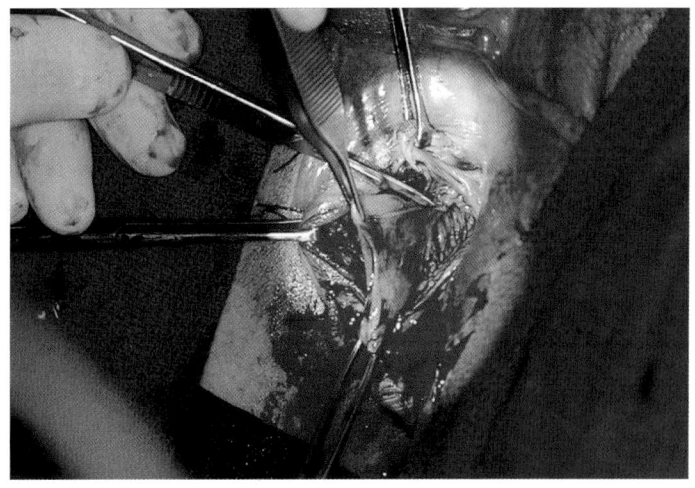

A

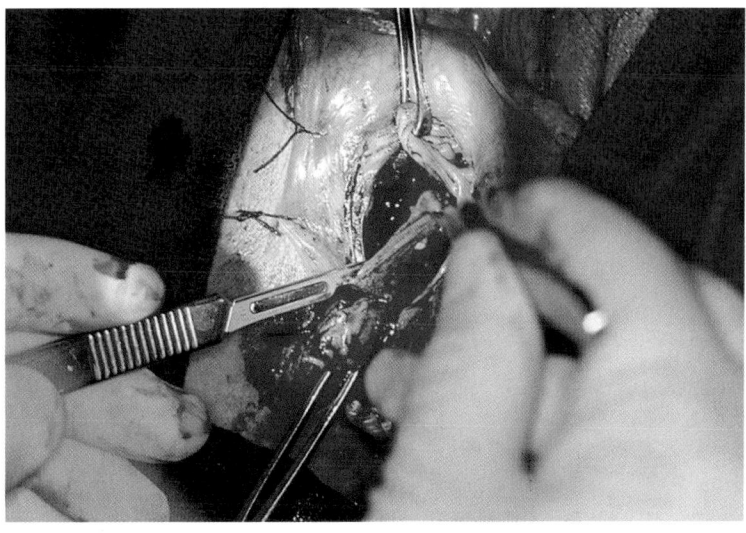

B

FIGURE 67–13 A. The lower vagina, hymen, and medial aspect of the vestibule are excised with a sharp scalpel. B. The lateral aspect of the vestibule (abutting the labium majus) is excised.

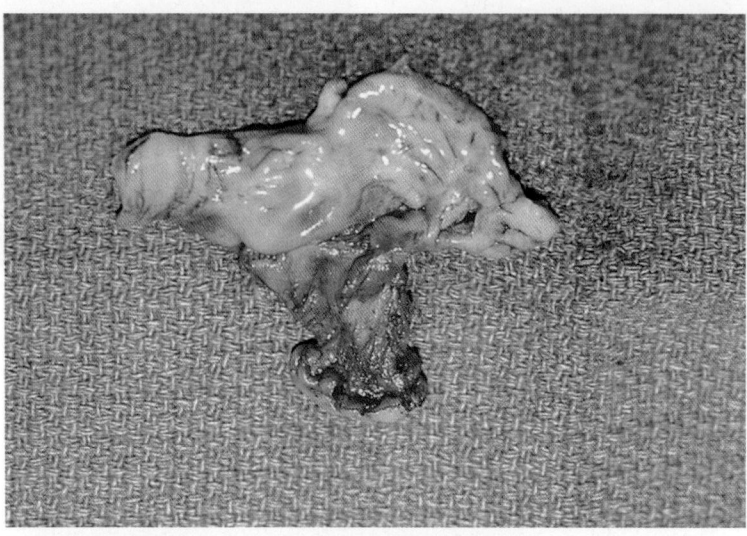

C

**FIGURE 67–13, cont'd   C.** The excised vestibular tissue is sent to pathology in a separate container from that used for the excised Bartholin gland.

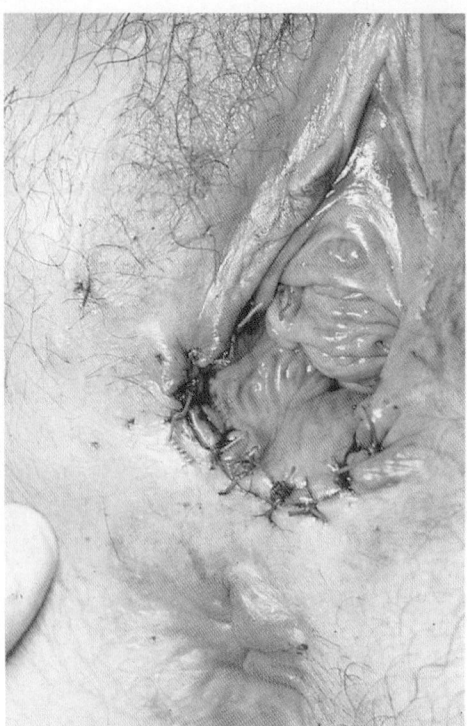

**FIGURE 67–14** The wounds have been closed bilaterally and the vagina advanced. The new introitus is enlarged.

# CHAPTER 68

# Wide Excision With or Without Skin Graft

## *Michael S. Baggish*

The treatment for vulvar intraepithelial neoplasia (VIN) varies depending on the extent of the disease process. Wide, local excision accomplishes therapeutic goals most simply and with the least disruption for the patient when the VIN is localized. On the basis of microscopic analysis of more than 1000 histologic sections of vulvar carcinoma in situ (CIS), the following data were obtained: (1) skin appendages (e.g., sebaceous glands, hair follicles, sweat glands) were involved (by extension) with neoplasia in 38% of all cases studied and in 60% of women older than 50 years of age; (2) skin appendages in hair-bearing areas extended to a mean depth of 1.53 ± 0.77 mm; (3) in the labia minora, extension of neoplastic cells into sebaceous glands plunged to a mean depth of 1.0 mm; and (4) the deepest skin appendage involvement (hair-bearing areas) was to a depth of 3 mm. Therefore, specifications for treatment required excision to a depth of 2.3 mm for labia majora and perineal and perianal skin; a depth of no more than 1 mm for the labia minora and periclitoral skin; and a peripheral margin of 3.0 mm (see Fig. 62–26).

Sharp excision may be performed with conventional instrument (knife, scissors) or by means of a superpulsed carbon dioxide ($CO_2$) laser. A basic tenet for surgical treatment of the vulva is limitation of deep tissue devitalization by energy devices (e.g., electrosurgical coagulation). After the excision is done, sufficient time and effort should be expended to obtain vigorous hemostasis. Bleeding vessels should be clamped and suture-ligated with 4-0 Vicryl (Figs. 68–1 through 68–4). When the latter is completed, the operative site is irrigated with normal warm saline. Primary closure without tension on the suture is the preferred method of closure. If the skin is tightly stretched to obtain closure, the edges may undergo necrosis and separate. Alternatively, wounds that are closed under tension are vulnerable to suture tear-out when inevitable postoperative tissue edema develops.

If primary closure is impossible or is tenuous, plans should be made to graft the operative site (Figs. 68–5A through 68–12B) either with a pedicle graft or a free graft (Fig. 68–13). The principle of the pedicle graft involves preservation of a plentiful blood supply to the graft. Therefore, the surgeon must know the source and direction of the blood vessels to avoid cross-cutting them. Second, the length of the graft should be approximately one-half the width of the base (i.e., if the height of the graft is 3 cm, then the pedicle width should be 6 cm) (Figs. 68–14 through 68–20). For small areas (i.e., 2 cm wide and 4 cm long), a full-thickness graft may be excised from the lower abdomen (see Fig. 68–11). This is carefully cleared of all fat and sutured into the wound. Finally, a split-thickness graft from the thigh or buttock may be obtained preoperatively and then grafted onto the wound. In actuality, this is the preferred method of treatment for large defect coverage. For all grafts, an evenly distributed pressure dressing is applied (Fig. 68–21).

When a large, deep resection or previous iatrogenic scar formation has compromised the blood supply and created massive tissue loss in the vulva or vagina, a myocutaneous graft should be considered. This type of graft provides tissue substance, as well as a blood supply to the graft. The graft utilizes the medially located gracilis muscle (see Chapter 70), which may be delivered via a tunnel from the thigh into the perineum or vagina (Figs. 68–22 through 68–24).

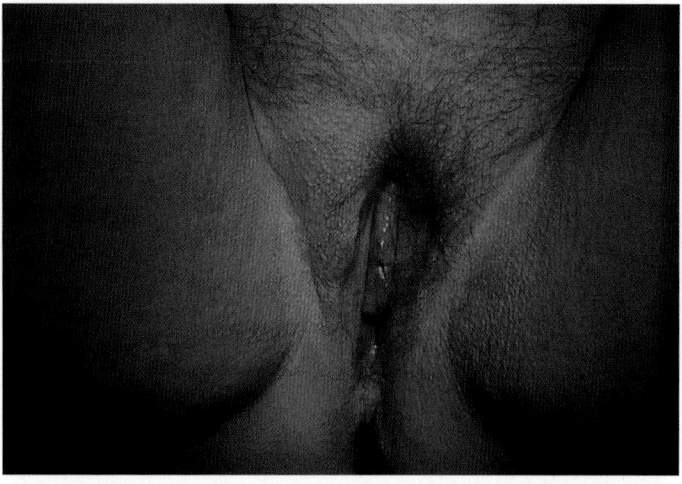

FIGURE 68–1  A lesion involving the entire right labium majus.

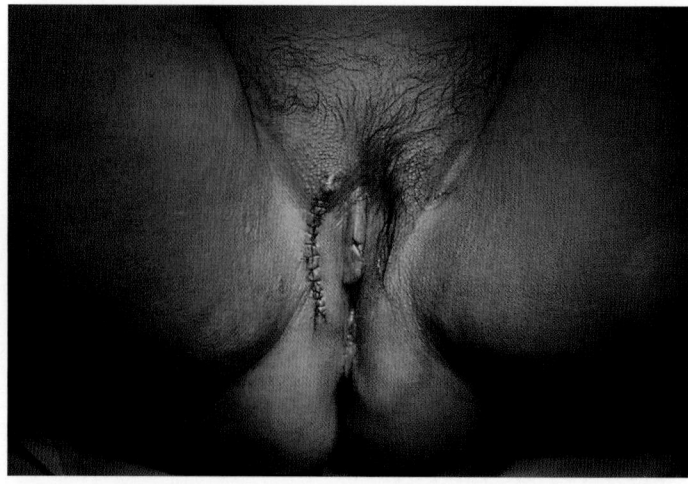

FIGURE 68–2  The labium has been excised with an adequate margin. The interlabial sulcus skin and the skin at the lateral margin of the labium majus have been approximated without excessive tension on the suture line.

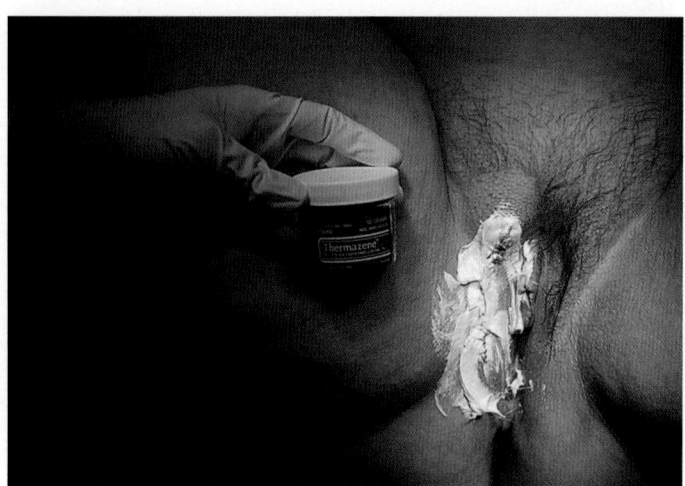

FIGURE 68–3  Silver sulfadiazine (Silvadene) is plentifully applied to the wound postoperatively.

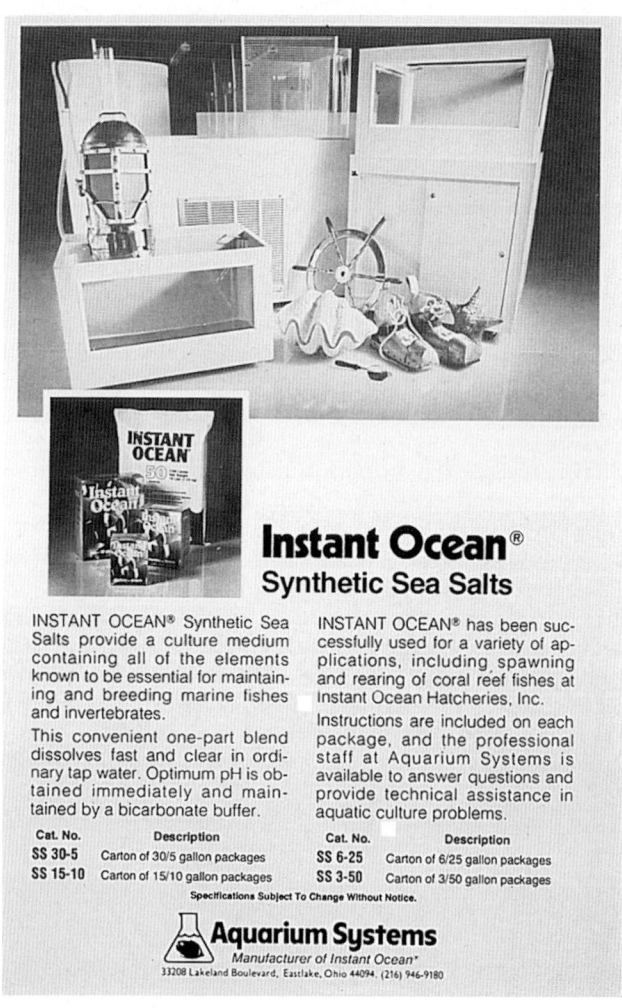

FIGURE 68–4  Instant Ocean tub baths are recommended on a daily basis during the recovery phase after vulvar surgery.

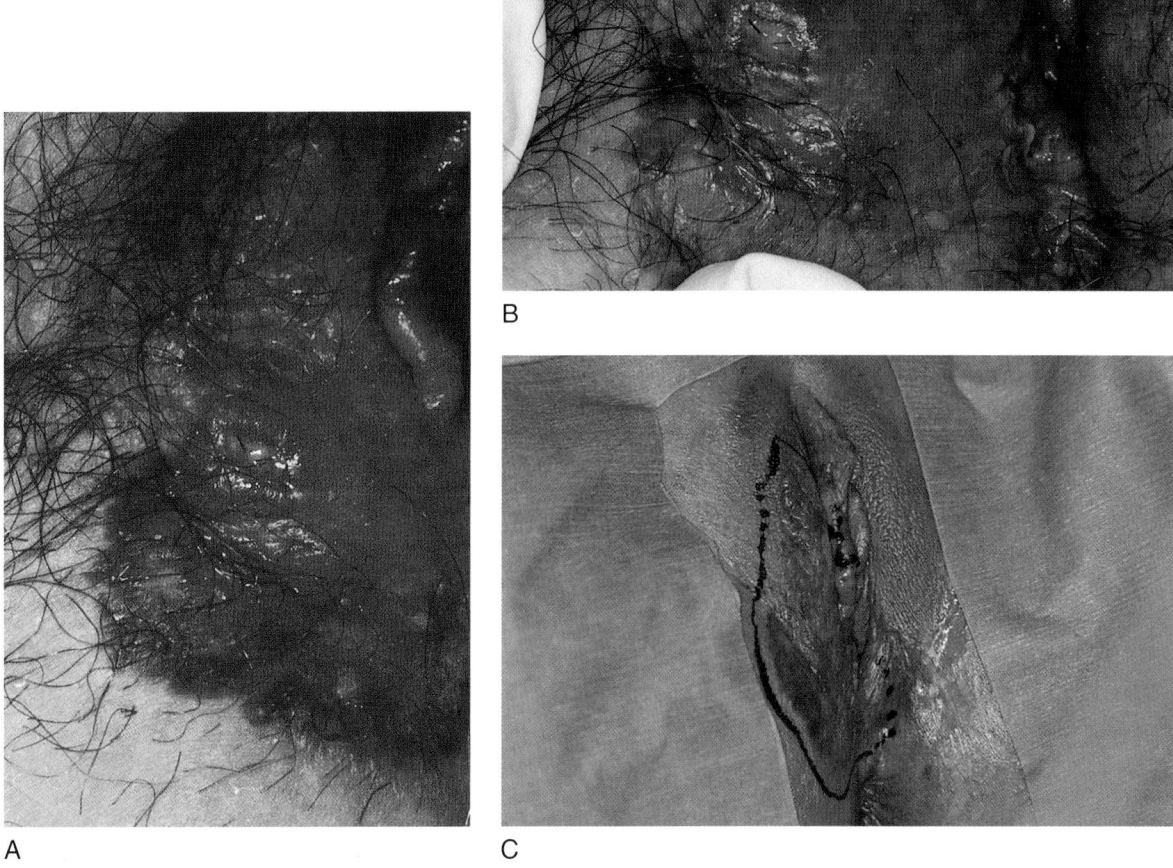

A

B

C

FIGURE 68–5 **A.** This patient has an extensive carcinoma in situ (CIS) of the right vestibule, labium minus, and labium majus. Note the recent biopsy wound in the lower labium majus. **B.** Another view of the red, dark brown, and raised areas of CIS. **C.** On the operating table, the extent of the area to be resected is sketched with a sterile marking pen.

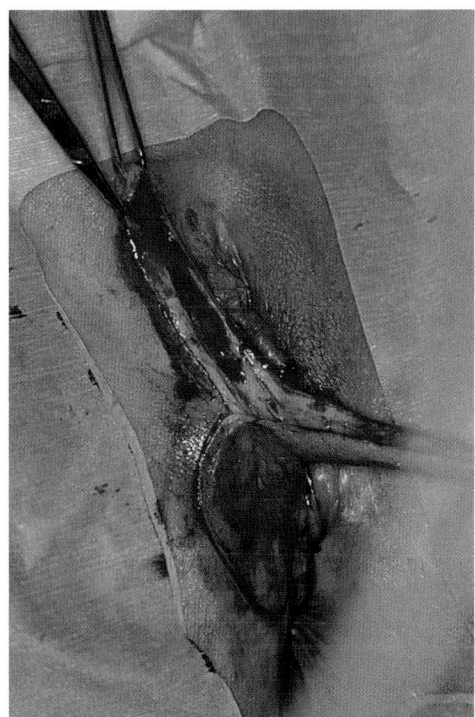

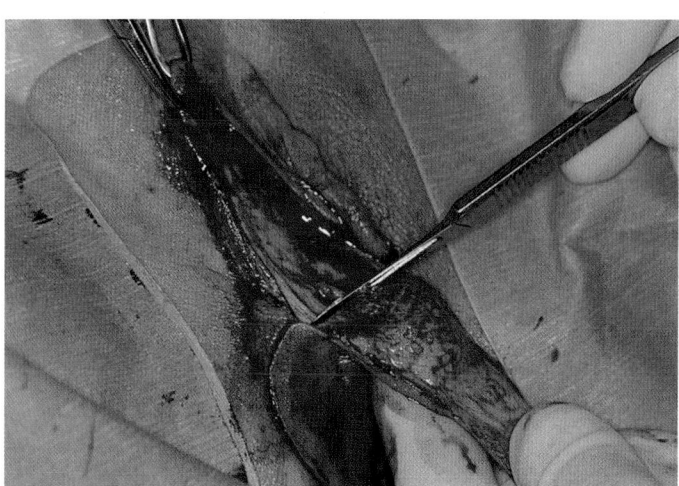

FIGURE 68–7 Hemostasis is obtained with the use of mosquito clamps and 3-0 or 4-0 polydioxanone (PDS) or Vicryl suture-ligatures. The proper depth of excision is maintained by the operator by stretching the skin inferiorly and pushing up on the skin with the index finger at the line of resection.

FIGURE 68–6 The skin containing the carcinoma in situ (CIS) is sharply excised en bloc. A full-thickness resection (i.e., extending into the subcutaneous fat) is done.

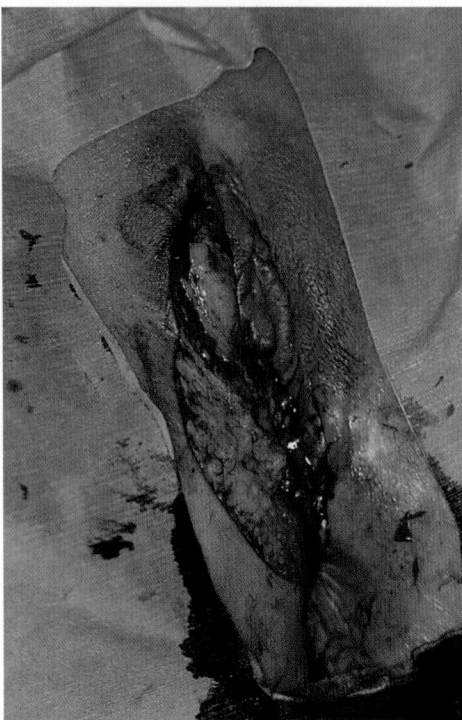

FIGURE 68–8 The entire right side of the vulva has been removed. Only a portion of the right labium minus (including the clitoris and its hood) remains.

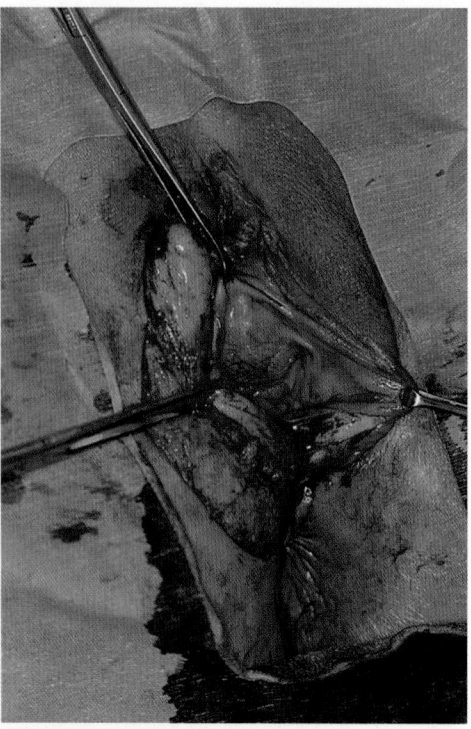

FIGURE 68–9 Allis clamps grasp the margins of the remaining portion of the right vestibule and the intact upper and left vestibular tissues.

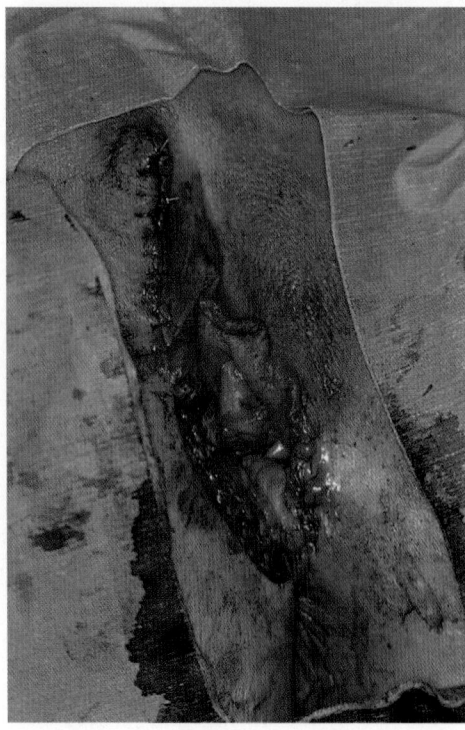

FIGURE 68–10 The upper portion of the wound has been closed with 3-0 Vicryl without excessive tension on the suture line.

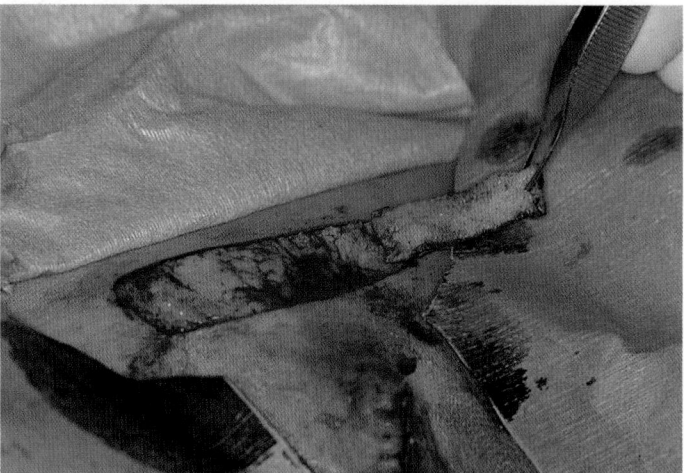

FIGURE 68–11 A graft is taken from the lower abdominal wall and is based on measurements of the vulvar wound defect. The skin is carefully defatted, moistened, and held in a sterile sponge until its use is required.

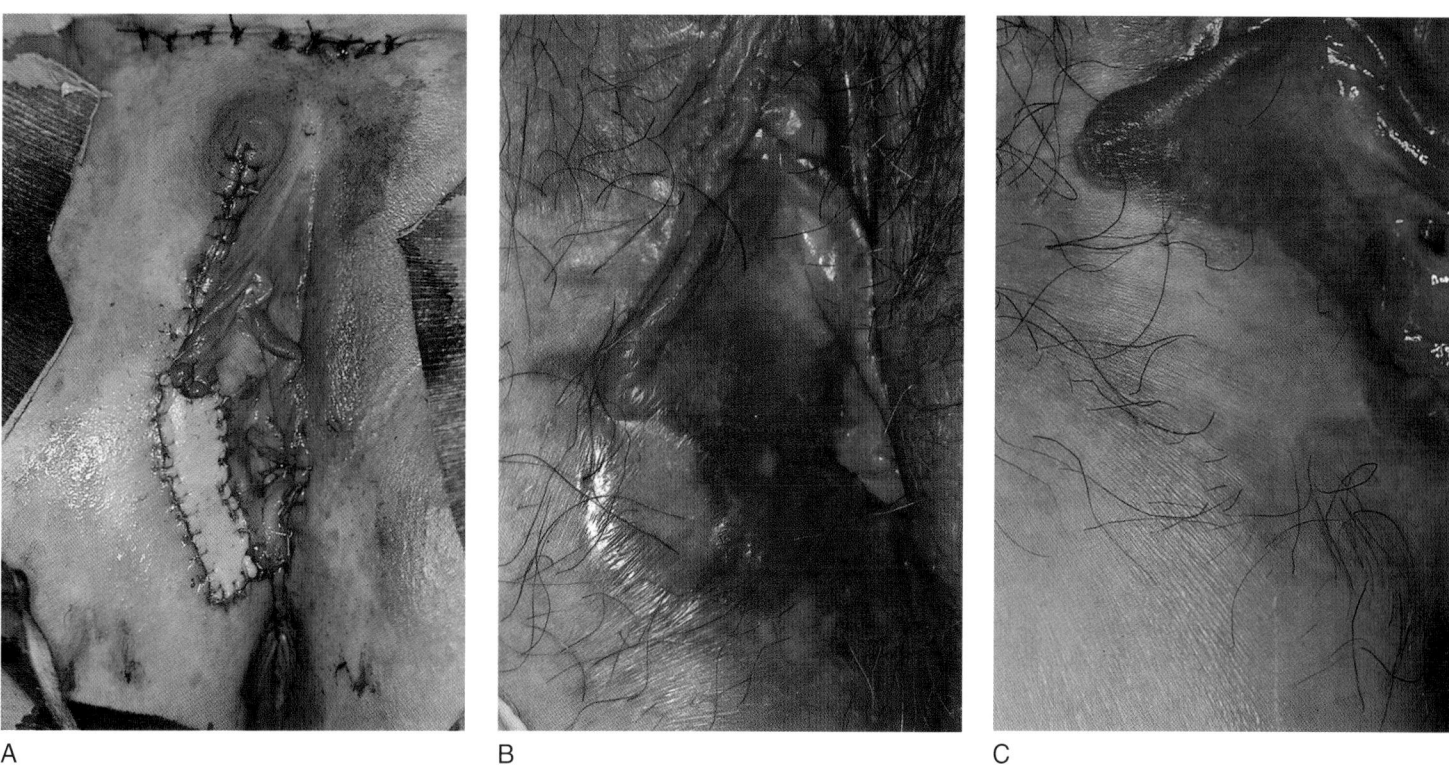

A                                    B                                    C

FIGURE 68–12  A. The graft seen in Figure 68–11 has been sutured into place to cover the defect left after extensive carcinoma in situ (CIS) resection of the right side of the vulva. B. View of part A shows the grafted site on the vulva 1 year postoperatively. Note that only one third of the right labium minus remains. C. Magnified view of the graft site at 1 year postoperatively.

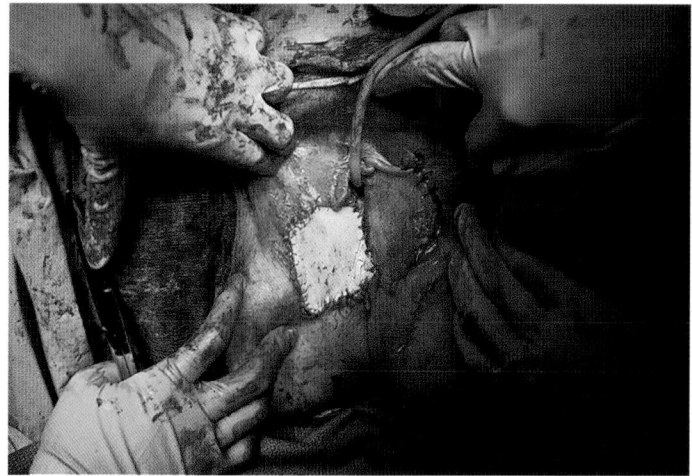

FIGURE 68–13  Extensive bilateral excision of the vulvar tissues was required to eliminate another patient's carcinoma in situ (CIS). A split-thickness graft was applied to the right side, whereas a pedicle graft was necessary on the left.

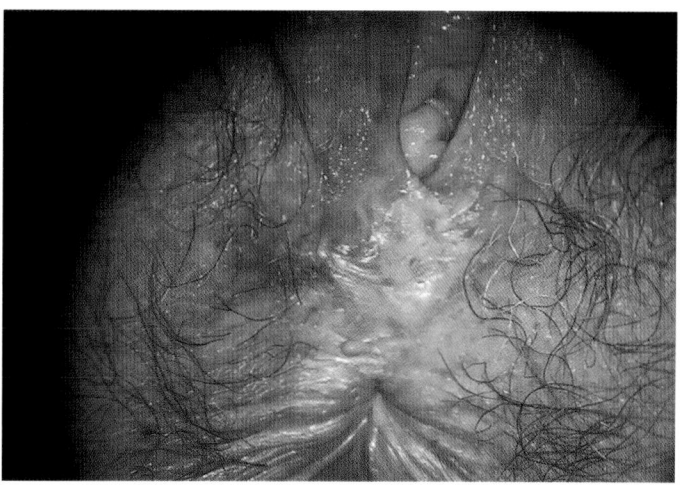

FIGURE 68–14  This patient had biopsy-proven carcinoma in situ (CIS) of the perineum and perianal skin.

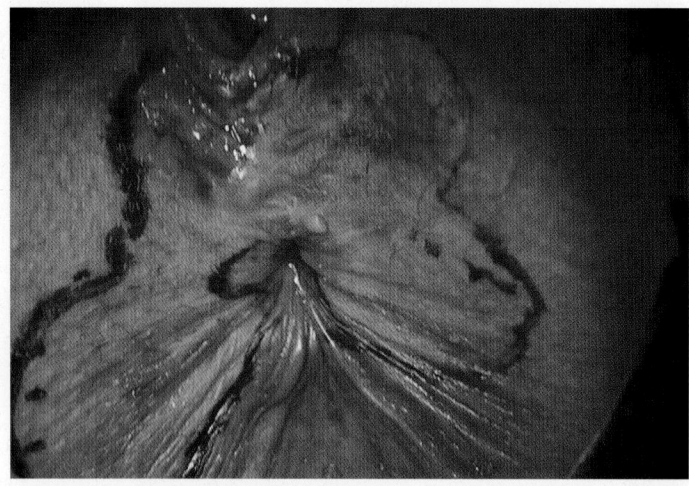

**FIGURE 68–15** The extent of the planned resection is outlined with a sterile marking pen.

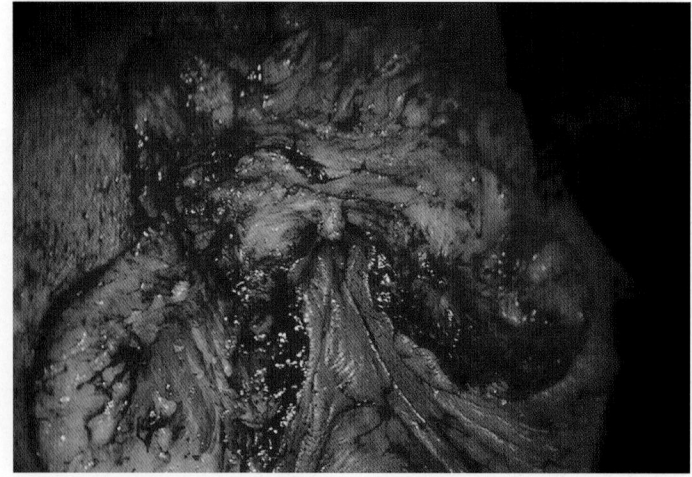

**FIGURE 68–16** The skin of the perineal and perianal area has been excised into the subcutaneous tissues.

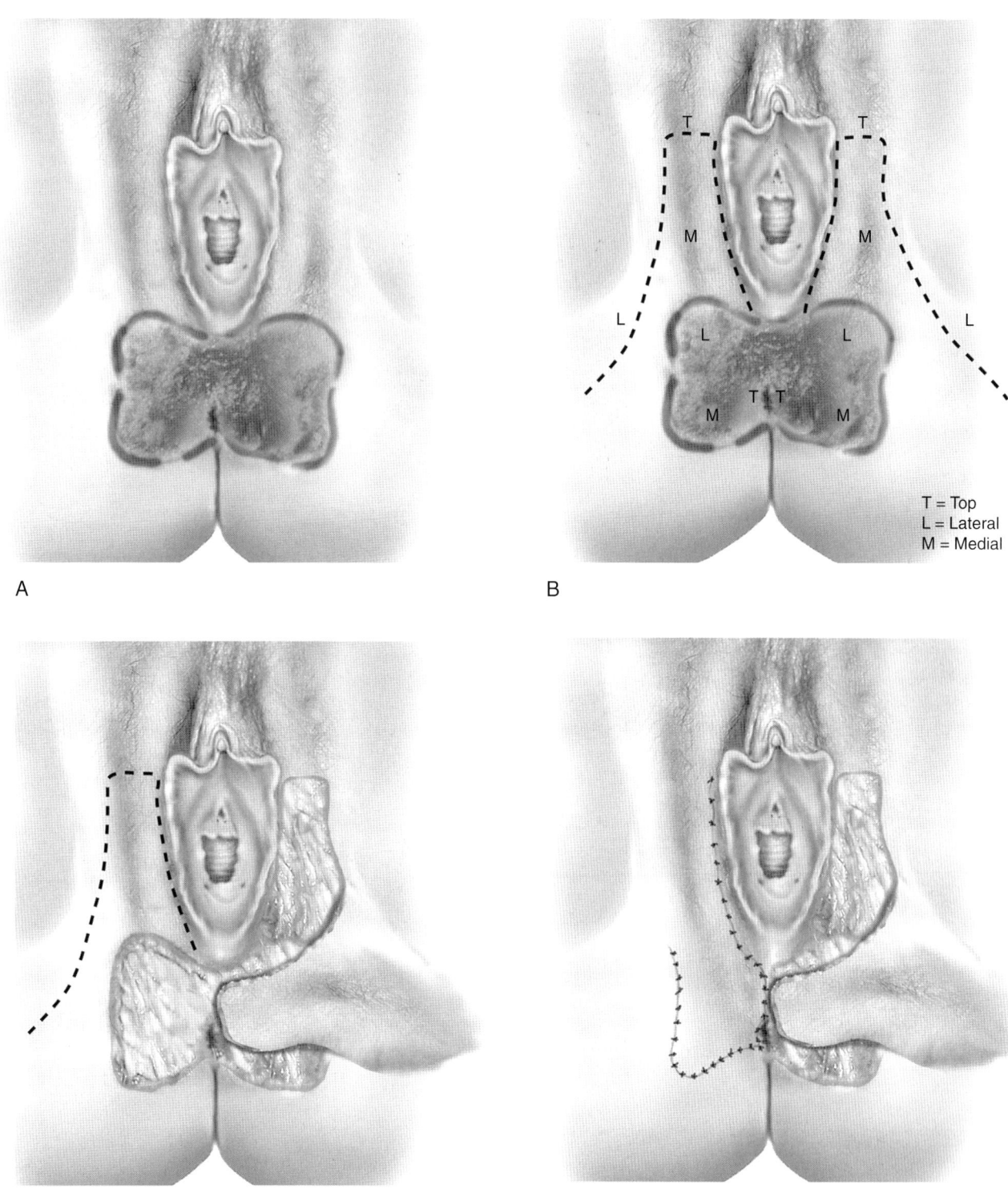

A

B

T = Top
L = Lateral
M = Medial

C

D

**FIGURE 68–17  A.** The perianal and perineal defect is clearly seen. The full-thickness resection was shown in Figure 68–16. **B.** A broad-based pedicle graft is outlined. The graft will be cut and freed from the underlying fat and rotated posteriorly (inferiorly) and medially. **C.** The left flap has been rotated into place. **D.** The right flap has been rotated and sutured into place with 3-0 Vicryl. The donor site has been closed on the right. No sutures have been placed into the left-sided graft.

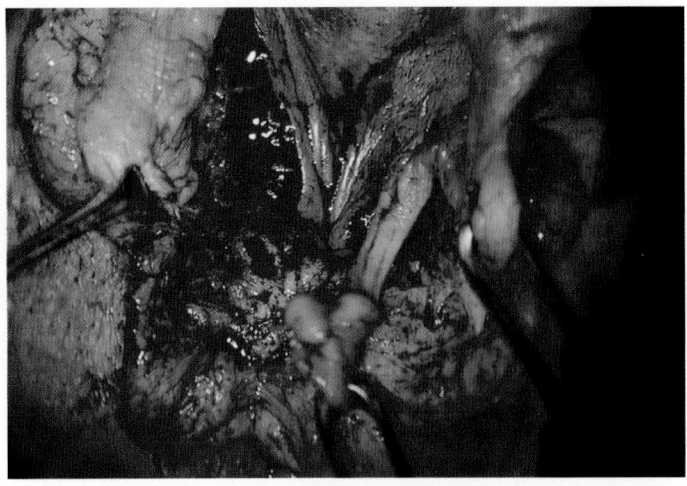

FIGURE 68–18 Allis clamps have been placed on the pedicle grafts to facilitate their rotation to cover the wound.

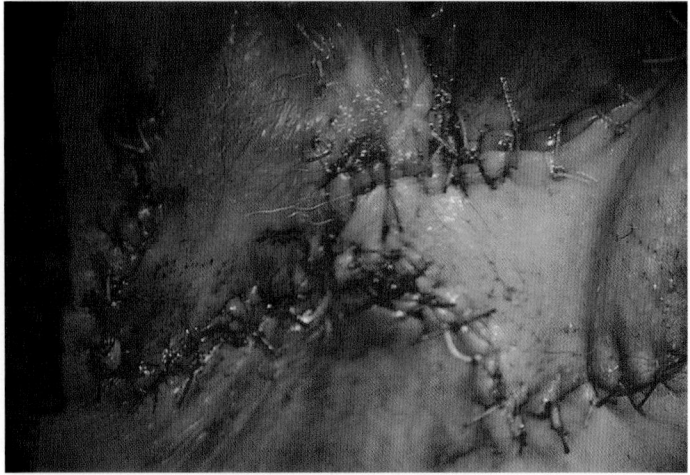

FIGURE 68–19 The grafts have been rotated, sutured into place, and secured.

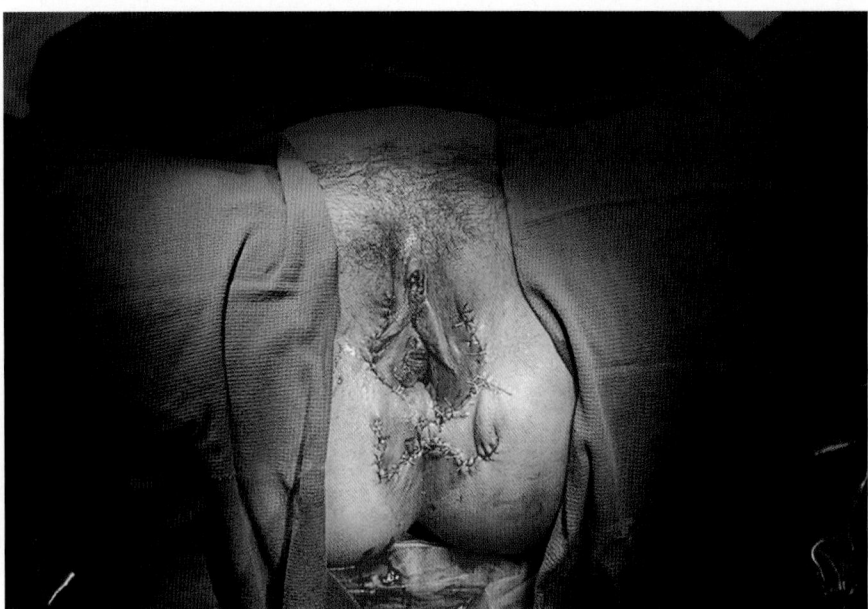

FIGURE 68–20 Both pedicle grafts have been sutured into the margins of and cover the wound totally. The distal edges of the graft are sutured to the anal mucosa.

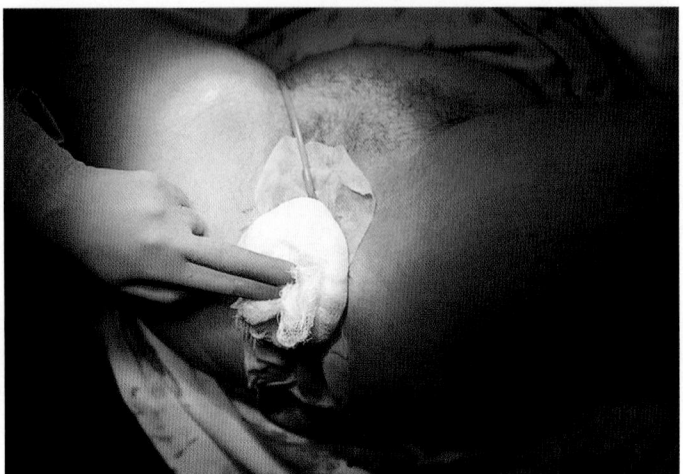

FIGURE 68–21 When the surgery has been completed, the wounds are thoroughly irrigated with sterile normal saline. Xeroform gauze is applied to the graft, and this is followed by the application of a pressure dressing. A Foley catheter has been placed in the bladder.

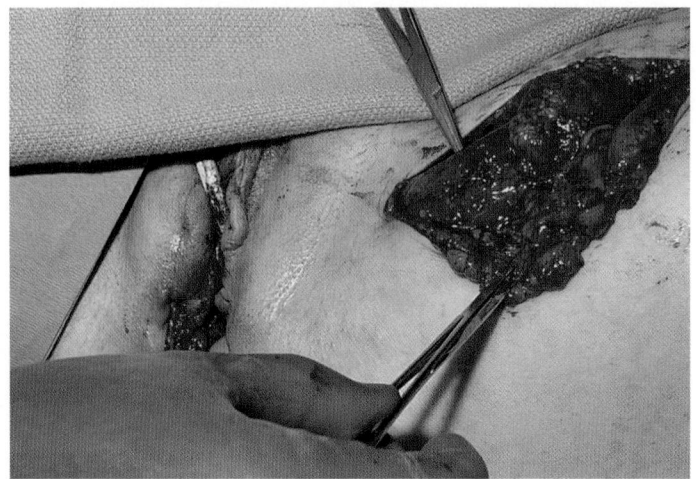

FIGURE 68–22 When an extensive mass of tissue is resected in the vulva or vagina, a myocutaneous graft is indicated. Here, the gracilis muscle and its posterior blood supply are secured.

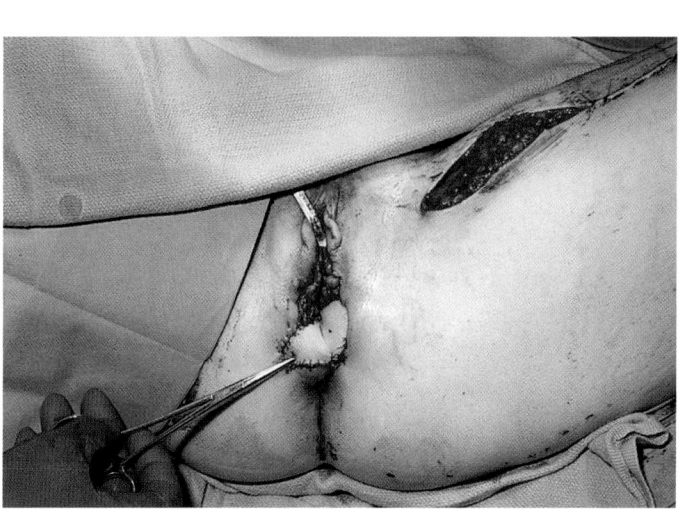

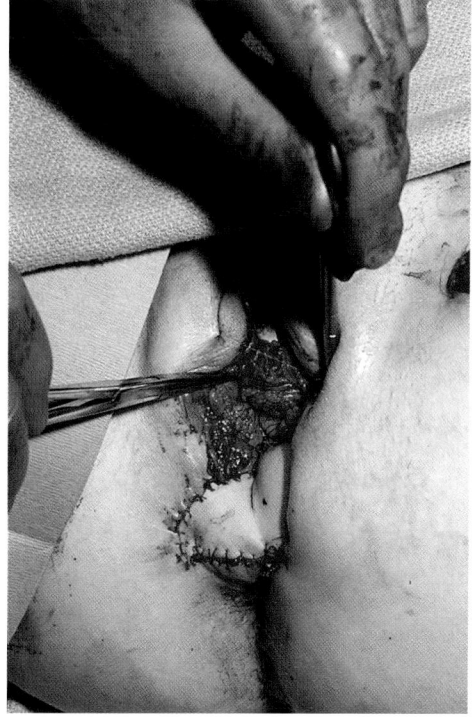

A

B

**FIGURE 68–23 A.** The muscle, together with the overlying skin and subcutaneous tissue, constitutes the pedicle graft. This graft is rotated and delivered via a tunnel through the thigh to the labial area. The graft is then sutured into place after testing for the adequacy of blood flow (using Doppler sonography). **B.** Detailed view of part **A.** The wound is being closed.

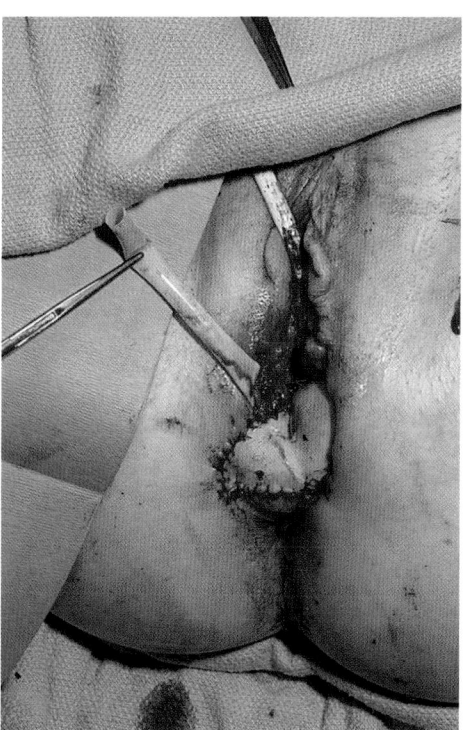

**FIGURE 68–24** A drain has been placed into a portion of the vagina. The left wall of the vagina and the perineum have been replaced and repaired with a gracilis myocutaneous flap.

# CHAPTER 69

# Laser Excision and Vaporization

*Michael S. Baggish*

Although carbon dioxide ($CO_2$) laser vaporization of vulvar intraepithelial neoplasia is an effective, quick, and cost-efficient method of treatment, it does present a significant disadvantage: No tissue specimen is available for histologic examination when tissue is ablated; therefore, no information relative to margins or the severity of the disease can be obtained. For obtaining a tissue specimen, laser excision is preferable to ablative techniques.

## Laser Excision by Thin Section

The laser "thin section" has three advantages: It (1) requires neither closure nor grafting, (2) heals rapidly without gross scar formation, and (3) provides a specimen for pathologic examination.

The lesion should be mapped preoperatively. The patient is positioned and prepared as for a knife resection (Fig. 69-1). A superpulsed (UltraPulse) $CO_2$ laser coupled to a micromanipulator is the instrument of choice. The area for resection is outlined with laser spots (Fig. 69-2). The laser power is set at 8 to 12 W, and a tracer cut is made around the lesion. Next, a 1:100 vasopressin solution is injected subdermally, completely circumscribing the lesion and infiltrating beneath the skin (Fig. 69-3). Next, laser power is increased to 15 to 20 W, and, with a tightly focused beam, a plane is created parallel to the surface of the skin. The cut is made beneath the papillary dermis into the reticular dermis (Fig. 69-4). Maintenance of the plane and the excision is facilitated by keeping constant tension on the skin that is to be excised (Fig. 69-5). Small bleeding vessels are directly sutured with 4-0 or 5-0 Vicryl (Fig. 69-6). Application of clamps is avoided to diminish trauma to the tissue.

The excised specimen is placed in fixative and sent to pathology (Figs. 69-7 and 69-8A, B). Postoperatively, the patient is instructed to take tub baths in salt water (Instant Ocean) twice daily and to apply silver sulfadiazine (Silvadene) cream to the wound site 3 times per day. Alternatively, a urethane dressing (OpSite) is applied to the wound (Fig. 69-9A, B). Healing is complete at 4 to 6 weeks (Fig. 69-10A, B).

## Laser Vaporization

$CO_2$ laser vaporization is performed by using specifications identical to those used for excision (i.e., vaporization in hair-bearing areas, perineum, and perianal skin to a depth of 2.3 mm with a 3-mm peripheral margin) (Figs. 69-11 through 69-16). For the labia minora, periclitoral lesion vaporization is carried to a depth no greater than 1 mm; again, wide peripheral margins are recommended to diminish the chance of recurrence (Figs. 69-17 and 69-18). Preoperative mapping with extensive preoperative tissue sampling is a requirement before any laser vaporization to (1) determine that the disease is *not* invasive carcinoma, and (2) predict the extent of the disease and the peripheral margins for vaporization. The medial and lateral margins of the neoplasia are outlined after the patient has been anesthetized, prepared, and draped (Figs. 69-19 and 69-20). Power is set at 20 W, and the beam is defocused to permit a 2-mm-diameter spot (Figs. 69-21 and 69-22). The laser places multiple impact spots, much in the manner of marking the lesion with a pen. The spots are then connected, producing a clear outline of the area to be vaporized (Figs. 69-23 and 69-24). Laser power is turned up to 30 to 40 W, and the entire zone is vaporized to a uniform 2-mm depth (note that vaporization between 0.5 and 1.5 mm is accounted for by thermal conduction injury) (Figs. 69-25 through 69-27). When the vaporization is complete, any char is washed away. The wound is covered with Silvadene cream. The patient is instructed to take salt water tub baths 3 times daily, followed by application of Silvadene cream (Fig. 69-28).

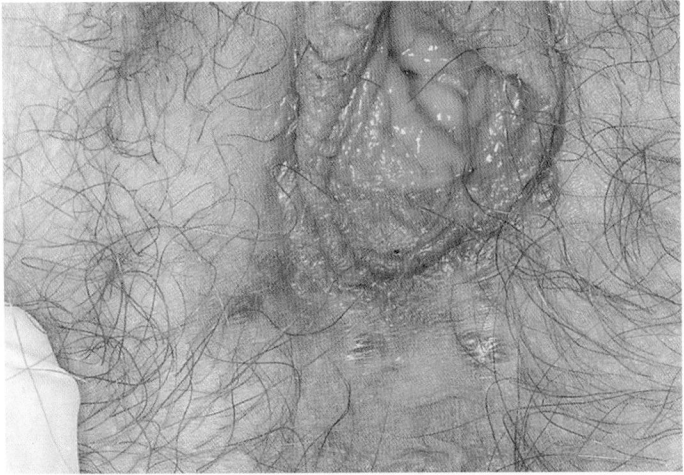

FIGURE 69–1  Raised, pigmented lesions characteristic of vulvar intraepithelial neoplasia (VIN) are clearly seen at the postcommissure, perineum, and lower labia majora.

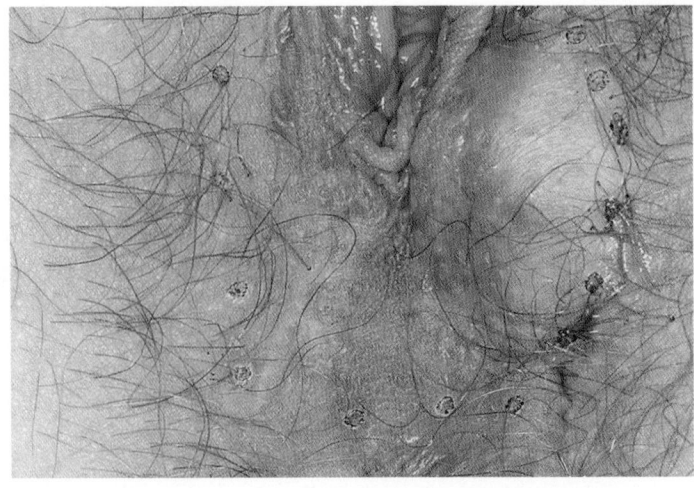

FIGURE 69–2  The area to be thin section–excised is outlined by carbon dioxide ($CO_2$) laser spots delivered by an UltraPulse $CO_2$ laser coupled to an operating microscope. Spot, 1.5 mm; power, 20 W.

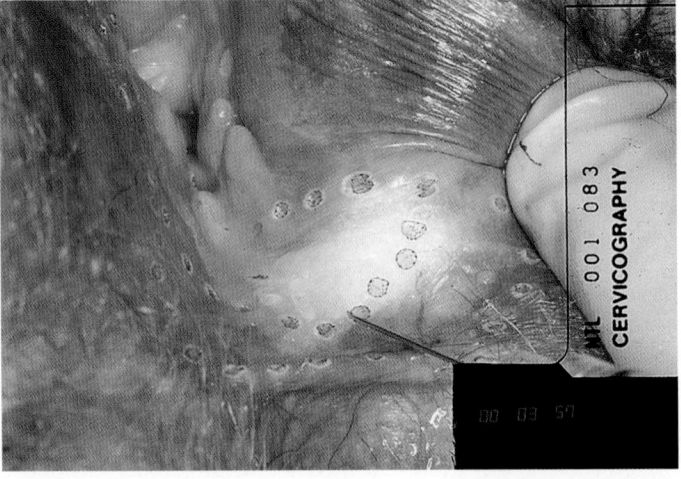

FIGURE 69–3  A 1:100 vasopressin solution is injected subdermally. This will serve a dual purpose: as a hemostatic agent and as a heat sink.

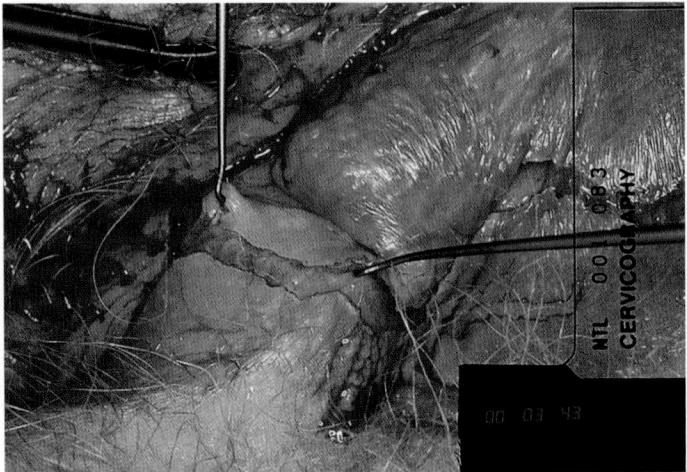

FIGURE 69–4  A shallow intradermal cut is made into the tissue with a highly pulsed, powerful laser cutting beam and a fine skin hook.

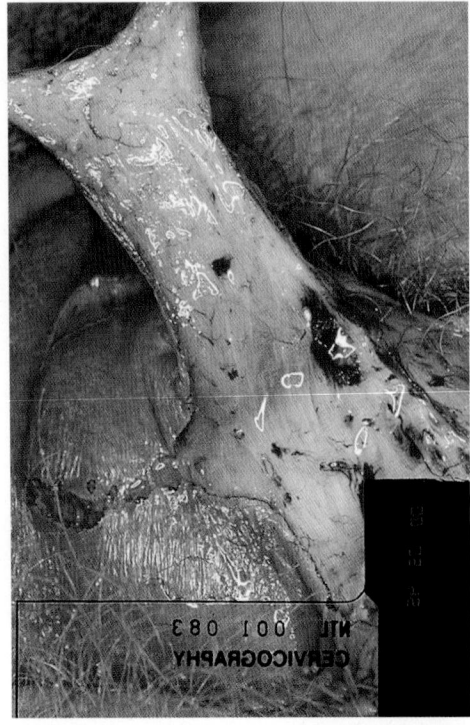

FIGURE 69–5  Tissue flaps are developed as the laser incision gains in area. Note the excellent hemostasis and the pink color of the skin to be excised, as well as the underlying dermis. The lack of thermal artifact is due to the superpulsed laser beam and the intradermal fluid.

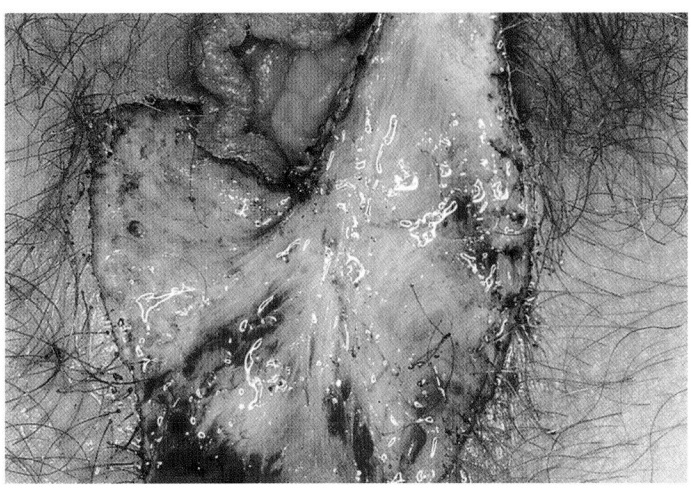

FIGURE 69–6 The "butterfly" area of laser excision is almost complete. The remaining skin on traction, seen on the left side, is ready to be cut off.

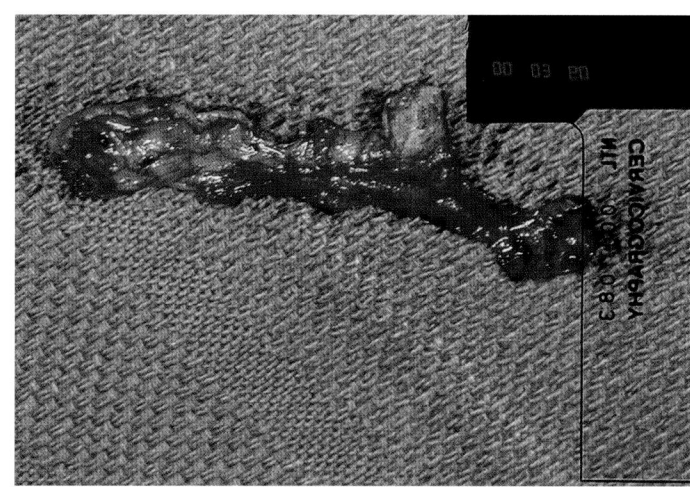

FIGURE 69–7 The excised specimen is sent to pathology. The surgeon will be assured that no invasion has occurred and will know the status of deep as well as peripheral margins.

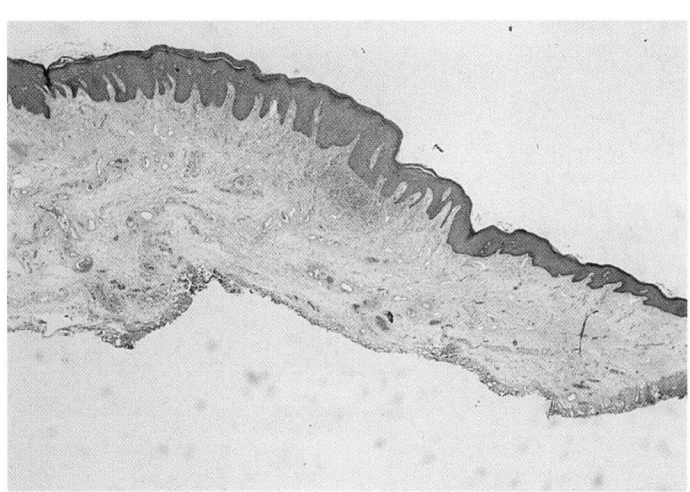

A

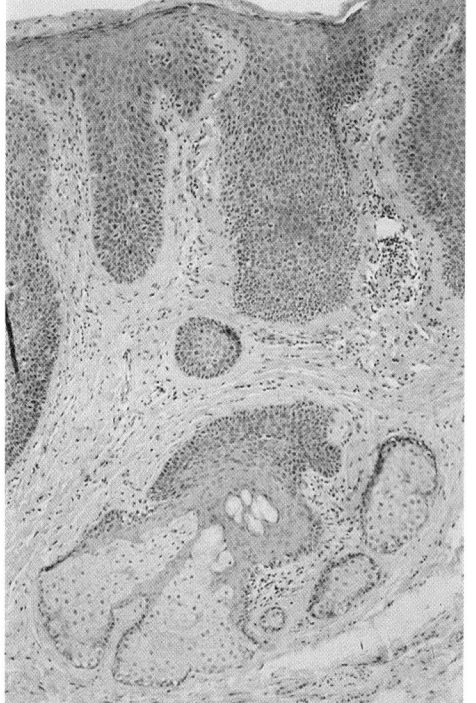

B

FIGURE 69–8 A. Microscopic section (magnification ×2) showing the excellent preservation and lack of cellular distortion of the thin-section sample. B. High-power view of Figure 69–8A shows the extension of neoplasia into underlying sebaceous glands. A hematoxylin and eosin stain has been used.

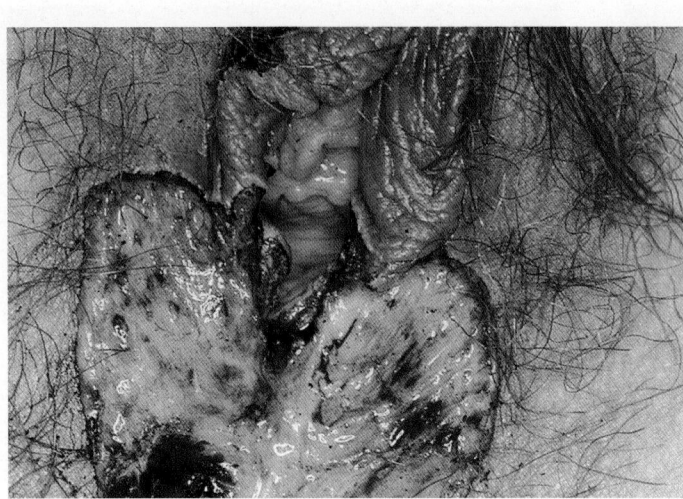
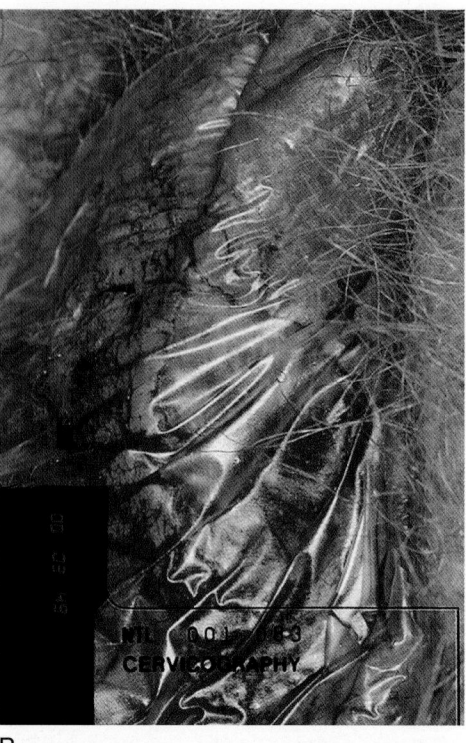

A                                                              B

**FIGURE 69–9  A.** Intraepithelial neoplastic tissues have been completely excised (by intradermal section). The wound has been thoroughly irrigated with normal saline. **B.** A urethane dressing has been applied to the wound.

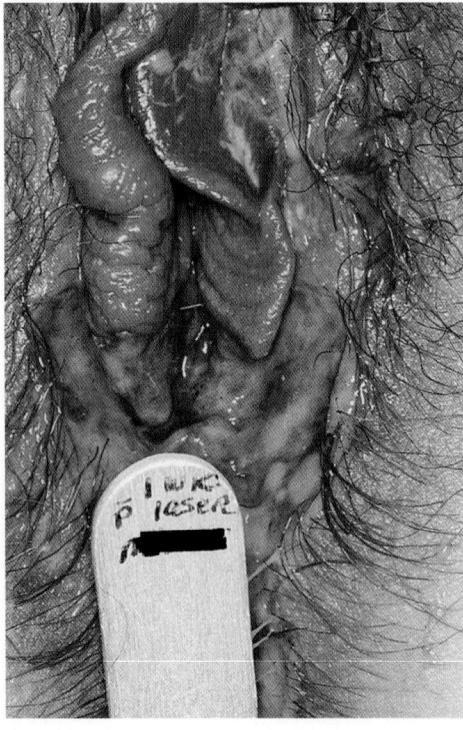
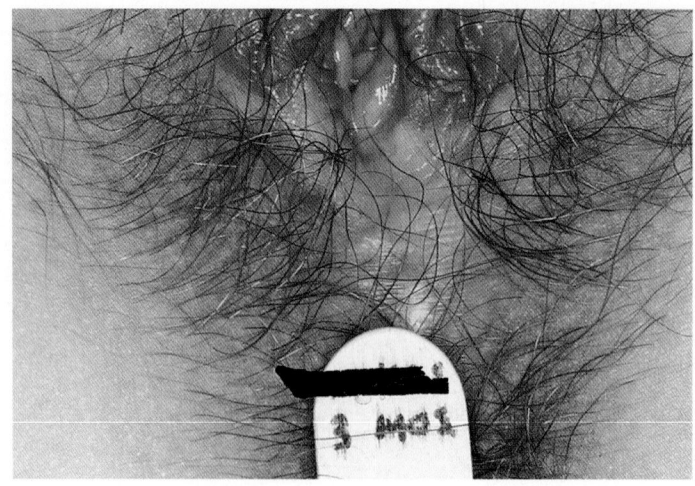

A                                                              B

**FIGURE 69–10  A.** The wound is clean and healing at 1 week postoperatively. **B.** At 3 months, the wound is completely healed with no gross scar formation and no evidence of persisting neoplasia.

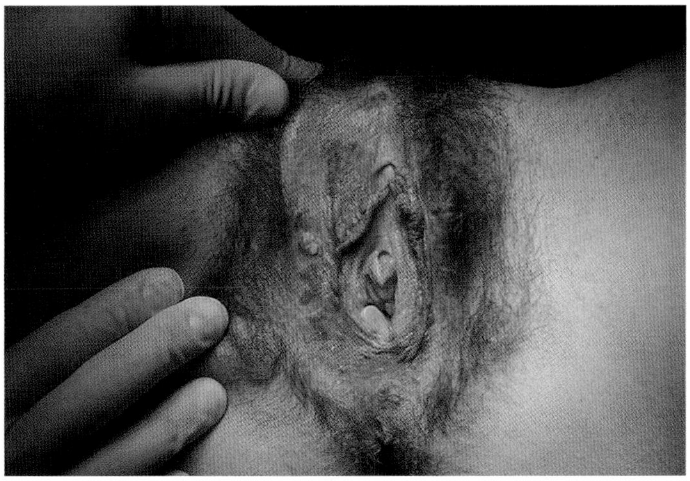

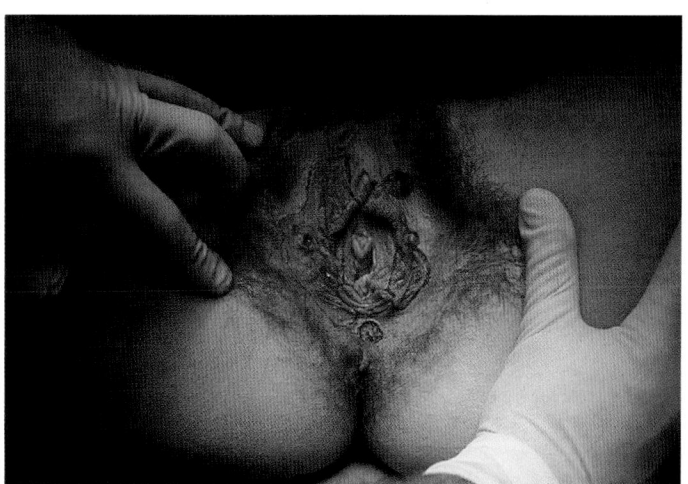

FIGURE 69–11 Extensive multifocal carcinoma in situ (CIS) of the vulva. The lesions were previously multiply biopsied and mapped. Note the darkly pigmented warty lesions.

FIGURE 69–12 The areas to be treated are outlined with the carbon dioxide ($CO_2$) laser beam and vaporized with the microscope and laser-coupled micromanipulator. Vaporization carries into the reticular dermis but not the fat.

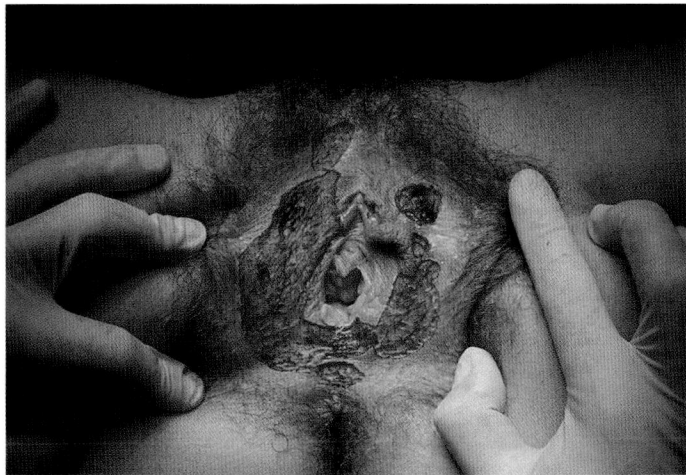

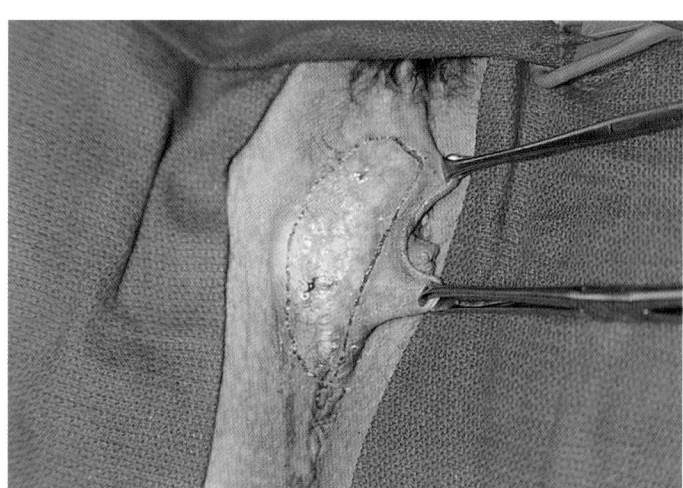

FIGURE 69–13 Vaporization is complete. Hair-bearing areas are treated to a depth of 2 mm. Non–hair-bearing areas are treated to shallower depths (1 mm).

FIGURE 69–14 The area of vulvar intraepithelial neoplasia (VIN) is outlined with the carbon dioxide ($CO_2$) laser beam at 20 W of power.

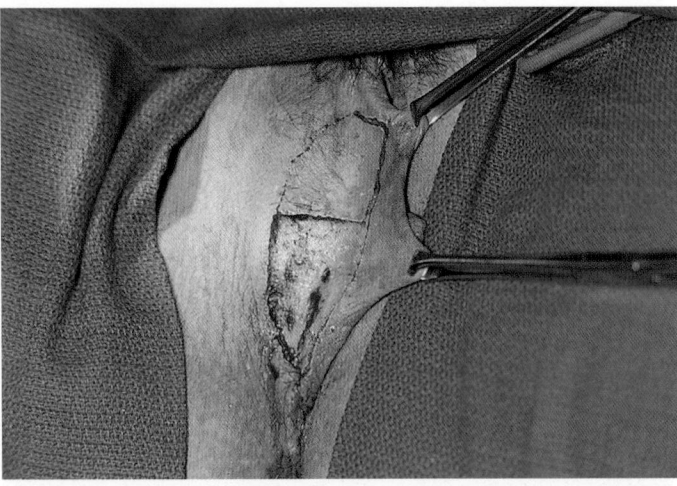

FIGURE 69–15 Vaporization with a 2-mm spot (beam diameter) is carried out uniformly to a 2-mm depth.

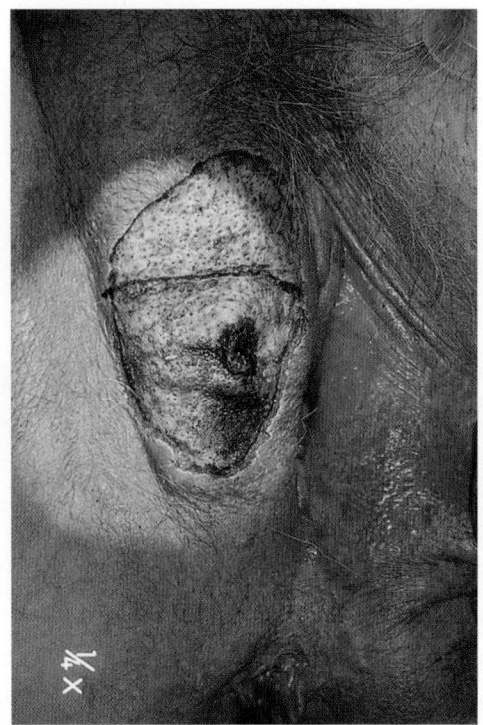

FIGURE 69–16 Vaporization is complete. The wound is cleansed with sterile water or saline to remove the char.

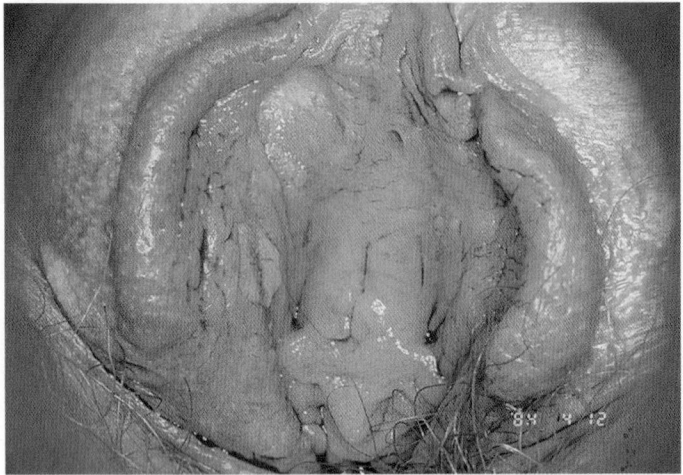

FIGURE 69–17 Typical flat, warty carcinoma in situ (CIS) of the vestibule and labia minora.

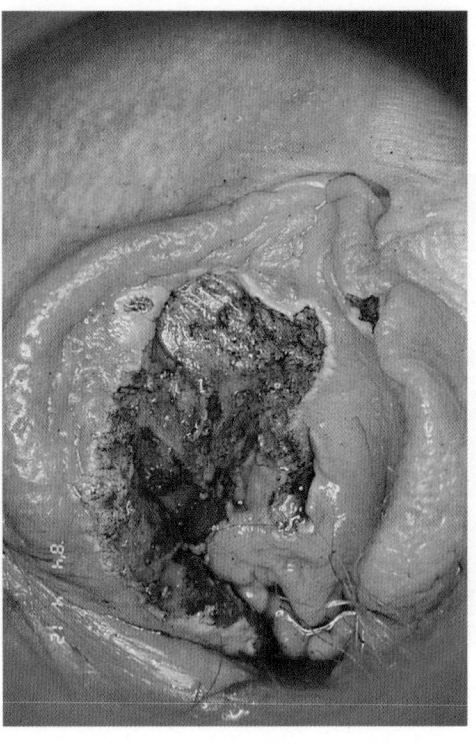

FIGURE 69–18 Carbon dioxide ($CO_2$) laser vaporization to a depth of 1 mm has been completed.

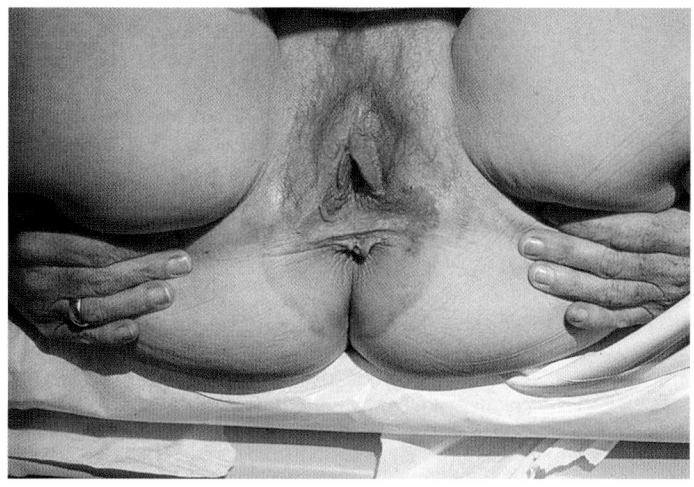

FIGURE 69–19 This patient has a parakeratotic (red) lesion consistent with carcinoma in situ (CIS) involving the left labium majus, perineum, and proximal buttock skin.

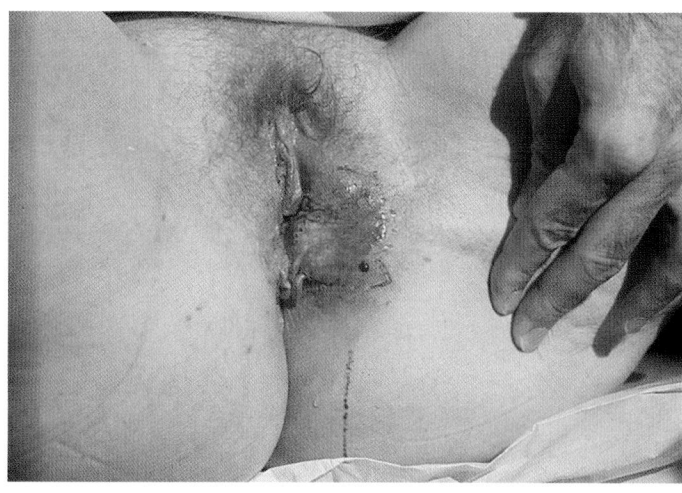

FIGURE 69–20 The lesion is trace-marked with the carbon dioxide ($CO_2$) laser after injection of a local anesthetic.

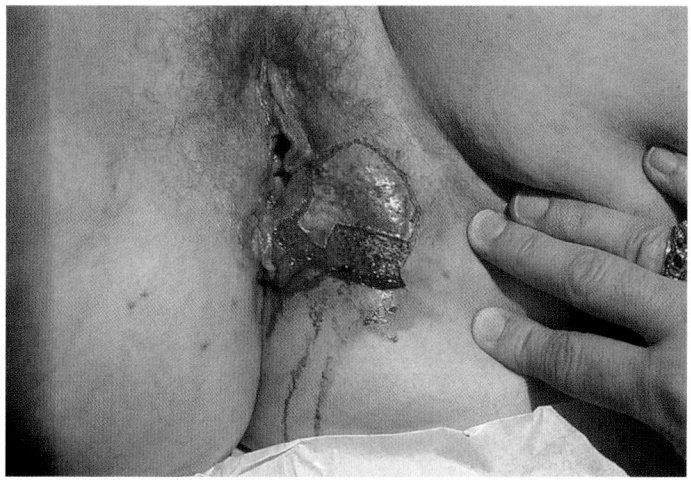

FIGURE 69–21 The area within the tracing is systematically vaporized to a 2-mm depth.

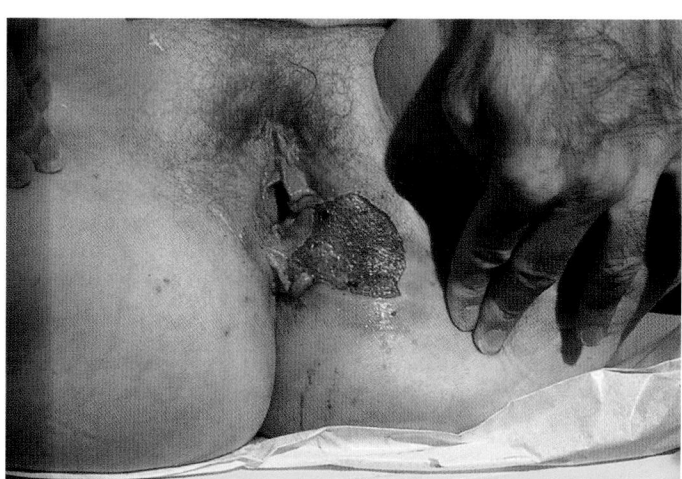

FIGURE 69–22 Vaporization is complete. The wound is irrigated with sterile water and covered with Silvadene cream.

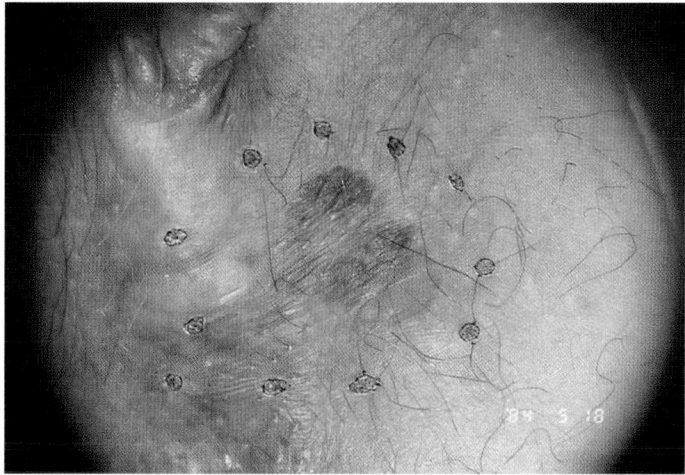

FIGURE 69–23 Typical pigmented, focal papular carcinoma in situ (CIS) of the perianal skin. The lesion has been trace-marked with the carbon dioxide ($CO_2$) laser. A 3-mm margin has been traced.

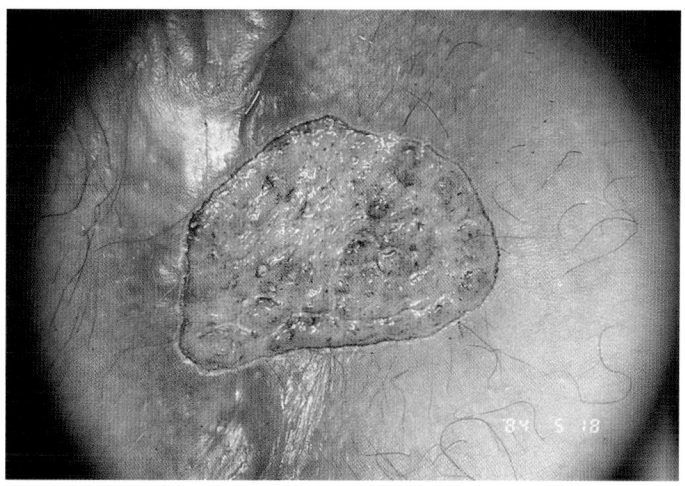

FIGURE 69–24 The lesion has been completely vaporized. The char has been irrigated away.

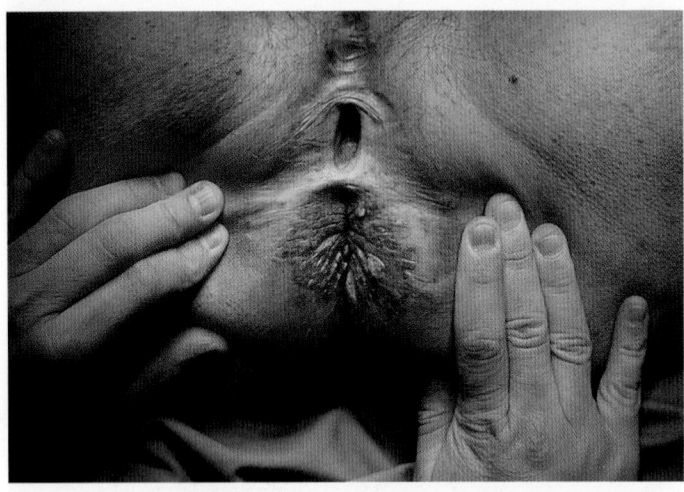

**FIGURE 69–25** This woman had a previous "simple" vulvectomy for carcinoma in situ (CIS). Extensive, diffuse anal and perianal recurrent lesions are clearly visible.

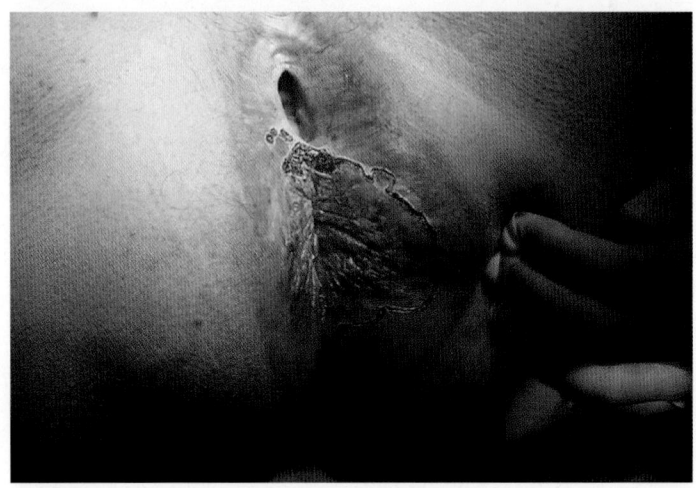

**FIGURE 69–26** With the patient under general anesthesia, the perianal carcinoma in situ (CIS) is outlined for vaporization.

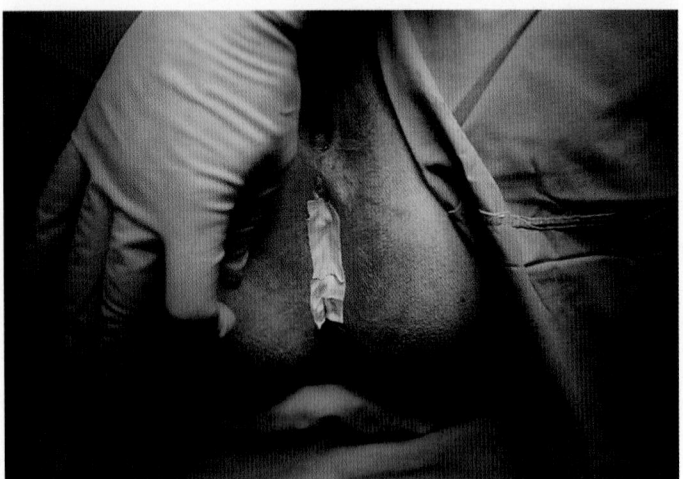

**FIGURE 69–27** The lesions have been completely vaporized to a depth of 1.5 to 2.0 mm, and the wound is covered with Xeroform gauze.

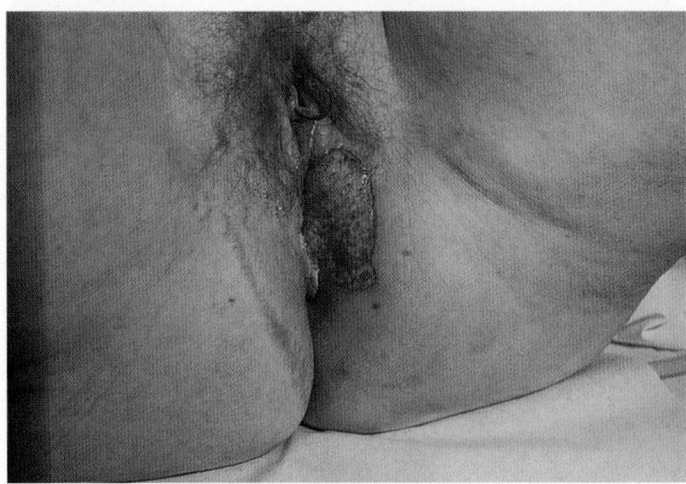

**FIGURE 69–28** The same patient depicted in Figure 69–19 at her 1-week postoperative visit. The wound is clean. Healing has begun from the deeper and peripheral skin appendages.

# CHAPTER 70

# Anatomy of the Groin and Femoral Triangle

*Michael S. Baggish*

Knowledge of inguinal anatomy is essential before vulvectomy is performed. The lymphatics of the vulva drain to the superficial inguinal lymph nodes and to the femoral and external iliac nodes. To expose the area, an incision is made on the thigh just below and parallel to the inguinal ligament (Fig. 70-1A). A second incision is made to intersect with the first at the anterior superior iliac spine and is continued caudally toward the apex of the femoral triangle. The flap created is dissected medially (Fig. 70-1B).

The triangular area is bordered laterally by the sartorius muscle and medially by the pectineus and adductor longus muscles (Fig. 70-2A). Traveling from below upward within the medial aspect of the fat above the aforementioned medial muscles is a large vessel, the saphenous vein (see Fig. 70-2A). The vein pierces the cribriform fascia overlying the fossa ovalis and the femoral vessels and joins the femoral vein below the fascia (Fig. 70-2B). The femoral vein lies in its own tough fascial compartment. Several small veins and arteries join to or branch from the femoral vein and artery: (1) the superficial circumflex iliac, (2) the superficial epigastric, and (3) the superficial external pudendal (Fig. 70-2D). Directly medial and slightly posterior is the femoral canal, which is a potential space juxtaposed medially to the pubic bone (Fig. 70-3A). This canal may contain the lowest node of the external iliac chain, Cloquet's node (Fig. 70-3B, C). Just lateral to the femoral vein, again within its own fascial compartment, lies the femoral artery, which accompanies the vein in a caudal and deep descending course (Fig. 70-4A, B). Finally, most lateral and again with a tough fascial compartment is the femoral nerve, which descends into the thigh as a series of branching, diverging fibers (Fig. 70-5A, B). The femoral nerve is vulnerable to injury during positioning of the inferior extremities for perineal operations (Fig. 70-5C). The inguinal ligament crosses the nerve perpendicularly, where the nerve probably is most exposed. The tight inguinal ligament therefore can put sufficient pressure on the underlying nerve to result in palsy. The nerve also may be injured by a hyperextended lithotomy position (high lithotomy) coupled with abduction at the thigh (Fig. 70-5D). This type of stretch injury occurs in the vicinity of the lumbar plexus, where the obturator nerve joins the lumbar plexus between the femoral nerve and the lumbosacral trunk (Fig. 70-5E). The obturator nerve and the relatively superficial genital femoral nerve are more susceptible to retractor injuries than is the femoral nerve, which is buried in the substance of the psoas major muscle (see Fig. 70-5D).

Farther lateral is the sartorius muscle, which in concert with the inguinal ligament takes its origin from the anterior superior iliac spine (Fig. 70-6A, B). It is useful to transplant this muscle over the exposed femoral vessels after a radical vulvectomy and inguinal lymphadenectomy (Fig. 70-6C).

The gracilis muscle is located at the medial side of the femoral triangle (i.e., medial and deep to the saphenous vein). This structure is useful as a myocutaneous flap for transplant to the vulva or vagina (Fig. 70-7A through C).

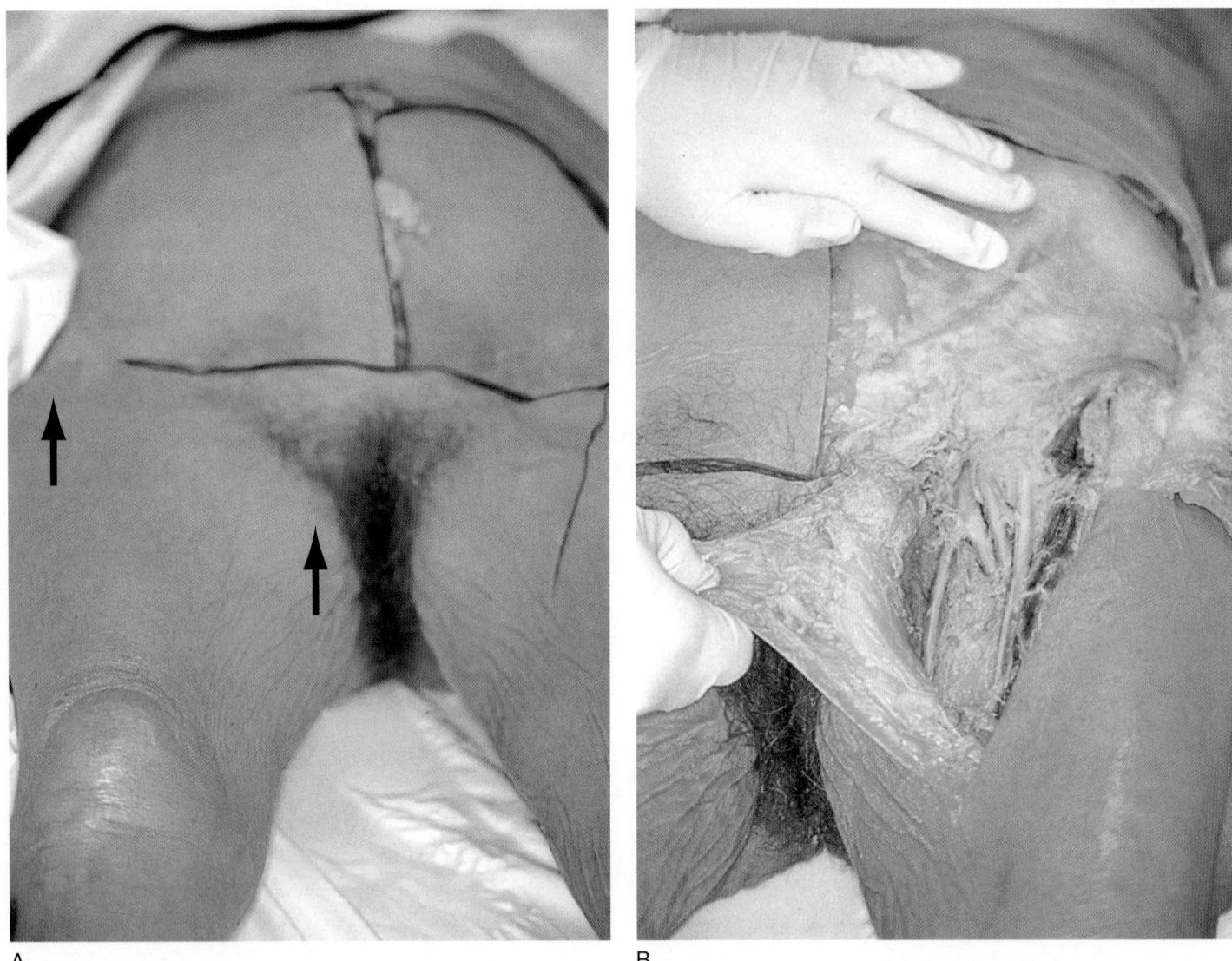

A

B

**FIGURE 70–1  A.** The inguinal area and the femoral triangle are located caudal to the inguinal ligament. The initial incision to expose the area is made in the thigh parallel to and below the inguinal ligament (*between the two arrows*). **B.** The second incision intersects with the first (see part **A**) at the anterior superior iliac spine and extends inferiorly toward the apex of the femoral triangle. The excision extends into the subcutaneous tissue. The flap is dissected medially.

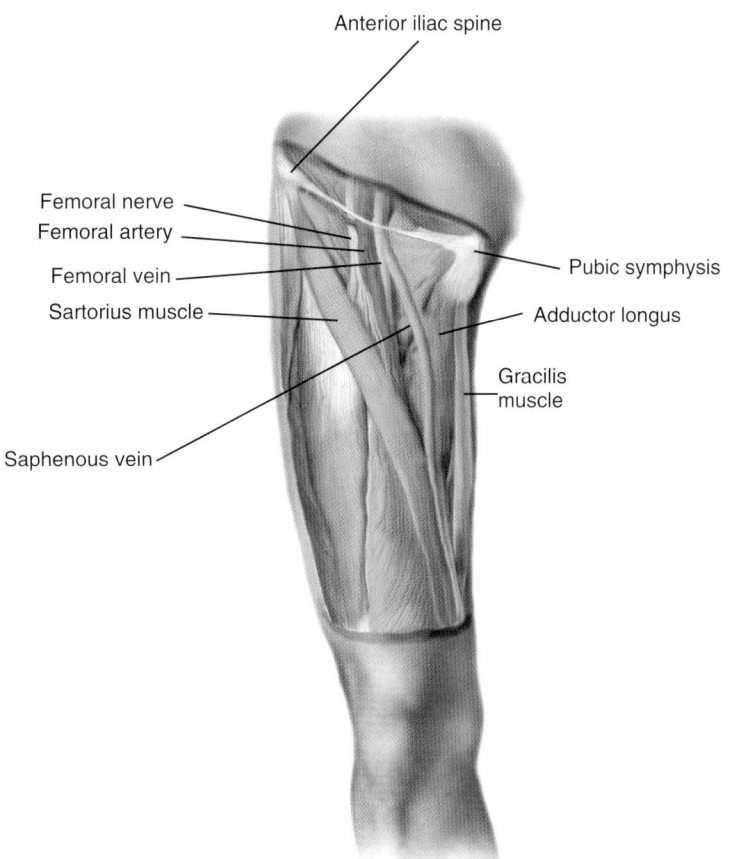

Anterior iliac spine

Femoral nerve

Femoral artery

Femoral vein

Sartorius muscle

Saphenous vein

Pubic symphysis

Adductor longus

Gracilis muscle

A

FIGURE 70–2  A. Overall schema of the femoral triangle. Medially is the gracilis muscle. Next to the gracilis is the adductor longus. The sartorius muscle is the straplike muscle extending from lateral to medial and forming the lateral side of the triangle. Behind the sartorius is the rectus femoris muscle.

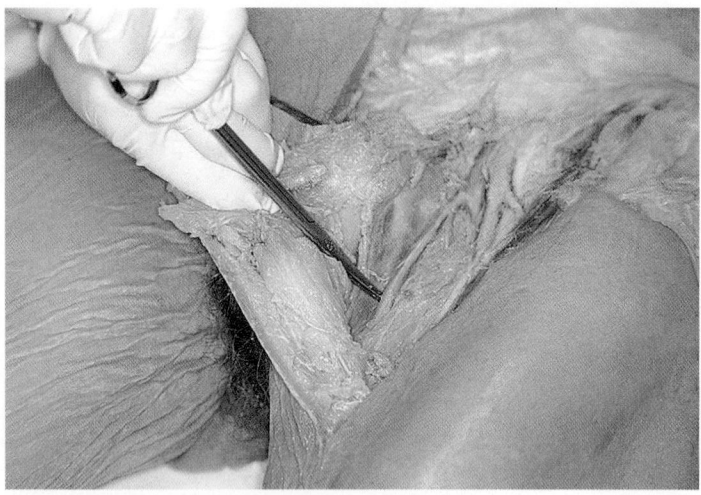

B

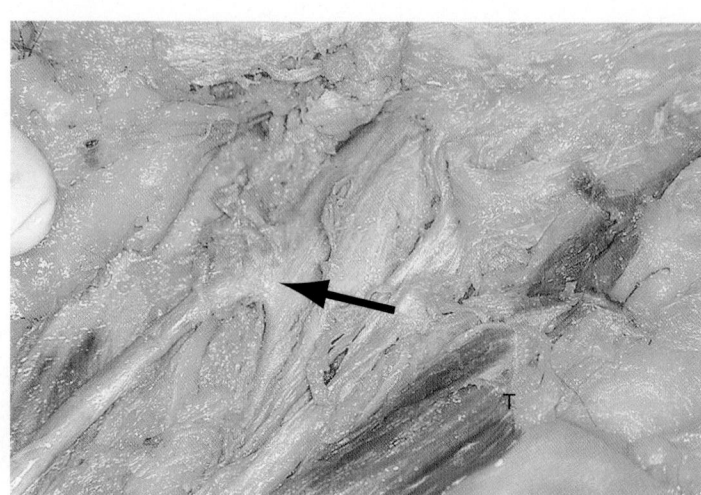

C

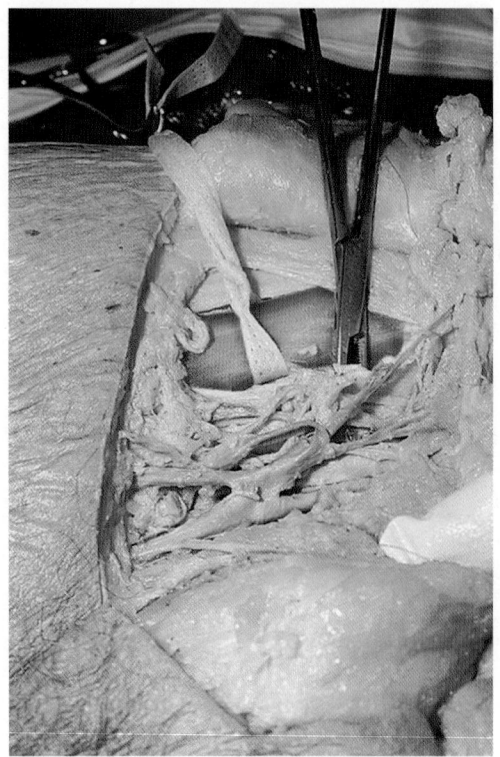

D

**FIGURE 70–2, cont'd** **B.** The saphenous vein is exposed (scissors are under the vein) as it sweeps through the fat, extending from a medial location in the thigh and vectoring toward the midpoint below the inguinal ligament. **C.** Close-up view of the saphenous vein penetrating the cribriform fascia and draining into the femoral vein (*arrow*). The sartorius muscle (*S*) is seen at the lateral margin of the femoral triangle. **D.** Several small veins can be seen to join the junction of the femoral and saphenous veins. These small tributaries include the superficial epigastric, superficial external pudendal, and superficial circumflex iliac veins. The umbilical tape has been placed around the sartorius muscle. The surgeon's gloved finger is on the pubic tubercle (i.e., at the medial insertion of the inguinal ligament).

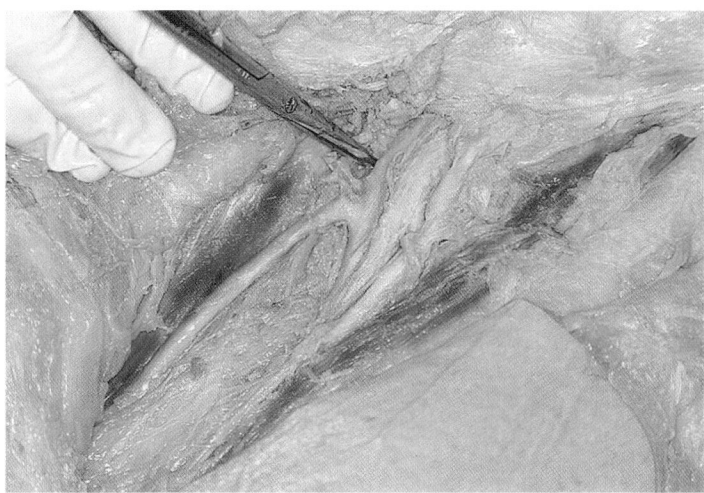

A

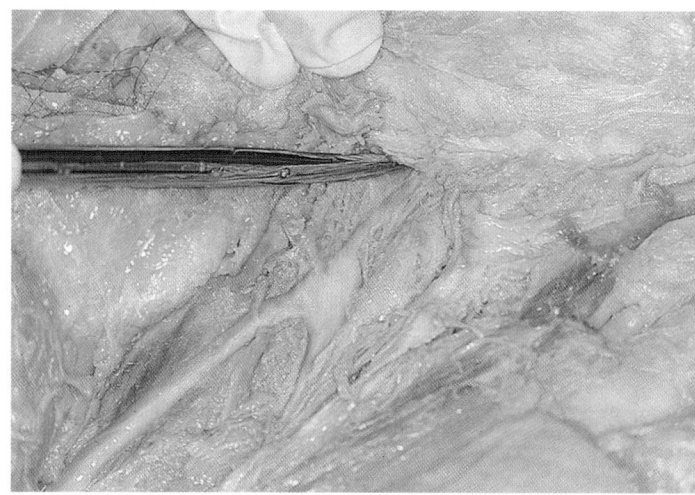

B

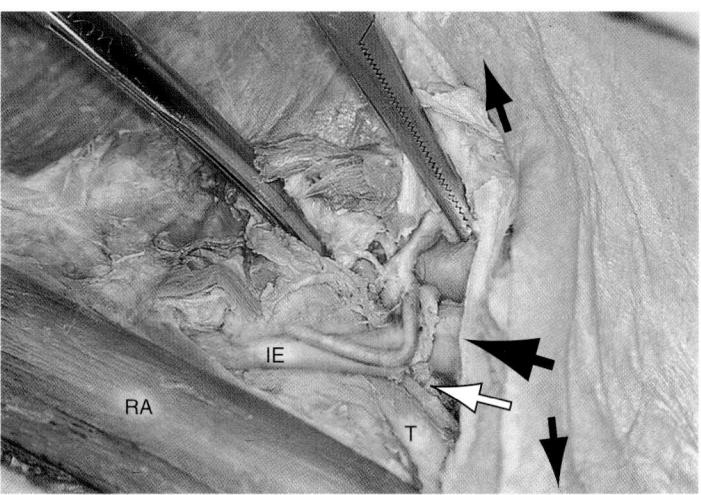

C

**FIGURE 70–3 A.** The scissors are dissecting the space medial to the femoral vein. This is the femoral canal. **B.** The scissors are lateral to the pubic bone and the lacunar ligament, beneath the terminal portion of the inguinal ligament, and medial to the femoral vein. The scissors are within the femoral canal. This canal is a potential space for the formation of a femoral hernia. **C.** Dissection above the inguinal ligament. The location of the inguinal ligament is shown by the small arrows. The medial border of the left rectus abdominis (RA) muscle is seen at the lower left-hand portion of the picture. The Kocher clamp points to the external iliac artery just cranial to the point where it crosses beneath the inguinal ligament. The external iliac vein is located medial to the artery (*large dark arrow*). The inferior epigastric (IE) crosses the femoral vein and travels cranially and medially to reach the lateral border of the rectus muscle. The bluish tissue on which these structures lie is the transversalis fascia (T). The open arrow points to the location of the lowest most external iliac node, Cloquet's node, which lies in the upper portion (cranial) of the femoral canal.

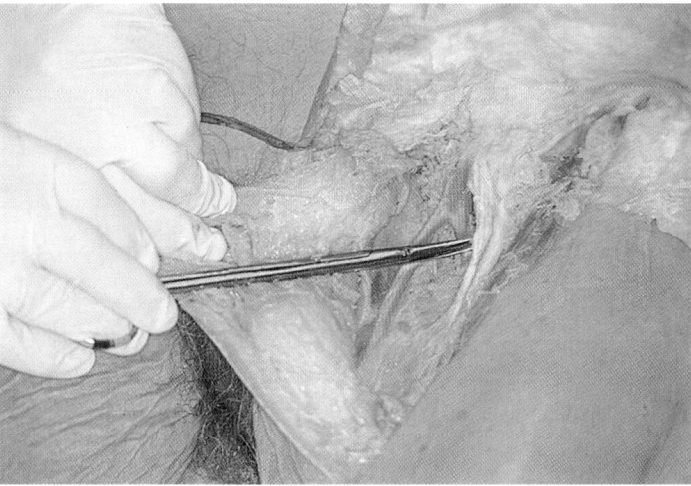

A

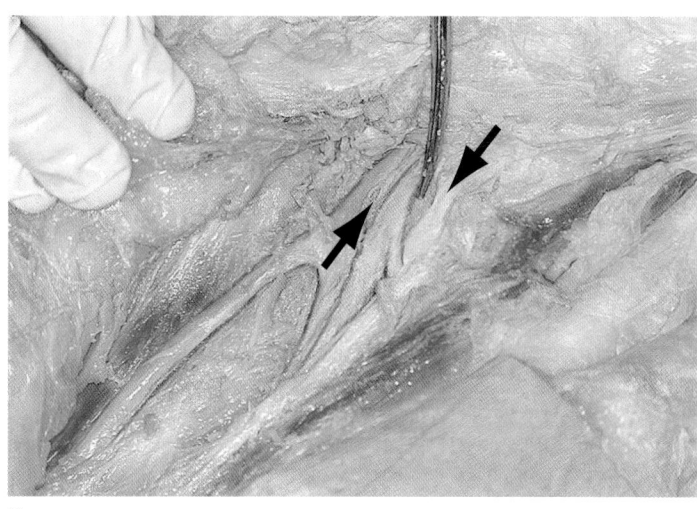

B

**FIGURE 70–4 A.** The scissors point to and are directly beneath the femoral artery. **B.** The probe points to the femoral artery. This vessel lies in its own fascial compartment and is separated from the femoral vein by tough connective tissue (fascia) (*arrows*).

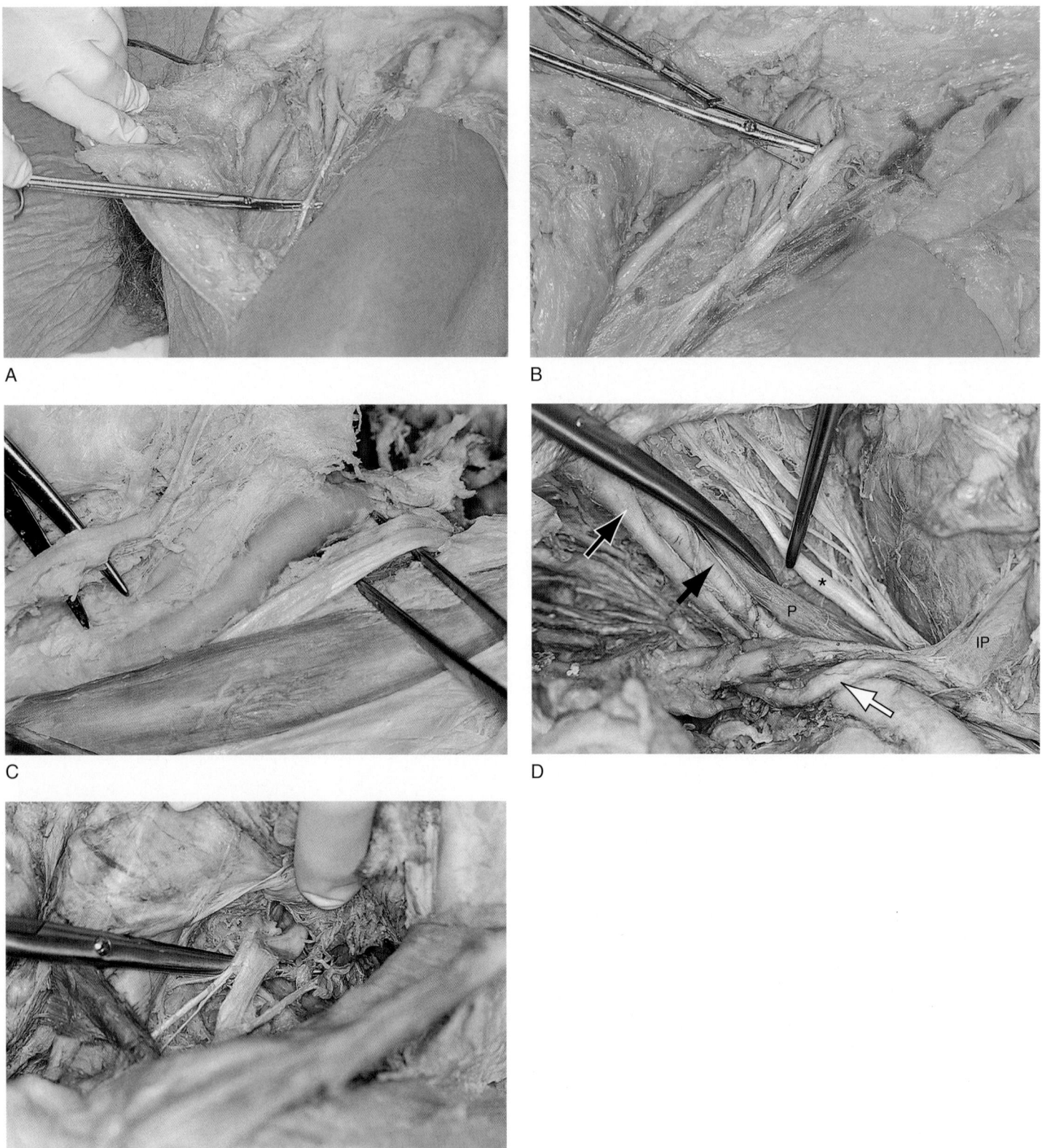

A

B

C

D

E

**FIGURE 70–5  A.** The femoral nerve is situated lateral to the femoral artery. The tip of the scissors lies beneath a branch of the main trunk of the nerve. **B.** The scissors are spread under the femoral nerve as it emerges from beneath the inguinal ligament. The sartorius muscle is lateral to the nerve. Pressure on the nerve by the inguinal ligament when the inferior extremities are severely flexed can result in femoral nerve palsy. **C.** Close-up view of the upper femoral triangle. The scissors are spread beneath the saphenous vein. The forceps are spread under the main trunk of the femoral nerve. The forceps arms lie on the sartorius muscle. **D.** This abdominal dissection demonstrates the upward course of the femoral nerve. The anterior portion of the psoas major muscle (P) has been cut away. The curved scissors sharply depress the medial aspect of the psoas major muscle (P). The tip of the forceps points to the femoral nerve (*), which was embedded within the substance of the psoas muscle. The infundibulopelvic ligament (IP) and the ureter (*open arrow*) cross the common iliac artery. The external iliac artery (*small arrow*) and the external iliac vein (*outlined small arrow*) below the artery are located medial to the retracted muscle. Below the external iliac vein is the dissected obturator fossa. **E.** Deep within the pelvis, above the sacrum, the femoral and obturator nerves join the lumbosacral trunk. The scissors are beneath the nerves.

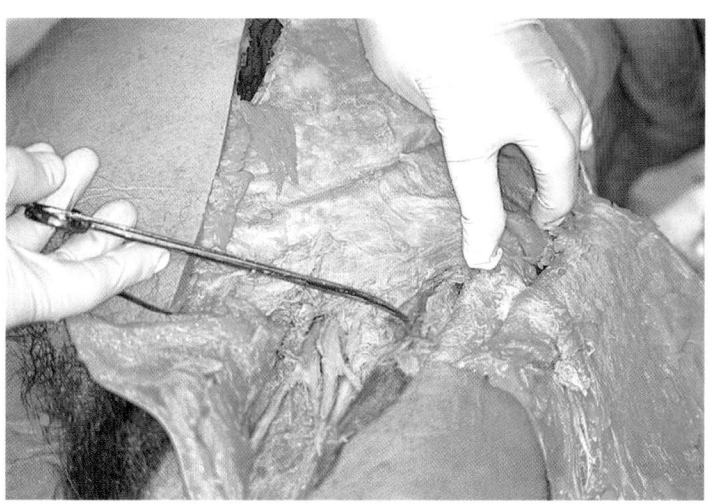

A

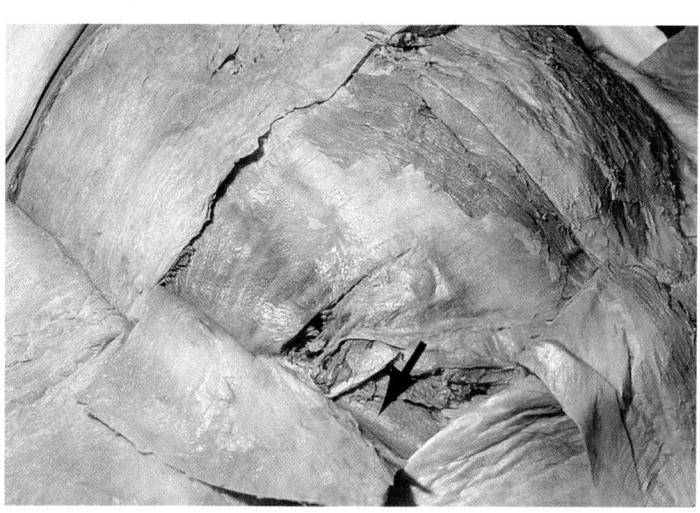

B

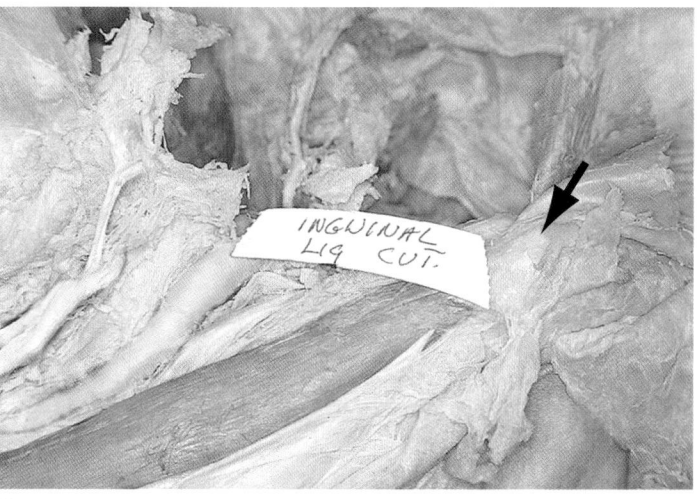

C

**FIGURE 70–6 A.** The scissors lie on the sartorius muscle. The surgeon's finger points to its origin on the anterior superior iliac spine. **B.** The upper portion of the sartorius muscle can be seen (*arrow*). Note its relationship to the muscles of the anterior abdominal wall. **C.** Close-up view of the sartorius muscle and the anterior superior iliac spine. The inguinal ligament has been excised.

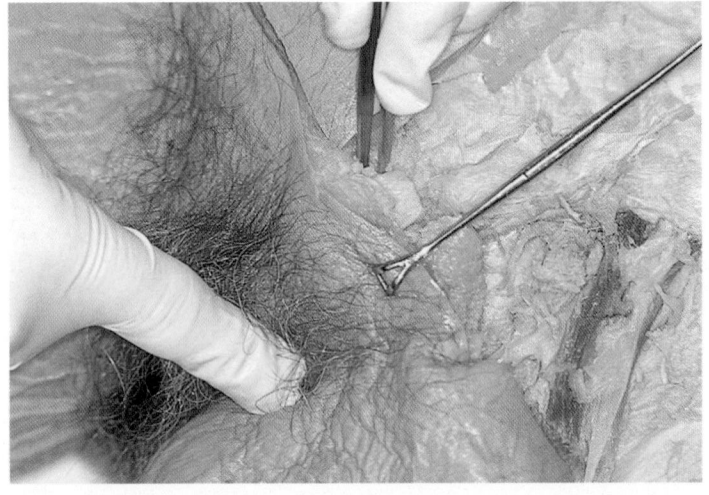

A

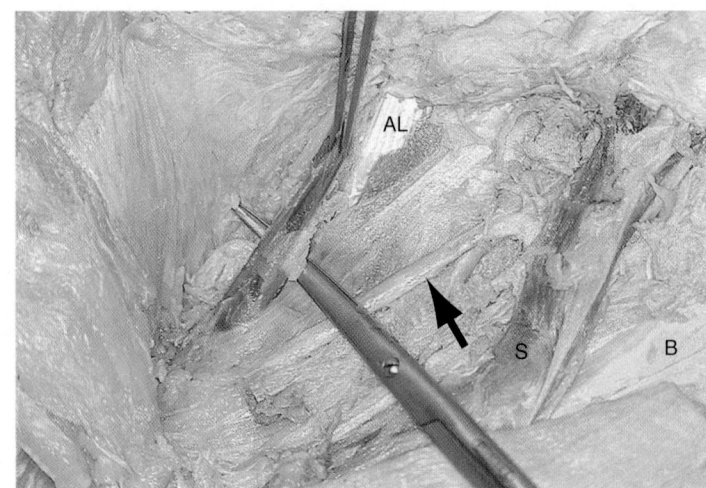

B

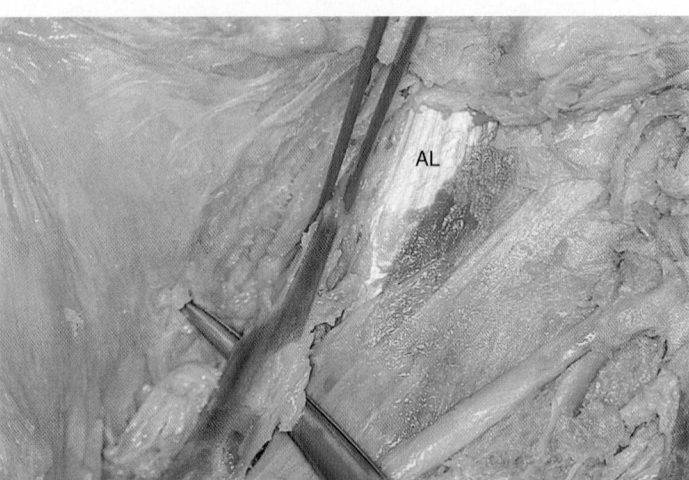

C

**FIGURE 70–7  A.** The clamp is on the cut edge of the upper margin of the mons. The finger of the surgeon points to the medial thigh and the location of the gracilis muscle. **B.** The medial thigh dissection exposes the fine, delicate gracilis muscle. Note that the blades of the scissors cross the saphenous vein. AL, adductor longus muscle; S, transplanted sartorius muscle (i.e., separated from the anterior superior iliac spine and sutured to the inguinal ligament); B, bed of the original site of the sartorius muscle; *arrow*, the saphenous vein. **C.** Magnified view of the gracilis muscle. The muscle arises from the lower portion of the symphysis pubis and pubic bone and inserts onto the medial surface of the tibia. The adductor longus muscle (AL) lies next to the gracilis muscle.

# CHAPTER 71

# Vulvectomy

*Michael S. Baggish*

## Simple Vulvectomy

Vulvectomy of any sort is not a simple operation because it destroys an important part of a woman's normal anatomy and psychologically is a significant blow to the individual's self-esteem. The vulva is an integral element of feminine sexual anatomy and physiology, and its loss seriously compromises an important day-to-day function. This operation therefore should be performed as a last resort when wide excision, laser excision, or laser vaporization cannot be performed, or when the end result of these procedures would produce a similar outcome—vulvectomy. A modification to simple vulvectomy is "skinning vulvectomy," which is a shallower excision. Logically, the need for very deep excision for intraepithelial disease is difficult to justify because the average thickness of involved mucosa (hair-bearing areas) ranges from 0.35 to 1.6 mm (mean thickness, 0.93 mm ± 0.37 mm). The depth of involved appendages ranges from 0.43 to 3.6 mm (mean depth, 1.53 mm ± 0.77 mm). Thus an excision of 2 to 3 mm will remove in excess of 95% of involved skin and appendages, predictably eradicating the disease. No justification is known for excising the vulva to a depth greater than 5 mm unless the operation is being performed for invasive carcinoma.

The patient is placed in the lithotomy position (not high lithotomy) (Fig. 71-1). After preparation, the extent of the incision should be sketched with a marking pen (Fig. 71-2). The incision is carried down from the lower mons to the lateral aspect of the labium majus with a 3-mm peripheral margin (from the lateral crease of the labium). This is continued to the lowest border of the labium majus, then across the perineum to the opposite side. The incision is brought upward on the opposite lateral margin of the labium to reach the starting point on the mons (Fig. 71-3). A vasopressin 1:100 solution is injected along the shallow cut edges of the incision. The incision then is carried into the fat to a depth of approximately 4 to 5 mm (from the surface) (Fig. 71-4A through C). If the clitoris and the labia minora are not involved, they should be preserved. Similarly, if the vestibule is not involved, it should be preserved. The defect created by excision of the labia majora and perineum is covered by a split-thickness skin graft, and a pressure dressing is applied.

If the labia minora, vestibule, and clitoris are involved in the intraepithelial neoplasia, then excision should include these structures. The depth of incision should *not* extend below Colles' fascia (Fig. 71-5). The dissection progresses from above downward and from lateral to medial (Figs. 71-6 through 71-8A). The body of the clitoris should be preserved. If the hood and glans are involved and have biopsy-proven carcinoma in situ, then the glans clitoris, the sheath, and the frenulum should be excised with the labia minora. The body of the clitoris is never exteriorized to simulate any part of the removed glans. Hemostasis is maintained by clamping off any and all bleeding vessels; this is followed by suture ligation with 3-0 Vicryl (Fig. 71-8B). Electrosurgical coagulation and dissection should be avoided in this area because it devitalizes tissue and increases the risk of necrotizing fasciitis. The dissection is carried to the vaginal margin, which is then circumscribed (Fig. 71-9). The specimen is removed (Fig. 71-10).

If primary closure can be accomplished without excessive tension on the suture line, then this type of closure is preferred; otherwise a split-thickness graft should be applied to the defect and sutured medially to the vaginal margins and laterally to the residual skin of the vulva and perineum (Fig. 71-11A through E). Care should be taken not to cause deviation of the axis of the urethra. It is obvious that the surgeon should dissect superficial to the external anal sphincter, perineal muscles, and levator ani muscles during the perineal portion of the vulvectomy. Exposure of muscle indicates that the surgeon has dissected unnecessarily too deep.

Unfortunately, these wounds cannot be practically dressed. The operative site should be covered with Silvadene cream 3 times per day and at bedtime when primary closure has been implemented. When a split-thickness graft has been applied, a pressure dressing consisting of fine-mesh gauze (Xeroform) followed by fluffed 4 × 4-inch sterile gauze pads should be applied and remain in place undisturbed for 1 week (Fig. 71-12). A Foley catheter must be inserted because voiding will be impossible (Fig. 71-13).

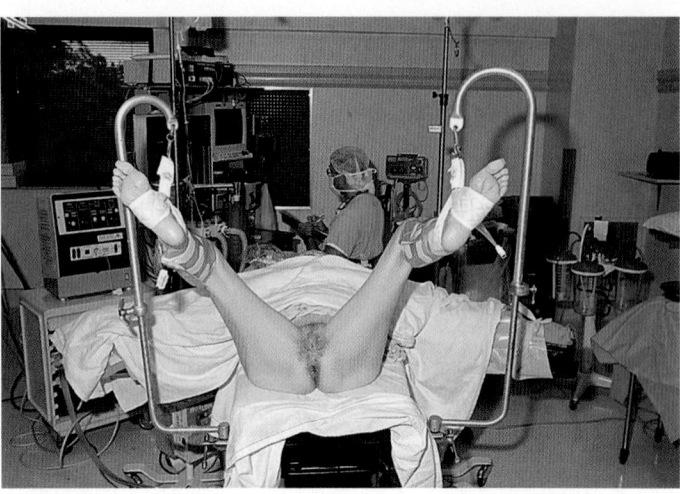

**FIGURE 71–1** The patient is placed in the lithotomy position. Pneumatic compression boots have been placed on both inferior extremities. The inferior extremities are lightly flexed and minimally abducted. Neither extremity touches the stirrups. The patient's buttocks are in firm contact with the operating table.

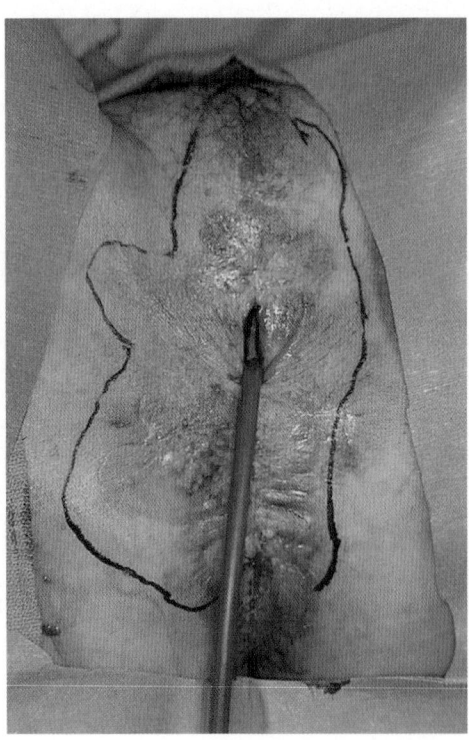

**FIGURE 71–2** The vulva is distorted from prior surgery and scar formation. The introitus is shrunken. The vulva shows the characteristic red appearance of Paget's disease. This diagnosis has been made by preoperative biopsies. A sterile marking pen has traced the outline of the intended excision.

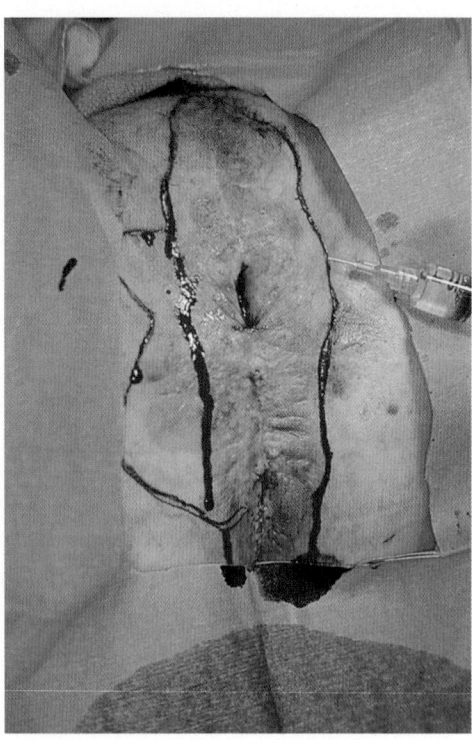

**FIGURE 71–3** Light scalpel pressure follows the trace pen lines to again outline the boundaries for excision. A 1:100 vasopressin solution is injected subdermally.

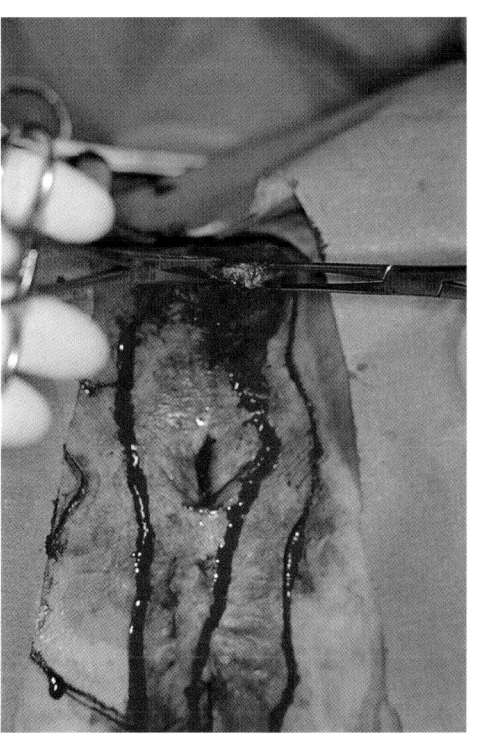
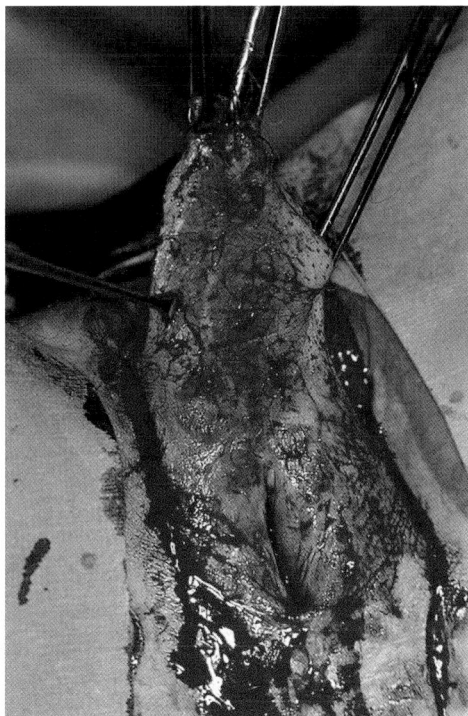
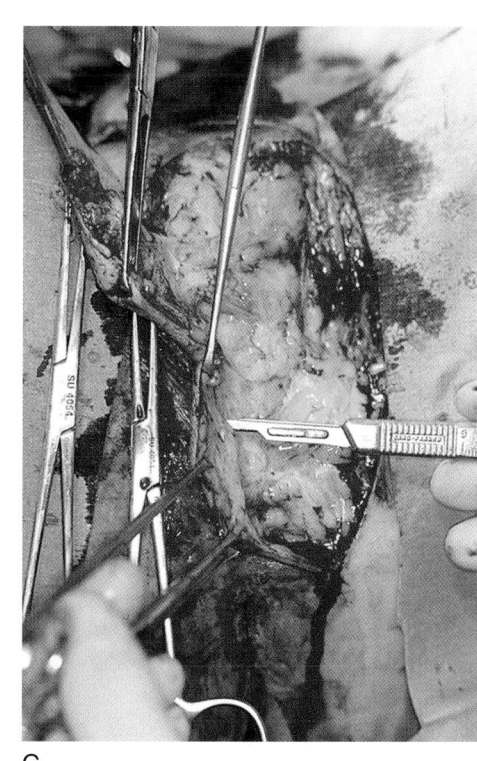

A                              B                              C

**FIGURE 71-4  A.** The scalpel cuts deeply at the 12-o'clock location into the subcutaneous fat. The edges of the specimen margins are grasped with Allis clamps, and the tissue is pulled outward and slightly inferiorly to create traction. **B.** The flap is rapidly developed. Hemostasis is maintained by applying mosquito clamps to any bleeding vessel. The margins of the excision are continuously checked. **C.** The depth of the excisional tissue plane is approximately 4 to 5 mm. Traction and countertraction are exceedingly important to ensure uniform thickness of the tissue that is to be removed.

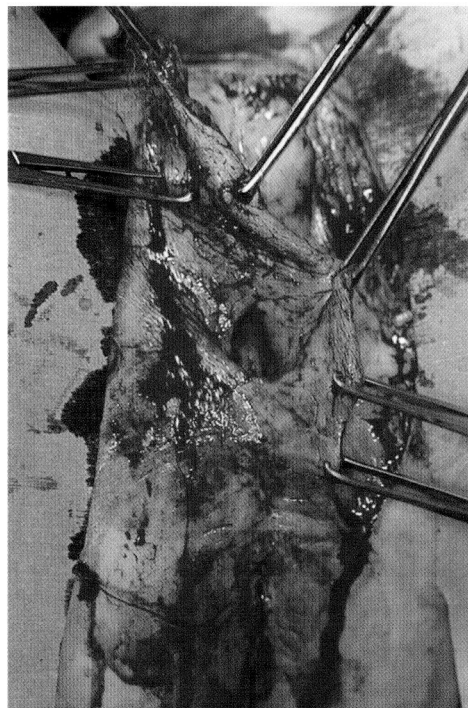
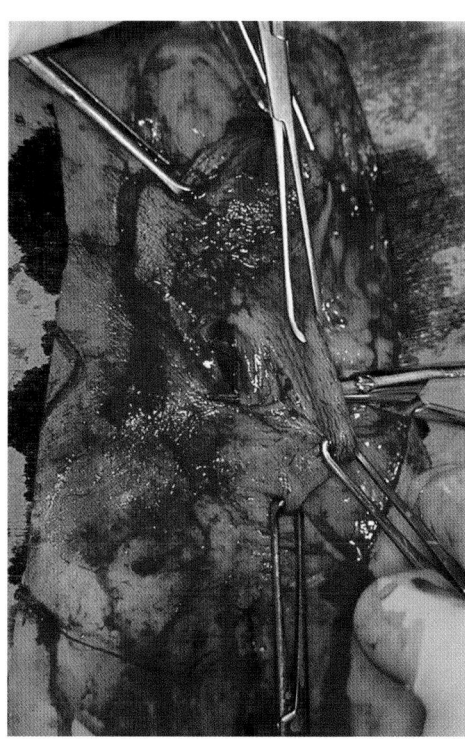

**FIGURE 71-5** The entire upper half of the vulva has been separated from the underlying connective tissue.

**FIGURE 71-6** An incision is made circumferentially around the lower vagina. The vestibule is cut away together with a 5-mm margin of lower vagina.

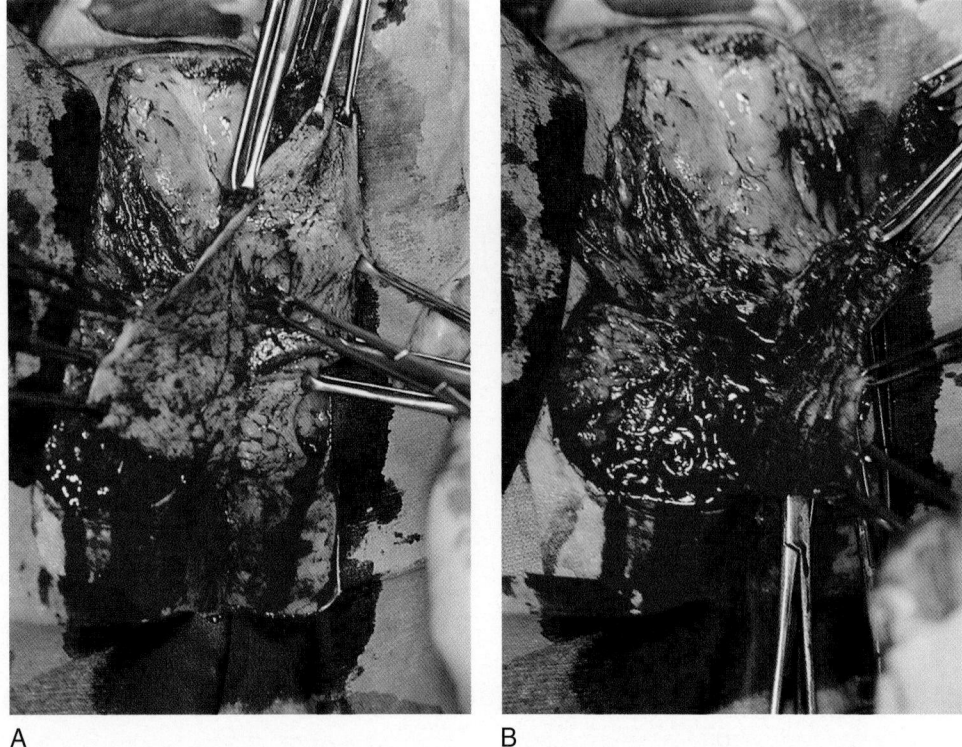

A    B

**FIGURE 71–7  A.** The lower right side of the vulva is dissected to the level of the anal verge. **B.** The lower left side of the vulva is dissected to the level of the anus.

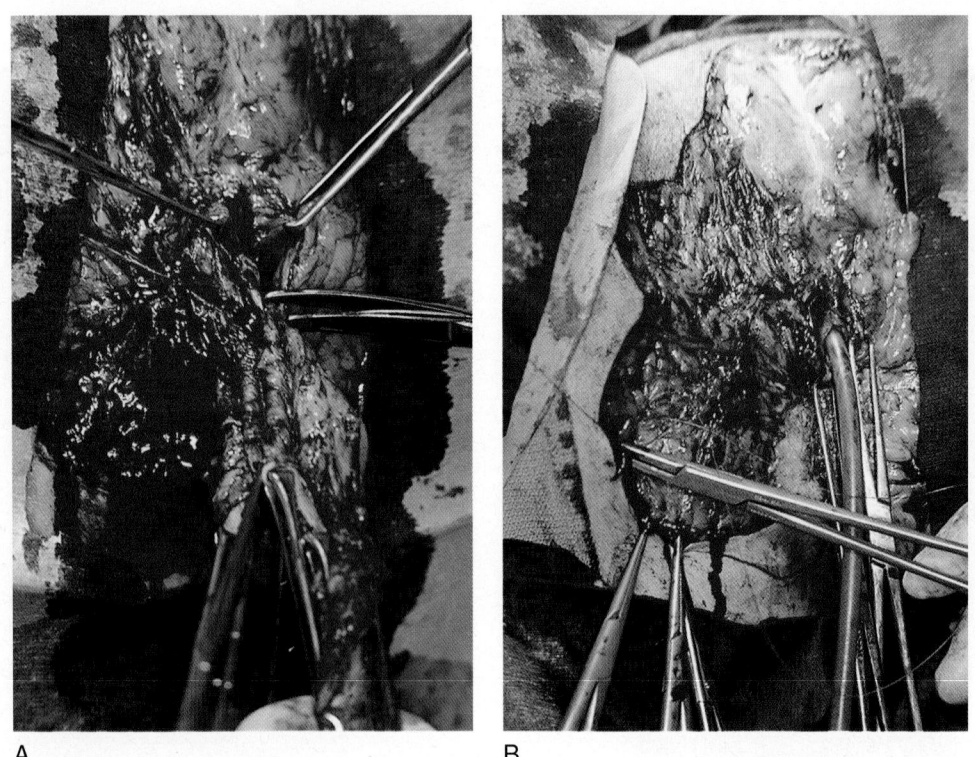

A    B

**FIGURE 71–8  A.** The last connections of the vagina to the vulva are cut. **B.** The specimen has been removed. Bleeding sites are sutured (figure-of-8 suture) with 3-0 Vicryl.

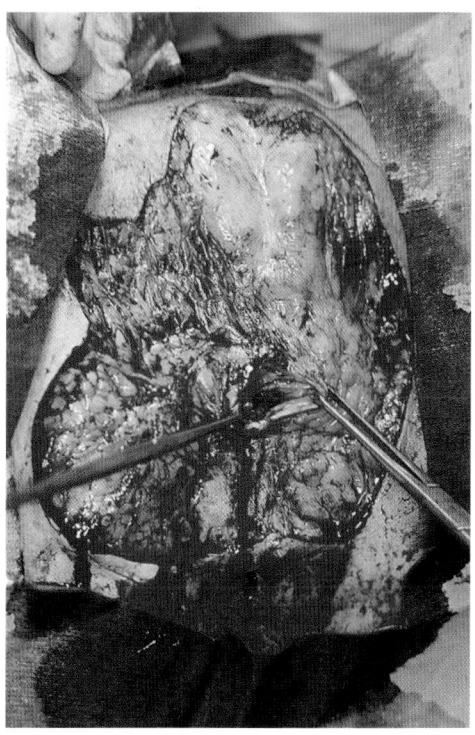

**FIGURE 71–9** The vagina is grasped with Allis clamps, and the margins are closely evaluated for adequacy.

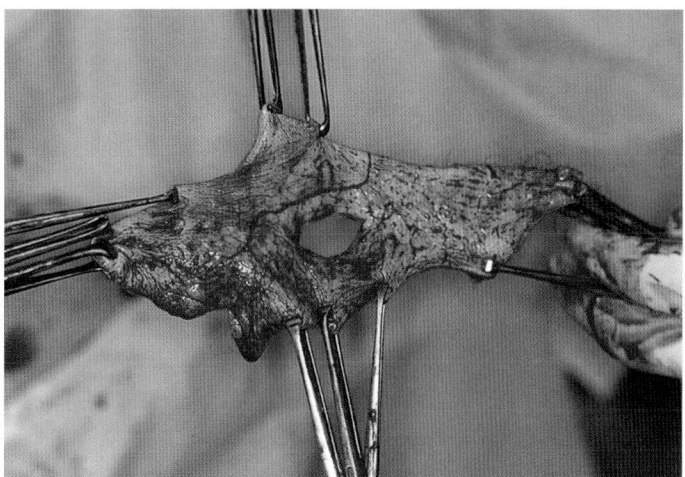

**FIGURE 71–10** The specimen is oriented and sent to pathology. The author prefers to wrap the specimen in a saline-soaked sponge and transport it immediately to the gross pathology laboratory.

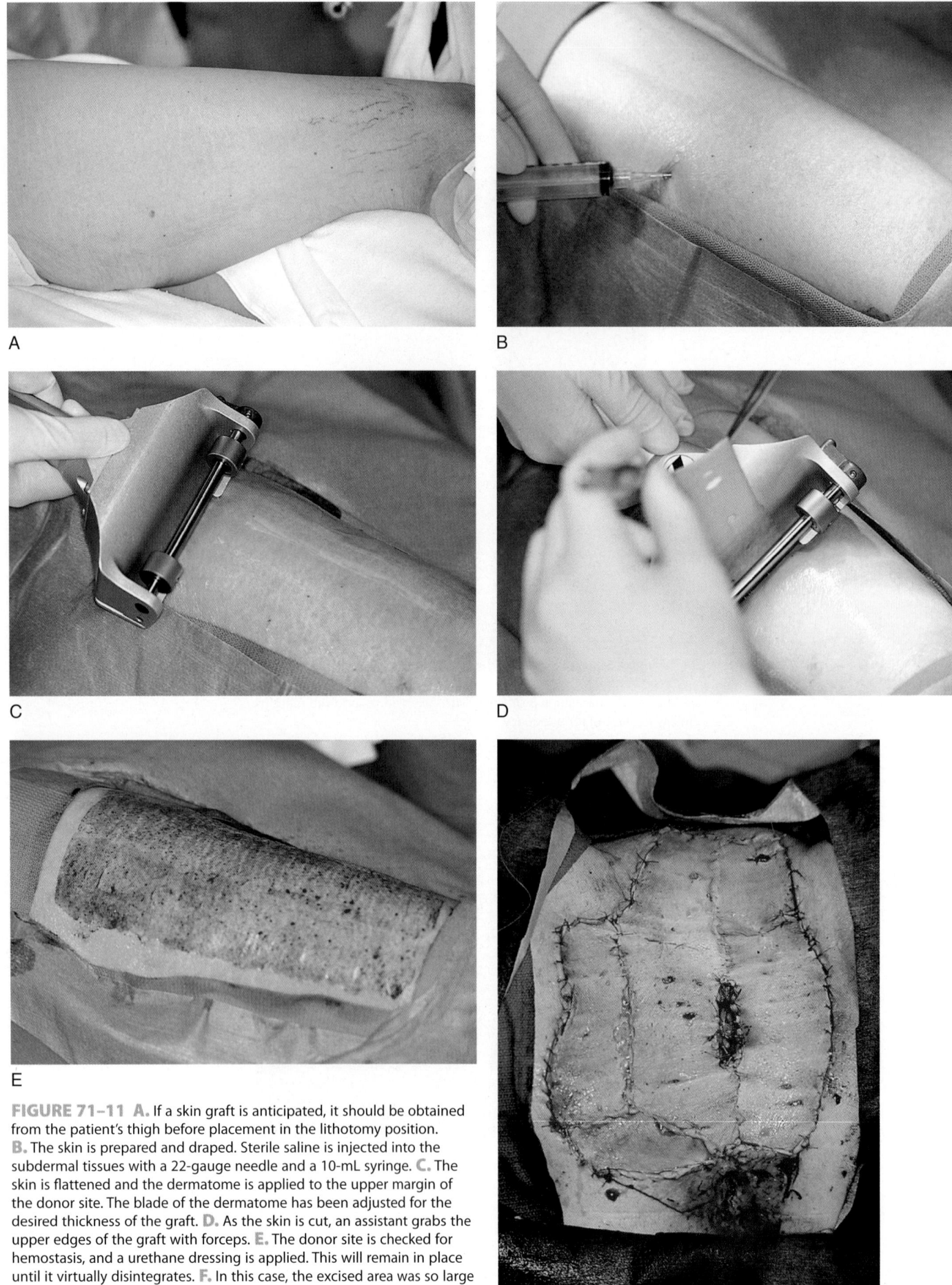

**FIGURE 71–11  A.** If a skin graft is anticipated, it should be obtained from the patient's thigh before placement in the lithotomy position. **B.** The skin is prepared and draped. Sterile saline is injected into the subdermal tissues with a 22-gauge needle and a 10-mL syringe. **C.** The skin is flattened and the dermatome is applied to the upper margin of the donor site. The blade of the dermatome has been adjusted for the desired thickness of the graft. **D.** As the skin is cut, an assistant grabs the upper edges of the graft with forceps. **E.** The donor site is checked for hemostasis, and a urethane dressing is applied. This will remain in place until it virtually disintegrates. **F.** In this case, the excised area was so large that four pieces of skin graft sutured together with 3-0 and 4-0 Vicryl were needed to cover the wound defect. The edges of the graft were sutured to vaginal, perineal, and anal margins.

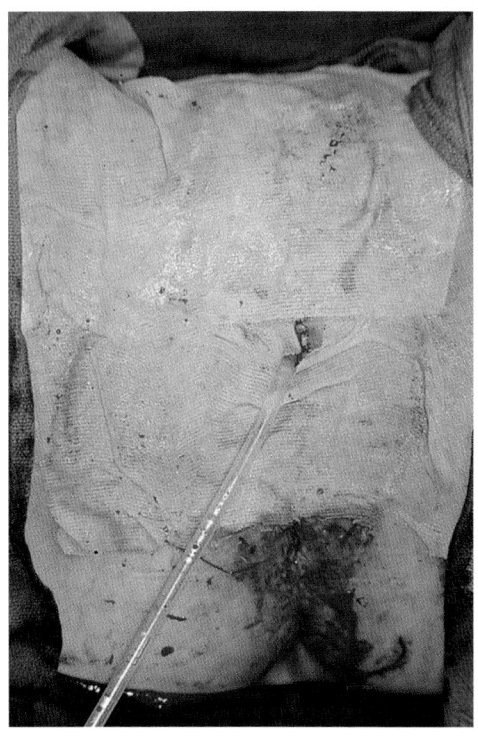

**FIGURE 71–12** A Foley catheter has been placed in the urinary bladder. Fine-mesh Xeroform gauze is applied directly to the grafted skin.

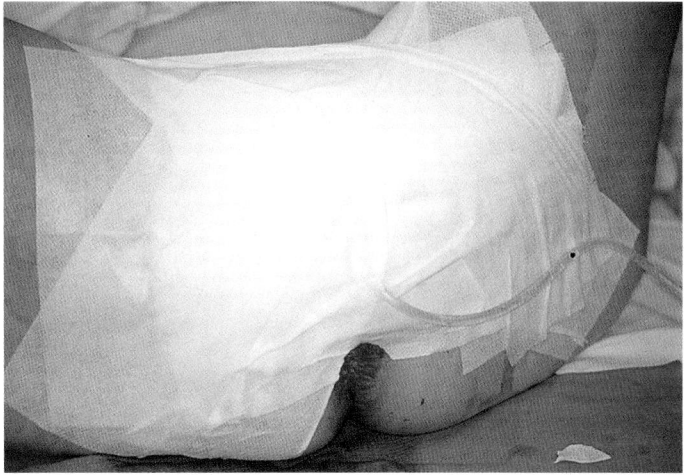

**FIGURE 71–13** A uniform pressure dressing consisting of fluffed 4 × 4-inch gauze pads and Corlex is taped into place. This will remain in place for at least 1 week.

## Radical Vulvectomy

Radical vulvectomy, which is usually combined with bilateral groin dissections (lymphadenectomy), is performed for the treatment of invasive cancer of the vulva (Fig. 71–14A through C). The principles of this operation are to deeply resect the tumor with wide peripheral margins and to extend the zone of resection to the vaginal and anal mucosa. This is coupled with an en bloc resection of the superficial inguinal and deep femoral lymph nodes. For large tumors, the iliac lymph nodes are also removed.

The patient is placed in Allen leg and foot supports in a position similar to that used for operative laparoscopy (Fig. 71–15). The inferior extremities are placed in compression boots. The

patient is given a prophylactic antibiotic 1 hour before surgery. With a marking pen, the margins of resection are traced (Fig. 71–16A, B). The incisions are cut transversely across the lower abdomen just above the symphysis and curving upward to the anterior superior iliac spine (i.e., parallel to the inguinal ligament) (Fig. 71–16C). Then the incision is carried downward and medially on the thigh side of the inguinal ligament and over the femoral triangle to the mons veneris (Fig. 71–17A). The incision is continued in a fashion identical to that described for simple vulvectomy (i.e., arcing peripherally around the lateral margin of the labia majora, perineum, and perianal skin). The inner margin of the cut is made into the vestibule at the hymenal ring (Fig. 71–17B).

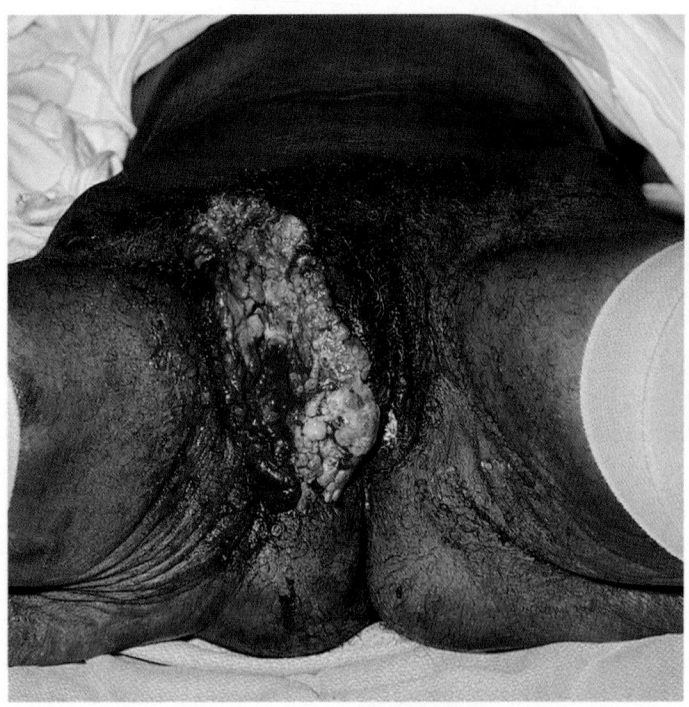

A

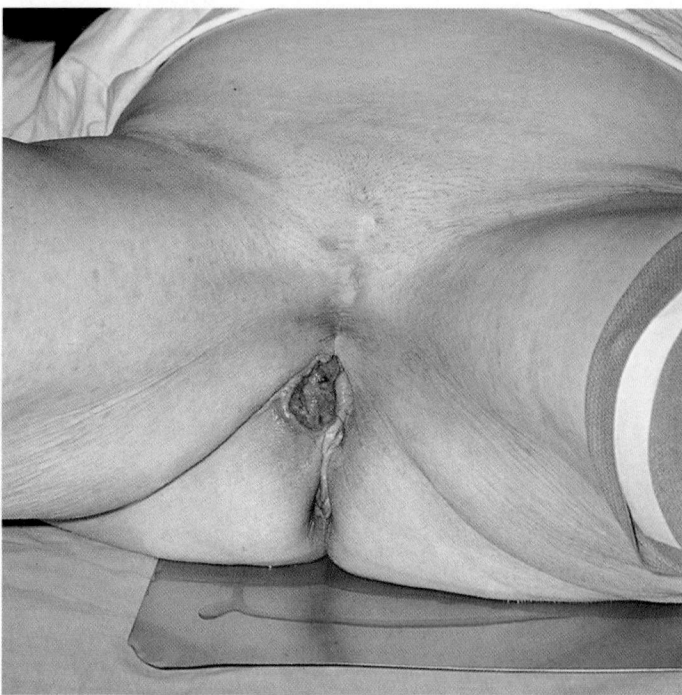

B

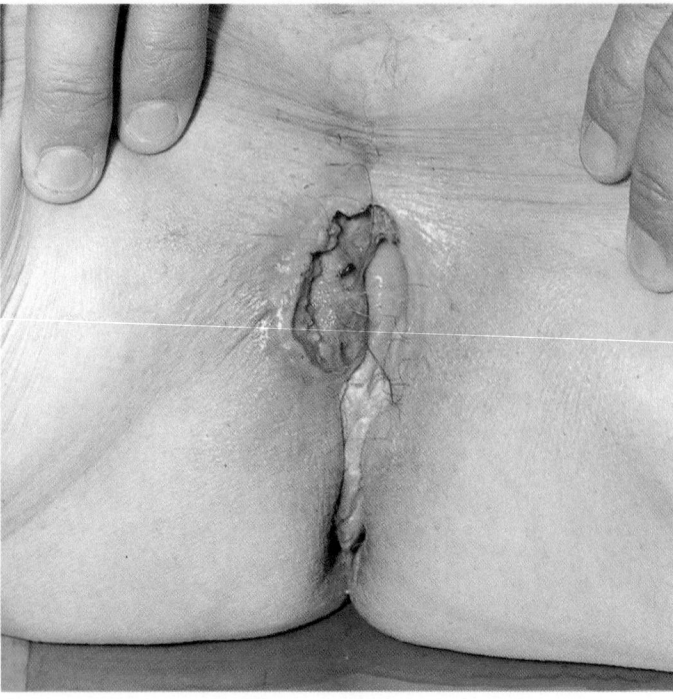

C

FIGURE 71–14 A. The large fungating mass destroyed the entire right labium majus and extended laterally to the crura (thigh) and inferiorly into the ischiorectal fossa. A biopsy of the lesion confirmed the diagnosis of invasive squamous cell carcinoma. B. Although less impressive than the cancer shown in Figure 71–14A, nevertheless this is a rather large malignancy involving the right side of the vulva and the clitoris. In this case, the entire clitoris must be removed. C. A magnified view of Figure 71–14B reveals that this lesion extended across the midline to involve the left side of the vulva as well as the right side.

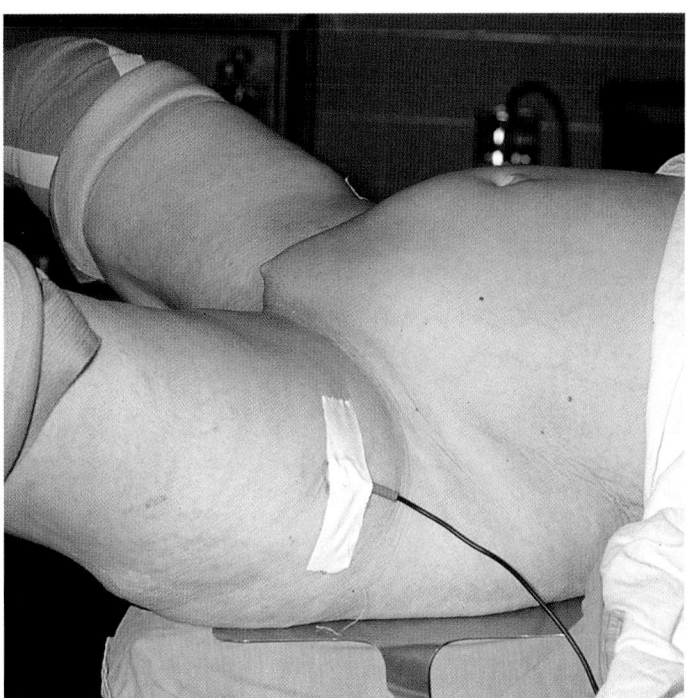

**FIGURE 71–15** The patient is positioned for a combined abdominal and perineal approach. Her inferior extremities are placed in Allen stirrups, and compression hose are applied to the legs.

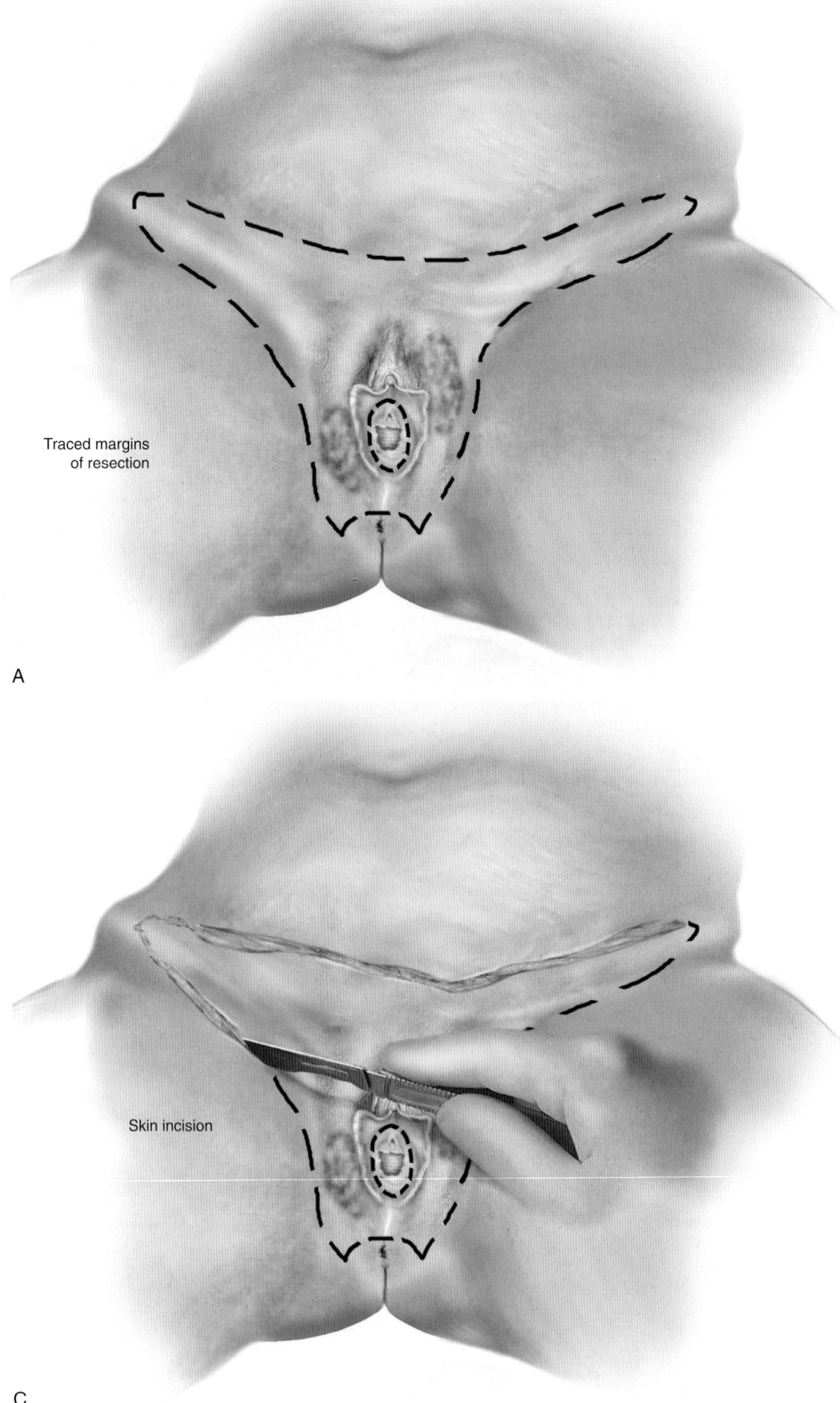

A

Traced margins
of resection

Skin incision

C

**FIGURE 71–16 A.** The extent of the dissection is traced with a sterile marking pen. **C.** A knife cut is made through the skin into the fat while following the tracing that was made previously. Flaps will be developed in the groin as the dissection progresses.

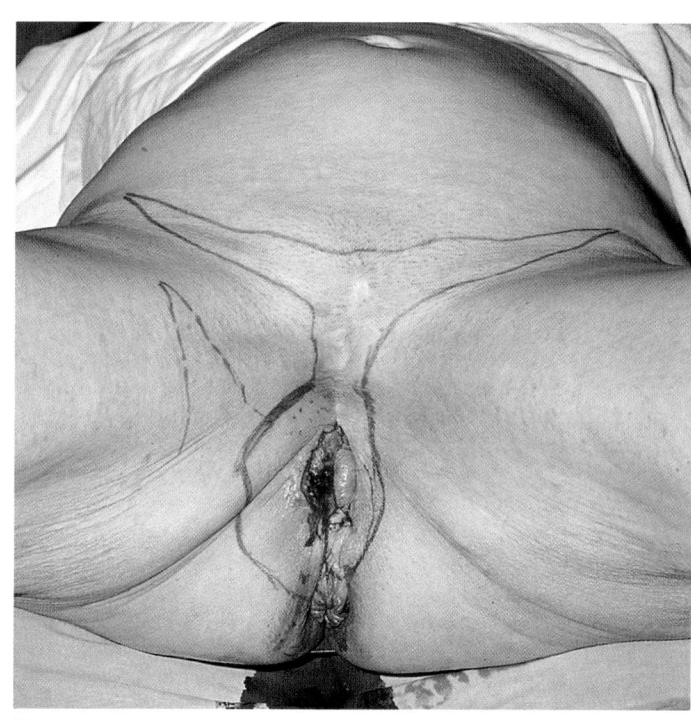

**FIGURE 71–16, cont'd   B.** The tracing encompasses incisions over the inguinal ligaments to the anterior superior iliac spine and circumscribes the vulva with generous margins, particularly around the gross lesion.

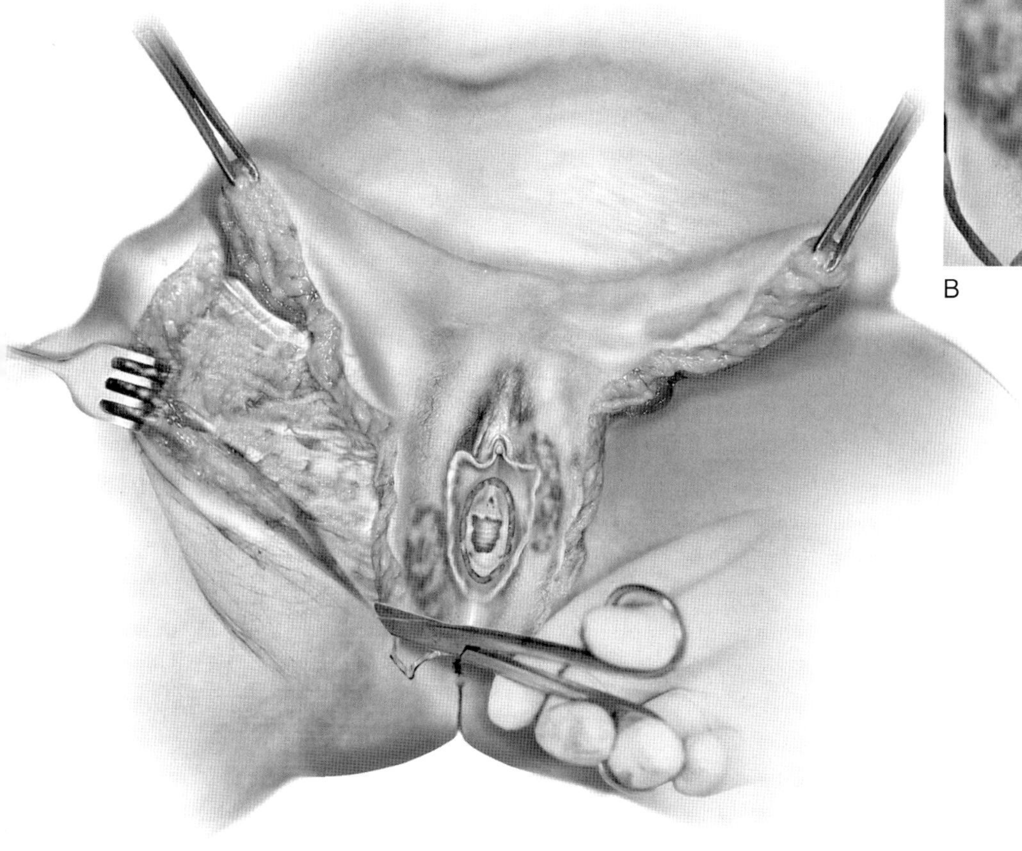

B

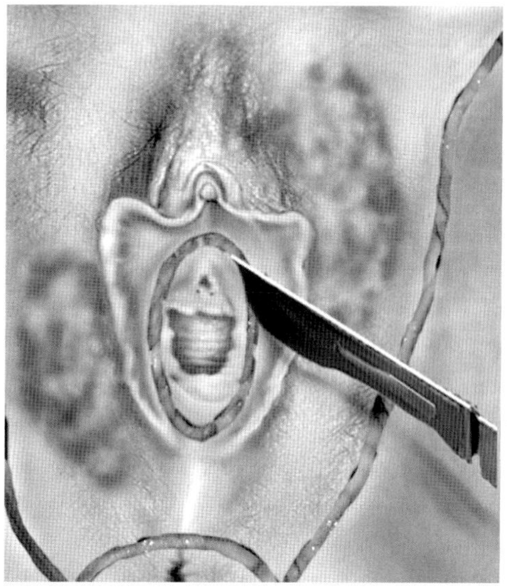

Inner margin
trace incision

B

A

**FIGURE 71–17 A.** The groin fat is excised from lateral to medial. The saphenous vein is located and traced cranially to the cribriform fascia and fossa ovalis. The femoral vein is located, and all nodal tissue overlying and between the femoral vessels is excised. **B.** At a convenient time, the margin of separation between the vulva and the vestibule or between the vulva and the vagina is gently marked with a shallow scalpel cut.

The deeper dissection is initiated at the level of the abdomen and is continued over the femoral triangle. The fatty tissue containing the superficial nodes is swept downward, clearing the fat from the investment fascia covering the rectus and external oblique muscles and exposing the inguinal ligaments (Fig. 71-18). The sartorius fascia (fascia lata) and muscle are exposed, and the node-bearing tissue is dissected downward (caudally) to the depth of the underlying fascia lata (Fig. 71-19A). The node dissection proceeds medially toward the saphenous vein. In turn, the femoral nerve, femoral artery, and upper saphenous vein are dissected free of fat, lymph nodes, and connective tissue (see Fig. 71-22). The cribriform fascia covering the fossa ovale has been exposed and dissected away. The saphenous vein is divided above its junction with the femoral vein (Fig. 71-19B). The vein again is ligated at the lower portion (apex) of the femoral triangle because a segment of this vein is included with the lymph node and fat specimens. The small branches of the femoral artery and the tributaries of the femoral vein have been clamped, cut, and suture-ligated with 3-0 Vicryl as they are encountered. If deep pelvic node dissection is to be performed, it is done at this point by excising over the inguinal ligament, locating the iliac vessels, and carrying out the dissection as described previously for radical hysterectomy (see Chapter 12) (Fig. 71-20A, B). When this has been completed, the incision above the inguinal ligament (at the level of the aponeurosis of the external oblique muscles) is closed with 0 Vicryl sutures (Fig. 71-21). Whether or not deep node dissection is carried out, the lowest external iliac node should be extricated and sampled. This is Cloquet's node (Fig. 71-22).

The femoral vessels are now completely exposed (Fig. 71-23). It is worthwhile to transplant the sartorius muscle to cover these vessels and provide a modicum of protection for them (Fig. 71-24A). The muscle is easily separated via curved Mayo scissors from its origin on the anterior superior iliac spine. Next, the muscle is freed from its bed for a distance of 2 or 3 inches and is swung medially to cover the femoral vessels (Fig. 71-24B through D). The free end of the sartorius muscle is sutured onto the inguinal ligament with 0 Vicryl or polydioxanone (PDS) sutures (Figs. 71-24E, F and 71-20A).

Attention is directed to excising the vulva proper (see Figs. 71-20 and 71-25). The incision at the superior portion of the mons is extended on the right and left sides. The mons fat, including the suspensory ligament of the clitoris, is dissected free and cut away from the symphysis pubis (see Fig. 71-20B). Care is taken not to injure the urethra, the clitoral crus, or the bulb of the vestibule. The deep plane of this vulvar dissection is carried out above the tough membrane covering the corpora cavernosa, the bulb, the levator fascia, and the clitoral body (see Fig. 71-25). The dissection will remove the bulbocavernosus, ischiocavernosus, and transverse perineal muscles, as well as Colles' fascia (Fig. 71-26A through C). A small portion of the clitoral body and the glans clitoris will be removed. The urethra and the lower vagina are left intact. Thus, the medial incision is made circumferentially around the vaginal outlet above the urethra and between the urethra and glans clitoris (see Figs. 71-25 and 71-27).

The final dissection is made to separate the vulva from the retained vestibule or vagina (see Fig. 71-25). The perineum is dissected with the specimen, but the anal sphincter and levator ani muscles are not disturbed. During this portion of the dissection, the pudendal vessels are secured and cut. These vessels are suture-ligated with 3-0 Vicryl sutures after adequate hemostasis has been obtained. The wound is now ready to be closed. The specimen is oriented and soaked in saline sponges and then is sent intact to pathology (Fig. 71-28). Closure is made per primum if possible but never under excessive tension. Tension closures result in wound separation and tend to then heal by granulation (i.e., secondary intention). This delayed healing is not optimal and results in prolonged hospitalization (Fig. 71-29).

The abdominal wall may be mobilized by bluntly dissecting along Scarpa's fascial plane up to the navel and pulling downward on the anterior abdominal wall (Fig. 71-30). If the vulvar wound cannot be closed adequately, a skin graft should be applied. Jackson-Pratt drains are placed under the groin flaps, anchored to the skin with 3-0 Vicryl, and attached to suction bags (Fig. 71-31). The subcutaneous tissue is sutured with 3-0 Vicryl interrupted sutures and is approximated above the drains. The skin is closed with 3-0 nylon or PDS interrupted sutures. The vestibule is sutured to the remaining perineal skin with interrupted 3-0 Vicryl sutures. The inferior extremities should be kept elevated to enhance lymphatic drainage (wrapped in elastic bandages or pressure stockings) during the postoperative course. If a graft is required, a pressure dressing should be placed. The Foley catheter is attached to a drainage bag to monitor urine output.

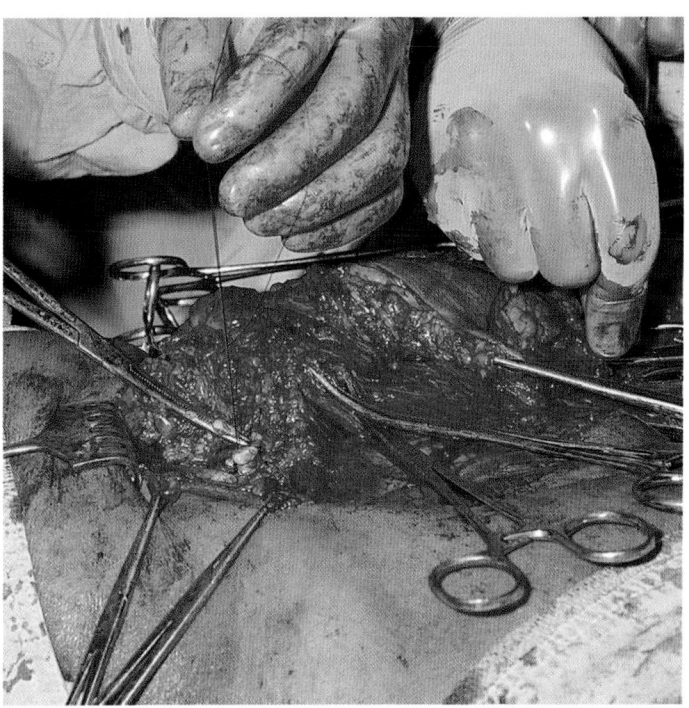

FIGURE 71–18 The superficial and deep nodes are dissected and swept inferiorly and medially. Small branches and tributaries of the femoral vessels are clamped with tonsil clamps and are suture-ligated with 3-0 Vicryl.

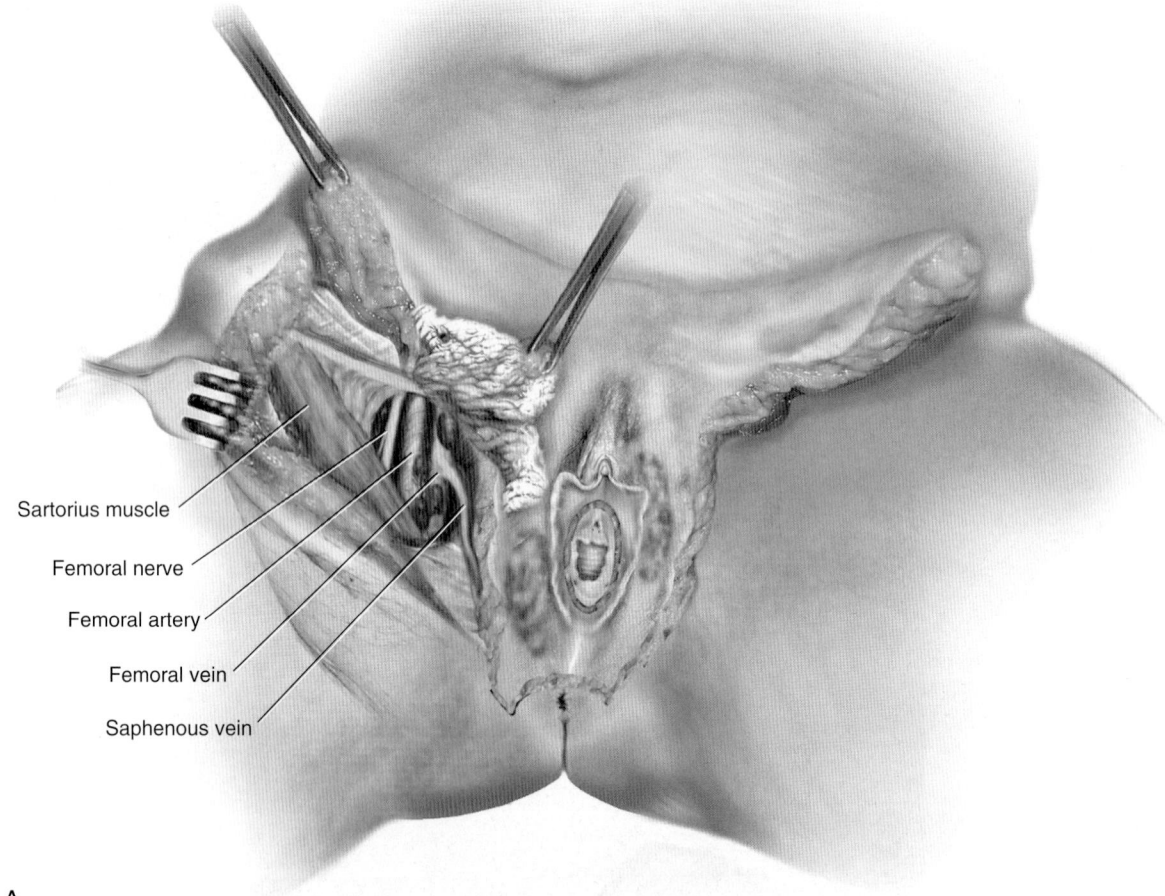

Sartorius muscle

Femoral nerve

Femoral artery

Femoral vein

Saphenous vein

A

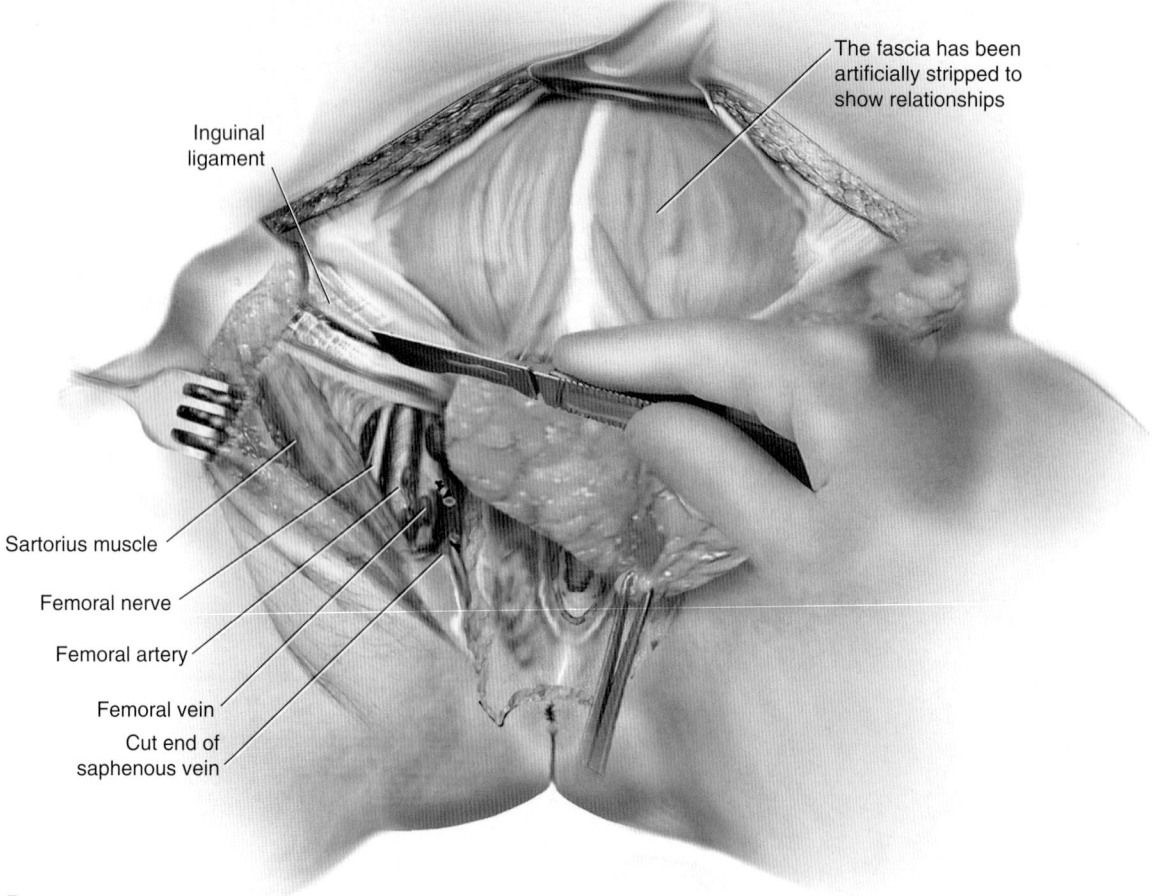

Inguinal
ligament

The fascia has been
artificially stripped to
show relationships

Sartorius muscle

Femoral nerve

Femoral artery

Femoral vein

Cut end of
saphenous vein

B

**FIGURE 71–19  A.** The sartorius muscle, femoral nerve, femoral artery, and femoral vein are cleared. The tough fascial sheaths are excised. **B.** The saphenous vein is clamped above the lower portion of the femoral triangle. It is excised with the fat to the point where it flows into the femoral vein. At this location it is clamped, double suture-ligated with 3-0 Vicryl, and cut.

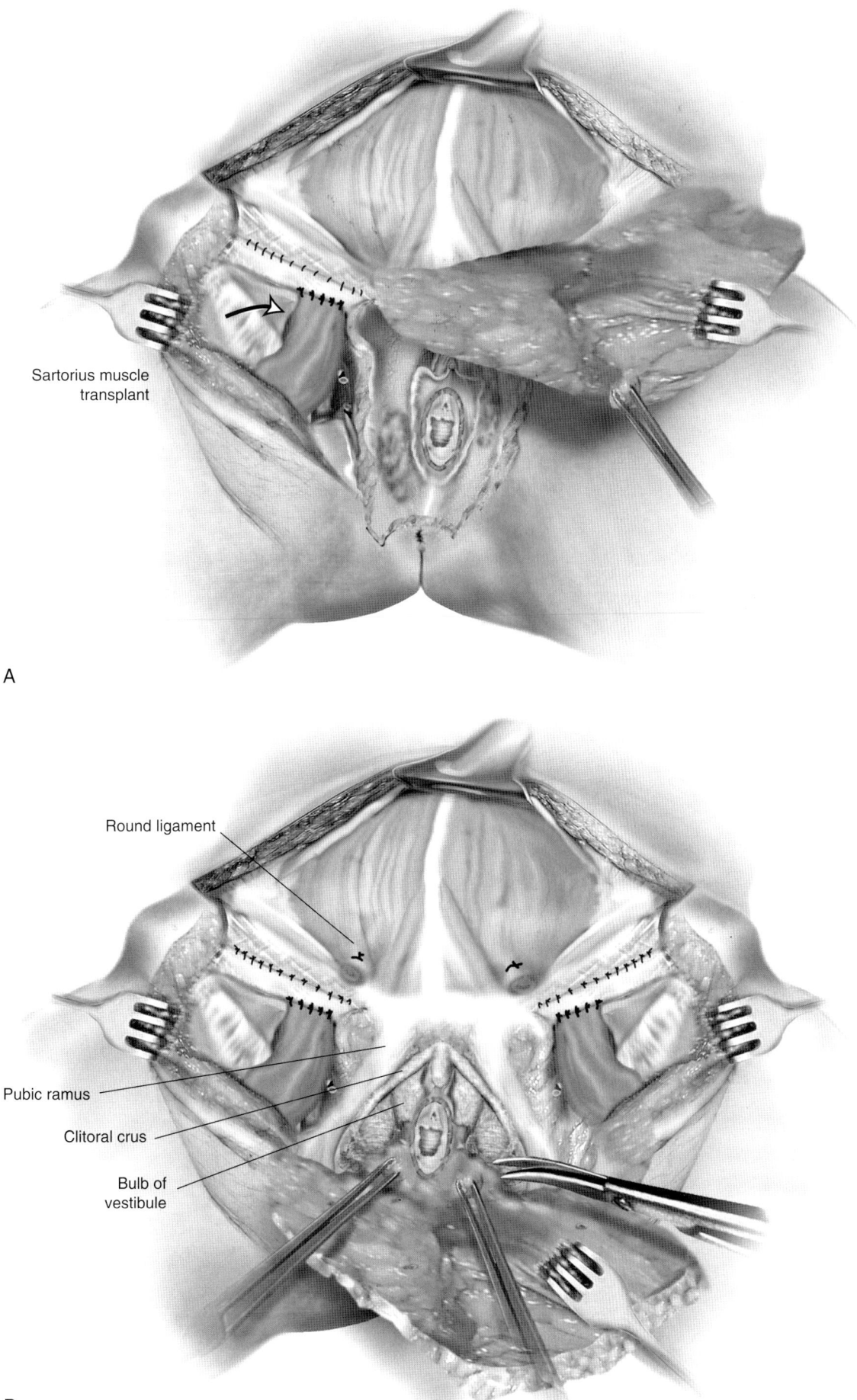

A

Sartorius muscle
transplant

B

Round ligament

Pubic ramus

Clitoral crus

Bulb of
vestibule

FIGURE 71–20  A. If a pelvic node dissection is to be performed, the aponeurosis of the external oblique is incised along the inguinal ligament. The external iliac vessels are located, and a lymphadenectomy is performed. B. The inguinal ligaments have been sutured. The sartorius muscles have been transplanted. Colles' fascia has been excised, exposing the tough membranes covering the "blood lake" (corpora cavernosa, clitoral body, and bulb of the vestibule). The vulva is in the process of being separated from the vestibular remnant.

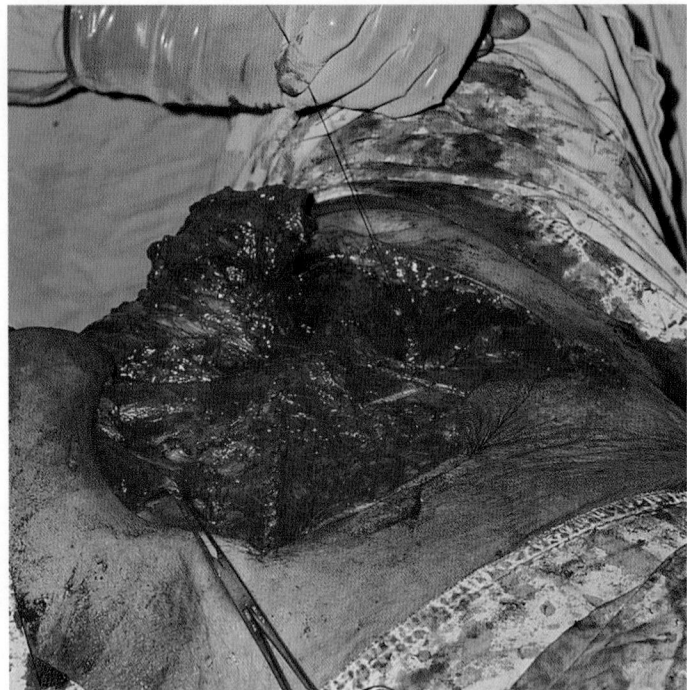

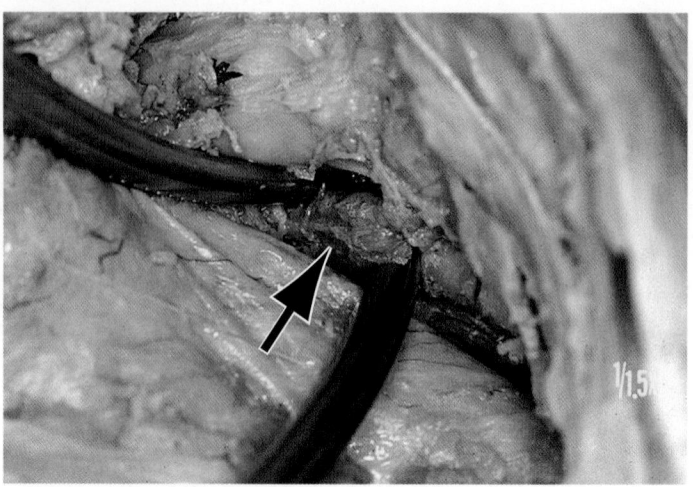

**FIGURE 71-22** Cloquet's node is seen at the *arrow*. The clamp is at the lower pole of the node. This would correspond to the upper part of the femoral canal. The scissors are under the femoral vein (bluish tint).

**FIGURE 71-21** The sartorius muscle is grasped with an Allis clamp. The deep node dissection is complete, and the inguinal ligament has been sutured.

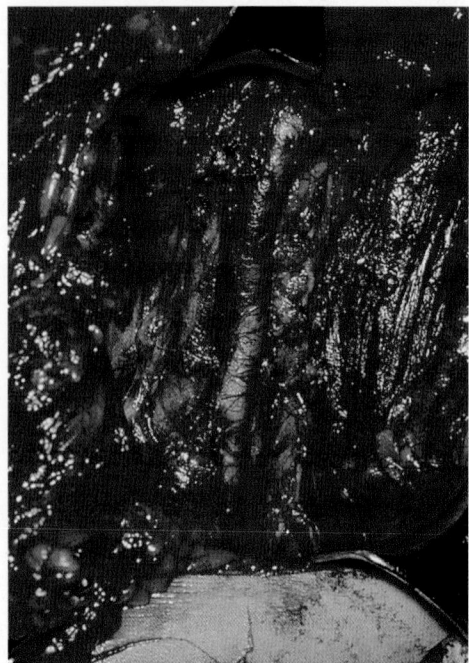

**FIGURE 71-23** The dissected femoral vessels devoid of fat and fascia are exposed and at risk for injury. The sartorius muscle is located to the right in this photo.

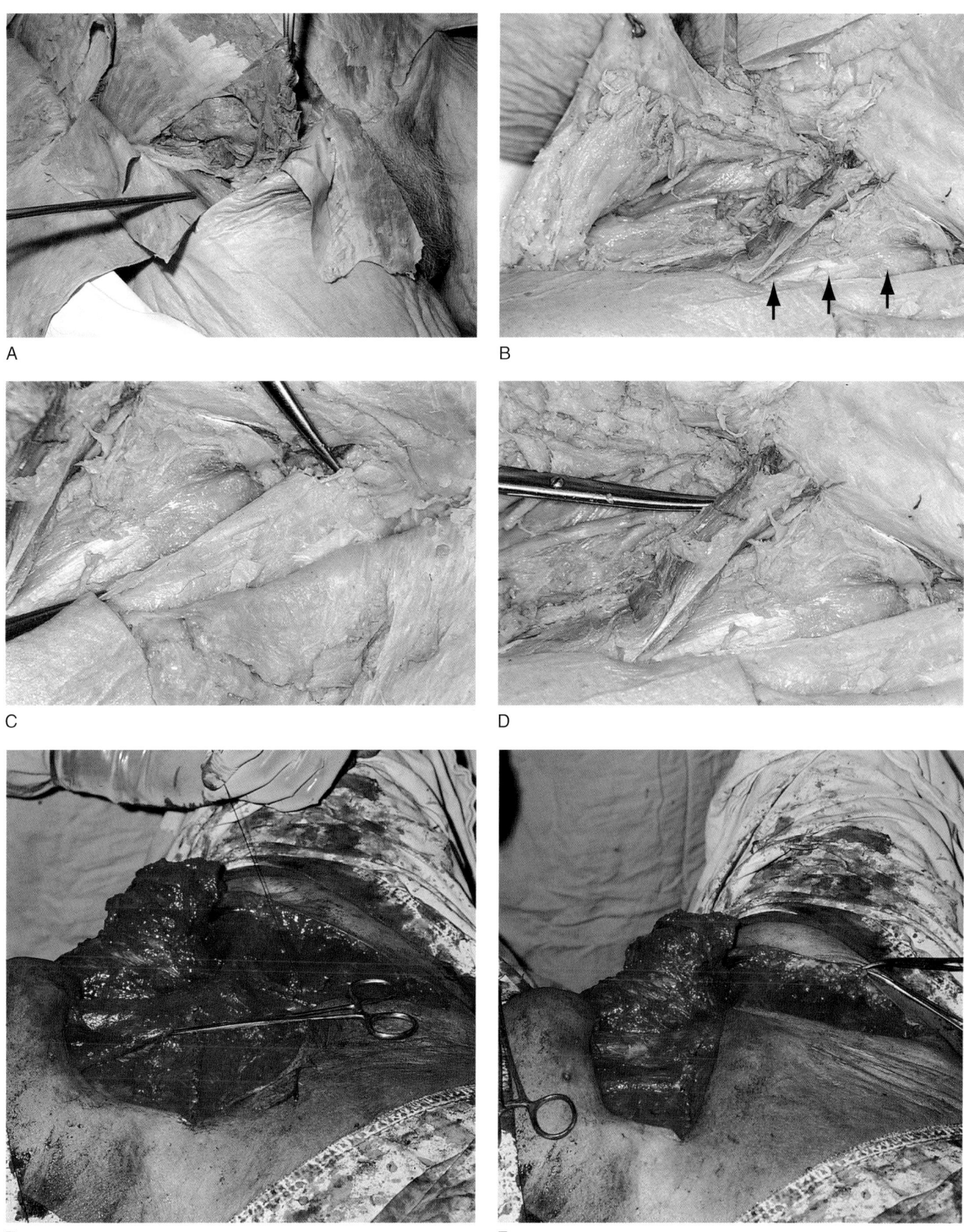

A

B

C

D

E

F

**FIGURE 71-24 A.** The instrument points to the sartorius muscle. The inguinal ligament is above it, coursing obliquely toward the pubic bone. **B.** The bed of the sartorius muscle is indicated by the arrows. The muscle has been detached from the anterior superior iliac spine and transposed to cover the femoral vessels. **C.** The original location of the sartorius muscle lies between the two instruments. The scissors (*upper*) point to where the muscle was cut free from its insertion on the anterior superior iliac spine. **D.** Magnified detail of the sartorius transposition to cover the femoral vessels. The cut end of the muscle will be sutured to the inguinal ligament. **E.** The sartorius muscle has been freed from its bed and insertion into the iliac spine. It has been moved medially and is held in the clamp. **F.** The sartorius muscle has been sutured to the inguinal ligament.

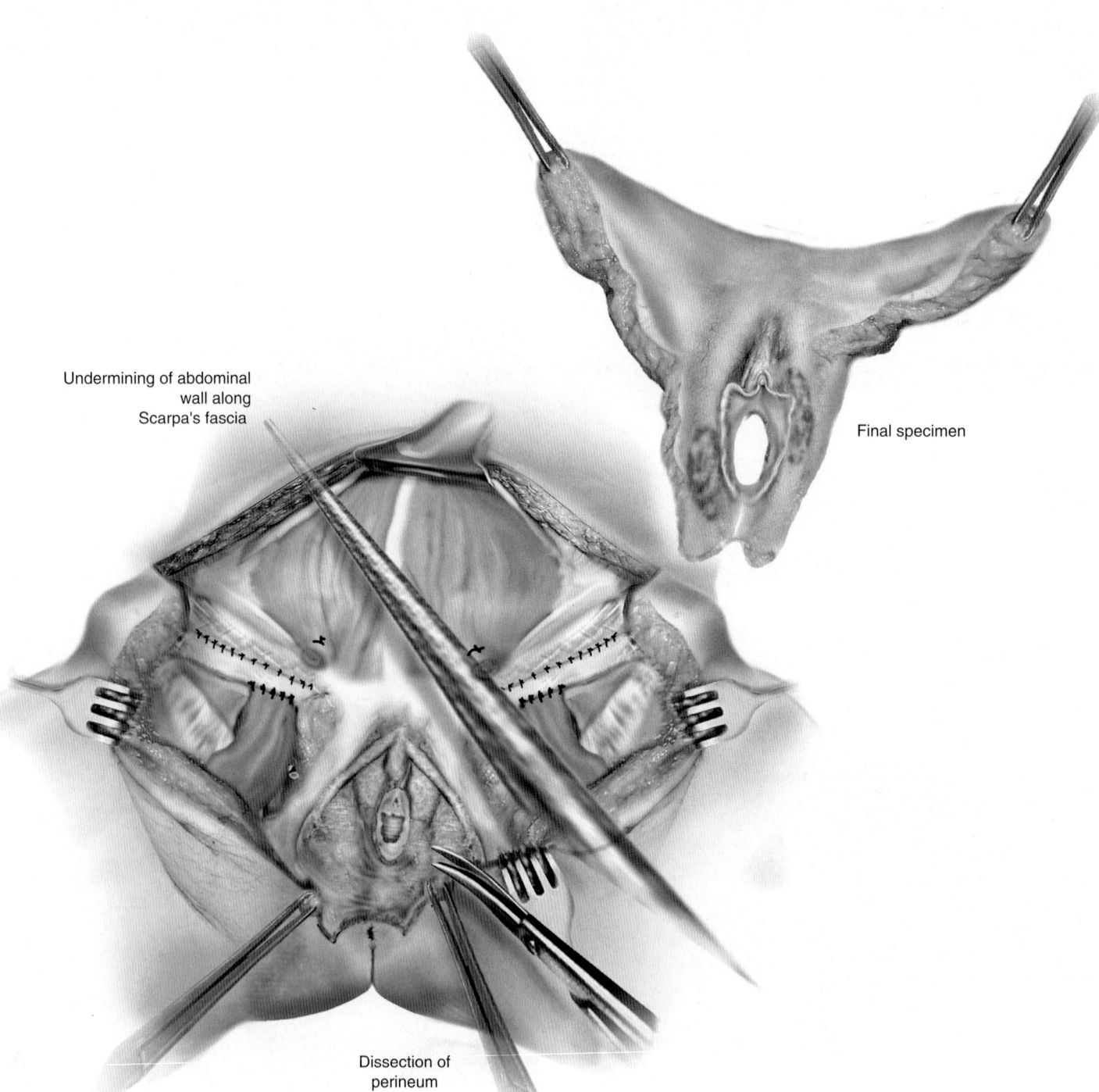

Undermining of abdominal
wall along
Scarpa's fascia

Final specimen

Dissection of
perineum

**FIGURE 71–25** The specimen has been excised. To facilitate skin closure, the abdominal wall is undermined over Scarpa's fascia. The abdominal wall can then be mobilized to approximate the cut groin and vulvar skin margins.

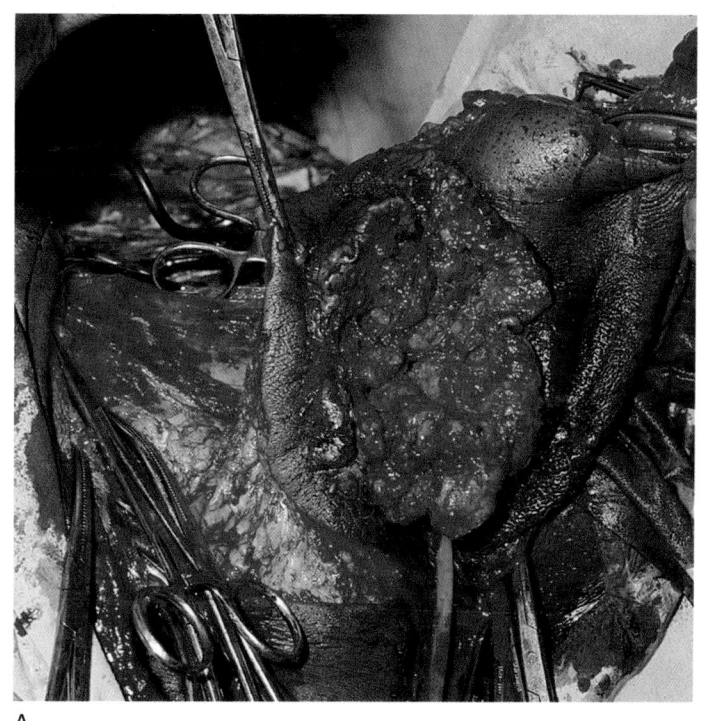

A

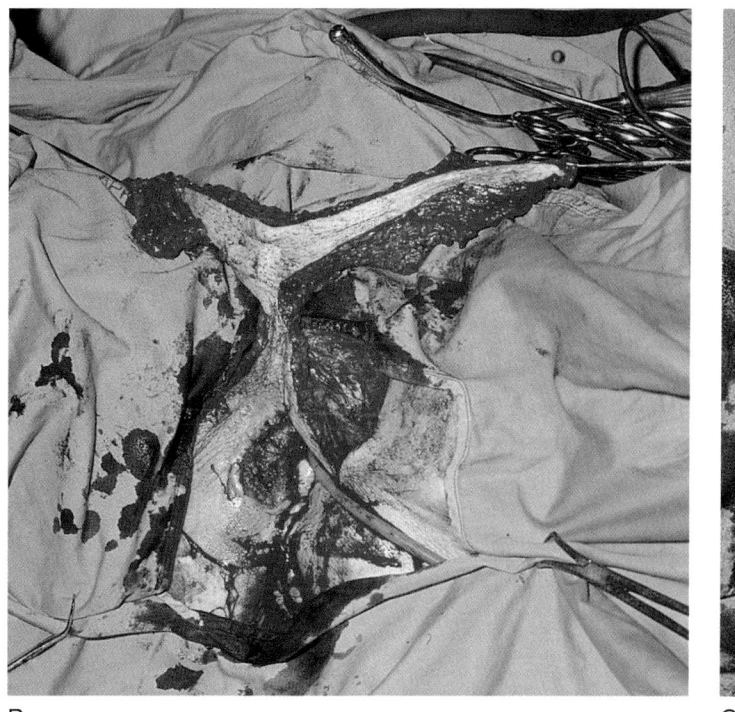

B

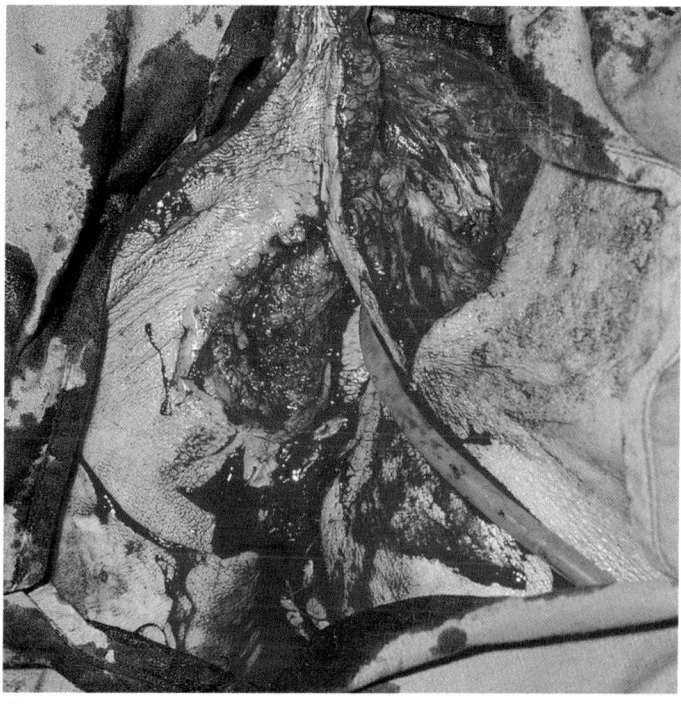

C

**FIGURE 71–26** **A.** This details the final steps in separating the vulva from its underlying attachments and cutting the vestibule (or vagina) free. **B.** The specimen is held up for orientation. The vulva must be freed from the perineal skin and connective tissue. **C.** This details the final stages of the vulvectomy. The vulva has been separated superiorly and laterally.

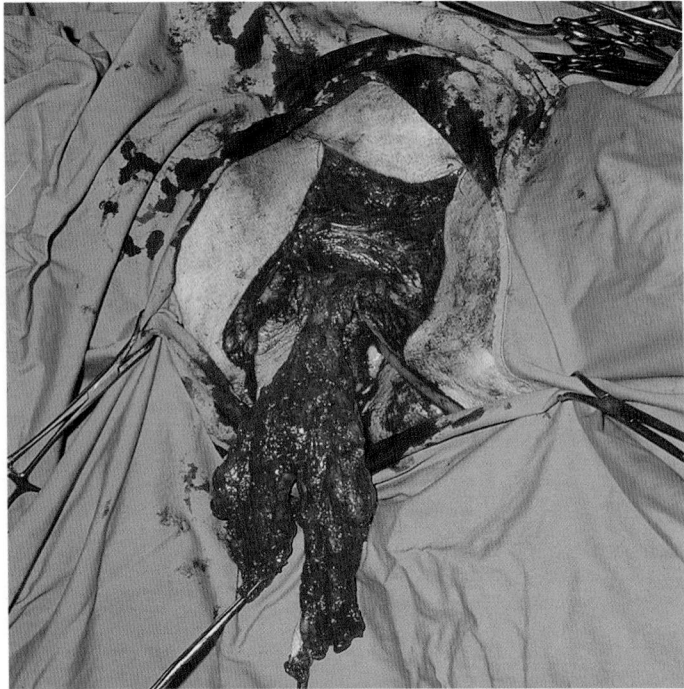

**FIGURE 71–27** The specimen hangs to the perineum by a thin bridge of tissue.

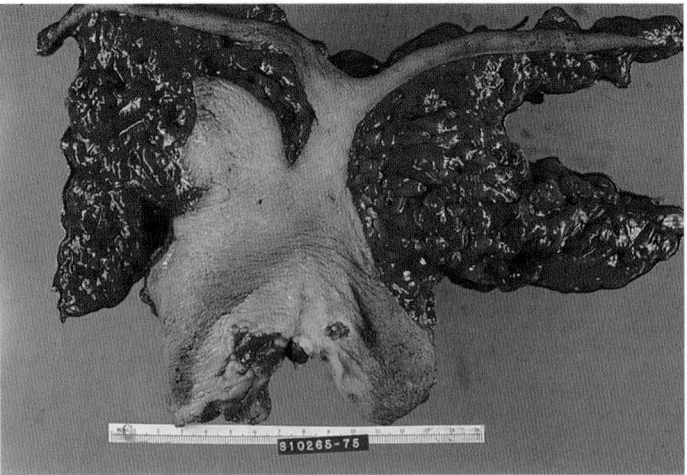

**FIGURE 71–28** The specimen has been deeply and widely excised. The node-bearing fat is attached, and the specimen is sent en bloc to pathology.

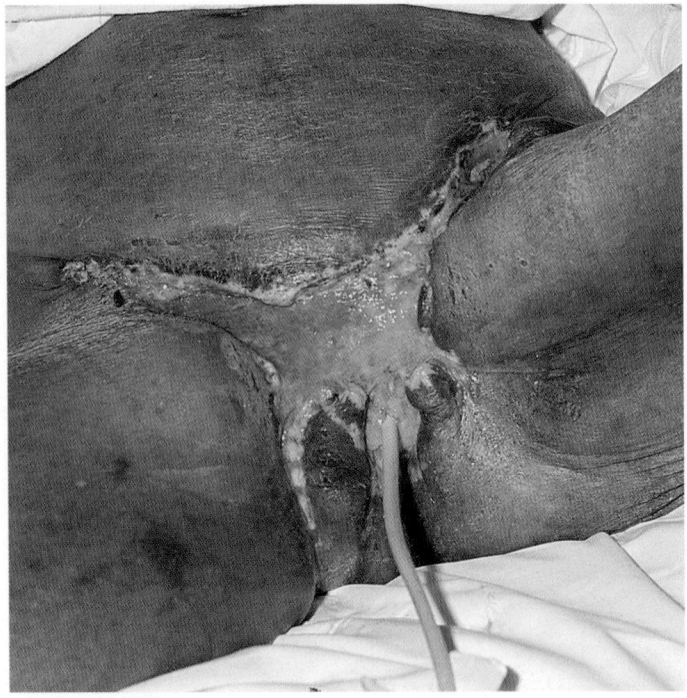

**FIGURE 71–29** If the wound edges are approximated under tension, the edges will separate, resulting in prolonged healing by second intention.

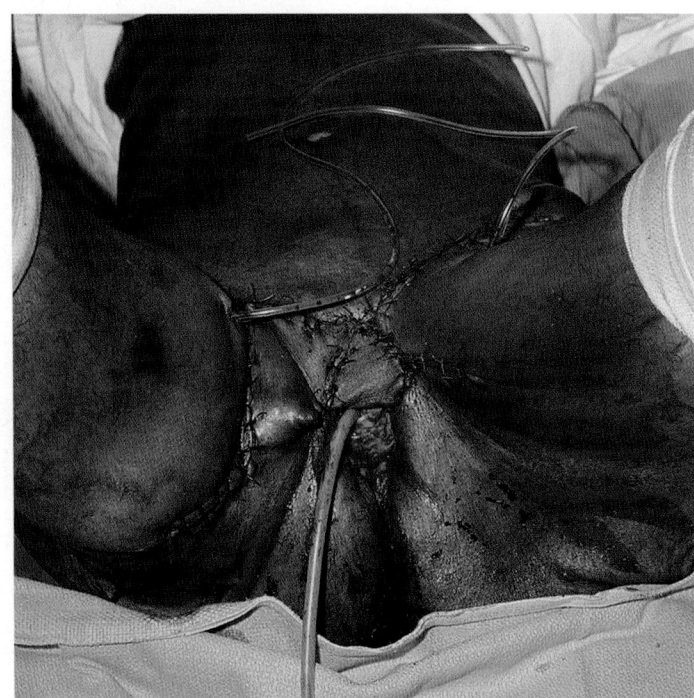

**FIGURE 71–30** The wound edges are approximated. The vaginal margin has been sutured to the perineal and thigh skin margins.

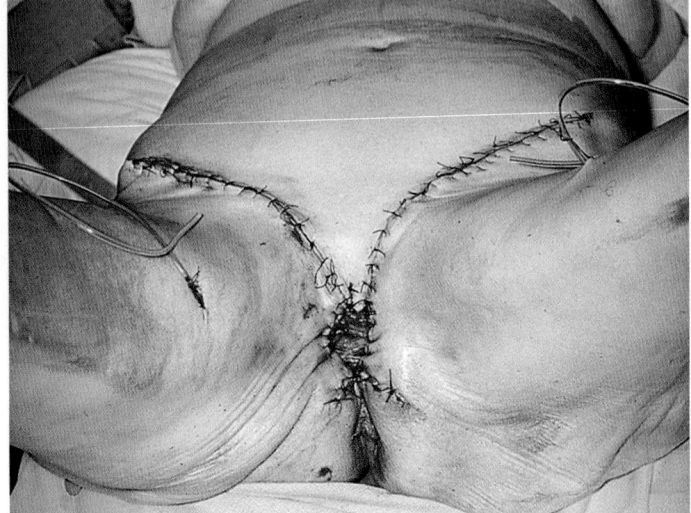

**FIGURE 71–31** The flaps came together nicely in this case. Jackson-Pratt drains have been placed under the flaps.

# CHAPTER 72

# Radical Vulvectomy With Tunnel Groin Dissection

*Helmut F. Schellhas*

A retrograde "tunnel" en bloc groin dissection commenced at the labial-crural fold is described (Fig. 72–1A). The procedure spares conventional inguinal incisions such as the "Texas Longhorn" incision (Fig. 72–1B) or the separate less radical groin incisions (Fig. 72–1C). Advantages include preservation of the groin skin layer, avoidance of incisional groin infection, and lymphedema of the legs. In our experience, operating time and hospitalization are markedly shortened.

This technique approaches easily the vulvar sentinel nodes because the fossa ovalis and the junctions of the femoral and greater saphenous veins are in close proximity to the labial-crural fold. The skin flap is raised from the labial-crural fold (Fig. 72–2) and is developed by sharp and blunt dissection (Fig. 72–3) until the underlying area of the fossa ovalis is reached. Sentinel groin nodes can then be removed from the fossa ovalis with adequate exposure (Fig. 72–4).

A classic en bloc specimen radical vulvectomy with bilateral groin dissection is outlined in Figure 72–5. Covering gauze is stapled over the tumor. The radical vulvectomy incision is started anteriorly. The skin flap is raised (Fig. 72–6) and developed by sharp and blunt dissection (Fig. 72–7). The surgical field is exposed by Deaver retractors. Vessels are transected by an electrosurgical device (Fig. 72–8). The fat pad is dissected from lateral to medial over the femoral triangle (Fig. 72–9).

Photographs show the exposure of the surgical field. The groin skin is exposed for assessment of thickness of the skin flap, although a groin incision is not made (Fig. 72–10). The specimen is rapidly developed from the area above the pubis and inguinal ligaments (Fig. 72–11). Dissection of the nodal fat pad over the femoral triangle is more delicate and is performed in traditional fashion with excellent exposure (Fig. 72–12). Tunnel groin dissection allows adequate surgical resection (Fig. 72–13).

The surgical field is tightly reapproximated (Fig. 72–14). Only one wound suction drain is inserted. We choose to use postoperative pressure dressings secured by stay sutures placed through the groin and anchored to the underlying fascia.

Because the pressure dressings are not covering an underlying wound, they do not get soiled and can remain in place for 1 week; they usually are removed in the office (Fig. 72–15). Postoperatively, the closed wound is covered with an antibiotic ointment.

Tunnel groin dissection is used mainly in T1 and T2 lesions. The operation avoids groin incision complications.

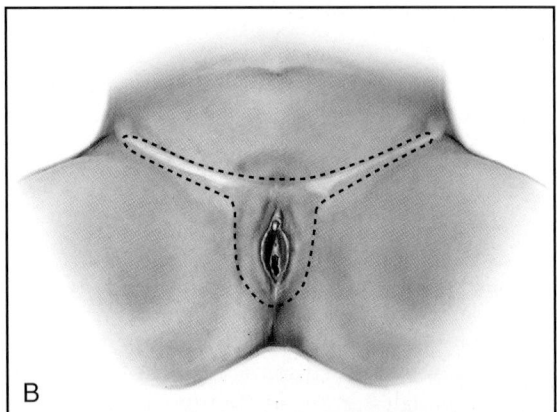

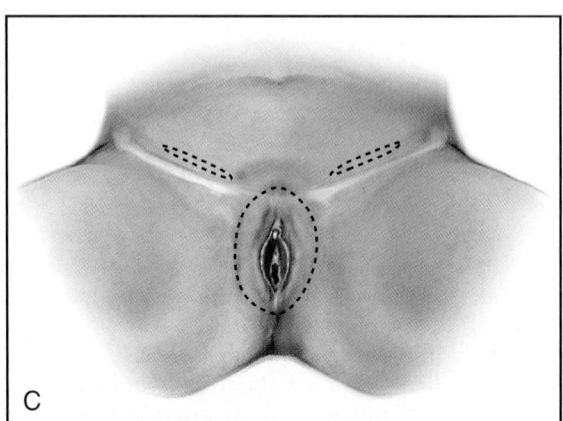

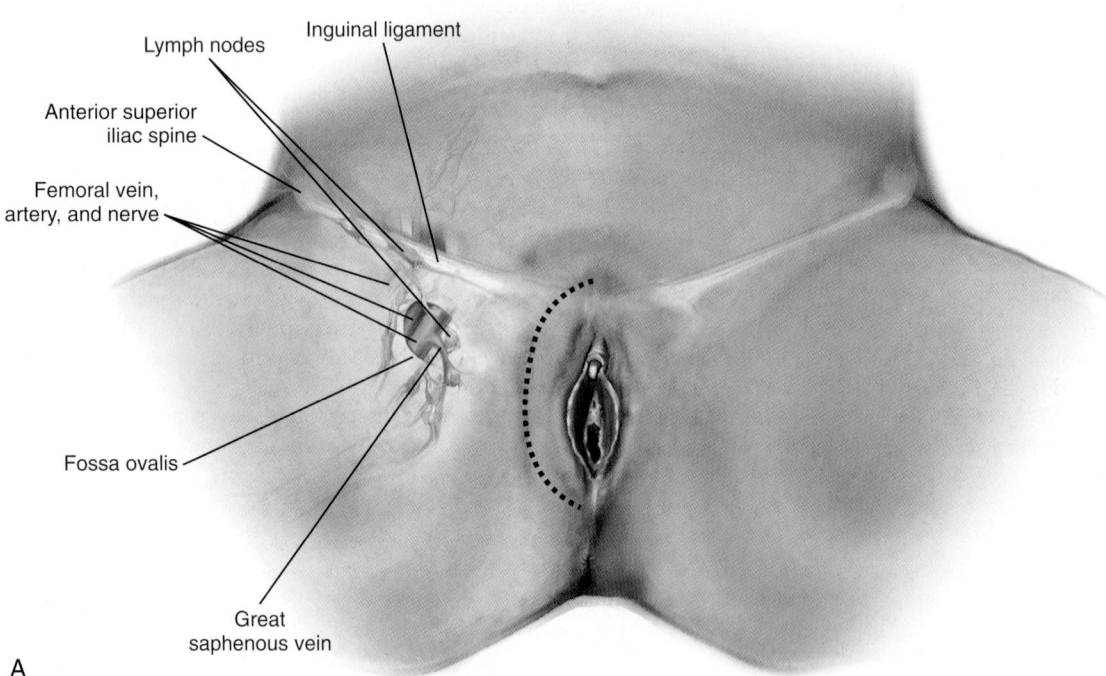

FIGURE 72–1  Different incisional approaches to radical vulvectomy with groin dissection are outlined. **A.** The lateral incision along the labial-crural fold used for the radical vulvectomy is also used to develop the skin flap over the femoral triangle with extension of the dissection above the inguinal ligaments and pubis. The proximity of the fossa ovalis and its vascular structures to the labial-crural fold is emphasized. **B.** The single Texas Longhorn incision, which is illustrated, is a more skin-sparing technique than the historical butterfly incision. **C.** A conservative three-incision technique is presently the preferred approach to groin dissection (see Fig. 72–1B); however, it does not allow en bloc dissection.

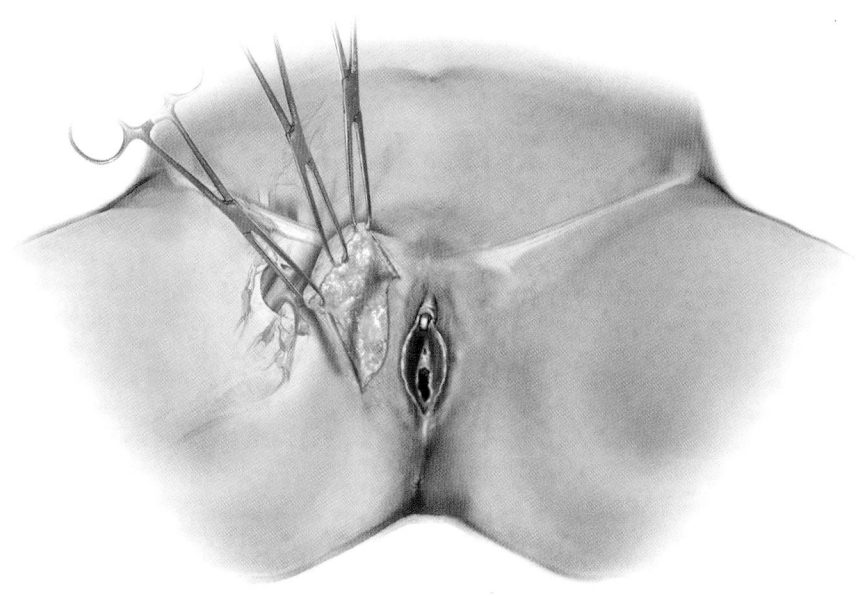

FIGURE 72-2 The skin flap for groin node dissection is raised.

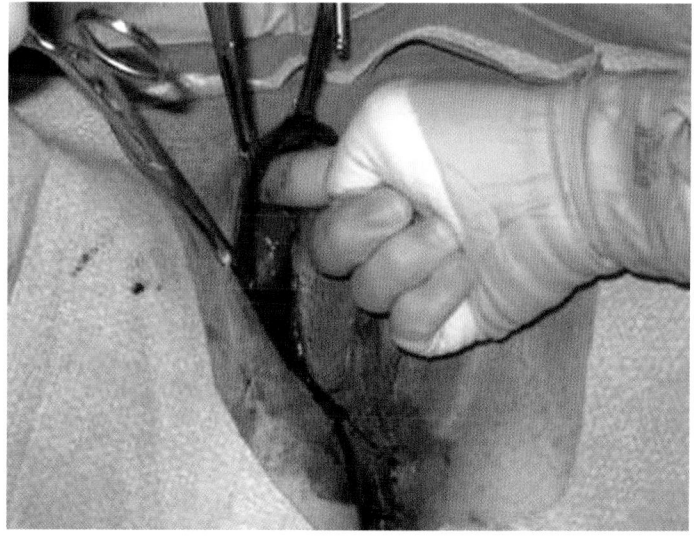

FIGURE 72-3 Much flap development is performed by finger dissection.

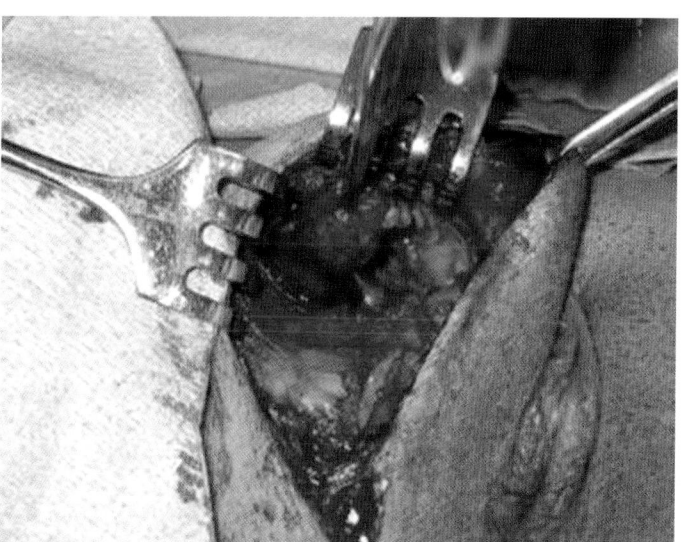

FIGURE 72-4 The fossa ovalis is exposed and lymph nodes are removed in a patient who underwent biopsy of the sentinel nodes only.

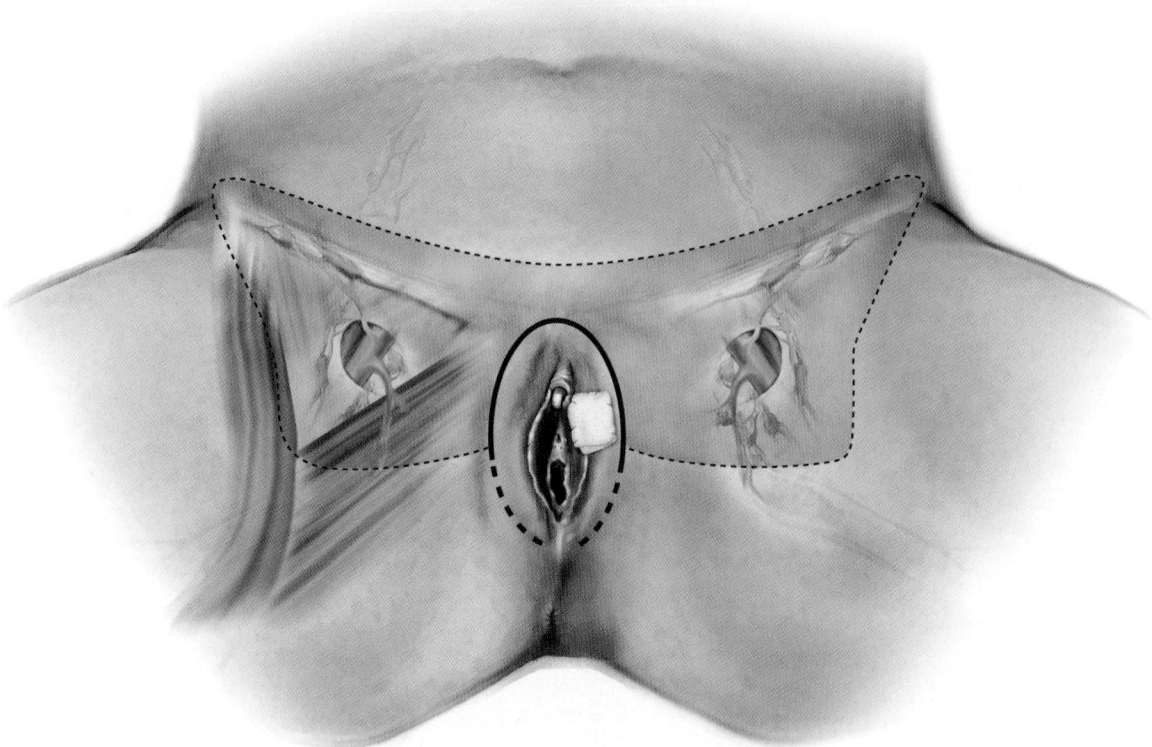

**FIGURE 72–5** The extent of the bilateral groin dissection is outlined in the shaded area. The vulvar lesion has been covered with gauze. Initially, only the upper part of the radical vulvectomy incision is used to develop the groin skin flaps.

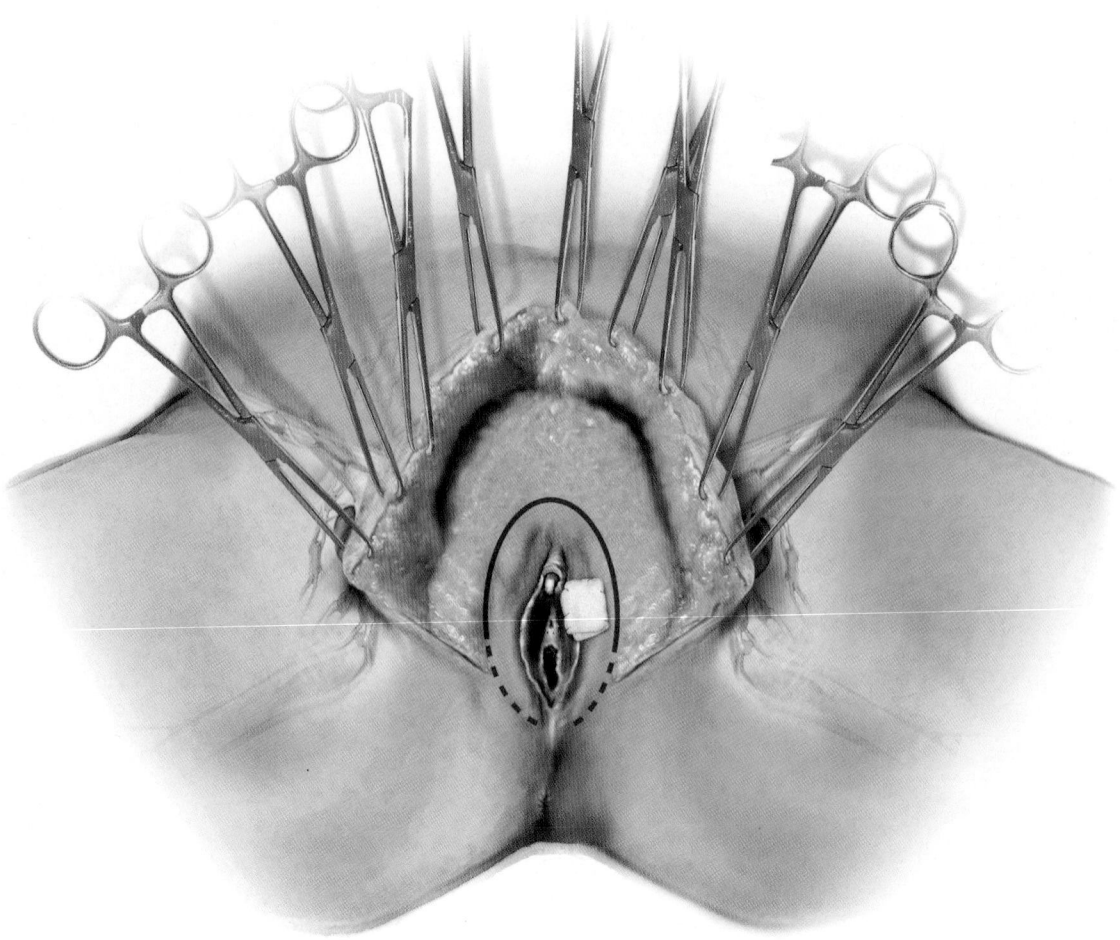

**FIGURE 72–6** The skin flaps are raised from the upper groin dissection.

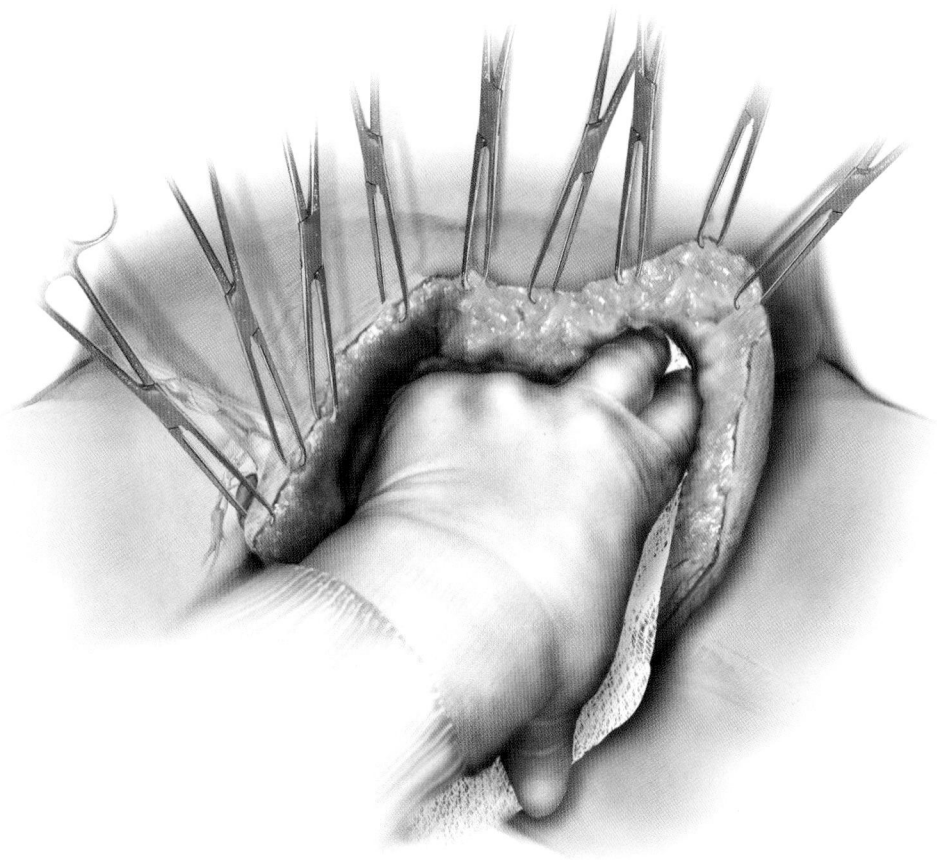

**FIGURE 72–7** Much of the skin flap is performed by full dissection. Use of dry gauze facilitates the dissection of fatty tissue.

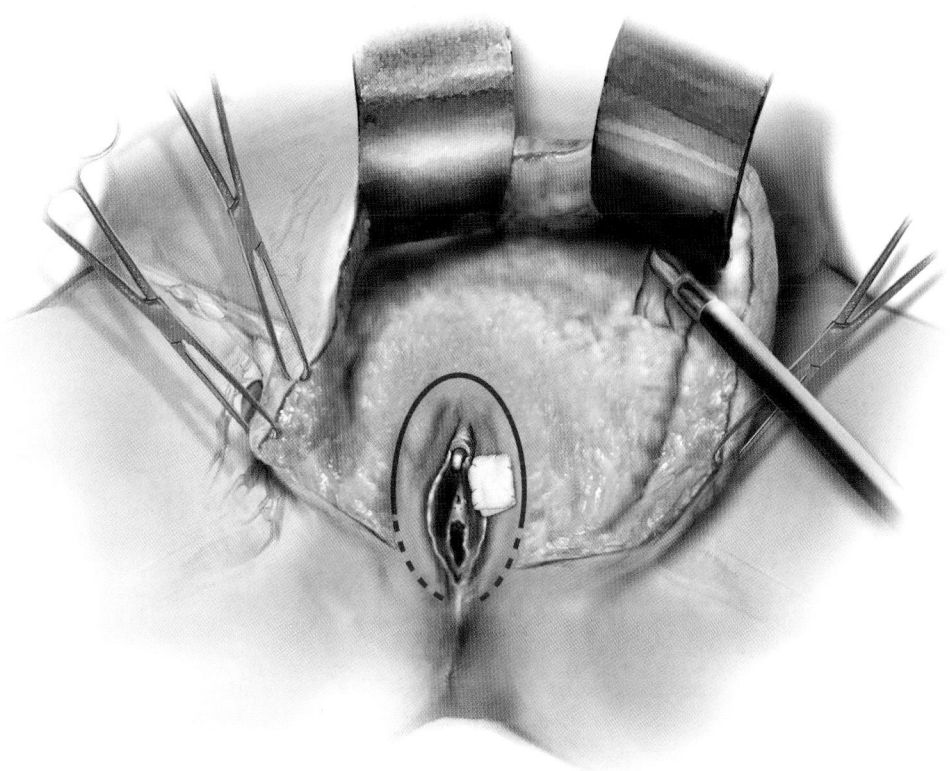

**FIGURE 72–8** Both flaps are raised in continuity. Vascular structures are transected and cauterized with an electrosurgical device.

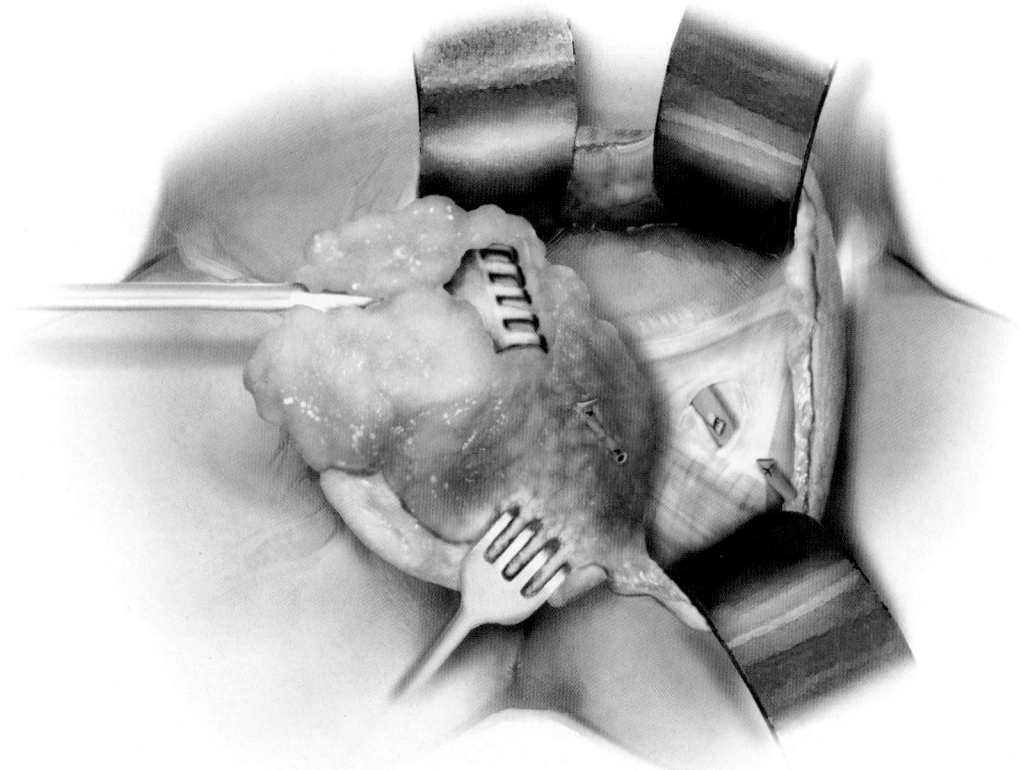

FIGURE 72–9  The fat pad is dissected from lateral to medial over the tunnel triangle. The greater saphenous vein is transected at the fossa ovalis.

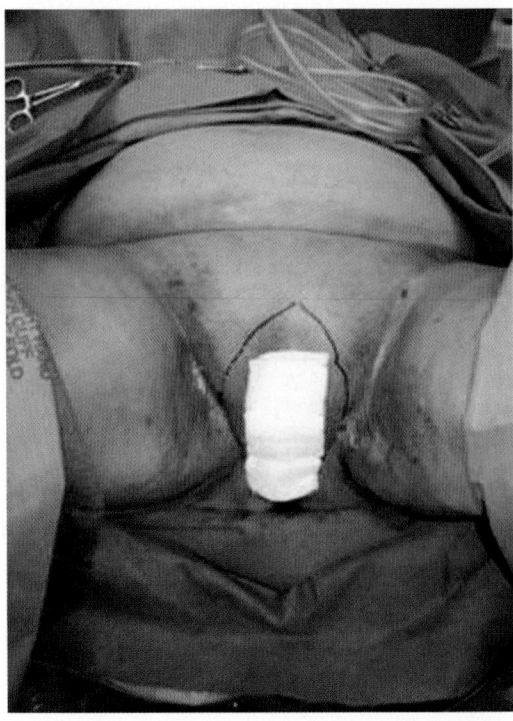

FIGURE 72–10  Illustration of a case before surgery. Gauze is stapled over the tumor.

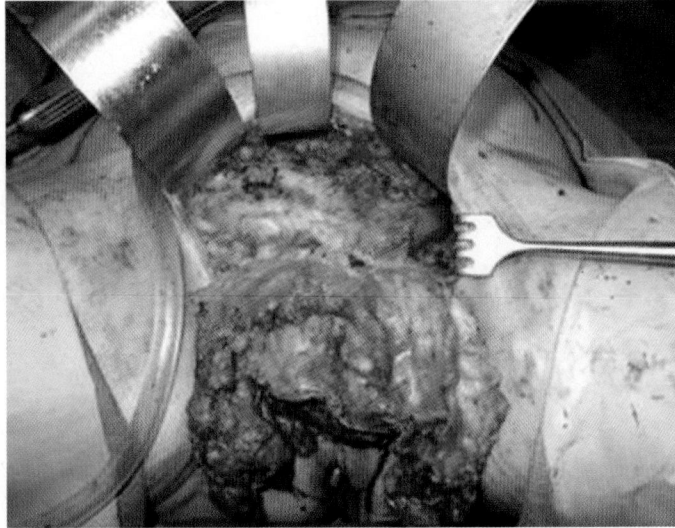

FIGURE 72–11  En bloc development of the surgical specimen over the lower abdominal fascia.

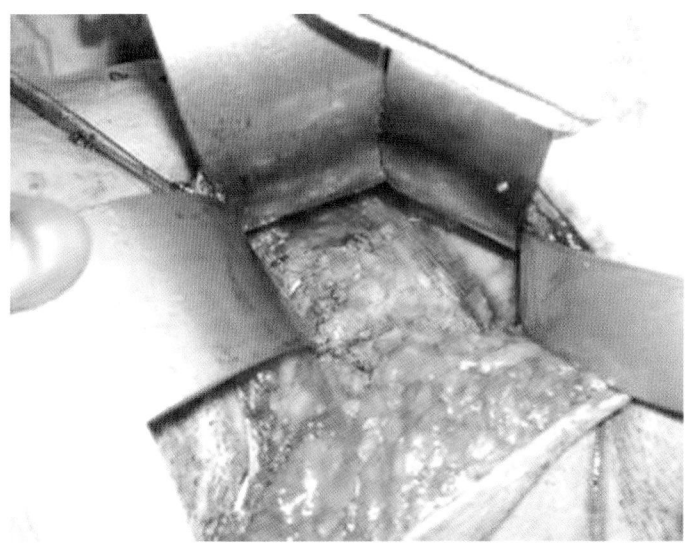

FIGURE 72–12 The femoral triangle is exposed with the femoral vein after transection of the greater saphenous vein.

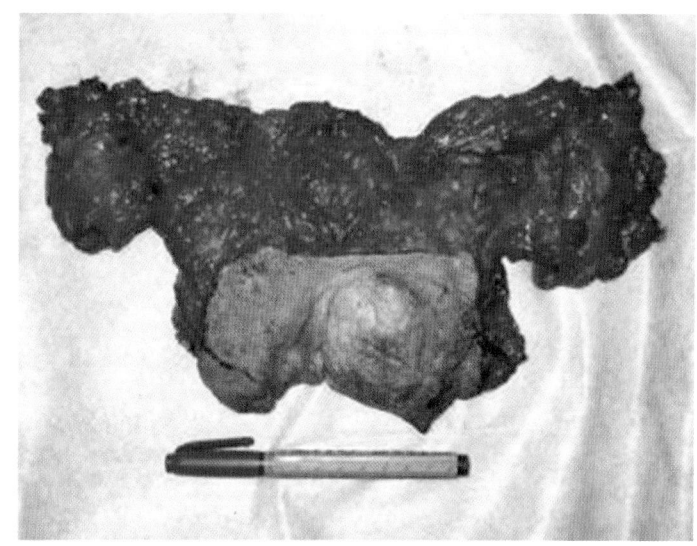

FIGURE 72–13 Radical vulvectomy specimen.

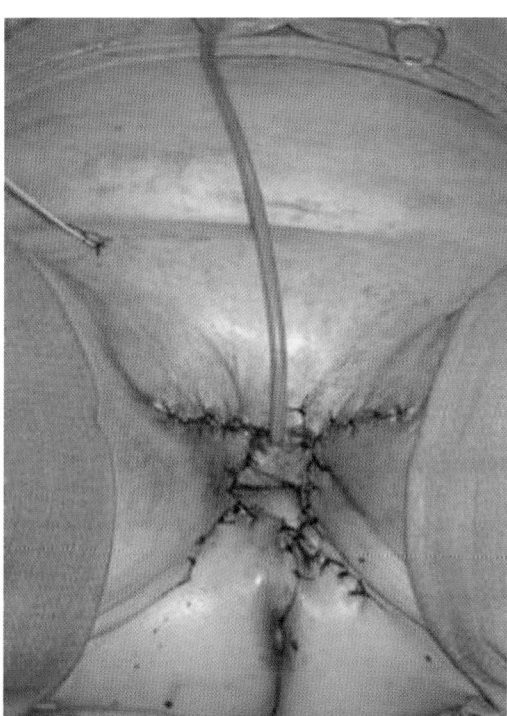

FIGURE 72–14 The reapproximated wound bed. One suction catheter drains the surgical beds of both groins.

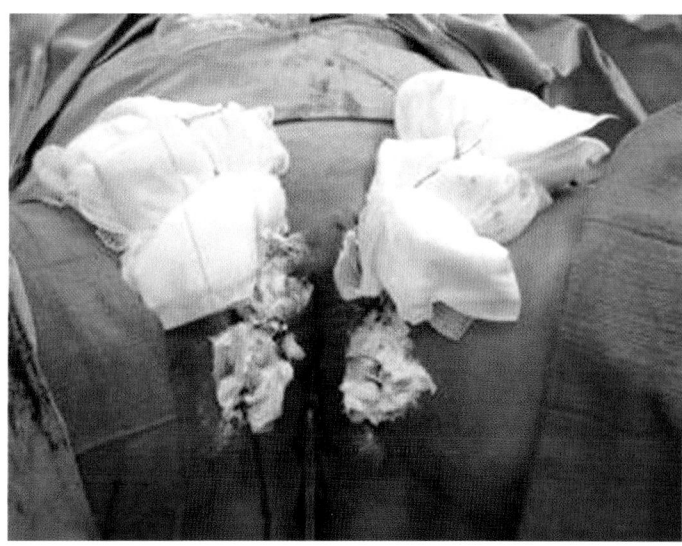

FIGURE 72–15 Pressure dressings are tied with stay sutures over both groins. Wide mattress sutures are anchored to the underlying fascia. The incision is covered with an antibiotic ointment.

# CHAPTER 73

# Vulvar Hematoma

## *Michael S. Baggish*

Hematomas occurring in the vulva may result from a variety of causes: episiotomy, traumatic forceps delivery, therapeutic vulvar or lower vaginal injection, vulvar surgery, and vulvar trauma, to mention a few.

Regardless of the cause(s), the end result may be the deposit of a massive amount of blood subcutaneously, typically along the plane of Colles' fascia or below it (Fig. 73–1). Coupled with the factors previously noted may be disruption of one of the structures forming the "blood lake" situated between Colles' fascia and the fascia encompassing the levator ani muscles. These cavernous structures (clitoris, bulb and vestibule, and corpora cavernosa) can and will bleed without remission for long periods, as manifested by a constant slow ooze.

Pressure of the blood on the vulvar skin may compromise its blood supply, causing actual necrosis. Therefore, when this condition occurs, the hematoma must be drained to relieve the pressure. Before it reaches a state necessitating surgical intervention, bleeding may be controlled by the timely application of an ice pack to the lesion, as well as by postural drainage. After the first 6 to 8 hours, the patient will benefit from warm salt water tub soaks (Fig. 73–2A, B).

Drainage may be implemented by a small incision at the most dependent portion of the hematoma. After the incision is made, the edges of the wound are sutured with a running stitch of 3-0 Vicryl. The hematoma is compressed every 3 to 4 hours to promote drainage (Fig. 73–3).

Exploration to locate the bleeding site should be done only as a last resort because it is exceedingly difficult to find the bleeding vessel in the midst of the substantial clot and tissue edema.

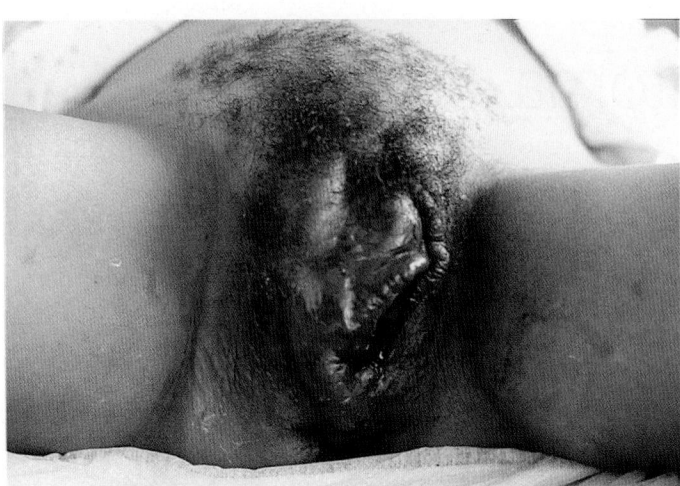

**FIGURE 73–1** Massive vulvar hematoma. Note that the blood has dissected so as to involve the right labium minus, labium majus, perineum, and mons. It has in fact extended to the contralateral labium majus. Dissection has progressed along a plane above Colles' fascia.

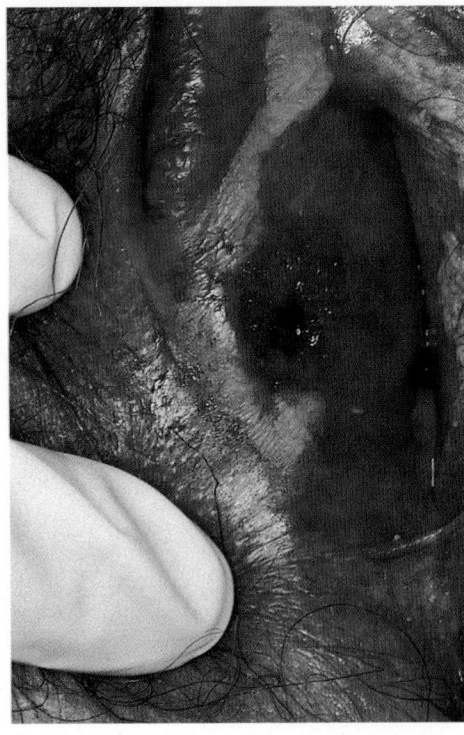

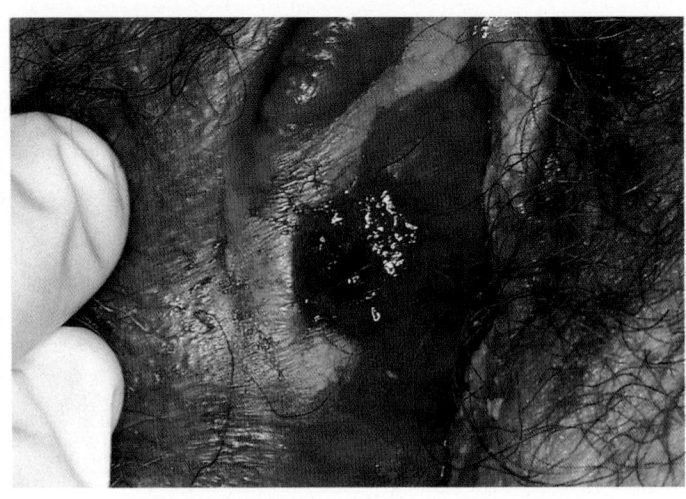

A                                                                    B

**FIGURE 73–2  A.** This hematoma occurred after a vestibular injection with a 27-gauge needle. The blood created tremendous swelling of the vestibule, perineum, and labium majus. The drainage site is noted in the lower right vestibule. **B.** Magnified view of drain site. The Penrose drain was removed 72 hours after drainage. The patient was admitted and catheterized for 24 hours. She was sent home with instructions to take salt water tub baths 3 times daily.

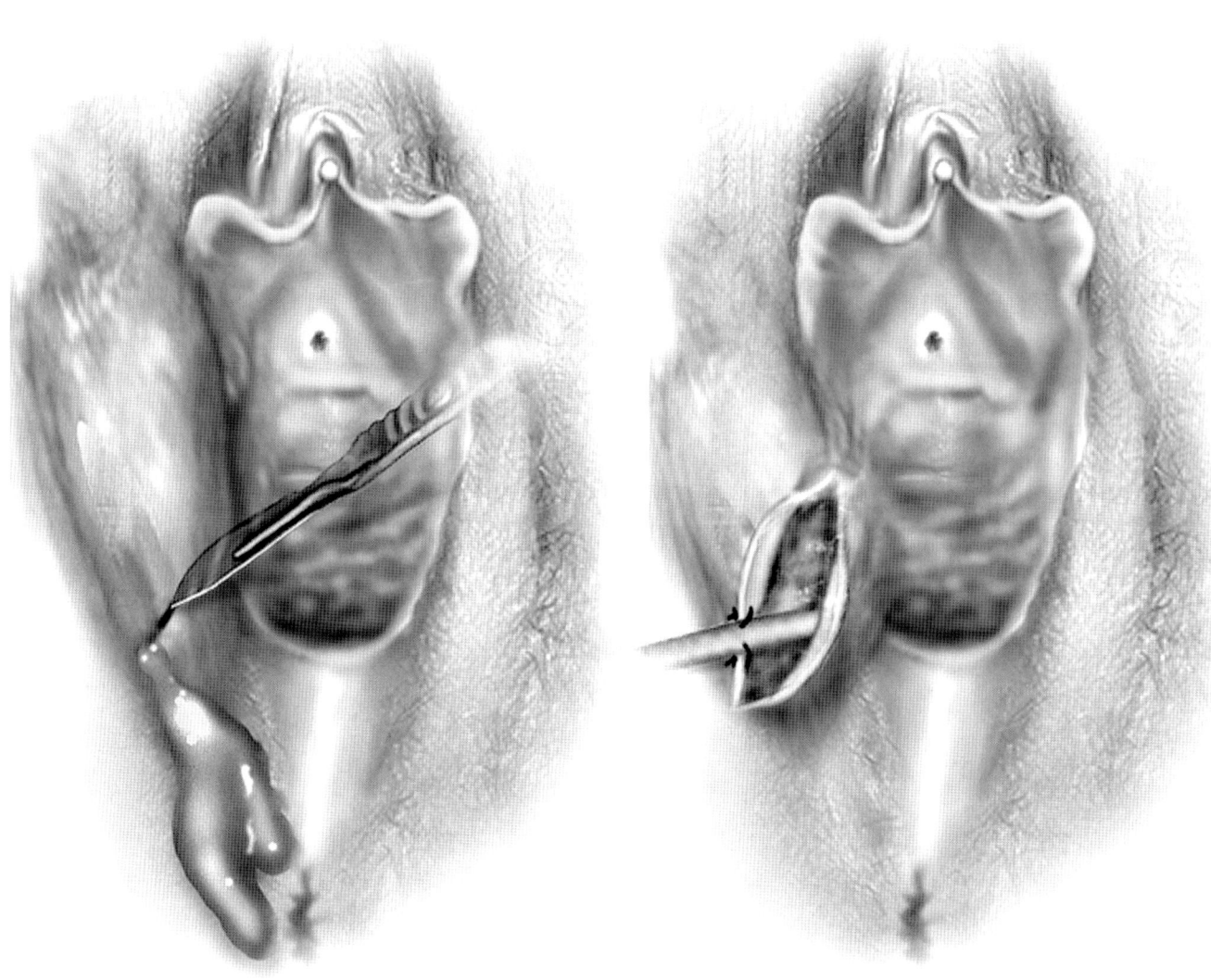

A

B

**FIGURE 73–3  A.** The drawing illustrates a hematoma that is drained at its dependent portion. A 1.5- to 2-cm hole is placed through the skin into the hematoma. **B.** A 0.25-inch Penrose drain is placed in the space, and its margins are anchored to the skin edges with 3-0 chromic catgut sutures. A large safety pin is placed through the terminal portion of the drain.

# CHAPTER 74

# Correction of Clitoral Phimosis

*Michael S. Baggish*

Severe clitoral phimosis is an end result of long-standing and suboptimally managed lichen sclerosus (Fig. 74–1A, B). In this circumstance, the skin of the frenulum and the clitoral hood fuse as a result of inflammation and subsequent scar formation (Fig. 74–1C). This creates persistent, severe itching, as well as outright pain. Because drainage is poor, smegma builds up, which may lead to abscess formation. The goal of surgery is to remove the scarred tissue and preserve the clitoris. Removal of the clitoris is unnecessary and should not be done.

Examination with an operating microscope (colposcope) will reveal a tiny opening in the sheath or complete incarceration of the glans (Fig. 74–1D). Identifying an opening gives the surgeon the advantage of being able to insert a probe in close proximity to the clitoris (Fig. 74–2). The entire operation should be performed with use of the microscope. With a 27-gauge needle, a 1:100 vasopressin solution is injected on either side of the clitoris through the mass of tissue that was once the clitoral hood (Fig. 74–3). A knife incision is made to one side of the palpated clitoris. The incision should be made on the side with the least amount of scar tissue (Fig. 74–4A).

Dissection proceeds from lateral to medial (Fig. 74–4B). The skin edges are retracted with Allis clamps. Stevens tenotomy scissors are ideal for sharply dissecting and separating the clitoral body from the scar tissue (Fig. 74–5). The scar is dissected anteriorly and posteriorly to completely mobilize the clitoris (Fig. 74–6). Next, the sheath and the remains of the frenulum are cut away from the glans clitoris (Fig. 74–7). The junction of the frenulum to the glans is highly vascular and must be clamped, cut, and suture-ligated with 4-0 or 5-0 Vicryl (Fig. 74–8). When this is completed, the entire hood complex is removed. Bleeding vessels are suture-ligated with 5-0 Vicryl. When all scar tissue has been excised, the clitoris is placed in the hemostatic bed beneath the subcutaneous tissue, which then is closed with 4-0 Vicryl (Fig. 74–9). The skin is closed with interrupted 3-0 or 4-0 Vicryl sutures. The wound is cleansed with sterile water, dried, and covered with silver sulfadiazine (Silvadene) cream (Fig. 74–10).

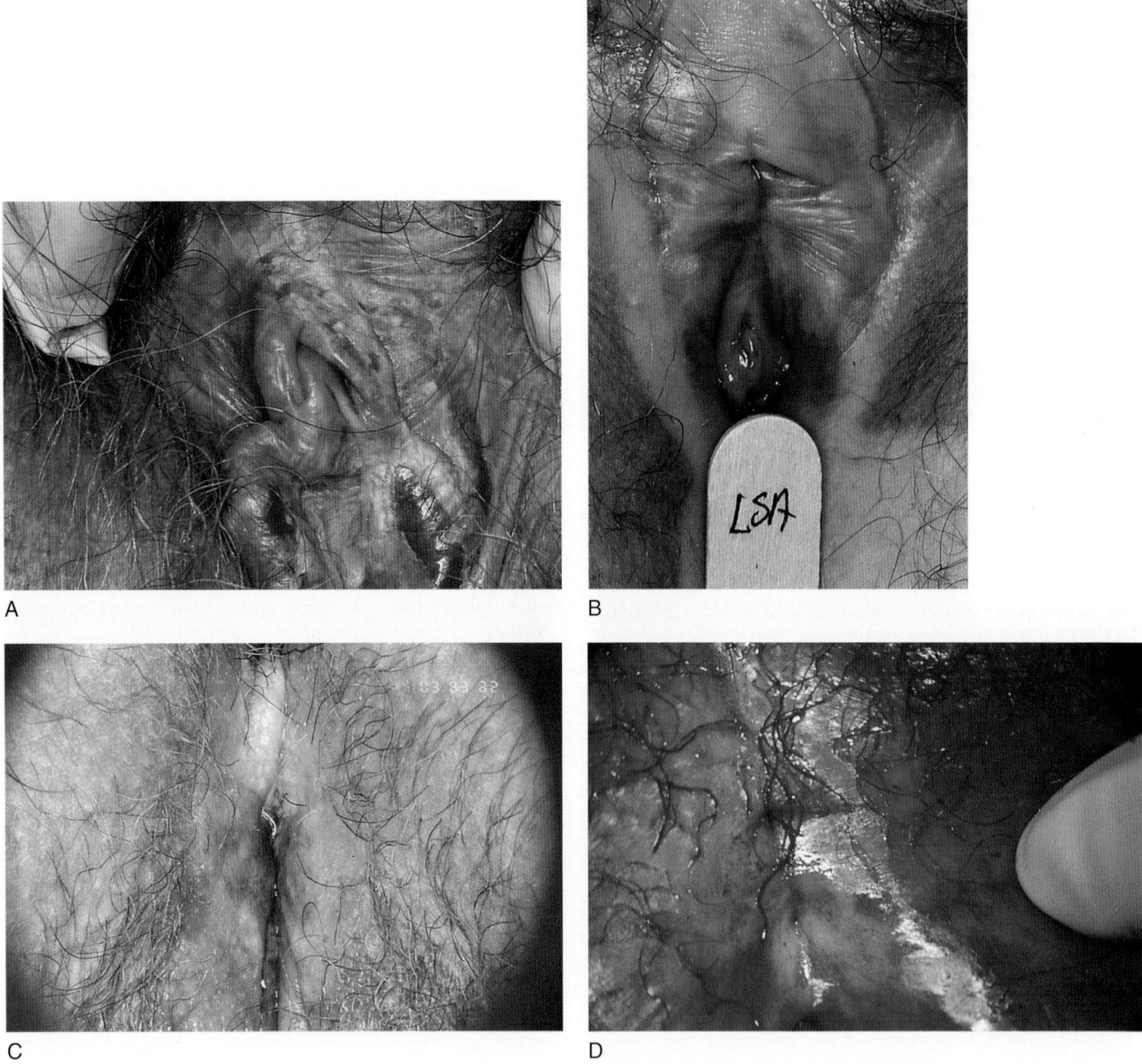

**FIGURE 74–1 A.** Severe lichen sclerosus et atrophicus (LSA) creates intense pruritus. The patient's scratching results in excoriation of the skin. The pallor of the vulvar skin is characteristic of LSA. Note the labial fusion, clitoral hood fusion, and puckering of the skin of the vulva. In this early case, the clitoris is relatively free. **B.** This more advanced case of LSA illustrates clitoral fusion, labial fusion, and introital stenosis. **C.** The clitoral hood and the frenulum are totally fused. The clitoris is tightly locked into its hood, which is adherent to the glans. The patient experienced painful swelling of the clitoris. **D.** This colposcopic view of a phimotic clitoris reveals a small opening. The location of the opening corresponds to the point where the frenulum joins the clitoral hood.

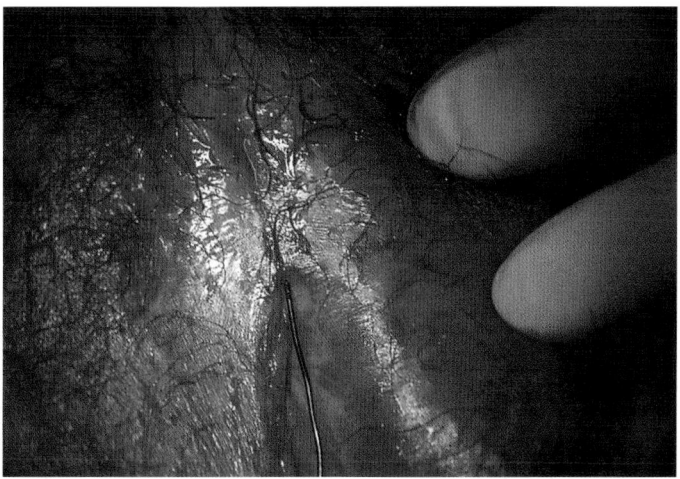

**FIGURE 74–2** A lacrimal probe is engaged into the opening (see Fig. 71–1D) and is used to break up and probe adhesions between the glans clitoris and the inner aspect of the hood. It also serves as a useful orientation marker.

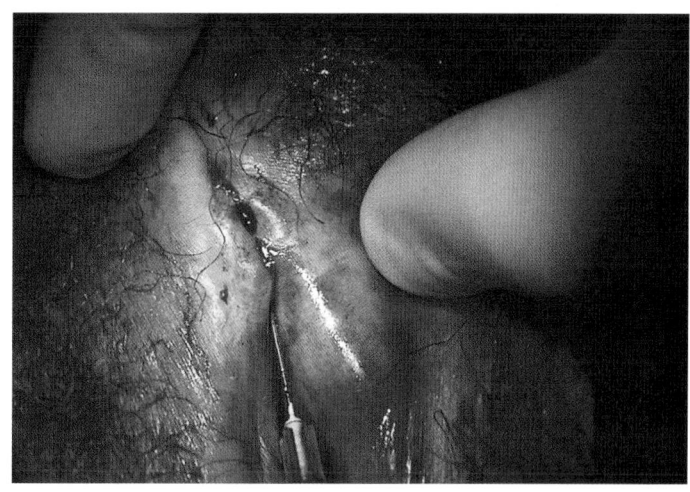

**FIGURE 74–3** Surgery for clitoral phimosis is best performed by utilizing the operating microscope. A 27-gauge needle is inserted via the opening seen in Figure 71–1D. A 1:100 vasopressin solution is injected into the hood. Additionally, the vasopressin is injected on either side of the palpated clitoral body.

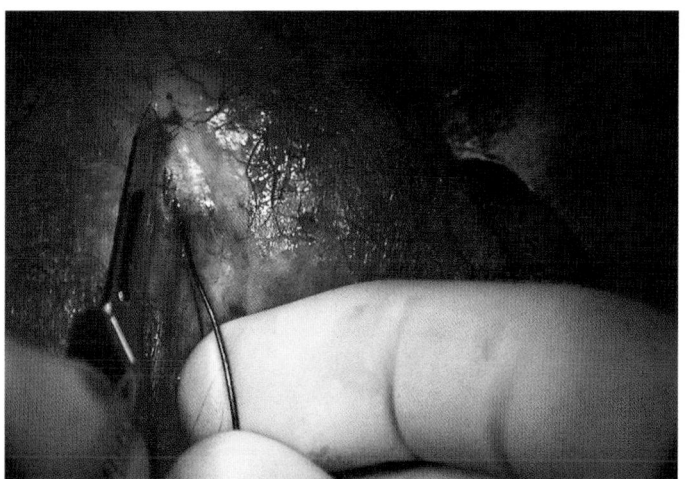

A

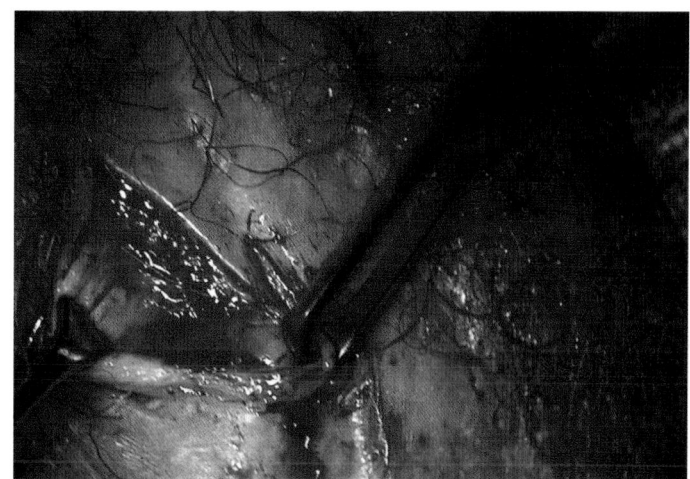

B

**FIGURE 74–4 A.** A scalpel cut is made through the skin to the level of Colles' fascia. This cut is located parallel but lateral to the body of the clitoris. Care must be taken not to go deeper than Colles' fascia. The clitoral corpora cavernosa (crus) are located beneath Colles' fascia in this view. **B.** The margins of the wound are placed on traction with Allis clamps. The dissection proceeds from lateral to medial with the use of mosquito clamps and Stevens scissors.

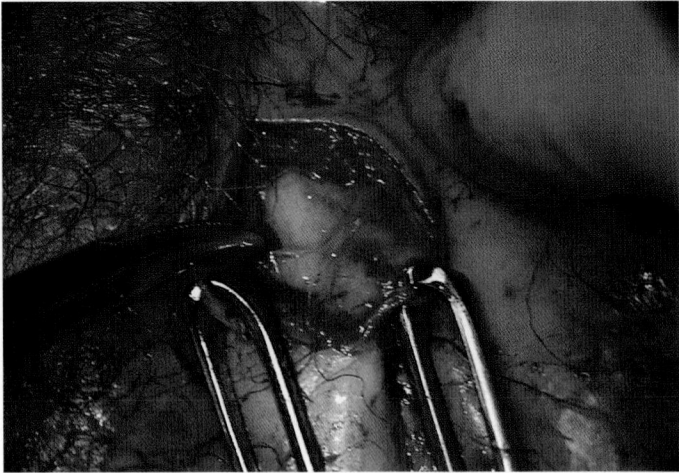

**FIGURE 74–5** The body of the clitoris is located. The entire length of the clitoris is dissected free from the surrounding scarred connective tissue and clitoral hood.

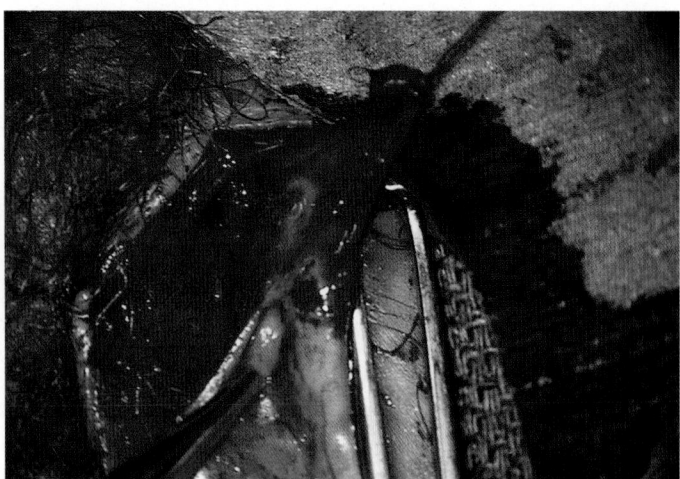

**FIGURE 74–6** The dissection proceeds from the root of the clitoral body to the terminal glans. All scar tissue is removed.

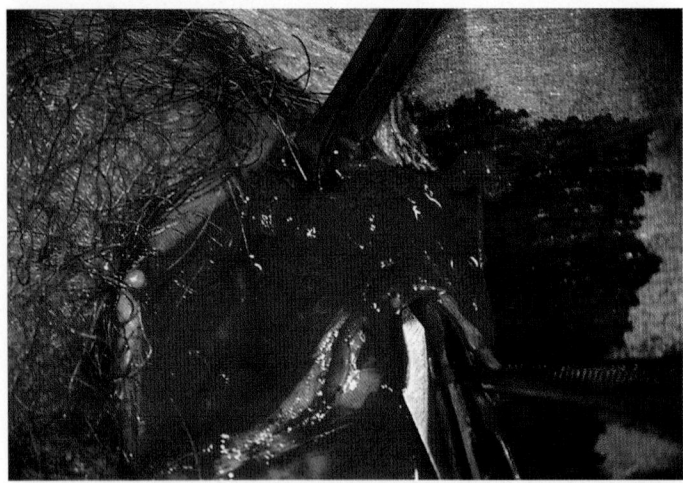

**FIGURE 74–7** The clitoral frenula are located and dissected away from the glans. These are cut with Stevens scissors. In this photo, the edge of the left frenulum is held in the forceps. The tip of the Stevens scissors is dissecting a space between the frenulum and the glans. The Allis clamp is holding the tissue just superior to the clitoral body.

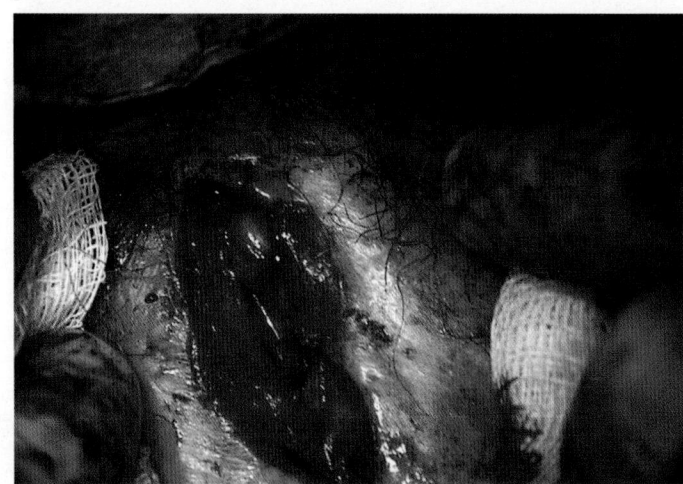

**FIGURE 74–8** The cut edges of the frenulum are sutured with 5-0 Vicryl. The unencumbered glans clitoris is clearly visible.

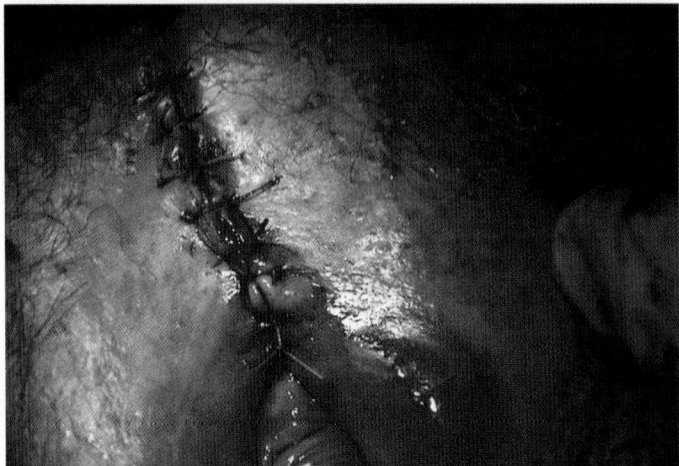

**FIGURE 74–9** All scarred tissue has been removed. The clitoris is located between normal subcutaneous tissue and Colles' fascia. No part of the clitoris has been excised or injured. The subcutaneous layer is closed with 4-0 Vicryl (interrupted) sutures. The skin margins are approximated without tension with 3-0 or 4-0 Vicryl sutures.

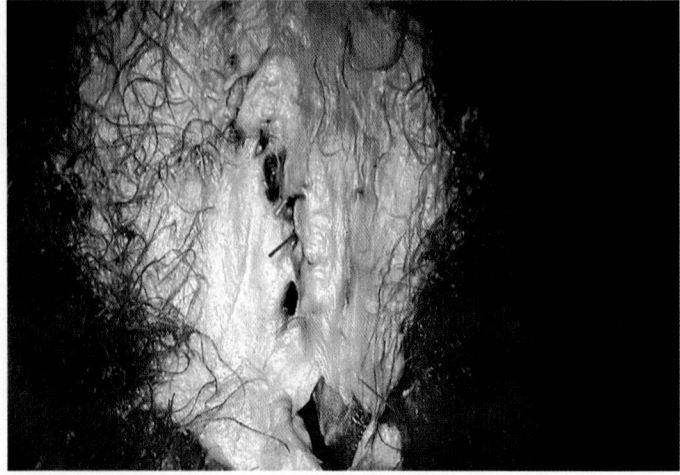

**FIGURE 74–10** The wound site is irrigated with normal saline or sterile water and then is covered with Silvadene cream. The cream is applied 3 times per day and at bedtime.

# CHAPTER 75

# Hymenotomy (Hymenectomy)

## *Michael S. Baggish*

Hymenectomy should be more accurately named *partial hymenectomy,* or *hymenotomy.* The operation is done primarily to diminish the discomfort of initial coitus in a virginal woman or to relieve dyspareunia for a woman already sexually active. The hymen is a point of constriction for intravaginal intercourse, and its stretching or tearing can be a significant source of discomfort during an ordinarily pleasurable physiologic act.

The patient is anesthetized, placed in the lithotomy position, prepared, and draped. The hymen is gently grasped with Adson-Brown forceps at the 1-o'clock position and with an Allis clamp at the 5-o'clock position. The hymen is placed on gentle traction with special care taken not to tear it by excessive force. A 1:100 vasopressin solution has been injected subdermally via a 27-gauge needle into the vestibule side just lateral to the hymenal attachment (Fig. 75-1A). The injection extends for the entire length of the hymen on the left side. The edge of the hymen is held with the Adson-Brown forceps and is placed on traction in the anterior direction. With the use of a scalpel (No. 15 blade), the hymen is cut free with a 2- to 3-mm margin from the vagina and vestibule, extending from the 1-o'clock position to just below 5 o'clock (Fig. 75-1B). The vagina is sutured with interrupted 3-0 Vicryl sutures to the vestibular margin (Fig. 75-1C). Next, Allis clamps are applied to the right side of the hymen at the 11-o'clock and 7-o'clock locations, and an identical procedure is performed. The operator's two fingers are placed in the vagina to check for introital capacity. They should enter without resistance, and the introitus should accommodate them without significant counterpressure. It is preferred to leave intact the small area of hymen between the 5-o'clock and 7-o'clock positions and the remnant beneath the urethra. For reassurance, the patient is given vaginal forms to insert into the vagina after the 6-week postoperative check. A small or medium form is given to the patient initially. The form is well lubricated with a water-based personal lubricant (Astroglide) and is inserted into the vagina. The patient is asked to remove the form and insert it while the gynecologist views her technique. The patient is then instructed to insert it twice daily for 10 minutes (supine position) while relaxing her pelvic floor muscles around the form. Two weeks later, she is fitted with a large form (the size of an average erect penis). She continues her relaxation exercises. After 2 weeks, she can be assured that intercourse will take place normally and will be comfortable for her. Lubricant should be used with every sexual exposure for at least 30 days after initiation of regular intercourse (e.g., during and after the honeymoon).

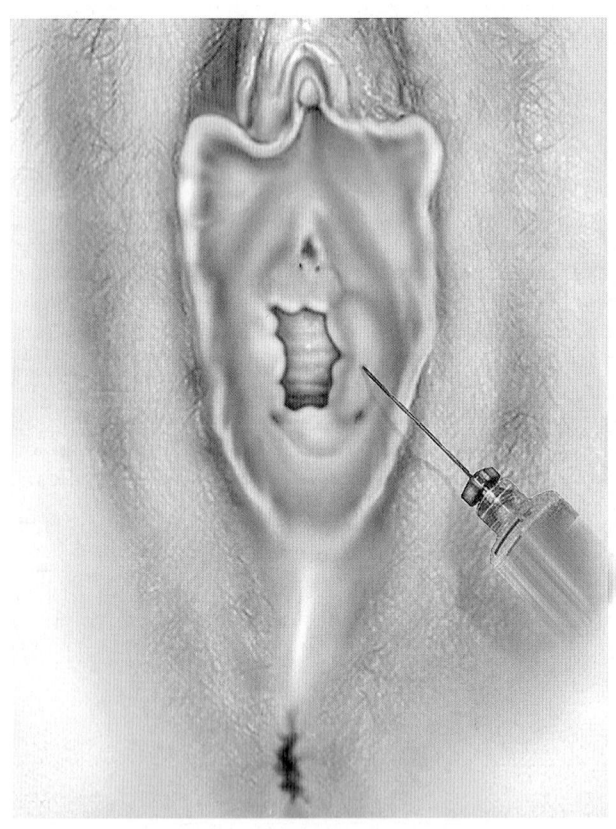

A

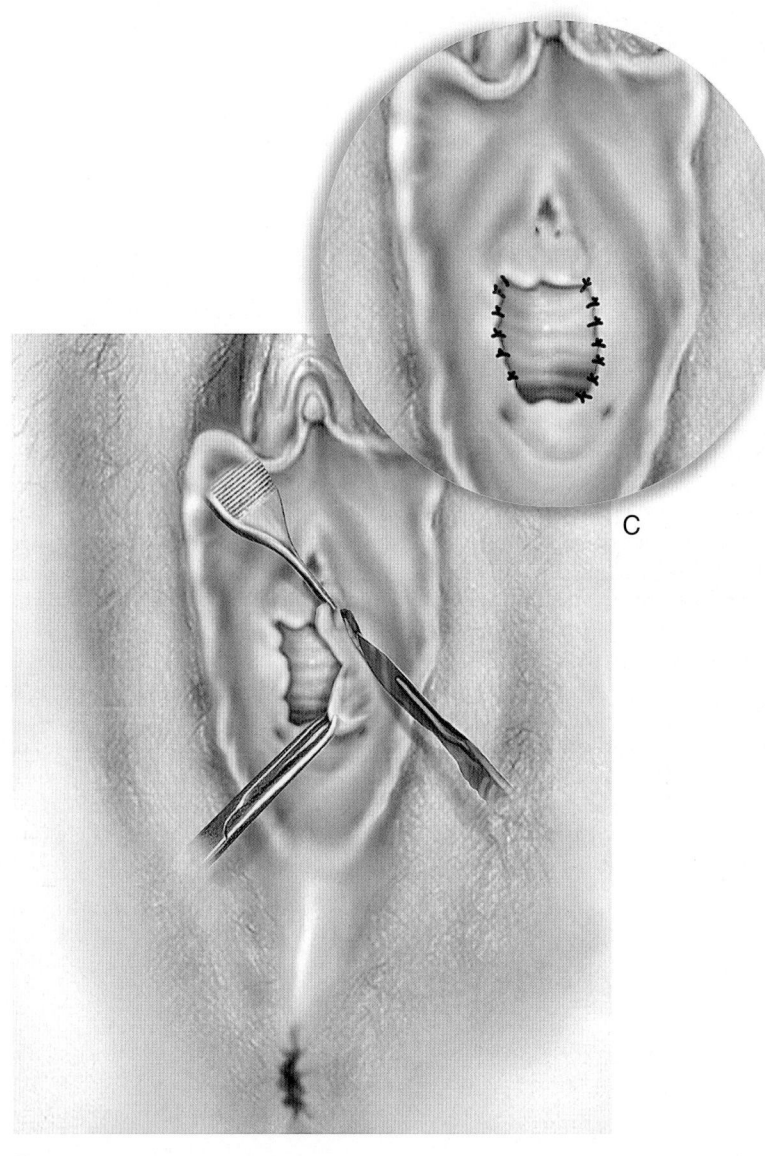

B

**FIGURE 75–1** **A.** Initially, with a 10-mL syringe and a 1½-inch, 27-gauge needle, a 1:100 vasopressin solution (20 units/mL) is injected immediately lateral to the hymen, beginning at 5 o'clock and extending the needle subdermally to the 1-o'clock position. The solution balloons the surrounding vestibular and vaginal tissue. **B.** The hymen is grasped with Adson-Brown forceps at the 1-o'clock position. The lower portion of the hymen is held with an Allis clamp at the 5-o'clock position. The hymen is excised with a straight vertical knife cut, leaving a margin of vestibule (outer) and vagina (inner). **C.** The vaginal and vestibular margins are sutured together with interrupted 3-0 or 4-0 Vicryl sutures. An identical procedure is performed on the right side. The wound is irrigated with normal sterile saline and is observed to ensure that complete hemostasis has been obtained.

# CHAPTER 76

# Plastic Repair of the Perineum (Perineorrhaphy)

*Michael S. Baggish*

Perineal reconstruction is indicated for patients who have dyspareunia associated with any number of causes, including, but not limited to, scar formation secondary to lichen sclerosus; tearing secondary to childbirth; excessively tight closure of an episiotomy; scar formation due to episiotomy breakdown, secondary infection, or suture reactive inflammation; faulty attempts at perineal repair; trauma; ulcer formation secondary to poor blood supply; burn scar formation due to electrosurgery, laser, or chemicals; chronic infection; and atrophy (Figs. 76–1 through 76–3).

Despite a long-held belief that tightening of the perineum and introitus will improve a woman's sexual response, invariably this action leads to dyspareunia. The anatomy of the vulva and vagina was described earlier; however, a few points should be considered here. First, the levator ani muscles do not cross the midline beneath (posterior to) the vagina. These muscles insert laterally into the wall of the lower vagina under the bulb. The levators insert lateral to and into the anterior anal sphincter. Second, the superficial muscles of the perineum are very thin structures and add little mass to the ill-defined perineal body. The bulk of that structure consists of the anterior external sphincter ani. Third, no well-defined fascial plane exists in the area of the perineum with the exception of Colles' fascia and the investment fascia overlying the external sphincter ani. Fourth, picking up muscle mass and plicating across the midline posterior to the lower vagina creates an unnatural hump; additionally, placement of a large number of absorbable sutures into the same tissue produces an inflammatory response, diminishes the blood supply to the overlying epithelium, and results in gross scar formation. These factors will result in painful intercourse because the normal anatomy is distorted. All of the procedures listed under the fourth point therefore should be avoided. Finally, unless the patient is symptomatic, surgery in this area should not be done. Even though the physical attributes of an individual woman's perineum may not be pleasing to an examiner's eyes, this is not an indication to perform surgery to "improve" it. Similarly, surgery to "tighten things up" based on the mindset of better sex for the patient's partner is unjustified. Perineal plastic and reconstructive surgery is based on the provision of easy vaginal ingress and the limitations of gross scar formation. Preservation or reconstruction of normal anatomy to restore physiologic function is the goal of perineal surgery.

The area of the vestibule or lower vagina that preoperatively has objectively demonstrated hypersensitivity and production of pain when provoked will be removed. Patients who have atrophy should be pretreated with topical and systemic estrogen at least 1 to 2 months before surgery. Testosterone topically applied does nothing whatsoever to nourish or improve the epithelium. More often, application of testosterone ointment produces an uncomfortable burning sensation.

The patient is placed in the dorsal lithotomy position, prepared, and draped. The area of the vagina, vestibule, or perineum to be excised is traced with a marking pen (Fig. 76–4A, B). The surgeon should check vaginal mobility with Allis clamps before excising the perineal tissue. Because the vagina will be advanced, the surgeon will need to estimate the distance between the advanced vagina and the perineal edge to avoid excessive tension during suture line closure. When the markings have satisfied the surgeon's eye, a 1 : 100 vasopressin solution is injected subdermally with a 1½-inch, 27-gauge needle. A transverse incision is made across the posterior vaginal wall with a No. 15 scalpel blade. This line will form the base of a triangle (see Figs. 76–4B, 76–5). The left and right lines of the triangle are equidistant and intersect at a central point on the perineum, as drawn previously by the surgeon. The skin and mucosa within the triangle are resected with the use of Adson-Brown forceps and Allis clamps for traction (Fig. 76–6). Cutting is done with Stevens or Metzenbaum scissors (see Figs. 76–4B, 76–7). The plane of dissection is the fascia between the anus and the vagina and the fascia underlying the vestibule and perineum. The triangular piece of tissue is dissected from apex to base until it is completely free; it is then removed with the accompanying cicatrix (Fig. 76–8). A second glove is placed over the surgeon's first glove, and a rectal examination is done to determine the position of the anus/rectum in relation to the plane of dissection. The removed tissue is placed into fixative and sent to pathology. The fascial edge underlying the vagina is grasped with forceps and elevated. Another 5 to 10 mL of vasopressin mixture is injected into it (Fig. 76–9). Next, the fascia is undermined with Stevens scissors for 5 to 10 mm superiorly (Fig. 76–10). The fascia is sutured transversely to the fascia underlying the perineal skin with interrupted 3-0 Vicryl sutures. Bleeding vessels are clamped with mosquito clamps and suture-ligated with 4-0 Vicryl. The vaginal mucosa is advanced without tension to the perineal skin edge (Fig. 76–11). The vaginal mucosa is sutured to perineal skin transversely along the line of the initial base incision with interrupted 3-0 Vicryl sutures (Fig. 76–12A through D). The wound is irrigated with normal saline. Ease of entry into the vagina is checked by inserting loosely approximated index and center fingers through the introitus (Fig. 76–13). The wound is covered with silver sulfadiazine (Silvadene). The final rectal examination is done to check the integrity of the bowel. Postoperatively, the patient takes daily salt water tub baths and applies Silvadene to the wound 3 times daily and at bedtime. A stool softener is prescribed because the patient is instructed to avoid bearing down. Nothing is placed in the vagina for 6 weeks. The final result of this operation is the excision of scar tissue, removal of poorly vascularized skin, and expansion of the vaginal opening.

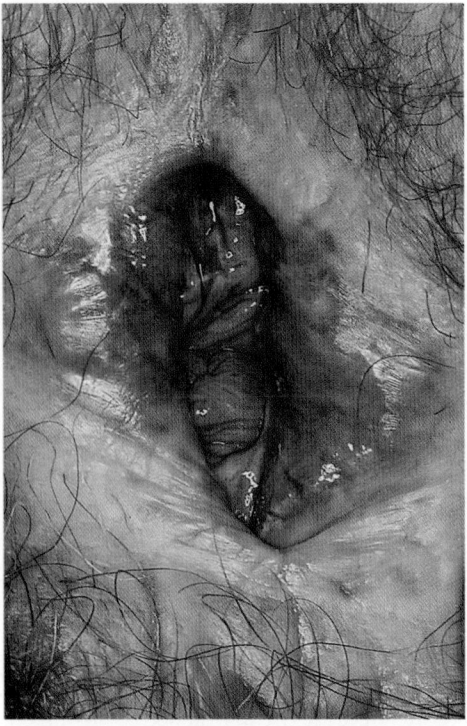

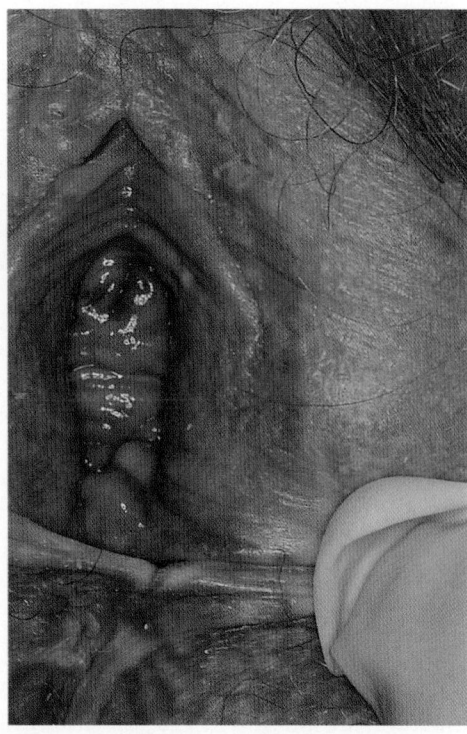

A

B

FIGURE 76–1  A. Severe and undertreated lichen sclerosus that has led to significant skin thickening and vulvar scarring. Elasticity in the affected areas has disappeared. B. This patient subsequently responded to serial, subdermal dexamethasone (Decadron) injections (see Chapter 79). Nevertheless, permanent scar formation at the posterior commissure and perineum led to significant dyspareunia.

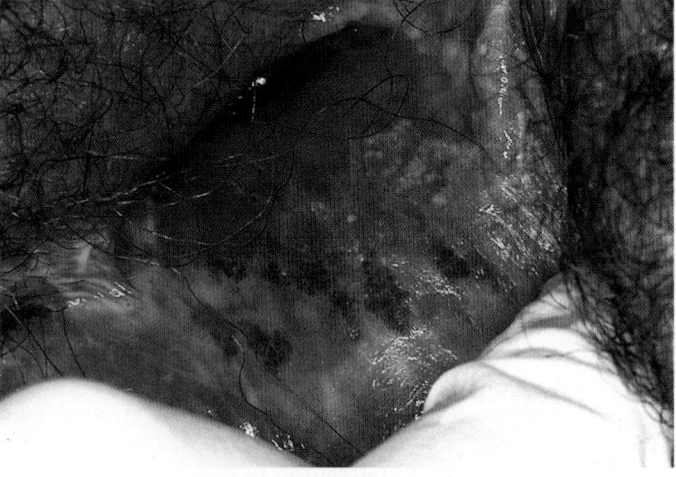

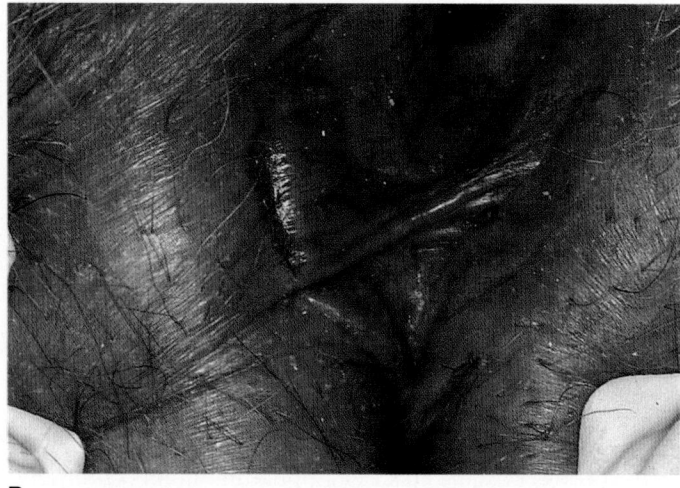

A

B

FIGURE 76–2  A. Chronic ulcer formation is evident in the fossa navicularis and posterior vestibule. The past history revealed prior excisions and laser vaporization, which were performed as attempts to "cure" the recurrent ulcers. The basic problem in this instance is atrophy secondary to a poor blood supply. Subsequent trauma results in ulcers that heal poorly and slowly. B. Scarring of the vulva secondary to prior injury. The inelastic tissue forms fissures when stretched.

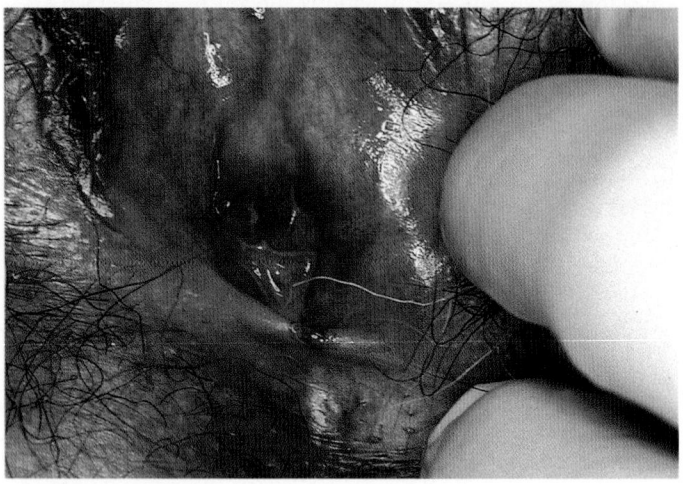

FIGURE 76–3  The posterior commissure tear in this atrophic vulva occurred acutely during examination.

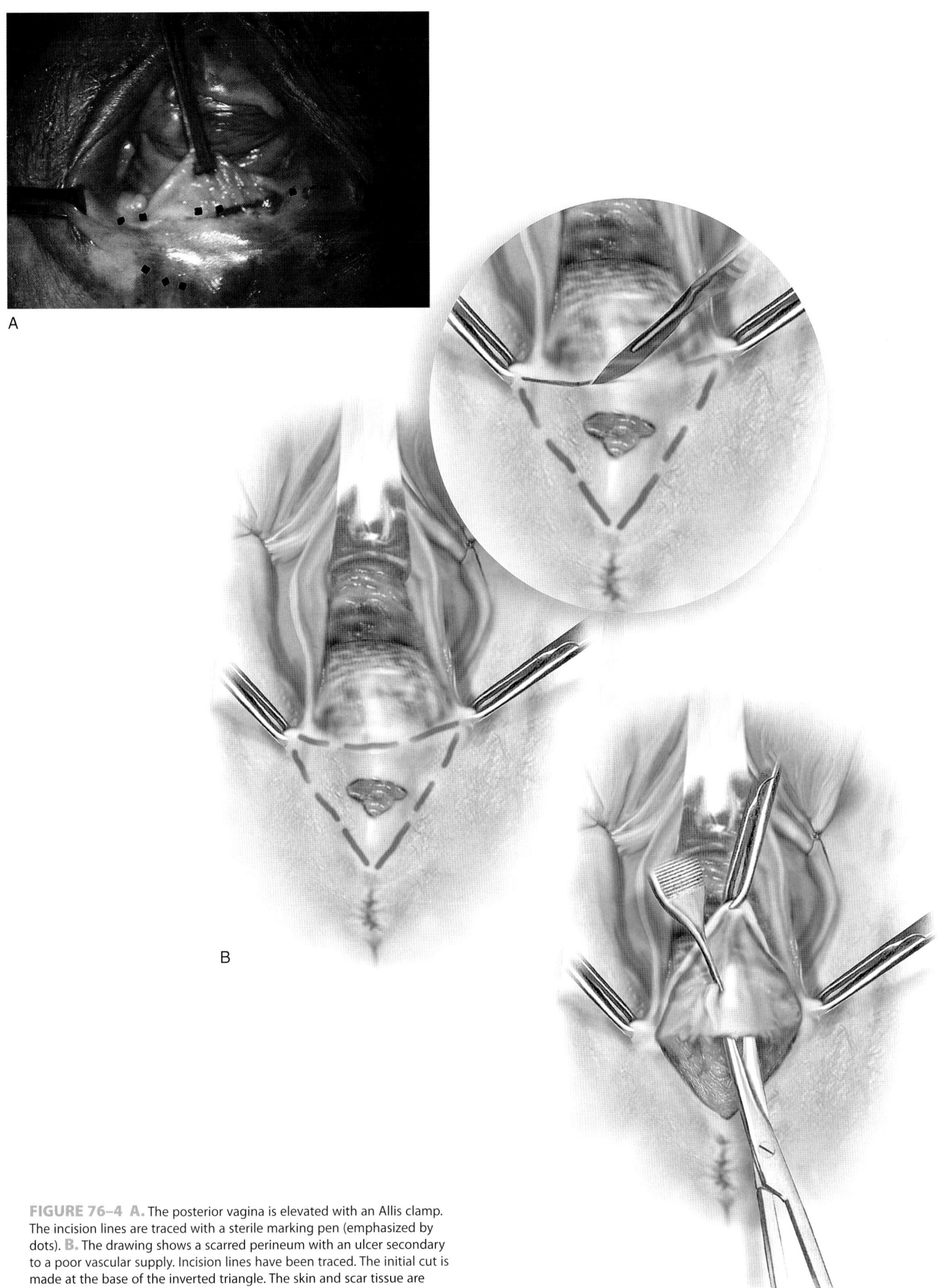

A

B

**FIGURE 76–4  A.** The posterior vagina is elevated with an Allis clamp. The incision lines are traced with a sterile marking pen (emphasized by dots). **B.** The drawing shows a scarred perineum with an ulcer secondary to a poor vascular supply. Incision lines have been traced. The initial cut is made at the base of the inverted triangle. The skin and scar tissue are dissected with Metzenbaum scissors.

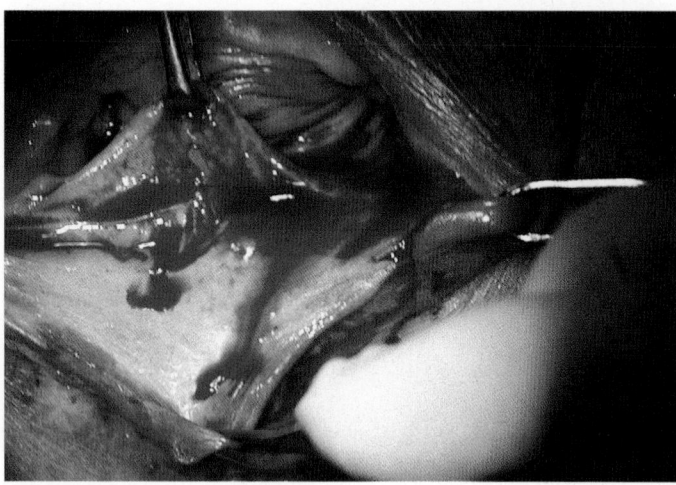

**FIGURE 76–5** The incision is made across the posterior, lower vagina. The area has been previously injected with a 1:100 vasopressin solution.

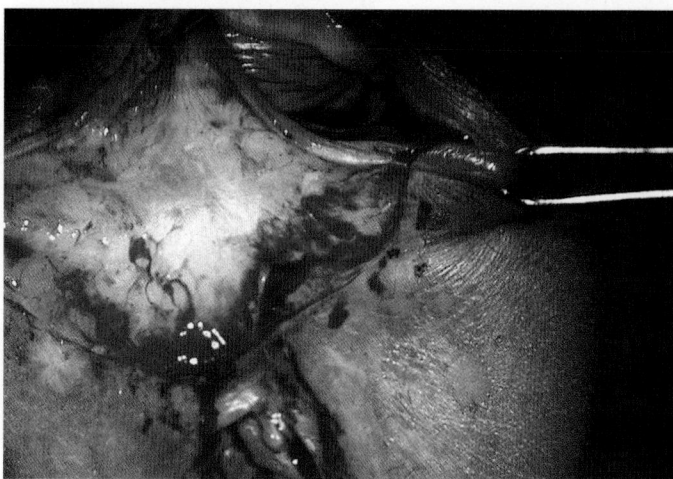

**FIGURE 76–6** Beginning at the apex of the triangle located on the perineum, the skin and underlying connective tissue are sharply dissected in a superior direction.

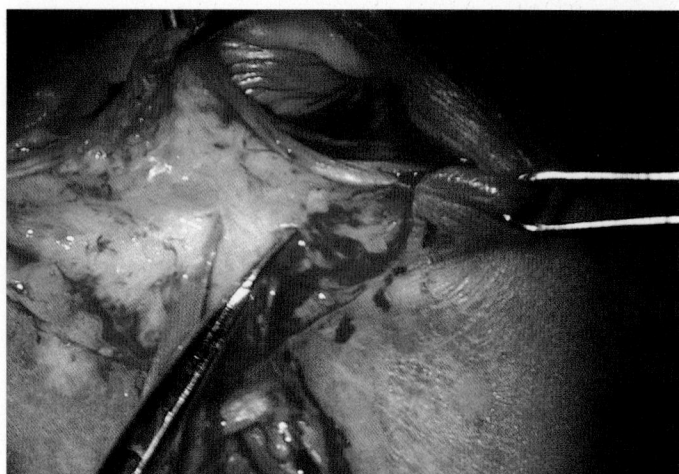

**FIGURE 76–7** Scar tissue is sharply dissected with the surrounding connective tissue with the use of Stevens scissors.

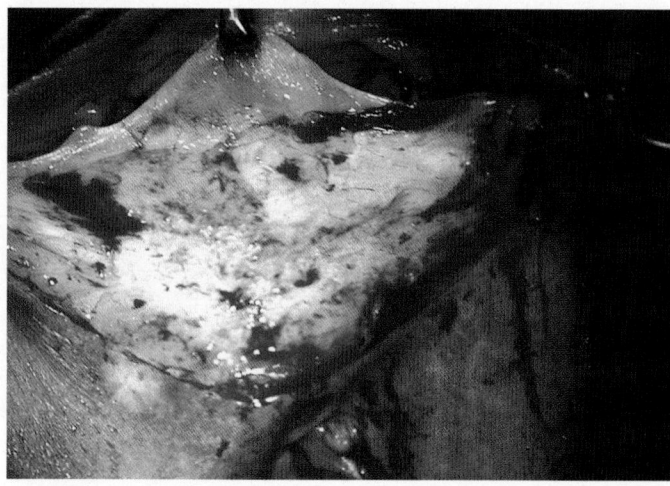

**FIGURE 76–8** The triangle of skin, connective tissue, and hard scar has been excised. Hemostasis is excellent. Any small bleeding points are suture-ligated with 4-0 Vicryl.

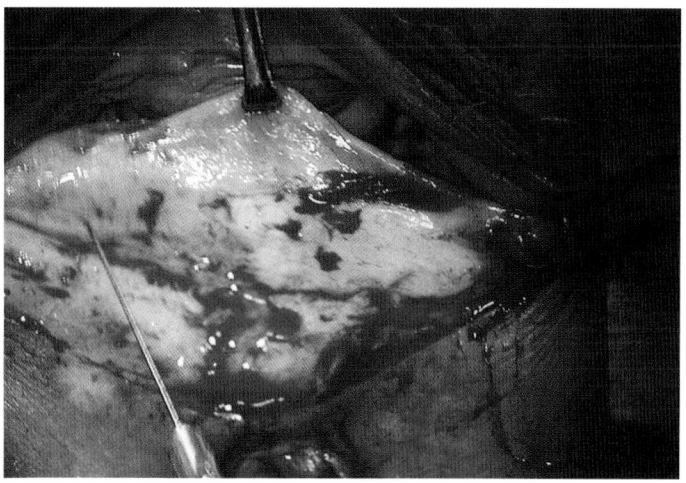

FIGURE 76–9 A second injection of 1:100 vasopressin (10 mL) is made into the vaginal margin and into the submucosa of the vagina.

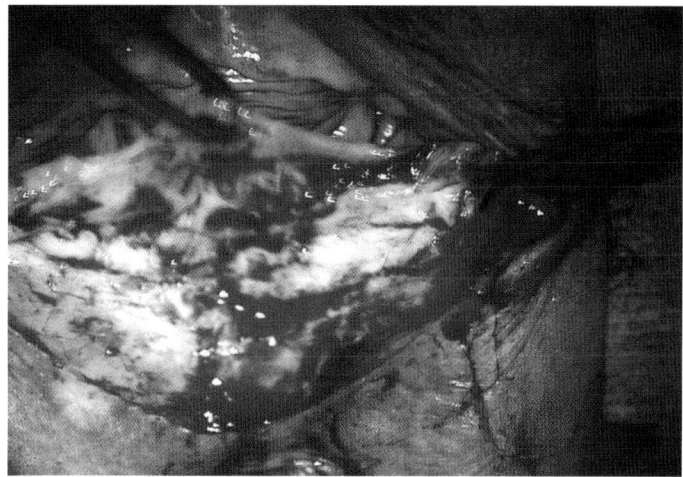

FIGURE 76–10 The vaginal margin is undermined with the use of Stevens scissors.

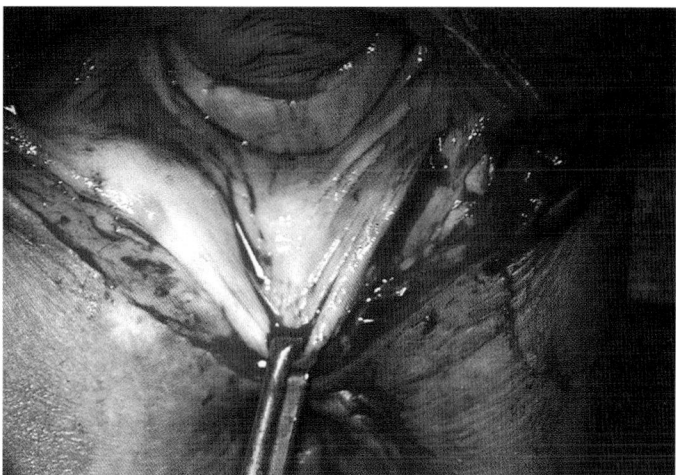

FIGURE 76–11 The mobility of the vagina is tested by applying an Allis clamp and advancing the vagina to the perineum. No tension should be required to mobilize the vagina.

UNIT 3 ■ SECTION C

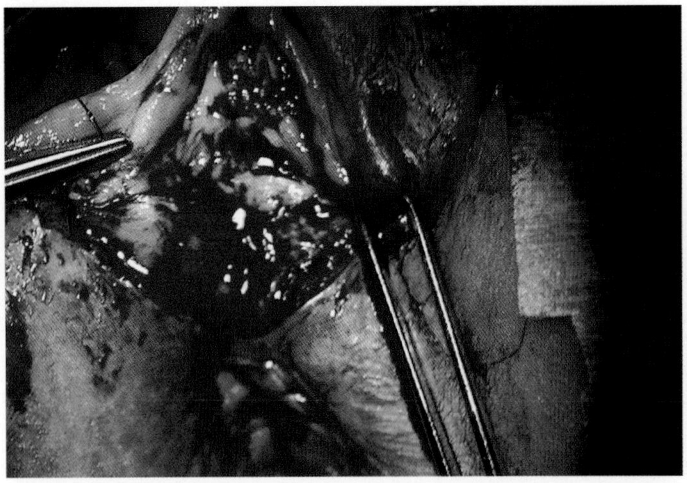

**FIGURE 76–12 A.** A layer of interrupted 3-0 Vicryl is placed through the perineal fascia and the vaginal submucosa. Closure is always transverse. **B.** When vaginal and perineal stromal sutures have been completed (i.e., extending across from right to left margin, side-to-side transverse closure), the wound is irrigated with sterile saline. **C.** Next, the vaginal mucosa is sutured to the perineal skin margin. Again, the orientation is similarly a transverse approximation without tension on the suture line. **D.** Final closure of the defect creates a smooth and wide entry into the vagina. The blood supply to this area is excellent (i.e., via advanced vaginal tissue).

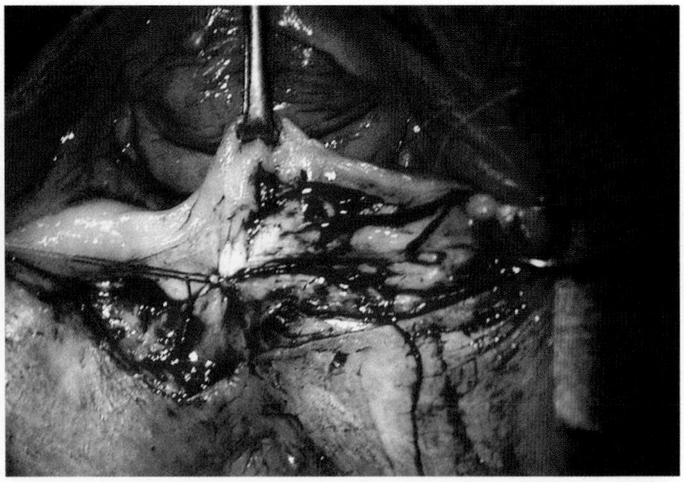

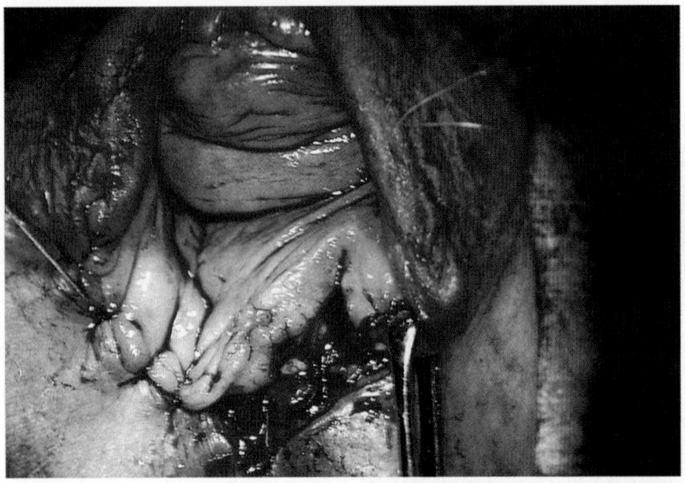

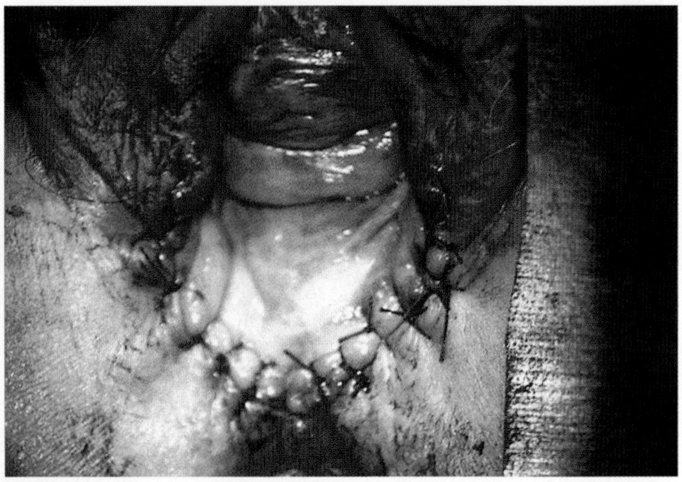

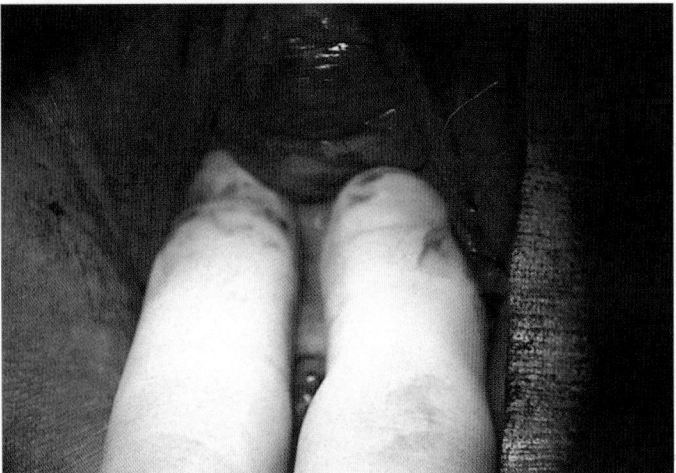

**FIGURE 76–13** The adequacy of the vaginal opening is checked at the end of the operative procedure.

# CHAPTER 77

# Benign Lesions of the Groin and the Canal of Nuck

*Michael S. Baggish*

## Hidradenitis and Other Groin Lesions

The most common lesions the gynecologist will encounter in the groin are enlarged lymph nodes, usually secondary to drainage from the inferior extremity or the neighboring vulva. These rarely require surgical treatment. However, an enlarging solitary mass in the groin, particularly without any identifiable cause, requires exploration and possible excisional biopsy. Differential diagnoses include enlarging lymph node(s), myoma, and femoral hernia. Here, knowledge of the precise anatomy of the femoral triangle is essential. Draining sinuses involving the vulva or the groin may be associated with a variety of disorders. Excisional biopsy may be required to make a diagnosis (Fig. 77–1A through D). Clearly, venereal causes should be excluded first by blood tests, smears, and punch biopsy. Disorders such as syphilis, lymphopathia venerea, and lymphogranuloma inguinale may be associated with sinus-like purulent drainage from matter and enlarged groin nodes. Treatment of these conditions is medical. Tuberculosis also may be associated with draining vulvar and inguinal sinuses. Again, this disorder may require that a generous excisional biopsy be performed and a portion of the tissue be sent for culture, while the remainder is sent to pathology for routine and acid-fast stains. Finally, infection of the apocrine sweat glands (hidradenitis) leads to persistent and chronic purulent draining sinuses in the vulva and groin (Fig. 77–2A through C). Additionally, this disorder may be seen in the axilla. These modified sweat glands may penetrate deeply into the underling stroma and typically plunge into the fat. Treatments for this disorder consist of antibiotics, retinoids, and/or surgery. Surgical excision is wide, with deep margins to eliminate the infected vulvar and inguinal tissues (Fig. 77–3A, B). The wounds may be left open after excision. In the latter instance, healing, of course, is by secondary intention (Fig. 77–3C through H). The wound site initially should be covered with wet-to-dry dressings. Longer term, the patient should sit in salt water (Instant Ocean) tub baths 3 times daily and should cover the operative site with silver sulfadiazine (Silvadene) cream. Alternatively, excised sites may be closed if the margins can be mobilized without undue tension (Fig. 77–4A through I). The patient should be placed on antibiotics (after the wound is cultured) and in Instant Ocean tub soaks 2 or 3 times daily.

## Lesions of the Canal of Nuck

Unilateral swelling of the labium majus may be due to a variety of nonsurgical disorders. The absence of inflammation and early pain selects out many nonsurgical causes. Several common surgical disorders should be borne in mind: cyst of the canal of Nuck, hernia into the canal of Nuck, myoma, and lipoma originating from structures in and around the canal. Transillumination may aid in the differentiation of a cystic from a solid mass preoperatively. Exploration, removal, and, in the case of hernia, correction are performed by making a vertical incision into the labium majus (Fig. 77–5A). The incision should be made above and to the lateral or medial side of the lesion. Once the subcutaneous tissue has been reached, 0 Vicryl traction sutures or Allis clamps are placed at the upper and lower margins of the mass. The anterior and lateral margins of the mass are completely dissected (Fig. 77–5B). Blood vessels are clamped and suture-ligated with 3-0 or 4-0 Vicryl. Next, the medial, posterior, and inferior margins of the mass are freed. The mass is carefully entered to ensure that no underlying intestine is present. If the mass is solid (e.g., a lipoma), it is simply excised (Fig. 77–5C). If the mass is cystic, the final upper margin of the mass is dissected and the upper opening is closed with a 3-0 nylon purse string suture, after which the entire cystic mass is excised. The wound is closed in layers with 3-0 Vicryl sutures (Fig. 77–5D, E). The skin likewise is closed with 3-0 Vicryl sutures. The wound is dressed with a nonadherent dressing covered by a pressure dressing and is taped.

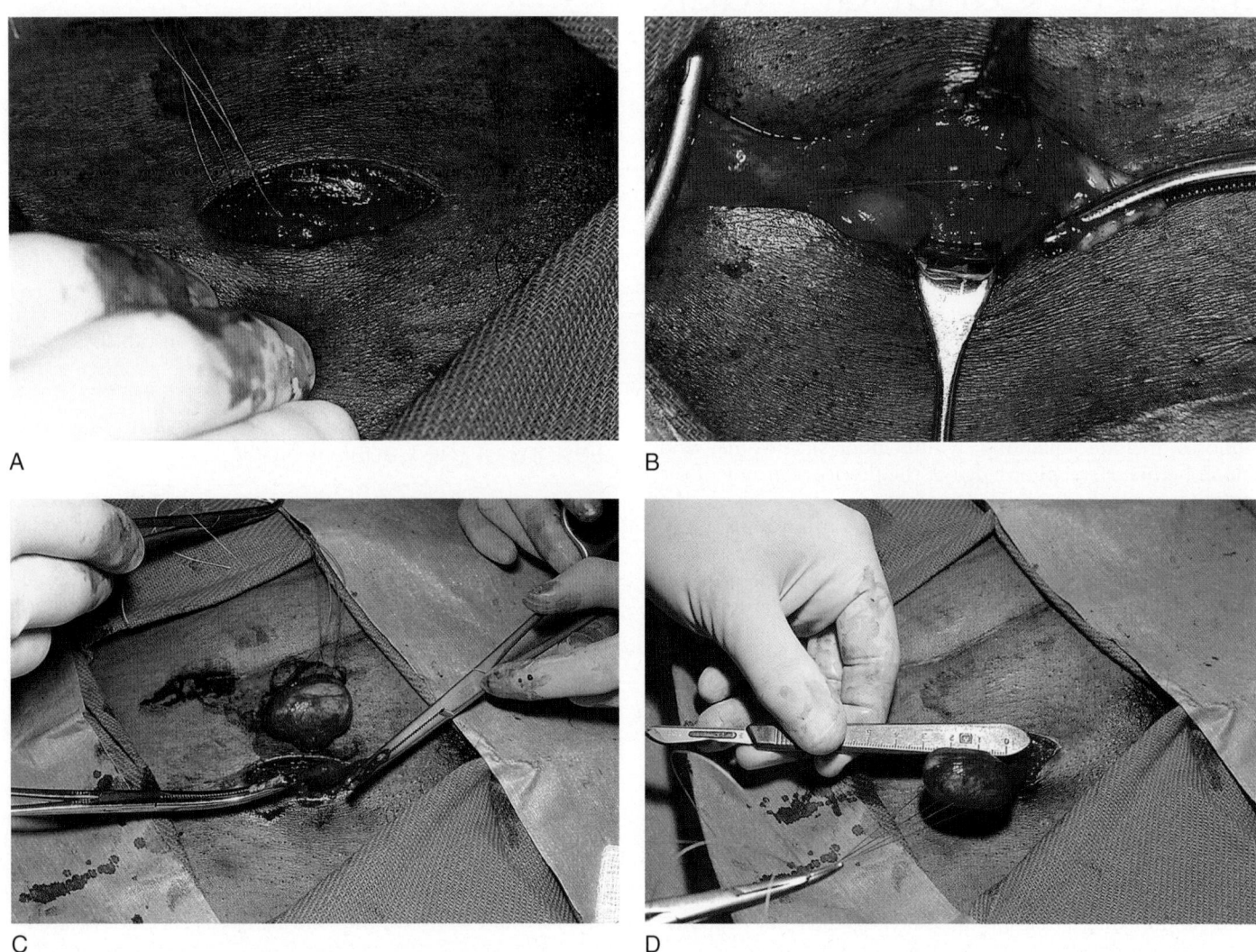

A

B

C

D

**FIGURE 77–1 A.** This patient presented with a painful, firm, 3-cm lesion in the left groin. Inspection revealed no vulvar or inferior extremity lesion to account for what was thought to be an enlarged inguinal lymph node. Exploration of the groin was indicated. A 3- to 4-cm incision is made in the groin over the lesion. **B.** The incision is carried deeply into the fat. Hemostasis is secured with mosquito clamps and 3-0 Vicryl suture-ligatures. Retraction is obtained with the use of vein retractors. **C.** The mass is isolated and cut out with Metzenbaum scissors. The base is clamped with mosquito clamps. It is obvious that the mass is not a lymph node but instead is a myoma. **D.** The myoma measures $2\frac{1}{2}$ cm and was proved by histologic evaluation to be benign. The wound is closed in layers with 3-0 or 4-0 Vicryl sutures in interrupted fashion.

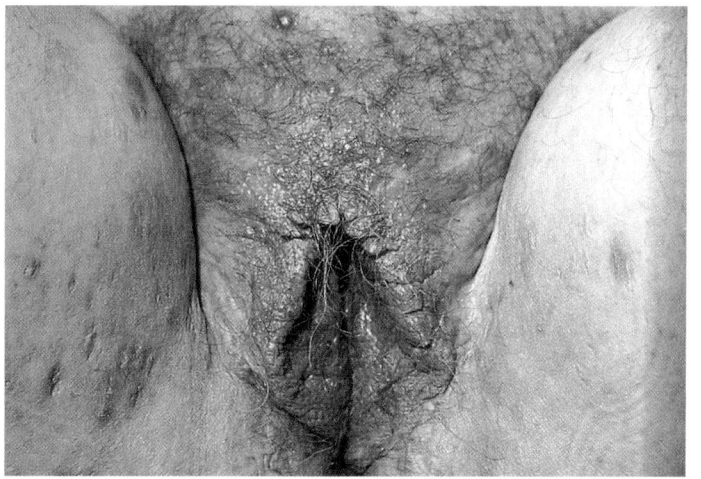

A

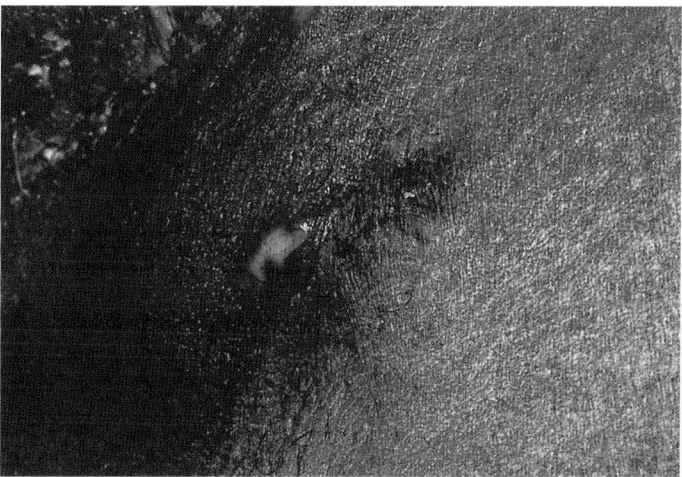

B

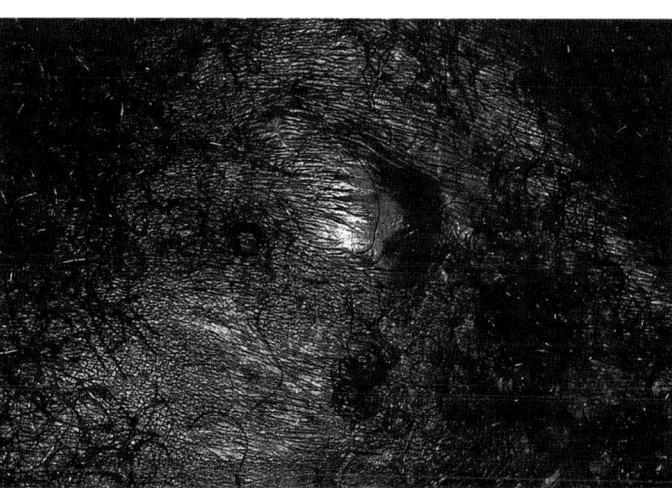

C

**FIGURE 77–2  A.** This patient suffered from persistent and recurring abscesses and draining sinuses through the mons and the groin. The appearance, together with the history, is highly suggestive of hidradenitis. A deep-wedge biopsy in the mons confirmed the diagnosis histologically. **B.** Close-up photo of the groin of another patient with hidradenitis. Note the pus draining from a deeply probed sinus. **C.** Another area in the groin of the patient shown in part **B.** The elevated "blister" of skin represents a sinus, which will shortly erupt and drain.

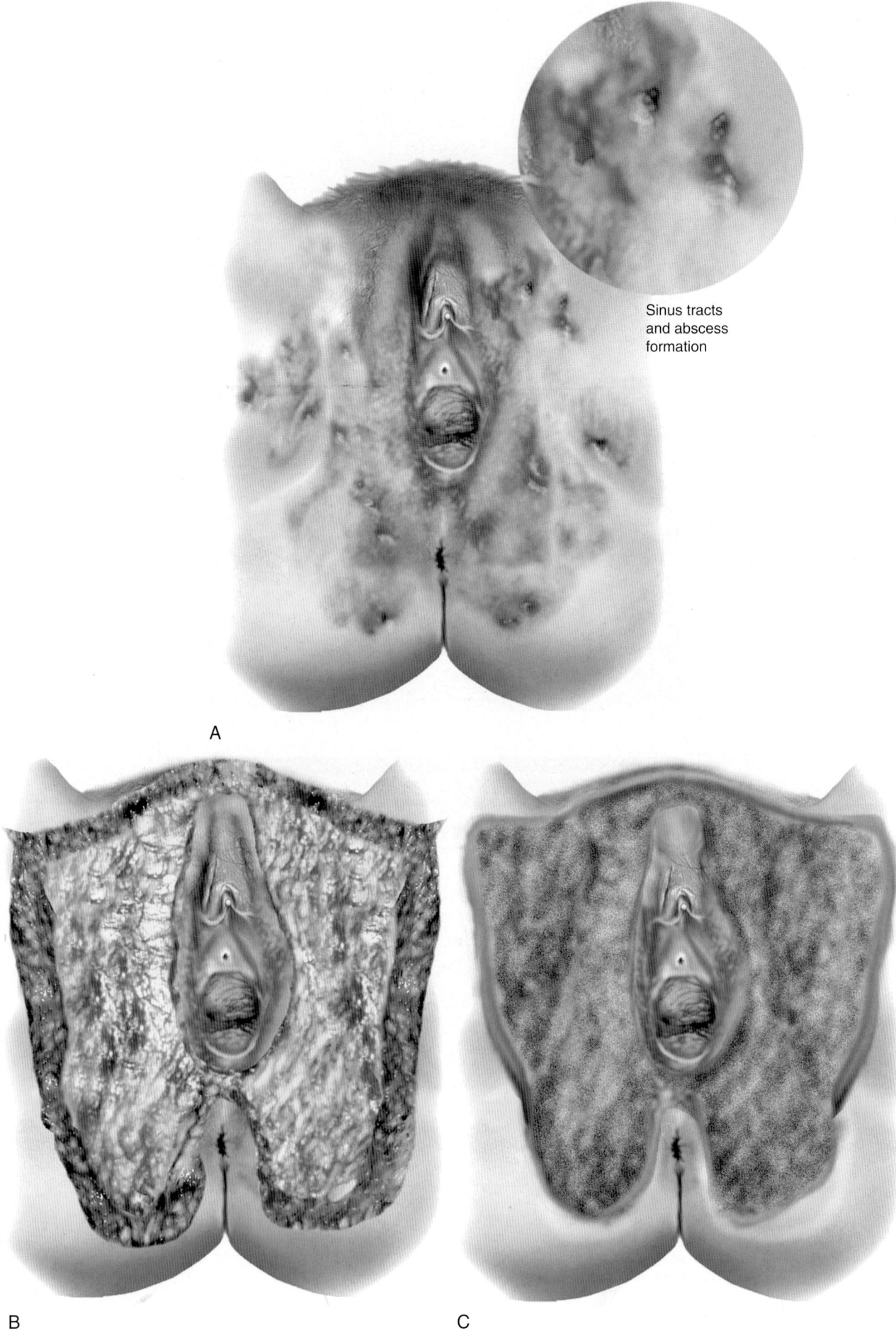

Sinus tracts
and abscess
formation

A

B                                        C

**FIGURE 77–3  A.** Hidradenitis must be widely and deeply excised. **B.** The entire affected area, including the mons and the groin, must be dissected, including the upper (ICM) layer of the subcutaneous tissue, and removed en masse. Less radical treatment invariably will result in recurrence. **C.** The wound must be carefully managed in the postoperative course. Because it cannot be grafted, it should heal from the bottom upward by granulation. All patients are covered with antibiotics administered first 1 hour preoperatively. Oral clindamycin is administered postoperatively for 1 week (300 mg every 6 hours).

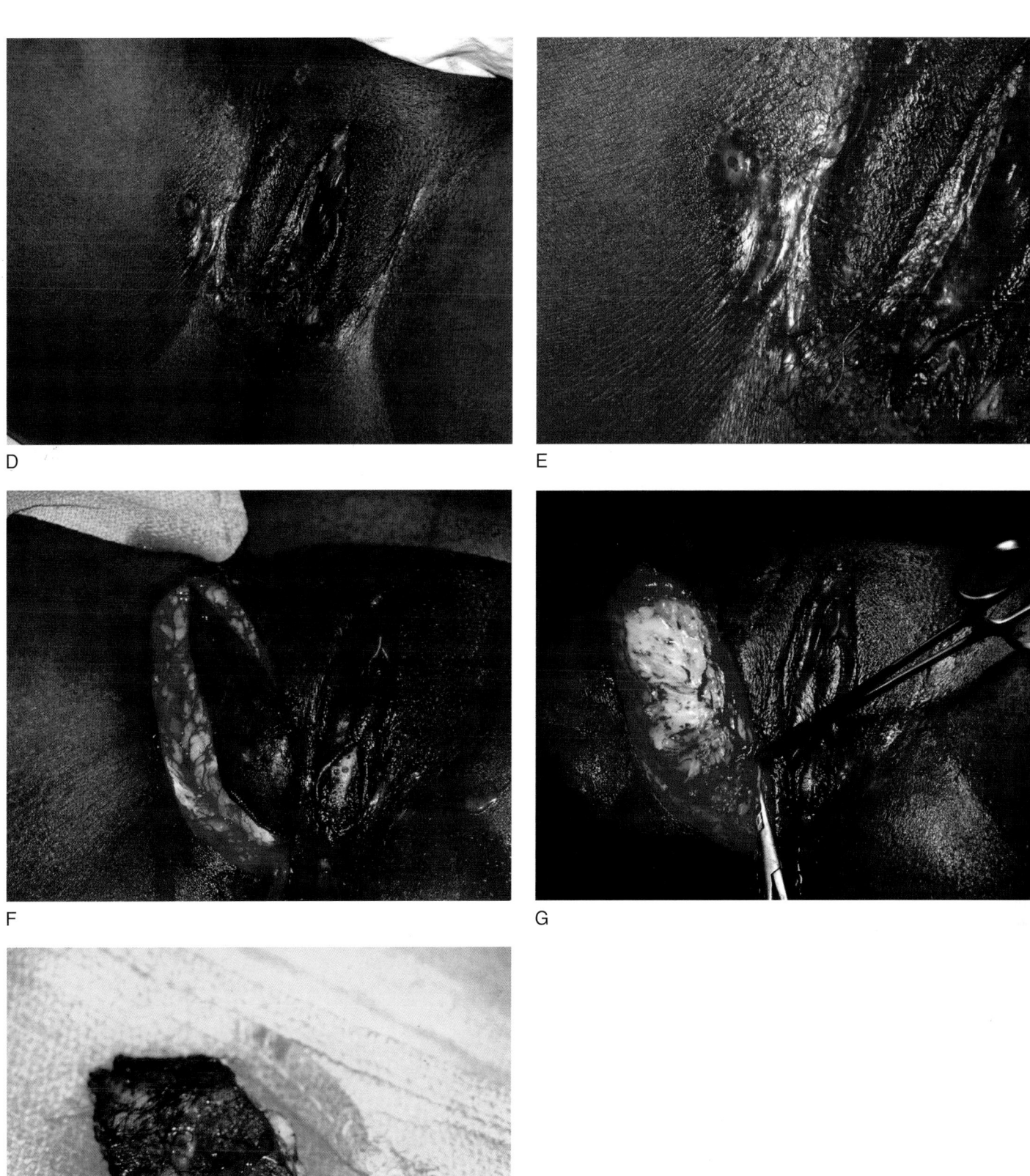

**FIGURE 77-3, cont'd** **D.** This patient presented with chronic draining sinuses emanating from the labia, mons, and groin. **E.** Close-up view of blebs, open lesions, and fissures. **F.** A deep initial incision is made into the right groin and is carried into the lower half of the right labium majus. **G.** The excision has been completed, thereby removing the sinus tracts and the underlying sweat glands. **H.** The large excised gross pathology specimen is shown here.

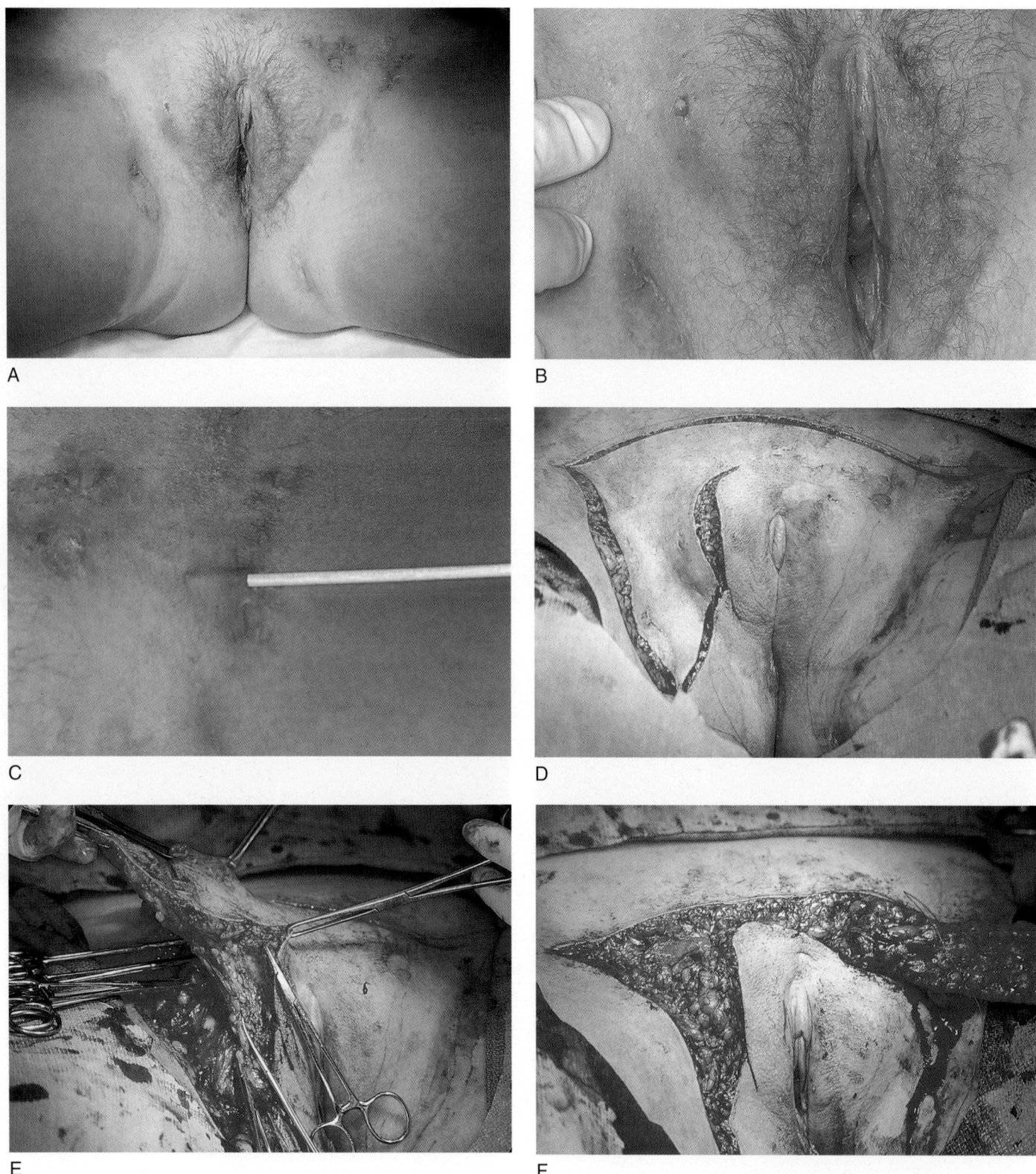

**FIGURE 77–4 A.** The patient in the lithotomy position shows scarring, sinus formation in the vulva, groin, and mons and buttock. **B.** Close-up view of a draining vulvar lesion and scar formation in the crural region. The pus tested positive for *Staphylococcus aureus*. **C.** A cotton-tipped application stick is placed into a draining sinus tract. **D.** The treatment plan calls for deep and wide excision of the recurrently infected tissues. The knife-cut outlines the wide margins of the proposed tissue resection. **E.** The resection begins in the right groin and proceeds from lateral to medial. **F.** The tissue resection is finished on the right side of the patient. Unaffected areas are spared.

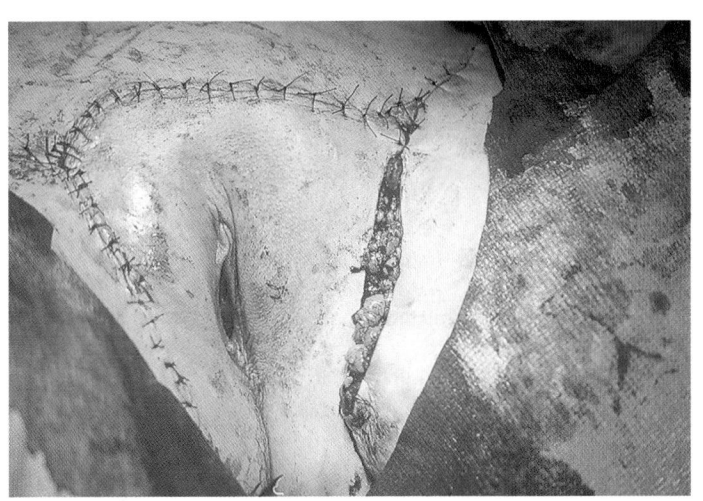

G

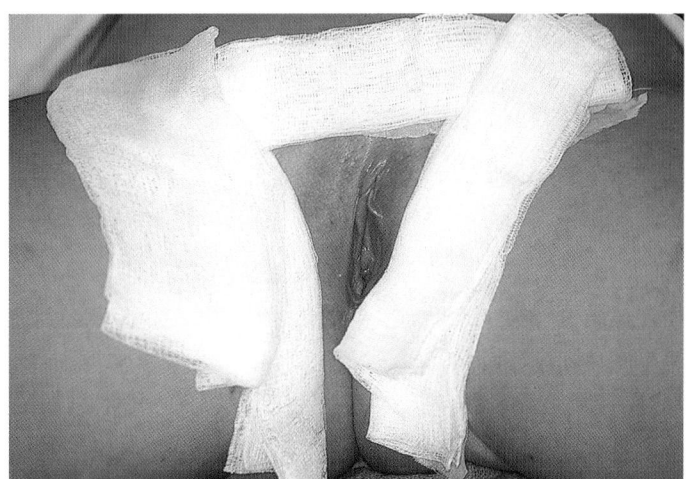

H

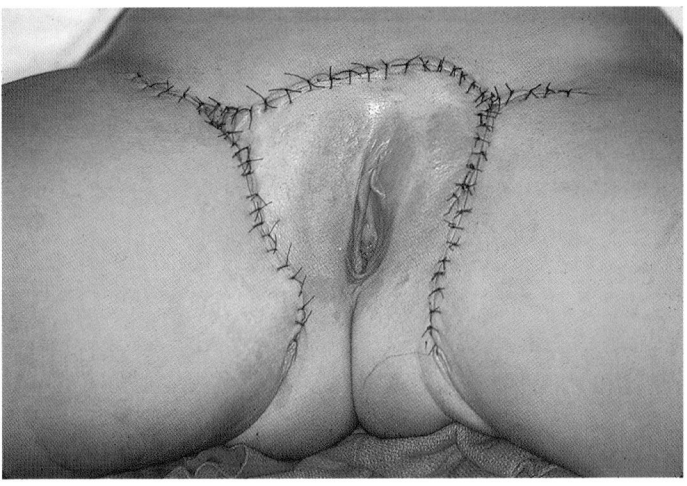

I

**FIGURE 77–4, cont'd   G.** The wound is partially closed without any skin edge tension. **H.** The closed wound is covered with Xeroform fine-mesh gauze, which, in turn, is covered with sterile gauze. **I.** The closure of this extensive excision is complete. All diseased tissue has been deeply cut away and sent to pathology.

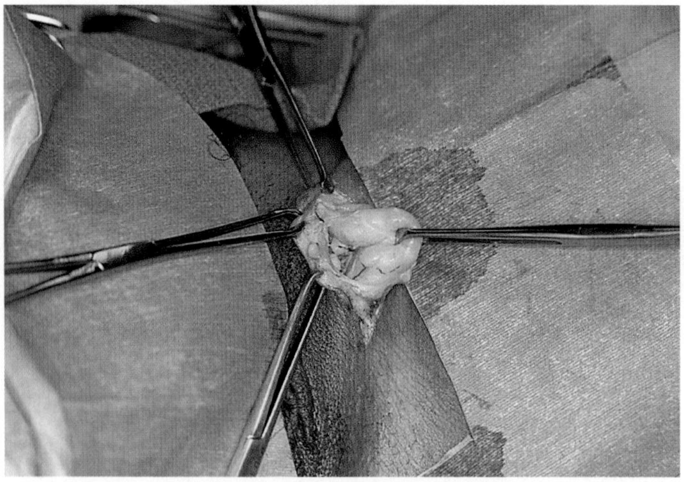

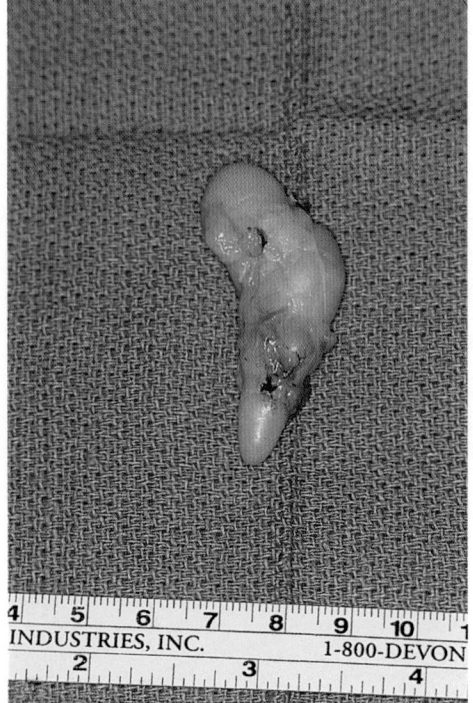

**FIGURE 77–5  A.** A deep, soft mass was palpated in the upper portion of the labium majus. A vertical incision is made above the mass and is carried deeply into the fat. The margins of the wound are retracted with 0 Vicryl traction sutures or with Allis clamps. An Allis clamp grasps the upper portion of the mass, and traction is placed on the mass. In this case, the lesion was not a cyst but rather a lipoma. **B.** The tissues surrounding the mass are clamped with tonsil clamps and are suture-ligated. The lesion is freed from the surrounding tissue by sharp dissection with the use of Metzenbaum scissors. **C.** The mass is delivered from the incision. Careful inspection reveals no herniated intestine. **D.** The fat is closed with interrupted 3-0 Vicryl sutures. The skin is likewise sutured with interrupted 3-0 Vicryl sutures. **E.** The lipoma is sent to pathology to ensure that it is benign.

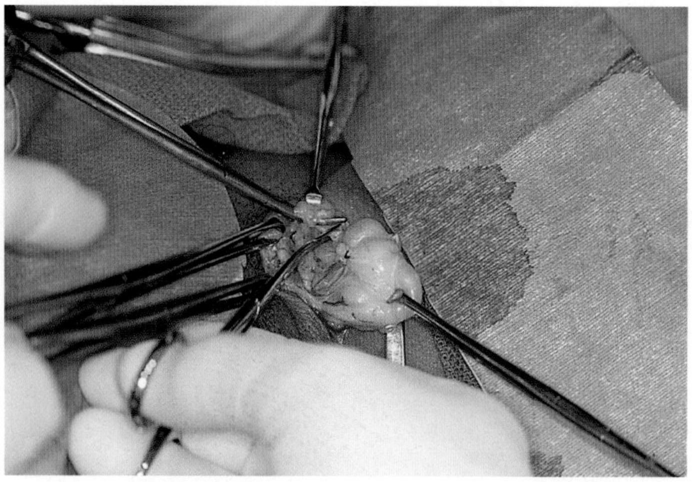

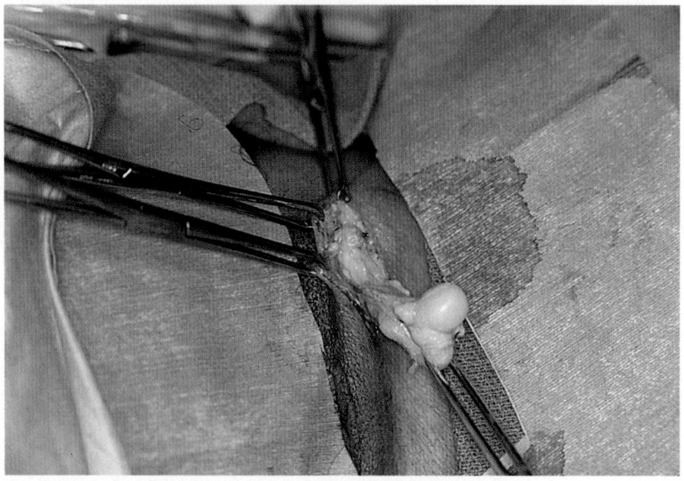

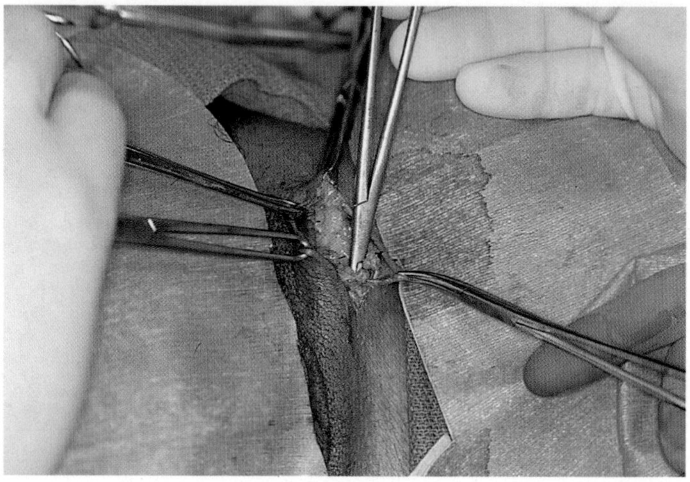

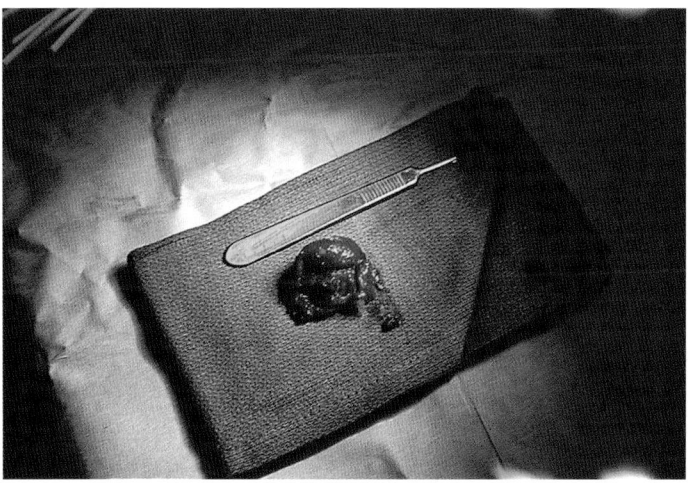

FIGURE 78–5  The cyst is completely excised. From the leaking foul-smelling material, it is identified grossly as a sebaceous cyst. The cyst is placed in fixative and sent to pathology.

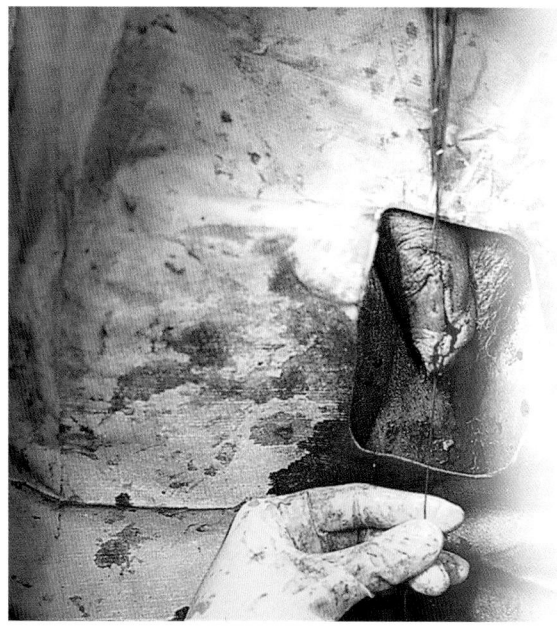

FIGURE 78–6  The wound is closed in layers with interrupted 3-0 Vicryl sutures.

## Hidradenoma

This usually benign sweat gland tumor creates a smooth, elevated, firm nodularity on the vulvar skin surface (Fig. 78-7). It looks like a firm sebaceous cyst. The tumor is small (i.e., <1 cm). The lesion should be excised by circumscribing an ellipse of skin with a margin of 2 to 3 mm around the mass and extending the incision deeper into the subcutaneous tissue. The skin and tumor are grasped with an Allis clamp, and traction is applied with the use of Stevens scissors. The deep subcutaneous fat is dissected free from the base of the tumor, and the entire small mass of tissue containing the lesion is removed. Histopathologically, the appearance of the tumor under the low-power lens of the microscope is ominous because of the glandular complexity (Fig. 78-8). However, higher-power lens inspection reveals the cells and nuclei to be clearly benign (Fig. 78-9).

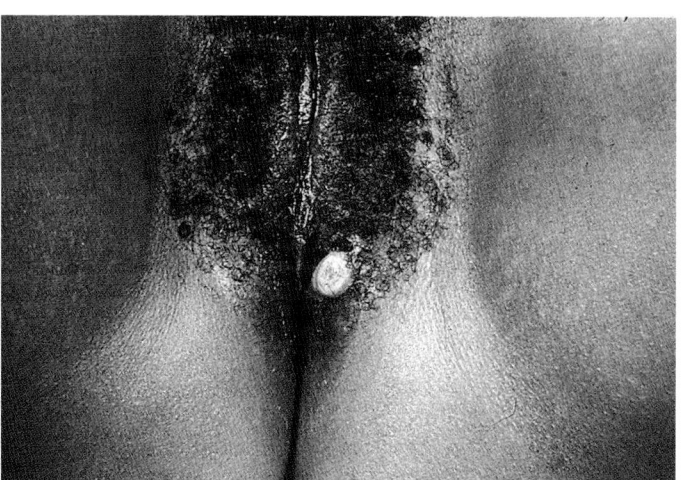

FIGURE 78–7  The hidradenoma is a solid, raised tumor originating in the sweat glands of the vulva. The lesion is fleshy and well circumscribed. It is also painless. The lesion may be excised in a manner identical to that described for sebaceous cysts.

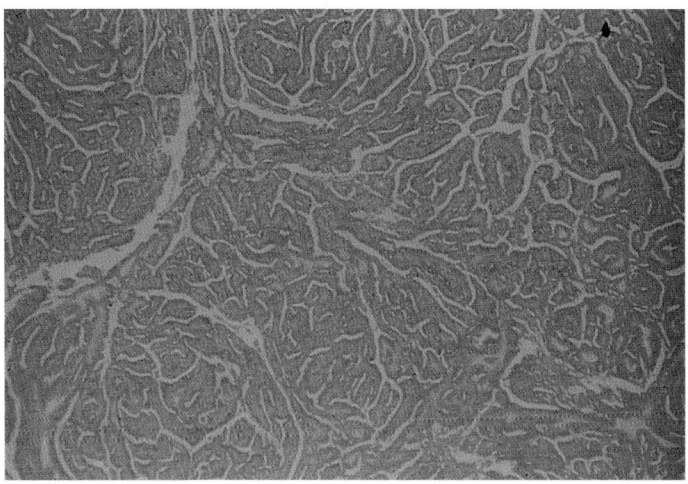

FIGURE 78–8  This low-power microscopic section shows a complex glandular proliferation; it appears to be atypical at least and at worst, malignant.

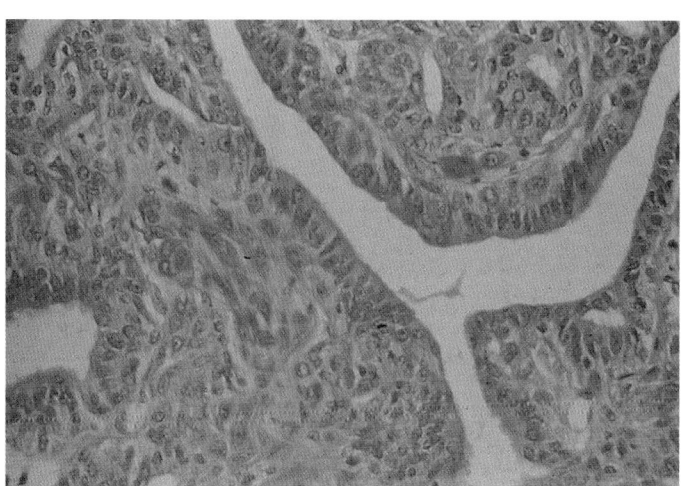

FIGURE 78–9  High-power microscopic study reveals well-organized glands and normal cytology. The diagnosis is benign hidradenoma.

## Labial Fusion

This problem occurs most commonly in the very young (pre-adolescent girls) (Fig. 78-10) or the elderly. Once firm fusion has occurred, it is unlikely that the application of topical estrogen will relieve the disorder. Surgical separation is usually required. The line of fusion *must* be accurately identified. This is accomplished with the aid of a magnifying loupe or an operating microscope. A small probe may be placed in the artificial pouch created by the fusion (i.e., the probe is placed behind [deep to] the fused labia). Pressure is exerted outward to stretch the surface of the labia; this in turn helps to identify the points of original fusion. A knife (No. 15 blade) cuts the stretched skin over the probe and down to the probe (Fig. 78-11). After the labia are separated, the edges are closed with a continuous 4-0 polydioxanone (PDS) suture on either side (Fig. 78-12). The suture line is covered with a topical estrogen cream, which is reapplied 2 or 3 times per day during the postoperative and recovery periods.

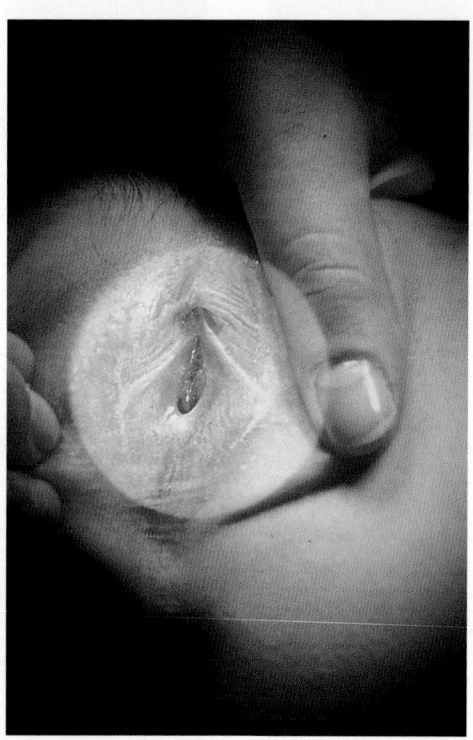

**FIGURE 78-10** This adolescent girl demonstrates fusion of the labia minora.

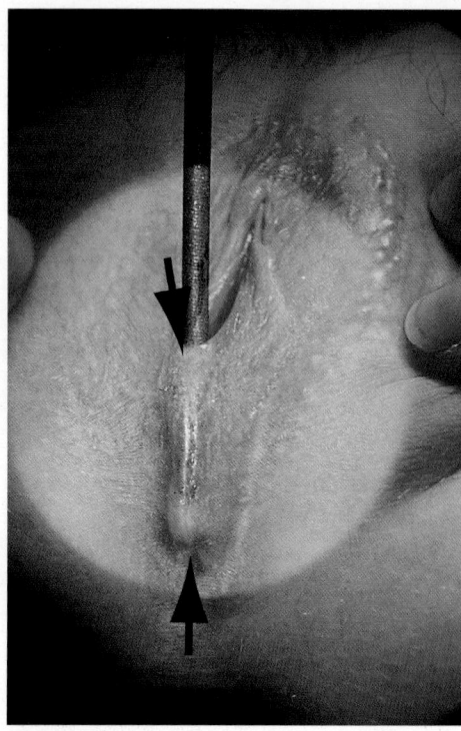

**FIGURE 78-11** A probe has been placed within the pocket created by the fusion. The arrows show the direction of the incision that will be made over the probe (i.e., with the probe used as a backstop).

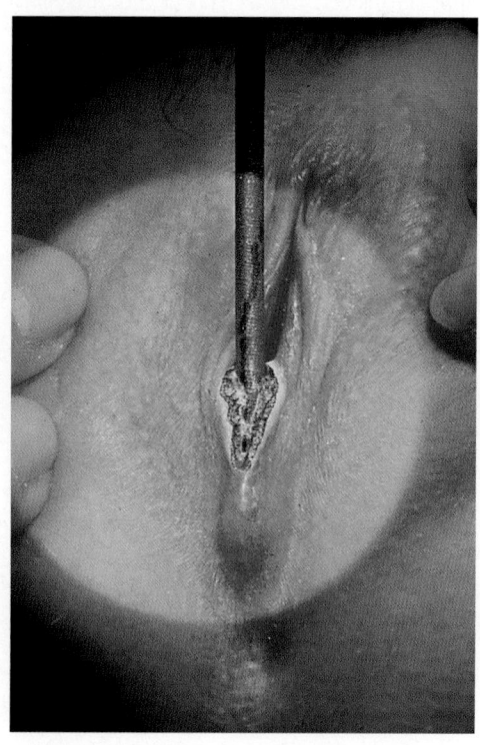

**FIGURE 78-12** An incision is made with a carbon dioxide ($CO_2$) laser; however, the same cut may be made with a scalpel. The edges are closed with a running 4-0 polydioxanone (PDS) suture. The wound is covered with topical estrogen to keep the respective edges from agglutinating.

## Draining Vulvar Lesions

Draining vulvar lesions cause a variety of pathologies, including venereal lesions and sinus tracts (Fig. 78–13). Although the first, nonsurgical approach consists of culture of the drainage for a variety of microorganisms (including fungi), diagnosis may be difficult. Drainage points should be explored with the use of lachrymal probes to determine whether a tract exists and where it goes. If a tract is identified, radiologic examination may be helpful in identifying a possible fistula. In this case, the patient should be scheduled for fluoroscopy. A small-gauge vascular catheter is engaged into the sinus opening and is manipulated through the tract. Water-soluble dye is injected during real-time fluoroscopic examination to determine whether a connection with the intestine or another structure exists.

If no fistulous tract is demonstrated and no diagnosis has been made on the culture, then a wide and deep excision of the lesion should be performed (Fig. 78–14). The patient is given a general anesthetic and is placed in the lithotomy position, the skin is prepared, and the operative field is draped. A skin pen is used to mark the boundaries for the excision. The traced area is shallowly circumscribed with a knife (No. 15 scalpel). The cut is extended more deeply into the fat, and the wound edges are grasped with Allis clamps for traction. A wedge-shaped incision is completed on all sides of the lesion margins, and the mass is removed. Tissue samples are placed in sterile containers to be cultured. Special stains are ordered for the pathologic specimen, including Giemsa, silver, acid-fast, and fungal stains. Draining wounds occurring in immigrants from developing countries should carry a high index of suspicion for tuberculosis (Fig. 78–15 through 78–17).

If initial probing reveals a sinus tract to the gastrointestinal tract (e.g., to the anus), then before excision, the patient must undergo a bowel prep (Fig. 78–18). The author recommends the following:

1. Three days before surgery: Begin a low-residue diet.
2. Two days before surgery: Begin a full liquid diet.
3. The day before surgery: Start a clear liquid diet, and take the following medications: neomycin 1 g by mouth at 11 AM, 12 PM, and 6 PM; metronidazole 500 mg by mouth at 11 AM, 12 PM, and 6 PM; Fleets Phospho-Soda 2.5 oz mixed with 4 oz of clear liquid (7-Up, lemonade, or water), followed by eight glasses of water to be completed by 1 PM; and metoclopramide (Reglan) 10 mg, one by mouth every 6 hours starting at 8 AM on the day before surgery (total, four tablets). The patient is anesthetized and is placed in the dorsal lithotomy position, and the skin and vagina are prepared. The operative site is draped. A probe is placed in the sinus tract, and the path of the tract is traced on the skin surface with a marking pen (Fig. 78–19). An incision is made on either side of the tract with a 5-mm margin on either side of the trace line. This cut is carried down deep to the palpable probe and is wedged inward below the tract. The entire sinus tract is excised (Fig. 78–20). The anal sphincter margins are grasped with Allis clamps. The anal mucosa is repaired with interrupted 2-0 chromic catgut sutures (Fig. 78–21). The sphincter is repaired inferiorly to superiorly with five or six 3-0 Vicryl sutures (Fig. 78–22). A Penrose drain is placed above the sphincter below the fat (i.e., superior to Colles' fascia). The fat is closed with interrupted 3-0 Vicryl sutures (Fig. 78–23). The skin is finally approximated with 3-0 Vicryl sutures. A large safety pin is placed into the terminal portion of the Penrose drain, and the edges of the drain are anchored to the skin with 3-0 chromic catgut sutures (Fig. 78–24). The wound is covered with silver sulfadiazine (Silvadene) cream, which the patient will apply 3 times daily and at bedtime during the postoperative recovery period. Crohn's disease may present with cutaneous vulvar fistulas. In this case, there may be multiple tracts, and wound breakdown is a significant risk. Consultation with the gastroenterologist should be carried out preoperatively and a therapeutic program instituted postoperatively if, in fact, the surgery proceeds at all.

## Vulvar Hemangiomas and Varicosities

Congenital hemangiomas and acquired varicosities may be troubling to patients not only because of their unsightly appearance but also because of their tendency to bleed as a result of even slight trauma (Fig. 78–25). The preferred treatment for these lesions is phototherapy with a selected-wavelength laser (Fig. 78–26A, B). The KTP laser coupled to a computer-controlled scanner is ideal for this type of surgery because the wavelength of this laser (532 nm) is very close to that of the light absorption of hemoglobin (Fig. 78–27). Similarly, the argon laser fits into this category. The scanner automatically exposes the laser energy (4 W) to the skin for a short time (30 to 60 msec) in several hundred pulses (Fig. 78–28). Thus, minimal surface skin effects are noted. In fact, the light skin of a white patient actually reflects away the laser energy. Because the selected absorption band corresponds to that of hemoglobin, the dilated vessels absorb the laser light selectively and undergo coagulation as well as slow obliteration. The end result consists of removal of the offending blood vessels and a nice cosmetic result with minimal discomfort, immediate recovery, low risk, and short hospitalization (Fig. 78–29). All cases may be performed with systemic analgesia and injection of local anesthesia. Postoperatively, the patient should cover the vulva with Silvadene or another suitable topical cream to keep the skin protected and moist. Treatments may be staged (i.e., three or four treatments over a period of months). The preferred interval between laser treatments is 1 month.

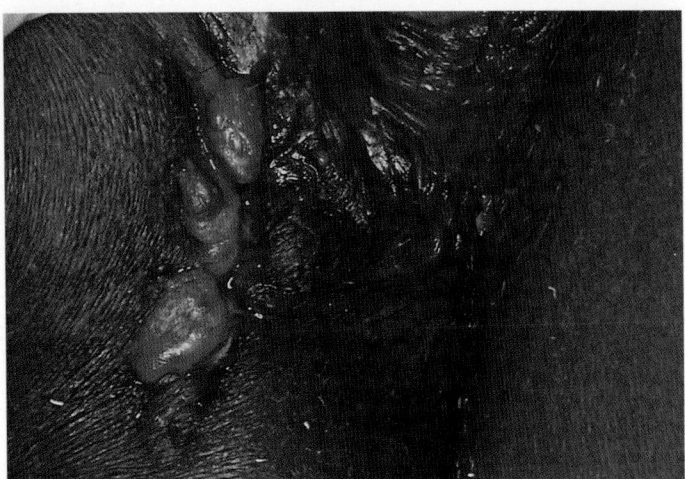

**FIGURE 78–13** This woman from Ethiopia presented with a fungating, draining lesion of the perineum. All cultures were negative.

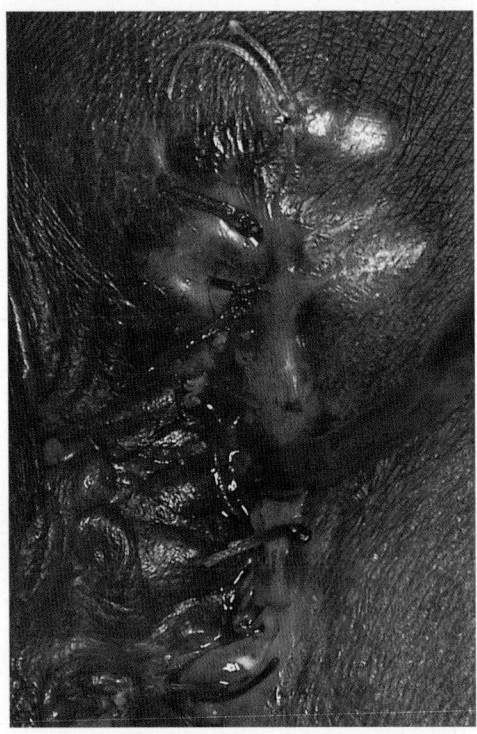

**FIGURE 78–14** A deep wedge biopsy excised the skin lesion and extended into the underlying fat. A fistulous tract was probed 8 cm deep, paralleling the colon. Fluoroscopic dye studies with the tract cannulated revealed no connection with the large or small intestine.

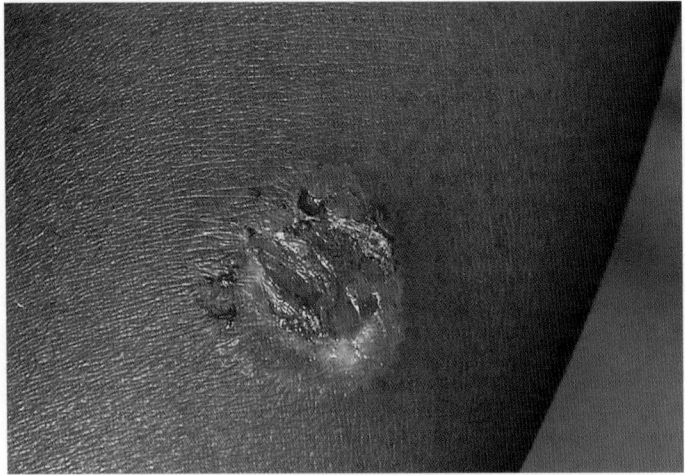

**FIGURE 78–15** The tuberculin skin test created 2 cm of induration and eventually ulcerated.

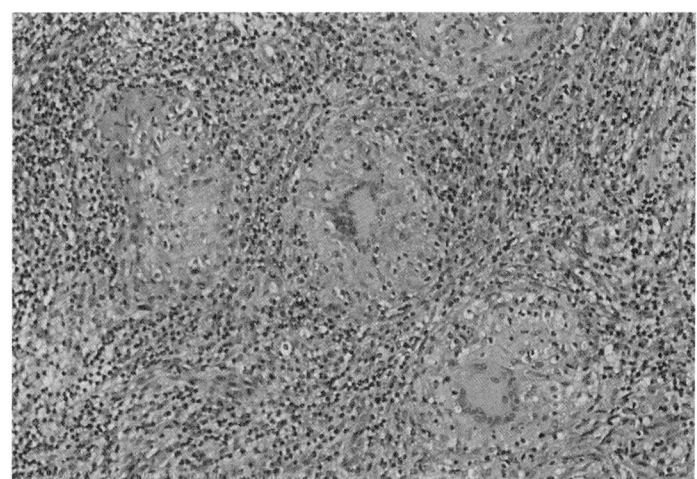

**FIGURE 78–16** Microscopic sections from the deep wedge excisional biopsy showed granulomas and Langerhans giant cells.

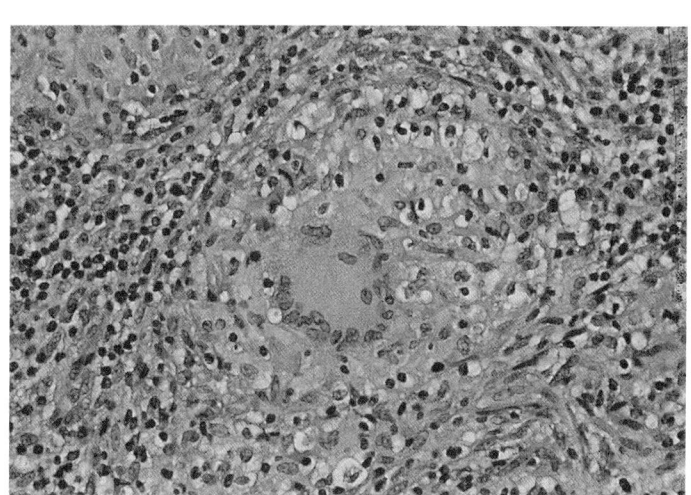

**FIGURE 78–17** High-power view of the giant cell within a granuloma. Note the peripheral arrangement of the nuclei. The patient was treated with antituberculosis medications.

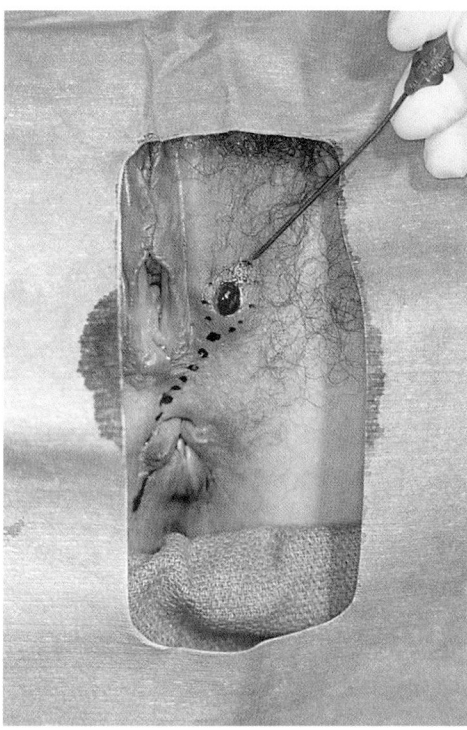

**FIGURE 78–18** The vulvar draining sinus was probed toward the anus. The marking pen dots indicate the direction of the sinus tract.

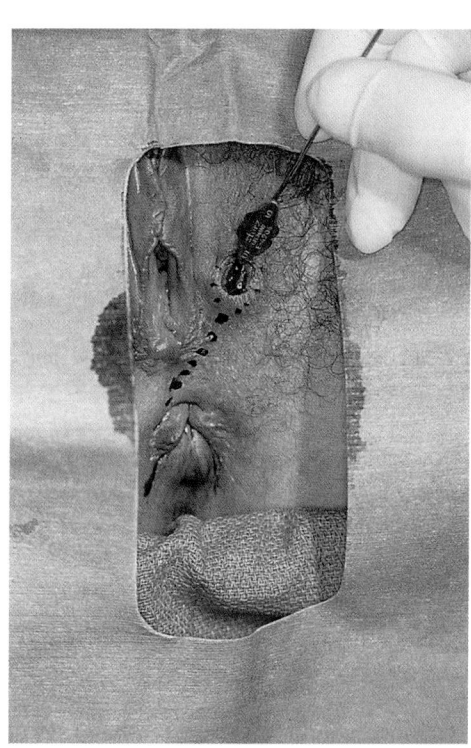

**FIGURE 78–19** The lacrimal probe has been engaged in the granulating sinus opening on the labium majus. The probe extends into the anus.

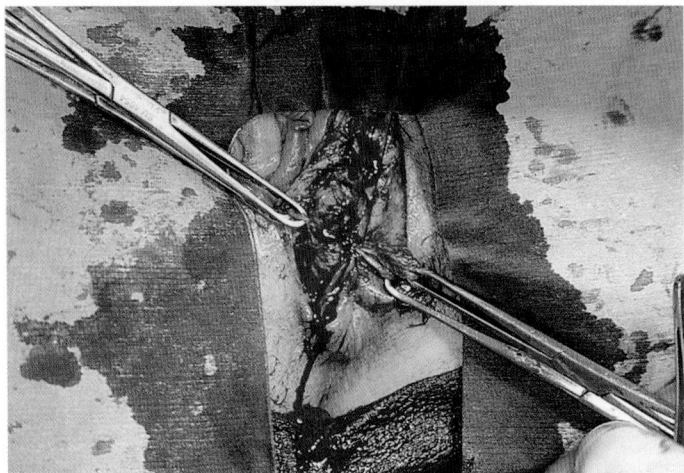

**FIGURE 78–20** The initial incision is made over the probe. The dissection continues through the external sphincter into the anus. The entire sinus tract is excised. The margins of the anus are held in the Allis clamps. Countertraction is produced by a single Allis clamp located at the vulvar skin margin.

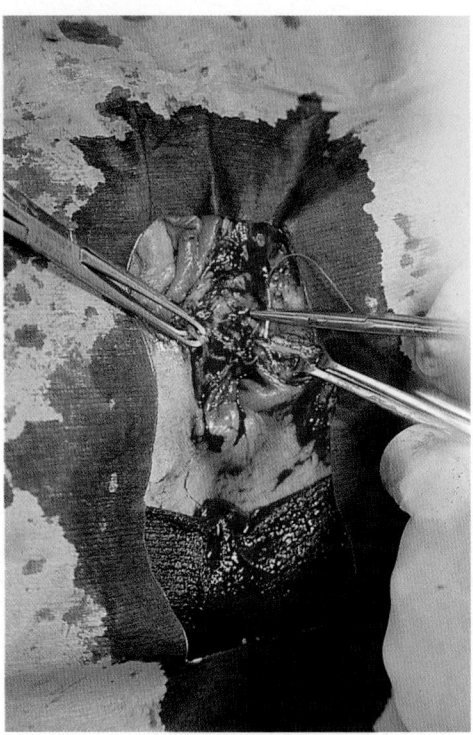

**FIGURE 78–21** The anal mucosa is repaired with interrupted 2-0 or 3-0 chromic catgut sutures.

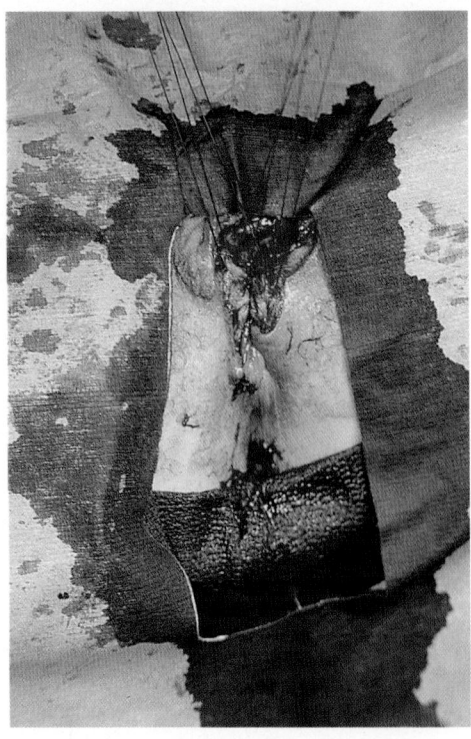

**FIGURE 78–22** The anal sphincter is repaired with 3-0 Vicryl sutures placed from the lowermost portion to the uppermost extreme of the sphincter.

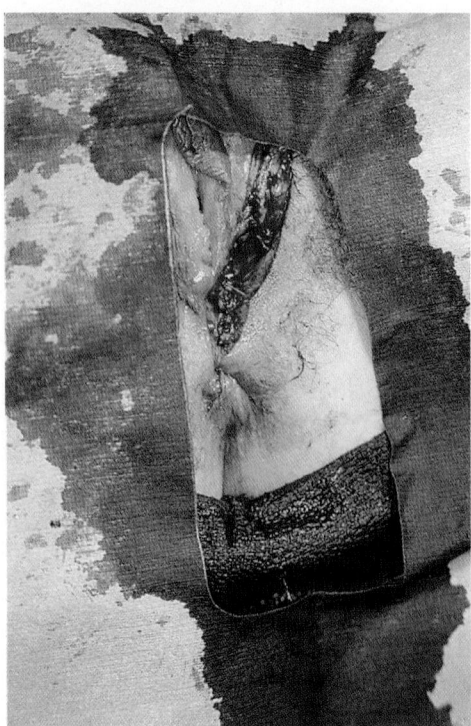

**FIGURE 78–23** The subcutaneous tissue is approximated with 3-0 Vicryl sutures.

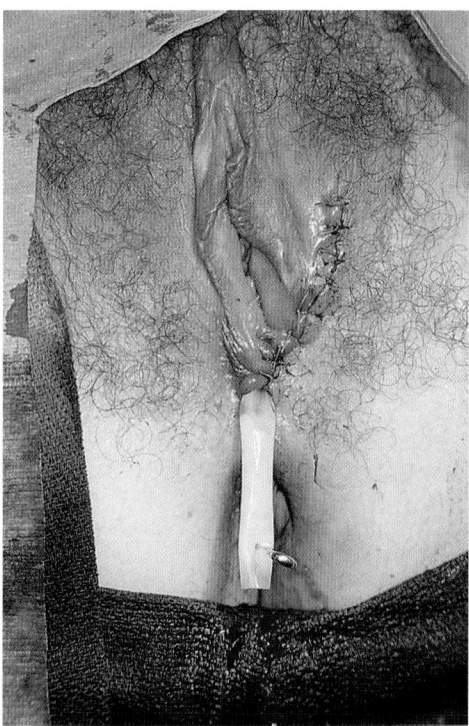

**FIGURE 78-24** A drain is placed above the sphincter repair below the fat but above Colles' fascial layer. The edges of the drain are sutured to the skin edges with two 3-0 catgut sutures. Note the large safety pin placed through the Penrose drain.

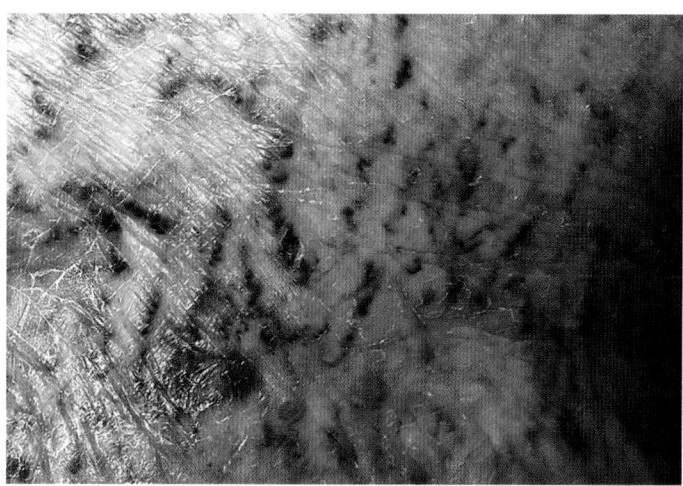

**FIGURE 78-25** Magnified view of vulvar skin demonstrating extensive varicosities. These lesions were acquired as a result of multiple childbearing episodes and a familial disposition to form varicosities.

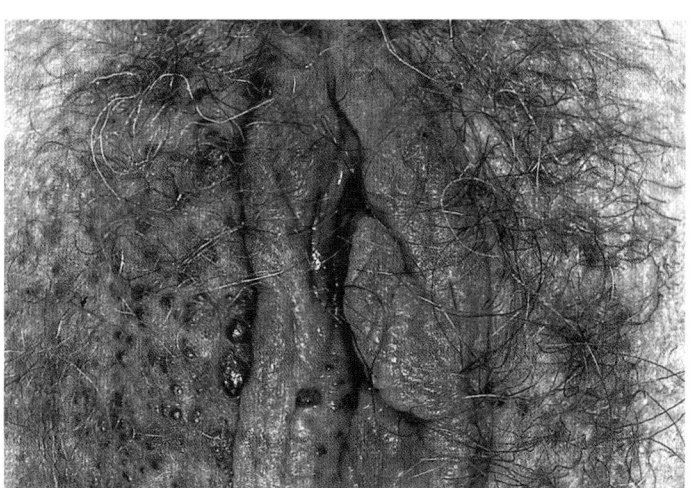

A

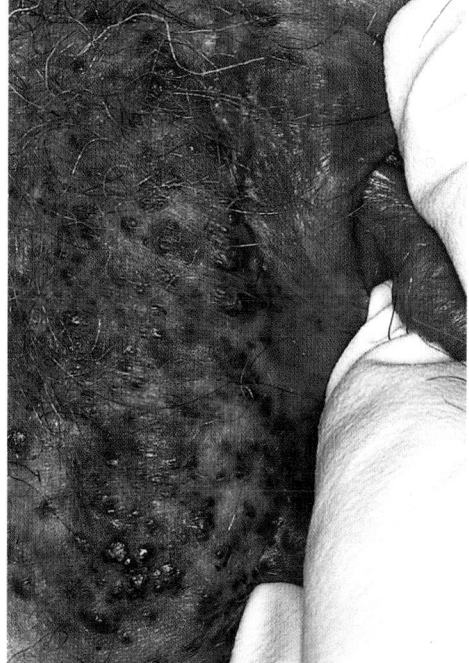

B

**FIGURE 78-26 A.** This young woman was afflicted with a congenital vulvar angioma affecting the labia minora and majora and the vestibule. The thin-walled vessels frequently burst, resulting in heavy vulvar bleeding. **B.** The labia majora were particularly affected. Note the grapelike cluster of vessels in the upper part of the picture.

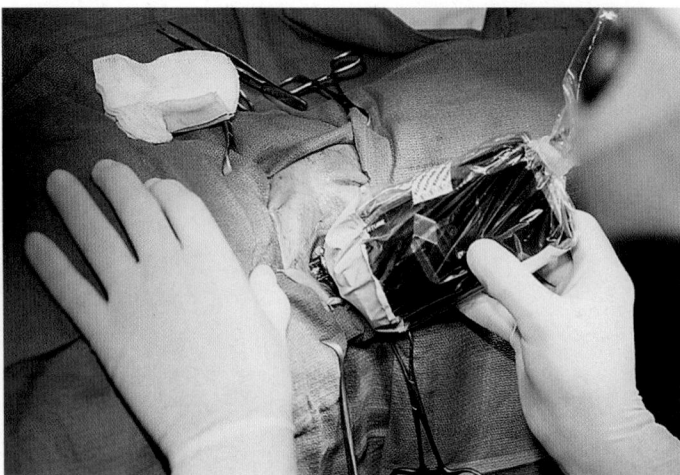

**FIGURE 78–27** The KTP-532 laser is connected to a computerized scanner. The handpiece controls the shutter. Attached to the end of this handpiece is a sterile quartz lens, which is pressed against the skin. The laser is set to deliver multiple pulses of 40- to 60-msec duration. The quartz lens is moved progressively over the field. In this case, the patient was staged for three treatment periods under local anesthesia.

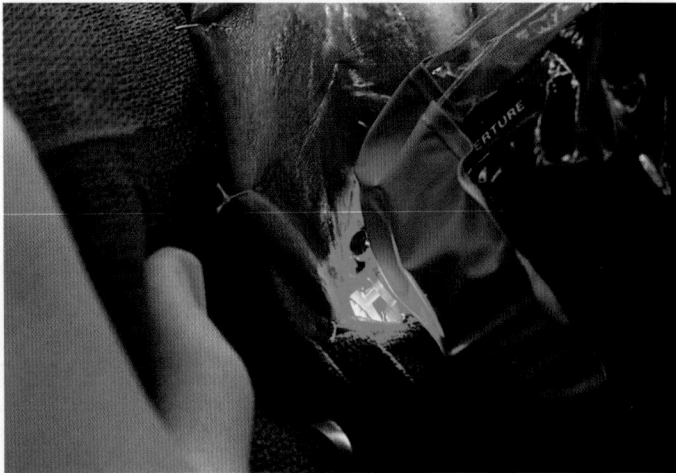

**FIGURE 78–28** The KTP-532 laser Hexascan photocoagulation system delivers intense pure green light to the angioma. The wavelength corresponds to the absorption spectrum of hemoglobin. The blood therefore selectively absorbs the laser light, whereas the surrounding skin reflects it.

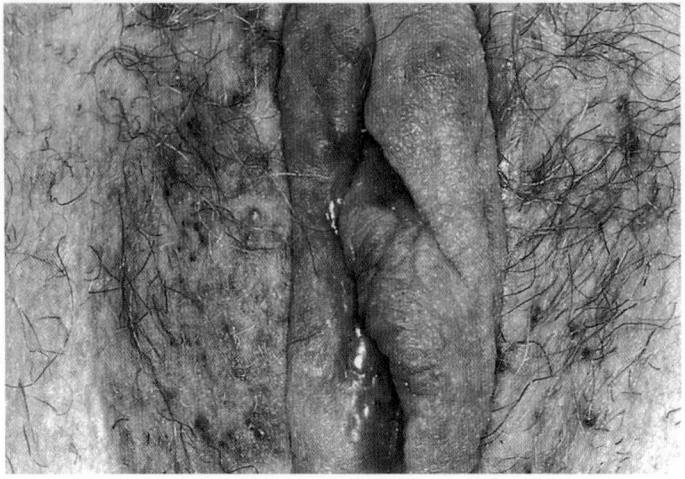

**FIGURE 78–29** In a comparison of this post-treatment photograph with Figure 78-26 (pretreatment), the vessels are shown to have been virtually erased with no skin damage and no scarring. Note the hair growth.

## Lymphangioma

Lymphangioma usually presents as a unilateral diffuse swelling of one labium majus (Fig. 78–30). The skin of the labium contains numerous bleblike surface lesions that are actually dilated subdermal lymphatics (Fig. 78–31). These are not infrequently misdiagnosed as condylomata acuminata. The lymphangioma causes a drawing type of discomfort and is clearly unsightly for the patient. The treatment for this disorder is excision of the labium majus. The patient is placed in the lithotomy position, prepared, and draped. The labial margins are outlined with a marking pen. The skin margins are cut and extended down to the level of Colles' fascia. The labium is placed on sharp traction by applying Allis clamps to the dorsum of the labium. Branches of the internal pudendal artery are clamped and suture-ligated with 3-0 or 4-0 Vicryl. After the labium has been removed and hemostasis attained, the wound is closed in layers with 3-0 Vicryl. The skin is approximated with interrupted 3-0 Vicryl with sutures or a subcuticular continuous suture (Figs. 78–32 and 78–33). Excellent healing with minimal deformity can be anticipated (Figs. 78–34 and 78–35).

## Condyloma Acuminata

This is a very common viral venereal infection. Venereal warts are caused by the human papillomavirus (HPV), types 6 and 11. Although these viral types have low malignant potential, several warts should be sampled and sent for pathologic evaluation before any surgical treatment is undertaken. Conservative topical treatment should be attempted for mild infections before surgical removal is considered. If these simple, conservative measures fail, then surgery under general anesthesia is indicated. Severe, widespread warts are unlikely to respond to simple measures (Fig. 78–36). Likewise, treatment with interferon has a poor response rate for numerous and widespread genital warts. Direct injection of warts with interferon is satisfactory for minimal disease but impractical and expensive for moderate or severe disease. A serum chorionic gonadotropin test should be performed to determine that pregnancy does not exist. Other venereal infections (e.g., human immunodeficiency virus, syphilis, gonorrhea, chlamydia) should be tested for (Figs. 78–37 and 78–38). If any of the aforementioned disorders is diagnosed, it should be treated. Preoperatively, condylomata lata or vulvar carcinoma in situ at first glance may be confused with condylomata acuminata. The surgeon also should take suitable precautions during surgery to protect himself or herself from contamination via vapor, blood, or body fluids. The treatment of choice for significant condylomata acuminata infestation is carbon dioxide ($CO_2$) laser vaporization followed by 3 to 6 months of systemic interferon-alfa injections. One million units of interferon is administered subcutaneously (self-injection) 3 times per week (Fig. 78–39). The patient is given a general anesthetic, placed in the lithotomy position, prepared, and draped (Fig. 78–40A, B). The $CO_2$ laser is coupled to an operating microscope and controlled by a micromanipulator. Power is set according to the skill and experience of the operator to a range of 20 to 60 W. A 2- to 3-mm spot diameter is set by first firing the laser into a wooden tongue depressor. The microscope objective lens is coupled to the laser lens at a 300-mm focal distance. Power is initially reduced to 20 W (i.e., power density of 500 $W/cm^2$), and a trace incision is made to encompass the field of vaporization. All warts and surrounding skin are then vaporized to a level *no deeper than the surrounding normal skin surface* (Fig. 78–40C, D). A 2- to 3-mm margin is "brushed" by reducing laser power to 5 to 10 W to simply blanch (lightly coagulate) the surrounding epithelium (Fig. 78–41). A laser speculum (with attached smoke evacuator) examination is carried out to detect and eliminate vaginal and cervical warts by spot vaporization (Fig. 78–42A). A narrow laser speculum is inserted into the anus to expose anal warts (Fig. 78–42B). These likewise are vaporized at 20 W of power (Fig. 78–42C). When the vaporization is complete, all char is washed away with sterile water, and the wound is covered with Silvadene cream (Fig. 78–43). Other skin lesions elsewhere on the body are carefully evaluated (Fig. 78–44). Postoperatively, the patient is instructed to soak in salt water (Instant Ocean) tub baths 3 times per day and to apply Silvadene cream liberally to the wound 3 times per day, as well as at bedtime (Fig. 78–45). The patient is examined frequently to ensure that the wound is clean and healing appropriately. Clindamycin (Cleocin) cream is applied twice daily into the vagina if that area has been involved (Fig. 78–46). In limited circumstances, urethane dressings may be applied to enhance healing and diminish postoperative pain (Fig. 78–47).

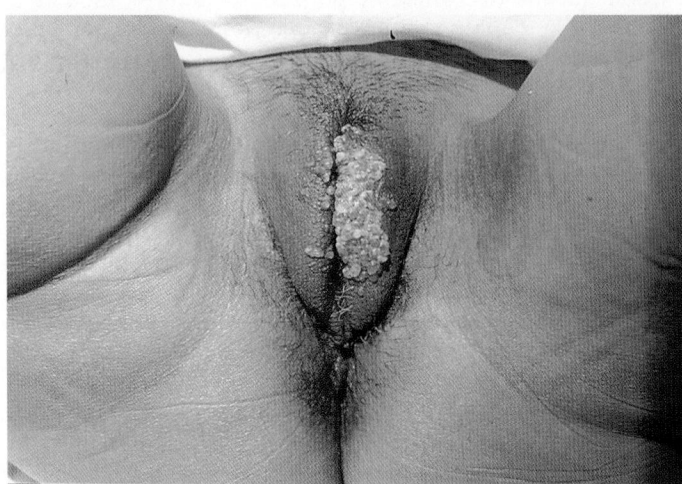

FIGURE 78–30 This Indian woman complained of "warts" on her genitalia. It is obvious that the lesions on the left labium majus are not warts but rather a type of angioma.

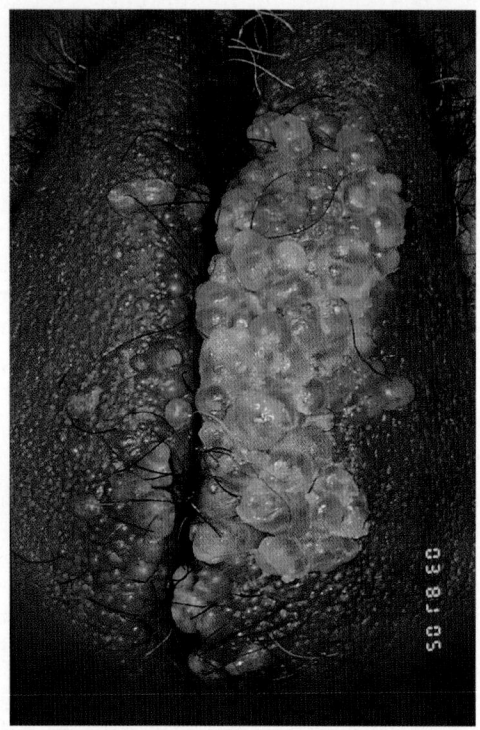

FIGURE 78–31 Close colposcopic evaluation under magnification reveals the lesion to consist of multiple blebs characteristic of a lymphangioma. The lesion extended deep into the labial fat pad.

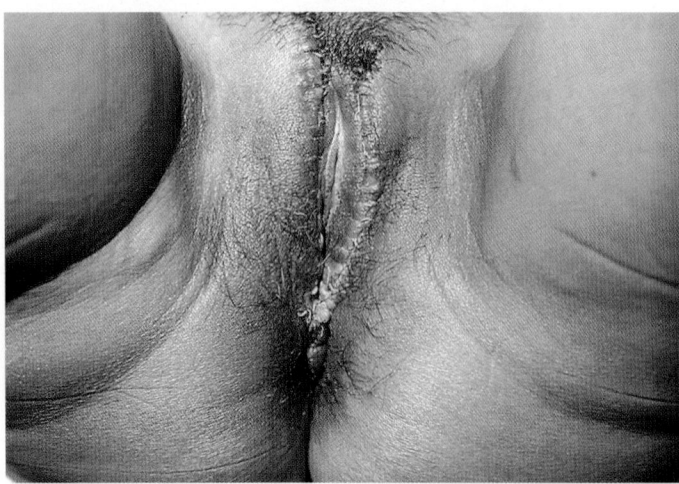

FIGURE 78–32 The left labium was excised, and the wound was closed in layers. The skin was approximated with a simple running 3-0 polydioxanone (PDS) suture.

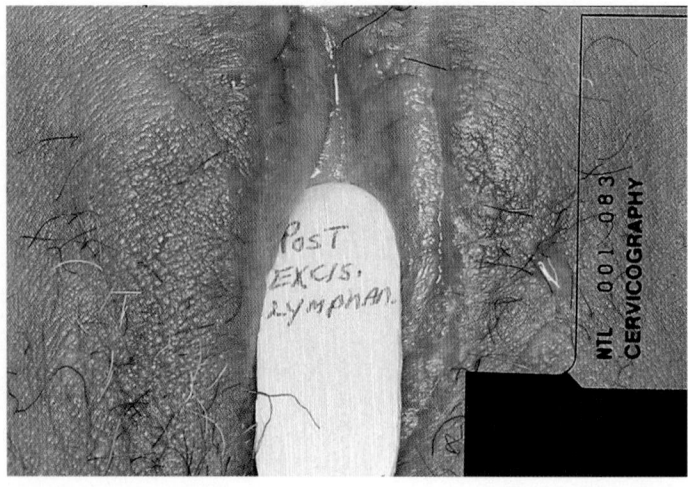

FIGURE 78–33 The healed wound at 6 weeks postoperatively reveals a good cosmetic result.

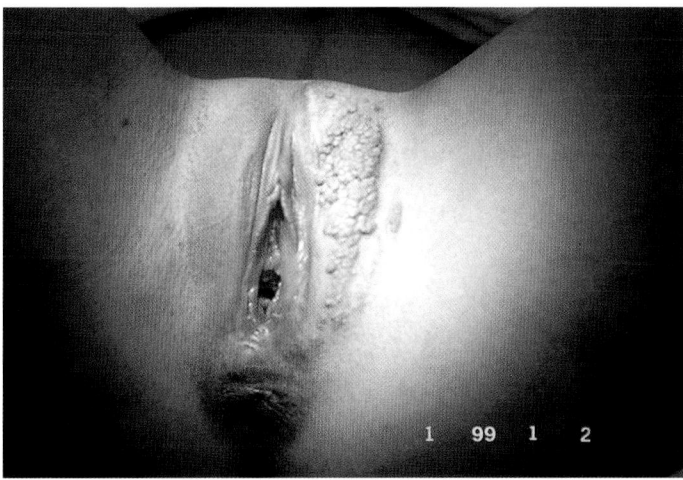

FIGURE 78–34 This lymphangioma in a white woman had approximately the same distribution as that of the patient in Figure 78-30.

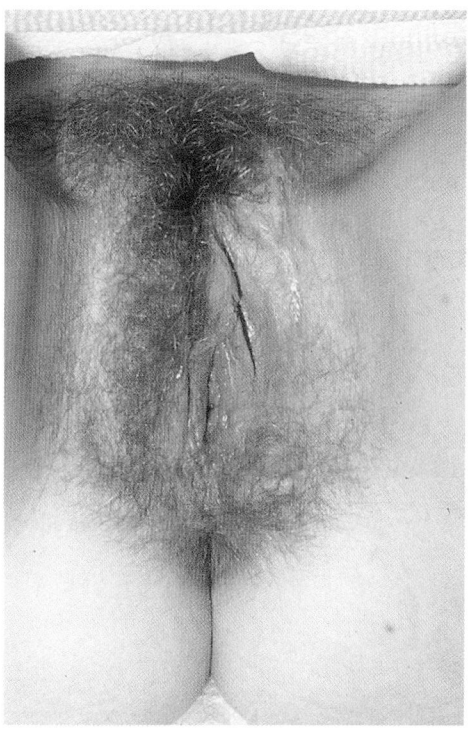

FIGURE 78–35 The postoperative result at 2 months' post excision is also quite satisfactory. Wide and deep excision to ensure clear margins will completely eradicate the angioma.

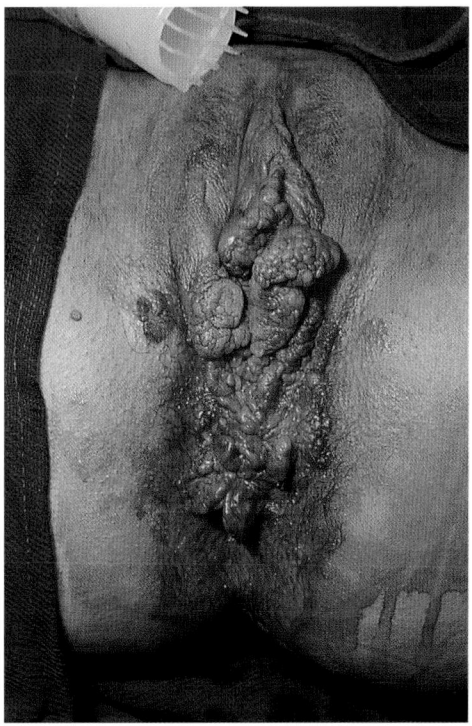

FIGURE 78–36 Severe, widespread genital warts (condylomata acuminata) as shown in this photograph are unlikely to respond to topical treatment regimens.

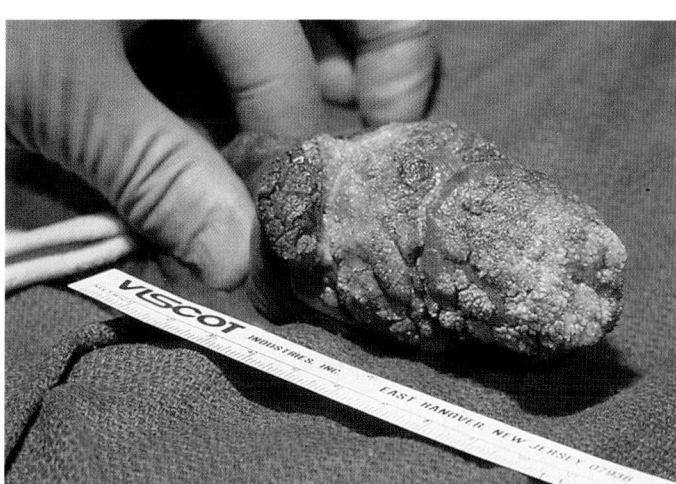

FIGURE 78–37 This man's penis is covered with warts. This degree of human papillomavirus (HPV) infection should set off warning signals to the gynecologist. The patient was human immunodeficiency virus (HIV)-positive and died 6 months after carbon dioxide ($CO_2$) laser treatment.

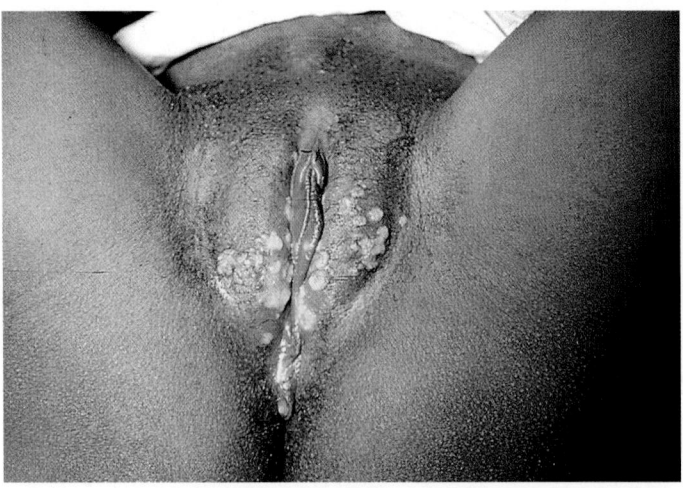

**FIGURE 78–38** Although these are warts, their appearance is flatter than that of condylomata acuminata. These are in fact condylomata lata. The serologic test for syphilis was positive, and the biopsy showed that the tissue was teeming with spirochetes.

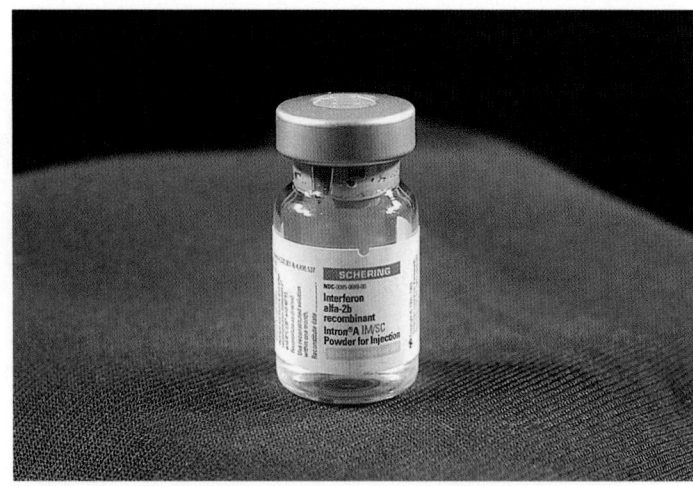

**FIGURE 78–39** Interferon-alfa is indicated for the prevention of recurrent warts. It is initially administered immediately after carbon dioxide ($CO_2$) laser eradication of the condylomata. One million units is injected subcutaneously 3 times per week for 6 months.

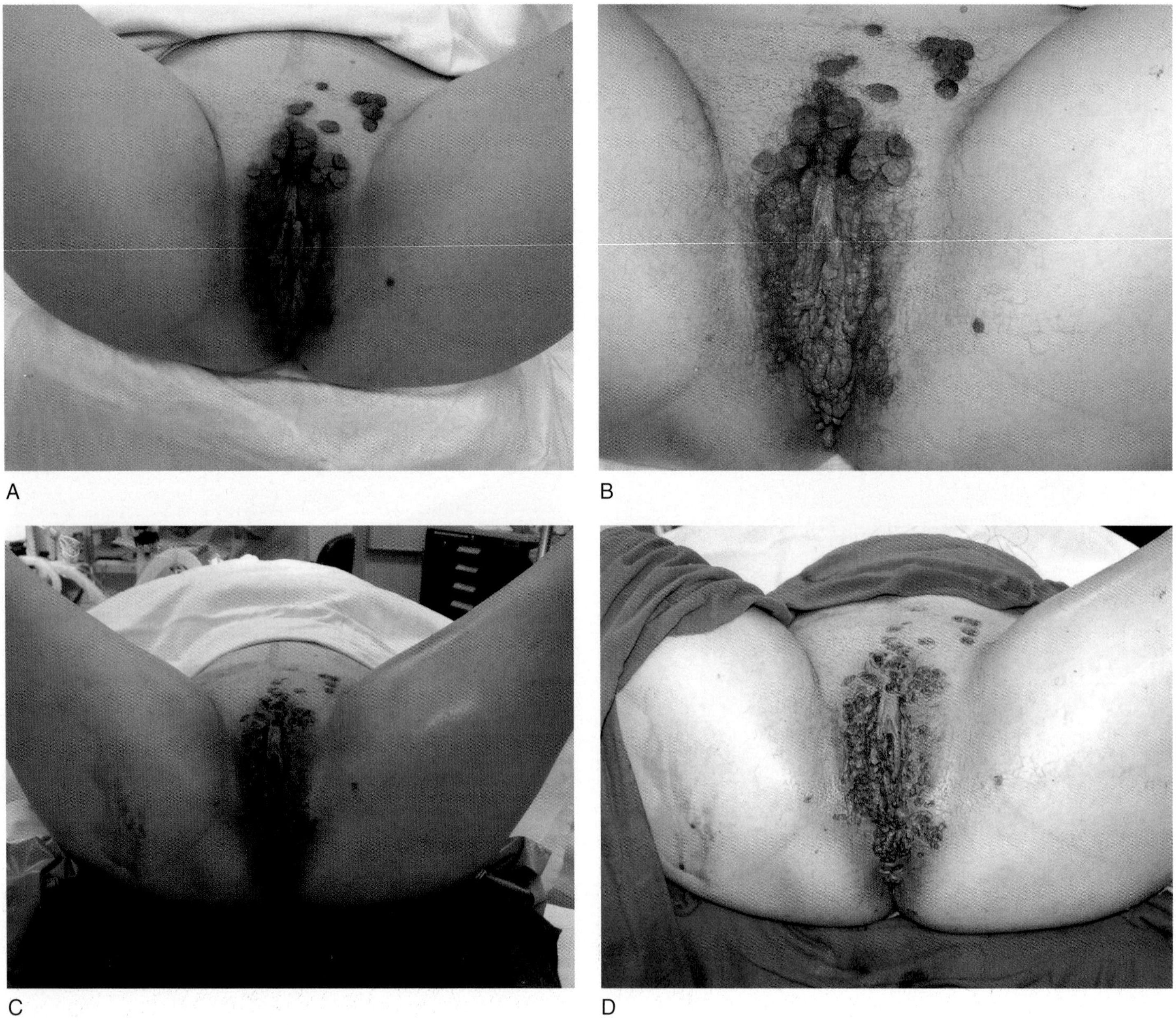

A

B

C

D

**FIGURE 78–40 A.** This insulin-dependent diabetic patient has extensive warts. Topical treatments have failed. **B.** The major distribution of these warts is located in the interlabial sulcus. The warts show typical bilateral involvement. **C.** Carbon dioxide ($CO_2$) laser ablation is performed with the patient under general anesthesia. The warts are carefully vaporized to the level of the surrounding skin surface and no deeper. **D.** The warts were vaporized with an UltraPulse $CO_2$ laser coupled to an operating microscope. Note the lack of char and the bright pink appearance of the underlying stroma. This is indicative of minimal heat conduction and likewise normal underlying dermis.

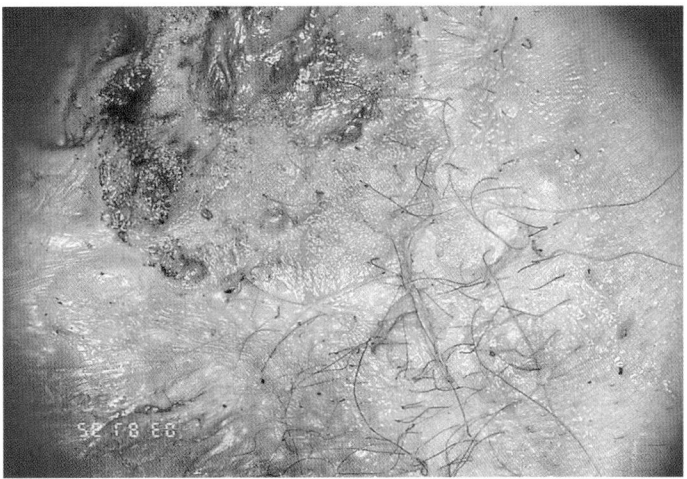

FIGURE 78–41 Another patient has undergone vaporization with a continuous-wave carbon dioxide ($CO_2$) laser. Note the char and stromal heat artifact. The surrounding white area has been brushed. This reduced-power technique only coagulates the surrounding epidermis, which is similar to the effect of laser dermabrasion.

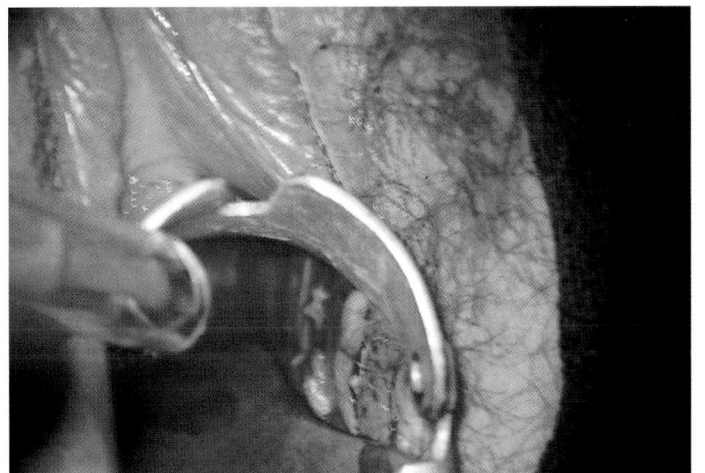

A

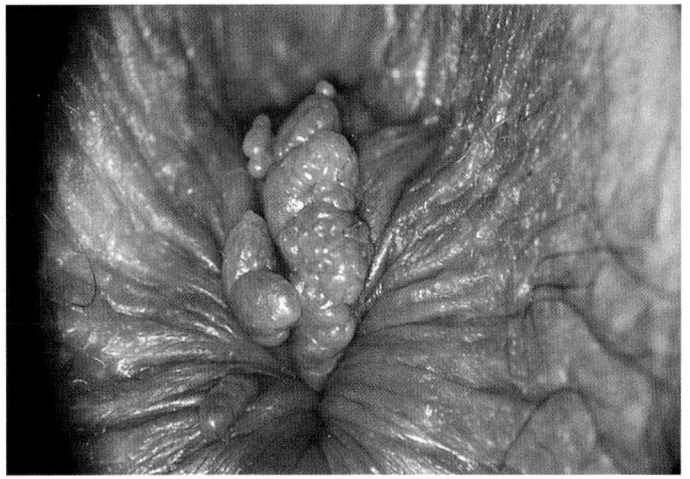

B

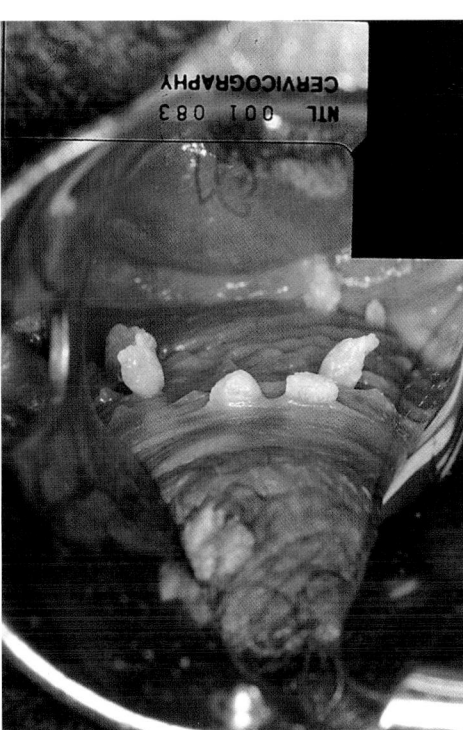

C

FIGURE 78–42 A. A laser speculum is placed in the vagina. The warts on the left vaginal wall are vaporized. B. Perianal warts are commonly present when a patient has significant vulvar condylomata acuminata. The presence of perianal warts requires inspection of the anus and rectum for warts. C. A thin-bladed speculum has been placed in the rectum. Numerous warts are seen on the intestinal mucosa. These must be vaporized.

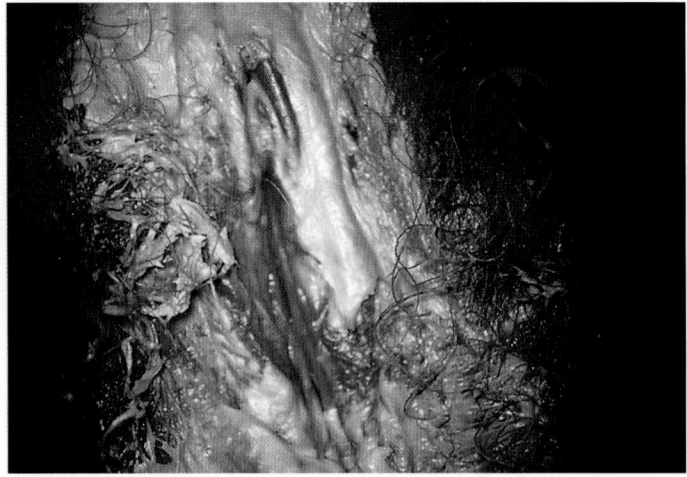

FIGURE 78–43 Upon completion of laser vaporization, the wound is covered with Silvadene cream. This treatment is continued until complete healing is observed.

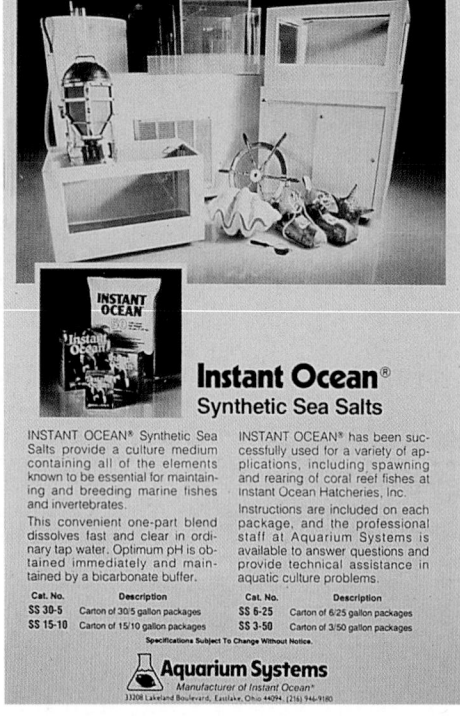

FIGURE 78–45 Every patient who undergoes carbon dioxide ($CO_2$) laser vaporization is instructed to take two or three salt water tub baths per day. Two cups of Instant Ocean are placed in a tub of comfortably warm water. After soaking for 10 minutes, the patient rinses off with fresh water, dries the wound, and applies Silvadene cream liberally over the wound.

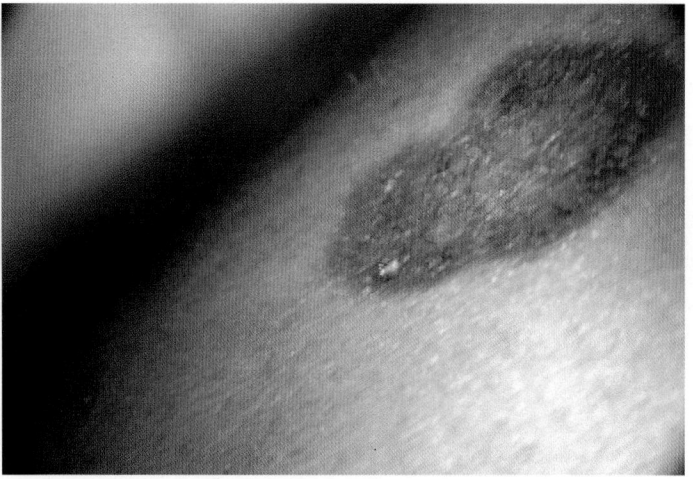

FIGURE 78–44 This forearm lesion in a diabetic woman (see Fig. 78-4A through D) treated for condylomata acuminata represents an area of necrobiosis.

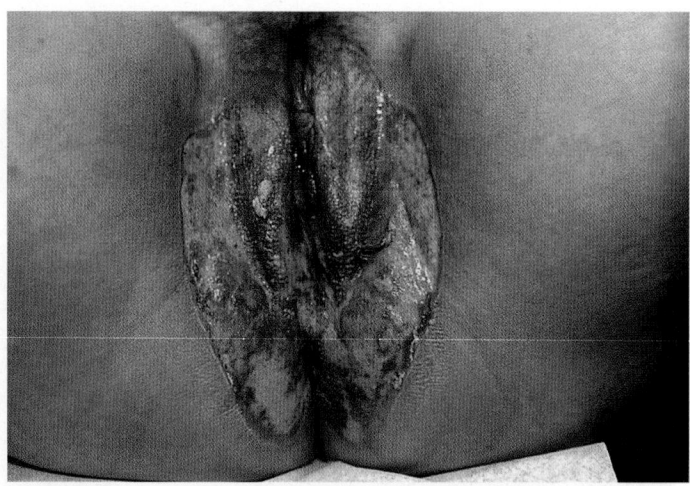

FIGURE 78–46 The patient shown in Figure 78-36 underwent extensive laser vaporization. At 2 weeks postoperatively, the vulva is beginning to reepithelialize.

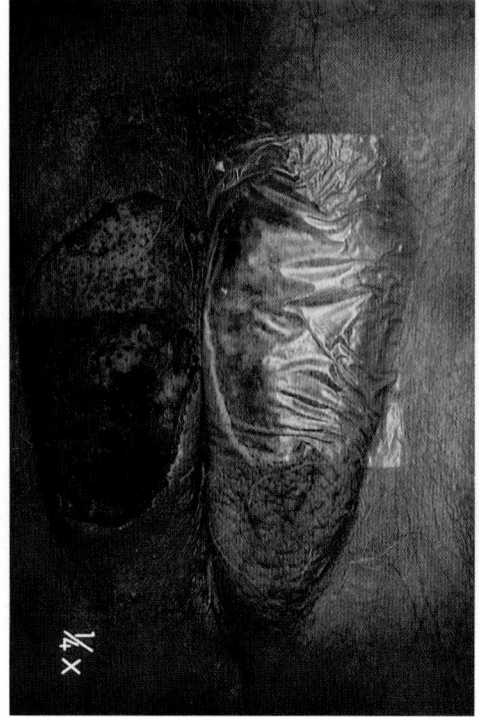

FIGURE 78–47 Alternatively, a urethane dressing (OpSite) may be applied to the treated vulva. This greatly reduces postoperative discomfort.

# CHAPTER 79

# Therapeutic Injection

## Michael S. Baggish

Two major categories of vulvar injections for the alleviation of debilitating symptoms associated with dystrophic disorders are as follows: (1) alcohol injection for the relief of pruritus (*not pain*), and (2) dexamethasone (Decadron) injection for the relief of chronic inflammatory conditions (e.g., lichen sclerosus) and for the relief of chronic pain (pudendal neuralgia).

## Alcohol Injection

Chronic pruritus that is unresponsive to topical medication (e.g., steroids) or retinoids is an indication for alcohol injection (Fig. 79-1). The criterion for injection to deaden the nerves is essentially the failure of conservative therapeutic measures to control vulvar itching. Patients should be warned that a complication of this type of treatment is neuropathy manifested by burning pain. Injection of an excessive volume of alcohol, as well as subcuticular injection, can and will cause tissue slough and possibly necrotizing fasciitis.

The patient is placed in the dorsal lithotomy position under general anesthesia. The area to be injected is divided into a grid, with all intersections 1 cm apart. The entire area may be large (i.e., encompassing the whole vulva) or limited to a single side. The grid is drawn after the vulva is prepared with hexachlorophene (Phisohex) or povidone-iodine (Betadine). A sterile surgical marking pen is the most convenient device for this task (Fig. 79-2). A 1-mL tuberculin syringe fitted with a 27-gauge needle is utilized for injection. Absolute alcohol is drawn up into the syringe. At each intersecting line, 0.1 mL of alcohol is injected into the subcutaneous fat (Fig. 79-3). The injection destroys the fine cutaneous branches of the perineal nerves, resulting in anesthesia to the vulva. The vulva is perceived by the patient as numb.

## Dexamethasone Injection

The current treatment of choice for the relief of pruritus associated with lichen sclerosus is 2 mg of dexamethasone diluted to 10 mL with 0.25% bupivacaine. Serial injections also appear to arrest the progress of the inflammatory reaction and subsequent scar formation associated with lichen sclerosus. Injections are given in the office weekly, then biweekly, then monthly.

All patients are prepared with the application of EMLA cream 30 minutes before injection (Fig. 79-4). This effectively numbs the skin and greatly reduces the discomfort of needle entry. A 10-mL syringe is fitted with a 1½-inch, 27-gauge needle or a short, 30-gauge needle. Needle selection depends on the relative distribution of disease. After the skin is prepared with Betadine, the needle is directed along the interlabial sulcus subdermally (in contrast with the alcohol injection, which is subcutaneous). Two milligrams of the dexamethasone mixture is injected on each side of the vulva (Fig. 79-5A, B). The needle is inserted into the tissue to its hub, and the injection is performed during slow withdrawal of the needle (Fig. 79-6A through D).

Pudendal neuralgia is associated with burning, sticking, or sharp pain that is more or less continuous and not restricted to the vestibule. The pain is aggravated most consistently by sitting. The disorder is more common in women 50 years of age or older but may occur as the result of surgery for vulvar vestibulitis syndrome. Injection of dexamethasone into the area of the specific pudendal nerve branch is analogous to injection of an anti-inflammatory drug into the foot for relief of Morton's neuroma. Most patients with pudendal neuralgia can pinpoint the area of hyperesthesia and pain instigation. A similar mixture of dexamethasone and 0.25% bupivacaine is utilized for these injections, as was described earlier for the treatment of lichen sclerosus. A 10-mL injection is made into a specific site (e.g., for clitoral pain, the injection is aimed at the clitoral crus). A finger into the vagina helps direct the needle to the specific site for injection. After the injection, which contains a long-acting local anesthetic, the patient should experience (on the table) immediate relief of her pain. These injections may be repeated at 1-, 2-, or 3-month intervals as required for pain relief.

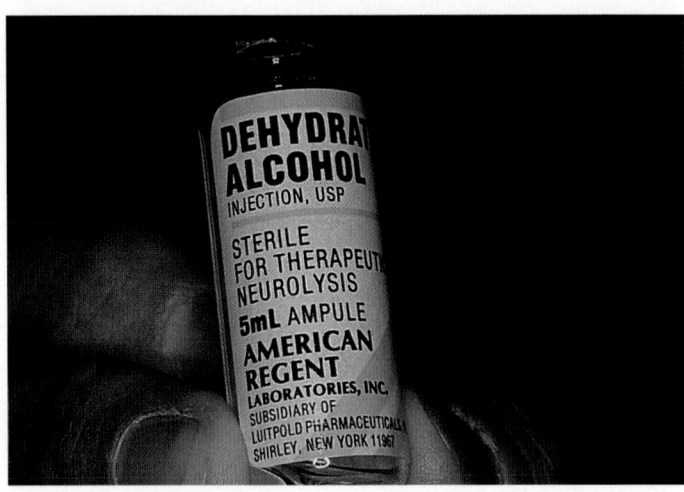

**FIGURE 79–1** Chronic pruritus of the vulva that is unresponsive to topical and systemic medications may be relieved by alcohol injection. Absolute alcohol is the only appropriate agent for this therapy.

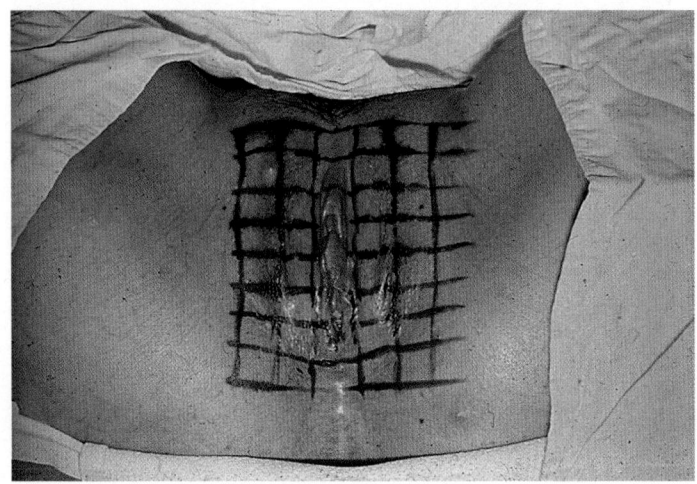

**FIGURE 79–2** A grid is marked on the vulva with a sterile pen after the site has been surgically prepared and draped. The intersecting lines are 1 cm apart.

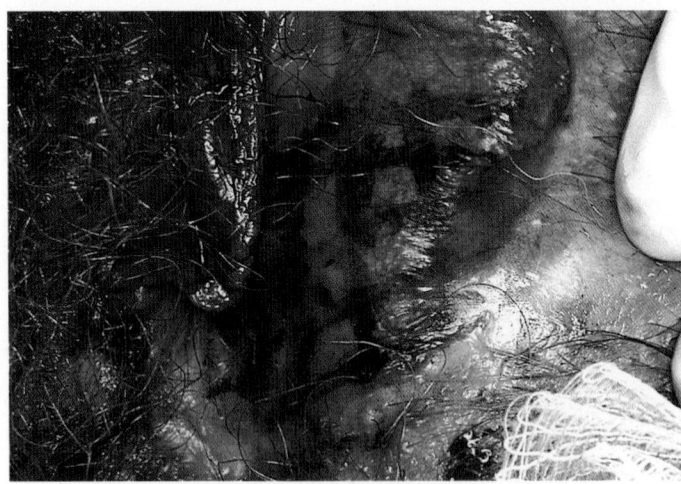

**FIGURE 79–3** The alcohol, which has been drawn into a tuberculin syringe fitted with a 27-gauge needle, is injected at each intersecting point. Only 0.1 mL is injected into the subcutaneous tissue at each point. Care should be taken not to inject intradermally because this will produce tissue slough.

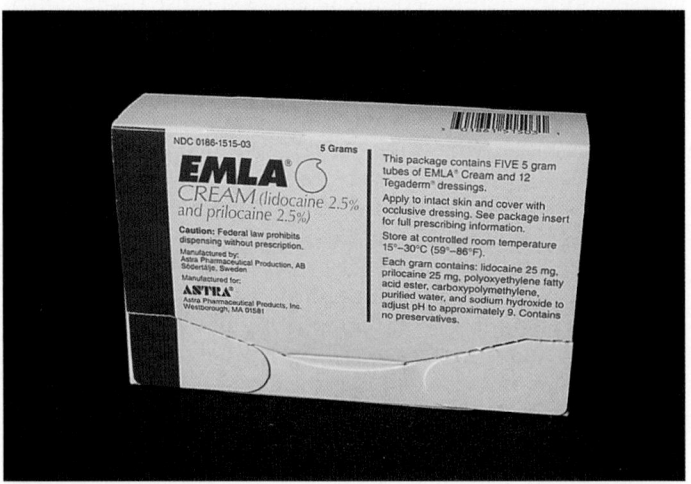

**FIGURE 79–4** EMLA cream is applied liberally to the vulvar skin 30 minutes before the anticipated injection. This preparation is by far the most effective topical anesthetic available. The discomfort of a vulvar needle stick is ameliorated by 80% to 90% via the application of EMLA.

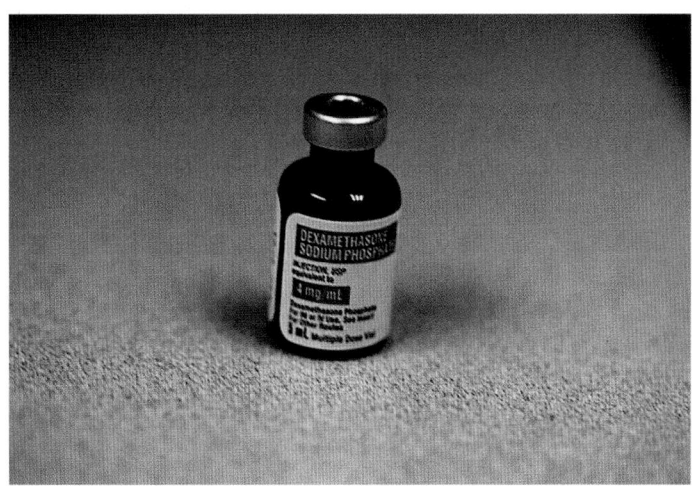

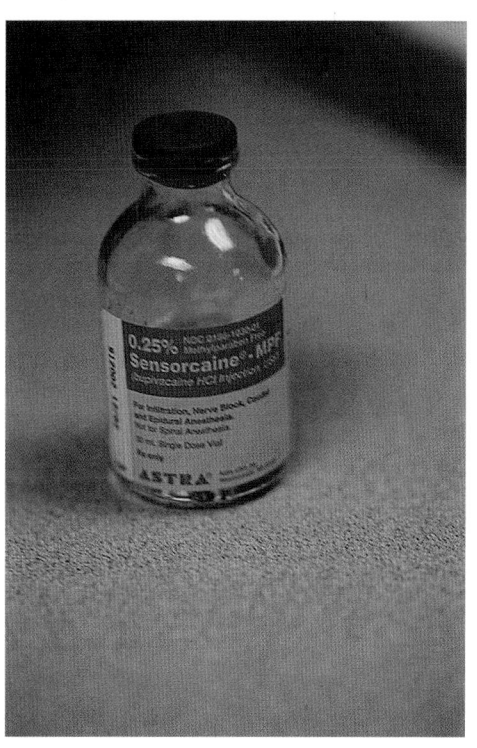

A                                                                                                    B

FIGURE 79–5  A. Dexamethasone is a very effective and potent anti-inflammatory agent. It is the drug of choice for the treatment of lichen sclerosus and pudendal neuralgia. Two milligrams is serially injected into each side of the vulva. B. Bupivacaine (Sensorcaine) 0.25% is an excellent agent to couple with dexamethasone. Typically, 10 mL of bupivacaine serves to dilute the dexamethasone. It simultaneously provides pain relief for 4 to 5 hours at the injection site.

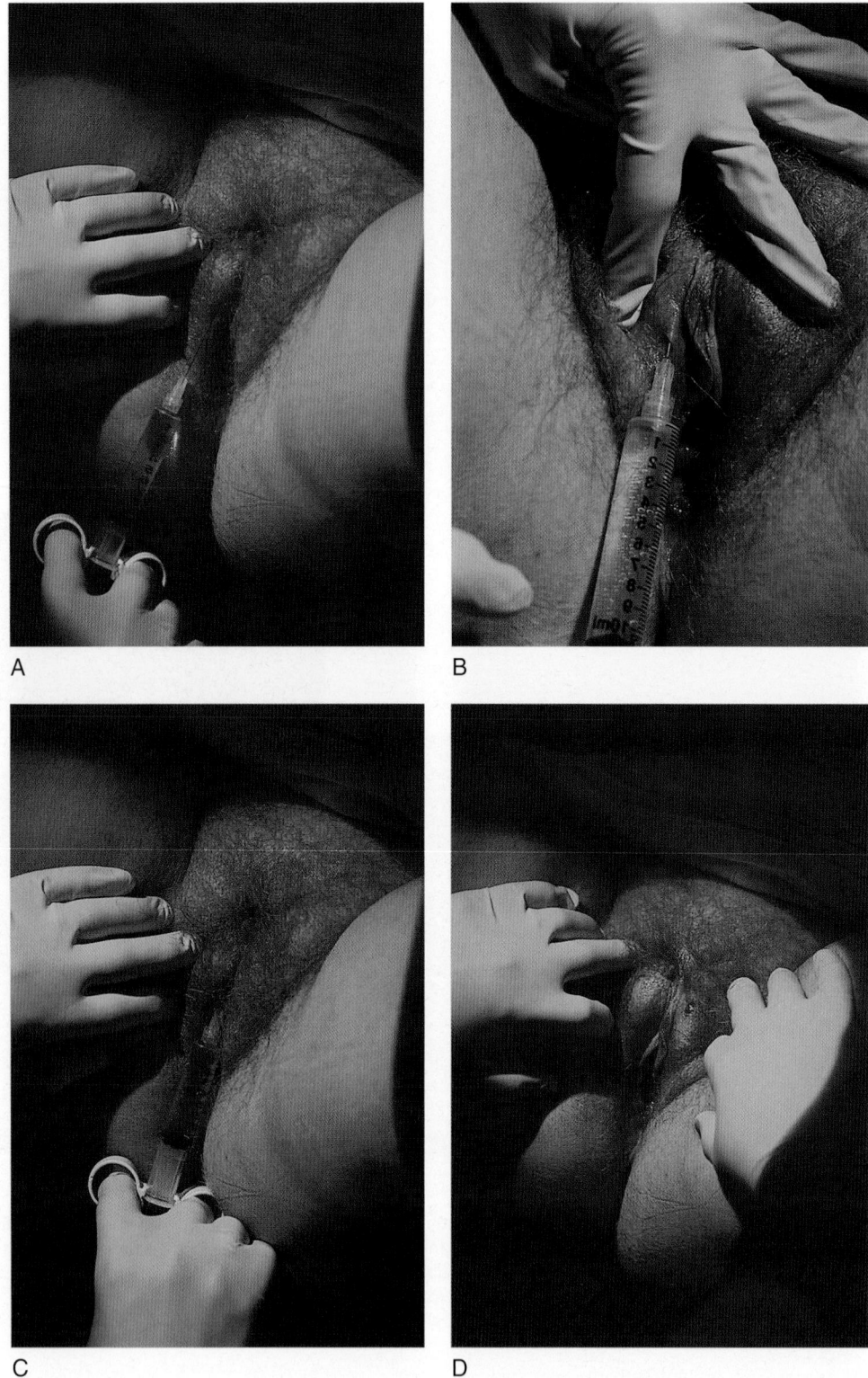

A

B

C

D

**FIGURE 79–6** **A.** For the management of lichen sclerosus, the needle (27-gauge) is aimed at the affected location, typically the interlabial sulcus, clitoral frenulum, and hood. **B.** The needle is advanced subdermally to its hub. **C.** The solution is slowly injected while the needle is withdrawn. The procedure is repeated identically on the opposite side. **D.** The injection has been completed bilaterally. The labial swelling disappears as the injected solution is absorbed.

# CHAPTER 80

# Episiotomy

## Michael S. Baggish

In the United States, episiotomy had been performed routinely when coupled with preterm or full-term obstetric delivery. Recently, the benefits of this operation have been questioned. The risk of third- or fourth-degree lacerations has been shown to be significantly greater, particularly with midline (median) episiotomies versus no episiotomy. No conclusive evidence has yet been published showing that routine (nonselective) episiotomy performance is associated with significantly diminished risks of later pelvic floor dysfunction. A large volume of data verifies that selective episiotomy is beneficial insofar as it avoids anal sphincter injury and diminishes later pelvic floor problems. Most recent reports favor mediolateral over medial (midline) episiotomy because of the decreased risk of third- and fourth-degree tears. Although cutting an episiotomy is an "operation," its historical performance at best can be described as rugged, and its repair most charitably depicted as casual. For this operation, acceptable precepts appropriate for every surgical procedure should be followed. The latter include knowledge of anatomy, sterile technique, careful tissue handling, sharp and minimally traumatic dissection, control of bleeding, avoidance of tissue devitalization, and anatomic-physiologic reconstruction.

The goal of the surgeon under all circumstances should be to cut an episiotomy when required to implement easy, atraumatic delivery while minimizing the risk(s) for third- or fourth-degree lacerations. The bizarre practice of purposely cutting a midline episiotomy and extending it into the rectum should be relegated to the archives of past history.

## Mediolateral Episiotomy

This procedure cuts or creates an incision directed from the right or left lower vagina (at the level of the hymenal ring), through the vestibule, and through the lowest margin of the labium majus, where it joins the perineum, and into the ischiorectal fossa. The operation may include any portion of the structures noted earlier. It is vectored in a direction approximately 45° to 50° from the midline and may include all of the previously mentioned structures (Fig. 80-1). The lower portion of the bulbocavernosus muscle is always cut, and if the incision is extended, the transverse perineal muscle will also be cut (Fig. 80-2). During pregnancy, every one of these structures has an excellent blood supply. Cut vessels in the subcutaneous tissues, fascia, and muscles can bleed briskly and therefore must be clamped and ligated to avoid moderate or even substantial blood loss.

The episiotomy cut is usually made with scissors. The operator's fingers should be inserted between the vagina/vestibule and the baby's head to protect the latter from injury.

The incision, if made correctly and according to previously cited instructions, will clearly avoid injury to the anal sphincter muscle and rectum. It is directed away from those structures.

Following delivery of the infant while placental separation is awaited, the incision should be tamponaded with pressure via an abdominal pad(s). Bleeding vessels should be clamped and suture-ligated with 3-0 Vicryl. The cut bulbocavernosus muscle margins should be secured with Allis clamps. Fascial edges at the level of the transverse perineal muscle should be secured with Allis clamps. After the placenta has been delivered, the wound is closed with 2-0 or 3-0 Vicryl sutures approximating the muscles and fascia; 3-0 Vicryl closes Colles' fascia and subcutaneous tissue, and 3-0 Vicryl is placed through the skin (Figs. 80-3 and 80-4).

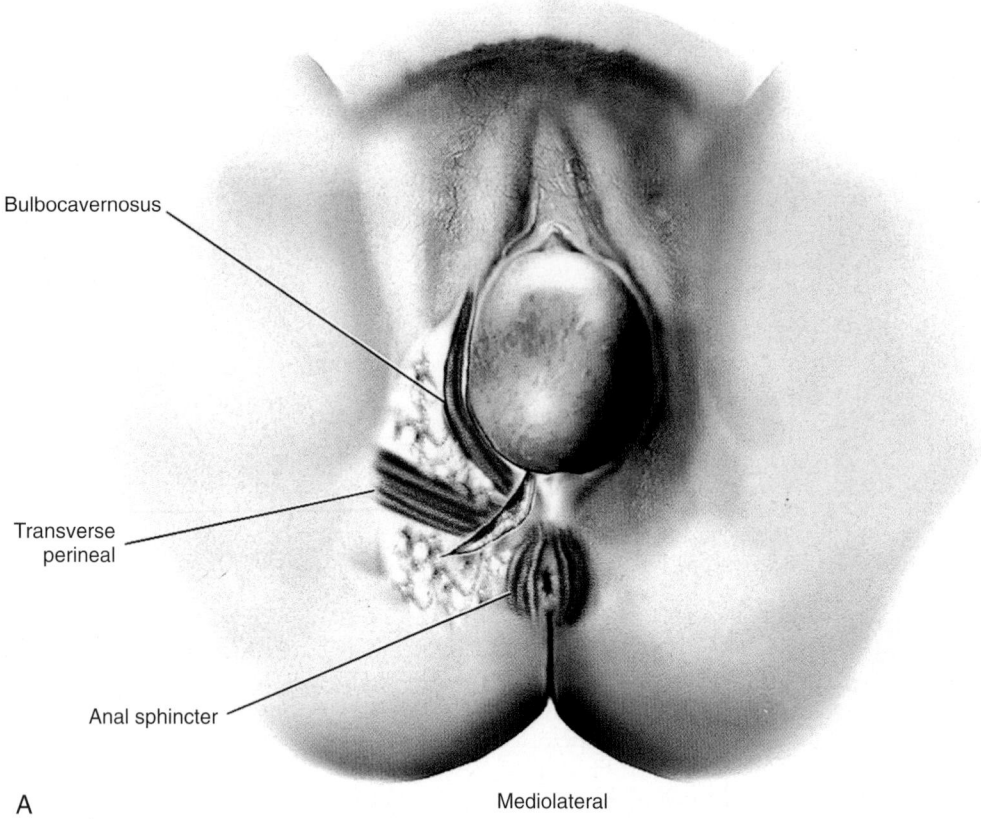

Bulbocavernosus

Transverse
perineal

Anal sphincter

A                                                Mediolateral

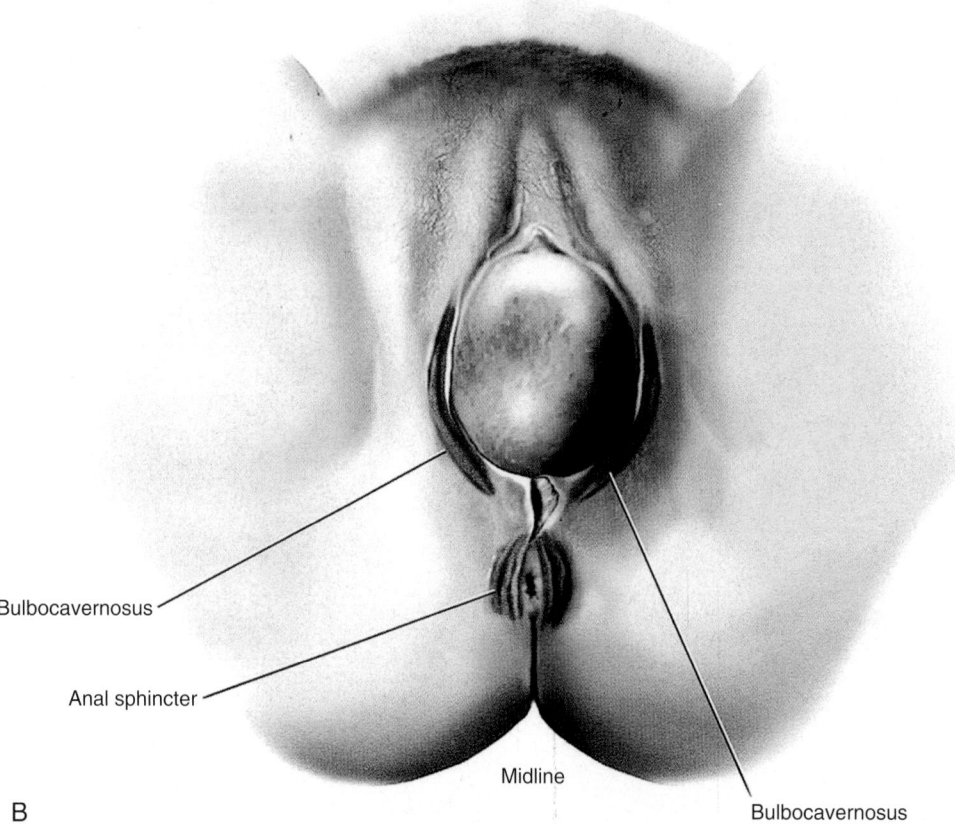

Bulbocavernosus

Anal sphincter

B                                                Midline                    Bulbocavernosus

**FIGURE 80–1**  The two types of episiotomy, which may be cut at the time of vaginal birth, are illustrated here. Key perineal muscles have been superimposed. **A.** Mediolateral approach. **B.** Midline approach.

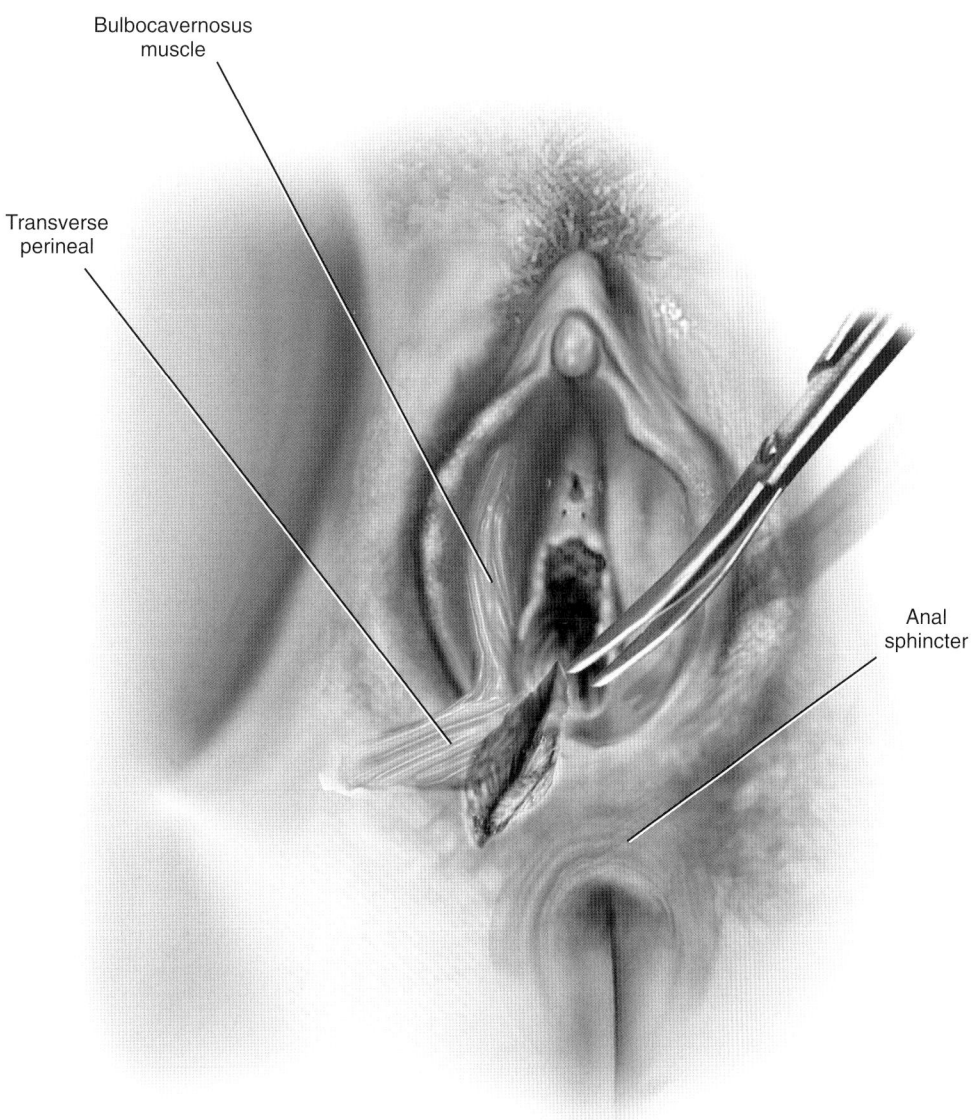

Bulbocavernosus
muscle

Transverse
perineal

Anal
sphincter

**FIGURE 80-2** A right mediolateral episiotomy has been cut. The superimposed bulbocavernosus and transverse perineal muscles have been cut as a result of the direction of the incision. If the episiotomy extends, it will be vectored into the ischiorectal fossa and not into the external sphincter ani.

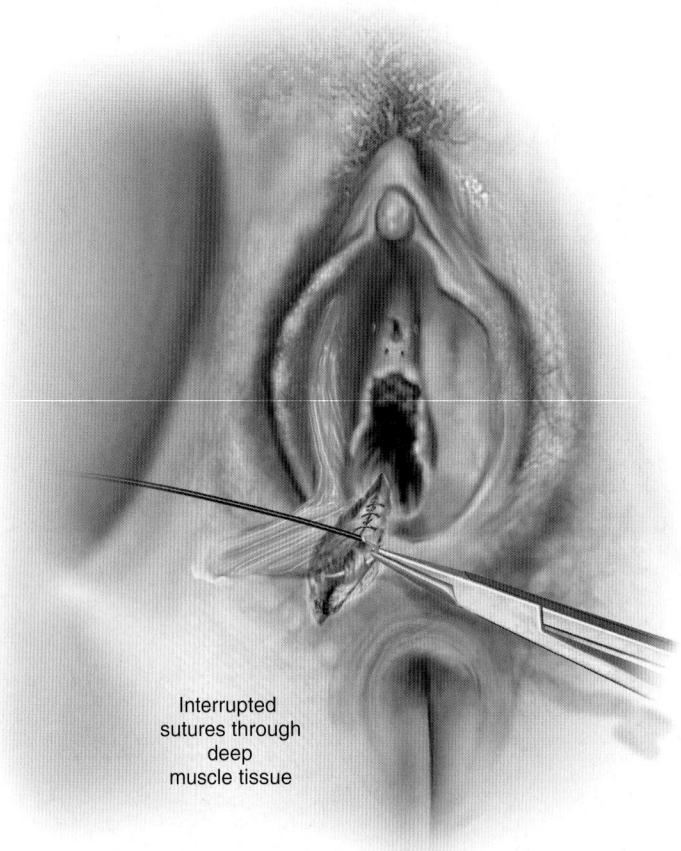

Interrupted
sutures through
deep
muscle tissue

FIGURE 80–3  The severed muscles are sutured with interrupted 2-0 Vicryl stitches.

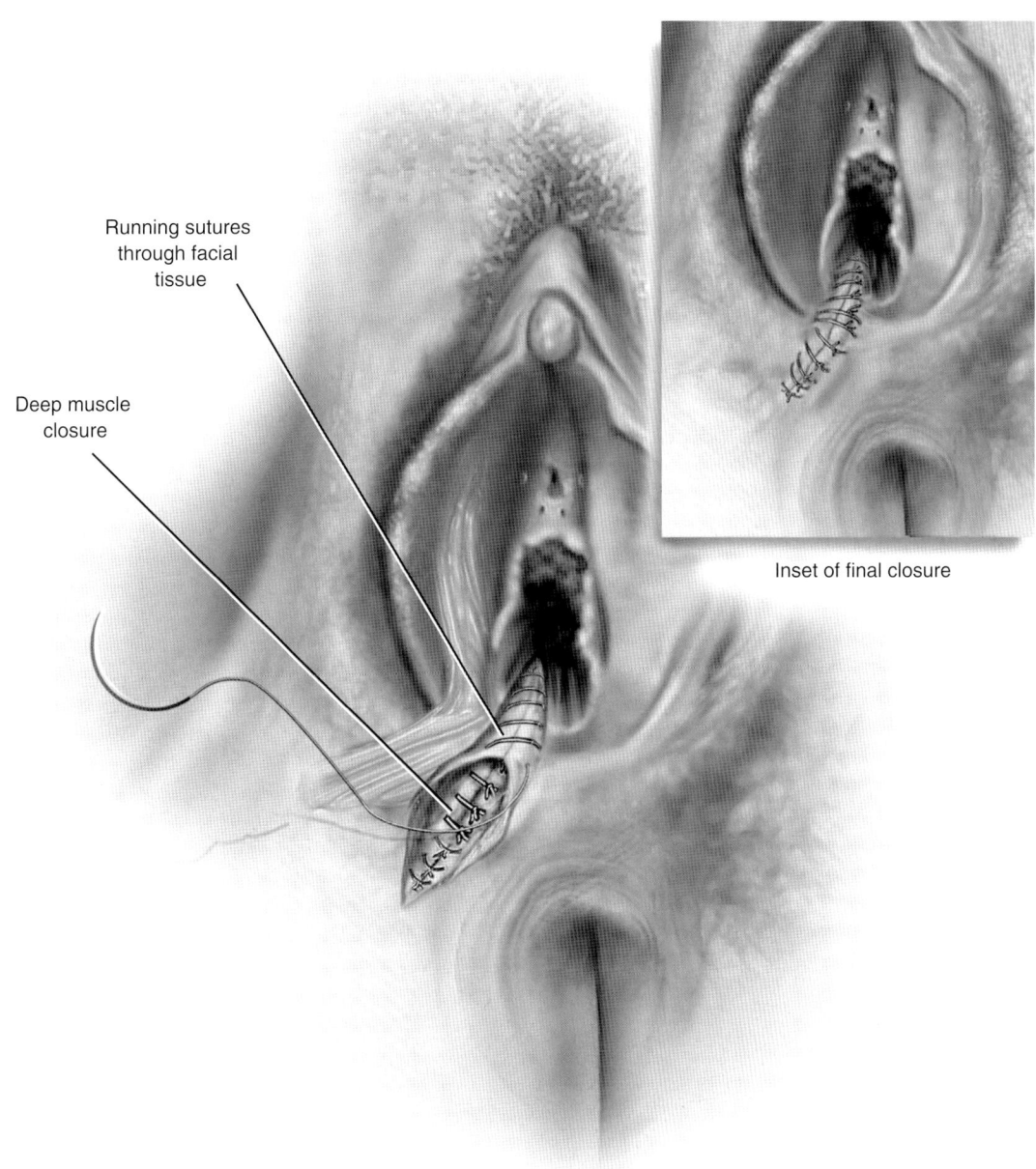

Running sutures
through facial
tissue

Deep muscle
closure

Inset of final closure

**FIGURE 80–4**  Colles' fascia is closed with a running 3-0 Vicryl continuous stitch. The skin is closed with an interrupted or running stitch of 3-0 Vicryl. Alternatively, a subcuticular stitch may be placed.

## Midline Episiotomy

The cut is made into the lower, posterior vaginal midline just superior to the hymenal ring and extends through the vestibule at the level of the fossa navicularis, through the posterior fourchette to the perineal-vestibular junction (see Fig. 80–1). In previous descriptions, the cut continues into the "perineal body," which older anatomy texts and drawings depict as a grand central terminus of various muscles into a defined structure ("tendon"). In fact, cadaver dissections utilizing both fixed and fresh specimens fail to show such a defined central tendon or body. These dissections demonstrate that the external sphincter and to some extent the levator ani structurally form the deeper perineal substructure lying beneath the skin, superficial fat, and Colles' fascia. Inevitably, a midline episiotomy will cut into some of the external sphincter ani. If this impingement is limited to a few fibers, then the functional outcome is minimal. If a quantitatively greater volume of external sphincter is cut, retracts, and remains unrecognized, then the patient suffers some impairment of anal sphincter control, for example, difficulty controlling flatus and leaking stool. If 50% or more of the sphincter is cut, the patient will have fecal incontinence of moderate to severe degree. Complete transection always translates to severe fecal incontinence.

Finally, the risk of severing the sphincter and extending through the anterior rectal wall is great with the midline episiotomy because significant pressure created by the head exiting the vagina can spread and uncontrollably extend the midline cut, which naturally vectors directly toward the external sphincter and the anorectum.

## Repair of Third-Degree Laceration

For this type of repair to be successful, the surgeon must have current and thorough knowledge of perineal anatomy. The external anal sphincter is a wide but relatively thin structure in vivo. The internal sphincter in reality is the most external portion of the rectal muscularis at the level of the anus and the lowest portion of the rectum. Anatomic dissection of the anal sphincter demonstrates that the mean width of the external sphincter is 1 inch.

Vital reconnaissance should be carried out before any repair is done. Hemostasis should be obtained with mosquito clamping and suture-ligatures of 3-0 Vicryl. A thorough inspection of the wound is performed to identify the degree of sphincter injury, and to ensure that the anal and rectal mucosa has not been entered or damaged.

Next, the retracted edges of the external sphincter are grasped and held with multiple Allis clamps (Fig. 80–5). The examiner should double-glove and place his or her index finger into the rectum while simultaneously having an assistant create countertraction with the Allis clamps. This examiner should feel the sphincter tightening as the assistant pulls the Allis clamps in a crossover-like maneuver. The sphincter is sutured while a finger is maneuvered in the anus (Fig. 80–6). Although some surgeons prefer mattress sutures, the author uses a simple wide bite with 3-0 Vicryl. Approximately five to six stitches are required to adequately approximate a completely torn sphincter (see Fig. 77–6). After sphincter repair, the operator's finger is withdrawn from the anus, and the outer double glove is removed and discarded. Colles' fascia is closed with interrupted 3-0 Vicryl. The fat is closed with 3-0 or 4-0 Vicryl running stitches, the skin with interrupted 3-0 Vicryl stitches (Fig. 80–7). Alternatively, the new skin may be closed with a subcuticular running suture.

Postoperatively, nothing is placed in the rectum. The patient is clearly advised to take no enemas, to insert no suppositories, and to avoid straining at stool. She should be instructed to take 1 oz daily of mineral oil or one capsule of docusate and casanthranol (Peri-Colace) twice a day and seawater (Instant Ocean) baths once or twice daily, and to apply Silvadene cream to the wound 2 or 3 times a day. The patient should drink a minimum of four to six glasses of water per day and should be placed on a diet high in fiber and fruit.

## Repair of Fourth-Degree Laceration

The occurrence of a fourth-degree perineal laceration creates a significant risk for fistula formation. A compulsive, precise repair is essential to avoid that complication.

As with the third-degree laceration, extensive and thorough pre-repair inspection is an essential step for successful repair (Fig. 80–8). Hemostasis should be complete before inspection is begun. Fine clamping and ligatures are the best way of achieving hemostasis and avoiding tissue devitalization. The cut edges of the anorectal mucosa are grasped with Babcock clamps, beginning at the anal verge and extending upward (cranially) to the junction of the intact rectal mucosa. A 2-0 or 3-0 chromic catgut stitch is placed through the rectal wall at this point as a marker stitch.

Next, the rectum is repaired with a single layer of or interrupted 2-0 chromic catgut sutures. Each stitch is placed through the entire rectal wall thickness and tied down (Fig. 80–9). When the rectal wall has been completely repaired, the external sphincter is grasped with Allis clamps and repaired as previously described with 3-0 Vicryl sutures (Fig. 80–10). Finally, Colles' fascia, fat, and skin are repaired with 3-0 Vicryl. A final finger examination rechecks the completeness of the repair.

Postoperatively, nothing is placed into the rectum. No enemas and no suppositories are ordered. Stool softeners and a high-fiber diet are prescribed. The author prefers that the patient take 1 oz of mineral oil by mouth once per day. Additionally, ciprofloxacin (Cipro) 500 mg twice daily is administered for 7 days. The patient should take a 10-minute Instant Ocean bath per day and cleanse her perineum and perianal area daily with Phisohex; Silvadene or Cleocin cream is applied to the wound 3 times a day.

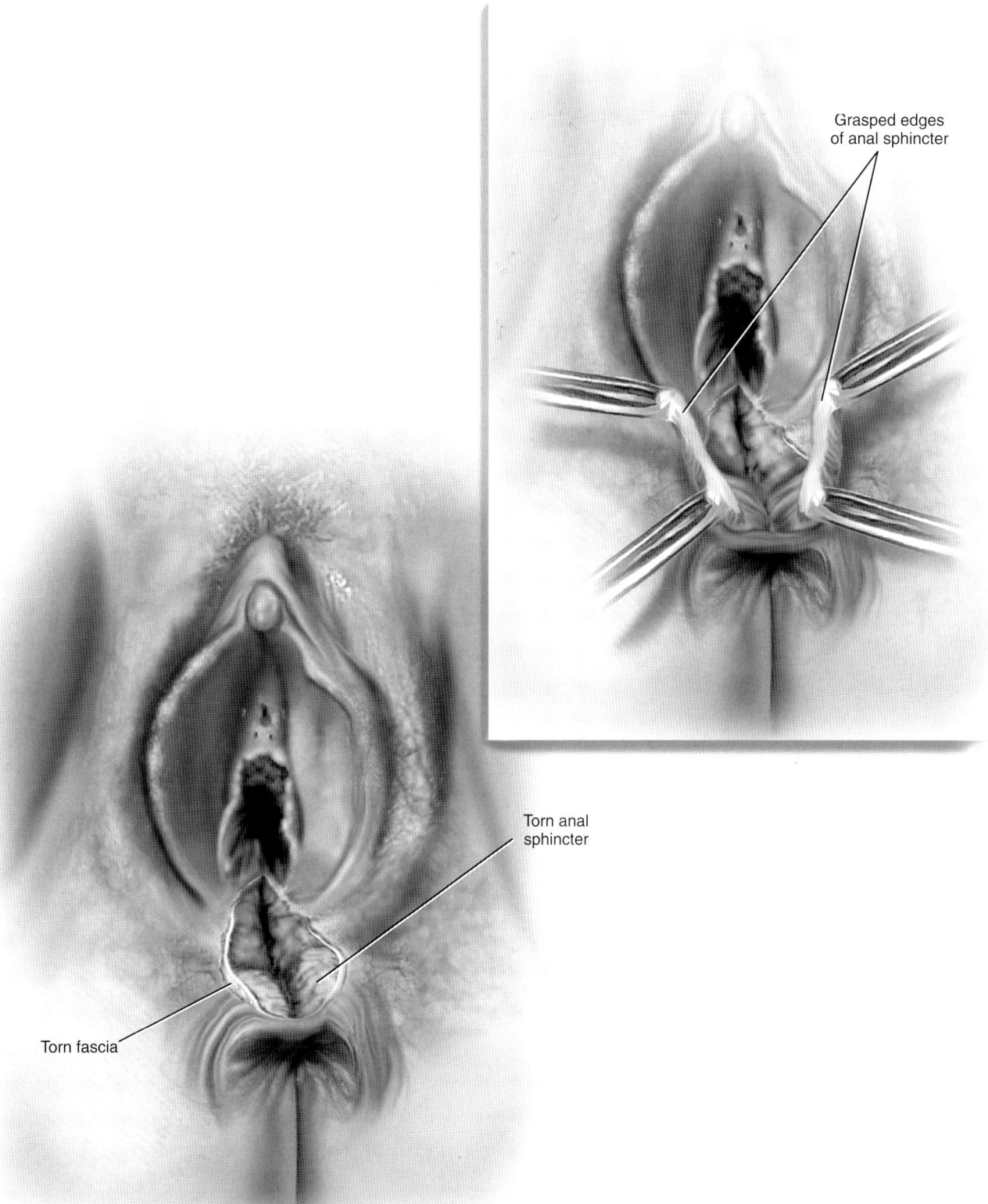

Grasped edges
of anal sphincter

Torn anal
sphincter

Torn fascia

**FIGURE 80–5** In this drawing, a midline episiotomy has extended through the external anal sphincter. The **inset** shows the application of Allis clamps and the upper and lower margins of the sphincter injury. Note that the anal mucosa is intact.

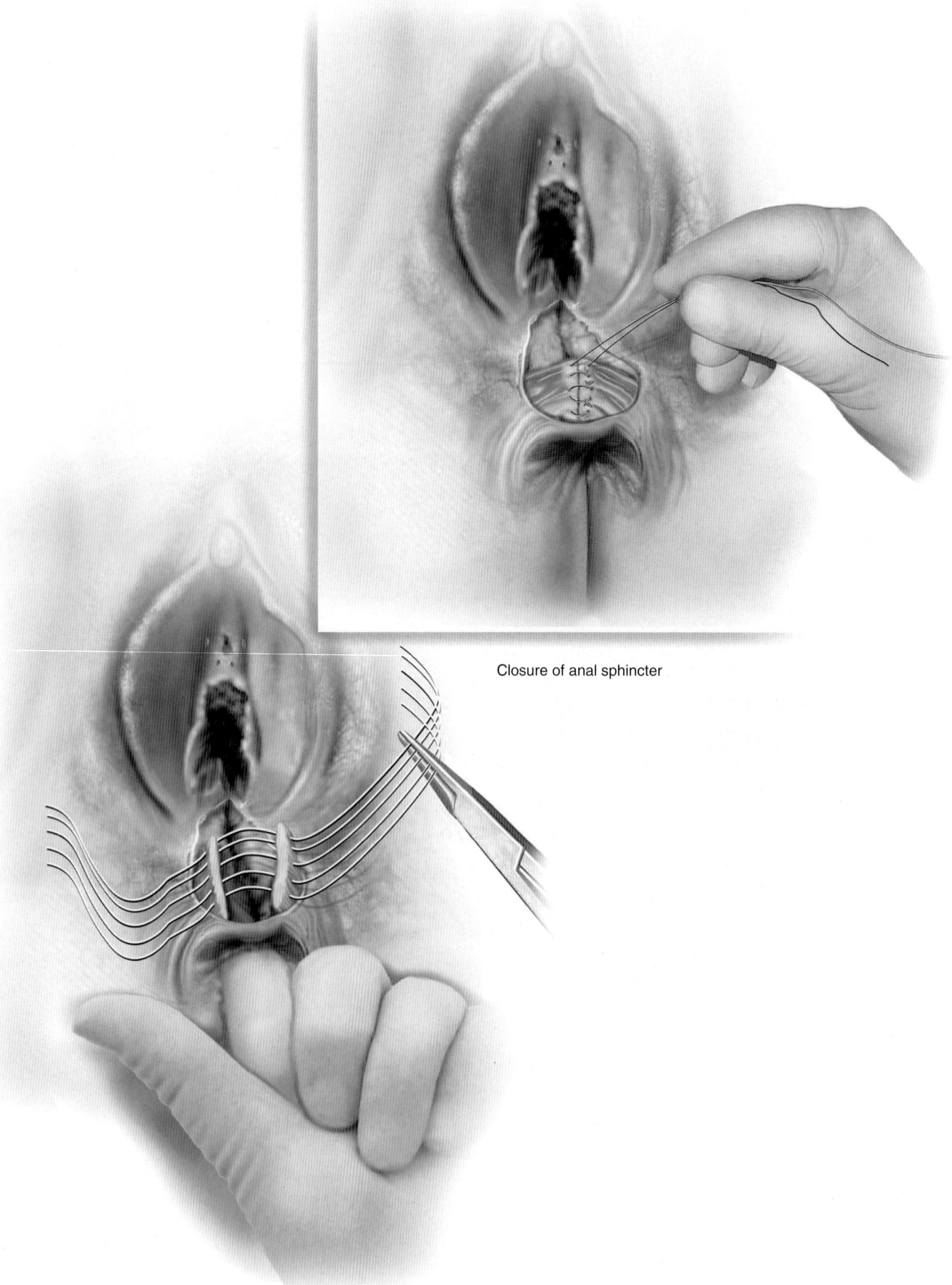

Closure of anal sphincter

**FIGURE 80–6** With a gloved finger in the rectum, interrupted 2-0 or 3-0 Vicryl sutures are placed through the entire width (in the case illustrated, a complete sphincter tear) of the external sphincter ani. Approximately five or six stitches are usually required. The stitches are tied into place, and a gloved finger in the rectum can feel the tightening of the sphincter after closure. This examination will ensure that overcorrection has been avoided.

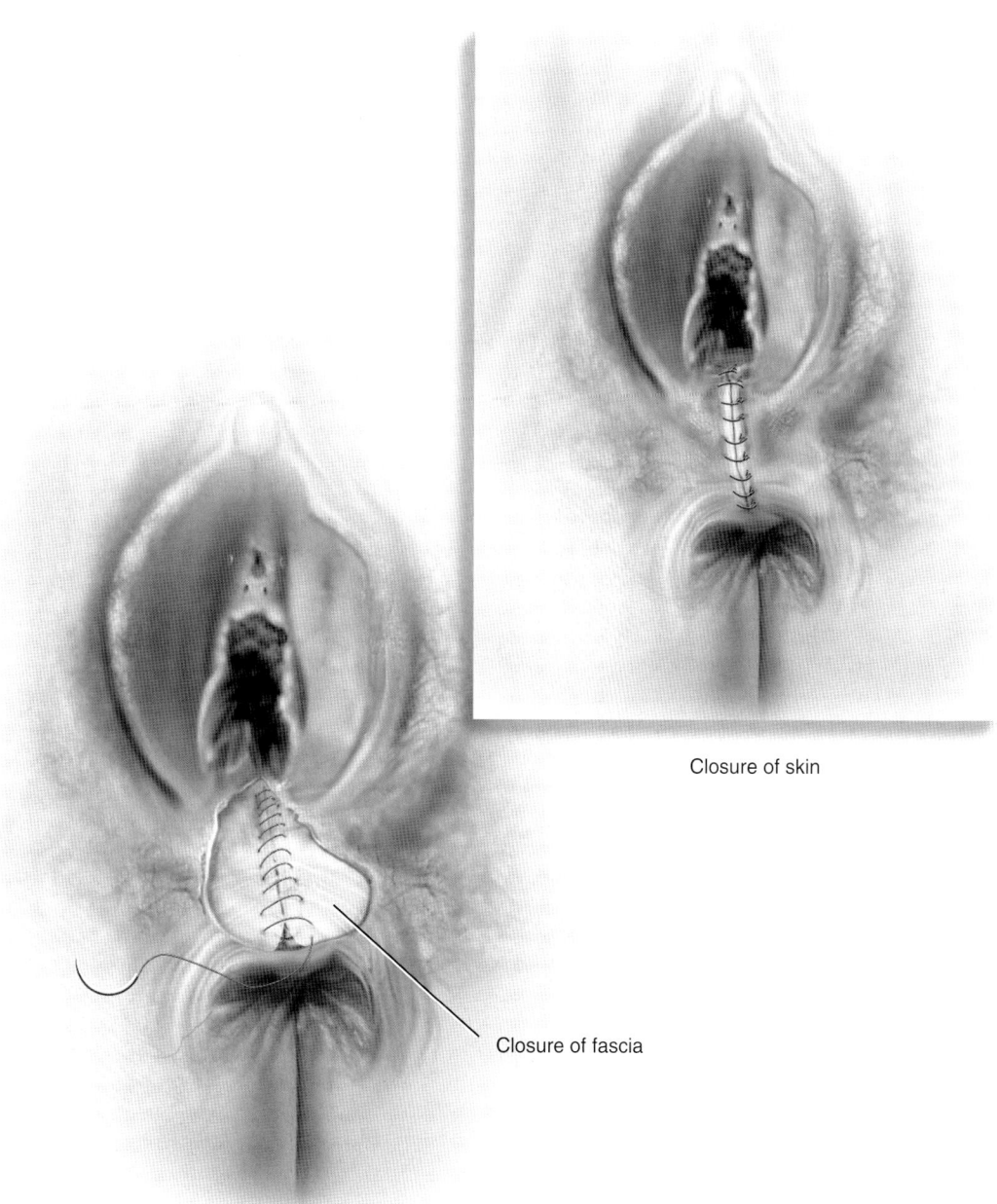

Closure of skin

Closure of fascia

**FIGURE 80–7** The fascia is closed with a running 3-0 Vicryl, and the vagina and vestibular and perineal skin are closed with running or interrupted 3-0 Vicryl sutures. Alternatively, a subcuticular closure may be performed with a 3-0 or 4-0 running Vicryl suture (see inset of Fig. 80–10).

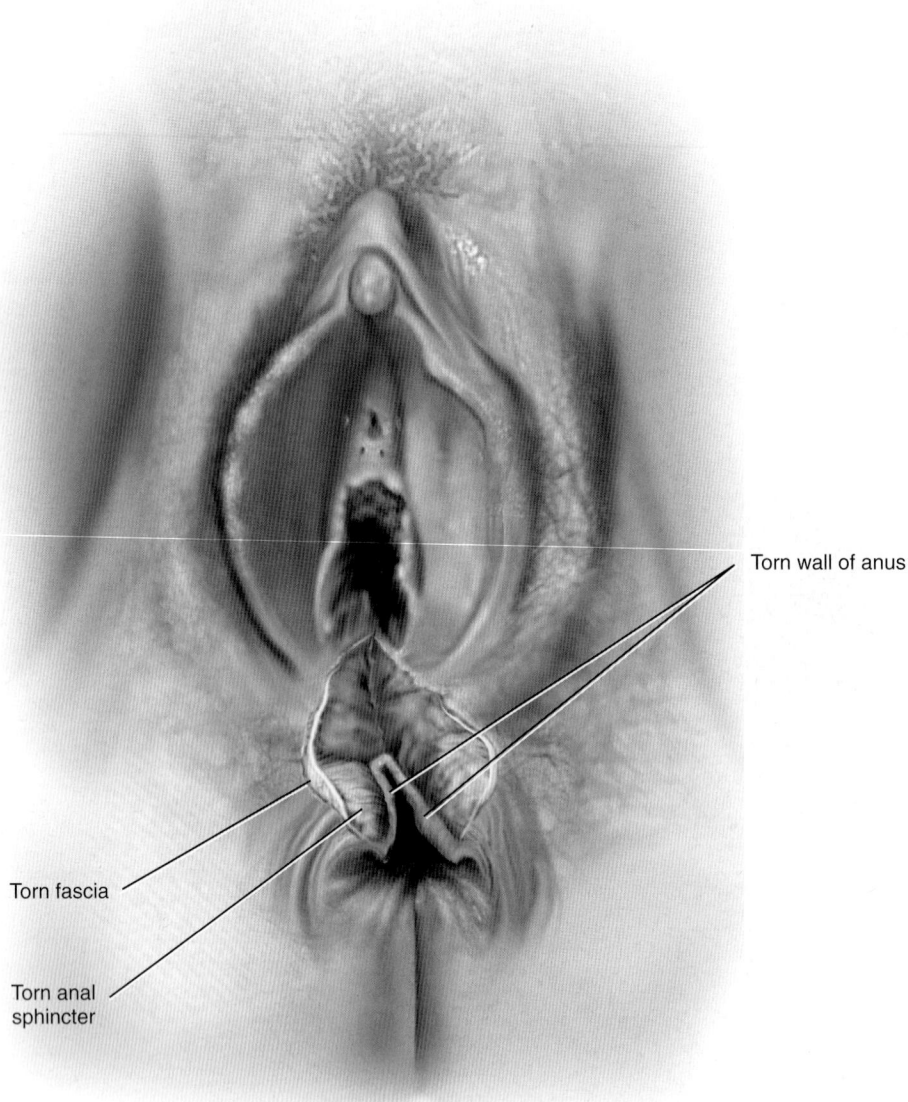

Torn wall of anus

Torn fascia

Torn anal
sphincter

**FIGURE 80–8** A complete perineal laceration is shown in this illustration. The anterior anal sphincter is completely separated, and the wound further extends through the anal wall with disruption of the anal mucosa.

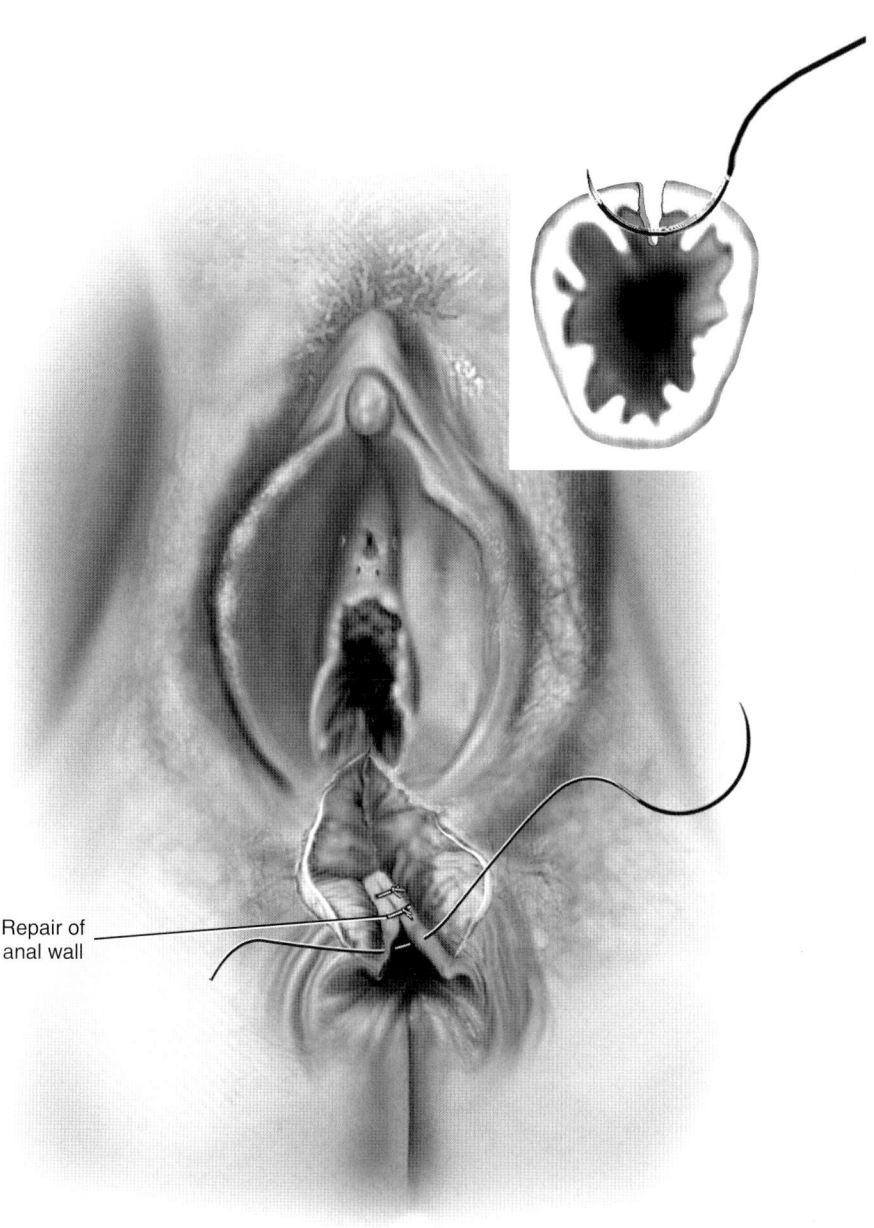

Repair of
anal wall

**FIGURE 80–9** After the upper and lower margins of the injury are secured, interrupted 2-0 chromic sutures are placed through the full thickness of the anorectal wall as illustrated. The wound is closed without tension on the suture line.

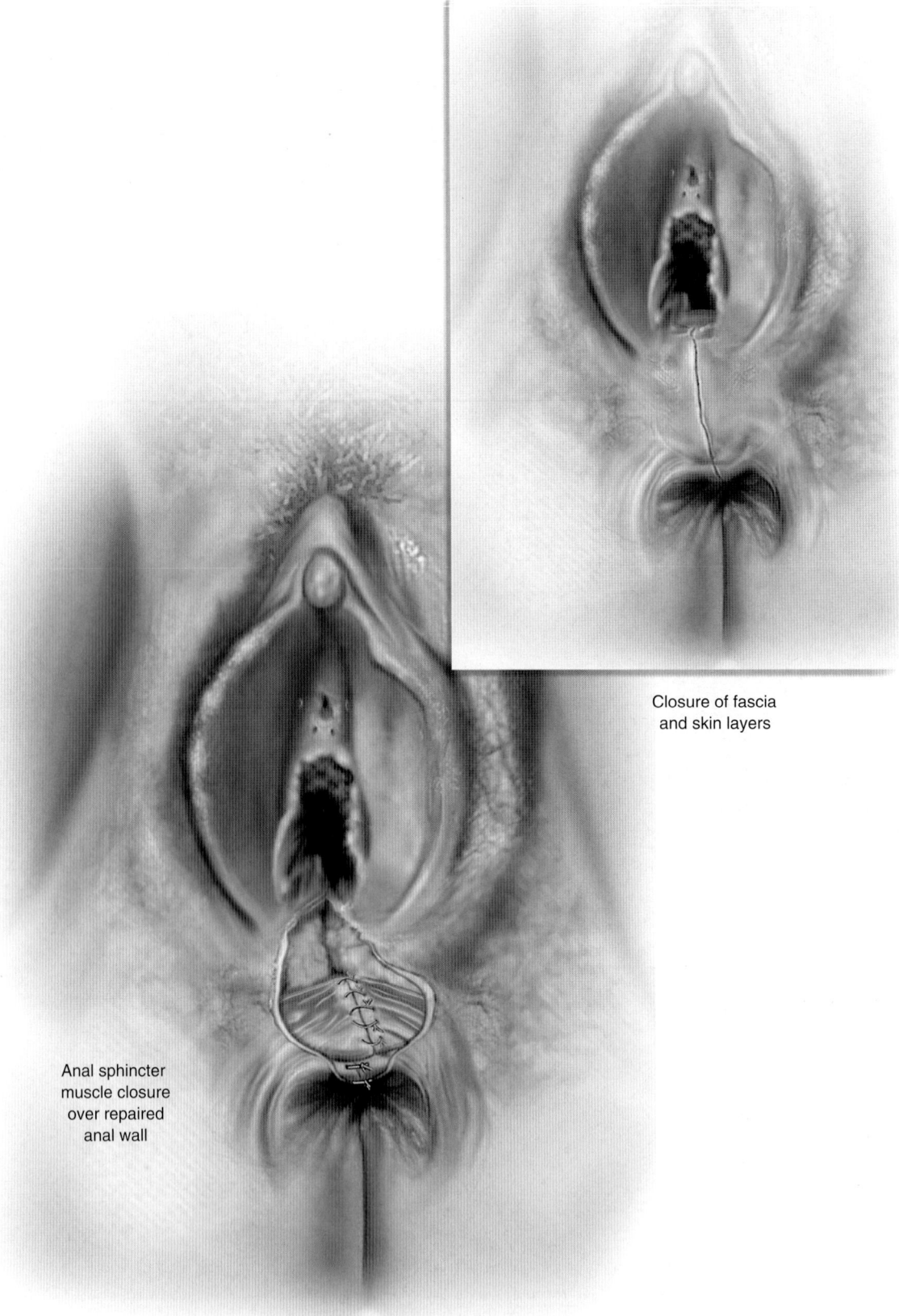

Closure of fascia
and skin layers

Anal sphincter
muscle closure
over repaired
anal wall

**FIGURE 80–10** The anal sphincter is closed as described in Figure 80-6. Although a gloved finger need not be placed into the repaired anus until the repair has been completed, it is preferable that the sphincter repair suture line not overlie the anal repair suture line.

# Other Related Gynecologic Surgery

# SECTION A

## Surgical Procedures Performed on the Lower Urinary Tract

UNIT 4 ■ SECTION A

# CHAPTER 81

# Anatomy of the Urethra

*Michael S. Baggish* ■ *Mickey M. Karram*

The female urethra is about 4 cm long and averages 6 mm in diameter. Its lumen is slightly curved as it passes from its internal position in the retropubic space, perforates the perineal membrane, and ends by opening into the vestibule directly above the vaginal opening. Throughout its length, the posterior urethra is embedded in the anterior vaginal wall.

The epithelium of the urethra is continuous externally with that of the vulva and internally with that of the bladder. It consists primarily of stratified squamous epithelium that becomes transitional near the bladder. The epithelium is supported by a layer of loose fibroelastic connective tissue—the lamina propria. The lamina propria contains many bundles of collagen fibrils and fibrocytes, as well as an abundance of elastic fibers oriented both longitudinally and circularly around the urethra. Numerous thin-walled veins are another characteristic feature. This rich vascular supply is thought to contribute to urethral resistance. Cross-sections of the urethra below the urethrovesical junction at 6 to 9 mm (distal) clearly show the cavernous vascularity that contributes more than 50% of the volume of tissue constituting the anterior and lateral walls of the urethra (Fig. 81-1A through D).

The smooth muscles of the urethra are composed primarily of oblique and longitudinal muscle fibers with a few circularly oriented outer fibers. This smooth muscle, along with the detrusor muscle in the bladder base, forms what can be called the intrinsic *urethral sphincter* mechanism. Longitudinally directed muscle probably shortens and widens the urethral lumen during micturition, whereas circular smooth muscle contributes to urethral resistance to outflow at rest.

Historically, striated muscle termed the *striated urogenital sphincter* has been divided into three muscles: the sphincter urethrae, which is described as a striated band of muscle that surrounds the proximal two thirds of the urethra, and the compressor urethrae and urethrovaginal sphincter, which consist of two straplike bands of striated muscle that arch over the ventral surface of the distal third of the urethra. The authors' recent dissections on multiple female cadavers with gross and microscopic examination of this area revealed no separate or distinct striated musculature of the urethra. The authors were unable to identify any striated musculature in the periurethral area that was not an extension of the levator ani muscle (Fig. 81-2A through G). In a series of 12 cadaveric dissections, the levator ani muscle was thought to extend over the anterior surface of the urethra. The authors were thus unable to identify the previously described separate and distinct striated urogenital sphincter. Figs. 81-3 through 81-6 are gross and microscopic sections showing the levator muscle over the urethra. In performing histologic sections throughout the length of the urethra, the authors also observed that most of the vascular contribution of the urethra stemmed from the bulb of the vestibule. The vascularity created an umbrella-type effect over the anterior and lateral walls of the urethra (Figs. 81-1B and 81-7).

Urethral support, which is thought to be important in the continence mechanism, has traditionally been thought to be provided by the inner action of the pubourethral ligaments, the urogenital diaphragm, and the muscles of the pelvic diaphragm. Numerous investigators have described the so-called pubourethral ligaments as extending from the inferior surface of the pubic bones to the urethra. More recently, it has become apparent that the urethra is not suspended ventrally by ligamentous structures, but instead the proximal urethra and bladder base are supported in a slinglike fashion by the anterior vaginal wall, which is attached bilaterally to the muscles of the pelvic sidewall at the arcus tendineus fasciae pelvis, or white line. The tissues previously described as pubourethral ligaments are in actuality made up of the perineal membrane and the most caudal portions of the arcus tendineus fasciae pelvis, which fix the distal urethra beneath the pubic bone (Fig. 81-8).

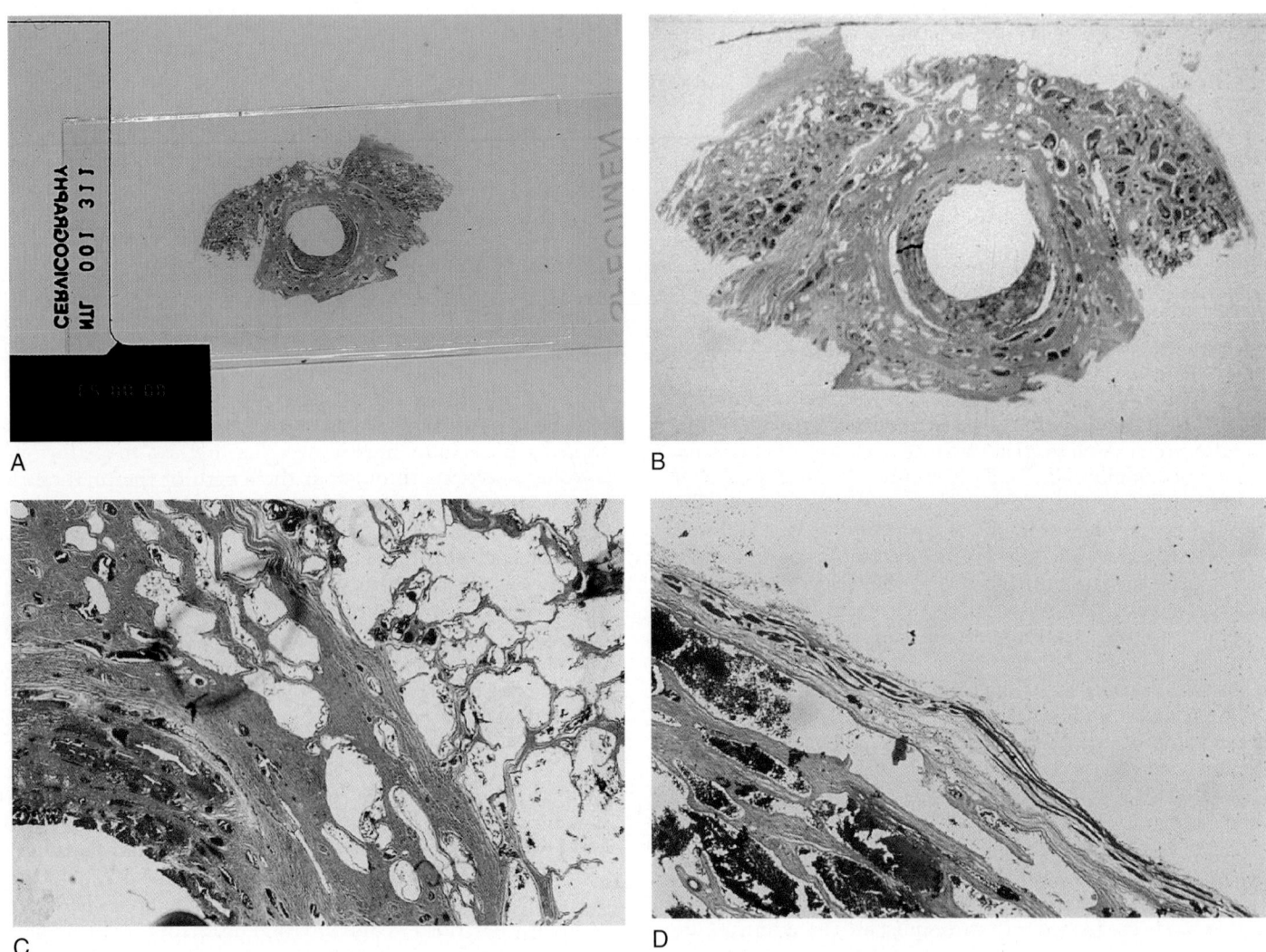

**FIGURE 81–1  A.** This section clearly shows the cavernous tissue making up an integral portion of the anterior urethral wall between 11 and 1 o'clock (6 to 9 mm distal to the urethrovesical junction) (H & E). **B.** This section at 9 mm below the urethrovesical junction shows the smooth muscle of the urethra, as well as the umbrella of cavernous tissue (*pink*) forming the major portion of the anterior and anterolateral wall of the urethra. **C.** High-power view of the anterolateral wall of the urethra. The cavernous bulb tissue is closely applied to the urethra. **D.** A thin layer of skeletal muscle probably derived from the bulbocavernosus muscle overlies the cavernous (bulb) tissue of the urethra.

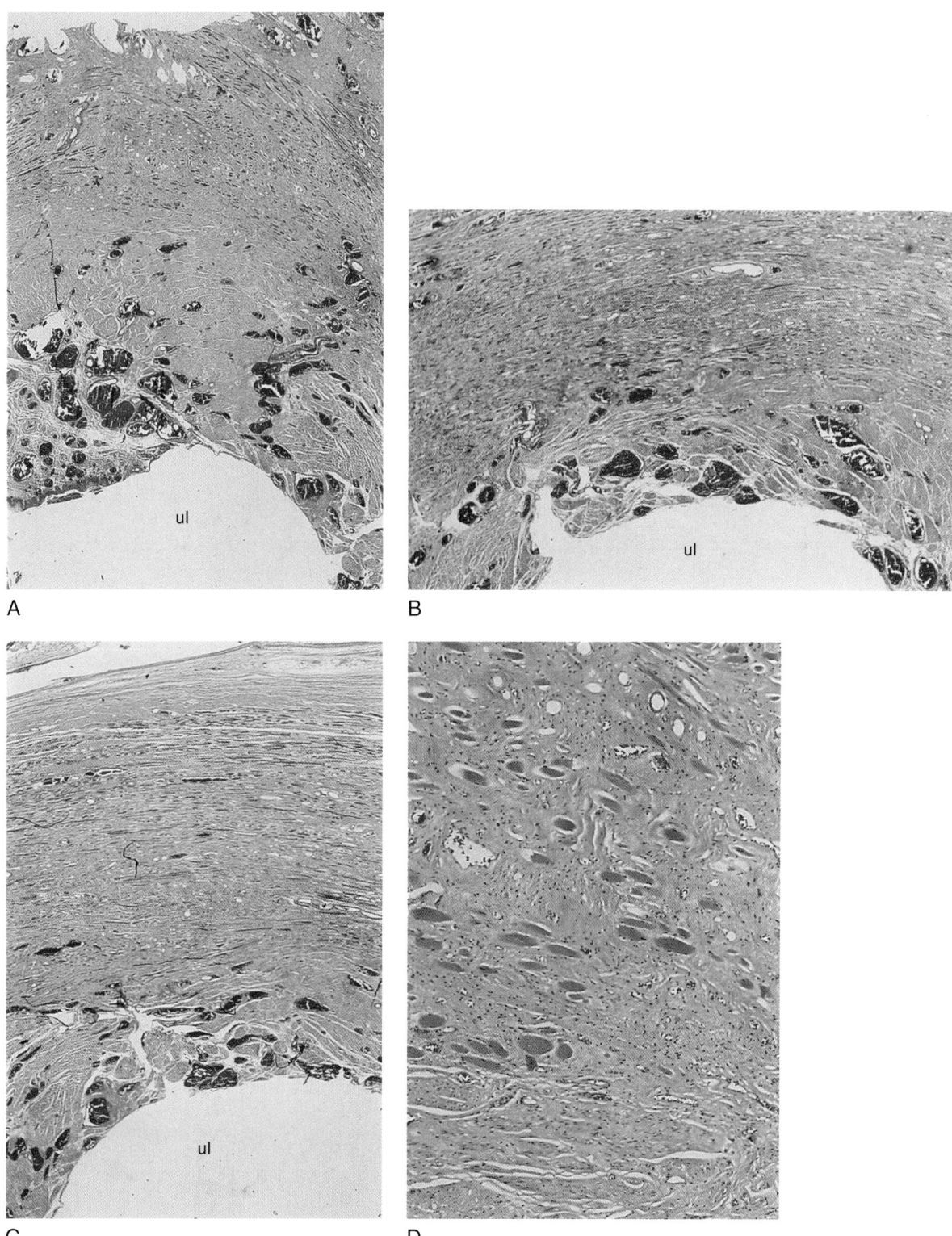

**FIGURE 81–2  A.** This section of the anterior urethra is obtained at 15 mm below (distal to) the urethrovesical junction. Anterior to (above) the lumen (ul), with its rich vascular submucosa, is the thickened anterior urethral wall. The deep pink tissue (outer half) is skeletal muscle derived from the levator ani muscles. **B.** This section is obtained at level 6, or 18 mm distal to the urethrovesical junction. The anterior urethral wall is dense pink tissue, and the upper three fourths of the wall consists of skeletal muscle. **C.** Another view at level 6 confirms the layers of skeletal muscle making up the greatest mass volume of the anterior urethra. **D.** High-power view of the deep pink skeletal muscle seen in parts **B** and **C.**

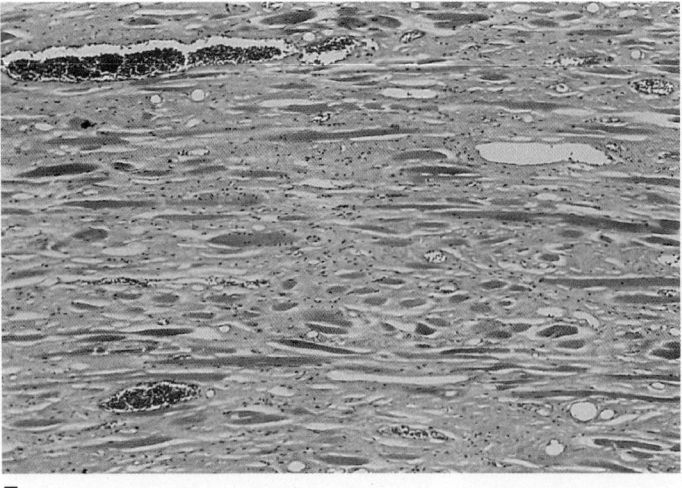

E

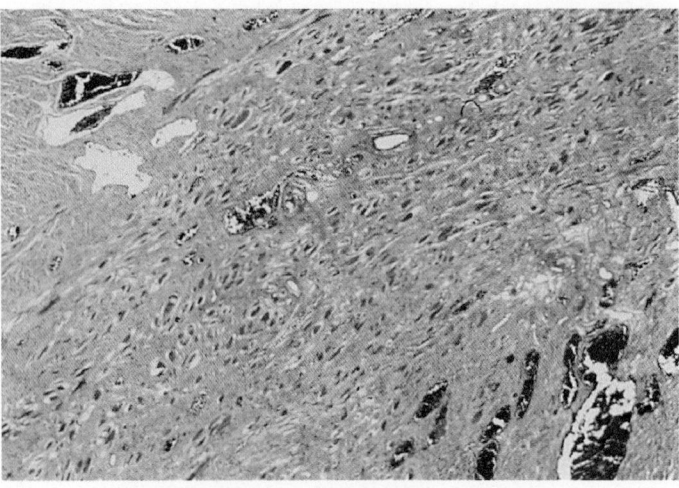

F

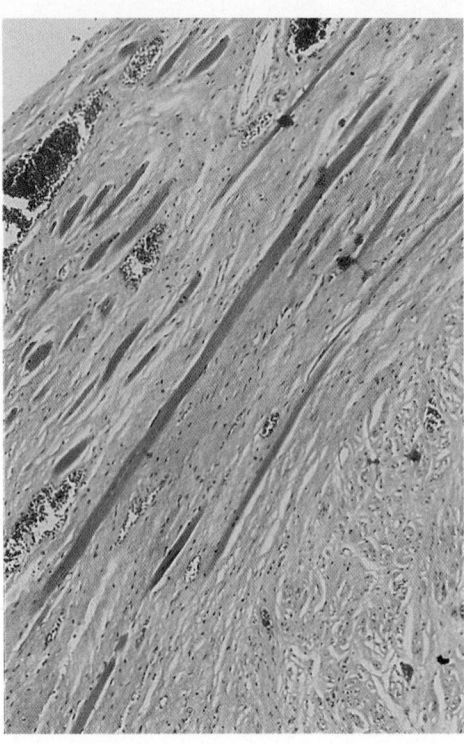

G

**FIGURE 81–2, cont'd E.** High-power view of the skeletal muscle of the anterior urethral wall (different cut level than part **D**). **F.** The anterolateral wall of the urethra similarly shows a mass of skeletal muscle (11 o'clock position). **G.** Similar cut at the lateral outer urethral wall shows the deep-pink staining skeletal muscle 20 mm distal to the urethrovesical junction. The muscle is derived from the levator ani muscle.

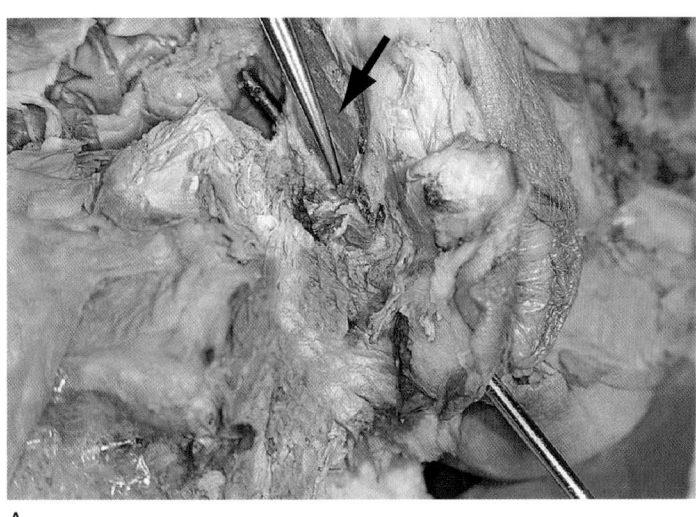

A

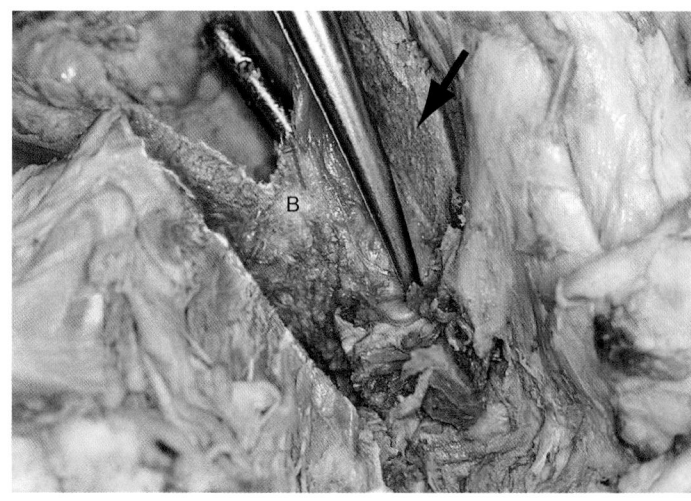

B

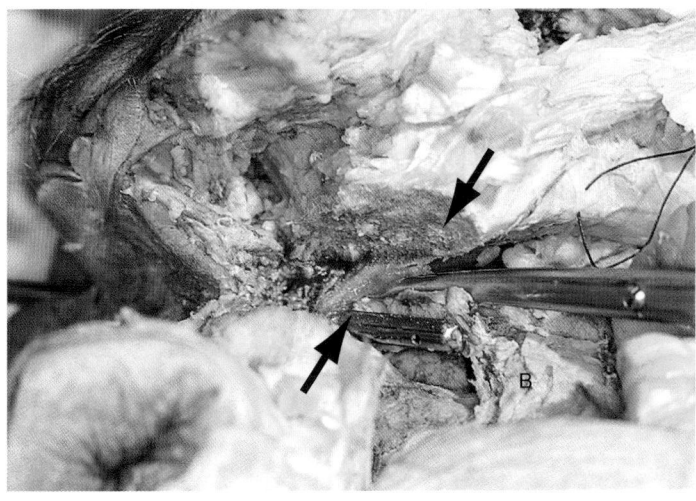

C

**FIGURE 81-3** **A.** A metal cannula is seen in the opened bladder. The arrow points to where the pubic bone was sawed away. A mass of skeletal muscle inserts into the urethrovesical junction and originates from the levator ani below the pubic ramus (tip of scissors). **B.** The bladder (B) is opened with a transurethral cannula seen protruding from the bladder (B) lumen. The arrow points to the sawed pubic bone. The scissors point to skeletal muscle at the urethrovesical junction. **C.** The lower arrow points to a continuation of the descending levator ani muscle from beneath the pubic bone, which is in continuity from the levator below the white line. It enters the urethrovesical junction laterally and anteriorly.

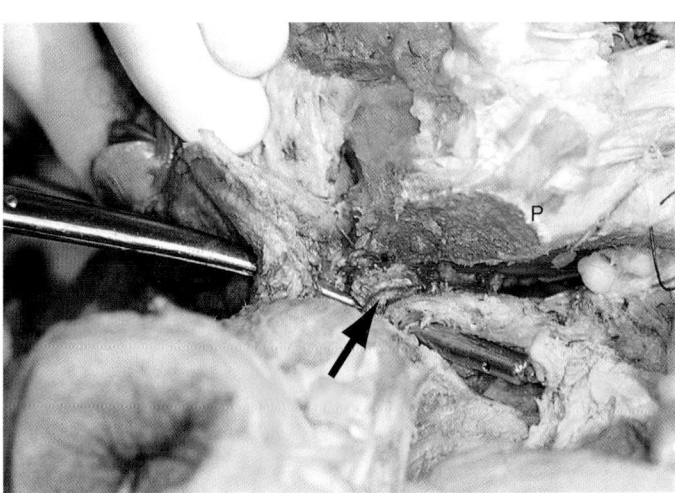

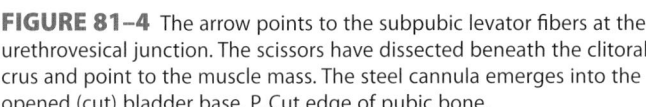

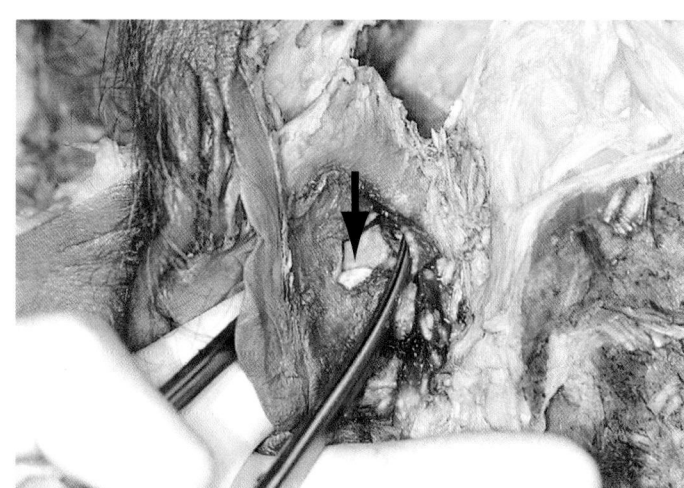

**FIGURE 81-4** The arrow points to the subpubic levator fibers at the urethrovesical junction. The scissors have dissected beneath the clitoral crus and point to the muscle mass. The steel cannula emerges into the opened (cut) bladder base. P, Cut edge of pubic bone.

**FIGURE 81-5** The operator's left index finger is inserted through the introitus into the vagina. The metal cannula on the gloved finger has been inserted into the external urethral meatus. The scissors point to the left vestibular bulb. The arrow points to the thin outer (but intact) wall of the urethra. The white gloved fingertip can be seen via an opening in the lateral vaginal wall.

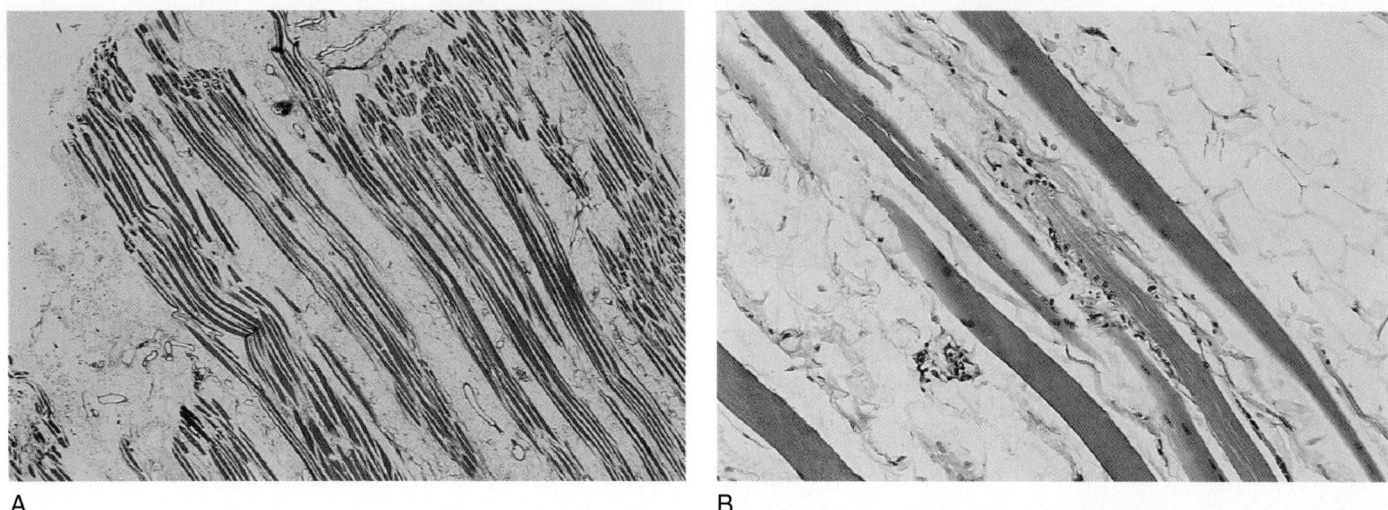

A                                                                                B

**FIGURE 81–6  A.** Sample of the muscle bundle descending from beneath the pubic ramus (see Figs. 55–3 and 55–4) to insert into the lateral and anterior urethral wall at the urethrovesical junction. The muscle is clearly skeletal. **B.** High-power view showing cross-striations of skeletal muscle.

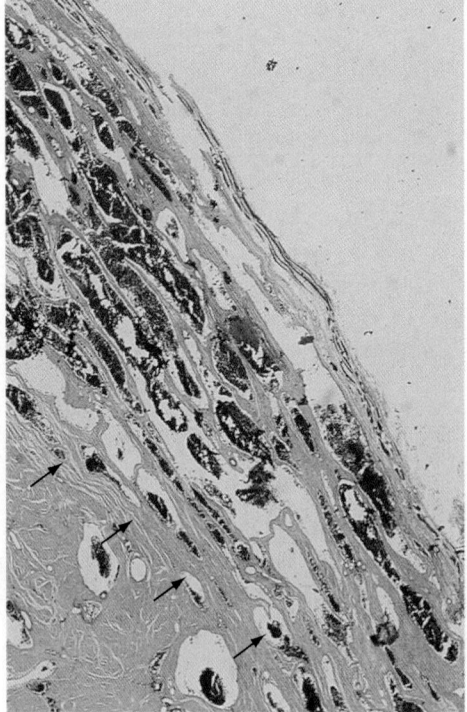

**FIGURE 81–7** This high-power view shows the relationship of the anterolateral cavernous bulb tissue to the vascularity above the urethral mucosa. The arrows indicate the boundary between the cavernous tissue and the smooth muscle of the urethral wall.

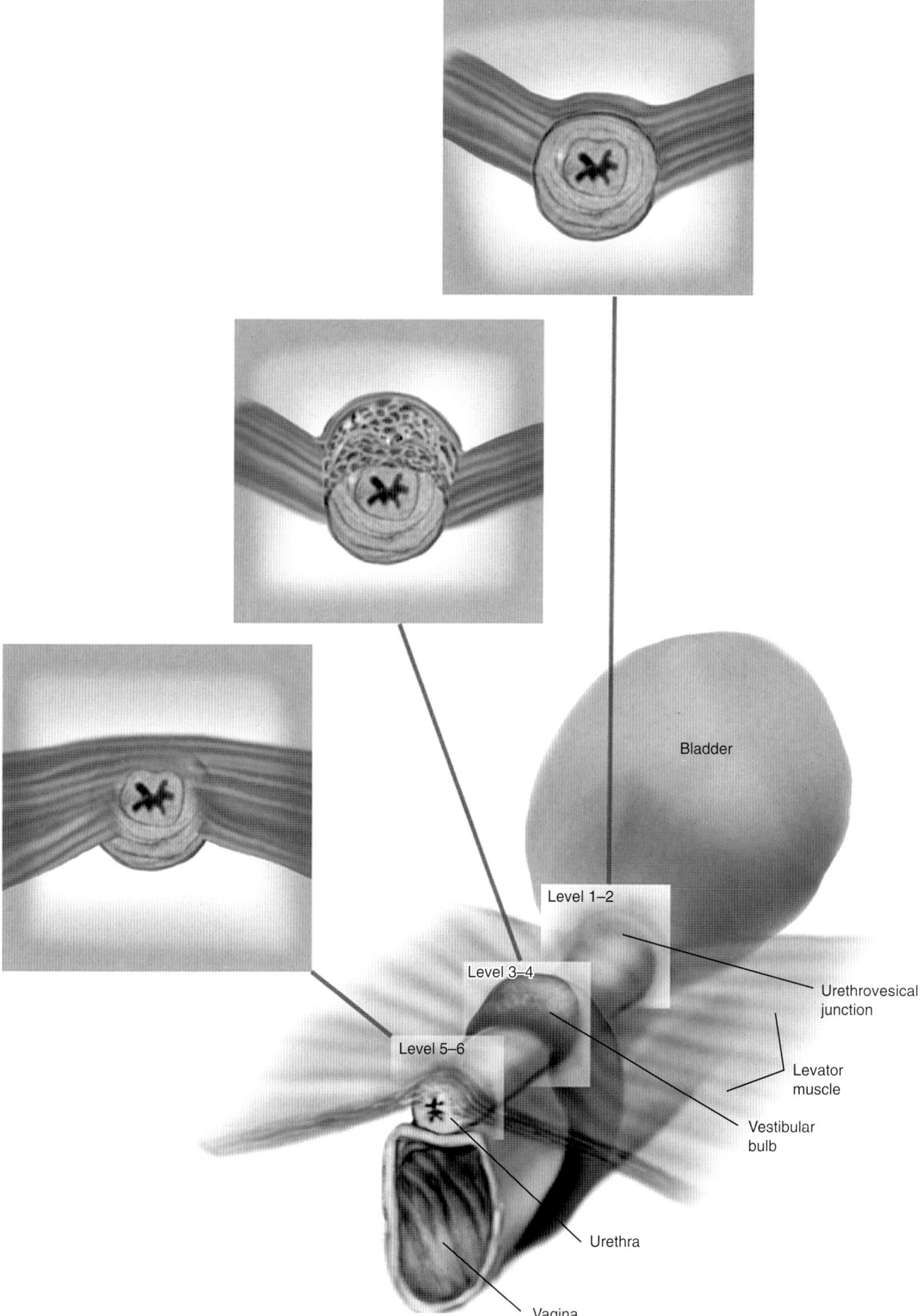

**FIGURE 81–8** Schematic view of the relationships of cavernous and skeletal muscle based on serial histologic cuts from the proximal to the distal urethra. The skeletal muscle is derived from the levator ani muscles on either side of the pelvis and descends from beneath the pubic rami. The cavernous tissue takes its origin mainly from the bulb of the vestibule but also from the clitoral body and crura (at the point of fusion to the clitoral body).

# CHAPTER 82

# Surgical Repair of Urethral Prolapse

*John B. Gebhart*

Prolapse of edematous urethral mucosa may be of sufficient degree to require surgical excision (Figs. 82–1 and 82–2). It is important to differentiate urethral prolapse from a urethral caruncle. The former is circumferential in nature, is less common, and is treated surgically, whereas the latter is much more common, usually requires only topical estrogen therapy, and usually is isolated to the posterior urethral meatus.

The procedure begins by identifying the urethral lumen (Fig. 82–3). Placement of a transurethral catheter is an option; however, it can be difficult to work around. The excision begins at the 12 o'clock position. A stay suture is placed to hold the tissue and provide traction. Working in a counterclockwise fashion, the redundant mucosa is trimmed with a scissors or is excised using needle-tip cautery (Fig. 82–4). During excision, each anchoring suture (usually 3-0 chromic or 4-0 Vicryl) is placed as the mucosa is freed (Fig. 82–5). This tissue is usually very edematous and friable. Failure to secure the mucosa with stay sutures as the mucosal prolapse is excised can result in retraction of the mucosa superiorly, making it much more difficult to reapproximate. A transurethral catheter may be left in place for a day if there is significant swelling.

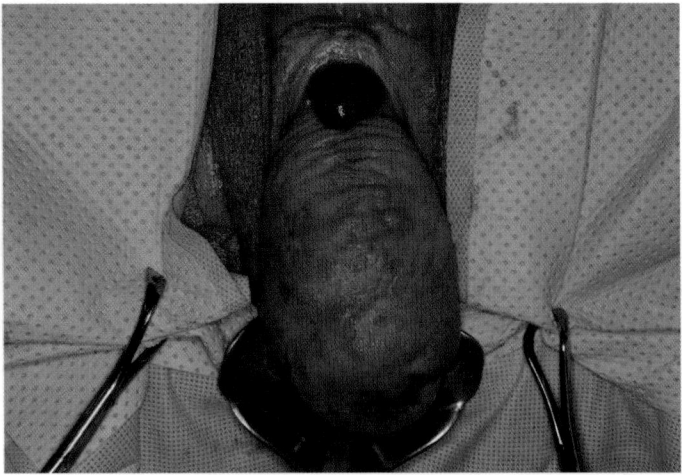

**FIGURE 82–1** Complete uterovaginal prolapse with urethral prolapse.

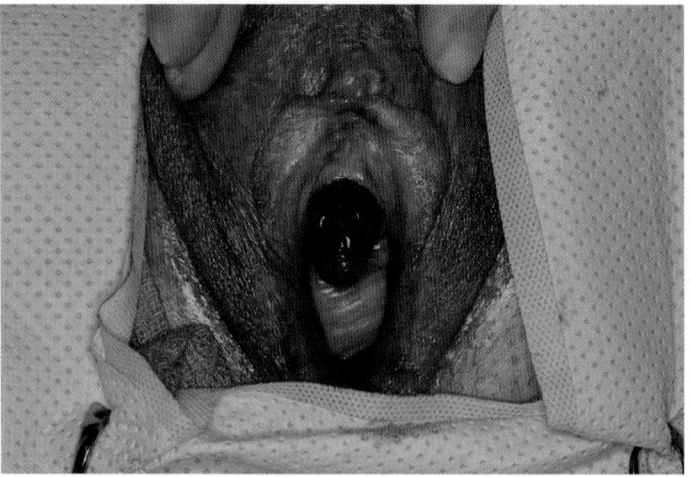

**FIGURE 82–2** Close-up view of the urethral prolapse once the uterovaginal prolapse has been reduced.

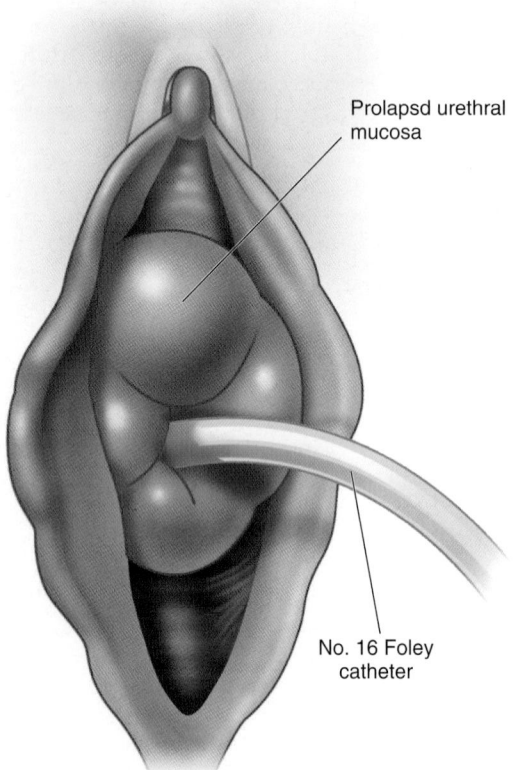

**FIGURE 82–3** Circumferential urethral prolapse with a transurethral catheter in place.

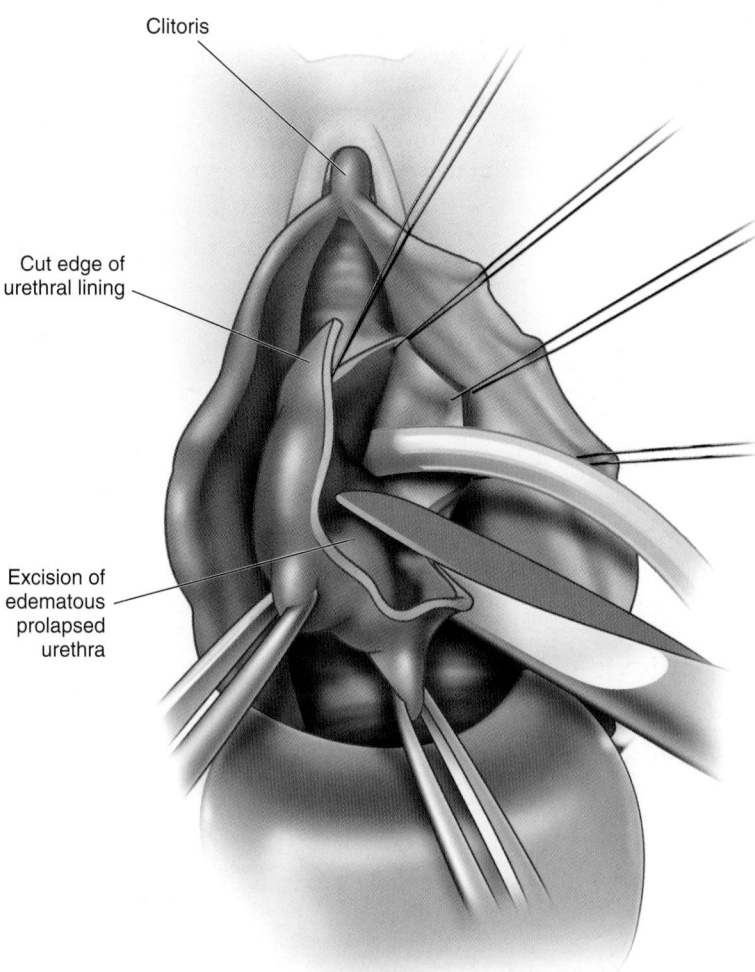

**FIGURE 82–4** Anchor sutures are placed as the urethral prolapse is trimmed.

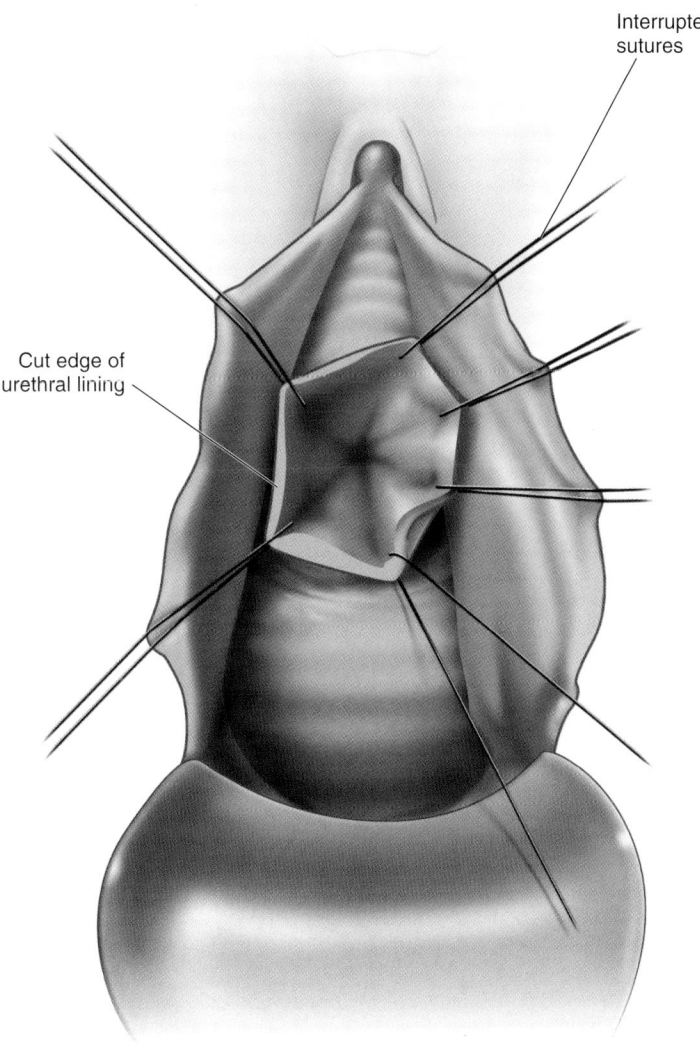

Interrupted
sutures

Cut edge of
urethral lining

**FIGURE 82–5** The urethral prolapse has been excised and the anchor
sutures are now ready to be secured in place.

# CHAPTER 83

# Repair of Urethrovaginal Fistula

*Mickey M. Karram*

Most urethrovaginal fistulas result in urinary incontinence and require surgical repair (Fig. 83–1). Rarely, a distal urethrovaginal fistula may be asymptomatic and not require repair. A non-irradiated primary fistula can usually be successfully repaired by a layered tension-free closure of the fistula (Figs. 83–2 through 83–4). If the surrounding tissue appears to be devascularized, the tissue has been irradiated, or the fistula is recurrent, it is probably best to interpose a labial fat pad between the urethra and the anterior vagina (see section on Martius Fat Pad Transposition) (Fig. 83–5). If the fistula is in the proximal urethra or at the bladder neck and the continence mechanism is thought to have been compromised, an anti-incontinence procedure, most commonly a suburethral sling, may be performed at the time of the fistula repair.

The repair begins with the placement of a transurethral Foley catheter. The anterior vaginal wall is then injected with a dilute hemostatic solution to facilitate dissection in the appropriate plane and decrease bleeding. A midline anterior vaginal wall incision or an inverted-U incision is made and extended on both sides of the urethral defect (see Fig. 83–2). The edges of the vagina are grasped with Allis clamps, and the vaginal wall is sharply separated from the underlying tissue (see Fig. 83–2C). This dissection should be extended laterally to the descending pubic rami and posteriorly until the urethra is mobilized as much as possible to allow a tension-free closure. Rarely, the retropubic space must be entered vaginally to facilitate this urethral mobility (see Fig. 83–5) (see section on Vaginal Urethrolysis). The edges of the wall of the urethra are then approximated with fine delayed absorbable interrupted sutures. The sutures should be placed in the extramucosal position (see Figs. 83–2 and 83–3). The initial suture line is then inverted with a second suture incorporating the pubocervical fascia (see Figs. 83–2E and 83–3). The vaginal incision is closed with interrupted 3-0 delayed absorbable sutures (see Fig. 83–2F). A Foley or suprapubic catheter should be left in place for 7 to 10 days.

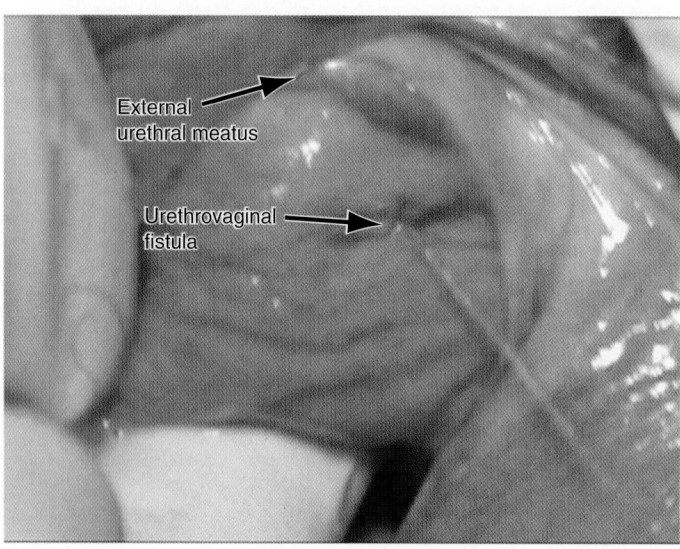

**FIGURE 83–1** Urethrovaginal fistula. Note the fistula is in the midportion of the urethra, and urinary incontinence is readily demonstrated through the fistulous tract.

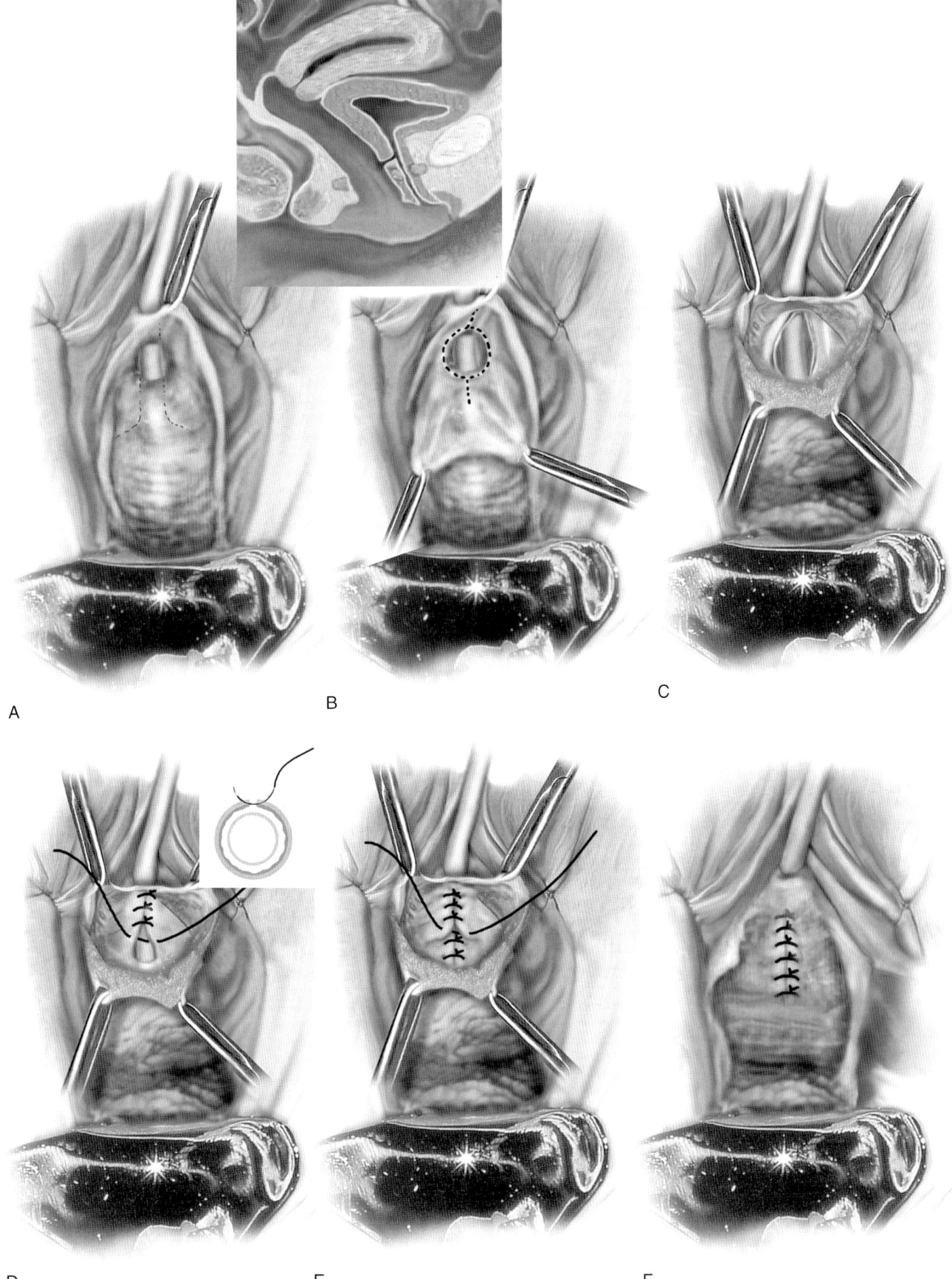

**FIGURE 83–2** Repair of urethrovaginal fistula. **A.** Urethrovaginal fistula. **B.** Anterior vaginal wall incision is made and extended on both sides of the urethral defect. **C.** Vaginal wall is sharply separated from the underlying pubocervical fascia. **D.** Fine delayed absorbable interrupted sutures are placed in an extramucosal fashion. **E.** The initial suture line is then inverted with a second suture incorporating the pubocervical fascia. **F.** Vaginal incision is closed with interrupted 2-0 delayed absorbable sutures.

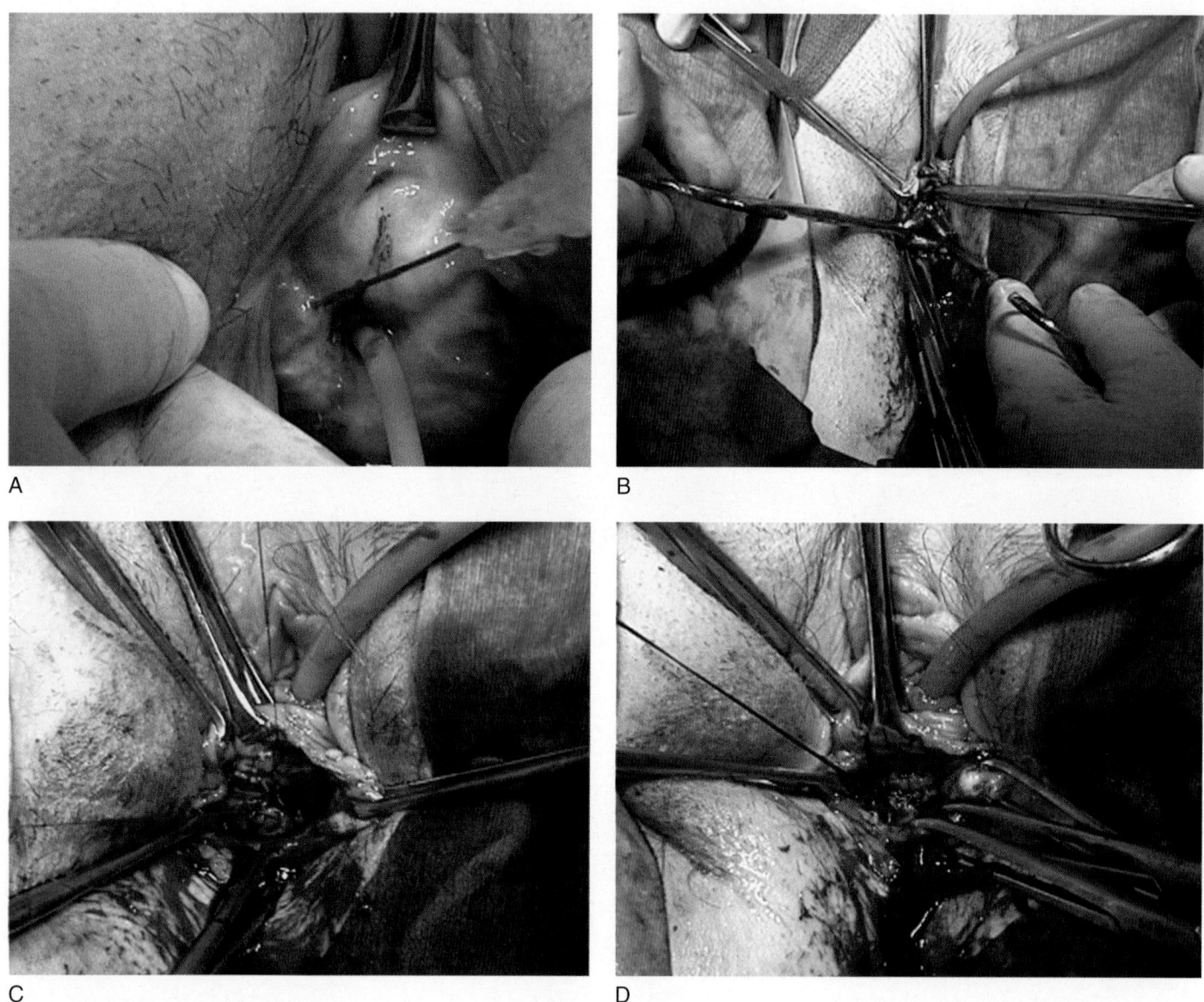

**FIGURE 83–3** Urethrovaginal fistula at the level of the proximal urethra. **A.** A pediatric Foley catheter has been placed in the urethrovaginal fistula, and a hemostatic solution is injected to hydrodistend the anterior vaginal wall. **B.** The anterior vaginal wall has been dissected off the posterior wall of the urethra, and the edges of the fistula are grasped with Allis clamps. **C.** An initial layer of 4-0 delayed absorbable sutures has been placed in an interrupted fashion approximating the edges of the urethra mucosa. **D.** A second layer of 3-0 delayed absorbable sutures has been placed, imbricating the muscular portion of the wall of the urethra over the initial layer.

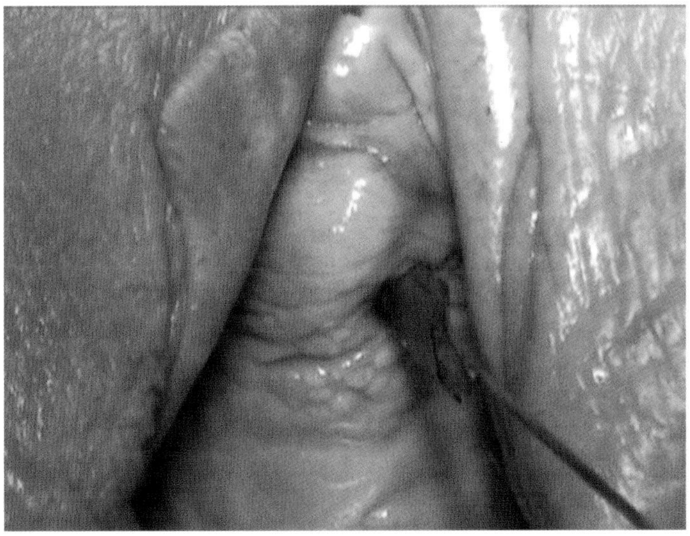

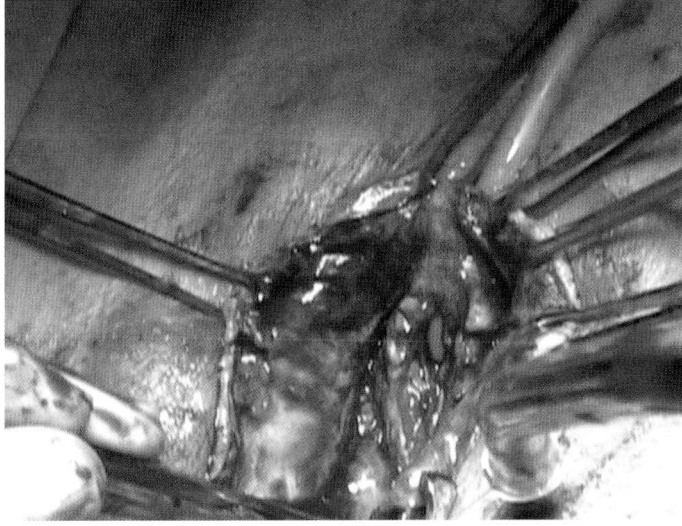

**FIGURE 83–4** Repair of a recurrent urethrovaginal fistula. **A.** A probe has been placed in the fistulous tract. **B.** A Foley catheter has been placed in the fistulous tract to facilitate the dissection. Note that excessive scarification is being sharply excised from the fistulous tract. **C.** A bridge of devascularized tissue is noted and will be excised. **D.** The fistulous tract is seen after excision of all of the devascularized, scarred tissue from the previous repair. **E.** The healthy edges of the fistulous tract are noted and will be closed in two layers as previously mentioned.

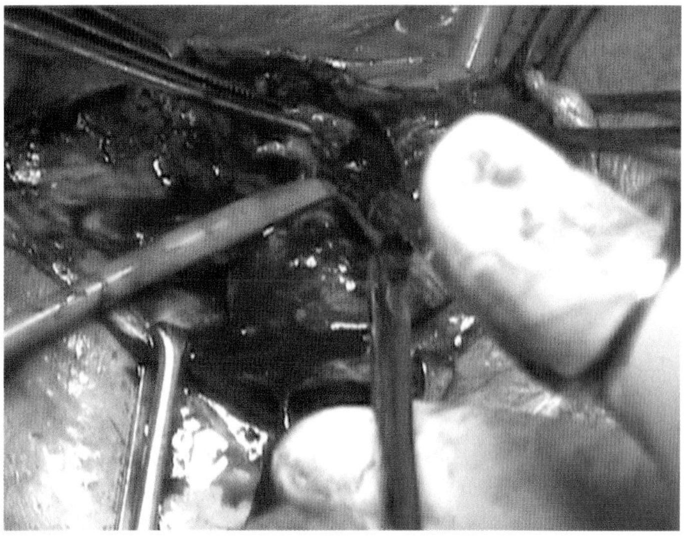

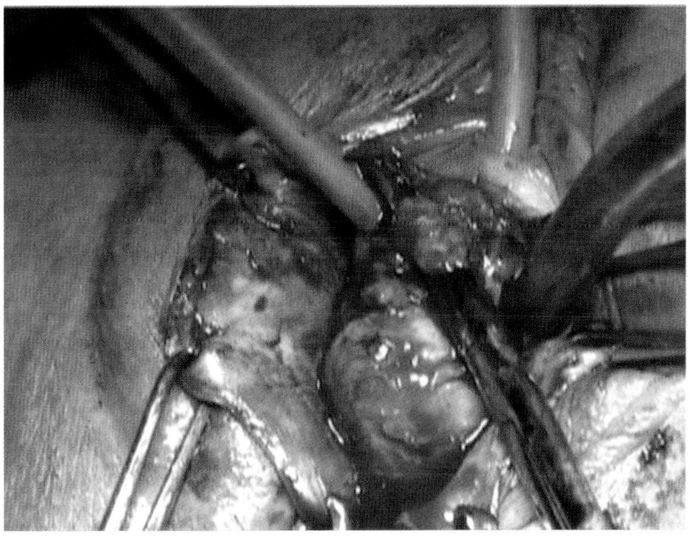

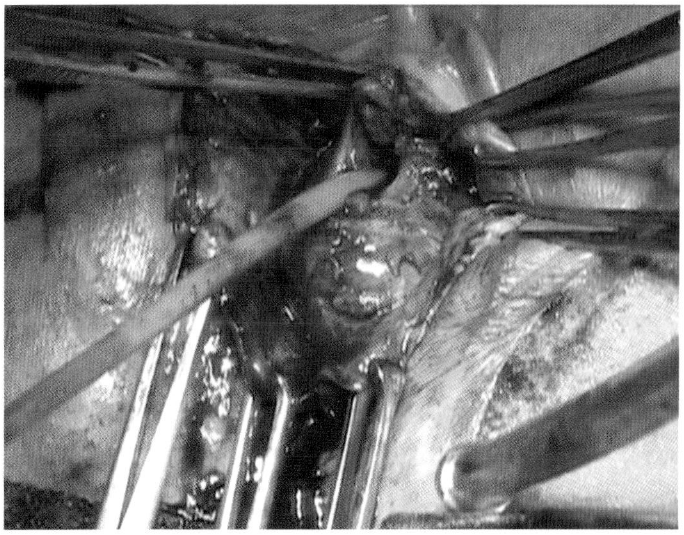

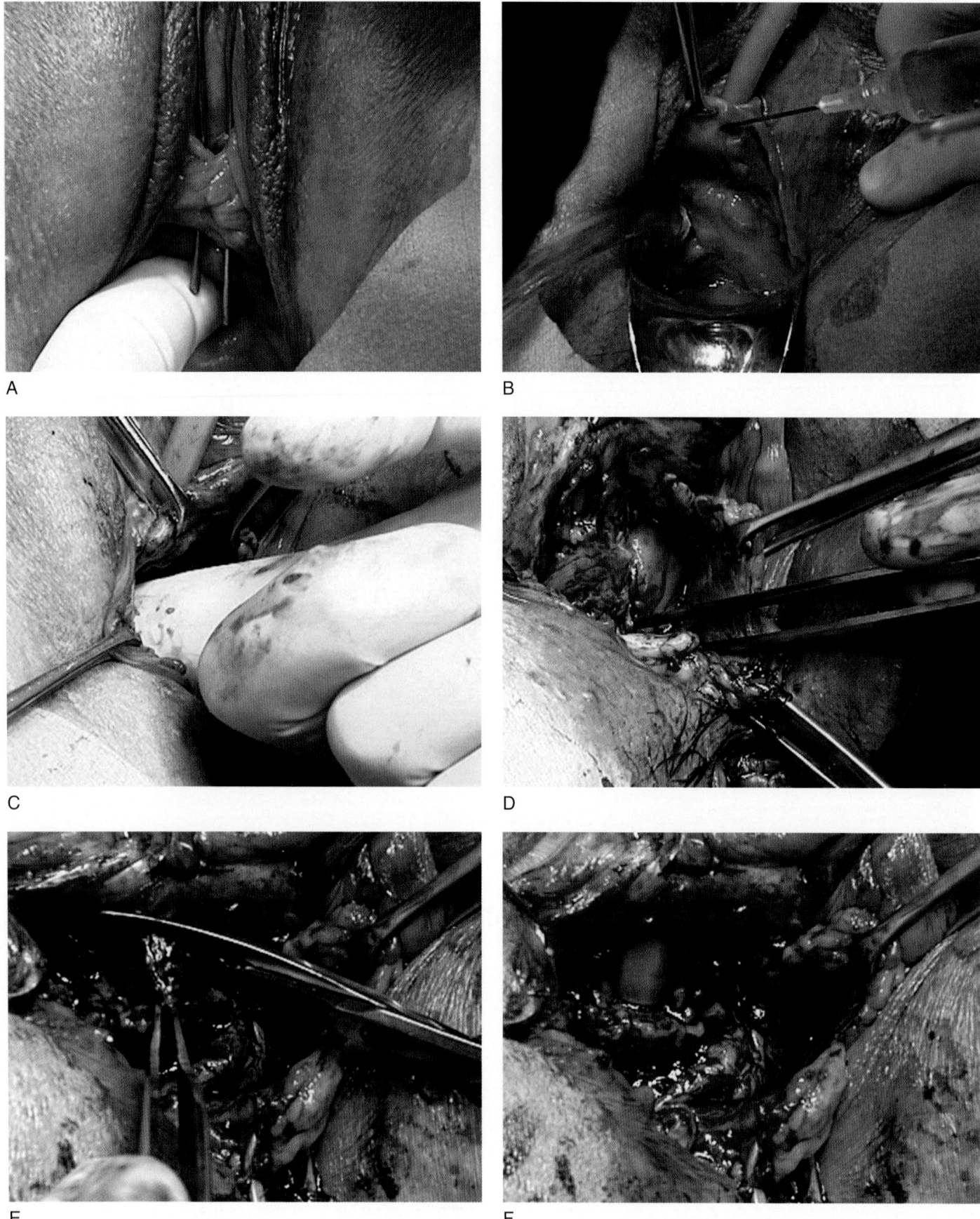

**FIGURE 83–5** Recurrent, multiple urethrovaginal fistulas are noted in a 27-year-old female. **A.** Probes are passed through two fistulous tracts. **B.** The anterior vaginal wall is injected with a hemostatic solution to be used for hydrodistention. **C.** An inverted-U incision has been made on the anterior vaginal wall, and the dissection is being extended laterally to the inferior pubic ramus. Because this is a recurrent case, the urethra must be completely mobilized, and thus the retropubic space will be entered on each side of the urethra. **D.** The retropubic space has been entered on the left side. Note the retropubic fat is seen. **E.** The scarred bridge of tissue between the fistulous tracts is being excised. **F.** The scar tissue has been excised, and the defect in the urethra is noted with fresh vascular edges of urethral tissue present.

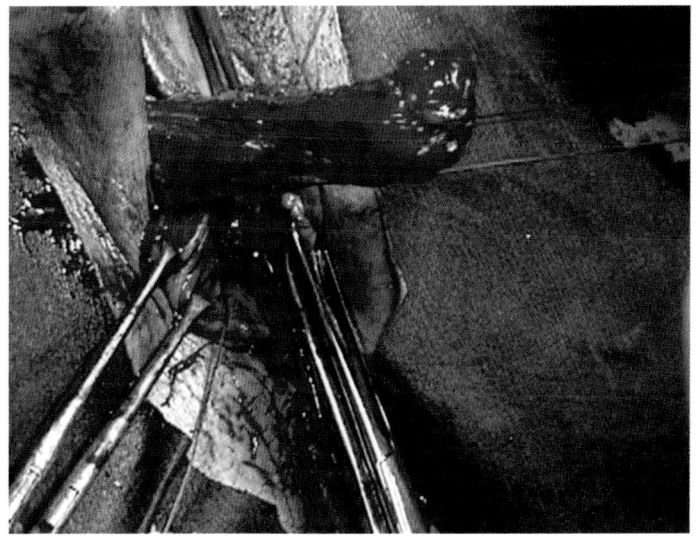

G

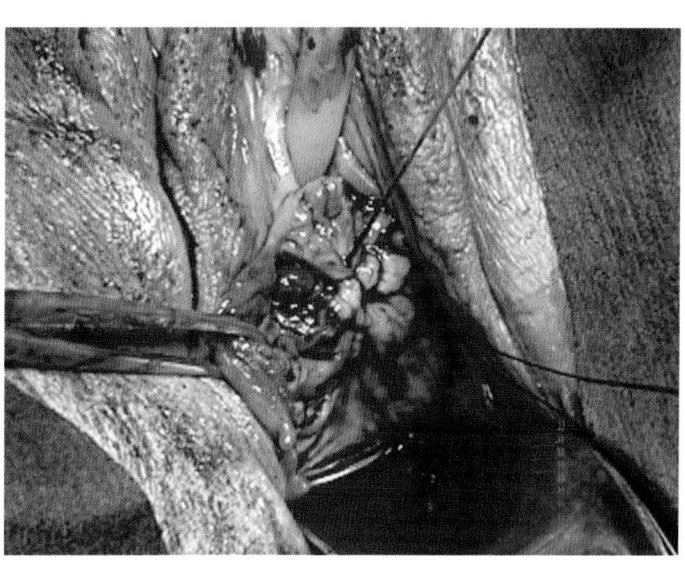

H

**FIGURE 83–5, cont'd G.** The fistulous tract has been closed in two layers as previously mentioned. Because this is a recurrent case, a Martius fat pad has been transposed and brought into the field to be placed between the repaired urethra and the anterior vaginal wall. **H.** The anterior vaginal wall has been mobilized and is being closed with 3-0 delayed absorbable sutures, thus completing the repair.

# CHAPTER 84

# Repair of Suburethral Diverticulum

*Mickey M. Karram*

For practical purposes, a suburethral diverticulum is any fluid-filled mass along the anterior lateral portions of the vagina that can be shown to have a direct communication with the urethra. Patients with a suburethral diverticulum may be asymptomatic or may complain of chronic recurrent cystitis, pain, burning and frequency, dyspareunia, voiding difficulty, postvoid dribbling, urinary incontinence, gross hematuria, or protrusion of a vaginal mass. Surgery should be considered only when the diverticulum becomes symptomatic.

A Tratner double balloon catheter (Fig. 84-1A, B) is specially designed to assist in the diagnosis of a diverticulum, as well as in the identification and location of the diverticulum at the time of surgery. The catheter is composed of a proximal balloon that inflates within the bladder neck, anchoring the catheter, and a distal balloon that occludes the external meatus (see Fig. 84-1B). Contrast fills the urethra through a slit between the balloons. With this catheter, the urethra basically becomes a closed tube that can be injected with contrast medium under moderate pressure, permitting radiographic visualization of diverticula even with minute

sinus tracts. This has been termed *positive-pressure urethrography* (Fig. 84-2).

The degree of difficulty associated with repair of diverticula depends on their size and number (Fig. 84-3), the position of the ostium in relation to the bladder neck and trigone, and the degree of inflammation. Very commonly pus or discharge can be seen at the urethral meatus (Fig. 84-4) or in the urethra (Fig. 84-5) when anterior vaginal wall massage is performed. Large *multiloculated* or saddle-shaped diverticula in the proximal urethra or bladder neck region may require extensive dissection extending under the trigone (see Fig. 84-3). In these situations, preoperative placement of ureteral stents may facilitate identification of ureters and reduce the risk of damage during dissection. Some surgeons will routinely perform a suburethral sling at the time of repair of a diverticulum if they believe that the incontinence mechanism is going to be significantly compromised. In these situations, transposition of the labial fat pad between the repaired diverticulum and the suburethral sling should be performed (see Chapter 85, Martius Fat Pad Transposition and Urethral Reconstruction).

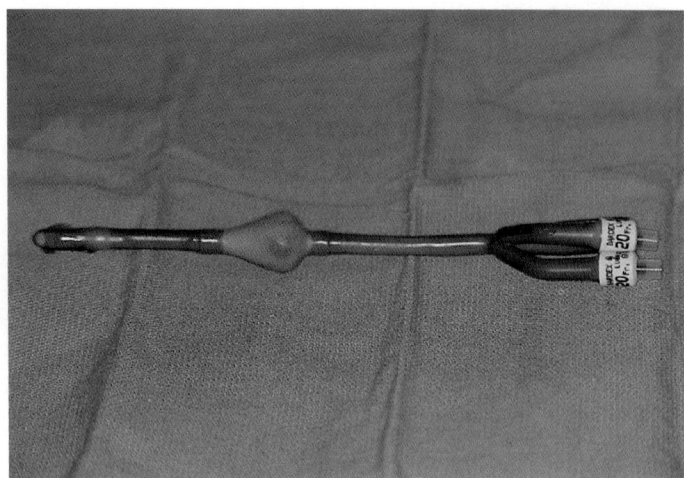
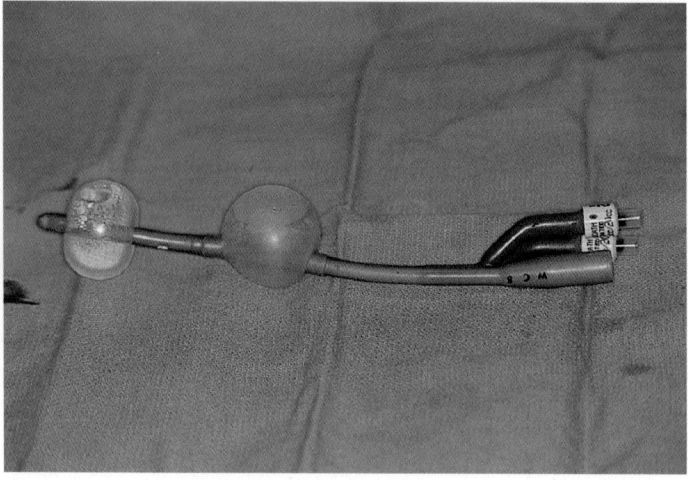

A   B

**FIGURE 84–1** Tratner double balloon catheter. **A.** Note the deflated proximal and distal balloons. **B.** Inflation of the proximal and distal balloons makes the urethra a closed tube that could be injected with contrast medium under moderate pressure, permitting radiographic visualization of diverticula even with minute sinus tracts.

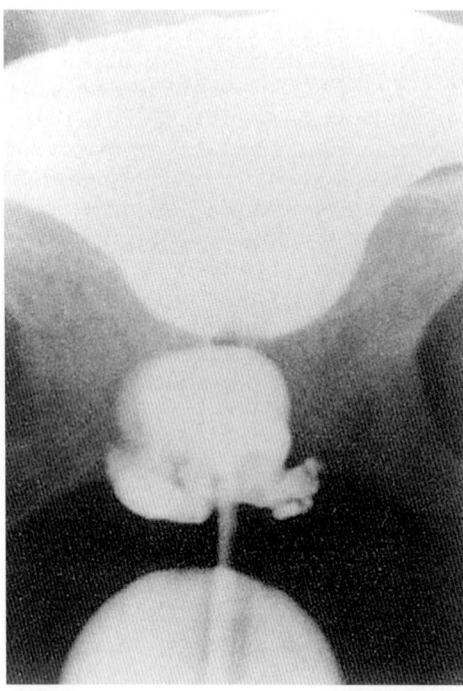

**FIGURE 84–2** Positive-pressure urethrogram showing a large, multiloculated suburethral diverticulum. (From Walters MD, Karram MM: *In* Urogynecology and Reconstructive Pelvic Surgery, 2nd ed. CV Mosby, St Louis, 1999, with permission.)

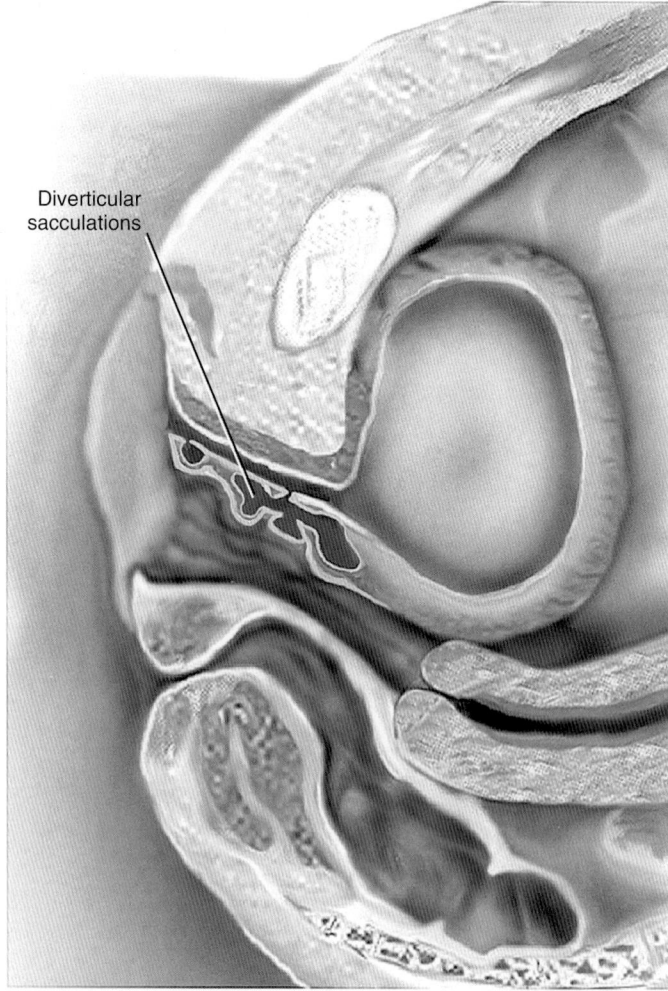

Diverticular sacculations

**FIGURE 84–3** The varied potential complexity of urethral diverticula. Note the small distal diverticulum, which if symptomatic could be treated with a Spence procedure, in contrast to a complex multiloculated proximal diverticulum.

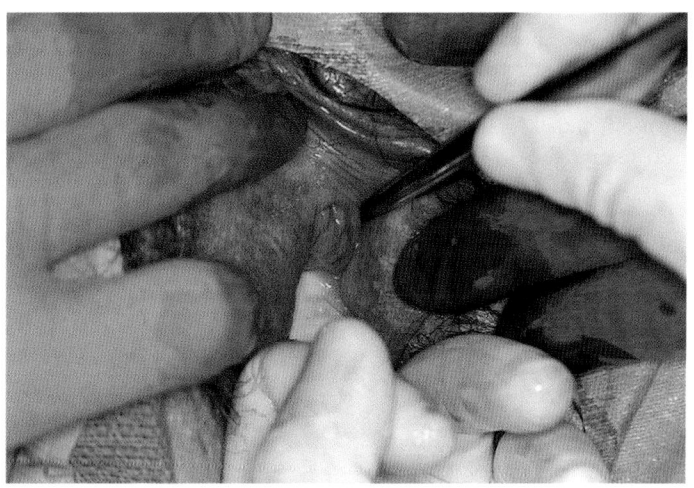

**FIGURE 84–4** Anterior vaginal wall massage in a patient with an infected diverticulum produces a discharge from the urethral meatus.

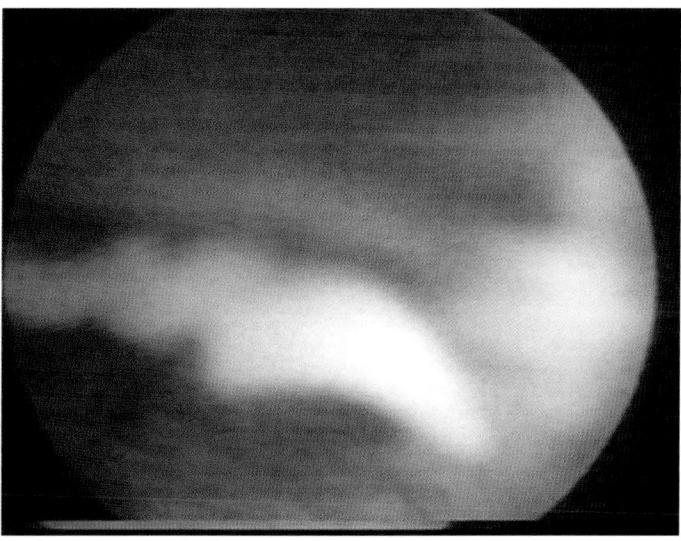

**FIGURE 84–5** Urethroscopic view of diverticular opening. Note that puslike discharge is seen exiting the opening when anterior vaginal wall massage is performed.

Multiple methods have been described to surgically correct the suburethral diverticulum. The two most commonly performed techniques are diverticulectomy and the partial ablation technique. With both techniques, a "vest-over-pants" closure of the periurethral fascia is utilized to avoid overlapping sutures and thereby reduce the incidence of urethrovaginal fistula (Figs. 85-6 through 85-8).

Following is a step-by-step description of the techniques utilized to repair a urethral diverticulum:

1. Usually regional or general anesthesia is utilized. Prophylactic antibiotics are generally given on call to the operating room. Cystourethroscopy is performed before surgery to localize the diverticular opening in the urethra and ensure that there are no other unsuspected findings. A double balloon catheter is placed, and the balloons are inflated proximally and distally. Sterile milk or methylene blue is injected into the catheter to inflate the urethra and the diverticulum. The author prefers to keep the catheter in place until the sac is entered, as it can be inflated periodically to assist in identification and mobilization of the sac off the vagina. Hydrodissection is utilized in the anterior vaginal wall to facilitate dissection in a proper plane.

2. An inverted-U incision is made over the diverticulum in the vaginal epithelium, and the vaginal wall is sharply dissected off the urethra and periurethral fascia.

3. A longitudinal incision is made carefully over the diverticular sac. The fascial tissue overlying and surrounding the diverticulum is completely dissected and mobilized, thus creating two flaps of fascia that will be utilized for the "vest-over-pants" closure of the diverticulum.

4. Dissection is continued around the sac until the neck is visualized. If the entire sac of the diverticulum is isolated, the diverticulum is excised from the urethra. If the sac cannot be mobilized, the sac is opened longitudinally and the inside of the diverticulum is explored to note the condition of the tissue and the presence of other diverticular openings, sacculations, or foreign bodies (see Figs. 84-5 and 84-6). If the base of the sac is firmly adherent to the urethra, a partial ablation technique is used to close off the opening of the urethra (see Fig. 84-6). If the sac can be completely excised at its neck, a complete diverticulectomy is performed and the urethral opening is closed longitudinally over a Foley catheter with interrupted fine delayed absorbable sutures (see Fig. 84-7).

5. The periurethral fascia previously developed into flaps bilaterally is closed in a "vest-over-pants" fashion over the urethra. This maneuver avoids suture lines that overlap the urethral repair (see Figs. 84-6 and 84-7).

6. The flap of the vaginal epithelium is repositioned, and the incision is closed with a 2-0 absorbable interrupted suture. The author generally will pack the vagina for 24 hours and will utilize continuous transurethral Foley drainage for 7 to 10 days. Fig. 84-8 reviews the entire procedure with illustrations. Figs. 84-9 and 84-10 demonstrate two cases in which a calculus had formed in the diverticulum.

Thus the partial ablation technique is identical to that of diverticulectomy except that no effort is made to enucleate the sac at its neck or at the juncture with the urethra. The base and neck of the diverticulum are closed side-to-side using fine interrupted sutures, and then a second layer of similar sutures is placed that imbricates the previous urethral defect. Periurethral fascia is then sutured down in a "vest-over-pants" fashion in both techniques (see Fig. 84-8).

A Spence procedure can be used for diverticuli present in the distal urethra (distal to the area of maximum urethral closure pressure). This is basically a distal marsupialization in that one blade of a pair of scissors is placed in the urethra and the other in the vagina. The scissors divide the floor of the diverticulum and the overlying vaginal epithelium, including the posterior urethra distal to the diverticulum. Redundant flaps of diverticulum and vaginal epithelium are trimmed, and a running interlocking delayed absorbable suture coapts the margins of the remaining lining of the sac and adjacent vaginal epithelium.

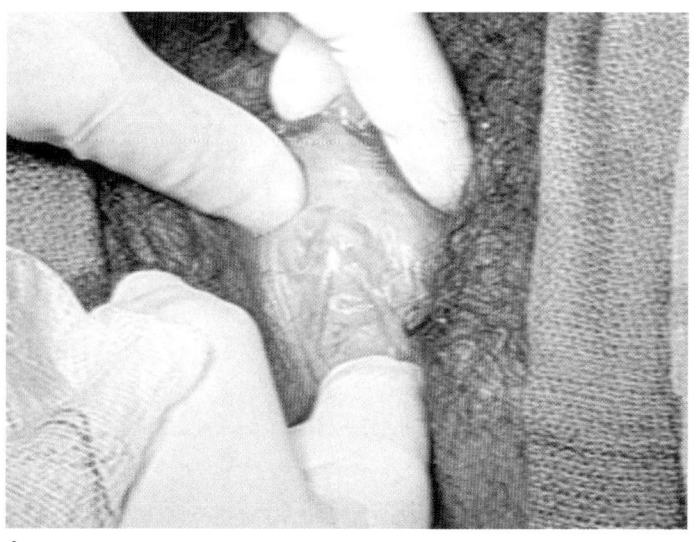

A

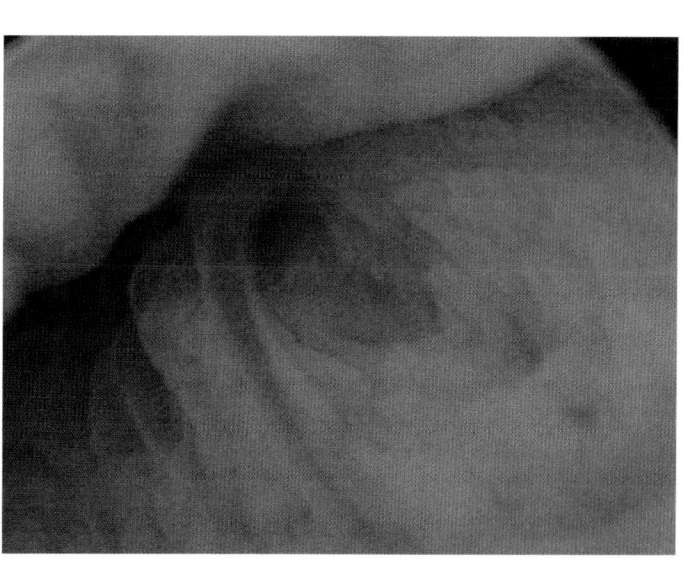

B

**FIGURE 84–6** Urethral diverticulum with a small orifice opening into the urethra in which a partial ablation technique is the preferred surgical repair. **A.** Note that discharge is readily seen from the external urethral meatus with massage of the anterior vaginal wall. **B.** Note the very small opening of the urethral diverticulum into the midportion of the urethra when viewed urethroscopically.

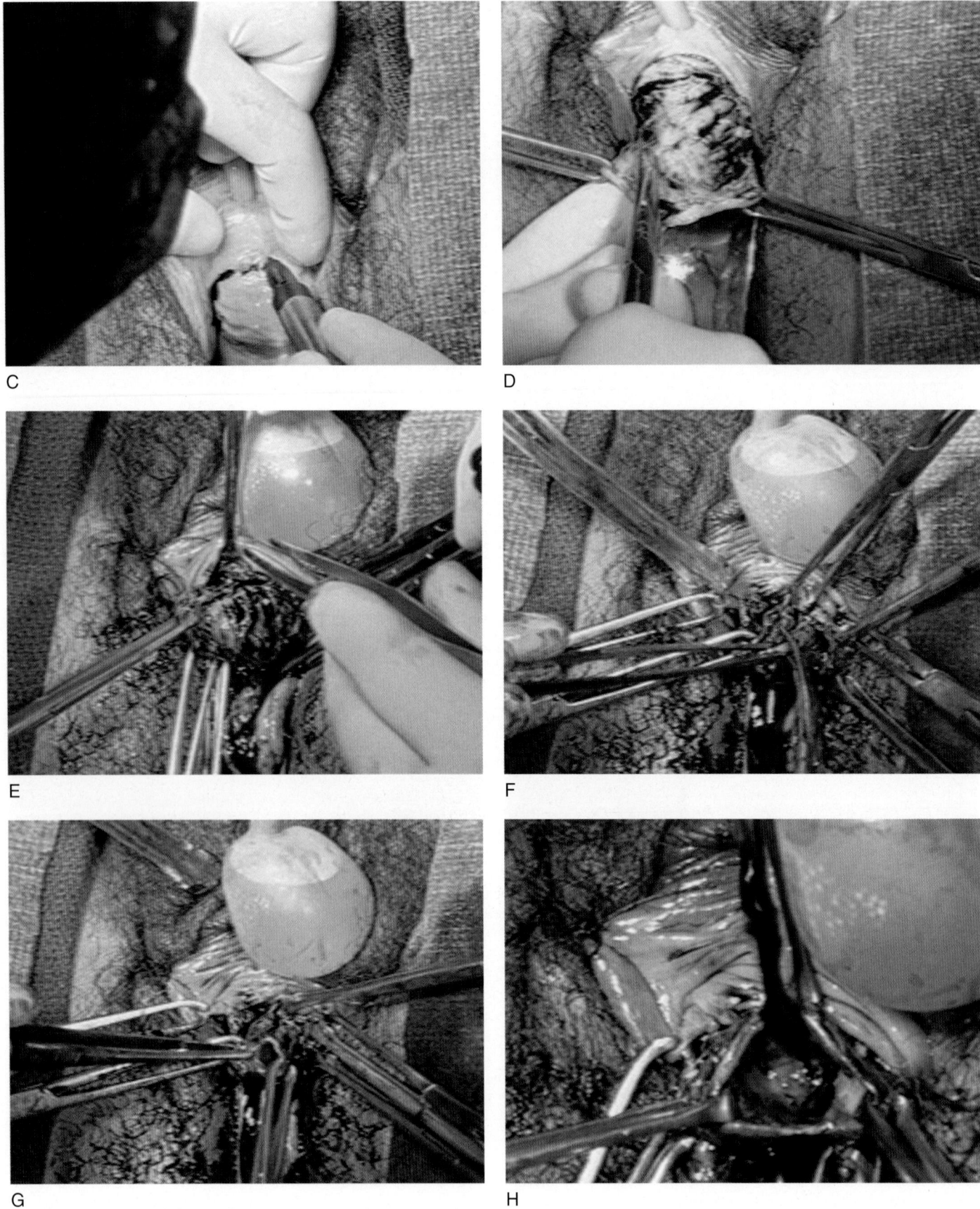

**FIGURE 84–6, cont'd C.** The large diverticulum is being outlined with a marking pencil. **D.** An inverted-U incision has been made on the anterior vaginal wall, and the vagina is sharply dissected off the underlying fascia. **E.** Periurethral flaps are being created that will facilitate closure of the defect in the urethra. **F.** The diverticular sac has been isolated and mobilized away from the periurethral fascia and is being sharply entered. **G.** The diverticular sac has been opened. **H.** Note the entire extent of the diverticular sac and a small diverticular opening into the urethra. Positive-pressure urethrography is utilized to demonstrate the spillage of dye from this orifice. Because the opening in the wall of the urethra is small, the sac will be excised and a partial ablation of the opening will be performed, followed by a "vest-over-pants" closure of the fascia that was previously mobilized.

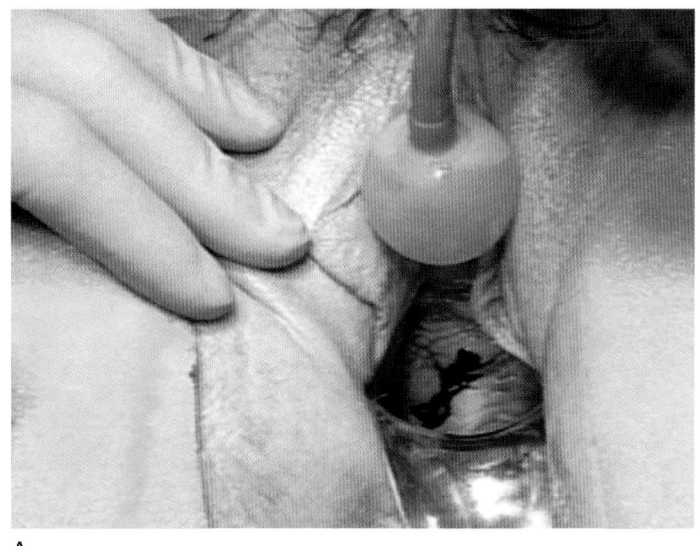

A

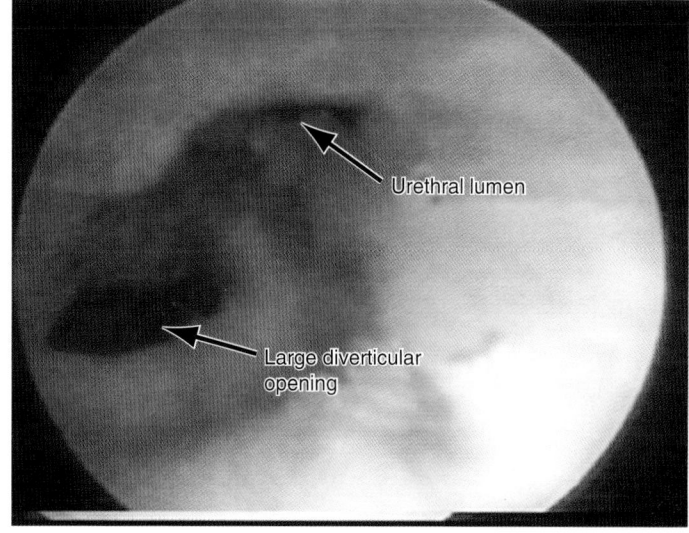

Urethral lumen

Large diverticular
opening

B

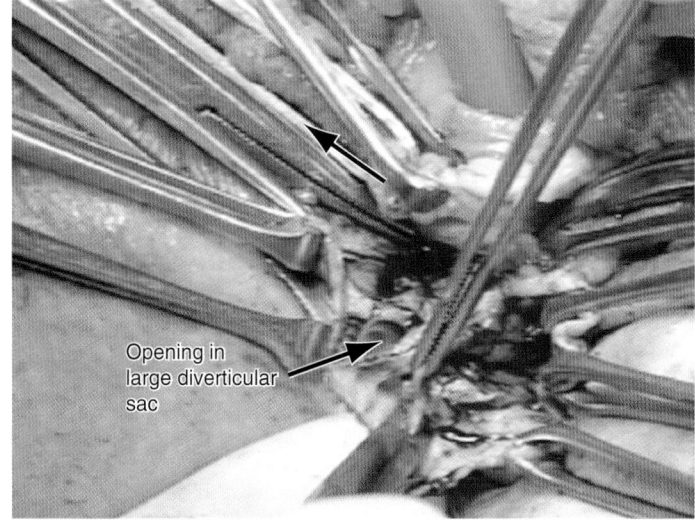

Opening in
large diverticular
sac

C

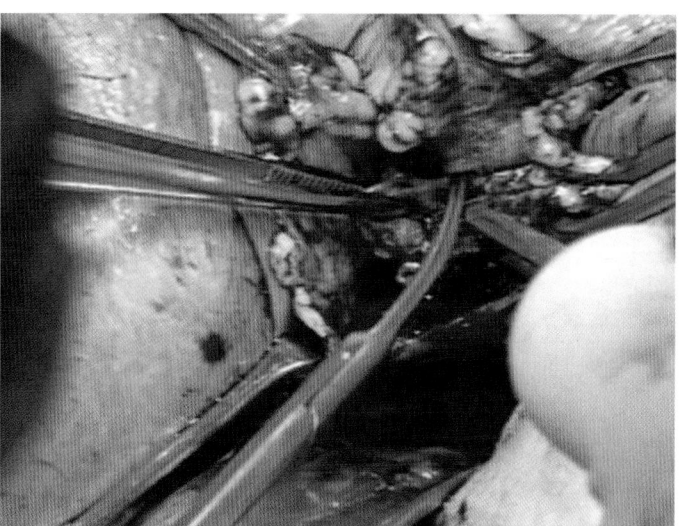

D

Inside lining of
large diverticular
sac

E

**FIGURE 84–7** Large midurethral diverticulum. **A.** With positive-pressure urethrography, the diverticulum spontaneously ruptures into the anterior vaginal wall. **B.** Urethroscopic examination demonstrates a very large diverticular opening. **C.** The anterior vaginal wall has been opened, and spontaneous rupture in the diverticular sac is noted. **D.** The diverticular sac has been mobilized off the anterior vaginal wall and is being excised back to the large diverticular opening. **E.** Inside lining of the diverticular sac. Excision of this will complete the diverticulectomy, and the urethra will then be closed in layers, followed by a "vest-over-pants" closure of the periurethral fascia.

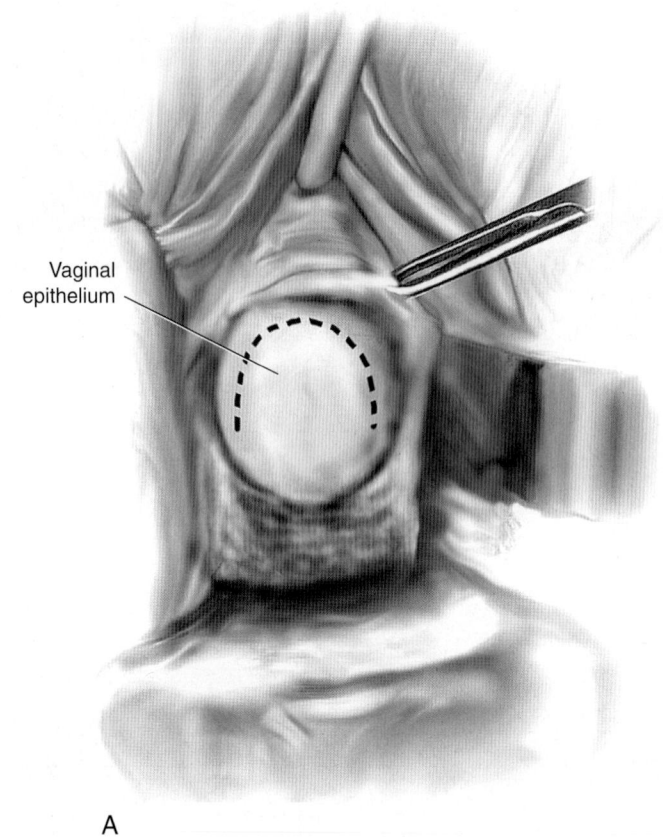

Vaginal
epithelium

A

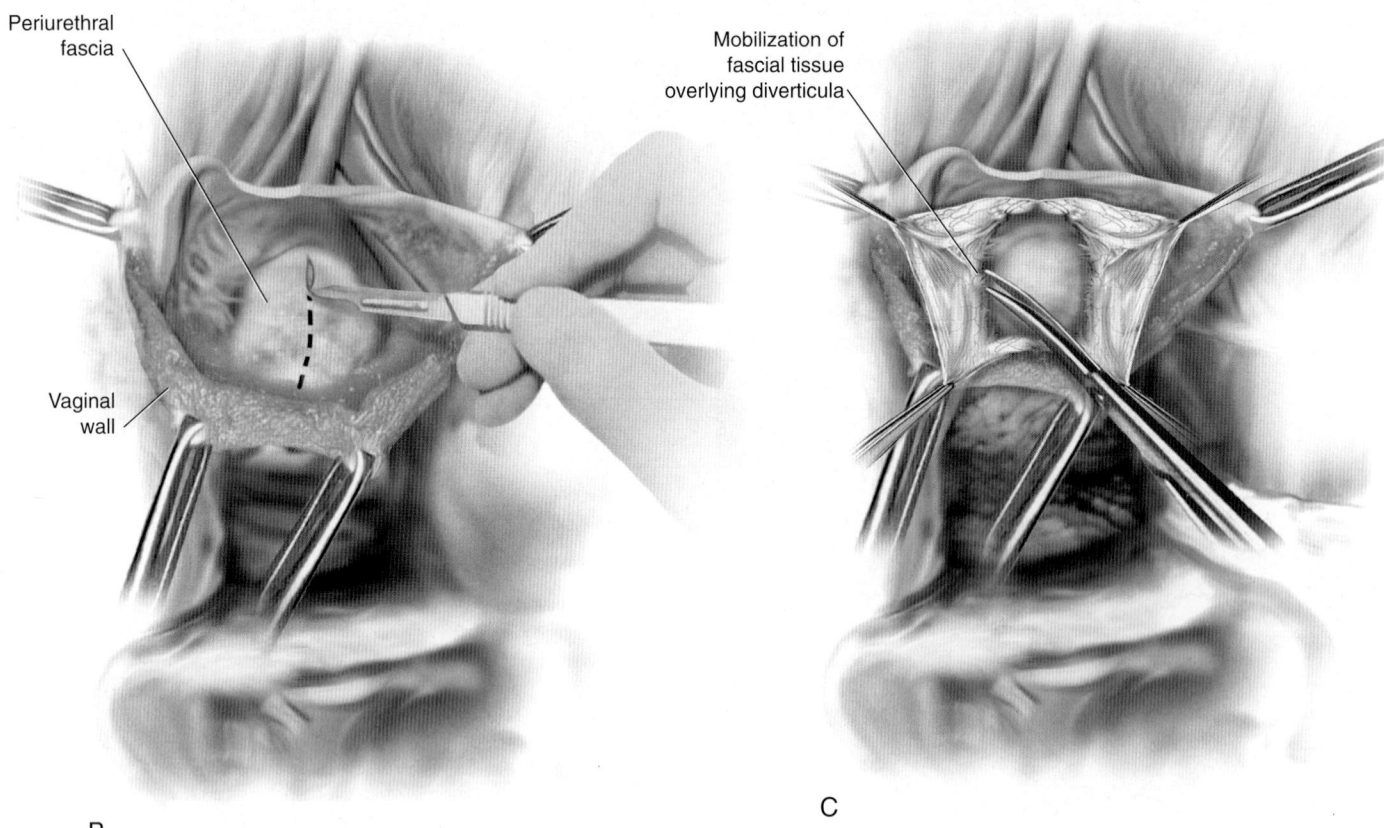

Periurethral
fascia

Vaginal
wall

B

Mobilization of
fascial tissue
overlying diverticula

C

**FIGURE 84–8** Technique of suburethral diverticulectomy with "vest-over-pants" closure of periurethral fascia. **A.** Inverted-U incision on the anterior vaginal wall. **B.** Complete mobilization of the anterior vaginal wall off the diverticular sac. A longitudinal incision is made in the wall of the diverticulum. **C.** Sharp dissection creates two flaps of periurethral fascia.

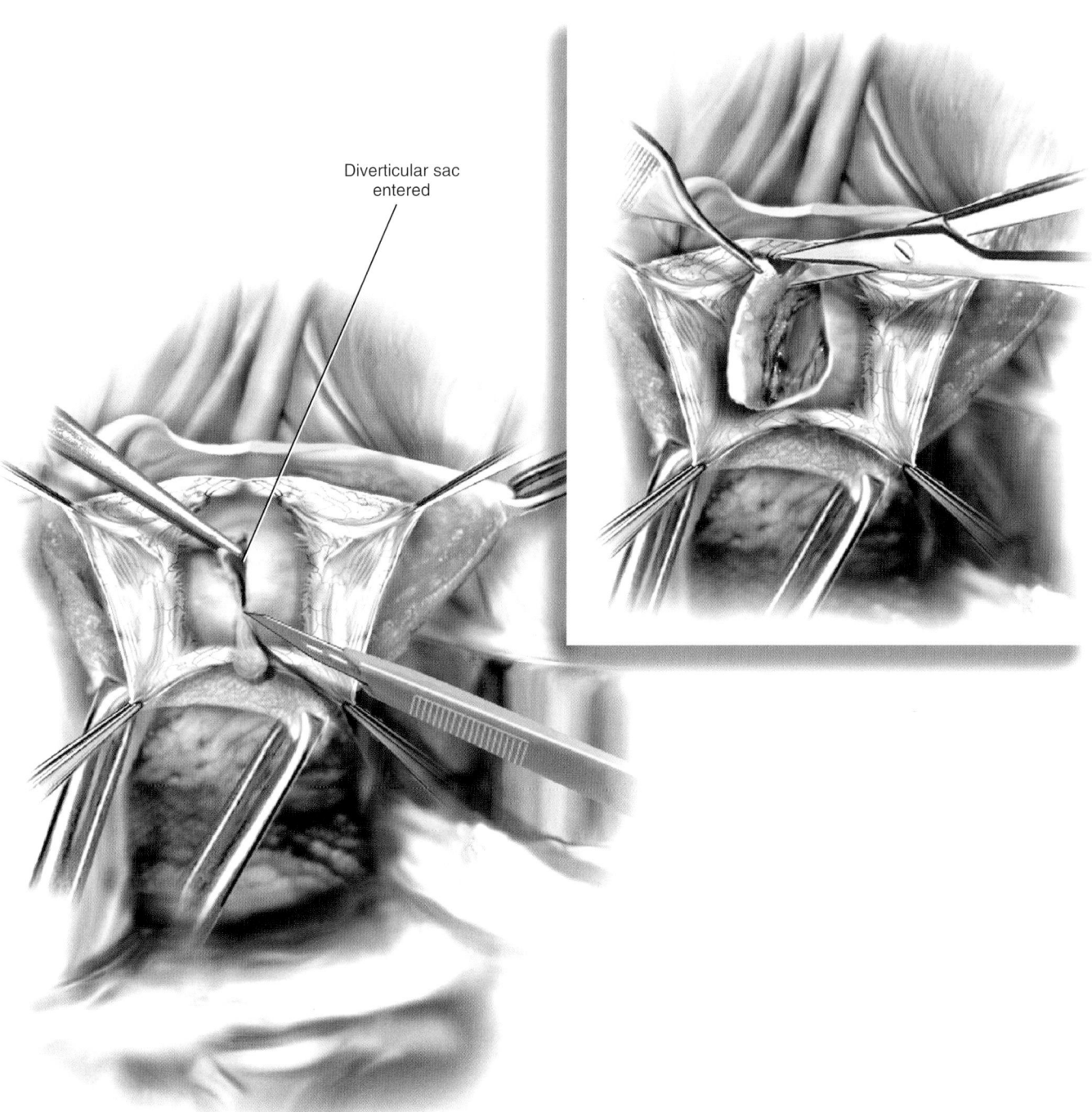

Diverticular sac
entered

D

**FIGURE 84–8, cont'd D.** The diverticular sac is sharply entered and the wall of the sac is trimmed.

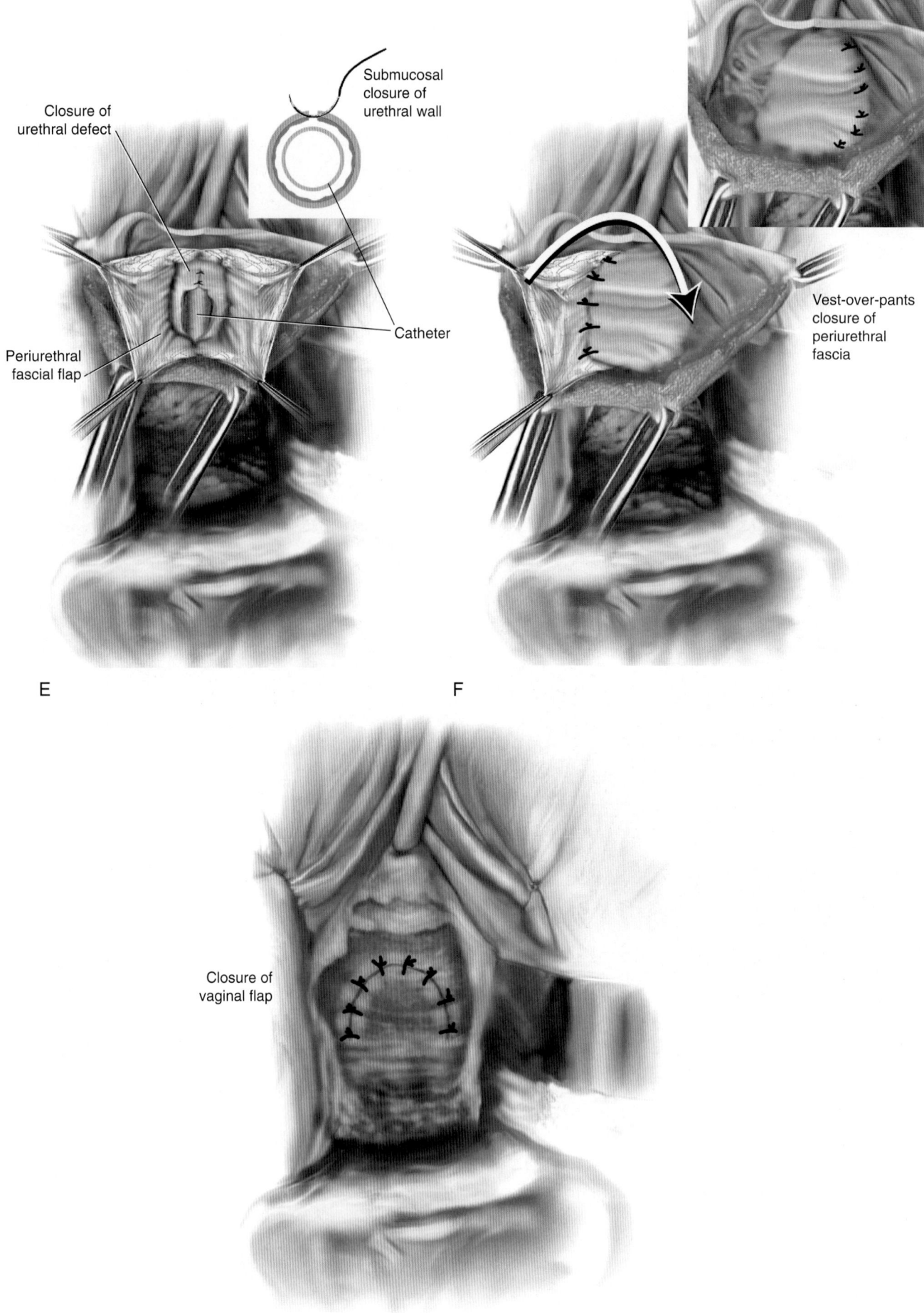

E

F

G

**FIGURE 84–8, cont'd  E.** The diverticular sac has been excised and the defect in the urethra is closed in a submucosal fashion with fine interrupted delayed absorbable sutures. **F.** Periurethral fascia is laid down in a "vest-over-pants" fashion. **G.** The anterior vaginal wall incision is closed.

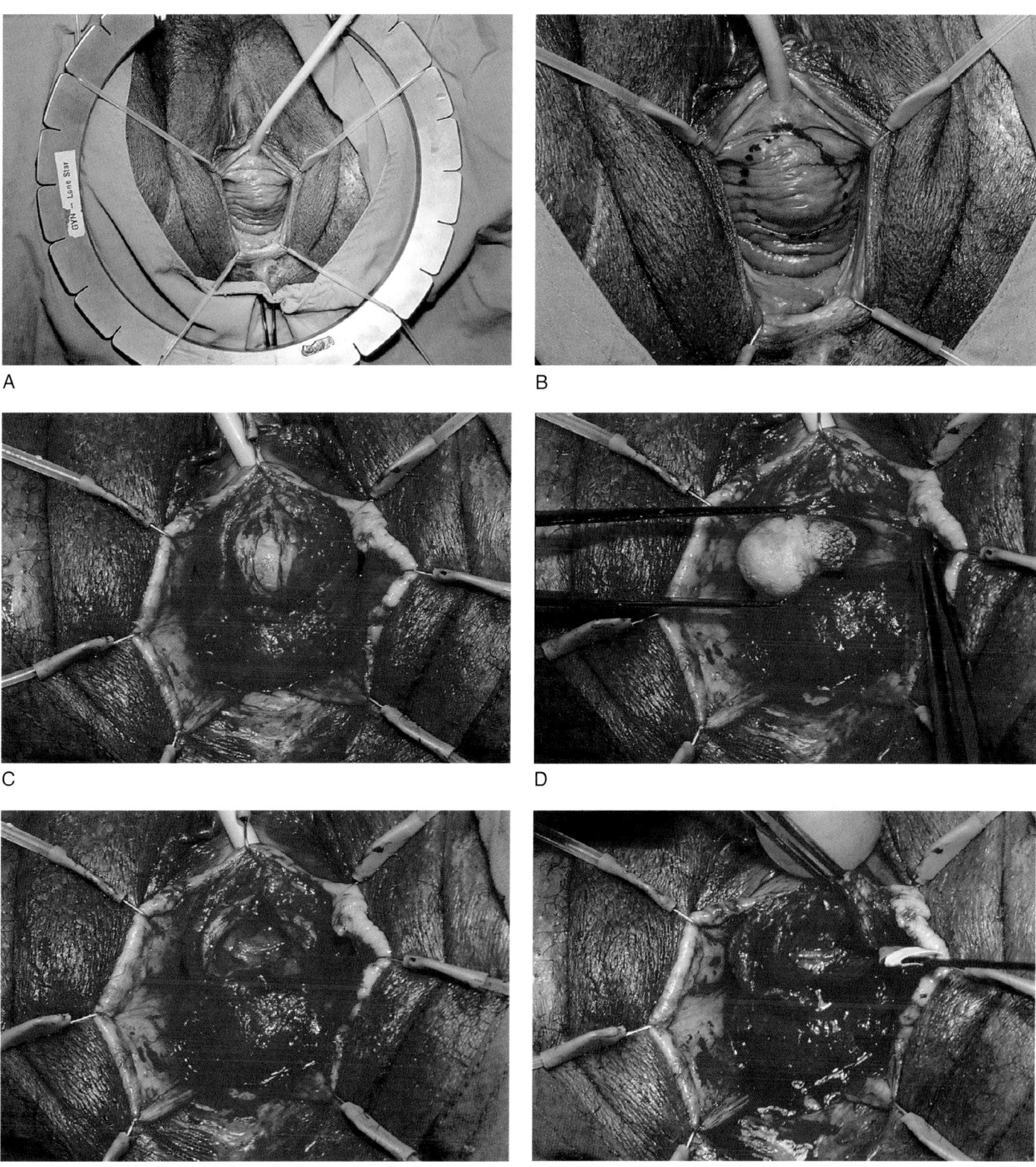

**FIGURE 84–9** Suburethral diverticulum in which a calculus has developed. **A.** Exposure of the anterior vaginal wall. **B.** The location of the diverticulum has been marked. **C.** The anterior vaginal wall has been mobilized off the diverticular sac, two flaps of periurethral fascia have been created, and the diverticulum has been opened exposing a calculus. **D.** The calculus is shown being removed from the diverticulum. **E.** The edges of the sac have been trimmed back in preparation for partial ablation closure of the defect. Note the dissected flaps of periurethral fascia, which will be laid down in a "vest-over-pants" fashion. **F.** Probe is passed into an opening in the diverticular sac that communicates with the urethra.

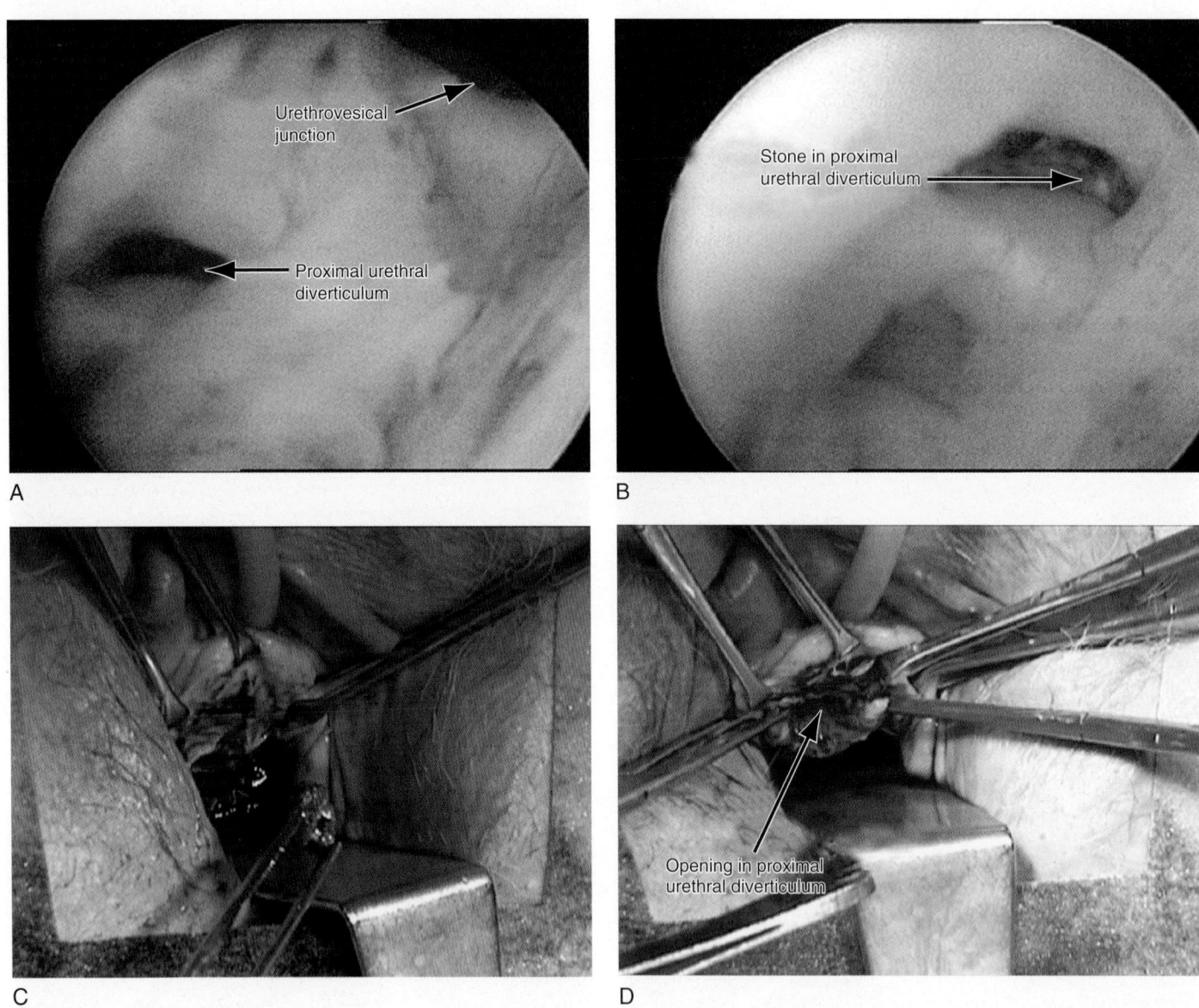

**FIGURE 84–10** Proximal urethral diverticulum with a calculus in the diverticulum. **A.** Note the proximal opening of the diverticulum as it relates to the urethrovesical junction. **B.** Urethroscopic view of the calculus in the diverticular sac. **C.** The diverticulum has been opened vaginally, and the stone has been removed. **D.** The opening in the proximal urethral diverticulum is noted.

# CHAPTER 85

# Martius Fat Pad Transposition and Urethral Reconstruction

*Mickey M. Karram*

## Martius Fat Pad Transposition

Transposition of a labial fat pad with or without the bulbocavernosus muscle has been used to facilitate closures of fistulas involving the anterior and posterior vaginal wall. The procedure yields tissues that can fill in dead space and provide an excellent blood supply. The fact that this operation does not alter the anatomy of the vulva and is cosmetically pleasing is also important.

Fig. 85–1A demonstrates the abundant blood supply to the labial fat. It has been empirically stated that the majority of the blood supply comes from the inferior direction (internal pudendal artery); thus the detachment of the fat should be anterior.

Our dissections and experience with the procedure would indicate that sufficient blood supply is present from both directions; thus detachment should be at the discretion of the surgeon and more related to the anatomic location of the defect in the vagina. The procedure begins by marking an incision over the labial fat. The fat pad is mobilized on each side. After the vaginal dissection has been completed, a long curved clamp is passed medially into the vaginal incision, thus creating a tunnel that the fat pad will pass through to reach the vaginal area. The fat pad is then detached either anteriorly or posteriorly and passed into the vaginal area and fixed with delayed absorbable sutures. The vaginal and labial incisions are closed without tension (see Figs. 85–1 and 85–2).

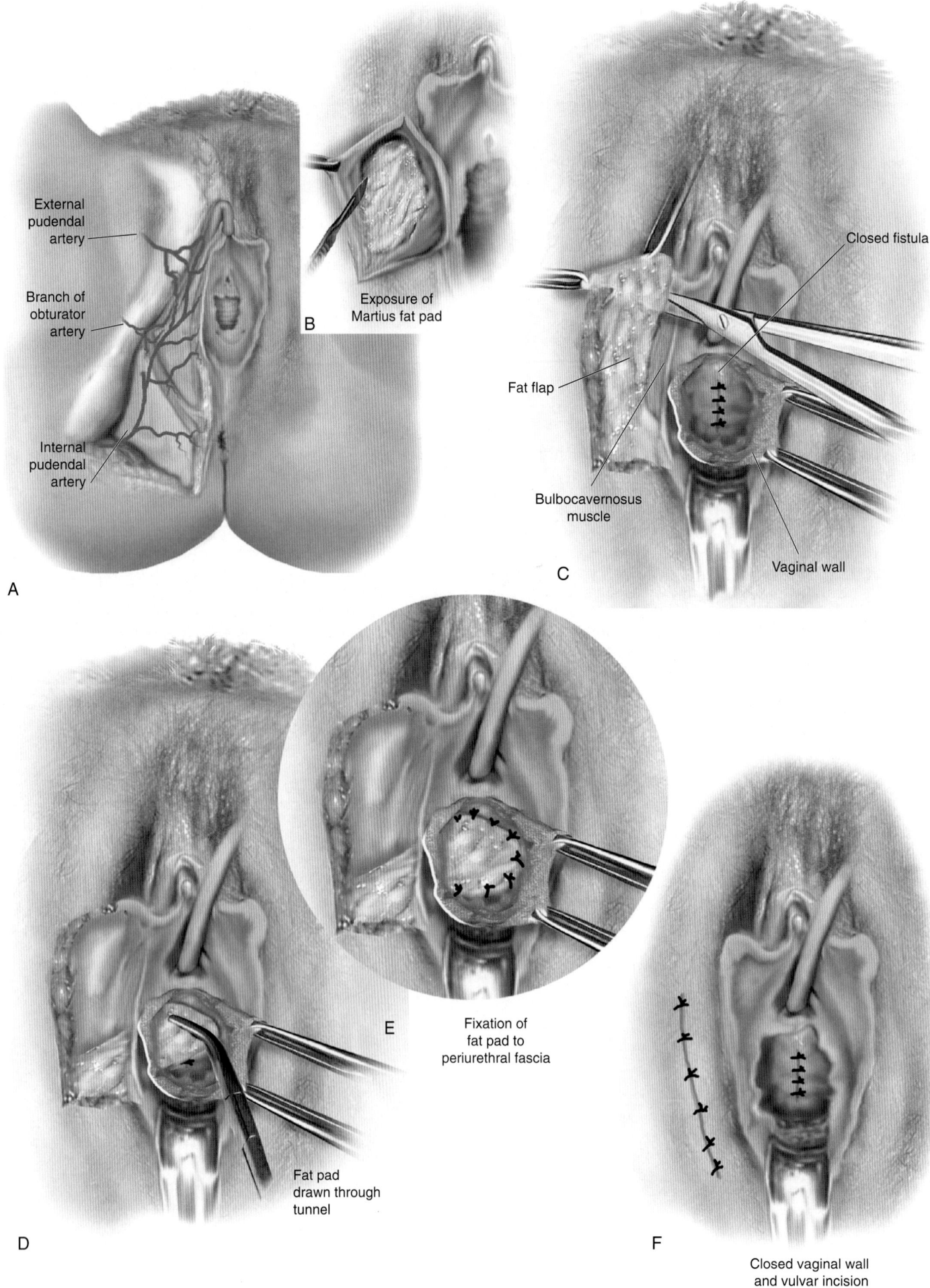

**FIGURE 85–1** Technique of Martius fat pad transposition. **A.** Blood supply to the labial fat. **B.** Exposure of the fat pad via labial incision. **C.** Mobilization of fat. **D.** Anterior detachment of the fat pad with tunneling into the vaginal incision and fixation of the fat pad over the closed urethrovaginal fistula. **F.** Closure of the vaginal and labial incisions.

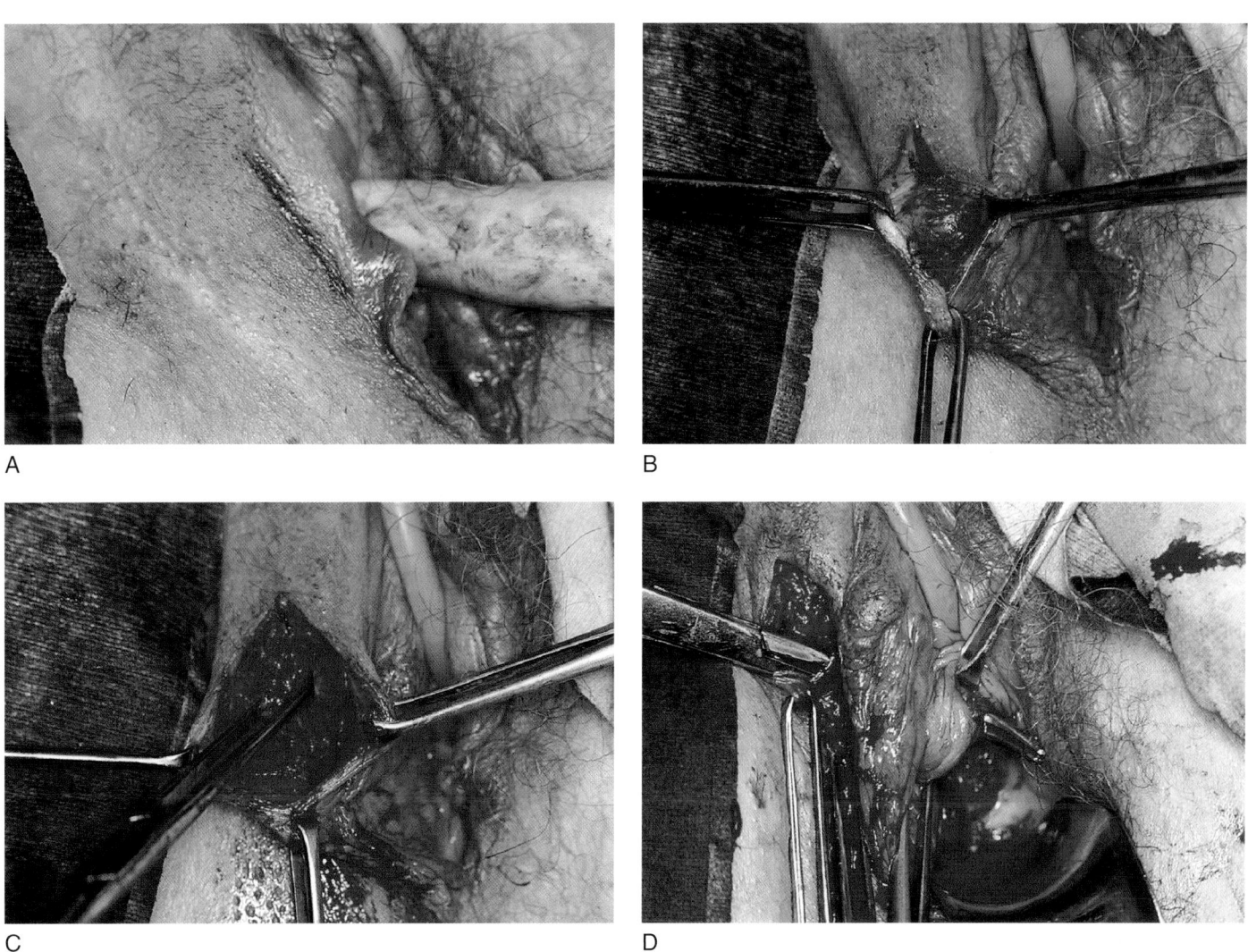

**FIGURE 85–2** Technique of labial fat pad transposition. **A.** Site of the labial incision. **B.** Mobilization of skin off of the fat pad. **C.** Mobilization of the fat pad. **D.** A long clamp is used to tunnel under the skin into the vaginal incision.

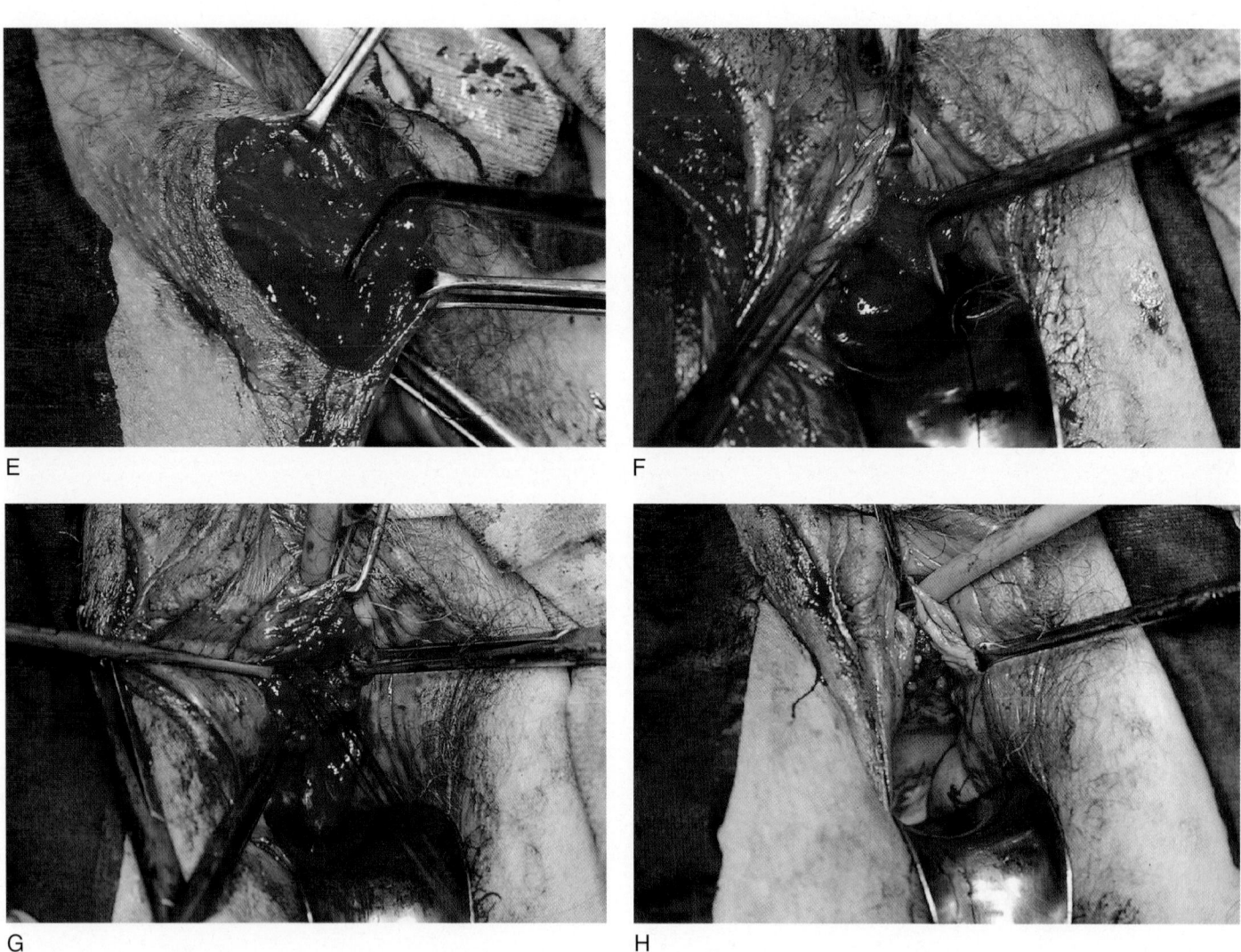

**FIGURE 85–2, cont'd  E.** The labial fat pad is detached posteriorly. **F.** The labial fat pad is transposed into the vaginal incision. **G.** The labial fat pad is fixed into place with delayed absorbable sutures. **H.** The labial and vaginal incisions are closed.

## Urethral Reconstruction

Repair of a damaged urethra is one of the most challenging problems in vaginal surgery. Indications for urethral reconstruction can include congenital abnormalities, radiation, multiple previous surgeries, and pelvic trauma. The goals of the surgical correction include creation of a continent sphincter mechanism, construction of a conduit for the urine to flow in a normal location, and covering the area with fresh vascularized tissue to avoid subsequent breakdown or fistula formation. In patients who have loss of a major portion of the posterior urethra, urethral reconstruction may be difficult, and normal urinary function, even in what appears to be a well-constructed urethral tube, is very unpredictable. The patient in Fig. 85–3 initially presented in her early thirties with a congenitally short urethral tube and an ectopic ureter implanting into the midportion of the urethra on the right side. The patient underwent a reimplantation of her right ureter (which was her only ureter) and a suburethral sling procedure. She presented approximately 2 years following this procedure with a complete breakdown of the anterior vaginal wall and loss of the entire posterior wall of the urethra, extending up into the region of the trigone (Fig. 85–4A, B). The basic principles of the repair are very similar to those of urethrovaginal fistula repair. In this situation an incision is made in the anterior vaginal wall adjacent to the margins of the defect. The vaginal wall is widely mobilized laterally to well beyond the pubic ramus. The retropubic space is entered bilaterally on each side to facilitate mobilization of the urethra. Once the vaginal mucosa has been mobilized laterally and the urethra has been mobilized as much as possible, the urethral tube is reconstructed. Usually the closure of the urethral tube is done over a No. 10 or 12 F urethral Foley catheter. This permits accurate approximation of the free edges of the roof of the urethra and the reconstruction of the tube. The sutures are placed in an interrupted fashion with 4-0 delayed absorbable sutures positioned extramuscosally. Ideally, the initial suture line should be followed by a second layer approximating the periurethral tissues to aid and support the initial suture line. A third layer of tissue, usually pubocervical fascia, is then mobilized from the inside of the vaginal wall. Since this is commonly very damaged tissue, a vascular pedicle in the form of a Martius fat pad is usually indicated. In patients who have a slough of the entire urethra including the bladder neck, it is necessary to attempt to preserve a continence mechanism, which is usually accomplished by the placement of a suburethral sling. Usually patients with a linear loss of the urethral floor also have loss of a significant portion of the anterior vaginal wall, and thus at the completion of the reconstruction it is impossible to cover the area with vaginal wall without creating significant unwanted tension. In these cases the size of the defect is accurately evaluated and an appropriate tongue of tissue from the labia minora is identified to be incised and swung into the vagina to replace the anterior vaginal wall. This fibro-fatty flap is usually hinged anteriorly. Usually a U flap is made and the base of the U is developed, mobilized and sutured to the edges of the vagina, thus covering the defect in the anterior vaginal wall. The site of the graft is then closed by approximating the skin edges with 4.0 delayed absorbable sutures (see Figs. 85–3 and 85–4).

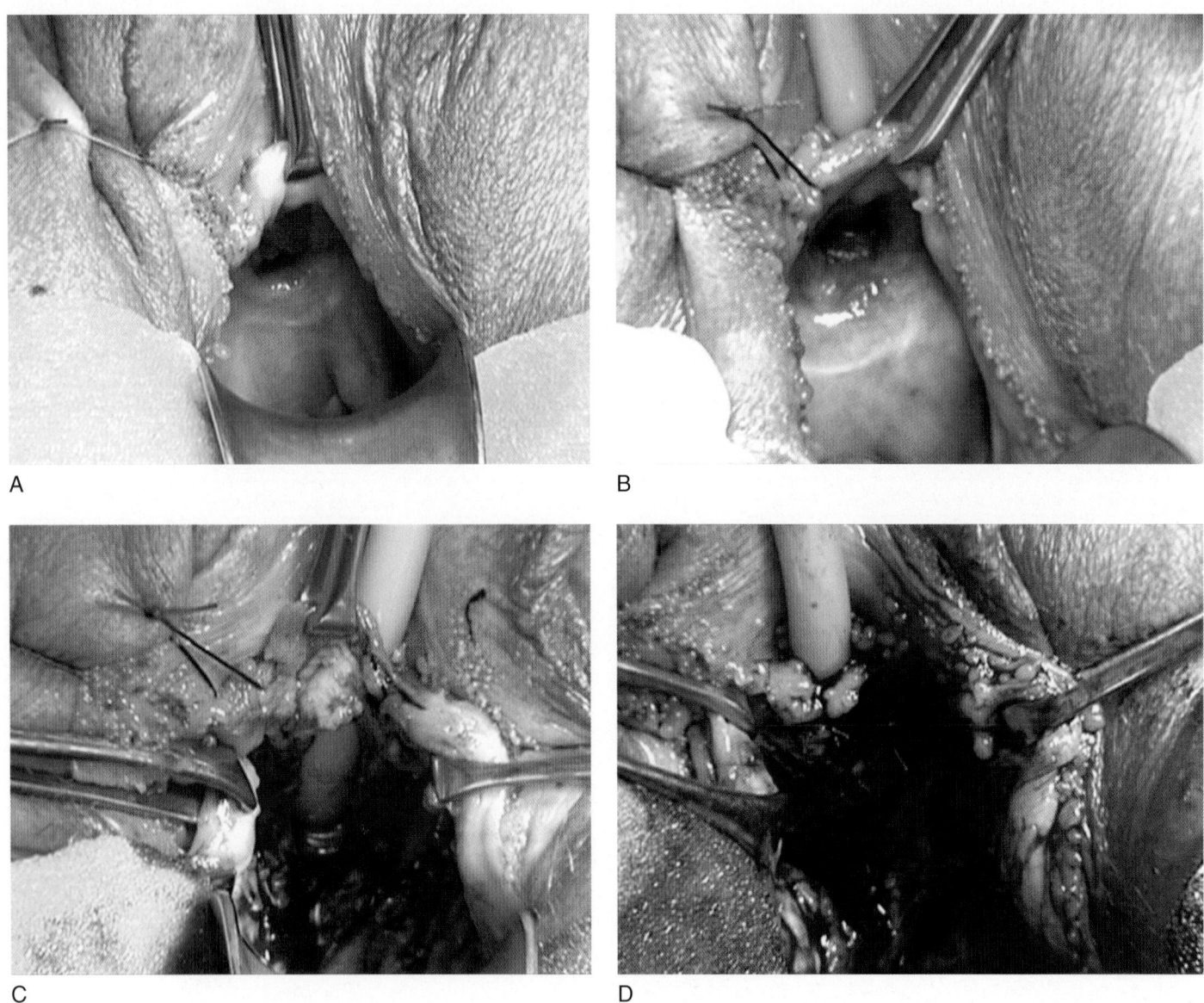

**FIGURE 85–3 A.** A vaginal view of a patient who has suffered complete linear loss of the posterior urethra. **B.** With a Foley catheter in place, one can see that the loss of tissue extends up into the trigone of the bladder. **C.** The initial dissection involves freeing and mobilizing the anterior wall of the vagina from the posterior wall of the urethra in preparation for layered closure of the posterior wall of the urethra. **D.** The urethra has been closed with interrupted 4-0 absorbable sutures, and the urethra has been mobilized completely to the inferior pubic ramus on each side to facilitate this closure in a tension-free fashion.

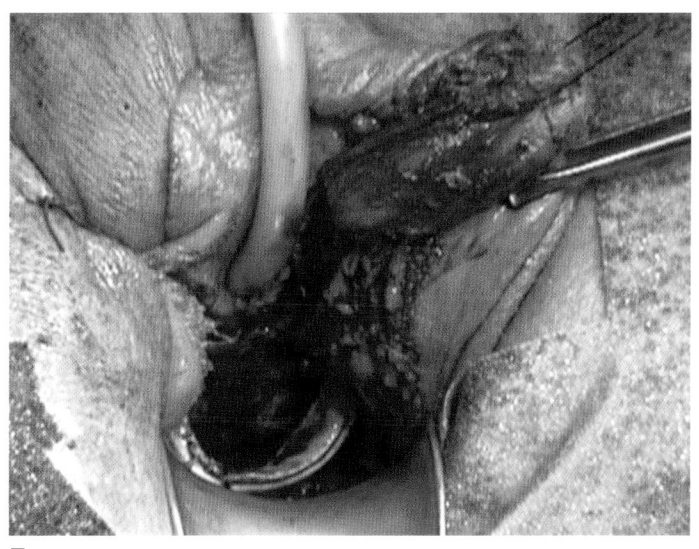

E

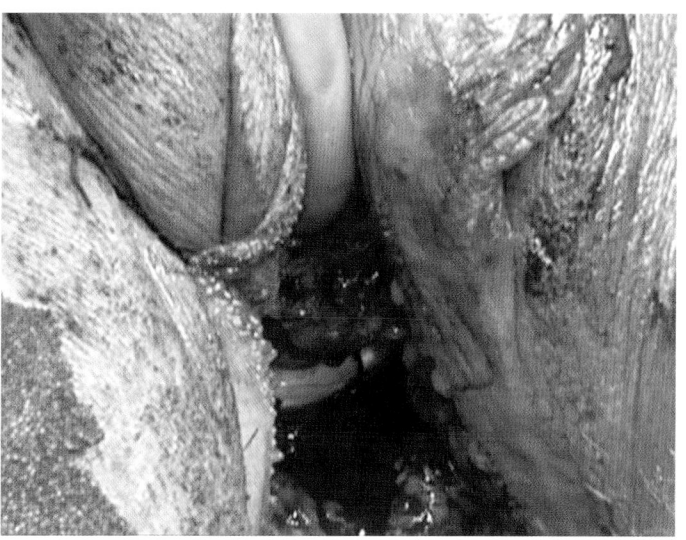

F

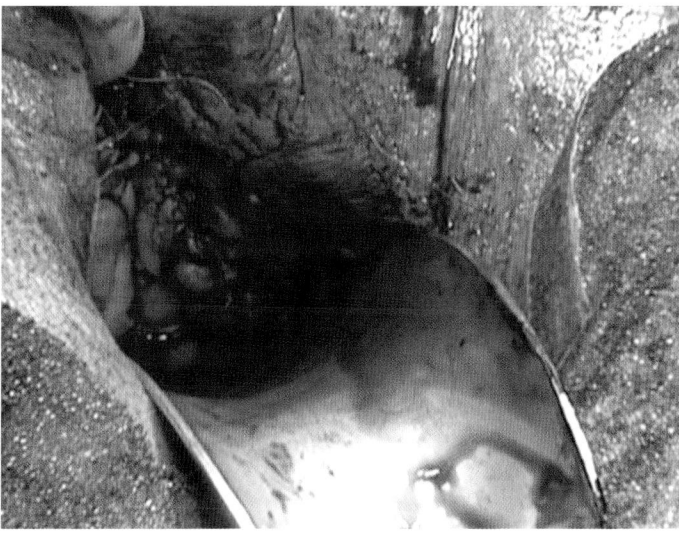

G

**FIGURE 85–3, cont'd E.** A layer of fascia has been mobilized off the vaginal wall, laid across the posterior urethra, and sutured in place. **F.** A Martius fat pad has been transposed from the right labial area. It is sutured in place across the entire posterior urethra. A cadaveric fascia lata sling has been placed at the anatomic level of the proximal urethra. **G.** A skin flap from the left labia has been mobilized and sutured into the anterior vaginal wall to close the defect.

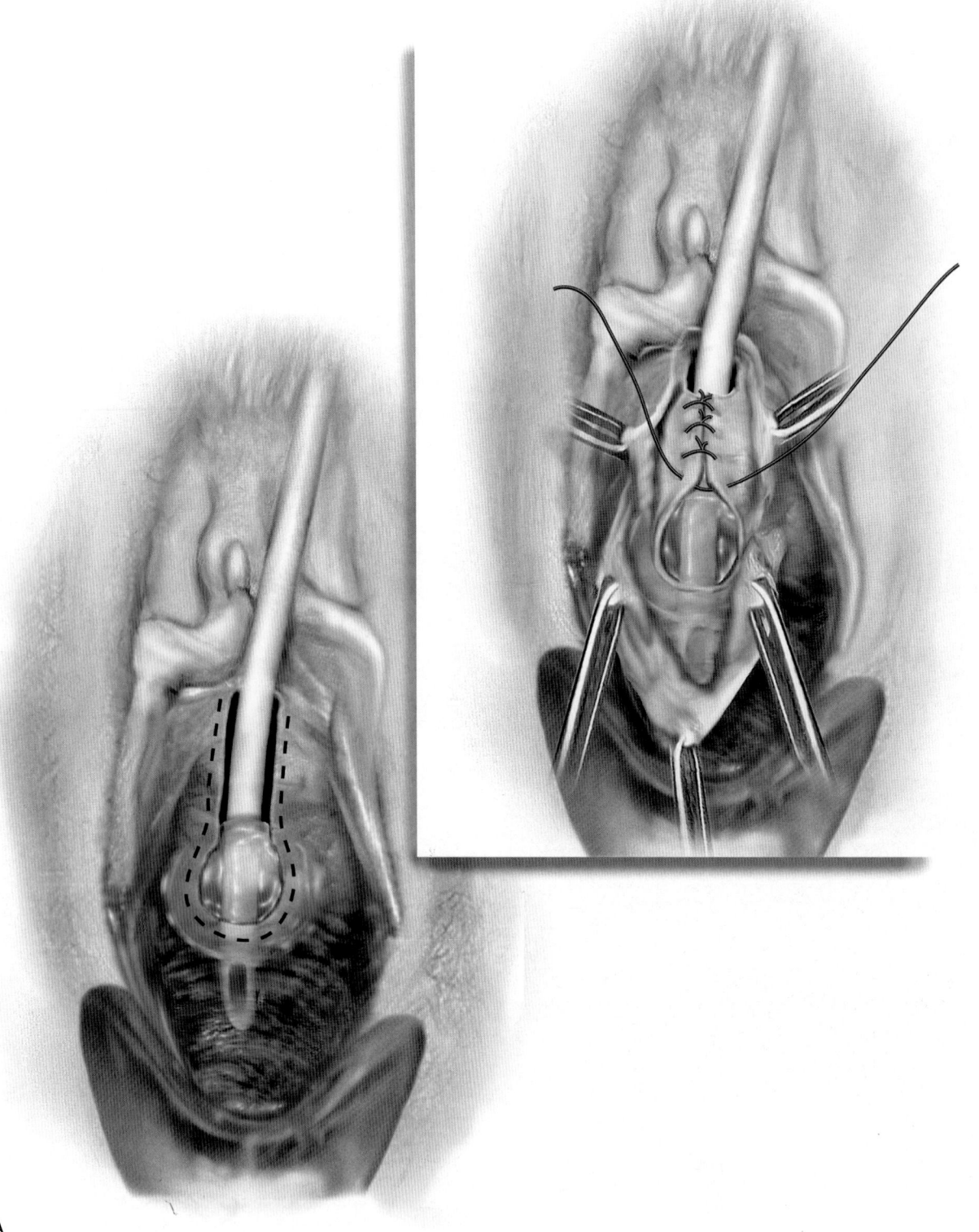

A

**FIGURE 85–4** Urethral reconstruction. **A.** The dashed line depicts the location of the initial incision. Once the vagina is completely mobilized off the urethra and bladder, the defect is closed over the catheter with interrupted 4-0 delayed absorbable sutures.

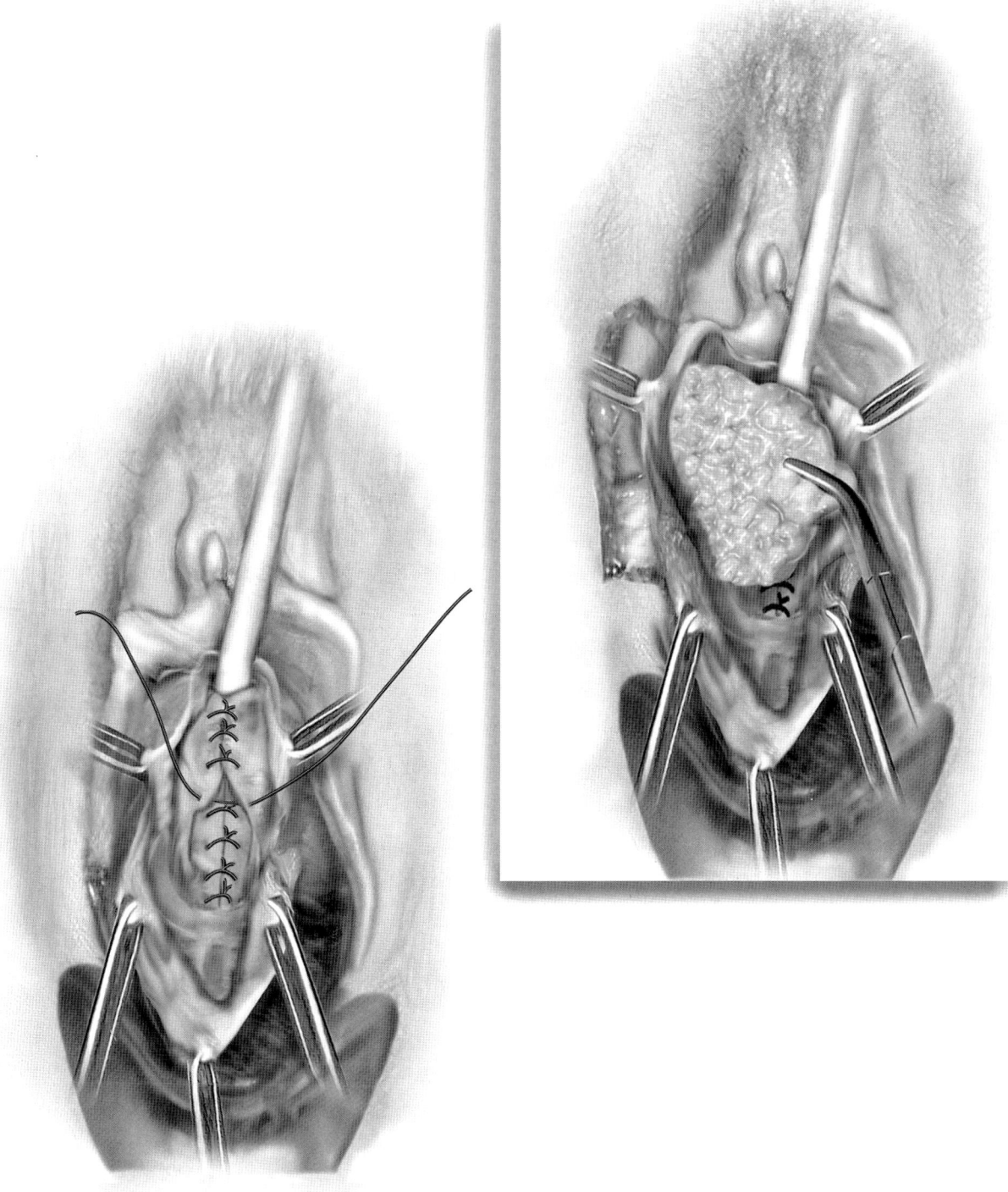

B

**FIGURE 85–4, cont'd B.** A second layer of interrupted sutures is placed to reinforce the initial layer. If possible, a third layer of pubocervical fascia is then placed over the urethral closure. This is followed by the placement of a Martius fat pad to act as a vascular pedicle for this damaged tissue.

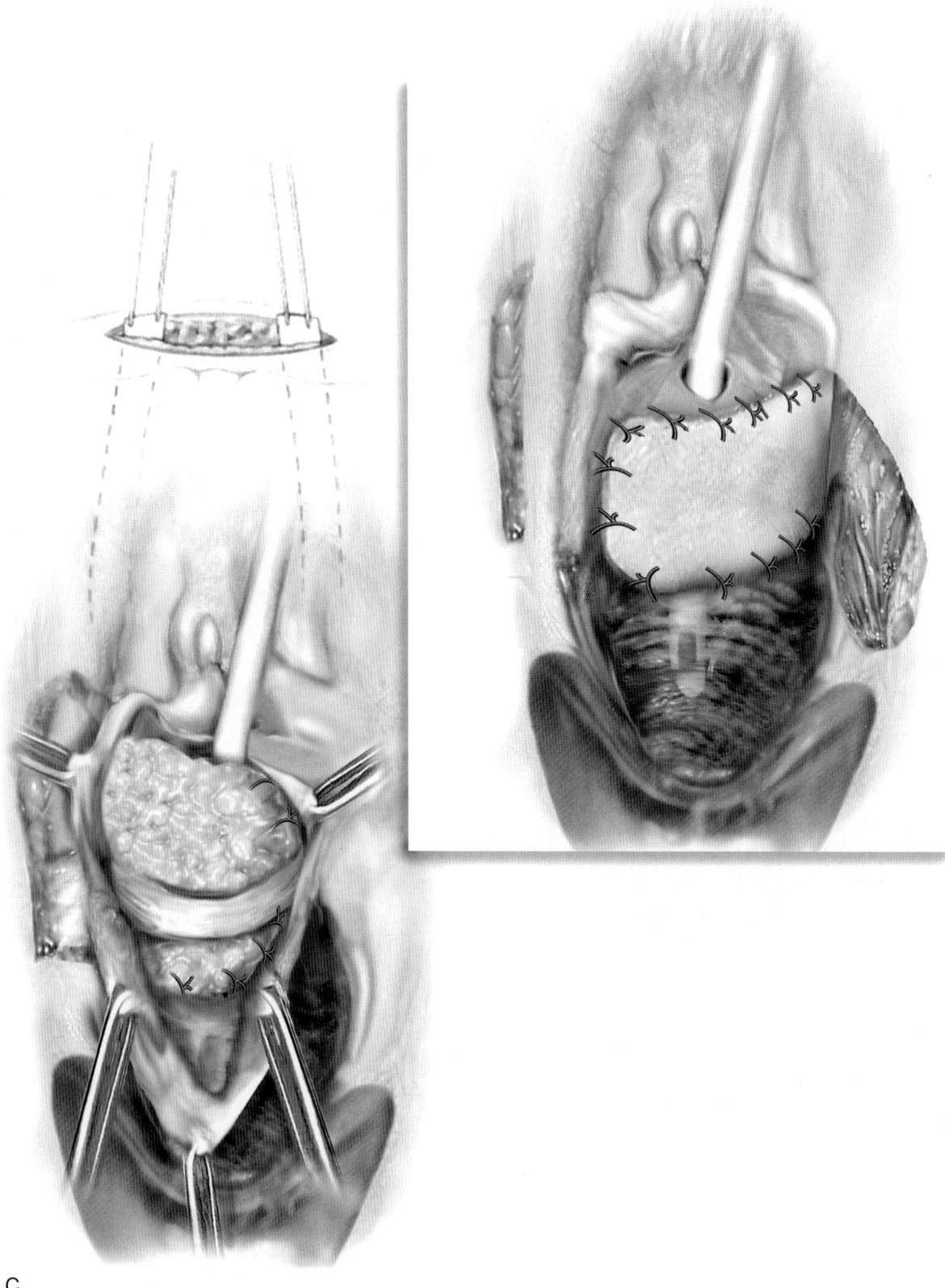

C

**FIGURE 85–4, cont'd  C.** A pubovaginal sling is commonly placed at the level of the proximal urethra in the hope of preserving continence. Because many of these cases are associated with loss of most of the anterior vaginal wall, it is not uncommon that a labial skin flap is required to close the defect in the anterior vaginal wall in a tension-free fashion.

# CHAPTER 86

# Surgical Anatomy of the Bladder and Ureter

*Mickey M. Karram*

The bladder is a hollow, muscular organ, its main function being that of a reservoir. Secondary to the distensibility of its muscular wall, it has the inherent ability to maintain a low pressure even when fully distended so as to maximum capacity. When empty, the adult bladder lies behind the pelvic symphysis and is a pelvic organ. When full, the bladder rises well above the symphysis and can readily be palpated and percussed. The empty bladder is described as having an apex, a superior surface, two anterior lateral surfaces, a base or posterior surface, and a neck (Figs. 86–1 and 86–2). The apex reaches a short distance above the pelvic bone and ends with a fibrous cord derivative of the urachus, which originally connects the bladder to the allantois. This fibrous cord extends from the apex of the bladder to the umbilicus between the peritoneum and the transversalis fascia. It raises a ridge of peritoneum called the median umbilical ligament. The superior surface is the only surface of the bladder covered by peritoneum. The superior surface of the bladder is in relation to the uterus and the ileum. The base of the bladder faces posteriorly and is separated from the rectum by the uterus and vagina. The anterior lateral surfaces on each side of the bladder are in relation to the obturator internus, levator ani muscles, and pelvic bone (Figs. 86–3 and 86–4). However, the bladder is actually separated from the pelvic bone by the retropubic space (see Chapter 31). The interior of the bladder is completely covered by several layers of transitional epithelium (see Fig. 86–1). A loose underlying connective tissue permits considerable stretching of the mucosa; for that reason, the mucosal lining is wrinkled when the bladder is empty but quite smooth and flat when the bladder is distended. This arrangement exists throughout except over the trigone area, where the mucous membrane is fairly adherent to the underlying musculature of the superficial trigone. This is why the trigone is always smooth whether the bladder is full or empty (see Fig. 86–4).

The ureter is about 28 to 32 cm long in the adult and runs half its course in the abdomen and half in the pelvis after it crosses the iliac vessels (Fig. 86–5). During abdominal or vaginal surgery, the ureter may be inadvertently bruised, lacerated, ligated, partially or completely transected, or mishandled in such a way that the blood supply is disturbed and necrosis develops at a later time. The anatomy of the entire ureter has been reviewed in Chapters 36 and 37.

The ureter enters the pelvis by crossing over the iliac vessels where the common iliac artery divides into the external iliac and hypogastric vessels. At this point, the ureter lies medial to the branches of the anterior division of the hypogastric artery and lateral to the peritoneum of the cul-de-sac. It is attached to the peritoneum of the lateral pelvic wall. The ureter passes beneath the uterine artery approximately 1.5 cm lateral to the cervix. As it proceeds more distally, the ureter courses along the lateral side of the uterosacral ligament and enters the endopelvic fascia of the parametrium (cardinal ligament) (Figs. 86–5 through 86–11). The ureter then enters the envelope of the endopelvic fascia and follows the lateral true ligament of the bladder, accompanied by a few vesical vessels and a component of the autonomic pelvic plexus, to run in front of the vagina and enter the bladder base. The intravesical ureter is about 1.5 cm long and is divided into an intramural segment that is totally surrounded by the bladder wall and a submucosal segment (about 0.8 cm long) directly under the bladder mucosa. All the ureteral muscles extend uninterrupted into the base of the bladder and continue as the trigone. The juxtavesical ureter (the distal 3 to 4 cm) as well as the intramural segment of the intravesical ureter is surrounded by a fibromuscular sheath—Waldeyer's sheath (Fig. 86–12). As this sheath is traced upward, its muscular element gradually fuses with the ureteral musculature and becomes an integral part of the ureteral wall. In this manner, Waldeyer's sheath proximally fuses with the intrinsic musculature of the ureter and distally acts as an added fixation linking the ureter proper and the detrusor (see Fig. 86–12).

The trigone is composed of superficial and deep layers (see Fig. 86–12). The longitudinal fibers of the intravesical ureter diverge at the ureteral orifice and continue uninterrupted at the base of the bladder as the superficial trigone. Some fibers run across the base of the trigone between one submucosal ureter and the other. The rest fan out and converge at the internal meatus to proceed downward into the urethra in the midline posteriorly. In the female, the same fibers terminate at the level of the external meatus. All the fibers forming Waldeyer's sheath continue downward uninterrupted into the base of the bladder, forming the deep trigone. The upper fibers proceed medially to meet those from the other side, forming the base of the trigonal structure—the interureteric ridge, or Mercier's bar. There is muscular communication between the superficial and deep trigone. They can be easily dissected from one another. The two layers of the trigone are in direct continuation with the lower ureter, with no interruption or loss of any of the musculature. One can say that the ureter does not end at the ureteral orifice but continues uninterrupted as a flat sheet instead of a tubular structure.

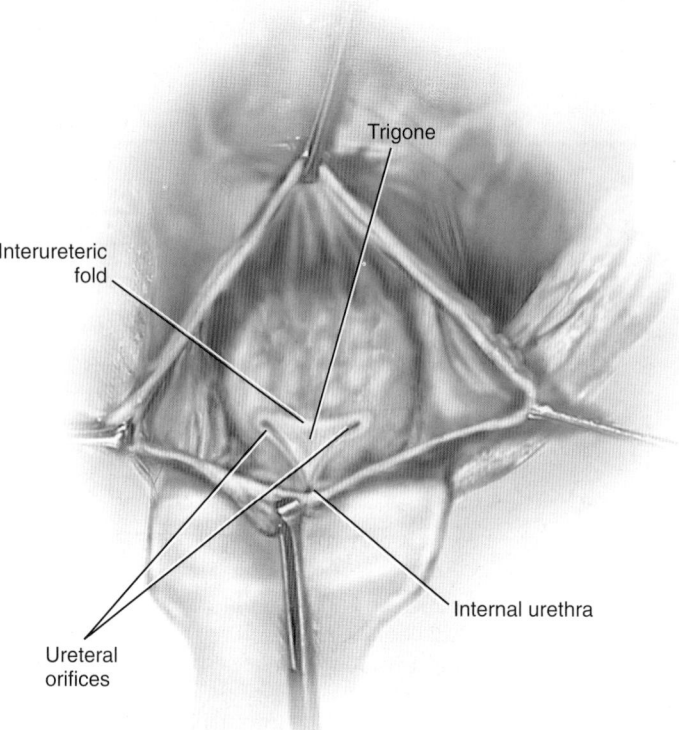

**FIGURE 86–1**  Abdominal view of the inside of the urinary bladder. Note the structure of the urinary trigone, ureteral orifices, and interureteric fold, or ridge. Also note the smooth appearance of the trigone and the wrinkled appearance of the mucosal lining of the bladder.

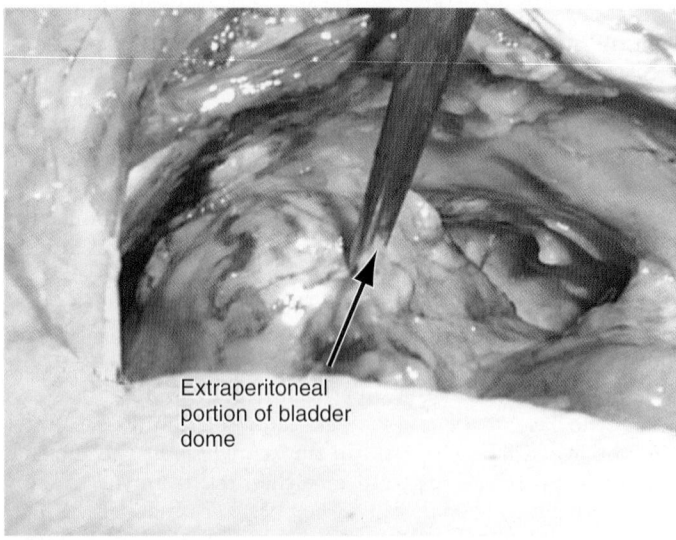

**FIGURE 86–2**  The bladder from the retropubic space is visualized. The pick-ups are holding the dome of the bladder in its extraperitoneal portion.

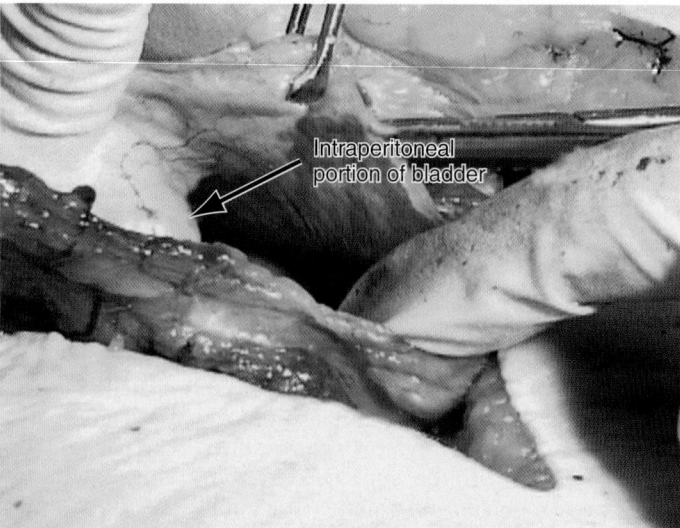

**FIGURE 86–3**  The peritoneum has been opened and the interperitoneal portion of the bladder is shown.

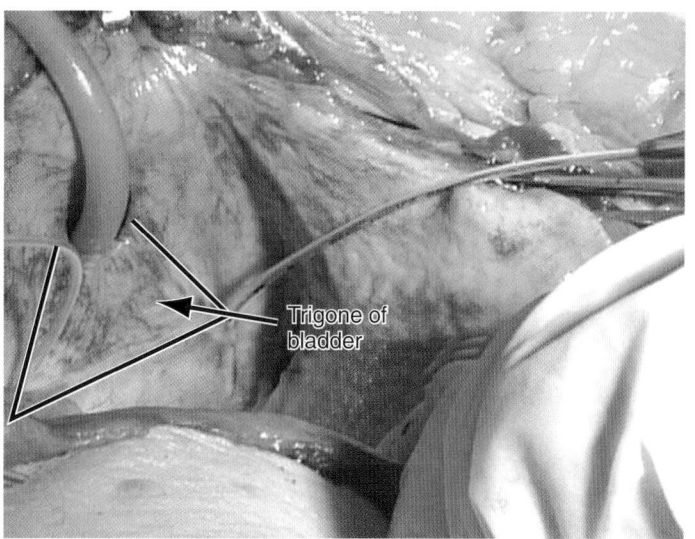

**FIGURE 86–4** The bladder has been opened and the trigone of the bladder is shown in this cadaver. *Note:* Both ureteral orifices have been threaded with a pediatric feeding tube. This figure depicts the normal intravesical anatomy of the bladder and the trigone.

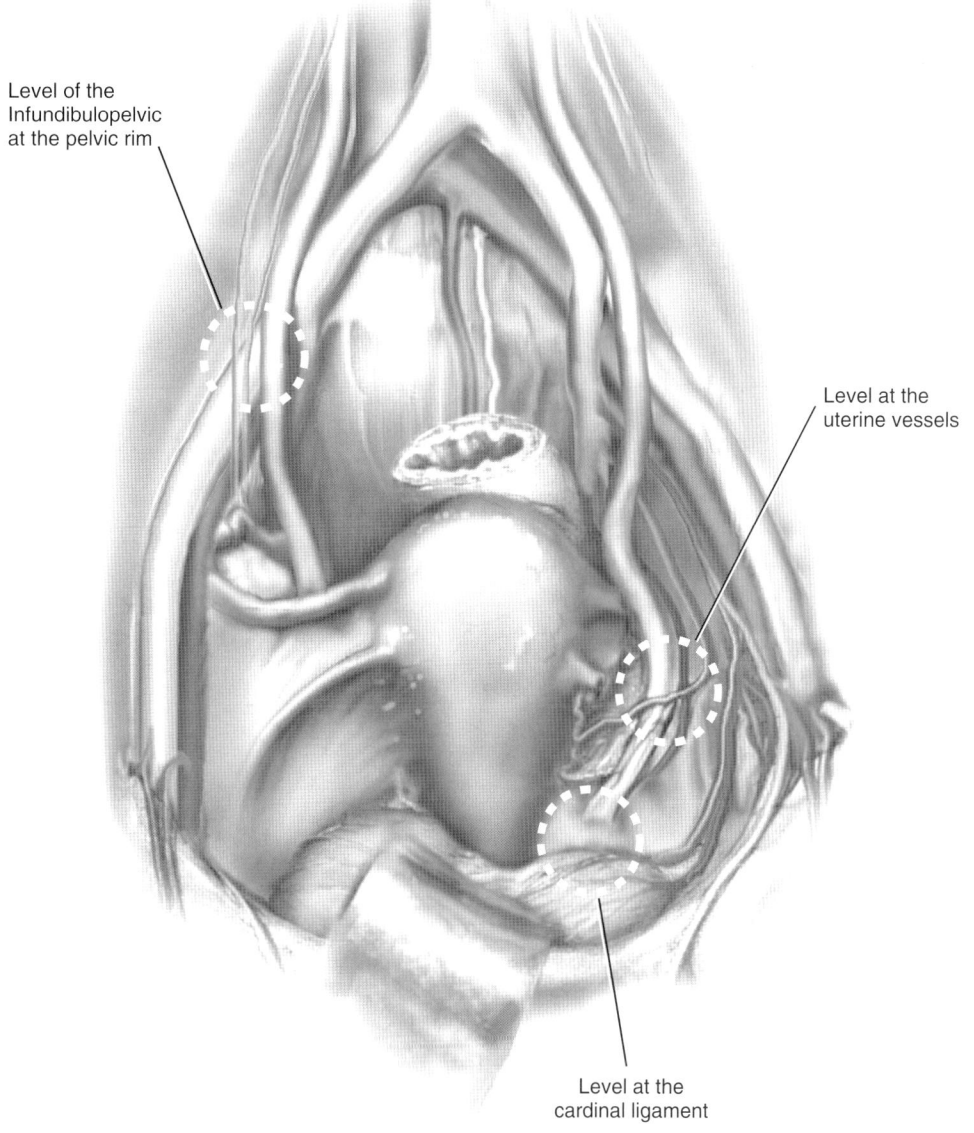

**FIGURE 86–5** This drawing shows the anatomy of the pelvic ureter. Circled areas are anatomic sites where the ureter is most likely to be injured during gynecologic surgery.

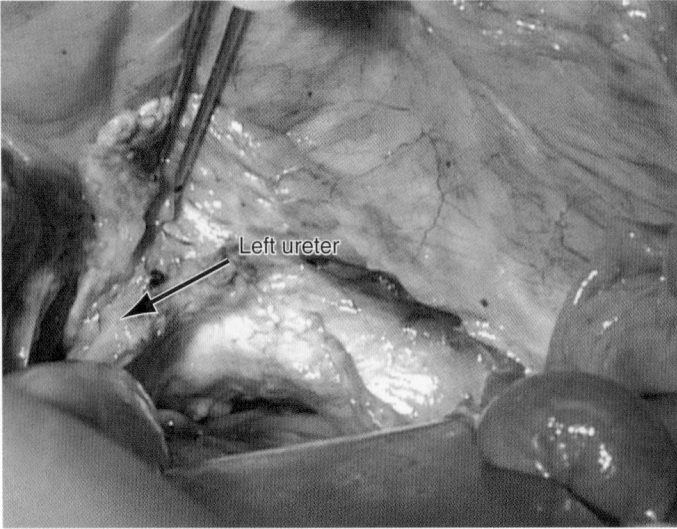

**FIGURE 86–6** The relationship of the left ureter to the apex of the vagina is shown.

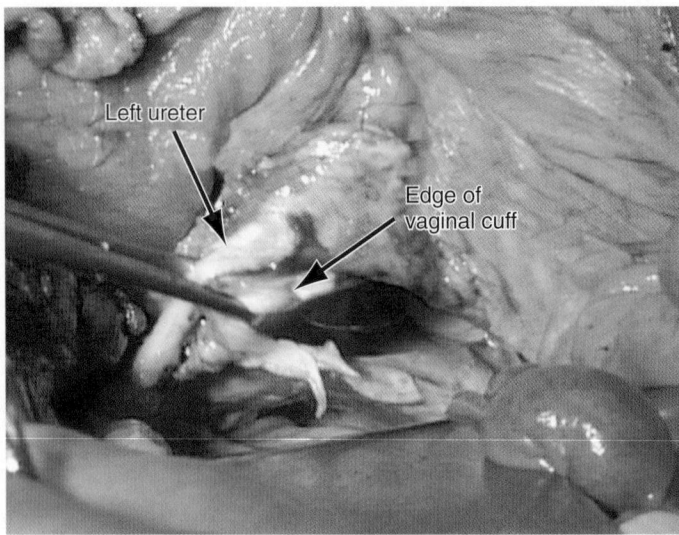

**FIGURE 86–7** The vaginal cuff has been opened, and pick-ups have been used to grasp the lateral edge of the vaginal cuff and the left ureter as it enters the urinary bladder. Note the close proximity of the ureter to the vaginal cuff at this anatomic location.

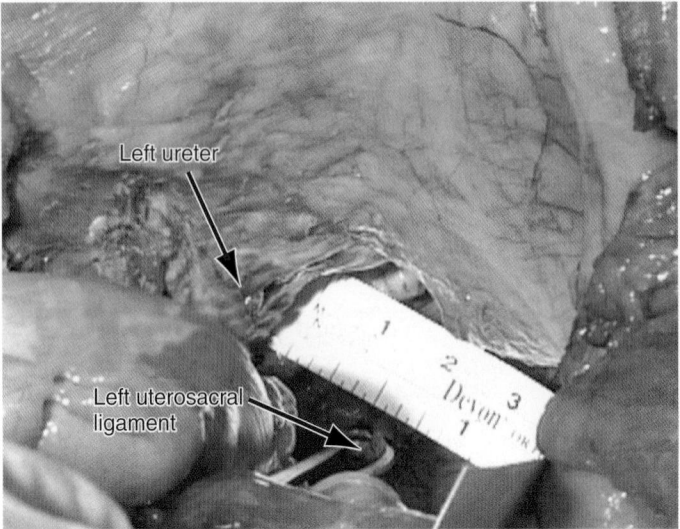

**FIGURE 86–8** This figure demonstrates the relationship between the left ureter and the left uterosacral ligament in the lower portion of the pelvis. Note that in this specific cadaver, the ureter was approximately 2 cm lateral to the left uterosacral ligament.

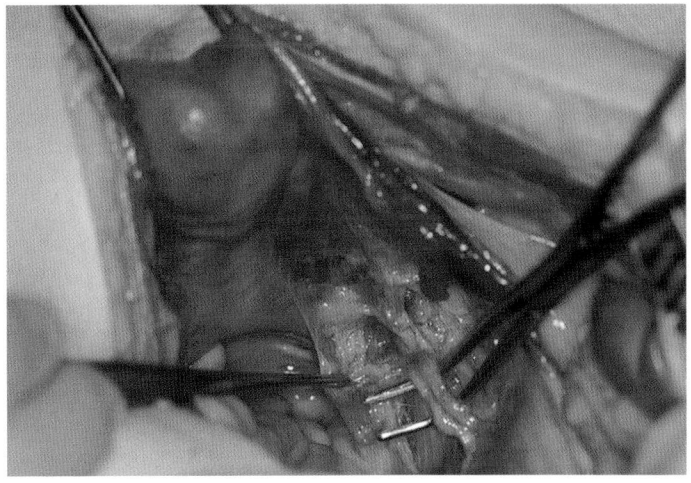

**FIGURE 86–9** The relationship of the right ureter to the right uterosacral ligament is shown.

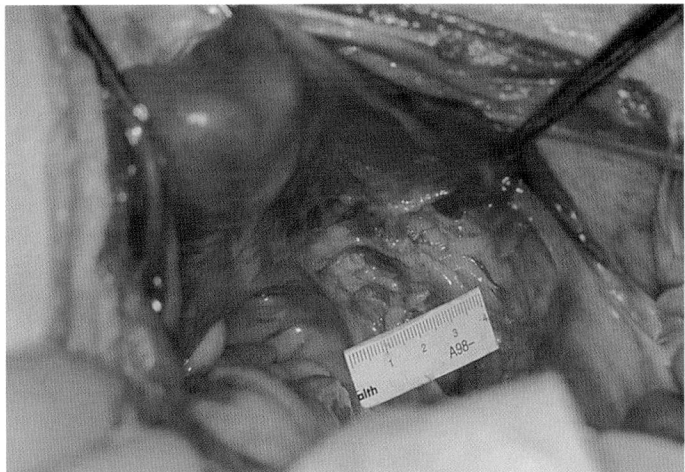

**FIGURE 86–10** This figure illustrates the relationship of the right ureter to the right uterosacral ligament at the level of the ischial spine. Note that the distance between the two structures was about 4 cm in this specific cadaver.

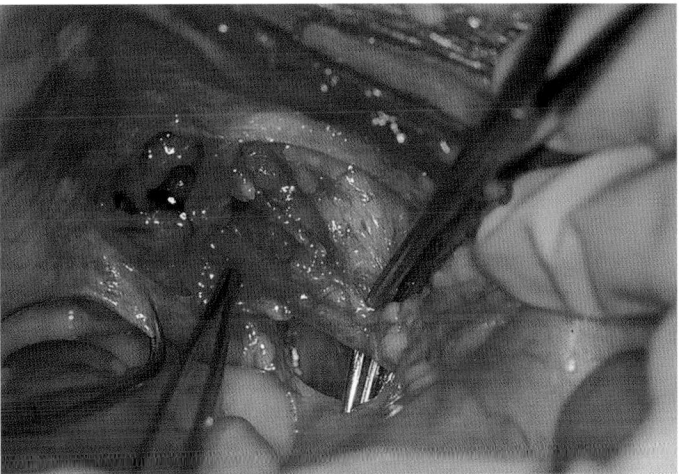

**FIGURE 86–11** The backs of pick-ups point to where the right ureter enters the fascial tunnel of the cardinal ligament. The right-angle clamp to the left of the pick-ups is on the right uterosacral ligament close to its insertion into the uterus.

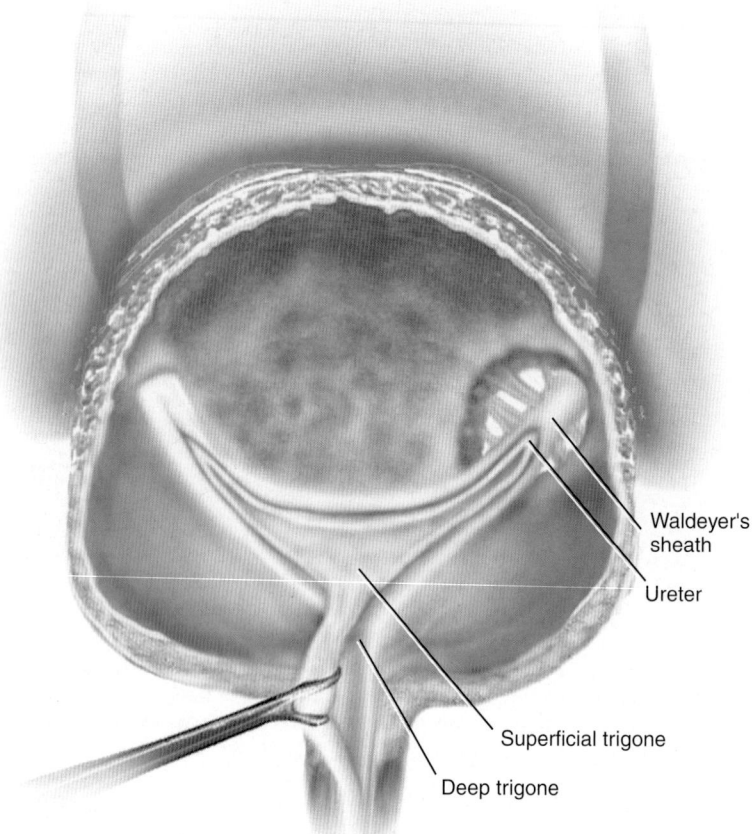

Waldeyer's
sheath

Ureter

Superficial trigone

Deep trigone

**FIGURE 86–12** Waldeyer's sheath connected by a few fibers to the detrusor muscle in the ureteral hiatus. This muscular sheath inferior to the ureteral orifice becomes the deep trigone. The musculature of the ureters continues downward as the superficial trigone.

# CHAPTER 87

# Suprapubic Catheter Placement

*Mickey M. Karram*

Suprapubic catheters are commonly placed after surgeries that may delay the return of normal, efficient voiding, such as anti-incontinence procedures and procedures for pelvic organ prolapse. Suprapubic catheters are thought to improve patient comfort and ease of nursing care; however, the real advantage is that they allow patients to control voiding trials, thus obviating repeated transurethral catheterizations to check postvoid residual volumes.

The major catheter types available are listed in Table 87-1 and shown in Fig. 87-1. Suprapubic catheters can be inserted using an open or a closed technique. Open techniques are commonly utilized at the time of abdominal surgeries, such as a retropubic urethropexy. Any of the catheter types listed in Table 87-1, as well as a Foley catheter, can be used. To perform the open technique of suprapubic catheter placement, the bladder is filled in a retrograde fashion with saline or water, usually through a three-way Foley catheter. A stab incision is made through the skin above or below a transverse skin incision or off to one side of the lower end of a vertical incision. If a Foley catheter is going to be used, a curved clamp is passed from the undersurface of the rectus muscle and fascia and then out the stab wound (Fig. 87-2A). The Foley catheter is then pulled into the field and is brought into close proximity to the extraperitoneal portion of the dome of the bladder (Fig. 87-2B). If a high extraperitoneal cystotomy has already been made to assess bladder integrity or ureteral patency, the Foley catheter is placed into the same incision of the bladder and the cystotomy is closed in two layers around the catheter (Fig. 87-3) (see description of opening and closing the bladder in Chapter 88). If suprapubic teloscopy has been performed (see Chapter 123), the catheter is placed through the same stab wound in which teloscopy is performed (Fig. 87-4). Otherwise, a stab wound is placed in the extraperitoneal dome of the bladder, the catheter is placed directly into the bladder, and a purse string suture is

placed and tied around the catheter (Fig. 87-5). If a commercially available suprapubic catheter is used, the catheter and an introducer are placed into the previously made stab wound in the skin and inserted through the skin muscle and fascia. The bladder is then punctured through the dome, taking care to avoid large vessels. The catheter is advanced through the sheath or over the needle guide, which is simultaneously withdrawn. Efflux of urine or saline should be ensured. If the catheter has a balloon, it is inflated and the catheter is sutured in place on the skin.

Closed insertion can be performed using a variety of catheters (see Table 87-1 and Figure 87-1) and is commonly done after vaginal procedures. The patient should be placed in a Trendelenburg's position and the bladder filled with at least 500 mL of sterile water or until the bladder is easily palpable abdominally. This positioning helps ensure that no bowel lies between the bladder and the anterior abdominal wall. After the usual skin prepping, the needle or trocar should be inserted through the skin and fascia and into the bladder at a point no more than 3 cm above the pubic symphysis. The trocar or needle is removed (peeled away) and the catheter secured (Fig. 87-6). The transurethral catheter can then be removed.

A third method of suprapubic insertion of a Foley or Malecot catheter is to insert a perforated urethral sound or Lowsley retractor transurethrally into the bladder. The tip of the sound is directed anteriorly into the bladder dome, and the abdominal wall is tented upward by the sound (Fig. 87-7). A suprapubic stab wound is made into the bladder right over the sound or retractor. The catheter is sutured to the sound in the suprapubic area and pulled backward through the bladder and out the external urethral meatus, where the suture is removed. The catheter is then withdrawn into the bladder and the balloon is inflated. This technique allows placement of very large Foley catheters (22F) to be used as suprapubic tubes.

**TABLE 87–1 ■ Types of Suprapubic and Self-Catheterization Catheters**

| Name of Catheter | Type and Size | Insertion Method | Manufacturer |
|---|---|---|---|
| Bonanno | Pigtail loop: 7 French (F) | Over a needle | Beckton Dickinson, Rutherford, NJ |
| Argyle-Ingram | Balloon: 12, 16F | Over a needle | Sherwood Med Co., St Louis, Missouri |
| Supraflex | Pigtail with or without balloon: silicone 12, 18F | Over a needle | Rusch Inc., Duluth, Georgia |
| Simplastic | Balloon: PVC plastic 10, 12, 16F | Over a needle | Rusch Inc. |
| Stamey | Malecot: 8, 10, 12, 14, 16F Loop: 10, 12, 14F polyethylene | Over a needle | Cook Urological Inc., Spencer, Indiana |
| Sof-Flex | Loop: polyurethane 8, 10, 12, 14F | Over a needle | Cook Urological Inc. |
| Rutner | Balloon: polyurethane 10, 12, 16F | Over a needle | Cook Urological Inc. |
| Pigtail | Pigtail: polyurethane 7F | Through a needle/cannula | Cook Urological Inc. |
| Cook Cystostomy | Silicone loop | Through steel sheath with stylet | Cook Urological Inc. |
| Cook–Cope Loop | Loop: polyurethane 8.2, 10, 12, 14F | Through dilators with trocar and wire guides | Cook Urological Inc. |
| Supra Foley inserter | Plastic trocar and sheath: 8, 10, 12 16F | Allows Foley insertion through peel-away | Rusch Inc. |
| Trocha Fix | Steel trocar and sheath: 8, 12, 14F | Allows Foley insertion through peel-away | Rusch Inc. |
| Suprapubic introducer | Steel stylet with TFE sheath: 15, 16F | Allows Foley insertion through peel-away | Cook Urological Inc. |
| Suprapubic | Needle introducer: 14F Foley set | Allows Foley insertion | Bard, Covington, Georgia |
| Self-Cath | Plastic: 5 to 18F | | Mentor Corp., Santa Barbara, California |
| Icath | Steel curve with mirror: 12F | | Cook Urological Inc. |

From Walters MD, Karram MM: Urogynecology and Reconstructive Pelvic Surgery. 2nd ed. St Louis, Mosby, 1999, with permission.

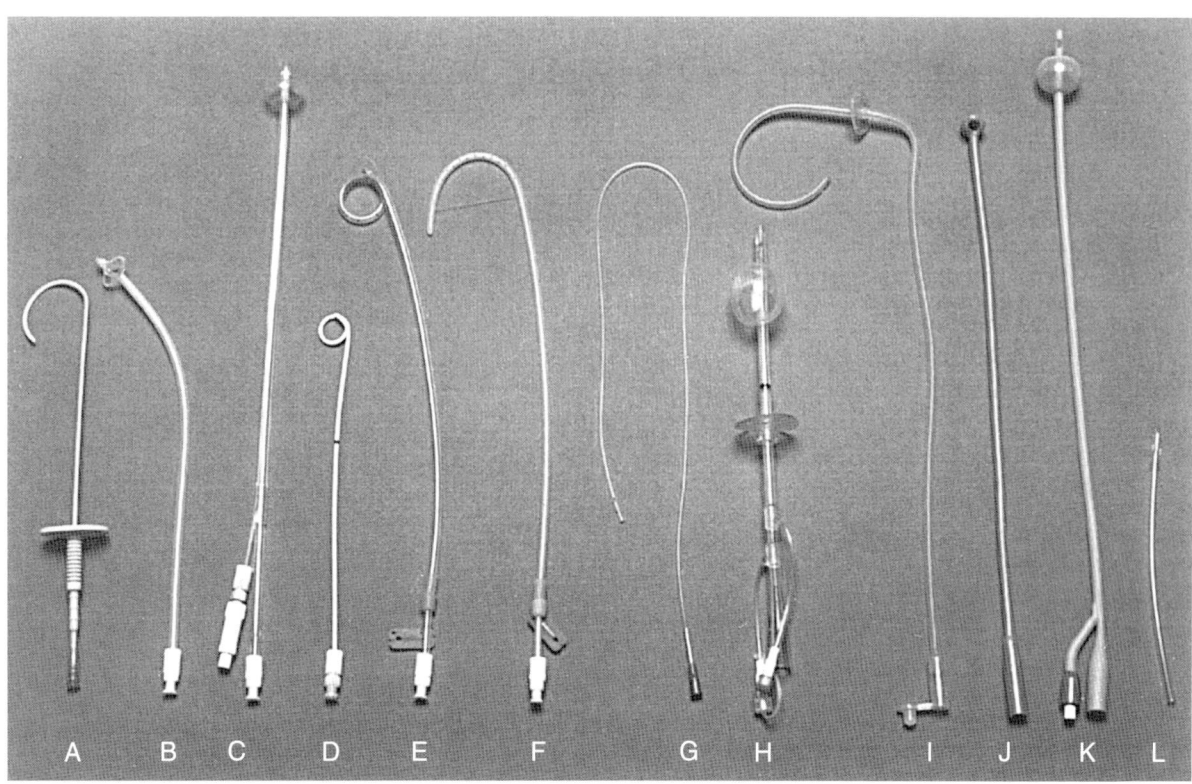

**FIGURE 87–1** Suprapubic and self-catheterization bladder drainage catheters. **A.** Bonanno, 7 French (F). **B.** Stamey Malecot, 12 or 14F. **C.** Rutner balloon, 16F. **D.** Pigtail, 7F. **E.** Sof-Flex loop, 14F. **F.** Stamey loop, 12F. **G.** Cystocath, 8F. **H.** Argyle-Ingram, 12 or 16F. **I.** Robertson, 15F. **J.** Malecot. **K.** Foley. **L.** Mentor Self-Cath, 14F. (From Walters MD, Karram MM: *In* Urogynecology and Reconstructive Pelvic Surgery, 2nd ed. St Louis, Mosby, 1999, with permission.)

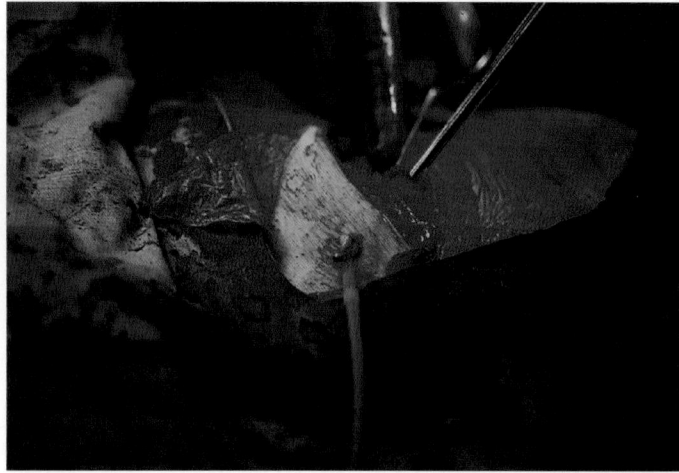

A

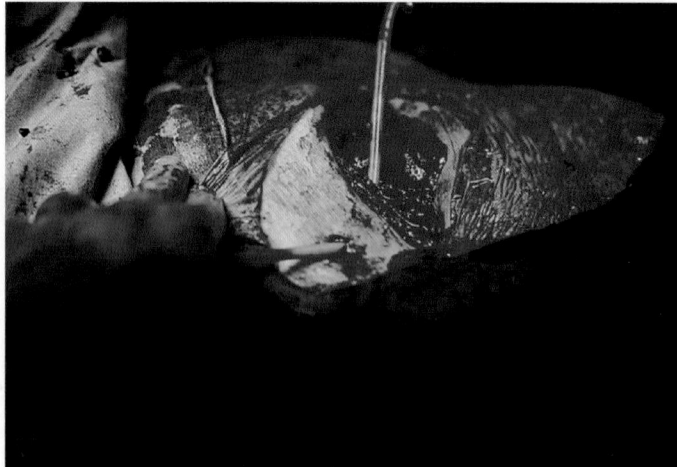

B

**FIGURE 87–2** The Foley catheter to be used as a suprapubic catheter is being brought through a separate skin incision at the time of abdominal surgery. **A.** A Kelly clamp is passed through a stab wound below the incision, and the catheter is grasped. **B.** The catheter is pulled through the stab wound.

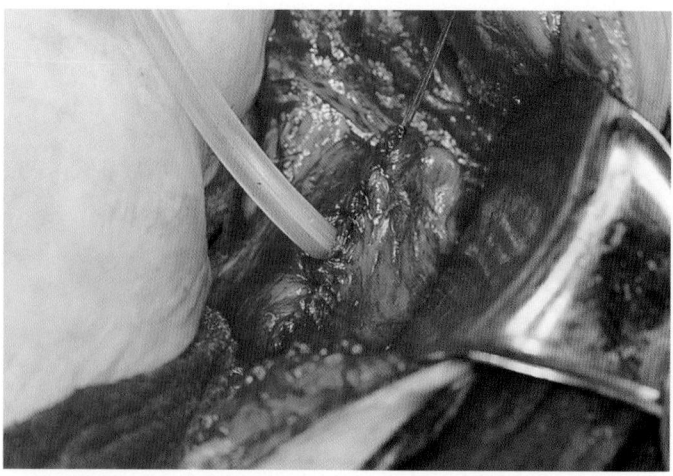

**FIGURE 87–3** The Foley catheter has been placed through an extraperitoneal cystotomy. Note that the bladder has been closed around the catheter in two layers.

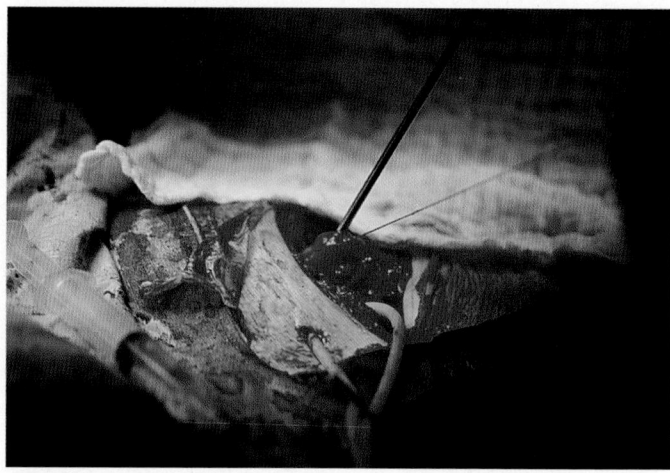

**FIGURE 87–4** Suprapubic teloscopy is being performed. Note that a purse string suture has been placed through the muscular portion of the bladder wall.

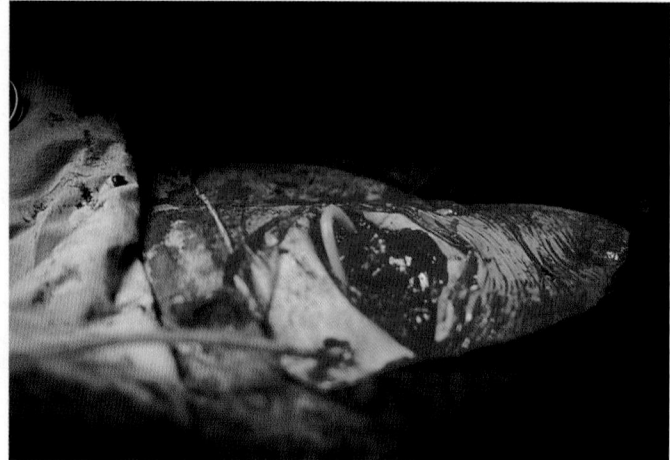

**FIGURE 87–5** The Foley catheter has been passed through a stab wound in the dome of the bladder. The purse string suture is tied and cut.

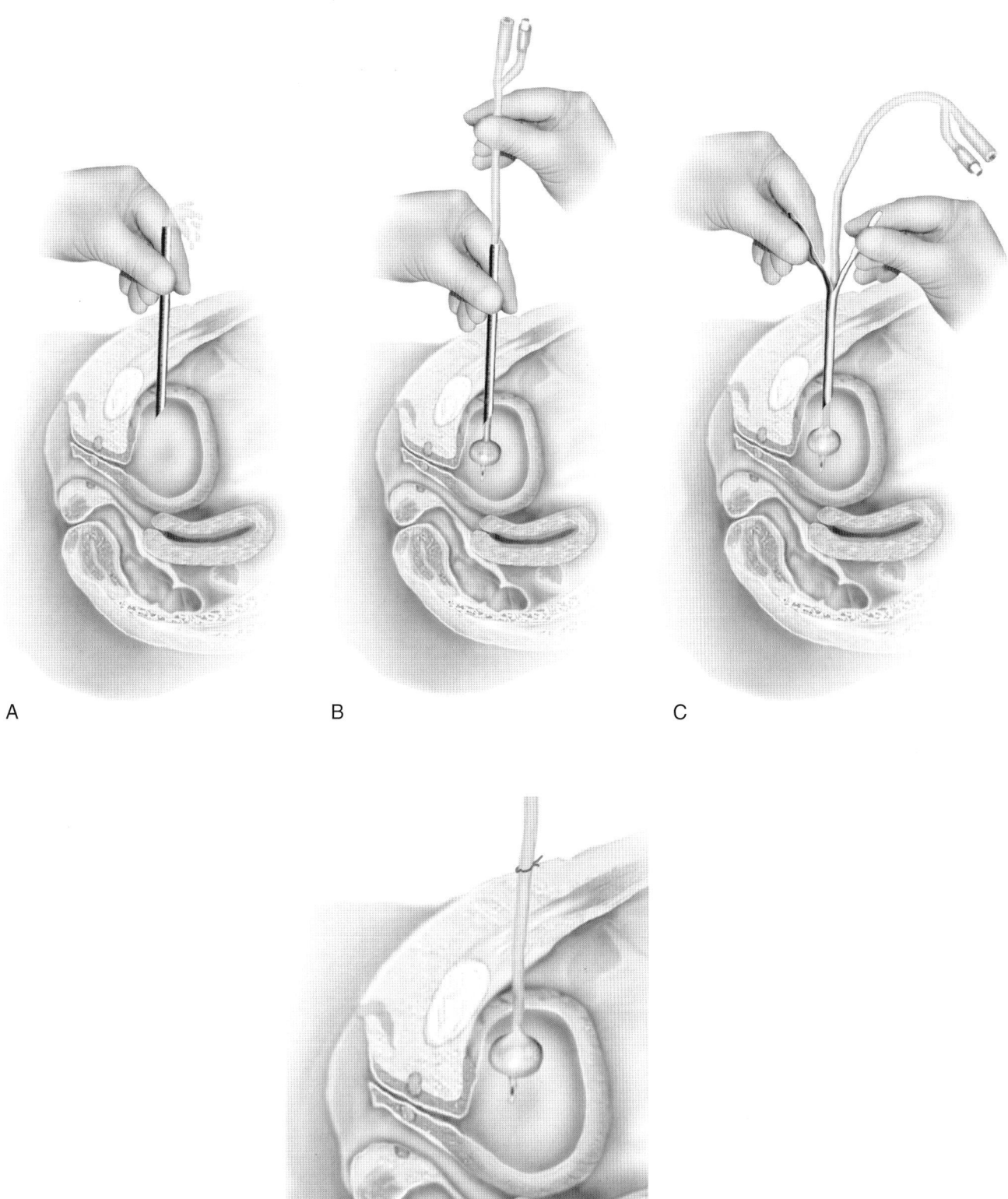

A

B

C

D

**FIGURE 87–6** Technique of closed insertion of a suprapubic catheter. **A.** With the patient in Trendelenburg's position, a stab incision in the skin is made approximately 3 cm above the symphysis. The trocar or the suprapubic tube is passed into the bladder, and efflux of urine is noted. **B.** A Foley catheter is passed down the trocar into the bladder, and the 5-mL balloon is inflated. **C.** The peel-away sheath is removed, and (**D**) the Foley catheter is fixed to the skin with a permanent suture placed in a purse string fashion.

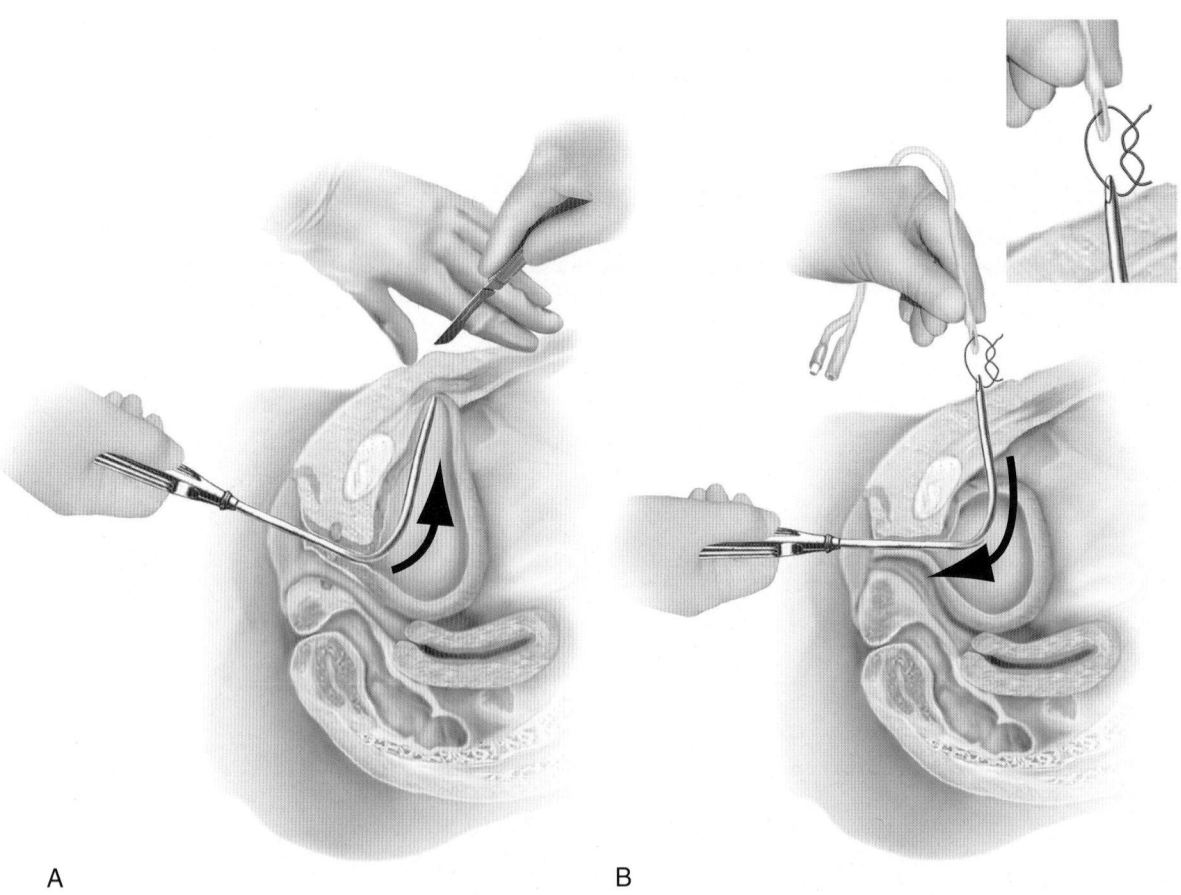

A                                                                          B

**FIGURE 87-7** Alternative method of insertion of a suprapubic catheter using a transurethral sound. **A.** Tenting of the anterior abdominal wall with a uterine sound in preparation for a suprapubic incision. **B.** The catheter is pulled into the bladder. The **inset** demonstrates the temporary suture used to secure the Foley catheter to the tip of the sound. This technique allows placement of very large Foley catheters to be used as suprapubic tubes.

# CHAPTER 88

# Repair of Advertent and Inadvertent Cystotomy

*Mickey M. Karram*

## Opening and Closing the Bladder

When performing abdominal surgery, the surgeon may encounter pelvic pathology that involves the lower urinary tract. The gynecologist should be comfortable with performing a cystotomy to assist in dissection of the bladder off pelvic organs such as the uterus or possibly off the back of the symphysis pubis in cases of retropubic urethropexy. Also, when ureteral injury has potentially occurred, it is reasonable to make a high cystotomy to assess ureteral patency. Making an incision into the urinary bladder is best done high up in the extraperitoneal portion of the dome of the bladder. An easy way of doing this is to mobilize the balloon of the Foley catheter up into the dome of the bladder (Fig. 88–1), go to the extraperitoneal portion of the dome of the bladder, and using cautery or a knife incise down onto the balloon until the bladder is penetrated (Figs. 88–2 and 88–3). Through a 4- to 5-cm incision in the dome of the bladder, one can assess the inside of the bladder for any potential suture penetration or injury and can visualize the ureteral orifices to ensure ureteral patency (Fig. 88–4). Also, if indicated, a ureteral stent or pediatric feeding tube can be passed in a retrograde fashion (Fig. 88–5). Ureteral stent placement may be very helpful when pelvic pathology such as endometriosis, pelvic inflammatory disease, or a pelvic mass distorts or involves the pelvic ureter. To close the bladder, delayed absorbable 3-0 sutures are utilized. The author prefers to use chromic catgut suture as it does not tear through the tissue and its short time of absorption will never allow stone formation. The first layer is a continuous suture that approximates the vesical mucosa (Figs. 88–6 and 88–7). A second layer is then placed to imbricate the muscular portion of the wall of the bladder over the mucosal closure (see Figs. 88–7 and 88–8). This is usually performed with a 3-0 absorbable suture in a continuous or an interrupted fashion.

## Repair of Bladder Lacerations

Even with extensive surgical expertise, injury to the urinary tract does occur. Most injuries to the bladder occur during abdominal hysterectomy, cesarean section, or retropubic urethropexy. When injury occurs, it is important to differentiate low intraperitoneal injury from high extraperitoneal injury. When a low intraperitoneal injury occurs, the injured bladder needs to be completely mobilized from surrounding tissue and closed in layers under no tension. On the other hand, a high extraperitoneal cystotomy utilizes the technique discussed in the previous section on opening and closing the bladder. With an increasing number of women undergoing cesarean section, it is relatively common to encounter some adhesions between the lower uterine segment and the bladder when performing a hysterectomy. For this reason, it is important to utilize sharp dissection when mobilizing the bladder off the lower uterine segment. Fig. 88–9 demonstrates how utilizing blunt dissection with a sponge stick in a patient with dense adhesions can at times result in an inadvertent tear into the bladder. Figure 88–10 demonstrates how sharp dissection allows appropriate mobilization of the base of the bladder off the lower uterine segment. This then allows a tension-free closure of inadvertent cystotomy. Figure 88–11 demonstrates how blunt finger dissection at the time of vaginal hysterectomy can result in an inadvertent cystotomy.

The duration of bladder drainage after cystotomy depends on the position and extent of the cystotomy. In general, high extraperitoneal cystotomies in a nondependent portion of the bladder require very little drainage time, whereas low intraperitoneal cystotomies in a dependent portion of the bladder usually require 7 to 10 days of bladder drainage. This can be performed via a suprapubic catheter or a transurethral catheter.

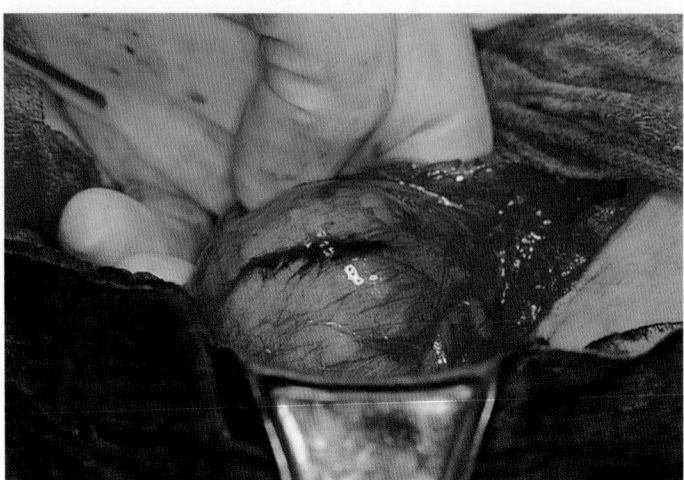

**FIGURE 88–1** The balloon of the Foley catheter is mobilized into the extraperitoneal portion of the dome of the bladder in preparation for cystotomy. A line has been drawn to indicate the location and size of the cystotomy.

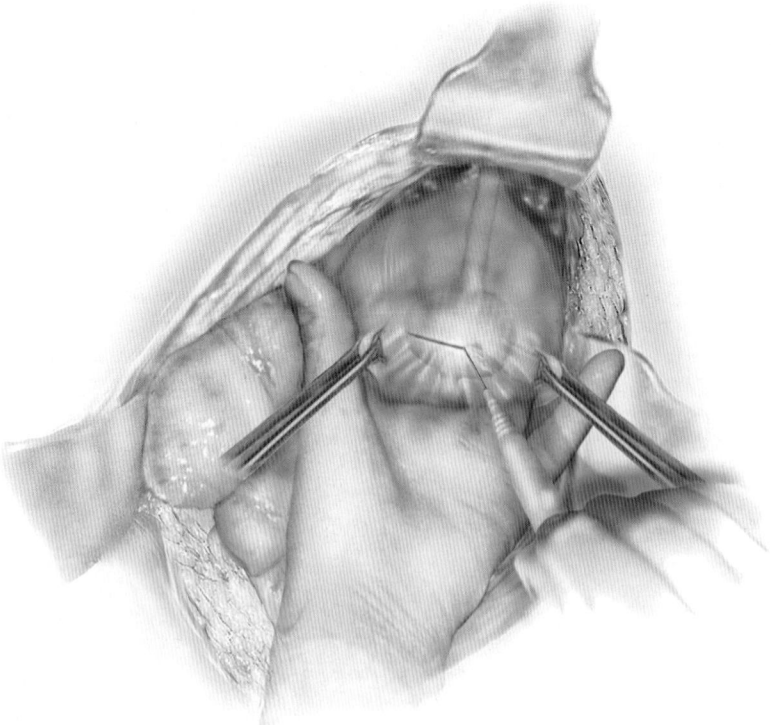

**FIGURE 88–2** Drawing showing the use of electrocautery to perform cystotomy.

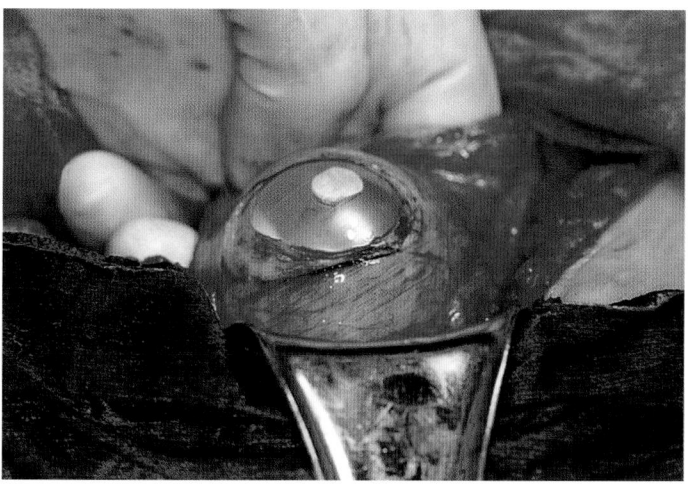

**FIGURE 88–3** Cystotomy has been made over the elevated Foley balloon in the extraperitoneal portion of the dome of the bladder.

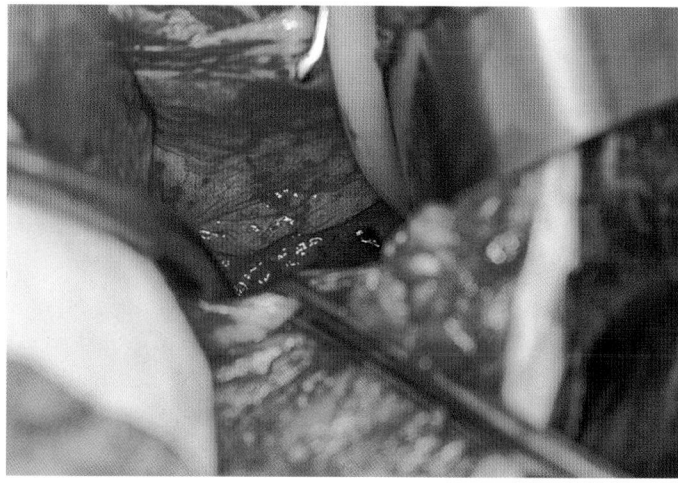

**FIGURE 88–4** The inside of the bladder is being assessed through the cystotomy. Note that the Foley catheter has been pulled up through the cystotomy, and intravesical placement of a small Deaver or malleable retractor aids in visualization of the lower portion of the bladder, trigone, and ureteral orifices. Dye-colored urine is seen effluxing from the left ureteral orifice.

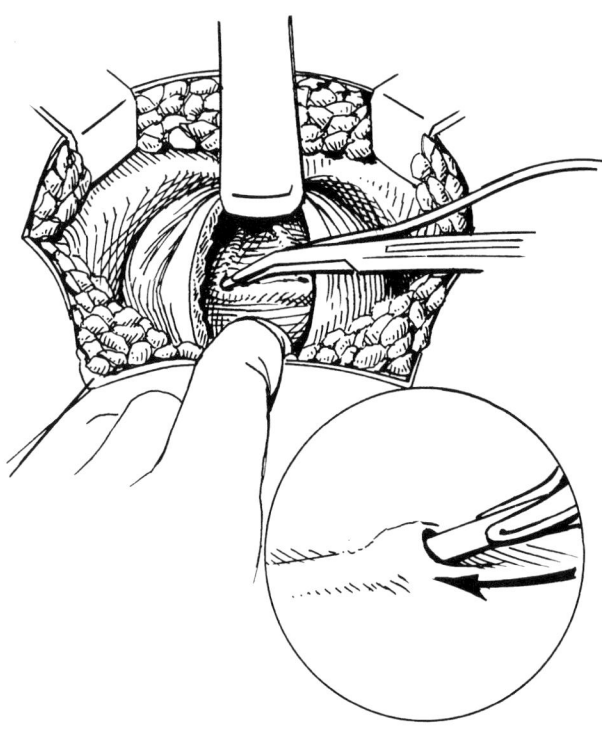

**FIGURE 88–5** Technique of retrograde passage of a ureteral stent or pediatric feeding tube through a high cystotomy. (From Walters MD, Karram MM: *In* Urogynecology and Reconstructive Pelvic Surgery, 2nd ed. St Louis, Mosby, 1999, with permission.)

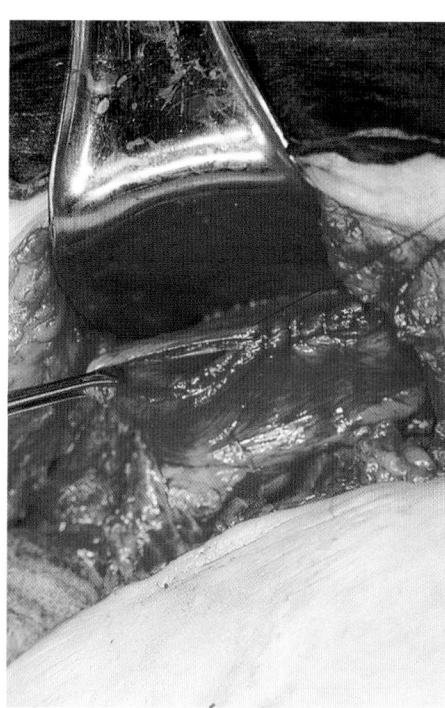

**FIGURE 88–6** Closure of a high cystotomy. Continuous 3-0 absorbable through-and-through suture in the bladder mucosa is being placed as the first layer of closure of a high cystotomy.

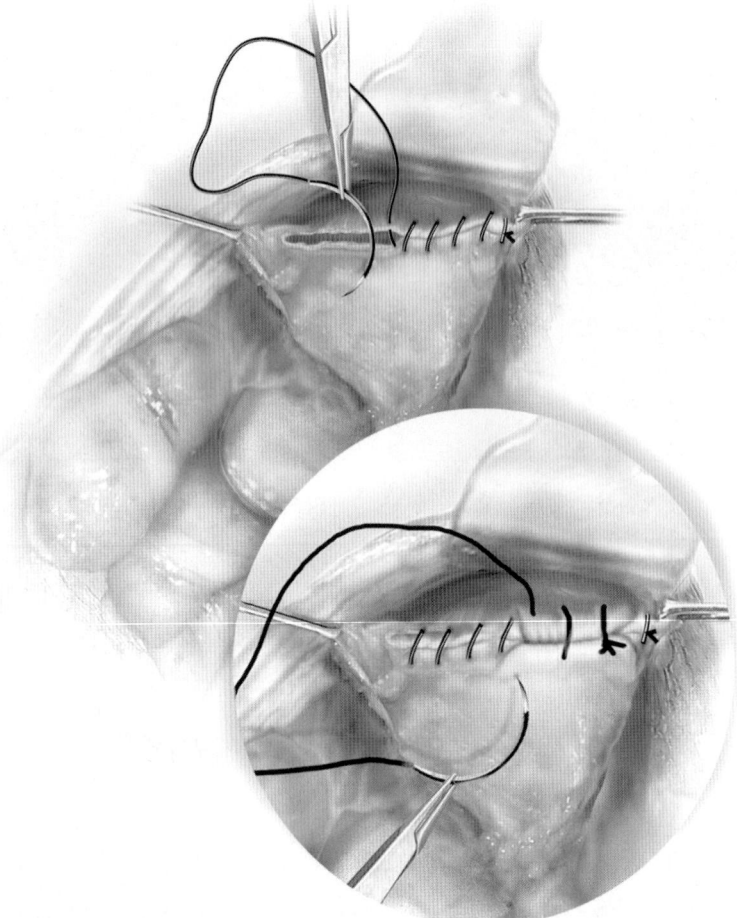

**FIGURE 88–7** Technique of two-layer closure of a high cystotomy. Note that the first layer is a running through-and-through suture that approximates the mucosa, and the second layer is a running suture that imbricates the bladder muscularis.

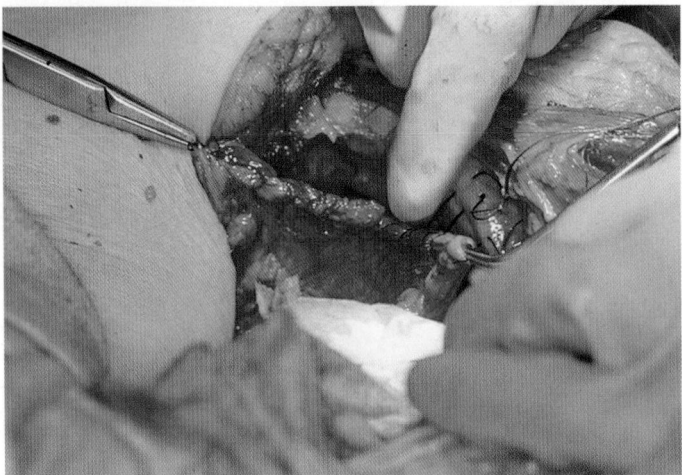

**FIGURE 88–8** The second layer of bladder closure demonstrating imbricating of the muscularis.

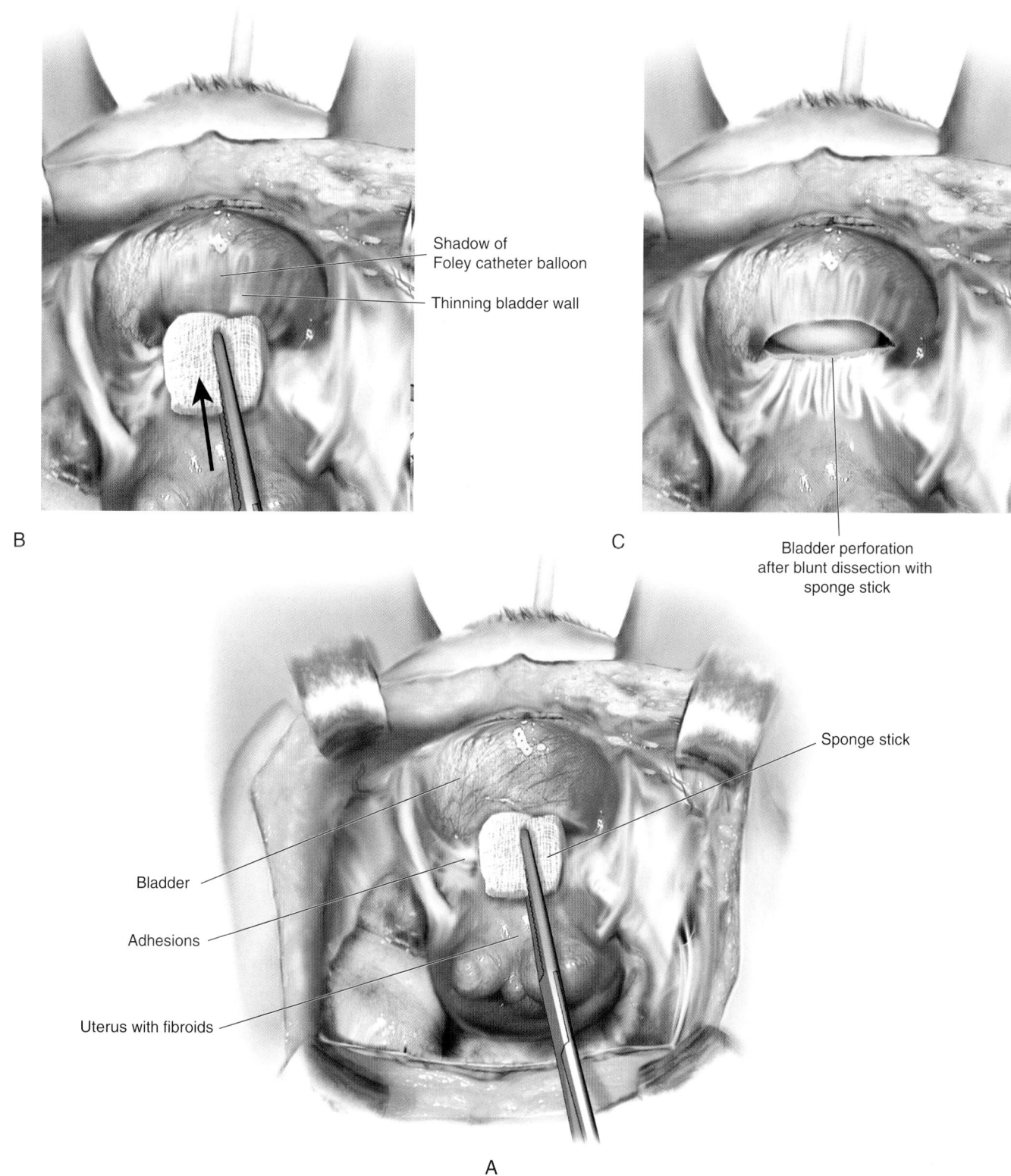

Shadow of
Foley catheter balloon

Thinning bladder wall

B

C

Bladder perforation
after blunt dissection with
sponge stick

Sponge stick

Bladder

Adhesions

Uterus with fibroids

A

**FIGURE 88–9  A.** Blunt dissection using a sponge stick is being performed at the time of an abdominal hysterectomy in a patient with dense adhesions between the base of the bladder and the lower uterine segment. **B.** As the sponge stick is aggressively advanced, it thins the wall of the bladder because this is the area of least resistance. **C.** The end result of inadvertent cystotomy due to aggressive blunt dissection with a sponge stick.

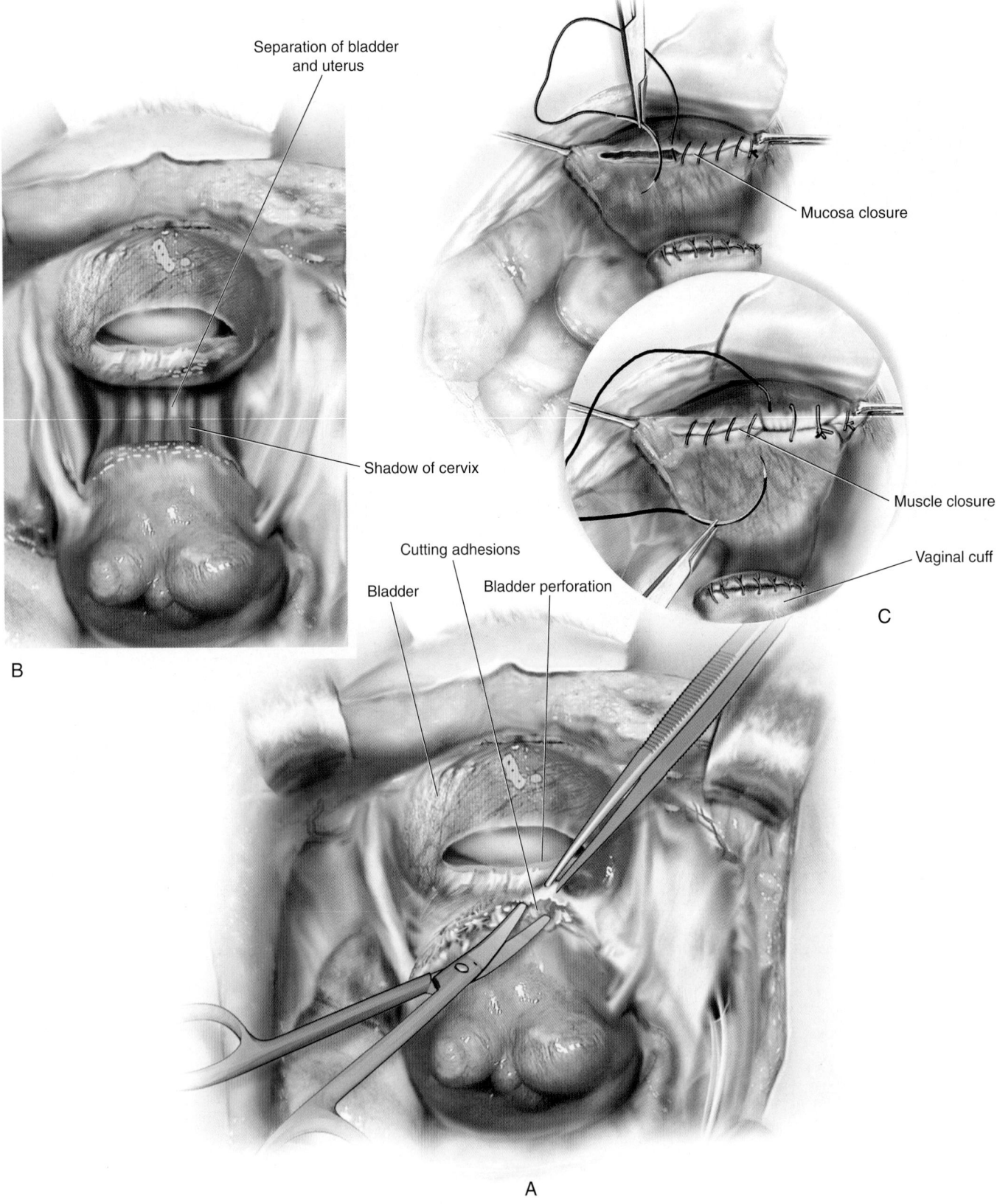

**FIGURE 88–10 A.** Sharp dissection is used to appropriately mobilize the base of the bladder off the lower uterine segments. **B.** Once the bladder is completely mobilized, a tension-free layered closure of the inadvertent cystotomy is performed (**C**).

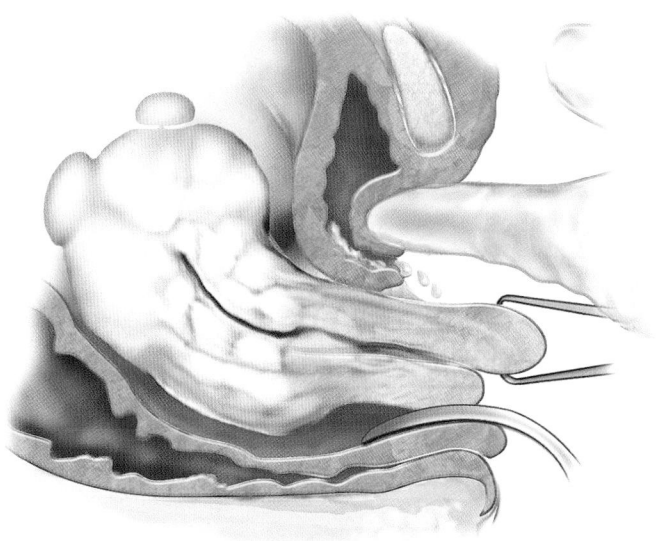

A

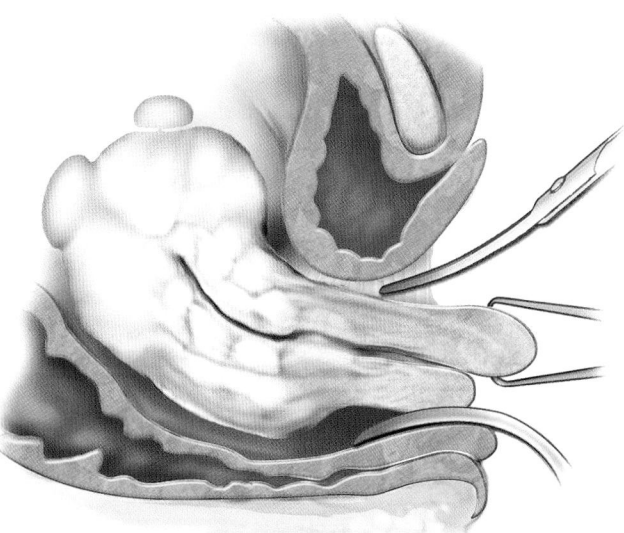

B

**FIGURE 88–11 A.** Blunt finger dissection utilized at the time of vaginal hysterectomy can result in an inadvertent cystotomy. **B.** Sharp dissection with scissors should be utilized to initially mobilize the base of the bladder off the lower uterine segment, allowing entrance into the vesicouterine space.

# CHAPTER 89

# Abdominal Repair of Vesicovaginal and Vesicouterine Fistula

*Mickey M. Karram*

## Abdominal Repair of Vesicovaginal Fistula

Lower urinary tract fistulas can communicate with the vagina or the uterus (Fig. 89–1). Although the indications for abdominal repair of vesicovaginal fistula are somewhat controversial, certain conditions involving the bladder are best approached via an abdominal route. These include high and inaccessible fistulas, multiple fistulas, involvement of uterus or bowel, and the need for ureteral reimplantation.

A midline or transverse skin incision can be made. A midline incision will allow easier access to the abdomen for retrieval and mobilization of omentum. If a transverse incision is utilized, often a muscle-splitting incision such as a Maylard or Cherney incision (Fig. 89–2) will facilitate exposure. Once the peritoneum has been opened, the bowel is packed posteriorly and usually a self-retaining retractor is placed. The bladder is then exposed, and a high extraperitoneal intentional cystotomy is made (see previous section on opening and closing the bladder). The fistulous tract is then visualized from the inside of the bladder (Figs. 89–3 and 89–4). If it is in close proximity to the ureteral orifices, ureteral stents should be placed (Fig. 89–5). They can be placed via a cystoscopic approach or intraoperatively via a transvesical approach. The bladder incision is then taken down along the back of the bladder all the way to the fistulous tract (Figs. 89–6 and 89–7). The fistulous tract is completely excised, and the vagina is sharply mobilized off the back of the bladder (Fig. 89–8). A pack or EEA (end-to-end anastomosis) sizer placed in the vagina will produce vaginal distention and facilitates countertraction, which assists the dissection. Traction and countertraction on the vagina and bladder facilitate sharp accurate separation of these two surfaces (Fig. 89–9). It is important to proceed with this dissection well beyond any scarification produced by the fistula (see Figs. 89–9 and 89–10). The vagina is then closed with interrupted 2-0 absorbable sutures, preferably in two layers (see Figs. 89–10 and 89–11). The bladder is closed with 3-0 absorbable sutures in a running fashion or with interrupted sutures. The bladder is also preferably closed in two layers (see Figs. 89–10 through 89–12). It is usually advantageous to mobilize a piece of omentum down to the site of the fistula repair. It is sutured to the anterior wall of the vagina or the posterior wall of the bladder to thus give additional blood supply and a tissue barrier between the suture lines (Figs. 89–13 and 89–14). Fig. 89–15 shows the inside of the bladder after closure and repair of the fistula. Fig. 89–16 is a drawing of the completed repair. Fig. 89–17 reviews again, in a stepwise fashion, the abdominal repair of a vesicovaginal fistula. Catheter drainage may be accomplished with a transurethral or suprapubic catheter (or both), depending on the extent and circumstances of the repair.

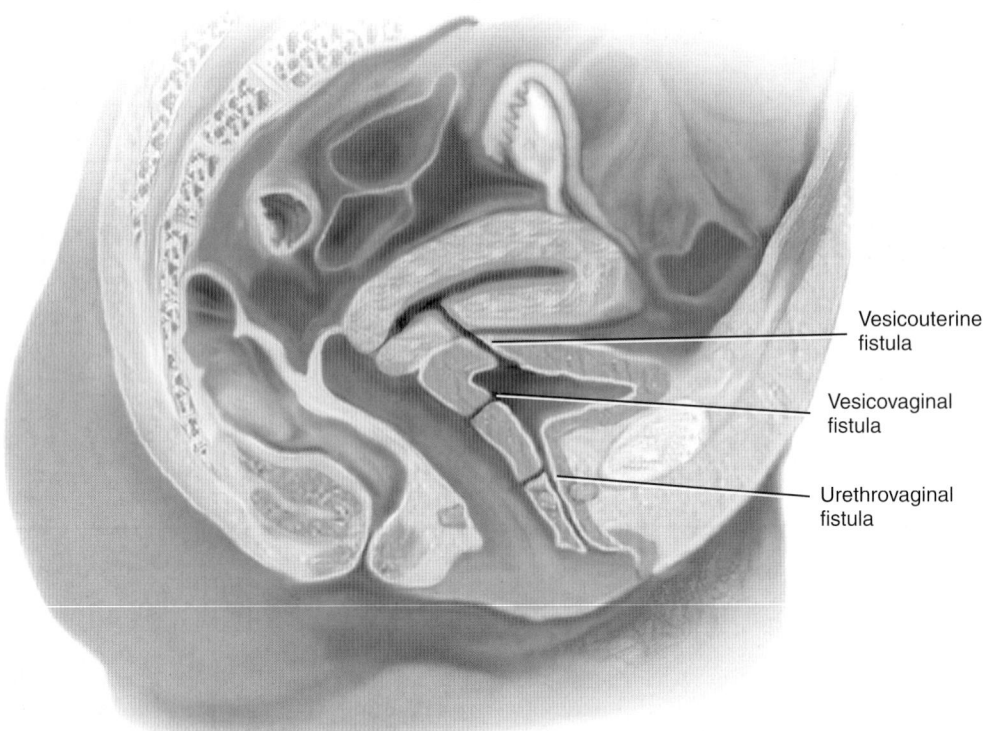

**FIGURE 89–1** Lower urinary tract fistulas can communicate with the vagina or the uterus. The extent of the fistula and the anatomic location are important factors to be considered when deciding whether to approach the repair vaginally or transabdominally.

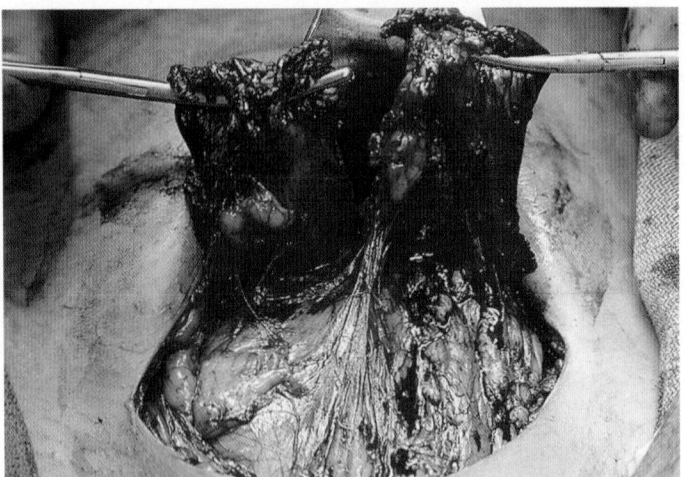

**FIGURE 89–2** Low transverse muscle-cutting incision of the Cherney variety. Note that the muscle is detached from the pubic bone very low near its insertion. The peritoneum is then usually opened transversely.

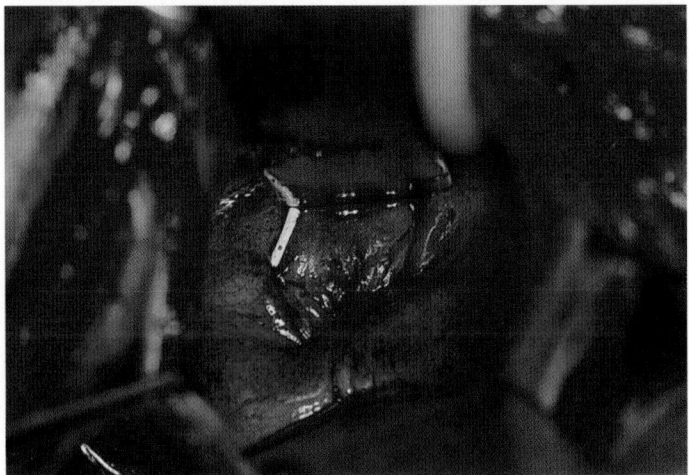

**FIGURE 89–3** View of the inside of the bladder in a patient with multiple vesicovaginal fistulas involving the lowest portion of the bladder base just above the trigone. These particular fistulas occurred after an abdominal hysterectomy for severe endometriosis in which the bladder wall was most likely included in the sutures utilized to close the vaginal cuff. Note the stent in the right ureter.

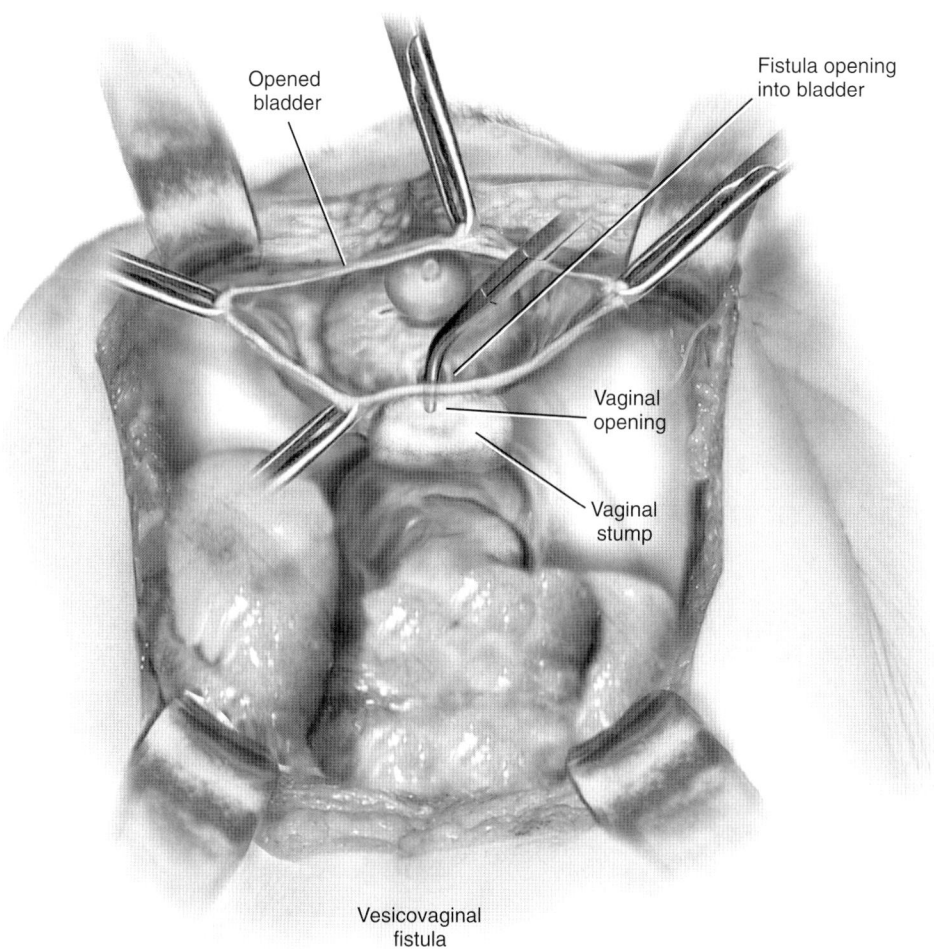

**FIGURE 89–4** Drawing showing the inside of the bladder with a fistulous tract into the vagina.

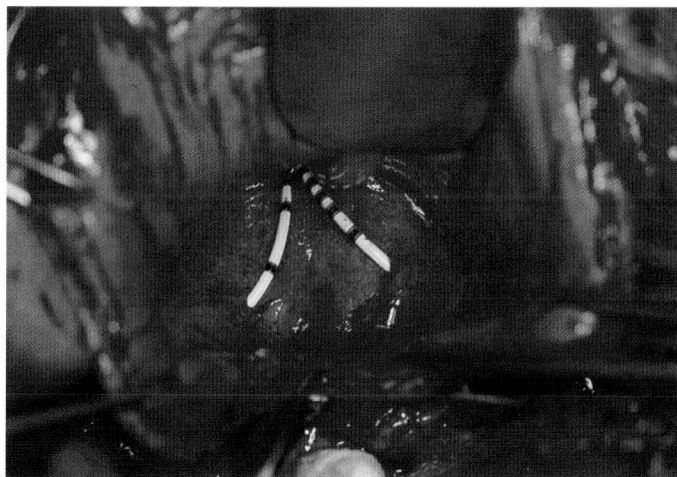

**FIGURE 89–5** Inside view of the bladder. Both ureters have now been catheterized secondary to the close proximity of the fistulous tracts to the trigone and ureteral orifices. An incision has been initiated down the back of the bladder toward the fistulous tracts.

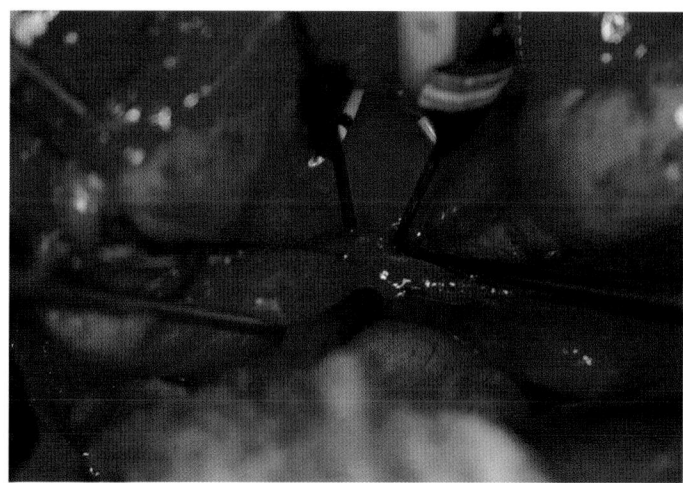

**FIGURE 89–6** The back wall of the bladder has been cut down to the level of the fistulous tracts. Note that two probes have been placed into the fistulous tracts.

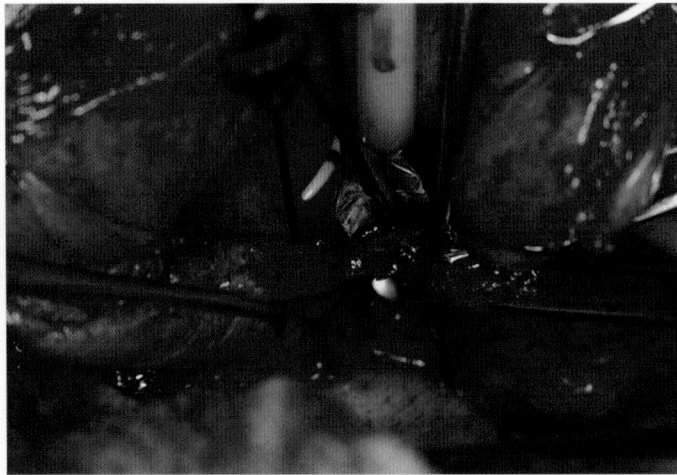

**FIGURE 89–7** Sharp dissection has been used to completely mobilize the vaginal cuff from the back of the bladder. Multiple probes demonstrate the fistulous tracts in this particular case. It is very important to continue the dissection of the bladder off the vagina wall beyond the lowest portion of scarification, thus allowing bladder closure without tension.

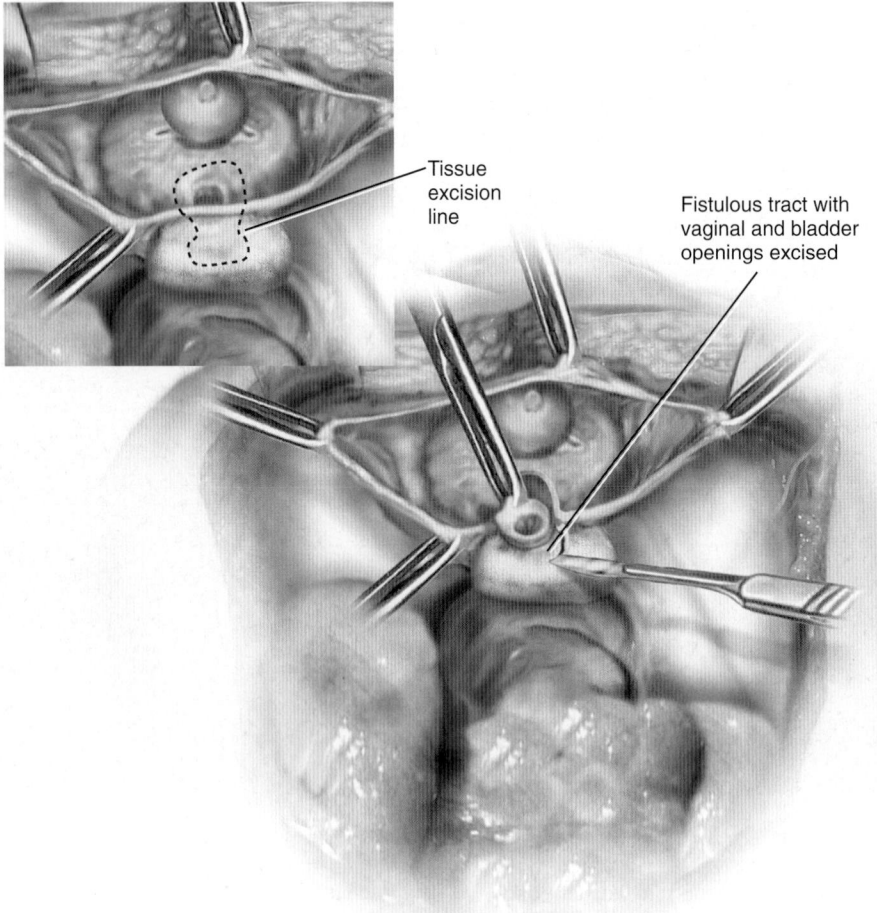

Tissue excision line

Fistulous tract with vaginal and bladder openings excised

**FIGURE 89–8** Fistulous tract and scarred vagina and bladder are excised.

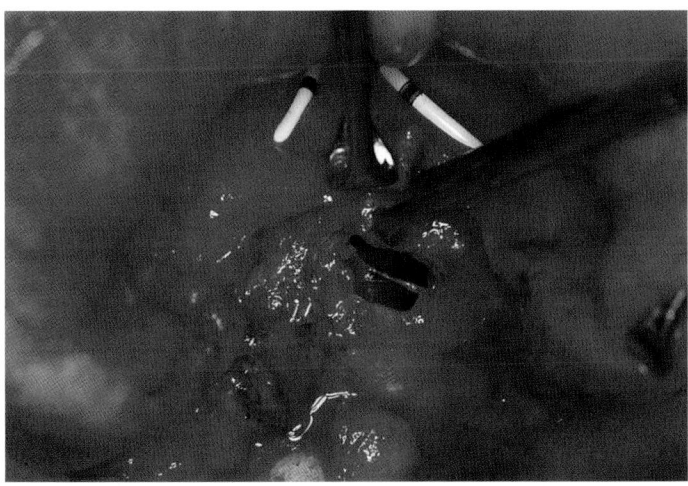

**FIGURE 89–9** Mobilization of the bladder and excision of the fistulous tract have been completed. An EEA sizer was placed in the vagina to facilitate sharp dissection of the bladder off the vagina. Note that dissection has been extended beyond the lowest portion of the fistulous tract.

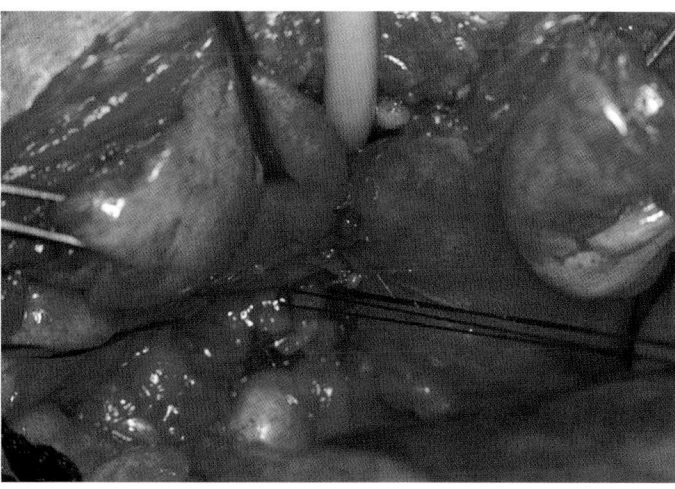

**FIGURE 89–10** The vaginal cuff has been closed with interrupted absorbable sutures, which are tagged in this photograph. The lowest portion of the bladder incision has been closed with interrupted 3-0 absorbable sutures.

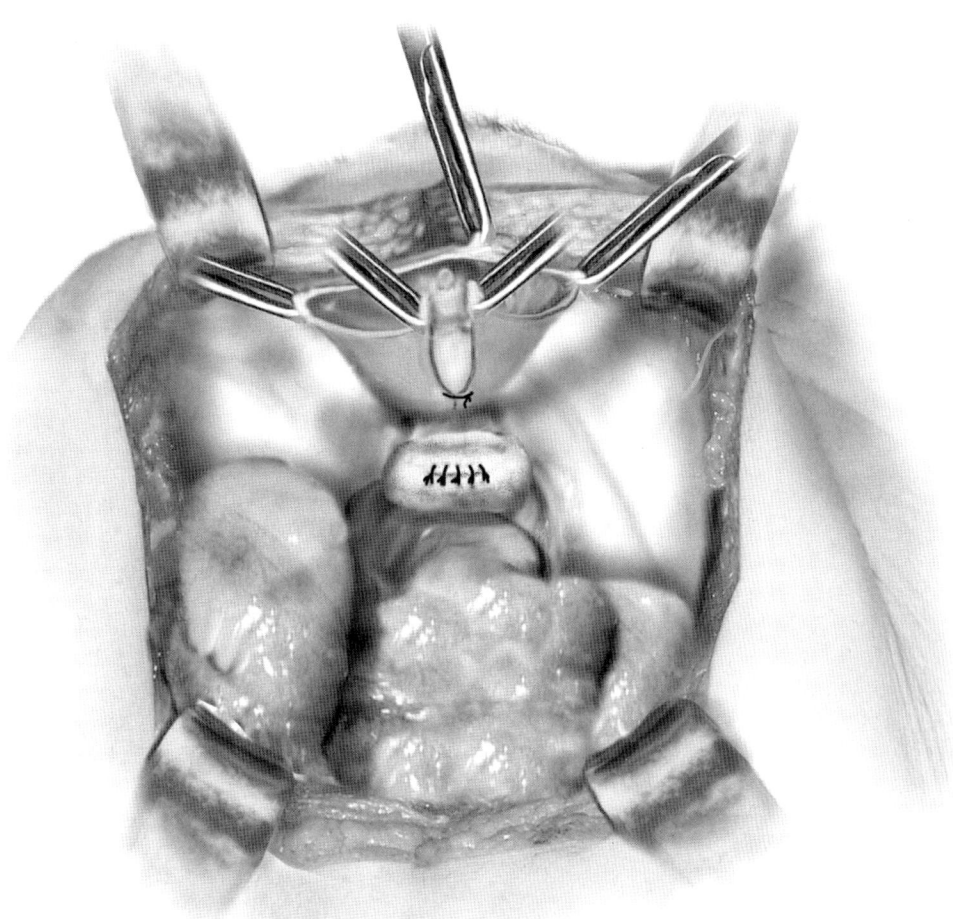

**FIGURE 89–11** Dissection has been completed, and the fistulous tract has been excised. The vagina has been closed, and closure of the back of the bladder has been initiated. Note that dissection has extended well below the level of the fistula.

UNIT 4 ■ SECTION A

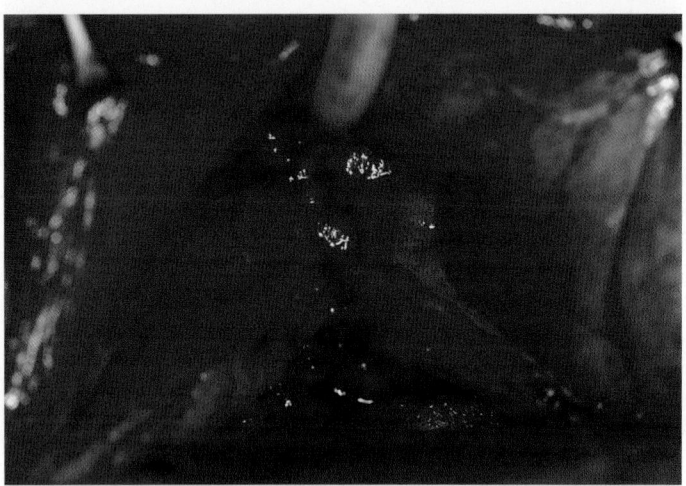

**FIGURE 89–12** Closure of the lower part of the bladder viewed from the inside. Because this is a very dependent portion of the bladder, it is probably best to place the sutures in the submucosa if possible.

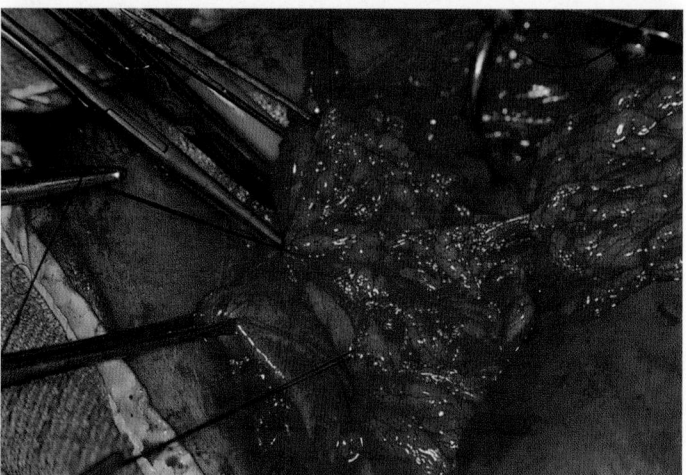

**FIGURE 89–13** Omentum is mobilized down into the pelvis.

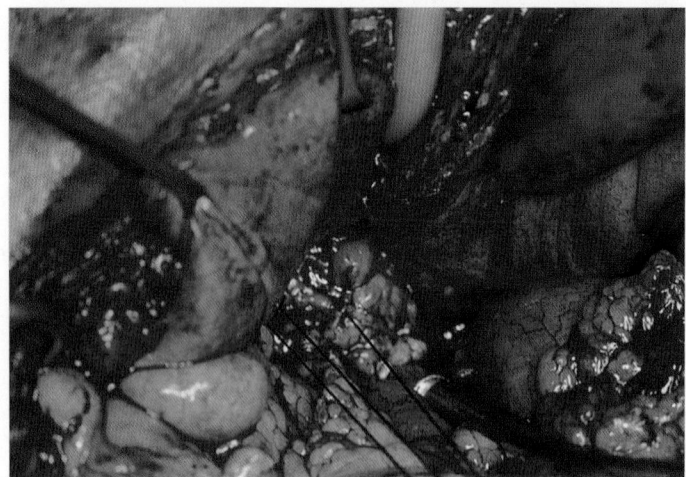

**FIGURE 89–14** Omentum is fixed to the top of the vagina and will act as interposition tissue between the vagina and the bladder.

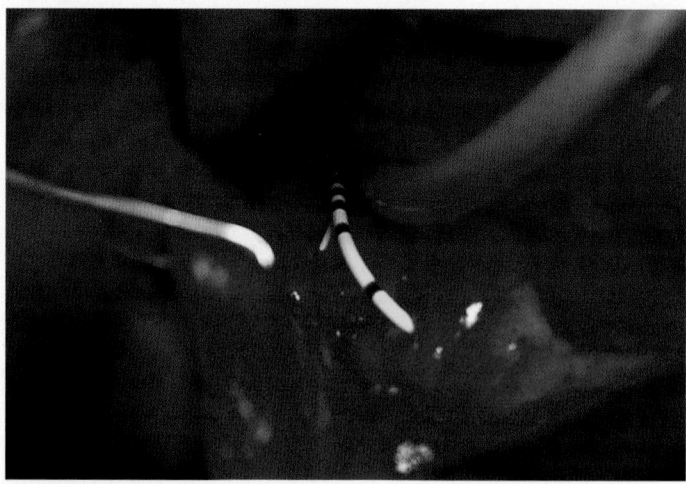

**FIGURE 89–15** Inside of the bladder viewed from the dome after completion of the repair. Note that the bladder has been repaired with very minimal distortion of the trigone.

Placement of
omental flap

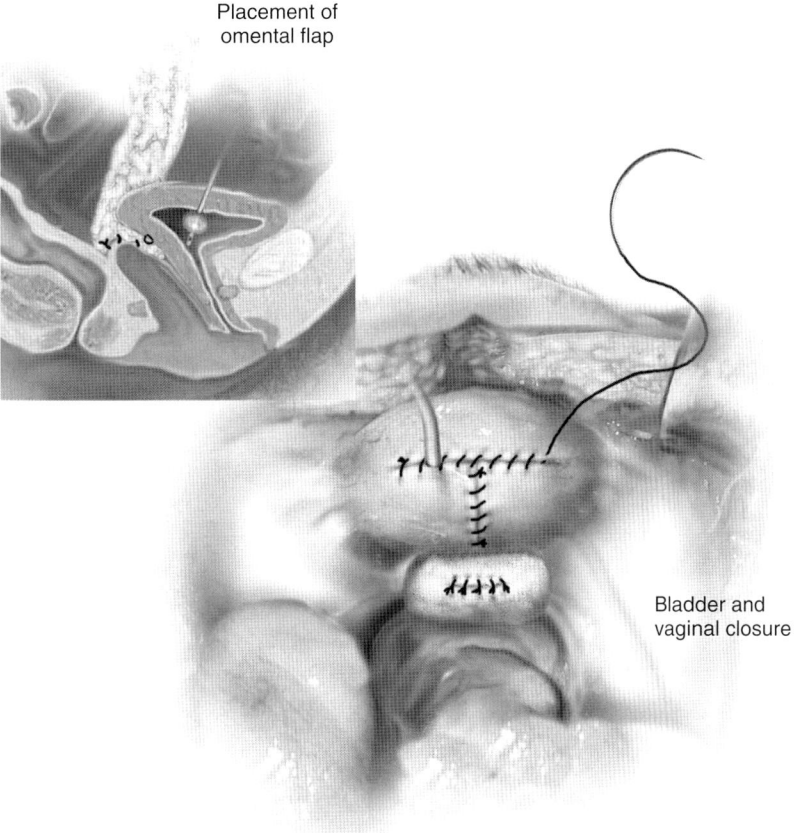

Bladder and
vaginal closure

**FIGURE 89–16** Drawing of the completed repair. Note the closure of the bladder and vagina with interposition of an omental flap (see **inset**).

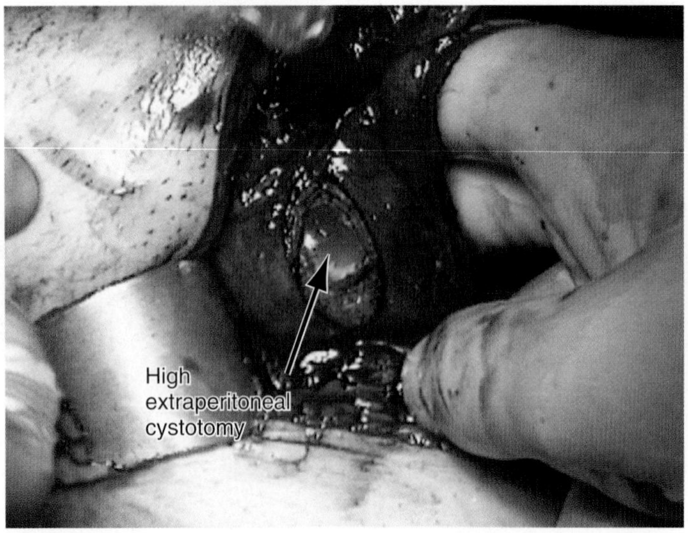

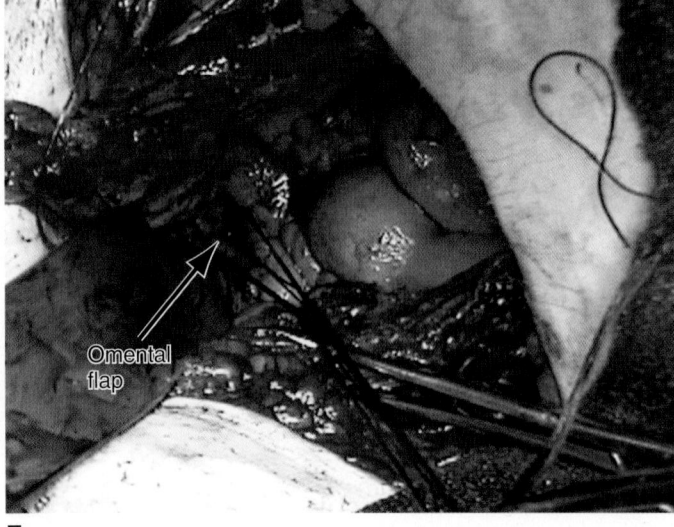

**A** High extraperitoneal cystotomy

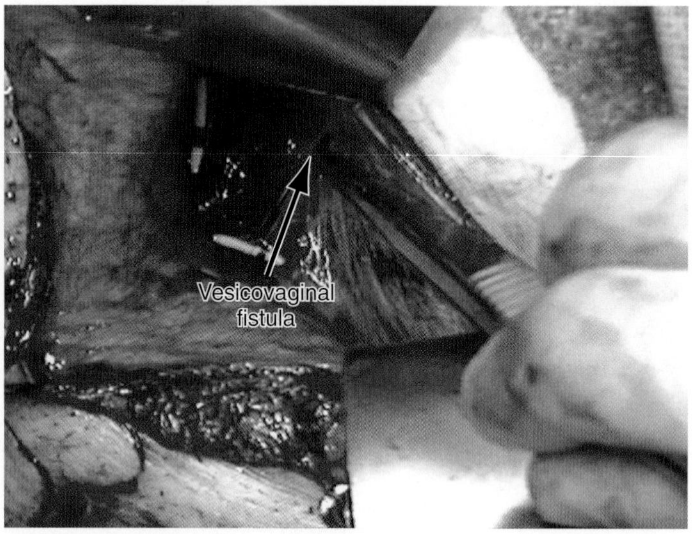

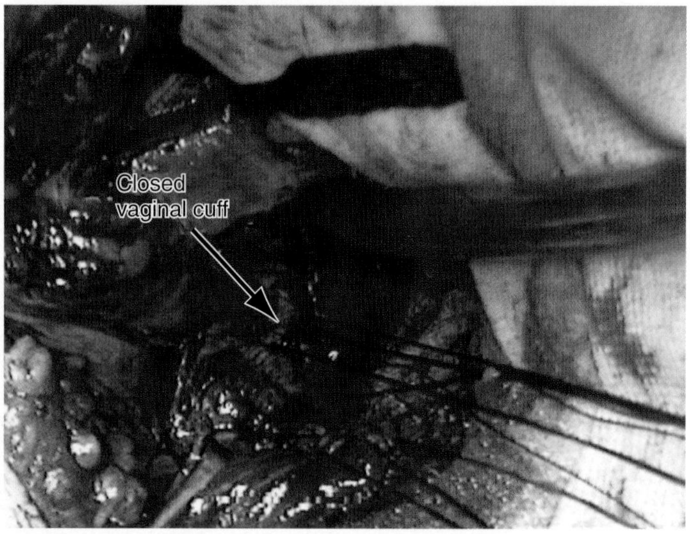

**B** Vesicovaginal fistula

**C** Vaginal cuff — Base of bladder

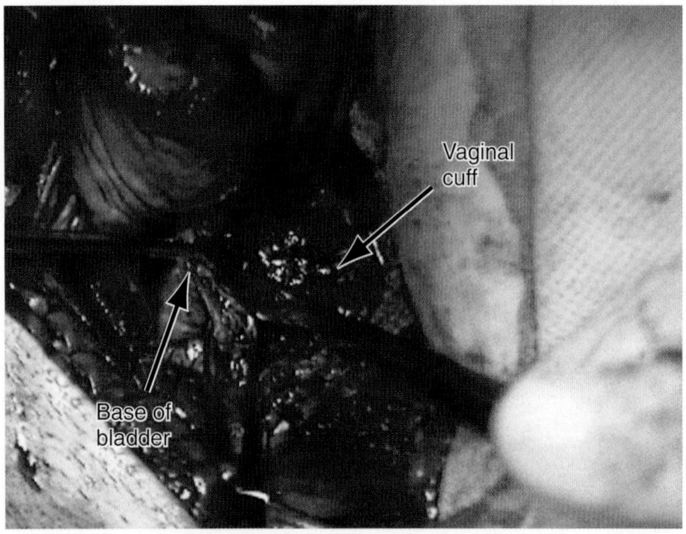

**D** Closed vaginal cuff

**E** Omental flap

**FIGURE 89–17** Abdominal repair of vesicovaginal fistula. **A.** The repair begins with high extraperitoneal cystotomy to visualize the inside of the bladder and identify the exact location of the fistula. **B.** The fistula has been identified at its intravesical portion. **C.** Sharp dissection with a scalpel is utilized to mobilize the scarred vagina away from the base of the bladder. It is very important to extend this dissection to a level well below the scarification to allow for appropriate healing of the bladder and the vaginal cuff. **D.** The vaginal cuff has been closed with interrupted 2-0 delayed absorbable sutures. **E.** The back of the bladder has been closed as has the vaginal cuff, and an omental flap has been brought down to be fixed to the anterior aspect of the vaginal cuff as an interposition between the vagina and the base of the bladder.

## Repair of Vesicouterine Fistula

Fistulas between the bladder and uterus usually result from obstetric trauma, particularly bladder injuries at cesarean section. Extravasation of urine, superimposed infection, and subsequent dehiscence of the uterine incision constitute the most likely sequence of events in formation of the fistula. Women with vesicouterine fistulas may have cyclic hematuria (menouria; Youssef syndrome). Incontinence or loss of urine through the cervix may at times be absent secondary to a valve mechanism. The tract between the bladder and the uterus is best demonstrated by hysterosalpingography. Small fistulas can heal spontaneously with long-term bladder drainage or hormonal suppression of menstruation for a few months.

Surgical repair of a vesicouterine fistula is very similar to abdominal repair of a vesicovaginal fistula. A transverse or longitudinal skin incision is made. The peritoneum is opened, and a high cystotomy is made in the extraperitoneal portion of the bladder (see Fig. 89-17A). The fistulous tract is then identified, and sharp dissection is used to dissect between the bladder and the uterus (Figs. 89-18 through 89-20). Once the bladder is completely mobilized off the uterus and the fistulous tract has been excised (Fig. 89-21), the bladder is closed in two layers with interrupted 3-0 absorbable sutures. This is followed by interrupted closure of the defect in the uterus. The repair is completed by the interposition of a piece of omentum between the two suture lines (Fig. 89-22). If the patient is not desirous of future fertility, abdominal hysterectomy with closure of the bladder defect is the definitive therapy for a vesicouterine fistula.

UNIT 4 ■ SECTION A

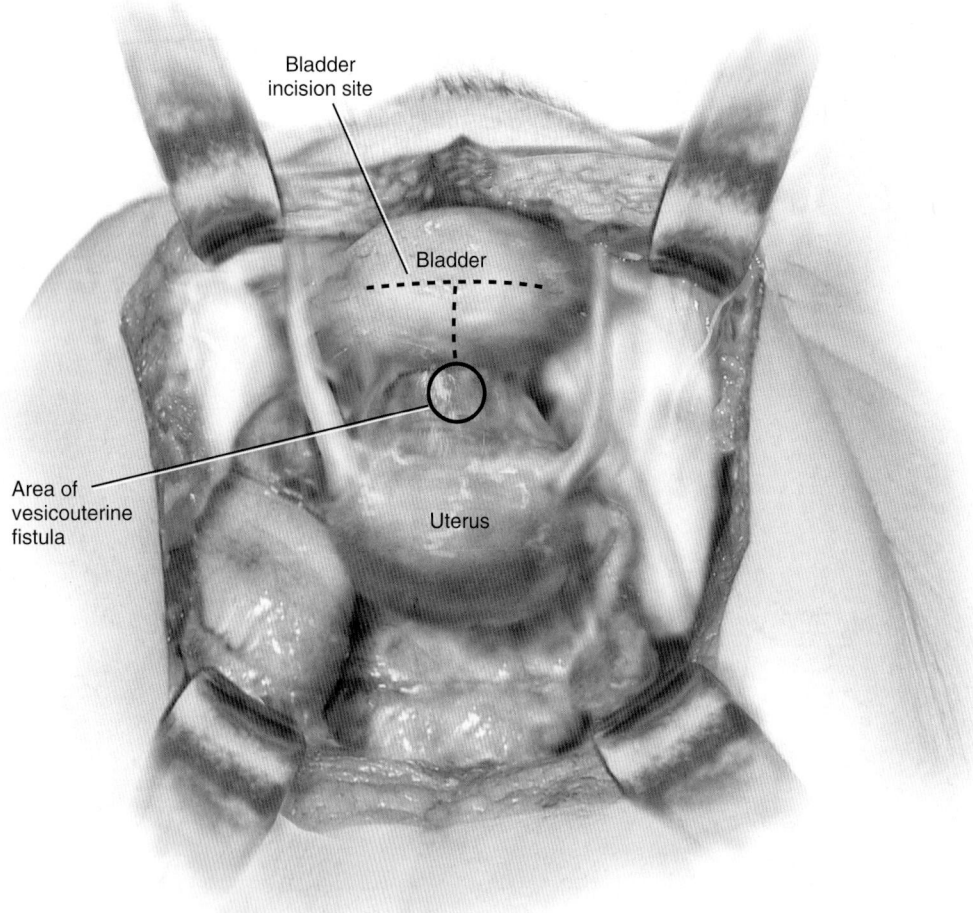

**FIGURE 89–18** Vesicouterine fistula between the lower uterine segment and possibly the upper cervix and the base of the bladder. Dotted line shows the bladder incisions used to expose the fistula.

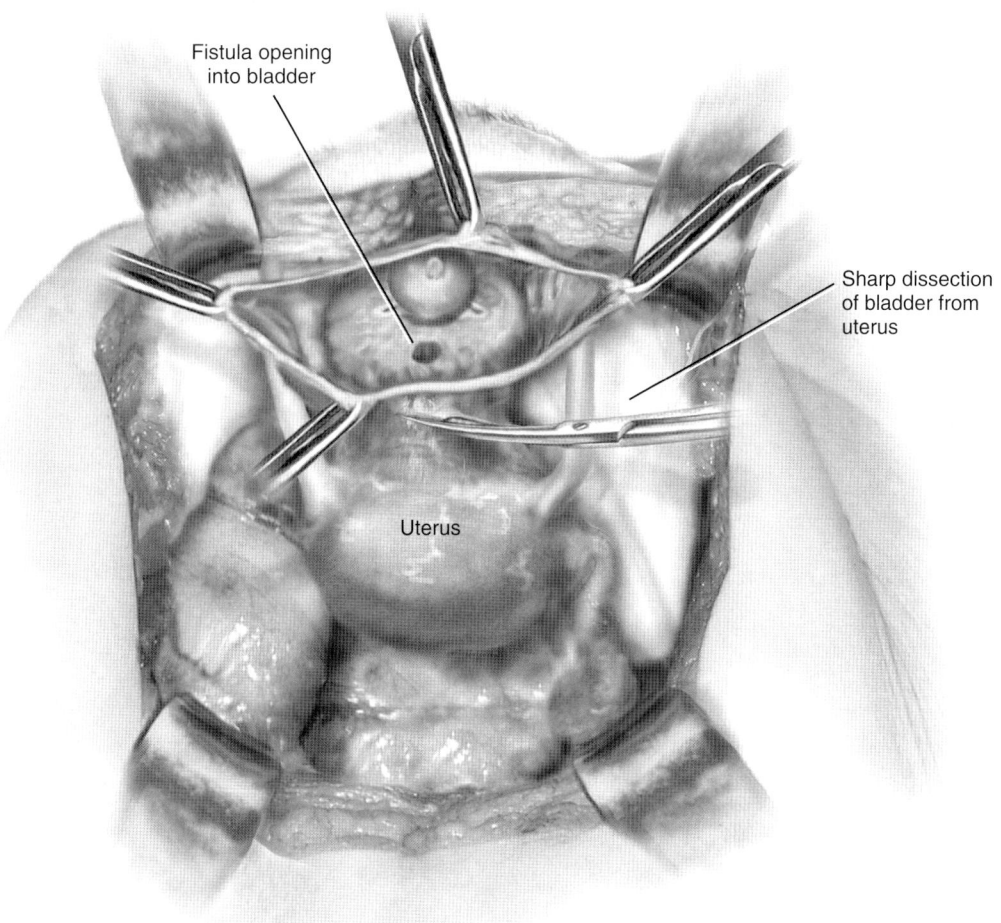

Fistula opening
into bladder

Sharp dissection
of bladder from
uterus

Uterus

**FIGURE 89–19** A high cystotomy has been made and sharp dissection used to separate the bladder from the uterus.

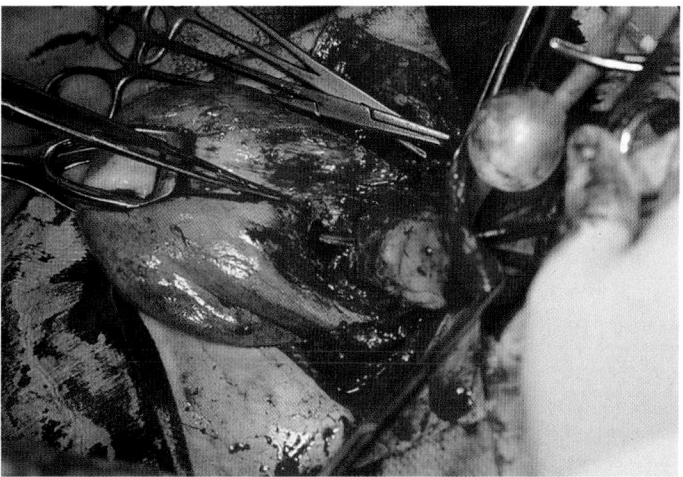

**FIGURE 89–20** Vesicouterine fistula. Note that a high cystotomy has been made and a probe has been placed from the inside of the bladder through the fistulous tract into the uterus.

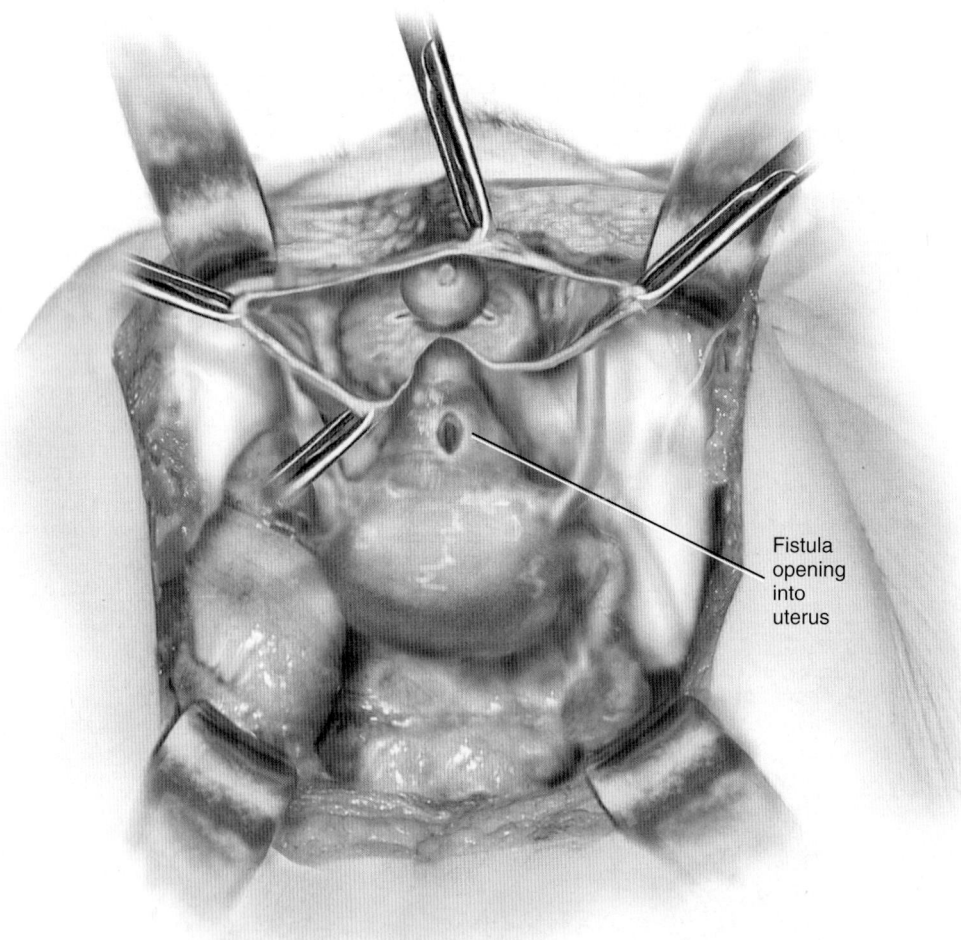

Fistula
opening
into
uterus

**FIGURE 89–21** Sharp dissection has been completed, as there is complete separation of the bladder and the uterus.

Placement of
omental flap

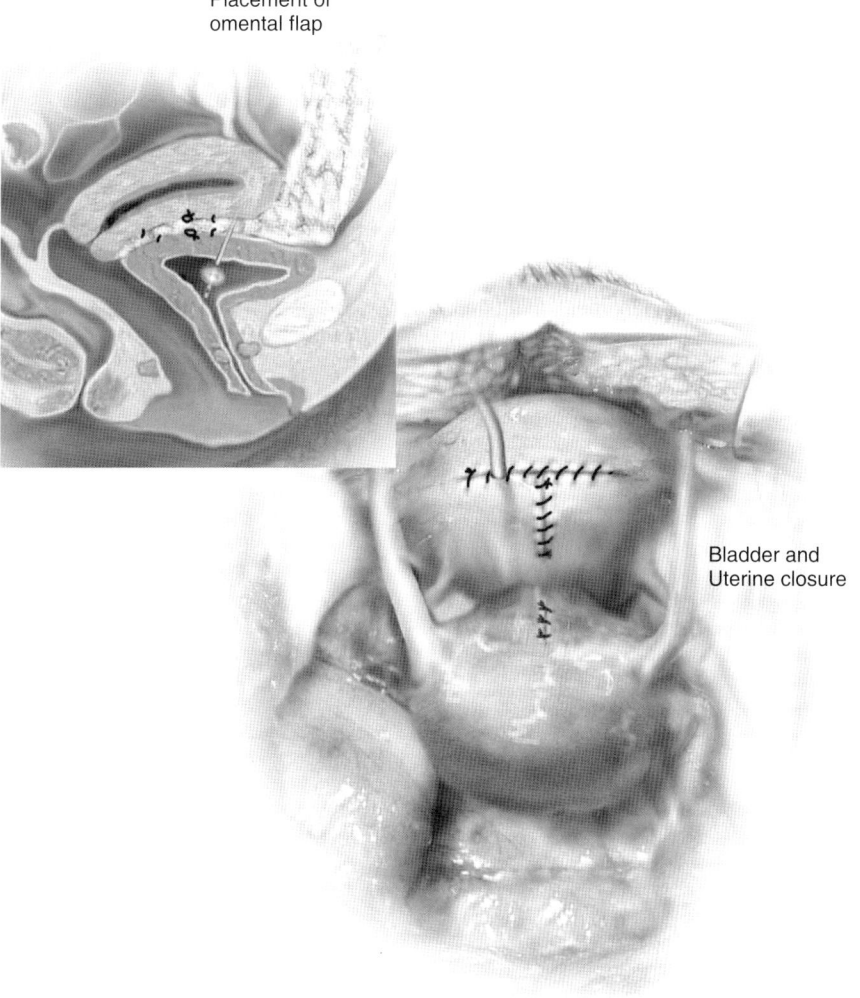

Bladder and
Uterine closure

**FIGURE 89–22**  Both bladder and uterus are closed in two layers. **Inset** shows omental flap interposed between the two structures.

# CHAPTER 90

# Vaginal Repair of Vesicovaginal Fistula

*Mickey M. Karram*

Surgical treatment of benign pelvic conditions causes approximately 90% of vesicovaginal fistulas, with total abdominal hysterectomy being the most common cause. The point at which the fistula first becomes symptomatic is determined to a major degree by its cause, its site of origin, and the method of catheter drainage. Immediate postoperative leakage probably represents an unrecognized perforation or laceration somewhere in the lower urinary tract. Many fistulas occur secondary to trauma, crushing injuries from clamps, or suture penetration into the lower urinary tract, which may result in devascularization, necrosis, and invariably fistulous development between the second and tenth postoperative days.

If a vesicovaginal fistula is diagnosed within 7 days of occurrence, is less than 1 cm in diameter, and is unrelated to malignancy or irradiation, bladder drainage alone for up to 4 weeks allows spontaneous healing in 12% to 80% of cases; however, the outcome is very unpredictable. Cystoscopic cauterization of small lesions may also be successful. Standard management of the vesicovaginal fistula dictates an interval from injury to repair of 3 to 6 months in surgical and obstetric fistulas, and up to 1 year in irradiation-induced fistulas, to ensure complete resolution of necrosis and inflammation. However, recently, some have championed the early closure of small fistulas with good results.

Most vesicovaginal fistulas can be closed transvaginally. Simple vesicovaginal fistulas are usually repaired with the Latzko technique (Fig. 90-1), whereas more complex procedures usually require excision of the tract and a layered closure of the defect (Fig. 90-2). If the fistula encroaches on one or both ureteral orifices (Fig. 90-3), the ureters should be catheterized at the onset of surgery. Intraoperative placement of a pediatric Foley catheter through the fistula and into the bladder helps to evert the fistula edge, thus improving descent and stability for dissection (Fig. 90-4).

The Latzko technique of partial colpocleisis may be used for repair of posthysterectomy vesicovaginal fistulas, with reported cure rates of between 93% and 100% after the first attempt. As a simple procedure, it offers the advantages of a short operating time, minimal blood loss, and low postoperative morbidity. Inadequate vaginal length is not a problem unless the vagina is already shortened. In the Latzko operation, the vaginal mucosa is mobilized around the fistula margin in the shape of an ellipse for at least 2.5 cm in all directions, with closure of the subvaginal tissue and vaginal mucosa in layers using 2-0 or 3-0 interrupted absorbable sutures (see Fig. 90-1). The vaginal wall in contact with the bladder reepithelializes transitional epithelium.

For complicated or larger fistulas, a classic technique is best. This involves circumscribing the vaginal mucosa in the region of the fistula (see Fig. 90-2A). Sufficient vaginal mucosa is separated from the underlying pubocervical fascia to permit a tension-free closure of the tissues. This usually requires a fair amount of mobilization of the vagina (Figs. 90-5 and 90-6). Traction is applied to the scar tissue of the fistula, and countertraction is placed on the edges of the vaginal mucosa to facilitate accurate undermining of the vagina. The subvaginal plane is dissected in all directions. At times, entering the peritoneum facilitates mobilization of the fistulous tract (see Fig. 90-6B). If the fistulous tract is small, it can be completely excised. If large and fibrotic, the edges should be freshened (see Fig. 90-5A). Overexcision of fistulous edges may enlarge the defect and increase the risk of hemorrhage from the bladder edges postoperatively. This can cause catheter blockage, bladder distention, and failure of the repair. If mobilization proves difficult, regular circumferential vaginal incisions made at a distance from the fistula may facilitate mobilization and low-tension closure. Once hemostasis is achieved, these incisions are left open to heal. Once the tract has been excised or the edges of the fistula have been converted to a fresh injury with healthy tissue and a healthy blood supply, a layered closure is performed (see Fig. 90-2). The first layer involves interrupted 4-0 delayed absorbable sutures placed in an extramucosal fashion extending lateral to the fistulous opening. All sutures are placed and then individually tied. The initial suture line is then inverted, and a second suture line of similar sutures is placed through the muscular portion of the wall of the bladder. This row of sutures will imbricate the first layer of sutures (see Fig. 90-2). The author prefers to test the integrity of the repair at this time by instilling methylene blue or sterile milk into the bladder. Care should be taken to avoid overdistention. This ensures that the entire fistula has been identified and approximated appropriately. An attempt is then made to place a third layer of pubocervical fascia over the fistulous closure. This is placed with interrupted 3-0 delayed absorbable sutures. At times, if the peritoneum has been entered, a J-flap of omentum or a peritoneal flap can be interposed between the repaired fistula and the vagina (see Fig. 90-5C). The vaginal epithelium is closed with delayed absorbable 2-0 sutures (see Fig. 90-2). A vaginal packing is usually inserted for 24 hours postoperatively, and the bladder is drained for 1 to 2 weeks. The author considers the transurethral Foley catheter the most efficient method of drainage.

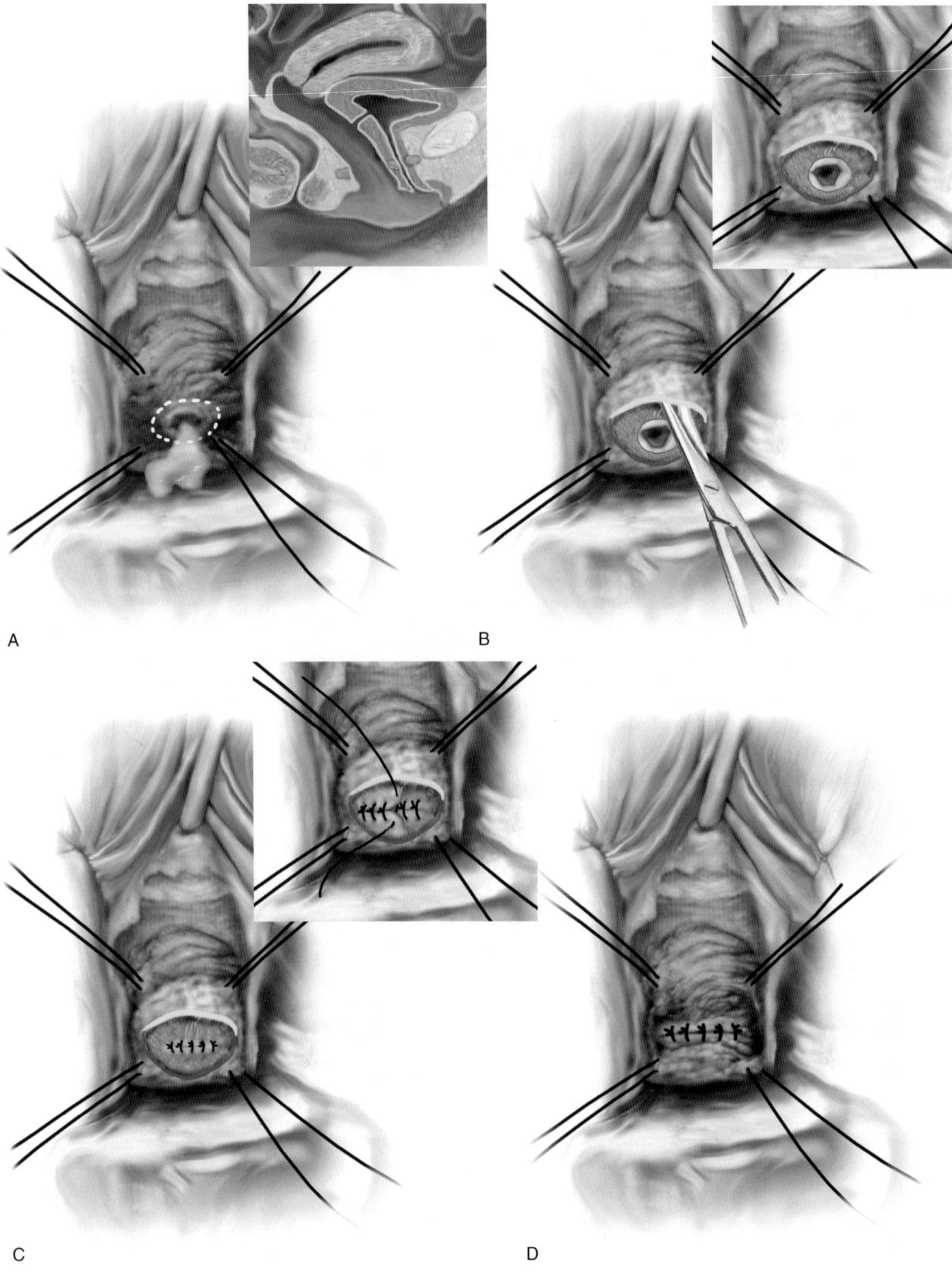

A

B

C

D

**FIGURE 90–1** The Latzko technique of partial colpocleisis. **A.** Stay sutures are placed in the vaginal wall to assist in exposing the fistula. An initial circumferential incision is made around the fistulous tract (*dashed white line*). **B.** Sharp dissection mobilizes the vaginal mucosa for a distance of 2.5 cm in all directions. **C.** The vaginal edges are then approximated with delayed absorbable sutures. Note that no attempt is made to excise the fistulous tract or freshen the edges of the fistula. If possible, a second layer of pubocervical fascia is approximated over the initial layer. **D.** The vaginal mucosa is closed, thus completing the repair.

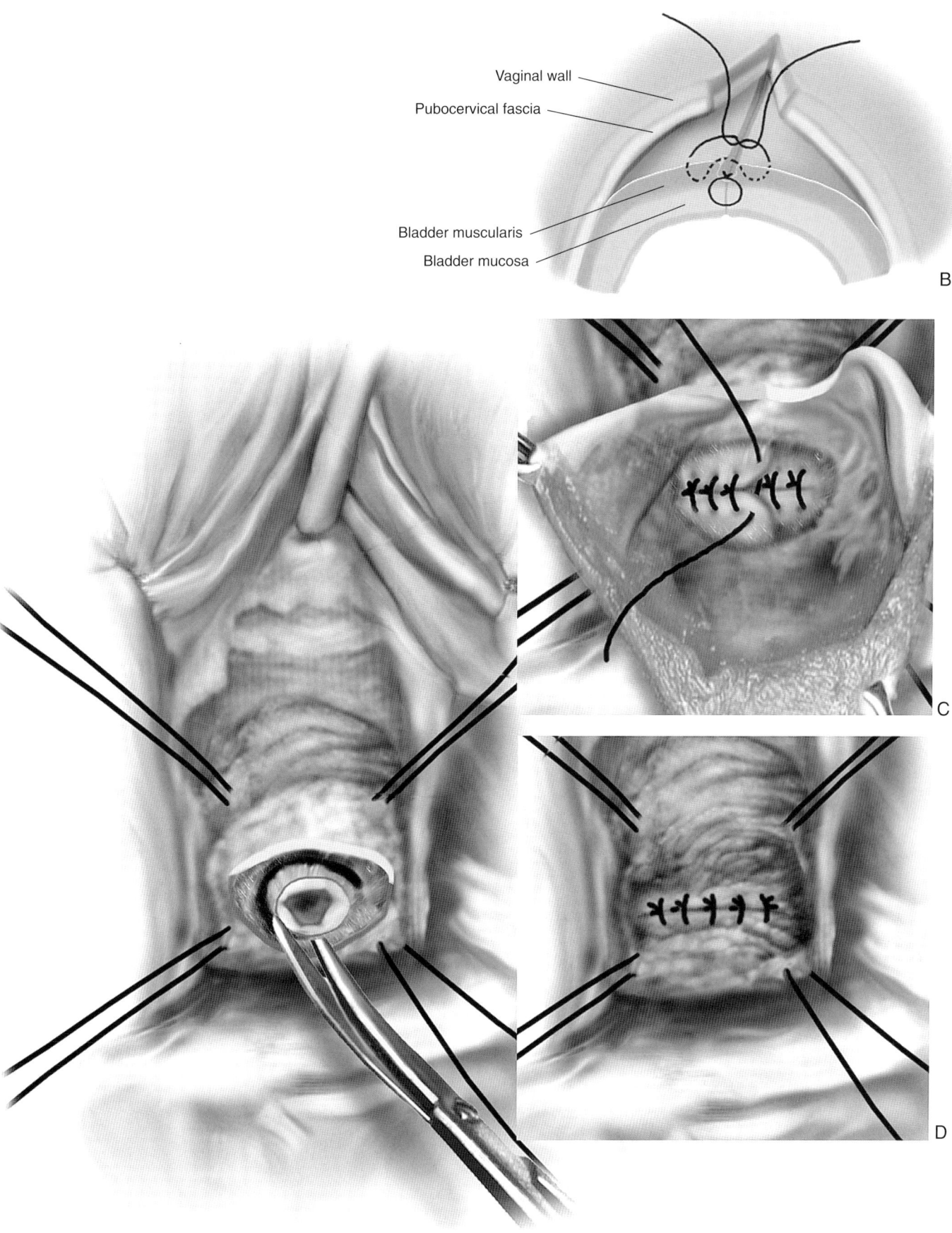

Vaginal wall

Pubocervical fascia

Bladder muscularis

Bladder mucosa

B

C

D

A

**FIGURE 90–2** The classic method of vaginal repair of a vesicovaginal fistula. **A.** Stay sutures are placed to help expose the fistula. After an initial circumferential incision is made around the fistula, the fistulous tract is excised completely (smaller fistulas) or the scarred edges are cut back until fresh vascular tissue is identified (larger fistulas). **B.** The vaginal mucosa is widely mobilized in all directions, and the fistula is closed in layers. The initial layer involves placement of 4-0 delayed absorbable sutures in the extramucosal portion of the bladder edge. The second layer is placed through the muscular portion of the bladder wall, imbricating the first layer. **C.** A third layer approximates the pubocervical fascia over the bladder closure. **D.** The repair is completed by closure of the vaginal epithelium.

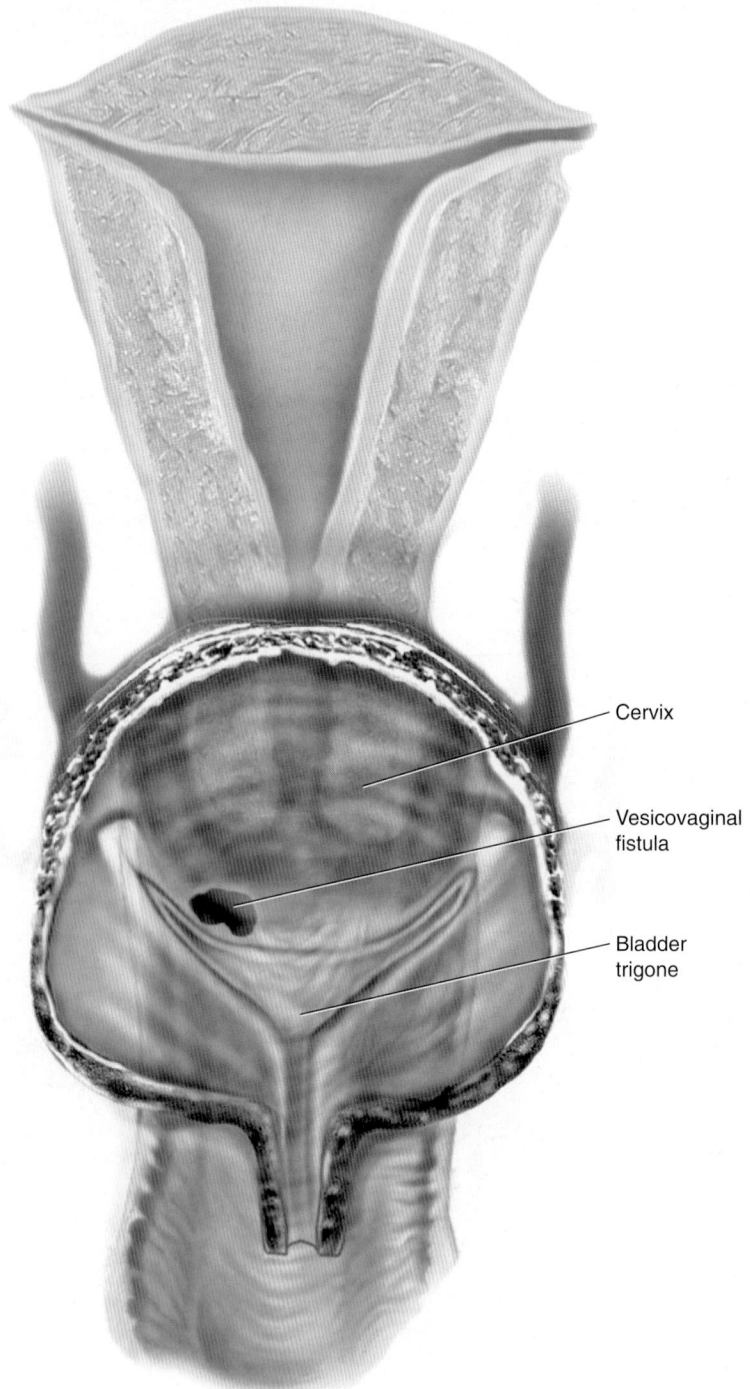

Cervix

Vesicovaginal
fistula

Bladder
trigone

Frontal view

**FIGURE 90–3** Intravesical view of a vesicovaginal fistula. Note that the
fistula extends very close to the opening of the right ureter.

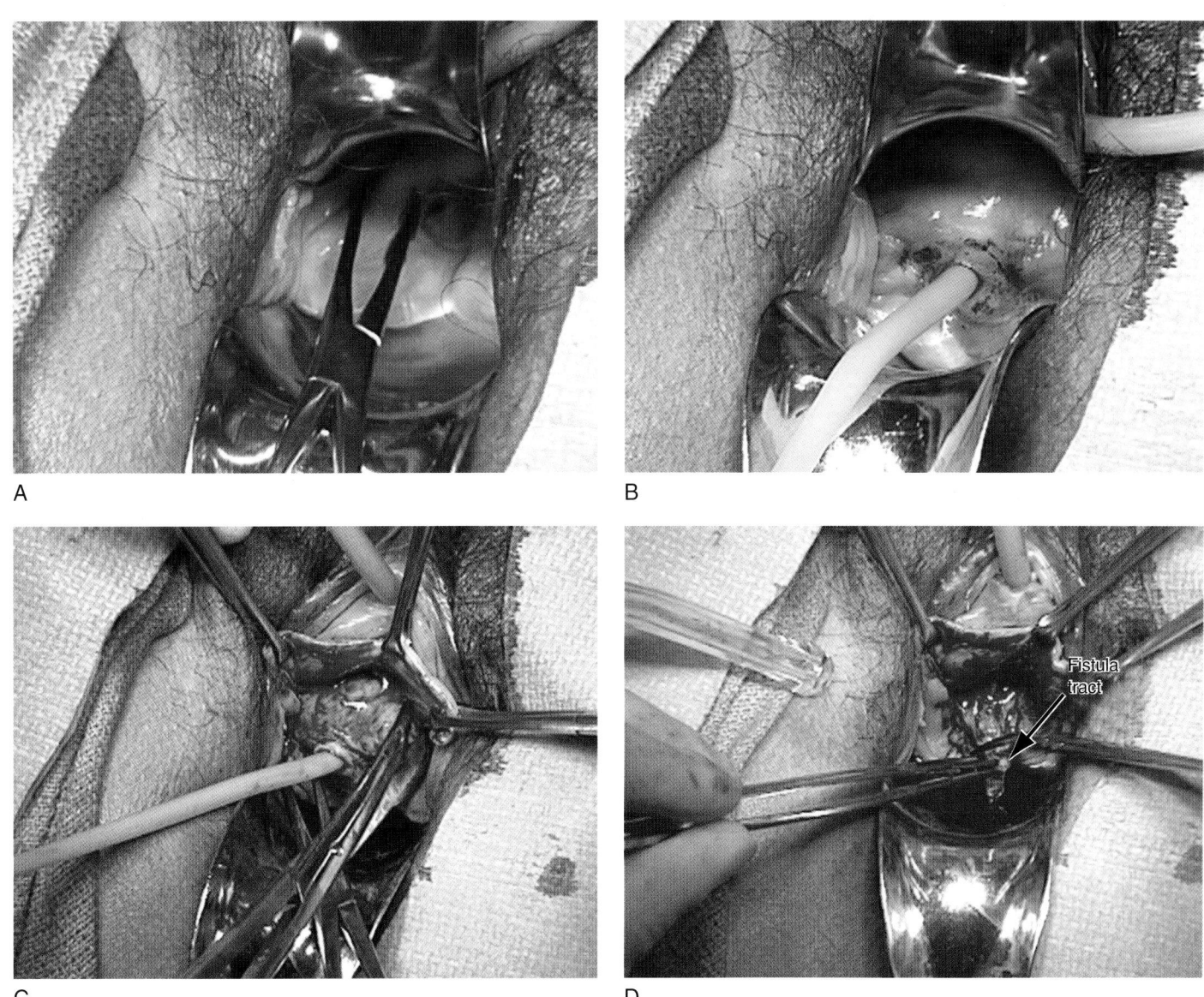

**FIGURE 90–4** Vaginal repair of a vesicovaginal fistula. **A.** The fistula is seen at the level of the vaginal cuff. **B.** A pediatric Foley catheter has been placed in the fistula to facilitate the dissection of the vagina away from the underlying bladder. **C.** Sharp dissection is used to completely mobilize the fistulous tract from the anterior vaginal wall. **D.** The fistulous tract is being excised in preparation for a layered closure of the defect in the bladder.

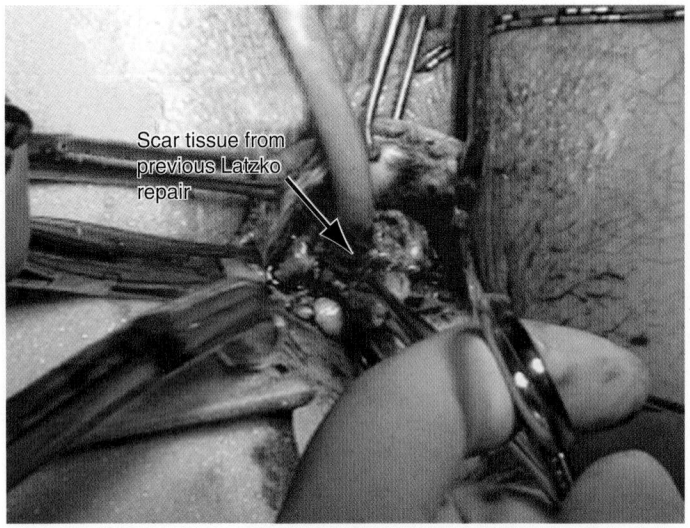

A

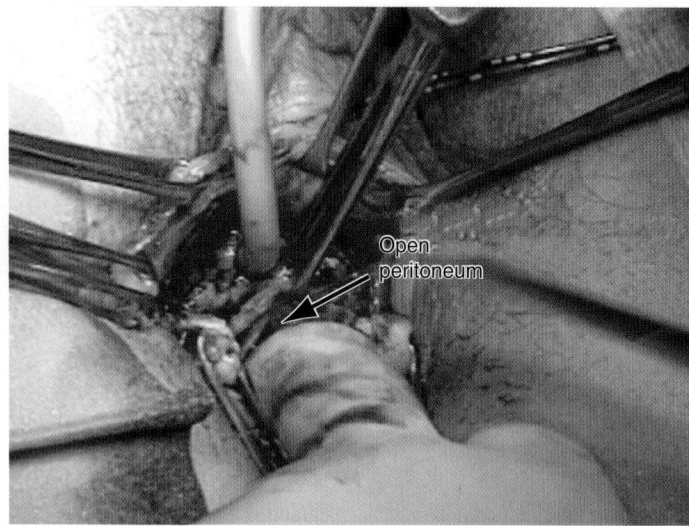

B

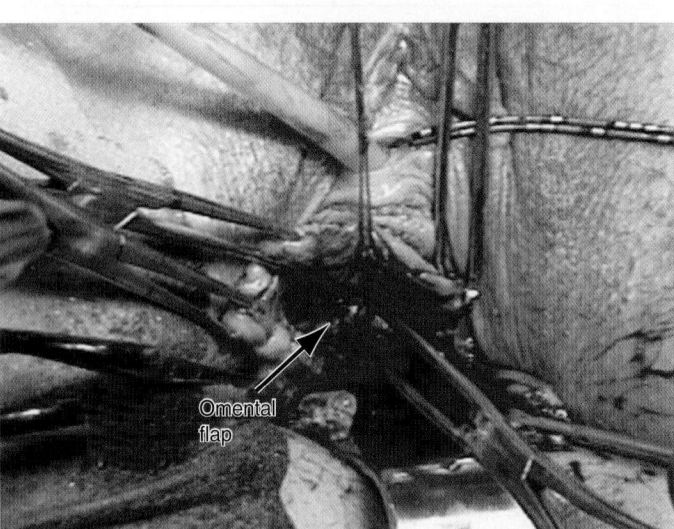

C

**FIGURE 90–5** Vaginal repair of a previously failed Latzko procedure. **A.** The scar tissue from the previous Latzko repair is grasped in preparation for excision. **B.** During dissection of the vagina off the anterior wall of the bladder, the peritoneum is entered, which will facilitate mobilization of the fistulous tract. **C.** The fistulous tract has been excised and closed in two layers. A J-flap of omentum is brought from the intraperitoneal area and interposed between the bladder and the vagina.

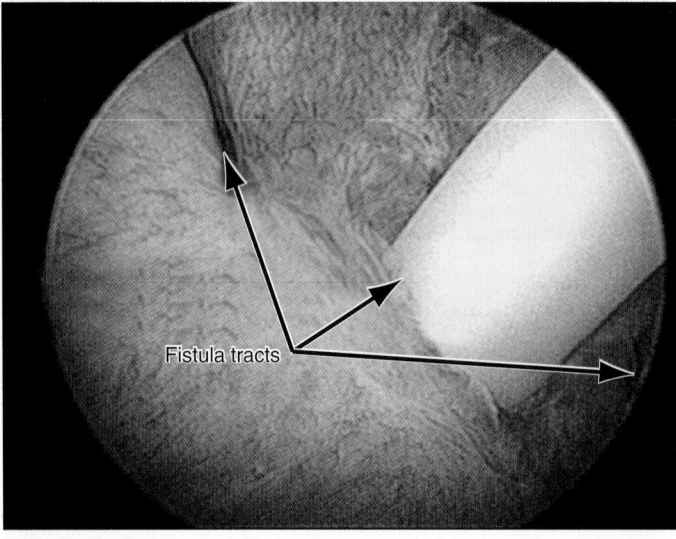

A

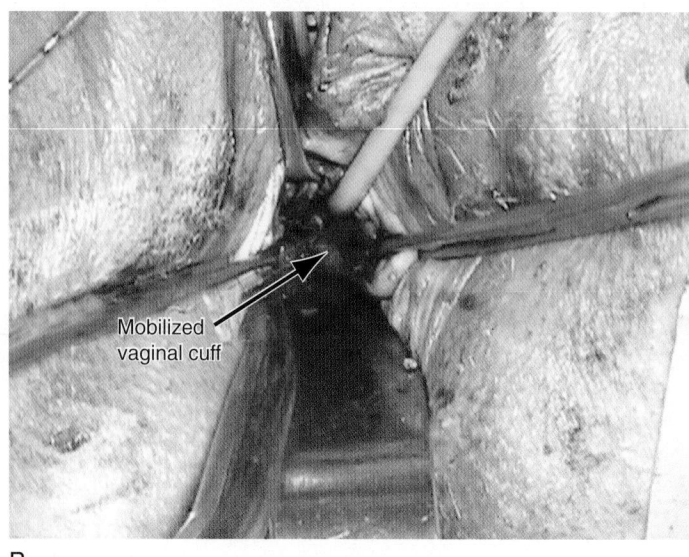

B

**FIGURE 90–6** Multiple vesicovaginal fistulas. **A.** An intravesical view of three separate and distinct fistulous tracts. **B.** A Foley catheter has been placed in the largest fistulous tract. Sharp dissection is utilized to completely mobilize the fistulous tract, and the peritoneum is entered at the level of the vaginal cuff.

# CHAPTER 91

# Managing Ureteral Injury During Pelvic Surgery

*Michael Maggio* ▪ *Emanuel C. Trabuco* ▪ *John B. Gebhart*

Injury to the lower urinary tract will occur in approximately 1% to 2% of women undergoing major gynecologic surgery. Although the risk of injury increases with increasing difficulty of the primary operation (e.g., large uterus, excessive bleeding, prolapse procedures, malignancy, endometriosis), more than 50% of injuries occur during uncomplicated procedures. Furthermore, in the absence of cystoscopy, most injuries are undetected during the primary operation, leading to increased morbidity and costs associated with diagnostic procedures, prolonged hospital stay, reoperations, return visits, and delay in diagnosis (e.g., ileus, urosepsis, fistula formation). The incidence of ureteral injury following gynecologic surgery ranges from 0.2% to 11.0%, depending on the type of study (historical vs. prospective) and the definition of injury (kinking from suspension vs. transaction/crush injury). Intraoperative techniques to avoid ureteral injury and the ability to ensure ureteral patency at the time of surgery should be in the realm of every gynecologic surgeon. During vaginal or laparoscopic surgery, cystoscopy after the administration of indigo carmine can be utilized to visualize the spill of blue dye from the ureteral orifices (see section on cystoscopy). During open abdominal surgery, advertent cystotomy with visualization of the ureteral orifices is an option that will avoid repositioning of the patient required for cystoscopy (see Chapter 88). Ureteral catheters can be placed at the time of cystoscopy to help avoid ureteral injury in selected cases (Figs. 91-1 and 91-2). Ureteral anatomy can be variable depending on the anatomy of the patient, as well as the anatomic distortion that can occur when the pelvic abnormality is addressed. Also, overzealous or inappropriate use of an energy source can result in ureteral injury (Figs. 91-3 through 91-5). The surgical procedure utilized to address an intraoperative or postoperative ureteral injury depends on the extent and location of the injury.

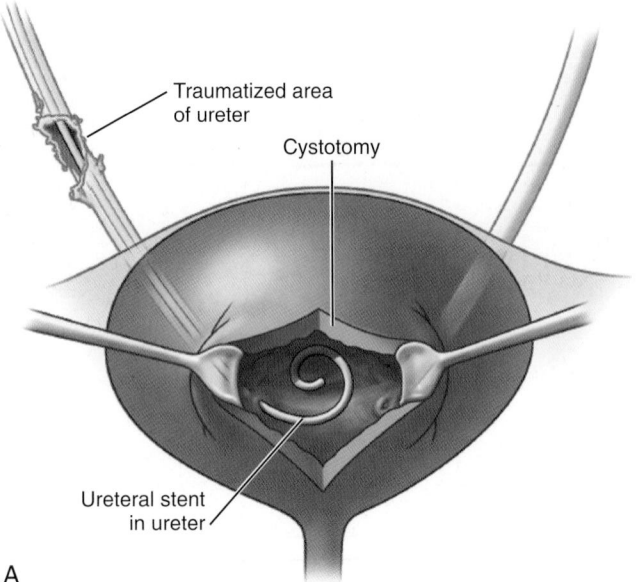

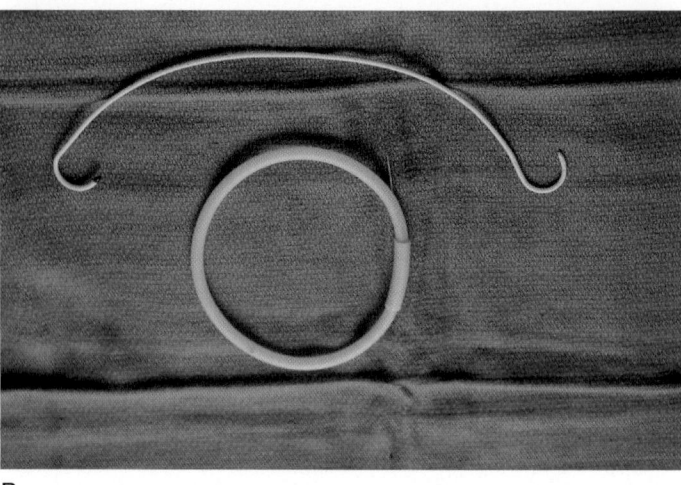

A

B

**FIGURE 91–1 A.** Schematic representation of a distal right ureteral serosal injury. Injuries of this type can be handled by retrograde stenting of the affected ureter via bladder dome cystotomy. **B.** 6 French × 26-cm double J stent and wire. The wire is used to make the stent rigid during placement.

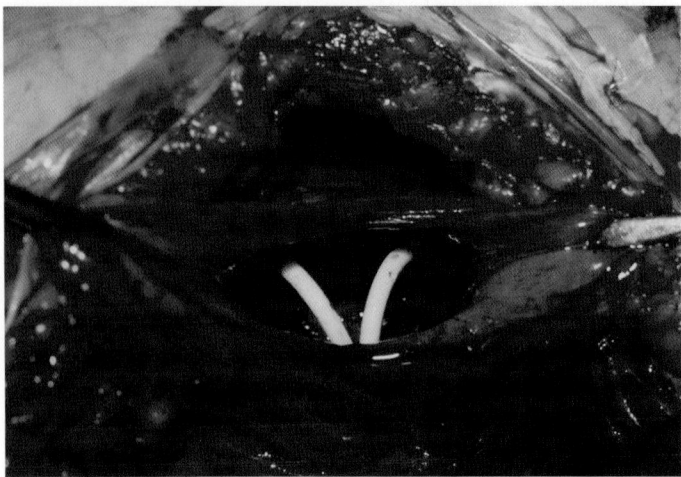

**FIGURE 91–2** Photograph of bladder dome cystotomy with two retrograde placed double J ureteral stents.

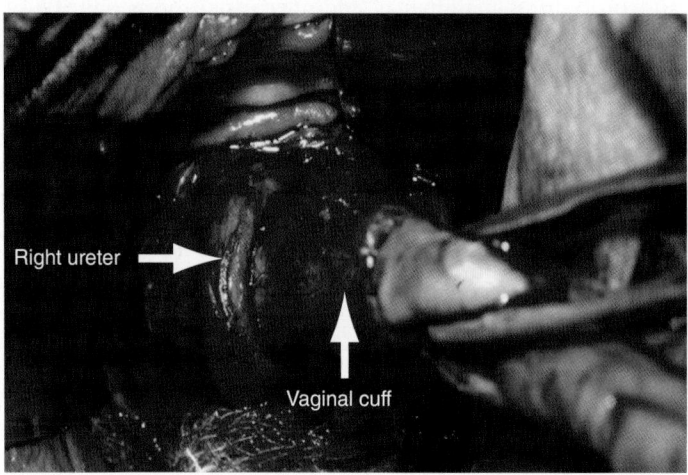

**FIGURE 91–3** Photograph of the right distal ureter entering the bladder (*left arrow*). The photo illustrates the close proximity of the ureter to the vaginal cuff during a posthysterectomy vault prolapse repair. Failure to identify the ureter before securing the uterosacral and cardinal remnant pedicles (*right arrow*) would have led to injury.

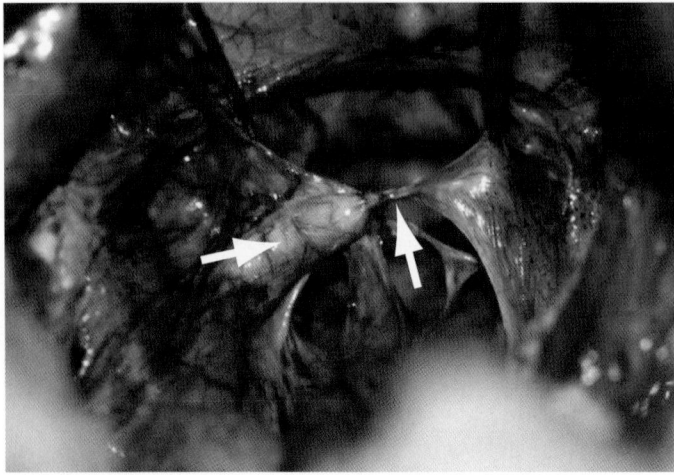

**FIGURE 91–4** Photograph of left ureteral obstruction following uterosacral vault suspension. Note the dilated proximal ureter (*left arrow*) and the offending suture (*right arrow*).

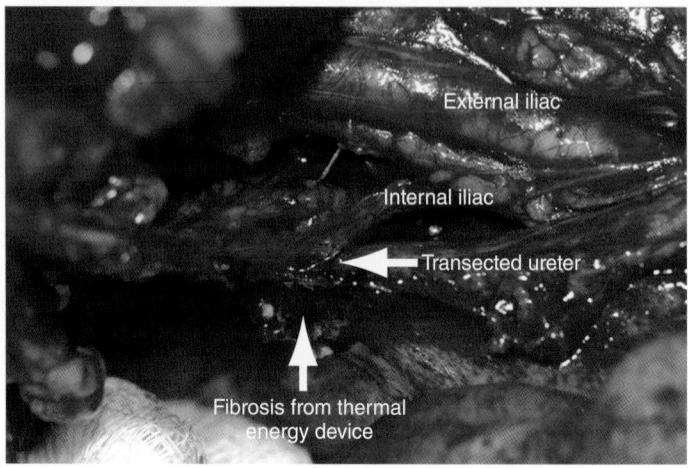

**FIGURE 91–5** Photograph of a transected ureter due to inaccurate placement of a thermal energy device at the time of radical hysterectomy.

## Ureterotomy and Catheterization

Excessive fibrosis or anatomic distortion of the ureter at times can be encountered intraoperatively. In these situations, it may be beneficial to perform a ureterotomy and pass a stent antegrade into the bladder or retrograde into the kidney. The procedure is performed as follows. Dissection of the ureter should be minimized to prevent ischemic injury by interrupting the blood supply to the ureter and the periureteral tissue. Stay sutures can be placed laterally before the incision is made, and a hook blade can be used for the ureterotomy. The authors prefer a longitudinal incision. The ureter then can be catheterized to ensure patency or determine the level of obstruction, or even to assist in dissection lower down near the bladder. Closure is accomplished with interrupted 4-0 or 5-0 absorbable sutures. Closure should include only the adventitia and superficial incorporation of the ureteral musculature. A double J stent is placed before closure, and a drain is left in place and removed after drainage subsides (Fig. 91–6).

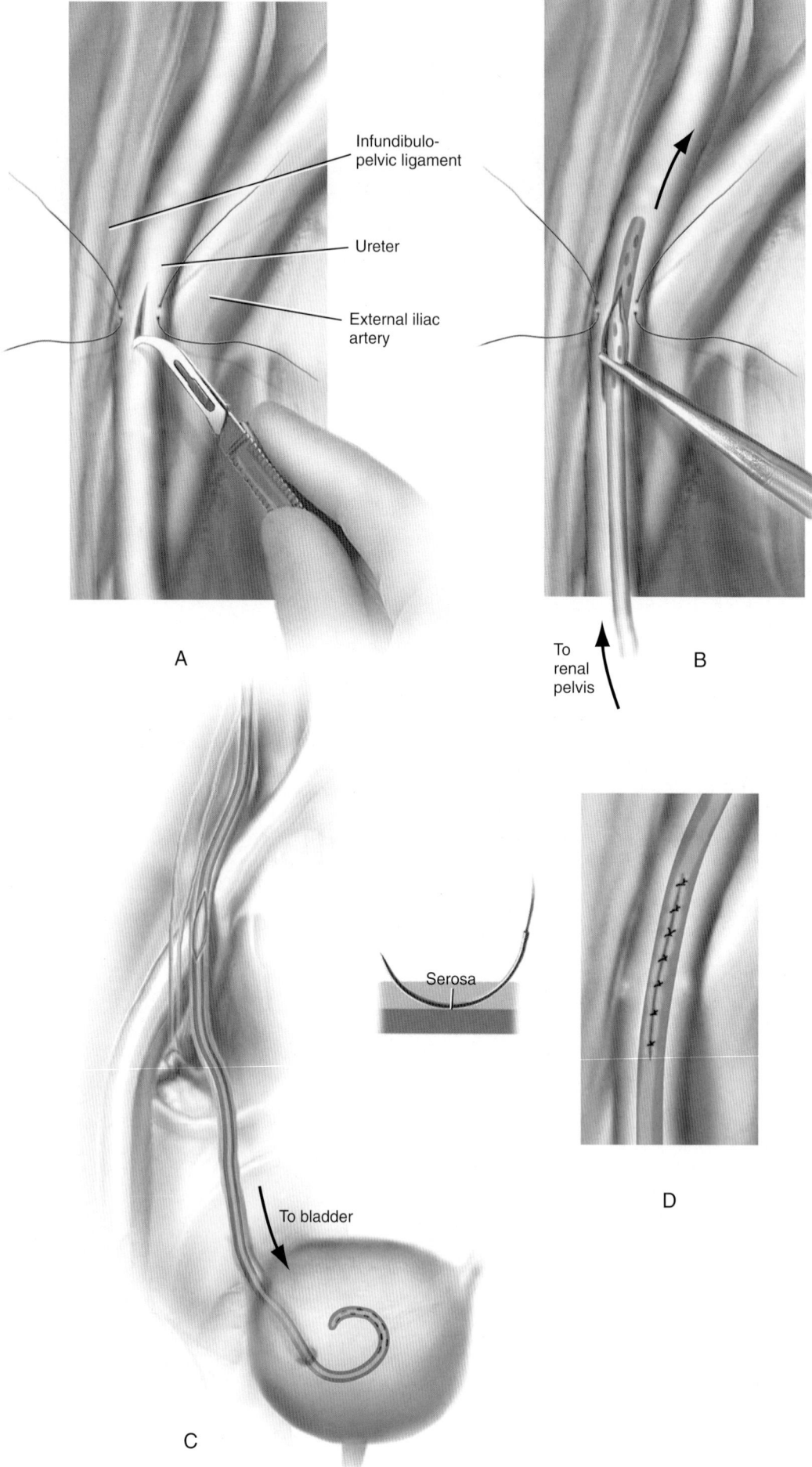

**FIGURE 91–6** Technique of ureterotomy. **A.** Stay sutures are placed laterally to facilitate traction on the ureter. A hook blade is used to make a longitudinal incision in the ureter. **B.** A double J stent is passed antegrade into the kidney and (**C**) retrograde into the bladder. **D.** Ureterotomy is closed with interrupted 4-0 or 5-0 absorbable sutures. Closure should include only the adventitia and a superficial incorporation of the ureteral musculature.

## Ureteroureterostomy

An end-to-end anastomosis of a lacerated or partially transected ureter is usually indicated when the lesion or injury is located above where the ureter crosses the iliac vessels. Most injuries below this area are best treated by ureteral implantation (see description of ureteroneocystostomy). Ureteral damage should not be viewed as an isolated anatomic problem. The danger of infection in the retroperitoneum, urinary extravasation, or the development of lymphoceles and possible damage from ureteral denudation and disturbance of the ureter's blood supply all must be appreciated. To perform an end-to-end anastomosis, the ureter should be mobilized to ensure a tension-free anastomosis, and damaged tissue needs to be resected. Both proximal and distal margins of the transected ureter are spatulated, and an end-to-end anastomosis is accomplished with interrupted sutures (Figs. 91-7 and 91-8). A double J stent is placed before the anastomosis is completed and is removed approximately 4 to 6 weeks after the repair. Periureteral drainage is accomplished with a Jackson-Pratt or a Penrose drain exiting from a separate stab wound in the skin.

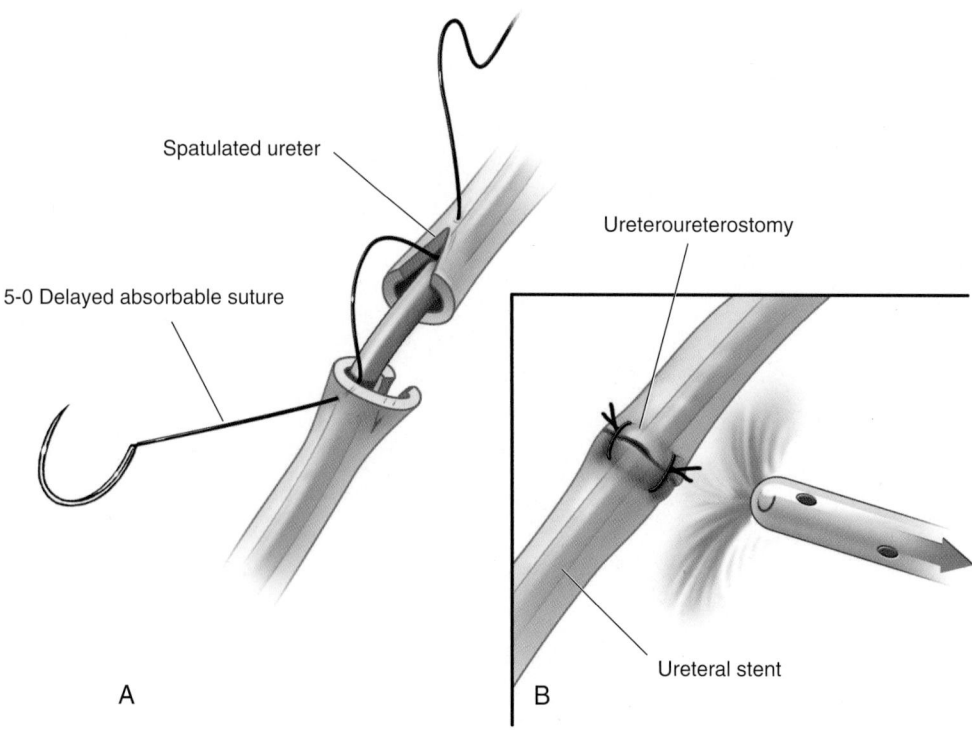

Spatulated ureter

5-0 Delayed absorbable suture

Ureteroureterostomy

Ureteral stent

A

B

**FIGURE 91–7** Schematic of abdominal ureteroureterostomy. **A.** Spatulation performed before anastomosis to increase surface area at the anastomosis. **B.** Completed anastomosis with protecting drain.

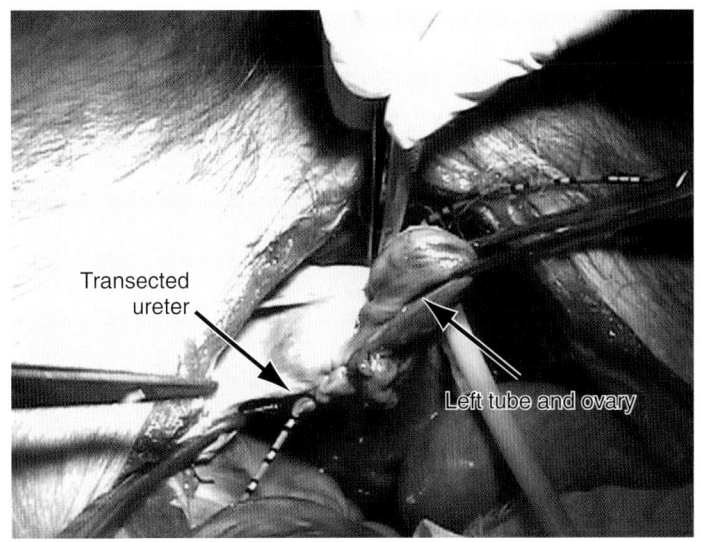

Transected ureter

Left tube and ovary

A

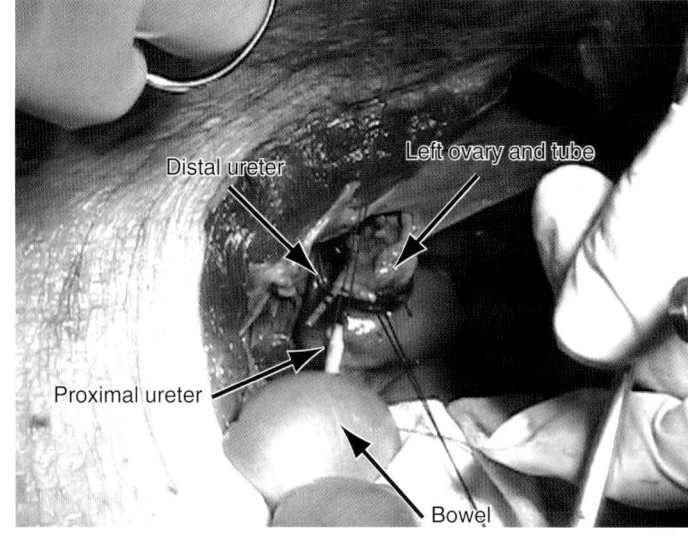

Distal ureter

Left ovary and tube

Proximal ureter

Bowel

B

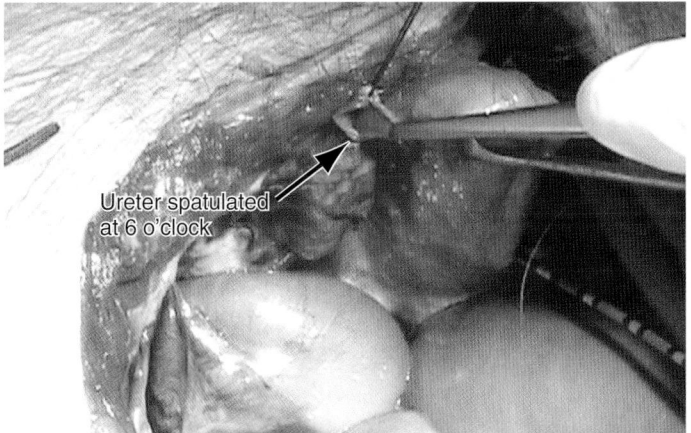

Ureter spatulated at 6 o'clock

C

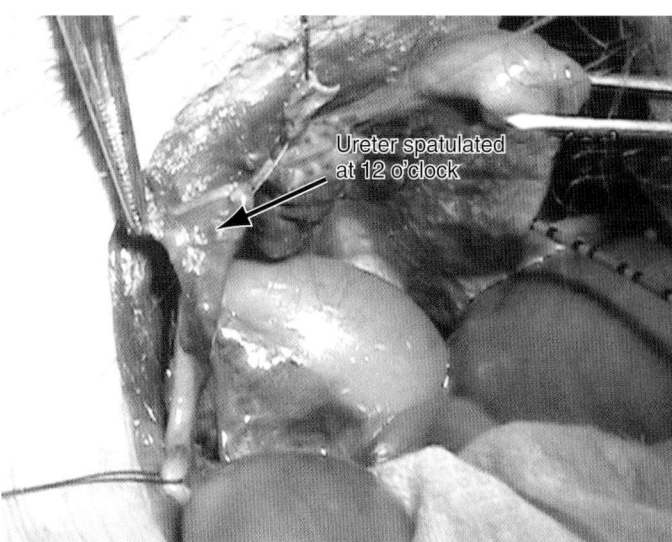

Ureter spatulated at 12 o'clock

D

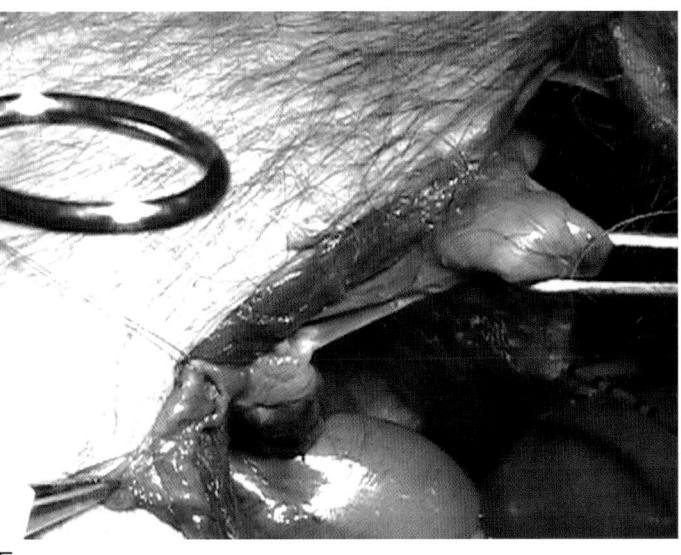

E

UNIT 4 ■ SECTION A

**FIGURE 91-8** Cadaveric dissection demonstrates the technique of ureteroureterostomy. **A.** Note the ureter has been transected and a ureteral stent has been passed through the transected distal end of the ureter. **B.** The proximal end of the ureter has been completely mobilized; note that the two ends of the ureter easily come together with minimal to no tension. **C.** In preparation for the end-to-end reanastomosis, the distal end of the ureter has been spatulated at 6 o'clock. **D.** The proximal end of the ureter has been spatulated at 12 o'clock. **E.** Reanastomosis of the ureters is shown here. The sutures are passed as demonstrated in Figs. 91–7). Fine absorbable sutures are used for the reanastomosis and are taken at right angles to each cut end and passed into the angle of the spatulated incisions on the opposing ureteral cut end. The suture at 6 o'clock has been passed and tied.

## Ureteroneocystostomy

Distal ureteral injuries requiring reimplantation can be approached with a combined intravesical and extravesical repair. The main goals of any reimplantation are to ensure a tension-free anastomosis and to create an adequate submucosal tunnel to maintain the antireflux mechanism. The bladder is approached retroperitoneally (Fig. 91–9), and a midline cystotomy is made. Stay sutures are placed lateral to the midline cystotomy in the region of the dome for cephalad traction. Lateral and caudal traction of the bladder exposes the trigonal area (Fig. 91–10). The ureter is mobilized as far down as possible (Fig. 91–11). The ureter is then transected in preparation for reimplantation (Fig. 91–12). Once adequate ureteral length is ensured, a site is identified for the new location of the ureteral orifice, preferably near the trigone. A submucosal tunnel is created utilizing a right-angle clamp or tenotomy scissors for an approximate length of 15 to 20 mm (Fig. 91–13). The transected ureter is then brought through the bladder wall musculature and under the submucosal tunnel (Fig. 91–14). It is sutured circumferentially at the site of the neoureteral orifice (Figs. 91–15 and 91–16). The first stitch placed at the 6-o'clock position should be a full-thickness stitch incorporating bladder muscularis and mucosa with the ureteral wall. The remaining circumferential stitches are placed from the ureteral cuff to the bladder mucosa (see Fig. 91–16). The anastomosis can be accomplished with interrupted 4-0 or 5-0 absorbable sutures. A double J stent is then placed across the anastomosis before the bladder is closed and is left in place for 4 to 6 weeks (Fig. 91–17). Fig. 91–18 reviews the entire technique of ureteroneocystostomy.

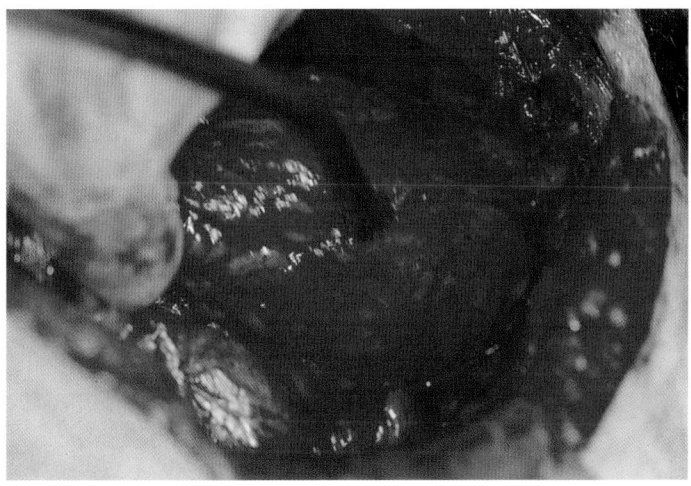

FIGURE 91–9 The bladder has been mobilized away from the pubic bone in preparation for cystotomy.

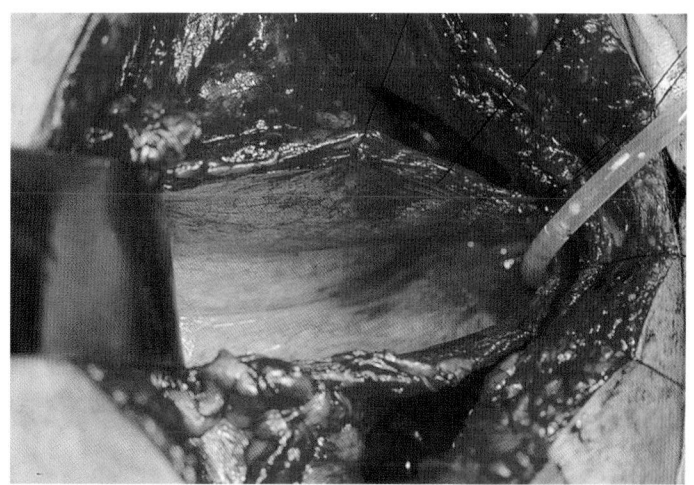

FIGURE 91–10 A high cystotomy has been made, and the trigone is exposed.

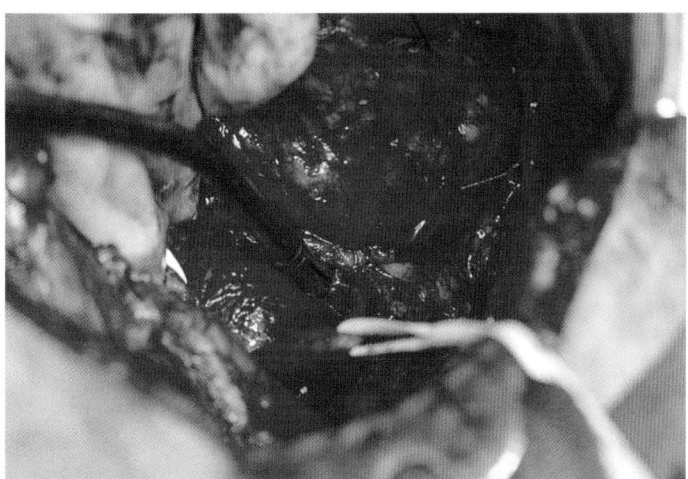

FIGURE 91–11 Umbilical tape is placed around the lower portion of right ureter to assist in mobilization.

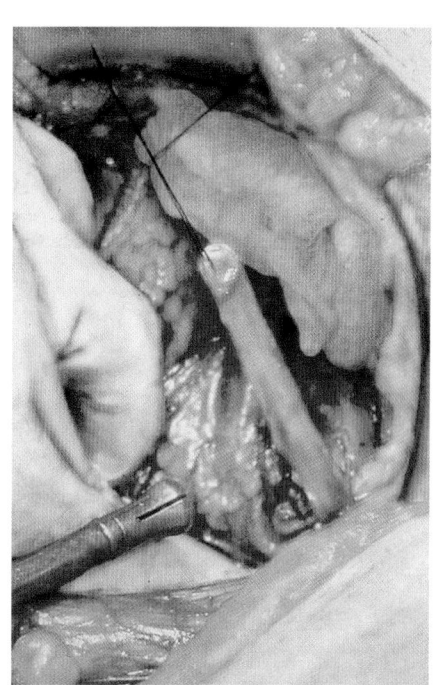

FIGURE 91–12 The ureter has been transected in preparation for reimplantation.

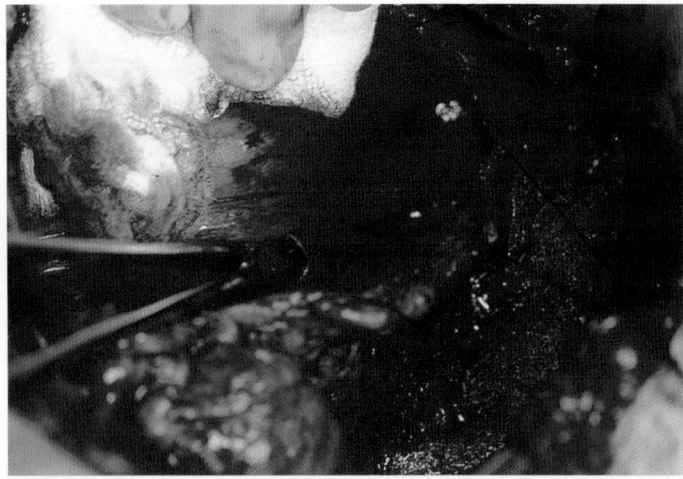

**FIGURE 91–13** A submucosal tunnel is created for a distance of 15 to 20 mm.

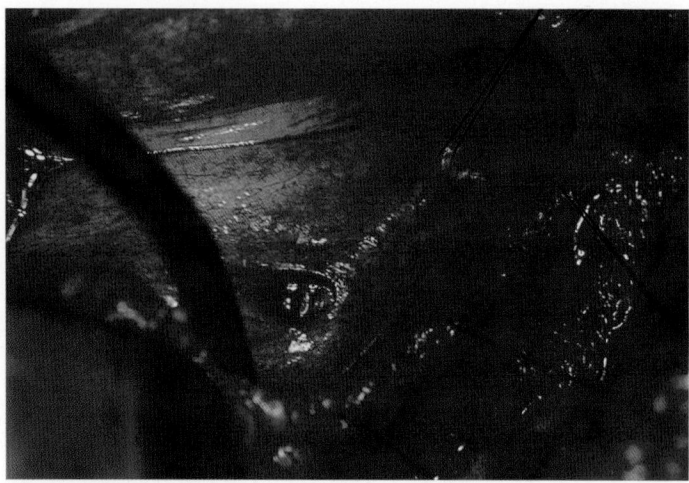

**FIGURE 91–14** The transected ureter is brought through the bladder wall musculature and under the submucosal tunnel.

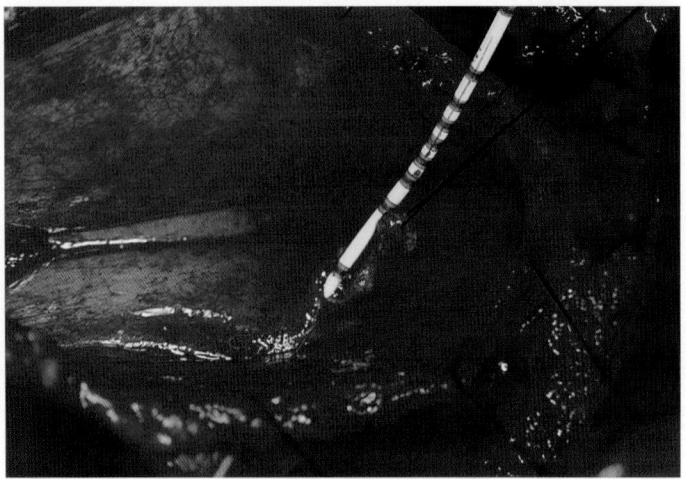

**FIGURE 91–15** A ureteral stent is placed to facilitate suturing of the ureter into the bladder.

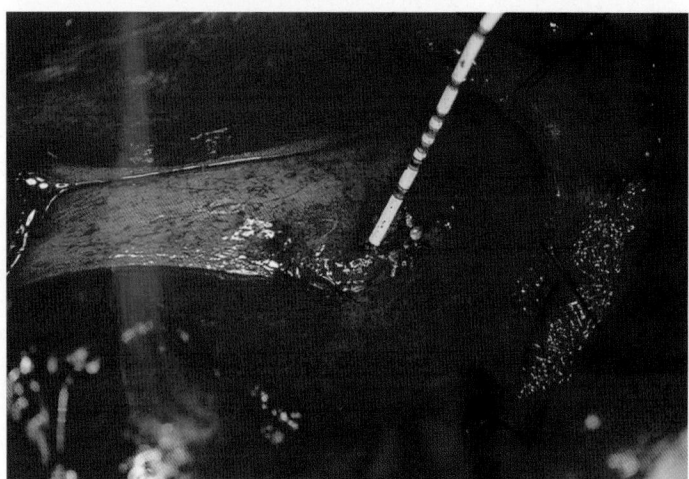

**FIGURE 91–16** The ureter has been circumferentially sutured into the bladder using 4-0 or 5-0 absorbable sutures.

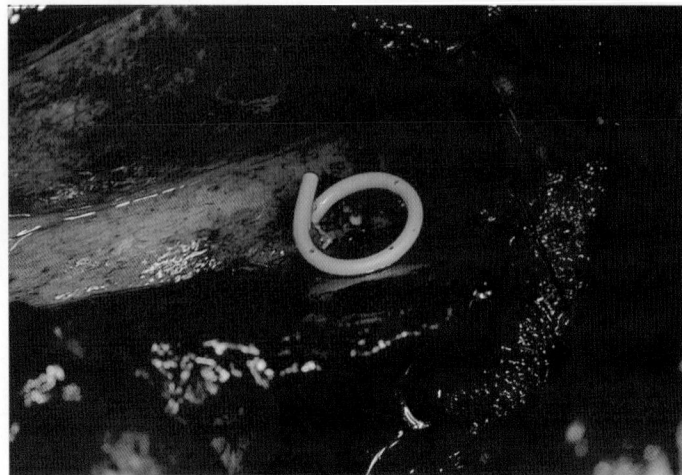

**FIGURE 91–17** A double J stent is placed across the anastomosis before the bladder is closed.

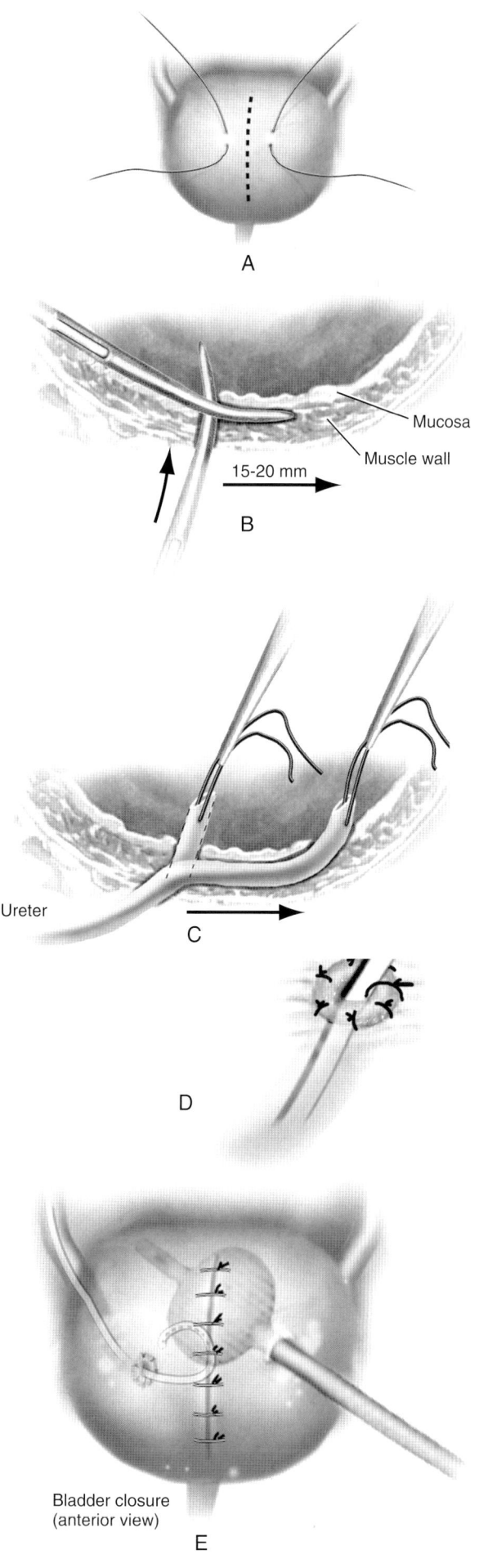

A

B

Mucosa

Muscle wall

15-20 mm

Ureter

C

D

Bladder closure
(anterior view)

E

**FIGURE 91–18** Technique of ureteroneocystostomy. **A.** Stay sutures are placed, and a high cystotomy is made. **B.** A submucosal tunnel is created. **C.** The ureter is passed through the tunnel. **D.** The ureter is fixed to the bladder with 4-0 or 5-0 interrupted, absorbable sutures. **E.** A double J stent is placed, and the bladder is closed.

## Ureteroneocystostomy With Bladder Extension

A psoas hitch is a relatively easy technique utilized to gain length for a successful ureteroneocystostomy (Fig. 91–19). The technique is based on the fact that distortion of the bladder does not usually interfere with function and gains the surgeon between 3 and 5 cm of additional length. Relative contraindications to this procedure are a contracted scarred bladder and previous pelvic surgery in which the blood supply to the bladder has been compromised. The anterior parietal peritoneum from the lower abdominal wall is incised, and the bladder is displaced posteriorly off the symphysis pubis. If additional length is needed, the parietal peritoneum can be divided laterally above the bladder. This approach thus completely mobilizes one entire side of the bladder. Through an anterior and vertical incision in the bladder, a finger can be placed into the dome of the bladder to elevate the bladder to the anterior surface of the ipsilateral iliopsoas muscle. Superior and middle vesical arteries can be ligated on the contralateral side to gain additional mobility of the bladder. The ureter can be reimplanted into the dome of the bladder, creating an antirefluxing submucosal tunnel. In older patients, in whom reflux may not be as much of a concern, a direct anastomosis to the dome can be performed. It is extremely important that the reimplantation be done without tension or angulation of the ureter. The reimplantation should be stented with a double J stent. The bladder mucosa is closed as previously described.

## The Boari-Ocherblad Flap

The Boari-Ocherblad flap is utilized to gain additional length to bridge a gap between the ureter and the bladder. In this situation, a flap of bladder is mobilized and tubularized (Figs. 91–20 and 91–21). The length of the flap depends on the particular deficit length between the posterior lateral wall of the bladder and the proposed site of the ureteroneocystostomy. The ureter is tunneled in the submucosal portion of the flap, which is then tubularized around the ureter. If adequate length does not allow for creation of a submucosal tunnel, the ureter can be anastomosed end to end to the tubularized Boari-Ocherblad flap. The anastomosis is then stented with a double J stent.

When ureteral injury occurs, the technique used to correct the injury depends on the location of the injury. Fig. 91–22 reviews available surgical options based on the level of the ureteral injury.

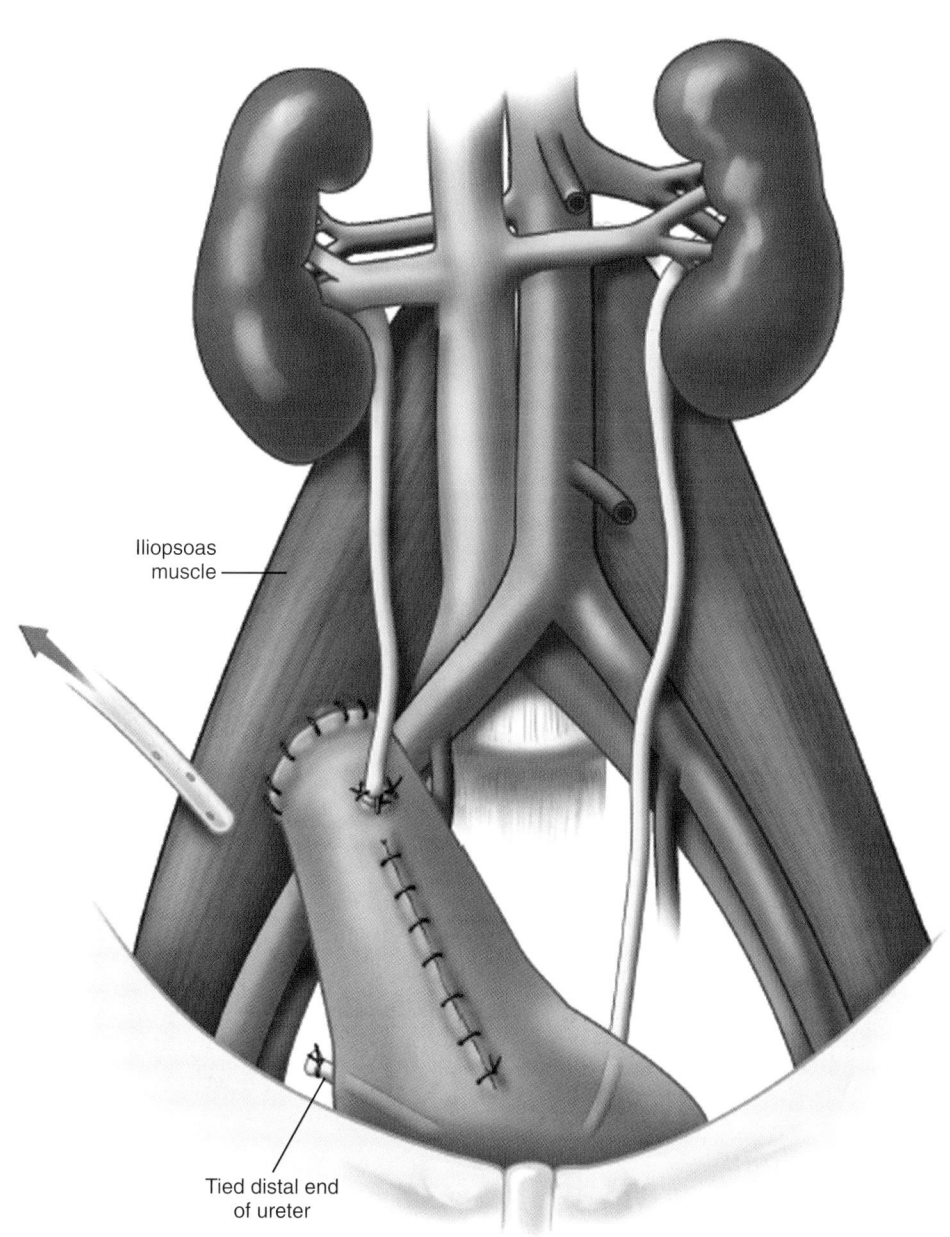

Iliopsoas
muscle

Tied distal end
of ureter

**FIGURE 91–19** Schematic representation of a completed psoas hitch. Note that reimplantation of the ureter is completed before the bladder is secured to the psoas muscle.

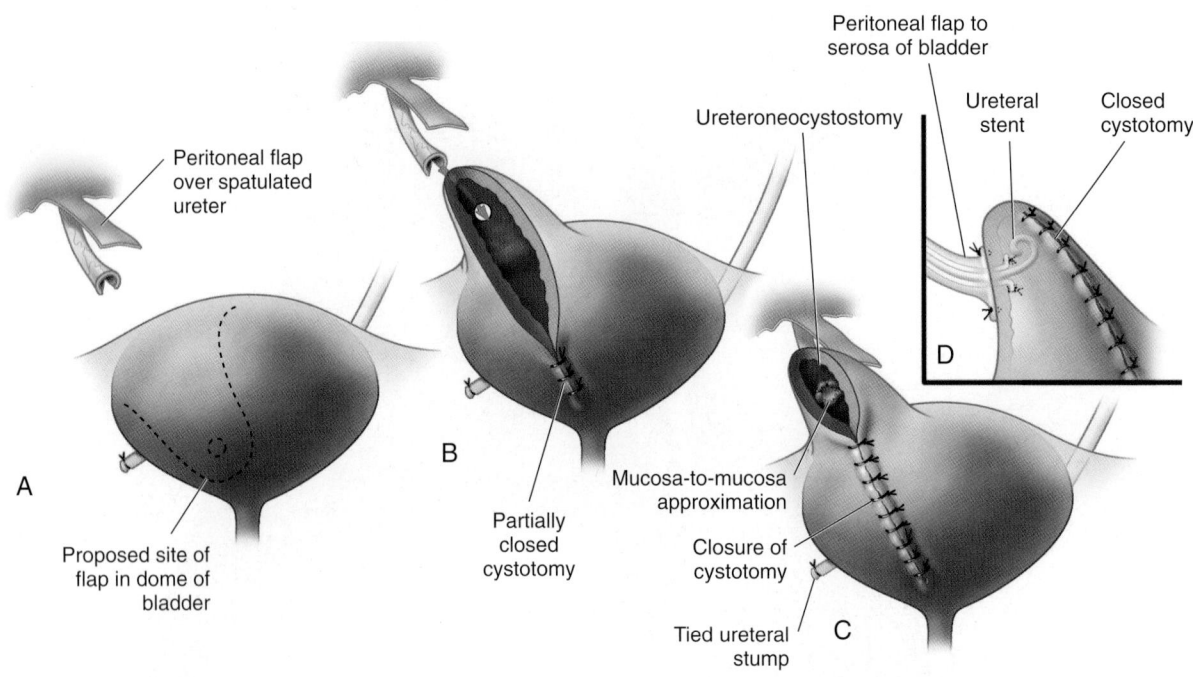

**FIGURE 91–20** Schematic overview of Boari bladder flap. **A.** Outline of oblique bladder incision used to construct the bladder bridge. Note the broad base (roughly 2 times the diameter of the apex) and the outlined (*dashed circle*) future site of ureteral implantation. **B.** Site of future ureteral implantation. **C.** End-to-side ureteral anastomosis completed, and double J ureteral stent placed. **D.** Cystotomy closure completed and (*not shown*) psoas hitch performed to keep anastomosis off tension.

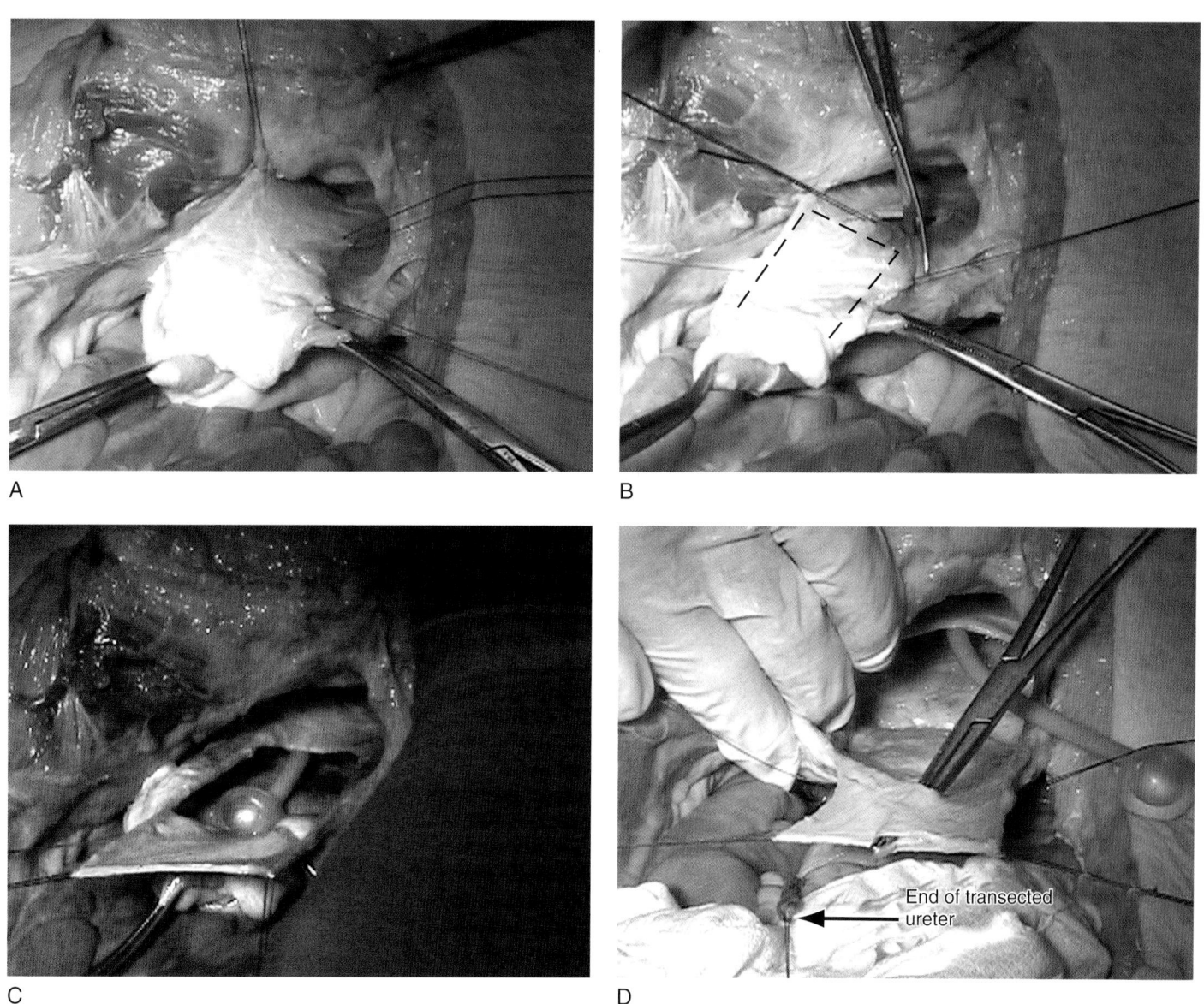

**FIGURE 91–21** Cadaveric dissection demonstrates the technique of creation of a Boari flap. **A.** Area of the bladder is identified and tagged with stay sutures. **B.** An anterior U-shaped incision is made in the anterior extraperitoneal portion of the bladder, as demonstrated by the dashed line. **C.** The flap is reflected in a cephalad direction. **D.** A submucosal tunnel is created.

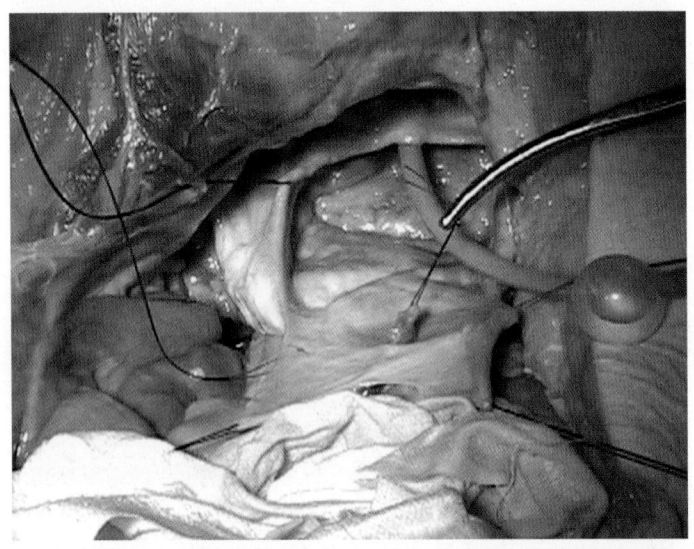

E

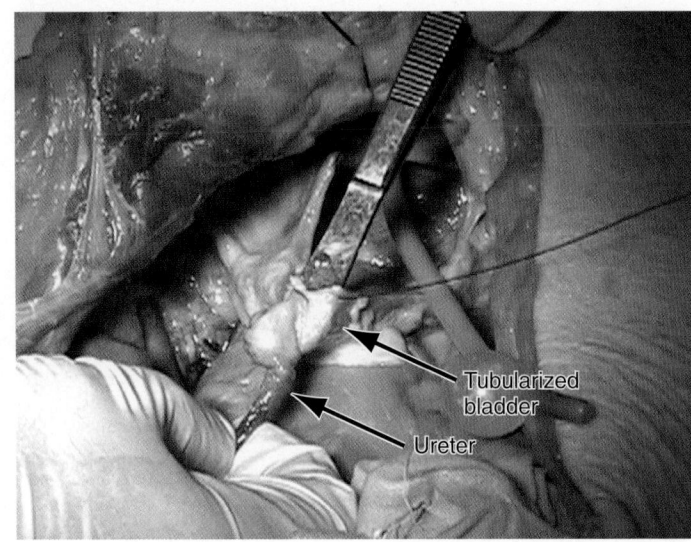

Tubularized bladder

Ureter

F

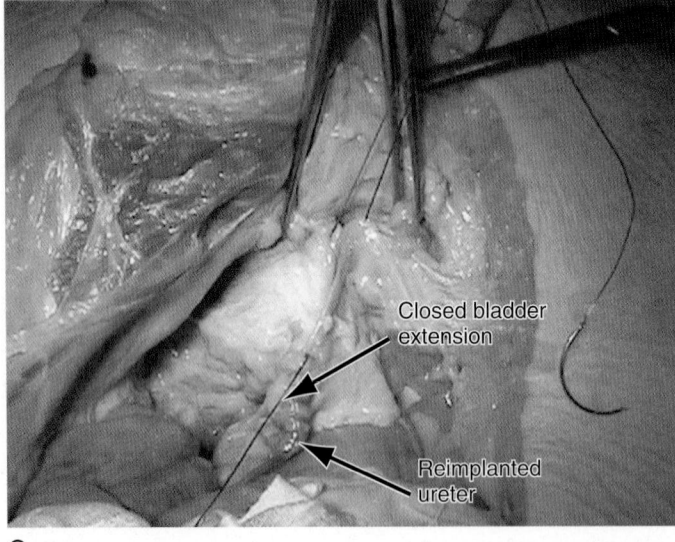

Closed bladder extension

Reimplanted ureter

G

**FIGURE 91–21, cont'd E.** The ureter is brought through the submucosal tunnel, spatulated, and sutured to the wall of the Boari flap. **F.** The flap is tubularized over the implant, thus closing the bladder extension. **G.** The remainder of the bladder is closed, completing the repair.

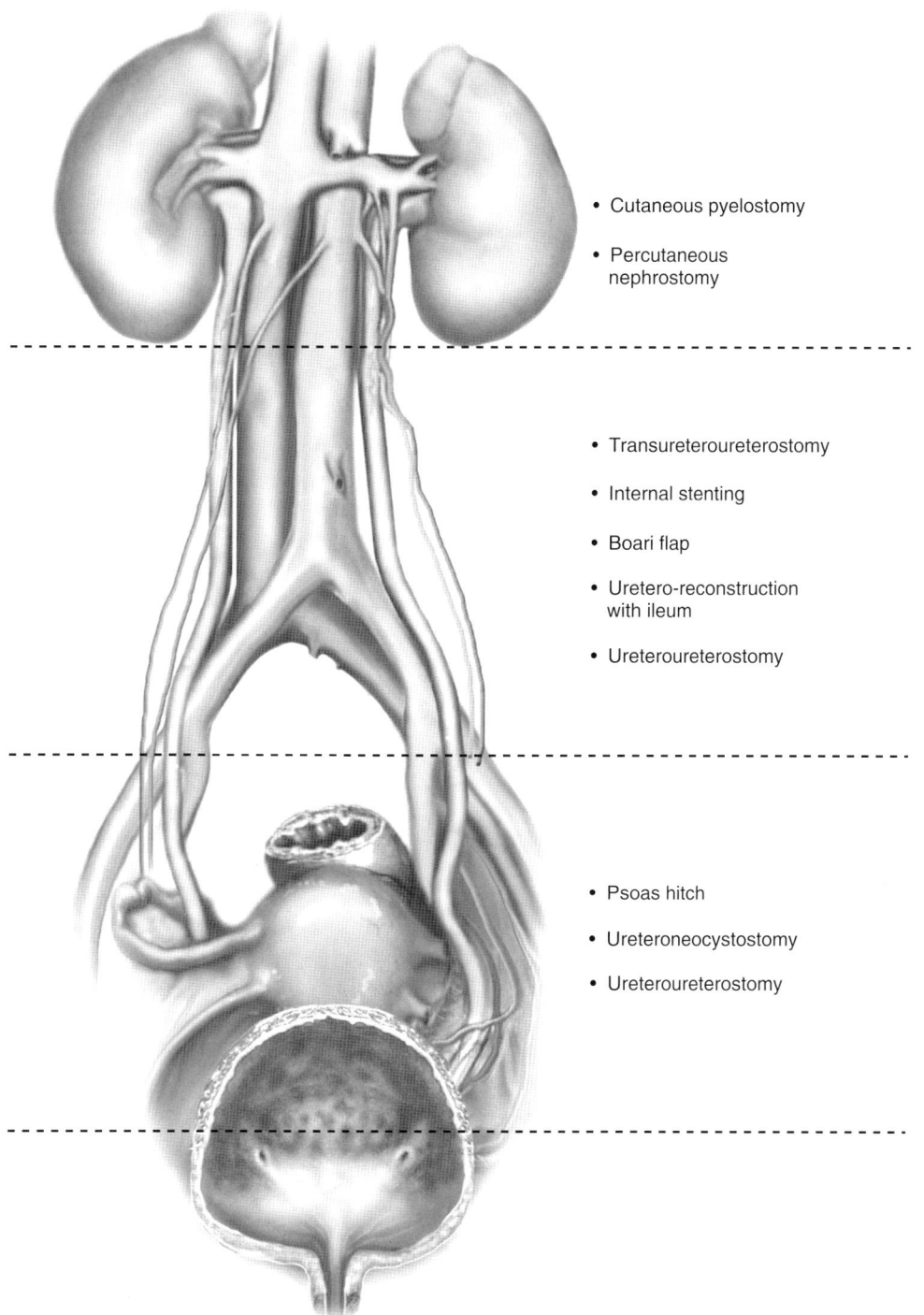

- Cutaneous pyelostomy
- Percutaneous nephrostomy

- Transureteroureterostomy
- Internal stenting
- Boari flap
- Uretero-reconstruction with ileum
- Ureteroureterostomy

- Psoas hitch
- Ureteroneocystostomy
- Ureteroureterostomy

**FIGURE 91–22** Illustration showing the entire length of the ureter. The various operations performed for ureteral injury are listed according to the anatomic level of injury.

# CHAPTER 92

# Surgical Management of Detrusor Compliance Abnormalities

## W. Stuart Reynolds ▪ Roger Dmochowski

When conservative and medical therapies for detrusor compliance abnormalities fail, few surgical options remain for "refractory" patients. Presently, there are three accepted modalities of surgical treatment: (1) sacral nerve stimulation (sacral neuromodulation [SNM]), (2) injectable bladder neuromodulation with neurotoxins, most notably botulinum toxin (BoTN), and (3) bladder augmentation. Uses, indications, and techniques for these three modalities continue to evolve as experience and understanding of each are gained. Patient selection, therefore, remains an important aspect of determining which surgical option is best for the patient; an appropriate patient evaluation is required.

## Evaluation of Patients

A full patient history is necessary to elucidate the character of urinary symptoms, to evaluate any previous attempts at medical or surgical treatment, and to identify concomitant medical conditions that may influence the success of treatment or provide contraindications to different therapies. In general, a patient who may be considered for surgical treatment of detrusor abnormalities will need to have failed more conservative treatment modalities, and a complete understanding of previous treatments is essential. A thorough physical examination is warranted that focuses on the lower abdomen and pelvis to note any structural abnormalities, including a vaginal speculum examination and bimanual physical examination in women to evaluate for any associated pelvic organ prolapse, as well as a prostate examination in men. Also, inspection and palpation of the lower back and spine can uncover signs of bony abnormality or scars from any previous spine surgery that may suggest a potential neurologic insult. Finally, the extremities should be examined for pedal edema and neurologic or musculoskeletal abnormalities.

A bladder or voiding diary can be considered to better quantify the degree of urinary dysfunction, not only for diagnostic purposes but also to serve as a baseline for subsequent post-treatment comparison. Similarly, patient self-reported quality-of-life and symptom severity questionnaires can provide a more objective, comparable picture of the degree of urinary dysfunction. Finally, in any patient who fails conservative or empirical therapy, multichannel urodynamics is warranted to objectively characterize the nature of the urinary dysfunction and to identify any negative or worrisome prognostic factors associated with the voiding complaints, including bladder capacity and compliance, the presence of detrusor overactivity, the magnitude of resting detrusor pressures, and the coordination of

detrusor and sphincter function, all of which may have negative implications for renal function. Combining fluoroscopy ("videourodynamics") can add important information regarding structural abnormalities of the bladder or ureters, including vesicoureteral reflux, bladder morphology, and bladder neck function.

## General Introduction to Three Modalities

Sacral neuromodulation has been available since FDA approval in 1997 (Interstim, Medtronic, Inc, Minneapolis, Minnesota) and is currently indicated for the treatment of urge urinary incontinence, frequency-urgency syndrome, and idiopathic urinary retention. Although the exact mechanism of action of SNM has not been fully determined, it appears to modulate bladder behavior through electrical stimulation of somatic afferent axons in the spinal roots, which in turn modulate voiding and continence reflex pathways in the central nervous system, likely by inhibiting interneuronal transmission in the bladder reflex pathway.

With the present configuration, the Interstim device (comprising a battery-powered neurostimulator, an extension cable, and a tined electrical lead) (Fig. 92–1A) is implanted via a staged, two-step process involving initial percutaneous placement of a semipermanent, tined electrical lead within close approximation of the third sacral nerve root (S3) by placement of the lead through the S3 spinal foramen (Fig. 92–1B). This is typically done with fluoroscopic guidance but may be done without. The tined lead is an insulated, electrical stimulation lead with four contact points near the tip and four plastic collapsible projections, which help to anchor the lead to the surrounding tissue. A temporary, external electrical stimulator is attached and a clinical trial period of 1 to 4 weeks ensues, during which the patient evaluates his or her response to therapy. If appropriate benefit occurs (defined as greater than 50% improvement in symptoms), then an implantable pulse generator (IPG) is connected to the previously placed lead and is surgically implanted in the upper buttocks during a second surgical stage procedure. If there is not a significant response, the implanted lead is removed without implanting an IPG. Adjustments to the impulse generator settings can be made with a remote programming device.

Interest in and use of BoTN injection into the bladder for treatment of voiding dysfunction have increased over the past several years, although BoTN is not currently FDA approved for use in the genitourinary system. The causative toxin for botulism, produced by the bacterium *Clostridium botulinum*, may be one of seven distinct toxins depending on the serotype of the organism (BoTN types A, B, C1, D, E, F, and G). Presently, only BoTN A (Botox, Allergan, Irvine, California; or Dysport, Ipsen, Luxembourg) and B (Myobloc or Neurobloc, Elan, Dublin, Ireland) are commercially available for clinical use. BoTN acts by cleaving a specific site (specific to each BoTN serotype) of a protein complex (soluble $N$-ethylmaleimide-sensitive factor attachment protein receptor [SNARE] complex) responsible for exocytosis of neurotransmitter vesicles from the neuron. In the case of BoTN A, the most well-studied toxin subtype, the specific substrate is the synaptosome-associated protein of 25 kD (SNAP-25), a component of the SNARE complex; this results in inhibition of synaptic release of acetylcholine from the peripheral motor neurons (Fig. 92–2).

At therapeutic doses used for the urinary system, BoTN is understood to inhibit the release of acetylcholine from the motor neuron end plant at the neuromuscular junction, inducing paralysis in the affected muscle, or the bladder in the case of bladder injections. Additionally, BoTN may directly inhibit sensory nerve activity and thus modulate bladder sensory input to the central nervous system. In cases of bladder overactivity or diminished bladder compliance, both mechanisms of action are exploited. Presently, no standardized technique or approach to cystoscopic bladder injections of BoTN is used: a wide range of doses have been used, and a number of different injection templates have been followed. In general, however, BoTN can be injected into the wall of the bladder under cystoscopic vision in an outpatient setting, with local or general anesthesia. The effects of BoTN injection are generally immediately apparent, and symptom improvement can be seen after the first day or so of injection. However, the effects are generally short-lived and wear off after approximately 6 months.

When more conservative or less invasive measures have failed in the treatment of bladder compliance abnormalities, the most aggressive management option is augmentation cystoplasty. The goal of bladder augmentation is to create a large-capacity, low-pressure (i.e., high-compliance) reservoir for urine storage. Larger volumes of urine may be stored for longer periods of time, which is beneficial for continence, while detrusor pressure remains low, protecting the urinary system upper tracts from dysfunction and ultimately from renal failure. This is generally achieved at the cost of bladder emptying, and many patients are dependent on intermittent catheter bladder drainage after augmentation.

Many different techniques have been developed for augmentation cystoplasty employing a variety of different tissues, including segments of detubularized bowel (ileocystoplasty, cecocystoplasty, sigmoid cystoplasty, and gastrocystoplasty), dilated ureter (ureteroplasty), autoaugmentation (removal of the overlying detrusor muscle of the dome of the bladder), and, more recently, biologic substitution using techniques of bioengineered tissue. The most common procedure involves the use of small intestine, specifically the ileum, and because it has been the best characterized, the ensuing discussion focuses on this technique.

Efficacy with use of any of the described techniques can be expected in the properly selected patient. Overall, 70% of patients with urgency, frequency, or urge incontinence achieve success with SNM, defined as "a greater than 50% improvement in symptoms." Furthermore, for many patients, outcomes are durable for longer than 5 years. Among patients treated with BoTN injection, up to 80% of those treated for overactive bladder symptoms will demonstrate symptom improvement, and up to 70% of those with neurogenic detrusor abnormalities will show improvement. Efficacy in general is limited to 6 months because the effects abate at that time. Repeat injection can be performed with similar efficacy anticipated. Among patients undergoing augmentation cystoplasty, improvement in continence can be expected in more than 75%, with 50% or more completely continent. In some reports, this occurs in 95% of patients. Upward of 80% of patients will experience resolution of preoperative urgency.

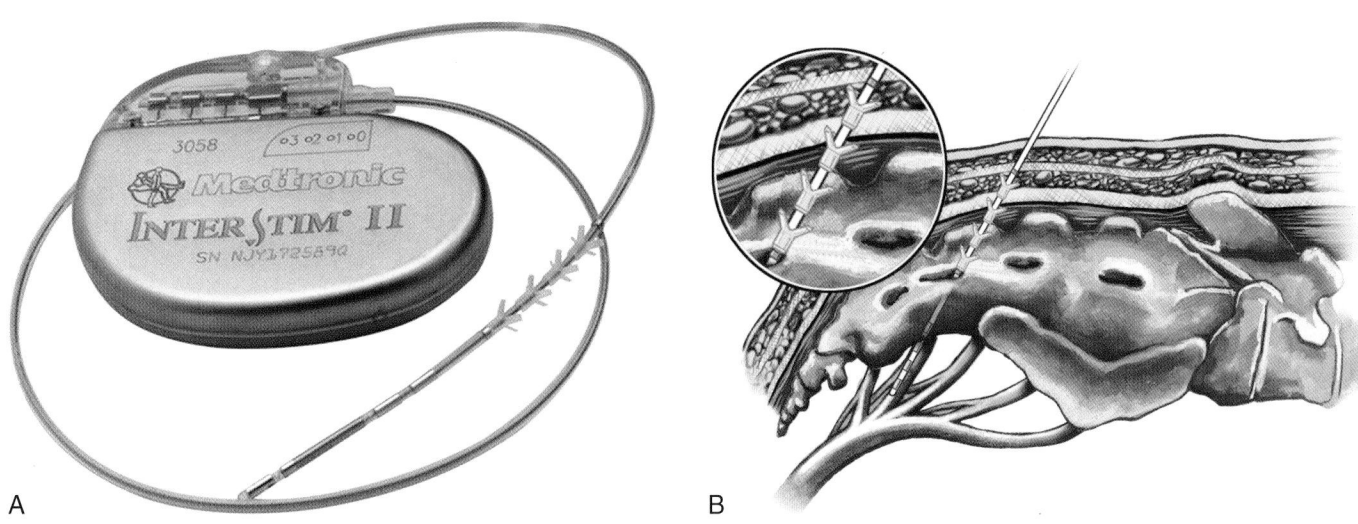

**FIGURE 92–1  A.** Interstim device (Medtronic, Inc, Minneapolis, Minnesota), composed of a battery-powered, remote-programmable neurostimulator (implantable pulse generator [IPG]), a semipermanent tined electrical lead, and an insulated extension cable. **B.** Illustration depicting the final position of the four electrical contact points of the stimulation lead in close proximity to the third sacral nerve root (S3) and the four plastic projections or tines embedded in and securing the lead to the tissue overlying the sacral foramen. (Images source: Medtronic, Inc.)

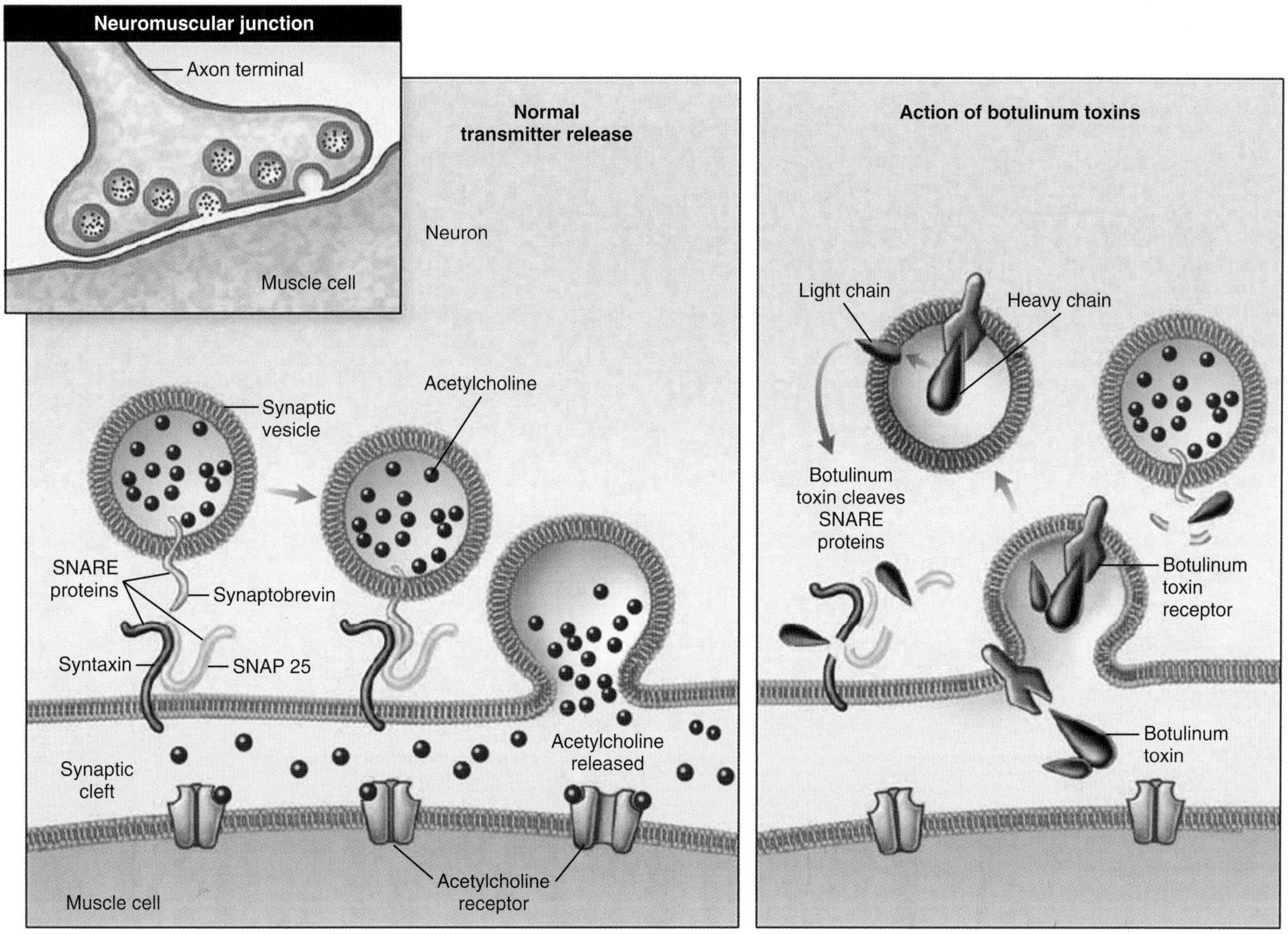

**Neuromuscular junction**

- Axon terminal

Neuron

Muscle cell

**Normal transmitter release**

- Acetylcholine
- Synaptic vesicle

SNARE proteins
- Synaptobrevin
Syntaxin — SNAP 25

Synaptic cleft

Muscle cell

Acetylcholine released

Acetylcholine receptor

**Action of botulinum toxins**

Light chain    Heavy chain

Botulinum toxin cleaves SNARE proteins

Botulinum toxin receptor

Botulinum toxin

**FIGURE 92–2**  Schematic depicting the molecular action of botulinum toxin. (Adapted with permission from Rowland LP. New Engl J Med 2002;347:382.)

UNIT 4 ■ SECTION A

## Surgical Techniques

### Sacral Neuromodulation

Surgical implantation of an SNM device proceeds by a two-stage process: during the first stage, the electrical stimulation lead is percutaneously placed and positioned in close proximity to the S3 nerve root via the S3 foramen; during the second stage, an IPG is surgically implanted in the upper buttocks, after a successful trial of an external device demonstrating clinical effectiveness.

For the first stage, percutaneous lead placement, the patient is placed prone on the operative table; the upper thighs, buttocks, and lower back are widely cleansed, and surgical drapes are placed to allow visualization of the buttocks and gluteal crease, as depicted in Fig. 92–3. With the use of fluoroscopy and a metal surgical instrument, the approximate location of the S3 foramen is noted at the skin level (Fig. 92–3D). A 20-gauge foramen needle is inserted at a 60-degree angle to the skin approximately 2 cm cranial to the actual location of the S3 foramen and is directed into the S3 foramen (Fig. 92–4A). The correct position is verified by electrical stimulation of the foramen needle with an external stimulator (Fig. 92–4B) and by examination for appropriate motor and sensory responses, which for S3 include a bellows response of the pelvic floor and ipsilateral great toe plantar flexion (Table 92–1). Bilateral foramen needles may be used to assess for better response on each side (see Fig. 92–4). Using the Seldinger technique concept, the directional guide wire (23 gauge) is placed through the foramen needle and the needle is removed, leaving the wire in place. A scalpel is used to nick the skin along the wire, and the introducer (composed of a 16-gauge dilator nestled in a 14-gauge introducer sheath) is then passed over the wire to an appropriate depth of insertion determined by lateral fluoroscopy (Fig. 92–4C). Radio-opaque markings on the introducer (one at the dilator tip and one at the introducer sheath tip) allow accurate positioning of the device within the S3 foramen. The introducer sheath marking should be at the level of the ventral S3 foramen, and the dilator tip marking just beyond (Fig. 92–4D). The introducer wire and dilator are removed, leaving the introducer sheath behind.

Next, the tined lead is inserted into the sheath (Fig. 92–5A) and is positioned such that electrical contact point #1 is straddling the ventral S3 foramen (Fig. 92–5B). The introducer sheath is withdrawn slightly to the level of a white marking on the lead, thereby exposing the lead contact points without deploying the tined plastic projections. Electrical stimulation confirms the position of the lead at the appropriate level; all four positions are tested for proper motor and sensory functions. After satisfactory positioning, the sheath is completely removed, deploying the tined plastic projections that anchor the lead to surrounding soft tissue.

At this point, a second 3-cm skin incision is made in the upper buttock on the contralateral side from the lead insertion, and a small subcutaneous pocket is developed (Fig. 92–6A). This will serve as the future implantation site for the IPG. A tunneling trocar device is used to pass the stimulation lead into the IPG pocket: the tunneler is passed to the pocket, the sharp trocar blade is removed, and the lead is passed through the remaining plastic sheath or tunneler (Fig. 92–6B, C). A temporary, external lead extension is connected to the stimulation lead within the IPG pocket, and the external extension is further tunneled to exit the skin superolaterally to the IPG pocket (Fig. 92–6D). The leads are tunneled to decrease the risk of infection to the IPG device with externalized wires. The externalized lead is connected to the external stimulator. The redundant lead wire and connection covers are buried in the subcutaneous pocket previously developed, and the subcutaneous tissue and overlying skin are closed with absorbable sutures. The percutaneous tined lead insertion site is also closed with simple interrupted absorbable sutures.

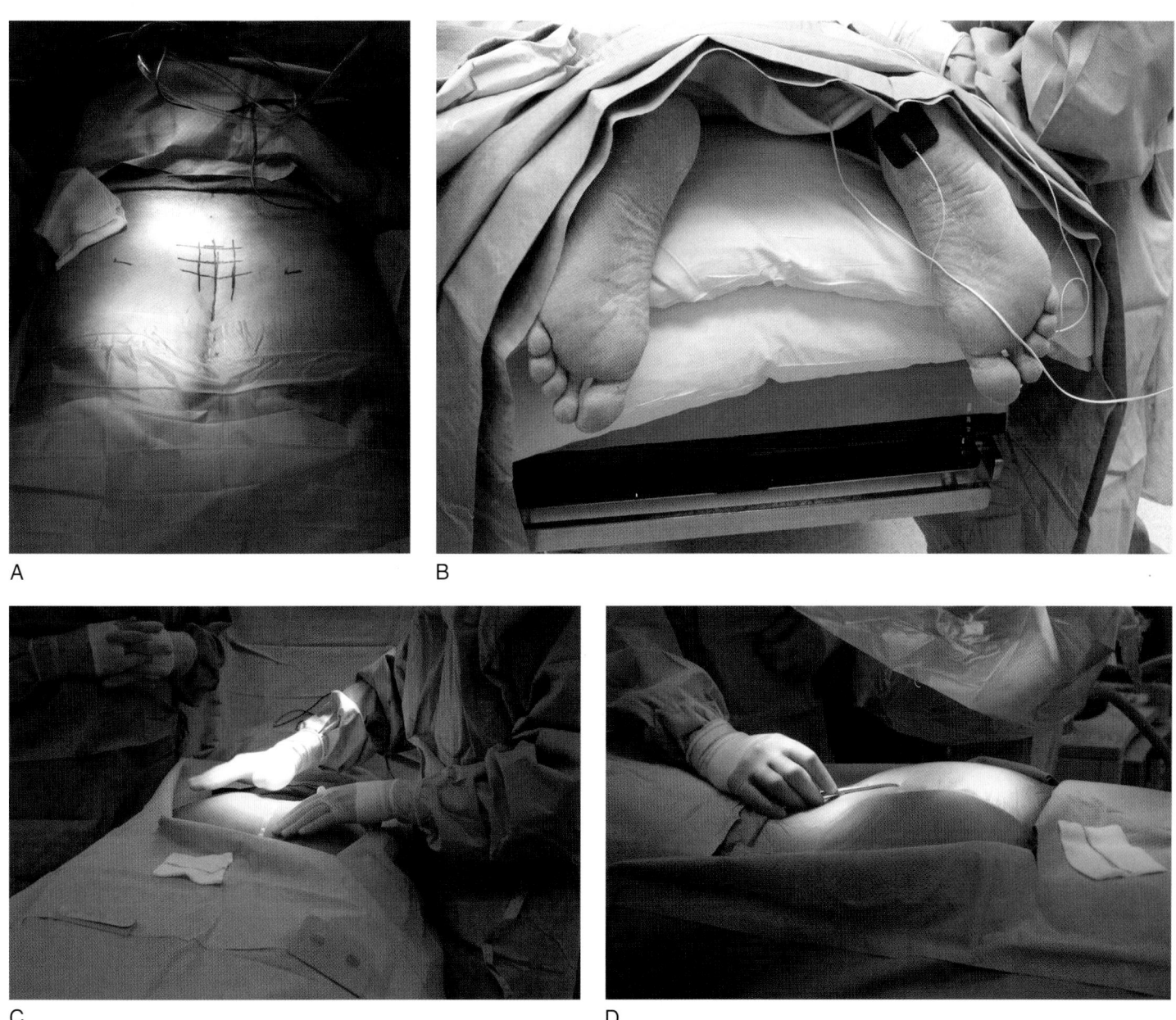

A

B

C

D

**FIGURE 92–3  A.** With the patient in the prone position, the posterior thighs, buttocks, and lower back are sterilely prepared and draped as depicted, allowing visualization of the buttocks and gluteal cleft, as well as the feet (**B**). Skin markings outlining the approximate location of the sacral foramen have been made using a combination of palpation (**C**) and fluoroscopic guidance (**D**).

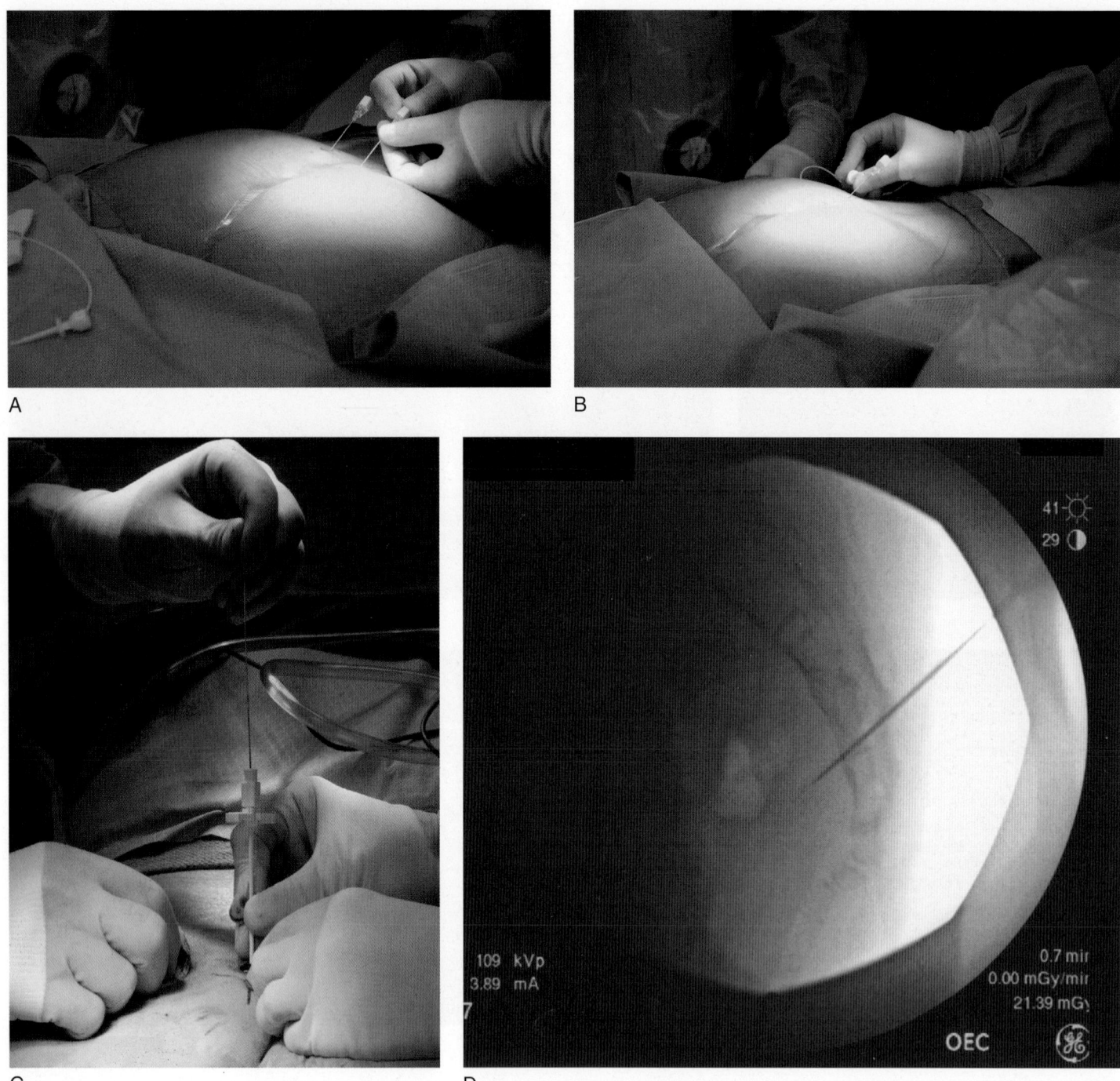

**FIGURE 92–4  A.** A foramen finder needle is inserted approximately 2 cm cranial to the actual location of the S3 foramen at a 60-degree angle to the skin and is blindly positioned in the foramen using palpation of the needle against the bone. **B.** Positioning of the needle within the correct sacral foramen is confirmed fluoroscopically and with the use of test stimulation and monitoring for the appropriate motor response (see Table 92–1). **C.** The foramen needle is exchanged for the directional guide wire by inserting the wire through the needle lumen and removing the needle over the wire. The introducer is then passed over the wire, after a small skin nick is made. **D.** Correct depth positioning of the introducer is confirmed by lateral fluoroscopy: the distal opaque marking should be positioned just below the S3 foramen, and the proximal marking at the level of the ventral foramen.

UNIT 4 ■ SECTION A

**TABLE 92-1 ■ Sacral Nerve Root Responses to Electrical Stimulation**

| Nerve Root | Pelvic Floor | Ipsilateral Lower Extremity | Sensation |
|---|---|---|---|
| S2 | Anal sphincter contraction | Lateral leg rotation, Plantar flexion of entire foot | Sensations in leg or buttock |
| S3 | "Bellows" response of pelvic floor (levator muscle contraction) | Great toe dorsiflexion | "Pulling" in rectum, scrotum, or vagina |
| S4 | "Bellows" response of pelvic floor | None | "Pulling" in rectum only |

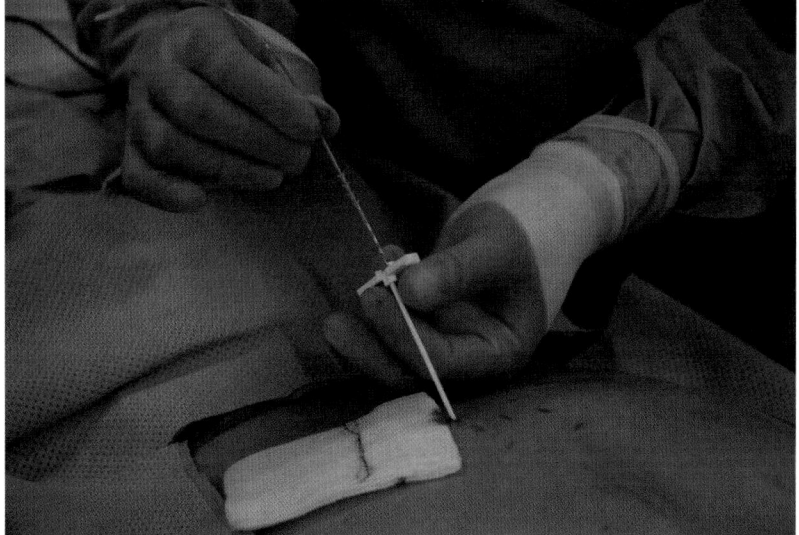

A

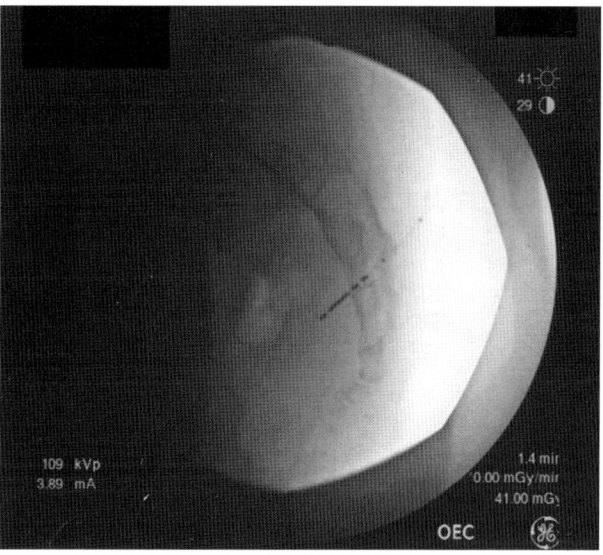

B

**FIGURE 92–5 A.** After the directional wire and dilator are removed from the inside of the introducer sheath, the tined lead is inserted through the lumen of the sheath and the sheath is backed out slightly to the level of a white marking on the lead, thereby exposing the lead contact points. **B.** On fluoroscopy, electrical contact point #1 should be straddling the S3 foramen. The sheath is then completely removed, deploying the tined projects and securing the lead to surrounding tissue.

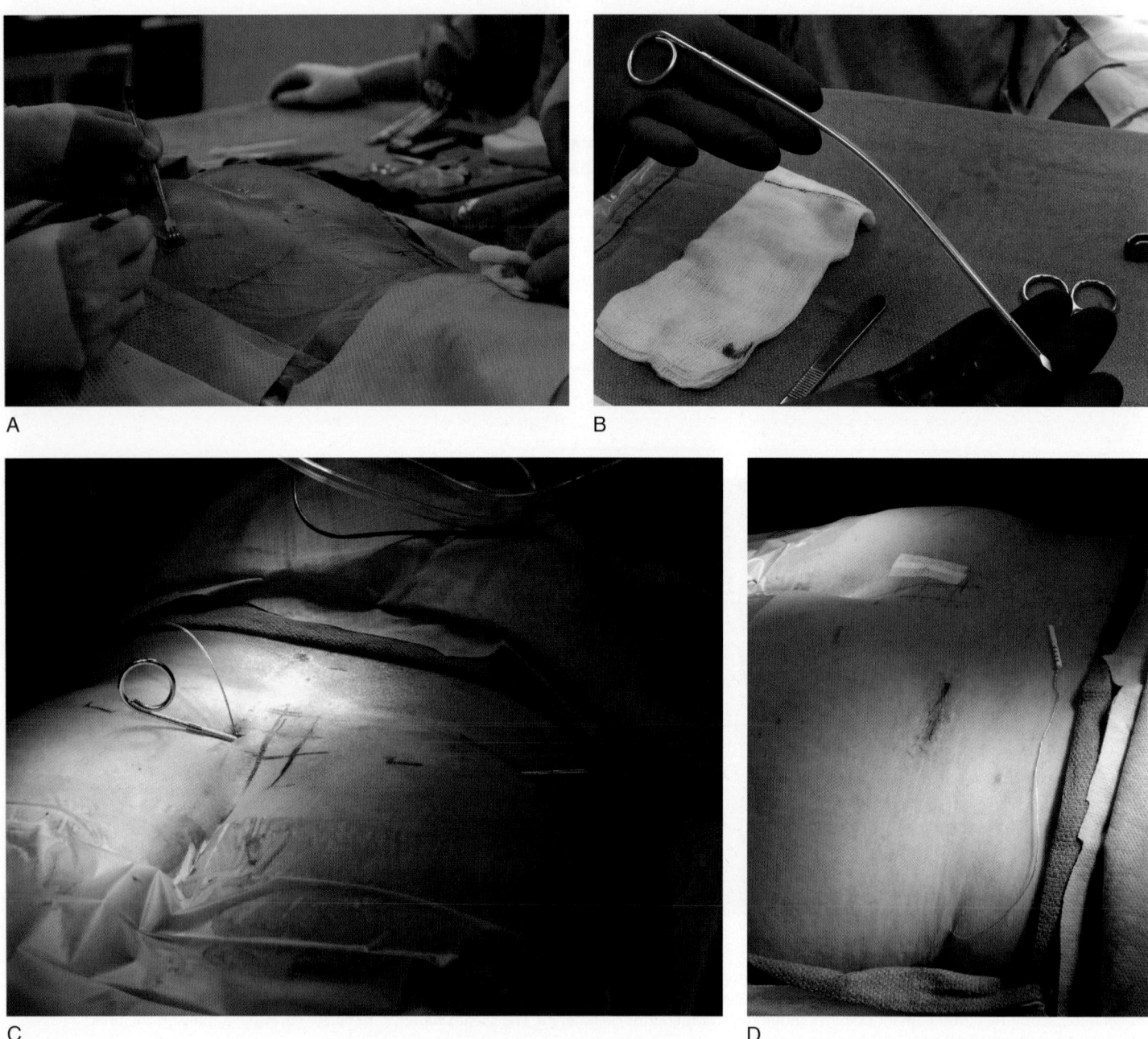

**FIGURE 92–6 A.** A 3- to 4-cm incision is made in the contralateral upper buttocks, while a subcutaneous pocket is developed at the future implantation site of the implantable pulse generator (IPG). **B.** The sharp-pointed tunneling trocar device is used to tunnel the stimulation lead to the IPG pocket. **C.** With the trocar in place, the sharp blade and obturator are removed, and the lead is passed through the tunneling sheath. **D.** A temporary, external lead extension is attached to the lead, the connection is buried in the IPG pocket, and the external end is further tunneled laterally to exit superolaterally to the IPG pocket site.

After a successful trial period with the external stimulator, defined as a "greater than 50% reduction of symptoms," the IPG is implanted during the second stage of the procedure. The previous incision over the buttocks is opened, and the buried electrical connection is exposed. The external lead extension is removed and the subcutaneous pocket enlarged to accommodate the IPG. The IPG is then connected to the tined stimulation lead, and the IPG is buried in the subcutaneous pocket (Fig. 92-7). Again, the skin incision is closed with absorbable sutures. Once the patient is awakened, the IPG is programmed using the remote programming device.

Few complications are seen with SNM, and they generally are related to lead migration and loss of clinical benefit, device malfunction, or infection. For lead migration and device malfunction, a revision procedure in which the lead or the IPG or both can be removed and reinserted can be curative. For infection, prompt surgical removal is warranted; a new device can be inserted at a later date. No neurologic complications have been reported. It is important to note that the safety and efficacy of SNM implants have not been established for use with magnetic resolution imaging (MRI), and patients who may require future or repeated MRI should not undergo SNM implantation.

## Botulinum Toxin Bladder Injections

Because most clinical experience involves the use of BoTN A (Botox), this discussion focuses on use of this toxin subtype. It is important to note that dosing of BoTN is defined by units of biologic activity, which are neither interchangeable nor directly comparable with those of other botulinum toxin types. BoTN A is supplied in 100-unit (U) vials as a desiccated powder (Fig. 92-8), which is reconstituted immediately before injection with injectable-grade, preservative-free normal saline. Dosing protocols are variable, and anywhere from 100 to 300 U may be injected at a single session. Depending on the desired concentration of injection solution, anywhere from 1 to 10 mL of injectable saline is used to dissolve each vial of BoTN A, and the solution is drawn up in appropriately sized syringes. The filled syringe is then attached to a long, 23-gauge needle for use with cystoscopic equipment.

Botulinum toxin bladder injections are performed via a cystoscopic approach. Injection may be performed in an outpatient setting with any level of anesthesia, including local, regional, or general. Local anesthesia typically involves the instillation of intraurethral 2% lidocaine jelly followed by intravesical 2% lidocaine solution. Additionally, a rigid or flexible cystoscope can be used for bladder injections of BoTN with an appropriately matched cystoscopic injection needle (Fig. 92-9). Typically, injection of BoTN proceeds with 20 to 30 submucosal injection sites spread across the base and posterior wall of the bladder, including or not including the trigone; 0.1 to 1 mL of BoTN solution is given, depending on the concentration (approximately 10 U per injection) (Fig. 92-10). Injecting at the appropriate depth is important so as to avoid extravasating BoTN through the bladder wall or depositing the BoTN too superficially within the bladder mucosa. Ideally, injecting the solution will raise the overlying mucosa only minimally, avoiding large blebs on the mucosal surface (Fig. 92-11).

Some controversy exists as to whether or not the bladder trigone should be included in the injection template because of theoretical concerns about inducing vesicoureteral reflux by injecting near the ureteral orifices. This has not been substantiated clinically, and indeed, because the trigone is thought to be densely innervated, many regularly include it in the template. The major adverse event related to BoTN bladder injection is urinary retention; although this is relatively uncommon, it occurs frequently enough that patients must be counseled on and/or instructed in clean intermittent catheterization (CIC) if retention ensues. This is typically transient and resolves with time. Minor complications of the procedure include transient dysuria, hematuria, and occasional urinary tract infection (UTI). More worrisome are rare reports of generalized weakness, malaise, and muscle weakness, possibly due to systemic effects of BoTN absorption. In general, any effect of BoTN injection diminishes and abates by approximately 6 months, and repeated injection is necessary to recoup any clinical benefit previously seen.

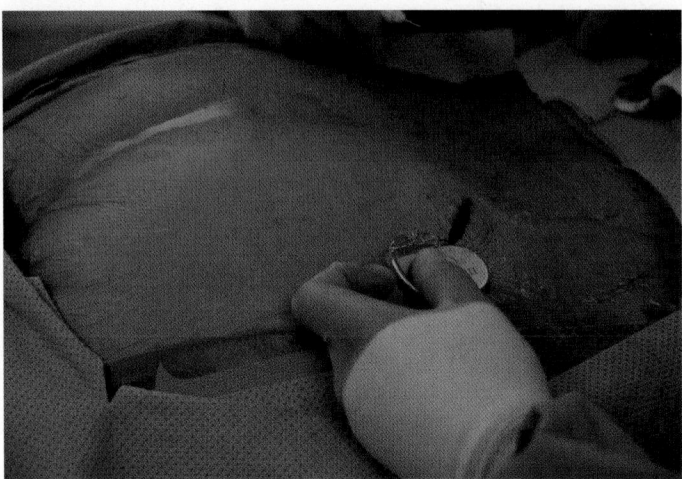

**FIGURE 92–7** During the second stage of implantation, the incision over the implantable pulse generator (IPG) site is incised and the tined lead–extension lead connection is disconnected. An IPG device is connected to the tined stimulation lead and is inserted into the subcutaneous pocket. The overlying skin is closed with absorbable sutures.

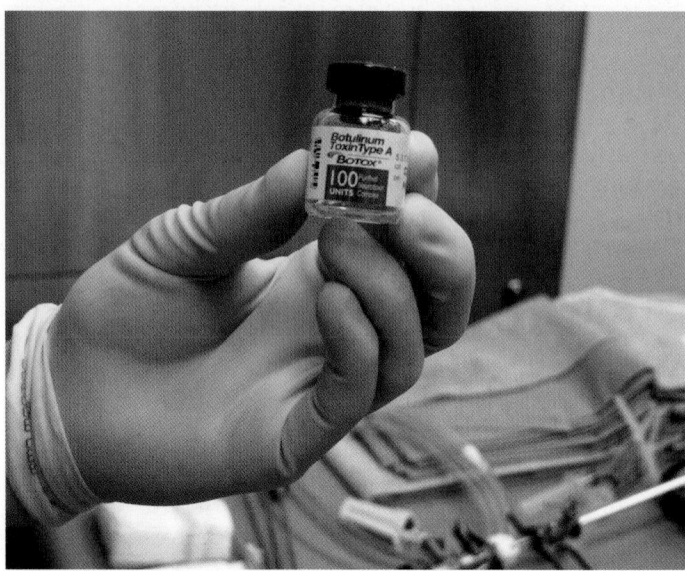

**FIGURE 92–8** Botulinum toxin A is supplied as a desiccated powder in 100-unit vials and must be reconstituted with preservative-free, injectable-grade normal saline.

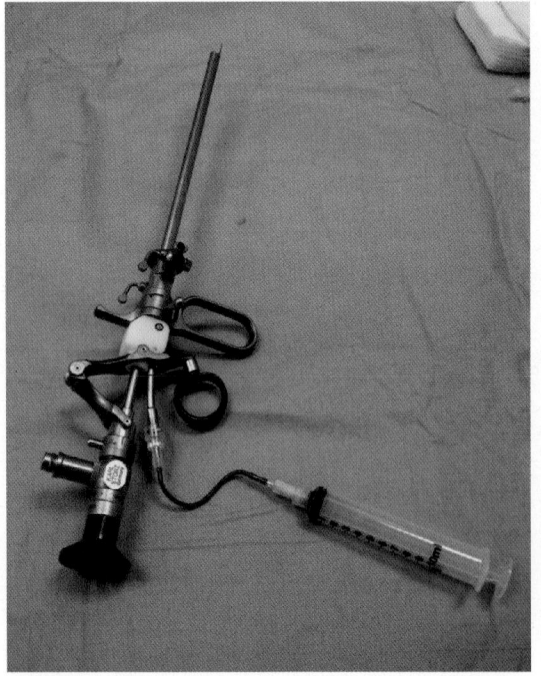

A

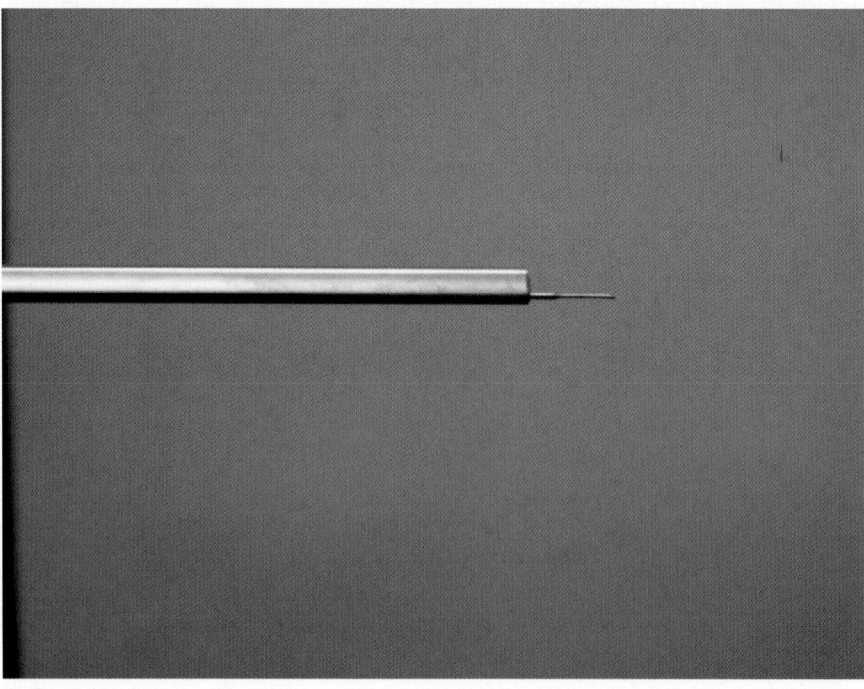

B

**FIGURE 92–9 A.** A 22-French rigid injection cystoscope with a 22-gauge injection needle is used to inject botulinum toxin A (BoTN A). **B.** Alternatively, a flexible cystoscope and corresponding injection needle can be used.

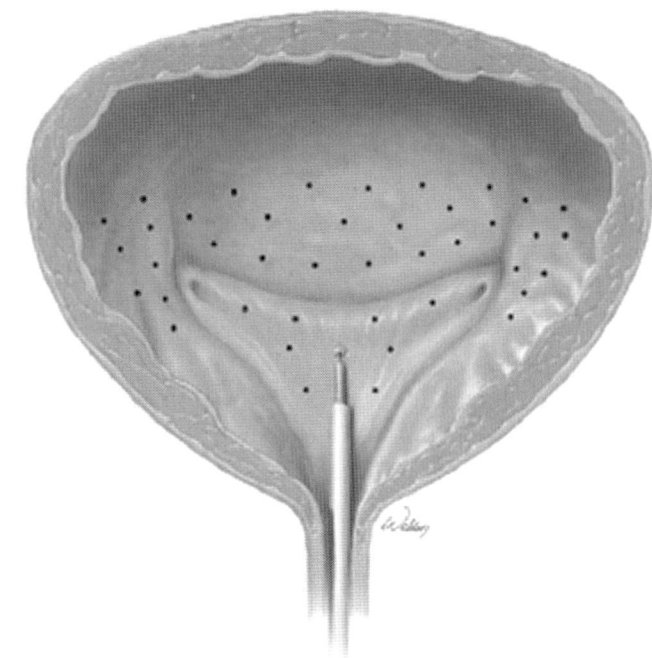

**FIGURE 92–10** Injection techniques vary, and many different injection templates have been described. A typical template involves 20 to 30 bladder injections spread over the posterior aspect of the bladder and dome and may or may not include the bladder trigone. (Image sources: Kim D et al: Urol Clin N Am 33:503-510, 2006.)

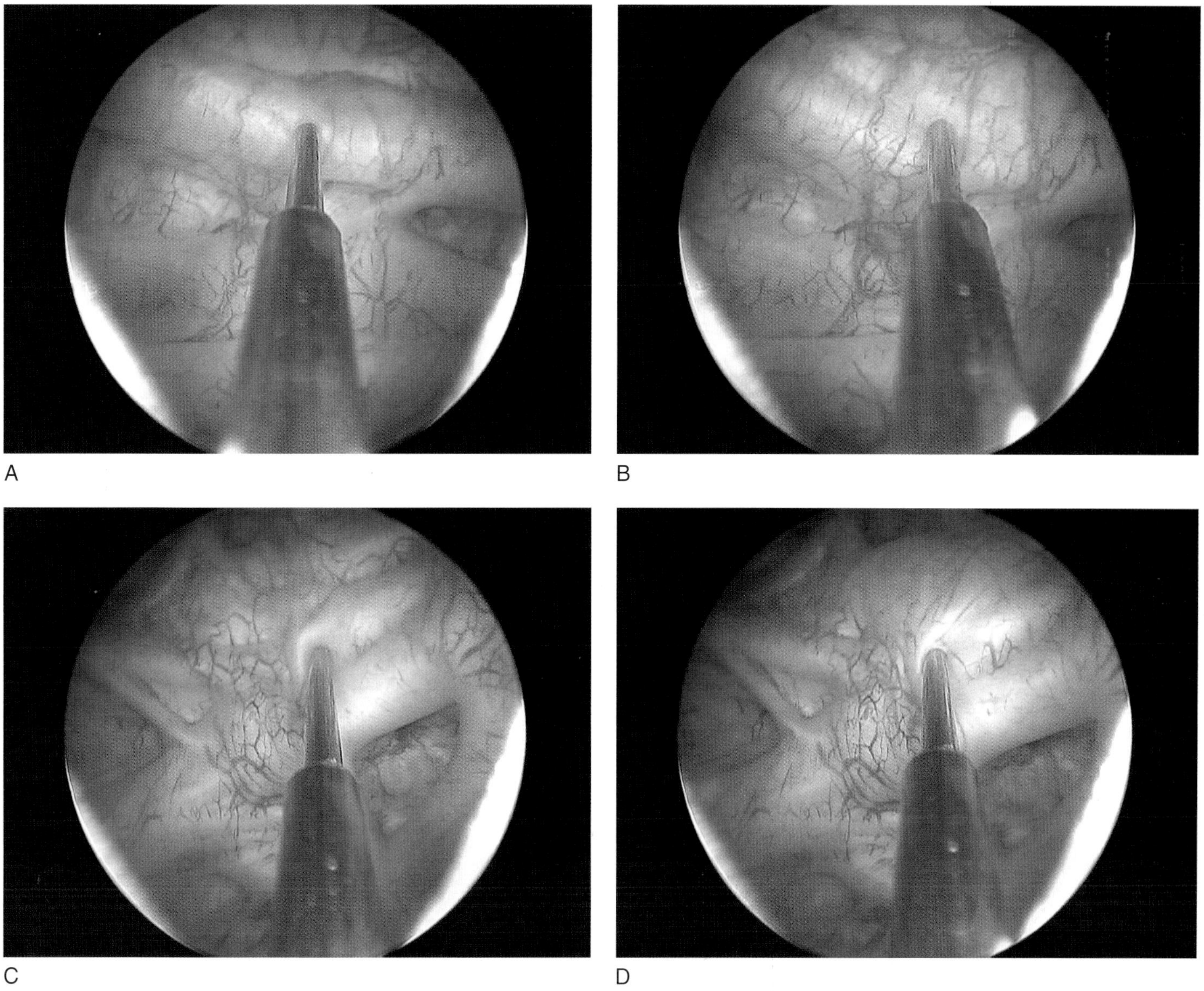

A

B

C

D

**FIGURE 92–11** To achieve the proper depth of injection, the needle should be inserted through the mucosa (**A** and **C**), typically with a slight "popping" feel, and the injected material should raise the overlying mucosa minimally, as demonstrated in the images by the "filling" of areas between bladder trabeculae (**B** and **D**).

## Augmentation Cystoplasty

The procedure for augmentation ileocystoplasty is generally illustrated by Fig. 92–12. The operation proceeds via a standard lower midline laparotomy incision. The patient typically is positioned supine on the operating room table or in the low lithotomy position with legs in stirrups. Although the genitalia are not necessarily needed as part of the surgical field, access to the urethral catheter to fill the bladder with saline during detrusororrhaphy can be helpful. A midline incision is made from the pubis to the umbilicus and is carried down through the anterior abdominal fascia, splitting the rectus muscles and opening the transversalis fascia and peritoneum. To prepare the bladder, a sagittal incision is made to almost completely bivalve the bladder, extending from 3 cm above the bladder neck anteriorly to 2 cm above the trigone posteriorly (see Fig. 92–13). Filling the bladder with saline before incising the detrusor can help to maintain a sagittal plane of incision.

To prepare the bowel segment, the terminal ileum is identified and a segment of ileum approximately 20 to 40 cm in length is isolated 15 cm or more proximal to the ileocecal valve. Care is taken to divide the mesentery so as to preserve blood supply to both the ileum segment and the eventual bowel anastomosis (Fig. 92–14A). Bowel division and subsequent anastomosis can be performed with handsewn sutures or with bowel anastomotic staplers (Fig. 92–14B). The isolated section of ileum is then opened longitudinally along its antimesenteric border (Fig. 92–15B). Typically, the bowel is then reconfigured in one of several ways, in a U-shape or S-shape, by folding the bowel and suturing the inner edges with full-thickness, running 3-0 absorbable suture (see Fig. 92–15).

The reconfigured bowel is then anastomosed to the bivalved bladder, starting at the posterior margin, with running 3-0 absorbable suture, along each of the sagittally incised bladder edges (see Fig. 92–12C). Before complete closure, a suprapubic tube is placed to exit through the native bladder wall; a urethral catheter is also placed. The bladder is then irrigated with saline to confirm water-tight integrity (Fig. 92–16); a closed-suction drain is placed, and both it and the suprapubic tube are brought out through the skin in separate stab incisions. The abdominal wall is finally closed in standard fashion.

The suprapubic tube and the urethral catheter are left in place for approximately 10 to 21 days, at which time a cystogram can be obtained to confirm that there is no extravasation. The urethral catheter is then removed, the suprapubic tube clamped, and the patient started with CIC. When the patient is comfortable with this, the suprapubic tube can be removed. Typically, the patient is instructed to CIC every 2 to 3 hours during the day and once or twice at night. The frequency of catheterizations can be increased to every 4 hours. If the patient demonstrates the ability to completely empty, then CIC can be discontinued.

Patients post augmentation should be followed with regular renal imaging (ultrasound, intravenous pyelography [IVP], or renal scan) during the first year and subsequently at regular intervals to monitor for upper urinary tract changes. Additionally, serum electrolytes and creatinine levels should be monitored regularly during this time to screen for electrolyte and metabolic abnormalities. Finally, because of the risk of tumor formation, surveillance should be performed regularly with cystoscopy.

Bacteriuria is a common finding after augmentation, particularly in patients on CIC. However, it need not be treated unless associated with a bone fide urinary tract infection, considered to be bacteriuria associated with symptoms of fever, suprapubic pain, hematuria, foul-smelling urine, incontinence, and increased production of mucus. Antibiotic therapy should be organism-specific and directed by urinary culture results. Other complications of bladder augmentation include bladder stone formation, thought to be related to urease-splitting bacterial UTI, uncleared mucus, hypercalciuria, residual urine or bladder foreign bodies, overproduction of mucus, metabolic acidosis due to abnormal reabsorption of urinary ammonium, and idiopathic bladder perforation.

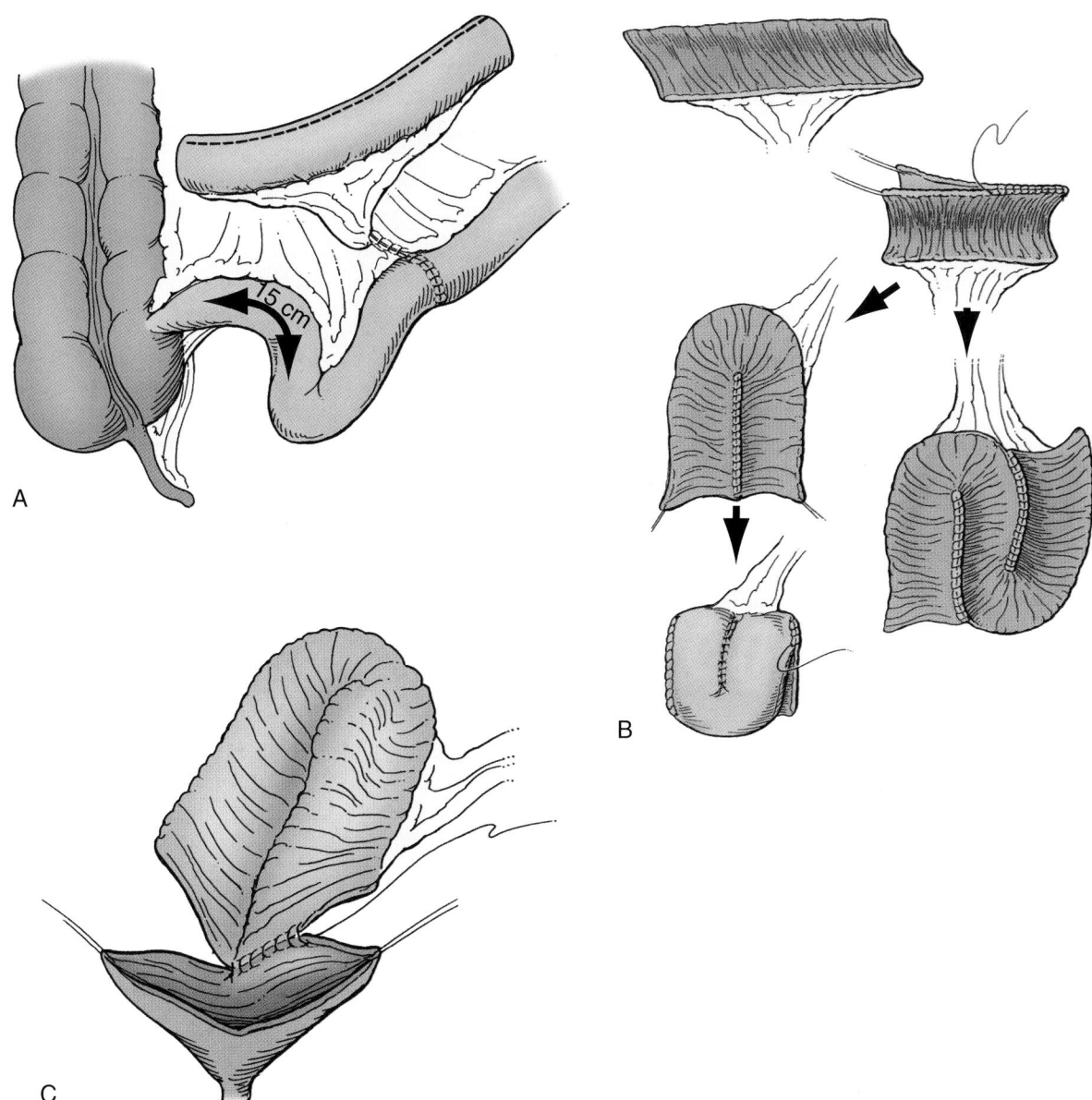

**FIGURE 92–12** As depicted in the illustration, augmentation ileal cystoplasty entails isolating a segment of distal ileum (while preserving the terminal ileum and ileocecal valve), opening the segment longitudinally, reconfiguring the ileal patch, and anastomosing the reconfigured patch to a sagittally bivalved bladder. (From Adams MC, Joseph DB: Urinary tract reconstruction in children. *In* Wein AJ, Kavoussi LR, Novick Andrew C, et al, eds: Campbell-Walsh Urology. 9th edition. Philadelphia, 2007, Saunders, p. 3674.)

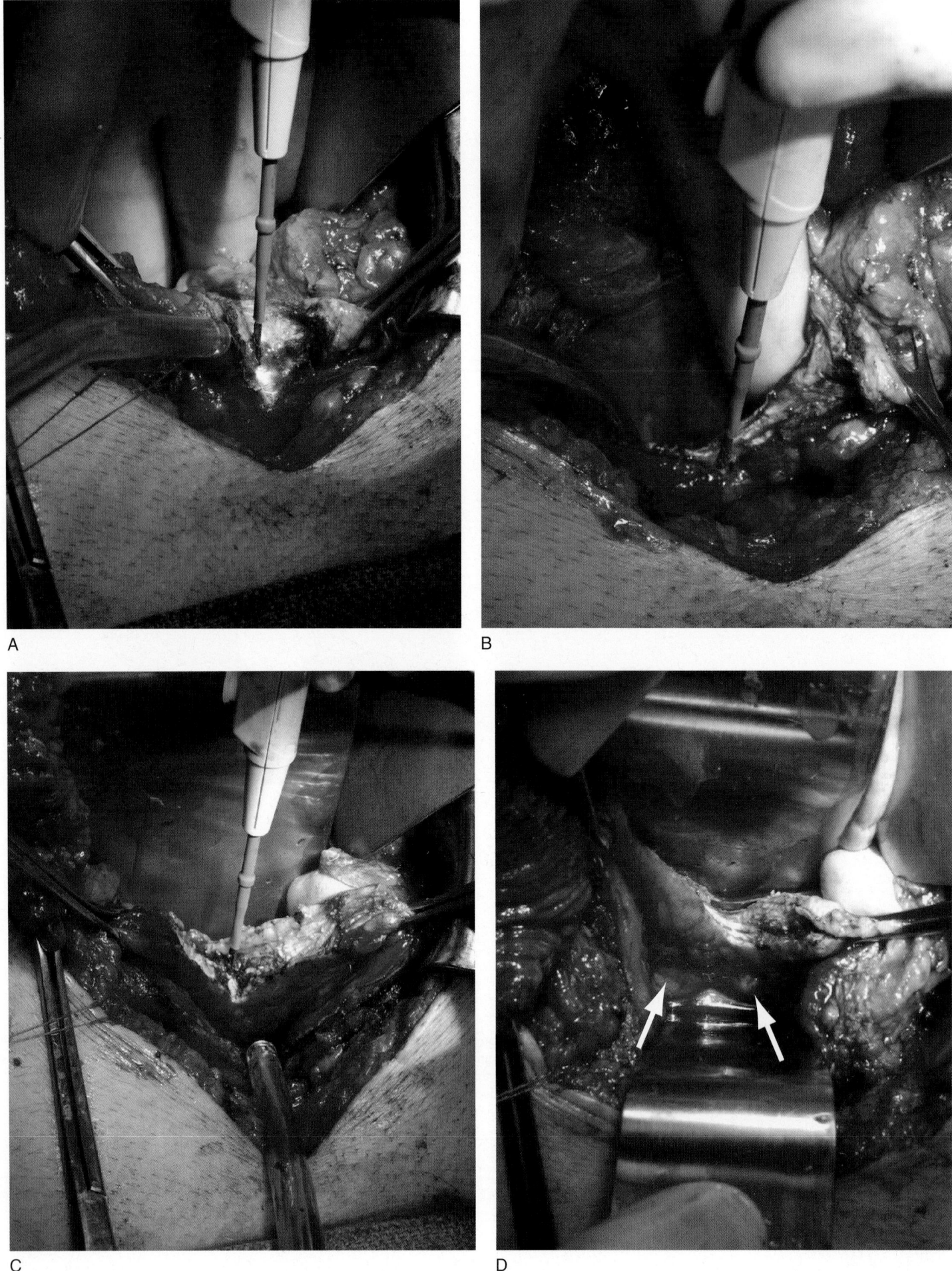

A

B

C

D

**FIGURE 92–13** **A.** To prepare the bladder, a sagittal cystotomy is made in the dome of the bladder. **B.** The cystotomy is carried anteriorly to 3 cm above the bladder neck and (**C**) posteriorly to 2 cm above the trigonal ridge. **D.** The prepared bladder is thus almost completely bivalved in the sagittal plane as depicted in the figure. The ureteral orifices are denoted by the arrows.

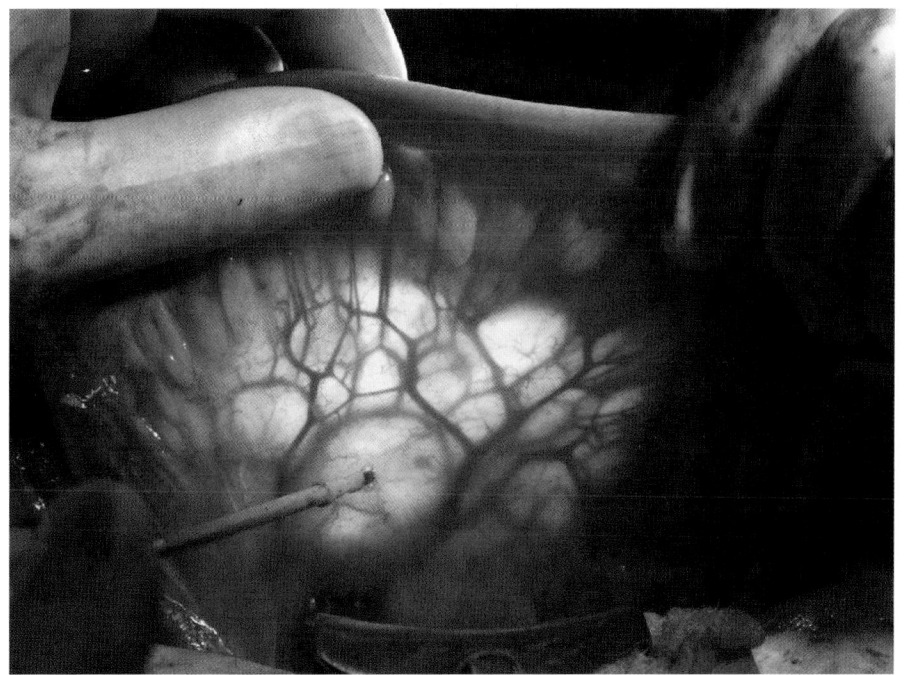

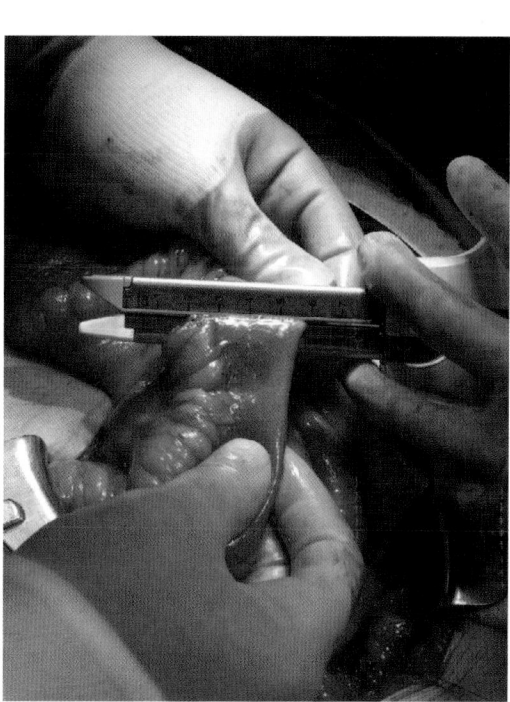

A

B

**FIGURE 92–14 A.** To isolate the bowel segment, the mesentery is divided so as to preserve blood supply to both the ileum segment and the eventual bowel anastomosis. **B.** Bowel division and reanastomosis may be performed using a handsewn technique or with bowel anastomotic staplers, as pictured in the figure. Here a 3.8-mm straight gastrointestinal stapler is used to divide the ileum.

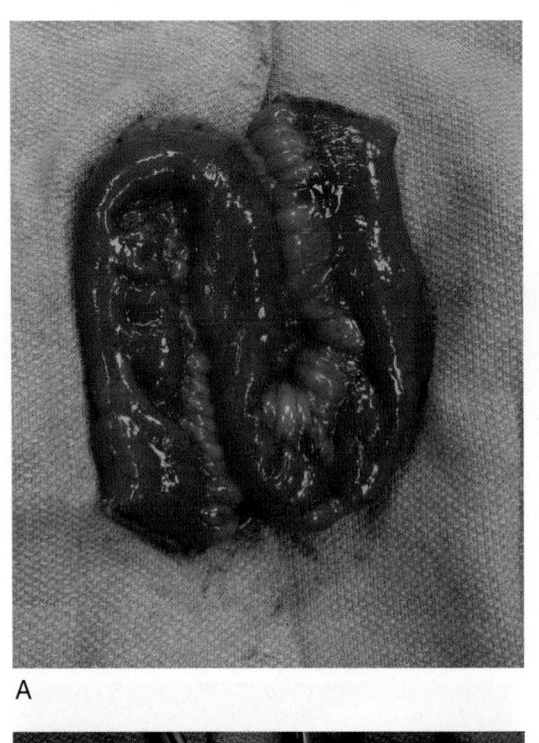

A

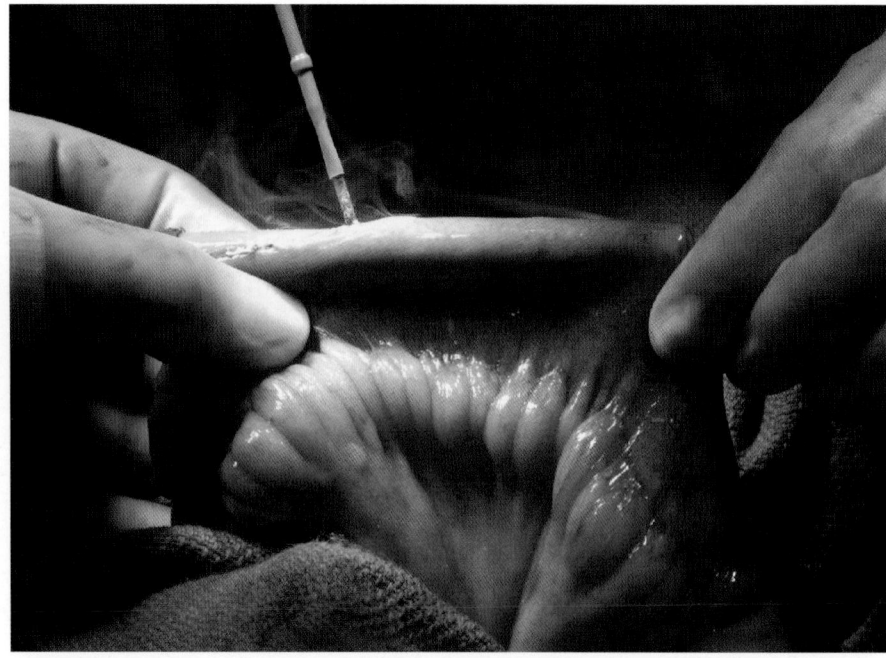

B

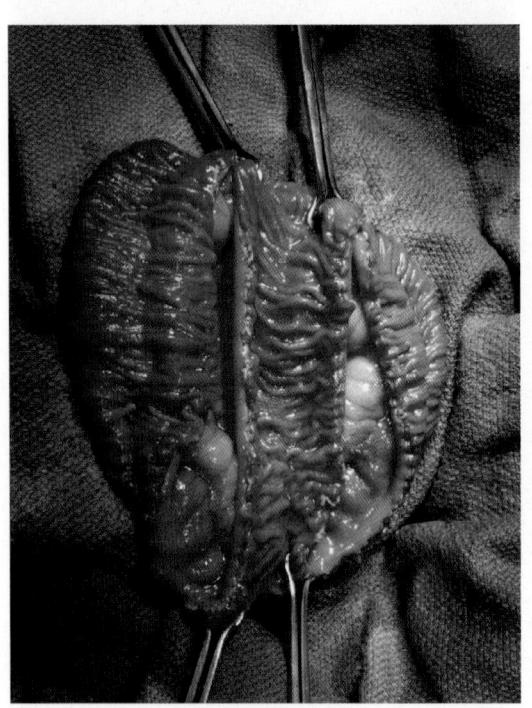

C

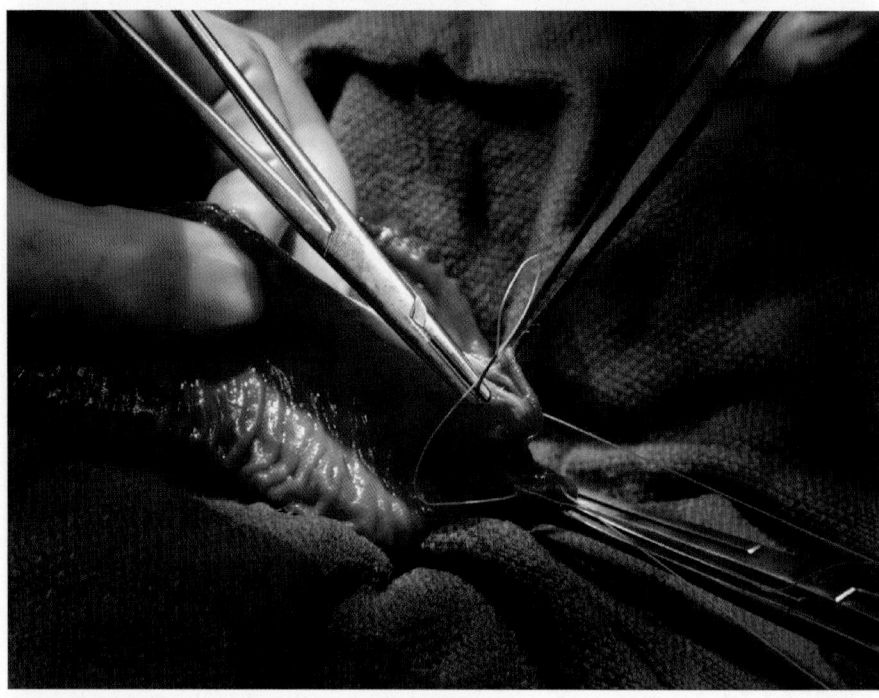

D

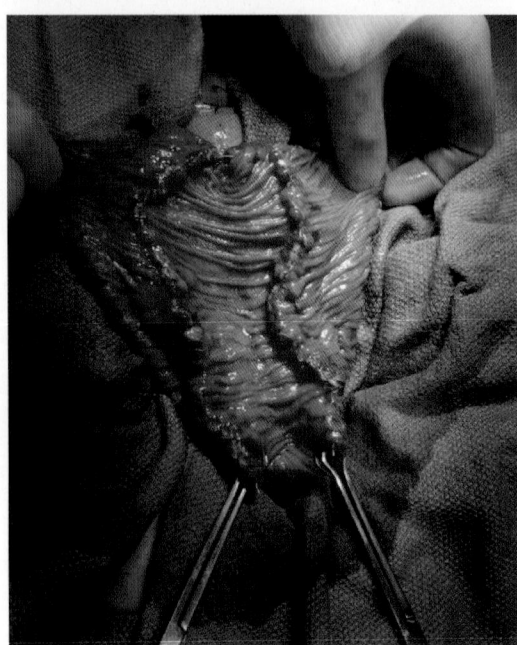

E

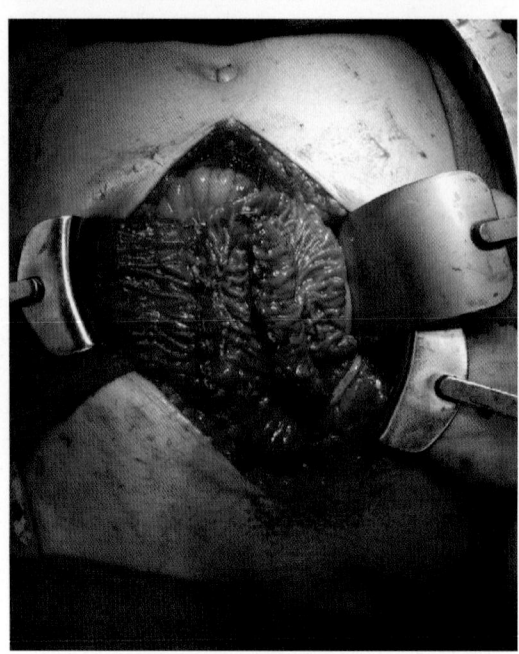

F

**FIGURE 92–15 A.** Typically, the bowel is reconfigured before anastomosing to the bladder to maximize spherical surface area; in this case, the bowel was arranged in an S shape as depicted. **B.** The bowel is incised longitudinally along the antimesentery border with electrocautery to completely detubularize the segment. **C.** This figure demonstrates the S configuration of the incised bowel before suturing. **D.** The two internal cut edges of the bowel are sutured longitudinally in a simple, running technique with 2-0 absorbable suture. **E.** The completely reconfigured ileal patch is shown aligned for anastomosis to the bladder. **F.** Beginning at the posterior apex of the bladder incision, the outer cut edges of the ileal patch and the bivalved bladder are sutured in a single layer with 2-0 absorbable suture, progressing in an anterior fashion until the entire patch is anastomosed to the bladder, effectively "clam-shelling" the ileal segment onto the dome of the bladder.

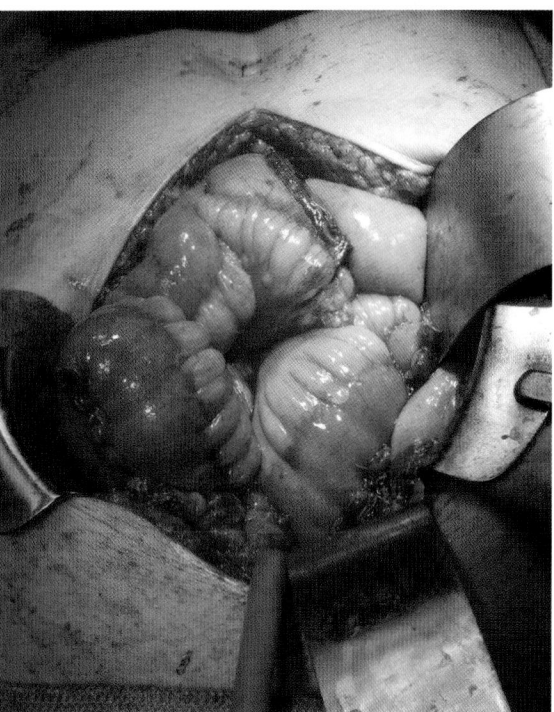

**FIGURE 92–16** The completed ileal augmentation is shown in the figure and is filled with saline, confirming the water-tightness of the closure. A suprapubic tube is placed before complete closure and is brought out to the abdominal wall through a separate stab incision.

# Bowel Surgery

# CHAPTER 93

# Intestinal Surgery

*Michael S. Baggish*

## Anatomy of the Small and Large Intestine

The intestines constitute the largest organ system within the abdominal cavity. Pelvic surgery always translates into some contact with the intestines. Although some individual variation may be noted, upon entering the peritoneal cavity of a person who has not previously been operated on, the greater omentum can be seen to cover the intestines (Fig. 93–1A). The omentum takes its origin from the greater curvature of the stomach and also attaches to the transverse colon (Fig. 93–1B). Beneath the omentum lies the small intestine (Fig. 93–2A). The small bowel measures $22\frac{1}{2}$ feet in length, and for the most part is completely covered with peritoneum and is suspended by a wide mesentery (Fig. 93–2B). The latter extends from the upper left abdomen to the lower right portion of the posterior wall of the abdomen (Fig. 93–3). The small intestine is divided into three portions: (1) duodenum, which is uncommonly related to gynecologic surgery; (2) jejunum; and (3) ileum; all three are frequently encountered (Fig. 93–4). The duodenal–jejunal junction is secured by a fibromuscular band on the upper left side of the abdomen. This band is called the ligament of Treitz. This is a convenient initial landmark for systematic examination of the entire small intestine for a suspected injury (Fig. 93–5A through C). Another important anatomic reference point is the ileocecal junction, where a valve connects the small to the large intestine (Fig. 93–6A, B). The small intestine receives its blood supply from the superior mesenteric artery via its mesentery (Fig. 93–7). The vessel branches into a series of arches, which terminate in a small straight artery that surrounds the segment of intestinal wall. The nerve supply emanates from the superior mesenteric plexus of nerves, which is in direct continuity with the celiac plexus.

The large bowel measures approximately 5 feet in length and can be distinguished from the small intestine by the presence of appendices epiploicae (three longitudinal bands of muscle fibers) and by its larger diameter (Fig. 93–8A). The large intestine forms a three-sided framelike structure (see Figs. 93–2B, 93–8B). On the right side, the cecum frequently dips into the pelvis and importantly terminates in the vermiform appendix. The ascending colon at its hepatic flexure imperceptively joins the transverse colon. The latter is located just beneath (inferior to) the stomach and connects to the left, or descending, colon at the splenic flexure.

The left (descending) colon joins the S-shaped sigmoid portion in the left iliac fossa. The sigmoid colon enters the pelvis by passing anterior to the sacrum and crossing it from the left to right side of the pelvis (Fig. 93–9). The sigmoid colon then curves back upon itself to the midline, descending just posterior to the uterus, where it joins the straight terminal portion of the colon (i.e., the rectum) (Fig. 93–9B). The sigmoid colon is completely surrounded by peritoneum and moves freely via its mesentery (sigmoid mesocolon). It is important to note that the sigmoid and the left colon are attached to the peritoneum along the lateral aspect of the abdominal wall. These attachments are not adhesions (Fig. 93–10A). The entire descending colon may be mobilized by cutting the peritoneum overlying the left gutter (Fig. 93–10B, C). At the lower pole of the aforesaid incision, the ovarian vessels and the psoas major muscle are encountered beneath the peritoneum (Fig. 93–10D). The inferior mesenteric artery supplies the left colon via three branches: the left colic, sigmoid, and superior hemorrhoidal arteries. This is an important area for collateral circulation between the middle and inferior hemorrhoidal branches of the hypogastric artery and the superior hemorrhoidal branch of the inferior mesenteric artery. The right side of the colon receives its blood supply from the ileocolic branch of the superior mesenteric artery (see Fig. 93–7).

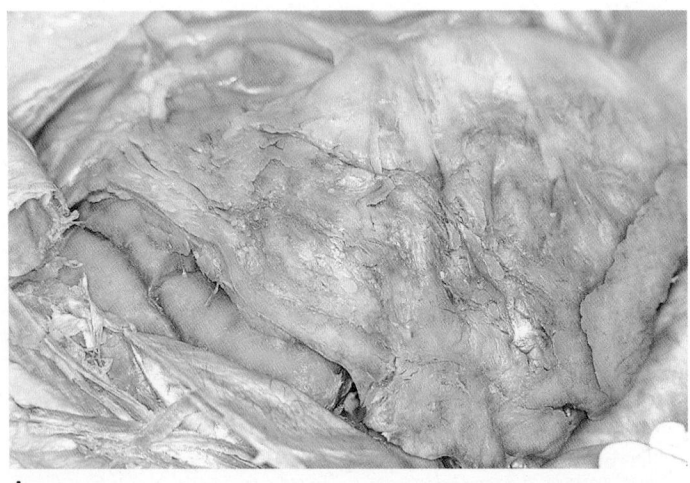

A

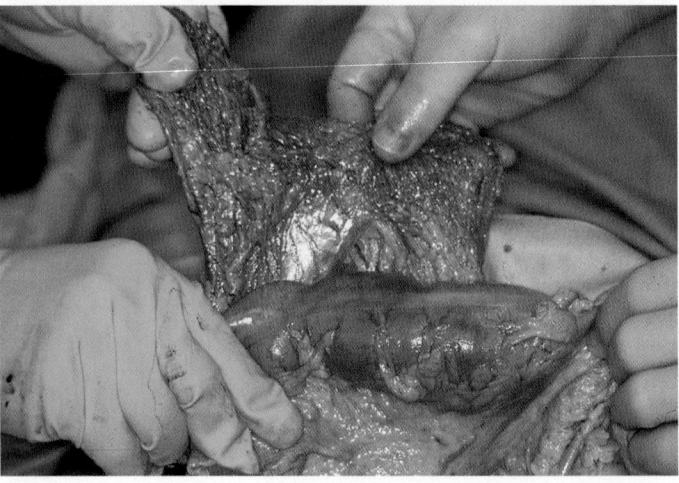

B

**FIGURE 93–1  A.** The abdomen has been opened and the peritoneal cavity entered. The greater omentum is draped over and, for the most part, covers the intestines. **B.** The stomach has been pulled out of the abdomen to demonstrate the omentum originating from the greater curvature and the transverse colon.

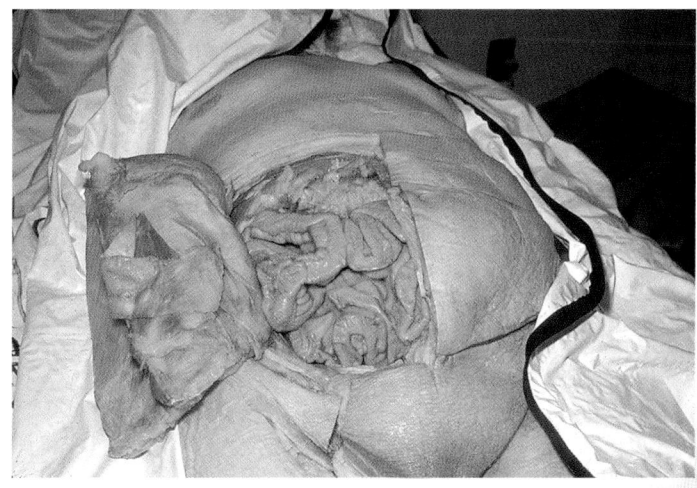

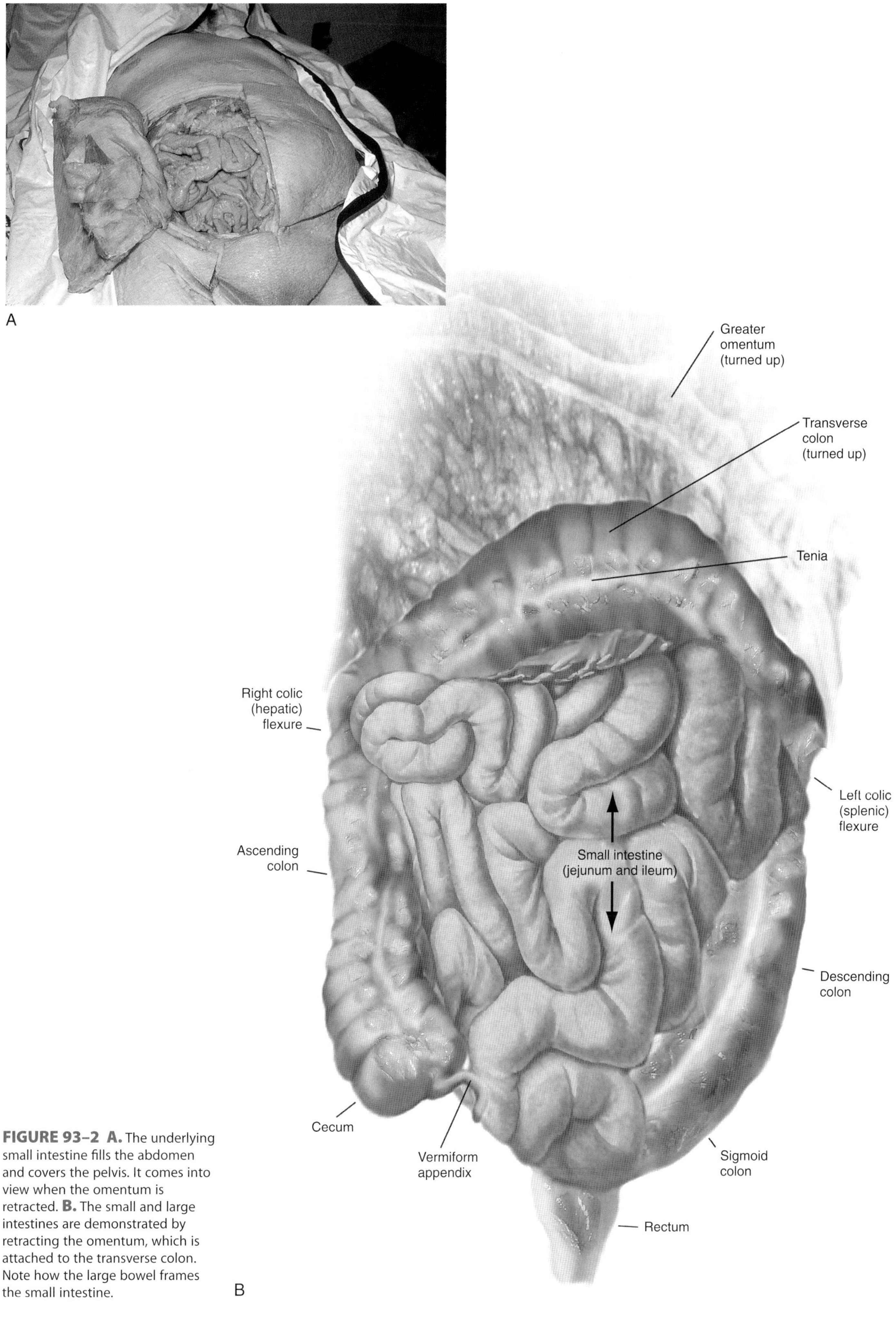

A

Greater
omentum
(turned up)

Transverse
colon
(turned up)

Tenia

Right colic
(hepatic)
flexure

Left colic
(splenic)
flexure

Ascending
colon

Small intestine
(jejunum and ileum)

Descending
colon

Cecum

Vermiform
appendix

Sigmoid
colon

Rectum

**FIGURE 93–2  A.** The underlying
small intestine fills the abdomen
and covers the pelvis. It comes into
view when the omentum is
retracted. **B.** The small and large
intestines are demonstrated by
retracting the omentum, which is
attached to the transverse colon.
Note how the large bowel frames
the small intestine.                        B

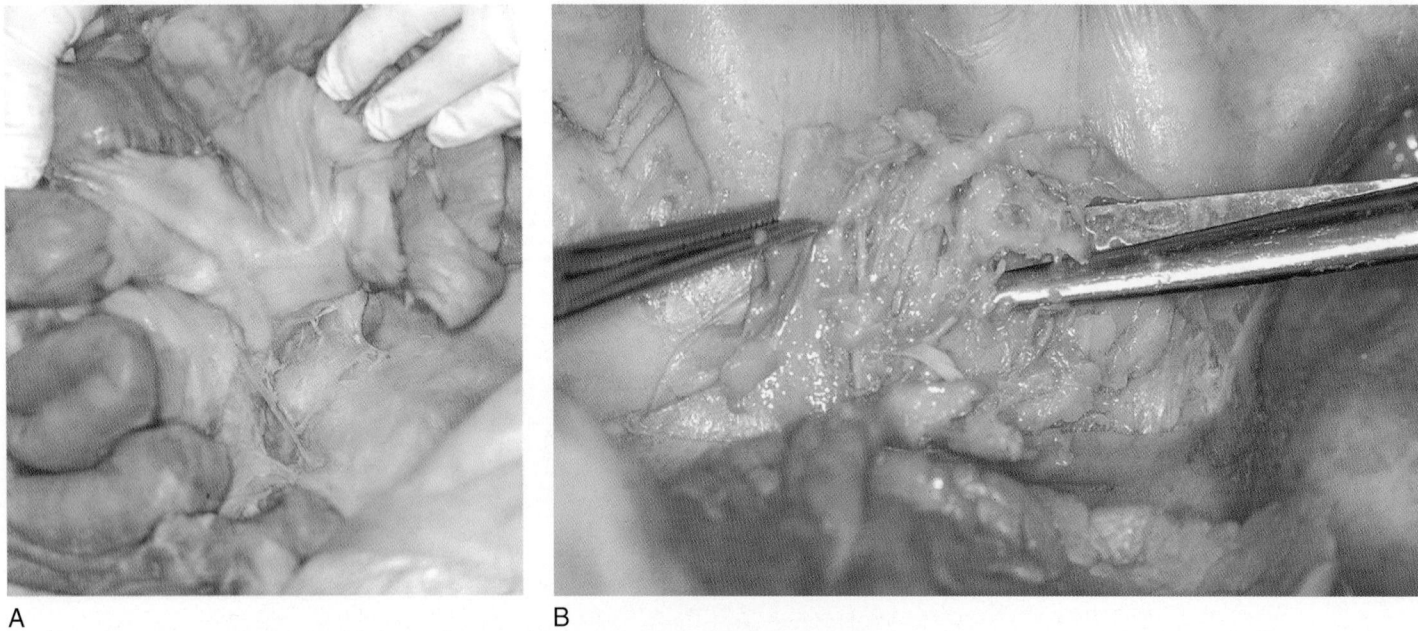

A                                                      B

**FIGURE 93–3 A.** The small intestine is supported by a mesentery, which sweeps from the upper left to the lower right quadrant. **B.** The mesentery contains the blood supply of the small bowel. The blood vessels are buried in the fat, which is sandwiched between the two layers of peritoneum.

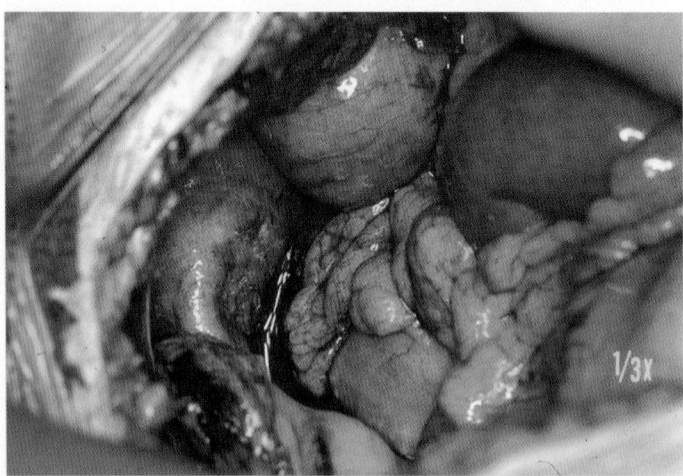

**FIGURE 93–4** The small bowel is divided into three portions; however, the duodenum is rarely encountered during gynecologic surgery. As can be seen here, the jejunum and ileum are commonly within the operative field.

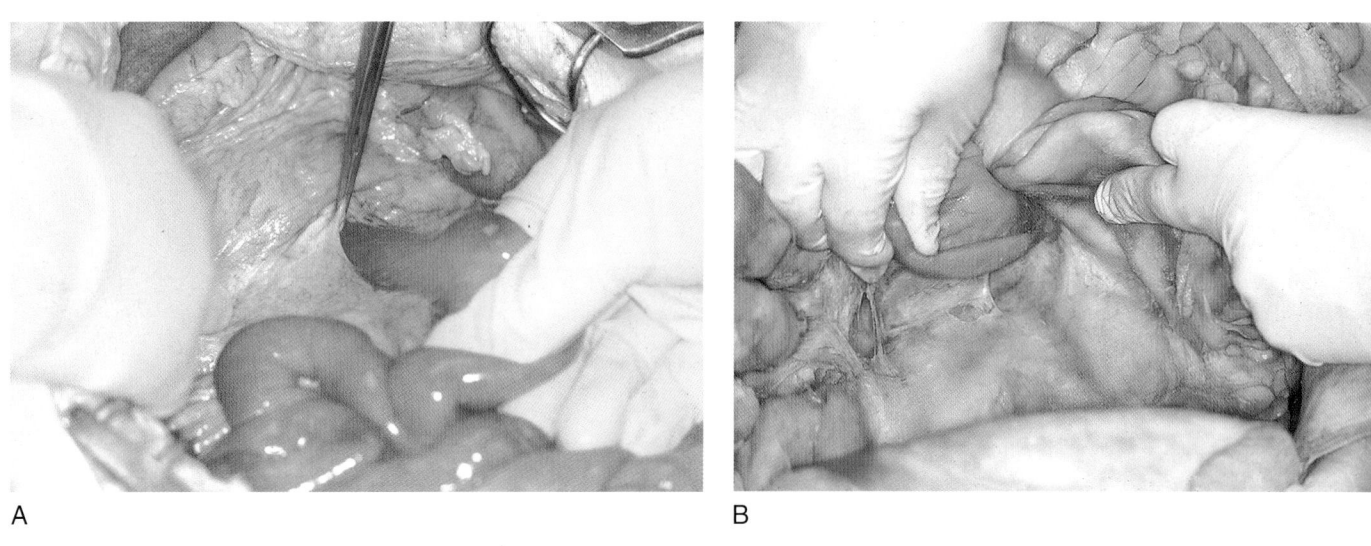

A

B

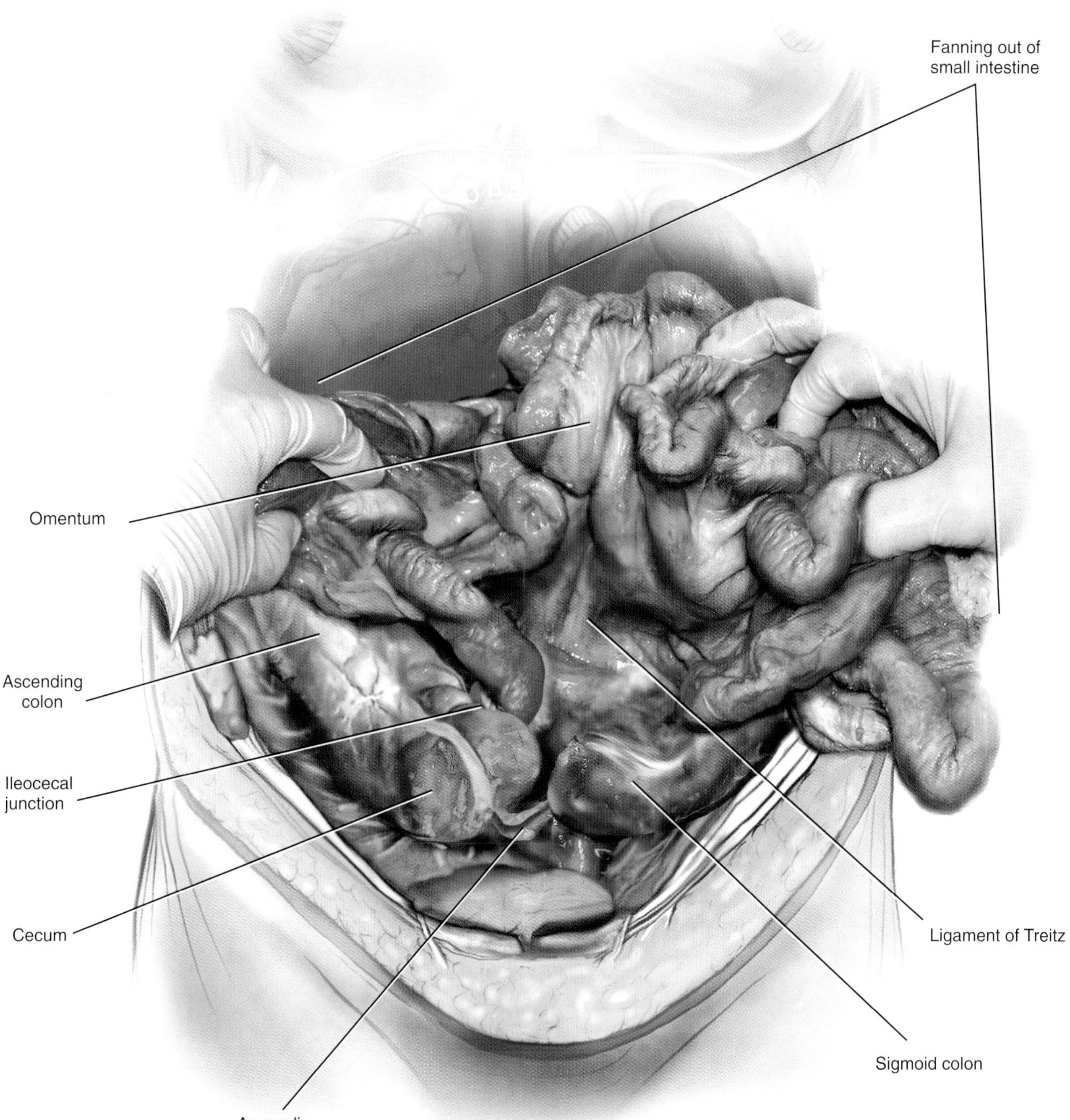

Fanning out of
small intestine

Omentum

Ascending
colon

Ileocecal
junction

Cecum

Appendix

Ligament of Treitz

Sigmoid colon

C

**FIGURE 93–5** **A.** At the junction of the jejunum and duodenum is a fibromuscular ligament attached to the intestine. This is the ligament of Treitz. **B.** Close-up view of the ligament of Treitz. The surgeon's finger points to the ligament. **C.** The small intestine is fanned out and anchored by its mesentery. The entire bowel is seen from the ileocecal junction to the ligament of Treitz.

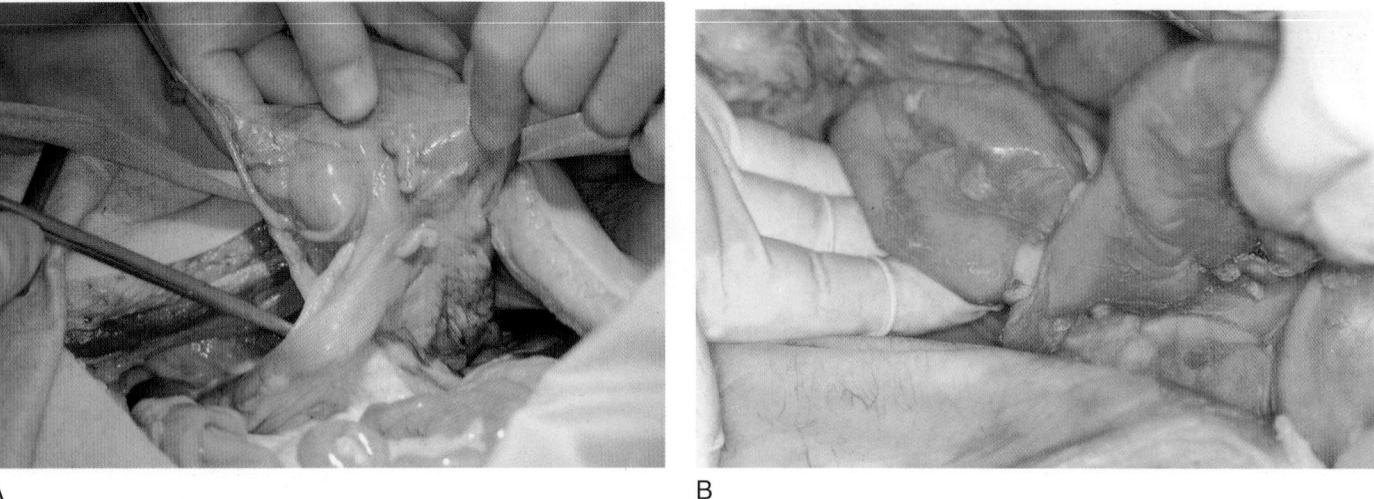

A    B

**FIGURE 93–6 A.** The surgeon is holding the cecum in his right hand and elevating the mobilized right colon. The ileum is tented up by a tonsil clamp. The ileocecal junction is clearly seen. **B.** The ileum joins the cecum at the ileocecal junction. The dissector's hand is resting under the cecum. The other hand is pulling on the terminal ileum.

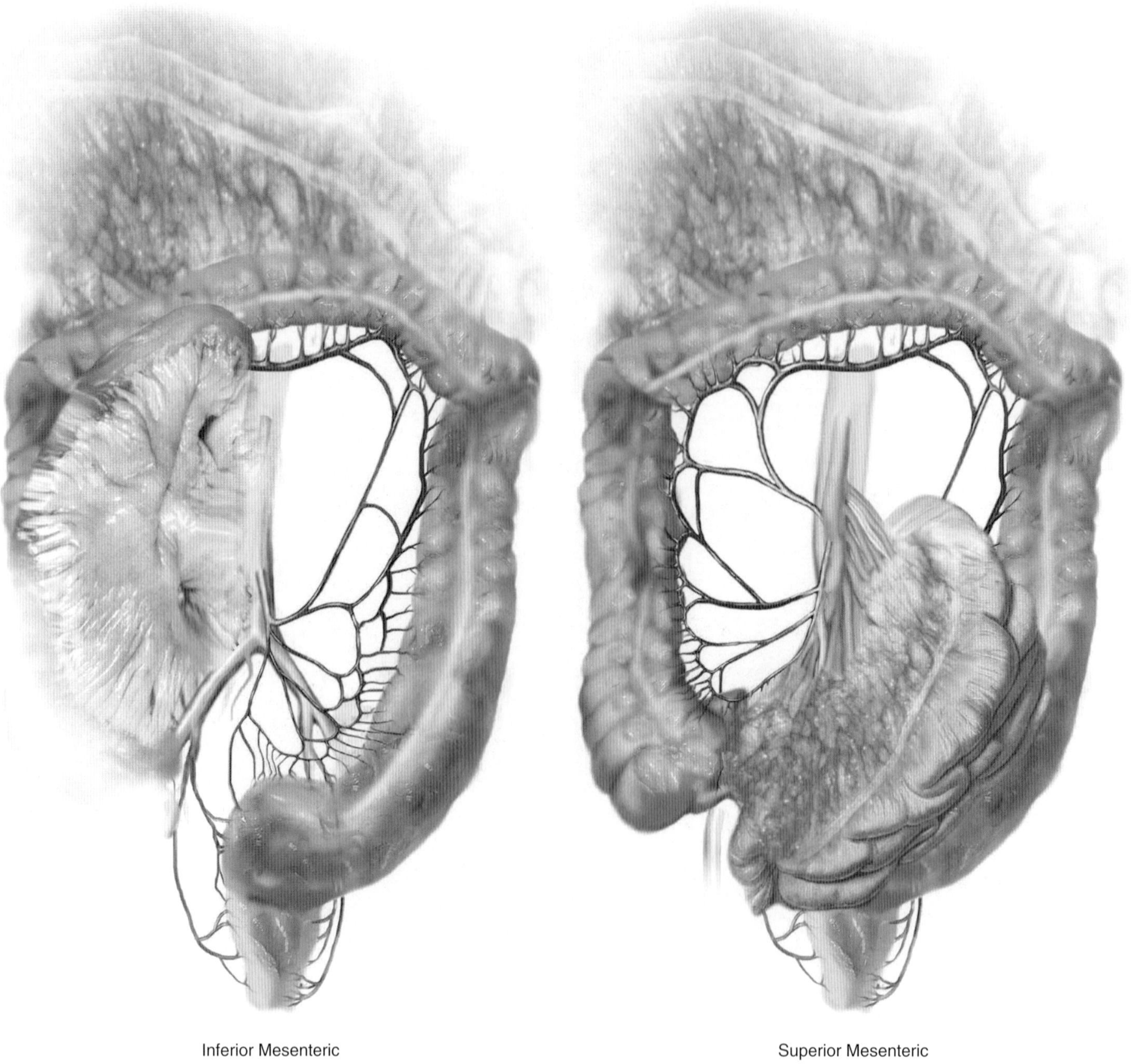

Inferior Mesenteric                                    Superior Mesenteric

**FIGURE 93–7** The small intestine is supplied by the superior mesenteric artery via a series of arcades. This major vessel also supplies the right colon and the right side of the transverse colon. The inferior mesenteric artery supplies the left transverse, left colon, sigmoid colon, and rectum.

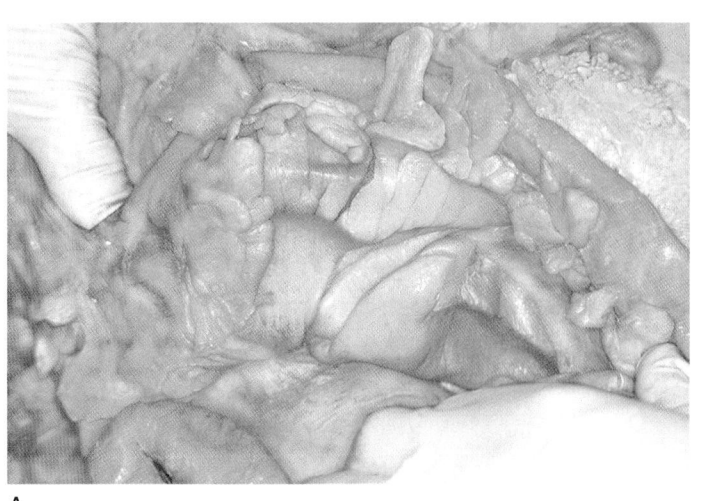

A

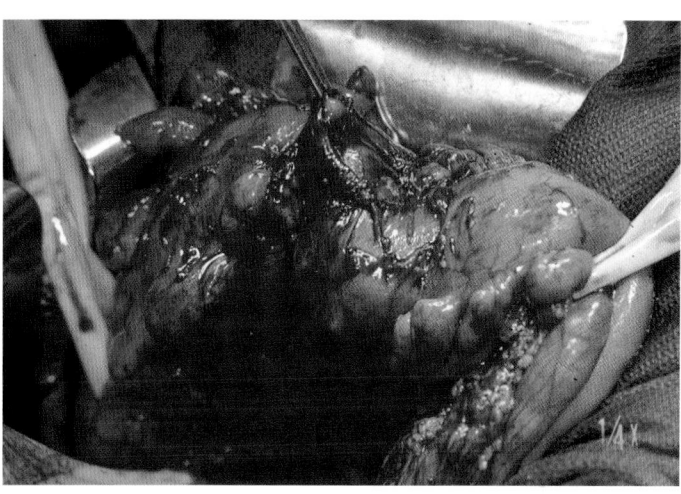

B

**FIGURE 93–8  A.** The transverse colon with its prominent appendices epiploicae and taeniae is shown here. **B.** The transverse colon is held by two rubber retractors. Note that the combined ascending, transverse, and descending colon frames the abdominal contents.

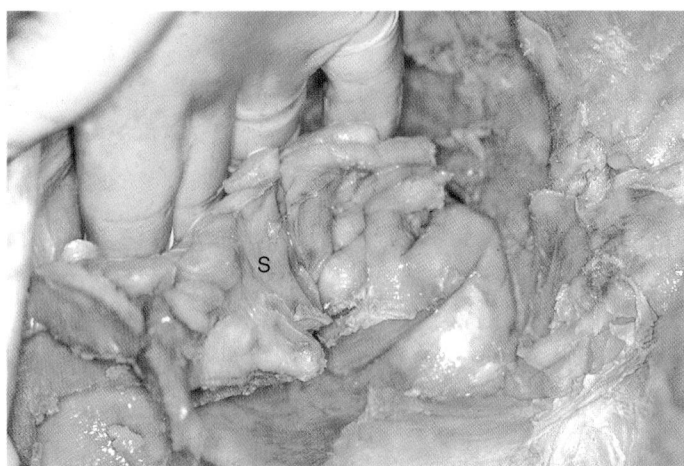

**FIGURE 93–9**  The sigmoid colon vectors from left to right over the sacrum, then turns upon itself back to the midline. The left colon is seen on the lower left side of the picture (l). The left colon joins the sigmoid (s), which veers to the right and descends into the pelvis.

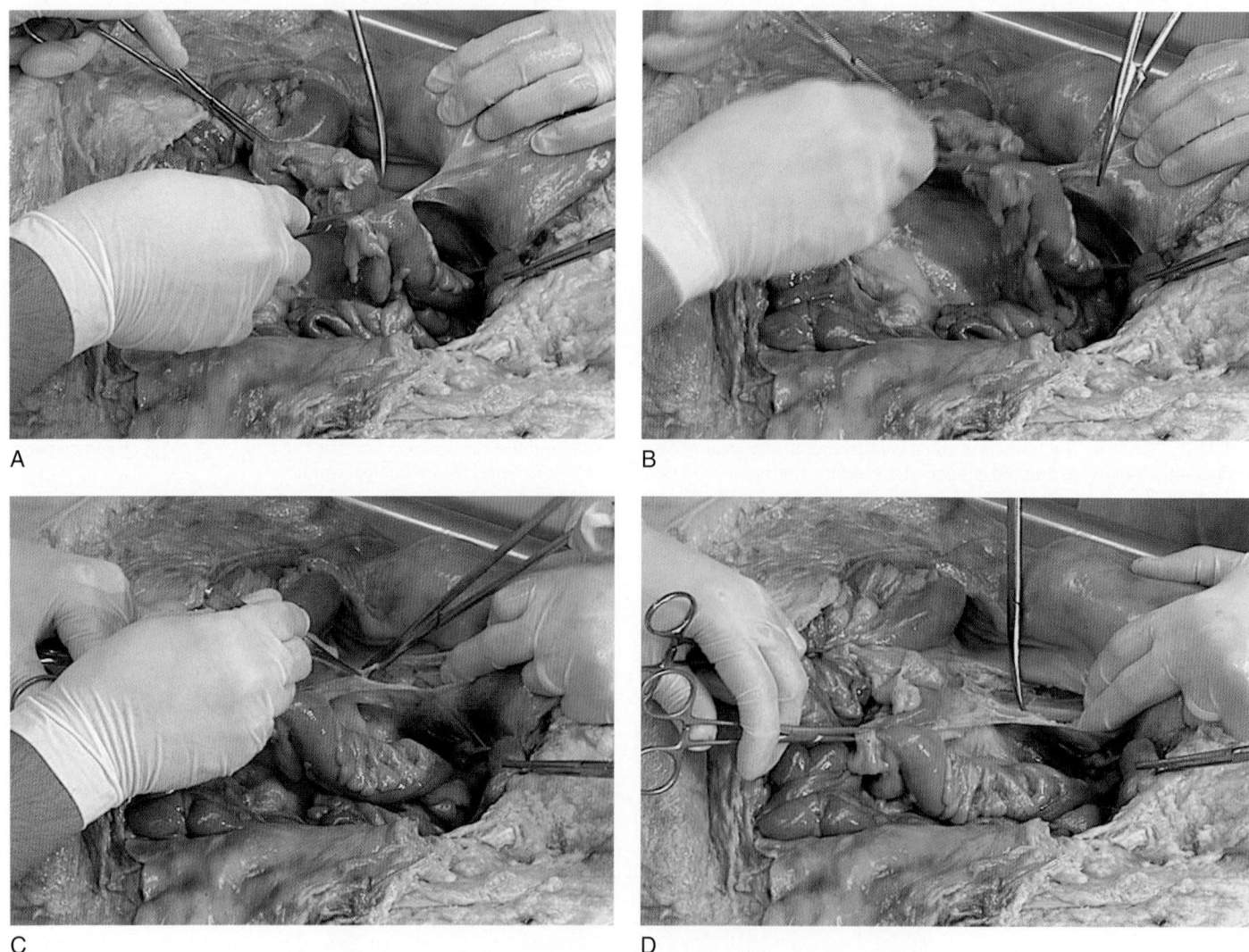

A

B

C

D

**FIGURE 93–10 A.** The left colon and the upper sigmoid colon attach to the lateral abdominal wall. These are normal peritoneal attachments.
**B.** The peritoneum at the left colonic gutter may be opened. **C.** The avascular plane may be opened along the entire length of the left colon.
**D.** The colon can be completely mobilized. Note the relationship of the sigmoid colon to the psoas major muscle, which is visible at the cut edge
of the peritoneum.

# CHAPTER 94

# Small Bowel Repair/Resection

*Brian J. Albers* ■ *David J. Lamon*

The small intestine is a continuation of the gastrointestinal (GI) tract, extending from the duodenal bulb to the ileocecal valve. It comprises the luminal mucosa, an inner circular layer and outer longitudinal layer of muscle, and the external serosa. For surgical purposes, the small bowel has two layers: the inner mucosa and the outer serosa. Blood is supplied by the mesentery, whose vessel of origin is the superior mesenteric artery and vein.

Isolation of the segment to be resected is done with noncrushing clamps across the bowel proximally and distally (Fig. 94–1). The mesentery is taken down with clamps and ligated with 2-0 silk free ties (Figs. 94–2 and 94–3). If a handsewn anastomosis is desired, the bowel is sharply divided along the edge of a noncrushing clamp. The injured segment is removed, and the two ends of remaining small bowel are opposed and held aligned with traction sutures of 3-0 silk (Fig. 94–4). Circumferential, single-layer, 3-0 silk, interrupted sutures are used for the anastomosis (Fig. 94–5) with inversion of the mucosa (Fig. 94–6). All sutures are placed under direct visualization (Fig. 94–7), with palpable confirmation of a patent anastomotic ring (Fig. 94–8). The mesenteric defect is then closed to prevent internal herniation (Fig. 94–9).

If a stapled anastomosis is planned, the resected segment is excised with successive firing of a GIA 75-mm stapling device.

The proximal and distal segments are then affixed in parallel with seromuscular sutures at the inner mesenteric border (Figs. 94–10 and 94–11). Enterotomies are created to admit the stapler (Fig. 94–12), which is fired as the bowel segments are rotated to oppose the antimesenteric borders of each segment (Fig. 94–13). The anastomosis is briefly inspected for significant mucosal bleeding. If none is found, the enterotomy is then grasped with Allis clamps. The edges are opposed perpendicular to the direction of the side-to-side anastomosis just created (Fig. 94–14). Firing the GIA across and under the clamps creates a functional end-to-end anastomosis (Fig. 94–15). The mesenteric rent is then closed.

Repair of a transmural injury may be performed on unprepped small bowel with minimal risk, as long as good technique is used. The edges of the perforated bowel should be trimmed before suturing. Simple transmural lacerations not involving the mesentery may be closed transversely (Heineke-Mikulicz operation closing the wound so as not to constrict the lumen) by placement of corner traction sutures and single-layer interrupted 3-0 silk (Figs. 94–16 and 94–17). Multiple focal injuries or devascularization requires resection with anastomosis. This can be handsewn or stapled, with similar results.

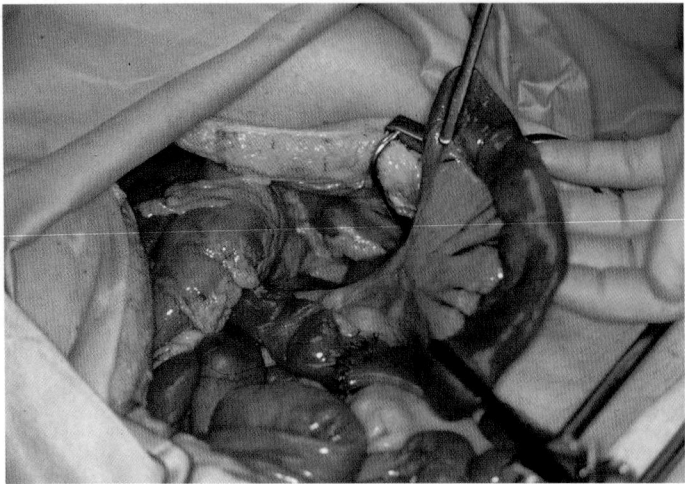

**FIGURE 94–1** The segment to be resected is isolated from enteric flow by application of proximal and distal noncrushing clamps to prevent further contamination.

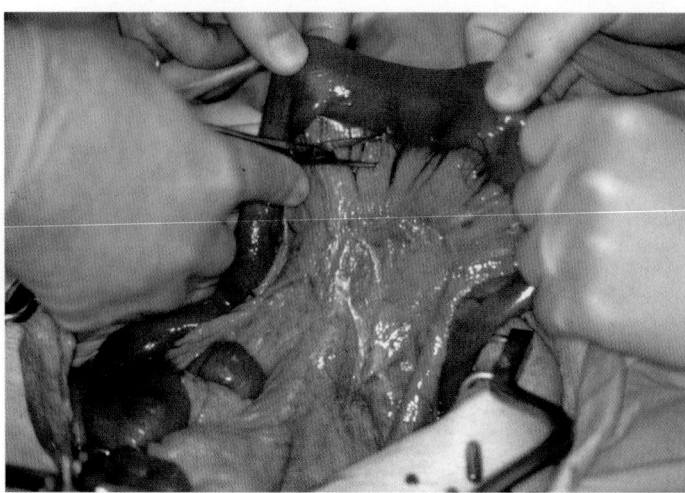

**FIGURE 94–2** A defect in the mesenteric border is created at the proximal and distal ends to be resected, staying close to the bowel wall.

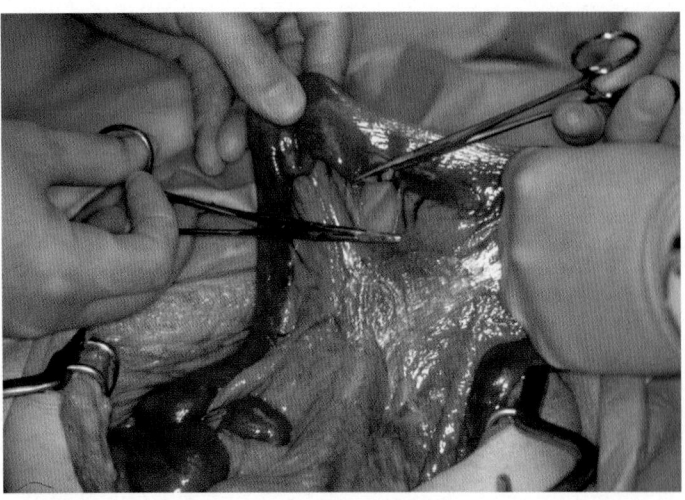

**FIGURE 94–3** The mesentery is then taken down between clamps and ligated with 2-0 silk suture.

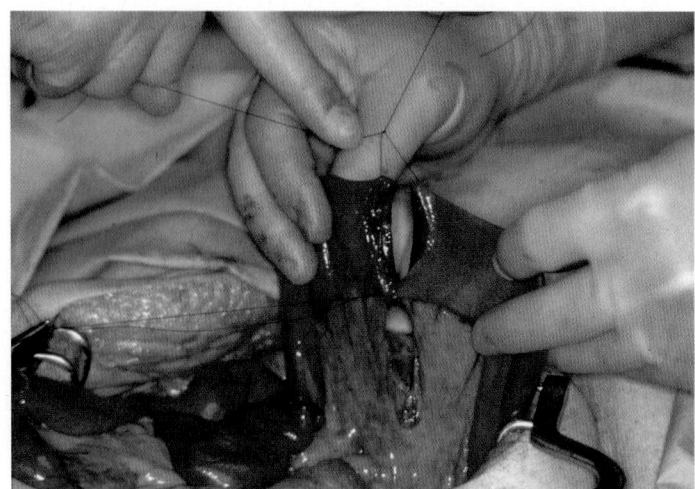

**FIGURE 94–4** Once devascularized, the bowel segment is excised sharply. Mucosal bleeding should be evident from the opposed ends to be anastomosed. Brisk mucosal bleeding can be controlled with judicious use of electrocautery. The ends of the bowel to be anastomosed are aligned and held in place with 3-0 silk traction sutures placed at the mesenteric and antimesenteric borders.

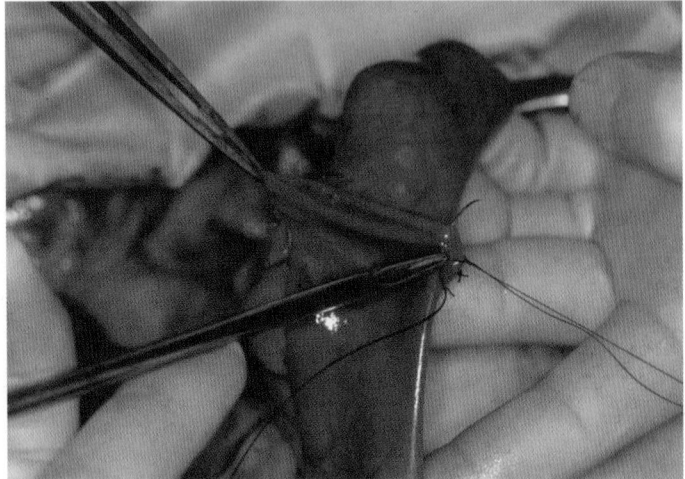

**FIGURE 94–5** Single-layer, interrupted 3-0 silk sutures are used to perform the anastomosis. Care is taken to incorporate 4 to 5 mm of serosa and just the edge of the mucosa with each needle throw through the bowel edges. Knots are tied on the outside and are spaced 4 mm apart.

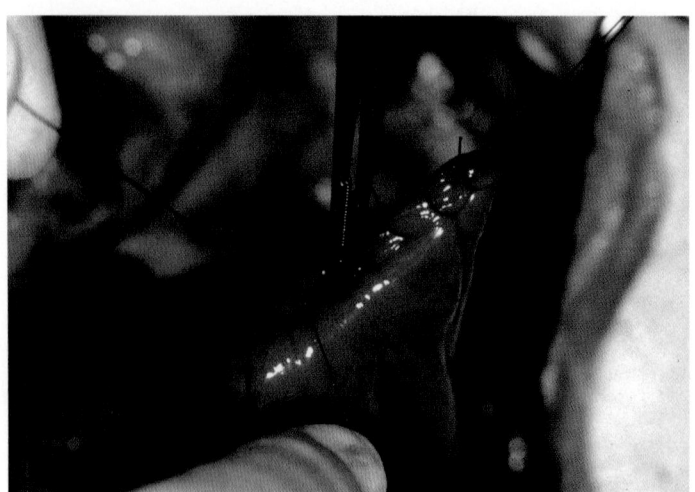

**FIGURE 94–6** When the anastomotic suture is tied, care is taken to invert the mucosa while setting the knot.

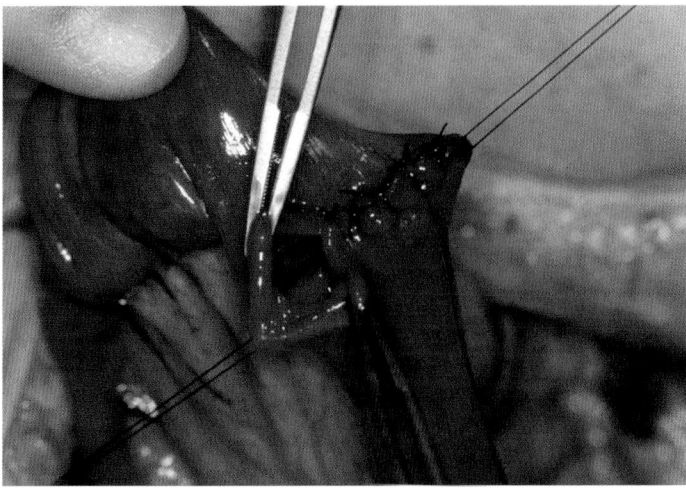

**FIGURE 94–7** Nearing completion of the anastomosis, the last several sutures are left untied until the last suture is placed to permit full visualization of each needle throw. Inspect the corner suture placement carefully to ensure there are no gaps.

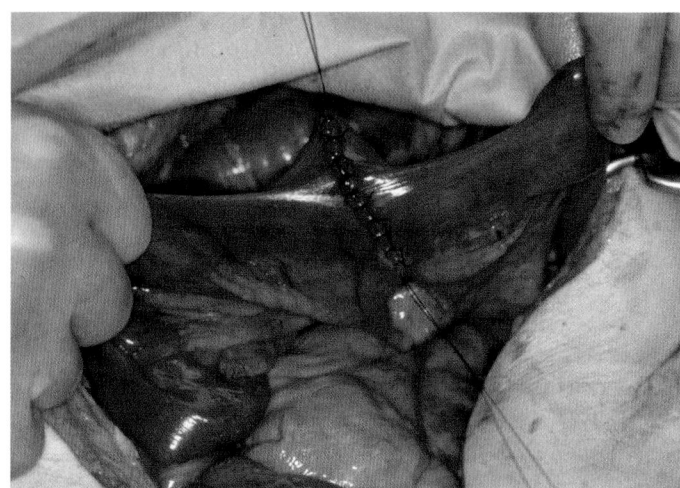

**FIGURE 94–8** Once completed, the anastomosis is inspected circumferentially. Any gaps between sutures are filled with 3-0 silk interrupted serosal sutures placed superficially, taking care not to encroach on the lumen. The anastomotic ring is palpated, and continuity is ensured by admittance of a fingertip through the ring. The traction sutures are then tied and cut.

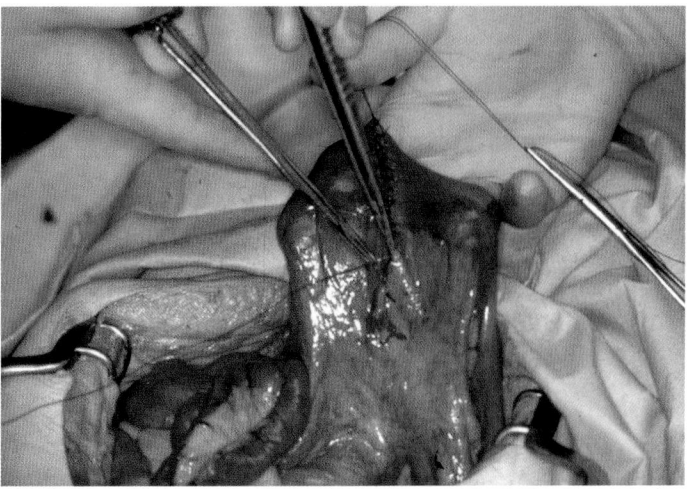

**FIGURE 94–9** The mesenteric defect is then closed with interrupted 3-0 silk sutures, incorporating only the peritoneum and avoiding the underlying vessels.

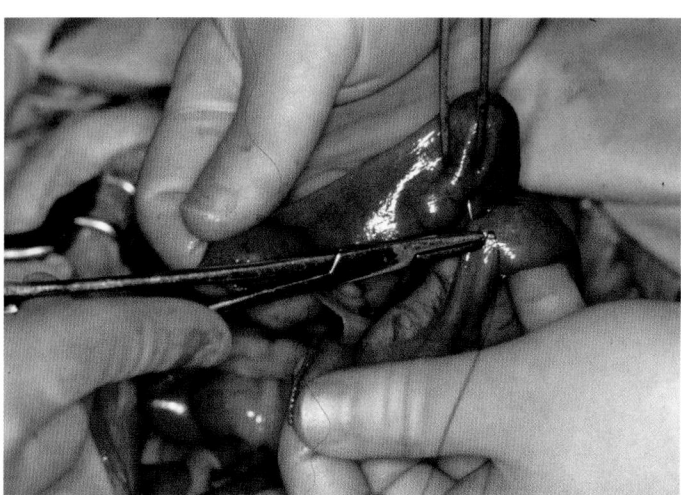

**FIGURE 94–10** The proximal and distal portions of divided small bowel are held parallel to each other. A single seromuscular 3-0 silk traction suture is placed at the inner mesenteric border, joining the two segments approximately 100 mm from the stapled edge.

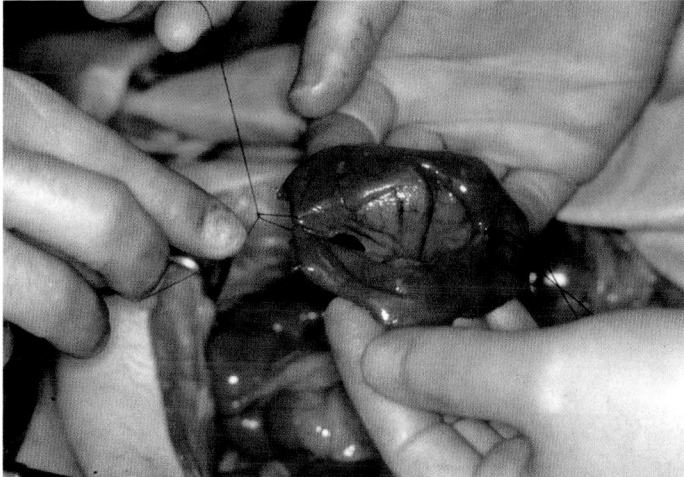

**FIGURE 94–11** Another seromuscular traction suture is placed at the inner mesenteric border, near the mesenteric side of the staple lines.

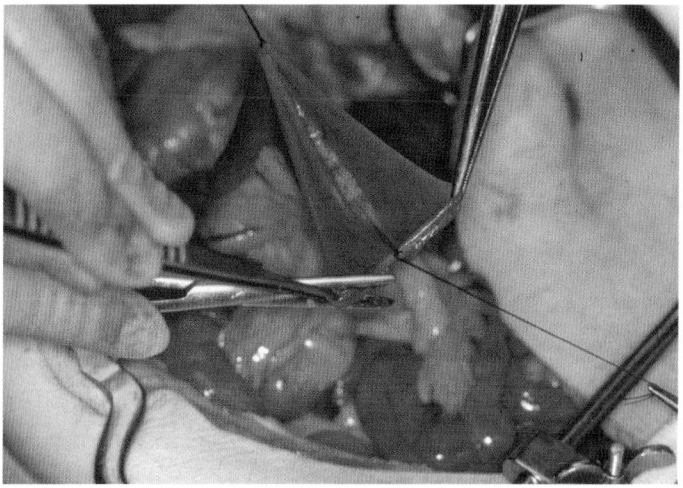

**FIGURE 94–12** The antimesenteric edge of each staple line is then sharply opened only enough to permit entry of the GIA stapling device (75 mm).

UNIT 4  ■  SECTION B

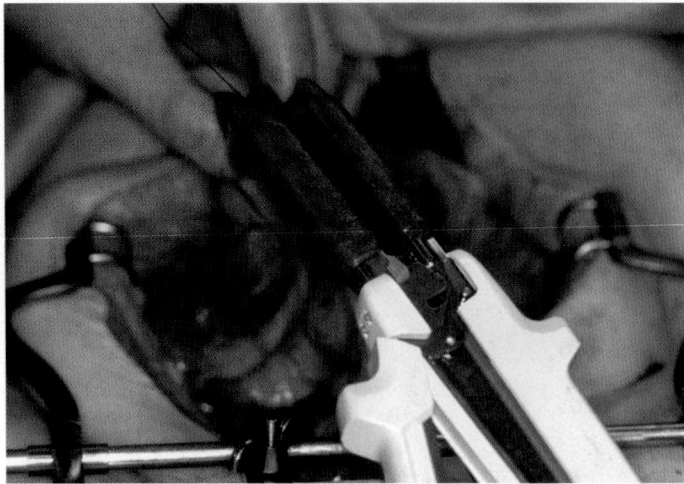

**FIGURE 94–13** The stapling anvil and cartridge are placed into each limb of the bowel as shown. Downward traction is then applied to the previously placed mesenteric traction sutures, thereby rotating the bowel so that the antimesenteric bowel borders are opposed between the jaws of the stapler. Once the operator is satisfied that no mesenteric fat is caught in the staple line, as evidenced by the ability to run a finger along both sides of the stapler while touching only serosa, the stapling device is fired.

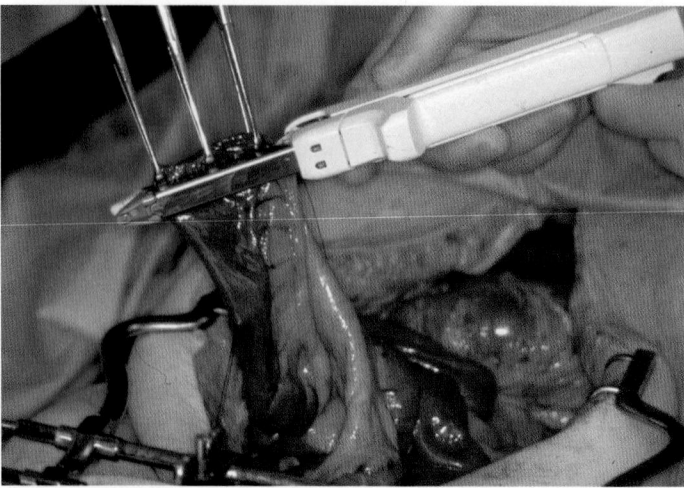

**FIGURE 94–14** Once the fired stapler is removed, the side-to-side small bowel anastomosis can be visually inspected for significant mucosal bleeding. If none is found, several Allis clamps are used to grasp the enterotomy edges in a fashion that incorporates generous amounts of serosa perpendicular to the direction of the side-by-side anastomosis. Ideally this should incorporate the staple lines from the original resection edges, as well as the traction sutures adjacent to these.

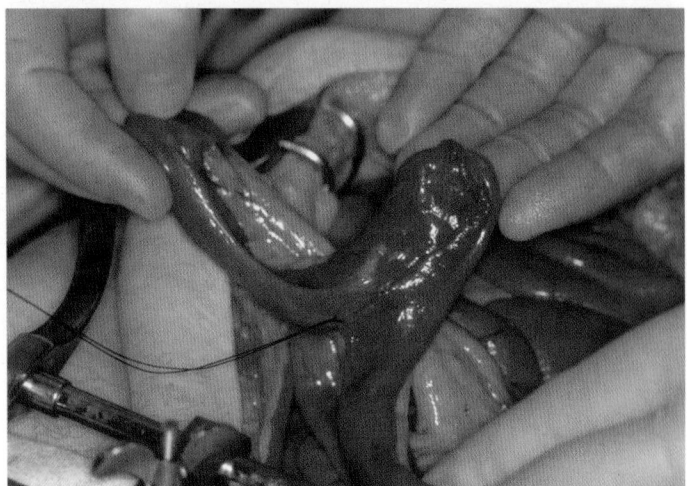

**FIGURE 94–15** The stapler is reloaded, positioned as described, and is fired, with the resulting side-to-side, now functional end-to-end anastomosis appearing like this. Inspect the stapled edges carefully, milking enteric contents through the anastomosis to check for leaks. Close the mesenteric defect as previously described.

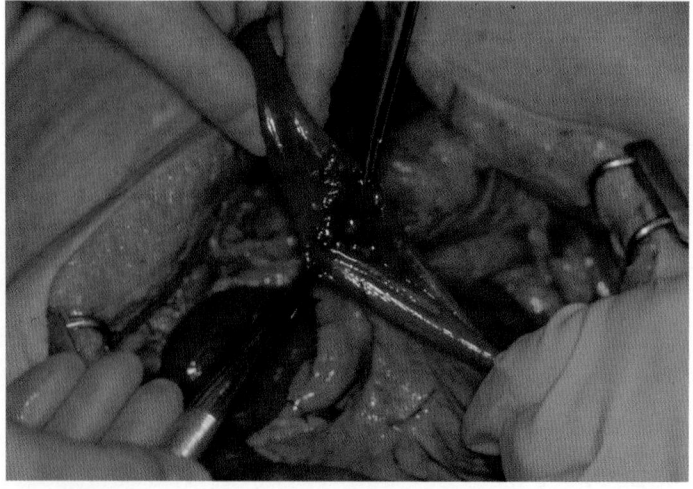

**FIGURE 94–16** A transmural laceration in the small bowel is shown. The mesentery is not involved. Simple closure is sufficient.

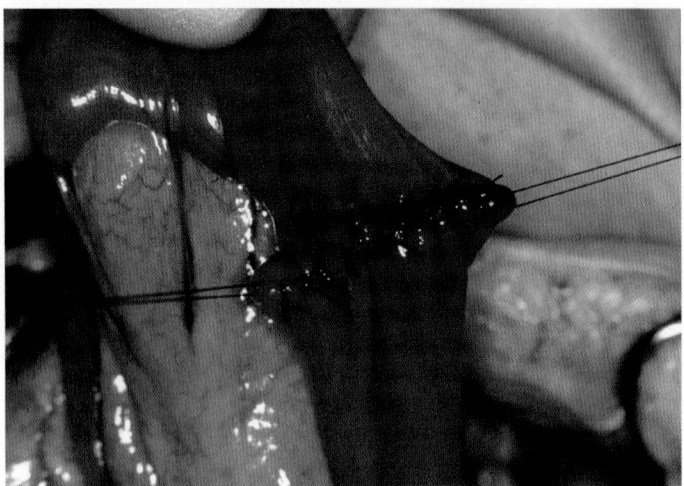

**FIGURE 94–17** Corner sutures of 3-0 silk are placed and are used to elongate the laceration in a transverse fashion to facilitate closure with interrupted 3-0 silk sutures placed approximately 4 mm apart, with bites encompassing 4 to 5 mm of serosa and just the edge of the mucosa on each side of the defect. The knots are tied as the mucosa is invaginated. The repair is then checked for leaks and luminal patency.

# CHAPTER 95

# Closure of a Simple Transmural Injury to the Small Intestine

*Michael S. Baggish*

An injury to the wall of the small intestine incurred during a pelvic dissection can be managed without resorting to an intestinal resection if the blood supply to the bowel segment has not been interrupted. Observation of the intestine will show the bowel to maintain a healthy pink color (Fig. 95–1). Next, the edges of the wound should be trimmed with a fine scissors (Fig. 95–2A, B). The cut edges should bleed to further indicate healthy intestinal tissue. Next, a through-and-through closure utilizing 2-0 or 3-0 chromic catgut is placed as interrupted sutures (Fig. 95–2C). A second imbricating layer of 2-0 interrupted silk is sutured into the muscularis and serosa (Fig. 95–2D through F). The suture line is irrigated and the bowel lumen is checked for adequacy between the surgeon's thumb and fingers.

Alternatively, contemporary surgical techniques utilize a simple single-layer closure consisting of 2-0 silk sutures. The needle and suture penetrate serosa, muscularis, and mucosa on one side of the defect, and mucosa, muscularis, and serosa on the other. Each extreme is tied first, followed then by the remaining ligatures. The wound is irrigated with normal saline, then the lumen is checked for adequacy (Fig. 95–3A through C).

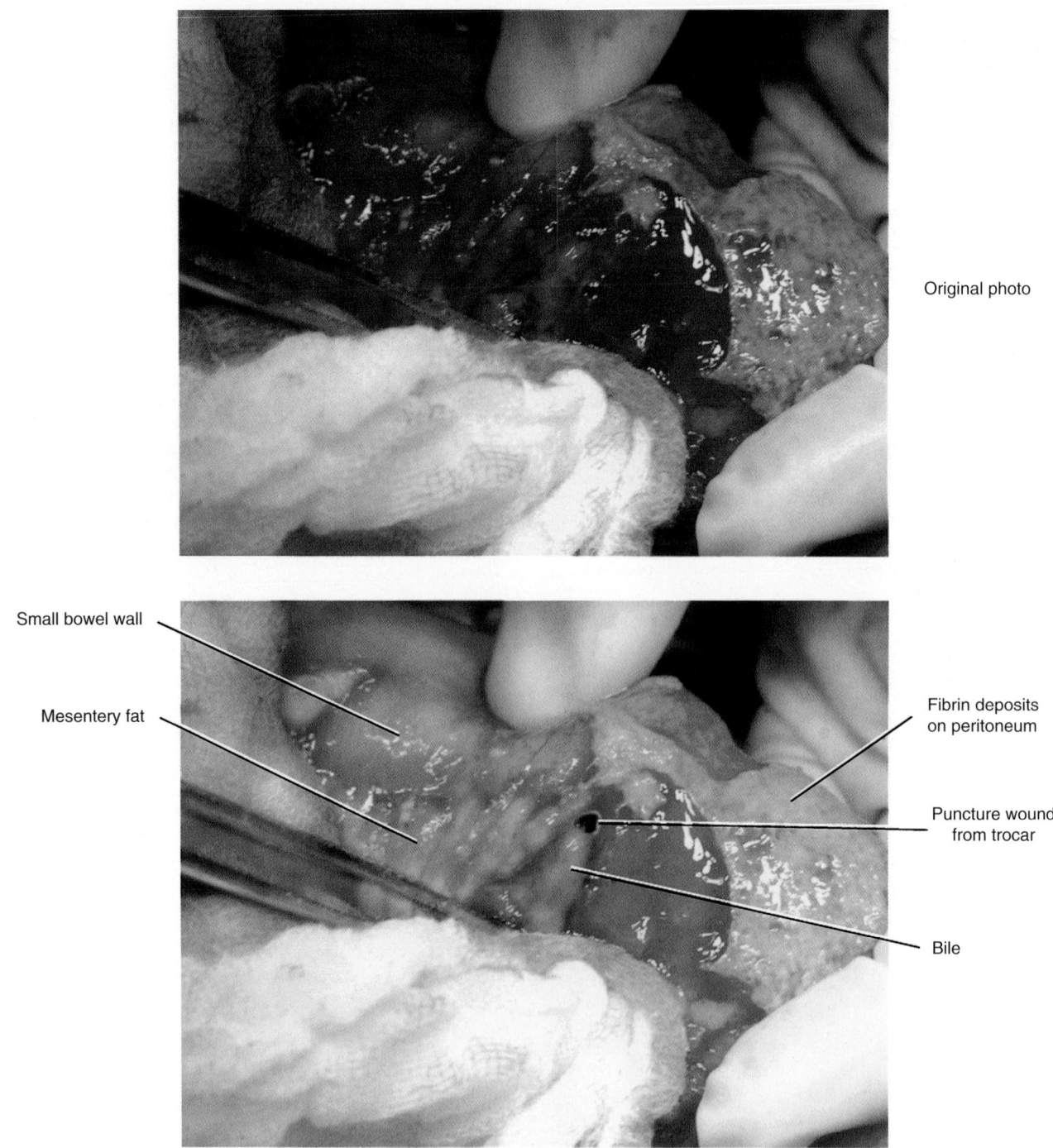

Original photo

Small bowel wall

Mesentery fat

Fibrin deposits
on peritoneum

Puncture wound
from trocar

Bile

**Decompress forcing out bowel
contents and collapsing bowel wall**

**FIGURE 95–1** The original actual photograph shows a bowel perforation just above the mesenteric border of the small intestine. Blood and fibrin are present on the bowel. Above the forceps, bile-stained intestinal contents spill from the wound. Note the bubbles of air. Below, the artist has drawn the same injury for emphasis.

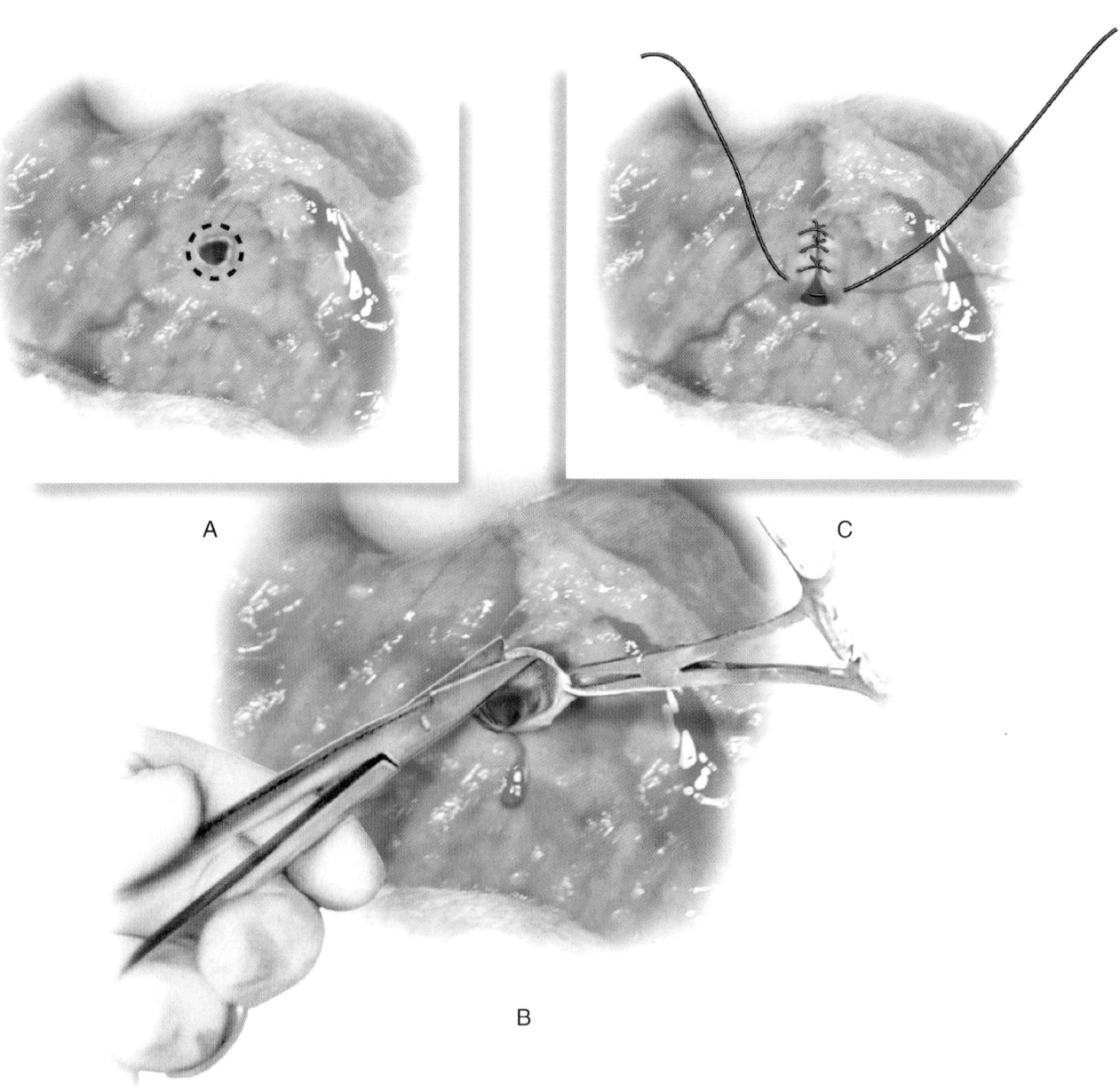

A

C

B

**FIGURE 95–2  A.** An outline of the portion of intestinal wall to be debrided. **B.** The surgeon cuts away devitalized tissue around the margin of the perforation. Good blood flow from the incision edges ensures viability. **C.** Chromic catgut sutures placed through serosa, muscularis, submucosa, and mucosa (through-and-through), and then vice versa in interrupted fashion, close the defect.

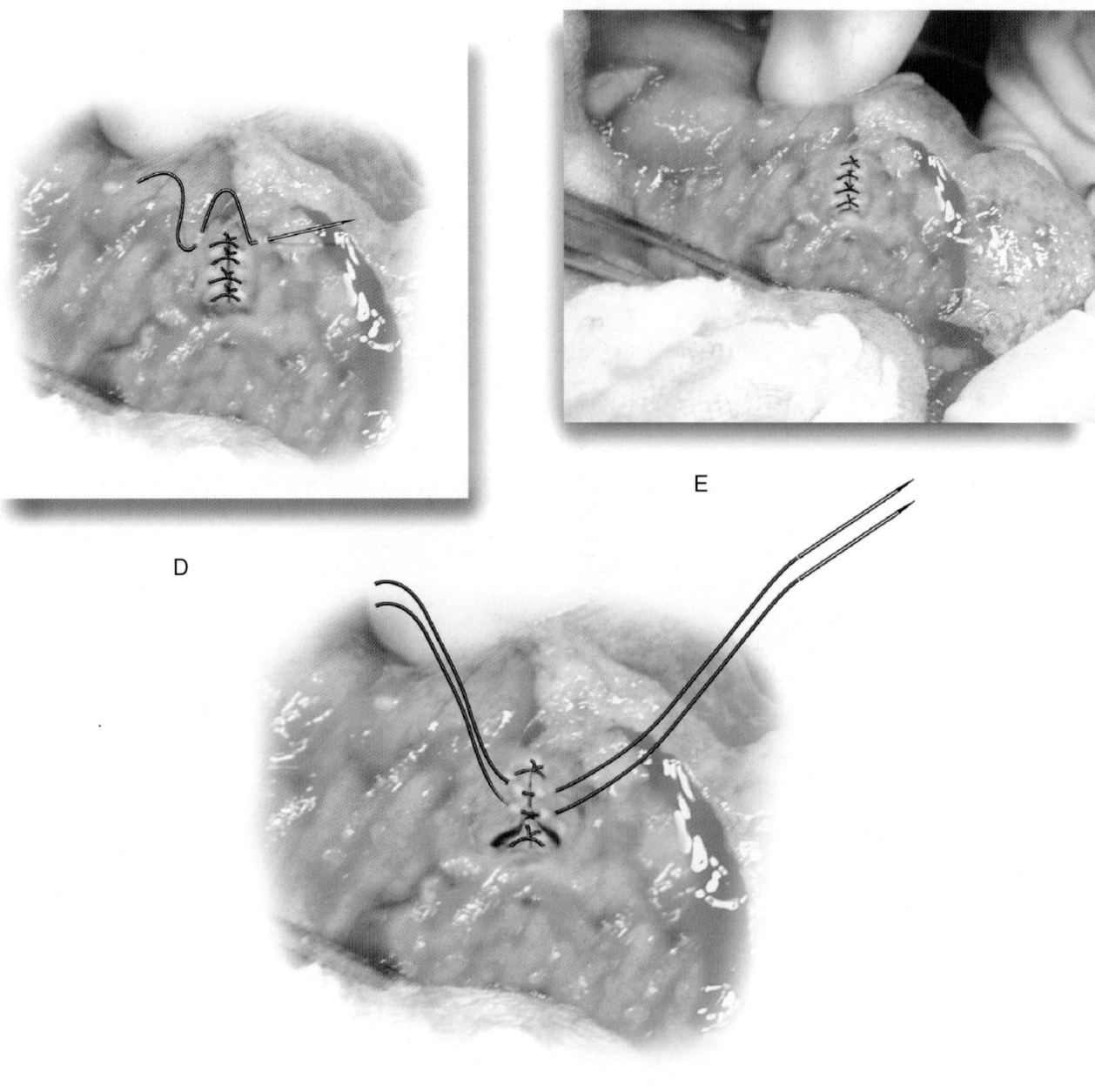

D

E

F

**FIGURE 95–2, cont'd  D.** A second layer of 2-0 silk is placed only through the serosa and muscularis via fine intestinal needles. **E.** The second line of silk sutures covers the first through-and-through layer. **F.** The wound is completely closed and is strongly sealed.

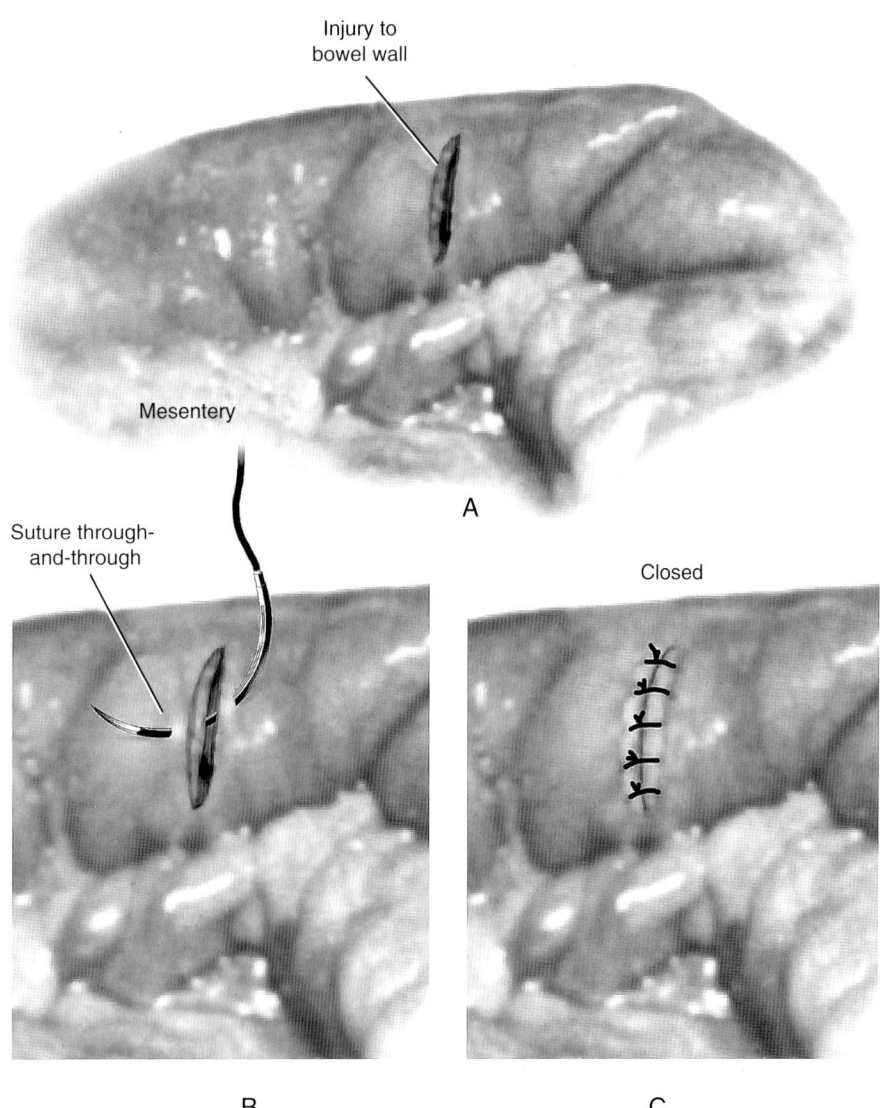

Injury to
bowel wall

Mesentery

A

Suture through-
and-through

Closed

B

C

**FIGURE 95–3 A.** An opening has been made in the small intestine. Investigation reveals
that the mucosa has been entered. **B.** The defect is closed by a series of simple (single-layer)
2-0 silk or polydioxanone (PDS) sutures. **C.** The completed closure is irrigated and checked for
fluid tightness. The lumen is also examined to determine its adequacy.

# CHAPTER 96

# Meckel's Diverticulum

*Michael S. Baggish*

Meckel's diverticulum is a common congenital anomaly affecting the small bowel. Typically, the diverticulum is located within 2 feet of the ileocecal valve and arises from the antimesenteric border of the ileum. The protrusion is about 2 inches long and occurs in 2% of the population (Figs. 96-1 through 96-3). The diverticulum may contain stomach, pancreas, and biliary and colonic tissue, which may create symptoms (e.g., peptic ulcer).

Significant intestinal hemorrhage, which manifests itself by rectal bleeding, may emanate from Meckel's diverticulum. Other complications include inflammation, obstruction, and fistula.

The diverticulum may be removed by clamping the base, cutting the diverticulum off, and suturing the bowel. Similarly, the base may be stapled and cut (Fig. 96-4).

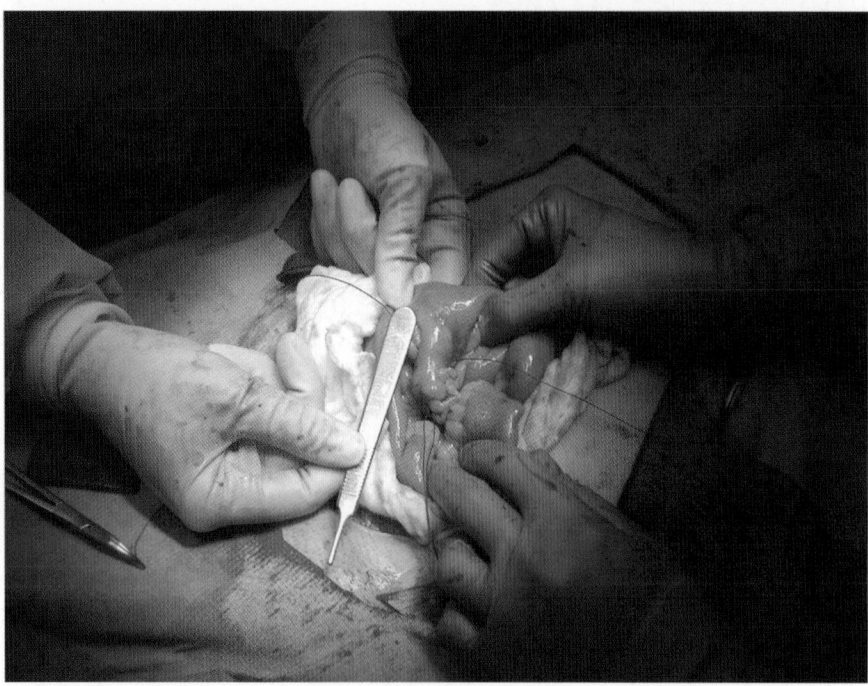

**FIGURE 96–1** Meckel's diverticulum located about 12 inches from the ileocecal junction. The diverticulum has a wide mouth and measures 2 inches in length.

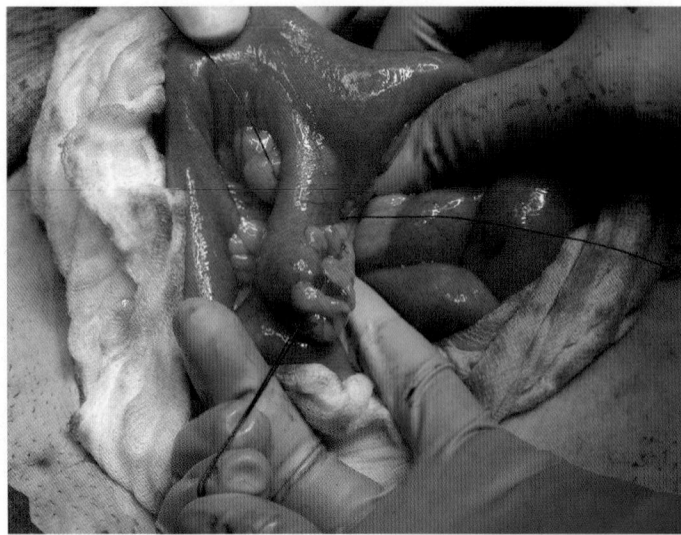

**FIGURE 96–2** Close-up view of the diverticulum. Note that traction sutures have been placed to facilitate manipulation.

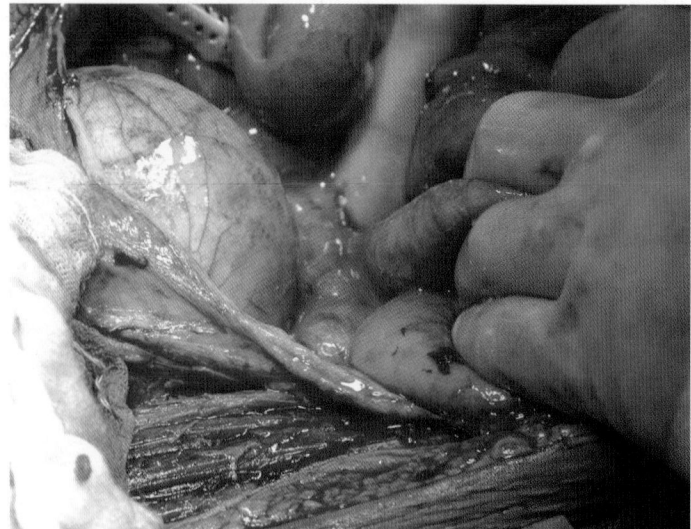

**FIGURE 96–3** A still more magnified view of the ileal diverticulum. Note the cecum in the foreground.

# CHAPTER 97

# Appendectomy

*Michael S. Baggish*

In the past, removal of the appendix was electively performed by gynecologists during laparotomy. Now, this practice is less commonly carried out for a variety of reasons, including medical liability risks, perceived advantage for retention of the appendix, lack of informed consent, and lack of technical know-how. Clearly, the latter two concerns can be remedied by explaining the advantages and disadvantages of the procedure to the patient preoperatively and obtaining permission for including the procedure during the proposed laparotomy. Lack of technical know-how requires that the gynecologist or resident be supervised and taught the technique of appendectomy. Obviously, the best scenario for teaching the appendectomy operation is during elective surgery. Patients who have undergone salpingostomy for tubal pregnancy, tubal reconstruction, or treatment for pelvic inflammatory disease and those who have severe adhesions are candidates for routine appendectomy. Similarly, fecoliths identified by computed axial tomography (CAT) scan or by palpation are reasonable indications for incidental appendectomy.

The cecum and ileocolic junction are identified. The cecum is elevated, and the appendix, together with its blood supply (in the mesoappendix), is noted. The terminal portion of the appendix is grasped with a Babcock clamp and placed on stretch. A window through the mesoappendix is tunneled between the cecum and the appendiceal artery. Usually an avascular clearing in the mesentery can be seen. Kelly clamps are placed in pairs along the axis of the appendix across the mesoappendix. The mesentery is progressively cut between the clamps until the base of the appendix and the cecum are reached (Fig. 97–1). Next, a purse string stitch of 2-0 silk or 3-0 Vicryl is stitched into the muscularis of the cecum surrounding the base of the appendix. Two Kelly clamps are placed across the proximal portion of the now freed appendix. The first clamp is juxtaposed to the cecum. A third Kelly clamp crushes the appendix between the point where the first and second clamps have been secured. A ligature is then applied across the appendix in the crush zone. The appendix is incised between the first and second clamps but above the ligature (Fig. 97–2A); it is placed in a formalin-containing specimen jar. A second ligature of 3-0 Vicryl is tied beneath clamp #1 (Fig. 97–2B). The doubly tied appendiceal stump is inverted into the center of the cecal purse string suture (Fig. 97–2C). The purse string is tightened, thereby burying the appendiceal stump. The purse string is tied (Fig. 97–2D). The surgical site is irrigated with normal saline and checked for bleeding. Alternatively, during laparoscopy or laparotomy, the appendix can be rapidly removed by using the surgical stapler (Fig. 97–3).

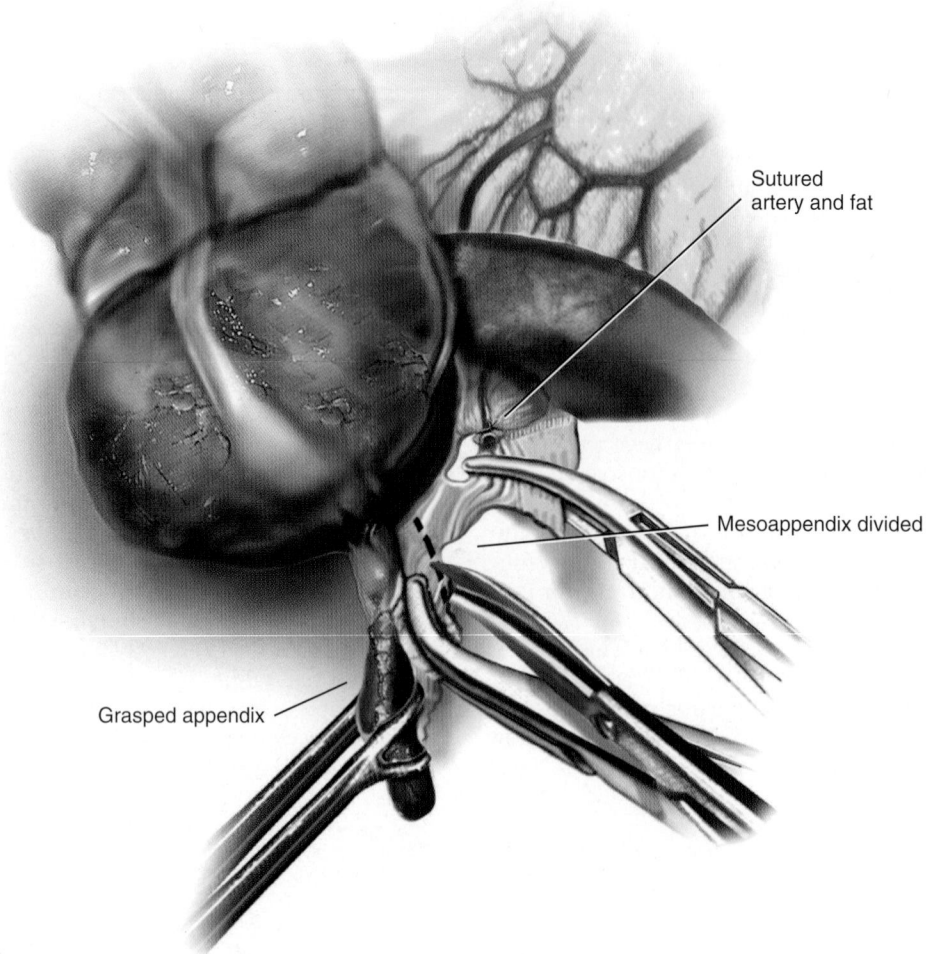

Sutured
artery and fat

Mesoappendix divided

Grasped appendix

**FIGURE 97–1** The distal portion of the appendix is secured with a Babcock clamp. A window has been developed in the mesoappendix, and a Kelly clamp has been placed along the mesentery to secure the blood supply. A 3-0 Vicryl suture ligature has been placed and tied. The Kelly clamp has been moved forward. Kelly clamps have been placed along the mesentery close to the appendix. The mesentery is cut between the clamps.

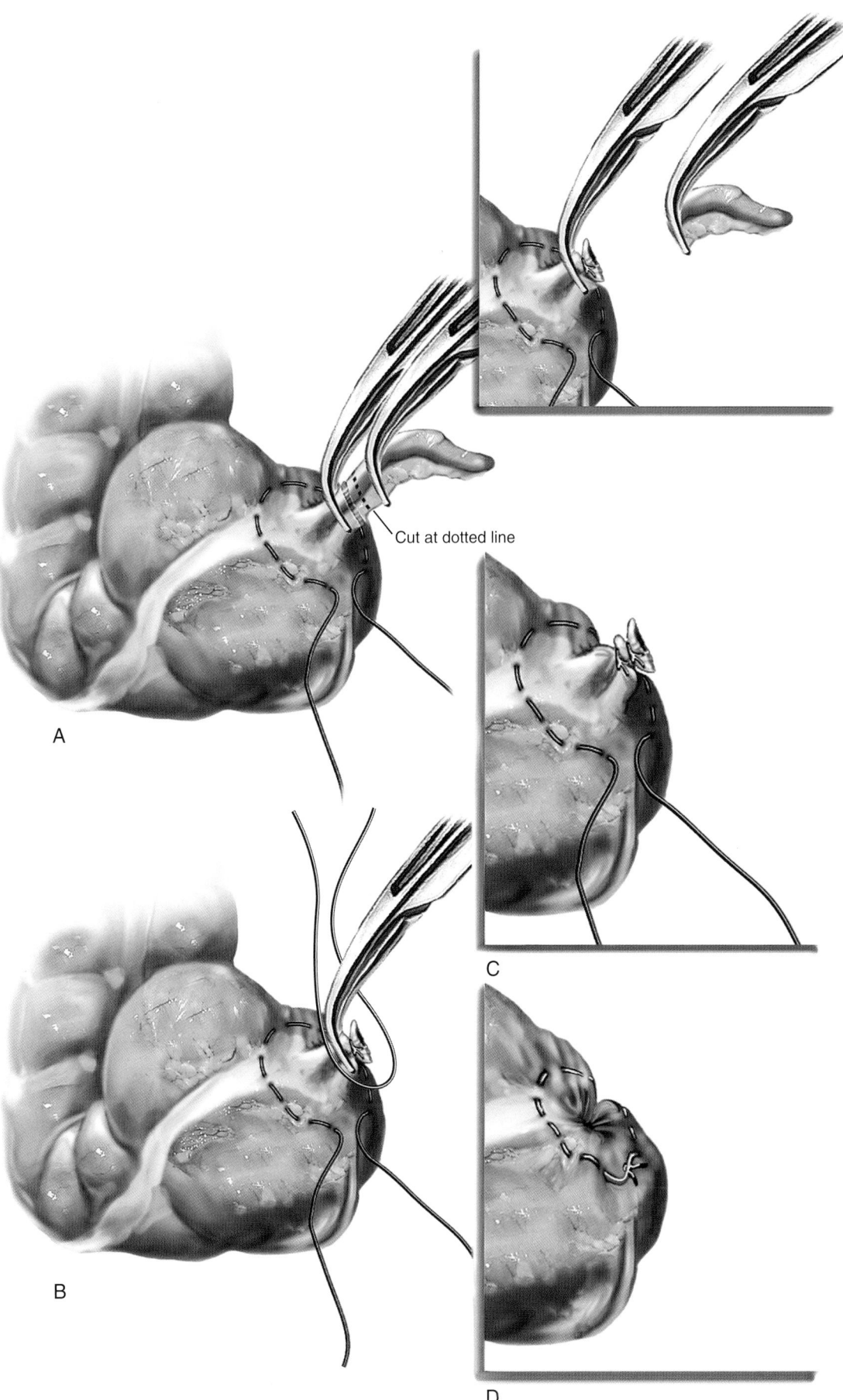

Cut at dotted line

A

B

C

D

**FIGURE 97–2  A.** Two (1 and 2) Kelly clamps have been placed across the proximal appendix. A third clamp has been removed and a 3-0 Vicryl ligature tied in the crushed area. Alternatively, the appendix could be cut between the clamps, and a single ligature could be tied beneath clamp #1. **Inset.** The appendix has been cut between the first ligature and the second applied clamp (clamp #2). **B.** A purse string suture of 2-0 silk is placed into the cecum at the base of the appendix. **C.** A 3-0 Vicryl ligature is tied beneath clamp #1. The appendiceal stump is now doubly ligated. Some surgeons prefer at this point to apply phenol to the end of the stump by using a cotton-tipped applicator. **D.** The stump is inverted into the purse string. The latter is tightened and tied.

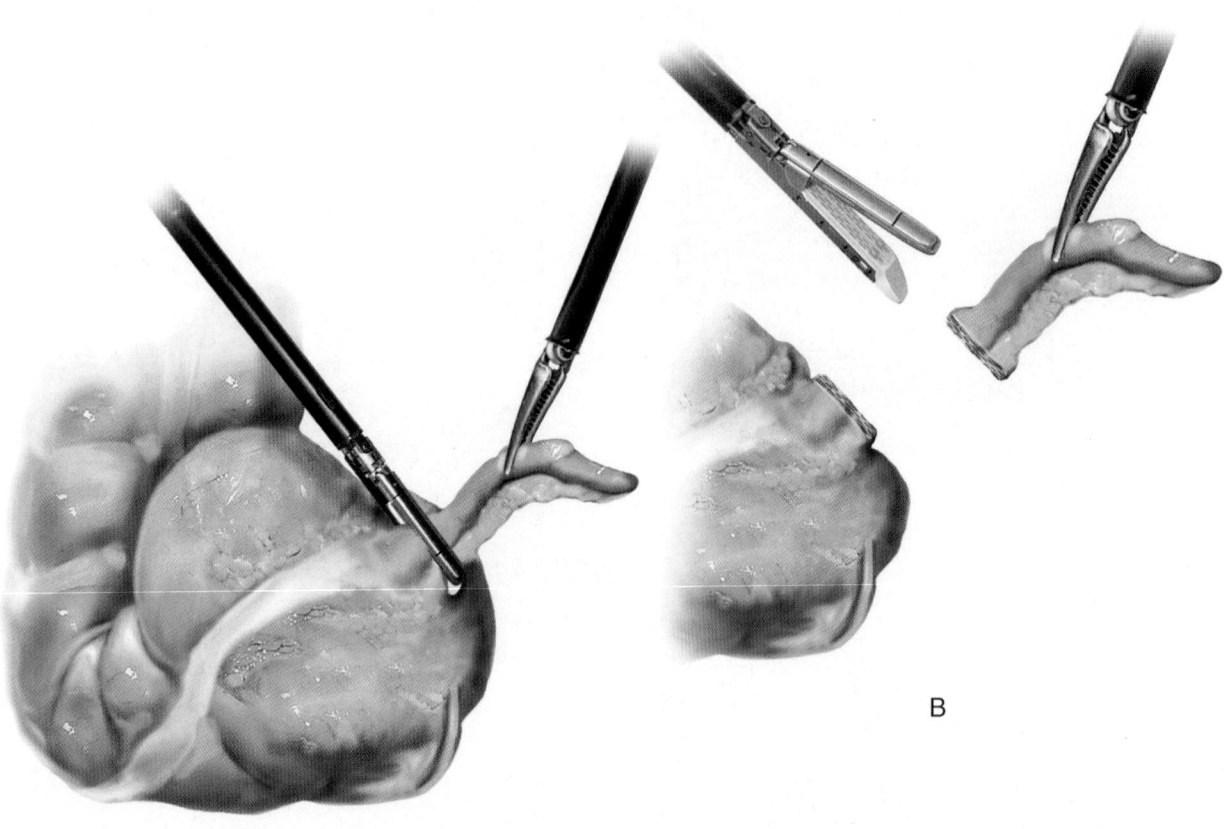

A

B

**FIGURE 97–3  A.** A laparoscopic curved clamp grasps the appendix. **B.** A laparoscope stapling device seals and cuts the appendix at the base.

# CHAPTER 98

# Colon Repair/Colostomy Creation

*Brian J. Albers* ■ *David J. Lamon*

The colon is the distal continuation of the gastrointestinal (GI) tract, extending from the ileocecal valve to the distal anal canal. It measures 4.5 to 6 feet in length and functions to reabsorb sodium and water and to provide temporary storage for enteric wastes.

Operating on the colon mandates knowledge of its segmental blood supply. The right colon is supplied by the ileocolic and right colic branches of the superior mesenteric artery. The hepatic flexure to midtransverse colon is supplied by the middle colic artery. The distal transverse, splenic flexure, and descending and sigmoid colon are perfused by the left colic and sigmoidal branches of the inferior mesenteric artery. The region of the splenic flexure is known as a "watershed" area of marginal arterial supply, requiring extra caution during surgery. In addition, the ascending and descending colon have retroperitoneal attachments that must be divided during mobilization.

Areas of the colon most susceptible to injury during gynecologic procedures are the cecum, the sigmoid colon, and the rectum. Primary repair of injuries to the cecum and proximal sigmoid colon without prior bowel preparation can be performed if soilage is minimal and the mesentery is *not* involved. Seemingly minor injuries to the mesentery can result in delayed ischemia with transmural infarction and perforation of the affected segment. In addition, there should be no hemodynamic shock or more than 1 L of blood loss from the primary procedure. The repair is performed in a manner similar to that previously described for small bowel injuries—interrupted 3-0 silk suture closure in a transverse fashion so as not to encroach on the lumen. Copious field irrigation with normal saline should follow. A 5% to 7% incidence of postoperative localized abscess is reported. This is often amenable to percutaneous drainage.

Injuries of the distal sigmoid colon and rectum without previous bowel preparation are best treated with repair of the injury as described, but with proximal division of the colon and end sigmoid colostomy construction. If the injury involves the mesentery and there is a question of bowel viability, it is always safest to divide the colon distal to the point of injury using a gastrointestinal anastomosis (GIA) stapling device (Fig. 98–1A). Then, the proximal limb is brought out through the abdominal wall as a colostomy. Some degree of judgment is required in managing these injuries, and when available, an experienced general surgeon's assistance should be obtained.

Performance of sigmoid colostomy begins with adequate exposure. Lower abdominal transverse incisions often do not permit adequate visualization for colonic mobilization. If the real possibility of requiring a postoperative colostomy exists, a midline or midabdominal transverse incision is more desirable and permits the use of a larger retractor such as a Buchwalter or Balfour device. The small bowel is carefully packed off to the right side and moved with a wide Deaver retractor. The sigmoid colon is then grasped and retracted medially, exposing the lateral retroperitoneal attachments. The membrane ("white line") of Toldt is incised along the length of the descending colon down to the level of the pelvic brim. Once the white line is incised, further lengthwise dissection can often be carried out bluntly with the fingers (Fig. 98–1B). Care must be taken to visualize the path of the ureter during all parts of the dissection; it is usually found medial and posterior to the colon. In addition, it is important to locate and preserve the nutrient vessels within the colonic mesentery. The left colic and sigmoidal branches of the inferior mesenteric artery are necessary for colonic function and healing.

Depending upon the location of the injury, the colon should be divided distal to the left colic artery to ensure good perfusion to the stoma. The location of division is chosen, and a rent is created between the colon wall and the mesentery large enough to admit the GIA stapling device (Fig. 98–2). The stapler is then fired, resulting in division of the colon. The distal end is dropped into the pelvis. Further mobility of the proximal sigmoid is gained by scoring the peritoneum of the mesentery on both medial and lateral sides parallel to the length of the colon. Gentle blunt dissection with a sponge stick while upward retraction is applied to the colon should increase usable length. Care is taken not to avulse major mesenteric nutrient vessels. Small mesenteric bleeders may be controlled with electrocautery or suture ligation. Once sufficient length is gained so as to easily reach the anterior abdominal wall, an exit site is chosen. Traversal of the lateral rectus sheath just below or above the umbilicus is preferred because of a lower incidence of subsequent peristomal herniation. The skin is grasped with an Allis clamp (Fig. 98–3), and a circular wound is created (Fig. 98–4). The rectus fascia is incised in a cruciate fashion so as to admit two fingers snugly (Fig. 98–5). The proximal stapled end of the colon is then grasped with a Babcock clamp through the stoma site and is brought out through the fascial defect. The clamp is left on while the primary incision is closed to prevent retraction of the colon back into the peritoneal cavity. There should be enough redundancy so the colonic staple line extends several centimeters above the skin level with minimal tension. With the primary wound now closed and protected, the stoma is "matured" by sharply excising the staple line to open the colonic lumen (Fig. 98–6). Mucosal bleeding should be evident; if brisk, it is controlled with pinpoint electrocautery. A 3-0 absorbable suture is then used to circumferentially evert the colonic stoma. This is best performed in an interrupted fashion by a generous mucosal/serosal "bite" at the cut edge (Fig. 98–7A) and another smaller serosal bite 3 cm proximal with the needle (Fig. 98–7B). A small skin edge is then included, and the knot is tied (Fig. 98–7C). The finished result should be as shown with no exposed mesentery (Fig. 98–8). A lubricated finger should easily pass through the fascial portion of the stoma lumen. An ostomy appliance is then applied.

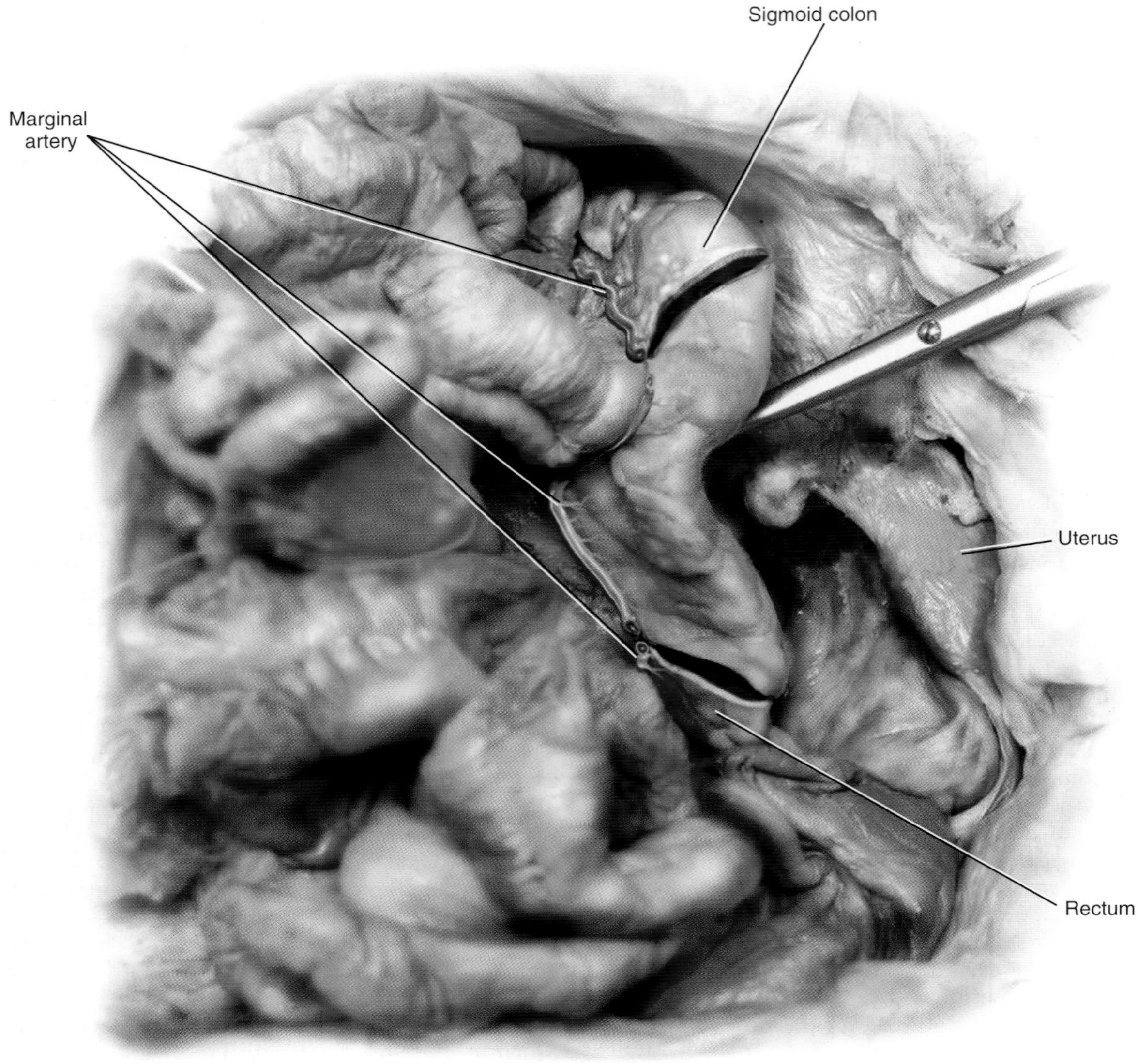

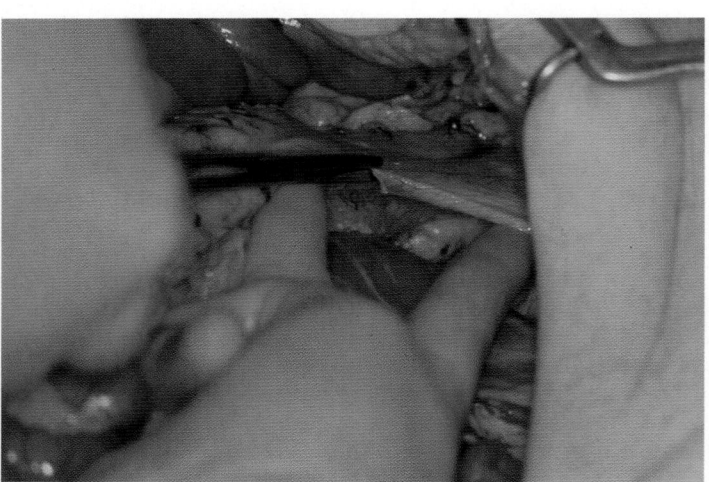

Sigmoid colon

Marginal
artery

Uterus

Rectum

A

B

**FIGURE 98–1  A.** Injury to the sigmoid mesocolon can lead to devascularization of the large intestine (sigmoid colon). Here the marginal branches of one of the sigmoid branches of the inferior mesenteric vessels were disrupted, leading to complete necrosis and perforation of a segment of the sigmoid colon. **B.** The sigmoid colon is visible to the left of the scissors. The lateral peritoneal attachments are sharply incised while the colon is reflected medially.

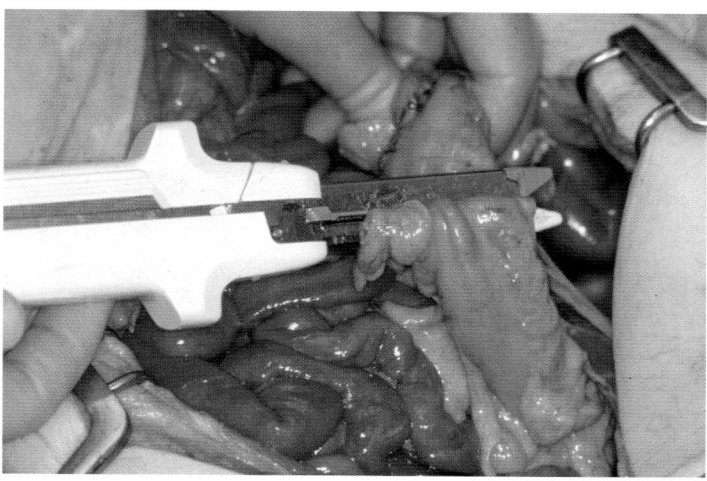

**FIGURE 98–2** The gastrointestinal anastomosis (GIA) 75-mm stapling device is used to divide the colon proximal to the injury. The mesenteric edge of the colon is cleared to admit the stapler.

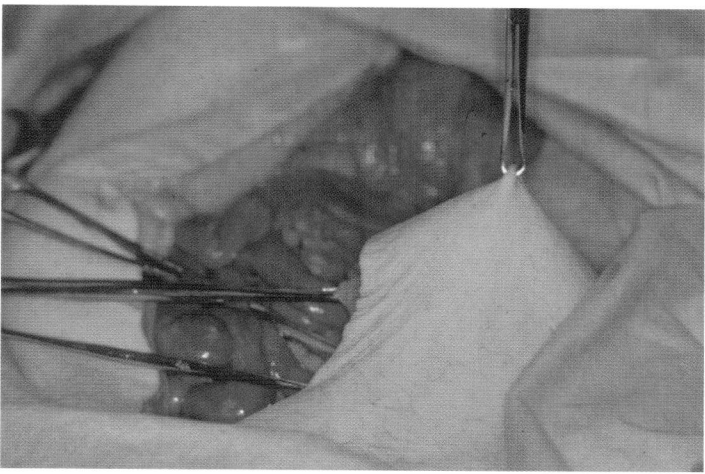

**FIGURE 98–3** The site for stoma placement is chosen. Often this can be marked preoperatively by the institution's enterostomal therapist if a colostomy is planned. A site at the lateral aspect of the rectus sheath traversing both anterior and posterior layers is best.

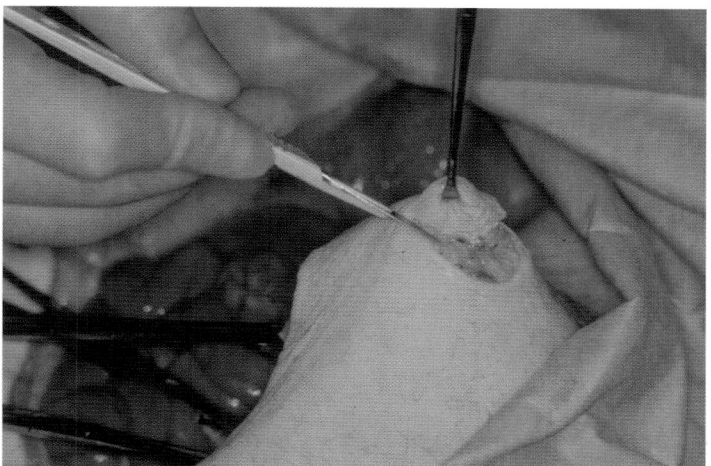

**FIGURE 98–4** A 3-cm circular ellipse of skin and subcutaneous fat is excised down to the level of the anterior fascia.

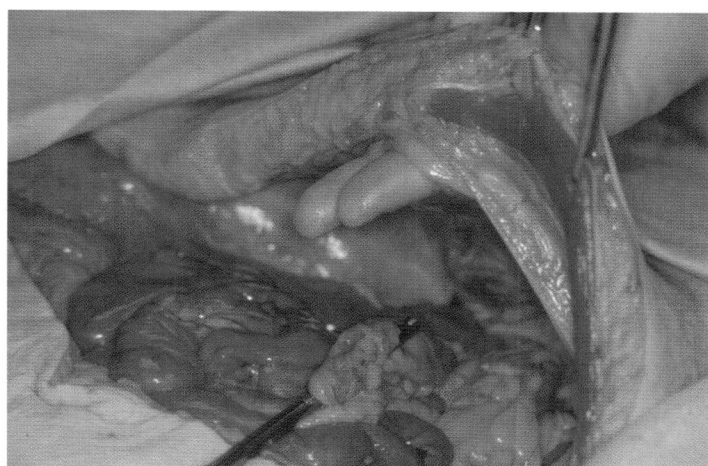

**FIGURE 98–5** A cruciform incision is made in the anterior and posterior fascia through which two fingers may fit snugly.

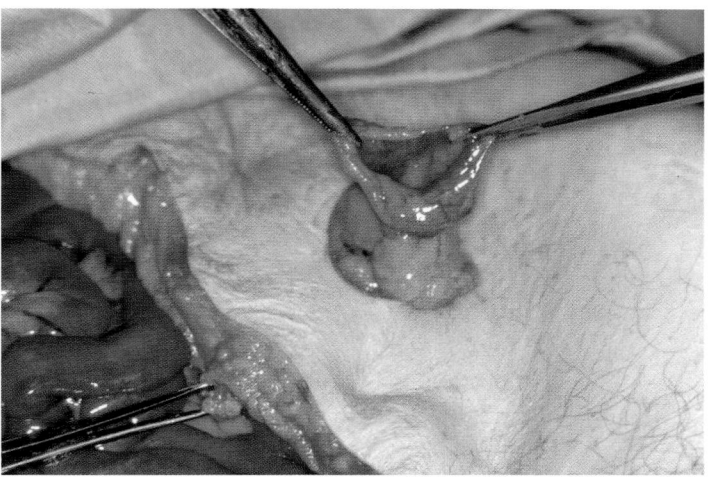

**FIGURE 98–6** The proximal colonic staple line is grasped with a Babcock clamp and brought through the abdominal wall. Once the surgical incision is closed, the colon is opened.

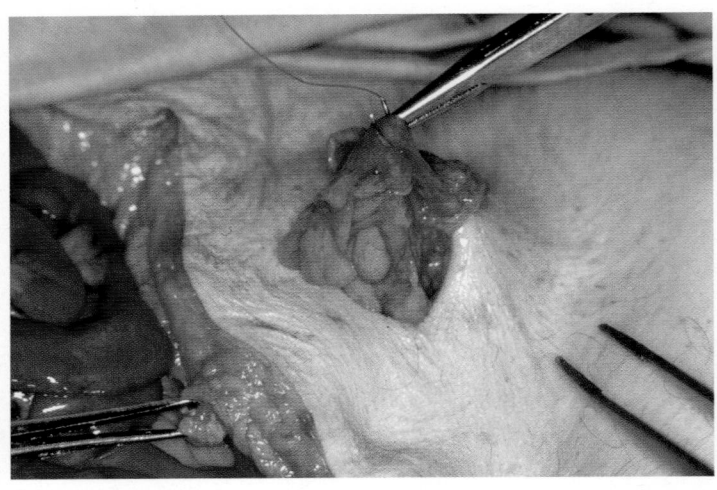

A

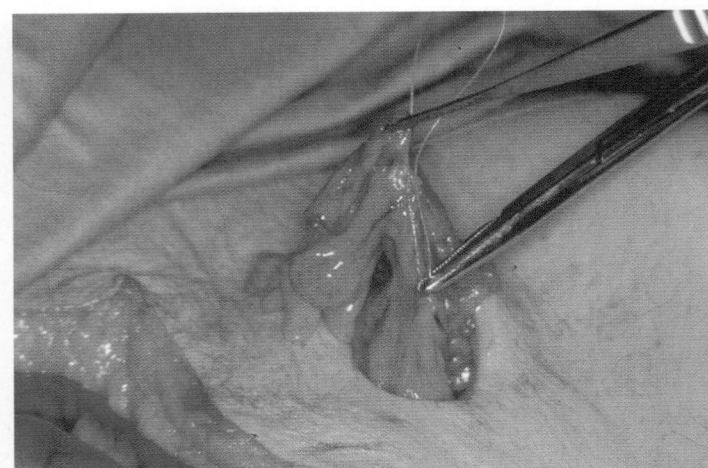

B

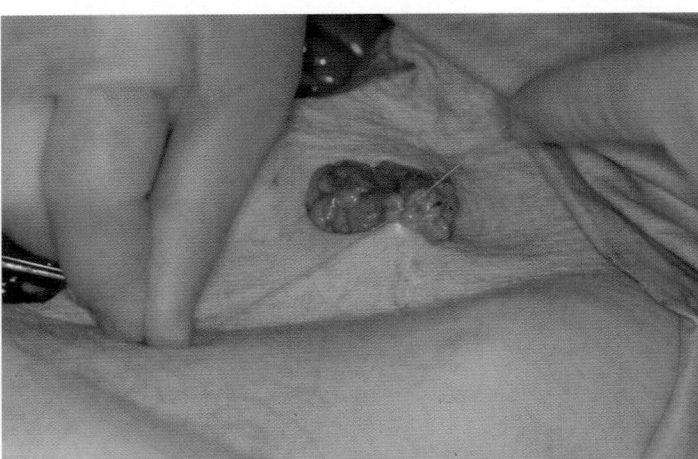

C

**FIGURE 98–7** The stoma is matured by interrupted circumferential 3-0 absorbable sutures encompassing the cut edge (**A**), a 3-cm proximal serosal bite (**B**), and the skin edge (**C**).

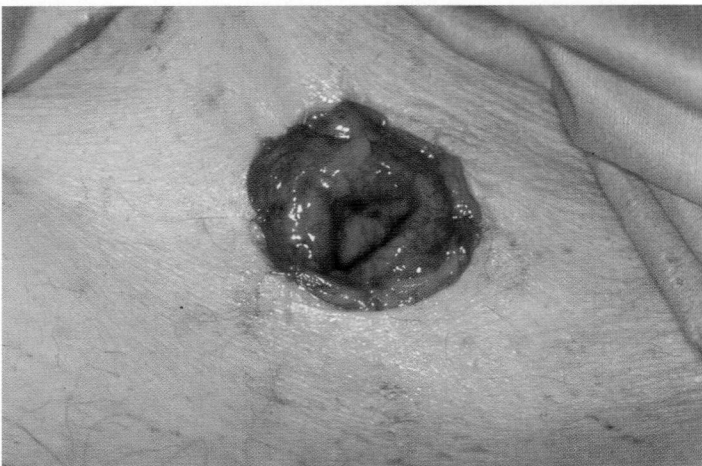

**FIGURE 98–8** Finished stoma shown with everted colonic wall and central lumen.

# CHAPTER 99

# Repair of Rectovaginal Fistulas

*Mickey M. Karram*

Most rectovaginal fistulas seen by the obstetrician/gynecologist are secondary to obstetric injury. These fistulas are usually in the distal third of the vagina. The key to successful repair of a rectovaginal fistula is excision of the fistulous tract with tension-free approximation of the edges of the defect. There should be excellent hemostasis, and perioperative antibiotics should be administered to decrease any potential for infection.

Most fistulas are easily visualized and can be palpated on rectovaginal examination. At times, the passage of a probe helps delineate the fistula and its tract (Fig. 99–1).

Following is a description of a repair of a primary nonirradiated rectovaginal fistula:

1. The surgeon's nondominant index finger is placed in the rectum to aid in identification of the fistula and to assess the extent of scarification. A rectal finger will also facilitate dissection in the appropriate plane.
2. The initial incision depends on the anatomic location of the fistula. Many fistulas are best approached with an inverted-U perineal incision (Fig. 99–2). This allows easy mobilization of the posterior vaginal wall from the anterior rectal wall, as well as rebuilding of the perineal body. If the external anal sphincter is intact, there is no reason to disrupt it. If the fistula is higher in the vagina and the perineum is intact, an incision can be made directly into the posterior vaginal wall over and around the fistula.

3. With traction of the vaginal wall and a finger in the rectum to provide support of the rectal wall, sharp dissection is used to widely mobilize the posterior vaginal wall from the anterior rectal wall (Figs. 99–3 and 99–4).
4. Once the vaginal walls are widely mobilized from the underlying rectum, the entire fistulous tract is excised. After the scar tissue is removed, the defect in the anterior rectal wall will enlarge. The rectal wall is cut back until fresh edges are encountered (see Fig. 99–4).
5. With the surgeon's index finger elevating the anterior rectal wall, an initial row of 3-0 or 4-0 absorbable sutures is placed (Fig. 99–5). These sutures are best placed extramucosally and should include a portion of the muscularis and submucosa.
6. A second layer of inverted sutures is then placed (Fig. 99–6). This inverts the first suture line into the rectum; ideally, no suture penetrates the rectal lumen.
7. If possible, a third layer of sutures is placed by plicating the fascia of the posterior vaginal wall over the rectal closure (Fig. 99–7).
8. The vaginal skin is closed, and the perineum is reconstructed if necessary (Fig. 99–8).

Fig. 99–9 reviews the steps for rectovaginal fistula repair with an intact perineum.

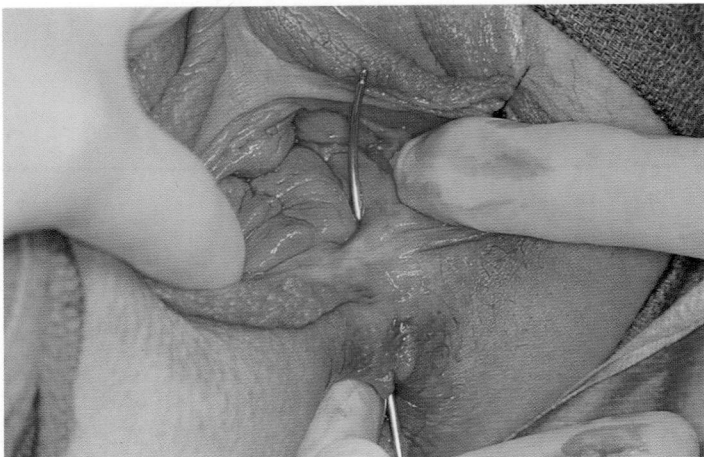

**FIGURE 99–1** Example of a rectovaginal fistula in which a probe helps delineate the fistula and its tract, which notes a very distal fistula opening at the posterior fourchette.

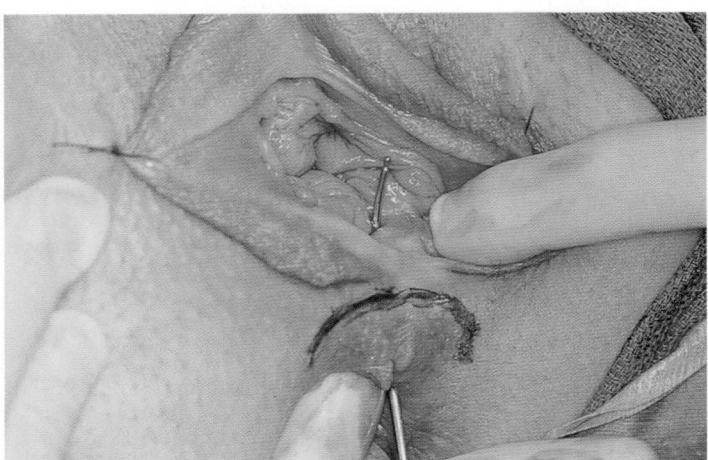

**FIGURE 99–2** Usually an inverted-U incision is made on the perineum for distal fistulas. If the external anal sphincter is intact, there is no reason to disrupt it.

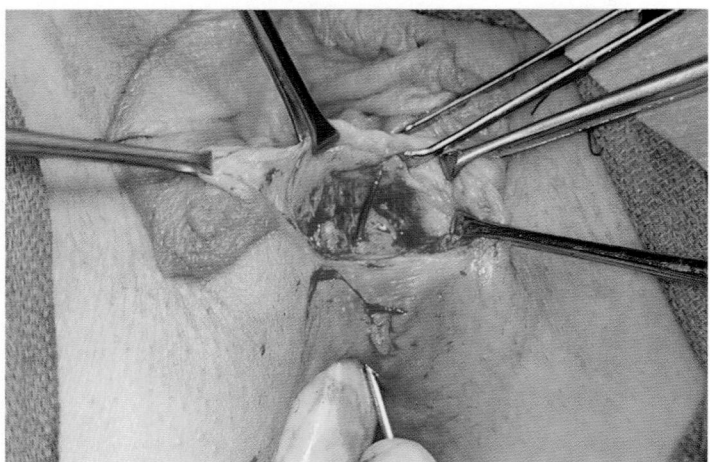

**FIGURE 99–3** Sharp dissection with a finger in the rectum exposes the fistulous tract and begins development of the rectovaginal space.

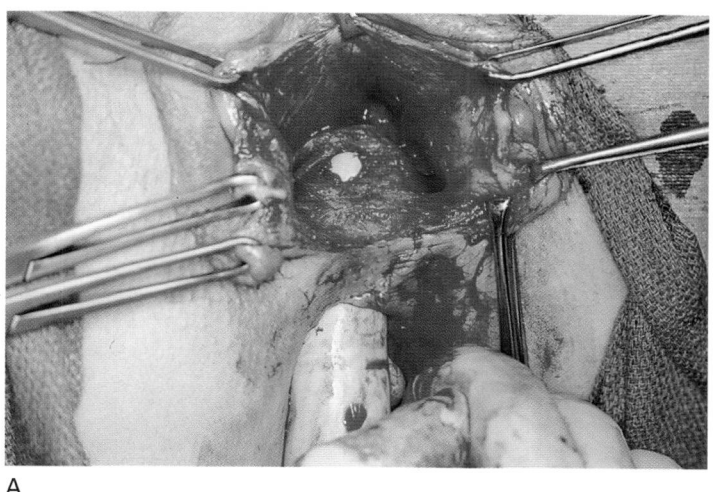
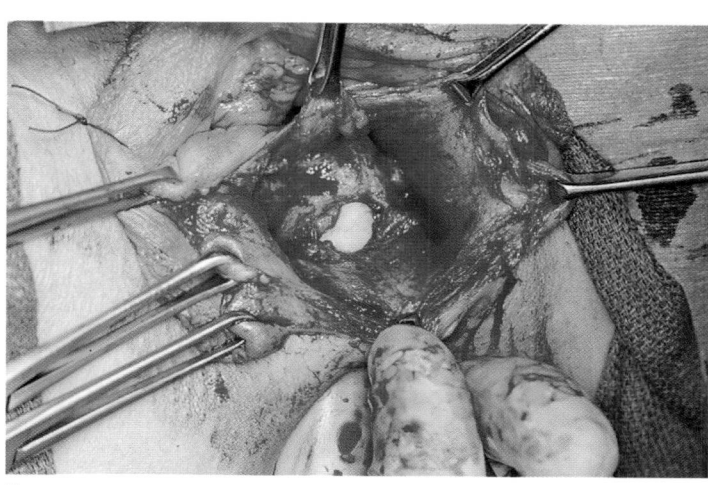

A

B

**FIGURE 99–4  A.** Sharp dissection completely mobilizes the posterior vaginal wall from the anterior rectal wall. The dissection must be extended well beyond the edges of the fistula to provide tension-free closure. **B.** Note that the fistula will enlarge as more scar tissue is excised.

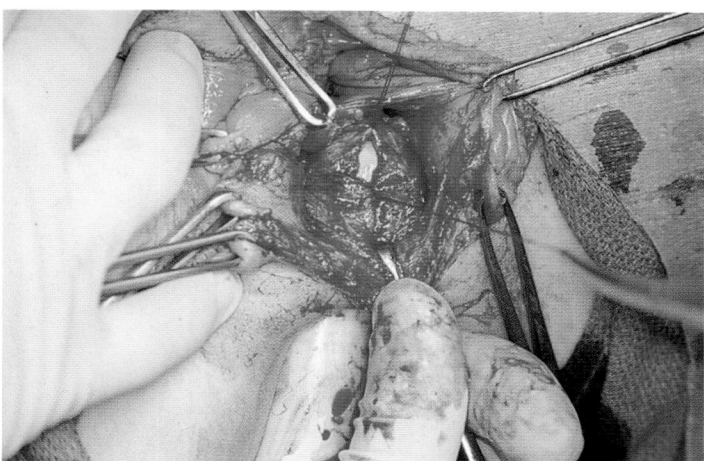

**FIGURE 99–5** Once the dissection is completed and the scarred edges of the fistulous tract have been excised, closure of the anterior rectal wall is initiated with a fine absorbable suture. The author prefers a 4-0 chromic catgut suture. The distal and proximal edges of the fistula have been tagged. Sutures should be passed extramucosally if at all possible.

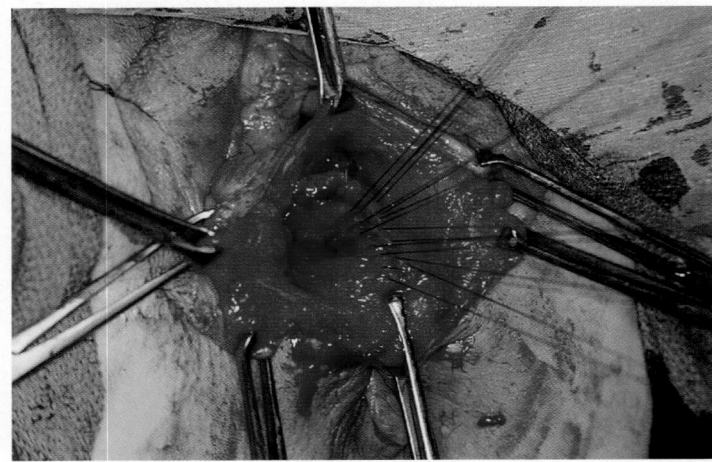

A

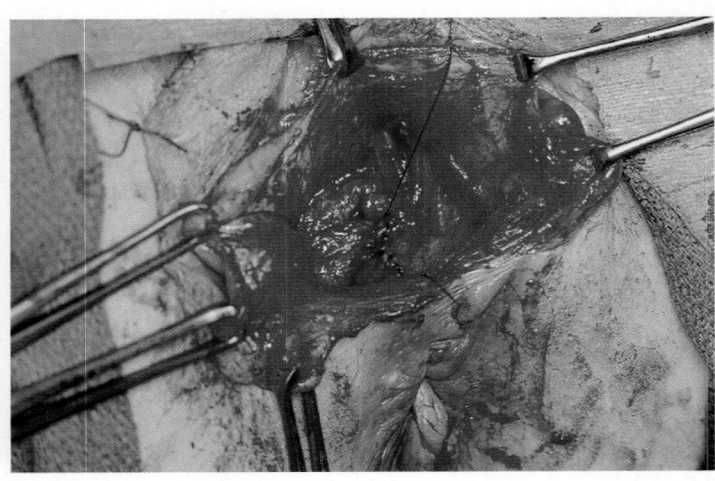

B

**FIGURE 99–6  A.** The initial layer of interrupted extramucosal sutures has been passed, approximating the anterior rectal wall. **B.** This layer is followed by a second layer of imbricating sutures.

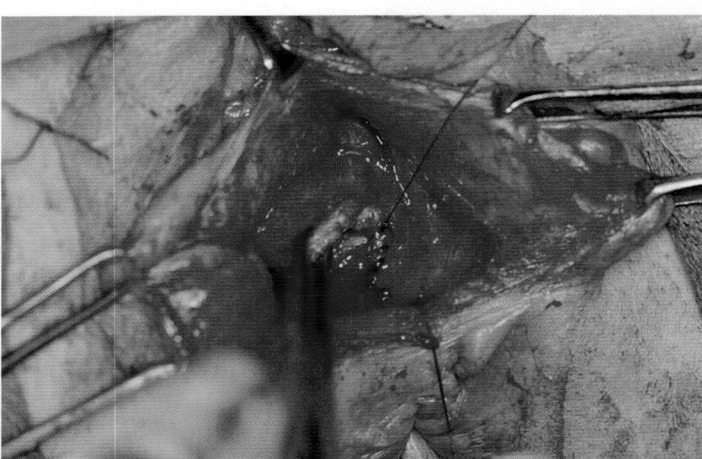

**FIGURE 99–7** The rectovaginal fascia is identified and grasped with an Allis clamp. If possible, this tissue is then approximated over the initial closure of the fistula.

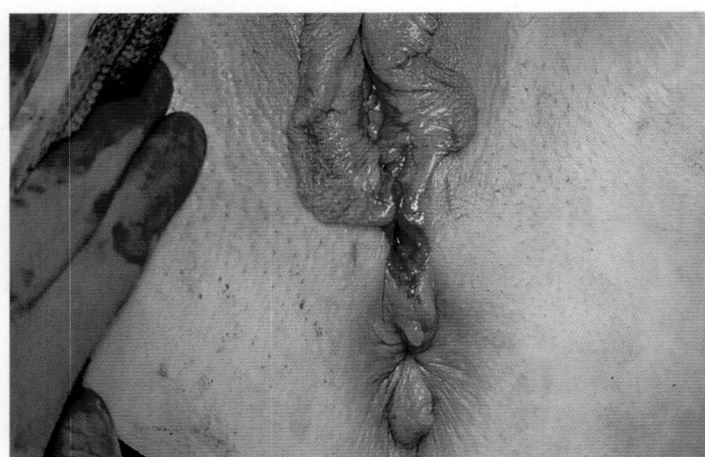

**FIGURE 99–8** The posterior vaginal wall is closed and the perineum is reconstructed if necessary.

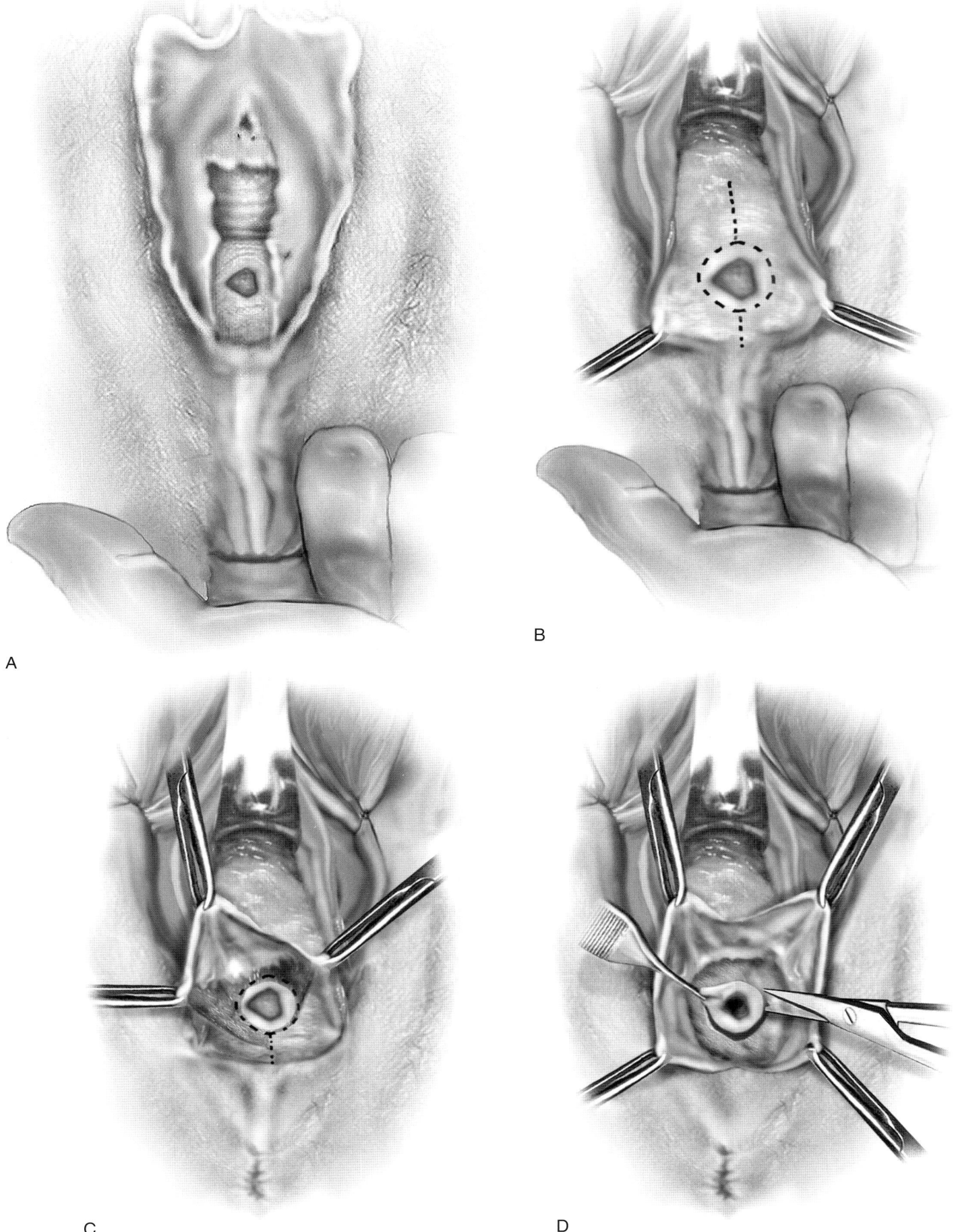

A

B

C

D

**FIGURE 99–9** Rectovaginal fistula repair in a patient with an intact perineum. **A.** A rectovaginal fistula present in the midportion of the posterior vaginal wall. **B.** The dashed line demonstrates the site of the posterior vaginal wall incision. **C.** The vaginal wall is mobilized off the anterior rectal wall. **D.** The fistulous tract is excised. The rectal wall is cut back until fresh edges are encountered.

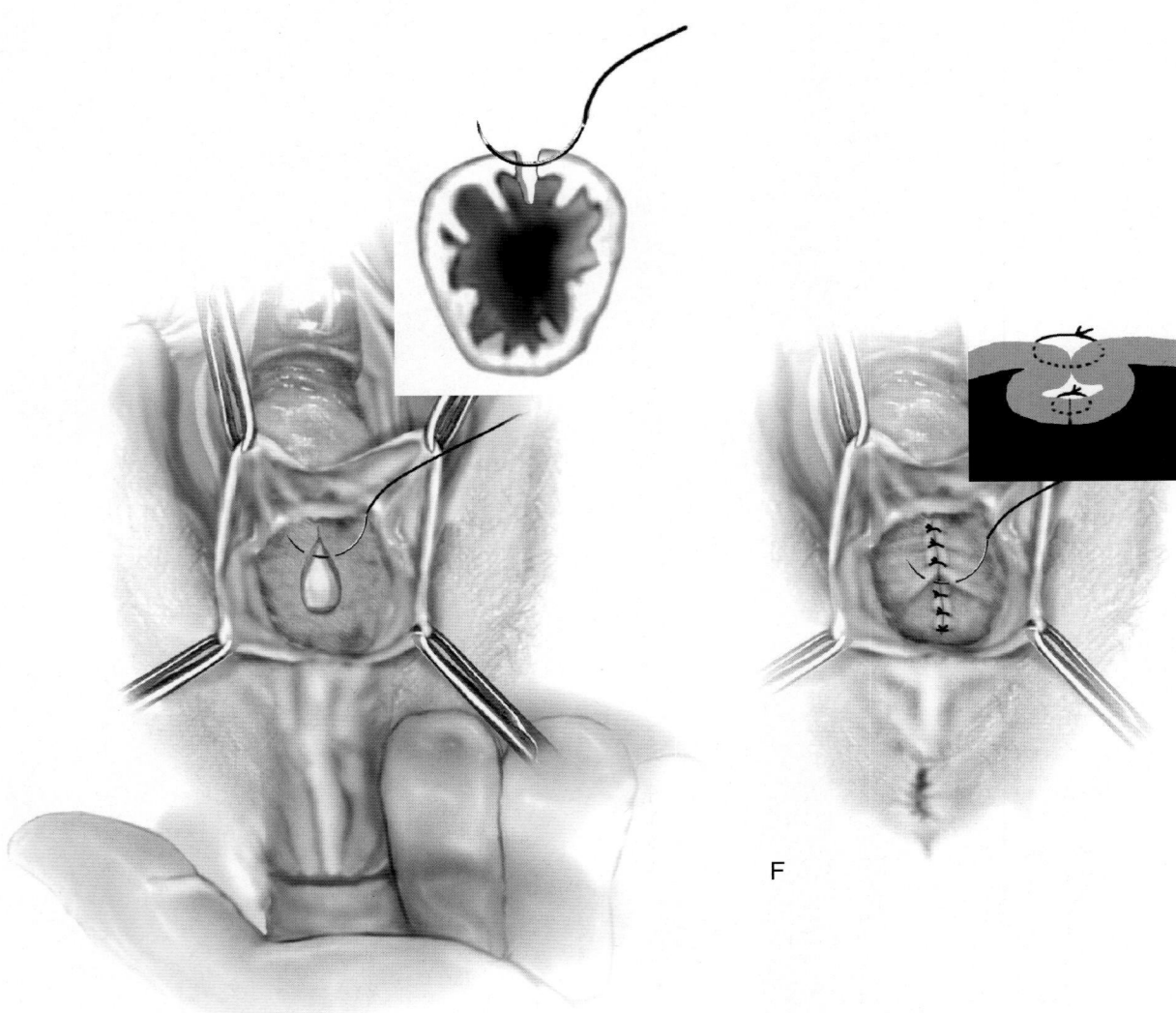

E

F

**FIGURE 99–9, cont'd  E.** Extramucosal closure of the anterior rectal wall with interrupted fine delayed absorbable sutures. **F.** The second layer imbricates the muscular portion of the wall of the rectum over the initial layer. The repair is completed by plicating the rectovaginal fascia and closing the posterior vaginal wall.

# Surgery for Anal Incontinence

*Mickey M. Karram*

## Anatomy of the Rectum and Anal Sphincters

Fecal control is a complex process that involves an intricate interaction between anal function and sensation, rectal compliance, stool consistency, stool volume, colonic transit, and mental alertness. Alteration of any of these can lead to incontinence of gas, liquid, or solid stool. Disruption of the normal anatomy of this area, usually secondary to obstetric trauma, may result in some degree of incontinence. The intact anatomy of the internal anal sphincter, external anal sphincter, and puborectalis division of the levator ani muscle must be understood to fully appreciate anatomic abnormalities that may lead to anal incontinence (Fig. 100–1).

The rectum extends from its junction with the sigmoid colon to the anal orifice. The distribution of smooth muscle is typical for the intestinal tract, with inner circular and outer longitudinal layers of muscle. At the perineal flexure of the rectum, the inner circular layer increases in thickness to form the internal anal sphincter. The internal anal sphincter is under autonomic control (sympathetic and parasympathetic) and is responsible for 85% of resting anal pressure. The outer longitudinal layer of smooth muscle becomes concentrated on the anterior and posterior walls of the rectum, with connections to the perineal body and coccyx, and then passes inferiorly on both sides of the external anal sphincter. The external anal sphincter is composed of striated muscle that is tonically contracted most of the time and can also be voluntarily contracted. The external anal sphincter functions as a unit with the puborectalis portion of the levator

ani muscle. The anal sphincter mechanism comprises the internal anal sphincter, the external anal sphincter, and the puborectalis muscle portion of the levator ani (see Fig. 95–1). A spinal reflex causes the striated sphincter to contract during sudden increases in intra-abdominal pressure. The anorectal angle is produced by the anterior pole of the puborectalis muscle. This muscle forms a sling posteriorly around the anorectal junction. The two sphincters are somewhat separated by the conjoint longitudinal layer formed by a merger of the longitudinal layer of the smooth muscle of the rectum and the pubococcygeal fibers of the levator ani muscle. These sphincters encircle the anal canal just distal to the anorectal angle. As was previously mentioned, the internal sphincter is thought to exert most of the resting pressure. The external sphincter, which is innervated by the inferior rectal branch of the pudendal nerve and the perineal branch of the fourth sacral nerve, exerts most of the maximal squeeze pressure. It is felt that a more anatomic repair and perhaps better restoration of a high-pressure zone will result if the repair incorporates both internal and external anal sphincters. These structures are approximately 2 cm thick and 3 to 4 cm long. The actual role of the puborectalis muscle in the incontinence mechanism is somewhat controversial. It has been thought that it supports the rectum above the level of the anorectal angle, keeping the pressure of the enteric contents as well as changes in intra-abdominal pressure away from the sphincteric complex. Recent studies suggest that fecal incontinence is often related to denervation of the pelvic diaphragm and to disruption and denervation of the external anal sphincter.

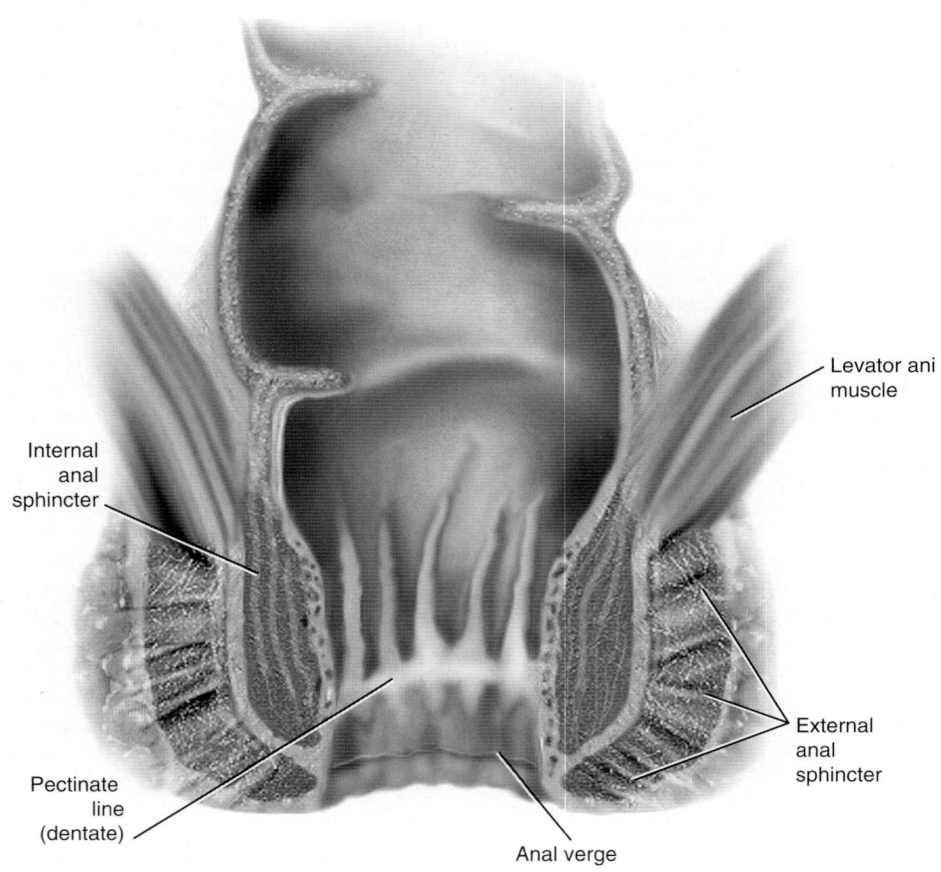

**FIGURE 100–1** Normal anatomy of the distal anal region.

## Repair of the Anal Sphincter

When a defect in the sphincteric complex is identified and testing reveals that this is the major factor contributing to the patient's incontinence of gas, liquid stool, or solid stool, reapproximation of the sphincter should dramatically improve the condition.

Following is a description of an overlapping sphincteroplasty repair for fecal incontinence:

1. The author prefers to perform this repair with a finger in the rectum. An initial inverted-U incision is made above the anal opening from the 9- to the 12- to the 3-o'clock position, followed by a midline incision extending up the remainder of the perineum and into the vagina (Figs. 100–2 through 100–5).

2. The mucosa of the vagina is separated from the anterior wall of the rectum sufficiently laterally and superiorly to provide access to the retracted muscles. Also, the dissection should extend almost to the level of the ischiorectal fossa because most of these patients have a very attenuated perineum, and a perineorrhaphy will need to be performed in conjunction with the anal sphincter repair (see Fig. 100–5).

3. Lateral dissection is performed until the ends of the sphincters can be identified. Many times it is helpful to utilize a nerve stimulator or low-power cautery to identify viable muscle, as frequently the viable muscle will be surrounded by scar tissue (Fig. 100–6). The author prefers to divide the scar in the middle, leaving the two ends of the sphincter with the scar attached. It is important to divide the scar but not to trim it from the ends of the sphincter because it will provide tensile strength when the repair is done.

4. The sphincter ends are sufficiently mobilized to allow overlapping of the muscle and are grasped with Allis clamps. If both internal and external muscles are injured, it is prefera-

ble to repair them as one unit. This is best performed by incorporating small bites of the anterior wall of the rectum into the sphincteroplasty. Some advocate merely approximating the muscles, but if possible, the author prefers to overlap the muscle ends, thus performing an overlapping sphincteroplasty. This is done by placing numerous mattress sutures through the entire length of the sphincter on each side (Fig. 100–7). Approximately six sutures (three on each side) are used. Mattress-type sutures are utilized to overlap the edges of the sphincter (Figs. 100–8 through 100–10). During the repair, irrigation of the wound is carried out with an antibiotic solution.

5. Frequently a perineorrhaphy needs to be performed (see Fig. 100–9). Also, if necessary, a distal levatorplasty may be performed to decrease the size of the vaginal introitus. At the completion of the repair, the anal canal should be tightened so that it allows just an index finger to be admitted.

6. The skin edges are then closed with interrupted 3-0 absorbable sutures. The author does not routinely place a drain in this area. Patients are maintained on stool softeners throughout the postoperative period.

If the ends of the anal sphincter are significantly refracted, then it becomes impossible to perform an overlapping sphincteroplasty. This is commonly seen when there is complete breakdown of a third- or fourth-degree episiotomy repair. Fig. 100–11A portrays a 28-year-old patient who is approximately 3 months postpartum after breakdown of a fourth-degree episiotomy repair, who presented with significant fecal incontinence. Note that there is complete loss of the perineal body with significant retraction of the external anal sphincter. The technique of an end-to-end sphincteroplasty with incorporation of the internal anal sphincter is demonstrated in Figs. 100–11 and 100–12.

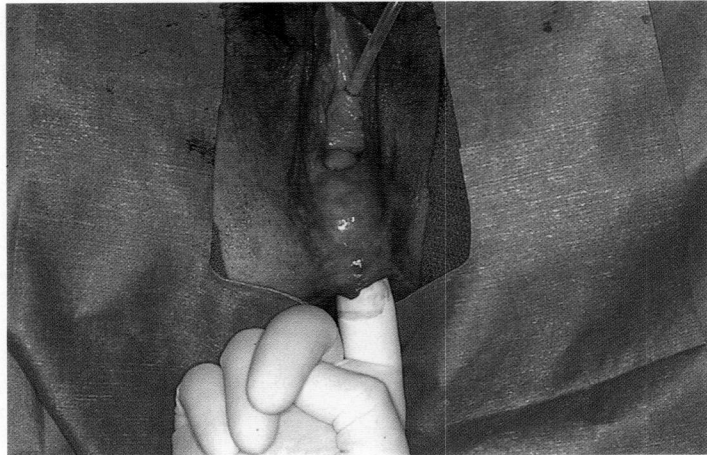

**FIGURE 100–2** Examination demonstrated an attenuated perineal body with a deficient anal sphincter anteriorly.

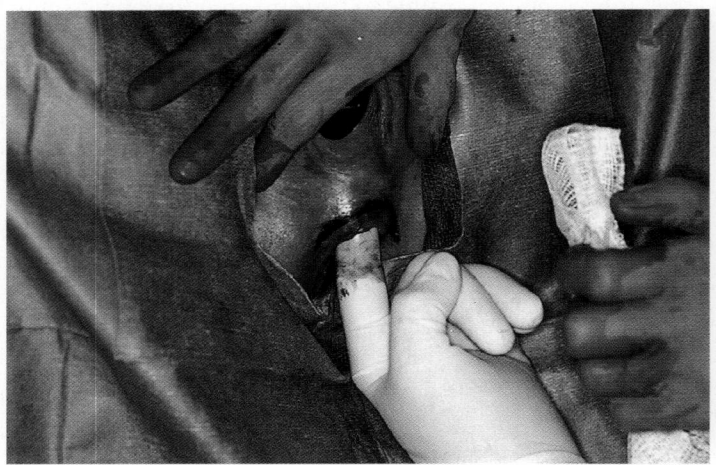

A

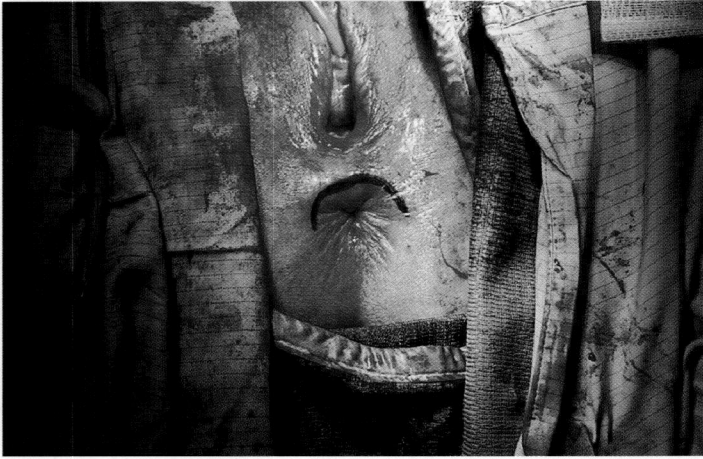

B

**FIGURE 100–3 A** and **B.** An inverted-U incision is made from approximately 9 o'clock to 3 o'clock to allow exposure and identification of the retracted edges of the external anal sphincter.

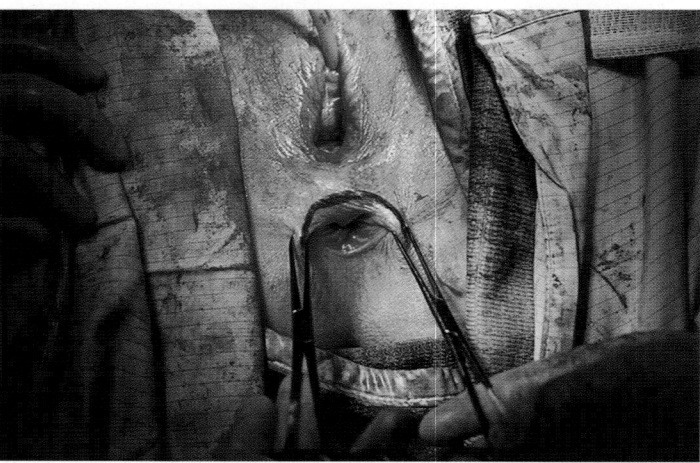

**FIGURE 100–4** Allis clamps are used for traction and indicate the approximate location of the retracted edges of sphincter.

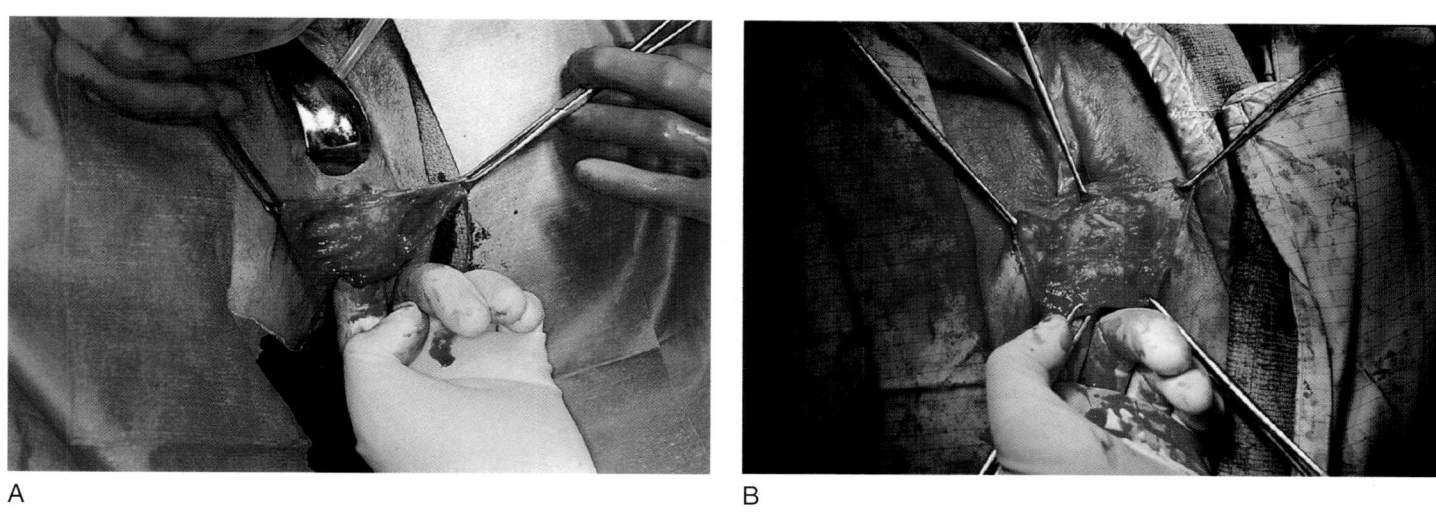

**FIGURE 100–5  A** and **B.** Sharp dissection mobilizes the perineal skin off the anterior rectal wall.

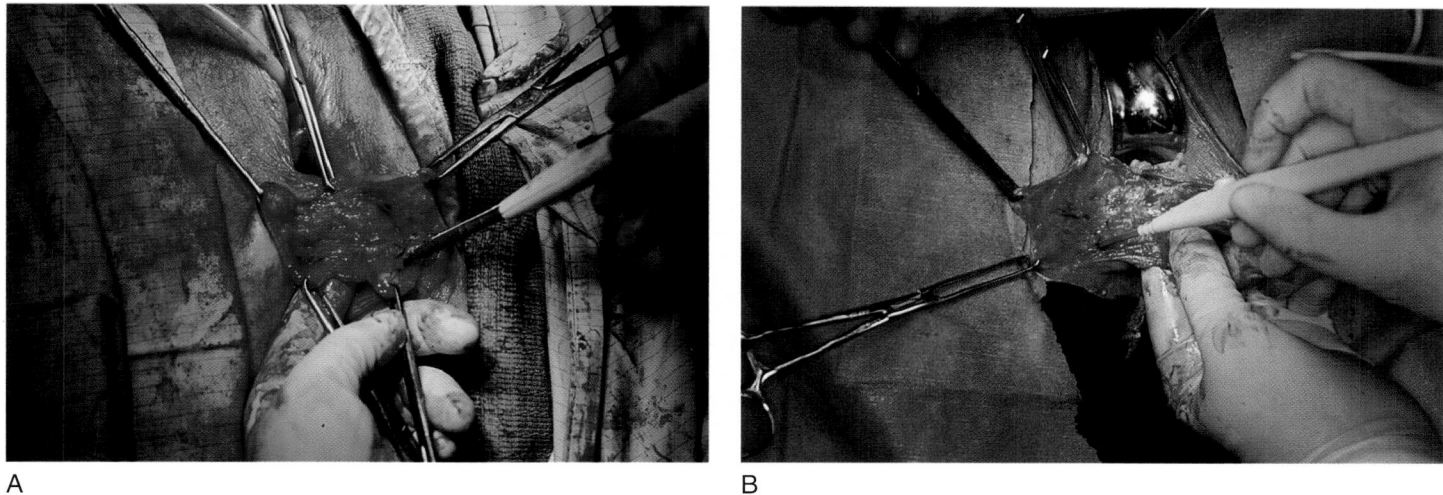

**FIGURE 100–6  A.** Dissection is extended laterally to expose the external sphincter. A nerve stimulator is used to identify viable muscle on the left side. **B.** Low-voltage cautery is used to identify viable muscle on the right side.

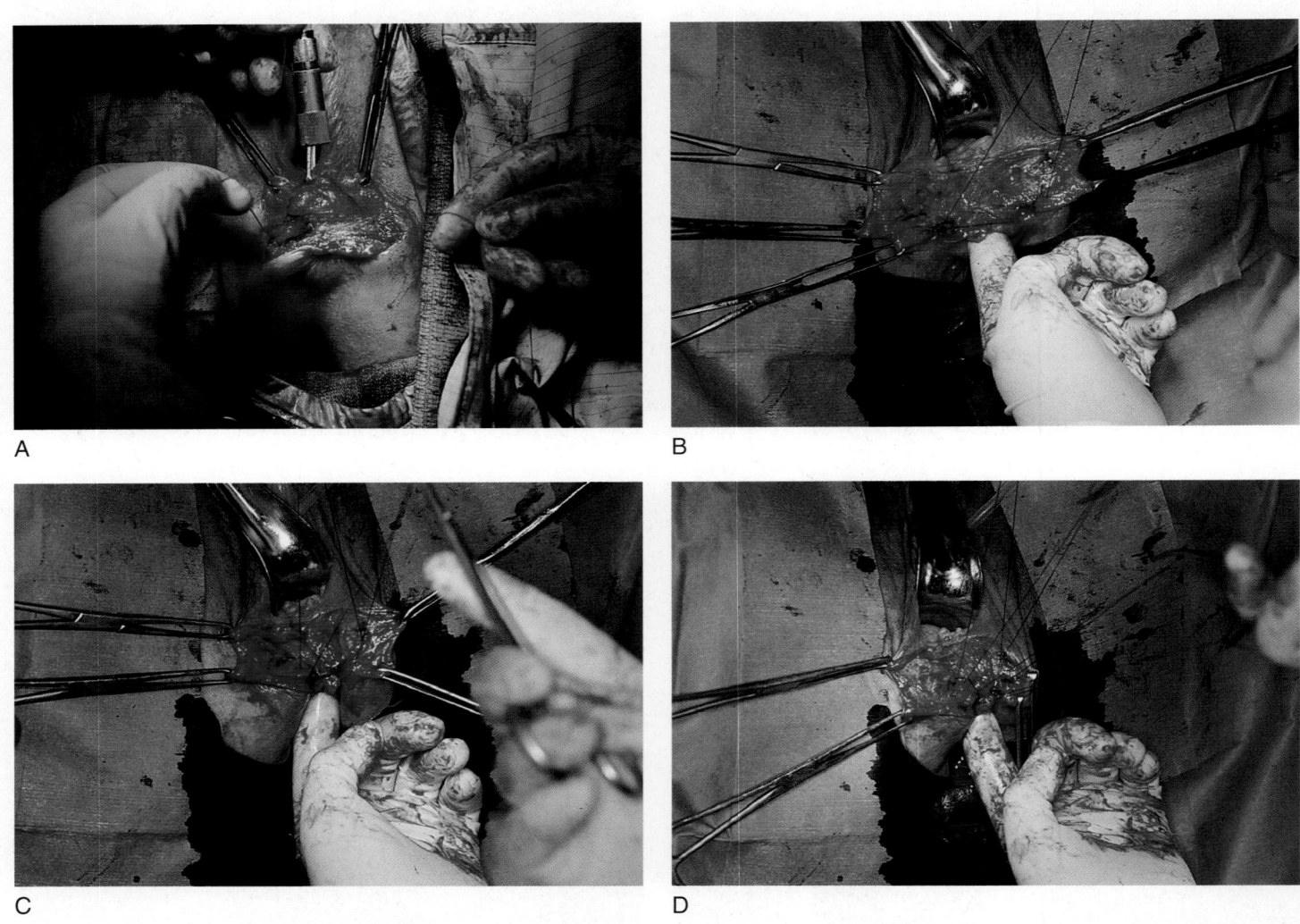

A

B

C

D

**FIGURE 100–7 A** through **D.** Sutures are passed through the retracted edges of the external anal sphincter on each side. Numerous sutures are placed over a 3- to 4-cm distance up the anal canal. Note that small bites incorporate the anterior rectal wall into the repair.

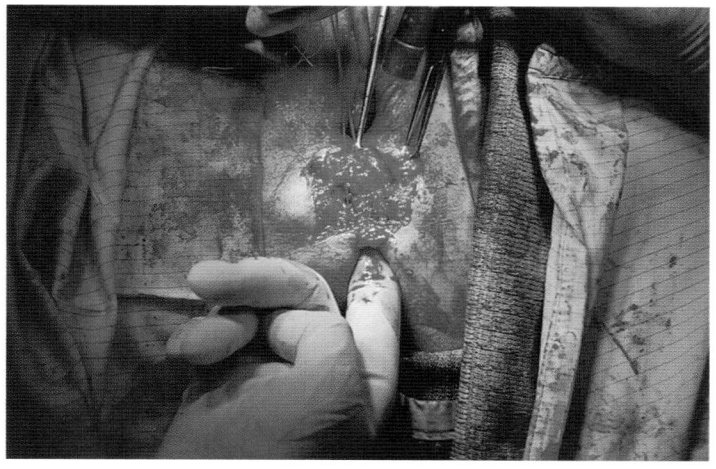

**FIGURE 100–8** Note that tying of the sutures approximates the ends of the external anal sphincter. Whenever possible, an overlapping sphincteroplasty is performed in a "vest-over-pants" fashion.

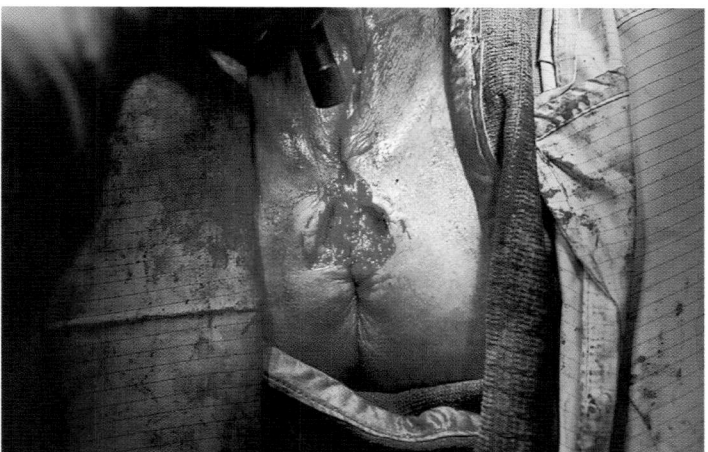

A

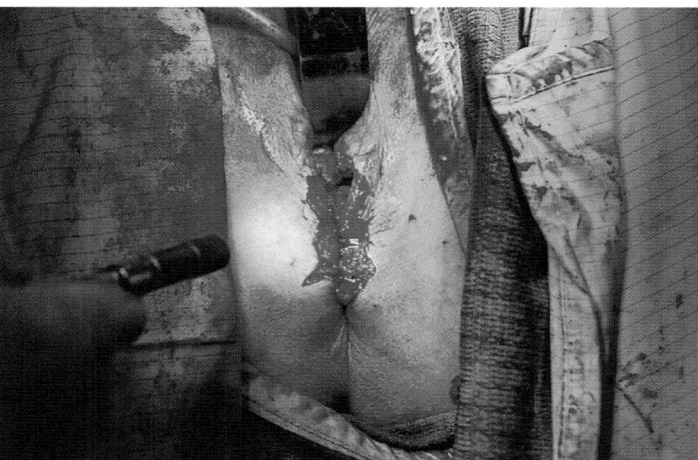

B

**FIGURE 100–9** The perineal body is rebuilt, and the perineal skin is approximated at the midline. Upon completion of the repair, the diameter of the anal canal should allow tight placement of an index finger.

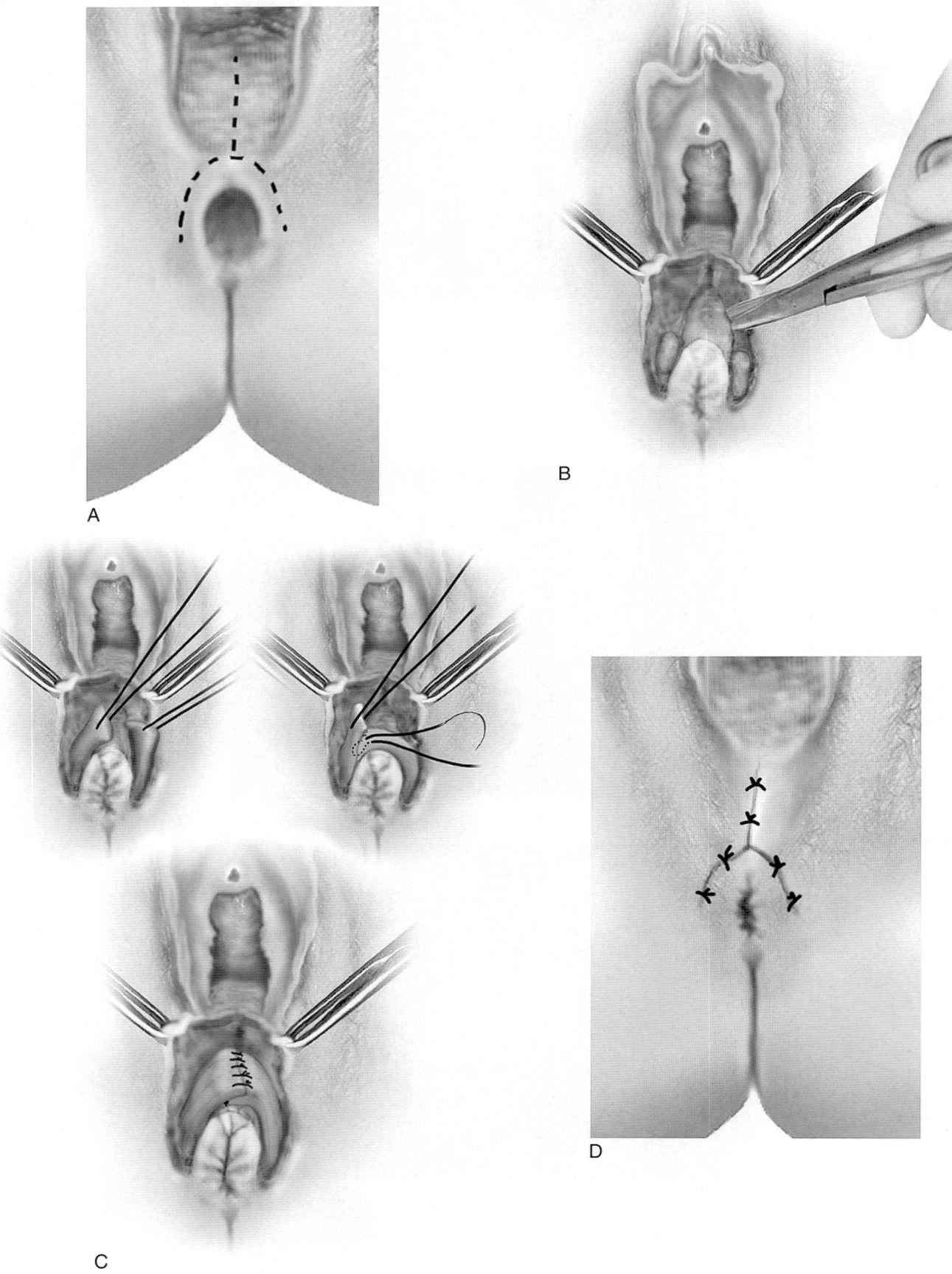

**FIGURE 100–10  A** through **D.** Technique of overlapping sphincteroplasty.

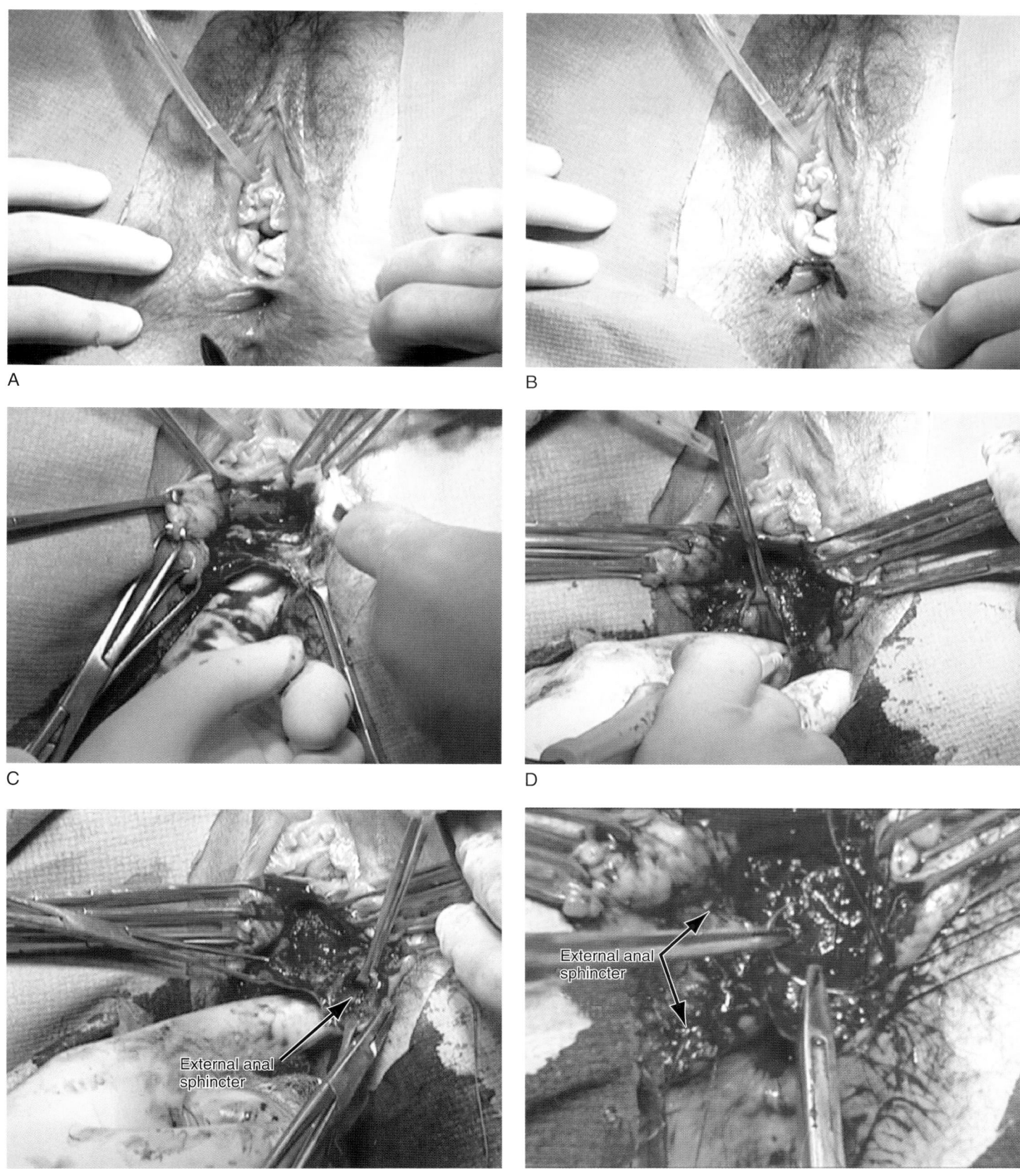

**FIGURE 100–11** Technique of an end-to-end sphincteroplasty in a patient who sustained a breakdown of a fourth-degree episiotomy repair. **A.** Note the widened vaginal hiatus, the patulous anal opening, and complete loss of the perineal body with significant retraction of the ends of the anal sphincter. **B.** An inverted-U incision is made. **C.** The incision is extended laterally and inferiorly to identify the retracted ends of the external sphincter. **D.** Viable muscle is identified at approximately 3 o'clock on the left side. **E.** The retracted end of the external anal sphincter is identified on the left side. **F.** The external anal sphincter on the right is demonstrated. Note that the dissected sphincter is approximately 4 cm wide. Numerous sutures have been passed through the left end of the external sphincter. As each suture is passed to the opposite side, small bites are taken through the internal anal sphincter.

UNIT 4 ■ SECTION B

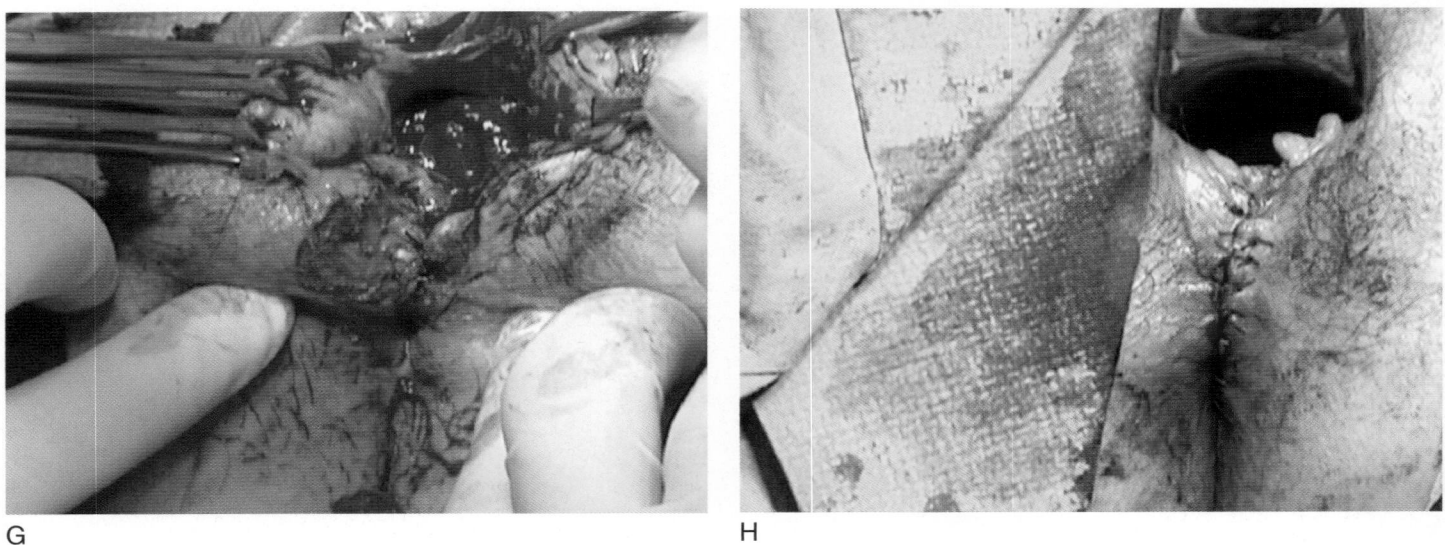

G          H

**FIGURE 100–11, cont'd G.** Sutures have been tied across the midline, completing the end-to-end sphincteroplasty. **H.** The perineal body has been rebuilt, and the completed repair is shown.

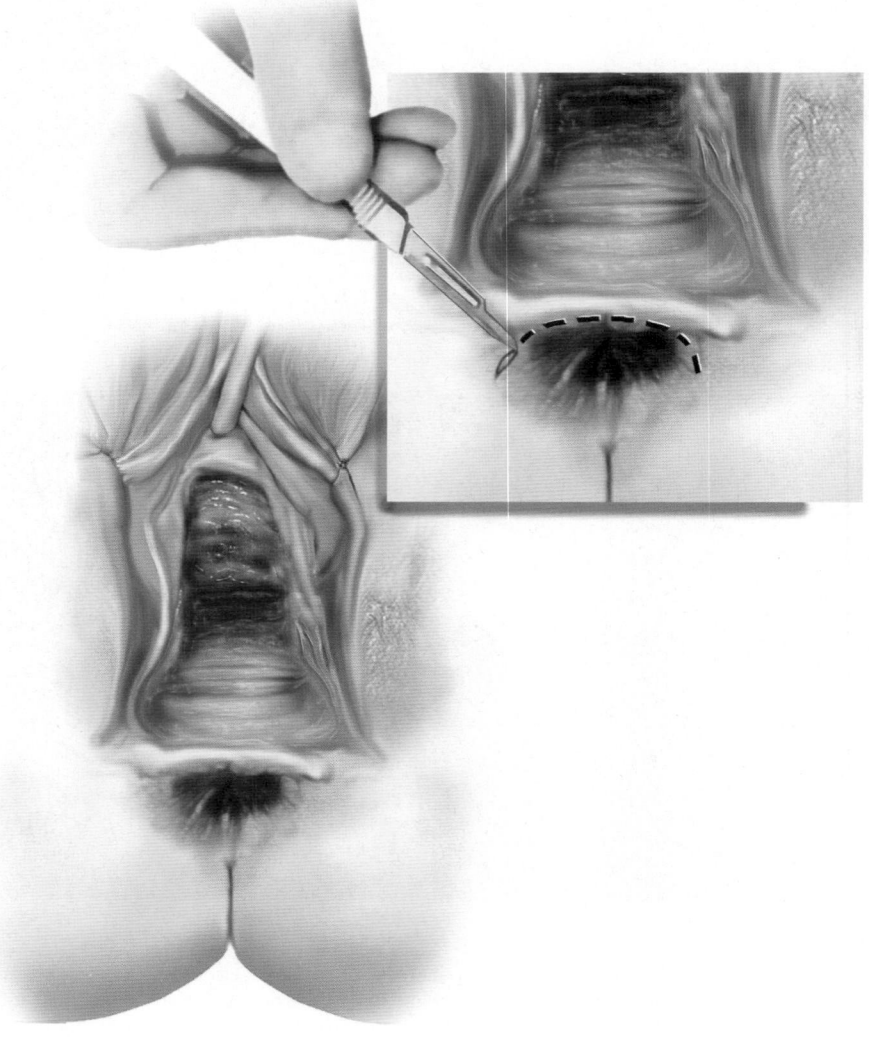

A

**FIGURE 100–12** Technique of end-to-end sphincteroplasty with perineal reconstruction. **A.** A cloacal perineal defect is noted in which the posterior vaginal wall and the anterior rectal wall are fused. An inverted-U or transverse incision is made (**inset**).

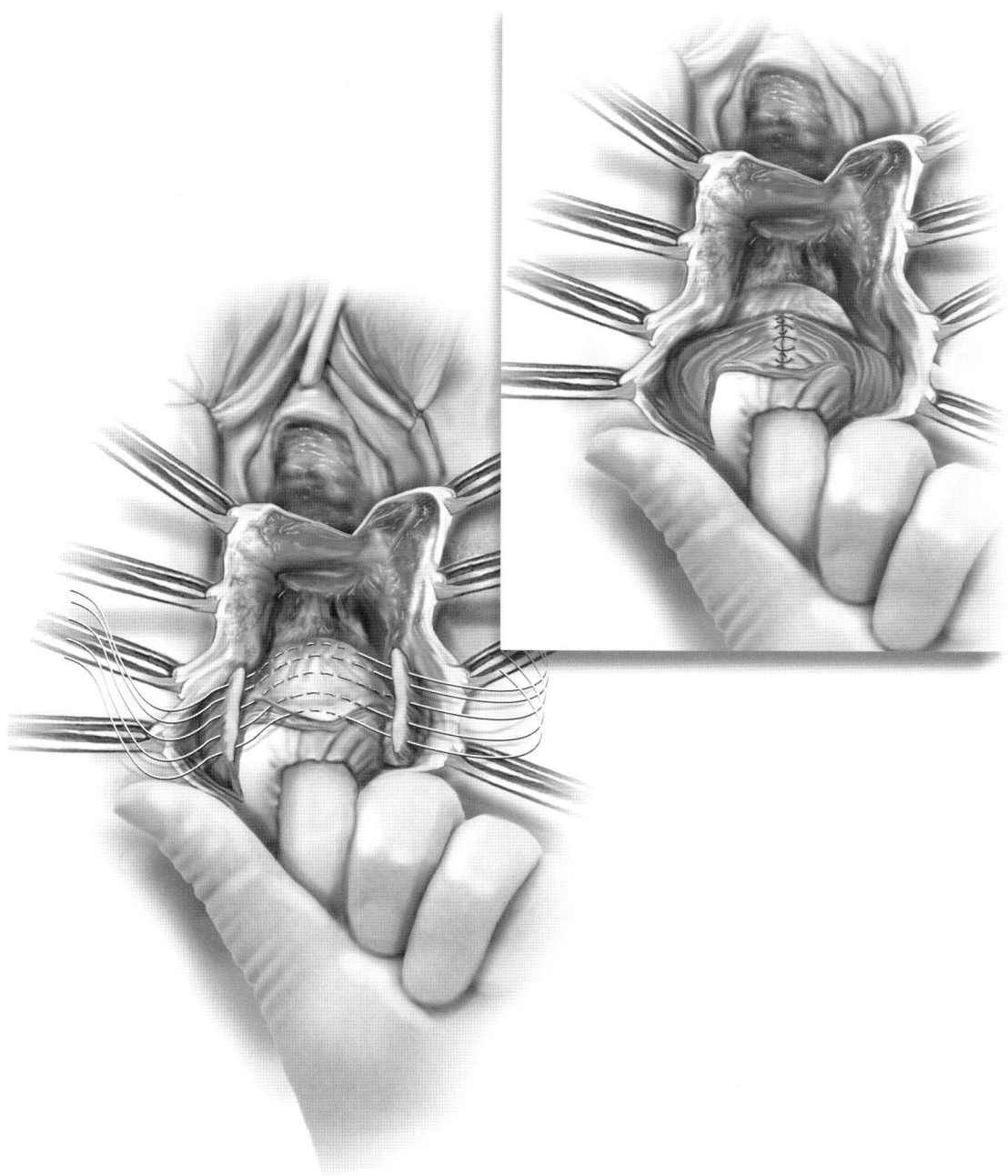

B

**FIGURE 100–12, cont'd   B.** The rectovaginal space has been opened, along with the posterior vaginal wall of the rectum. The retracted ends of the external anal sphincter have been identified. Sutures incorporate small bites through the internal anal sphincter as they are passed to the opposite side. The completed end-to-end sphincteroplasty is shown (**inset**).

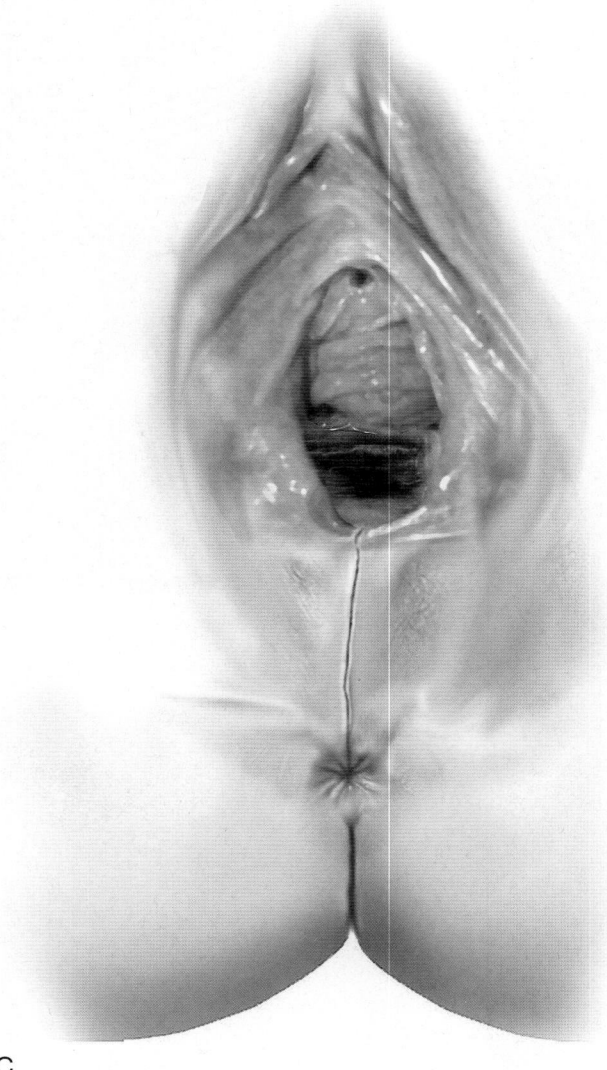

C

**FIGURE 100–12, cont'd  C.** The perineum has been completely reconstructed. The completed repair should show a perpendicular relationship between the posterior vaginal wall and the rebuilt perineum. Note that the anal opening becomes puckered and is no longer patulous.

# CHAPTER 101

# Transperineal Repair of Rectal Prolapse

*Bradley R. Davis*

Rectal prolapse is characterized by a circumferential full-thickness protrusion of the rectum from the anus. It is believed to represent the culmination of a series of events leading to a sliding hernia through the levator hiatus (Fig. 101–1). This includes loss of sacral fixation, redundancy of the sigmoid colon and its mesentery, a deep anterior cul-de-sac, and a patulous anus. Treatments for rectal prolapse attempt to correct these problems and either restore the rectum to the pelvis or remove the hernia and redundant rectum. Although a number of options are available for the surgical correction of rectal prolapse, they can be broadly classified as transabdominal or transperineal.

Transabdominal repairs (laparoscopic or open) are better suited for most patients as they provide a more durable repair with a lower incidence of recurrence and improved functional outcomes when continence and overall bowel function are assessed.

This chapter addresses transperineal repairs, which are performed more often in elderly patients, who are poor candidates for general anesthesia or an abdominal incision. These patients tend to be older, to reside more frequently in nursing homes or assisted living, and to have a significantly greater number of comorbidities. In all transperineal approaches, the redundant rectum and any redundant sigmoid colon are resected, the cul-de-sac is obliterated, and the levators can be plicated posteriorly. The decision to perform a full-thickness resection (perineal proctectomy or the Altemeier procedure) or a partial-thickness resection (Delorme procedure) is based mainly on the surgeon's preference, as these procedures seem to result in similar functional outcomes and recurrence rates.

## Perineal Proctectomy (Altemeier Repair)

1. Spinal anesthesia is adequate for this procedure, but general anesthesia is acceptable if deemed safe. Most colorectal surgeons prefer to position the patient in a prone jackknife position under a spinal anesthesia with the buttocks taped apart. However, if the patient requires a vaginal procedure concomitantly, then a lithotomy position (Fig. 101–2) is preferred, so there is no need to reposition the patient. It is important to point out that in any type of combined procedure, the rectal prolapse should be addressed first, as it will be difficult to prolapse the rectum once the posterior colporrhaphy is performed.

2. Once positioned, the rectum is prolapsed and a retractor is used to evert the anal canal (Fig. 101–3A, B), exposing the dentate line and the anal transition zone (zone between the rectal mucosa and the squamous mucosa of the anus). It is important to retain the transition zone, as it is important in discriminating gas from liquid and solid stool.

3. Electrocautery is then used to divide the rectal wall circumferentially (Fig. 101–4). With a finger in the rectum, folding of the rectal wall creates several layers, and the incision should be deep enough to expose the mesorectal fat on the inner tube of the rectum (Fig. 101–5).

4. Between the anterior rectal wall and the vagina (Fig. 101–6A), the hernia sac or enterocele sac can be found and should be opened to facilitate lateral and posterior dissection (Fig. 101–6B).

5. The author's preference is to divide the mesorectum with a bipolar energy device (Fig. 101–7A), but it can be clamped and ligated just as effectively with heavy Vicryl ties (Fig. 101–7B). The dissection should be continued until there is no more laxity in the bowel, which now should be tethered only by the sigmoid or descending colon mesentery at the top of the sacral promontory (Fig. 101–8).

6. Before the anastomosis is conducted, a posterior levatorplasty can be performed (Fig. 101–9) in an effort to restore the anorectal angle, which is believed to be important in the overall continence of the patient.

7. The redundant rectum is then resected (Figs. 101–10 and 101–11A, B) and sewn to the distal remnant with a series of interrupted 3-0 Vicryl sutures (Figs. 101–12 through 101–14).

8. Once completed, the anastomosis should be located at the top of the transition zone (Fig. 101–15), and the prolapse should be corrected (Fig. 101–16).

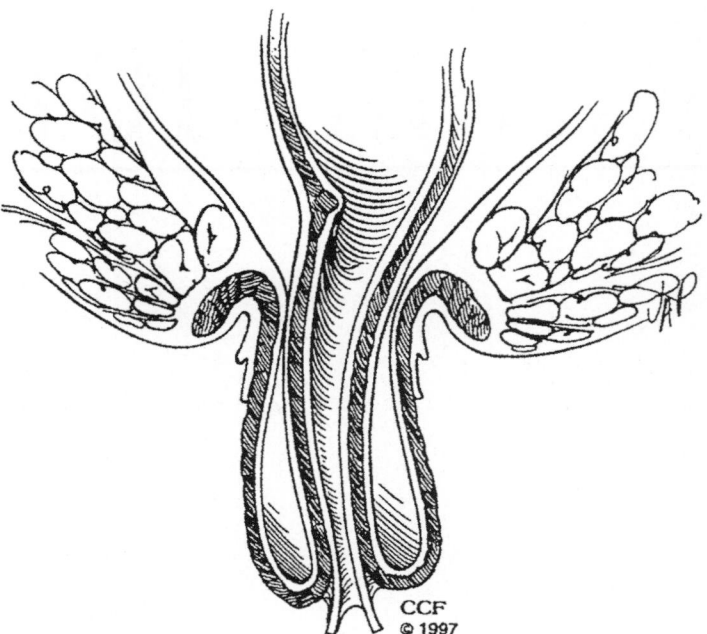

**FIGURE 101–1** This illustrates the sliding hernia through the levators and sphincters, creating the full-thickness prolapse. Note the two distinct tubes with mucosa being exposed overlying the muscularis propria, which when divided will expose the outer layer of the inner tube (mesorectal fat).

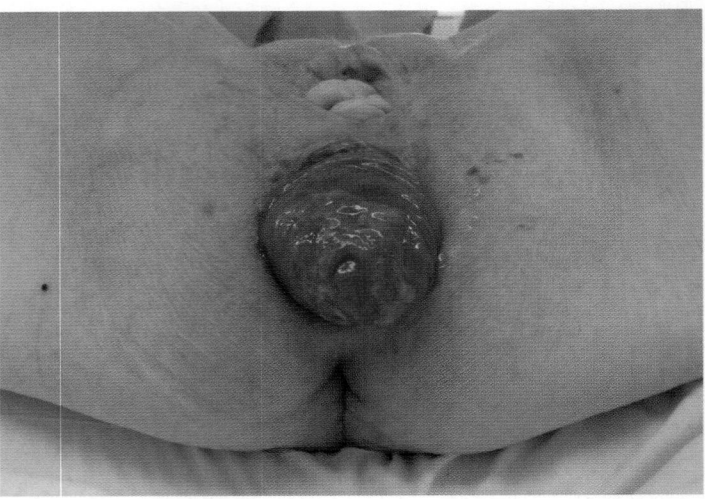

**FIGURE 101–2** The patient is in lithotomy with the rectum prolapsed. Note also the significant vaginal prolapse.

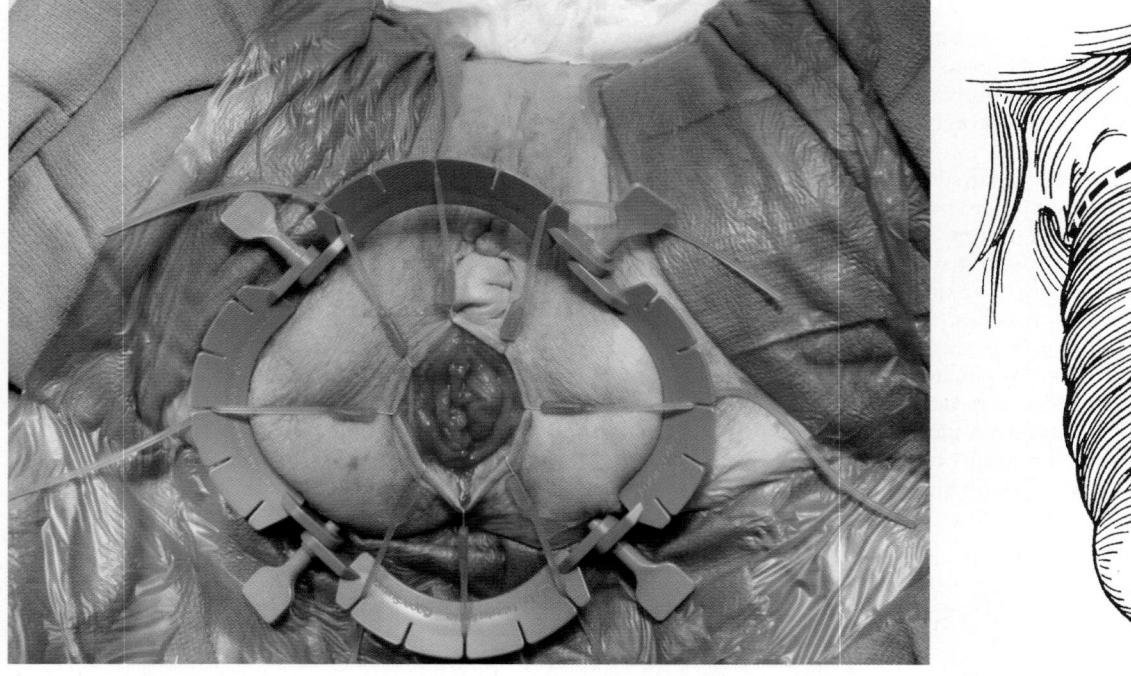

A                                                                                              B

**FIGURE 101–3  A.** The Lone Star Retractor (CooperSurgical, Trumbull, CT) is very useful in everting the anus while exposing the rectal mucosa and the anal transition zone. The characteristic patulous anus of patients with prolapse is evident. **B.** The dotted line shows the point of transection.

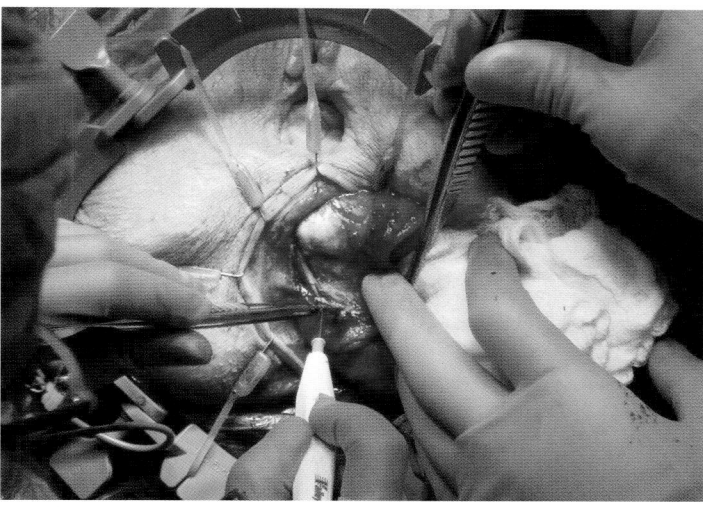

**FIGURE 101–4**  The rectal wall is divided circumferentially by means of electrocautery. All layers of the rectal wall need to be divided if the prolapse is to be resected successfully.

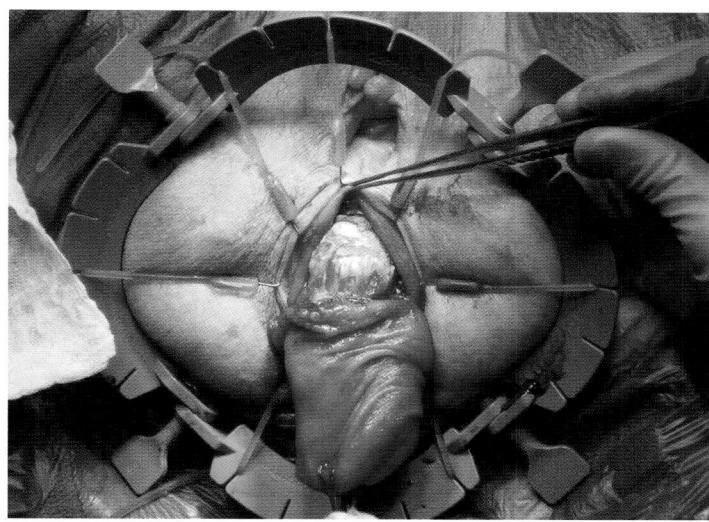

**FIGURE 101–5**  This picture demonstrates the division of the muscularis propria of the rectal wall, exposing the underlying fat layer referred to as the *mesorectum*. This contains the lymphatics and the blood supply to the rectum and needs to be divided. Once through this layer, the muscularis propria of the inner tube will be exposed.

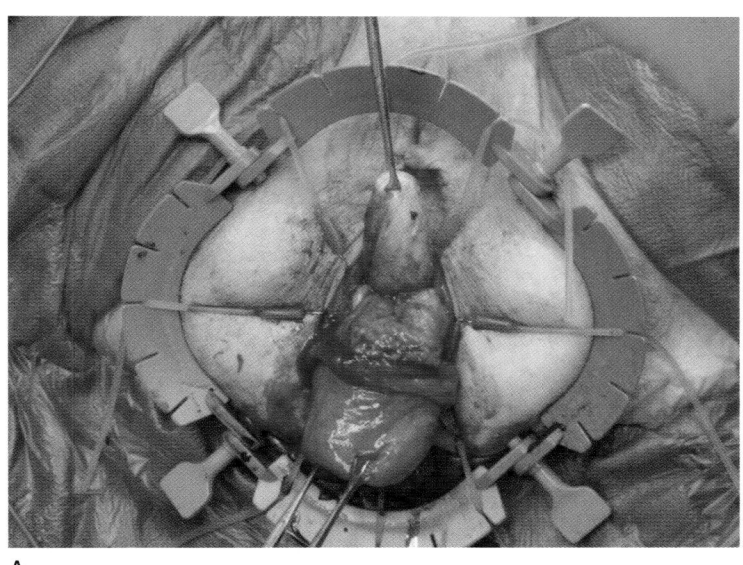

A

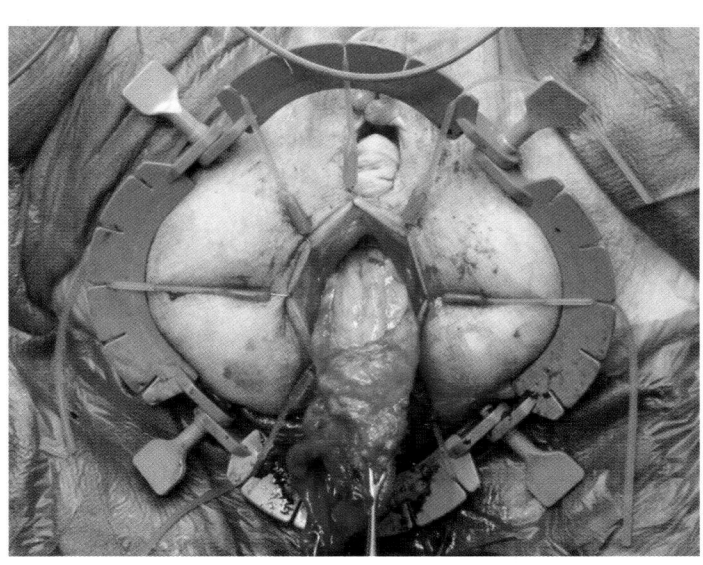

B

**FIGURE 101–6 A.** The vagina is prolapsed and is being lifted up off the anterior wall of the rectum. The enterocele or hernia sac will be found by continuing to dissect in this plane. If seen from an abdominal approach, this dissection would open the pouch of Douglas. **B.** Once the sac is opened, the rectum is delivered and the extraperitoneal rectum becomes evident.

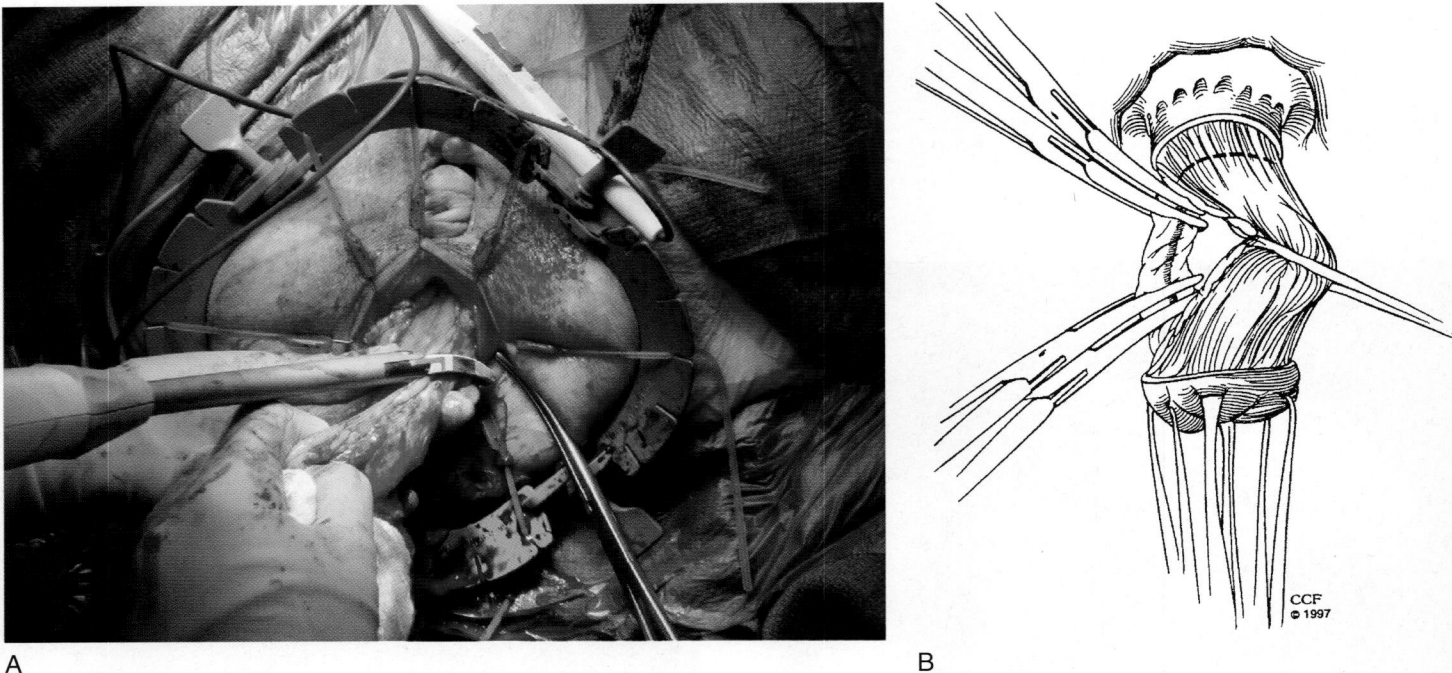

A                                                              B

**FIGURE 101–7** To resect the redundant rectum, the mesorectum must be divided. This (**A**) can be done with an energy or bipolar device or (**B**) can be ligated between Kelly clamps and tied.

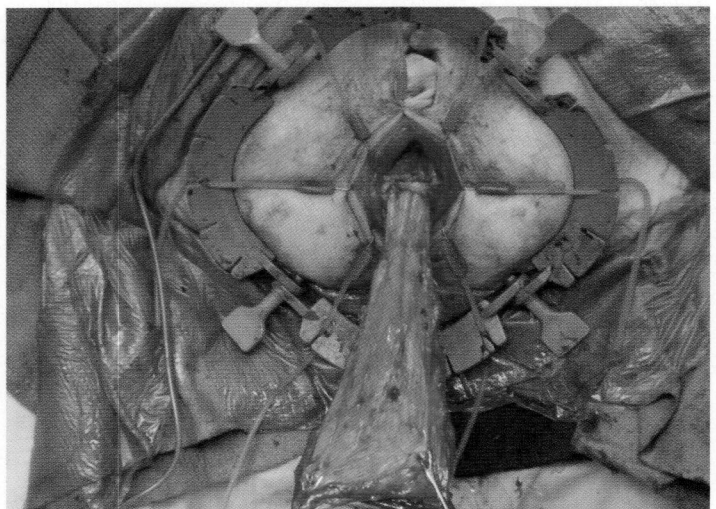

**FIGURE 101–8** Once the rectal mesentery is fully divided, the prolapse becomes fully everted, exposing the top of the rectum and not infrequently the sigmoid colon. If there is still redundancy, the sigmoid mesentery can be divided at the sacral promontory. Great care must be taken when dividing the mesentery very proximally, as bleeding can be difficult to manage in the pelvis. Additionally, if the mesentery is taken too proximally, the colonic wall can become ischemic, resulting in an unsafe anastomosis.

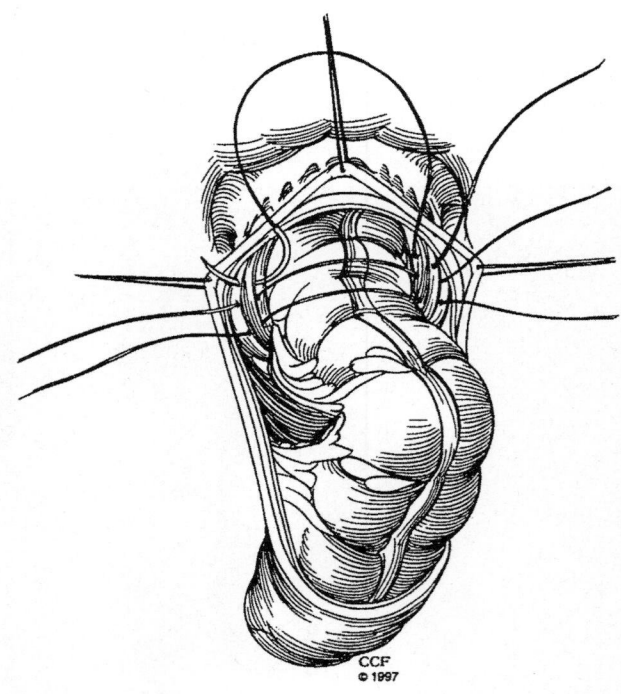

**FIGURE 101–9** Before performing the anastomosis, the levators can be plicated together using a nonabsorbable suture. This step can help restore the anorectal angle if placed posteriorly and reduce the size of the rectal hiatus. This may help to prevent recurrent prolapse. Care should be taken not to narrow the rectum, and at least one finger should be able to easily pass between the levators and the rectum.

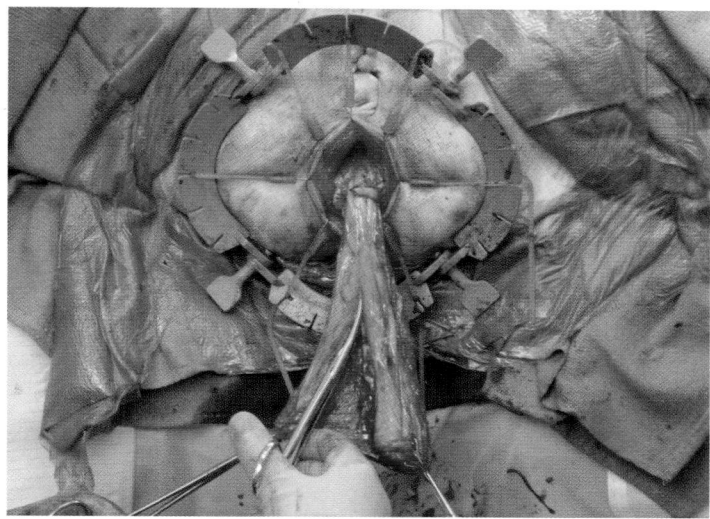

**FIGURE 101–10** The rectum is placed on stretch and the orientation is established so that there is no twisting. To maintain this orientation, the muscular tube is divided longitudinally along its anterior surface to the point where it will be cut off. The goal is to remove as much of the rectum or colon as is safe so that there is a good residual blood supply and the anastomosis is not under tension. A stitch is placed at the apex of the incision to the distal cuff of the transition zone.

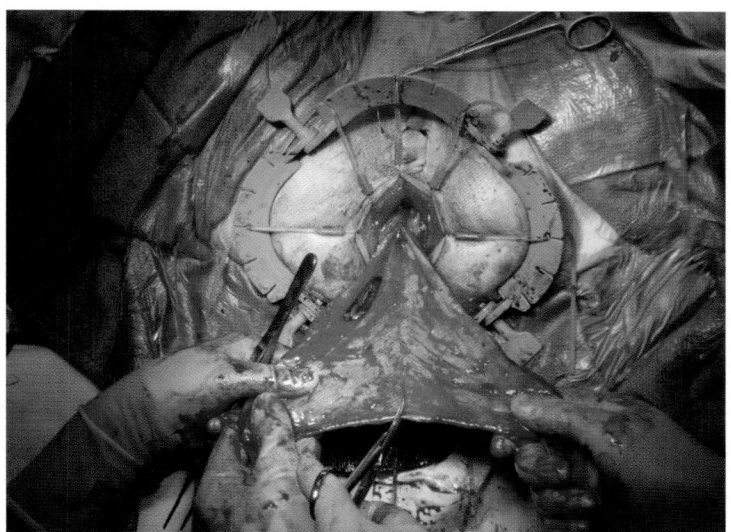

A

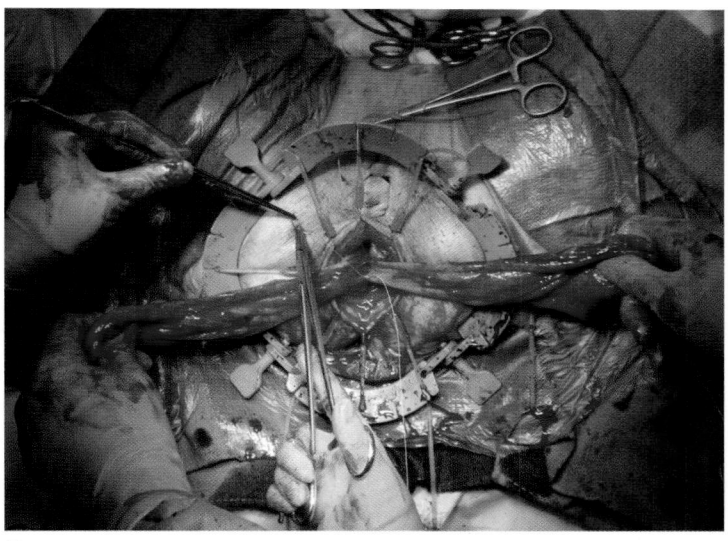

B

**FIGURE 101–11 A.** The anterior stitch can be seen at the top of the picture, and a second longitudinal incision is made along the posterior aspect of the muscular tube. By approaching the anastomosis in this way, there is no risk of losing the proximal segment into the pelvis, and orientation is maintained. **B.** A second stitch is then placed posteriorly, much like the first stitch.

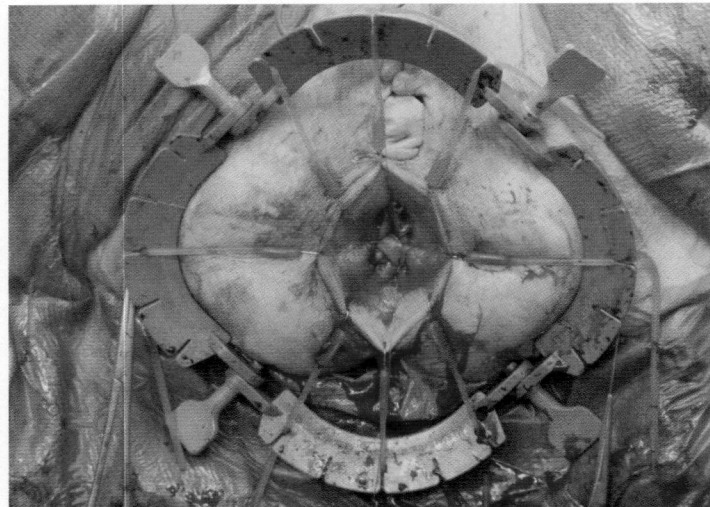

**FIGURE 101–12** The two halves of the muscular tube are then resected circumferentially right and left, with stitches placed right lateral and left lateral.

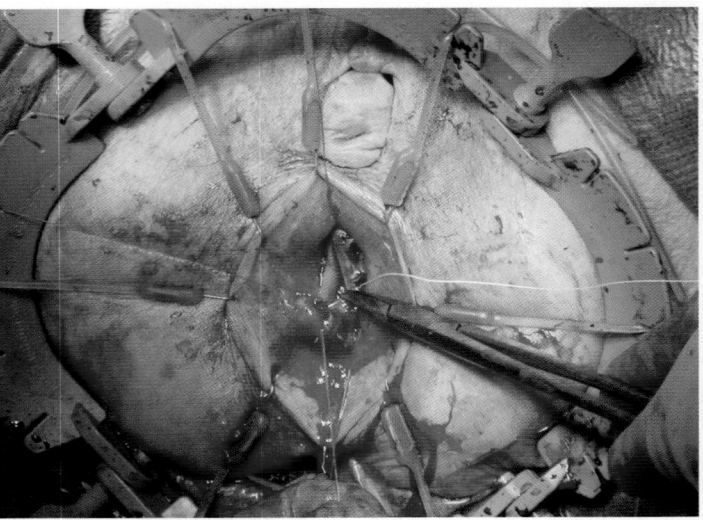

**FIGURE 101–13** Additional sutures are then placed in each quadrant. Two to three usually suffice. Often there is a size mismatch between the proximal colon and the rectal cuff, which can be dealt with by approaching the anastomosis through this stepwise approach.

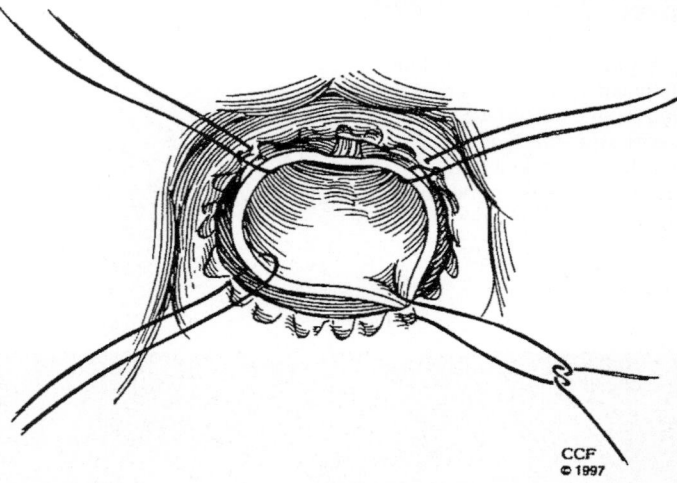

**FIGURE 101–14** The completed anastomosis should be tension-free and should show no evidence of ischemia. A gentle digital examination will reveal any defects remaining that can be repaired with additional sutures and will confirm a patent anastomosis.

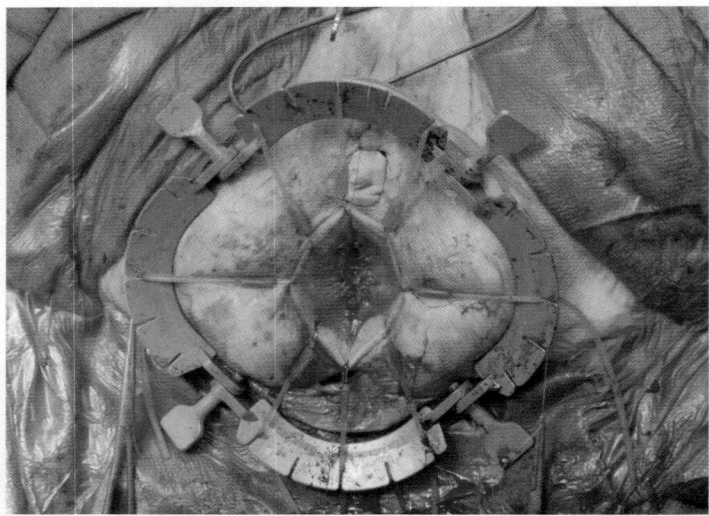

**FIGURE 101–15** Anastomosis is complete between the proximal colon and the transition zone (remnant rectal cuff). The transition zone allows for the discrimination of gas, liquid, and solid stool. Although this does not guarantee that the patient will be continent, most will experience improvement.

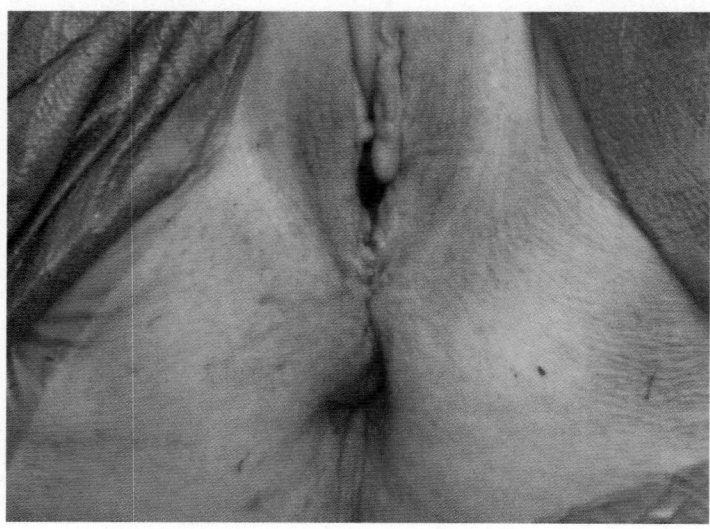

**FIGURE 101–16** At the conclusion of the procedure, the rectal prolapse is no longer evident. One can see that there is little trauma to the anal margin skin and anoderm, which means that patients will have very little pain postoperatively—a key goal of this procedure.

# SECTION C

## Cosmetic and Gender Reassignment Surgery

UNIT 4 ■ SECTION C

# CHAPTER 102

# Surgery for Labial Hypertrophy

*Michael S. Baggish* ■ *Mickey M. Karram*

The labia minora range in size and configuration from individual to individual. These small labia play a significant anatomic role in controlling under normal circumstances ingress and egress to and from the vestibule. These labia keep the vestibular skin moist and prevent external detritus from entering the lower vagina and vestibule.

Occasionally, the labial configuration is greatly exaggerated so as to create hygienic problems (Fig. 102–1). Labial hypertrophy can also damage the tissue by snagging on clothing and tearing. Likewise, chronic irritation may create fissures and/or ulcers. For the previous circumstances, labial reduction may be indicated (Figs. 102–2 and 102–3). The procedure removes excessive tissue, leaving behind sculpted but reduced labia (Fig. 102–4). Complete amputation is rarely if ever indicated.

Other indications for labial reduction may be solely aesthetic and/or psychological. Any woman requesting labial reduction requires education about variations in vulvar anatomy and symmetry, as well as the normality of these variations. An alternative technique for simplifying excision of excess labial tissue is wedge resection, which incorporates flap advancement. The advantage of the flap advancement technique relates to the fact that the free margins of the labia minora are preserved. Therefore, the likelihood of alteration in skin color and texture is reduced. Fig. 102–5A through C schematically illustrates a Z-plasty technique. Figs. 102–6 through 102–16 show the details of a wedge-type labial plasty in a woman who desired labial reduction. The young woman complained about pulling irritation and embarrassment related to the size of her labia minora.

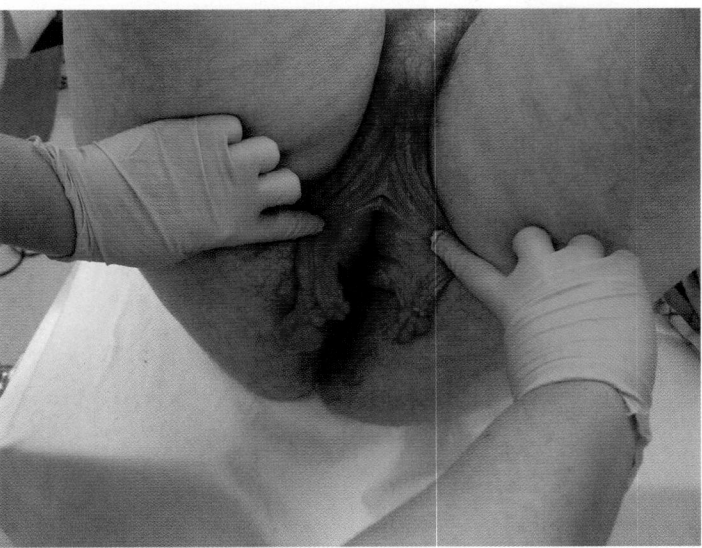

**FIGURE 102–1** Massive hypertrophy of the labia minora in a young woman with cerebral palsy.

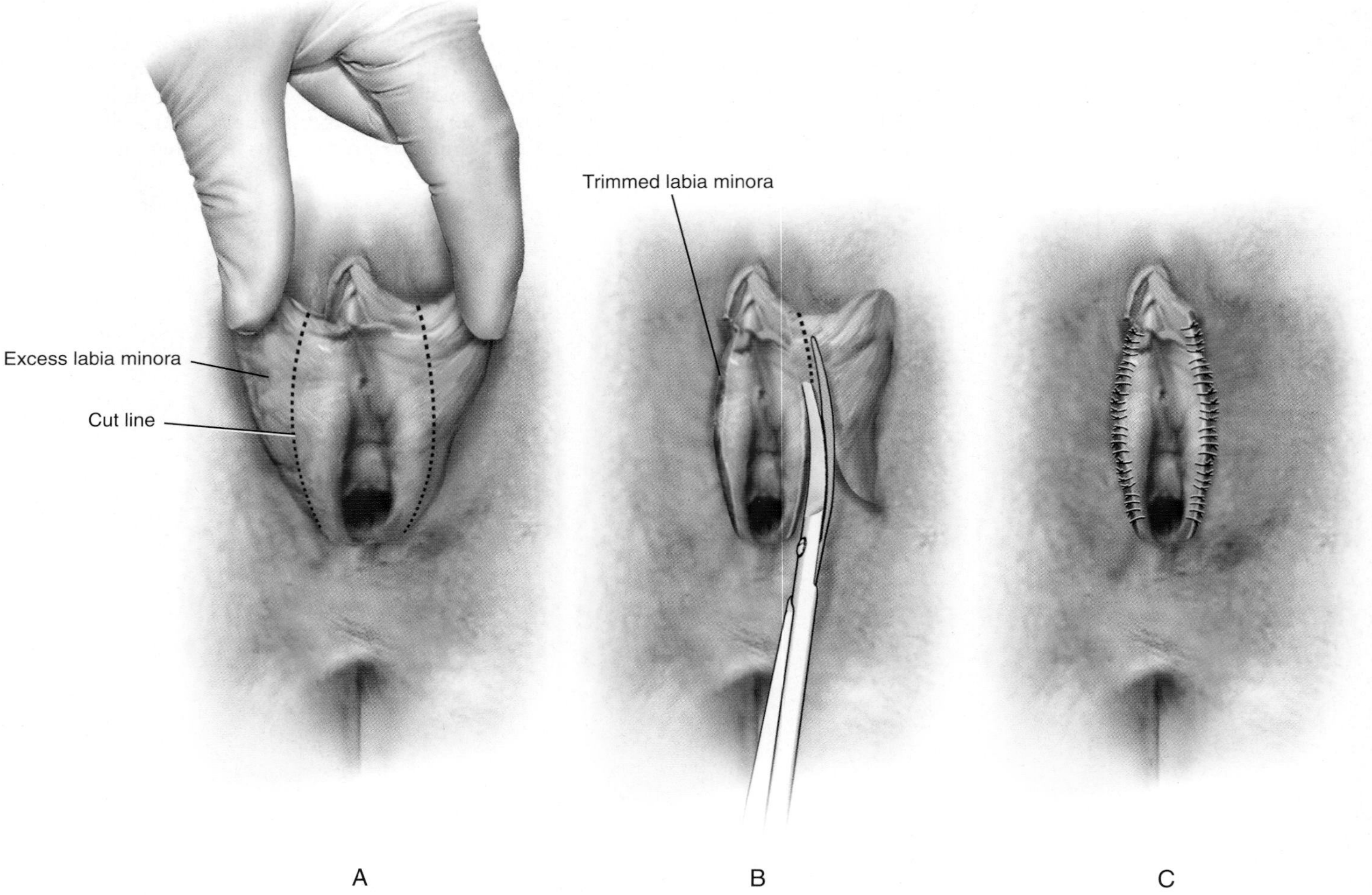

Excess labia minora

Cut line

Trimmed labia minora

A

B

C

**FIGURE 102–2** The technique for simple excision of enlarged or hypertrophied labial skin. **A.** Excess skin to be removed is marked. **B.** Skin is excised. **C.** Interrupted sutures reapproximate the edges of the labia.

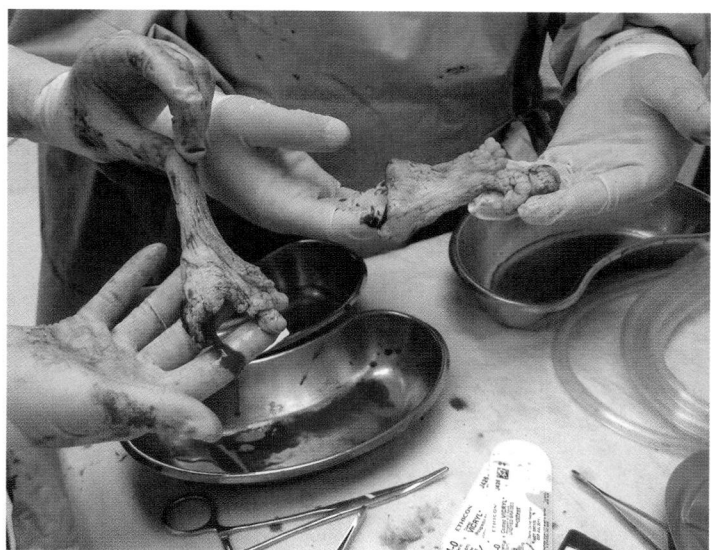

**FIGURE 102–3** Specimens obtained after resection of the redundant labial tissue.

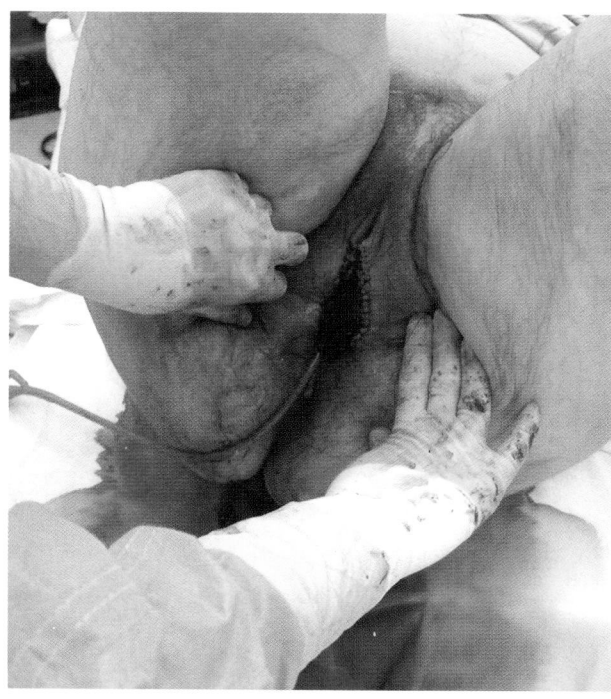

**FIGURE 102–4** The repairs leave sculpted labial tissue, which will not impinge on hygiene, and maintain the appearance and function of the labia minora.

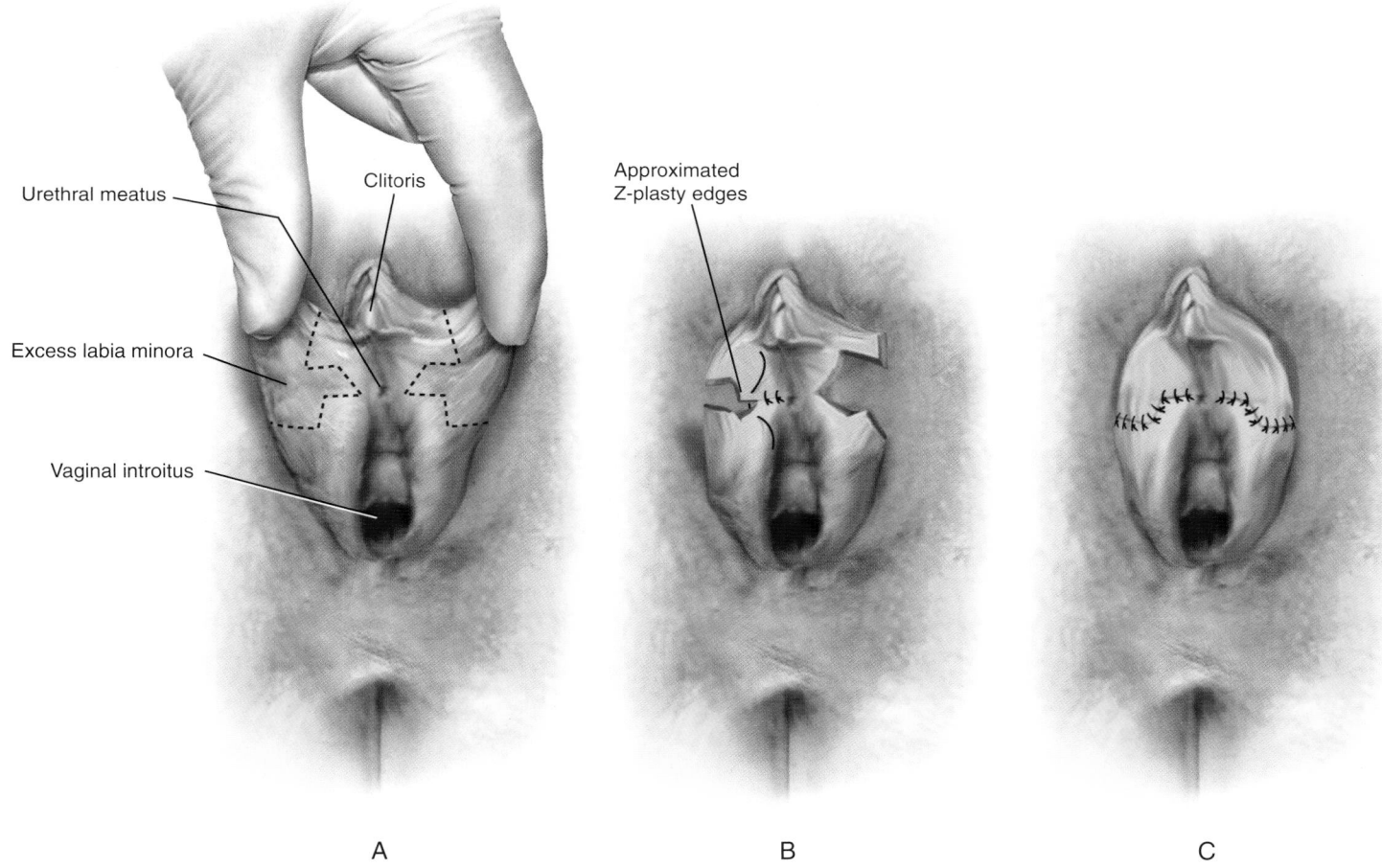

A

B

C

**FIGURE 102–5** Technique for Z-plasty. **A.** Skin is to be excised. **B.** Skin is excised and is reapproximated transversely with fine interrupted sutures. **C.** Completed repair.

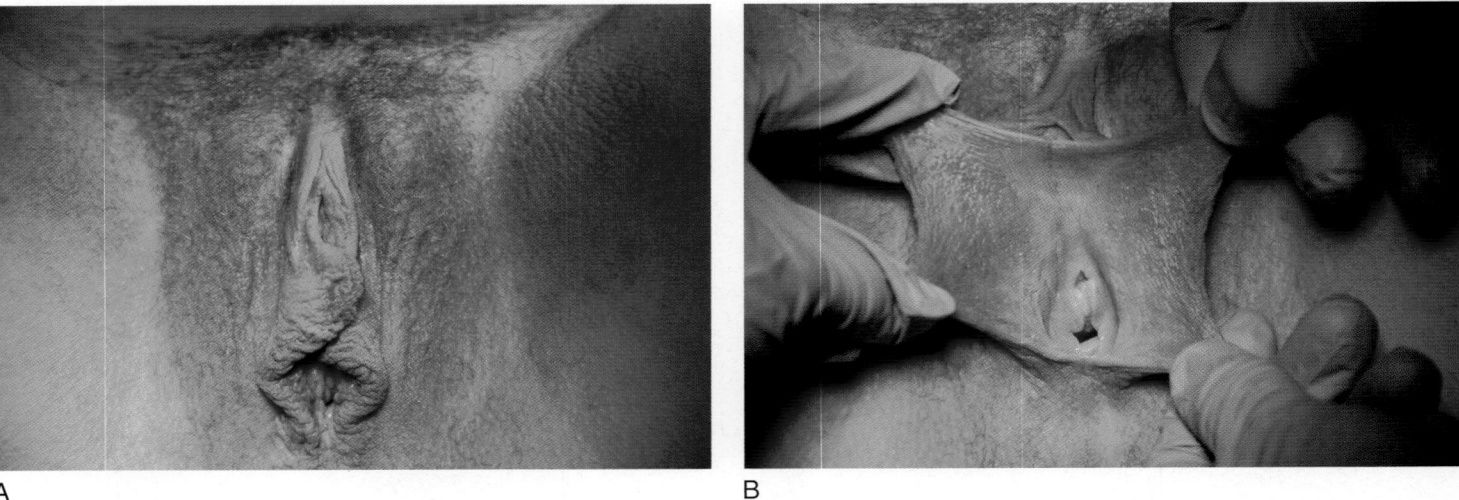

A                                                                                                                                B

**FIGURE 102–6  A.** A moderate degree of labial hypertrophy is seen in this photo. **B.** The degree of labial enlargement is more apparent when placed on stretch.

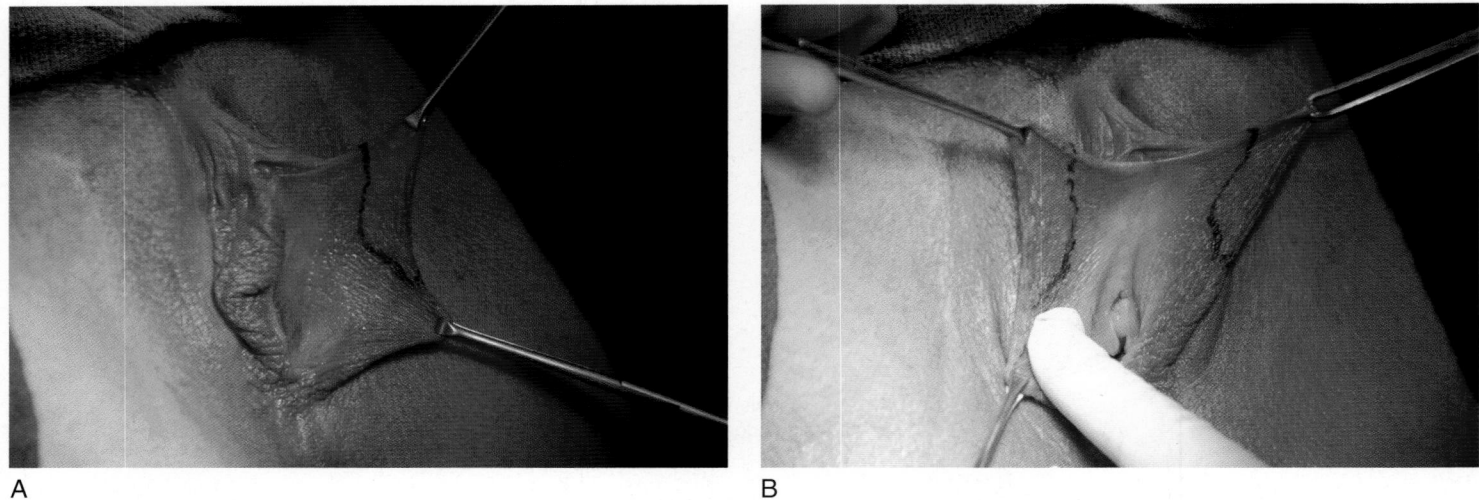

A                                                                                                                                B

**FIGURE 102–7  A.** The boundaries of the wedge to be resected are marked carefully with a pen on the left labium minus. **B.** The wedge configuration is likewise traced on the opposite labium.

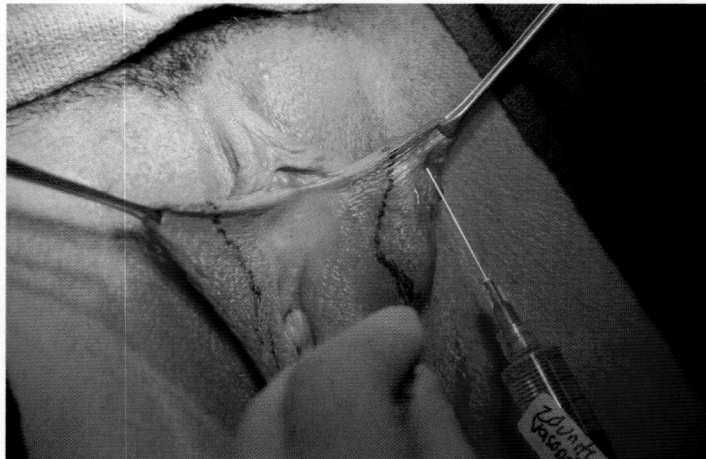

**FIGURE 102–8**  A 1:100 diluted vasopressin solution is injected into the labium for hemostasis.

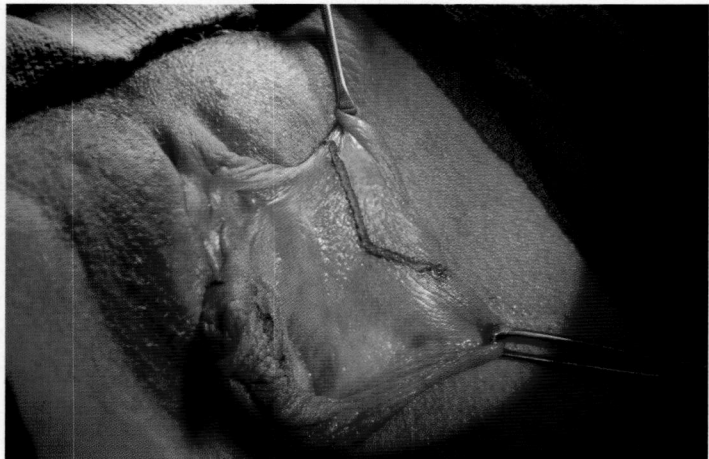

**FIGURE 102–9**  The wedge of tissue is sharply incised on the medial aspect of the left labium minus.

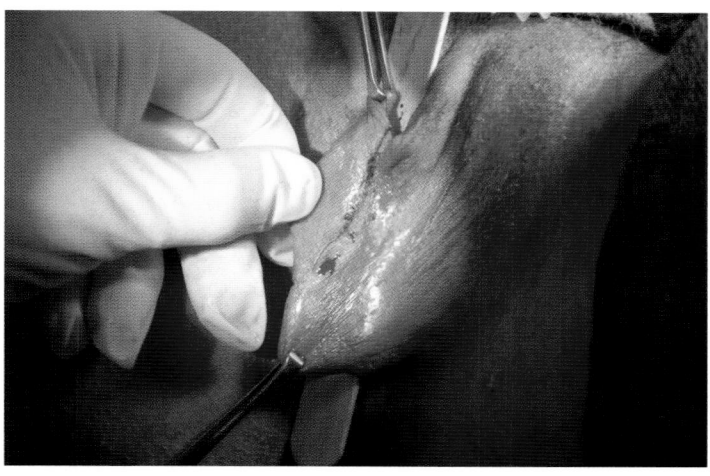

**FIGURE 102–10** A similar cut is made on the lateral surface of the left labium. The two cuts are connected at a precise intersection.

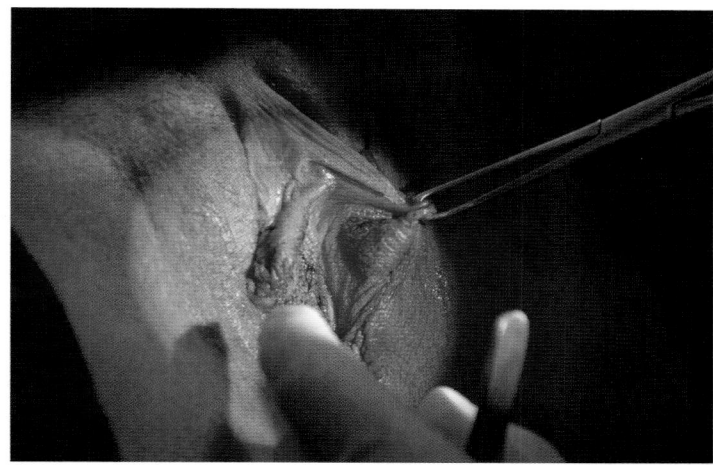

**FIGURE 102–11** The wedge of labial tissue has been removed. The lower portion of the residual labium is mobilized upward to precisely meet the upper flap, which is marked by the application of an Allis clamp.

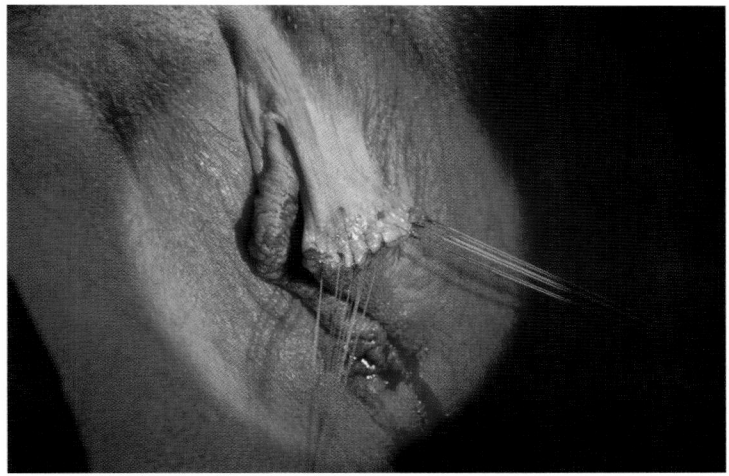

A

B

**FIGURE 102–12 A.** The lateral aspects of the approximated incision are sutured with 4-0 Vicryl sutures. **B.** The medial aspects of the wound are similarly secured.

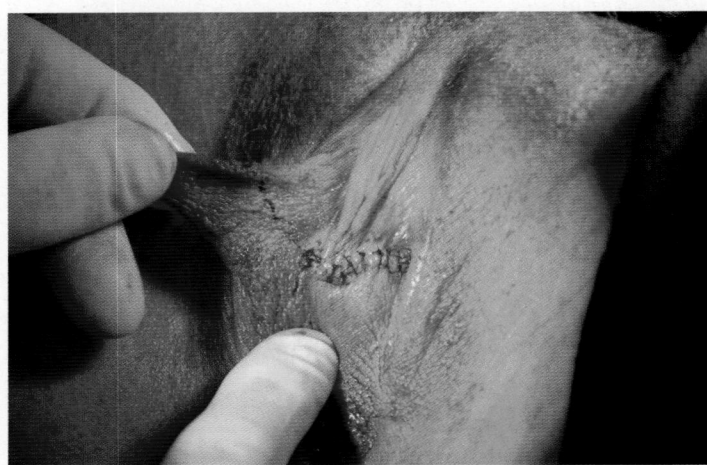

**FIGURE 102–13** Attention is now focused on the right labium minus.

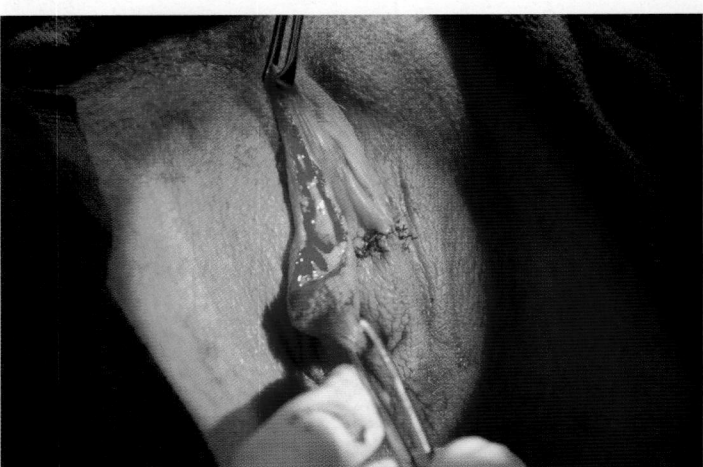

**FIGURE 102–14** In a fashion identical to that performed on the left side, a wedge of tissue has been excised from the right labium minus.

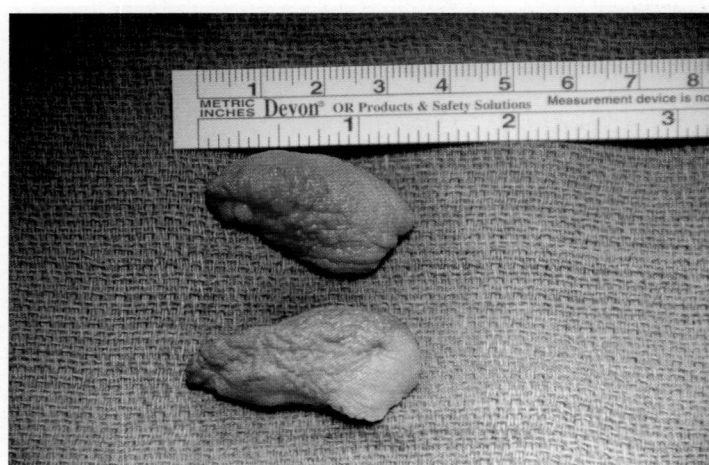

**FIGURE 102–15** The excised wedges are shown here before they were sent to pathology.

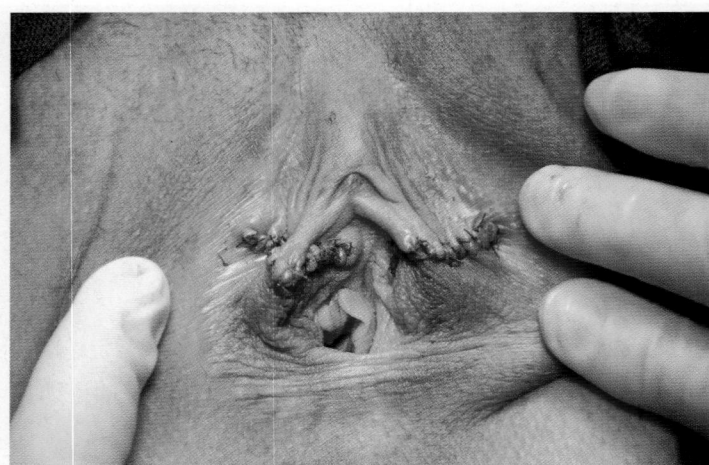

**FIGURE 102–16** The reduction is complete.

# CHAPTER 103

# Vaginoplasty With Perineal Reconstruction (Cosmetic Gynecologic Surgery)

*Mickey M. Karram*

The term *vaginoplasty* has been used to describe any reconstructive procedures performed on the vagina. This chapter specifically addresses the use of vaginoplasty with perineal reconstruction to tighten the introitus and vaginal lumen or to reconstruct the perineum for aesthetic or functional reasons.

Vaginoplasty often includes anterior and/or posterior colporrhaphy, in which portions of the mucosa are excised and the vaginal lumen and introitus are reconstructed. Unfortunately, no standardization for these types of procedures currently exists. The goal of all reconstructive procedures performed on the vagina should be to create a well-supported vagina of appropriate length and caliber. The axis of the vagina should not be deviated, with the vaginal vault having a slightly posterior direction toward the hollow of the sacrum. At the completion of any repair, the vaginal lumen should easily accept two fingers, and the posterior vaginal wall and perineum should have a perpendicular relationship. This usually is best accomplished by removing a diamond-shaped piece of tissue from the perineum and the posterior vaginal wall (Fig. 103–1). Every repair needs to be individualized to the patient's specific anatomy.

Figs. 103–2 through 103–5 provide examples of a variety of patients undergoing vaginoplasty and perineal reconstruction. Fig. 103–2 shows a patient with a symptomatic rectocele and dyspareunia secondary to a large buildup of the skin of the labia minora at the level of the introitus. Note that the completed repair re-creates an appropriate relationship between the perineum and posterior vaginal wall while creating posterior vaginal wall support and decreasing vaginal caliber. Fig. 103–3 presents a patient with a widened genital hiatus, as well as a perineal defect. Figs. 103–4 and 103–5 both show young patients who required extensive perineal reconstruction after vaginal birth. In both cases, a xenograft (Surgisis; Cook Medical, Bloomington, Indiana) is used to fill in a perineal skin defect.

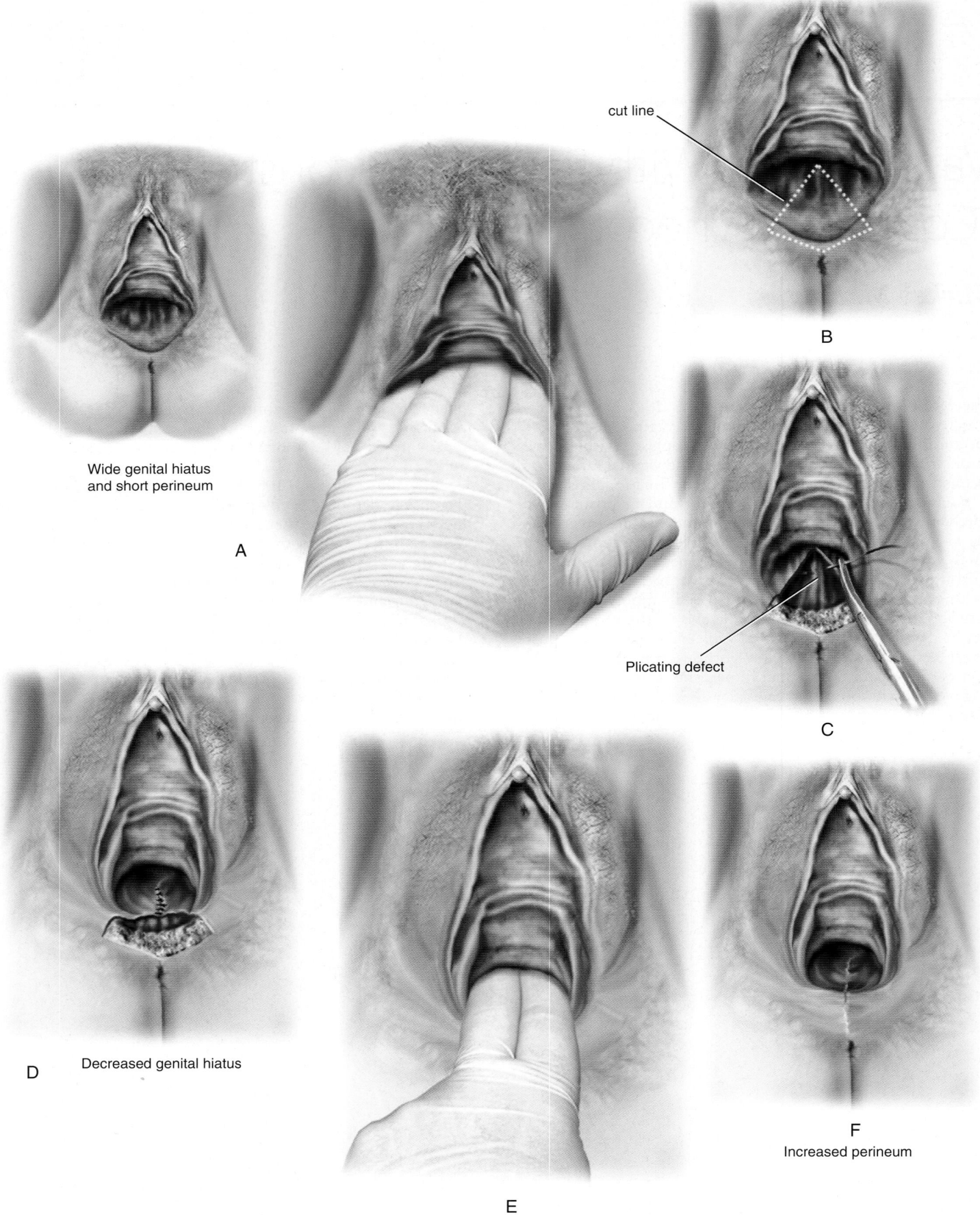

cut line

Wide genital hiatus
and short perineum

A

B

Plicating defect

C

Decreased genital hiatus

D

E

Increased perineum

F

**FIGURE 103–1**    Technique of vaginoplasty and perineal reconstruction with the sole aim of tightening the vaginal introitus. **A.** Note the wide genital hiatus, which easily allows the insertion of four fingers. **B.** A diamond-shaped piece of tissue to be excised is marked. **C.** The tissue has been removed, and deep stitches are taken through the perirectal fascia and levator muscles to build up the posterior vaginal wall. Great care is taken to avoid the creation of a posterior vaginal wall ridge. **D.** The upper portion of the posterior vaginal wall is closed in preparation for perineal reconstruction. **E.** After perineal reconstruction, the introitus allows the insertion of only two fingers. **F.** Completed repair; note the perpendicular relationship between the posterior vaginal wall and the perineum.

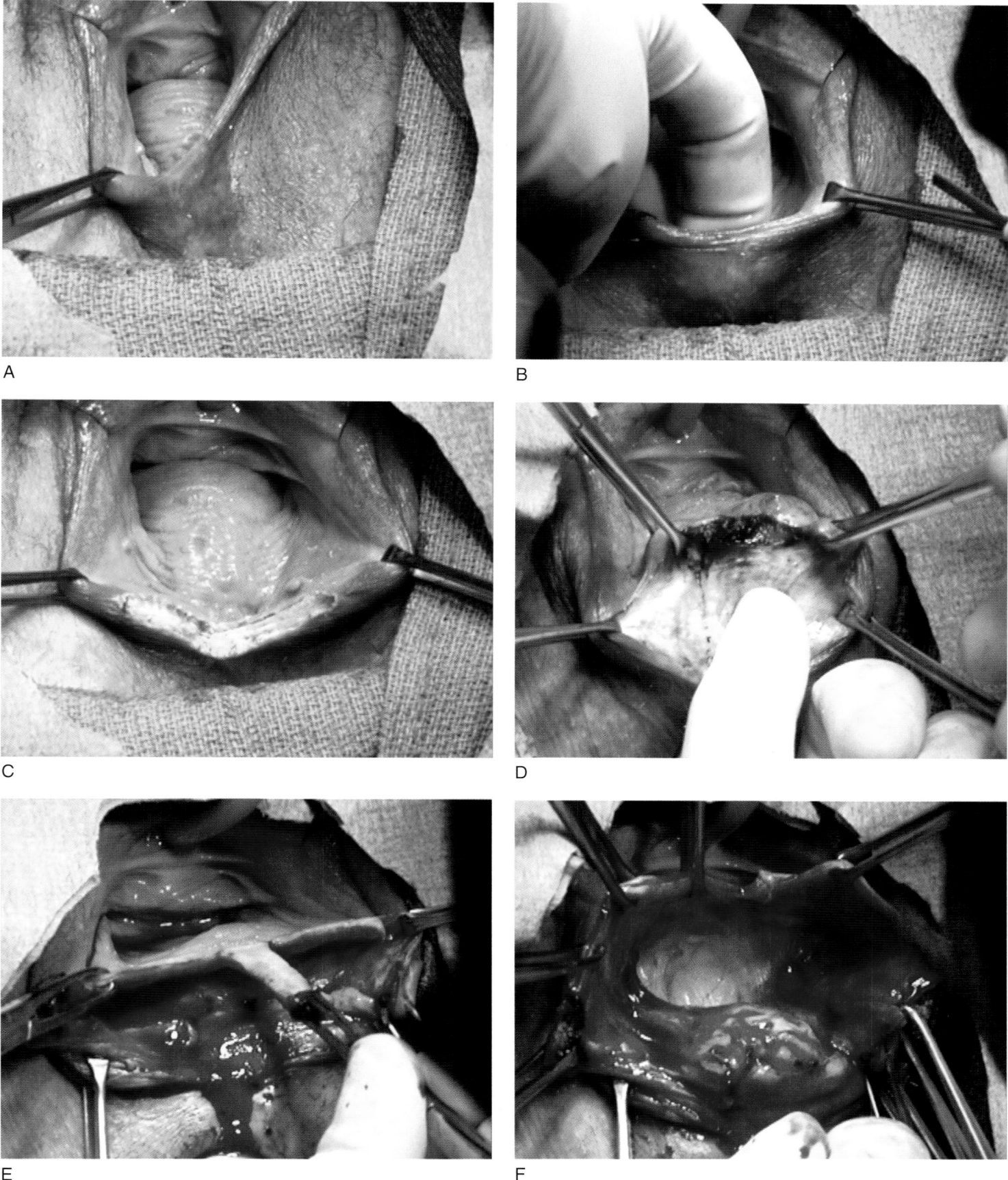

**FIGURE 103–2   A.** A patient with a large symptomatic posterior vaginal wall defect who also complains of dyspareunia secondary to an aggressive buildup of perineal skin. **B.** The skin of the labia minora has been previously sewn across the midline, most likely at the time of repair of a midline episiotomy. **C.** A longitudinal incision is made in the midline, taking down the built-up perineal skin. **D.** Sharp dissection is used to separate the distal posterior vaginal wall from the perineal muscles. **E.** The dissection is extended cephalad with removal of a midline tongue of vaginal mucosa. **F.** The dissection is extended to the pre-peritoneal space of the posterior cul-de-sac.

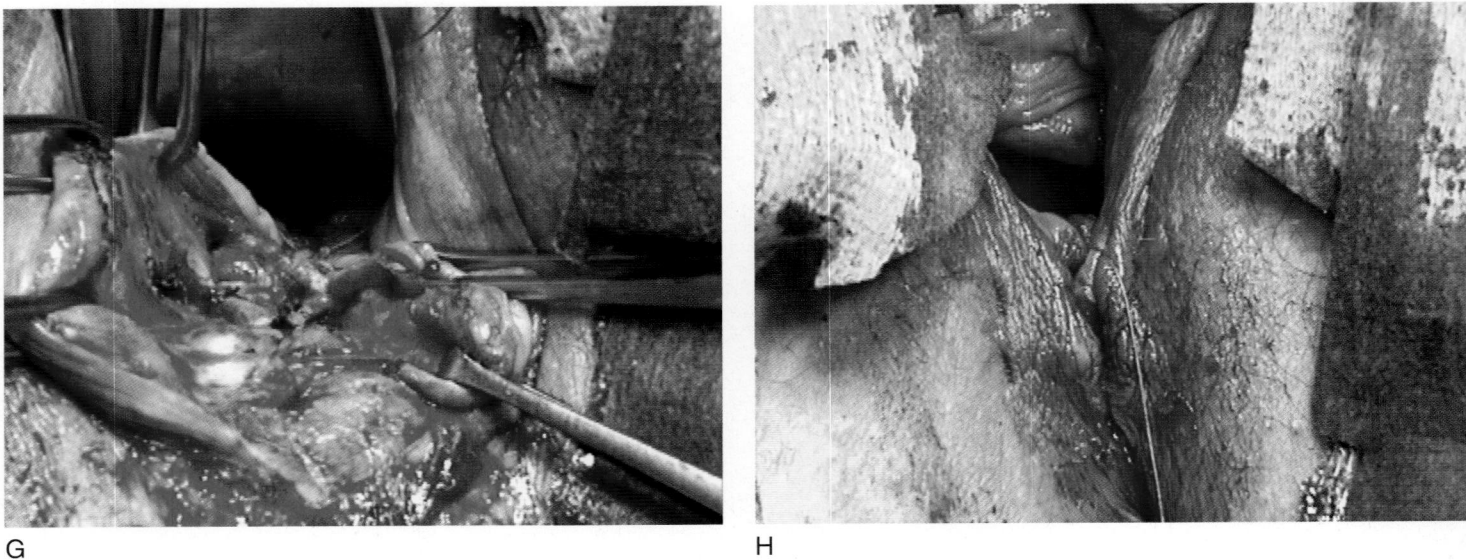

G          H

**FIGURE 103–2, cont'd  G.** A vaginal rectocele and enterocele have been performed, and the upper portion of the vaginal wall incision has been closed. **H.** The perineal body has been reconstructed and the vaginal introitus tightened. Note the perpendicular relationship between the perineum and the posterior vaginal wall.

A          B

C          D

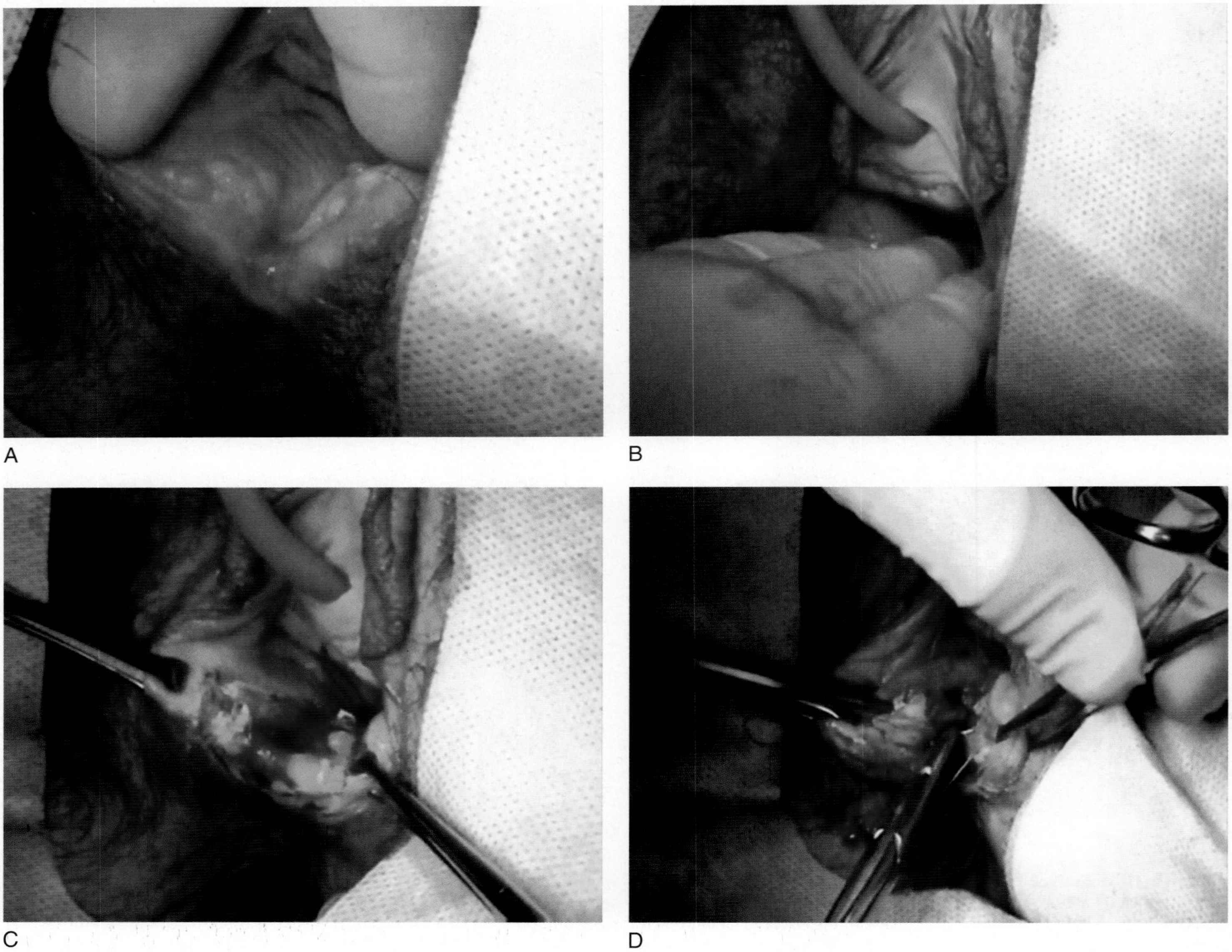

**FIGURE 103–3    A.** Patient with a widened genital hiatus and a small perineal defect. **B.** Note that the vaginal opening easily allows three fingers. **C.** A diamond-shaped piece of tissue is removed from the perineum and the posterior vaginal wall. **D.** Deep 2-0 absorbable sutures are placed to close off the defect, thus decreasing the vaginal caliber.

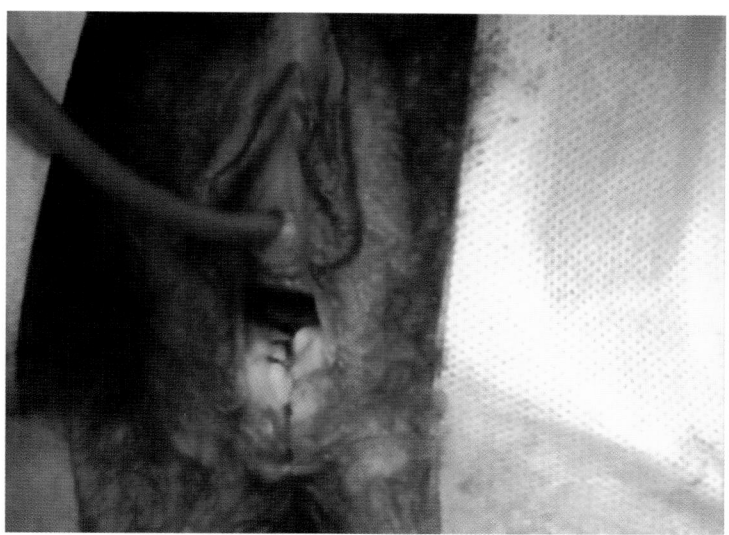

E

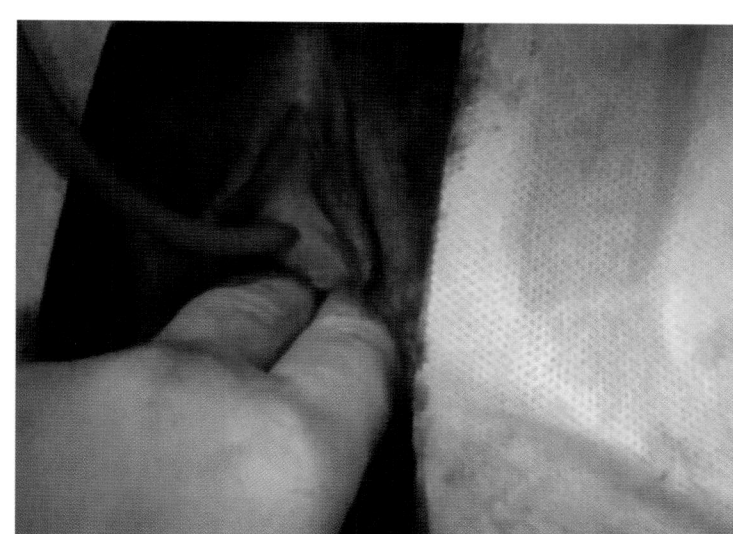

F

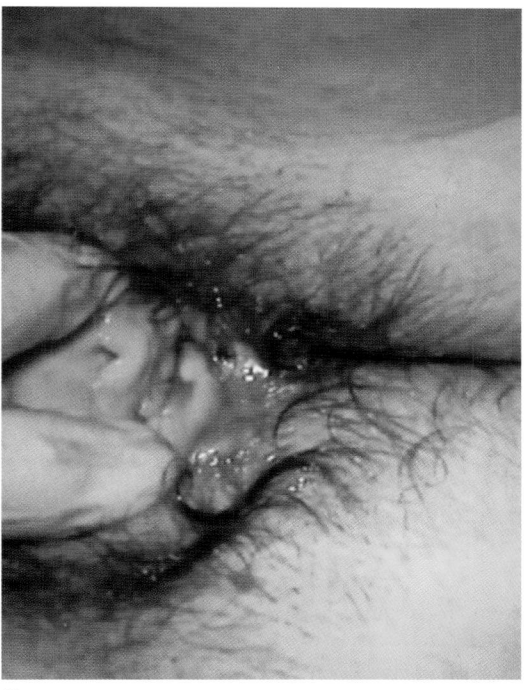

G

**FIGURE 103–3, cont'd  E.** The vaginal and perineal incisions have been closed using a fine delayed absorbable suture. **F.** Note after completion of the repair that the introitus allows only two fingers. **G.** Completed repair 6 weeks postoperatively.

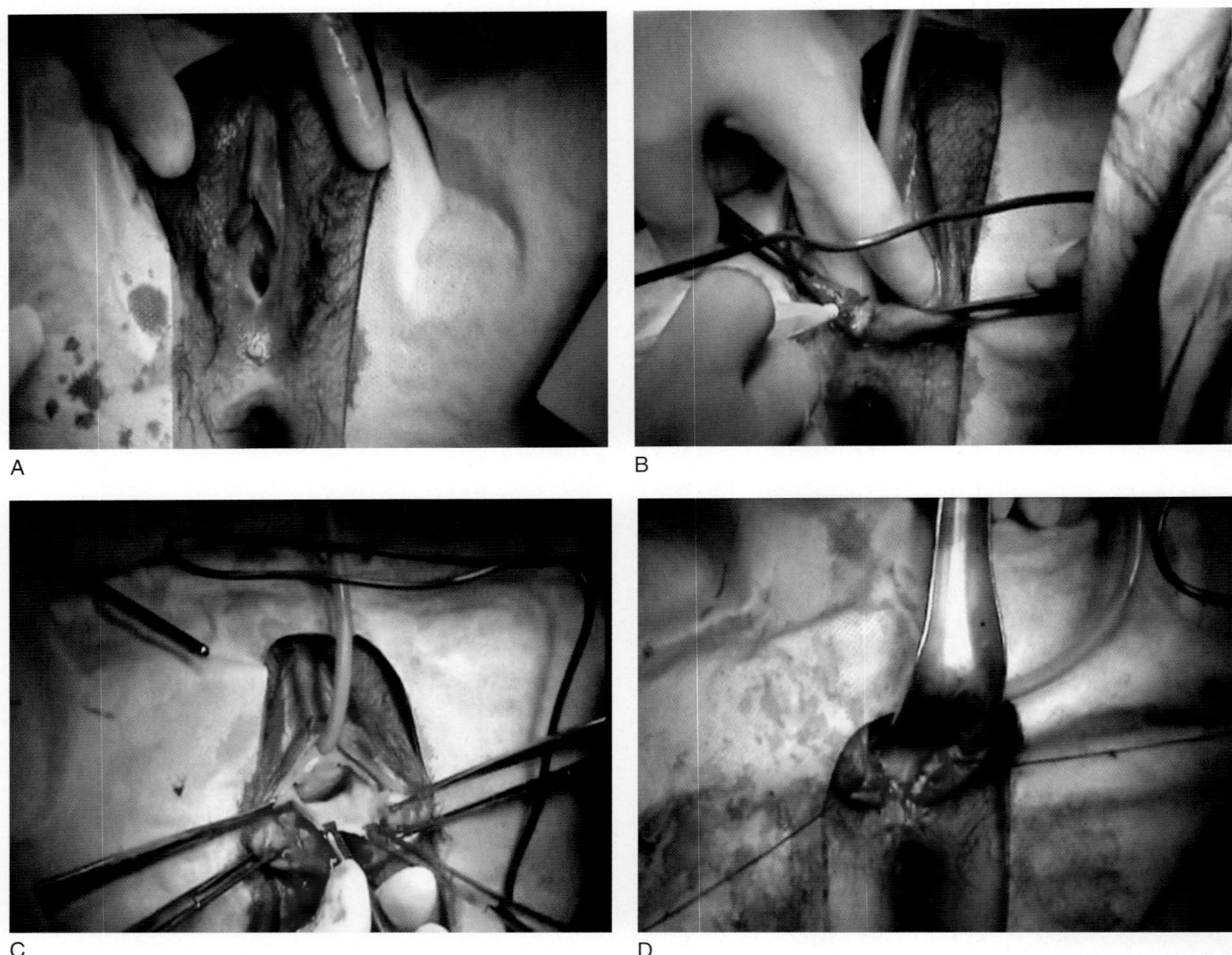

**FIGURE 103–4    A.** A young patient with a nonfunctional vagina secondary to a very tight introitus after an overaggressive repair of a midline episiotomy. **B.** Monopolar cautery is used to take down perineal construction at the midline. **C.** Sharp dissection is used to mobilize the posterior vaginal wall off the anterior wall of the rectum to allow for a vaginal advancement procedure. **D.** The incision has been closed transversely with interrupted delayed absorbable sutures. A defect in the perineal skin has been covered with a piece of Surgisis (Cook Medical).

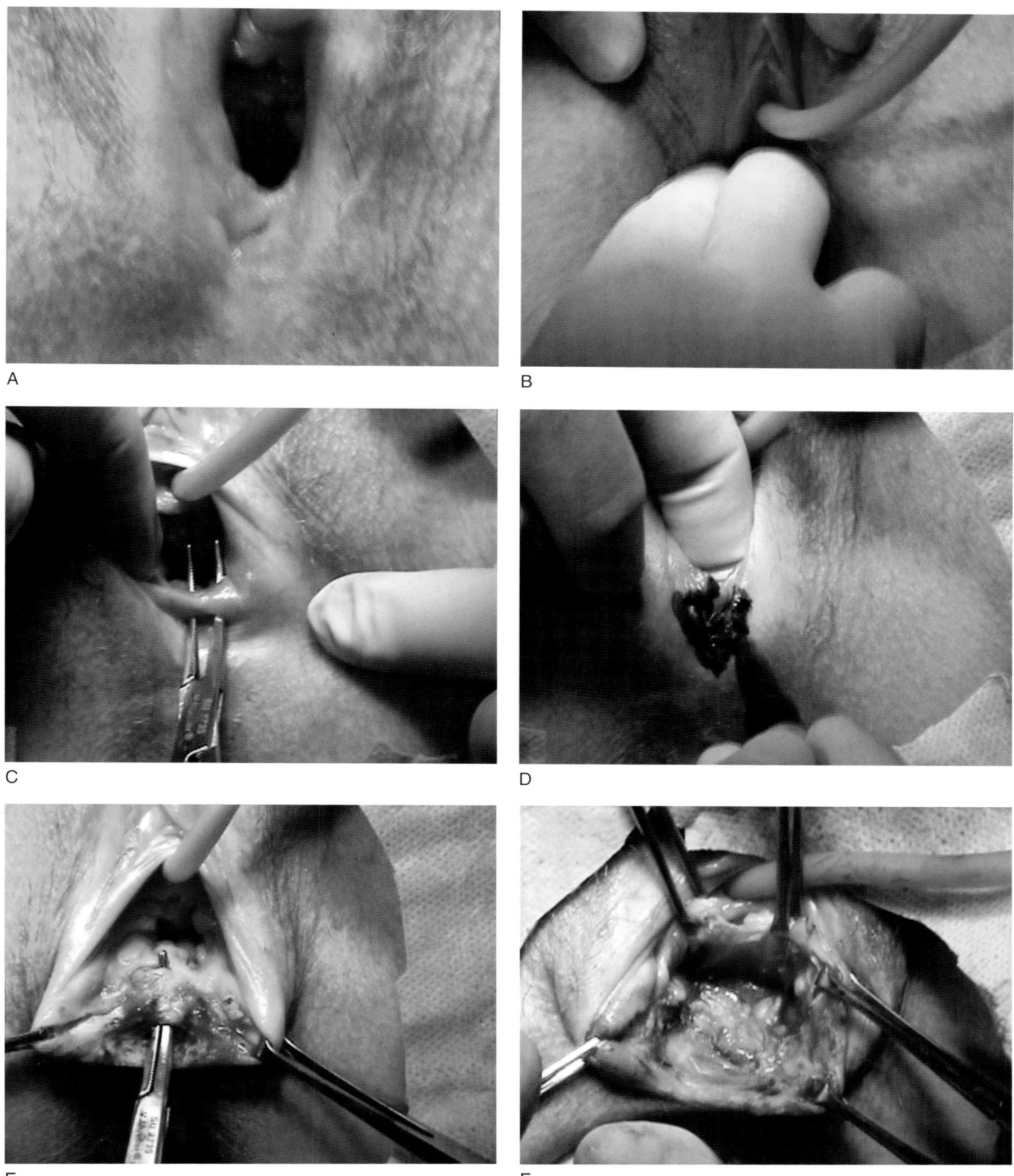

**FIGURE 103–5    A.** A young patient with excessive perineal scarring after repair of a perineal laceration. **B.** The introitus is noted to be very tight, allowing the insertion of only one finger. **C.** Band of perineal scar tissue. **D.** The area of perineal skin to be excised is marked. **E.** Perineal skin has been excised; note the extent of scar tissue. **F.** Scar tissue has been removed, and the posterior vaginal wall has been dissected off the anterior wall of the rectum.

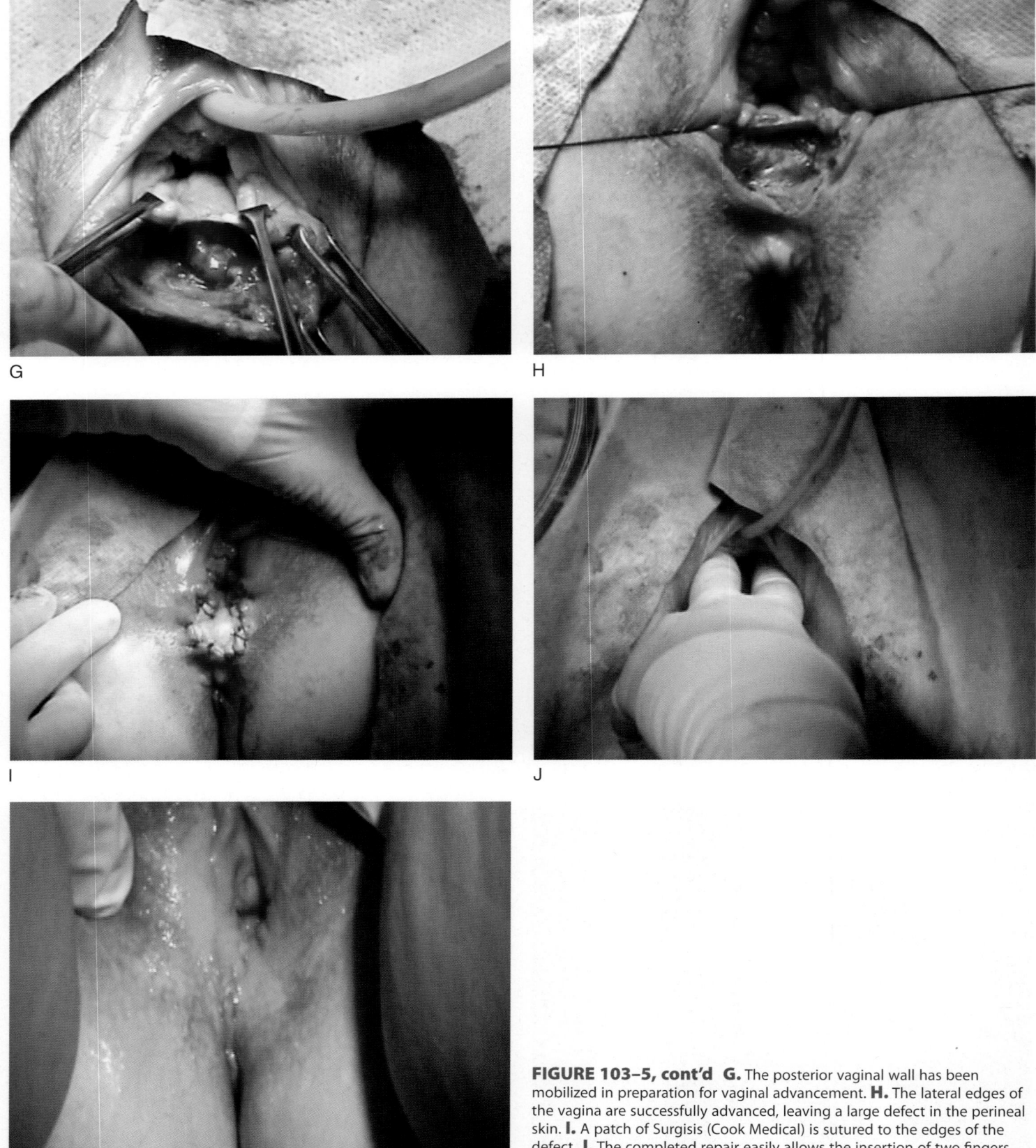

**FIGURE 103–5, cont'd  G.** The posterior vaginal wall has been mobilized in preparation for vaginal advancement. **H.** The lateral edges of the vagina are successfully advanced, leaving a large defect in the perineal skin. **I.** A patch of Surgisis (Cook Medical) is sutured to the edges of the defect. **J.** The completed repair easily allows the insertion of two fingers. **K.** Completed repair 3 months postoperatively. Note successful conversion of the Surgisis to what appears to be normal perineal skin.

# CHAPTER 104

# Gender Reassignment Surgery

*Michael S. Baggish*

Transsexualism is a bona fide psychosexual disorder in which a dissociation exists between the individual's morphologic sex and the brain's innate perception of that person's gender identity. Over the past 50 years, attempts to correct the central nervous system abnormality have been totally unsuccessful; thus surgery designed to change the morphologic sex has been performed to correct the paradox. This surgery typically is done within centers that specialize in these unusual sexual disorders. No operative procedure should ever be performed without proper screening, including thorough psychological, psychiatric, and sociologic testing followed by medical evaluation and hormonal therapy (Fig. 104–1). Additionally, and most important, every surgical candidate must successfully complete at least a year's trial of living and dressing in the desired sex of choice. At the end of the 1-year test period, the candidate again is thoroughly evaluated by a multidisciplinary team, which must unanimously agree that surgery is the appropriate therapy for that individual. Finally, the patient must be given an extensive and detailed informed consent, which explains that the surgery once performed is irreversible. Other persons (e.g., hermaphrodites) may undergo similar types of surgery. As in the case of transsexuals, the screening and evaluation process should be similarly stringent. Before surgery is conducted, as with transsexuals, a multidisciplinary committee, including the patient and the patient's immediate family, should be included in the informed decision to perform gender reassignment surgery. The type of surgery in which the gynecologist will be involved is the male-to-female reassignment procedure. All patients will have been feminized by more than 12 months' treatment with injections of estradiol (Fig. 104–2). Every patient also undergoes bowel preparation.

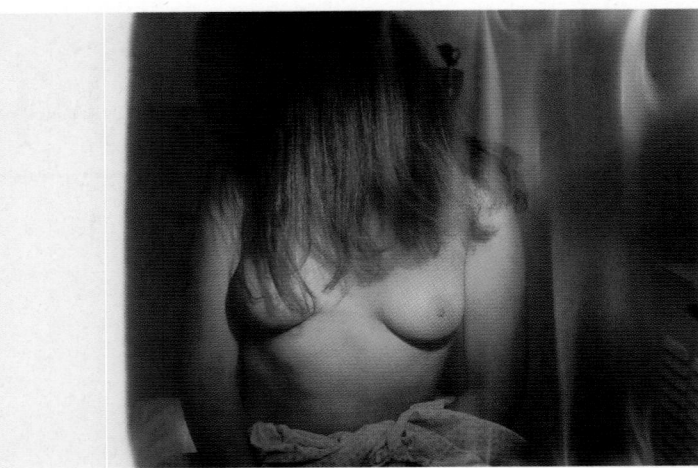

**FIGURE 104–1** Excellent breast development may be seen in the majority of male-to-female transsexuals through the administration of injectable estrogen. Maximal action is observed between 3 and 6 months after injections are begun.

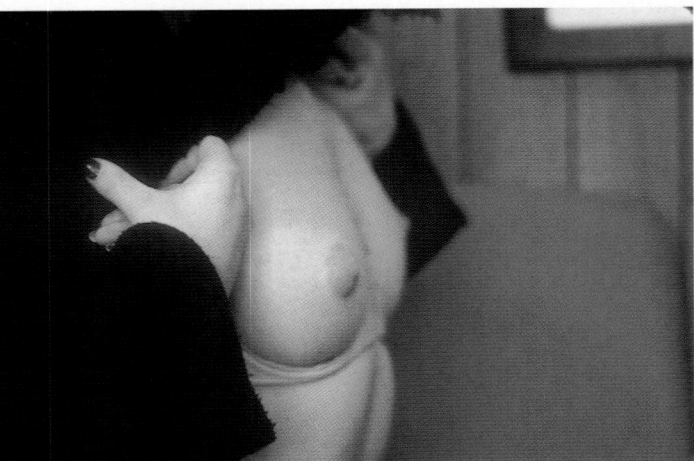

**FIGURE 104–2** After cross-dressing, receiving hormonal therapy, and living as a woman for a period of a year, candidates for surgery are evaluated by a multidisciplinary committee. This person presents as an authentic-looking female.

The surgery is performed with the patient in the lithotomy position (Fig. 104–3). However, before positioning, a split-thickness graft is obtained utilizing a drum-type dermatome (Fig. 104–4). The full-drum graft is obtained from the buttock or thigh (Fig. 104–5). The donor site is then covered with a polyurethane-type dressing (Opsite). The external genitalia and abdomen are completely shaved of hair, and a Foley catheter is placed via the penile urethra into the urinary bladder. A hemispheric incision is made into the mons at the junction of the penile root and the mons. This is carried down to the upper lateral portion of the scrotum (Fig. 104–6). The incision alternatively may comprise a short vertical incision into the scrotum and ventral surface of the penile skin (Fig. 104–7). The incision is carried down to Colles' fascia. By careful, non-traumatic sharp and blunt dissection, the penile skin is separated from the entire penile shaft to the level of the glans (Fig. 104–8A, B). The testes are dissected free from the scrotal skin (Fig. 104–9). The spermatic cords are doubly clamped, cut, and suture-ligated with 0 Vicryl, and the testes removed (Fig. 104–10A, B). The penile shaft proximal to the glans is clamped with a straight Zeppelin clamp, and the glans, together with the penile skin, is separated from the shaft (Fig. 104–11A, B). The urethra is recatheterized and is dissected from the bulb and shaft of the penis (Fig. 104–12A through C). On either side, the corpora cavernosa penis is isolated close to the pubic and ischial rami, clamped with two Zeppelin clamps, cut, and suture-ligated with 0 Vicryl or polydioxanone (PDS) (Fig. 104–13A, B). The entire corpora cavernosa penis is removed after it is sharply

dissected from the urethral bulb (Fig. 104–14A, B). Next, a transverse incision is made between the base of the urethral bulb and the rectum (Fig. 104–15). By very careful dissection, a space is developed between the aforementioned structures and deeper internally between the prostate gland and the rectum. The space must accommodate the width of the operator's index and center fingers loosely and must extend to a depth of 7 cm. Frequent rectal exams are performed during the critical tunneling phase. The full-thickness penile skin pedicle graft is inverted into the space, creating a full-thickness neovagina (Fig. 104–16A, B). The glans penis will be located at the vault and creates a pseudocervix (Fig. 104–16C). The urethra is shortened to approximately 3 to 4 cm and is recatheterized (Fig. 104–17A, B). The neovagina is packed with gauze (Fig. 104–18). The scrotum is sutured upward peripheral to the neovagina into Colles' fascia (Fig. 104–19A, B). At a second stage of the operation, the scrotum will be sectioned and separated centrally at its lower pole to create two labia majora. At the 2-month interval (second-stage operation), it will have gained sufficient collateral circulation to obviate slough (Fig. 104–19C). The split-thickness graft is cut to cover the large mons defect and is sutured to the margins of the abdominal, penile, and scrotal skin (Fig. 104–20). A hole is cut above the neovaginal introitus, and the urethra is brought out through this orifice. The edges of the terminal urethra are sutured circumferentially to the margins of the previously described opening in the skin graft with 4-0 Vicryl (Fig. 104–21). The operation is now finished. A pressure dressing is placed over the graft site and is taped into place (Fig. 104–22).

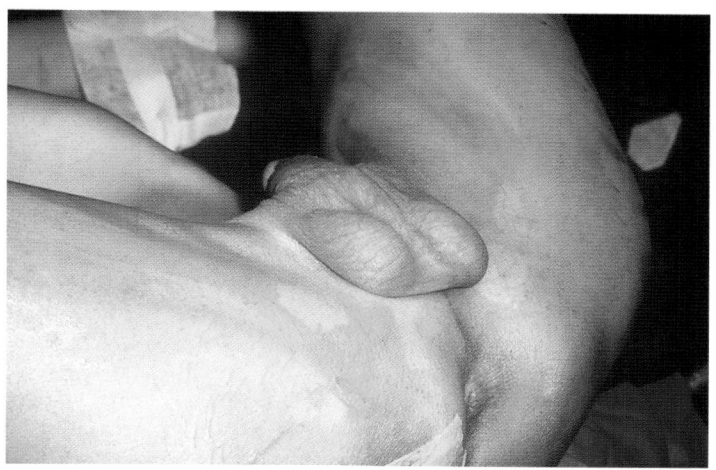

**FIGURE 104–3** Surgery is performed with the patient in the dorsal lithotomy position by a team consisting of a gynecologist, a plastic surgeon, and a urologist.

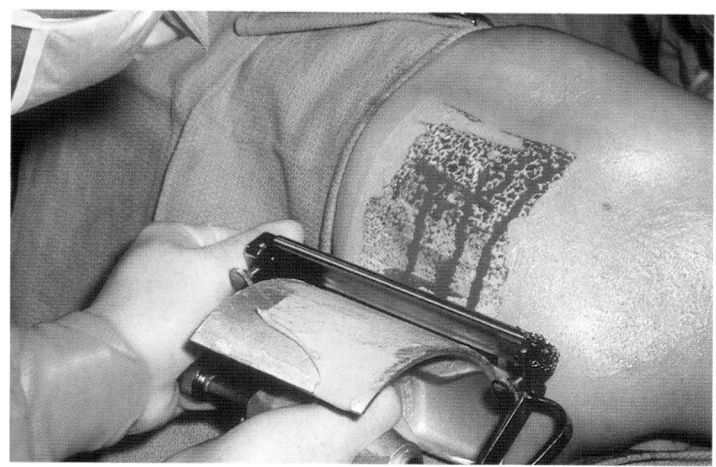

**FIGURE 104–4** Before the patient is placed in the lithotomy position, a split-thickness graft is obtained using a drum-type dermatome.

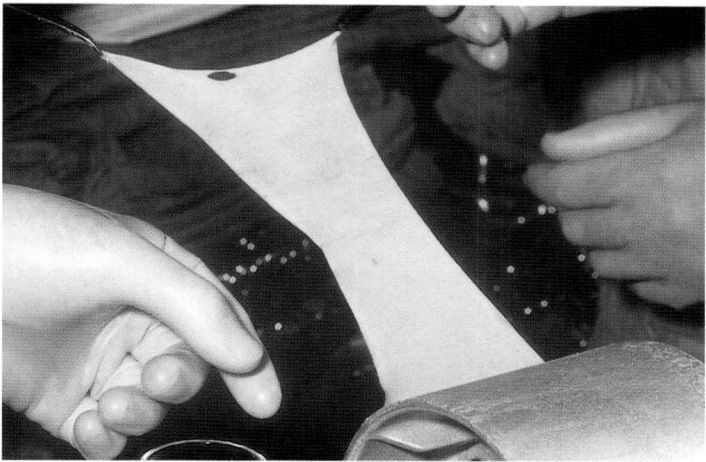

**FIGURE 104–5** A large split-thickness graft is retrieved from the drum. It is carefully wrapped in a moistened sterile gauze sponge and is placed in a secure location on the nurse's instrument back table for later use.

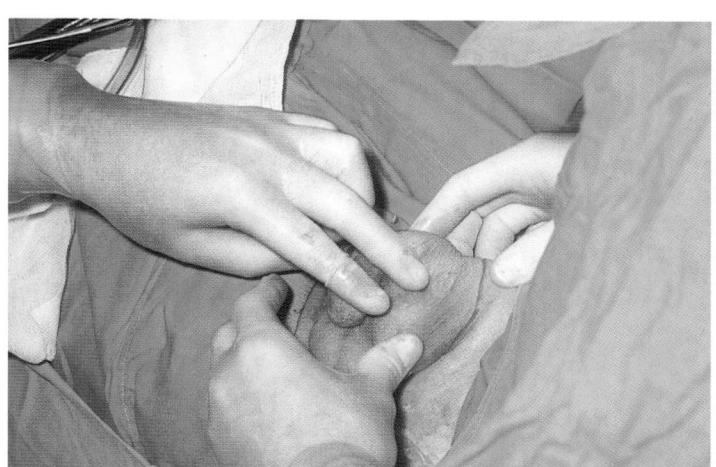

**FIGURE 104–6** A curved incision is made above the root of the penis and is carried laterally to the lateral lower margin of the scrotum. The incision is carried to the level of Colles' fascia.

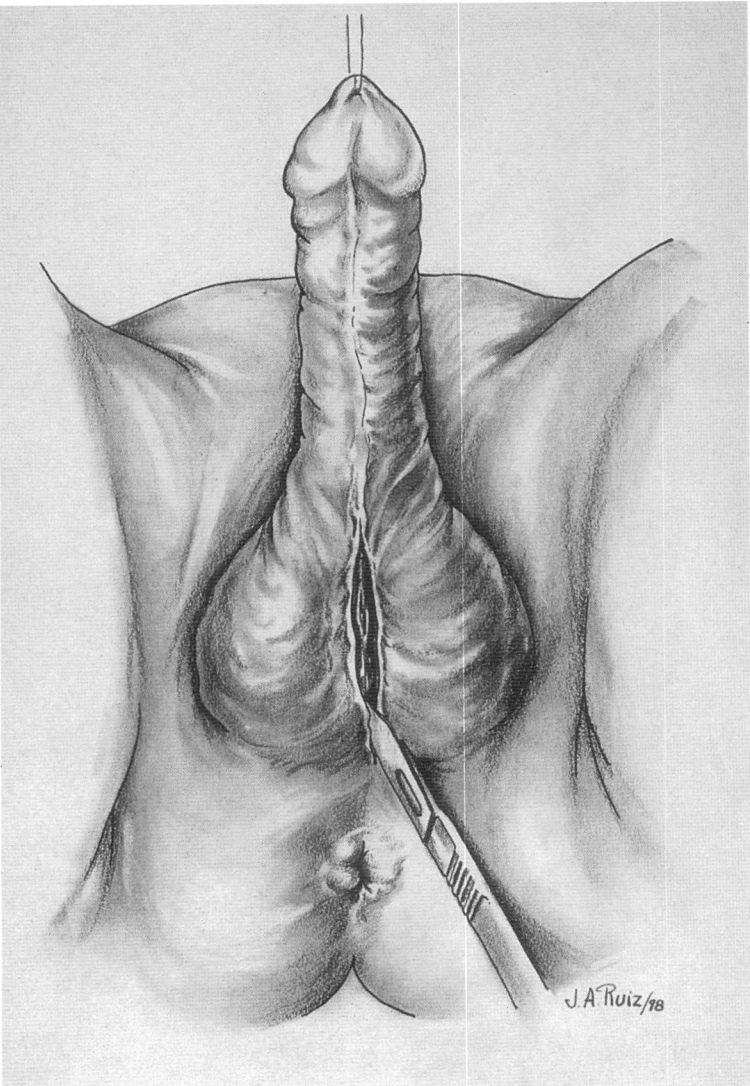

**FIGURE 104–7** Alternatively, a midline incision bisecting the scrotum and into the lower ventral skin of the penis may be made (optional).

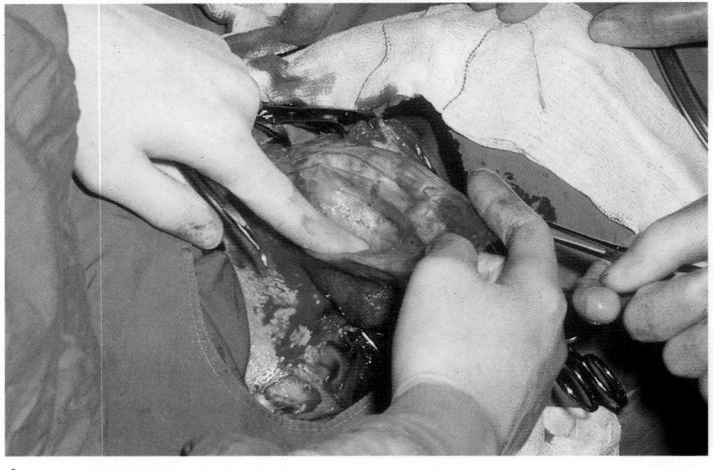

A

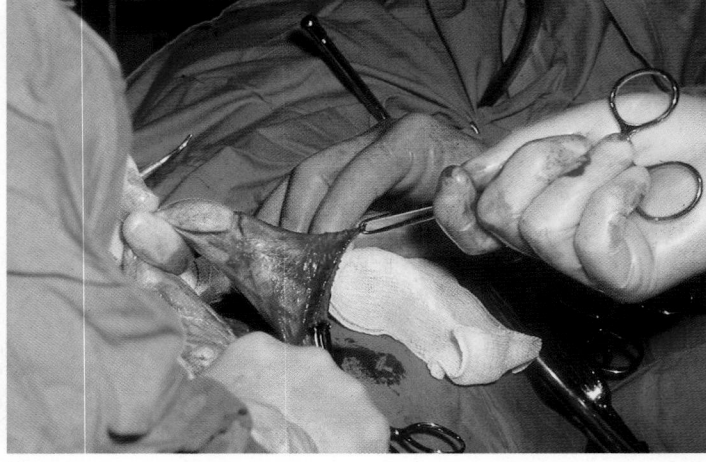

B

**FIGURE 104–8 A.** By blunt dissection, the penile skin is carefully separated from the fascia covering the penile shaft and scrotum. **B.** The skin is pulled downward to the level of its firm attachment to the glans penis.

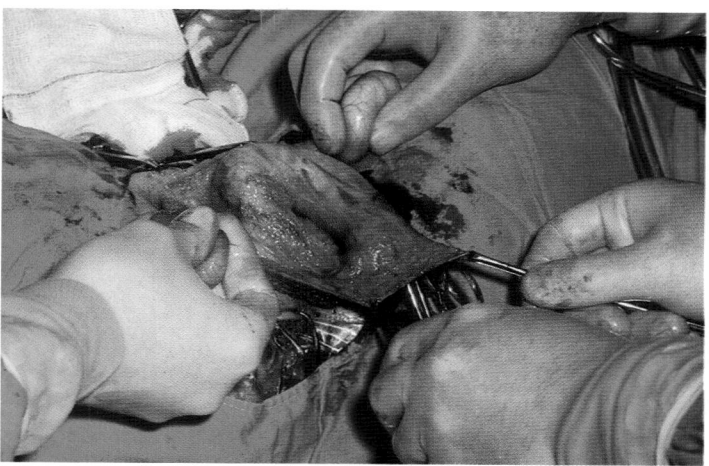

**FIGURE 104–9** The scrotal skin is bluntly pushed inferiorly. The testes are separated from the scrotum.

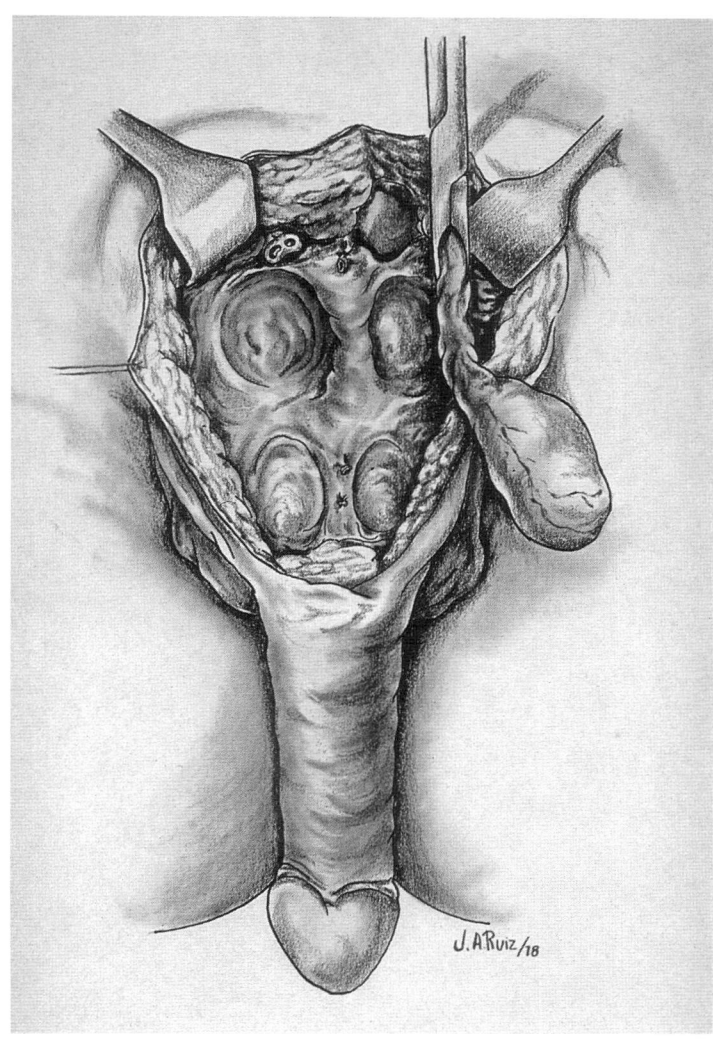

A

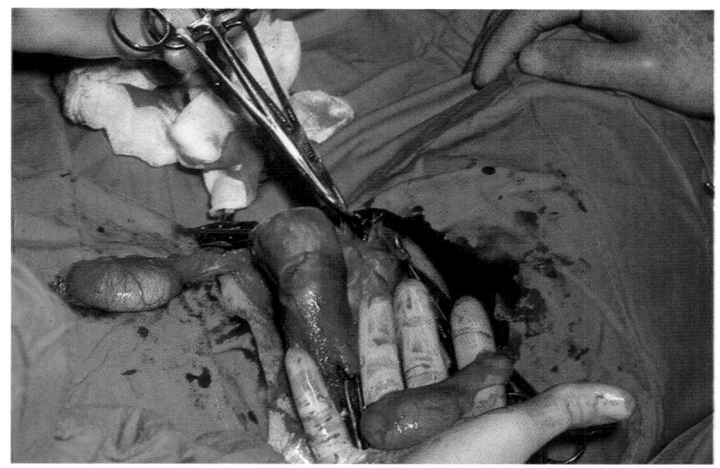

B

**FIGURE 104–10 A.** The spermatic cord is isolated, clamped, and cut. **B.** The testes are excised, and the cord is suture-ligated with 0 Vicryl.

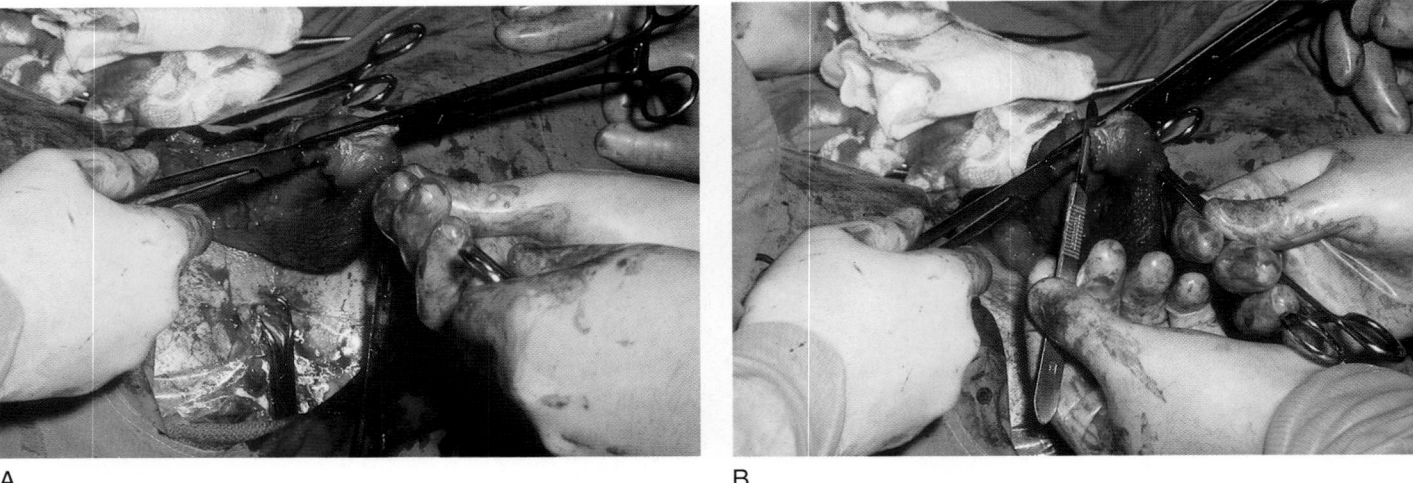

**FIGURE 104–11  A.** Zeppelin clamps are placed across the terminal part of the penile shaft below the glans and retracted penile skin. **B.** The penile shaft is cut distal to the applied clamps separating the glans, which remains attached to the penile skin.

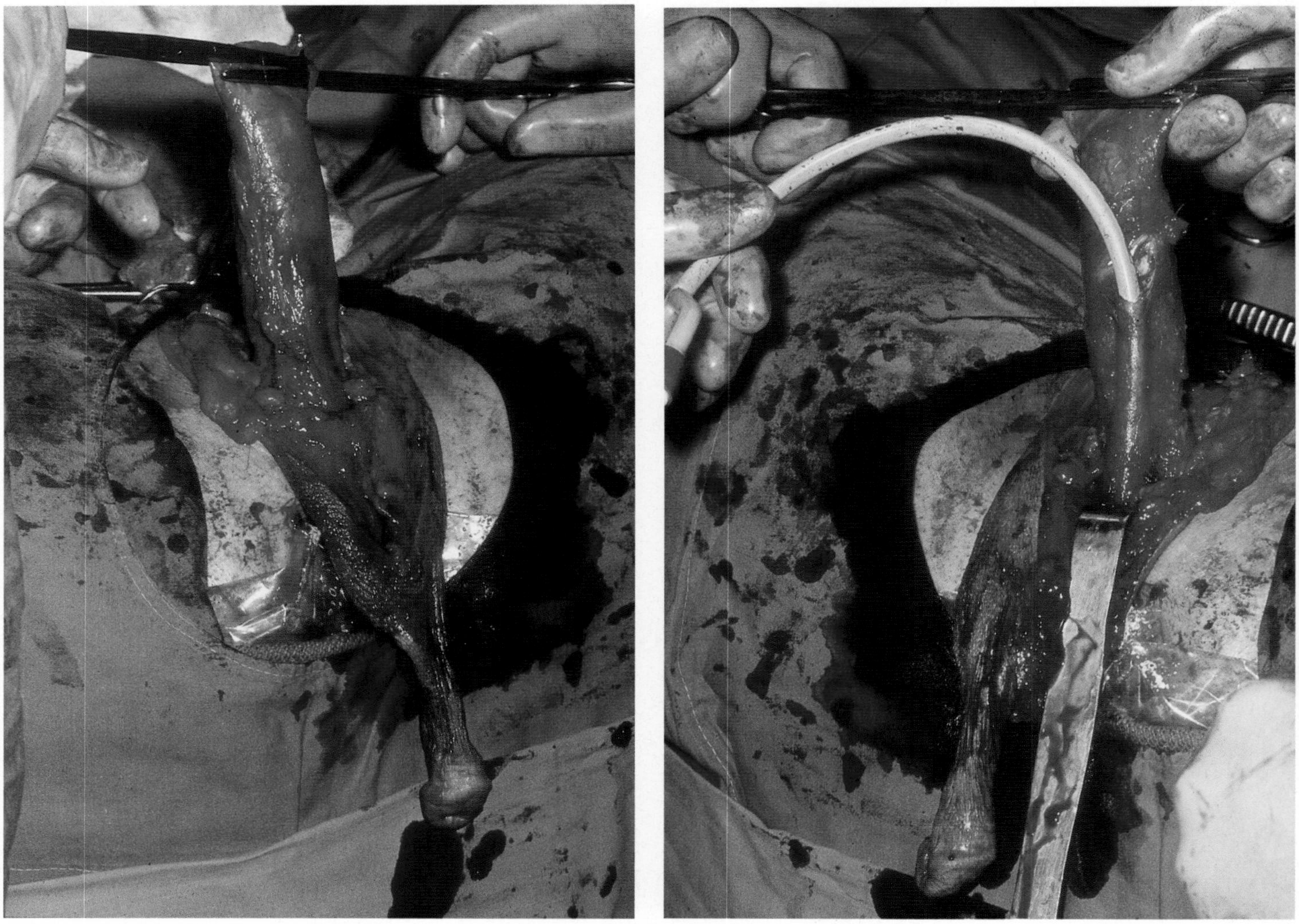

**FIGURE 104–12  A.** The penile shaft, now free from its skin and glans, is stretched to reveal the urethra and bulb groove. **B.** The urethra is dissected by means of Metzenbaum scissors from the corpora. A catheter is placed into the urethra and bladder.

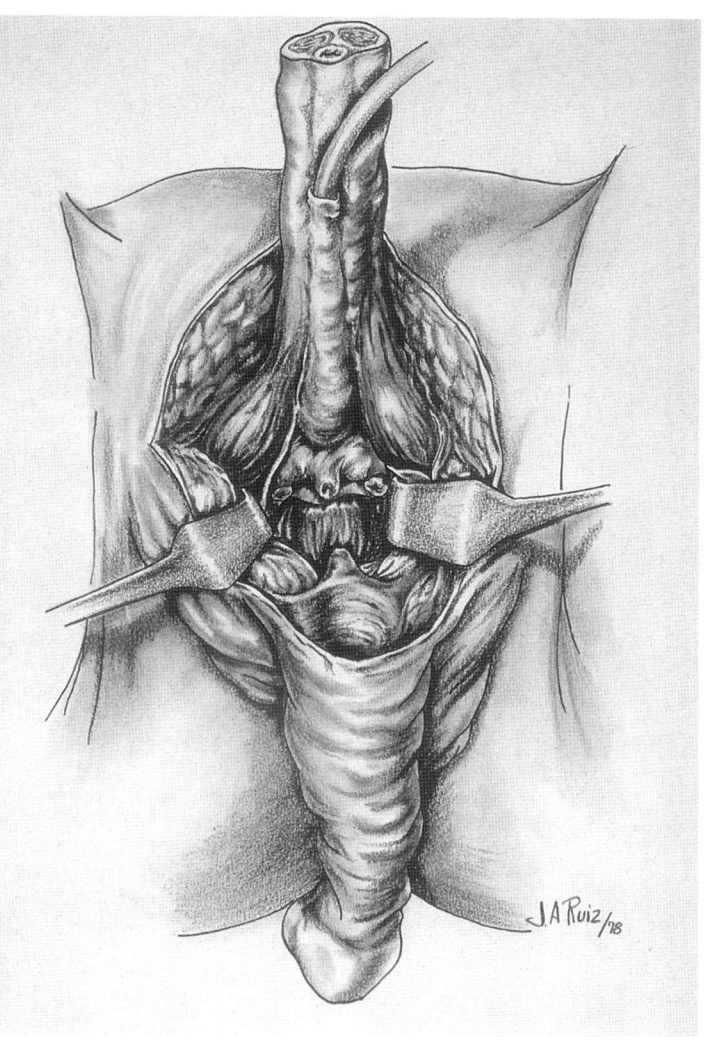

C

**FIGURE 104–12, cont'd  C.** The drawing shows the empty sheath of penile skin with attached glans. The corpora cavernosa and the catheterized urethra and bulb are seen above the skin sheath.

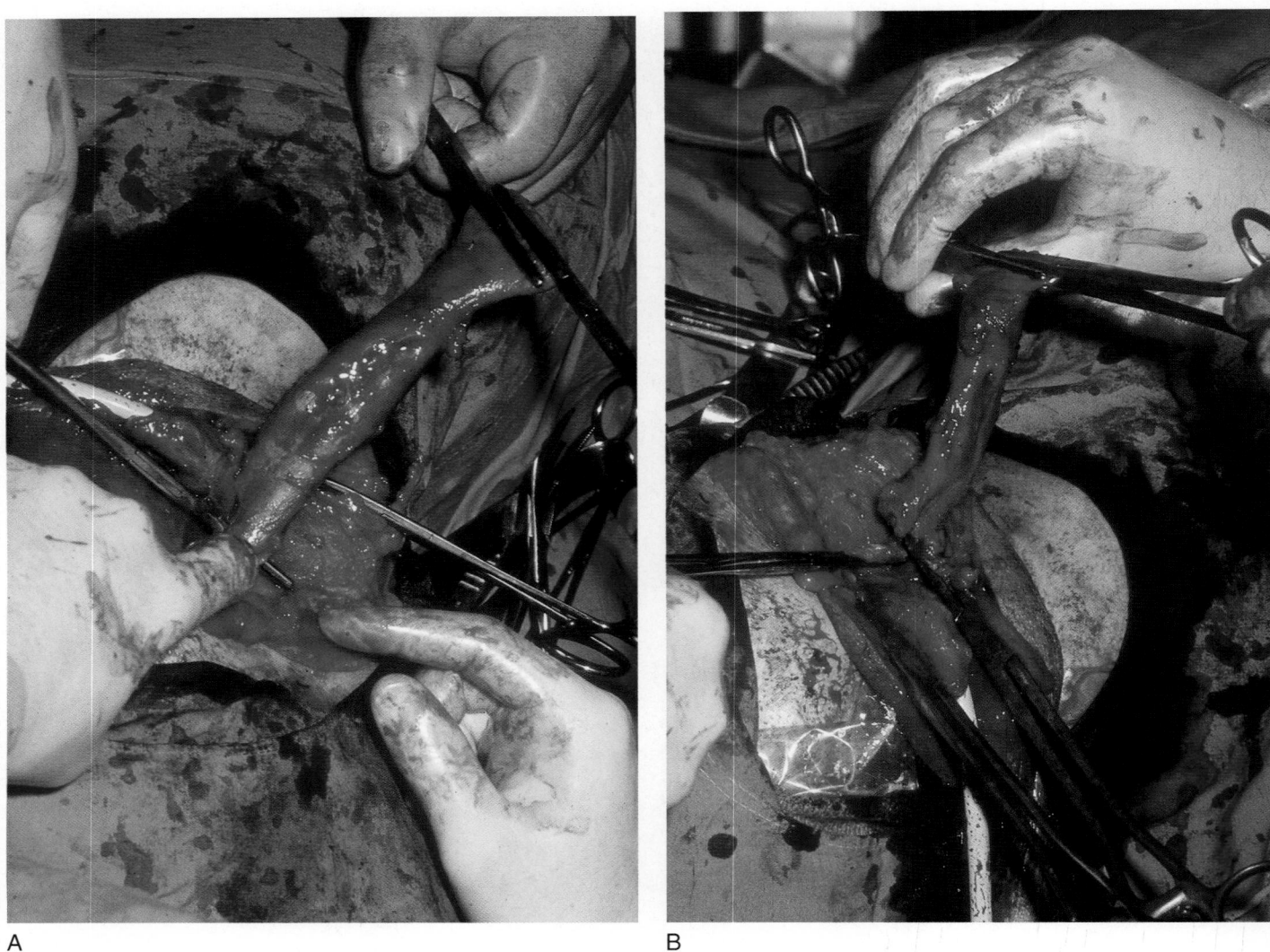

A                                                             B

**FIGURE 104–13 A.** Each corpus cavernosum is isolated at the ischiopubic ramus. Using a straight tonsil clamp, a tunnel is dissected between the corpora. Zeppelin clamps are applied over the bone, securing the right and left corpora cavernosa penis. **B.** The right and left corpora are cut over the clamp.

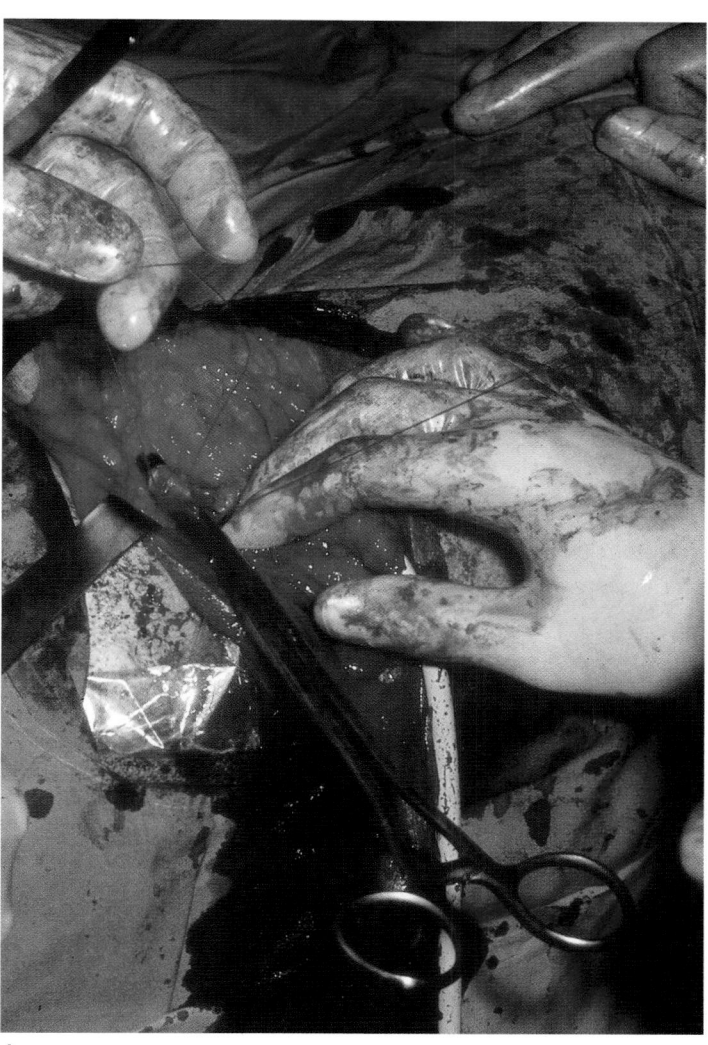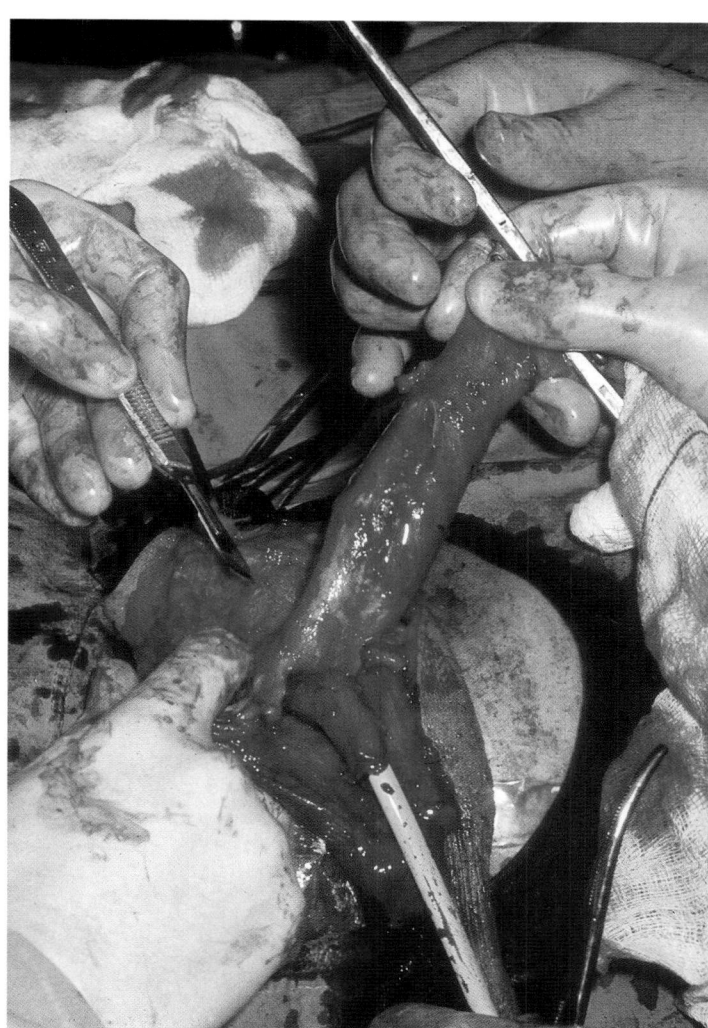

A
B

**FIGURE 104–14  A.** The corpus stump on the right is suture-ligated twice with 0 Vicryl. **B.** The urethra is shortened to the level of the bulb.

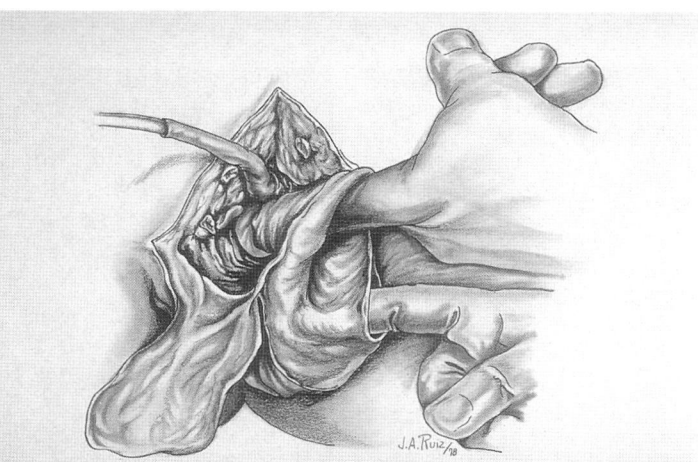

**FIGURE 104–15**  The levator ani is carefully cut between the bulb (anteriorly) and the rectum posteriorly, and the neovagina is tunneled bluntly. The cavity is dissected posteriorly to the atrophied prostate gland.

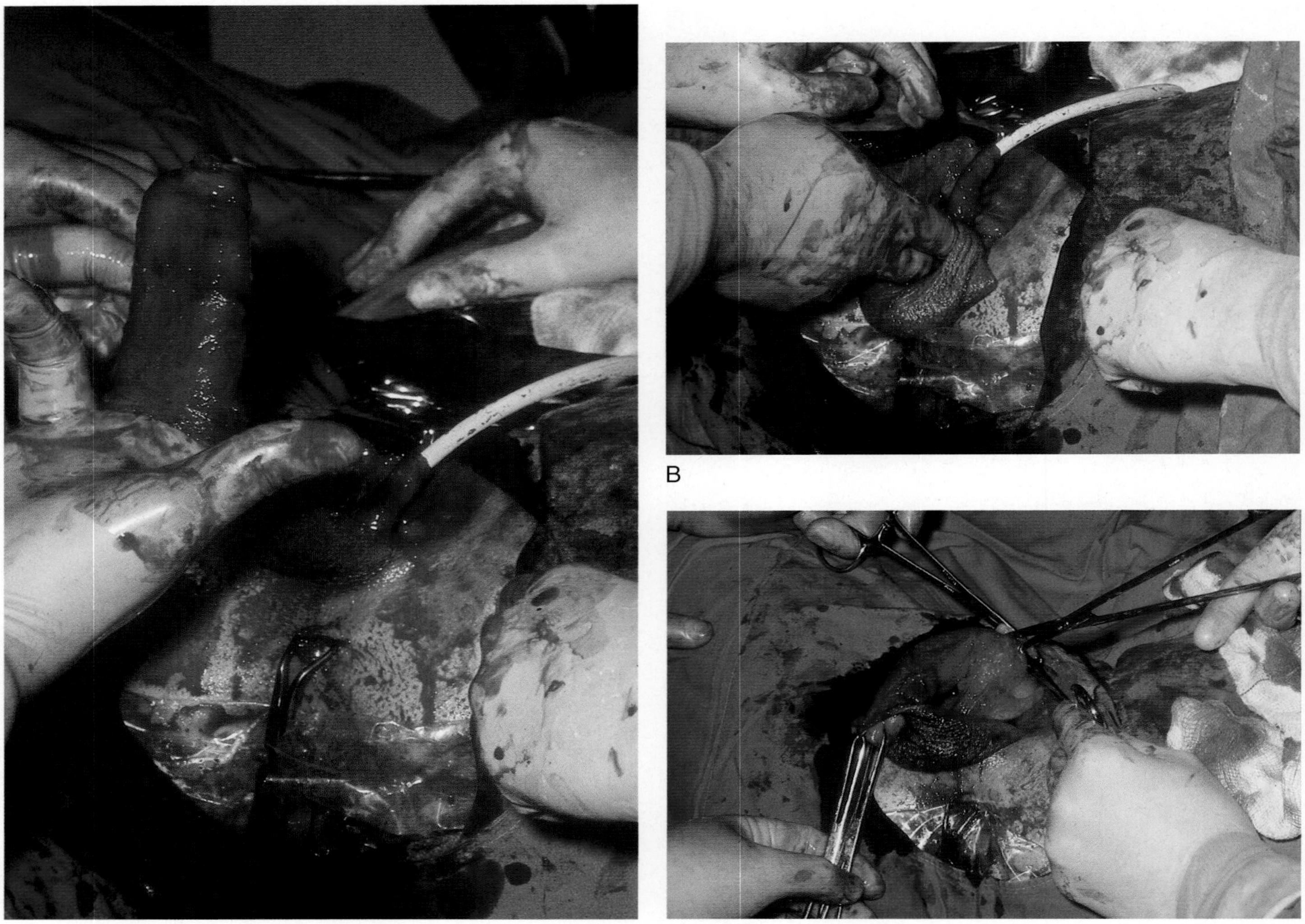

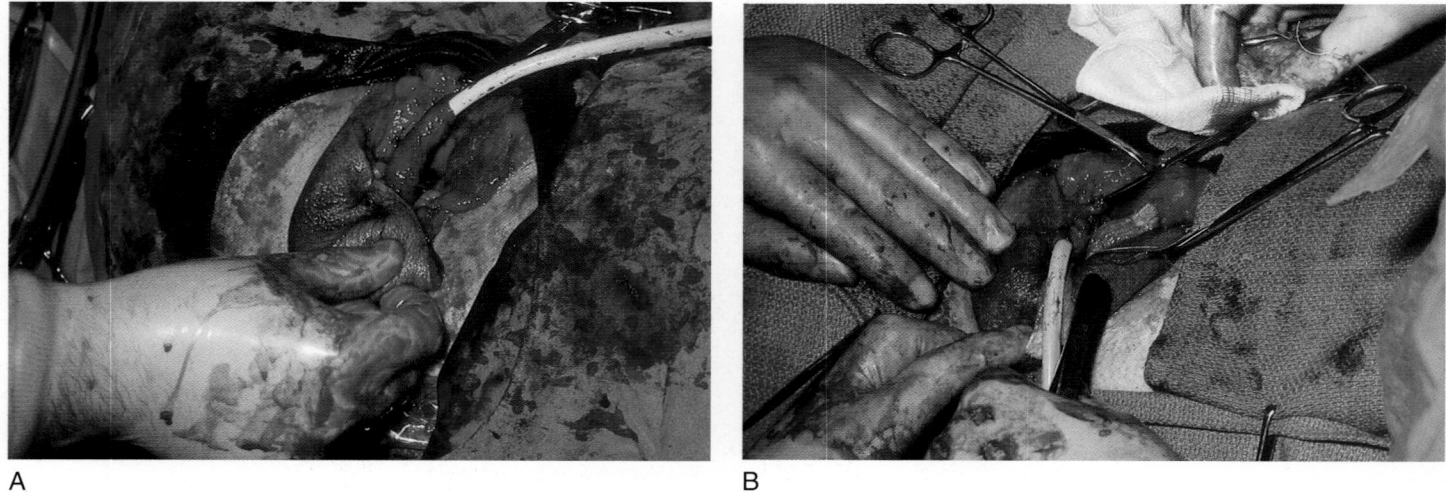

**FIGURE 104–16 A.** The full-thickness tube of penile skin is inverted and will form the neovagina. **B.** The penile skin tube is pushed into the space created through the levator ani muscles. The entire length of penile skin is pushed into the space. **C.** The glans penis sits at the deep end of the pedicle graft (penile skin tube). The glans will simulate a female cervix. On speculum exam, it looks and feels like a genuine cervix.

**FIGURE 104–17 A.** The urethra is further shortened and sculpted. **B.** The urethra is anchored to the connective tissue above the graft. Later, it will be brought through the split-thickness graft.

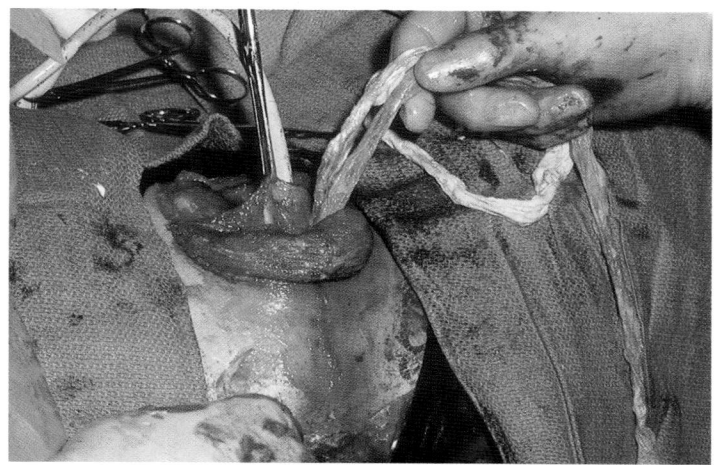

**FIGURE 104–18** The neovagina is packed with petroleum gauze.

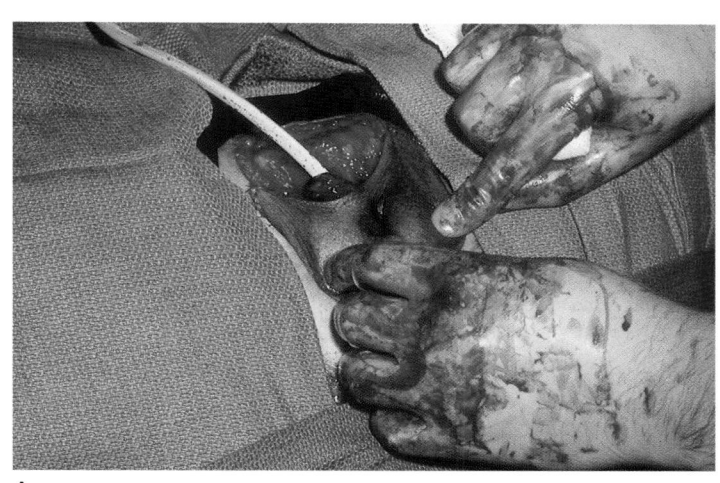

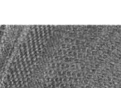

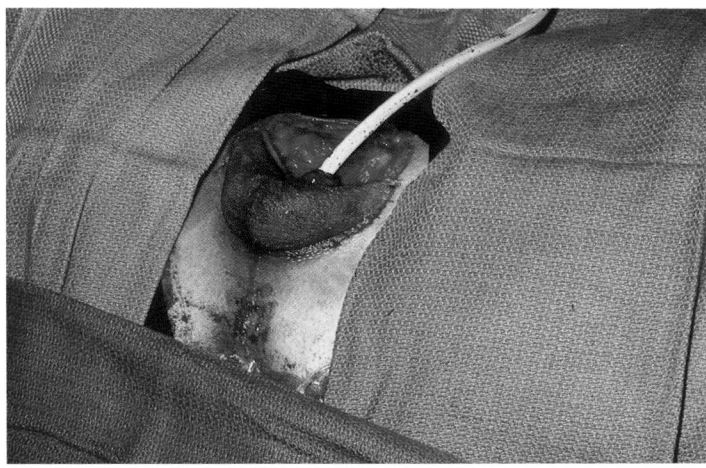

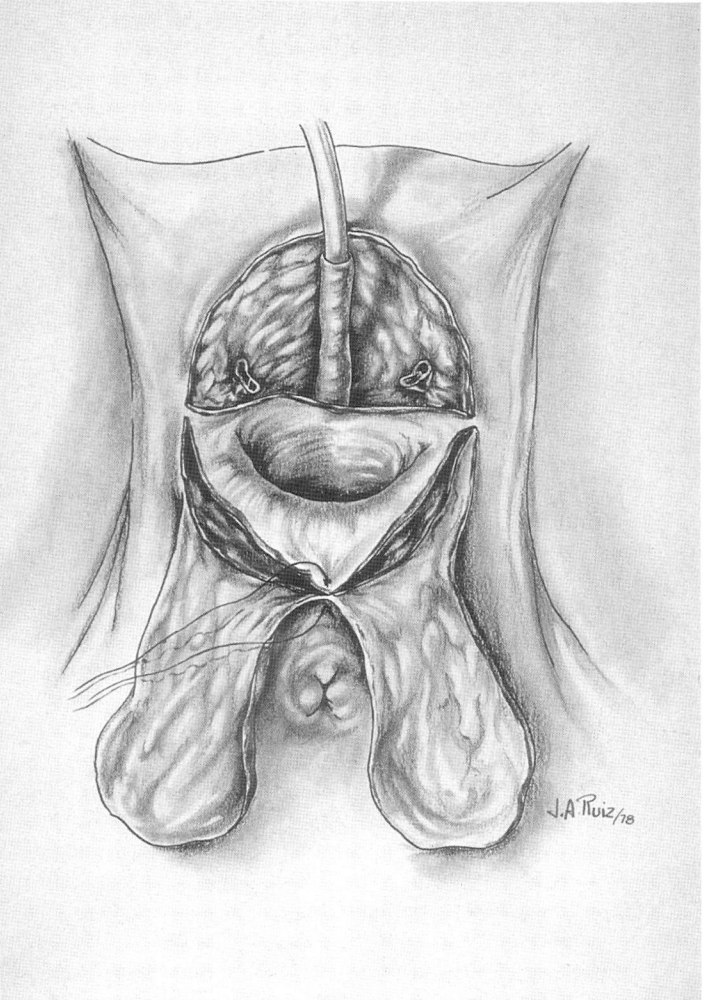

**FIGURE 104–19 A.** The empty scrotum is sutured around the entrance of the neovagina to the connective tissue (Colles' fascia). **B.** The scrotum if not split will be left intact for 2 months and separated to form two labia at a short second operation. This delay is required to ensure an adequate blood supply to the skin. **C.** Alternatively, if the midline cut was made into the scrotum (see Figure 104–7), the two halves of the scrotum will become the labia majora.

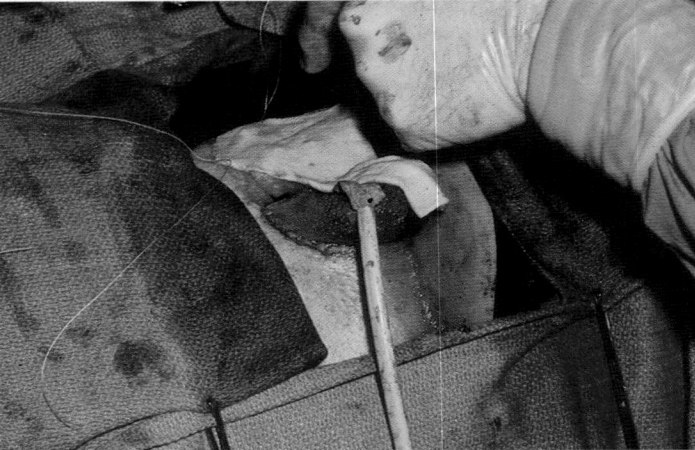

**FIGURE 104–20** The split-thickness graft obtained at the beginning of the surgery covers the denuded area above the neovagina. The urethra is brought through a cut made in the graft, and the edges of the terminal urethra are sutured to the skin graft (around the slit) with 3-0 or 4-0 Vicryl. Care is taken to make the skin opening large enough to prevent urethral stricture.

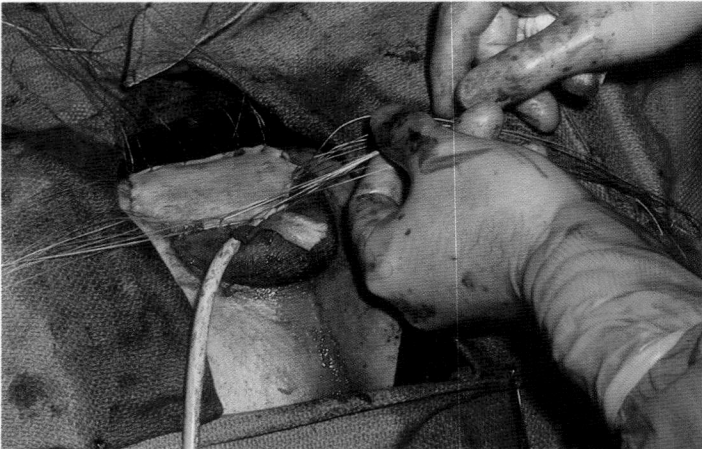

**FIGURE 104–21** The graft is secured to the surrounding skin margins with interrupted 3-0 Vicryl stitches. The excess skin is trimmed.

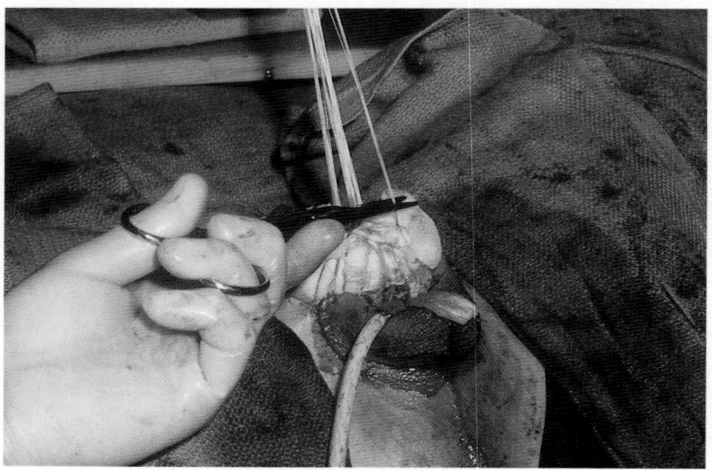

**FIGURE 104–22** Xeroform gauze and a uniform pressure dressing are secured over the graft by tying the long suture ends over the dressing.

During this time, the patient is placed on a low-residue diet, and a retention catheter remains in the bladder. The patient remains on ciprofloxacin (Cipro) 500 g twice a day for the 2-week period. Essentially, the operation recapitulates embryonic sexual differentiation, creating an unfused (female) status from a previously fused (male) condition. At 4 weeks postoperatively, the patient is fitted with a Silastic vaginal stent, which she must wear continuously until beginning actual intercourse (Fig. 104-23A through C). Healing is complete at 6 to 8 weeks. The cosmetic appearance after this surgery is very good (Fig. 104-24A through C). Similar surgery may be performed for hermaphrodites; however, the enlarged clitoris is too small for a full-thickness graft (Fig. 104-25).

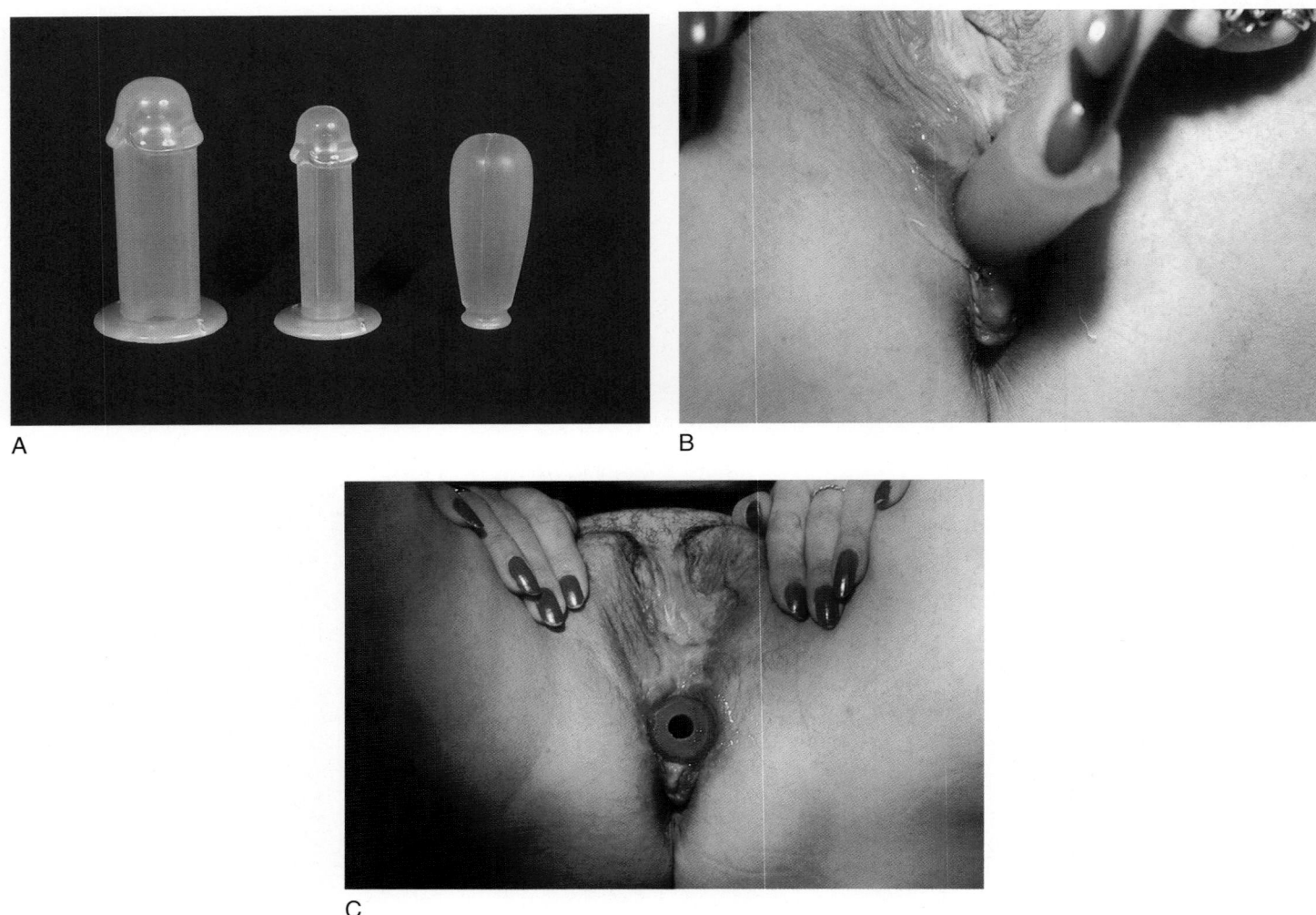

A

B

C

**FIGURE 104–23  A.** Various sizes of Silastic vaginal stents will be placed into the neovagina after the wounds have healed, usually 6 weeks postoperatively. **B.** The patient is taught to lubricate the vagina and the stent and place the latter in the vagina. **C.** The stent remains in the vagina continuously until regular intercourse ensues. The stent is removed and is cleaned once or twice daily.

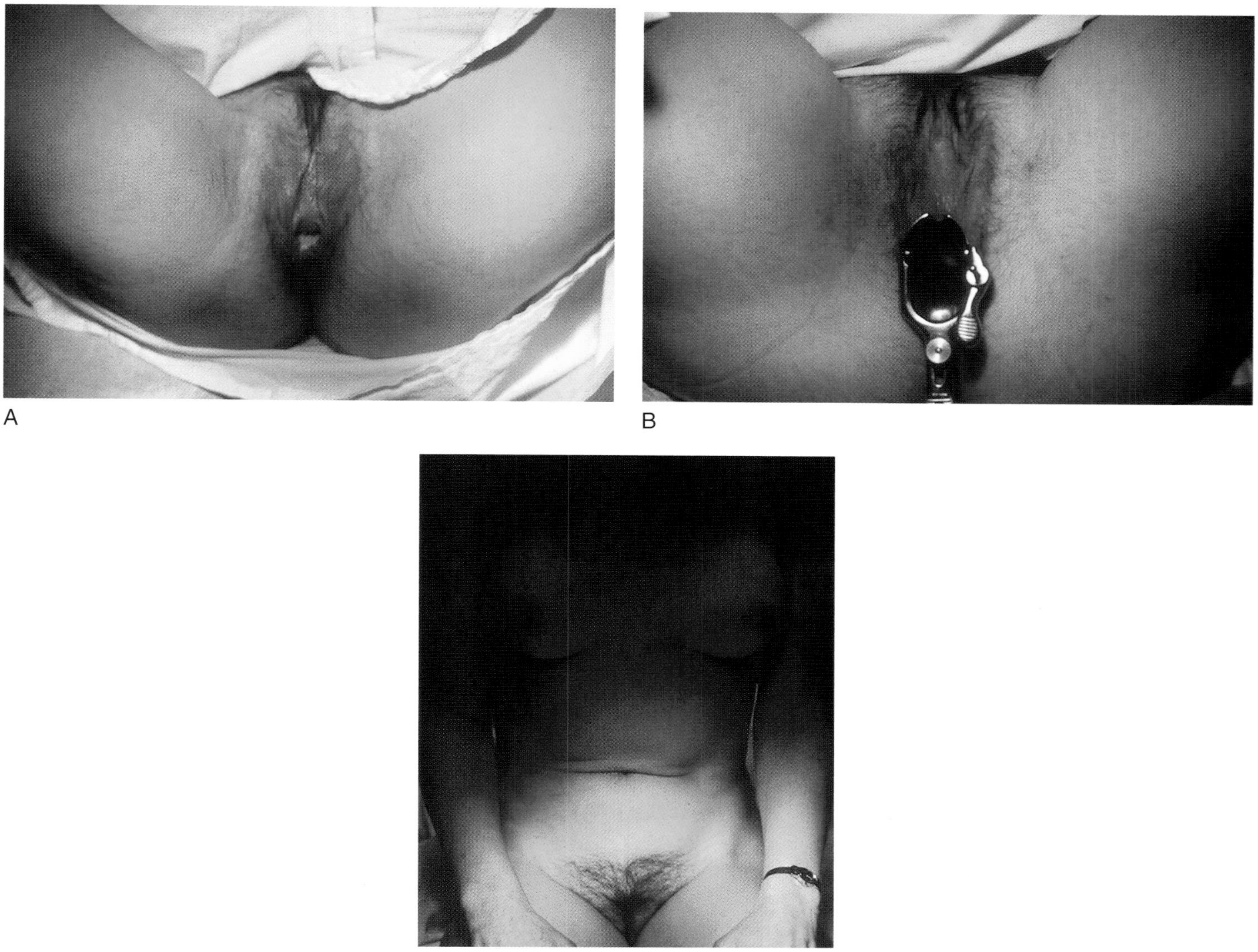

A

B

C

**FIGURE 104–24 A.** At 12 weeks postoperatively, the vulva and vagina appear cosmetically authentic. **B.** This standard Graves speculum easily negotiates the neovagina. **C.** This male-to-female transsexual appears to be a morphologically normal female.

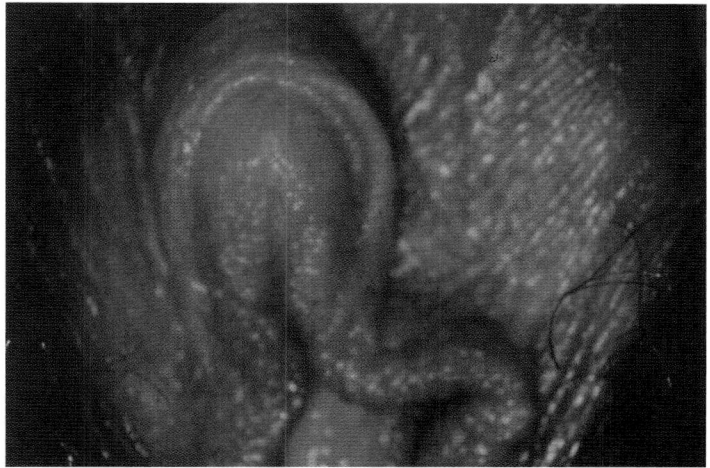

**FIGURE 104–25** The hermaphrodite pictured here has a micropenis (clitoris). This individual's karyotype is XY. The urethra opens at the base of the micropenis.

# SECTION D

## The Breast

# CHAPTER 105

# The Breast

*Donna L. Stahl* ■ *Karen S. Columbus* ■ *Michael S. Baggish*

## Anatomy of the Female Breast

The breasts are modified sweat glands and specifically function as modified apocrine glands. They represent significant gender-identifying structures, which society and the individual connote as phenotypically female. Mature adult breasts occupy a prominent position on the anterior chest wall between the second and sixth ribs (Fig. 105–1A). The "average" breast measures 10 to 12 cm in diameter and is 5 to 7 cm in thickness. Across the chest wall, the breast extends from the margin of the sternum to the midaxillary line. A portion of breast tissue projects into the axilla. This entity is known as the tail of Spence (Fig. 105–1B). Anatomically, the entire breast lies between the superficial and deep layers of the superficial pectoral fascia. The latter is contiguous with Scarpa's fascia of the anterior abdominal wall. Thus, the breast is roughly hemispherical in shape and sits on top of the deep pectoral fascia, which in turn encompasses the pectoralis major muscle (Fig. 105–2). A significant factor in the maintenance of the structure and shape of the breasts is attributed to fibrous bands that course between the deep and superficial layers of fascia. These dense Cooper's ligaments form the so-called suspensory ligaments of the breast, which are particularly prominent at its lower portion (inframammary fold).

The tissues lying between the deep and superficial layers of the superficial pectoral fascia consist mainly of fat but additionally of breast parenchyma and connective tissue (stroma). The relative amount of natural fat content contributes to the bounce of the breast with movement. As the volume of fat increases, so does the motion of the breasts, but only to the point where the quantity of fat produces such a large mass that it results in drooping, pendulous breasts. Scarring secondary to artificial augmentation of the breasts also diminishes the natural movement of the breasts on the chest wall (Fig. 105–3).

The breast parenchyma is divided into 15 to 20 segments or glandular units or lobes, which are radial in arrangement and converge to a series of ducts on the nipple. Approximately 5 to 10 major collecting ducts open at the nipple. Each duct drains a segment or lobe of the breast. Each lobe contains 20 to 40 lobules. Each lobule in turn consists of between 10 and 100 alveoli (Figs. 105–3 and 105–4).

Mounted on each breast is a more deeply pigmented circular area measuring an inch or more in diameter—the areola. The nipple caps the center of the areola. The dermis of the areola contains longitudinal and circular smooth muscle, which creates a wrinkled appearance when the muscles contract (see Fig. 105–1B, **inset**).

Several elevated openings may be observed on the periphery of the areola. These are the termini of the ducts of Montgomery's glands. The latter are modified sebaceous glands whose secretions keep the areolae lubricated and supple. During pregnancy, these same glands may secrete a milklike substance (see Fig. 105–1B, **inset**).

The functioning unit of the breast is the lobular unit. This consists of small glands lined by cuboidal and myoepithelial cells surrounded by a vascular stroma. Small interlobular terminal ducts lead to extralobular terminal ducts, which in turn lead to larger collecting ducts and then lead to still larger lactiferous ducts that drain entire lobes. Before draining into the nipple, these ducts dilate to form a lactiferous ampulla or sinus. Contraction of the myoepithelial cells as well as the smooth muscle of the areola aids in emptying the lactiferous sinuses of milk (see Fig. 105–4, **inset**).

Breast volume changes during the menstrual cycle. The breast parenchyma responds to stimulation with estrogen and progesterone. Similarly, water content within the fat (edema) parallels that seen within the endometrium, with peaks between days 22 and 25. The least amount of hormonal alteration occurs during the 4 to 5 days after the onset of menstrual flow.

Finally, although most breasts appear roughly symmetrical in size (volume), differences between the left and right breasts are common (Fig. 105–5).

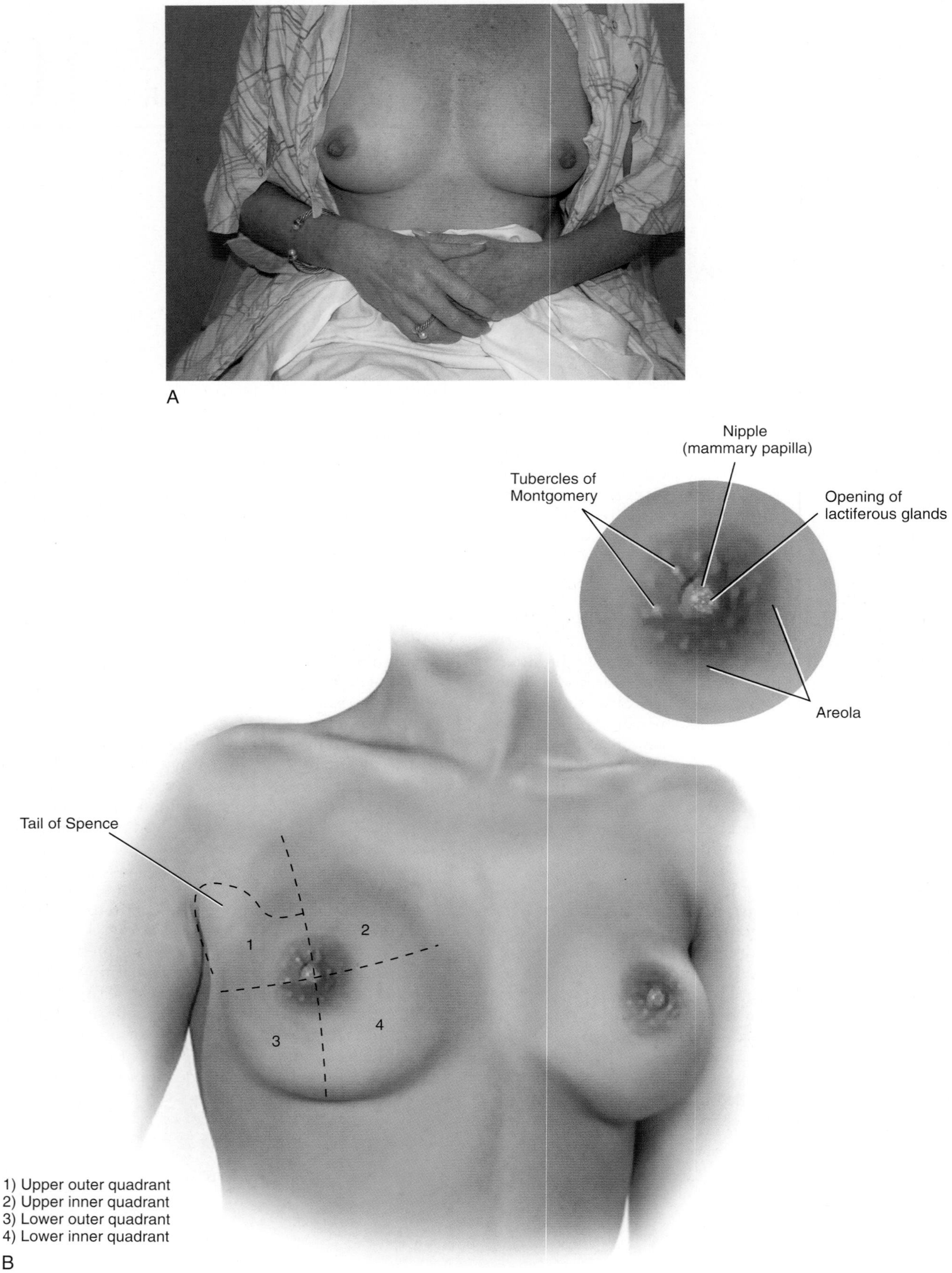

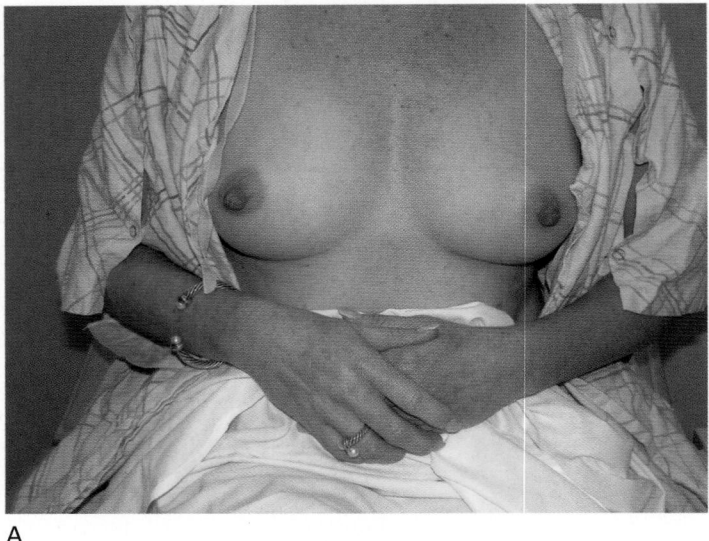

A

Nipple
(mammary papilla)

Tubercles of
Montgomery

Opening of
lactiferous glands

Areola

Tail of Spence

2

1

3

4

1) Upper outer quadrant
2) Upper inner quadrant
3) Lower outer quadrant
4) Lower inner quadrant

B

**FIGURE 105–1  A.** The mammary glands occupy a prominent location on the female chest wall. Phenotypically, they connote female gender to the individual. **B.** The breasts occupy space on the anterior chest wall between the second and sixth ribs. For purposes of description, the breasts are divided into four quadrants—two upper and two lower. The sculpted lower edge of the hemispheric breast is formed by the inframammary ridge. A portion of the breast tissue in the upper outer quadrant extends into the axilla (tail of Spence). The **inset** shows details of the areola, which encompasses the nipple, the tubercles of Montgomery, and the pigmented skin highlighting this area.

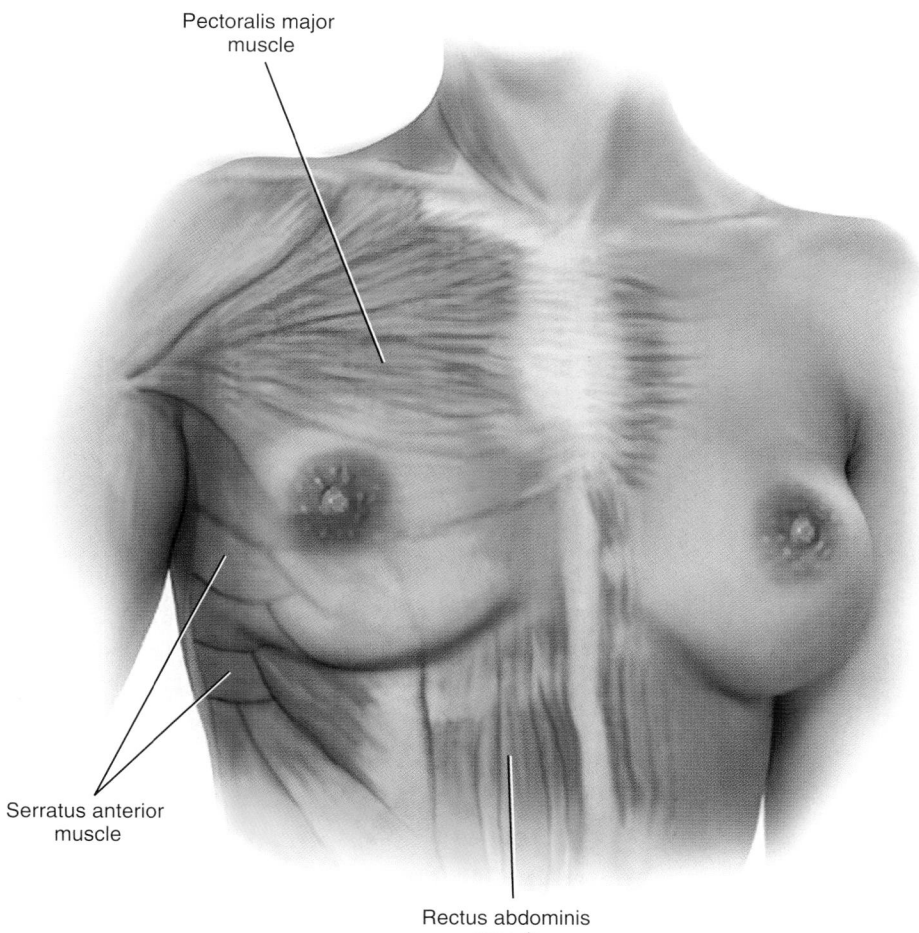

Pectoralis major
muscle

Serratus anterior
muscle

Rectus abdominis
muscle

**FIGURE 105–2** The breasts are contained within the superficial pectoral fascia and lie on the deep fascial layer that encloses the pectoralis major muscle. The breast encroaches inferiorly on the deep fascia of the serratus anterior, external oblique, and rectus abdominis muscles. The superficial pectoral fascia is subdivided into superficial and deep layers. The deep superficial layer is distinctly separated from the deep pectoral fascia by loose fat.

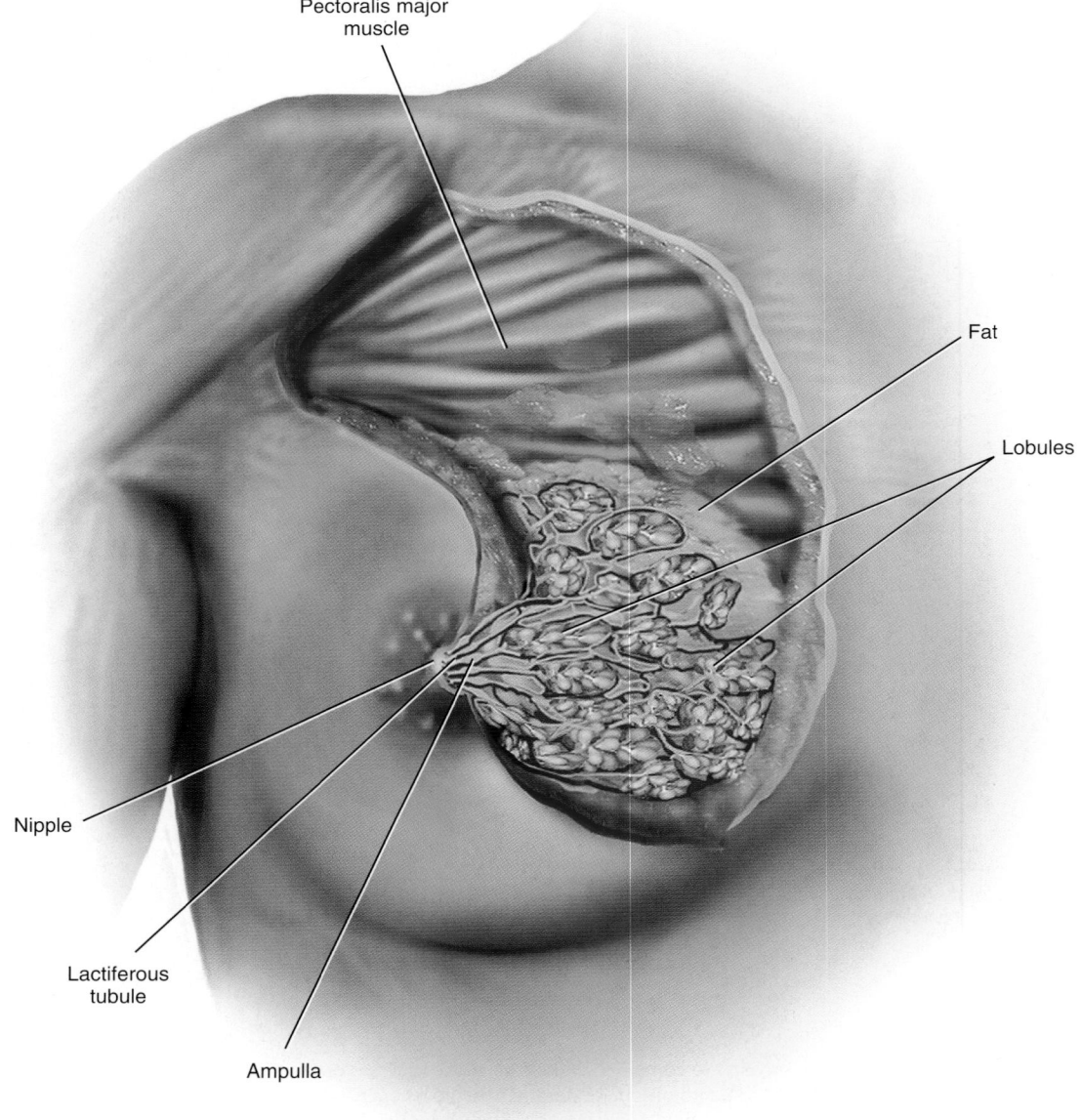

**FIGURE 105–3** The breast consists of fat and breast tissue. The latter is made up of lobules, ducts, and fibrous connective tissue. The apocrine glandular tissues or lobules secrete milk, which is collected and transported via a series of ducts to the nipple. The structural architecture of the breast is maintained by fibrous bands traveling between the deep superficial fascia and the dermal component of the breast's skin. These connective tissue bands or Cooper's ligaments largely account for the breast's spherical shape.

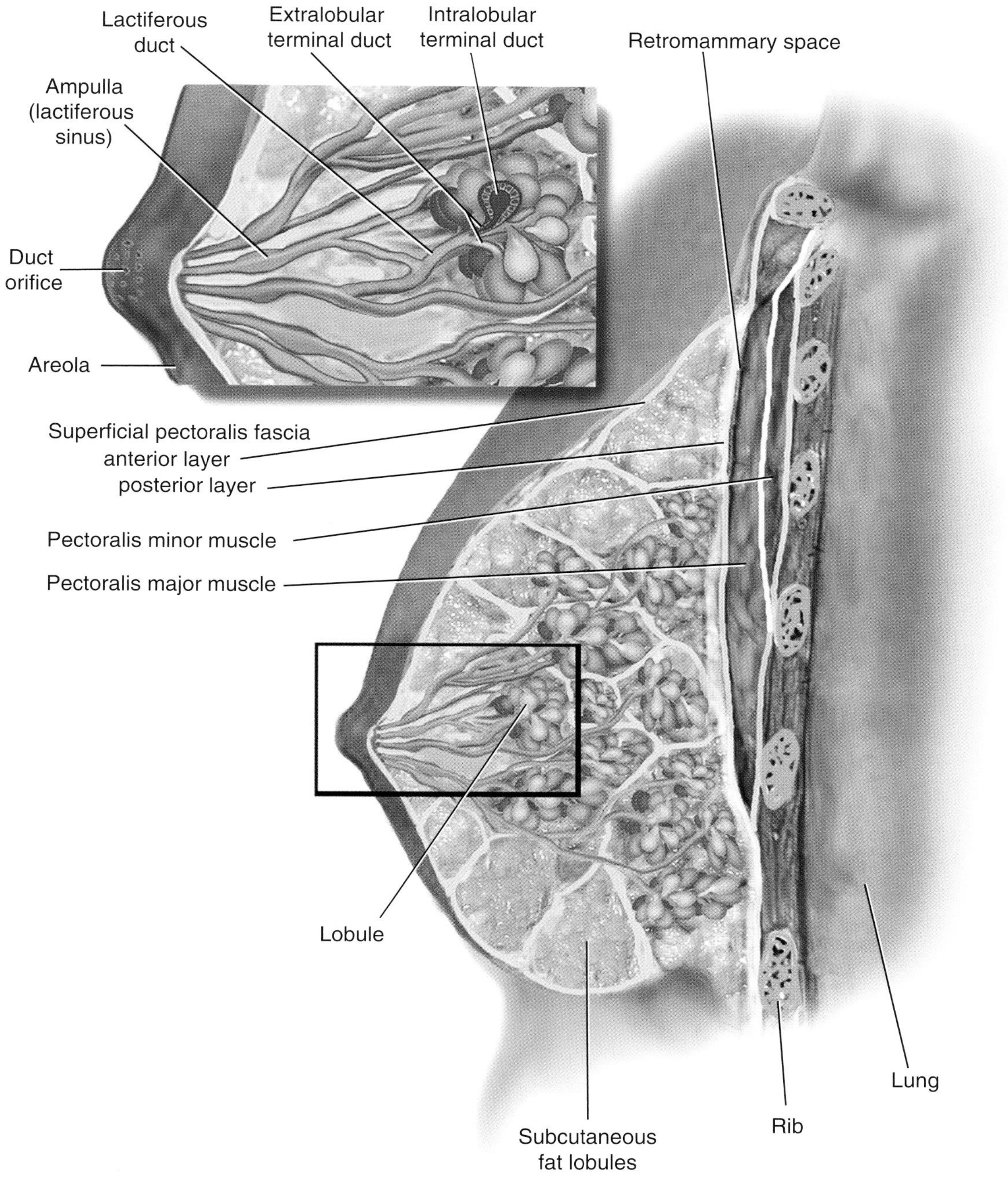

Lactiferous
duct

Extralobular
terminal duct

Intralobular
terminal duct

Retromammary space

Ampulla
(lactiferous
sinus)

Duct
orifice

Areola

Superficial pectoralis fascia
anterior layer
posterior layer

Pectoralis minor muscle

Pectoralis major muscle

Lobule

Subcutaneous
fat lobules

Rib

Lung

**FIGURE 105–4** The functioning unit of the breast is made up of small glands lined by cuboidal and myoepithelial cells, which elaborate a milky secretion. The secretion is propelled through intralobular and extralobular terminal ducts to larger lactiferous collection ducts. Before draining into the nipple, the secretions are stored in ampullary ducts (sinuses). Each duct drains a lobe consisting of 20 to 40 lobules.

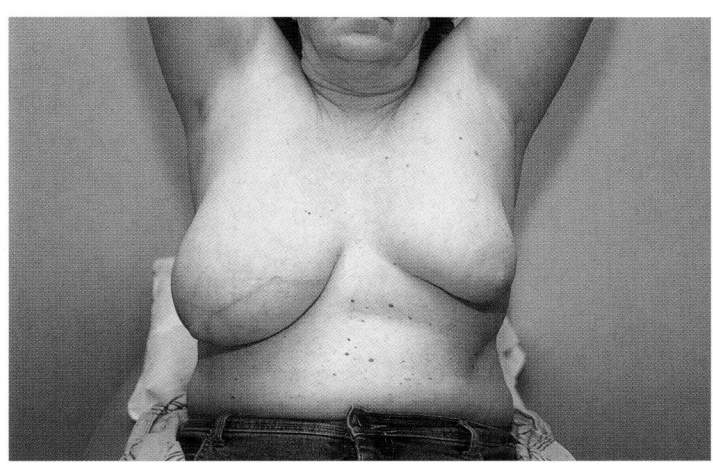

**FIGURE 105–5** This picture demonstrates rather extreme developmental asymmetry between the right and left breasts. Some slight size difference between the two breasts is not uncommon, and in contrast to the case illustrated here, the left breast is usually mildly larger than the right.

## Clinical Breast Examination

The breast examination is an integral part of the annual gynecologic examination for all women. This portion of the examination is an important screening tool for the detection of breast cancer. As with any physical examination, the end result, that is, early detection of a breast lump, depends on the quality and thoroughness of the examination. Sufficient time must be allocated to its performance, so the physician does not rush through this important component.

The ideal time period for the performance of a breast examination is during the early proliferative phase of the menstrual cycle. For a woman receiving hormonal replacement, the best time for the examination is 4 to 5 days after the last pill is taken.

The examination begins with the patient sitting at the end of the examination table facing the examiner (Fig. 105-6). With the patient's hands at her side, the breasts are observed for symmetry, retraction, and dimpling (Fig. 105-7). The color of the skin of the breasts is observed, inspecting particularly for redness, fixation, and scar formation. The areola and nipples are checked for inversion, dimpling, discoloration, and ulceration. The patient is asked to lean forward, which frees the breasts from the chest and accentuates pendulousness (see Fig. 105-7).

Next, the patient is asked to place her hands on her hips (Fig. 105-8). This move causes the pectoralis major muscle to contract. The patient next stretches her arms overhead, which elevates the breasts against the chest wall (Fig. 105-9). Similar observations are made in this position.

As noted in the anatomy section, most often the difference in breast volume is small; occasionally, the size difference between left and right breasts (i.e., asymmetry) is extreme (see Fig. 105-5).

While the patient remains seated, the axillary exam is performed on the right and left sides (Fig. 105-10). The patient's right arm is supported by the examiner's right arm, and the left hand palpates the axillary lymph nodes. The supraclavicular area is likewise palpated for adenopathy (Fig. 105-11). The procedure is then carried out on the left side. Next, the examiner stands behind the patient and compresses the breast and nipple for discharge (Fig. 105-12).

The patient is instructed to lie down on her back (supine position), and the end of the examination table is extended. Utilizing the flat of the hand while supporting the breast with the opposite hand, the examiner palpates the breast against the chest wall. A variety of techniques may be used. A convenient procedure is to divide the breast into three zones from top to bottom, beginning first with the upper third. Palpate beginning below the midaxillary line, and progress medially to the sternum. This is repeated until all three zones have been thoroughly examined. The nipples and areolae are separately examined by palpation and then by compression (Figs. 105-13 and 105-14).

For the sake of completeness, the inframammary ridge is checked separately (Fig. 105-15). The supraclavicular area may be examined in the sitting or supine position (see Fig. 105-11).

Because approximately 5% of breast cancers appear during pregnancy or the postpartum period, it is unwise to delay breast examination during these times. If the woman is lactating, the breasts should be pumped before the examination is performed.

Documentation is exceedingly important. Negatives as well as positives should be written into the patient's record. Differences in nodularity or lumpiness between the two breasts should be noted. Any mass must be described by size, shape (measured in centimeters), location (precise anatomic), mobility versus fixation, consistency (hard, soft, rubbery), and sensitivity (painful vs. nontender). Nipple discharge should be localized to the compressed quadrant and described as to color and consistency. A guaiac test should be done, and the material placed on a slide, fixed, and sent to pathology.

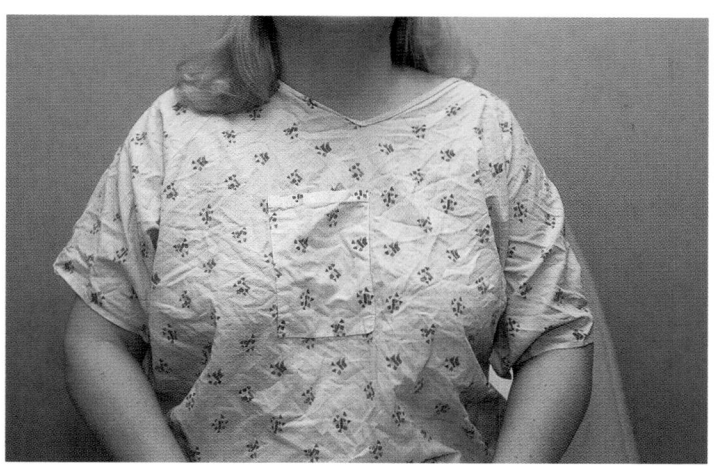

**FIGURE 105–6** The clinical breast exam (CBE) begins with the patient sitting on the end of the examination table facing the examiner.

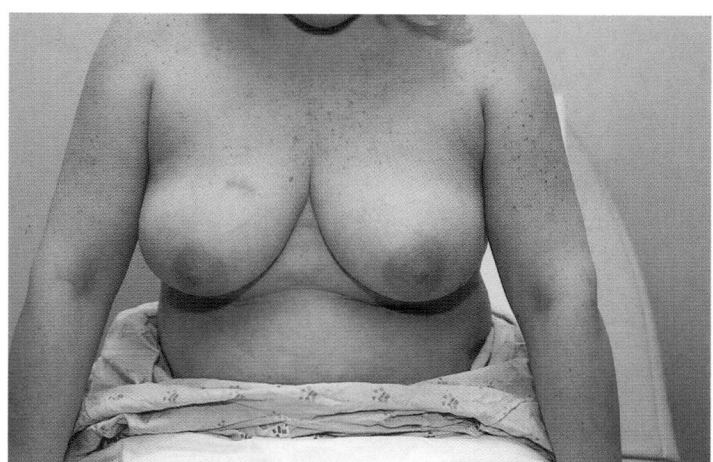

**FIGURE 105–7** The breasts are allowed to relax and hang free by having the patient bring her arms to her sides and lean slightly forward.

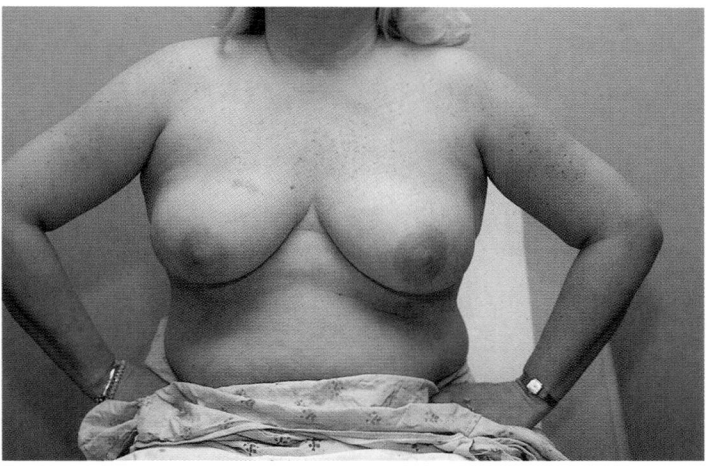

**FIGURE 105–8** The patient sits erect with her hands on her hips. The breasts are visually examined for symmetry, retraction, nipple location, and appearance. Note the scar in the upper inner quadrant of the right breast.

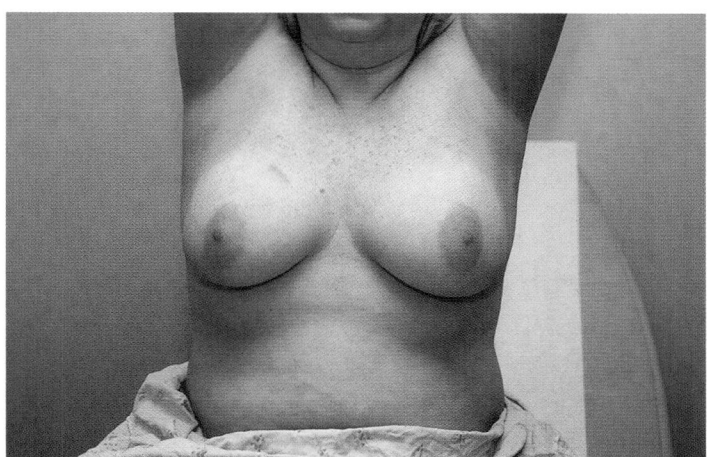

**FIGURE 105–9** The patient is instructed to raise her hands high above her head to place the breast tissue on tension. The skin of the breast is inspected for color changes, edema, thickening, ulceration, or dimpling. The nipples are described as erect, inverted, or distorted.

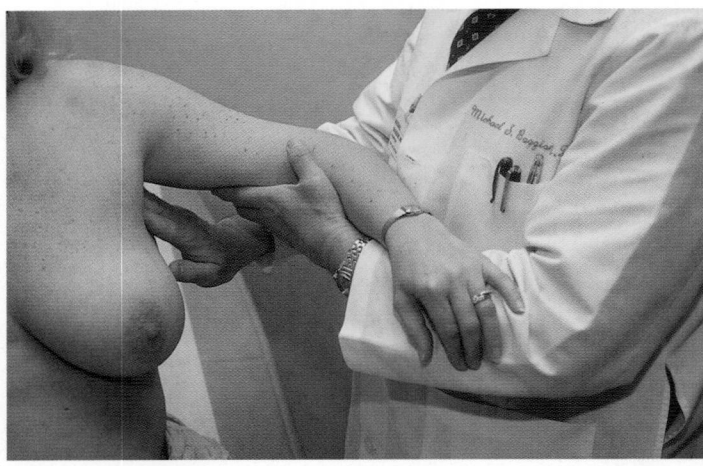

**FIGURE 105–10** The axilla is examined to determine whether there is adenopathy or tenderness. The ipsilateral arm is supported by the examiner to relax the pectoral muscle, while the other hand palpates into the axilla and against the chest wall.

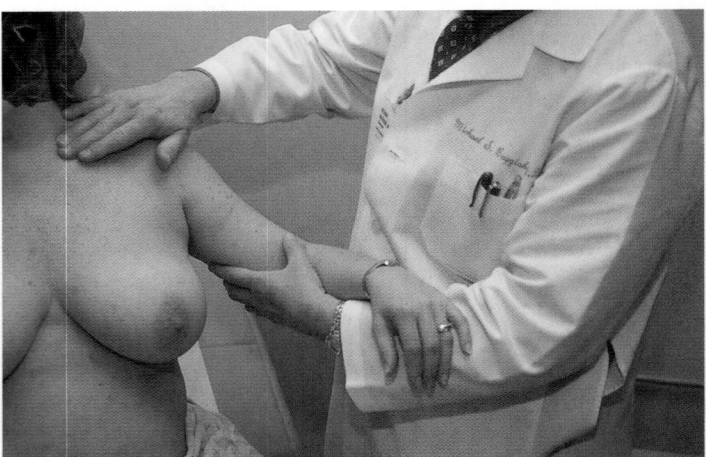

**FIGURE 105–11** Next, the supraclavicular area is examined for the presence of lymphadenopathy.

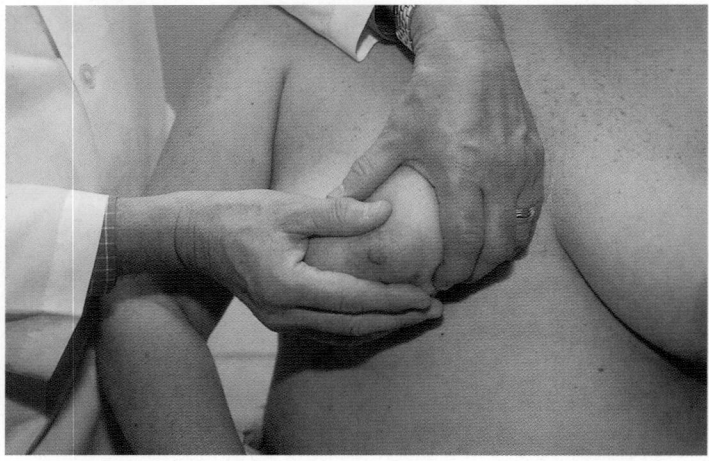

A

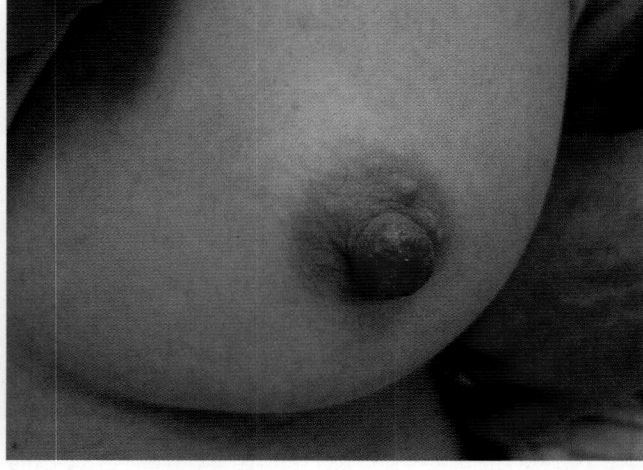

B

**FIGURE 105–12** Standing to the side and in back of the patient, the examiner compresses the areola and nipple to determine whether a discharge is present. By milking the individual quadrants, the examiner can determine the relative location from which the discharge is elicited.

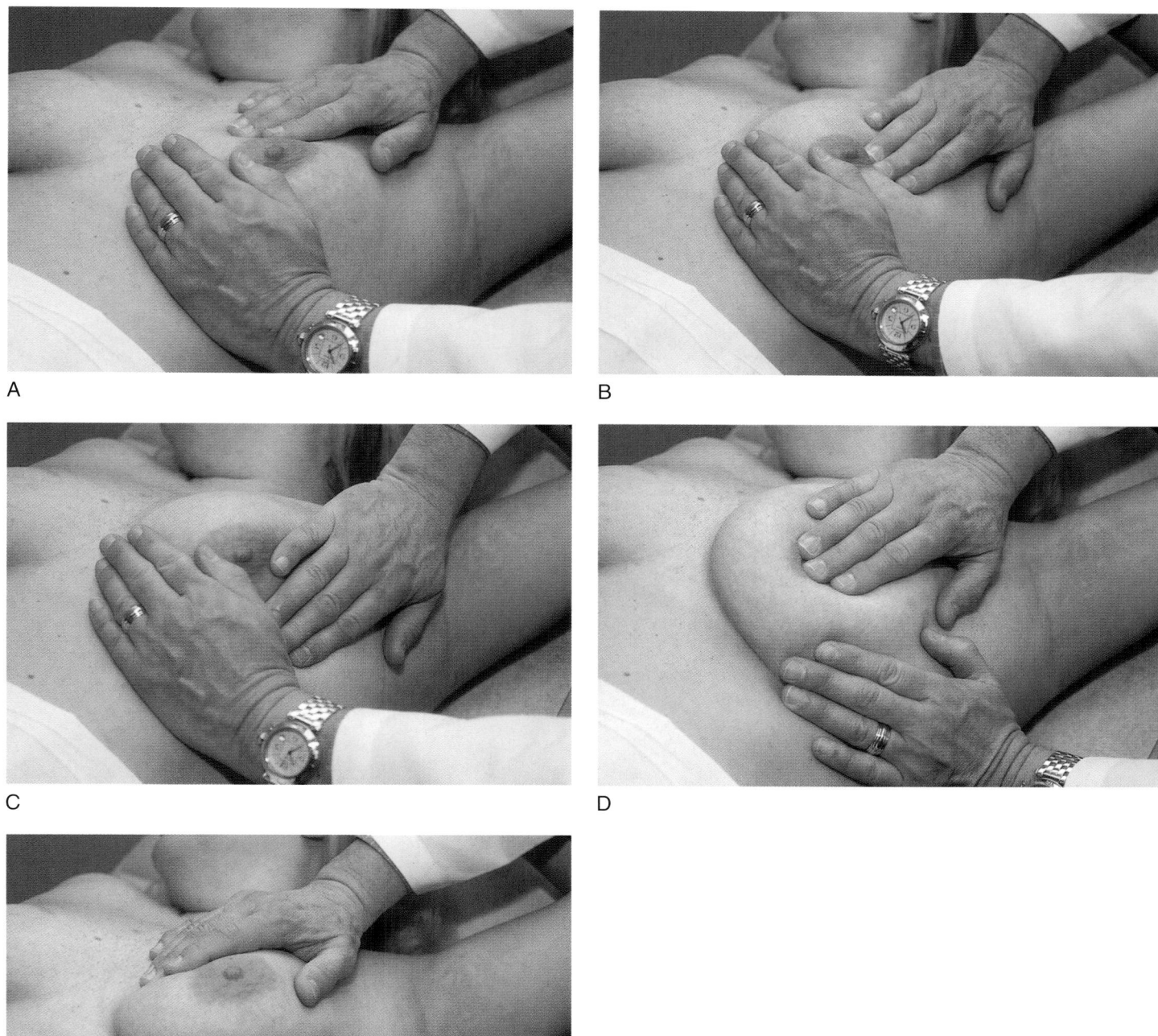

A

B

C

D

E

**FIGURE 105–13 A** through **E.** The patient is placed in the supine position, and the ipsilateral arm is extended above her head. The examiner palpates the breast with his or her flattened fingers against the chest wall. The author prefers to divide the breast into three or four horizontal zones. Palpation begins at the sternum and continues in a lateral direction until the midaxillary line is passed. The exam is repeated for each zone and covers the area from the clavicle above to the lower rib cage below. The nipples and areolar areas are separately compressed.

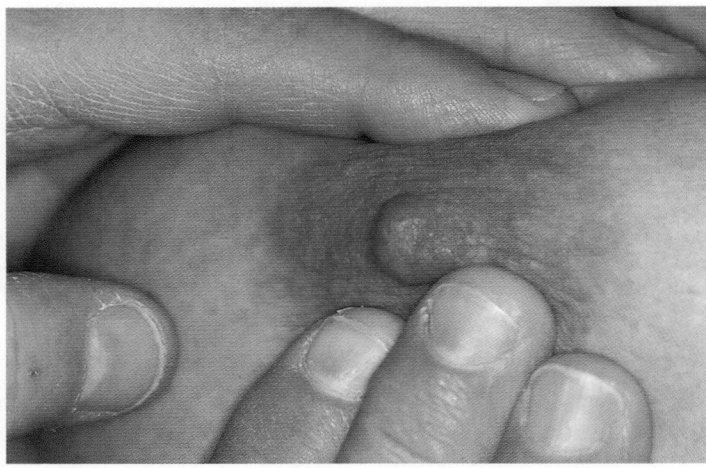

**FIGURE 105–14** The nipple and the areola are squeezed to determine whether any discharge can be identified.

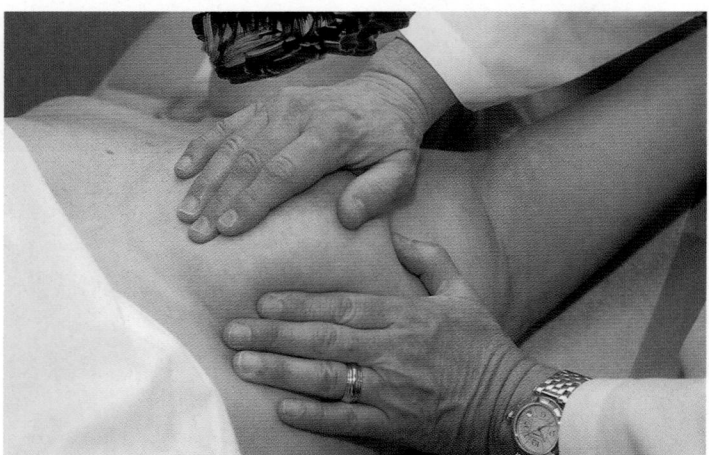

**FIGURE 105–15** The inframammary ridge is carefully palpated to finish the examination.

## Fine-Needle Aspiration

Fine-needle aspiration (FNA) coupled with cytology is a diagnostic technique that can be performed safely in the office setting. This may be performed by direct insertion or by ultrasound-guided insertion. A solid mass is unlikely to be differentiated from a breast cyst on the basis of clinical breast exam (CBE) alone. On the other hand, FNA can be used to differentiate between cystic and solid lesions. A diagnostic mammogram is likely to have been ordered before a breast aspiration (Fig. 105–16).

The diagnostic accuracy of FNA can be 95%. This accuracy depends on obtaining a sufficient amount of aspirate and on the proficiency of the cytopathologist. Remember, a negative FNA result should not dissuade one from doing a biopsy.

The technique for aspiration is simple. The breast, over the site of the mass, is prepped with an alcohol preparation. The tissue containing the mass is stabilized with one hand. Next, a 10-mL syringe with a 22-gauge needle attached is inserted into the mass while withdrawing on the plunger. If a cyst is present, the contents are aspirated and sent for cytology. Palpation after aspiration (if the lesion is a cyst) should reveal complete collapse and disappearance of the mass. If the mass remains, prompt breast biopsy is indicated (Figs. 105–17 through 105–25).

Specific training is required for gynecologists who wish to perform fine-needle aspiration biopsy.

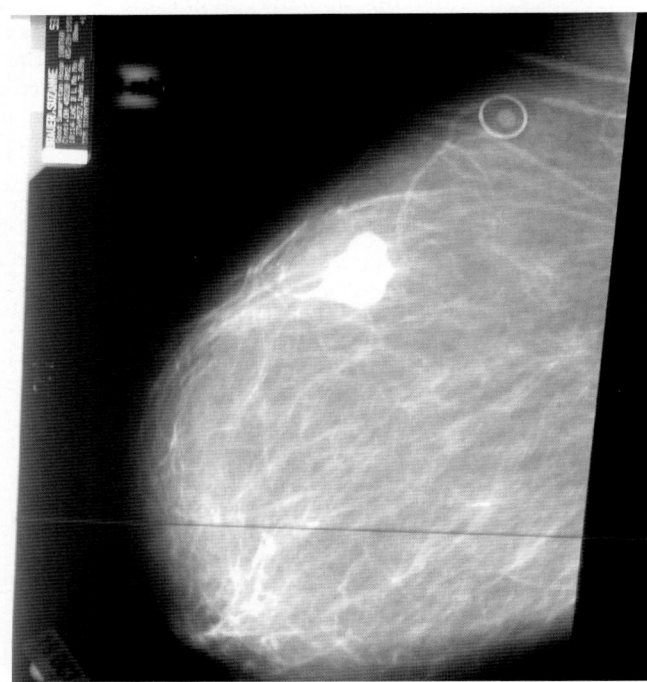

**FIGURE 105–16** This mammogram shows a mass in the upper quadrant, which represents a possible malignant lesion. A biopsy needs to be performed on this mass.

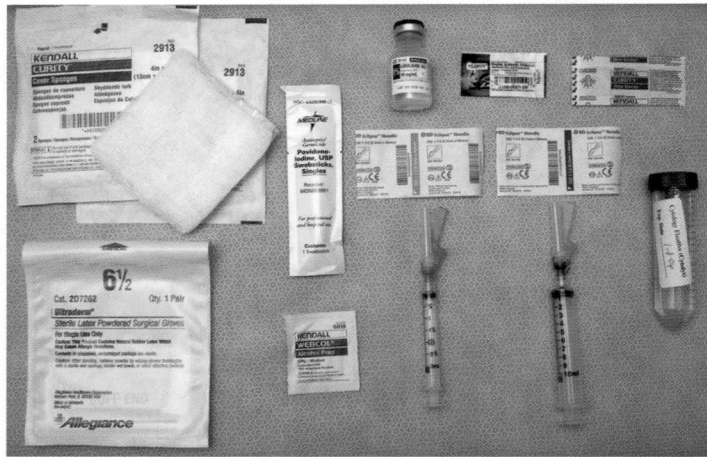

**FIGURE 105–17** This photograph illustrates the tools necessary for the performance of fine-needle aspiration. These items include iodine or alcohol skin prep solution, local anesthetic, syringes for anesthesia and aspiration, needles, syringes, cytologic vehicle, antibiotic topical ointment, and adhesive bandages.

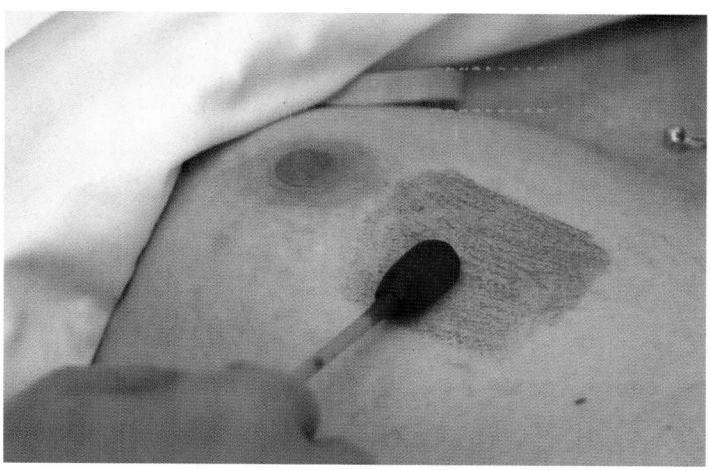

**FIGURE 105–18** The skin of the breast above the site of the suspected cyst is cleansed with iodine or alcohol. The surgeon must observe sterile technique.

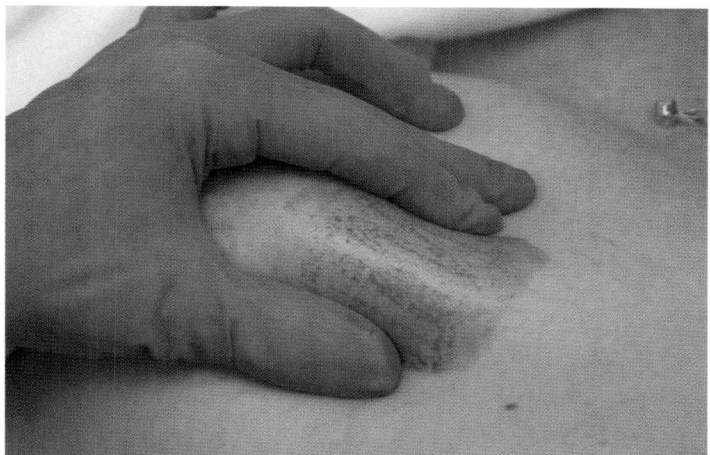

**FIGURE 105–19** The location of the breast mass *must* be stabilized with the fingers of one hand. This position must not be released until the aspiration has been completed.

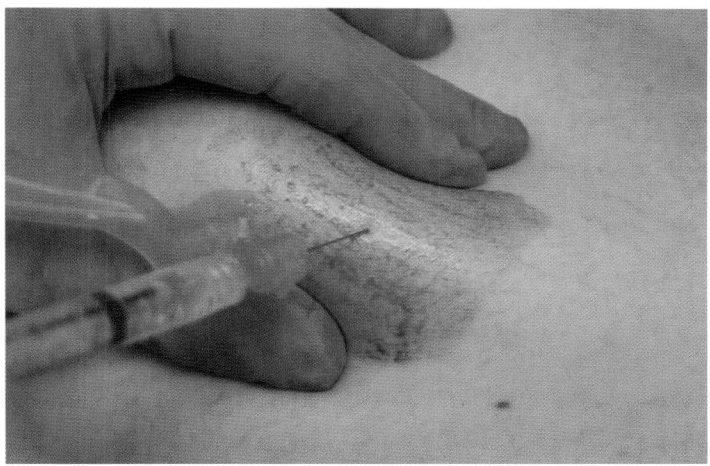

**FIGURE 105–20** The skin overlying the aspiration site is anesthetized by using a 25-gauge needle coupled to a 3- to 5-mL syringe with injection of 1% lidocaine (Xylocaine).

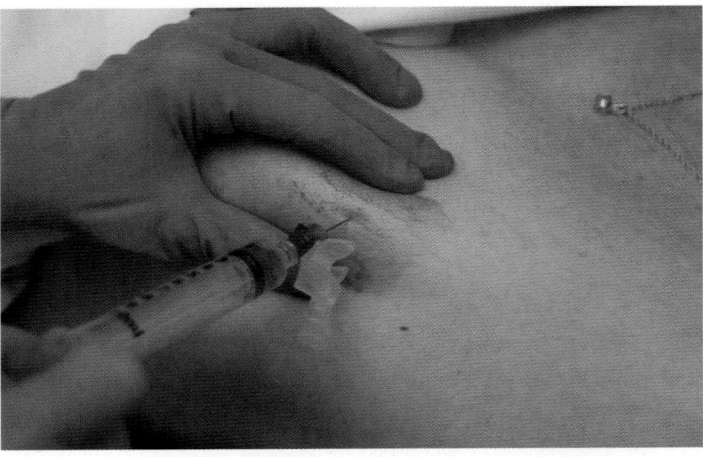

A

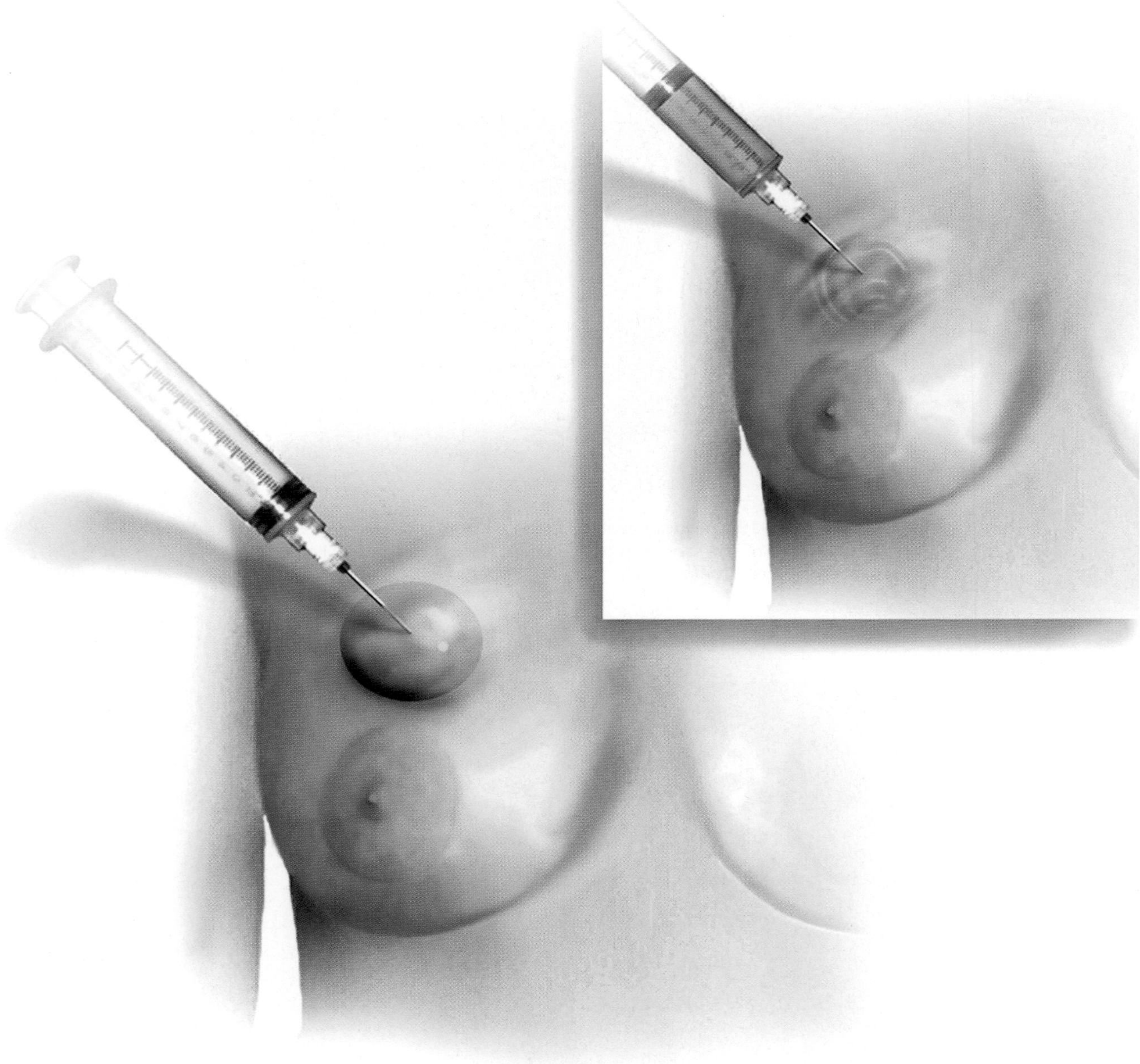

B

**FIGURE 105–21 A.** The fine-needle aspiration is performed via a 22-gauge needle and a 10-mL syringe. One cubic centimeter of air may be placed into the syringe before the aspiration. If *fluid* is obtained, the cyst should be completely emptied. Cytologic examination should be performed if the fluid is bloody (nontraumatic) or cloudy. Additionally, fluid should be sent for cytologic evaluation if the lesion does not disappear. For solid masses, several passes should be made into the lesion at different angles, while the operator firmly holds the lesion in place. During each pass of the needle, suction is maintained on the plunger of the syringe. **B.** The lesion is aspirated. In this illustration, a "blue dome" cyst is shown. The lesion is cystic, and it will collapse as the fluid is withdrawn (**inset**).

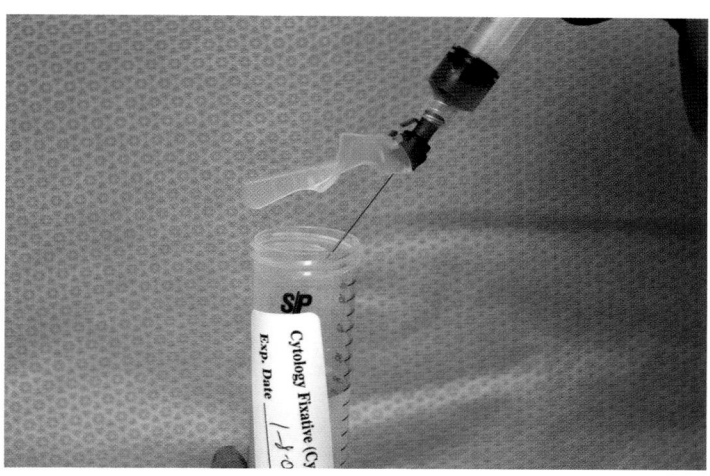

**FIGURE 105–22** The aspirate may be placed into cytology fixative or alternatively spread on a glass slide as a smear. The method for retrieval should be chosen by the surgeon, the gynecologist, and the pathologist.

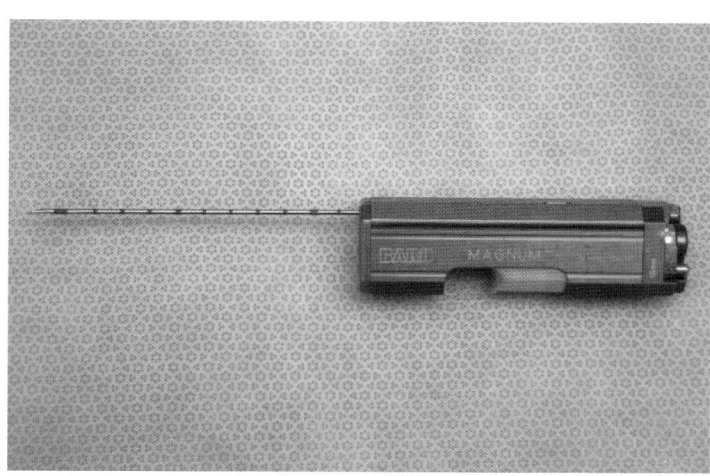

**FIGURE 105–23** The core needle is used for sampling solid lesions. The apparatus pictured here is a full-core biopsy instrument.

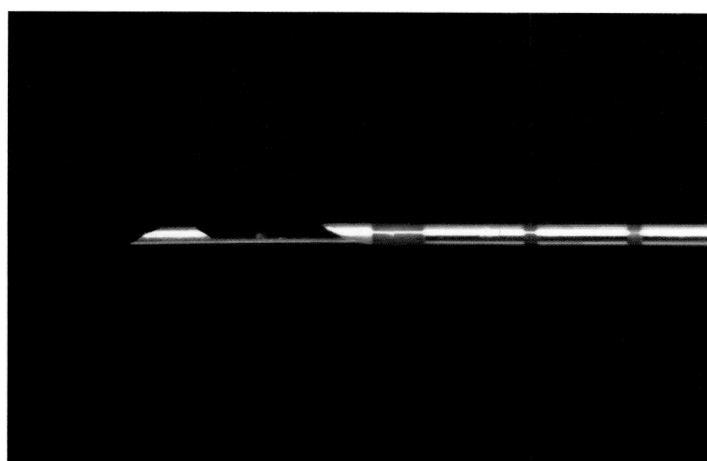

**FIGURE 105–24** The detail of the large-gauge core needle shows its sharp, beveled cutting tip.

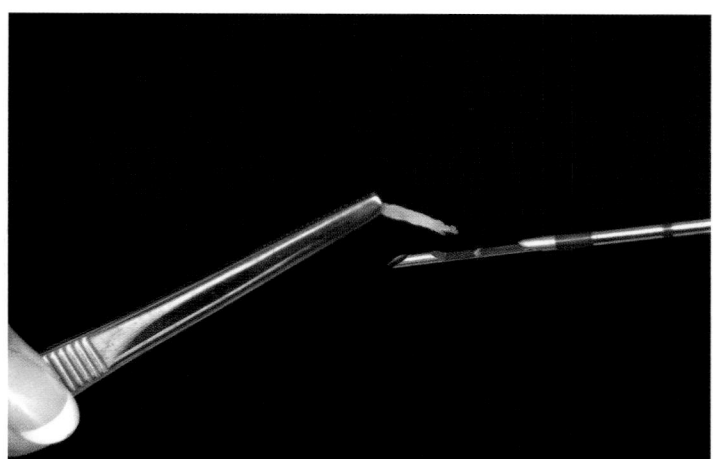

**FIGURE 105–25** The core needle makes a single pass into the suspected solid tumor. The fragment of retrieved tissue is sent to pathology, where it is embedded and blocked.

# Endoscopy and Endoscopic Surgery

# Hysteroscopy

# CHAPTER 106

# Hysteroscopic Instrumentation

*Michael S. Baggish*

To perform operative hysteroscopy as well as panoramic diagnostic hysteroscopy, the potential uterine cavity must be distended to allow the operator to see. Although a large number and variety of instruments are available, the critical implements required to perform manipulative hysteroscopic examinations and procedures are few.

The first and most important device is the telescope, which permits vision within the uterine space. Typically, rigid telescopes measure 4 mm in outer diameter (O.D.) and contain optical rod lenses as well as fiberoptic light–transmitting elements (Fig. 106–1A through C).

The second element is the hysteroscopic sheath, which transmits the distention medium into the uterine cavity. For simple viewing, the sheath measures 5 mm O.D.; however, larger sheaths ranging in size from 7.5 to 9.0 mm O.D. are required for operative hysteroscopy (Fig. 106–2A, B). Contemporary sheaths should have isolated inflow and outflow channels to properly and continuously flush the uterine cavity (Fig. 106–3A through D). Some sheaths are specialized, for example, the resectoscopic sheath is specifically designed for electrosurgery (Fig. 106–4A through C).

Third, a high-powered (and preferably xenon) light generator is required to provide high-intensity light (Fig. 106–5). Coupled with the light generator is a video camera and monitor, because most if not all modern hysteroscopy is performed with the surgeon and assistants viewing the operative field via a video monitor (Fig. 106–6A, B). Recording equipment for still, video, or digital photography should be available to memorialize findings and to supplement the dictated operative report (Fig. 106–7).

Accessory instruments may be divided into conventional devices and energy-delivered implements. Among the conventional tools are scissors, grasping forceps, biopsy forceps, and suction cannulas (Fig. 106–8A, B). The energy devices include bipolar and unipolar needles, coagulating ball electrodes, and laser fibers (Fig. 106–9A, B). A specialized sheath commonly utilized for hysteroscopic surgery is the resectoscope. This consists of a flushing sheath, a number of double-armed monopolar electrodes, and a spring-loaded trigger mechanism to move the electrode out of the sheath and then return it back to the sheath (Fig. 106–10). The most convenient consolidation of the myriad pieces of equipment is the mobile, multilevel, storage cart (see Fig. 106–5).

Finally, hysteroscopic infusion media (e.g., 32% dextran-70 [Hyskon], glycine, mannitol, saline) are vasoactive substances, which, because of pressure differentials, gain entry into the patient's vascular space (Figs. 106–11 and 106–12). Therefore, every operative hysteroscopy performed must be accompanied by an accurate accounting of **fluids in** versus **fluids out.** The most accurate method of quantifying fluid outflow is to employ a drape fitted with a waterproof pouch in which to collect the exiting medium (Fig. 106–13).

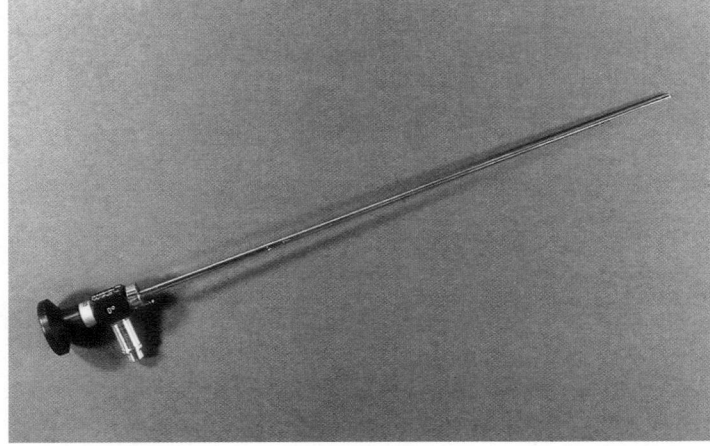

A

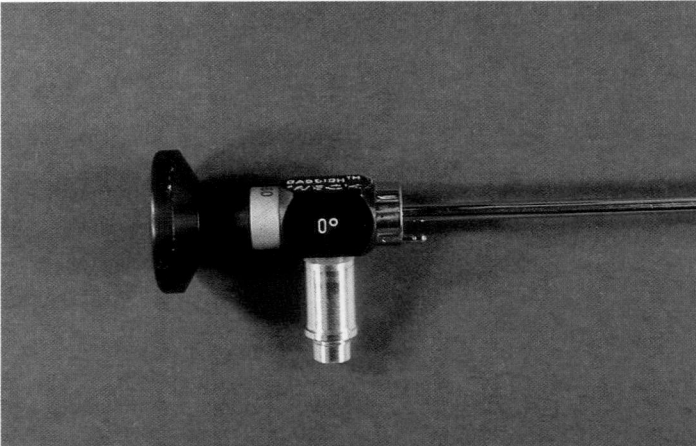

B

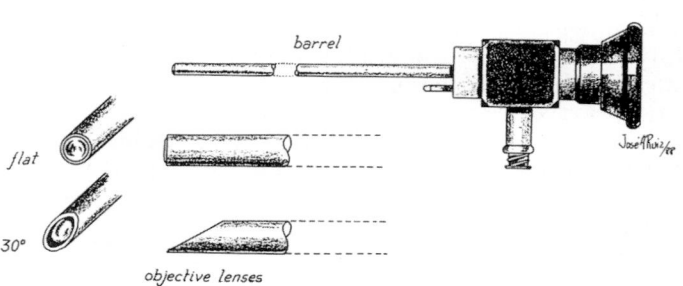

C

**FIGURE 106–1 A.** The telescope measures 4 mm O.D. and consists of an optic (viewing) and glass fibers that transmit light. **B.** Magnified view shows the magnifying eyepiece of the telescope and the connection for the fiberoptic cable that carries light from a remote generator to the telescope. **C.** This schematic drawing illustrates the components of the telescope. The objective lens is 0°, which produces a straight-on view, and the 30° scope gives an offset or angulated view of the object. From the objective, the image is transmitted by a series of rod lenses to the eyepiece.

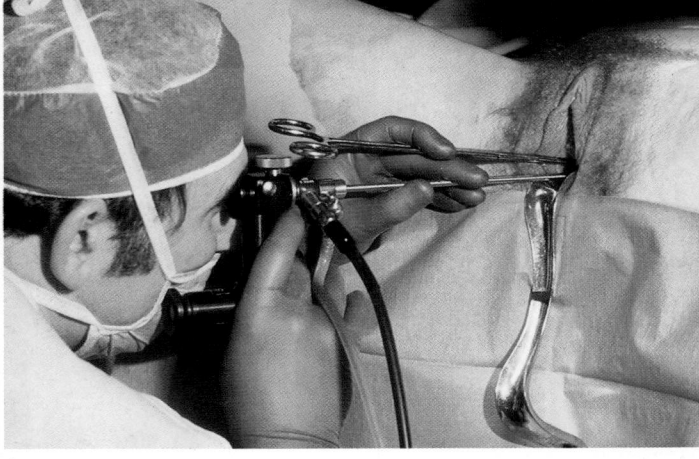

A

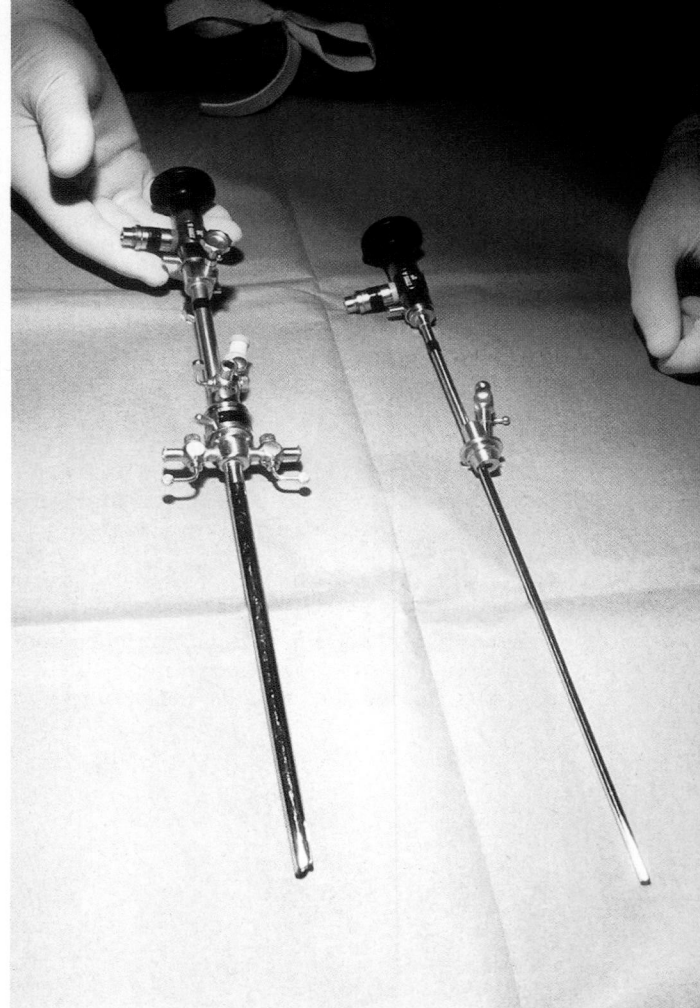

B

**FIGURE 106–2 A.** The telescope is fitted to a 5-mm diagnostic sheath, and the chosen medium is injected via the sheath to distend the cervix and corpus. The operator engages the scope at the external os and enters the cavity via direct vision. **B.** Operative (*left*) and diagnostic (*right*) sheaths are displayed side by side. The telescopes fitted to the sheaths are identical (4 mm O.D.).

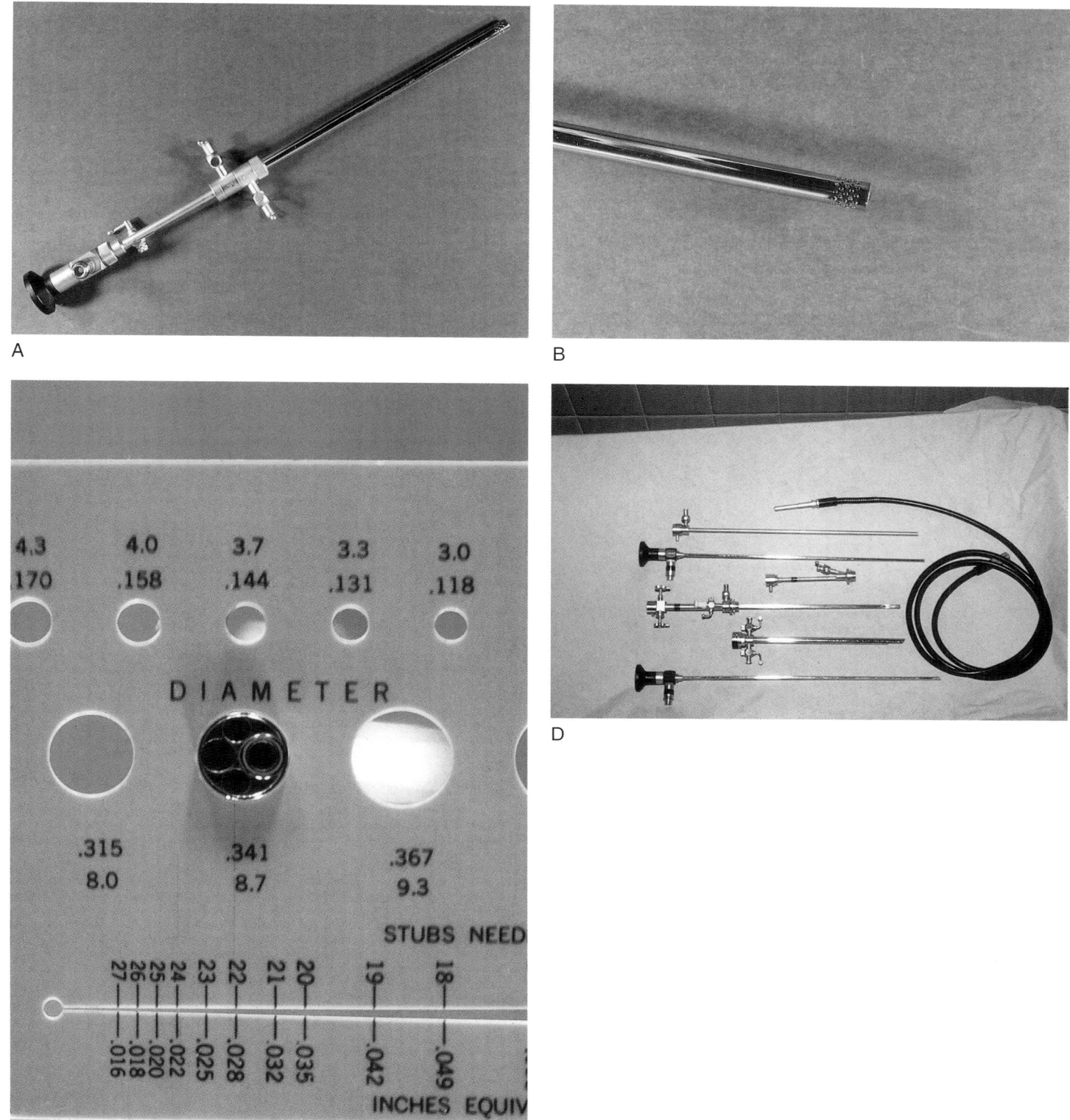

**FIGURE 106–3 A.** An isolated channel hysteroscope with a double sheath to allow return flow of the medium. The forward stopcock is for inflow; the aft stopcock is the outflow channel. **B.** The distal aspect of the sheath illustrated in Figure 106–3A. Perforations are present in the outer sheath and are the portal through which returning fluid enters the exterior sheath. **C.** The operative sheath is illustrated protruding through a measuring device. Note that the diameter of the hole is 8.7 mm. **D.** A complete instrument set includes diagnostic and operative sheaths, telescope, and fiberoptic light cable.

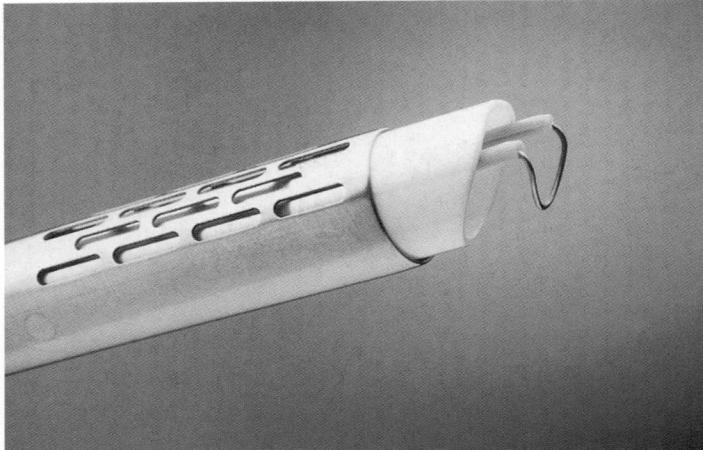

A

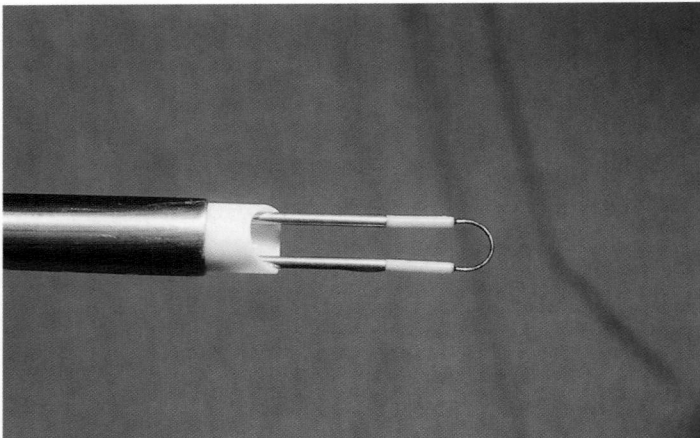

B

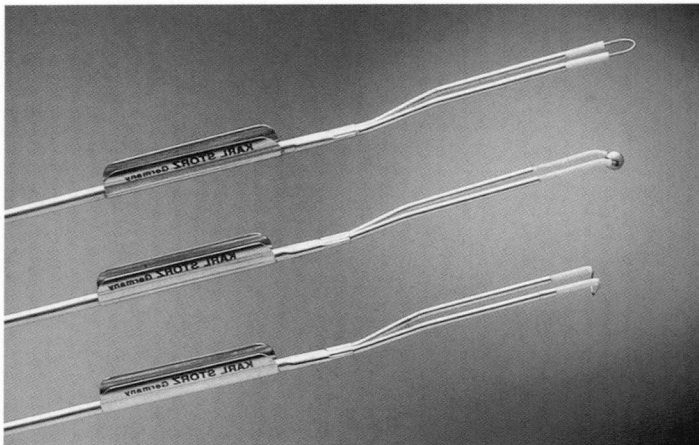

C

**FIGURE 106–4  A.** The resectoscope is a specially modified operative sheath that is suitable for monopolar electrosurgery. The sheath is a flushing type (double sheath). The electrode is an angulated loop supported by a double arm. **B.** The straight resectoscopic loop electrode is ideal for shaving or cutting lesions located at the fundus. **C.** A variety of electrodes are available for cutting, ablation, or coagulation.

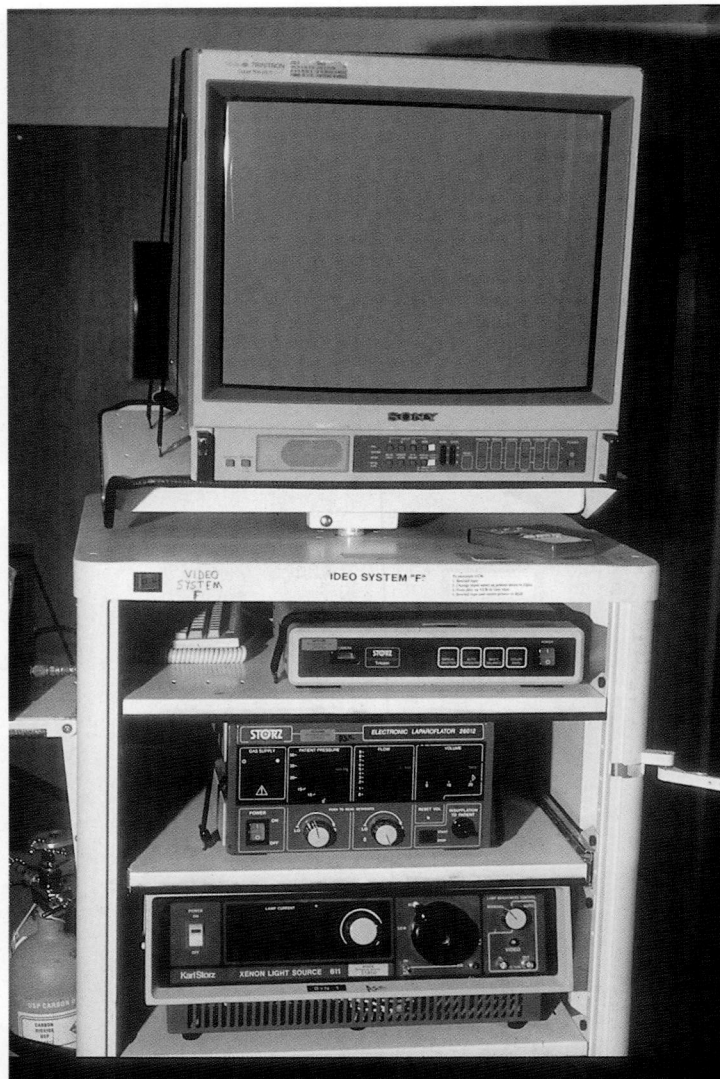

**FIGURE 106–5**  The large mobile instrument accessory cabinet contains a video monitor, a video control device, a fiberoptic light source, and a video recorder.

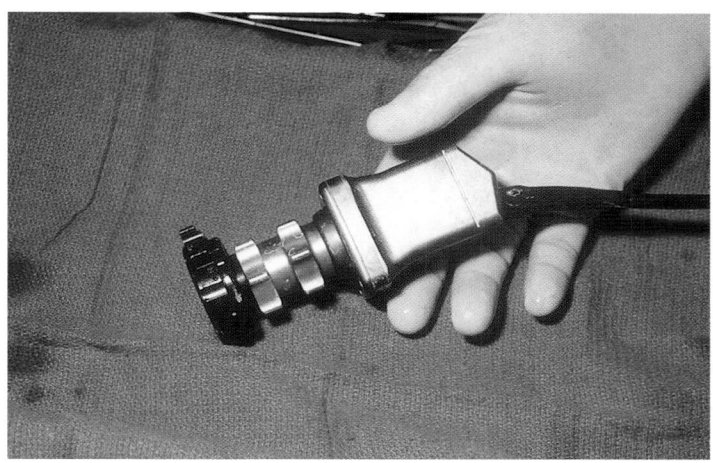

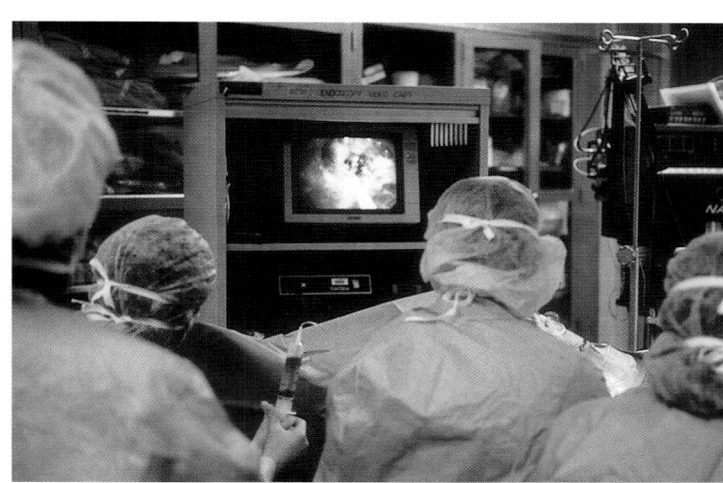

A                                              B

**FIGURE 106–6 A.** All contemporary hysteroscopic surgery is performed by viewing the field indirectly via the video screen. A small endoscopic TV camera attaches to the eyepiece of the telescope. **B.** The surgeon can sit up straight during hysteroscopic surgery because the operative field can be viewed via a TV monitor. The assistants have, of course, the same view as the surgeon.

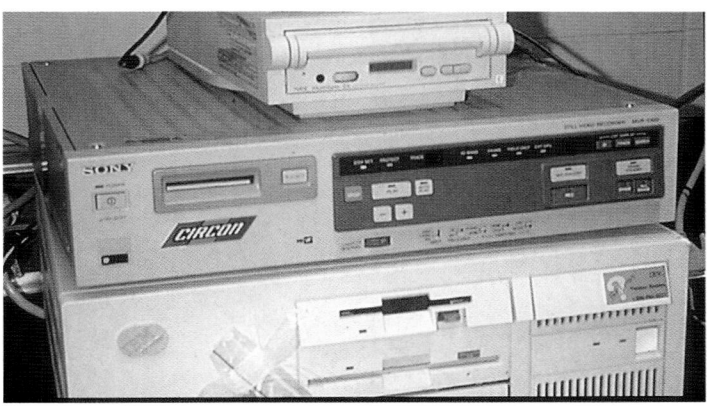

**FIGURE 106–7** The digital printer permits permanent still picture records and slides to be produced from the operation.

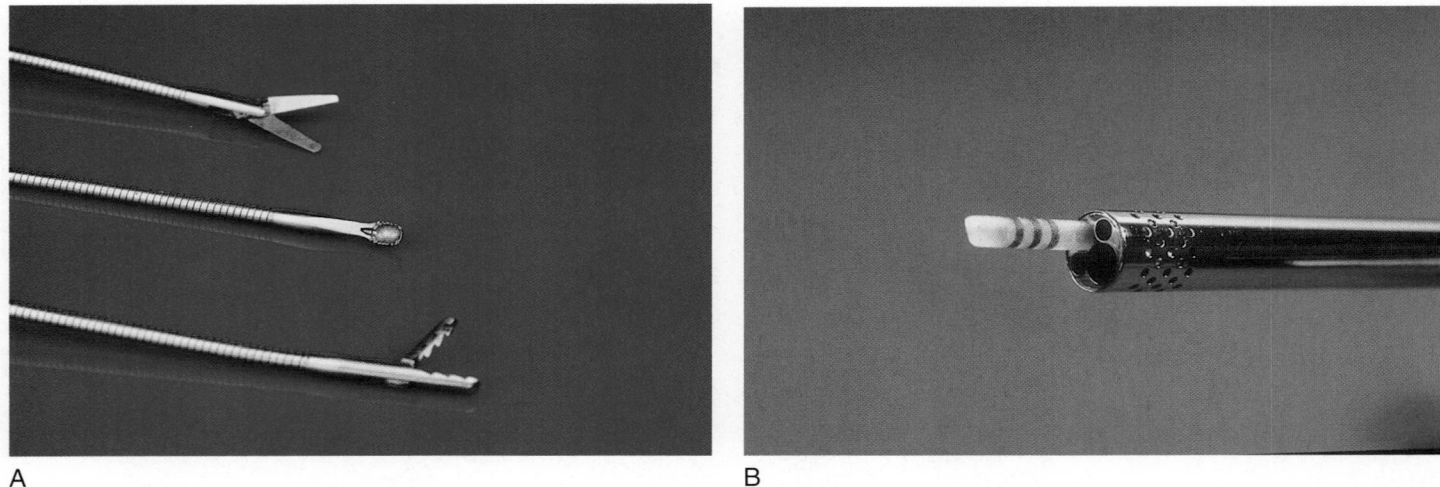

A                                                              B

**FIGURE 106–8  A.** These conventional tools are inserted via the operative channel of the hysteroscopic sheath into the uterine cavity. At the top are scissors, in the middle is a direct-sampling curette, and at the bottom are alligator grasping forceps. **B.** A 3-mm aspirating cannula is useful for evacuating blood and debris from the uterine cavity.

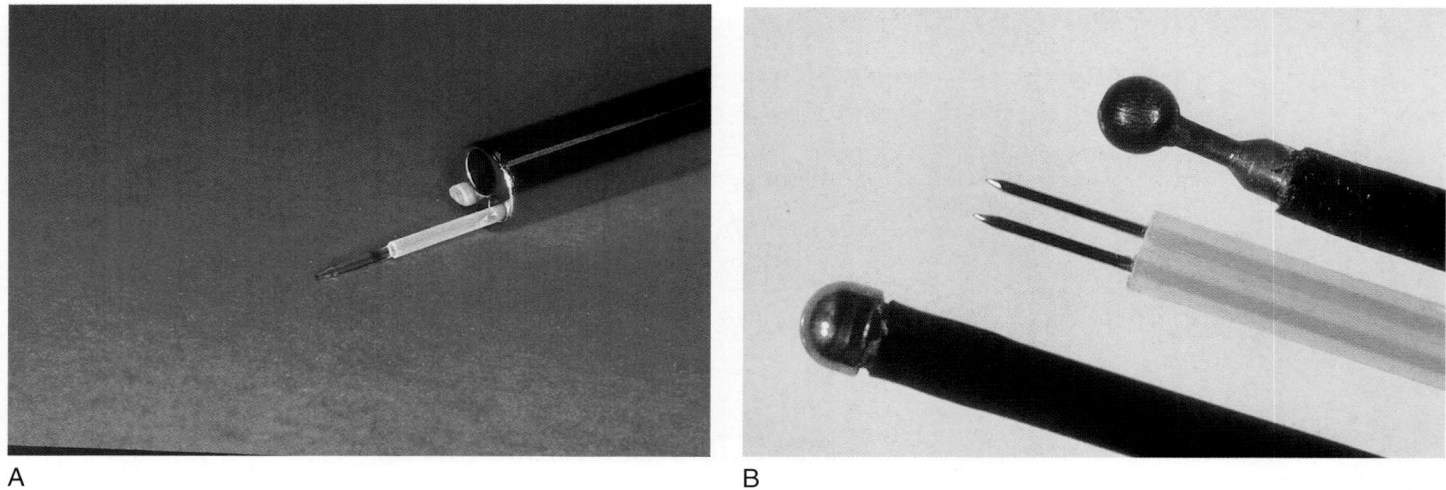

A                                                              B

**FIGURE 106–9  A.** A 1000-μm laser fiber is a useful tool for cutting, ablating, and coagulating. **B.** These three electrosurgical devices can be inserted through the operating channel. They are (*from top to bottom*) a 3-mm monopolar ball electrode, a bipolar two-prong needle electrode, and a 3-mm monopolar button electrode.

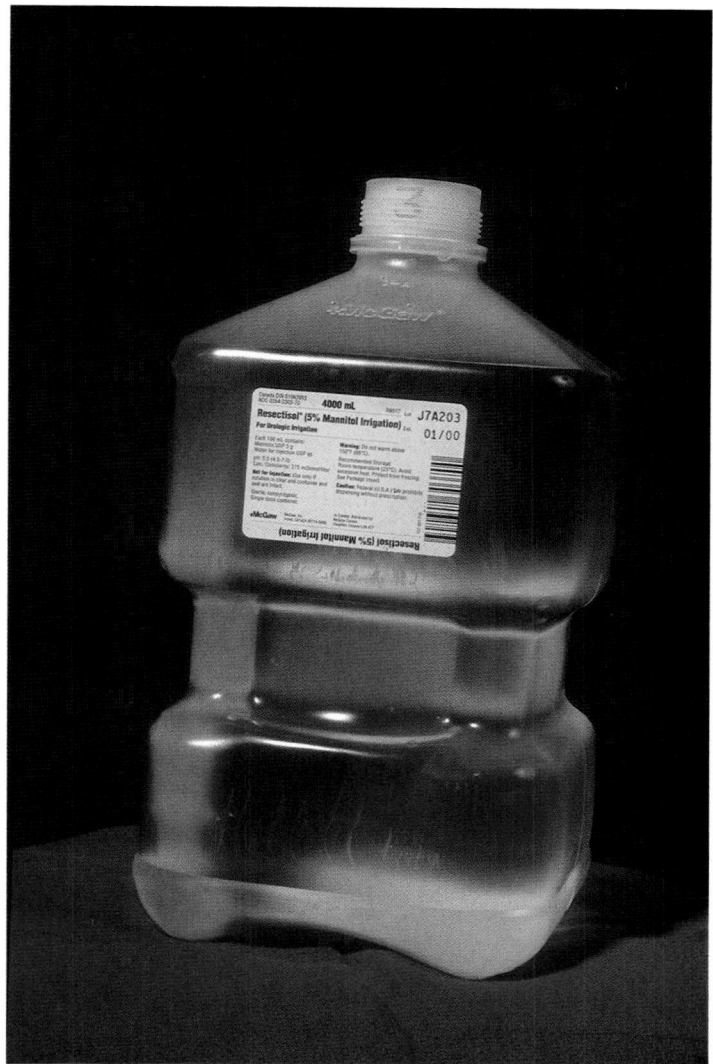

**FIGURE 106–11** A variety of hysteroscopic media are available to distend the uterus. When monopolar devices are to be used, the safest medium to employ is 5% mannitol because it is iso-osmolar.

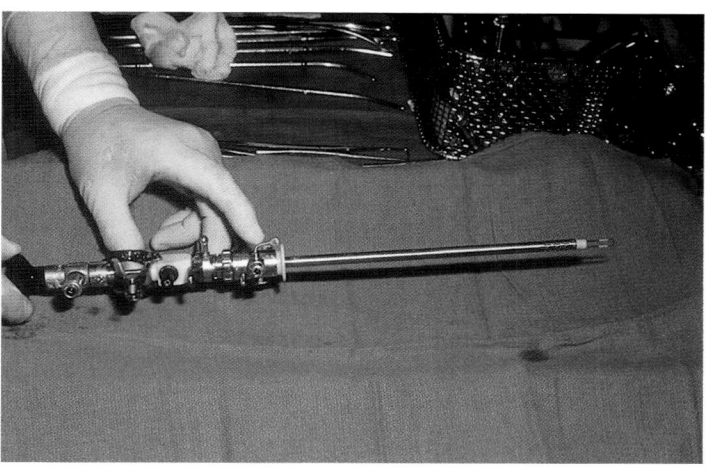

**FIGURE 106–10** The trigger mechanism for advancing and retracting the resectoscopic electrode is shown here.

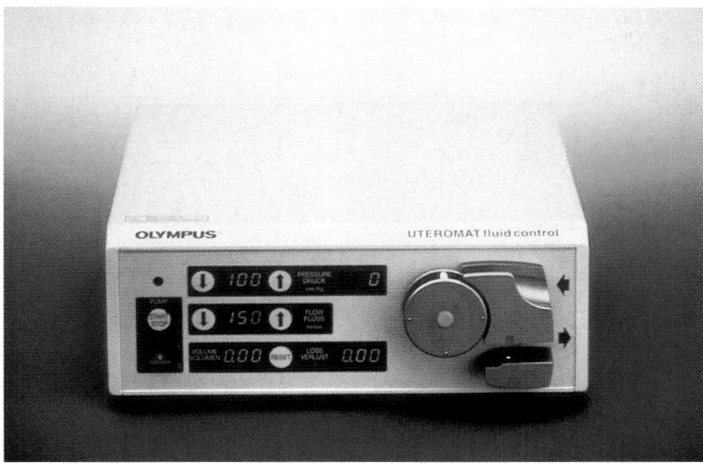

**FIGURE 106–12** A uterine pump may be utilized to infuse fluid. The newer pumps will record pressure, fluid infused (mL), and fluids remaining in the reservoir.

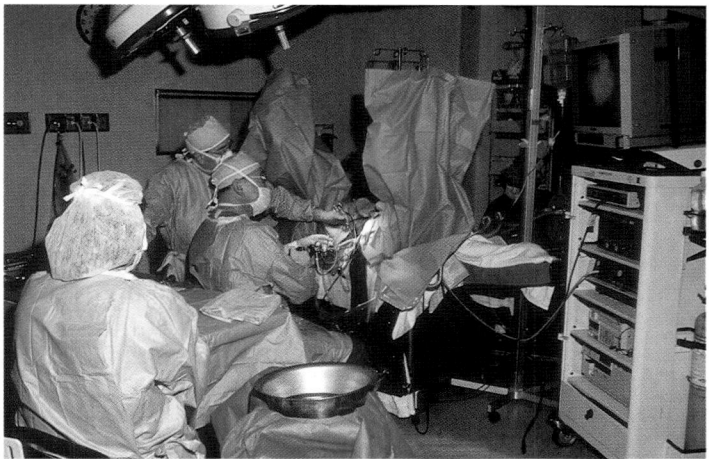

**FIGURE 106–13** The pouch drape shown here collects fluid returning via the outflow valve of the hysteroscope. It likewise collects fluid flowing retrograde via the cervix.

# CHAPTER 107

# Indications and Techniques

## *Michael S. Baggish*

Operative hysteroscopy is performed for the treatment of organic disease with one exception. That exception is the operation of endometrial ablation, which is done to treat abnormal uterine bleeding in the absence of organic disease (e.g., endometrial hyperplasia or cancer). Table 107-1 lists the most frequent indications for hysteroscopy and Table 107-2 for abnormal uterine bleeding by age-related diagnosis.

Certain principles prevail for all hysteroscopic surgery. In Chapter 103, the quantification of medium intake and outflow was already mentioned. No hysteroscopic surgery should be performed in an unclear visual field. The best example of the latter is one in which the bleeding is so brisk that it discolors the flushing medium, creating a pink or red field of view. No energy device should be activated on the forward thrust movement of an electrosurgical or laser-energized tool. Power should be applied only during the return stroke, that is, when the device is moving away from the uterine fundus (Fig. 107-1).

Another dictum involves loss of uterine distention and cessation of the surgical procedure. Loss of distention translates into a diminished view of the operative field. A cause for the loss of distention must be identified. Perforation of the uterus must be the first thing ruled out (Fig. 107-2).

Dilation of the cervix is typically required for the insertion of an operative sheath as compared with a diagnostic sheath (Fig. 107-3). The diagnostic sheath's diameter does not exceed 5 mm, whereas the average operative sheath measures 8 mm.

The surgeon must never overdilate the cervix because the fluid medium will leak out retrograde, resulting in the inability to properly distend the uterine cavity.

Certain procedures require simultaneous laparoscopy to avoid or immediately diagnose uterine perforation (Fig. 107-4). These include large submucous myoma resection and uterine septum section. Difficult cases of intrauterine adhesiolysis may benefit by viewing the uterus from above.

Clearly, proper preparation of the patient preoperatively will facilitate the performance of surgery. Evaluation of the endometrial cavity by endometrial sampling is required before an ablative operation is performed to rule out cancer. Administration of gonadotropin-releasing hormone (GnRH) is advised before a myomectomy or an endometrial ablation is performed. A septum should be preferentially cut during the proliferative phase of the cycle.

The gynecologist who undertakes to perform operative hysteroscopy must be prepared to manage bleeding from the operative site. Coagulation via energy devices may be used; however, when these methods fail, an intrauterine balloon should be placed into the uterine cavity (Fig. 107-5). Typing and holding blood beforehand is suggested to anticipate possible emergency transfusion for hemorrhage.

Finally, the orientation of nursing personnel, equipment, patient, anesthesiologist, and surgeon is key to a well-organized operating theater and subsequently the safe, expeditious utilization of operative time (Fig. 107-6).

**TABLE 107–1 ■ Indications**

1. Abnormal uterine bleeding
2. Suspected neoplasia
3. Malformations
4. Infertility and pregnancy wastage
5. Pregnancy conditions
6. Hormonal monitoring
7. Retained intrauterine device
8. Sterilizations
9. Accompanying dilatation and curettage
10. Adenomyosis

**TABLE 107–2 ■ Hysteroscopic Findings in 768 Patients With Abnormal Uterine Bleeding**

| Findings | Age Classification | |
| --- | --- | --- |
| | Reproductive Age | Postmenopausal |
| Myomas | 93 | 27 |
| Endometrial hyperplasia | 91 | 27 |
| Endometrial polyps | 82 | 70 |
| Endocervical polyps | 20 | 13 |
| Normal cavity | 68 | 38 |
| Placental polyps | 58 | 0 |
| Decidua (ectopic pregnancy) | 6 | 0 |
| Endometrial atrophy | 7 | 25 |
| Adenomyosis | 8 | 2 |
| Endocervical carcinoma | 4 | 4 |
| Endometrial carcinoma | 3 | 38 |
| Other | 47 | 37 |
| TOTAL CASES | 487 | 281 |

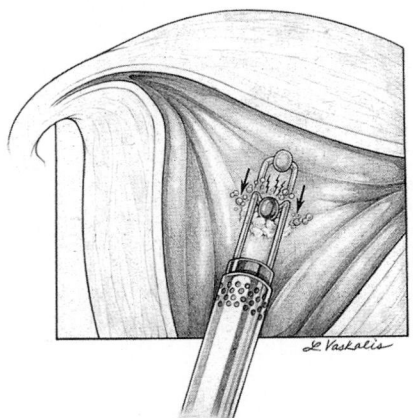

**FIGURE 107–1** During electrosurgery or laser surgery, the energy source is not activated while the electrode or the fiber is advanced. Power is applied only as the ball electrode (in this case) is retracted toward the sheath.

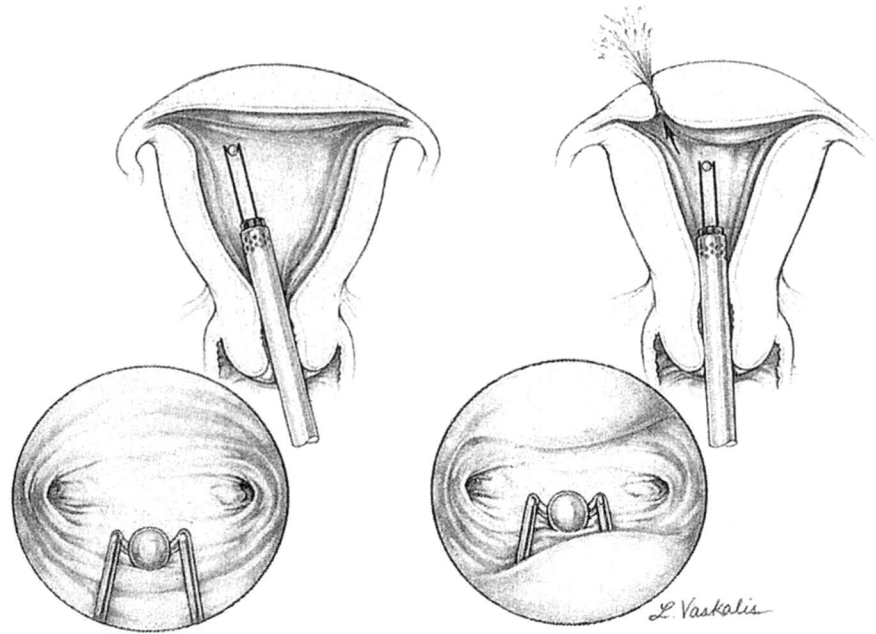

**FIGURE 107–2** All surgery should stop when uterine distention is lost. The figure and inset on the left illustrate the resectoscope within a properly distended cavity. On the right, a perforation has occurred and the cavity is collapsing around the resectoscope.

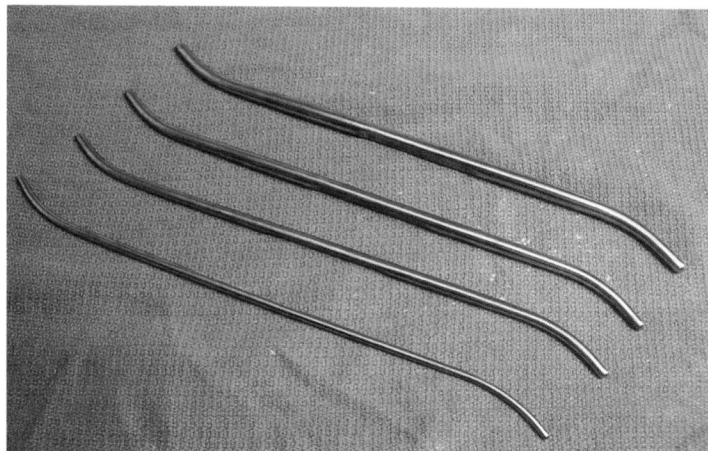

**FIGURE 107–3** Dilation, when required, should be performed with Pratt dilators because they are tapered and gentler on the cervix. Dilation always creates some bleeding within the uterus. Overdilation results in retrograde leakage of the hysteroscopic medium and loss of uterine distention. In fact, departure of the medium may force the hysteroscopy to be cancelled.

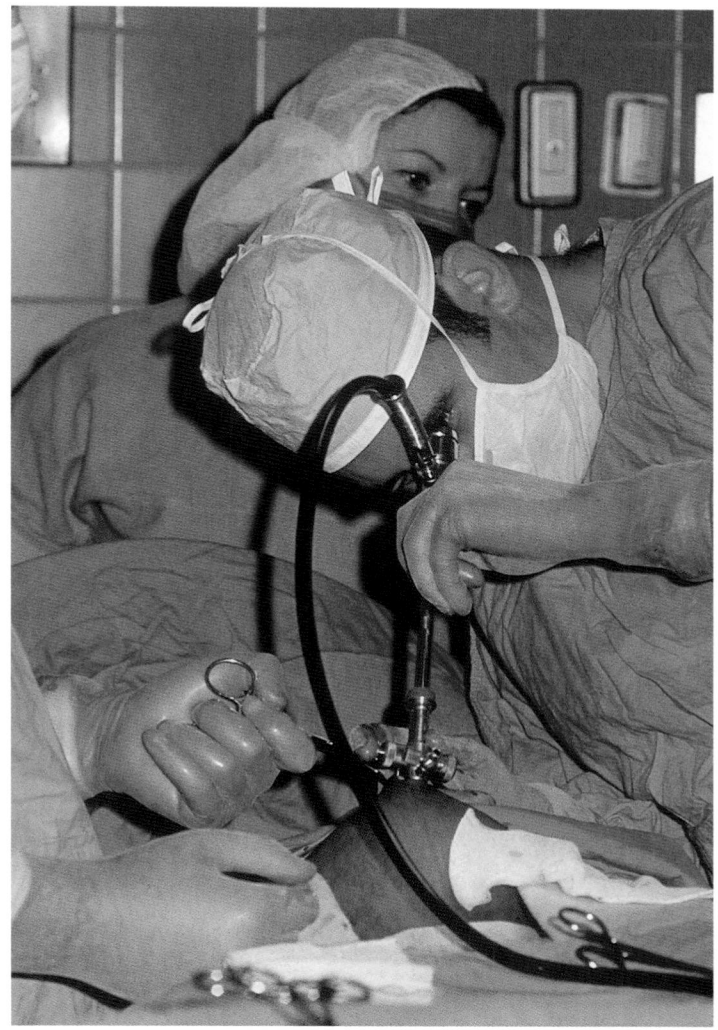

**FIGURE 107–4** Laparoscopy is an important adjunct to hysteroscopy, especially to prevent or at least recognize perforation. The uterus should be elevated via the hysteroscope from time to time to allow the laparoscopist to examine the posterior and fundal portions of the uterus.

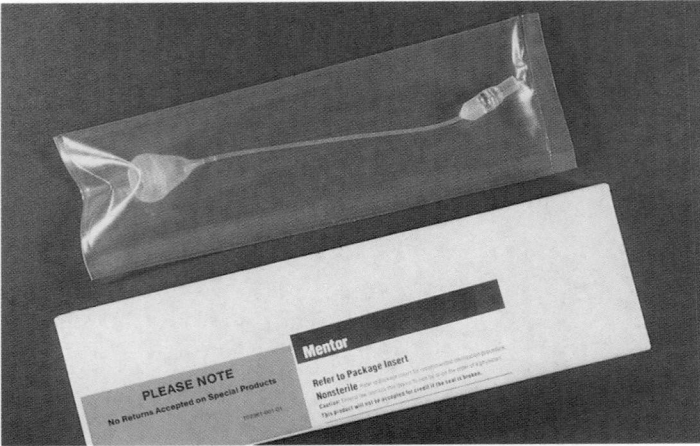

**FIGURE 107–5** If bleeding occurs after completion of operative hysteroscopy, an intrauterine balloon is inserted and inflated initially to 3 cm³. For a normal-sized cavity, the balloon inflation volume should be limited to 5 cm³. The balloon stem is pulled sharply down to close off the uterine canal at the level of the internal os. A vacuum bag is attached to the catheter to record blood loss.

## Operating Room

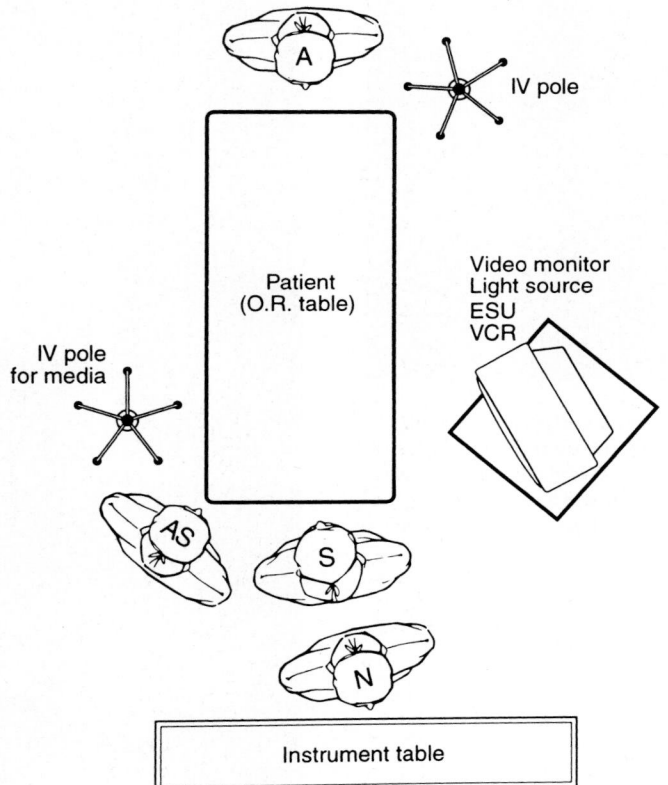

**FIGURE 107–6** This schematic drawing illustrates the arrangement of personnel in the operating room for operative hysteroscopy.

# CHAPTER 108

# Removal of Uterine Septum

*Michael S. Baggish*

The uterus develops during intrauterine life as a result of fusion of the right and left müllerian ducts. When the fusion process fails to happen or occurs incompletely, a uterine septum results. The septum divides the usually capacious corporeal cavity into two smaller spaces. A complete septum extends to the level of the cervicocorporeal junction. An incomplete septum extends variable distances downward from the fundus toward the cervix. Total nonfusion results in a didelphic uterus, that is, completely separate bodies and cervices.

The diagnosis of a septate uterus is suspected unexplained preterm labor occurs. The condition does not lead to infertility. The diagnosis can be objectively made by a variety of techniques, including hysteroscopy. The hysteroscopic examination is conclusive. The cavity is divided by a vertical pillar of tissue extending from anterior to posterior walls (Fig. 108-1). The finding is analogous to viewing the end of a double-barreled shotgun head-on.

A diagnostic laparoscopic examination must always precede hysteroscopic takedown of the septum. The intra-abdominal aspect of the uterus is viewed to exclude the diagnosis of a bicornuate uterus. Finding the latter contraindicates hysteroscopic septum resection. The surgical procedure required to correct a bicornuate uterus is described in Unit II (Chapter 16). Similarly, laparoscopy is simultaneously performed during the septal surgery.

Hysterosalpingography will memorialize the septum's structural presence and will document tubal patency (Fig. 108-2). Postoperative imaging will similarly document the adequacy of the surgery.

When the investigation has been completed, the septum is cut. The preferred tool to accomplish this is hysteroscopic scissors (Fig. 108-3). Thermal devices, such as resectoscope electrode, needle electrode, or laser, may be utilized; however, these devices all produce tissue necrosis and result in a greater potential for scar formation. The greatest risk for use of scissors is bleeding. This can be avoided by maintaining the incision through the septum at midpoint and avoiding cutting into the myometrium at the level of the fundus (Fig. 108-4). As the septum is incised, the hysteroscopist should regularly reorient to ensure that he or she is not drifting anteriorly or posteriorly (Fig. 108-5). Pulsatile bleeding indicates intrusion into the myometrium and should signal the operator to cease cutting. The assistant observing through the laparoscope can and should signal the operator as the intensity of the light on the hysteroscope increases (Fig. 108-6). The cold fiberoptic light of the hysteroscope transluminates through the uterine wall.

Upon completion of the procedure, the inflow and outflow ports of the operative sheath should be closed to decrease intrauterine pressure. This maneuver permits the surgeon to assess for any gross bleeding.

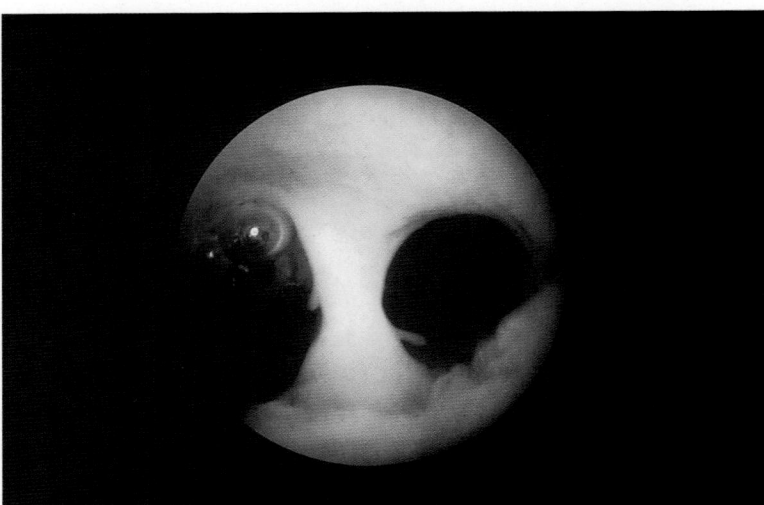

A

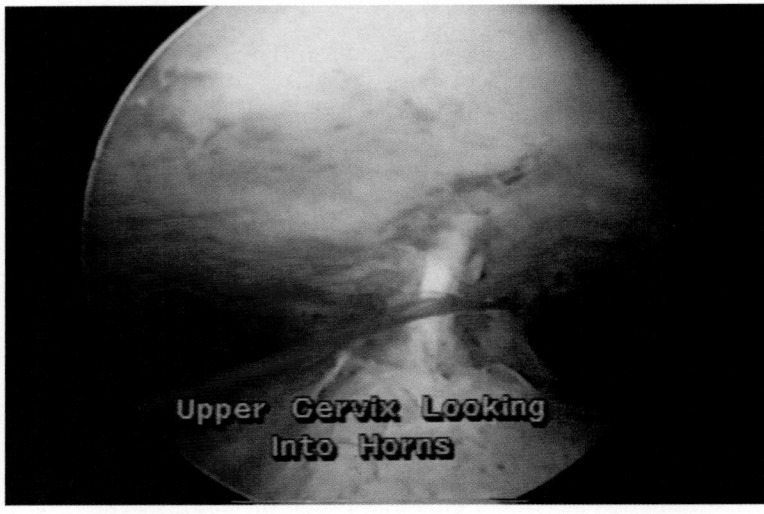

B

**FIGURE 108–1  A.** View of a subseptate uterus from a point just above the internal os of the cervix. **B.** View of a bicornuate uterus from the upper portion of the cervix. *Note:* Without a laparoscopic exam, the bicornuate and subseptate uterus would be difficult to segregate.

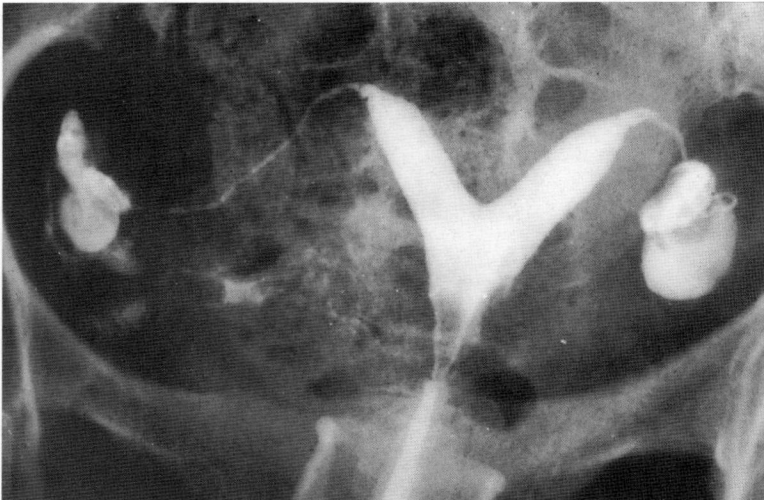

**FIGURE 108–2**  Hysterosalpingogram showing a fusion defect and a rather broad septum.

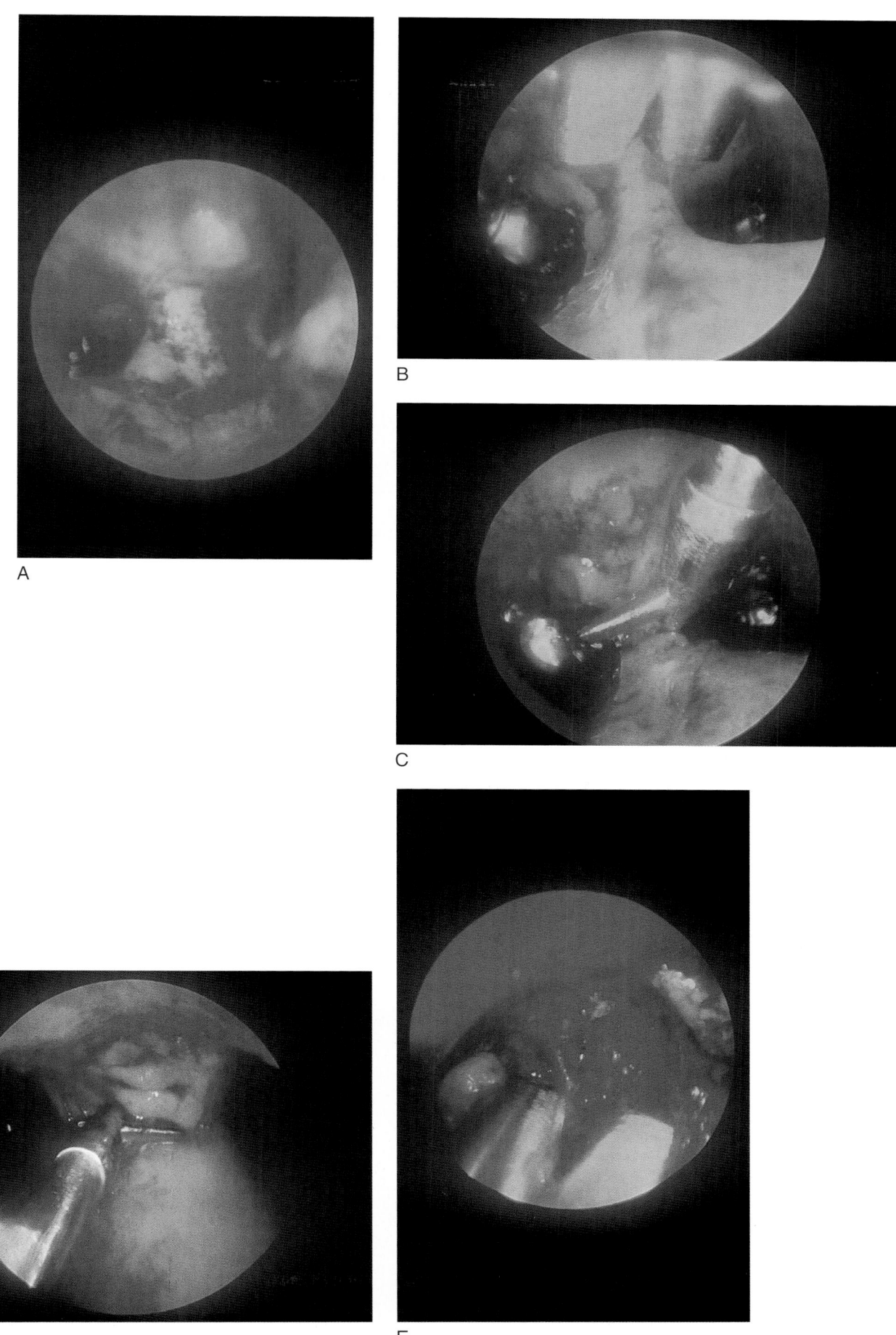

A

B

C

D

E

**FIGURE 108–3  A.** Subseptate uterus just before resection. **B.** The hysteroscopic scissors are seen at 12 o'clock approaching a midpoint of the septum between the anterior and posterior walls of the uterus. **C.** The scissors cut the septum, which rarely bleeds because it is largely avascular. **D.** Panoramic view showing the scissors cutting in the midplane, that is, at the correct location. **E.** The septum has been completely incised. As the top of the septum is reached, bleeding is encountered because of a better blood supply.

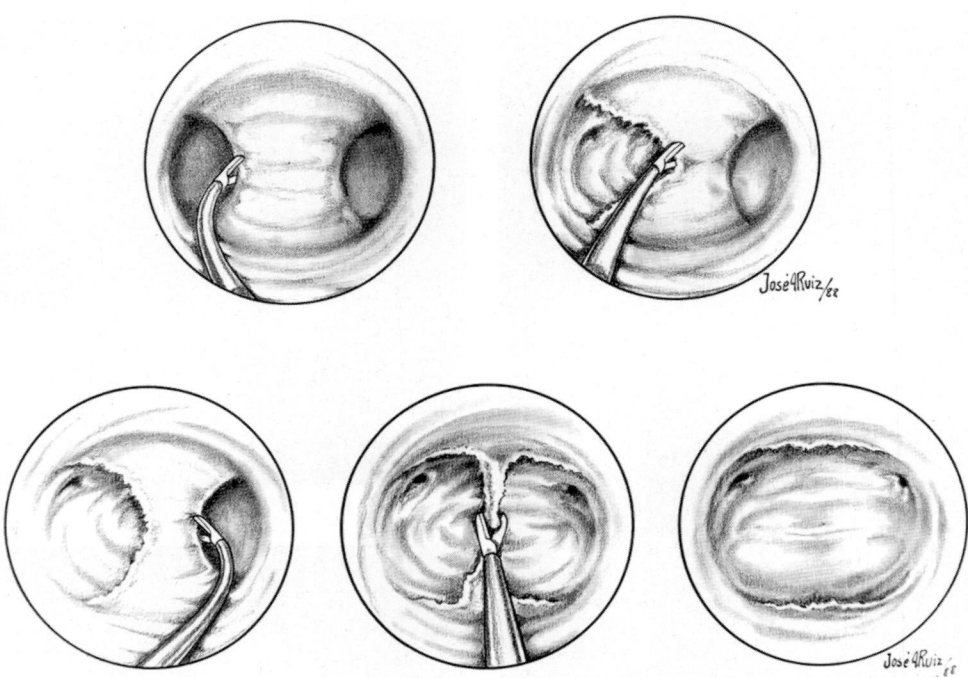

**FIGURE 108–4** Technique for incising a broad septum. The peripheral edges are cut, causing the thick septum to be whittled down.

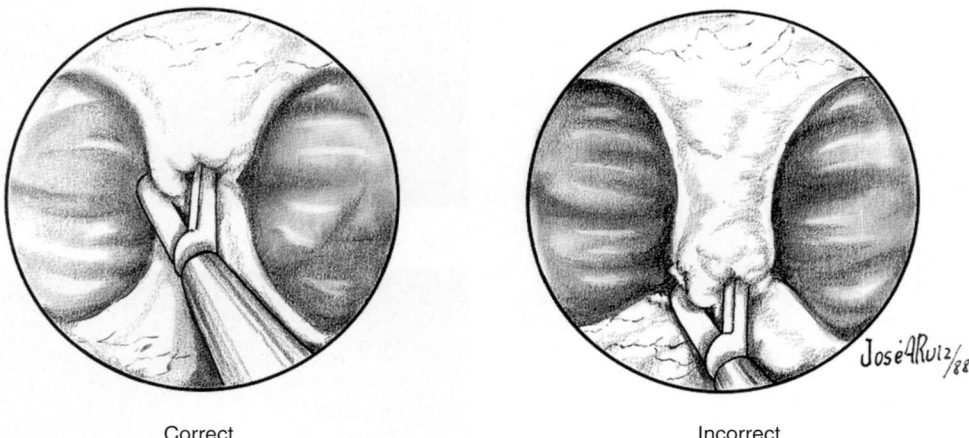

Correct                    Incorrect

**FIGURE 108–5** Schematic illustrating the correct location (*left*) versus the wrong location (*right*) at which to cut a septum. Drifting too low will invariably lead to bleeding.

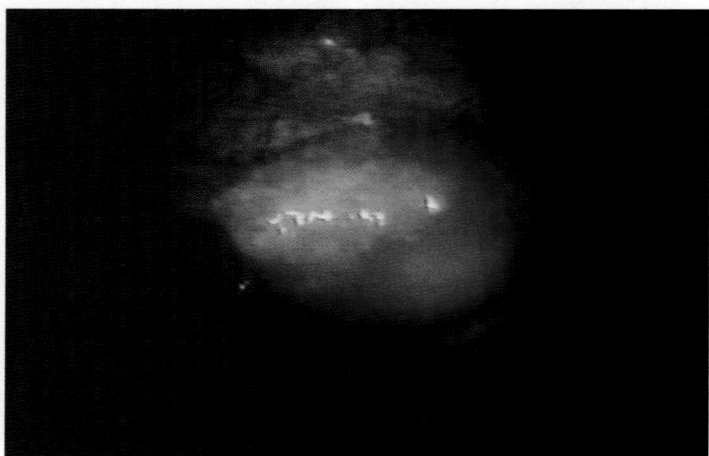

**FIGURE 108–6** An assistant observing via a laparoscope can alert the hysteroscopist that the septum incision should cease based on observing the relative brightness of the light on the hysteroscope, which transluminates through the uterine wall.

# CHAPTER 109

# Ablation Techniques

*Michael S. Baggish*

The application of minimally invasive hysteroscopic techniques to surgically manage intractable uterine bleeding has been well documented as an efficacious and cost-effective alternative to hysterectomy.

The indication for the operation is abnormal uterine bleeding in a woman who wishes to preserve her uterus or in whom a hysterectomy would be judged too risky. The contraindications for surgery would include the presence of adenocarcinoma of the endometrium, atypical hyperplasia, nonreverting benign hyperplasia, dysmenorrhea, or concurrent adnexal mass.

The term *ablation* has specific meaning. Ablation translates into vaporization of tissue, which is typically accomplished by thermal methods. When tissue cells are heated to 100°C, cell water is converted from a liquid to a gaseous state (steam). This change results in physical volume expansion within the intracellular space and a resultant explosive evaporation of the cell and its contents, that is, the cell virtually disappears. The most consistent and rapid vaporization is witnessed when the 100°C temperature is rapidly attained. For the aforementioned reasons, the best ablation procedures employ laser or radiofrequency (RF) electrosurgery techniques (Fig. 109–1A, B).

The laser used most commonly for endometrial ablation is the neodymium yttrium-aluminum-garnet (Nd-YAG) laser. This laser penetrates liquid media, exerts a supplementary coagulating action, is delivered by a 1-mm fiber via the operating channel of a hysteroscopic sheath, and passes through the endometrium to exert its principal action within the superficial myometrium (Fig. 109–2A through C).

The electrosurgical device of choice is the ball electrode, which alternatively may be delivered to the operative site by a hysteroscopic operative sheath or by a specially constructed sheath designed with an "in-and-out" sliding mechanism. The electrode is a monopolar, double-armed ball, cylinder, or cutting loop (Fig. 109–3).

The final common path (i.e., tissue heating) is identical regardless of whether an Nd-YAG laser fiber or a monopolar electrode is used. The most important factor related to the efficiency of the ablation is the power density, that is, the power absorbed by a unit of tissue ($W/cm^2$) or the energy density ($J/cm^2$), or the product of power density and time in seconds (Table 109–1). For example, the energy density for laser action on tissue over a period of 10 seconds (referring to parameters shown in Table 109–1) would be $8333 \times 10$, or $83,333\ J/cm^2$.

The technique for ablation utilizing an Nd-YAG laser begins with preparation of the endometrium 1 month before ablation by the administration of gonadotropin-releasing hormone (GnRH) agonist (Lupron). The endometrium has been preoperatively sampled and has shown to be benign (Fig. 109–4A, B). The patient is placed in the dorsal lithotomy position, prepared, and draped. The cervix is dilated, and the operative hysteroscope, to which an endoscopic video camera has been attached, is inserted into the uterine cavity via the transcervical route with the medium intake channel wide open. In this instance, normal saline (0.9%) is the medium of choice (Fig. 109–5).

After inspection of the cavity, the 1200-μm laser fiber is inserted through the operating channel and makes light contact with the endometrium (Fig. 109–6A, B). Beginning on the anterior wall, ablation is initiated. The fiber is advanced under direct panoramic view. As the fiber is drawn toward the hysteroscope, power is effected by depressing the foot pedal of the laser. The operator views the field from the video screen (Fig. 109–7). Row upon row of endometrium is ablated as the laser fiber is dragged over it, analogous to mowing a lawn (Fig. 109–8A, B). After the anterior wall has been ablated, the fundus and the cornua are treated via a side-to-side motion. Finally, the posterior and lateral walls are destroyed (Fig. 109–9). The ablation is carried from the top of the uterus (fundus) to the level of the internal cervical os (Fig. 109–10). The cervix is *not* ablated. Upon completion of the operation, medium inflow is restricted and the outflow channel is shut off. These latter maneuvers decrease intrauterine pressure. The surgeon observes the cavity for any sign of bleeding. Finally, the instruments are completely removed.

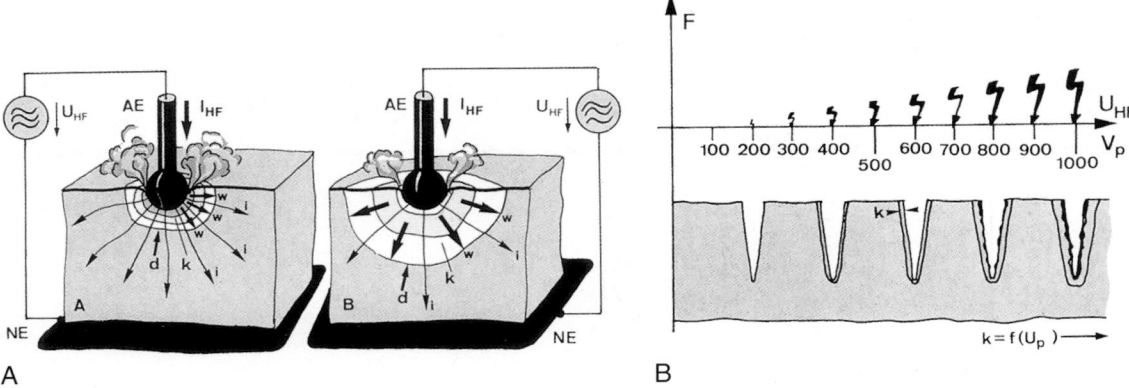

A

B

**FIGURE 109–1  A.** The ball electrode on the left attains vaporization temperature more rapidly than the electrode on the right. On the right, lower temperatures (i.e., coagulating) produce a larger area of thermal conduction. **B.** Electrosurgical (RF) cutting occurs when vaporization temperatures are rapidly reached and the electrode produces high power densities. This may be demonstrated by the relative size of the spark. As greater voltages are reached, a corresponding high level of coagulation accompanies the vaporization. AE, active electrode; f, intensity of arcs; $I_{HF}$, current concentrated at one point; K, depth of coagulation; NE, neutral electrode; $U_{HF}$, voltage; $V_p$, peak voltage.

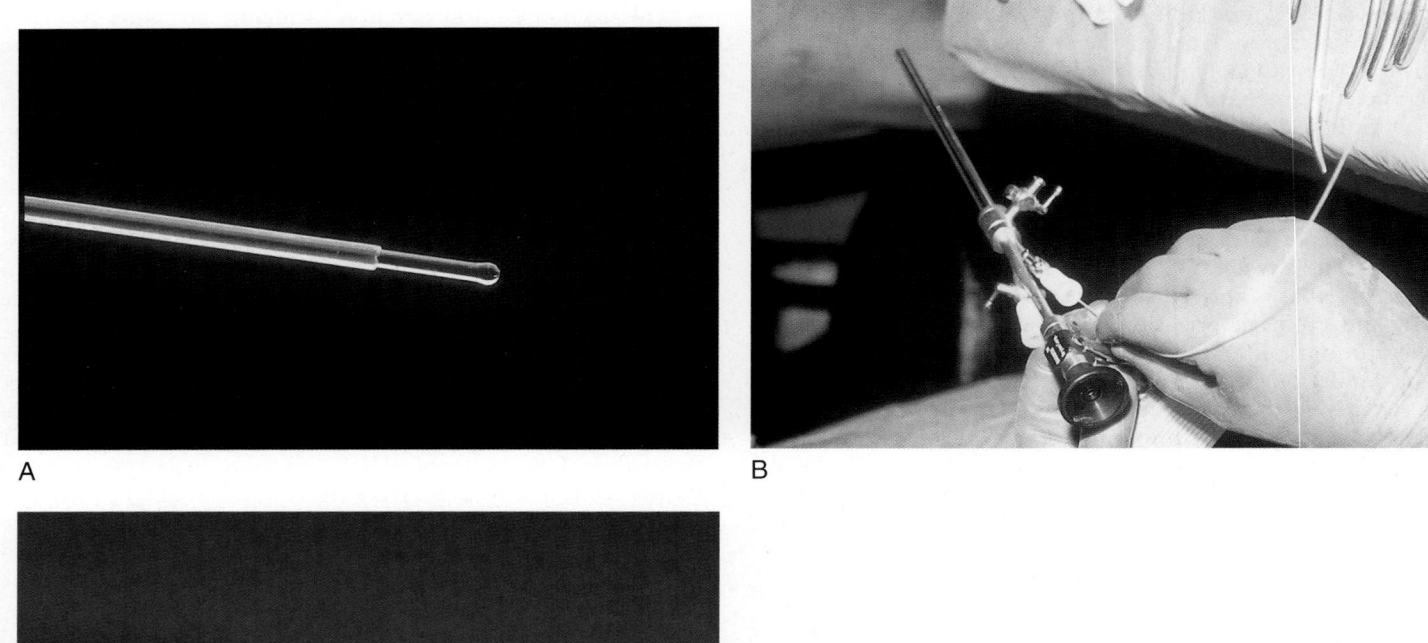

A

B

C

**FIGURE 109–2  A.** The tip of a 1000-μm, sculpted laser fiber (Nd-YAG) is shown. The bulbous tip is ideal for ablation of the endometrium. **B.** The fiber is being fed into one of two available operating channels of the hysteroscopic sheath. **C.** The sculpted point of a 1000-μm laser fiber protrudes from the end of the isolated hysteroscopic sheath. A suction cannula protrudes from a second operating channel.

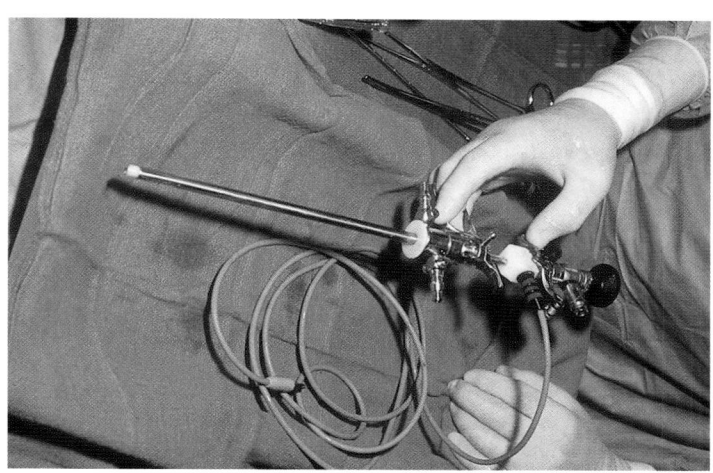

**FIGURE 109–3** Currently, most practitioners employ the resectoscope to ablate the endometrium. As illustrated, the advantage of this tool lies in easy manipulation of the sliding trigger operation.

**TABLE 109–1 ■ Energy Density for Laser Action on Tissue**

Watts: 30

Fiber diameter: 600 microns

$$\text{Power density} = \frac{30 \times 100}{(0.6)^2} = \frac{3000}{0.36}$$

$8333 \text{ W/cm}^2 = \text{PD}$

$8333 \text{ W/cm}^2\text{sec} = \text{work (Joules)}$

10 seconds of elapsed time produces $10 \times 8333 \text{ J/cm}^2$ or $83,333 \text{ J/cm}^2$

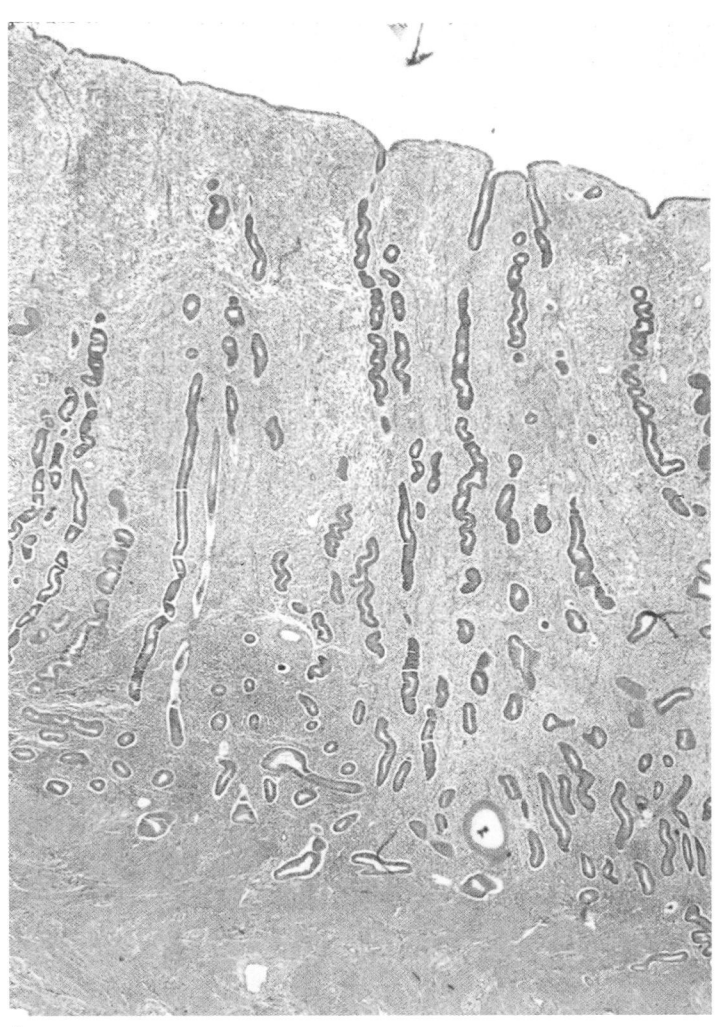

A

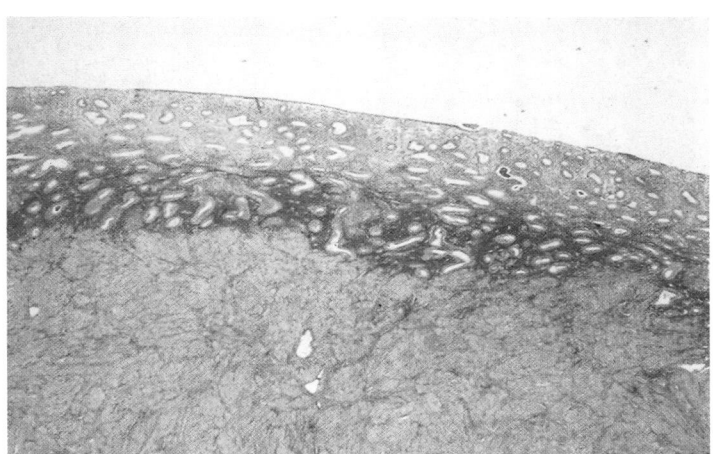

B

**FIGURE 109–4 A.** The tall, vascularized, unprepped endometrium is in stark contrast to (**B**) the thin, inactive endometrium, which is produced by hormonal suppression.

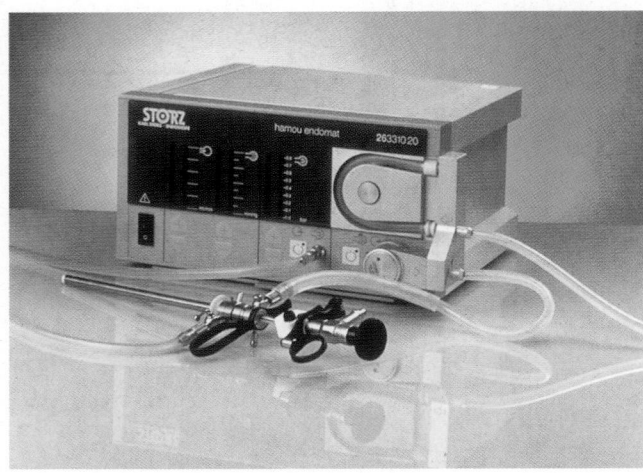

**FIGURE 109–5** A pump may be useful for delivering the distending medium to the uterine cavity because it propels the fluid at a constant rate.

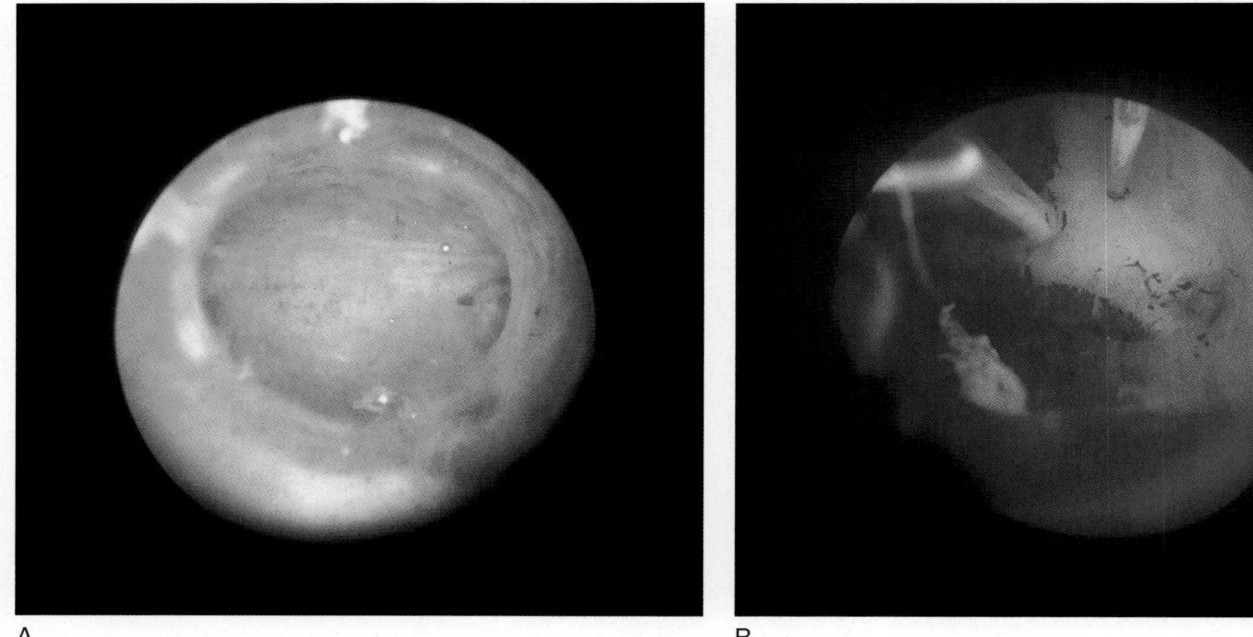

A                                                    B

**FIGURE 109–6 A.** A well-prepared thin endometrium is seen just before the operative equipment is inserted. **B.** The laser fiber is seen above at 12 o'clock. The suction cannula is located to the left of the laser fiber.

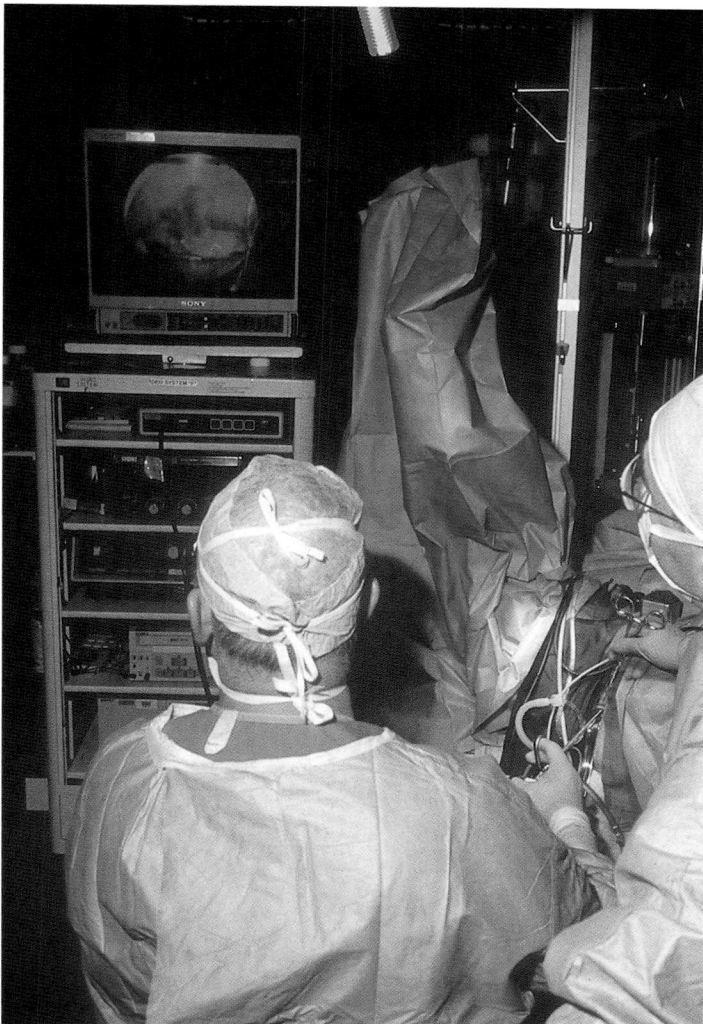

**FIGURE 109–7** The operator performs hysteroscopic surgery via a video monitor. The assistant sees what the surgeon sees.

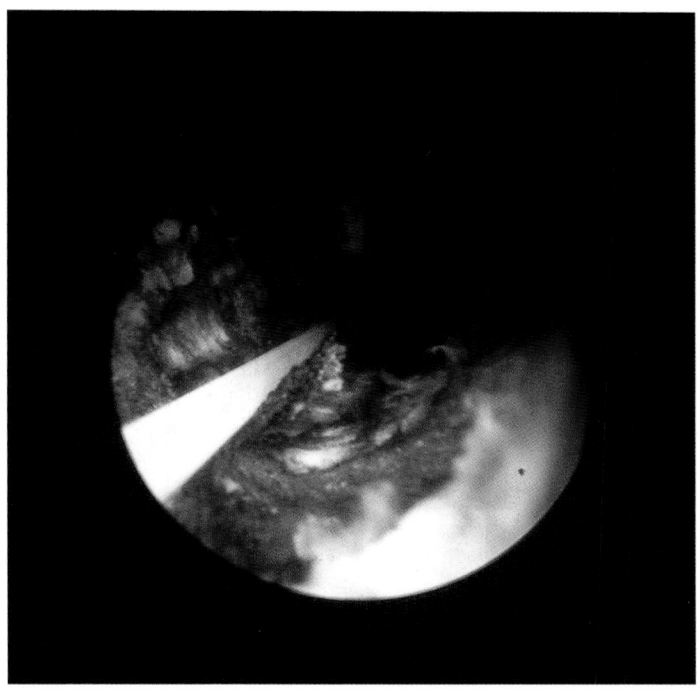

A

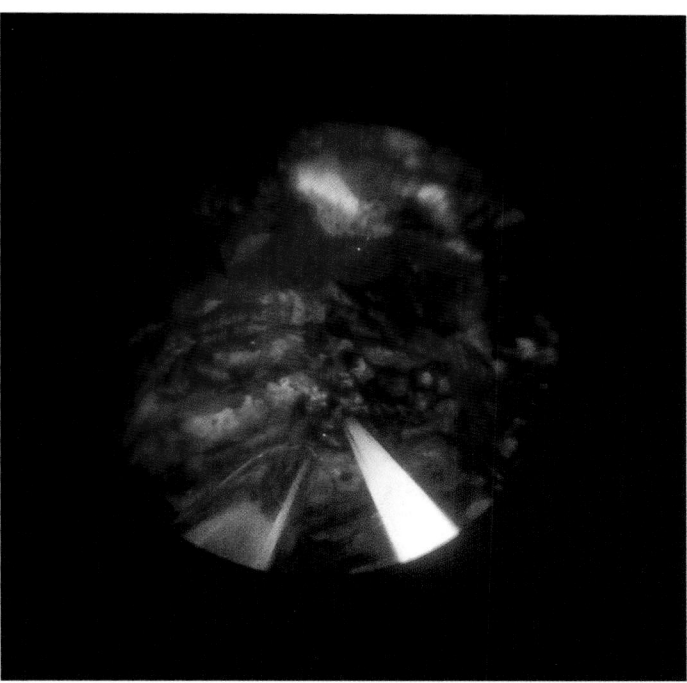

B

**FIGURE 109–8 A.** The ablation (with an Nd-YAG laser) is well under way. The cavity is 80% destroyed. **B.** The ablation is complete. The suction cannula is used to clean debris and blood from the field.

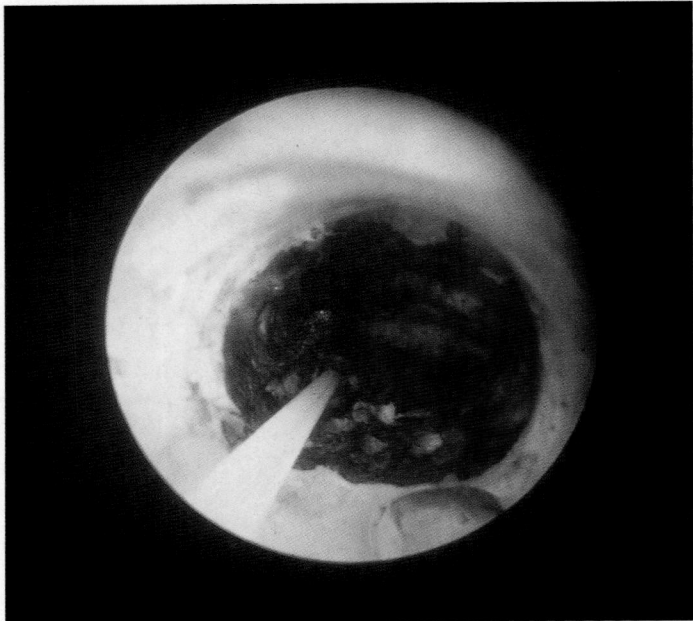

**FIGURE 109–9** The hysteroscope views the field from the upper cervical canal.

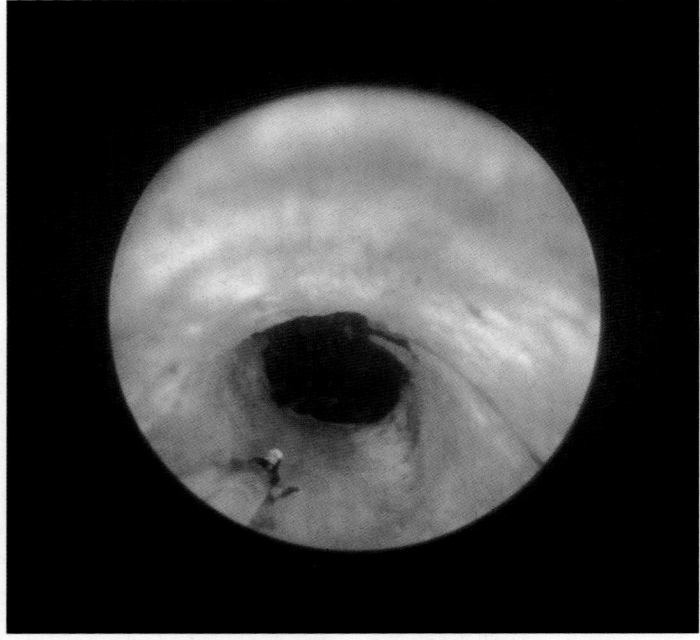

**FIGURE 109–10** The hysteroscope is withdrawn. *Note:* No ablation is done within the cervix.

When the resectoscope and radiofrequency electrosurgically powered electrodes are employed, the general procedure is similar to that described for the Nd-YAG laser, except that the distending medium must be nonelectrolytic, that is, not saline (Fig. 109–11). The safest of these media is 5% mannitol, which is iso-osmolar and permits concentration of current density sufficient to effect ablation. As with the laser, a systematic plan is followed to accomplish a complete endometrial ablation. It is most convenient that the fundus and the cornua are treated first because the entire resectoscope (with the electrode extended) must be gingerly moved from side to side (from right to left or vice versa) (Fig. 109–12). Next, the anterior and finally posterior walls are ablated (Fig. 109–13A, B). The technique for anterior and posterior walls is to extend the electrode away from the objective lens of the hysteroscope, make contact with the endometrium, and apply power as the electrode makes its controlled return to the sheath (see Fig. 104–1).

Endometrial resection has gained limited popularity in the United States; however, it is practiced widely in the United Kingdom and in Europe. In this case, a wire-loop electrode is substituted for the ball. Strips of endometrium are cut out and retrieved (Fig. 109–14). The procedure is otherwise identical to the previously described ablative technique. The risk with this operation involves resecting too deeply with resultant bleeding or perforation (Fig. 109–15A through C).

An exceedingly important part of any operative hysteroscopy is the accurate management of infused and returned medium. Fluid deficits or lack thereof must be determined continuously from the beginning to the end of the procedure. Immediately postoperatively, the patient is observed for bleeding and fluid overload. The author prefers to give a second injection of Lupron to discourage endometrial regeneration.

The final goal of endometrial ablation/resection is total destruction of the tissue lining the uterine cavity to the level of the inner aspect of the myometrium. Histologic sampling should be able to document the destruction (Fig. 109–16). A 4-month hysterogram should show a small, shrunken cavity with or without adhesions (Fig. 109–17).

UNIT 5 ■ SECTION A

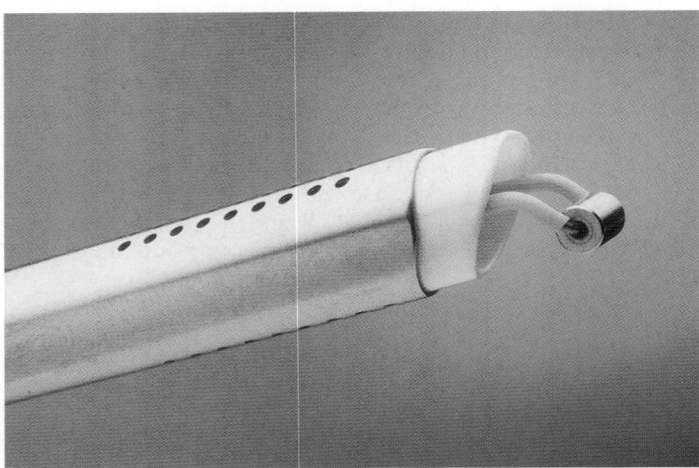

**FIGURE 109–11**  The roller ball electrode is large and creates a low power density even at high power. Therefore, to ablate rather than coagulate, the time on tissue must be increased.

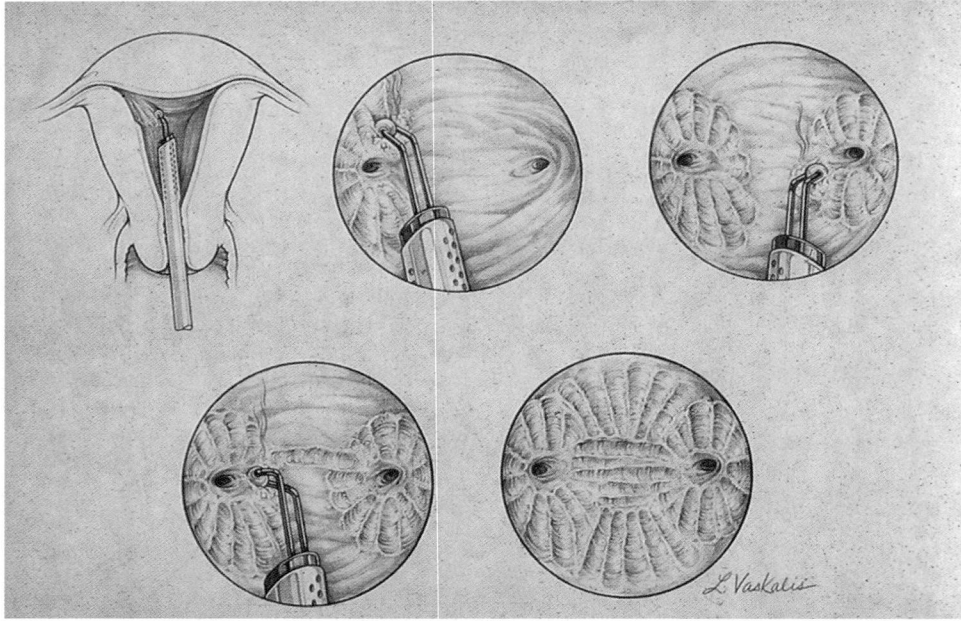

**FIGURE 109–12**  The technique for resectoscopic ablation is illustrated. The power is lowered for ablation of the cornua and fundus. It is increased for the anterior and posterior walls.

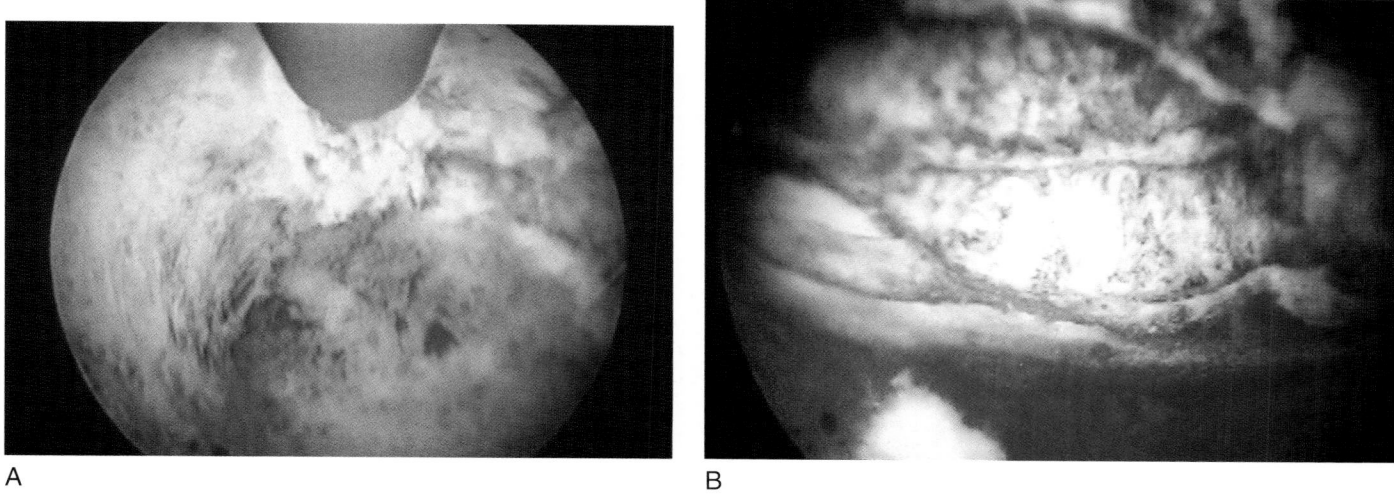

A                                                        B

**FIGURE 109–13 A.** A ball electrode is shown in contact with the anterior uterine wall. The current has just been activated; the white area is coagulated; the yellow area (myometrium) has been ablated. **B.** The sharp demarcation between ablated tissue (anterior wall and upper half of the fundus) and intact endometrium is shown here.

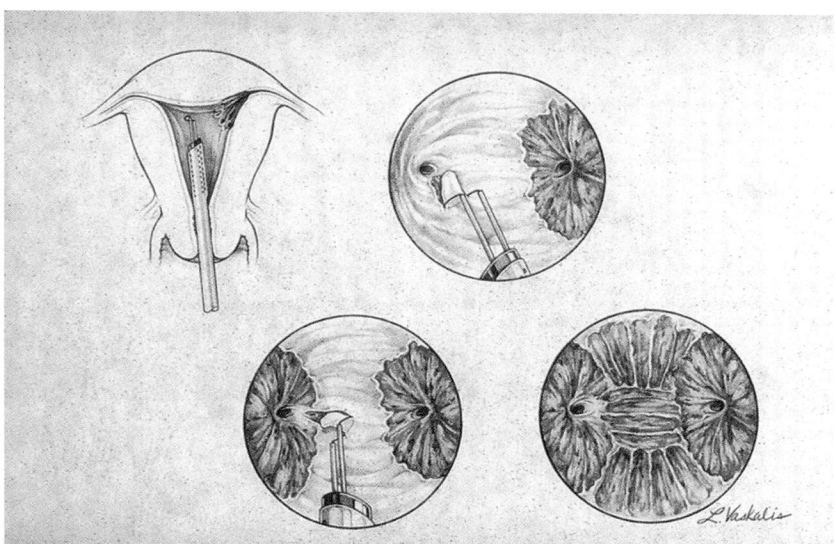

**FIGURE 109–14** This drawing shows an endometrial resection performed with the cutting loop electrode of the resectoscope.

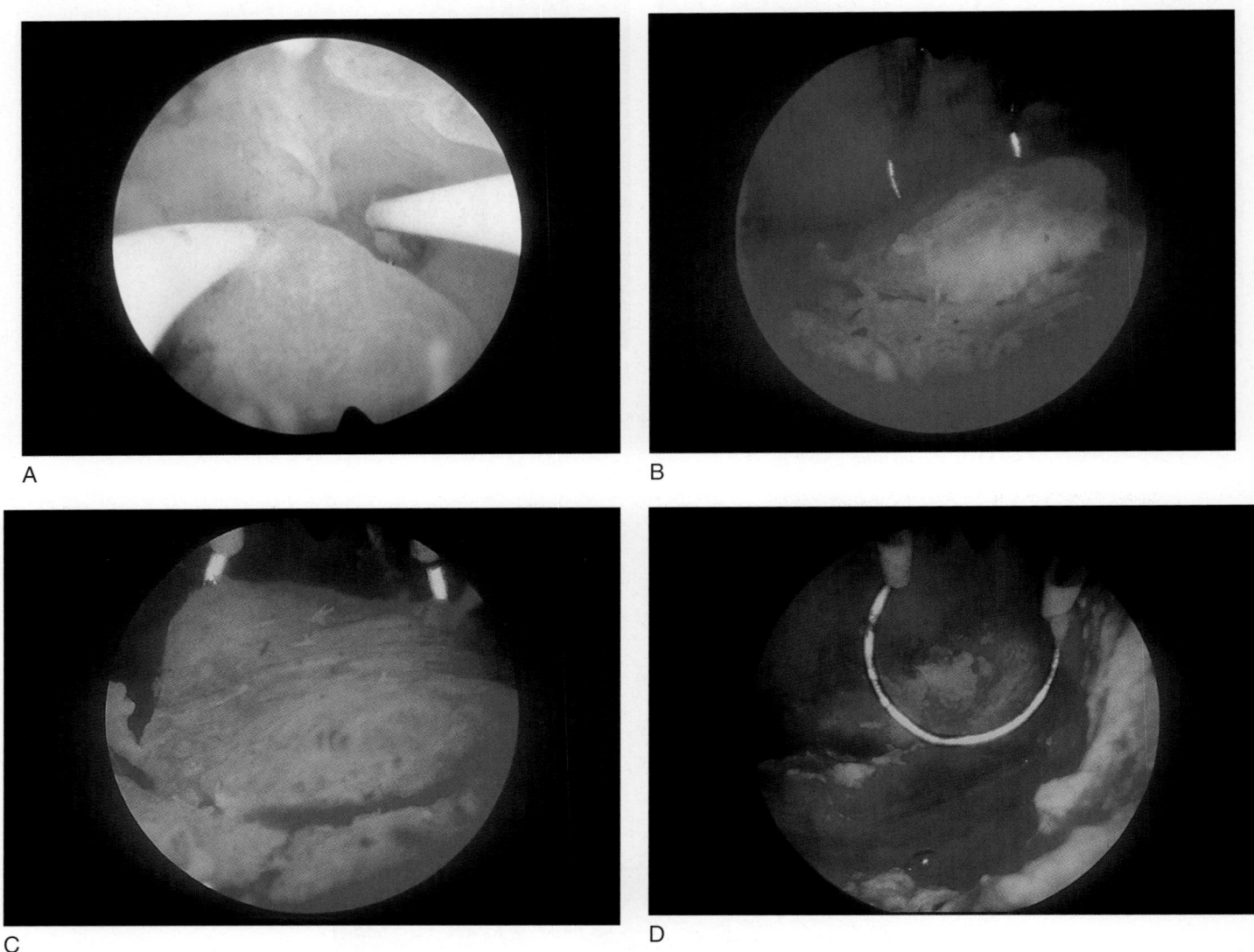

A

B

C

D

**FIGURE 109–15  A.** The double-armed loop electrode has been extended away from the objective lens of the hysteroscope. **B.** As the electrode returns toward the sheath, the electric current is activated and the loop cuts through the endometrium. **C.** Close-up of a piece of endometrium shaved by the loop electrode. **D.** The tissue has been sliced away.

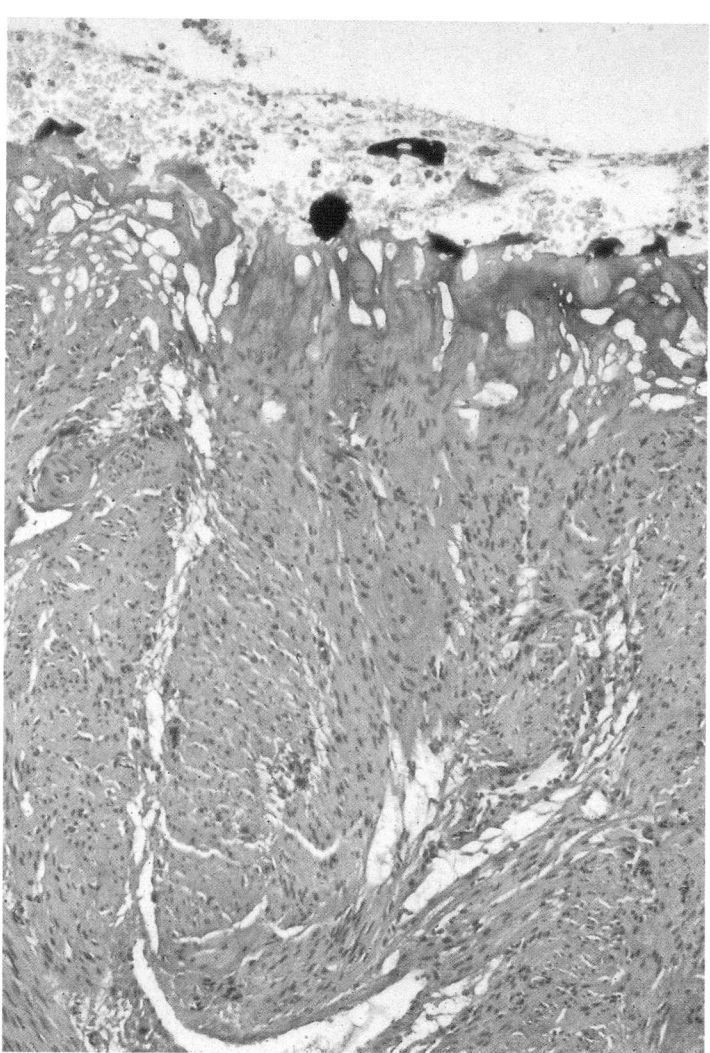

**FIGURE 109–16**  Charred and thermally damaged endometrium after hysteroscopic ablation.

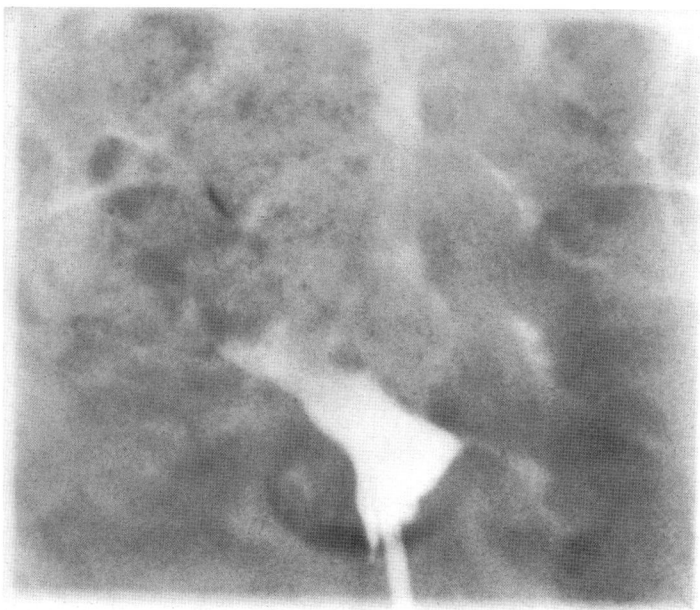

**FIGURE 109–17**  Four-month postoperative hysterogram reveals a shrunken, deformed uterine cavity.

# CHAPTER 110

# Minimally Invasive Non-Hysteroscopic Endometrial Ablation

*Michael S. Baggish*

Minimally invasive non-hysteroscopic techniques have largely replaced hysteroscopic endometrial ablation. The reasons for the gynecologist's preference for these minimally invasive procedures relate to the following: minimal skill required, no distension medium needed, and rapid performance time expected. The results of these minimally invasive ablations have been generally good if one uses a final common path of reduced or normal bleeding. Amenorrhea rates are generally lower than with direct vision hysteroscopic endometrial ablation. Disadvantages of the minimally invasive techniques include that the techniques are mainly blind (the exception being the hydrothermablator [HTA] device), and they typically rely on low intrauterine volume and pressure to ensure safety.

The more commonly used devices are described below.

**Hydrothermablator (Boston Scientific, Natick, MA)** (Fig. 110-1A, B). A modified hysteroscope is placed into the uterine cavity. A bag of normal saline serves as a reservoir, and the entire system is fluid filled. The uterine cavity is distended, and any leaks are detected by drops in the reservoir. The saline is heated outside of the uterus and is flushed through the uterine cavity at low pressure. The ablation can be directly viewed via the telescope.

**Microsulis (microwave endometrial ablation; Microsulis, Hampshire, UK)** (Fig. 110-2). This electrosurgical device consists of a monopolar probe, which functions as a microwave because the radiofrequency generator delivers frequency in the megahertz operational range. The endometrium is ablated via conversion of electrical to thermal energy. This is one of the oldest non-hysteroscopic devices, dating back to 1991. High power outputs (e.g., 200 watts) are required to maintain a constant probe temperature of 65°C. The probe is rotated intraoperatively to obtain even dispersal of heat. The patient must wear a large neutral electrode throughout the procedure.

**NovaSure (Hologic Inc., Marlborough, MA)** (Fig. 110-3A, B). Consists of a bipolar mesh bag, which is inserted into the uterus collapsed via an applicator. The device must be oriented so that the kitelike frame can accommodate to the inverted triangular uterine cavity. A dial that reads the cavity width and depth is obtained from a device display. Carbon dioxide gas pressurizes the cavity to determine whether leakage is or is not occurring. Radiofrequency biopolar electrical energy coagulates the endometrium at 180 watts of output.

**Thermachoice (Gynecare-Ethicon, Somerville, NJ)** (Fig. 110-4). This is a balloon device. A collapsed balloon is inserted into the uterine cavity via an applicator. The balloon is distended with sterile water or saline. Based on the pressure reading, the gynecologist can determine that the balloon is intact. Approximately 15 mL of saline within the balloon is heated in situ, creating thermal destruction of the endometrium. The cavity must be normal in configuration for the balloon to deploy properly.

## Complications

Table 110-1 (after Ob-Gyn Management Volume 19[9], 2007) depicts complications reported via the U.S. Food and Drug Administration (FDA). Each device has a peculiar footprint.

The principal complication associated with Thermachoice was perforation with balloon rupture (Fig. 110-5A, B). The HTA device was associated with retrograde leakage of hot fluid via the cervix (Fig. 110-6A). The company has recently developed a new sheath with a better cervical seal (Fig. 110-6B). The NovaSure device has a high propensity for uterine perforation as well as transmural thermal injury (Fig. 110-7). The microwave device is associated with high-frequency electrical leakage and thermal injury (Fig. 110-8).

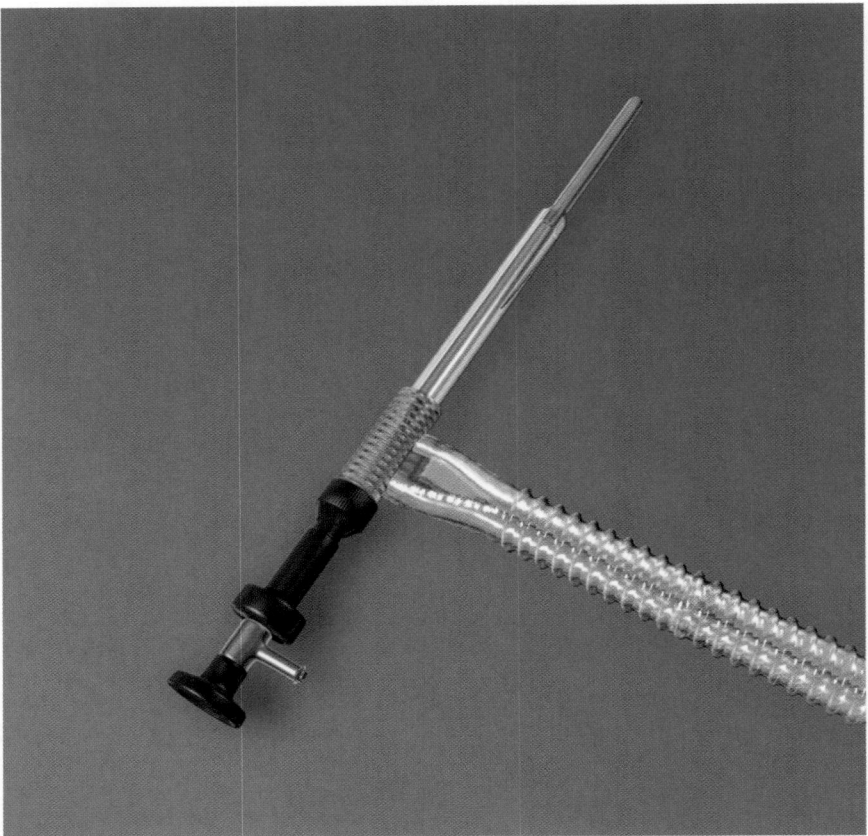

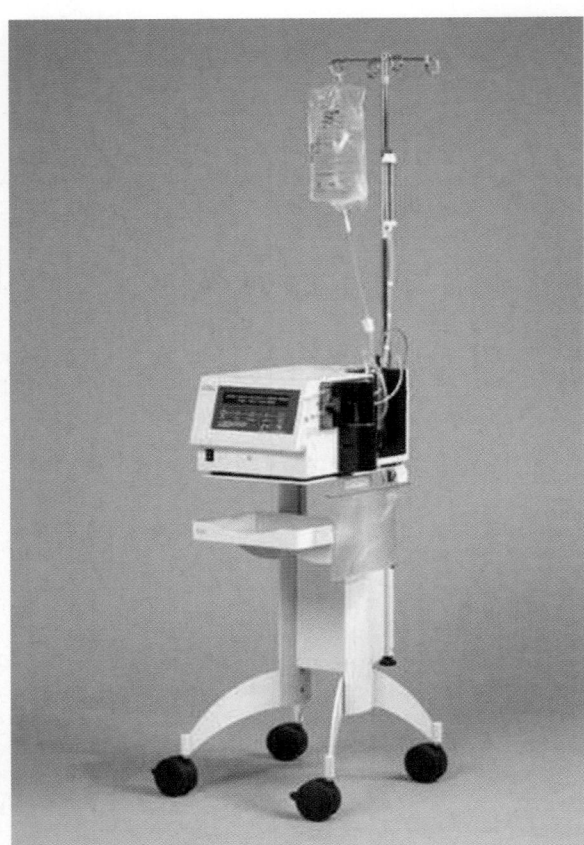

A

B

**FIGURE 110–1 A.** The hydrothermablator (HTA) sheath is shown with entry and return tubing for the circulation of hot saline within the uterine cavity. The telescope permits the surgeon to view the process. **B.** The HTA unit consists of a control device, a heater, and a reservoir. The bag of saline fills the entire system with fluid.

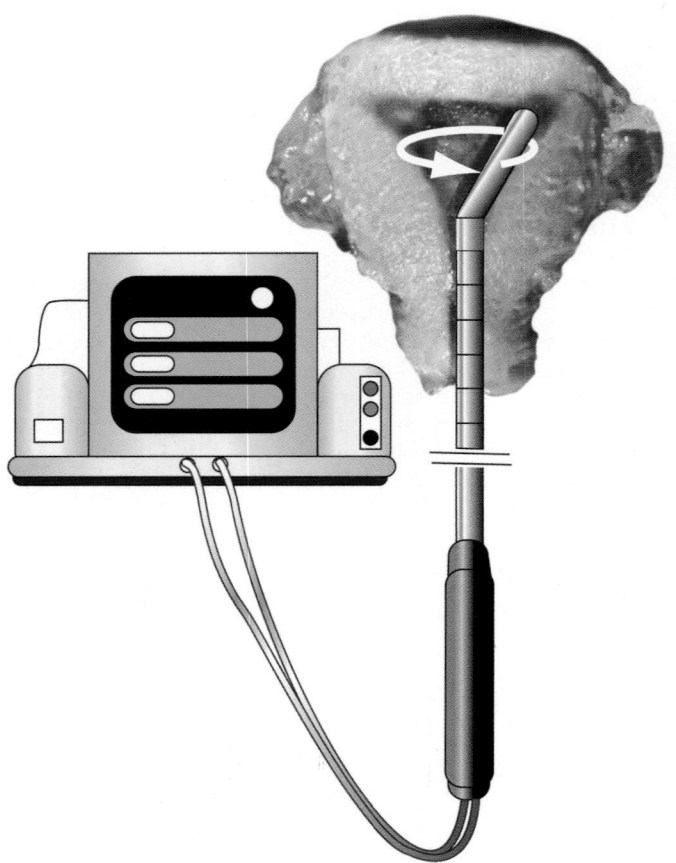

**FIGURE 110–2** The microwave probe and control unit are shown here. A neutral electrode belt is attached to the patient. The active electrode (probe) is rotated during the ablation procedure to obtain an even distribution of energy.

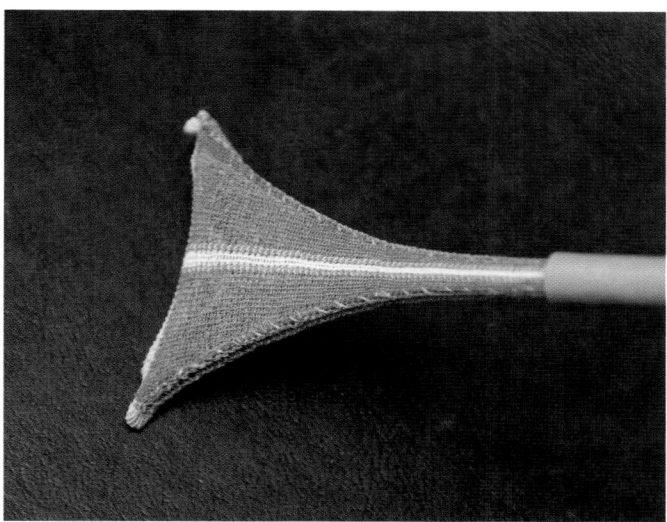

A

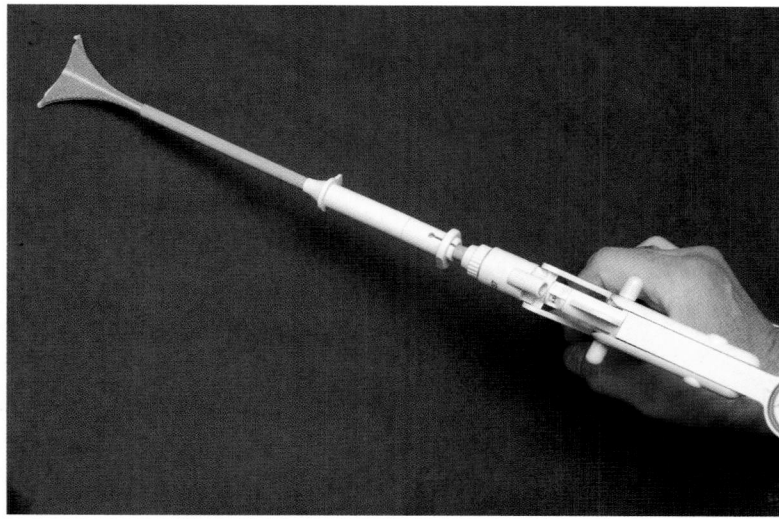

B

**FIGURE 110–3 A.** The NovaSure device consists of a mesh triangular framework with an underlying bipolar electrode. One portion of the electrode is the active electrode and the other, the neutral electrode. **B.** The device is folded within the application and is pushed open within the uterine cavity. A measurement of the opened width is indicated on a dial above the application grip.

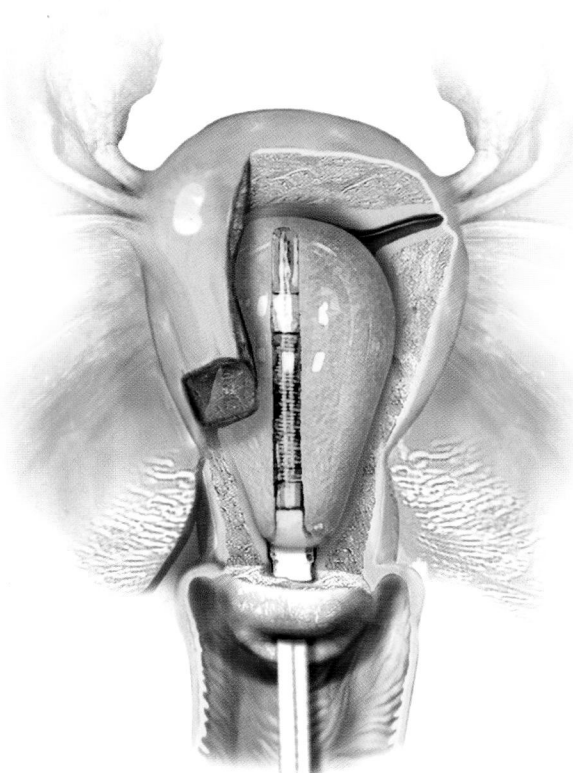

**FIGURE 110–4** The Thermachoice balloon is inserted into the uterus in a collapsed state. The balloon is distended with saline, which, in turn, is heated in situ. The hot distended balloon transmits heat to the surrounding endometrium, creating coagulation necrosis. (From Baggish MS, Valle RF, Guedj H: In Hysteroscopy: Visual Perspectives of Uterine Anatomy, Physiology, and Pathology. 3rd ed. Lippincott, Williams and Wilkins, Philadelphia, 2007.)

**TABLE 110–1 ■ Complications Associated With Four Endometrial Ablation Devices**

| Complication | Hydrothermablator* | Thermachoice | NovaSure | Microsulis |
|---|---|---|---|---|
| Uterine perforation | 2 | 3 | 26 | 19 |
| Intestinal injury | 1[†] | 1[†] | – | 13[†] |
| Retrograde leakage burn | 19 | 6 | – | – |
| Infection/sepsis | – | 1[†] | 2 | 1 |
| Fistula/sinus | – | 1[†] | 1 | – |
| Transmural uterine burn | – | 1 | – | – |
| Cervical stenosis | – | 8 | 1 | – |
| Cardiac arrest | 1 | – | 1 | – |
| Death | – | 1 | – | – |
| Other major | – | 3 | 1 | 4[†] |
| Total | 22 | 22 | 32 | 20 |

*Includes author's data; 6 retrograde leaks.
[†]From Baggish MS: Endometrial ablation devices: How to make them truly safe. Ob-Gyn Management Volume 19(9), 2007.

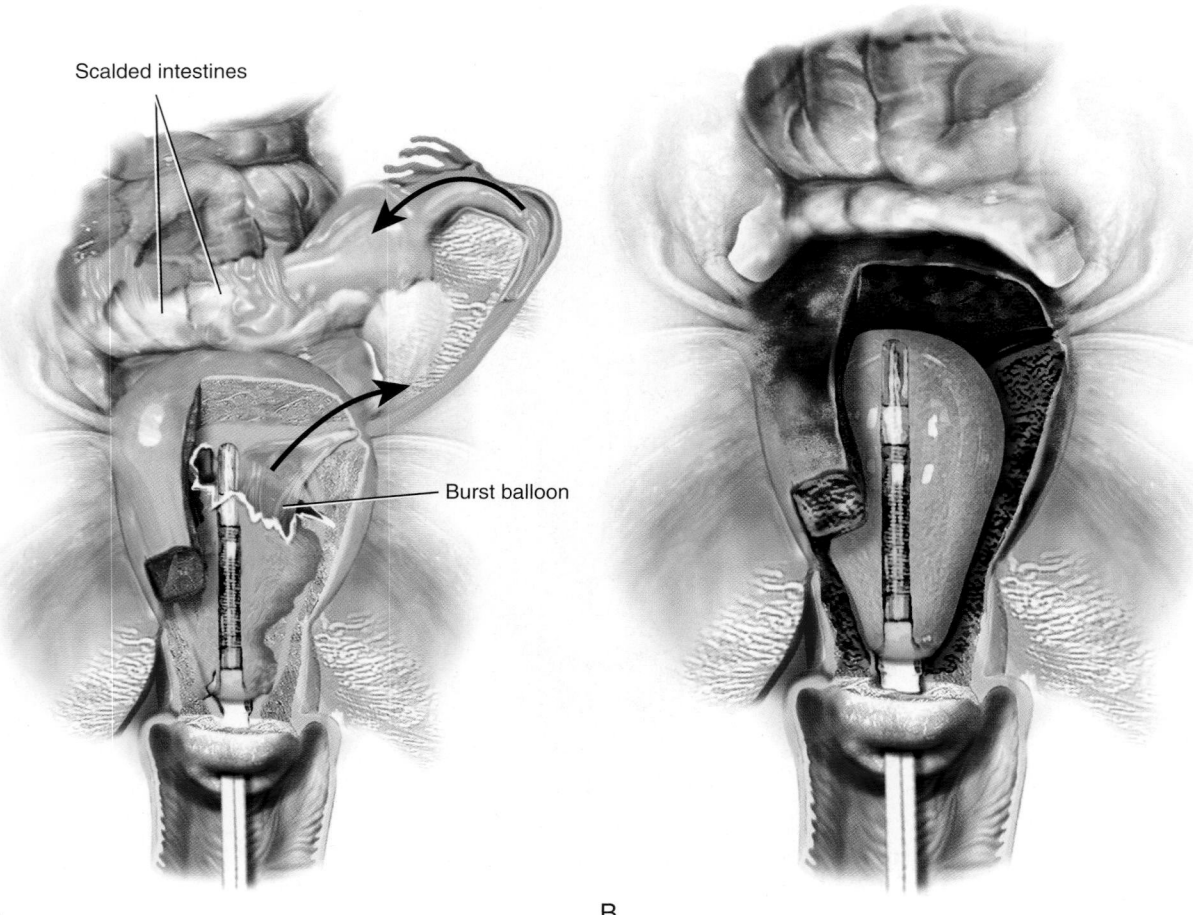

A                                                                                    B

**FIGURE 110–5 A.** A ruptured balloon containing hot water or saline can spill into the abdominal cavity via the oviduct or into the vagina via the cervix. **B.** Transmural thermal injury to the uterine wall (through and through burn) can additionally create a bowel burn if the intestine is in contact with the serosal surface of the uterus. (From Baggish MS, Valle RF, Guedj H: *In* Hysteroscopy: Visual Perspectives of Uterine Anatomy, Physiology, and Pathology. 3rd ed. Lippincott, Williams and Wilkins, Philadelphia, 2007.)

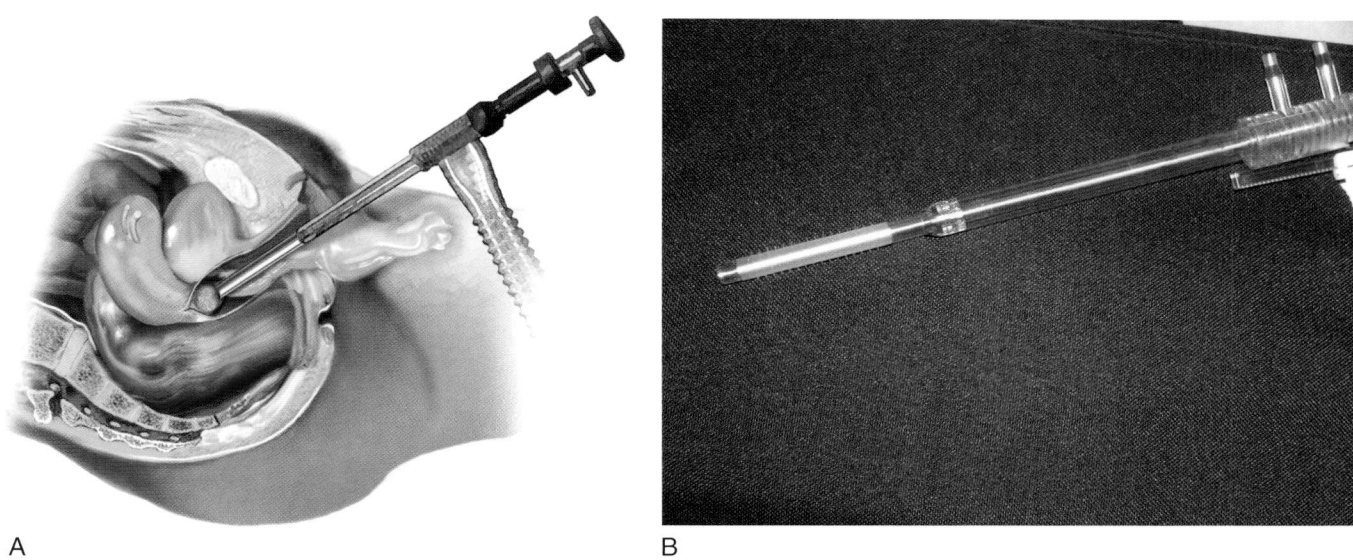

A                                                                                          B

**FIGURE 110–6  A.** A loose seal between the hydrothermablator (HTA) sheath and the cervix can result in retrograde leakage of scalding saline or water. **B.** An improved sheath permits a tighter cervical seal. Note the fine contact discs of Silastic-type construction. (From Baggish MS, Valle RF, Guedj H: *In* Hysteroscopy: Visual Perspectives of Uterine Anatomy, Physiology, and Pathology. 3rd ed. Lippincott, Williams and Wilkins, Philadelphia, 2007.)

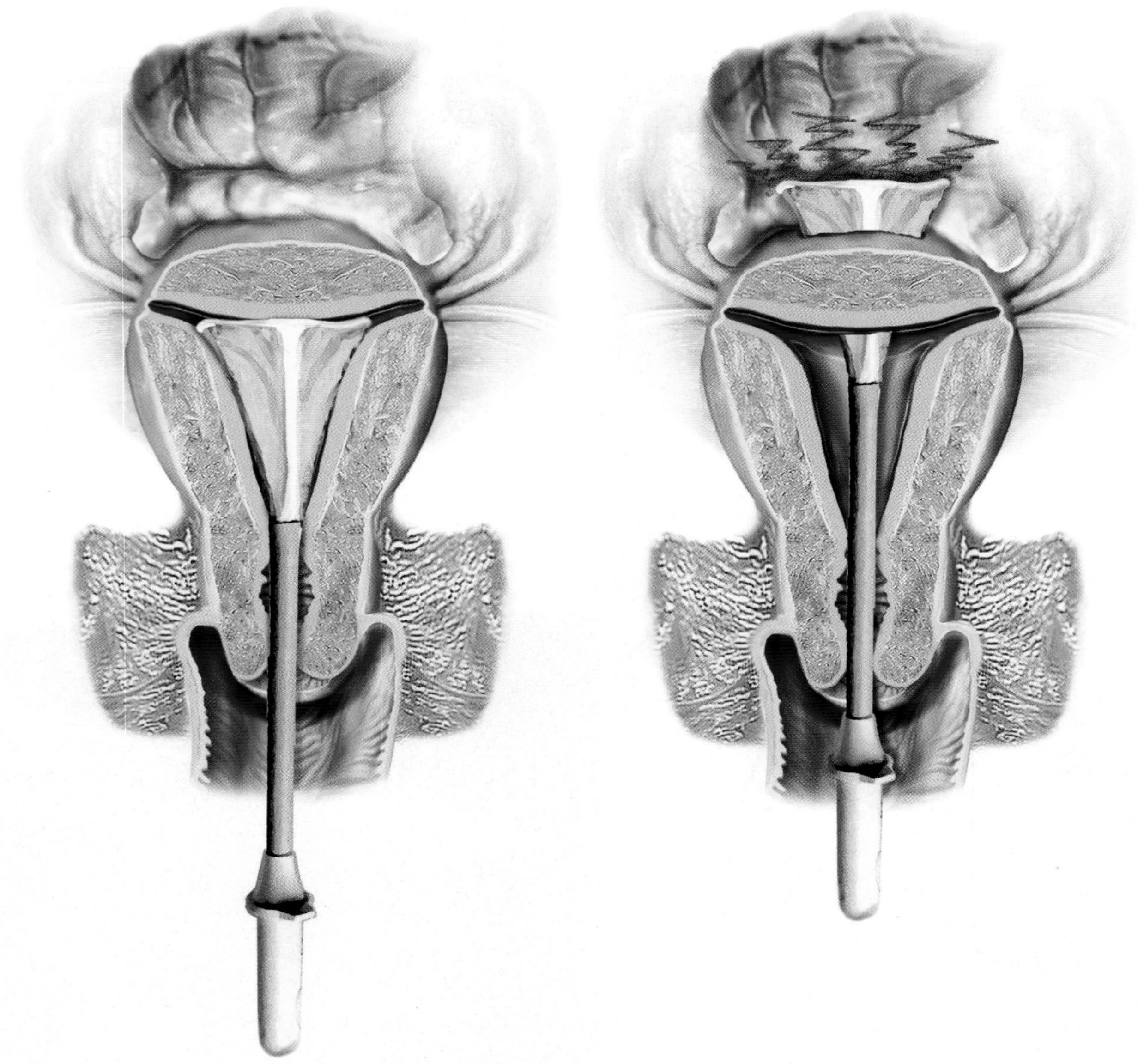

**FIGURE 110–7** The figure on the left shows the NovaSure device in proper position. The figure on the right shows the device perforating the uterus. If the electrode is activated, it will coagulate not only the uterine myometrium but also the surrounding intestine. (From Baggish MS, Valle RF, Guedj H: *In* Hysteroscopy: Visual Perspectives of Uterine Anatomy, Physiology, and Pathology. 3rd ed. Lippincott, Williams and Wilkins, Philadelphia, 2007.)

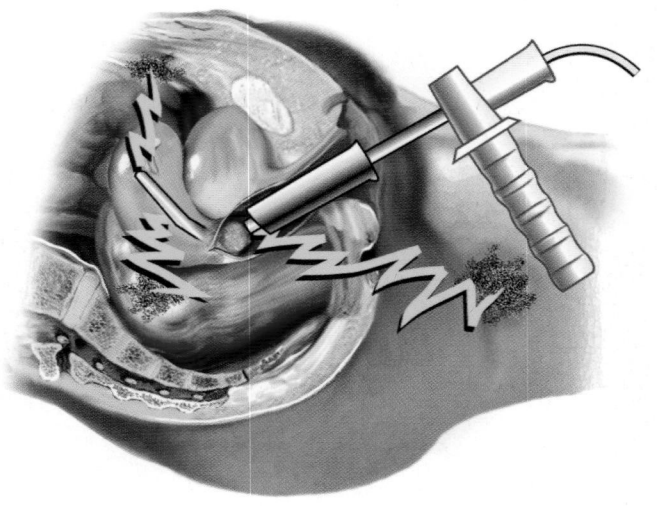

**FIGURE 110–8** The microwave electrode has perforated the uterus just above the cervix. The activated electrode can cause thermal damage to neighboring structures (e.g., bowel, bladder). (From Baggish MS, Valle RF, Guedj H: *In* Hysteroscopy: Visual Perspectives of Uterine Anatomy, Physiology, and Pathology. 3rd ed. Lippincott, Williams and Wilkins, Philadelphia, 2007.)

# Resection of Submucous Myoma

## *Michael S. Baggish*

Although uterine myomata may occur at any location within the uterus, the submucous variety accounts for most clinical symptoms. The usual clinical presentation for these lesions includes heavy and prolonged bleeding. The diagnosis is made most commonly by diagnostic hysteroscopy and less commonly by radiographic imaging procedures (Fig. 111–1A, B). The hysteroscopic appearance of a submucous myoma is consistently recognizable. A rounded mass lesion is seen (Fig. 111–2). Myomata are white or pink (Fig. 111–3). Their contour may be spherical or hemispherical, and they always project into the uterine cavity. Close-up scrutiny reveals numerous thin-walled, sinusoidal vessels branching upon the surface. Areas of ecchymosis or adherent blood clots are commonplace (Fig. 111–4). If a viscid medium is used to distend the uterus, the actual site(s) of hemorrhage may be viewed as the blood spews from the ruptured, surface, sinusoidal vessel (Fig. 111–5).

The treatment of choice for a submucous myoma is hysteroscopic destruction, preferably by resection. Alternative treatments include myolysis utilizing laser fiber or bipolar needles, or arterial embolization performed by invasive radiology. The obvious advantages of hysteroscopic resection are that it is less invasive than radiologic embolization, which entails arteriography; additionally, the physical removal of the myoma provides a specimen for the pathologist. Although leiomyosarcoma is not common, it is a risk and is associated with the presence of what may appear to be an otherwise benign myoma.

Candidates for hysteroscopic treatment should be prepared with the intramuscular administration of a gonadotropin-releasing hormone (GnRH) agonist (Lupron), 3.75 mg monthly for 3 months before the anticipated surgery. Lupron will reduce the size of the myoma, will reduce its vascularity, and will atrophy the surrounding endometrium. For large submucous myomata, the hysteroscopy should be accompanied by a simultaneous laparoscopy.

The patient is positioned as described in Chapter 106. The instruments of choice are the resectoscope fitted with a cutting-loop electrode, a fine electrosurgical needle, or a neodymium yttrium-aluminum-garnet (Nd-YAG) laser fiber (Fig. 111–6A, B). Most hysteroscopic surgeons will excise the myoma by shaving it with the resectoscope loop (see Fig. 111–6A). Therefore, a nonelectrolytic distending medium is required. Typically, the most appropriate medium in this case will be 5% mannitol. The medium is infused via tubing through the intake port of the operative sheath. Before the instrument is inserted, all the air is purged from the connecting tubing and the operating sheath. An endoscopic television camera is attached to the eyepiece of the optic, and the instrument is inserted transcervically into the uterine cavity under direct vision.

The myoma is located, and the cavity is flushed to remove blood and debris. The myoma is carefully mapped by circumnavigating around it with the hysteroscope. The pedicle of the myoma is identified. The relative width of the attachment is noted, as is its site of attachment. The uterine cornua and the tubal ostia are similarly located. The objective lens of the resectoscope is withdrawn away from the lesion to give the best panoramic view of the field (Fig. 111–7A). The cutting loop of the resectoscope is extended outward to the superior and posterior surfaces of the myoma, making contact with the lesion. The electrosurgical generator pedal activates the flow of electricity and cuts the myoma as the electrode is brought back toward the sheath of the resectoscope (Fig. 111–7B). The piece of tissue is shaken loose from the electrode and spins away into the uterine cavity. The loop electrode is again advanced and placed onto the myoma next to the place where the previous cut was made into its substance. The electrosurgical generator is again activated, and another piece of the myoma is sliced away. This process continues until the topmost part of the myoma has been reduced to a flat plateau (Fig. 111–7C). The next layer of the myoma is cut in a similar fashion; finally the entire mass has been reduced to a series of tissue chips, which are removed from the uterine cavity. Care is taken not to dig into the myometrium, that is, to reduce the projecting myoma only to the level of the surrounding tissue (Fig. 111–8).

Pressure is decreased by closing the outflow valve on the hysteroscope (resectoscope) sheath and partially closing the intake valve. This allows the surgeon to assess bleeding from the operative bed. Any brisk bleeding sites should be coagulated with a ball electrode. Finally, the cavity is flushed and re-distended to ensure complete integrity of the uterine wall.

The technique of myolysis is relatively easy to perform. The instrument of choice is an Nd-YAG laser fiber or a hysteroscopic bipolar needle (Fig. 111–9). The end result of this procedure is equivalent to an arterial embolization. The myoma is identified and mapped. The needle or fiber is jabbed into the myoma to a depth of 3 to 4 mm, and the laser or electrosurgical energy is simultaneously activated (Fig. 111–10). This procedure is repeated 20 to 40 times or more to coagulate and destroy the interior of the myoma. The myoma is left in situ to die "on the vine." The technique is enhanced by first coagulating the surface sinusoidal vessels. This technique diminishes bleeding from the surface of the myoma as the fiber or needle is withdrawn. At the terminus of the procedure, the myoma is studded with multiple blanched holes.

Pedunculated myomata with a narrow pedicle may be managed by cutting via a needle point electrode. After the myoma is mapped, the hysteroscope is insinuated between the myoma and the uterine wall immediately above the point of attachment of the pedicle to the uterine wall. The needle electrode is extended to make contact with the midportion of the pedicle (Fig. 111–11A). The electric current is activated as the entire hysteroscope is moved down, while the tip of the electrode incises the pedicle of the myoma. This may be repeated three or four times until the myoma is freed from its attachments to the uterine wall (Fig. 111–11B, C). The myoma is extracted by dilating the cervix and inserting a sponge forceps, which in turn grasps and compresses the myoma before withdrawing it via the dilated cervical canal. Alternatively, if the myoma is small (<2 cm) and the pedicle narrow, then scissors may be used to cut the myoma free (Fig. 111–12A through D).

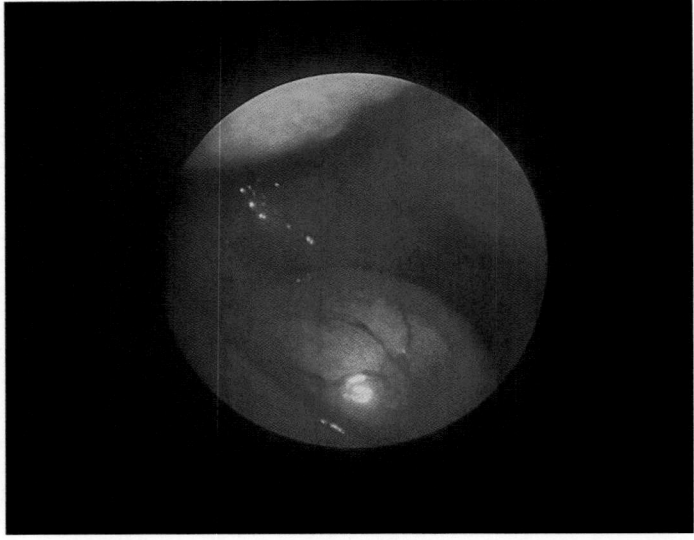

A

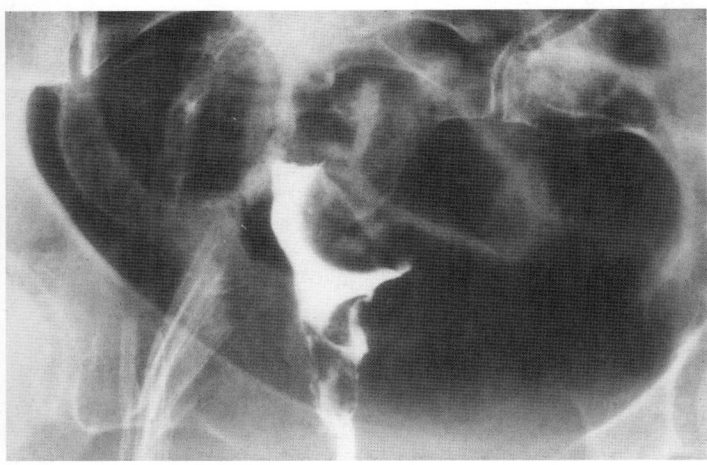

B

**FIGURE 111-1 A.** Panoramic hysteroscopic view of a submucous myoma. Hysteroscopy is the most accurate method for making this diagnosis. **B.** Hysterogram shows a filling defect consistent with submucous myoma. The smooth contour favors the myoma diagnosis but is not precise.

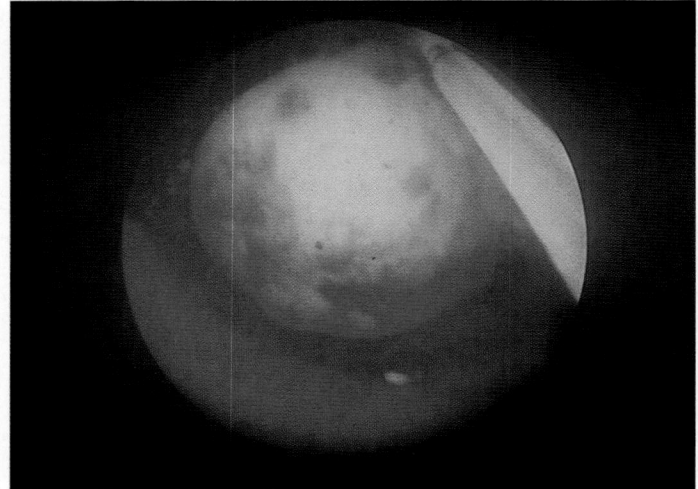

**FIGURE 111-2** The typical round appearance associated with some ecchymotic areas is diagnostic of a myoma with recent hemorrhage.

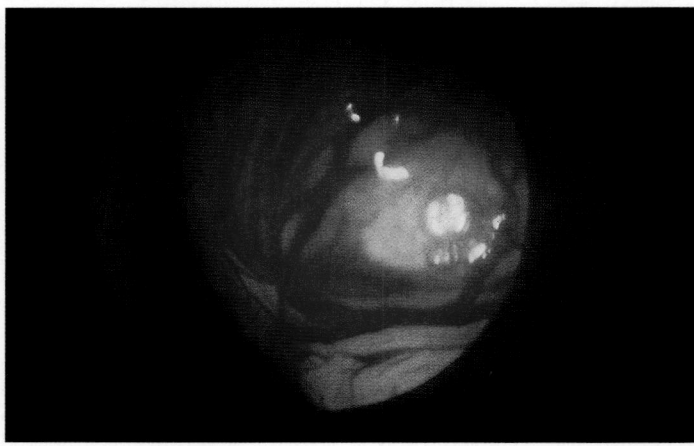

**FIGURE 111-3** The surface vascular pattern is also characteristic of submucous myoma.

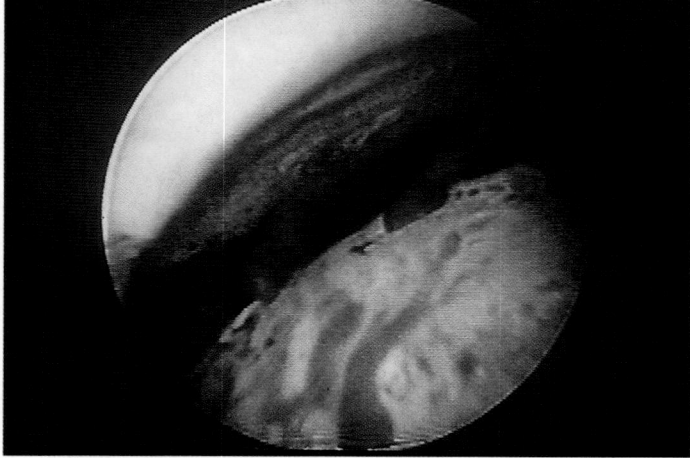

**FIGURE 111-4** Close-up view of the surface vessels confirms their composition. The thin-walled and fragile sinusoidal channels are engorged with blood.

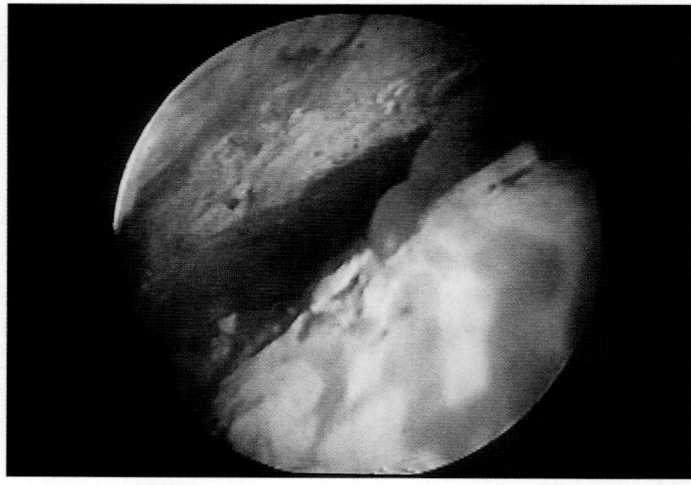

**FIGURE 111-5** Eruption of one of these channels. The 32% dextran-70 (Hyskon) medium (which does not mix with blood) permits a clear view of the spontaneous hemorrhage.

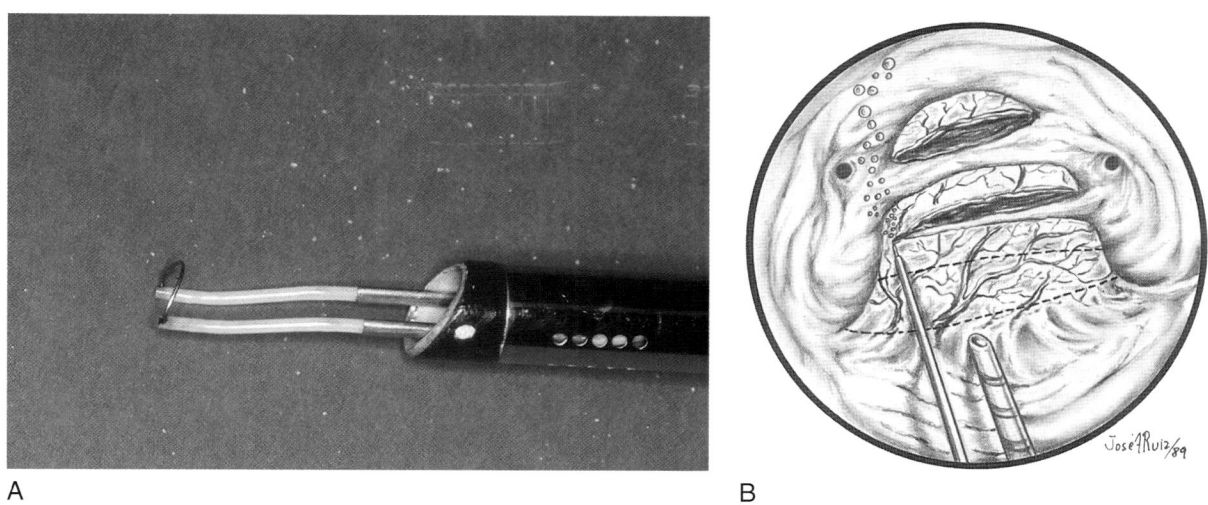

A                                                                    B

**FIGURE 111–6 A.** The most commonly used tool to treat submucous myoma is the resectoscopic shaving-loop electrode. This thin wire develops very high power densities, thereby permitting rapid vaporization (cutting) of the tissue. **B.** The neodymium: yttrium-aluminum-garnet (Nd-YAG) laser fiber is an alternative technique for sectioning a submucous myoma.

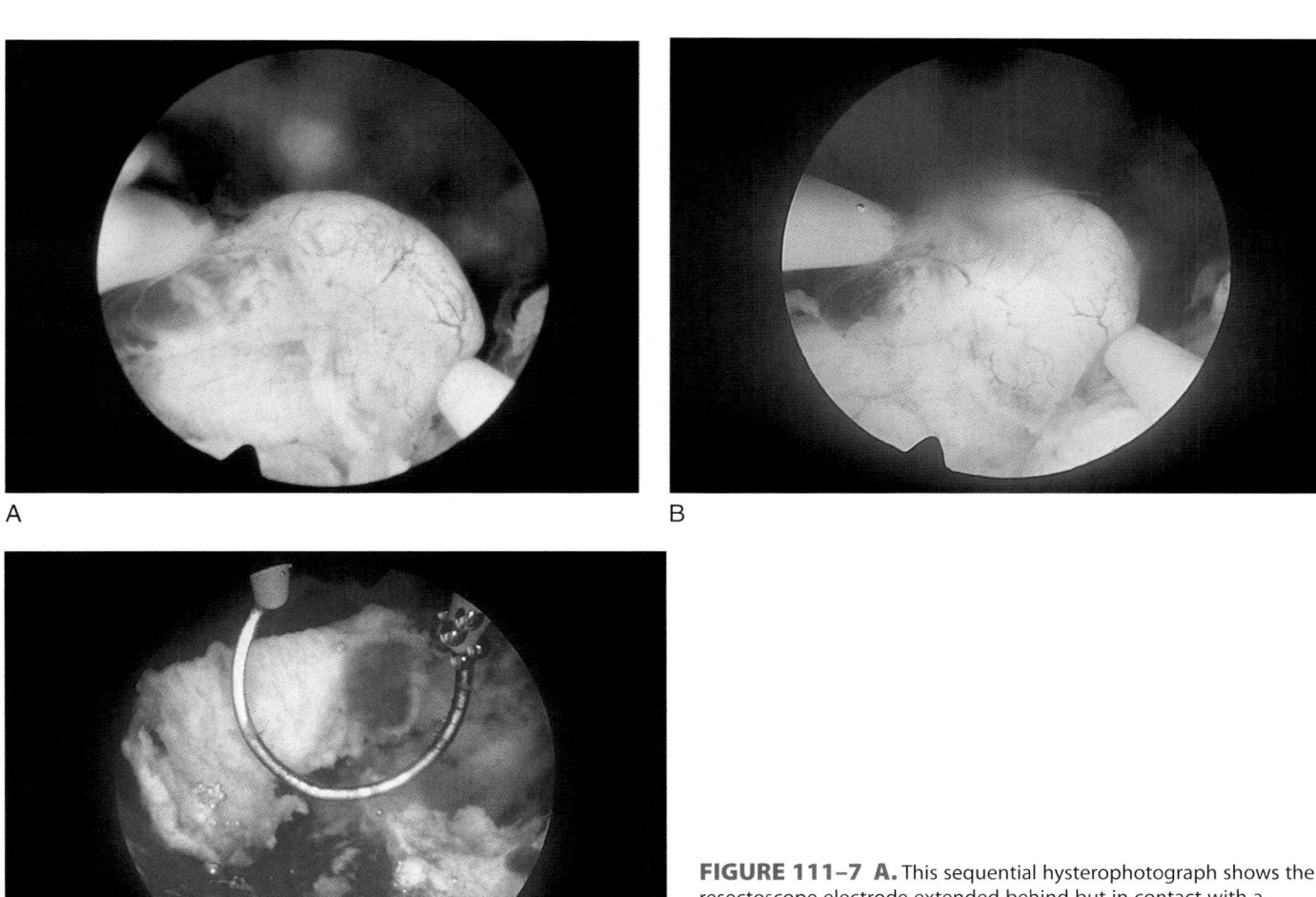

A

B

C

**FIGURE 111–7 A.** This sequential hysterophotograph shows the resectoscope electrode extended behind but in contact with a posterior wall submucous myoma. **B.** The electric current is activated, and the loop electrode cuts into the myoma. Note the blood spray to the left as the electrode is drawn back toward the hysteroscope. **C.** Most of the myoma has been resected. A few "chips" of tissue are floating in the medium.

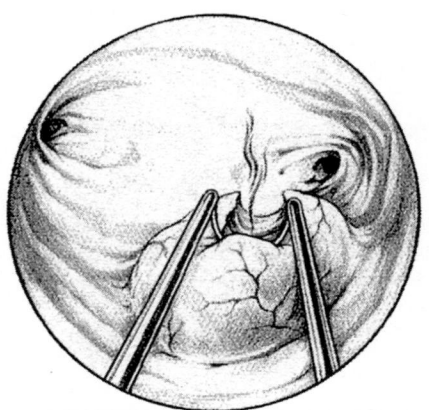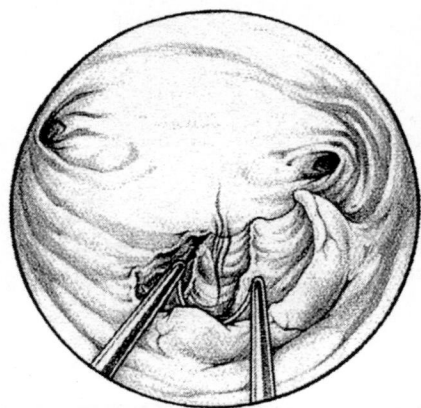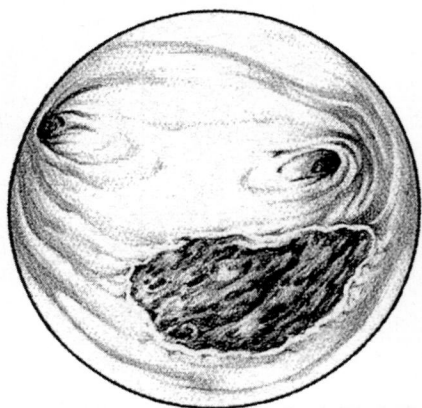

**FIGURE 111–8** Schematic illustrating the events shown in Figure 111–7A through C. Note that the myoma is systematically shaved away until the surface is flush with the surrounding endometrium. It is not advisable to dig into the surrounding myometrium to extract that portion of the myoma within the uterine wall.

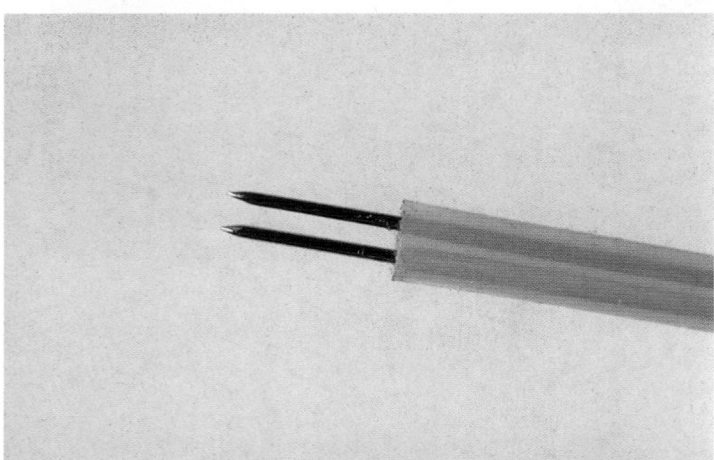

**FIGURE 111–9** Double-prong, bipolar needle electrode. One needle is the active electrode; the other is the return (neutral) electrode. This 3-mm instrument is inserted through the operating channel of the hysteroscopic sheath.

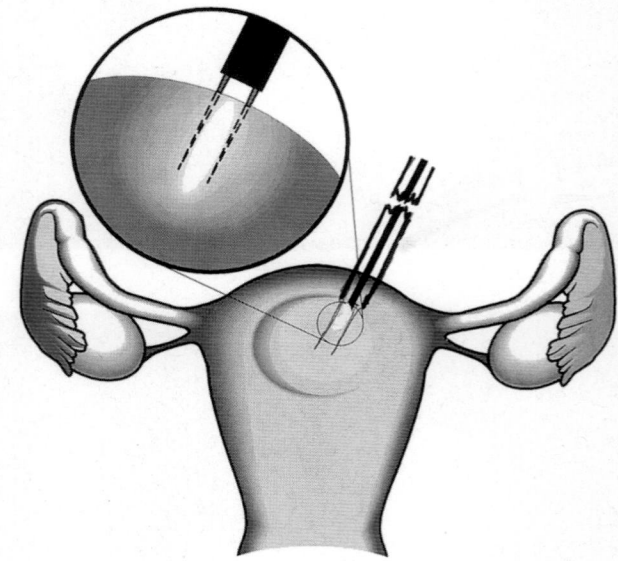

**FIGURE 111–10** Schematic view of myolysis. The bipolar needle jabs the myoma multiple times. Each jab is associated with coagulation of the interior of the myoma. Ultimately, the entire myoma is coagulated from within and undergoes necrosis and devascularization.

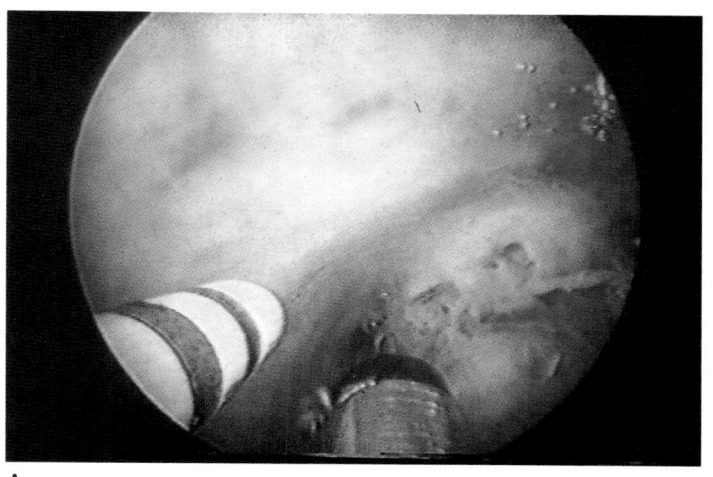

A

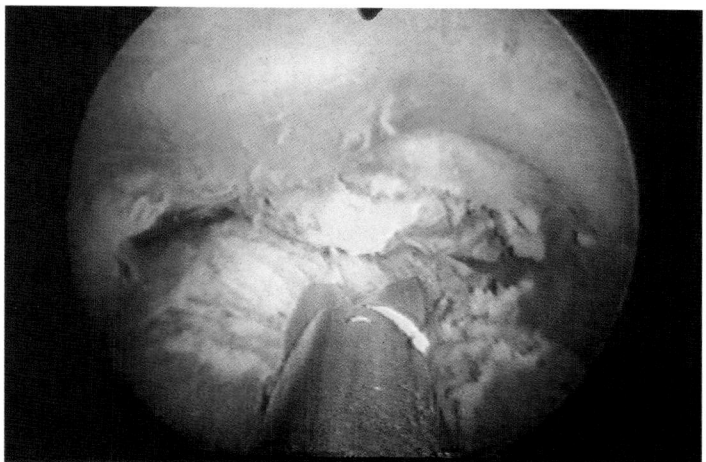

B

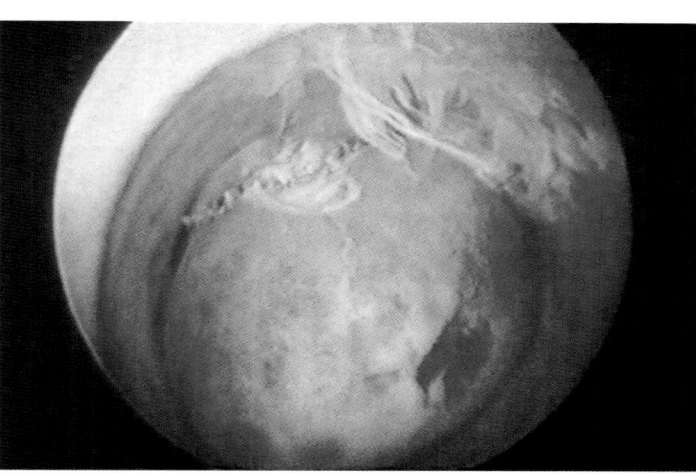

C

**FIGURE 111–11 A.** This large myoma is attached to the anterior uterine wall by a pedicle. A needle electrode contacts the right (patient) extreme of this attachment. **B.** The pedicle has been partially cut through with the electrode. It is now finished with hysteroscopic scissors. **C.** The myoma is completely detached and floats freely in the uterine cavity.

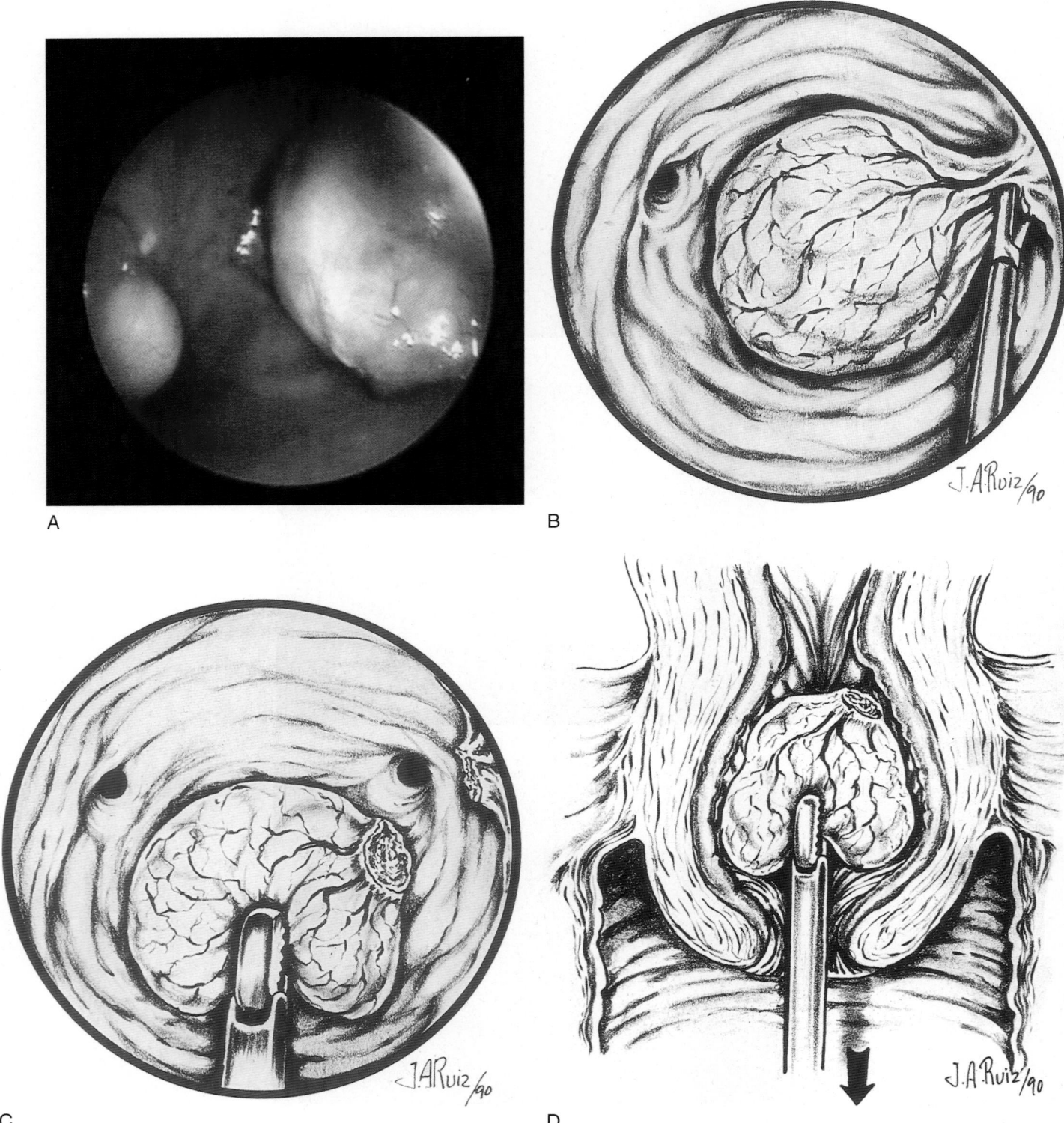

A

B

C

D

**FIGURE 111–12 A.** A small but well-defined submucous myoma. This has a rather broad-based (sessile) attachment to the uterine wall. An even myoma is seen on the opposite wall. **B.** A small myoma is attached to the left uterine wall by a narrow pedicle. The pedicle is cut under direct vision with hysteroscopic scissors. **C.** The myoma is grasped with alligator forceps. **D.** The myoma is delivered via a dilated cervix.

# CHAPTER 112

# Complications of Hysteroscopy

*Michael S. Baggish*

At any phase of operative hysteroscopy, a complication can occur. Obviously, it is best to avoid complications; however, if such an event happens, then recognition is mandatory. Because operative sheaths are large, cervical dilation is required to permit entry of the hysteroscope into the uterus. Perforation of the uterus may happen during dilation (Fig. 112–1). A diagnostic laparoscopic exam will allow the surgeon to determine whether to repair the injury. If bleeding continues after a reasonable clotting time, then the uterine wound should be sutured. Perforation may occur during intrauterine operations. If the injury results from the use of conventional tools (e.g., hysteroscopic scissors), then a laparoscopic view of the injury and surrounding viscera is acceptable (Fig. 112–2). If no continuing bleeding is observed, then no repair is required. If bleeding continues or is pulsatile in nature, then the wound must be hemostatically sutured (figure-of-8). When an energy device perforates the uterus (laser fiber or electrosurgical device), then laparotomy is necessary (Fig. 112–3). The surrounding intestine must be carefully and methodically inspected to determine whether a hole has been made in the small or large bowel (Fig. 112–4A, B). Similarly, the urinary tract and great vessels should be examined for injury.

A variety of complications result from the intravascular uptake of hysteroscopic media. These include fluid overload with resulting pulmonary edema. The latter can happen with any distending medium. Careful attention therefore is required to keep track of fluid deficits (the volume of injected fluid/the volume of returned fluid). The infusion of hypo-osmolar fluid can result in an even more serious complication, hyponatremia. Fluids such as glycine and sorbitol are hypotonic, whereas mannitol is iso-osmolar (Figs. 112–5 and 112–6).

A number of pumps have been employed to facilitate delivery of the distending medium to the uterus. Several of these pumps have utilized carbon dioxide ($CO_2$) gas or air as the driving force to push fluid into the uterus. These pumps are dangerous and should be avoided because patients have been killed or injured when high-pressure gas inadvertently entered the vascular space (Figs. 112–7 and 112–8). Roller-type pumps are safe and effective.

A common complication with hysteroscopic surgery is bleeding from the operative site. This can be managed by placing a balloon within the uterus. The balloon is inflated carefully with up to 5 mL of sterile water to tamponade the bleeding vessels. If the uterine cavity is enlarged, a balloon of greater capacity may be placed with it (Fig. 112–9).

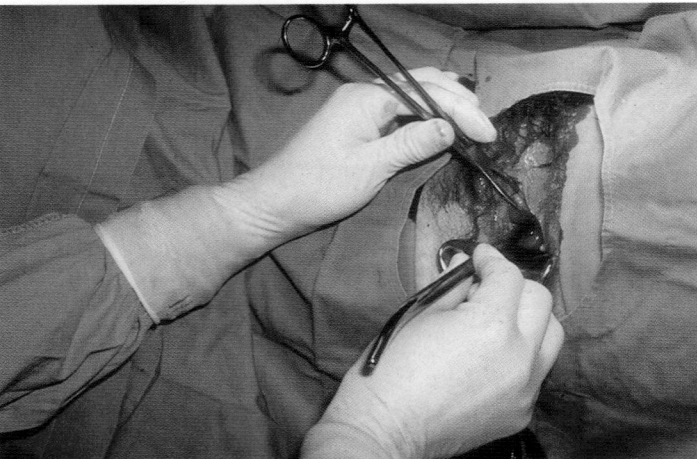

**FIGURE 112–1** The cervix is undergoing dilation to allow passage of the operating sheath. Perforation of the uterus may occur; however, operative interventions and long-term adverse sequelae are uncommon.

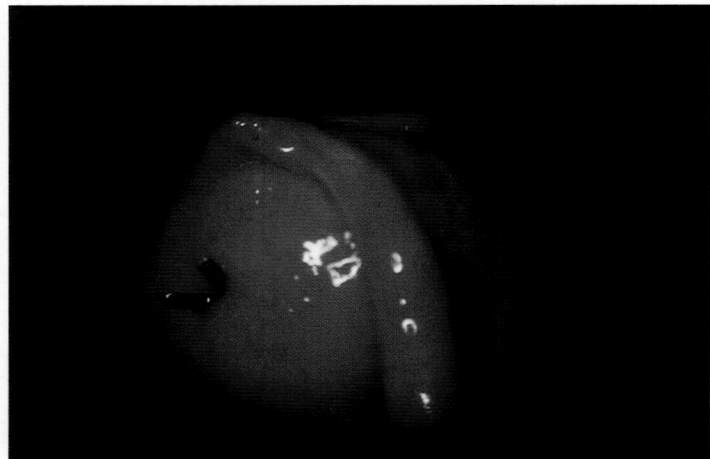

**FIGURE 112–2** Hysteroscopic scissors are seen via the laparoscope as it perforates the uterus. As with the dilator, unless persistent bleeding is observed, no treatment is required.

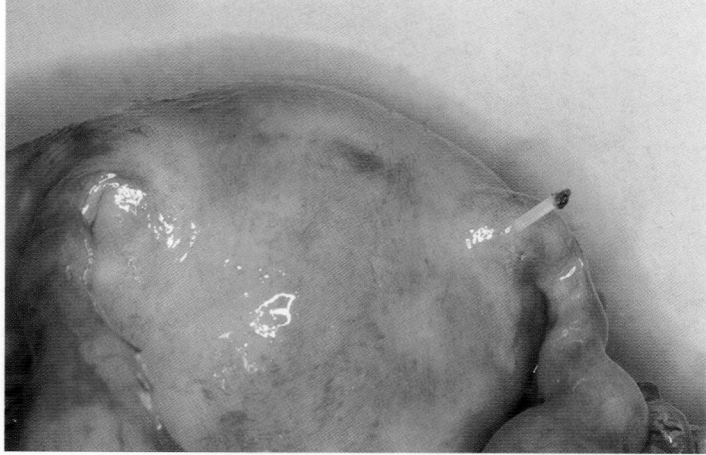

**FIGURE 112–3** When a laser fiber or electrode perforates the uterus, a laparotomy is needed to determine whether adjacent structures have been injured.

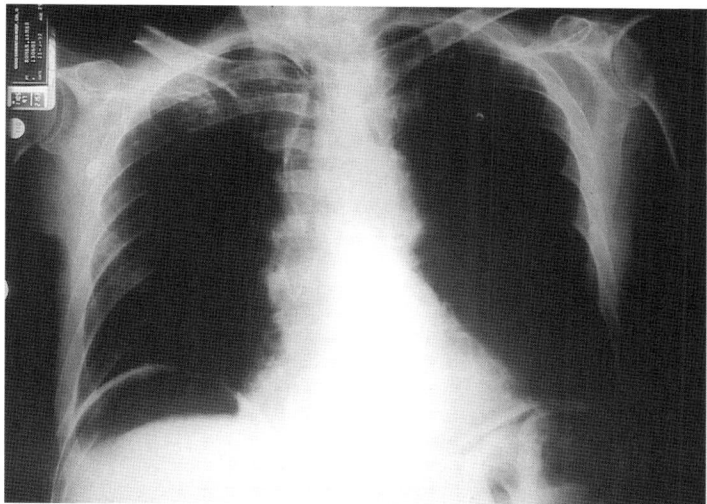

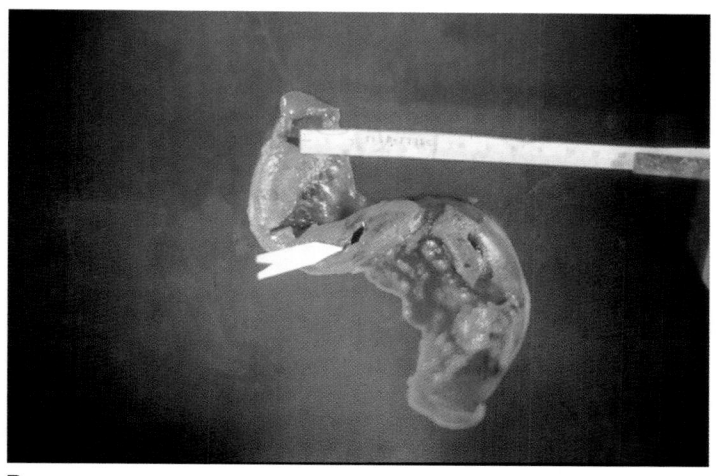

A                                                              B

**FIGURE 112–4 A.** This abdominal upright film illustrates free air under the diaphragm after perforation of the uterus with an energy device. The radiograph was taken 3 days after hysteroscopic surgery associated with perforation. **B.** A piece of resected small intestine obtained after hysteroscopic perforation with a monopolar electrode. Note the extensive thermal injury to the bowel. The intestinal injury was responsible for leakage of contents and air into the abdominal cavity.

**FIGURE 112–5** Glycine (1.5%) used for uterine distention has an osmolality of 200 mOsm/L. This hypotonic solution also is subsequently degraded to urea and ammonia.

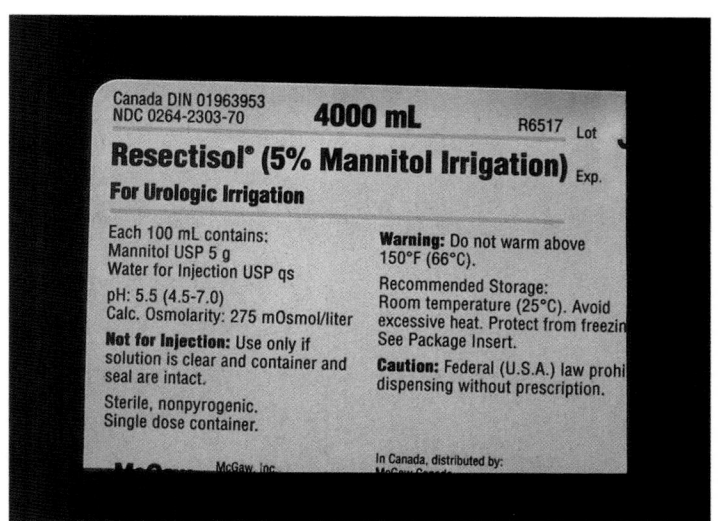

**FIGURE 112–6** Mannitol (5%) is iso-osmolar at 275 mOsm/L. It is a significantly safer distention medium than glycine.

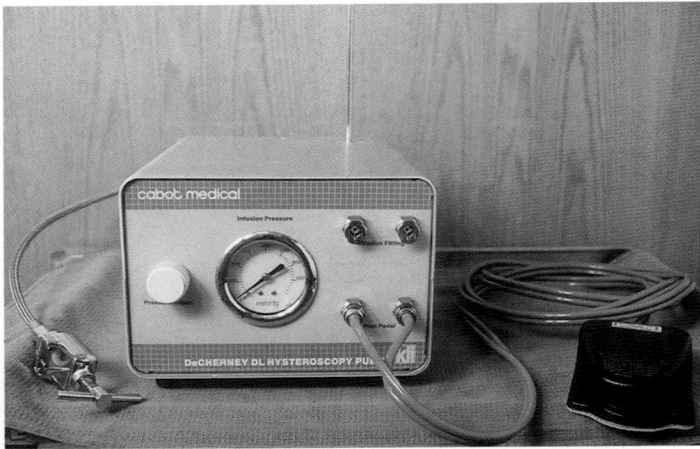

**FIGURE 112–7** This Hyskon pump utilized carbon dioxide ($CO_2$) gas to drive Hyskon into the uterus. When the Hyskon reservoir became exhausted and the ball valve failed, high-pressure $CO_2$ gas was infused into the uterus.

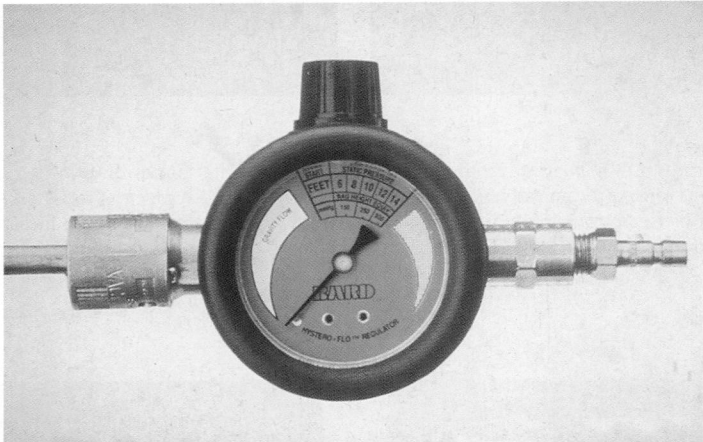

**FIGURE 112–8** This nitrogen-driven, low-viscosity, hysteroscopic-medium pump was withdrawn from the market. Air embolism can occur via valve failure after the liquid medium has emptied into the uterus.

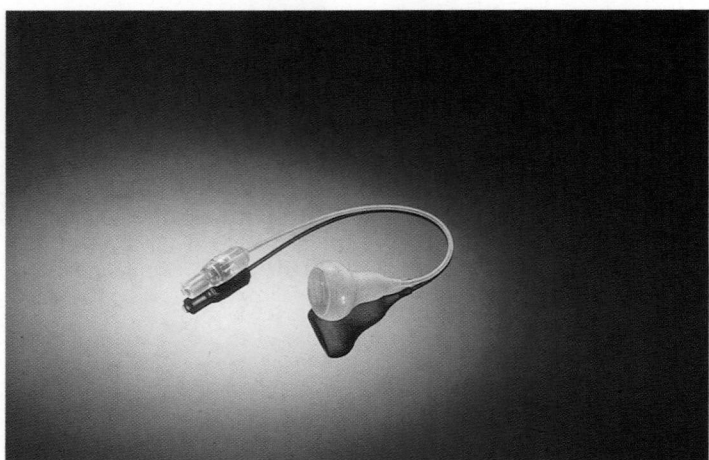

**FIGURE 112–9** This specially designed balloon (Mentor) is placed into the uterus and filled with 2 to 5 mL of sterile water. Pressure from the balloon on the uterine wall tamponades the bleeding vessel(s).

# SECTION B

# Laparoscopy

UNIT 5 ■ SECTION B

# CHAPTER 113

# Pelvic Anatomy From the Laparoscopic View

## *Tommaso Falcone* ■ *Mark D. Walters*

The anatomic view of the pelvis through a laparoscope can be somewhat disorienting to the pelvic surgeon. However, the same basic principle of understanding the relationship between important structures can be a guide. This chapter is an overview of some of the most commonly seen anatomic structures that should be visualized during most pelvic laparoscopic procedures.

An understanding of the anterior abdominal wall anatomy is critical for proper placement of the trocars required for laparoscopy. The anatomy of the inferior epigastric vessels and their relationship to the placement of accessory ports are covered in the chapter on trocar placement. The external iliac artery has two branches: the inferior epigastric artery and the deep circumflex iliac artery. The inferior epigastric artery branches from the external iliac artery at the level of the inguinal ligament. It is seen medial to the insertion of the round ligament at the deep inguinal ring and then courses medially anterior to the peritoneum toward the rectus muscle. It can easily be seen because of the lack of fascia at this level (Fig. 113–1). It forms a fold of peritoneum called the lateral umbilical fold. Two veins usually accompany the inferior epigastric artery

(Fig. 113–2). It then ascends behind the muscle and anterior to the posterior rectus sheath to anastomose with the superior epigastric vessel.

Two important nerves can be injured by the introduction of the trocar or closure of the port sites: the iliohypogastric and ilioinguinal nerves (Fig. 113–3). The iliohypogastric nerve originates from L1 and traverses through the abdominal muscles; its anterior cutaneous branch pierces the internal oblique muscle 2 cm medial to the anterior superior iliac spine (ASIS). It then travels between the internal and external oblique aponeurosis until it pierces the latter aponeurosis about 3 cm above the superficial inguinal ring. The ilioinguinal nerve also originates from L1 and traverses the internal oblique aponeurosis approximately 2 cm medial to the level of the ASIS. It travels between the external oblique and internal oblique aponeurosis and enters the inguinal canal to emerge from the superficial inguinal ring. These nerves are sensory to the ipsilateral mons pubis and labia majora; injury to them can cause paresthesia. Entrapment can cause pain over the nerve distribution. Insertion of accessory trocars above the ASIS usually avoids this injury.

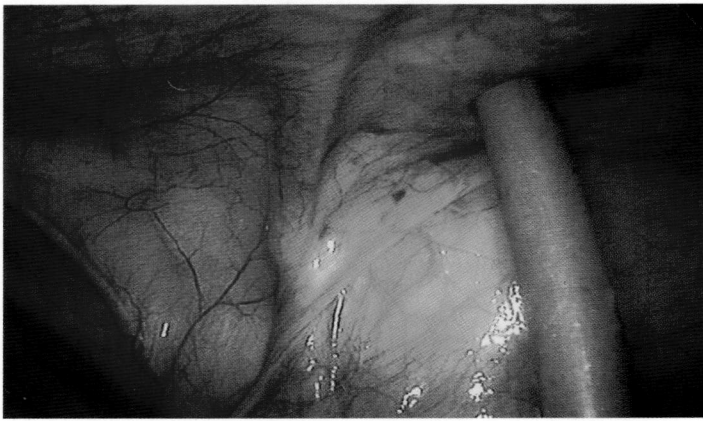

**FIGURE 113–1** The trocar is lateral to the right inferior epigastric vessels seen within the peritoneal fold.

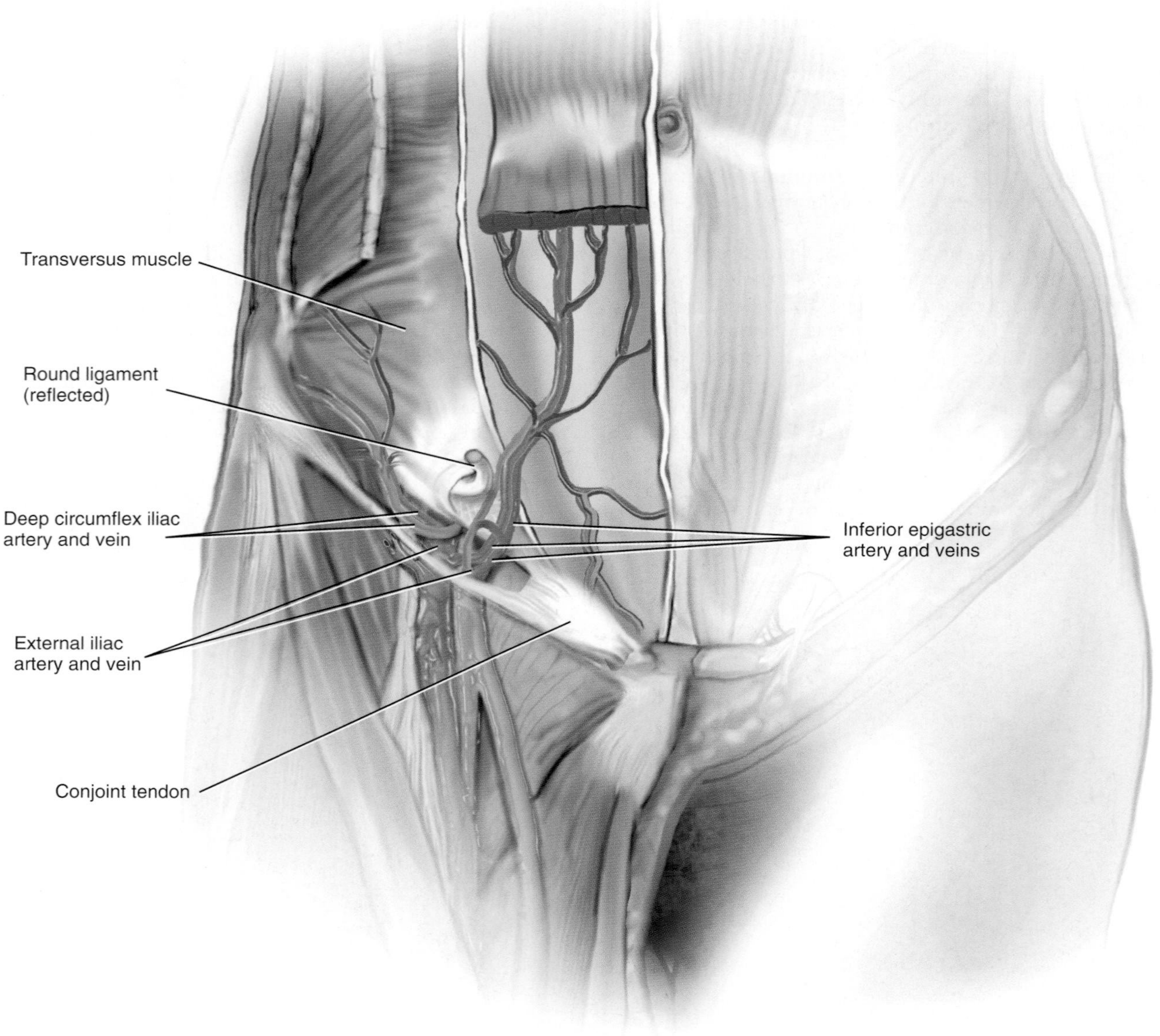

Transversus muscle

Round ligament (reflected)

Deep circumflex iliac artery and vein

External iliac artery and vein

Conjoint tendon

Inferior epigastric artery and veins

**FIGURE 113–2** The right round ligament has been transected, and the inferior epigastric vessels (one artery and two veins) are seen medial to it.

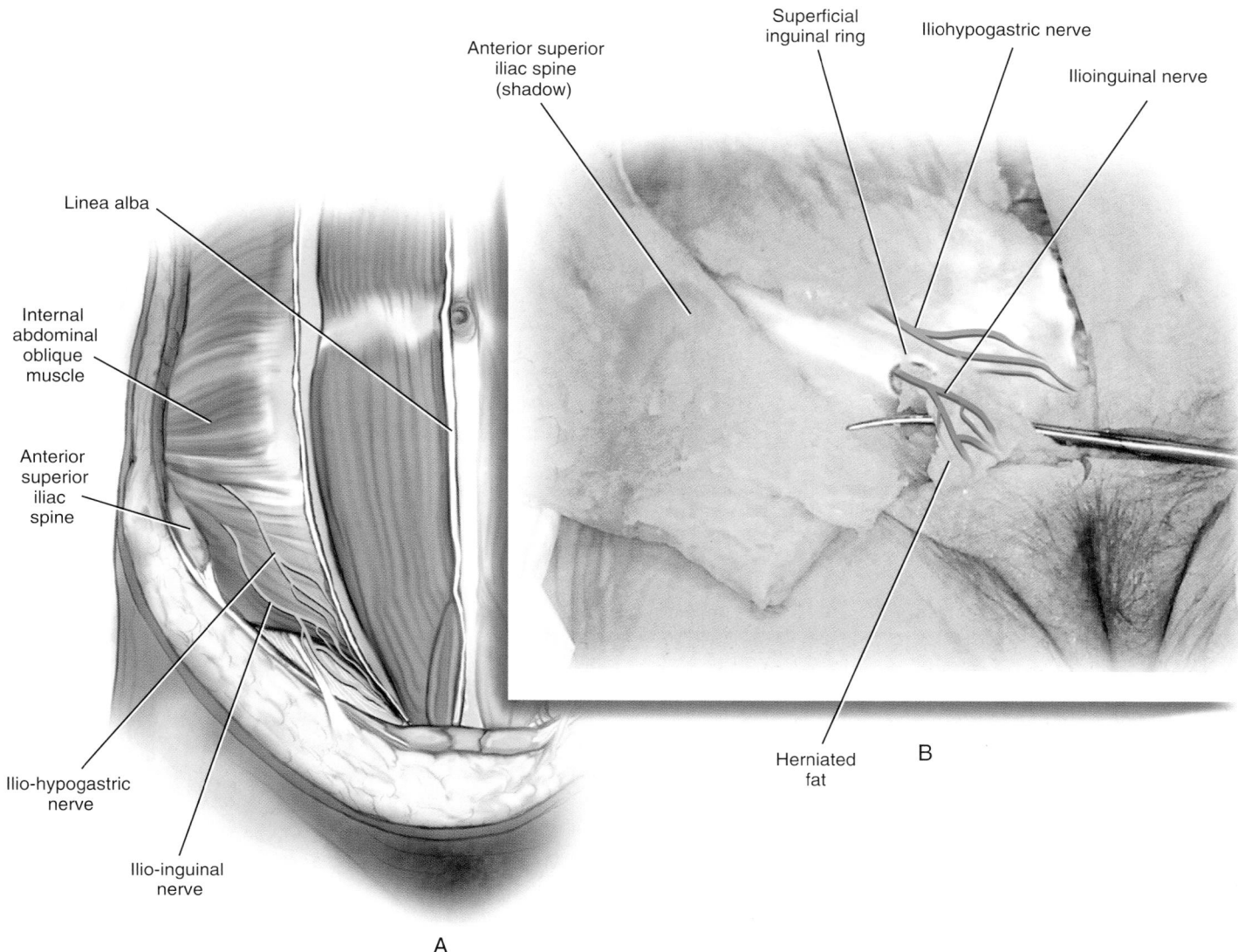

**FIGURE 113–3  A.** The external oblique aponeurosis has been removed, and the two nerves are seen on the internal oblique muscle arising 2 cm medial to the right anterior superior iliac spine. **B.** The terminal branches of the two nerves are seen. The ilioinguinal nerve exits the superficial inguinal ring.

The aortic bifurcation occurs approximately at the level of L4. In nonobese patients, this is found at the level of the umbilicus. With increasing weight, the umbilicus is located more caudad to the bifurcation. Typically, a trocar or pneumoperitoneum needle is angled at 45° to avoid the aorta. However, the major vessel that is seen below the bifurcation of the aorta is the left common iliac vein, which can be injured when the primary umbilical instrument is introduced (Figs. 113–4 and 113–5). This vessel is actually the most inferior large vessel in the midline and lies approximately at the level of the fifth lumbar vertebra. This area also contains the presacral nerve. The presacral nerve or superior hypogastric plexus is actually a plexus of nerves rather than a single nerve (Fig. 113–6). It lies anterior to the aortic bifurcation and left common iliac vein and therefore more prelumbar than sacral. It is retroperitoneal but can easily be stripped off the overlying peritoneum. It contains mostly sympathetic nerve fibers.

Knowledge of pelvic sidewall anatomy is critical for safe gynecologic surgery. Excision for treatment of endometriosis or hysterectomy usually involves some dissection around the ureter. Adnexal masses are occasionally adherent to the pelvic sidewall and also require dissection of the ureter. The anatomy of the ureter is often viewed in relationship to the pelvic sidewall vessels. The first view of the ureter is a panoramic one from the laparoscope (see Fig. 113–4). This view easily identifies the right ureter over the pelvic brim. The ureter is a retroperitoneal structure that descends medial to the psoas muscle. It is loosely attached to the peritoneum but will be drawn into any peritoneum that is tented upward. It enters the pelvis anterior to (crosses over) the external iliac artery or occasionally the common iliac artery (Fig. 113–7). At this level, the ovarian vessels lie in close proximity to the ureter and cross it as the vessels descend toward the ovary (Fig. 113–8). Injury to the ureter can occur at this level when the ovarian vessels are cauterized during adnexal surgery. After it enters the pelvis, it lies anterior to the internal iliac artery. On the left, clear visualization of the ureter at the pelvic brim is obscured by the sigmoid colon or its mesentery.

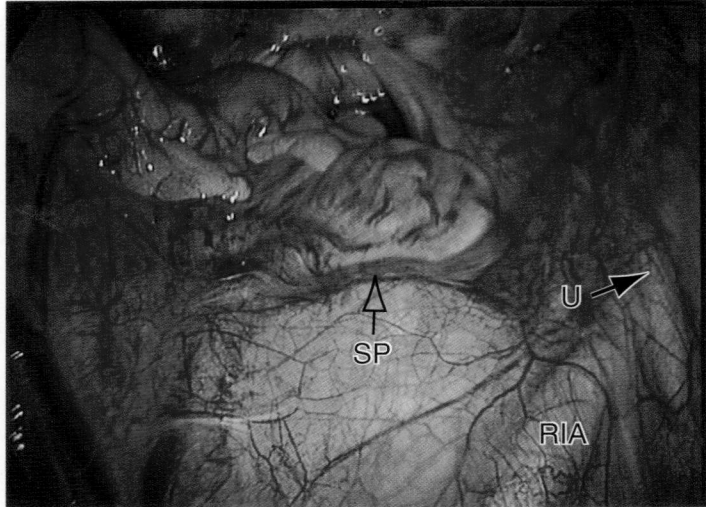

**FIGURE 113–4** Panoramic view of the pelvis and sacral promontory. The right common iliac vessel is seen with the right ureter crossing it. The inferior mesenteric vessels (*open arrow*) are seen on the left. Between these two structures is the left common iliac vein.

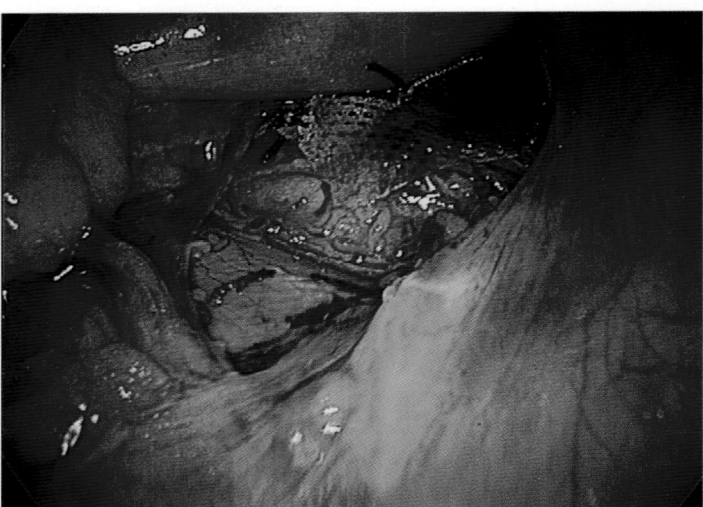

**FIGURE 113–5** The peritoneum has been removed from the presacral space in Figure 113–4, and the left common iliac is easily seen. It lies superior to the mesh that has been sutured into the sacral promontory.

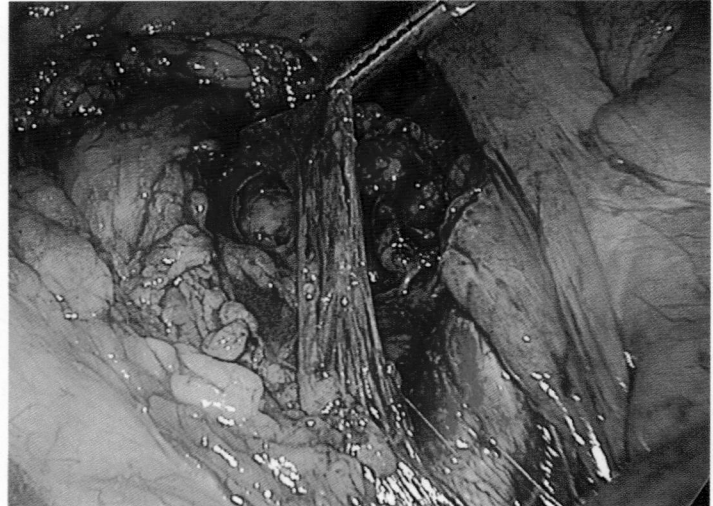

**FIGURE 113–6** The presacral nerve has been dissected and is grasped by an instrument. The right common iliac artery is seen.

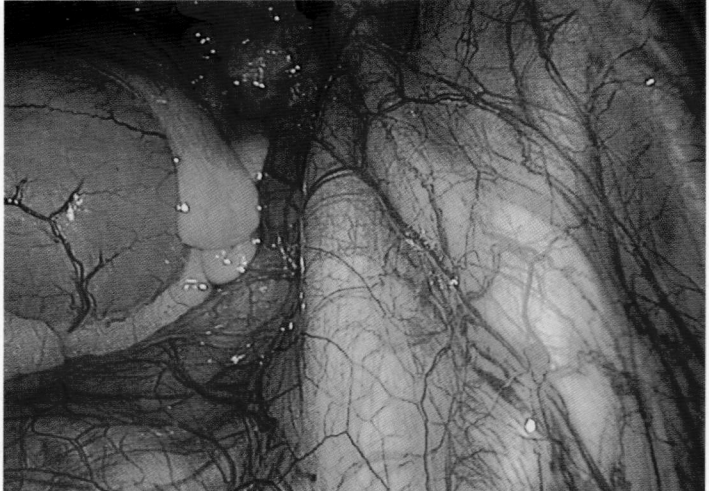

**FIGURE 113–7** The right ureter is seen crossing the right external iliac artery to lie anterior to the right internal iliac artery as it enters the pelvis.

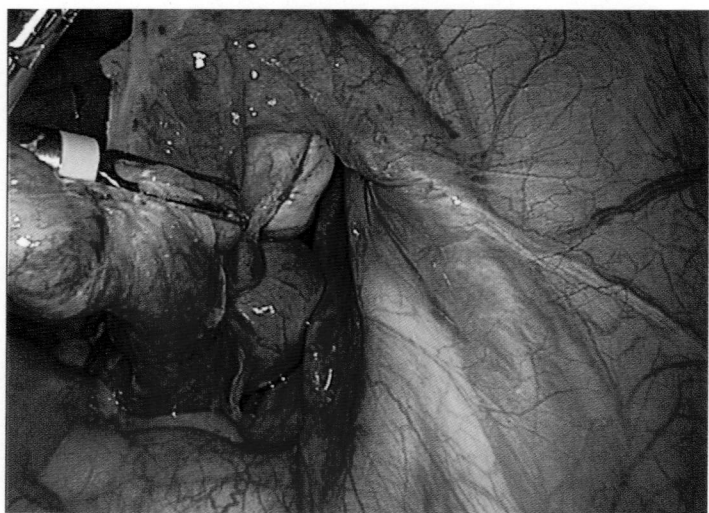

**FIGURE 113–8** The right ovarian vessels are seen close to the ureter as it crosses the pelvic brim.

The ureter descends from the pelvic brim in loose areolar extraperitoneal tissue. It lies anterior to the internal iliac and the anterior division of this vessel. Laterally, it lies on the fascia of the obturator internus muscle. The ureter can easily be identified after an incision is made in the peritoneum under the ovarian vessels in the midpelvis. It commonly stays attached to the medial leaf of the broad ligament (peritoneum) (Fig. 113–9). It lies medial to the branches of the anterior division of the internal iliac artery, notably the uterine, inferior vesical, and umbilical arteries (Figs. 113–9 and 113–10). The uterine artery lies lateral to the ureter until it crosses it to reach the uterus (Fig. 113–11).

The anatomy of the pelvic wall is encountered in procedures performed for vaginal prolapse and urinary incontinence. The main structures that are visualized are represented in Fig. 113–12. These include the obturator vessels and nerve and Cooper's ligament. The relationship of the obturator nerve and vessels to the branches of the internal iliac artery can be visualized from an intraperitoneal approach during dissection of the pelvic wall to obtain pelvic nodes (Fig. 113–13). The obturator nerve originates at L2-4 and descends in the psoas major muscle to the pelvic brim, whereupon it emerges medially to lie lateral to the internal iliac artery and its branches (see Fig. 113–13). It descends on the obturator muscle to enter the obturator foramen and exit in the thigh. It is sensory to the medial side of the thigh and motor to most of the adductor muscles.

The obturator nerve and vessels in the anterior pelvis are often seen during dissection of the bladder and vagina for pelvic support or urinary incontinence surgery (Figs. 113–14 and 113–15). The obturator vessels are branches of the anterior division of the internal iliac artery. However, many variable accessory branches stem from the inferior epigastric vessels (see Fig. 113–12). The obturator vessels lie on the obturator internus muscle and enter the foramen. During a Burch procedure, a suture is placed from the perivaginal tissue into Cooper's (pectineal) ligament. The accessory branches often lie on this ligament and can be injured easily. Cooper's ligament is a strong fibrous band attached to the pectineal line of the pubic bone (see Fig. 113–15). In the fat lateral to this ligament lie the external iliac vessels, which can be injured if a needle entering Cooper's ligament accidentally exists too laterally.

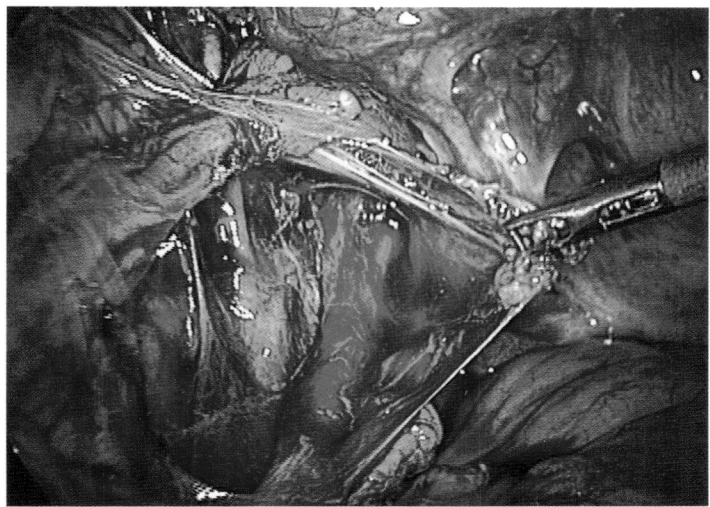

**FIGURE 113–9** The left broad ligament (peritoneum) is pulled by the instrument, and the left ureter is seen attached to it. Lateral to the ureter is the anterior division of the internal iliac artery with the umbilical artery branching off toward the anterior abdominal wall.

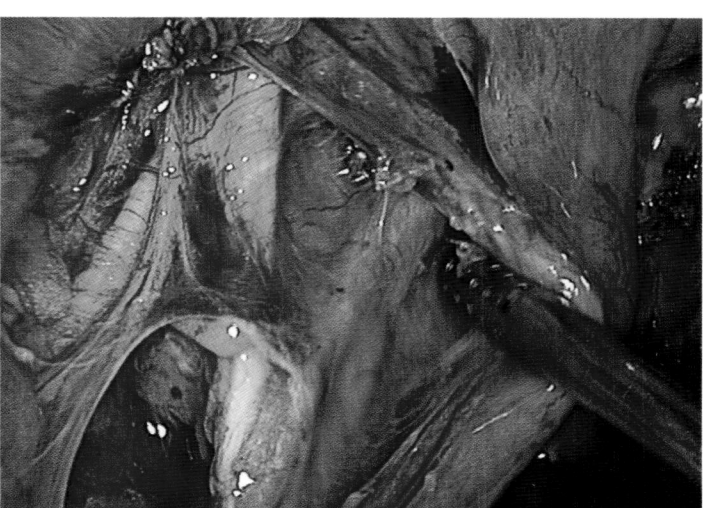

**FIGURE 113–10** The left ureter is retracted by the instrument, and the anterior division of the internal iliac and its two main branches (umbilical and uterine arteries) are seen. The left obturator nerve is seen lateral to the umbilical artery.

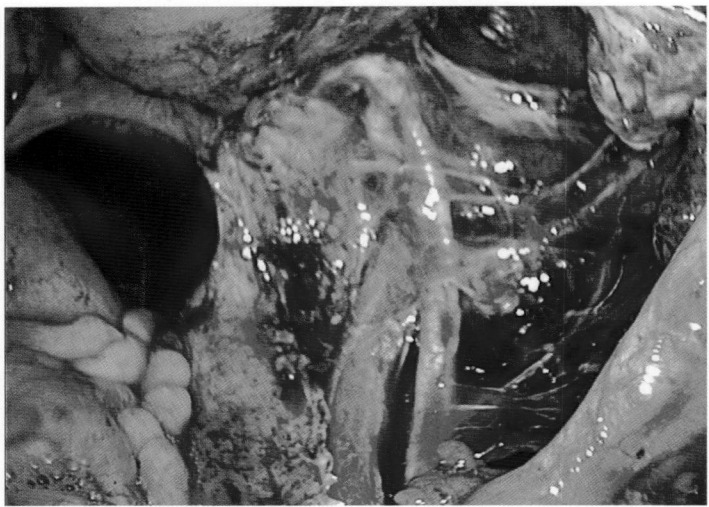

**FIGURE 113–11** The peritoneum has been removed; the right uterine artery is seen lateral to the ureter and then crosses over toward the uterus.

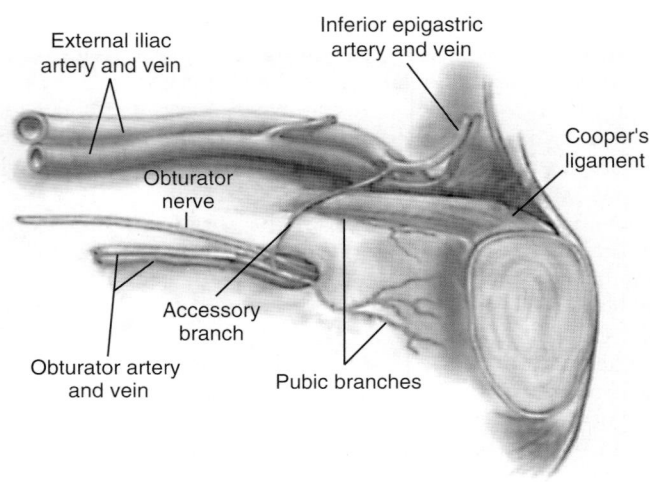

**FIGURE 113–12** This figure shows the important anatomy of the area where incontinence surgery is performed.

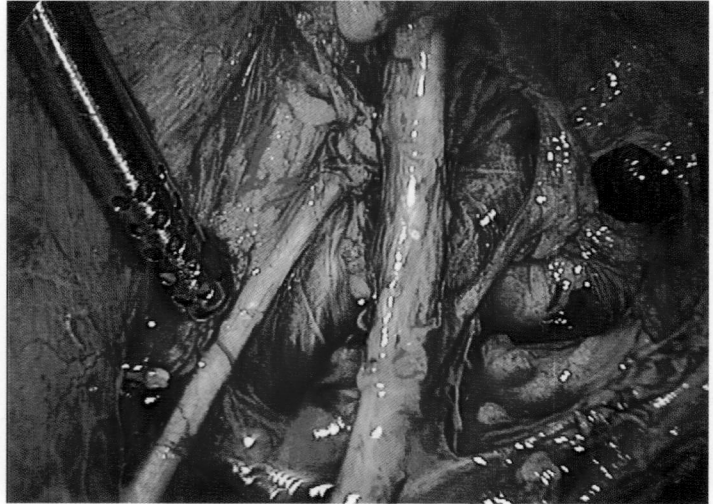

**FIGURE 113–13** The instrument that is pointing to the obturator nerve retracts the left external iliac vein. The umbilical artery is lateral to the nerve.

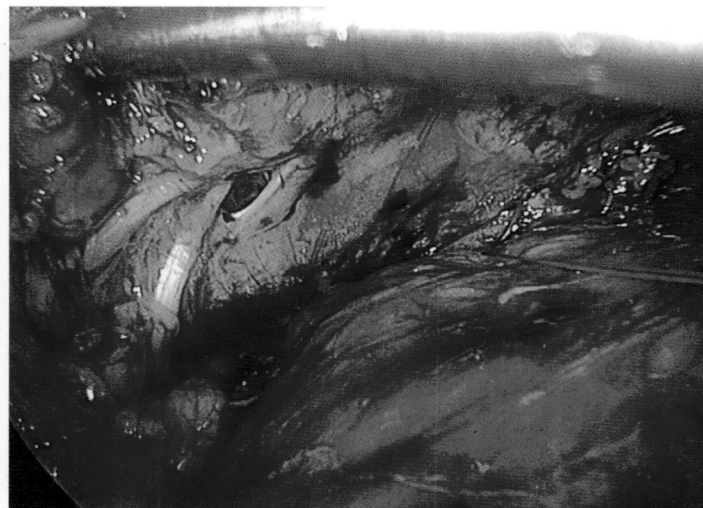

**FIGURE 113–14** The left obturator bundle is seen entering the obturator canal. A stitch has been placed into the paravaginal space.

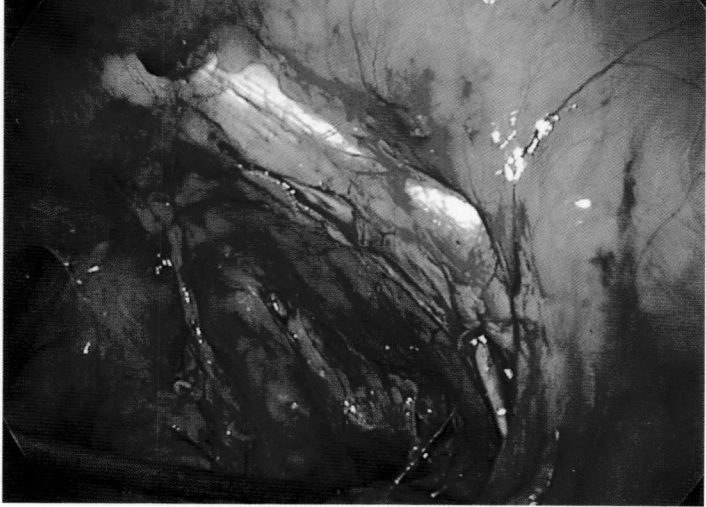

**FIGURE 113–15** Right Cooper's ligament is seen as a thick band of tissue. The fat lateral to this tissue includes the external iliac vessels. The nerve is seen inferior to Cooper's ligament.

# The Operating Room Suite and Instrumentation

*Tommaso Falcone* ■ *Mark D. Walters*

Many functional, uncluttered, and multidisciplinary systems are available to help organize an operating room suite. Most instruments can be placed on carts or booms, which can be moved to accommodate the surgical site (Figs. 114–1 and 114–2). An operating suite does not have to contain all commercially available instruments to function properly. The basic instruments that are required for safe laparoscopic surgery can be divided into three groups: the electronic cart, the laparoscopic instrument table, and the vaginal instrument table.

## Electronic Cart

The following instruments are usually placed on the electronic cart (Fig. 114–3):

- Monitor
- Light source
- Camera and camera control unit
- High-flow insufflator
- Electrosurgical unit
- Image recording device

The monitor can be on the cart as shown. Recently, the flat screen monitors are separate units.

A three-chip camera will give higher resolution than a one-chip camera. This will be noticed only if the monitor has the same number of lines of resolution. A xenon light source (300W) gives better illumination and color duplication than a halogen (150W and 300W) one. All insufflators have flow and pressure controls. The pressure should always be set at less than 15 mm Hg. Higher settings are rarely needed and should be used for brief periods of time. High-flow insufflators will render small leaks less important. An electrosurgical unit that has both unipolar and bipolar systems should be used. The unipolar system should generate both nonmodulated (cutting) and modulated (coagulation) current. The bipolar instruments will have the source current on a prong of the forceps or scissors and the return electrode on the other prong. In the unipolar system, the instrument is the source of the current, and the return electrode is the grounding pad.

Surgical instruments that are used for laparoscopic procedures are usually kept on one or two separate tables, depending on whether the operation will have a vaginal component.

## Laparoscopic Instrument Table

- Laparoscopes: three sizes (2/3, 5, and 10 mm) (Fig. 114–4)
- Light cables
- Trocars (2, 5, and 10/12 mm) and Veress needle
- Graspers and dissectors
- Scissors
- Needle holders, needle assist, and knot pushers
- Aspiration and injection instruments
- Bipolar forceps and cords
- Introducer for introducing a pretied suture

The laparoscopes used in gynecology have a 0° deflection. You see what is straight ahead. Several sizes of laparoscopes are useful (see Fig. 114–4). The larger the diameter of the laparoscope, the greater is the brightness. A 10-mm laparoscope with a working channel will decrease the brightness. The decrease in luminosity will depend on the size of the working channel (3 to 8 mm). The authors use a 5- to 12-mm laparoscope for operative laparoscopy, a 5-mm laparoscope for diagnostic laparoscopy under general anesthesia, and a 2- to 3-mm laparoscope for diagnostic laparoscopy under conscious sedation. A 12-mm laparoscope is used for robotic surgery, but a 5-mm laparoscope is used for all other operative procedures, including single port surgery.

A variety of graspers are available, but we use the following:

- Allis graspers when a firm purchase is required, as when the ovarian cortex or the myometrium is grasped
- Atraumatic graspers for grasping delicate tissues
- Soft bowel grasper for placing traction on the bowel
- Maryland dissector for blunt dissection or precise tissue grasping

All accessory instruments go down a 5-mm port. The scissors should be disposable because the reusable ones often are not sharp. An aspiration-suction device is mandatory for gynecologic laparoscopic surgery. The fluid bags should be warmed because hypothermia is a significant problem during prolonged surgery. The suction canisters and fluid bags are usually placed off to one side. The tips are reusable (5 and 10 mm), but the tubing and the handle are often disposable.

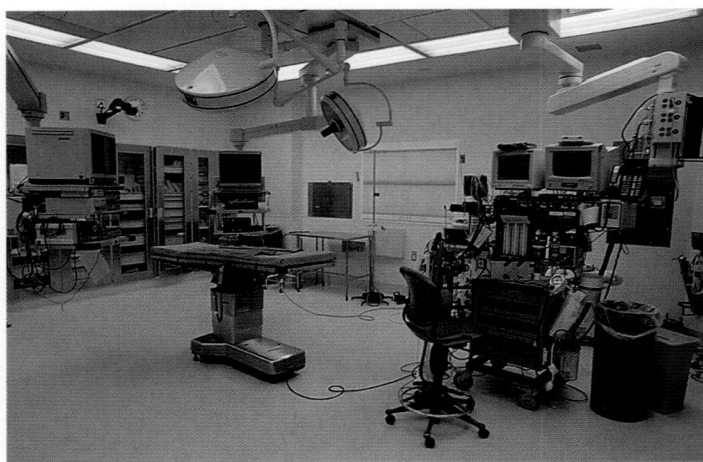

**FIGURE 114–1** An operating room can be structured so that equipment does not take up an inordinate amount of space.

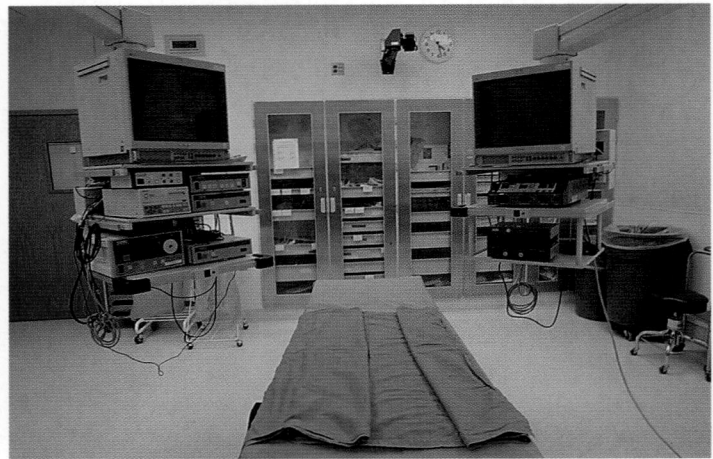

**FIGURE 114–2** Operating room setup. Note that there are two booms. Each has a monitor, so that all physicians can view the surgical field from a comfortable position.

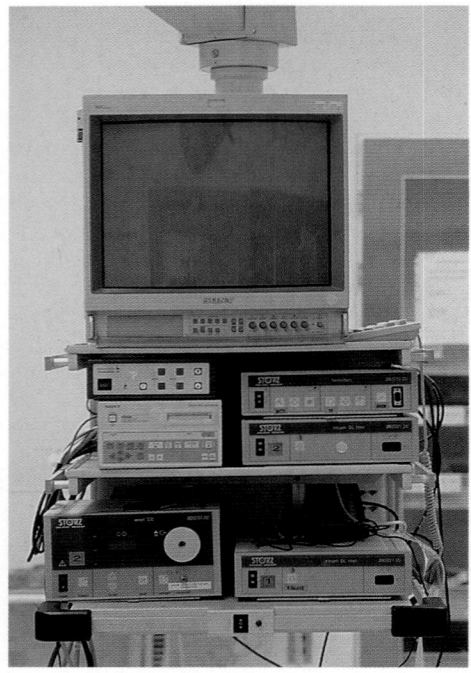

**FIGURE 114–3** Equipment placed on a cart or boom (Bertchold Co, Charleston, South Carolina).

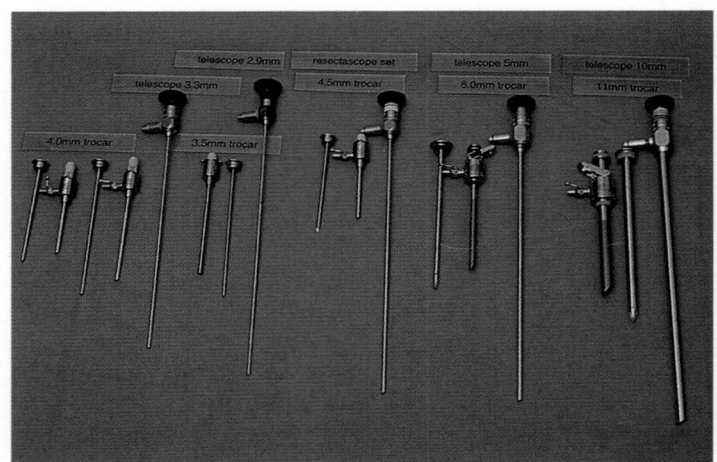

**FIGURE 114–4** Laparoscope sizes.

## Vaginal Instrument Table

- Open-sided speculum
- Single-toothed tenaculum
- Foley catheter
- Cervical dilators
- Uterine manipulators: Cohen cannula (Eder Instruments, Oak Creek, Wisconsin), RUMI manipulator (Cooper Medical, Oklahoma City, Oklahoma), Hulka uterine forceps (Rocket, Wolf, California)

The vaginal table may have other instruments if there is a significant vaginal component, such as with laparoscopic hysterectomy.

A variety of other instruments or energy forms may be useful in specific cases. These are described in the appropriate chapters. We do not routinely use other energy forms such as an ultrasonic scalpel or a carbon dioxide ($CO_2$) laser because they have never been shown to be safer or to cause less tissue injury or adhesion formation than electrosurgery.

# CHAPTER 115

# Trocar Placement

## *Tommaso Falcone* ■ *Mark D. Walters*

The most important prerequisite for proper trocar placement is knowledge of abdominal wall anatomy. Patient position is critical for a safe procedure. The patient is placed in the dorsal lithotomy position with foam-padded leg stirrups (Allen Medical Systems, Acton, Massachusetts), in which the calves and heels are supported and can be elevated for the vaginal portion of the surgery. The legs are checked for pressure points, and the arms are placed at the side wrapped in sheets and with cushions placed at pressure points.

An examination is performed with the patient under anesthesia, and the bladder is catheterized. For operative laparoscopy, a Foley catheter is left in the bladder. A uterine manipulator is inserted. For infertility cases, we use a RUMI (Cooper Medical, Oklahoma City, Oklahoma) or a Cohen manipulator (Eder Instruments, Oak Creek, Wisconsin).

## Veress Needle Insertion

A local anesthetic, such as an equal mixture of 1% lidocaine without epinephrine and 0.25% bupivacaine, is infiltrated into the umbilical area. A 20-gauge, 2-inch needle is used so that the skin and fascia are infiltrated. The abdominal skin should be elevated while this procedure is performed.

An orogastric tube should be inserted if intubation has been difficult or ventilation prior to intubation has been prolonged. A dilated stomach can be punctured easily under circumstances that result in gastric dilation. It is mandatory that the patient be kept in a horizontal position. An incision is made intraumbilically in the natural folds. It is a matter of preference whether a pneumoperitoneum is created before insertion of the primary trocar. Several articles have documented the safety of a direct trocar insertion without a pneumoperitoneum. Injuries to intraperitoneal structures such as the bowel and blood vessels have been clearly associated with Veress needle insertion. The abdominal wall should be elevated prior to insertion. If the bowel is adherent to the anterior abdominal wall, it will not move away with elevation. If the bowel is not adherent, it will be farther away from the needle. Vascular structures also will be farther away. The Veress needle should be aimed toward the uterus at a 45° angle and in the midline (Fig. 115–1). Before insufflating, correct intraperitoneal placement of the needle should be performed by one of these techniques:

■ A drop of fluid placed on the needle hub will trickle downward, especially if the anterior abdominal wall is elevated.
■ A syringe of fluid can be attached to the needle and easily injected. This fluid can then be aspirated. If there is no return, the needle has been placed correctly. If there is return of blood or bowel content, there is a problem.
■ Gas flow can be started at 1 L/min. Pressure should be less than 10 mm Hg.

High-flow insufflators that deliver 9 to 15 L/min are necessary to compensate for the constant irrigation and suction of fluids, as well as the leaking of gas that may occur. Intraperitoneal pressure should not exceed 15 mm Hg. Higher pressures can cause decreased venous return or ventilation problems.

## Primary Trocar Insertion

The primary trocar can be inserted with or without a pneumoperitoneum. If the direct trocar technique is used, correct placement is easily confirmed with introduction of the laparoscope. Either way, the abdominal wall should be grasped and elevated maximally, and with the other hand the trocar should be directed at a 45° angle and in the midline (Fig. 115–2). The patient must be kept in a horizontal position. In Trendelenburg's position, the anatomic relationship of the major vessels to the angle of insertion is altered, which may increase the risk of injury. We usually use a blunt-tipped optical trocar for this step. A pyramidal tip incises the fascia, whereas the conical tip dilates it. More force is required for the latter trocar. Excessive force reduces control of the angle and depth of the trocar tip, increasing the risk of injury to internal structures. Resistance to trocar insertion also occurs if the skin incision is too small, or if the instrument is dull. Optical access trocars were recently introduced into the market. Two commercially available trocars are the Excel (US Surgical, Norwalk, Connecticut) and the OptiView (Ethicon, Somerville, New Jersey). Several small case series but no large randomized studies have shown that these trocars are associated with fewer injuries than are conventional techniques.

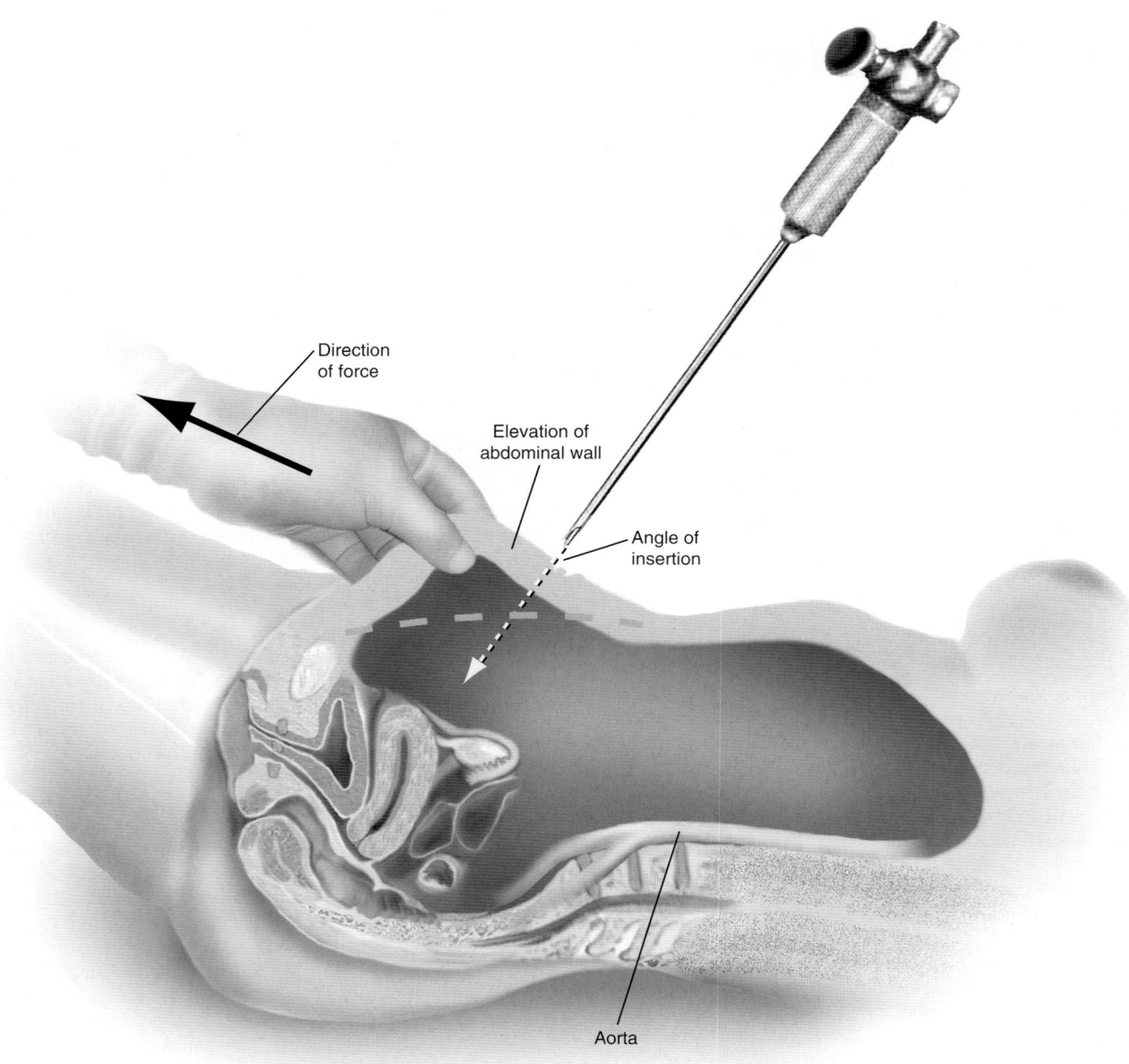

**FIGURE 115–1** Insertion of the Veress needle should be performed with elevation of the anterior abdominal wall. The angle should be at 45° and in the midline.

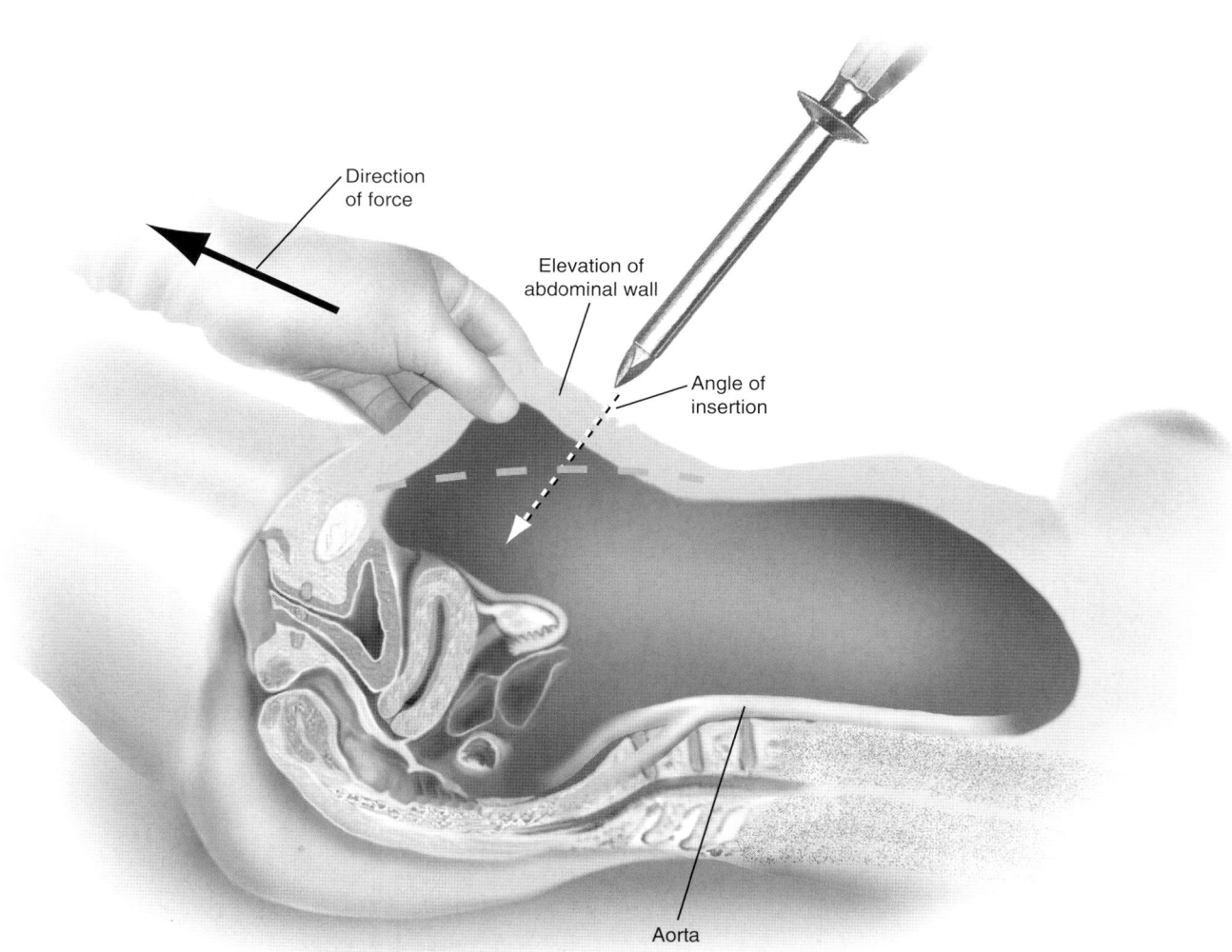

Direction
of force

Elevation of
abdominal wall

Angle of
insertion

Aorta

**FIGURE 115–2** Insertion of the primary trocar requires elevation of the abdominal wall. The other hand inserts the trocar at a 45° angle and in the midline.

## Open Laparoscopy and Alternative Techniques

Open laparoscopy is the only technique demonstrated to eliminate large-vessel injury. However, bowel injury has been reported with this technique as well. A 2- to 3-cm horizontal infraumbilical incision is made, and the fascia is exposed. An incision is made horizontally, and a suture is placed at each angle (Fig. 115-3). A blunt-tipped Hasson-type trocar is then inserted (Fig. 115-4). With the advent of single port laparoscopy, several disposable devices are available and can be placed through this incision.

Alternative methods should be utilized in patients who have midline scars from previous abdominal surgery. An open technique with a Hasson trocar at the umbilicus or at a left upper quadrant site should be utilized. In the left upper quadrant technique, an incision is made 2 cm below the costal margin at the left midclavicular line. A Veress needle or a small trocar can be inserted. The angle should be 45° and in a longitudinal plane without deviation toward the midline. The closest organs that may be injured are the stomach and the left lobe of the liver. This procedure should not be performed in patients with hepatomegaly, splenomegaly, or left upper quadrant surgery. An orogastric tube should be placed before the trocar is inserted.

## Secondary Trocar Insertion

Secondary trocars for pelvic surgery are placed lateral to the rectus muscle or suprapubically under direct vision. Knowledge of the anterior wall anatomy is essential for proper accessory port placement (Fig. 115-5). The most important vessels to visualize are the inferior epigastric arteries and veins. Transillumination will not help to delineate these vessels. They are lateral to the obliterated umbilical vessels and medial to the deep inguinal ring, which can be found by following the entry of the round ligament into the inguinal canal (Fig. 115-6). We recommend placing trocars 8 cm from the midline and 4 to 5 cm above the symphysis pubis. Conical-tipped trocars are probably better for these secondary sites because they have been associated with decreased risk of vessel injury. The tip of the trocar should be aimed toward the cul-de-sac. At the end of the procedure, the trocar sites should be inspected for bleeding. All lower quadrant incisions of 7 mm or greater should be closed (Fig. 115-7).

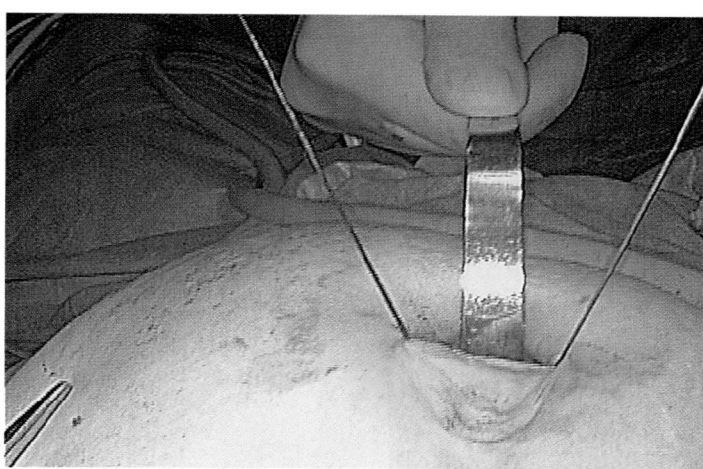

**FIGURE 115–3** Open laparoscopy technique: the skin and fat can be retracted with small S retractors. The fascia is incised, and a suture is placed at each angle.

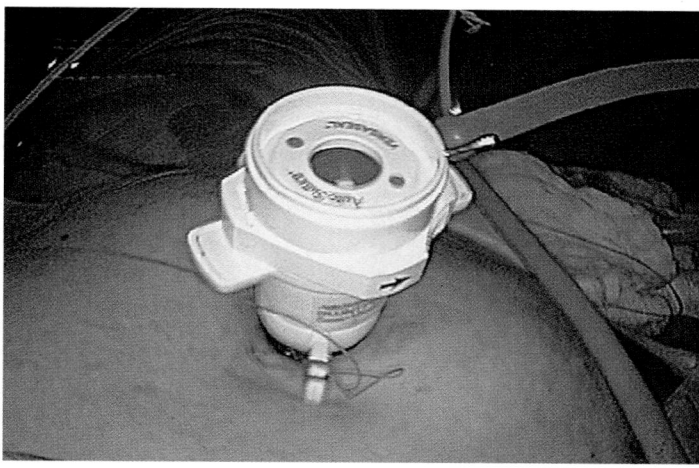

**FIGURE 115–4** The peritoneum is incised and the peritoneal cavity entered. A blunt-tipped trocar is inserted. The suture is then wrapped around the special grooves of the trocar.

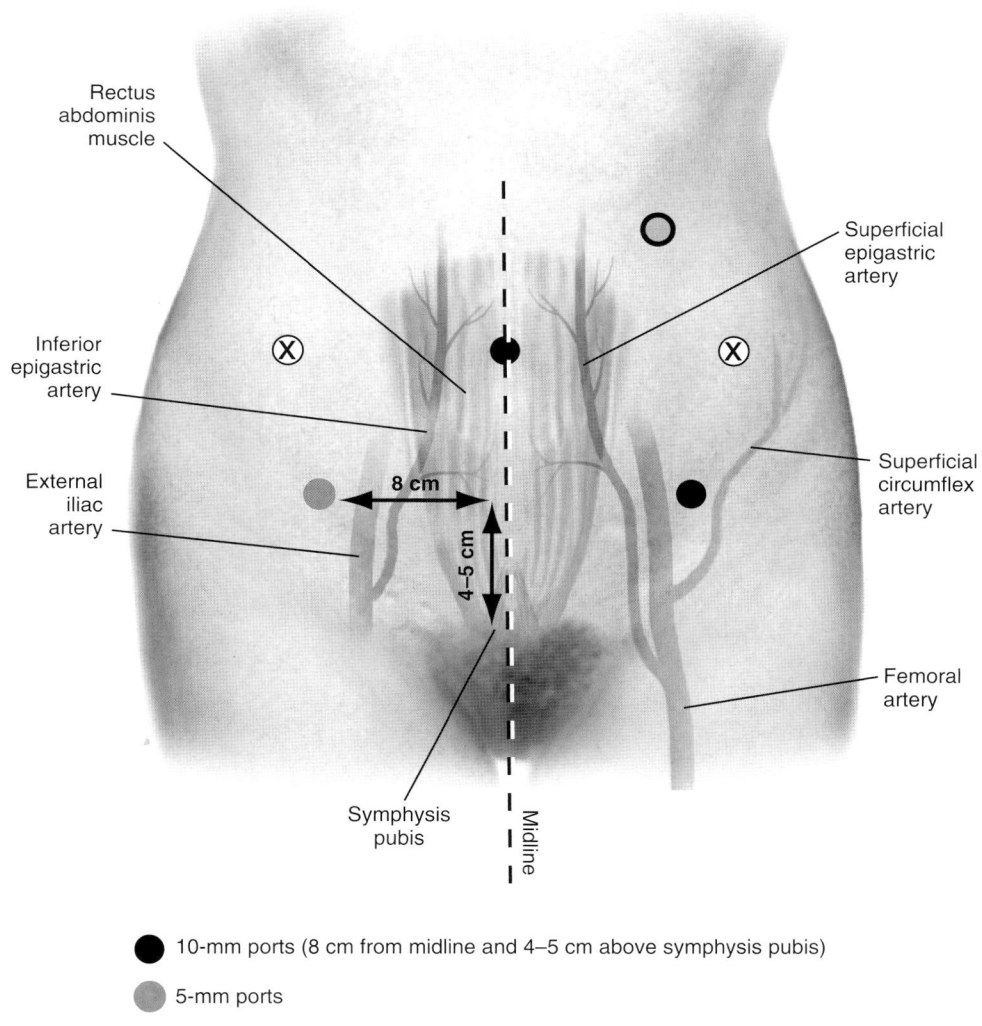

● 10-mm ports (8 cm from midline and 4–5 cm above symphysis pubis)

● 5-mm ports

Ⓧ 5-mm ports, as required

○ Left upper quadrant access

**FIGURE 115–5** Relationship of accessory port sites and the vessels of the anterior abdominal wall.

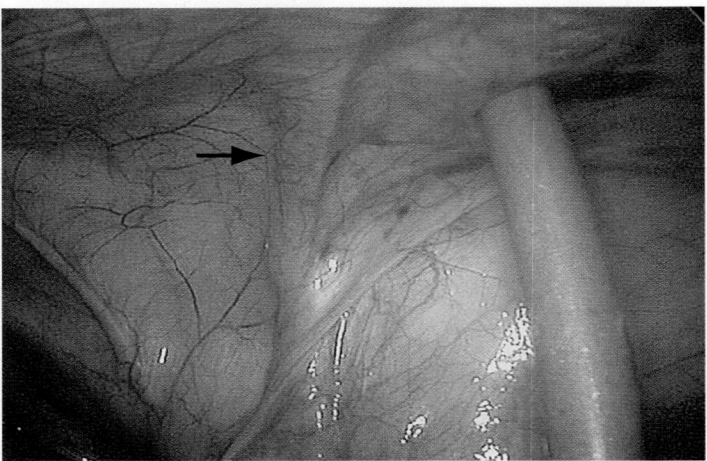

**FIGURE 115–6** Correct placement of a trocar lateral to the inferior epigastric vessels (*arrow*).

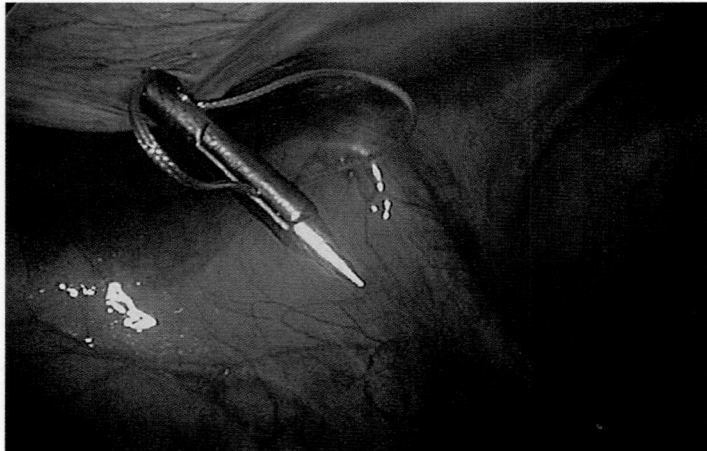

**FIGURE 115–7** This figure demonstrates the insertion of a fascial closure device (Karl Storz GmbH & Co KG, Tuttlingen, Germany) to close the defect. The suture is grasped within the instrument and is pushed through the superior part of the fascial defect.

# CHAPTER 116

# Diagnostic Laparoscopy

*Tommaso Falcone* ■ *Mark D. Walters*

## Standard Diagnostic Laparoscopy

Diagnostic laparoscopy should be performed at the beginning of all endoscopic procedures; therefore a systematic evaluation of the peritoneal cavity should be performed. This is especially important prior to laparoscopic management of an adnexal mass.

Generally, a right-handed surgeon should stand to the left of the patient (Fig. 116–1). The assistant stands on the right, and the scrub nurse or technician stands in between the legs. After insertion of the primary trocars, the patient is placed in Trendelenburg's position, and the peritoneal cavity is inspected to confirm that there is no contraindication to a laparoscopic procedure. If excrescences appear on the peritoneal surfaces or if an adnexal mass is present that is suspicious for malignancy, a laparotomy should be performed. If there is any active bleeding that is not clearly identified and easily controlled, a laparotomy should be performed.

It is difficult to perform a complete diagnostic evaluation without an accessory port. A suprapubic site is adequate for most diagnostic pelvic procedures. A suggested order of evaluation is:

- Panoramic view of the pelvis (Fig. 116–2)
- Cecum, appendix, and ascending colon (Fig. 116–3)
- Liver, gallbladder, and right hemidiaphragm (Fig. 116–4)
- Transverse colon, omentum, small bowel, and peritoneal surfaces (Fig. 116–5)
- Stomach, left hemidiaphragm, and descending colon and spleen (Fig. 116–6)
- Sigmoid and rectum (Fig. 116–7)

The spleen usually is not seen except in thin women or when traction is placed on the omentum.

A detailed view of the pelvic organs is obtained. A probe should be used to lift the ovaries so that a view of the ovarian fossa is obtained as well (Fig. 116–8).

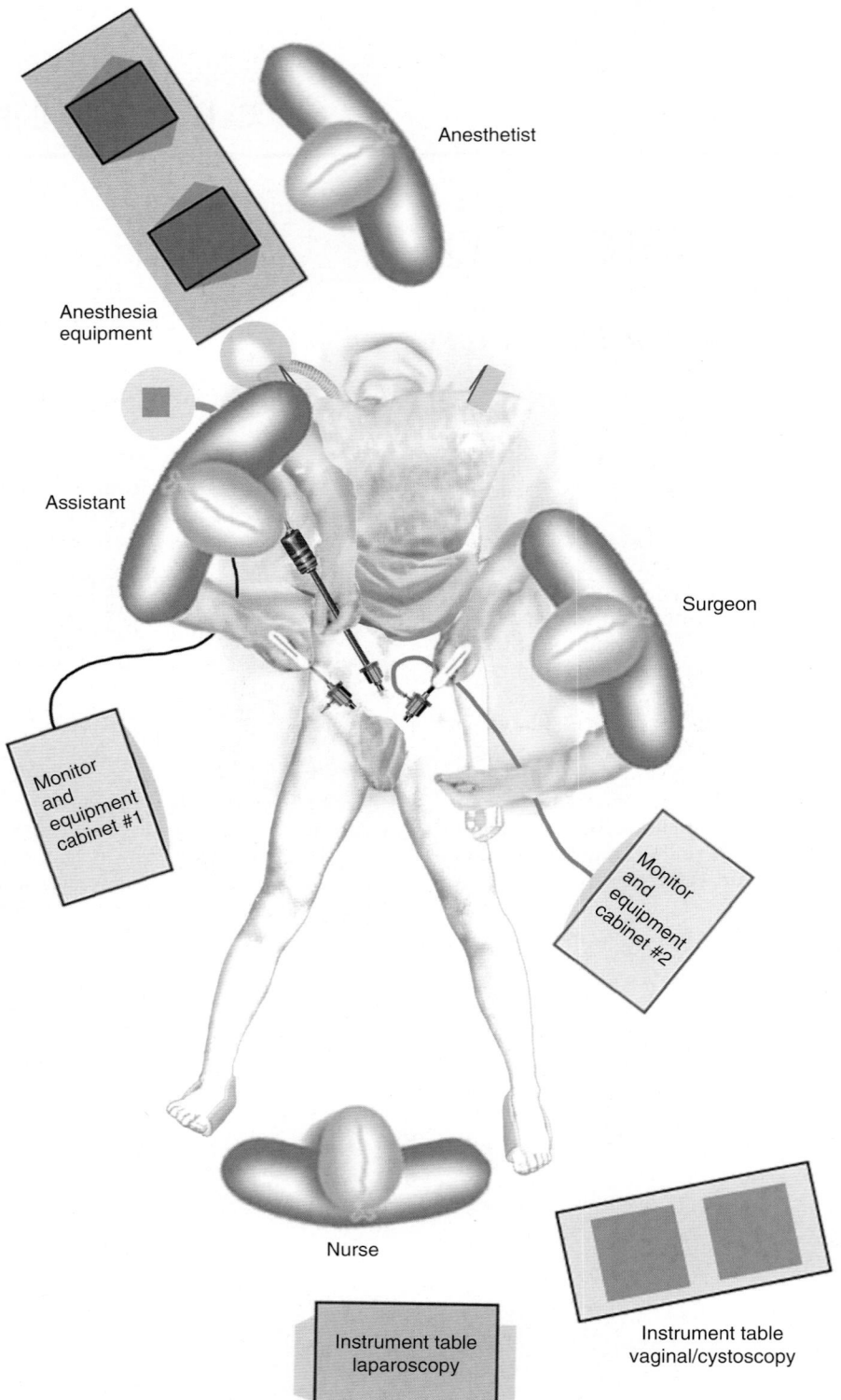

**FIGURE 116–1** Personnel placement during diagnostic laparoscopy.

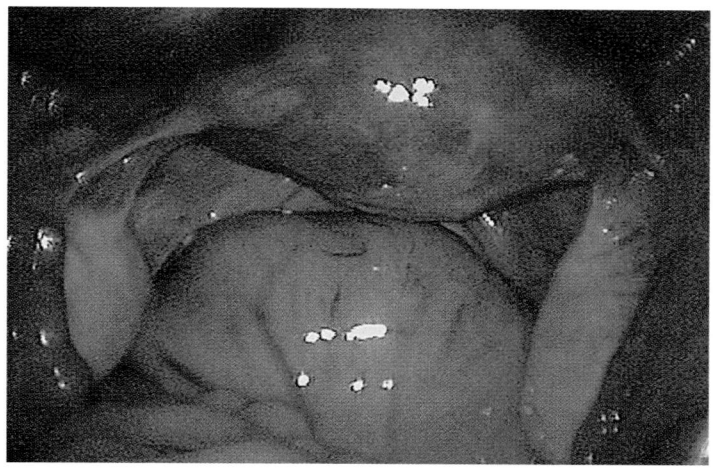

**FIGURE 116–2** Panoramic view of the pelvis.

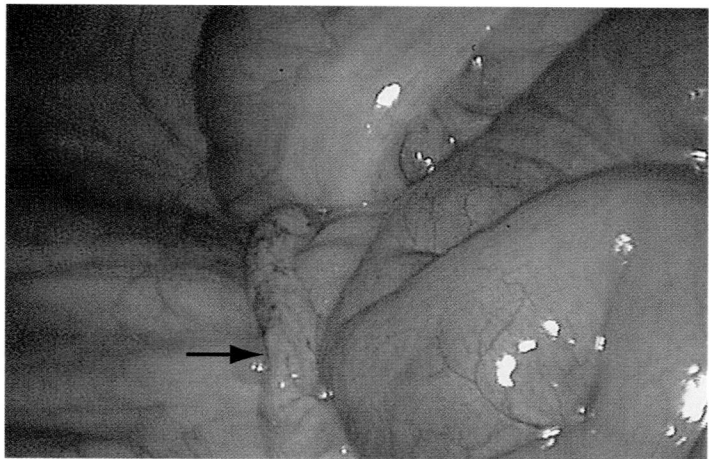

**FIGURE 116–3** Cecum, appendix (*arrow*), and ascending colon.

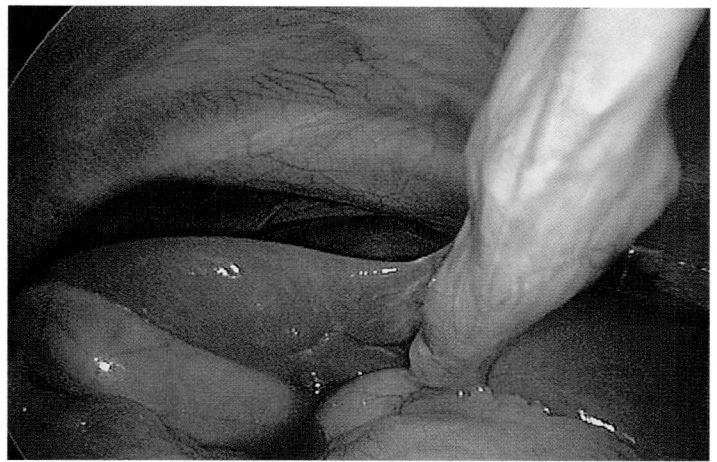

**FIGURE 116–4** Liver, gallbladder, and right hemidiaphragm.

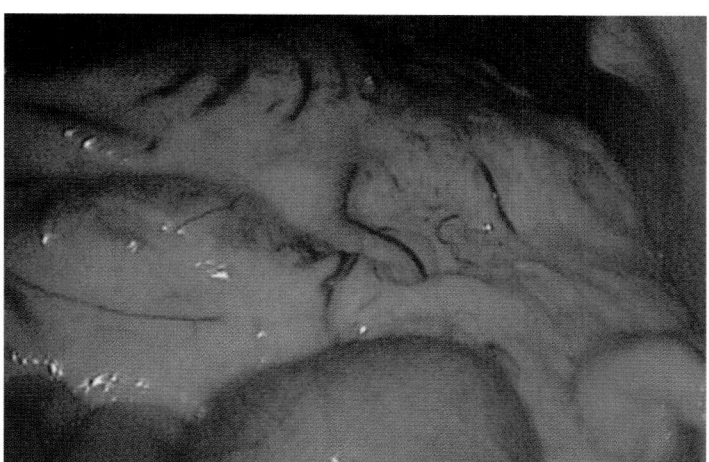

**FIGURE 116–5** Transverse colon, omentum, small bowel, and peritoneal surfaces.

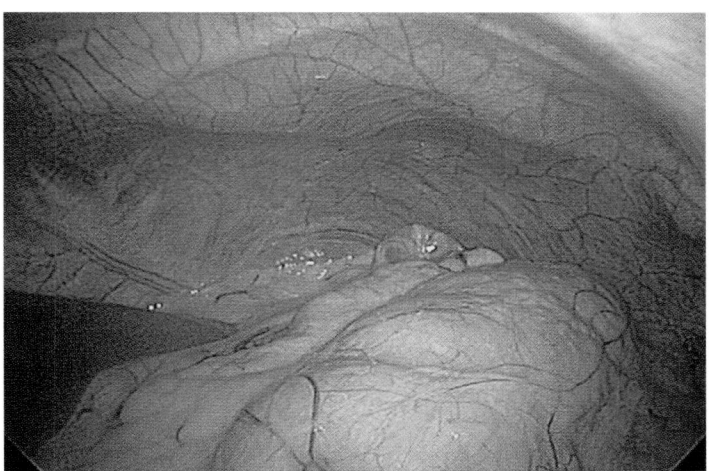

**FIGURE 116–6** Stomach, left hemidiaphragm, and descending colon; the spleen usually is not seen except in thin women or when traction is placed on the omentum. In this patient, the tip of the spleen is seen.

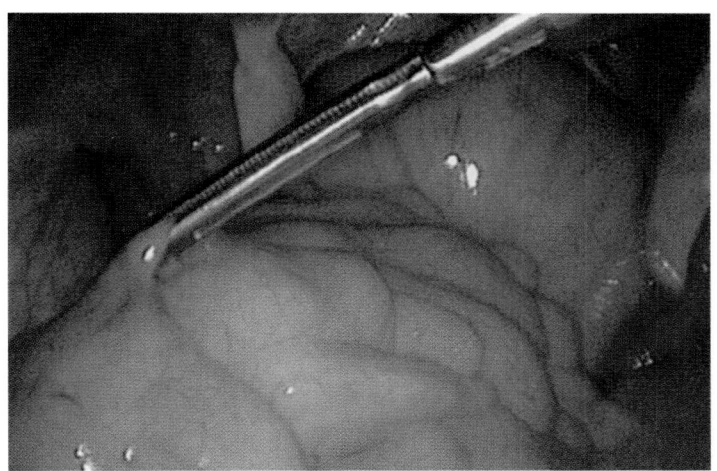

**FIGURE 116–7** An atraumatic clamp grasps the fat around the sigmoid colon.

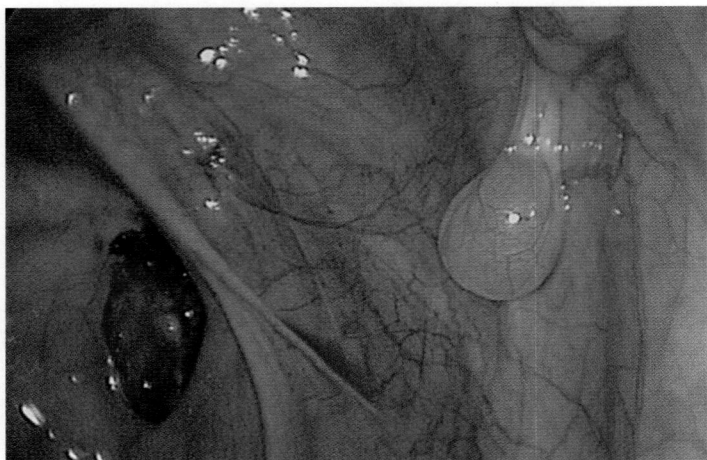

**FIGURE 116–8** A probe should be used to lift the ovaries to obtain a view of the ovarian fossa. An endometriotic lesion can be seen on the peritoneum, and a paratubal cyst on the fallopian tube. The ureter can be identified transperitoneally.

## Microlaparoscopy

The evolution of surgery toward a more minimally invasive approach has promoted technology that emphasizes smaller-caliber instruments. *Microlaparoscopy* refers to some of the applications of this technology; the most widely used of these is for diagnostic procedures, especially for infertility and chronic pelvic pain. These procedures can be performed with the patient under local anesthesia or conscious sedation.

Instruments used for this procedure range from 1.3 to 4 mm in diameter. The diagnostic accuracy of these smaller laparoscopes has received mixed reviews. A 5-mm laparoscope was found to give the best visualization. If this procedure is performed in an office setting, then a thorough knowledge of local anesthetic agents and sedatives is mandatory. We currently perform this procedure in an operating room setting with an anesthesiologist administering the sedation. The patient is conscious throughout the procedure. The following steps are required:

- The patient applies a local anesthetic cream (like EMLA cream) to the umbilical and suprapubic areas 2 hours before surgery.
- The patient empties her bladder before coming into the room.
- Intravenous access is obtained.
- The patient is brought into a procedure/operating room. The lights are dimmed.
- The abdomen and the vagina are prepared and draped in the usual manner.
- A paracervical block is performed, and a uterine manipulator is inserted.
- Local anesthesia is infiltrated in the umbilical area.
- The abdominal wall is elevated, and the primary trocar is inserted (Fig. 116–9).
- Insufflation is performed so as to maintain an adequate field. In this way, the carbon dioxide ($CO_2$) is insufflated with a pressure range of 15 mm Hg but is turned on and off to establish and maintain the appropriate visual field (Fig. 116–10).

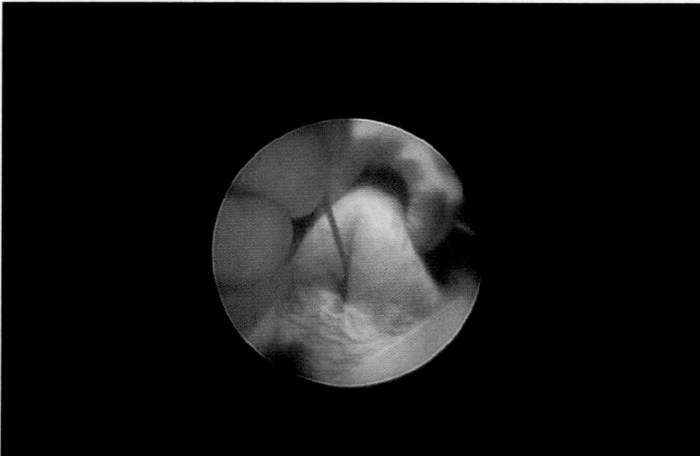

**FIGURE 116–9** The abdomen is elevated and a 2-mm introducer (Autosuture MiniPort Disposable Introducer, US Surgical, Norwalk, Connecticut) is inserted.

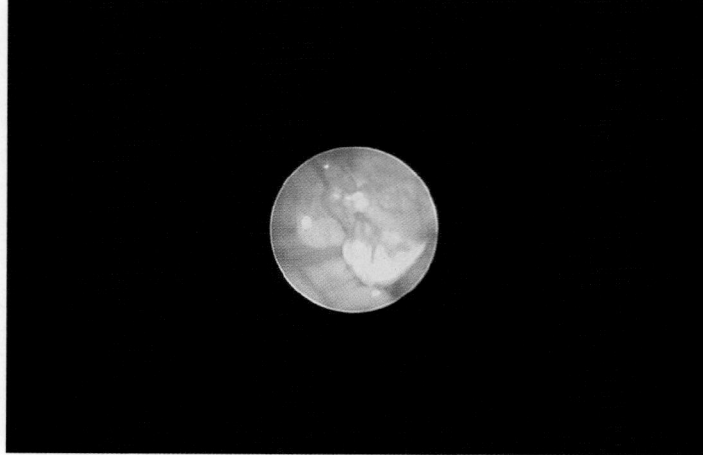

**FIGURE 116–10** View of the pelvis from a 2-mm laparoscope (Autosuture).

# Laparoscopic-Assisted Vaginal Hysterectomy

*Tommaso Falcone* ■ *Mark D. Walters*

Laparoscopic-assisted vaginal hysterectomy (LAVH) was introduced in the past 20 years as an alternative to abdominal hysterectomy. LAVH is a safe alternative to abdominal hysterectomy when a vaginal hysterectomy is contraindicated. In a prospective randomized clinical trial of LAVH versus abdominal hysterectomy at the Cleveland Clinic Foundation, LAVH was shown to be associated with less postoperative pain, shorter hospital stays, and a more rapid return to normal activities and work than abdominal hysterectomy.

There are several classifications of laparoscopic hysterectomy. The laparoscopic ligation of the uterine artery appears to be the critical step that differentiates a laparoscopic procedure from a laparoscopic-assisted one. In fact, this division is arbitrary. In practice, the procedure is continued laparoscopically until the surgeon is confident that the procedure can be completed vaginally. Ligation of the uterine artery by laparoscopy does not necessarily imply a more difficult case or one requiring more skill. Often the term is meant to convey to the operating room staff whether a vaginal table should be ready for the case.

We do not give oral antibiotics or preoperative bowel preparation. The patient is given a single dose of intravenous antibiotic, usually a cephalosporin, before the procedure. Pneumatic compression stockings are placed on the calves. An orogastric tube is used if stomach distention is suspected. Examination under anesthesia is carried out, and a Foley catheter is inserted.

A standard three-port technique is used: one umbilical and one in each lower quadrant. One of the lower ports is a 10-mm site for introduction of an electrocoagulating/cutting device such as a Seitzinger tripolar cutting forceps (Cabot Medical, Langhorne, Pennsylvania). We use the electrosurgical device set at 50W pure cut current.

We use a Hulka tenaculum as our uterine manipulator. A useful instrument for a total laparoscopic hysterectomy is a Koh colpotomizer (CooperSurgical Inc, Trumbull, Connecticut). This rigid cone fits on the RUMI uterine manipulator (CooperSurgical) and fits snugly on the cervix. It serves to delineate the fornices of the vagina that will be incised laparoscopically. This apparatus also has a balloon that will prevent escape of carbon

dioxide through the vagina. The vaginal table should include vaginal wall retractors and long instruments. At the end of the case a cystoscopy is performed. The bladder should be distended to check for injury. Intravenous indigo carmine also can be used to verify the integrity of the ureters.

The technique of LAVH is as follows: The round ligament is electrocoagulated and transected (Fig. 117-1). The uterus is pulled to the opposite side. The incision from the round ligament is carried cephalad to open the retroperitoneal space lateral to the ovarian vessels (Fig. 117-2) and caudad to incise the bladder peritoneum. The ureter is then identified and kept in view. A peritoneal window is made (Fig. 117-3). The ovarian vessels are grasped and electrocoagulated (Fig. 117-4). The bladder peritoneum is then dissected downward until the vagina is identified (Figs. 117-5 and 117-6). The uterine artery is identified and electrocoagulated (Figs. 117-7 through 117-9). The process is repeated on the opposite side. A sponge forceps is placed in the vagina in the anterior fornix, and the vagina is tented upward (Fig. 117-10). An incision is made circumferentially around the vagina (Fig. 117-11). After removal of the uterus through the vagina, carbon dioxide ($CO_2$) may escape through the vagina. If the Koh colpotomizer is used, the balloon will prevent this. If not, the vagina can be packed. The vault is then sutured with 0 Vicryl on a CT-1 needle (Fig. 117-12). Three to four interrupted stitches are placed and tied extracorporeally. A McCall's culdoplasty is generally performed.

The patient is usually discharged within 24 hours. Some patients can return to work as early as 1 week after surgery, but most require 4 weeks of convalescence.

If the ovaries are conserved, surgery starts with occlusion and transection of the utero-ovarian ligaments. This can be accomplished with bipolar energy or with a stapling device (Figs. 117-13 and 117-14). However, the use of a stapling device is not cost effective.

If a supracervical hysterectomy is performed, the specimen will require morcellation (Fig. 117-15). The morcellator device usually requires a 10/12-mm port. The cervical stump is closed, and the bladder peritoneum is sutured over it (Fig. 117-16).

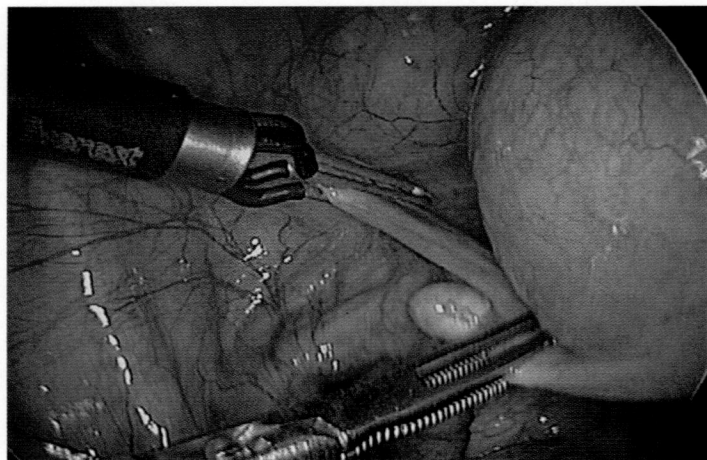

**FIGURE 117–1** The round ligament is grasped, electrocoagulated, and cut.

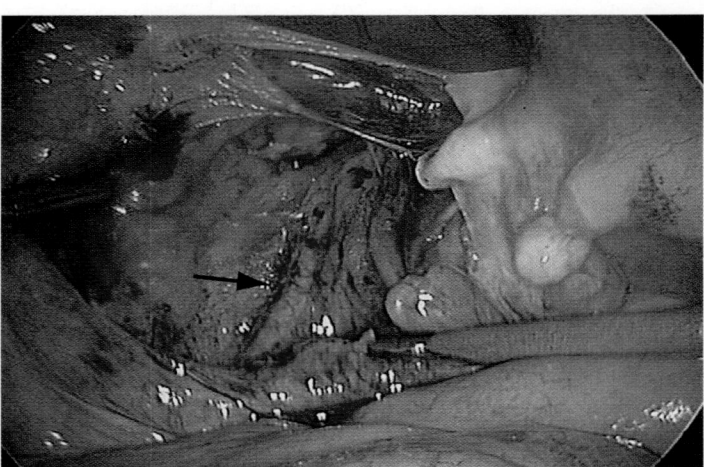

**FIGURE 117–2** The retroperitoneal space is dissected, and the ureter is identified (*arrow*).

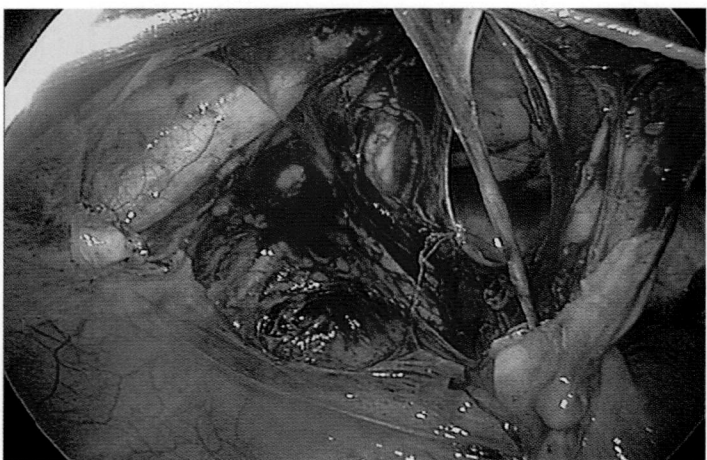

**FIGURE 117–3** A window is made in the medial leaf of the broad ligament above the ureter.

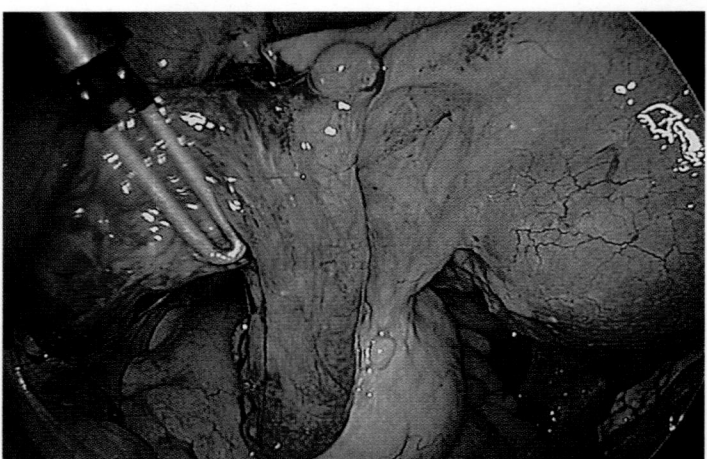

**FIGURE 117–4** The ovarian vessels are grasped and electrocoagulated.

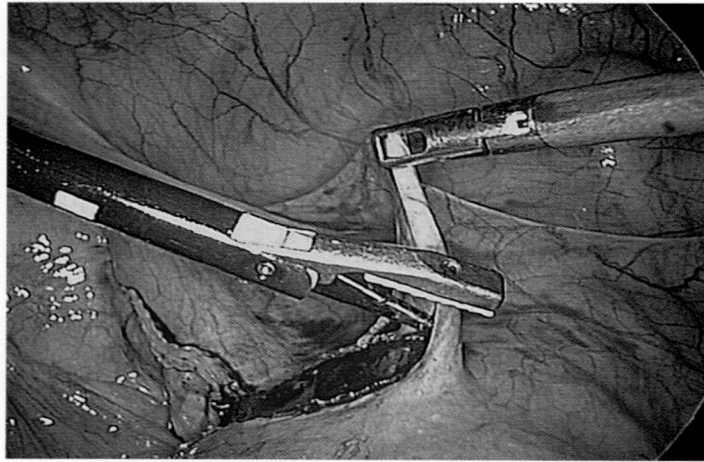

**FIGURE 117–5** The bladder peritoneum can be dissected downward with a harmonic energy device (Ultrashears, US Surgical, Norwalk, Connecticut).

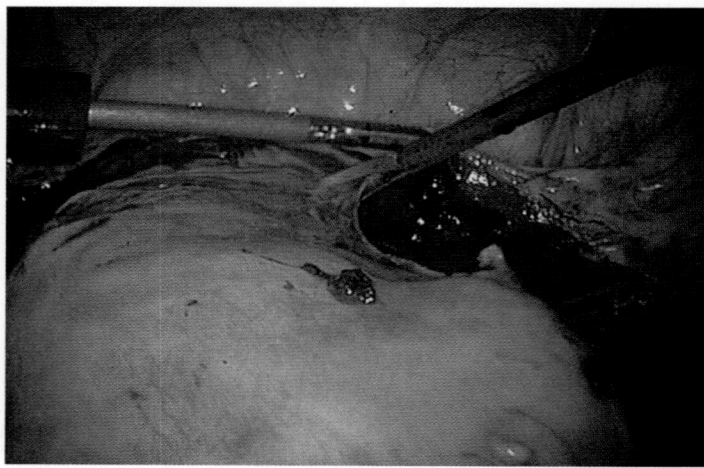

**FIGURE 117–6** The bladder peritoneum can be dissected downward with scissors using electrosurgery.

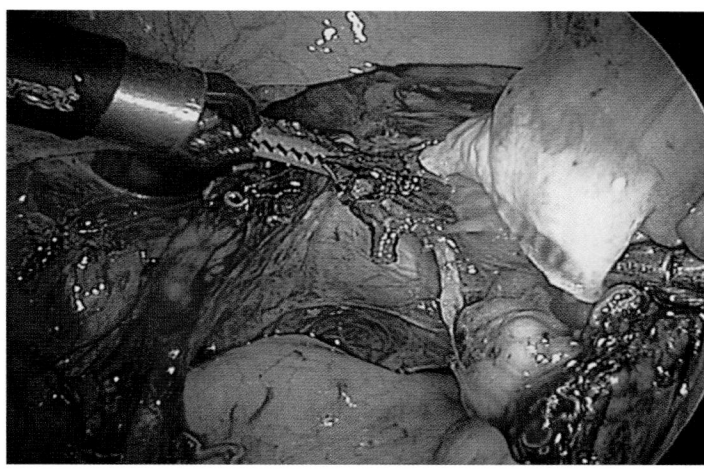

FIGURE 117–7 The uterine artery is identified along the uterus and is electrocoagulated and cut.

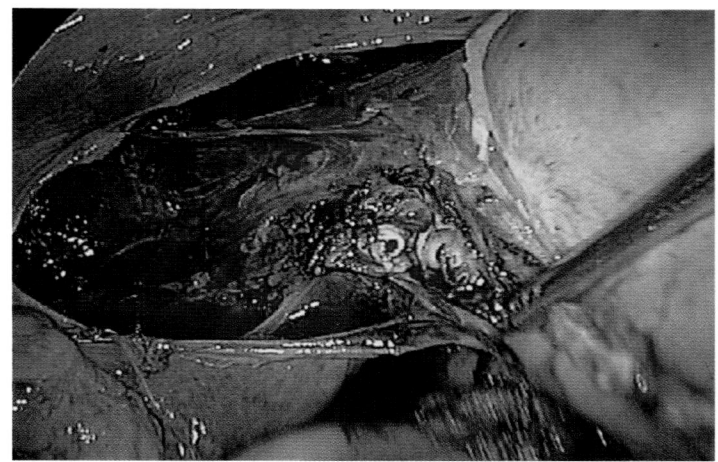

FIGURE 117–8 The transected uterine artery is seen.

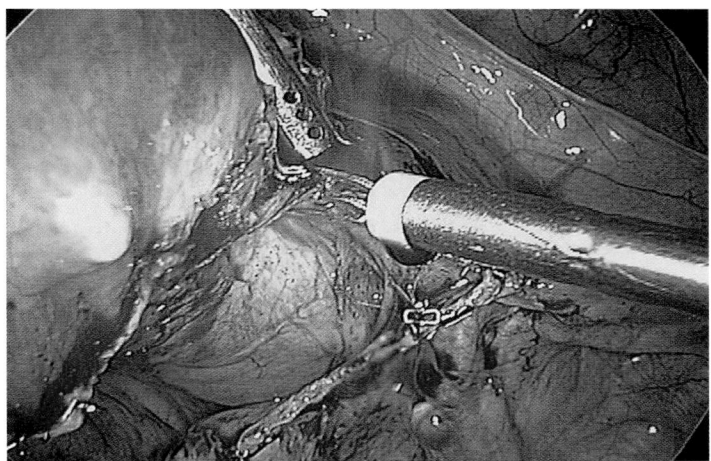

FIGURE 117–9 The procedure is repeated on the other side using a bipolar cautery.

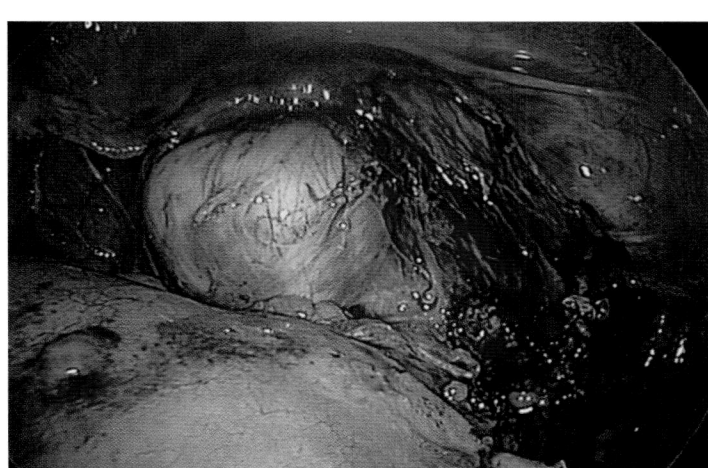

FIGURE 117–10 The vagina is tented upward with a sponge stick in the vagina.

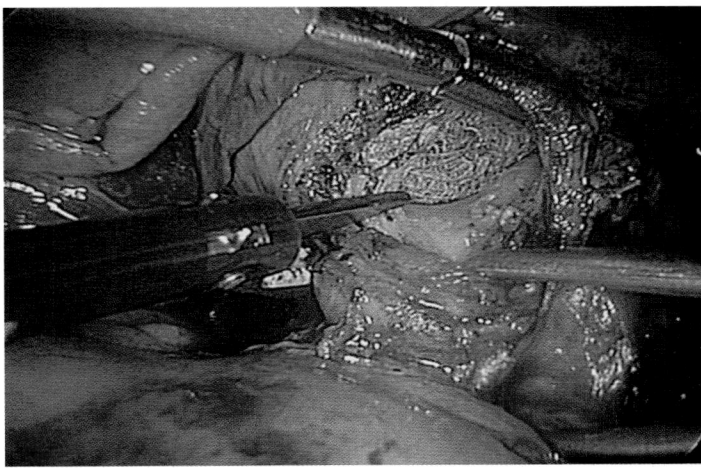

FIGURE 117–11 The vagina is then incised. In this case, harmonic energy is used (Ultrashears, US Surgical, Norwalk, Connecticut). Note that a laparoscopic tenaculum on the cervix moves the specimen around. Note the sponge in the vagina to prevent escape of carbon dioxide.

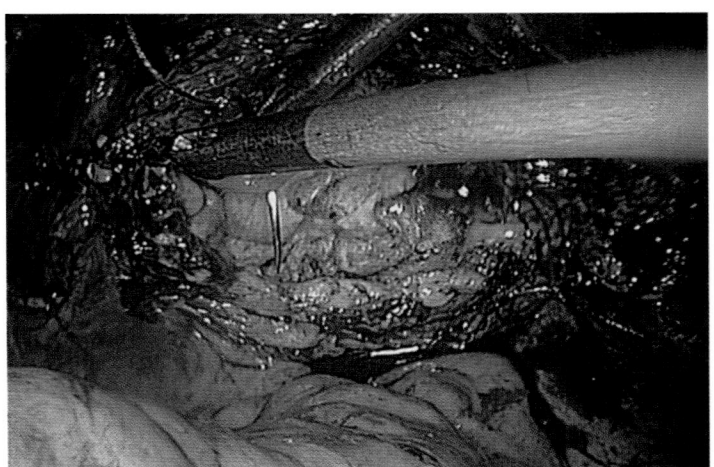

FIGURE 117–12 The vagina is closed with 0 Vicryl on a CT-1 needle. Note the sponge in the vagina to prevent gas from escaping.

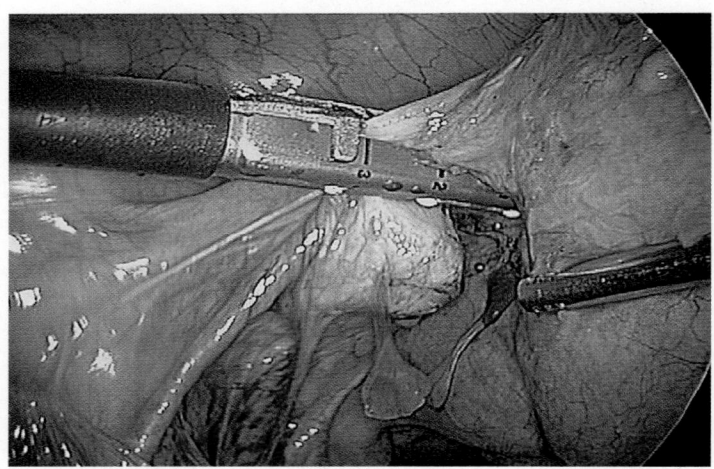

**FIGURE 117–13** A multifire Endo GIA (US Surgical, Norwalk, Connecticut) stapling device with a vascular cartridge has been applied across the utero-ovarian and round ligaments.

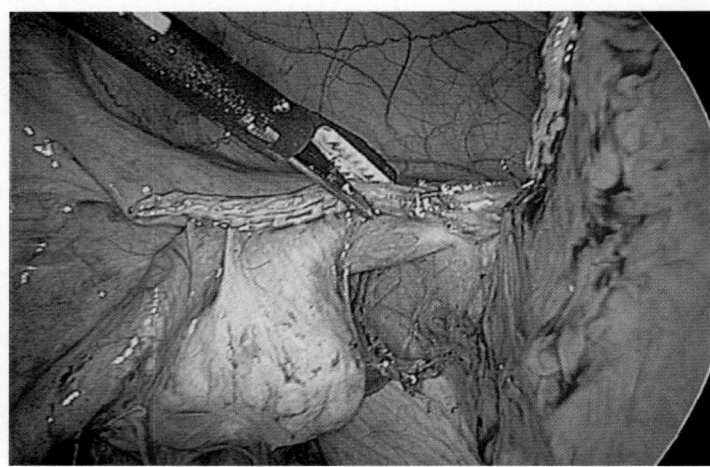

**FIGURE 117–14** The instrument has been fired and the transection site is examined for bleeding.

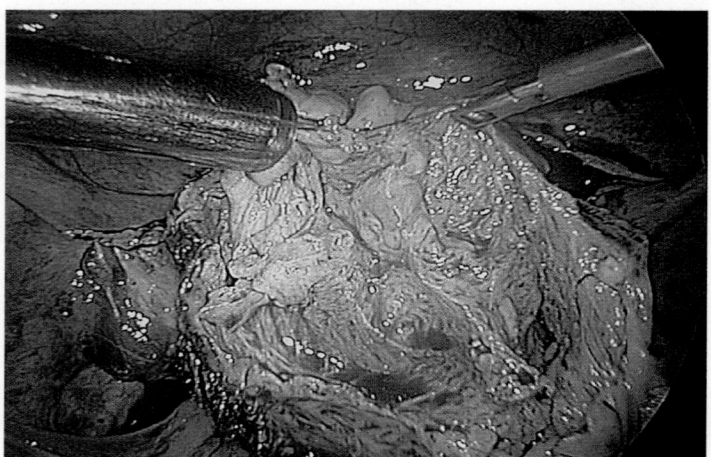

**FIGURE 117–15** A morcellator (Steiner Electromechanic Morcellator, Karl Storz GmbH & Co KG, Tuttlingen, Germany) has been introduced through a 10/12-mm port. The uterus is morcellated and is removed in pieces.

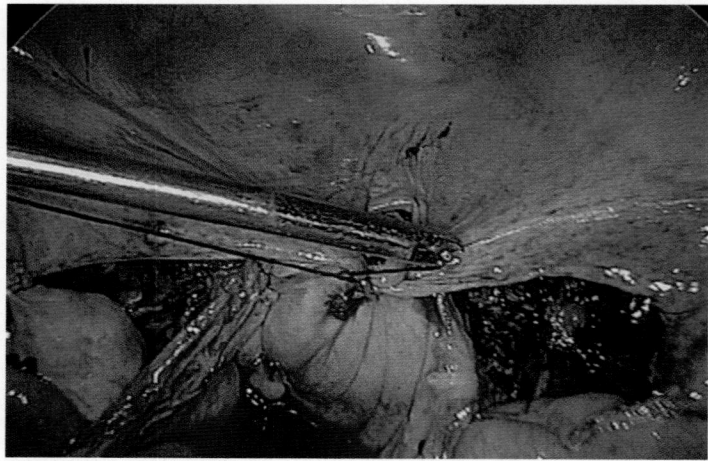

**FIGURE 117–16** The cervical stump is sutured closed and the bladder peritoneum is sutured to the peritoneum behind the cervix. A knot pusher is used for extracorporeal tying.

# CHAPTER 118

# Laparoscopic Adnexal Surgery

*Tommaso Falcone* ■ *Mark D. Walters*

## Ovarian Cystectomy

Ovarian cystectomy is the treatment of choice for the conservative management of ovarian cysts presumed to be benign. Simple aspiration is associated with a high recurrence rate, and cyst fluid cytology is unreliable. Transvaginal ultrasonography is used to evaluate an ovarian cyst. High-risk criteria on ultrasonography for predicting the pathologic diagnosis, such as a cystic-solid mass or ascites, are a contraindication to laparoscopic surgery unless a dermoid or endometriosis is suspected. A preoperative CA-125 level is useful in postmenopausal, but not in premenopausal, women. The same principle applies to Doppler flow assessment. Magnetic resonance imaging (MRI) does not help in distinguishing a malignant from a benign mass.

An attempt should be made to remove the cyst without rupture. Equivalent rates of rupture are found with laparotomy and laparoscopy. Rupture of a dermoid cyst does not appear to be associated with any short-term complications if copious irrigation is used. Intraoperative rupture of stage I ovarian carcinomas does not appear to affect prognosis.

The patient should have consented to a laparotomy if a cancer is found. Pneumatic compression stockings are placed on the calves. An orogastric tube is used if stomach distention is suspected. An examination is carried out with the patient under anesthesia, and a Foley catheter is inserted.

To perform ovarian cystectomy, the standard three-puncture technique is used. The peritoneal cavity is systematically assessed as described in Chapter 116. Peritoneal fluid should be obtained for cytology. If no excrescences or peritoneal signs of malignancy are present, the surgeon can proceed with the cystectomy.

The ovarian cortex is coagulated, and an incision is made (Fig. 118–1). The edge of the cortex is grasped with an Allis forceps and dissected from the cyst. The cyst can be separated from the cortex with blunt dissection using the suction-irrigation device (Fig. 118–2). The cyst is then enucleated from the ovary (Fig. 118–3) and is placed into the anterior cul-de-sac (Fig. 118–4). Bipolar cautery is used to achieve hemostasis from any blood vessels encountered. Once the cyst is ready to be removed from the peritoneal cavity, it is placed in a bag (Fig. 118–5). The bag is then brought up to the skin, and the cyst decompressed within it (Fig. 118–6). The cyst can then be morcellated out of the bag. The ovarian cortex is not usually closed, but a simple suture can be applied to close a deep defect.

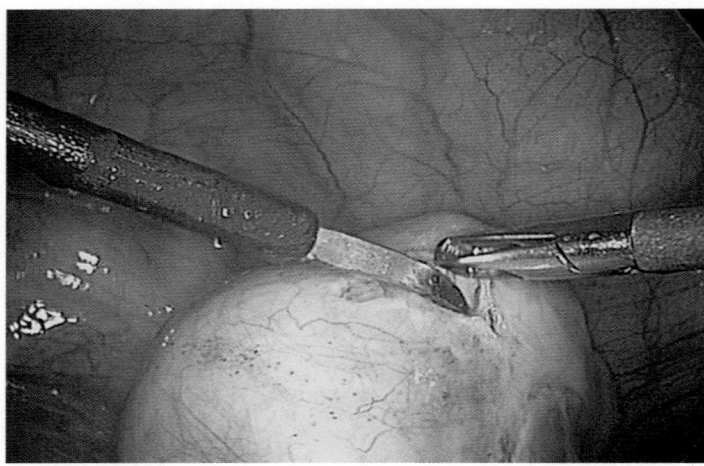

**FIGURE 118–1** The ovarian cortex is coagulated and incised.

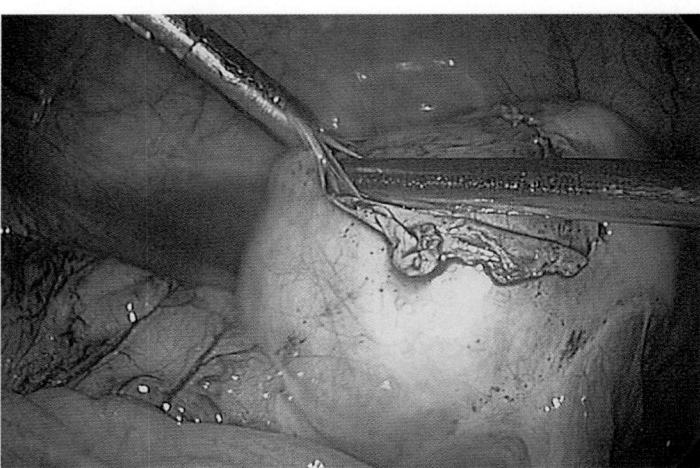

**FIGURE 118–2** A suction-irrigation device is used to get a plane of dissection between the cortex of the ovary and the cyst.

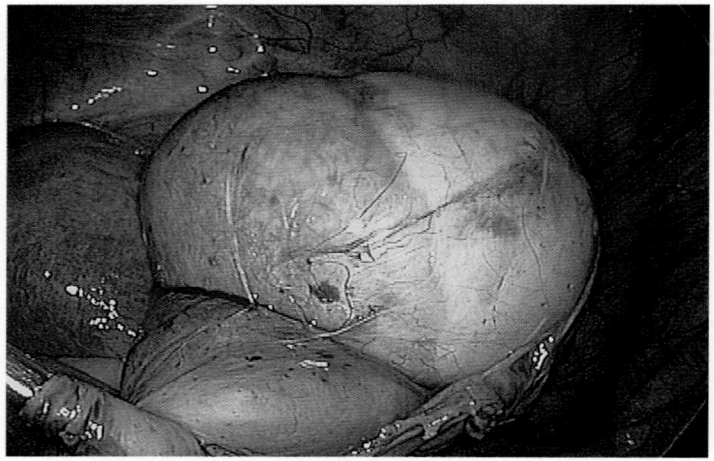

**FIGURE 118–3** The cyst is dissected from the ovary with a traction-countertraction technique.

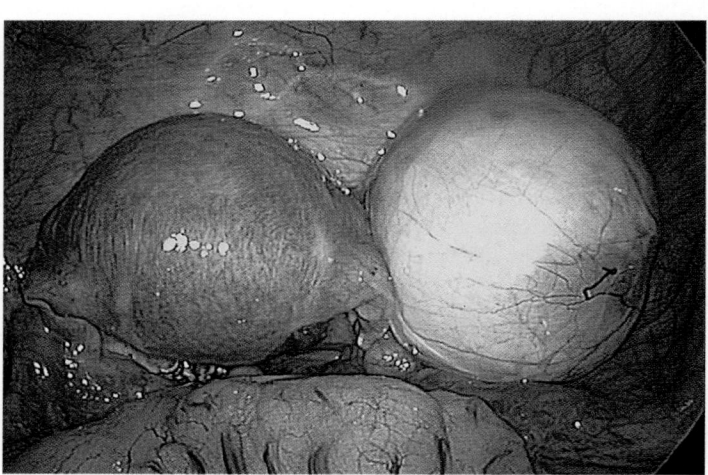

**FIGURE 118–4** The cyst is placed in the cul-de-sac so that the ovary can be inspected for bleeding.

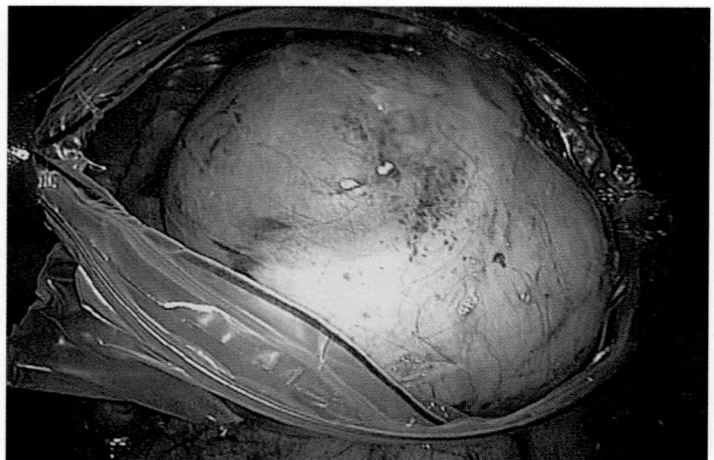

**FIGURE 118–5** The cyst is placed in the bag prior to removal.

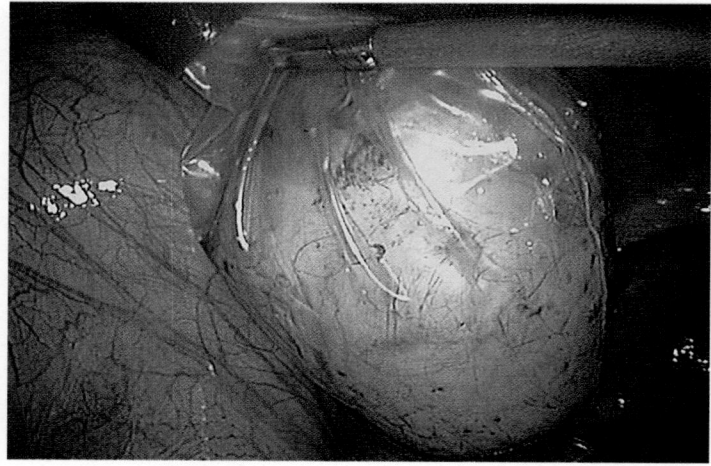

**FIGURE 118–6** The bag is brought through a port site. Most of the bag remains within the peritoneal cavity. The cyst is ruptured within the bag, the contents suctioned, and the solid parts removed in pieces.

## Salpingo-oophorectomy

A salpingo-oophorectomy is the treatment of choice for ovarian cysts found in perimenopausal and postmenopausal women because the chance of rupture is reduced substantially. The same preoperative and intraoperative preparation as for the cystectomy is performed prior to a salpingo-oophorectomy. A retroperitoneal approach is recommended.

The technique of ovarian salpingo-oophorectomy is as follows. The peritoneum is incised lateral to the ovarian vessels, and the retroperitoneal space is identified (Fig. 118–7). Blunt dissection is used to identify the ureter that is attached to the medial leaf of the broad ligament (Fig. 118–8). A window is then made in the broad ligament above the ureter. The ovarian vessels are coagulated and cut (Fig. 118–9). The ureter is always identified before any coagulation is performed (Fig. 118–10). The utero-ovarian ligament is then coagulated and cut (Fig. 118–11). The specimen is placed in a bag. The anatomy of the retroperitoneal space is clearly seen at the end of the dissection (Fig. 118–12).

## Ectopic Pregnancy

Prospective randomized clinical trials have demonstrated an advantage of laparoscopy over laparotomy for treatment of ectopic pregnancy. Tubal rupture can make surgery for salvage of the tube more difficult; however, no preoperative criteria can predict tubal rupture, and therefore the surgeon should be prepared to proceed appropriately.

The use of dilute vasopressin helps ensure hemostasis and reduces the need for electrocautery; however, it should not be used in hypertensive patients. Salpingostomy can be performed for ampullary ectopic pregnancies. Closure of the tube is not required. An exclusively isthmic ectopic pregnancy is usually managed with partial salpingectomy and anastomosis. A total or partial salpingectomy is performed if the tube is damaged beyond repair, if the patient has had prior tubal surgery or previous ectopic pregnancy within the ipsilateral tube, or if fertility is no longer desired.

The technique of salpingostomy is as follows. A standard laparoscopy with three ports is used. If a large quantity of blood is present in the peritoneal cavity, a larger port (10 mm) should be inserted to aspirate with a 10-mm suction cannula.

If it is an unruptured ectopic pregnancy, dilute vasopressin (10 IU in 100 mL of saline solution) is injected subserosally into the mesosalpinx beneath the mass, as well as where the incision will be made (Fig. 118–13). The serosa on the antimesenteric side is coagulated. The tubal wall is incised with scissors (Fig. 118–14). Hydrodissection is used to facilitate removal of the products of conception (Fig. 118–15). The implantation site is irrigated and observed for hemostasis. Bleeding is controlled with bipolar cautery. The specimen is extracted through the 10-mm port (usually umbilical) with a 5-mm laparoscope inserted through a lower port.

For salpingectomy, a standard three-port technique is used. Adhesiolysis is performed and the tube freed. The proximal tube is electrocoagulated and cut (Figs. 118–16 and 118–17). The mesosalpinx is then serially coagulated and cut, staying close to the tube to avoid compromising the blood supply to the ovary (Fig. 118–18A, B). The specimen is removed through the 10-mm port.

Follow-up serum human chorionic gonadotropin (hCG) levels should be obtained weekly until the level is less than the threshold for the lab. Rh-negative patients should receive RhoGAM.

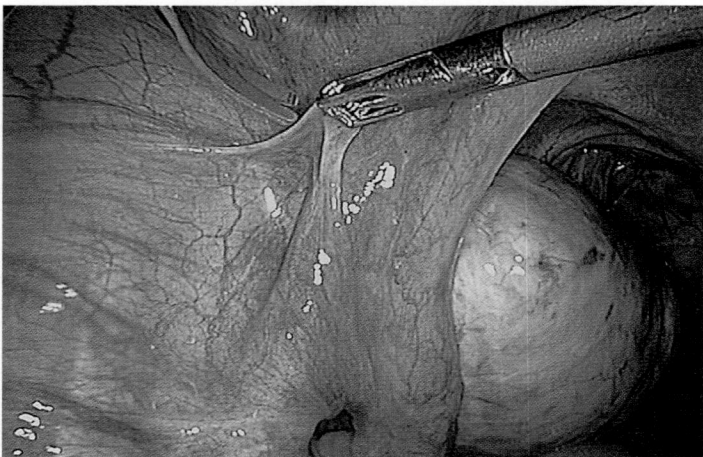

**FIGURE 118–7** The peritoneum lateral to the ovarian vessels and cephalad to the round ligament is grasped and incised.

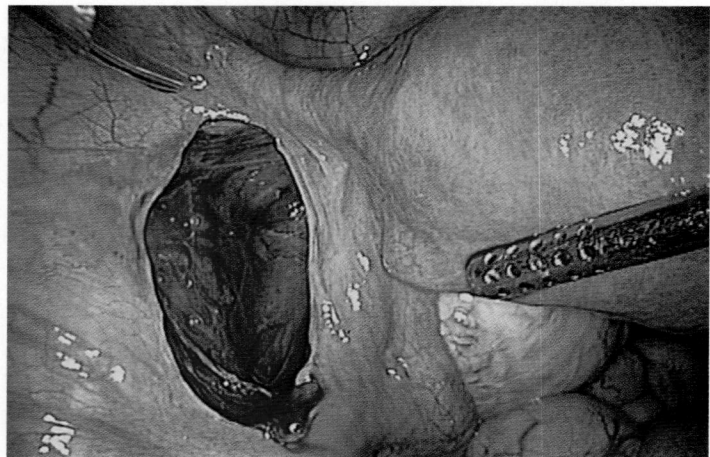

**FIGURE 118–8** The retroperitoneal space is dissected, and the ureter is identified.

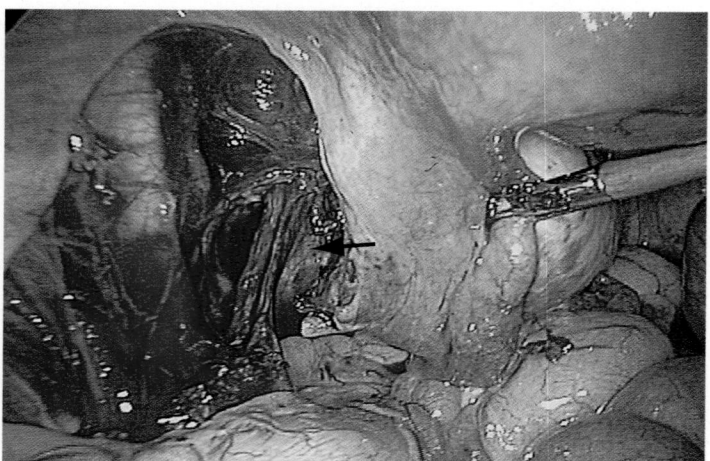

**FIGURE 118–9** The ovarian vessels are cauterized with bipolar cautery.

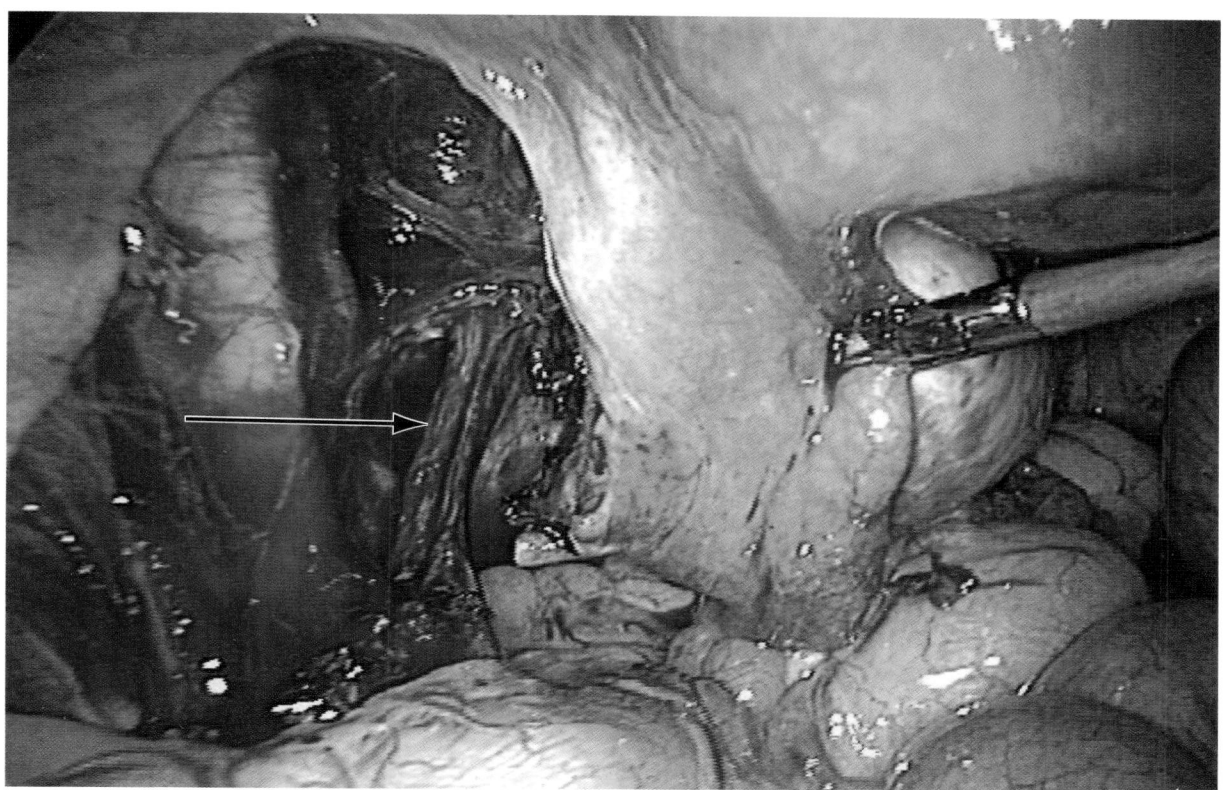

**FIGURE 118–10** The ureter (*arrow*) is always in view throughout the procedure.

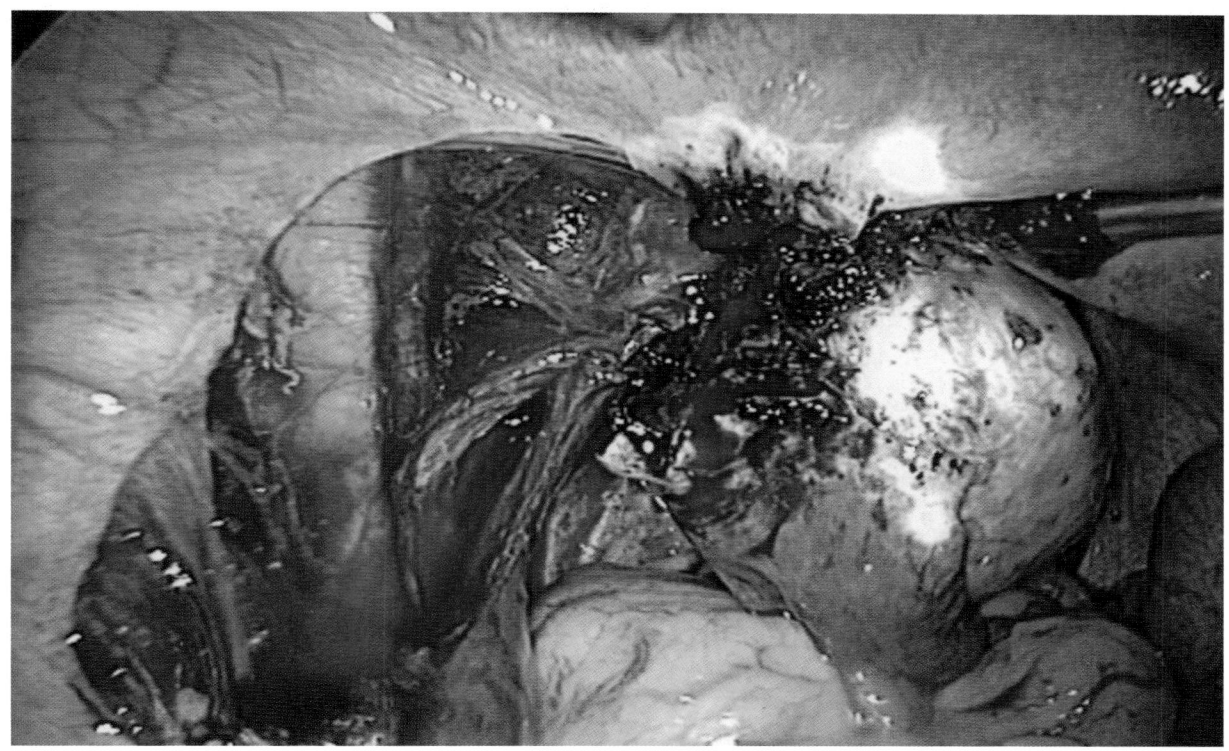

**FIGURE 118–11** The utero-ovarian ligament is coagulated.

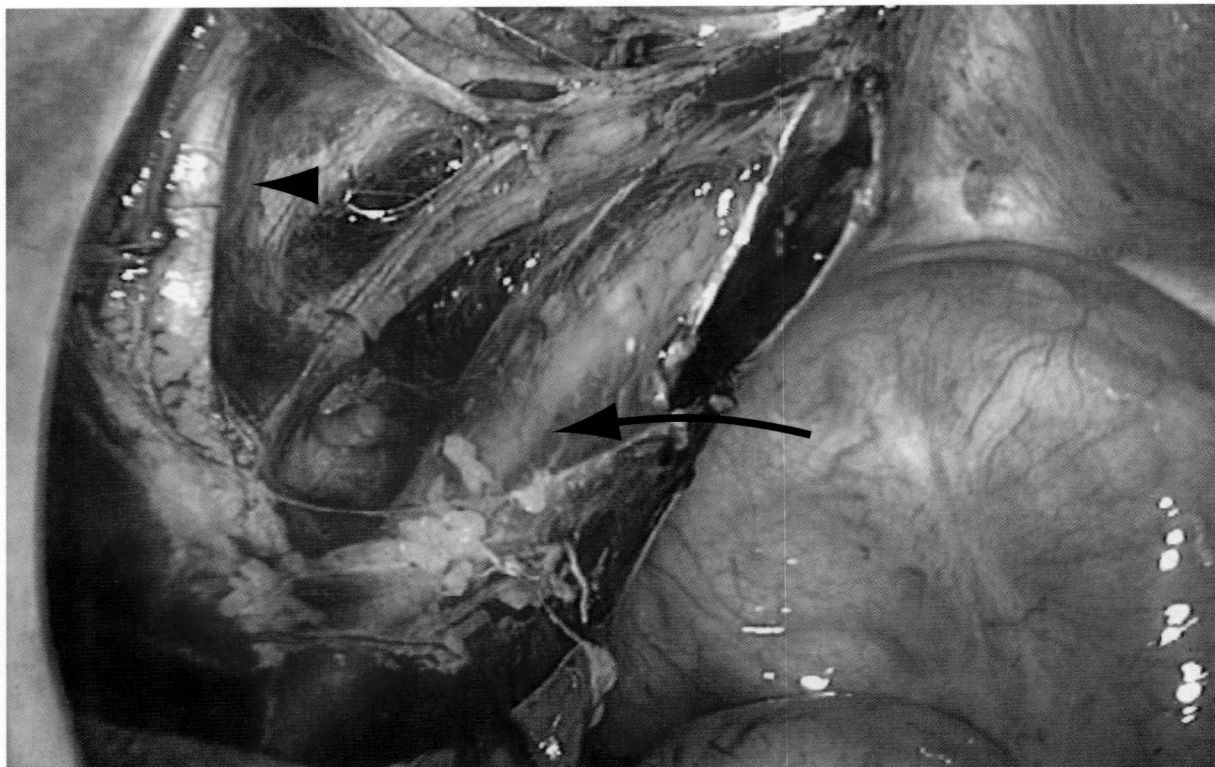

**FIGURE 118–12** The ureter is clearly seen (*arrow*). The internal iliac artery giving off the umbilical artery (*arrowhead*) and the uterine artery are seen. The uterine artery runs parallel to the ureter before crossing over it.

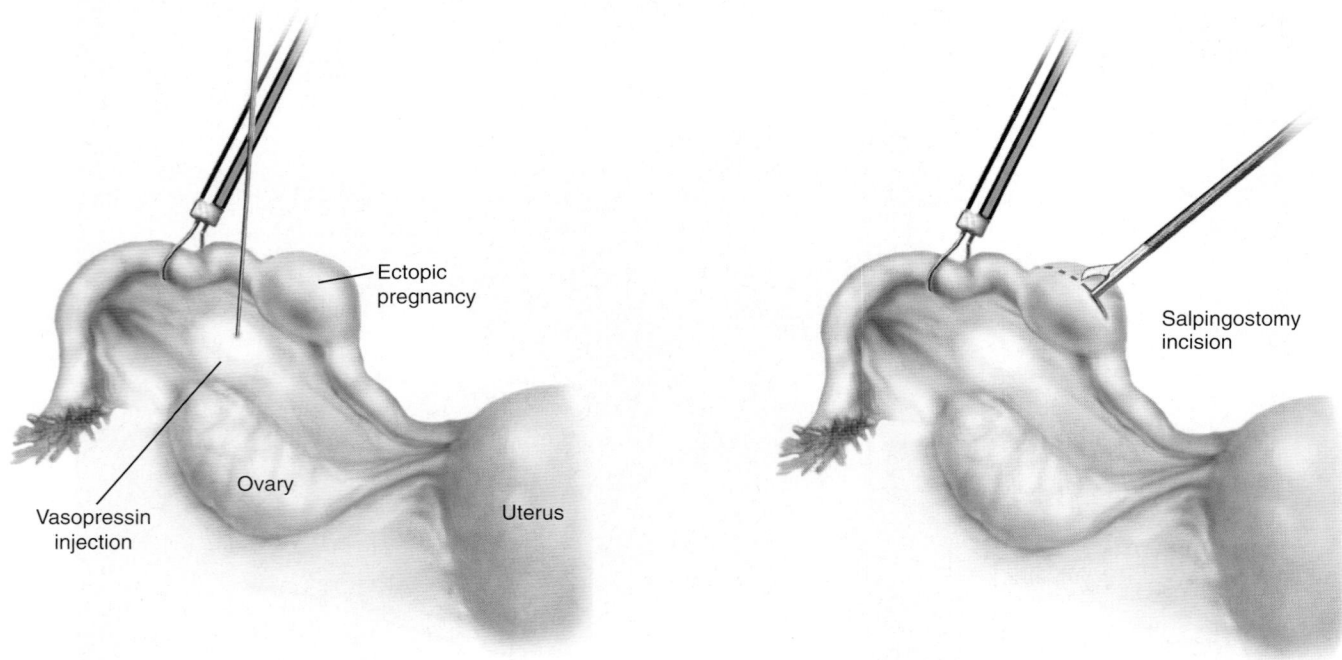

**FIGURE 118–13** Dilute vasopressin is injected into the mesosalpinx.

**FIGURE 118–14** An incision is made with scissors.

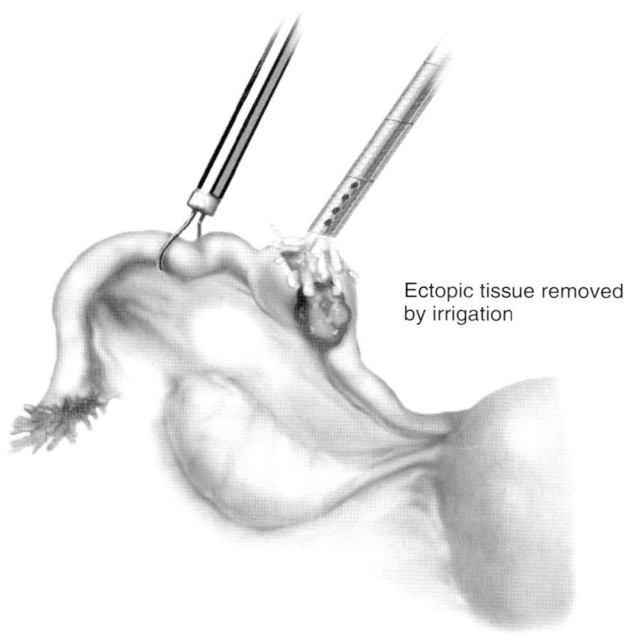

Ectopic tissue removed by irrigation

**FIGURE 118–15** An irrigation cannula is inserted into the ectopic area, and using hydrodissection, the pregnancy is delivered through the incision.

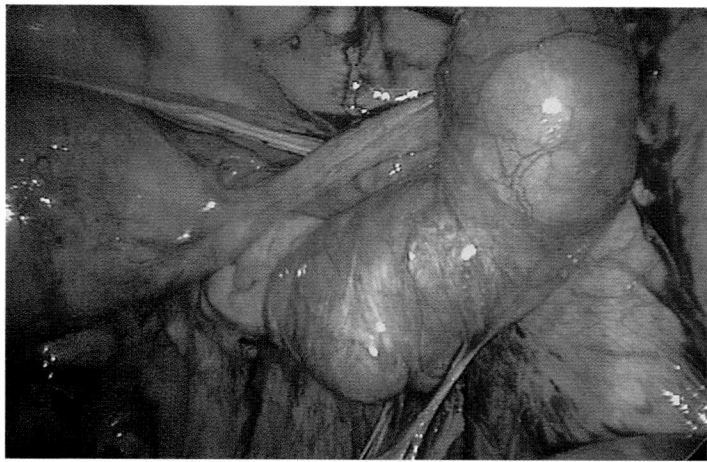

**FIGURE 118–16** A large tube is distended with an ectopic pregnancy.

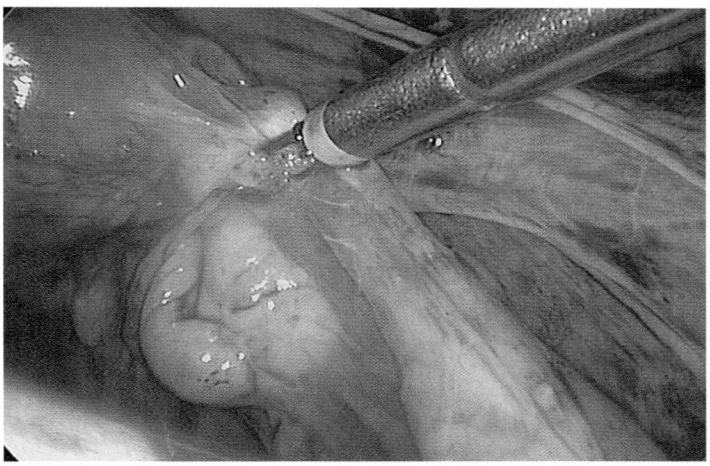

**FIGURE 118–17** The proximal tube is coagulated.

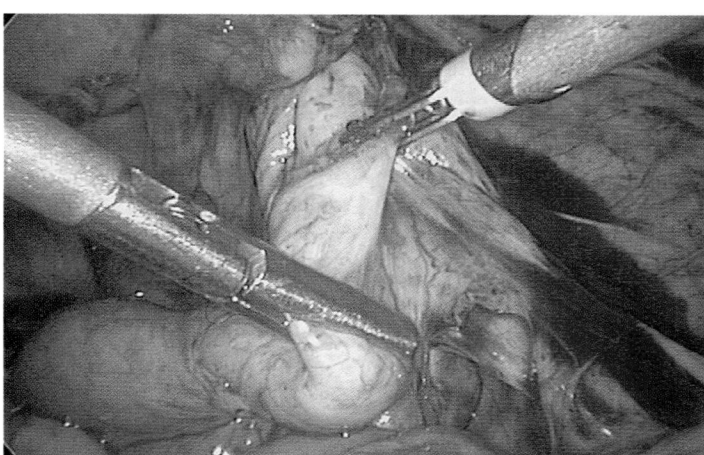

A

B

**FIGURE 118–18 A** and **B.** The mesosalpinx is serially coagulated and cut.

## Tubal Ligation

A tubal ligation can be performed with electrocautery, with the application of Silastic, Hulka, or Filshie clips. The fallopian tube is identified at the fimbriated end before proceeding with the tubal ligation.

For the electrocautery technique, the fallopian tube is cauterized 2 cm from the junction with a 40W cutting current. Two or three contiguous areas are cauterized (Fig. 118–19).

For the Falope ring technique, the tube is grasped 2 cm from the uterus with the applicator. The tube is drawn into the cylinder, and the band applied across a loop of it (Fig. 118–20). The applicator should be moved forward as the tube is brought into it, or the tube could be transected. At the end of the procedure, the loop of tube is inspected to ensure that two complete lumina are distal to the band.

With the clip technique, the tube is grasped 2 cm from the uterus with the applicator that has a clip already in place (Fig. 118–21). Once it is clear that the clip is applied across the entire tube, it is clamped down firmly. One clip per tube is sufficient.

## Tuboplasty

Patients with moderate to severe tubal disease by the American Fertility Society classification should usually be treated with in vitro fertilization rather than surgery. Infertility patients who are candidates for tubal surgery should have an assessment of the tube during hysterosalpingography or at the time of surgery. These criteria should be met:

- Thin-walled hydrosalpinges with mild dilation
- Minimal peritubal adhesions
- Preservation of mucosal folds

A fimbrioplasty is performed when fimbrial phimosis, a constriction of the distal tube, is present. A tuft of fimbriae may be extruding from the distal lumen. A neosalpingostomy is performed when the distal end of the tube is totally occluded.

Scissors should be used with no energy. Bipolar and microbipolar electrocautery should be used.

The technique for neosalpingostomy is as follows. The procedure is started with lysis of adhesions. The principles of traction and countertraction are used to develop tissue planes (Fig. 118–22). Chromotubation will dilate the distal tube. Dilute vasopressin is injected into the distal end. This will decrease the need for use of electrocautery. The tube is opened with scissors (Fig. 118–23). A cruciate incision is formed. A 4-0 to 5-0 reabsorbable suture is used to evert the edges. The suture goes through the mucosa from inside out and then through the serosa again distally (Fig. 118–24). It is tied intracorporeally. Usually two to three sutures are sufficient.

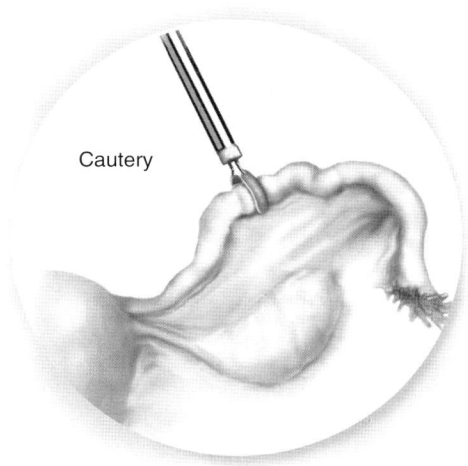

**FIGURE 118–19** A bipolar cautery grasps the tube and cauterizes two or three contiguous areas.

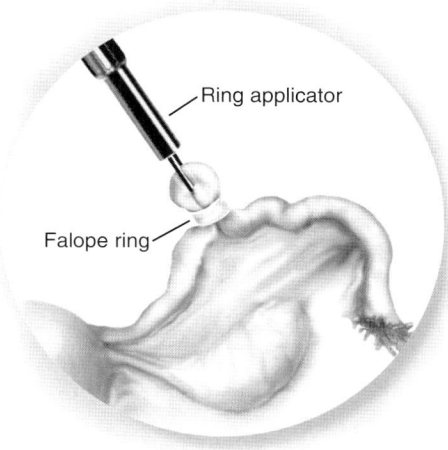

**FIGURE 118–20** A band is placed across a loop of tube.

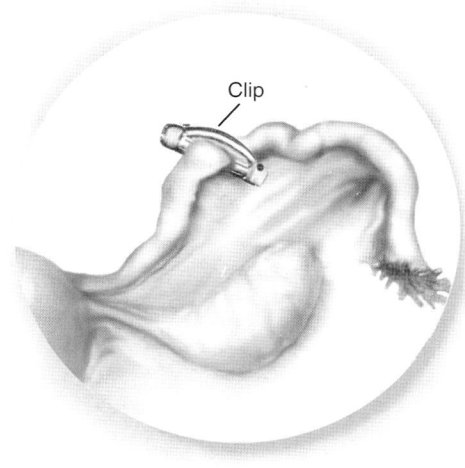

**FIGURE 118–21** A clip is placed across the entire tube.

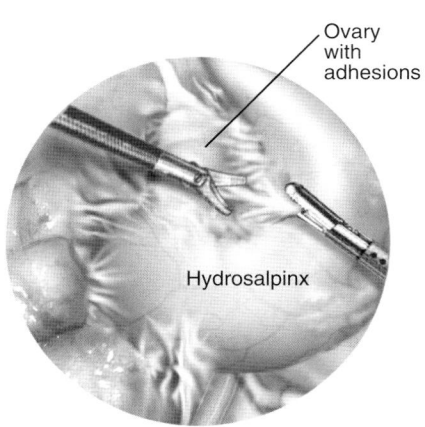

**FIGURE 118–22** Adhesions are excised with fine scissors using the principles of traction and countertraction.

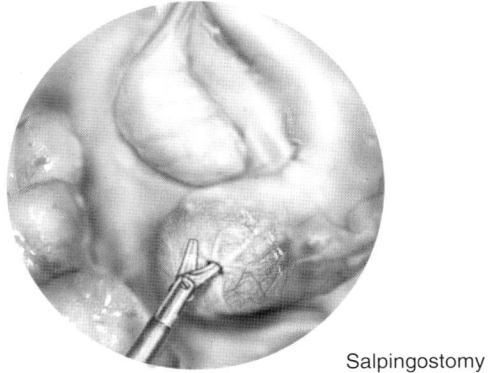

**FIGURE 118–23** The tube is distended with fluid, the vasopressin is injected, and a cruciate incision is made with scissors.

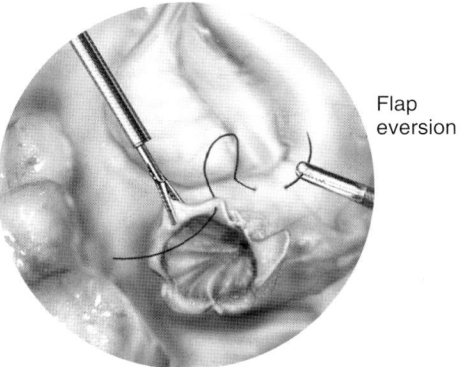

**FIGURE 118–24** The stitch goes from inside the lumen and out through the serosa; then the needle is inserted through the serosa of the tube a few millimeters away.

# CHAPTER 119

# Laparoscopic Surgery for Stress Urinary Incontinence (Burch Colposuspension)

*Mark D. Walters* ■ *Tommaso Falcone*

Laparoscopic Burch colposuspension is one of the primary surgical treatment options for stress urinary incontinence. Cure rates appear to be similar to open Burch colposuspension in most studies, although studies with long-term follow-up are not available. Several reviews of the literature on laparoscopic Burch colposuspension have been published.

Laparoscopic Burch colposuspension can be done using an extraperitoneal or an intraperitoneal approach. The intraperitoneal approach to the Burch colposuspension begins with insertion of the laparoscope through a 5- to 10-mm intraumbilical trocar, followed by intra-abdominal insufflation. Inspection of the peritoneal cavity is performed, delineating the inferior epigastric vessels, abdominal and pelvic organs, and any abdominal or pelvic pathology. Two additional trocars (5 mm and 5/12 mm) are placed under direct vision, one on each side in the lower abdomen.

The bladder is filled with 200 to 300 mL sterile water or saline. A probe can be used to press the base of the bladder upward so that the upper margin of the bladder is easily delineated (Fig. 119-1). Using sharp dissection with electrocautery or a harmonic scalpel, a transverse incision is made 2 cm above the bladder reflection between the median umbilical ligaments (Fig. 119-2). Blunt and sharp dissection aiming toward the posterior/superior aspect of the pubic symphysis decreases risk of bladder injury. Identification of the areolar tissue at the point of incision confirms a proper plane of dissection (Fig. 119-3). Blunt dissection is then carried out inferolaterally on both sides to identify the pubic symphysis, Cooper's ligaments, obturator internus muscles, arcus tendineus fasciae pelvis, and bladder neck (Fig. 119-4). Midline dissection over the urethra should be avoided.

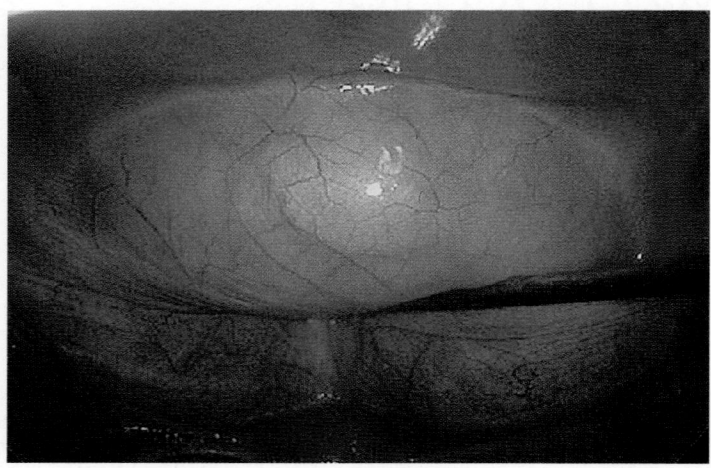

**FIGURE 119–1** The bladder is filled before the Burch colposuspension is begun. The upper margin of the bladder can be delineated by pressing up on the base of the bladder.

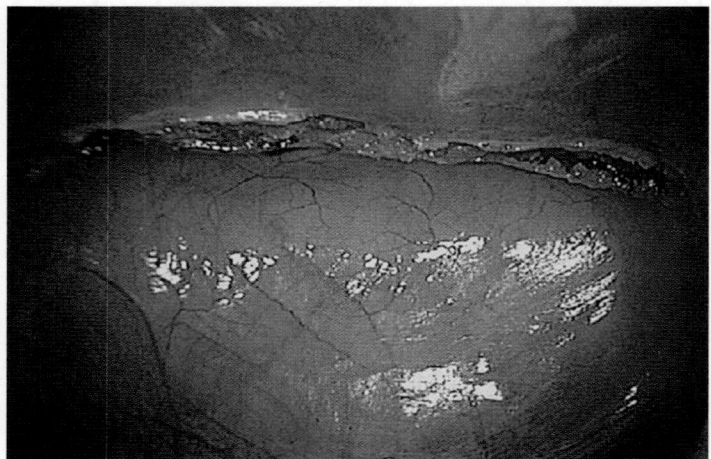

**FIGURE 119–2** Sharp dissection is used to incise the peritoneum 2 cm above the bladder reflection.

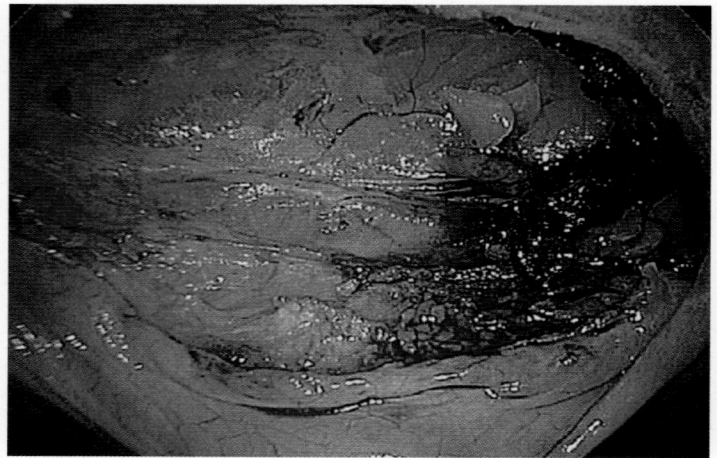

**FIGURE 119–3** Identification of areolar tissue at the point of incision confirms the proper plane of dissection.

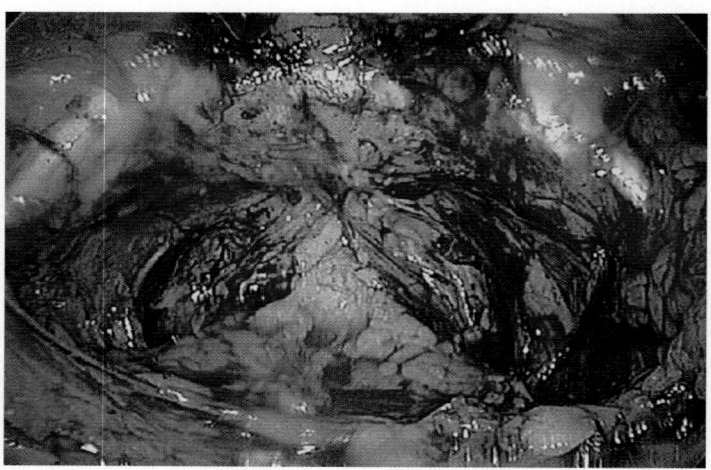

**FIGURE 119–4** The space of Retzius is visualized.

After the space of Retzius is exposed, the surgeon places two fingers in the vagina and identifies the urethrovesical junction by placing gentle traction on the Foley catheter. Using a vaginal finger to elevate the vaginal wall lateral to the bladder neck, we place stitches in the vaginal wall excluding the vaginal epithelium at the level of, or just proximal to, the midurethra and bladder neck (Fig. 119–5). A 0 nonabsorbable suture is placed in a figure-of-8 stitch, incorporating the entire thickness of the anterior vaginal wall. The needle is then passed through Cooper's ligament ipsilaterally (Fig. 119–6). If a double-armed suture is used, we make two passes through Cooper's ligament and subsequently tie above the ligament. We place Gelfoam between the vaginal wall and the obturator fascia before knot-tying to promote fibrosis. With simultaneous vaginal elevation, the suture is tied with six extracorporeal square knots. Two granny half-hitches and a flat square knot secure the stitch (Fig. 119–7).

Sutures are tied as they are placed to avoid tangling. Midurethral sutures are placed first, although this is a matter of preference. It is easier to place stitches from the contralateral low abdominal port. Fig. 119–8 shows the left bladder neck suture being placed from the right lower quadrant port, although it is possible to place it from either side. Both ends of the suture are then sutured into Cooper's ligament (Fig. 119–9) and tied. Two sutures are placed on each side to complete the operation (Fig. 119–10). The appropriate level of bladder neck elevation is estimated with the surgeon's vaginal hand. The goal is to elevate the vaginal wall to the level of the arcus tendineus fasciae pelvis bilaterally, so that the bladder neck is supported and stabilized by the vaginal wall. In tying the sutures, the surgeon should not reapproximate the vaginal wall to Cooper's ligament or place too much tension on the vaginal wall. A suture bridge of 1.5 to 2 cm is common.

If the patient has a large anterior vaginal wall prolapse, a paravaginal defect repair can be done in conjunction with a Burch colposuspension. When this is done, we bluntly dissect the paravaginal spaces on each side of the bladder. The dissection should identify bilaterally the lateral and lower edges of the bladder and urethra, the anterior vaginal wall and endopelvic fascia, the obturator internus muscle and fascia, and the arcus tendineus fasciae pelvis (Fig. 119–11). The arcus tendineus fasciae pelvis is a condensation of obturator fascia that runs from the pubic bone to the ischial spine. The ischial spine should be palpated or visualized as well as possible. Care should be taken to identify the obturator foramen and the neurovascular bundle to avoid damaging the obturator vessels and nerve. Starting at the vaginal apex, a single 2-0 nonabsorbable, 36- or 48-inch suture on a CT-2 needle is used to place a suture in the full thickness of the vagina, excluding the vaginal epithelium, and then into the arcus tendineus fasciae pelvis, which is 3 to 4 cm below the obturator fossa. This suture is then tied extracorporeally. An additional three to five sutures are placed through the vaginal wall and into the arcus tendineus fasciae pelvis or the fascia of the obturator internus muscle at 1-cm intervals until the defect is closed (Fig. 119–12). The same procedure is performed on the opposite side. If the procedure is performed concomitantly with the Burch colposuspension, the paravaginal defect repair should be performed first because exposure of the lateral defects decreases after the Burch sutures are tied. We place the stitch at the level of the ischial spine first and then place subsequent stitches as needed toward the pubic bone.

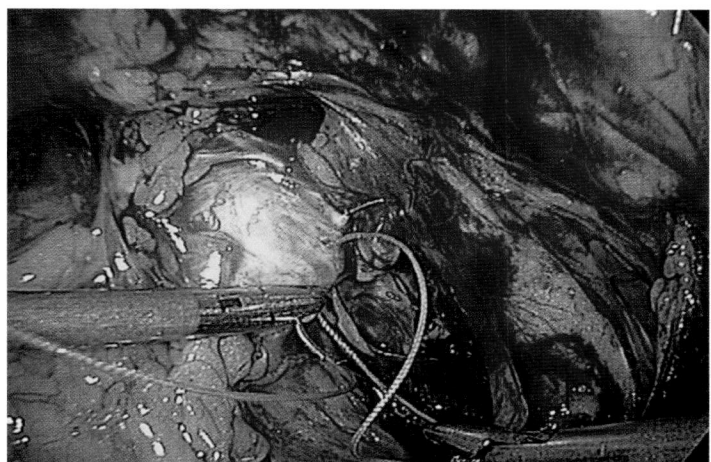

**FIGURE 119–5** Using laparoscopic suturing technique, a suture is placed in the right vaginal wall and endopelvic fascia at the level of, or just proximal to, the midurethra and bladder neck.

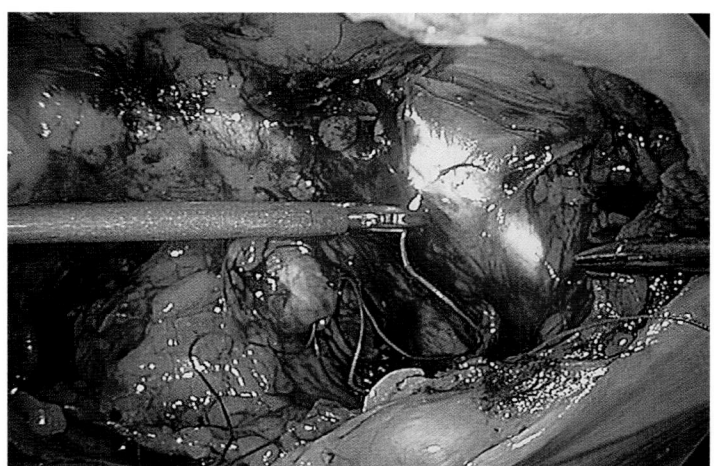

**FIGURE 119–6** The needle is passed through Cooper's ligament ipsilaterally.

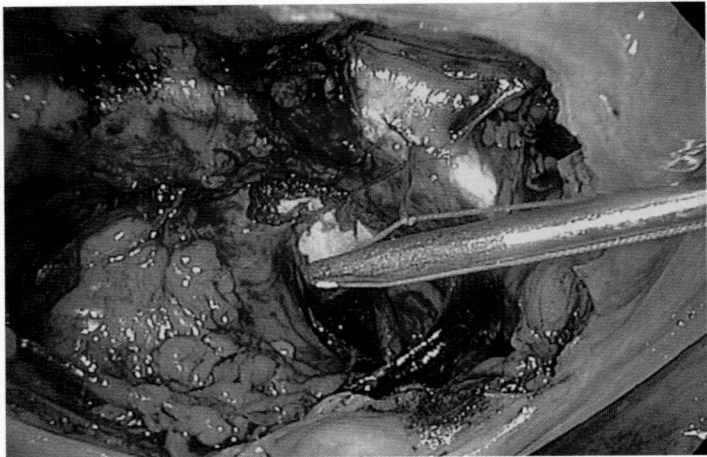

**FIGURE 119–7** The right Burch colposuspension suture is tied using extracorporeal knot-tying technique.

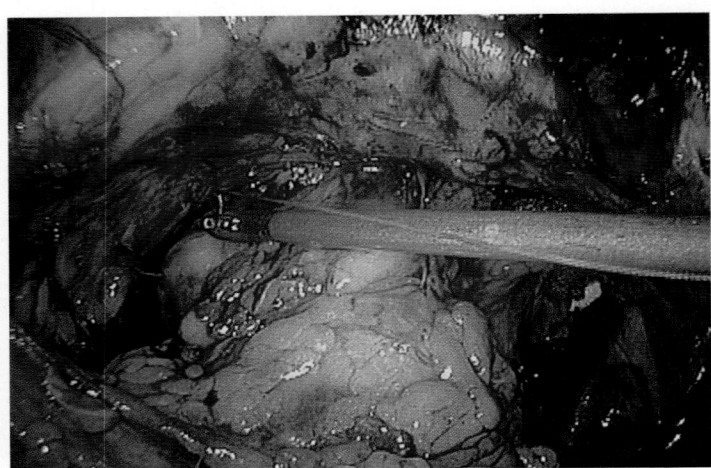

**FIGURE 119–8** The left periurethral suture is placed at the level of the bladder neck.

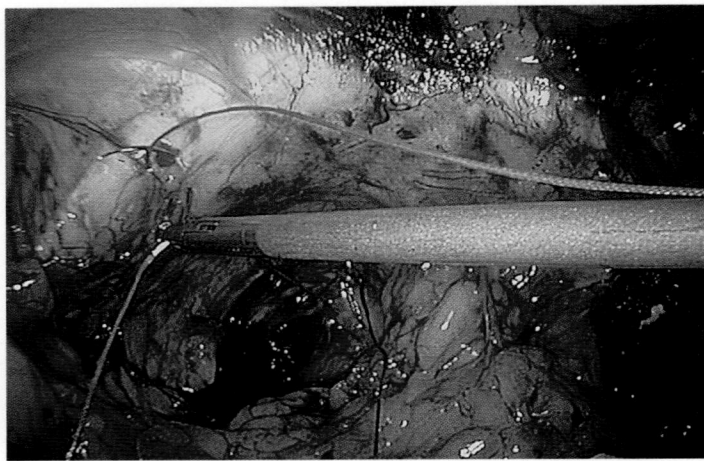

**FIGURE 119–9** Both ends of the left periurethral suture are placed through Cooper's ligament from the contralateral port.

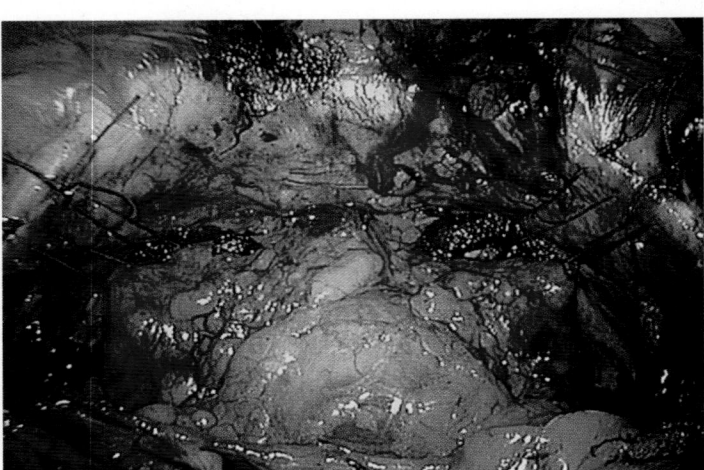

**FIGURE 119–10** The completed Burch colposuspension procedure is shown with two sutures on each side of the bladder neck.

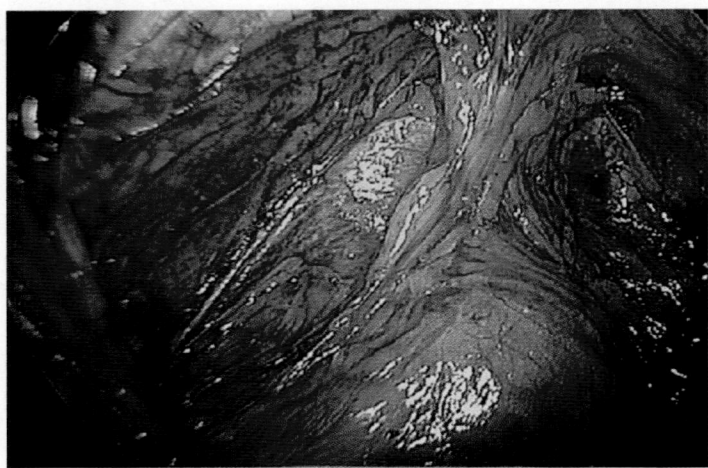

**FIGURE 119–11** The arcus tendineus fasciae pelvis with left paravaginal defect is shown.

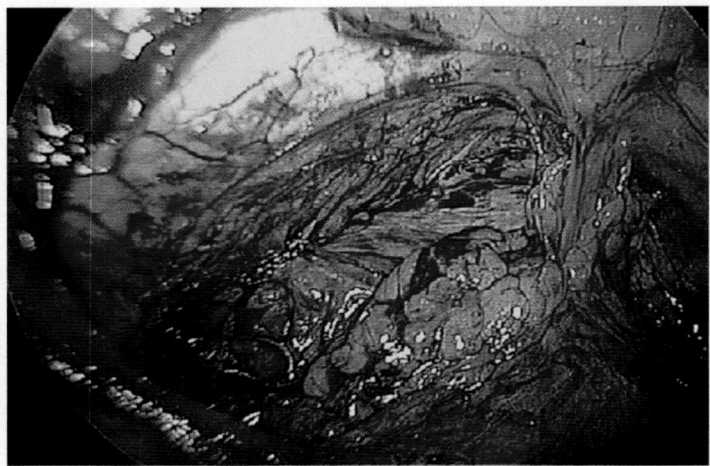

**FIGURE 119–12** The left paravaginal defect repair is completed with three sutures, before the Burch colposuspension sutures are placed on the left.

# CHAPTER 120

# Laparoscopic Surgery for Pelvic Organ Prolapse

*Mark D. Walters* ■ *Tommaso Falcone*

## Laparoscopic Sacral Colpopexy

In addition to the intraumbilical port, a 5/12-mm trocar should be placed in both lower quadrants for suture introduction. One or two additional 5-mm ports are placed at the level of the umbilicus lateral to the rectus muscle for retraction. The deep pelvis is then visualized, noting the pelvic structures and central enterocele (Fig. 120–1). A sponge stick or obturator is placed in the vagina to elevate the vaginal apex (Fig. 120–2). The peritoneum is dissected off the vaginal apex to delineate the vaginal wall and endopelvic fascia. Anterior dissection is performed as needed, taking care to avoid damage to the bladder (Fig. 120–3). We dissect the peritoneum from the posterior vaginal wall as deeply as possible in the rectovaginal space, sometimes extending almost to the perineal body. Occasionally, a lubricated sponge stick can be placed in the rectum, as well as in the vagina, to delineate both of these structures (Fig. 120–4). A 15 × 2.5-cm strip of polypropylene mesh is introduced through the 5/12-mm port. Three or four pairs of permanent sutures are placed to attach the mesh to the distal two thirds of the posterior vaginal wall (mesh should be attached as close to the perineal body as possible) (Fig. 120–5). An additional small strip of mesh is connected to the anterior vaginal wall near the apex using two pairs of permanent sutures. The posterior and anterior meshes can then be connected at the

vaginal apex, forming a Y- or T-shaped mesh. An alternative technique is to fashion the Y-shaped mesh extracorporeally and then bring it into the abdomen for suturing. Care should be taken to avoid twisting of the mesh and tangling of the sutures. Fig. 120–6 illustrates the completed vaginal mesh attachment. The mesh is then elevated, and the uterosacral ligaments are plicated in the cul-de-sac below the mesh using permanent sutures. One to three sutures may be necessary (Fig. 120–7). Alternatively, a Moschcowitz or Halban procedure can be done. The peritoneum over the sacral promontory then is examined, and key structures such as the aortic bifurcation, iliac arteries and veins, and right ureter are visualized. The peritoneum over the sacral promontory is carefully incised longitudinally, and, using elevation and blunt dissection, the sacral promontory is exposed (Fig. 120–8). The surgeon should identify the middle sacral artery and vein. A 3- to 4-cm section of anterior sacrum should be exposed if possible. The peritoneum running down the right pararectal space should be opened toward the cul-de-sac as well. Special care should, of course, be taken to avoid the ureter. Two to three permanent sutures are used to attach the mesh to the sacral promontory using extracorporeal knot-tying (Fig. 120–9). Alternatively, titanium tacks or hernia staples may be used to attach the mesh to the anterior longitudinal ligament of the sacrum. The peritoneum is then closed over the mesh using running or interrupted sutures (Fig. 120–10).

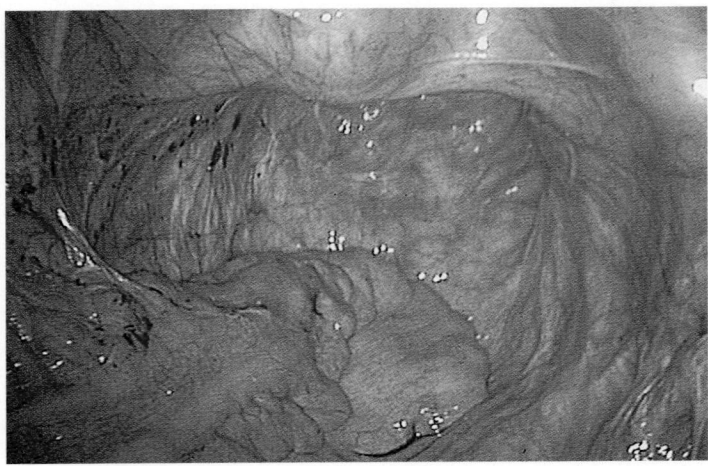

**FIGURE 120–1** The deep pelvis is visualized in a woman with vaginal prolapse and a central enterocele.

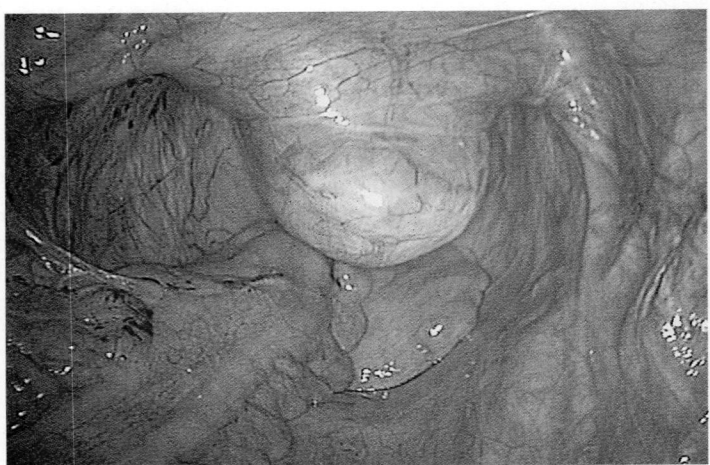

**FIGURE 120–2** A sponge stick or obturator is placed in the vagina to elevate the vaginal apex.

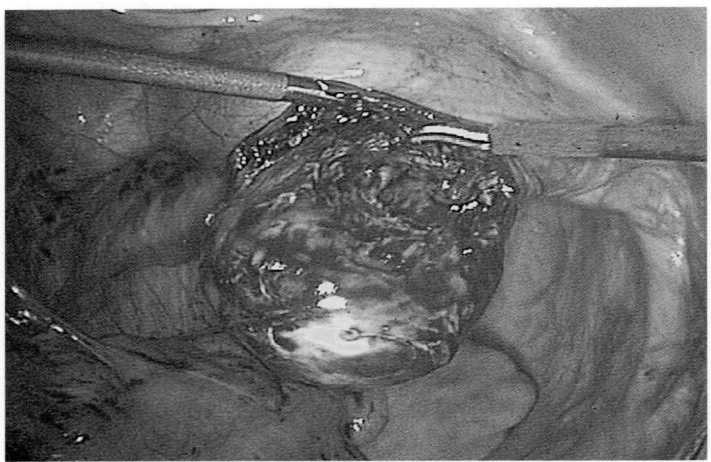

**FIGURE 120–3** The peritoneum is dissected from the vaginal apex, taking special care to avoid damage to the bladder.

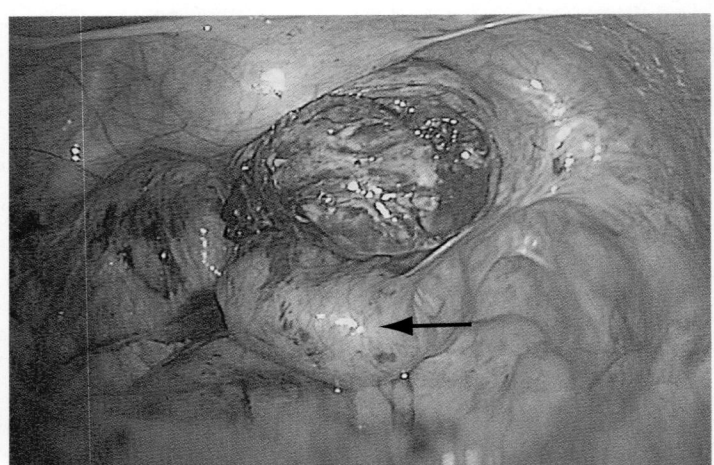

**FIGURE 120–4** A lubricated sponge stick is inserted in the rectum (*arrow*) as well as in the vagina to delineate both of these structures.

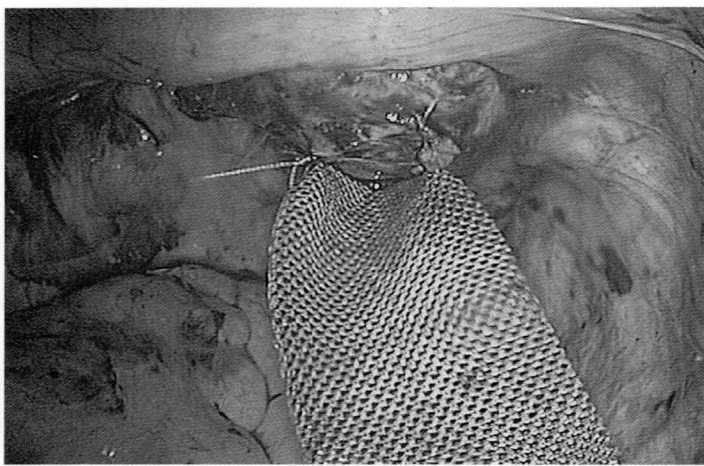

**FIGURE 120–5** The mesh used for the sacral colpopexy is sutured along the posterior wall of the vagina.

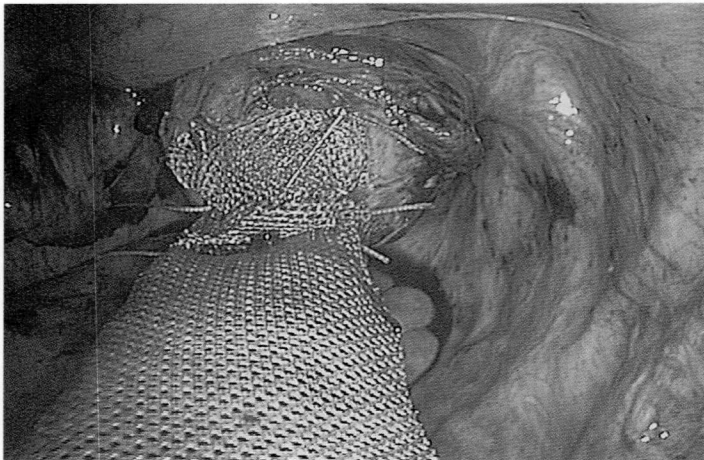

**FIGURE 120–6** The completed vaginal mesh attachment is ready for connection to the sacral promontory.

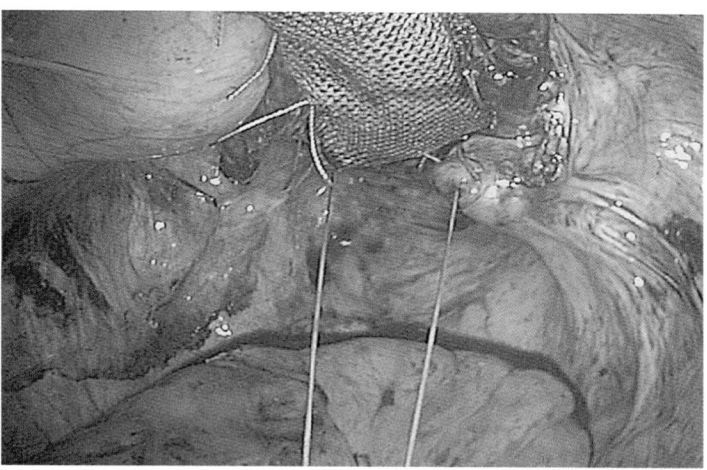

**FIGURE 120–7** A uterosacral ligament plication can be done to close the cul-de-sac below the mesh.

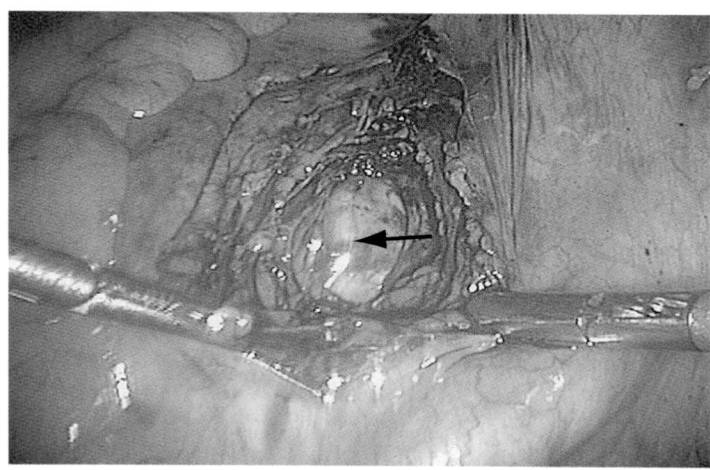

**FIGURE 120–8** The anterior longitudinal ligament (*arrow*) of the sacral promontory is exposed.

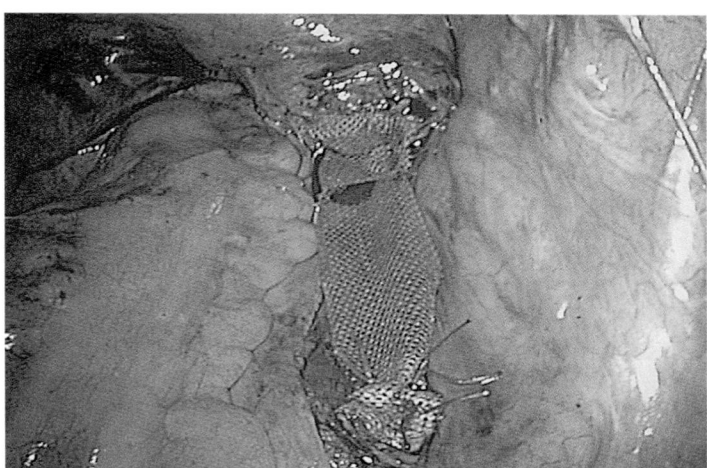

**FIGURE 120–9** The mesh is sutured to the sacral promontory, completing the sacral colpopexy procedure.

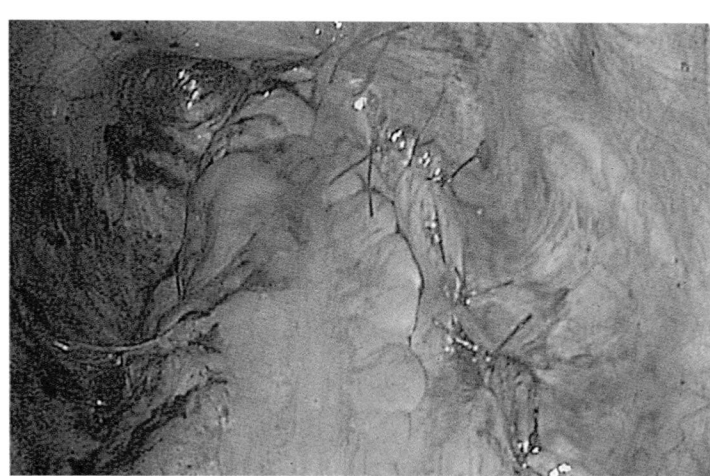

**FIGURE 120–10** The peritoneum is closed over the mesh.

## Laparoscopic Uterosacral Ligament Plication and Shortening

Occasionally, the uterus has a mild degree of prolapse or a very deep cul-de-sac, and the surgeon and the patient do not wish to have a hysterectomy done. This frequently occurs in women with stress urinary incontinence who are having a Burch procedure. It has been recommended that this be done prophylactically at the time of all Burch procedures, but the efficacy of this procedure to prevent future enterocele or uterine prolapse has not been established.

To perform uterosacral ligament plication and shortening, the posterior cervix, cul-de-sac, and uterosacral ligaments are identified. Pulling the uterus cephalad or ventral will place the uterosacral ligaments on stretch for easier identification. The uterosacral ligaments should be followed toward the sacrum bilaterally. Both ureters should be clearly visualized and avoided during the procedure. Permanent sutures are generally used. The first suture is placed near the insertion of each uterosacral ligament into the cervix, plicating these sites with an extracorporeal knot. This places the rest of the uterosacral ligaments under greater tension for easier identification. Two or three more sutures are placed and tied to bring the uterosacral ligaments together (Fig. 120–11). A suture is then placed into the proximal uterosacral ligament 2 to 4 cm from the sacrum. Again, care should be taken to avoid the ureter that lies several centimeters laterally. The suture is then placed into the uterosacral ligament near its attachment to the cervix and should be held until the second suture is placed. The second suture is placed, and both sutures are tied using extracorporeal knots to shorten the ligaments. The uterus can be elevated during this time to facilitate knot-tying.

## Laparoscopic Uterosacral Ligament/Vaginal Vault Suspension and Abdominal Enterocele Repair

As with the abdominal sacral colpopexy, the entire pelvis is inspected, and any adhesions are lysed. Fig. 120–12 shows an enterocele sac in association with vaginal prolapse. Both pelvic sidewalls are visualized, including the right uterosacral ligament (Fig. 120–13) and the left uterosacral ligament. The course of each ureter should be carefully identified lateral to each uterosacral ligament. A sponge stick or obturator is placed in the vagina to elevate the vaginal apex. The peritoneum is dissected off the vagina to delineate the vaginal wall and endopelvic (pubocervical and rectovaginal) fasciae (Fig. 120–14). Both the bladder anteriorly and the peritoneum posteriorly are dissected free. One should attempt to visualize the rectovaginal septum posteriorly and the pubocervical fascia anteriorly. There may be an area at the vaginal apex that is devoid of endopelvic fascia associated with the enterocele. The repair is begun by suturing the pubocervical fascia anteriorly (Fig. 120–15) to the rectovaginal septum posteriorly, then tying. Three to five sutures are placed across the vaginal apex to close any apical defects that are found (Fig. 120–16). A suture is then placed in the right uterosacral ligament approximately two thirds of the way up toward the sacrum. This suture is connected to the vaginal apex on the right. This procedure is repeated on the left (Fig. 120–17) and extracorporeal knot-tying is used. The ureters are again inspected, and any additional defects in the peritoneum can be closed. Fig. 120–18 shows the completed uterosacral ligament vaginal vault suspension.

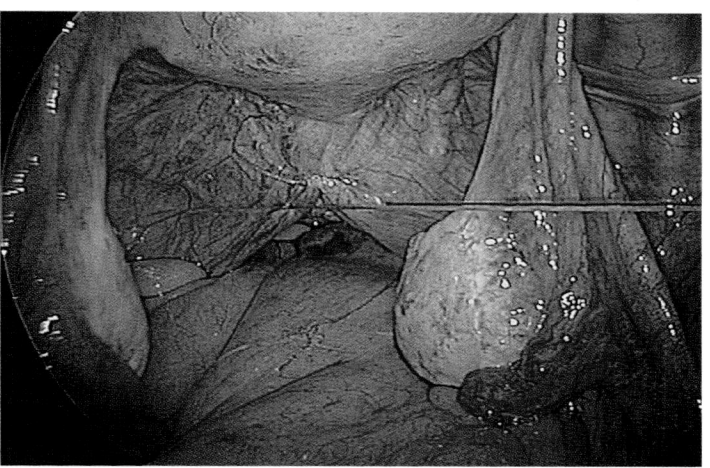

**FIGURE 120–11** Uterosacral ligament plication.

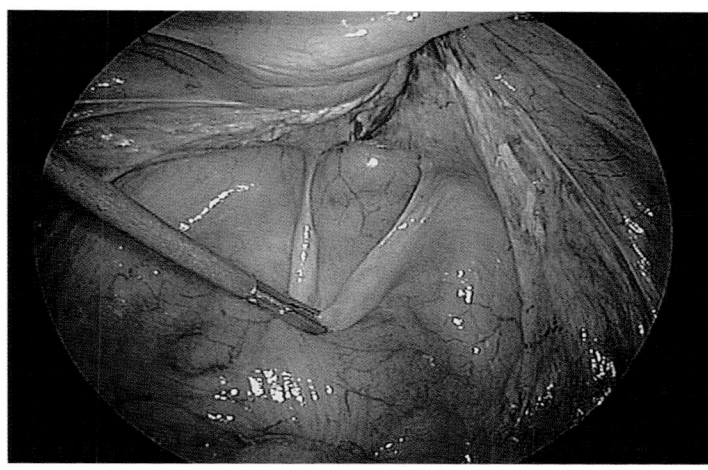

**FIGURE 120–12** A laparoscopic view of an enterocele sac in association with vaginal prolapse.

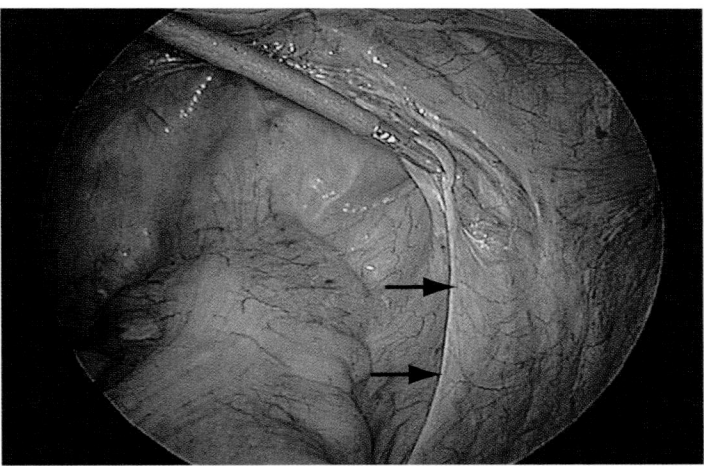

**FIGURE 120–13** The right uterosacral ligament (*arrows*) is grasped and placed under tension.

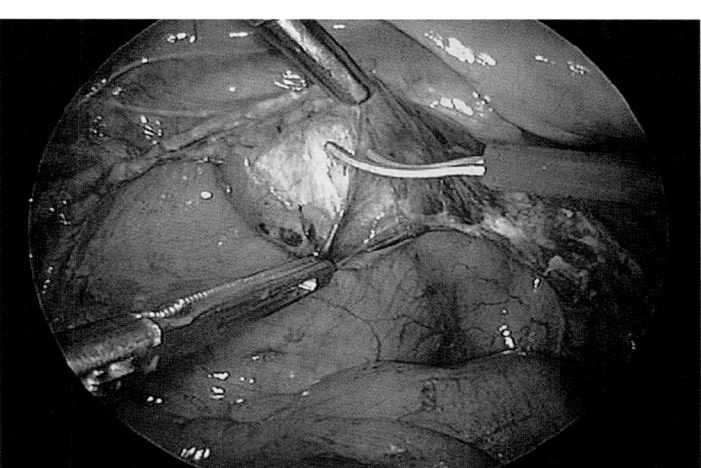

**FIGURE 120–14** The peritoneum is dissected off the vagina.

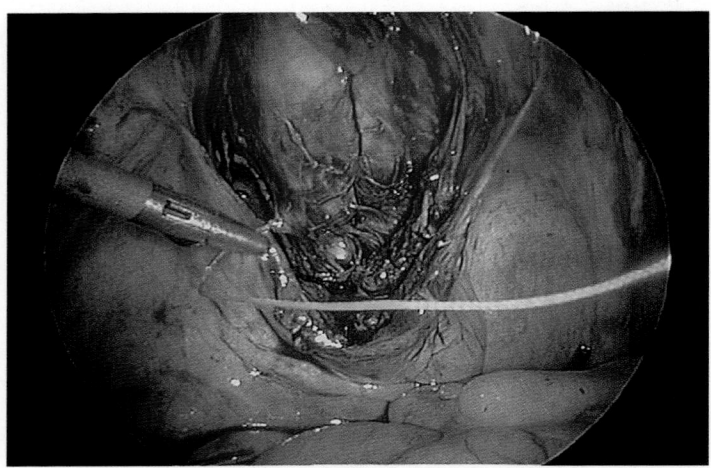

**FIGURE 120–15** The endopelvic fascia repair is begun by suturing the anterior pubocervical fascia (*as shown*) to the posterior rectovaginal fascia.

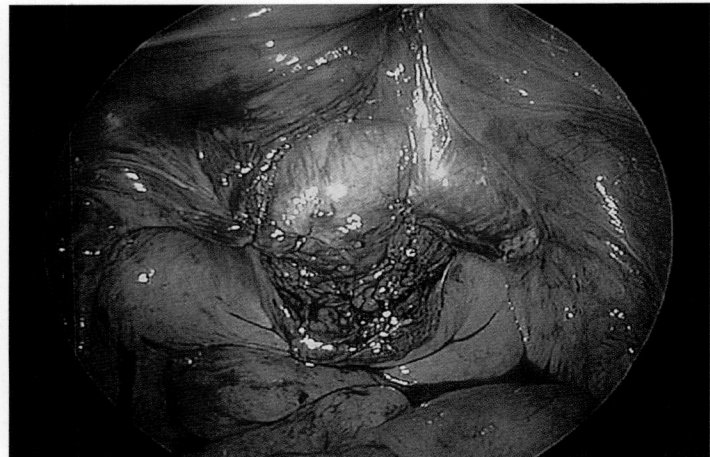

**FIGURE 120–16** The completed endopelvic fascia repair at the vaginal apex.

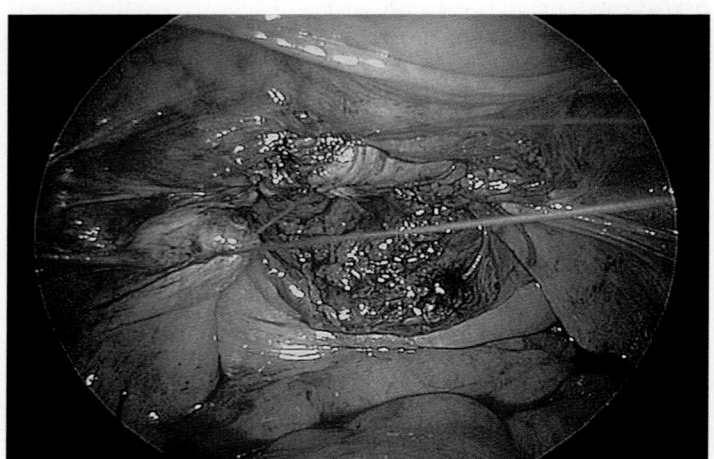

**FIGURE 120–17** The left uterosacral ligament is sutured to the vaginal apex.

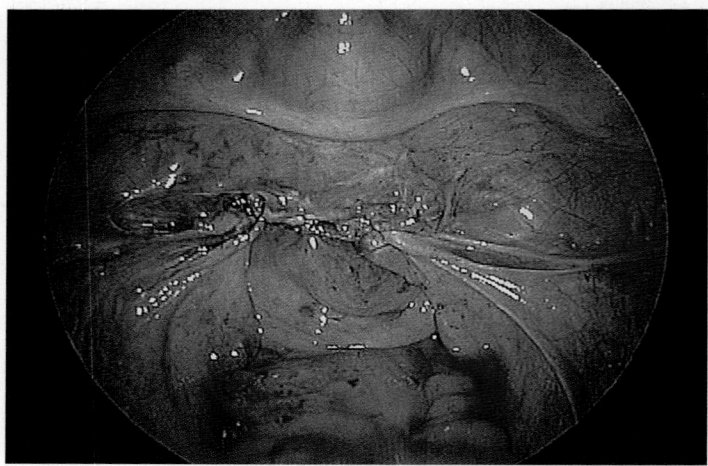

**FIGURE 120–18** Completed uterosacral ligament vaginal vault suspension.

# CHAPTER 121

# Robotic Gynecologic Surgery

*Jack Basil* ■ *James Pavelka*

The da Vinci surgical system (Fig. 121–1) is a minimally invasive robotic surgical platform approved by the FDA in 2005 for gynecologic surgeries. It is currently the only commercially available robotic surgical system. Utilization of robotic gynecologic surgery is rapidly increasing in the United States. Examples of gynecologic surgeries that can be performed with robot assistance include myomectomy, simple and radical hysterectomy, lymph node dissection, tubal reanastomosis, and sacral colpopexy. Robotic surgery was first conceived by the military, but it has evolved recently to enhance minimally invasive and laparoscopic surgery in the community.

Robotic surgery offers several advantages when compared with laparoscopic surgery. First, a magnified, three-dimensional, stereoscopic vision system is used (Fig. 121–2A, B). Second, EndoWrist instruments (designed with seven degrees of motion that mimic the human hand and wrist) provide hand movements with unparalleled precision, control, and dexterity (Fig. 121–3A through C). Last, the operating surgeon sits comfortably at an ergonomically designed surgeon console and controls the EndoWrist instruments and camera with hand controls and foot pedals (Fig. 121–4A, B).

The basic setup includes a robotic master console, a patient-side robot, and a vision tower with video screen. Once anesthetized, the patient is placed in dorsal lithotomy position in Allen stirrups and then is prepped and draped (Fig. 121–5). If a hysterectomy is to be performed, usually a uterine manipulator is placed (Fig. 121–6). Port placement varies, depending upon the surgeon and the operation to be performed. The da Vinci surgical system allows for two or three surgical arms and a camera port (all controlled by the operating surgeon at the console)

(Fig. 121–7). Additionally, one or two assistant ports are placed. Once the ports are placed, the patient is placed in Trendelenburg's position; the patient side cart (with robotic arms) is docked to the ports, and instruments are inserted through the robotic arms for console surgeon control at the bedside master console (Fig. 121–8). The surgery is then performed by the surgeon sitting at the master console with one or two assistants at the bedside (one for uterine manipulation and one for suction/irrigation, retraction, introducing suture, etc).

Potential patient benefits of minimally invasive robotic surgery compared with an open abdominal approach include shorter hospital stay, faster recovery, quicker return to normal activities, decreased incidence of wound infection, and less pain, blood loss, and scarring. Because robotic gynecologic surgery has been FDA approved only since 2005, data comparing it with open surgery and conventional laparoscopy are just becoming available. In general, gynecologic comparison of robotic hysterectomy (Fig. 121–9) versus conventional laparoscopic hysterectomy has shown a decreased need to convert to an exploratory laparotomy, reduced mean blood loss, and a similar rate of complications. In gynecologic oncology, lymph node counts (Fig. 121–10) have been shown to be higher with a robotic approach to both endometrial cancer and cervical cancer cases when compared with conventional laparoscopy and open surgery. Overall survival data comparisons are lacking at this time.

The number of gynecologic surgeries performed robotically in the United States is exponentially increasing. This advanced surgical technology offers potential benefit to both patients and physicians.

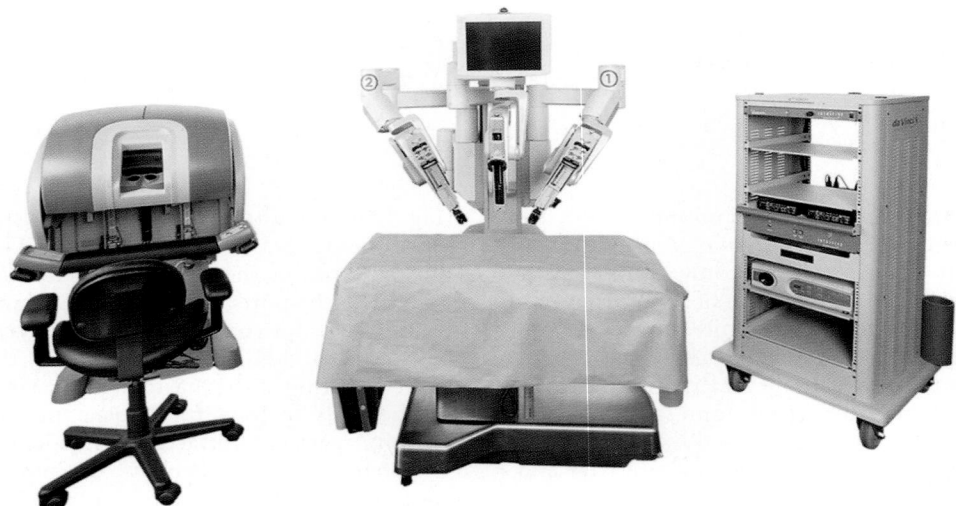

**FIGURE 121-1** The da Vinci surgical system consists of a surgeon console (*left*), a patient-side robot cart (*middle*), and a vision tower (*right*). (Copyright Intuitive Surgical, Inc. Reproduced with permission.)

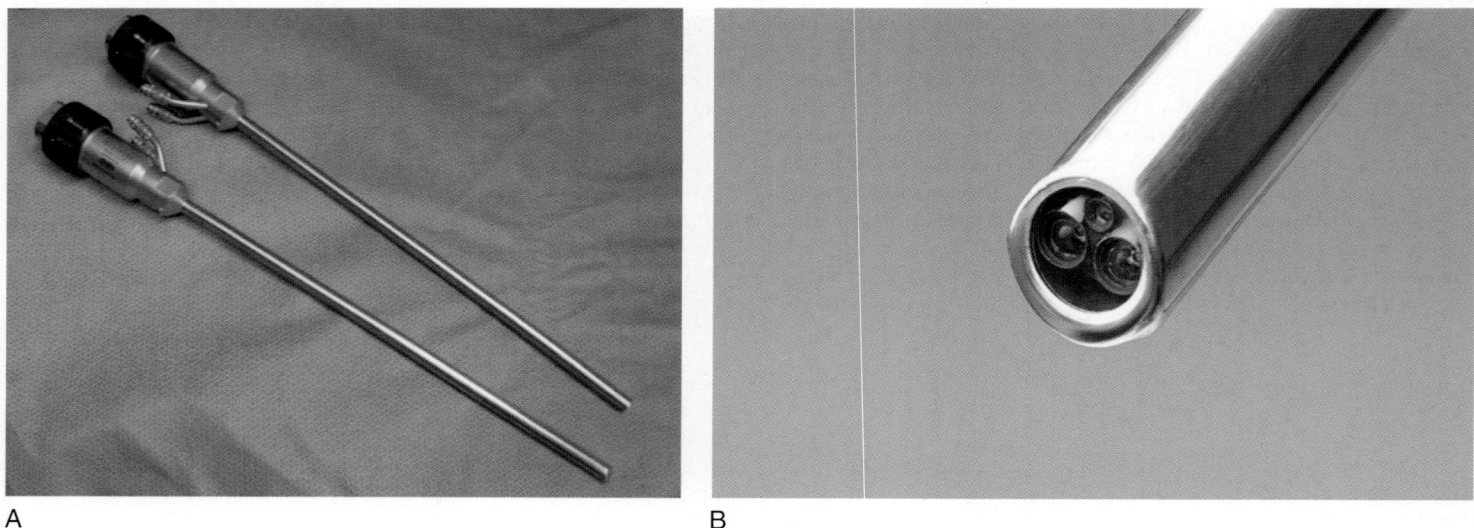

A

B

**FIGURE 121-2 A.** The endoscope vision system is available in both 0° and 30°. **B.** The 30° endoscope is pictured. (Copyright Intuitive Surgical, Inc. Reproduced with permission.)

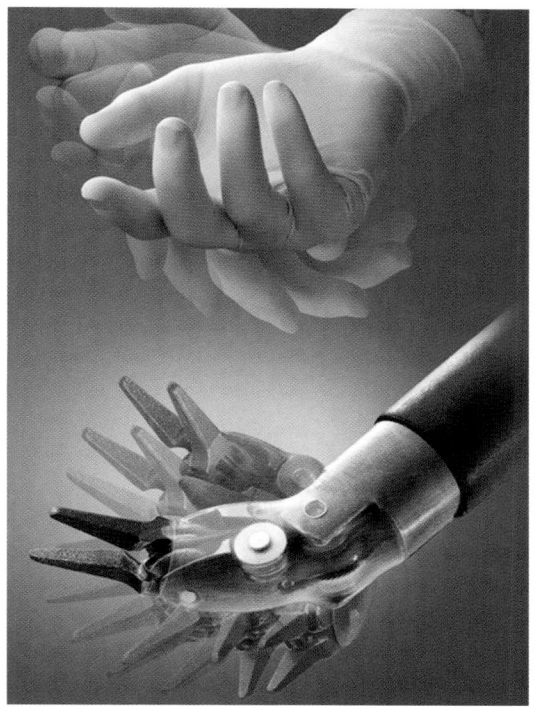

A

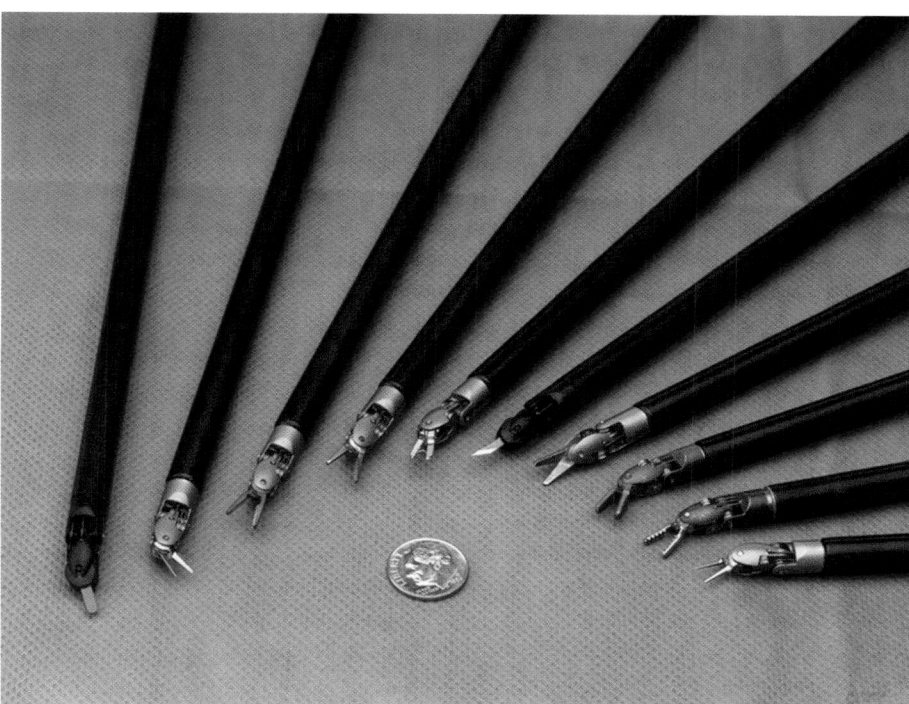

B

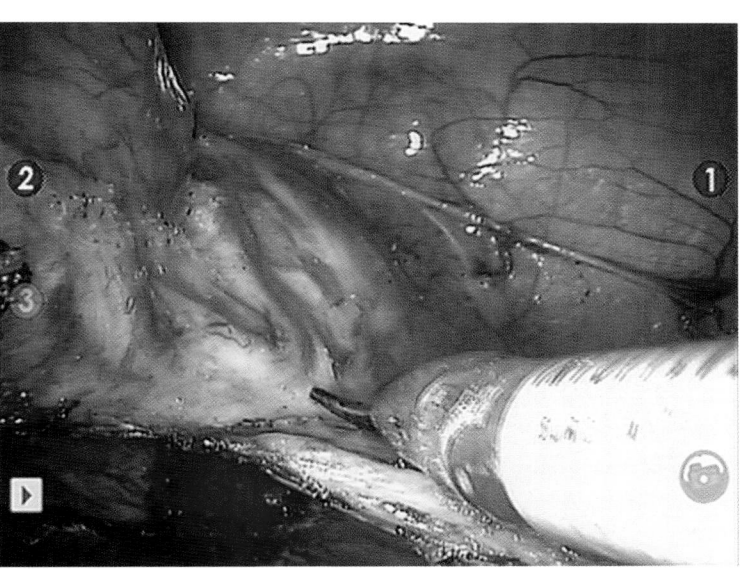

C

**FIGURE 121–3 A.** EndoWrist instruments with 7° of motion that provide greater precision control and dexterity when compared with laparoscopic instruments. (Copyright Intuitive Surgical, Inc. Reproduced with permission.) **B.** Comparison of EndoWrist instruments versus the size of a dime puts into perspective their small size. (Copyright Intuitive Surgical, Inc. Reproduced with permission.) **C.** This picture shows the precise dissection and superior visualization afforded with robotic gynecologic surgery. Pictured is the usage of monopolar scissors skeletonizing the right uterine artery during a hysterectomy.

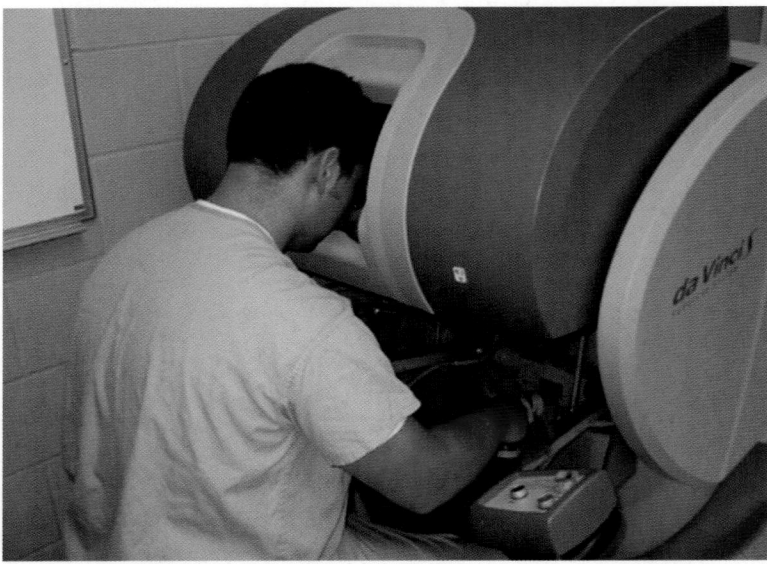

A

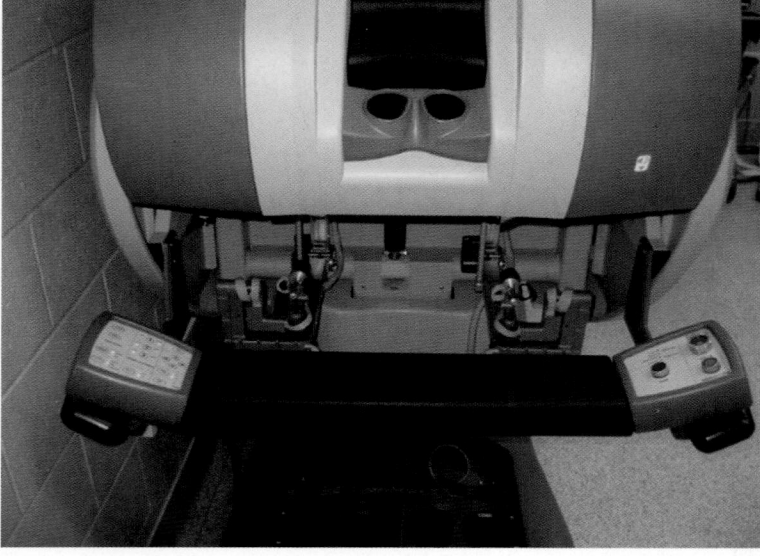

B

FIGURE 121–4 **A.** The operating surgeon sits at the surgeon console and controls the EndoWrist instruments with hand controls. **B.** The operating surgeon sits at the surgeon console and controls the camera with foot pedals.

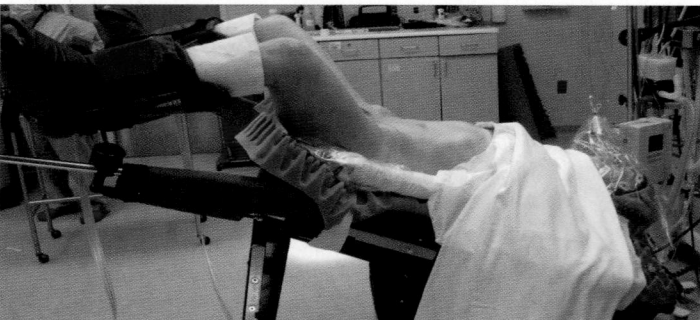

FIGURE 121–5 The patient is placed in Allen stirrups in steep Trendelenburg's position to facilitate robotic gynecologic surgery.

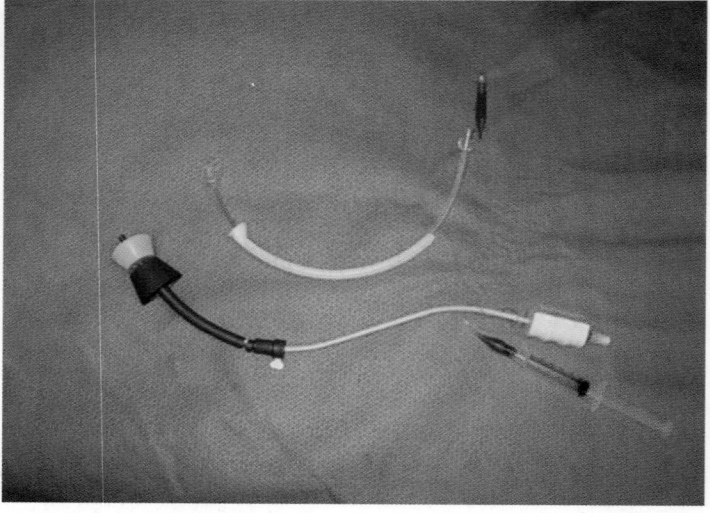

FIGURE 121–6 Several types of uterine manipulators can be used to facilitate gynecologic robotic surgery. The ZUMI (Zinnanti Uterine Manipulator Injector) clamp (CooperSurgical, Trumbull, CT) and CONMED VCare (Utica, NY) are shown here.

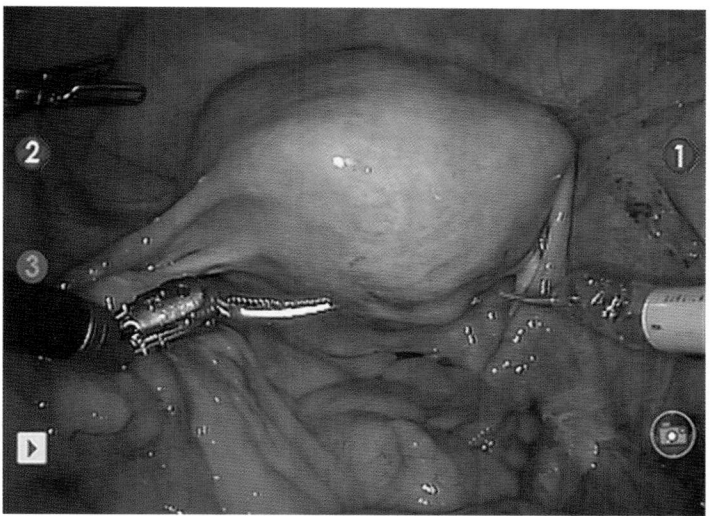

**FIGURE 121–7** The operating surgeon has control of three instruments (a prograsp, a PK dissector (Gyrus ACMI, Southborough, MA) with bipolar capabilities, and monopolar scissors with hand controls). The operating surgeon also controls the camera with a foot pedal.

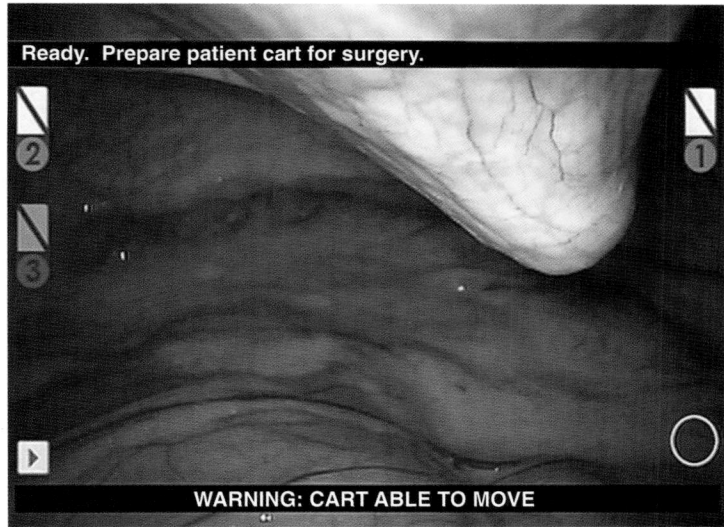

A

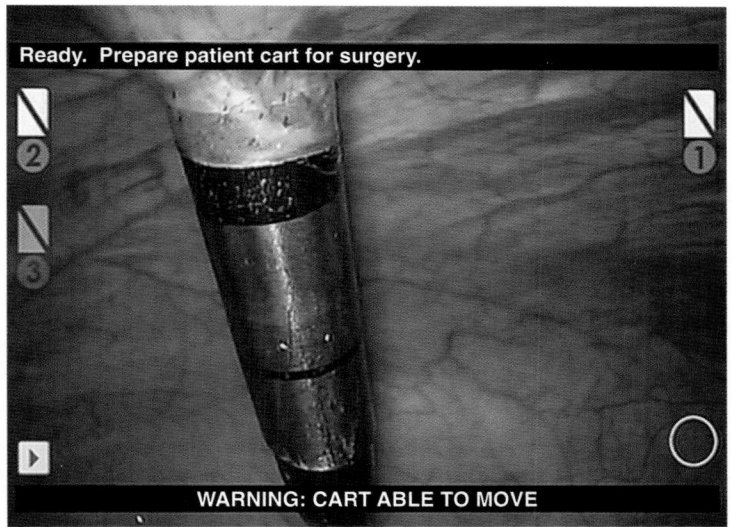

B

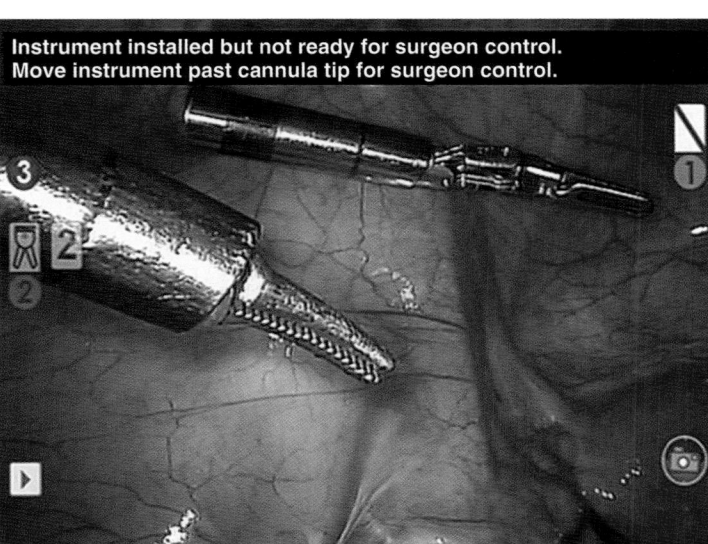

C

**FIGURE 121–8 A.** An 8-mm blunt tip trocar and cannula are being inserted under direct visualization to the left of the midline. The three robotic arms through which instruments are inserted are 8 mm in diameter. **B.** The 8-mm robotic cannula is inserted to the thick black line to provide maximum flexibility once the instrument is inserted. **C.** After insertion of the cannulas, two robotic instruments are placed by the bedside assistant. After insertion by the assistant, the operating surgeon takes control of the instruments.

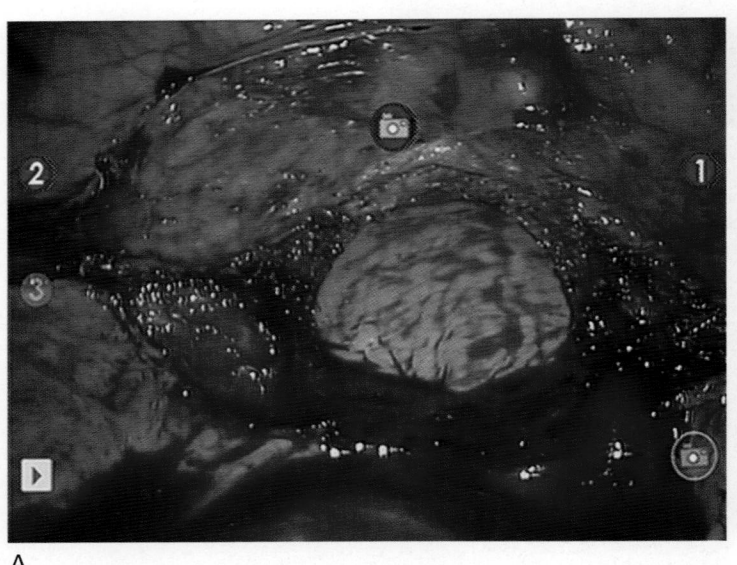

A

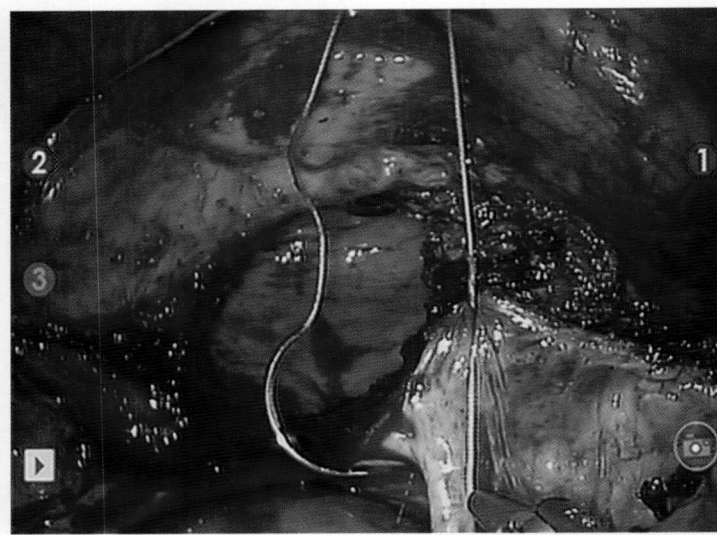

B

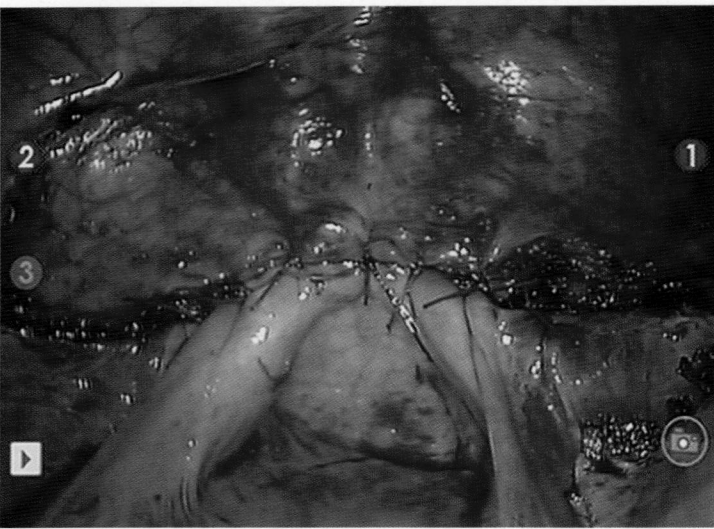

C

**FIGURE 121–9 A.** An open vaginal cuff is pictured after the removal of the uterus, cervix, ovaries, and fallopian tubes. **B.** Needle drivers have been inserted into two of the robotic ports, and the operating surgeon is now closing the vaginal cuff with 0 Vicryl interrupted sutures. Using robotic assistance facilitates suturing laparoscopically. **C.** The vaginal cuff has been reapproximated with sutures.

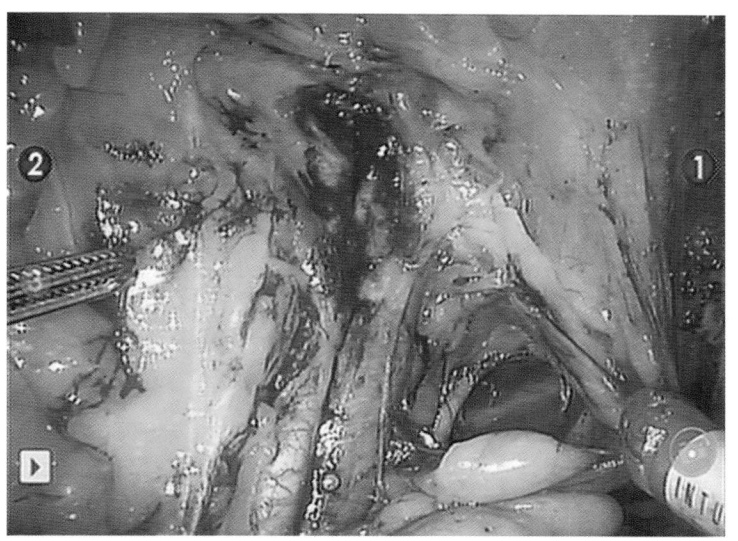

A

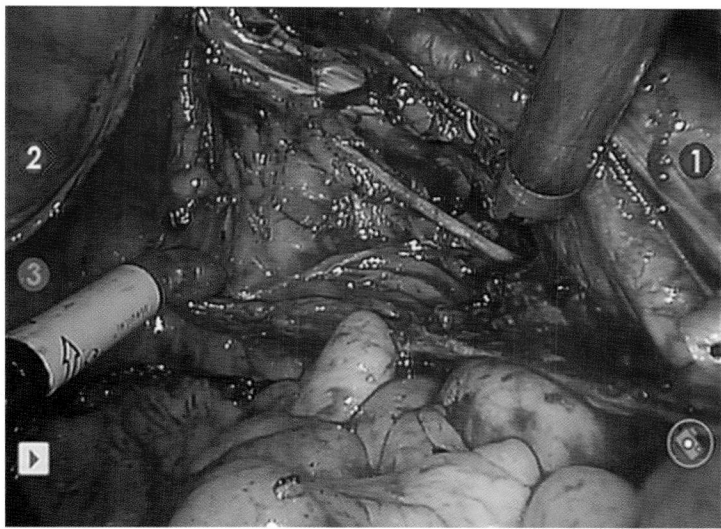

B

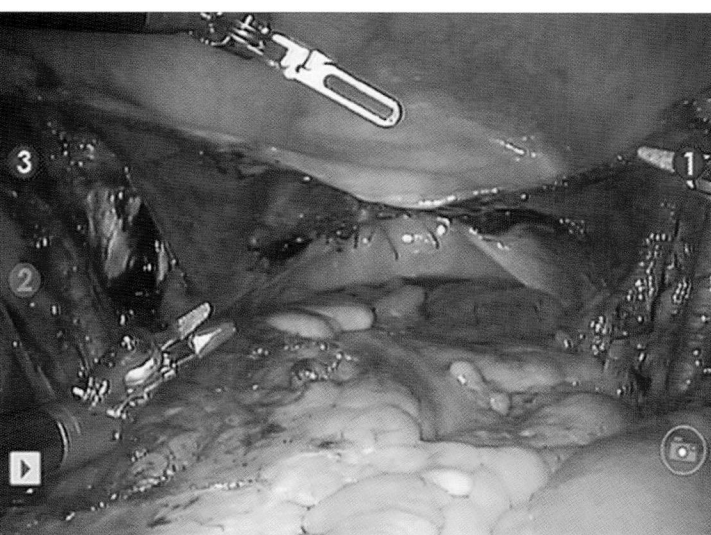

C

**FIGURE 121–10  A.** During endometrial cancer staging surgery, the left-sided external iliac lymph nodes are removed. After the paravesical and pararectal spaces are opened, the lymph nodes are removed from the bifurcation of the iliac vessel proximally to the recurrent circumflex vein distally. **B.** Exposure of the obturator nerve under the right external iliac vein is pictured. The right obturator lymph nodes have been removed. **C.** Endometrial cancer staging surgery has been performed with removal of the uterus, cervix, ovaries, fallopian tubes, and pelvic/para-aortic lymph nodes. The lymph nodes were placed in an endopouch bag and were taken out through the vagina before its closure.

# Major Complications Associated With Laparoscopic Surgery

*Michael S. Baggish*

A number of complications may be associated with laparoscopic surgery. Several of these iatrogenic injuries are unique and peculiar to the laparoscopic procedure itself (i.e., separate from the major surgical objective). For example, total abdominal hysterectomy is associated with the risk of a number of complications inherent to the surgical procedure, whereas laparoscopic hysterectomy has risks associated with the laparoscopic approach plus the hysterectomy portion of the operation.

## Vascular and Intestinal Injury

The two most serious laparoscopic complications are major vascular injury and intestinal damage. The former results in massive intra-abdominal hemorrhage and hypovolemic shock. This catastrophe must be managed in a timely, appropriate manner; otherwise, the patient will die (Fig. 122–1A through C). Small or large intestinal injury inevitably leads to immediate or delayed perforation (Fig. 122–2A, B). In some instances, significant damage to the bowel mesentery or directly to the blood vascular supply will result in ischemia followed by intestinal necrosis (Fig. 122–3A through D). As bowel contents spill into the abdominal cavity and then into the bloodstream, infection and sepsis follow. Sepsis syndrome is manifested by systemic inflammatory response syndrome (SIRS) (Tables 122–1 and 122–2). A cascade of events triggered by bacteremia and bacterial endotoxins and exotoxins eventuates in multiorgan failure. Necrotizing fasciitis may further complicate the picture in these cases. The condition progresses rapidly and is hallmarked by inordinate wound pain with cellulitis-like signs. Radiologic studies may show air within the abdominal wall (Fig. 122–3E, F). The bottom run of the downward spiral of events is septic shock (hypotension) and death. It is most convenient to subdivide these complications into those associated with the laparoscopic approach and those associated with the operative procedure (Table 122–3).

### Laparoscopic Approach

To gain access to the abdominal cavity, the laparoscope must be inserted through an appropriate sleeve or cannula (Fig. 122–4A through C). These generally range in size from 5 to 12 mm inner diameter. The sleeve is typically introduced directly by incision (usually infraumbilical) followed by dissection through the layers of tissue constituting the anterior abdominal wall. When the peritoneum is reached, it is tented up and incised or bluntly traversed. The sleeve is then introduced over a blunt trocar. This technique is described as open laparoscopy. An alternative technique introduces an inert gas (e.g., carbon dioxide) via a needle, which is thrust into the abdominal cavity. When sufficient gas has been introduced to create an adequate pneumoperitoneum, hallmarked by tympany on abdominal percussion, the sleeve is introduced into the peritoneal cavity over a sharp trocar. This is a de facto blind technique. Various alternations of the aforesaid technique have been described over the years, including a device that supposedly enables the operator to view each layer of the abdominal wall as the trocar is advanced (Fig. 122–5A, B).

The basis for a "safe" trocar thrust as described in an earlier chapter in this section depends on two rules. First, the trocar must be thrust into them midline without deviation to the right or to the left of the midline (Fig. 122–6A, B). Second, the angle of entry of the trocar must be made at 45° to 60° (i.e., in the direction of the uterus) (Fig. 122–7). Deviation from these key provisions will ultimately lead to disastrous consequences for the patient and her physician. Individuals at the extremes of body mass index (i.e., the very lean and the obese) are particularly at risk for iatrogenic injury (Tables 122–4 and 122–5). The obese patient is the most high-risk patient, particularly if she has had prior intra-abdominal surgery and is likely to have adhesions (Tables 122–6). Trocar entry for these women may be difficult (Fig. 122–8 and 122–9).

The surgeon should not resort to the use of extra long trocar devices (11 inches in length) (Fig. 122–10); these instruments are not necessary because a trocar of standardized length (8 inches in length) is more than adequate to gain entry (Fig. 122–11).

The surgeon is better advised to perform a laparotomy if a trocar of standard length is unable to provide entry into the abdominal cavity. A trocar that is thrust to the right or left of the midline may injure the iliac vessels or the vena cava (Fig. 122–12). A trocar that is thrust downward at 90° can and will injure the aorta or the left common iliac vein. Any primary trocar thrust has the potential for perforating the small intestines, whereas a deviant thrust may penetrate the large bowel (Fig. 122–13A). Because secondary trocars are placed under direct vision, injuries caused by these devices should not occur (Fig. 122–13B).

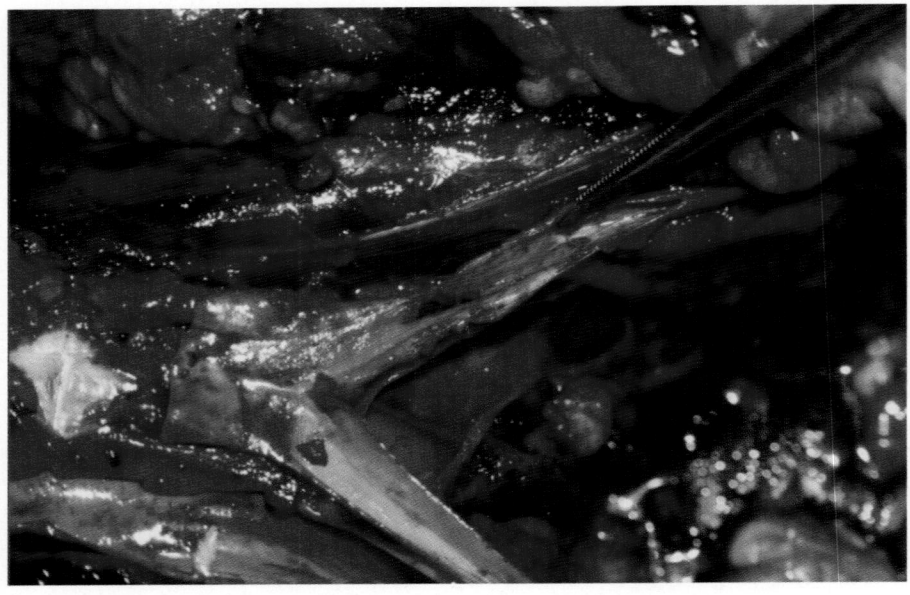

A

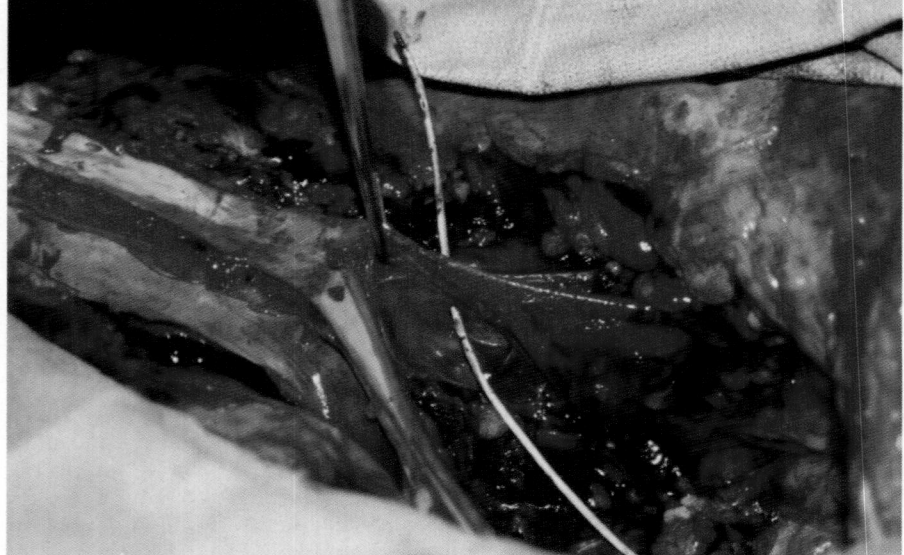

B

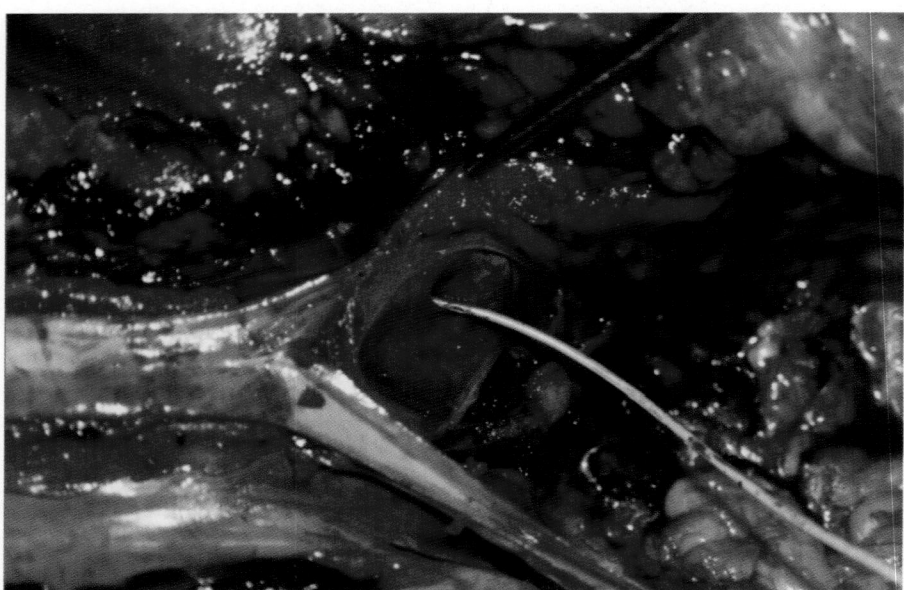

C

**FIGURE 122–1  A.** Autopsy of a young women who
sustained a through and through trocar injury of the left
common iliac artery and died of massive blood loss. The
area below the forceps shows the laceration on the
posterior wall of the artery. **B.** The probe passed by the
coroner enters the posterior wall of the artery and exits
through the anterior wall. Vascular clips can be seen on
the left common iliac vein. **C.** The probe points to a
laceration in the left common iliac vein. This was the
fatal wound.

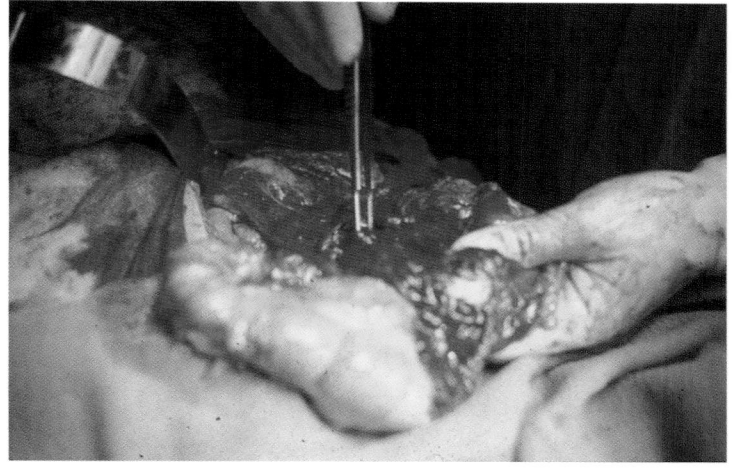

A

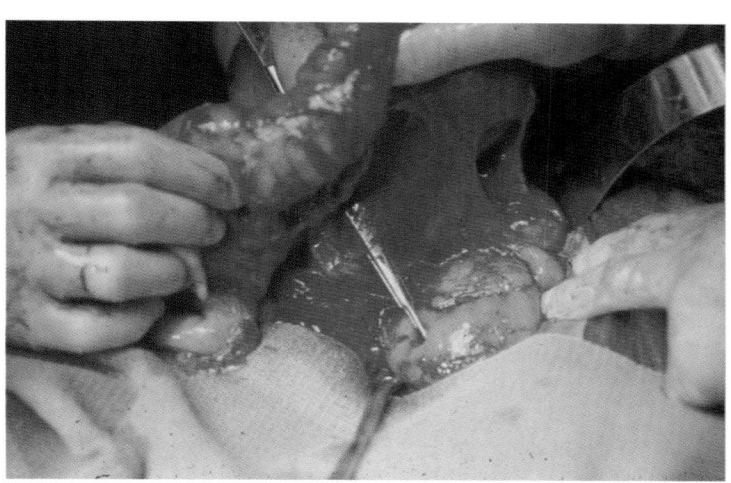

B

**FIGURE 122–2  A.** The forceps has been placed in a trocar wound of the omentum. **B.** The transverse colon has been elevated, permitting the scissors to trace the trajectory into a trocar-induced perforation of the duodenum.

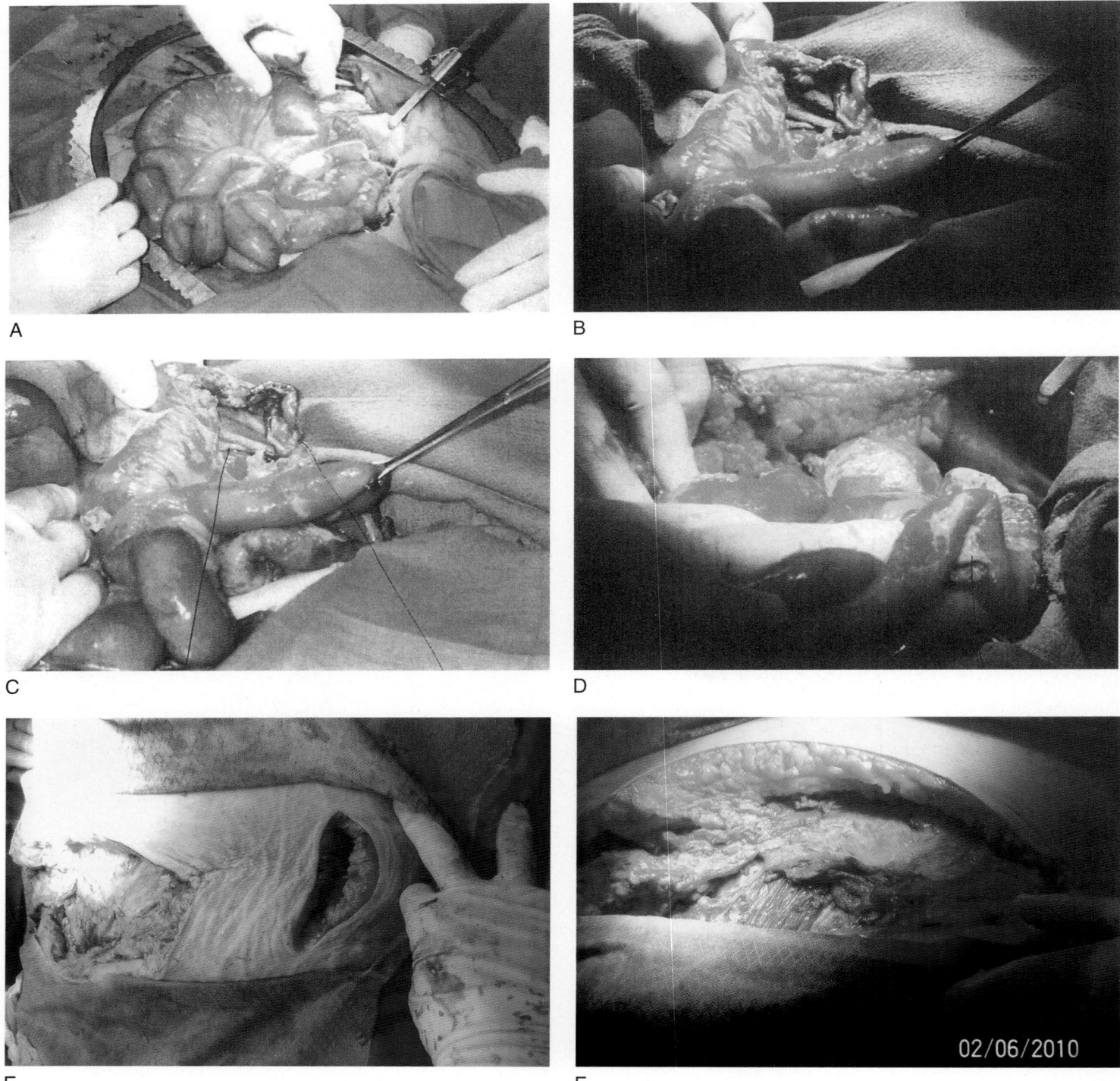

A

B

C

D

E

F

02/06/2010

**FIGURE 122–3 A.** This 28-year-old para 3-0-0-3 underwent a postlaparoscopy emergency laparotomy. At the time of the laparotomy, the patient had extensive peritonitis and multiple small-bowel interloop abscess formations. Note the swollen, edematous small intestine. The patient also exhibited clinical signs of septic shock. **B.** The mesentery of the small intestine had been coagulated by plasma kinetic forceps and torn away from the intestine by blunt dissection during attempted adhesiolysis. Note the extensive ischemic and necrotic small bowel. **C.** Close-up at the necrotic segment of the small intestine shown in Fig. 122–3B. **D.** The small bowel is covered with fibrin secondary to extensive peritonitis. **E.** Necrotizing fasciitis is a byproduct of intestinal perforation and sepsis, particularly in obese patients. Group "A" streptococci or methicillin-resistant staphylococci rapidly spread along tissue planes while their toxins digest fat and fascia. This is clearly shown in this photo. The fat becomes grayish as the tissue undergoes cell death. **F.** Treatment consists of radical debridement of all dead or dying tissue. Frequent returns to the operating room are the rule before the infection is terminated. In this photo most of the fat of the anterior abdominal wall is gone, including the rectus sheath.

## TABLE 122–1 ■ Definitions of Sepsis

**Infection:** Phenomenon characterized by an inflammatory response to the presence of microorganisms or the invasion of normally sterile host tissue by those organisms.

**Bacteremia:** Presence of viable bacteria in the blood.

**Systemic inflammatory response syndrome:** Systemic inflammatory response to a variety of severe clinical insults. The response is manifested by two or more of the following conditions:

Temperature >38°C or <36°C

Heart rate: >90 beats/min

Respiratory rate: >20 breaths/min or $PaCO_2$ < 32 mm Hg @ 4.3 kPa

White blood cell count: >12,000 cells/mm³, <4000 cells/mm³, or >10% immature (band) forms

**Sepsis:** Systemic response to infection. This systemic response is manifested by two or more of the following conditions as a result of infection:

Temperature: >38°C or <36°C

Heart rate: >90 beats/min

Respiratory rate: >20 breaths/min or $PaCO_2$ < 32 mm Hg @ 4.3 kPa

White blood cell count: >12,000 cells/mm³, <4000 cells/mm³, or >10% immature (band) forms

**Severe Sepsis:** Sepsis associated with organ dysfunction, hypoperfusion, or hypotension. Hypotension and perfusion abnormalities that may include, but not limited to, lactic acidosis, oliguria, or an acute alteration in mental status. Patients who are on inotropic or vasopressor agents may not be hypotensive at the time that perfusion abnormalities are measured.

**Hypotension:** Systolic blood pressure <90 mm Hg or reduction >40 mm Hg from baseline in the absence of other causes for hypotension.

**Multiple organ system failure:** Presence of altered organ function in an acutely ill patient such that homeostasis cannot be maintained without intervention.

From Goldman L, Ausiello D: Cecil Textbook of Medicine, 22nd ed. Philadelphia, 2004, Saunders; with permission.

## TABLE 122–2 ■ Effects of Intestinal Perforation: Infection, Fluid-Electrolyte Imbalance, Sepsis Syndrome

The principal derangements that arise as a result of bowel perforation include infection and fluid-electrolyte imbalance and their sequelae. Intestinal fluid and feces contain a variety of bacteria, such as *Escherichia coli, Enterococcus, Klebsiella, Proteus, Pseudomonas,* and *Clostridium,* to name a few. These bacteria produce toxins that facilitate entry of bacteria into the circulation and contribute to a downward spiral of events, referred to as sepsis syndrome, as well as intra-abdominal abscess:

1. Contamination of the abdominal cavity leads to inflammation of the peritoneum.
2. In turn, subperitoneal blood vessels become porous, causing interstitial fluid to leak into the third space.
3. Paralytic ileus and an accumulation of intra-abdominal fluid push the diaphragm upward, lowering the capacity for lung expansion within the thorax and contributing to partial lung collapse.
4. Fluid of inflammatory origin may accumulate in the chest as pleural cavity effusion.

A number of progressive complications are predictable but may occur at variable intervals after the initial perforation. The most frequent complications associated with colonic injury include the following:

■ Peritonitis (98% of cases)
■ Ileus (92%)
■ Pleural effusion (84%)
■ Colostomy (80%)
■ Intra-abdominal abscess (78%)

The most common sequelae after small-bowel perforation are as follows:

■ Peritonitis (100% of cases)
■ Intra-abdominal abscess (63%)
■ Ileus (89%)
■ Pleural effusion (59%)

Baggish MS: Ob-Gyn Management 20:47-60, 2008. With permission.

## TABLE 122–3 ■ One Hundred Thirty Cases of Intestinal Injury Associated With Laparoscopic Surgery

| Approach | Percentage | Small Intestine | Percentage | Colon |
|---|---|---|---|---|
| Entry related | 77% | 62 | 41% | 20 |
| Primary trocar | | (57) | | (18) |
| Secondary trocar | | (3) | | (1) |
| Other | | (2) | | (1) |
| Operative related | 23% | 19 | 59% | 29 |
| With energy | | (10) | | (11) |
| Without energy | | (9) | | (18) |
| Total | 100% | 81 | 100% | 49 |

Baggish MS: J Gynecol Surg 23:83-95, 2007. With permission.

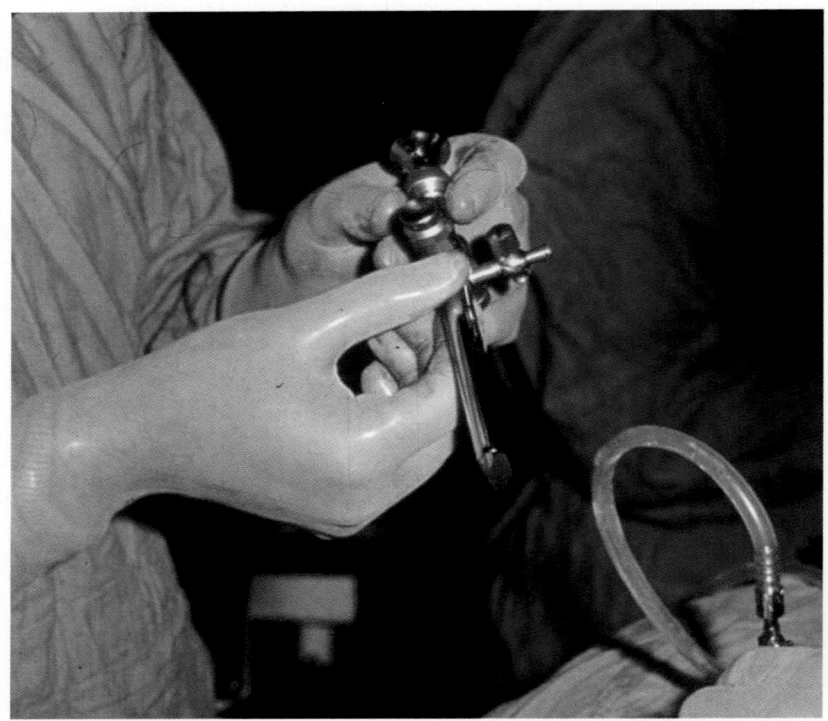

A

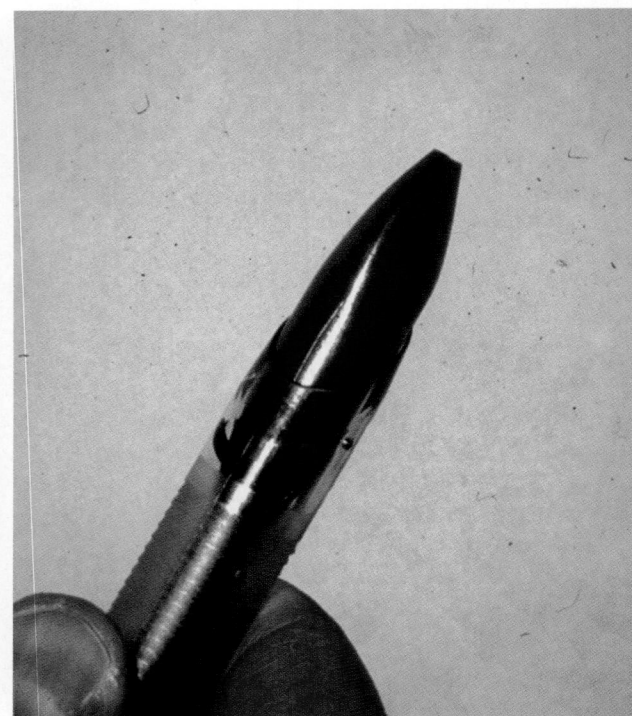

B

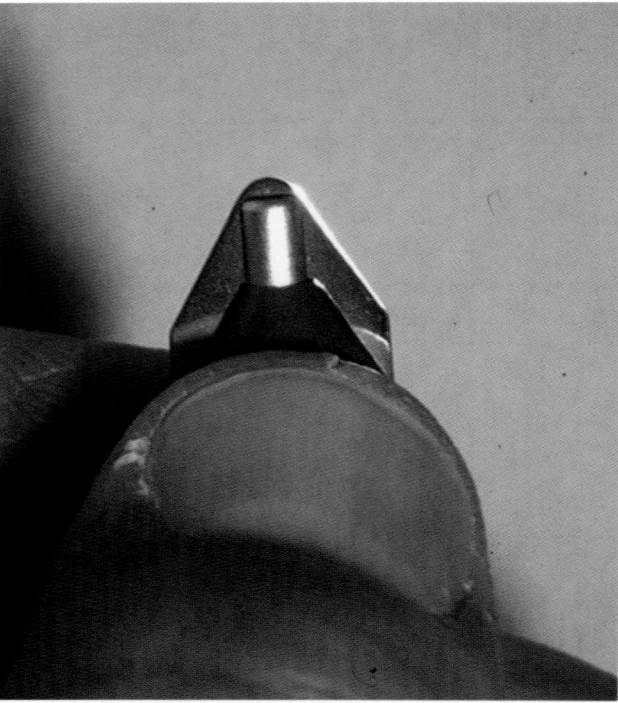

C

**FIGURE 122–4  A.** The 10-mm reusable trocar pictured here includes a pyramidal trocar fitted within the access sleeve. When properly sharp, this device can perforate bowel or one of the great retroperitoneal vessels. Frequently, the trocar is dull after multiple uses and is unlikely to create a major vessel injury. **B.** This figure illustrates the tip of a disposable trocar with the blade retracted (i.e., unarmed). **C.** In contrast to the trocar shown in Fig. 122–4A, the cutting blade of this disposable trocar (armed) is razor sharp. This device when misdirected can quite easily lacerate the wall of a major vessel.

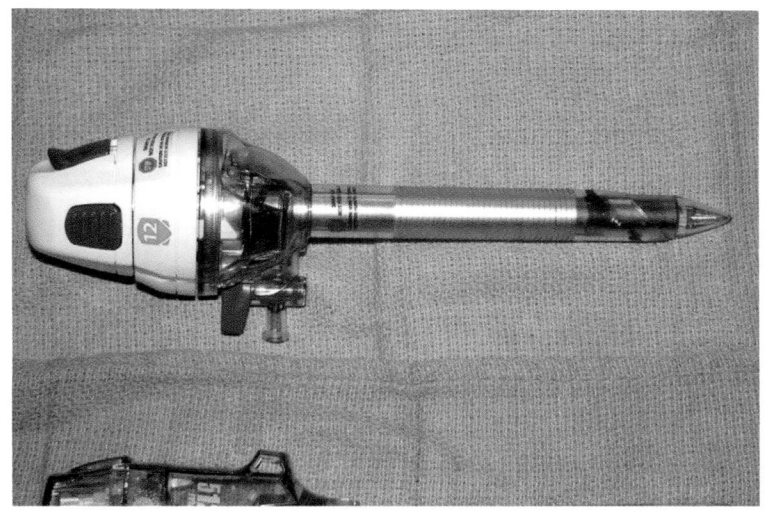

A

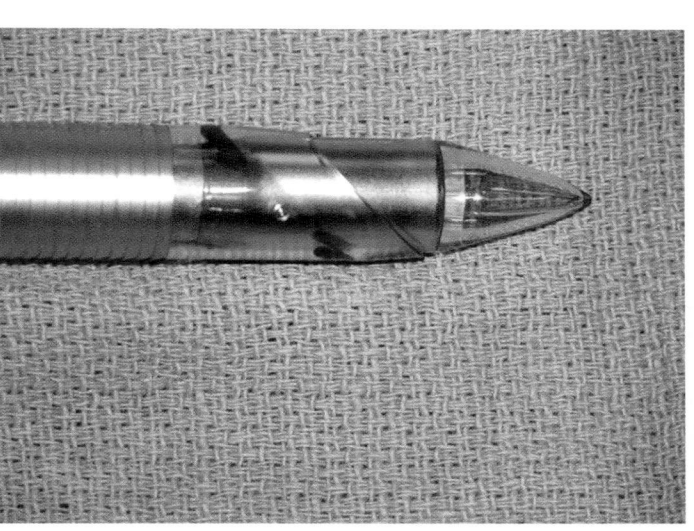

B

**FIGURE 122–5  A.** This specialized trocar hypothetically allows one to view the layers of the abdominal wall as the device is thrust into the abdominal cavity. **B.** The conical tip of the trocar shown in Fig. 122–5A is pointed but not sharp. The clear color permits a semblance of vision of the abdominal wall tissues.

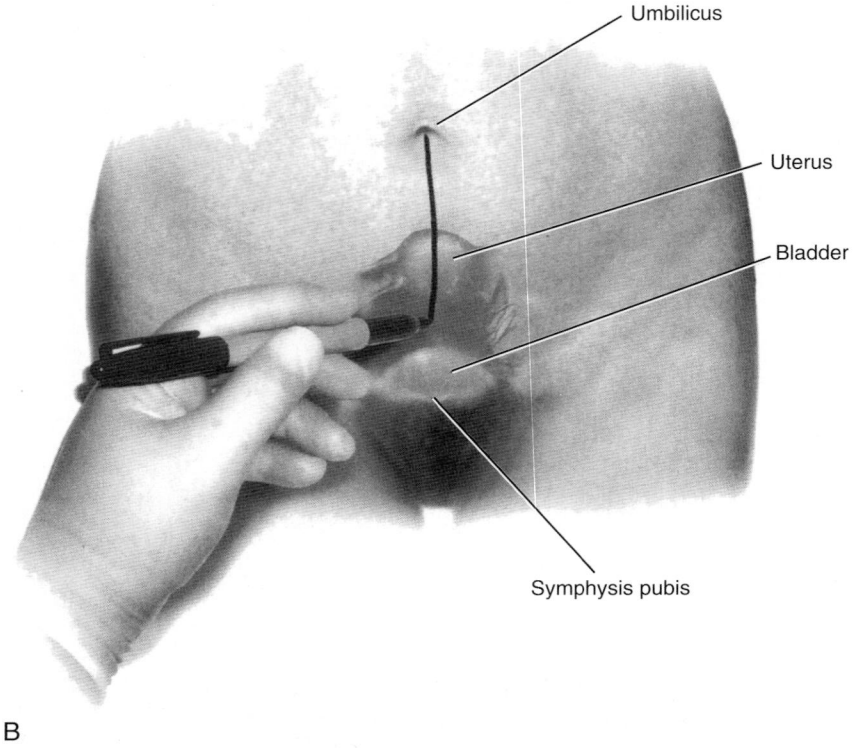

B

A

**FIGURE 122–6  A.** The trocar must be aimed at the midline to avoid injury to the iliac vessels. Deviation to the right or left places any and every patient at risk for major vessel injury. **B.** A convenient method to aid in the midline delivery of a trocar thrust is demonstrated here. A marking pen has been used to draw a straight line from the umbilicus to the symphysis pubis. (Baggish MS: J Gynecol Surg 19:63-73, 2003. By permission.)

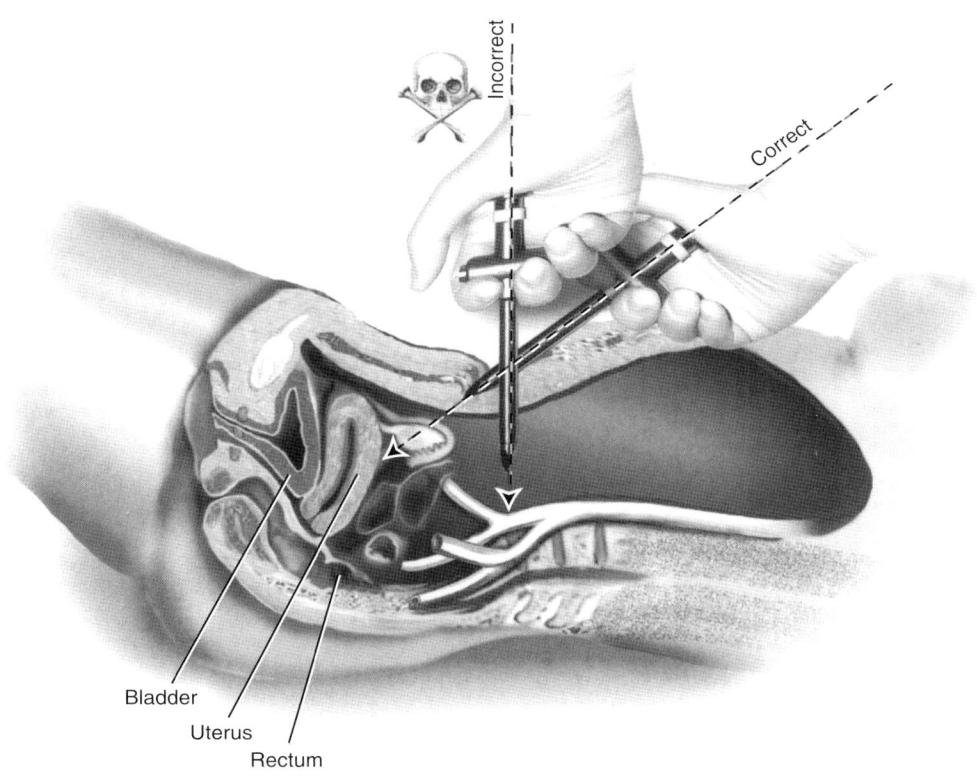

Bladder
Uterus
Rectum

**FIGURE 122–7** Equal in importance for safe trocar entry is the angle for vectoring the trocar into the abdominal cavity. The correct angle is 45° to 60°. This changes the aim of the device in the direction of the uterus. A thrust at 90° will target the aorta or the left common iliac vein. (Baggish MS: J Gynecol Surg 19:63-73, 2003. By permission.)

**TABLE 122–4 ■ Patients (n = 31) With Major-Vessel Injury by Body Mass Index (BMI)\***

| BMI* | Group | Number |
|---|---|---|
| <20 | Thin | 6 |
| <25 | Not obese | 3 |
| 25–30 | Overweight | 9† ⎫ |
| >30 | Obese | 13† ⎭ |

Baggish MS: J Gynecol Surg 19:63-73, 2003. With permission.
*Wt, kg/height, m².
†22 overweight or obese cases.

**TABLE 122–5** ■ **Critical Measurements From Primary Trocar Entry Point to the Great Retroperitoneal Blood Vessels**

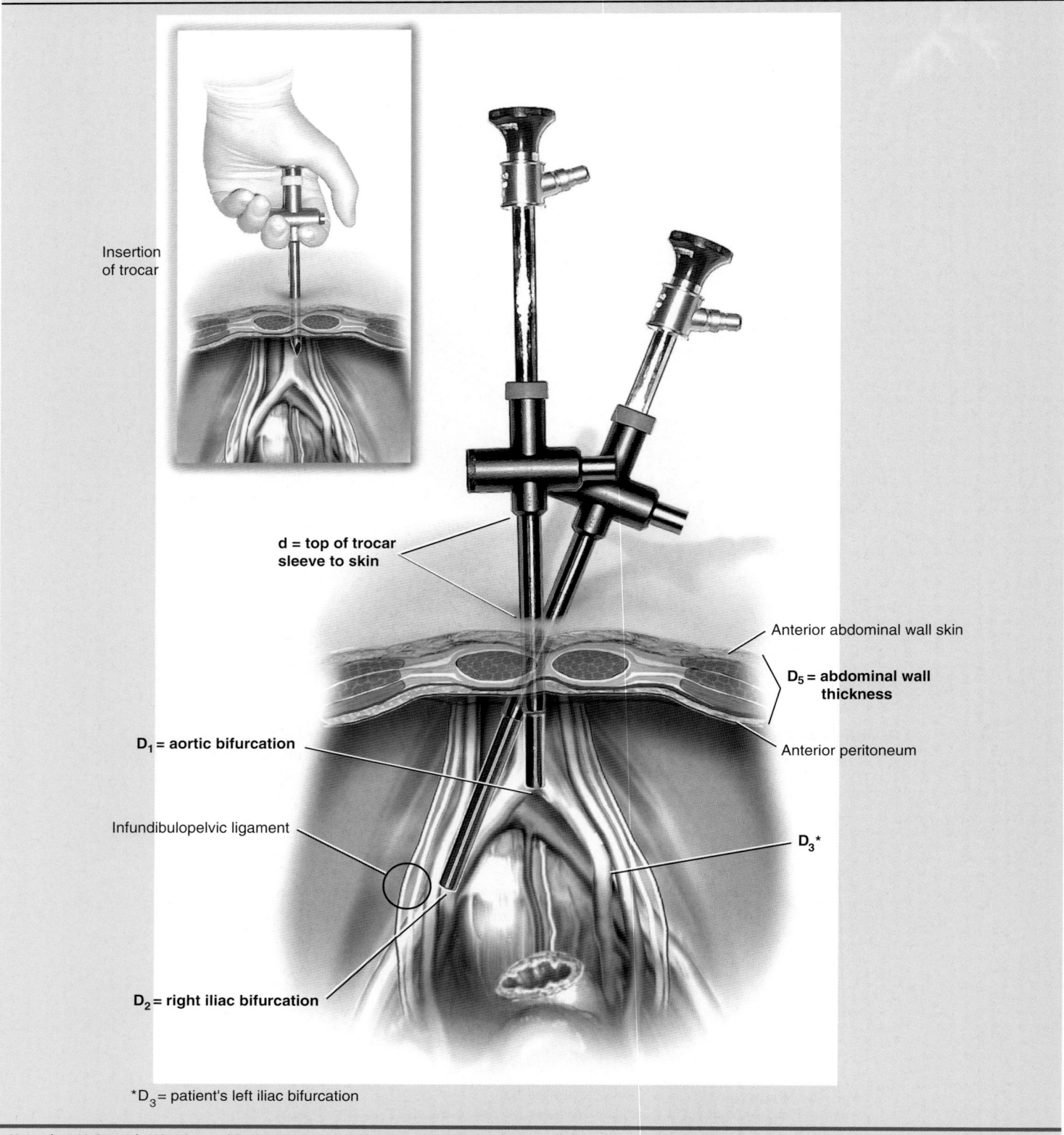

Insertion of trocar

d = top of trocar sleeve to skin

Anterior abdominal wall skin

$D_5$ = abdominal wall thickness

$D_1$ = aortic bifurcation

Anterior peritoneum

Infundibulopelvic ligament

$D_3$*

$D_2$ = right iliac bifurcation

*$D_3$= patient's left iliac bifurcation

Narendran M, Baggish MS: J Gynecol Surg 18:121-127, 2002. By permission.

**TABLE 122–6** ■ **Mean Distances (cm) Between Umbilical Trocar Entry and Large Retroperitoneal Vessels**

| Distance | Body Mass Index | | | | Height, m | | | |
|---|---|---|---|---|---|---|---|---|
| | <25 (n = 49) | 25.01–30 (n = 29) | >30 (n = 21) | *P* Value | 1.5–1.65 (n = 22) | 1.66–1.77 (n = 43) | 1.76–1.8 (n = 34) | *P* Value |
| Perpendicular distance to aortic bifurcation | 11.21 | 14.14 | 15.14 | .0006 | 12.60 | 12.56 | 13.78 | **NS** |
| Oblique distance to right common iliac vessels | 16.33 | 17.27 | 18.39 | NS | 16.49 | 16.24 | 18.41 | .02 |
| Oblique distance to left common iliac vessels | 16.49 | 17.36 | 18.53 | NS | 16.35 | 16.43 | 18.66 | .01 |
| Oblique distance to superior margin of bladder | 17.43 | 17.56 | 18.75 | NS | 16.18 | 17.41 | 19.13 | .04 |
| Perpendicular distance from peritoneum to skin at umbilicus (abdominal wall thickness) | 3.48 | 3.85 | 5.05 | .001 | — | — | — | — |
| Oblique distance from subumbilical peritoneal opening to right common iliac vessels | 12.69 | 12.96 | 13.12 | NS | — | — | — | — |
| Oblique distance from subumbilical peritoneal opening to left common iliac vessels | 12.93 | 12.91 | 13.39 | NS | — | — | — | — |

Source: Adapted with permission from Narendran M, Baggish MS: J Gynecol Surg 18:121-127, 2002.
NS, Nonsignificant.

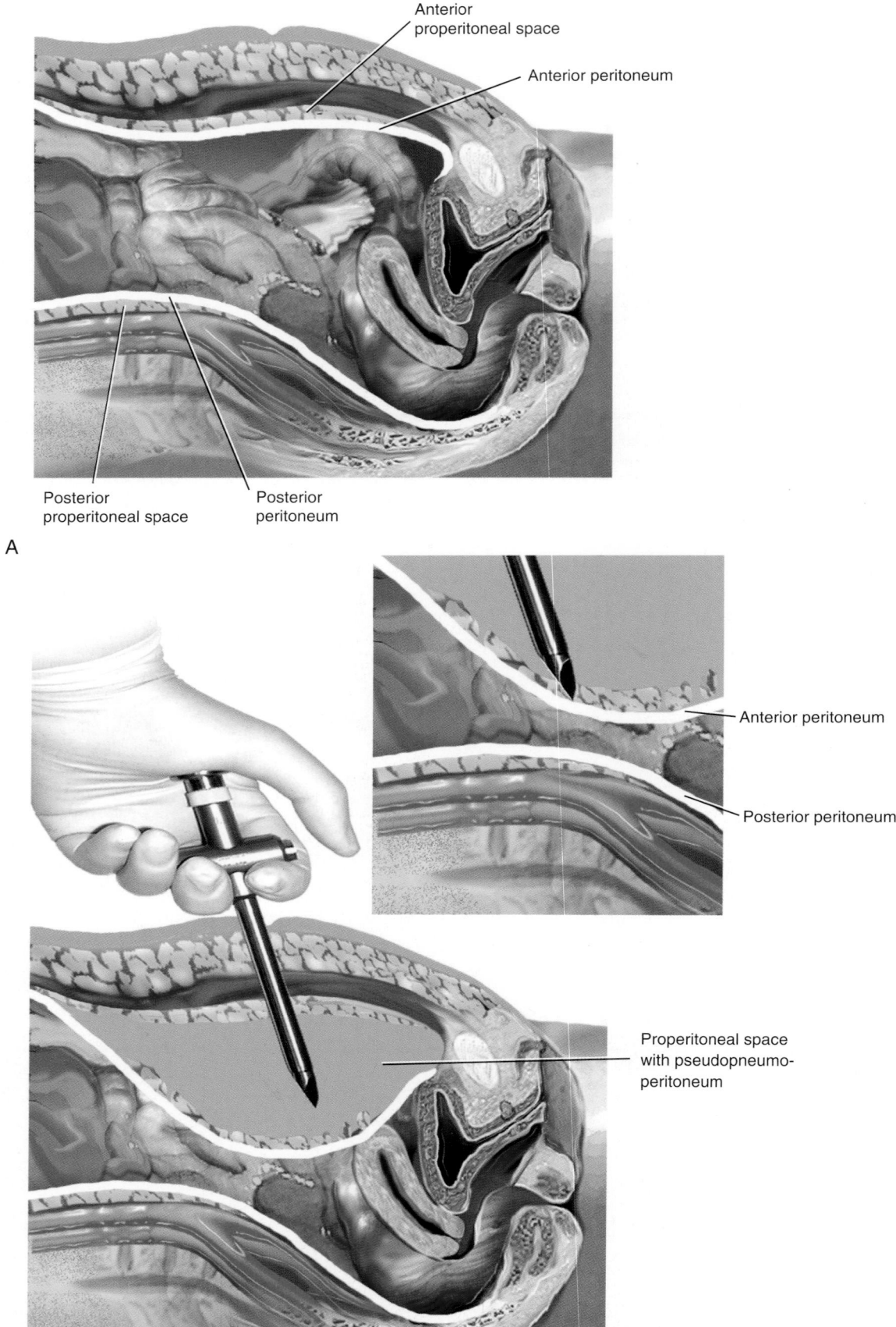

**FIGURE 122–8 A.** Creation of a pneumoperitoneum in an obese woman may be difficult. Not infrequently, the pneumoperitoneum needle is placed into the peritoneal fat of the anterior abdominal wall. **B.** Gas inflated outside the peritoneal cavity creates a pseudopneumoperitoneum. A reusable trocar, if dull, will not penetrate the anterior peritoneum toward the posterior wall. A dull trocar usually will not injure the large retroperitoneal vessels.

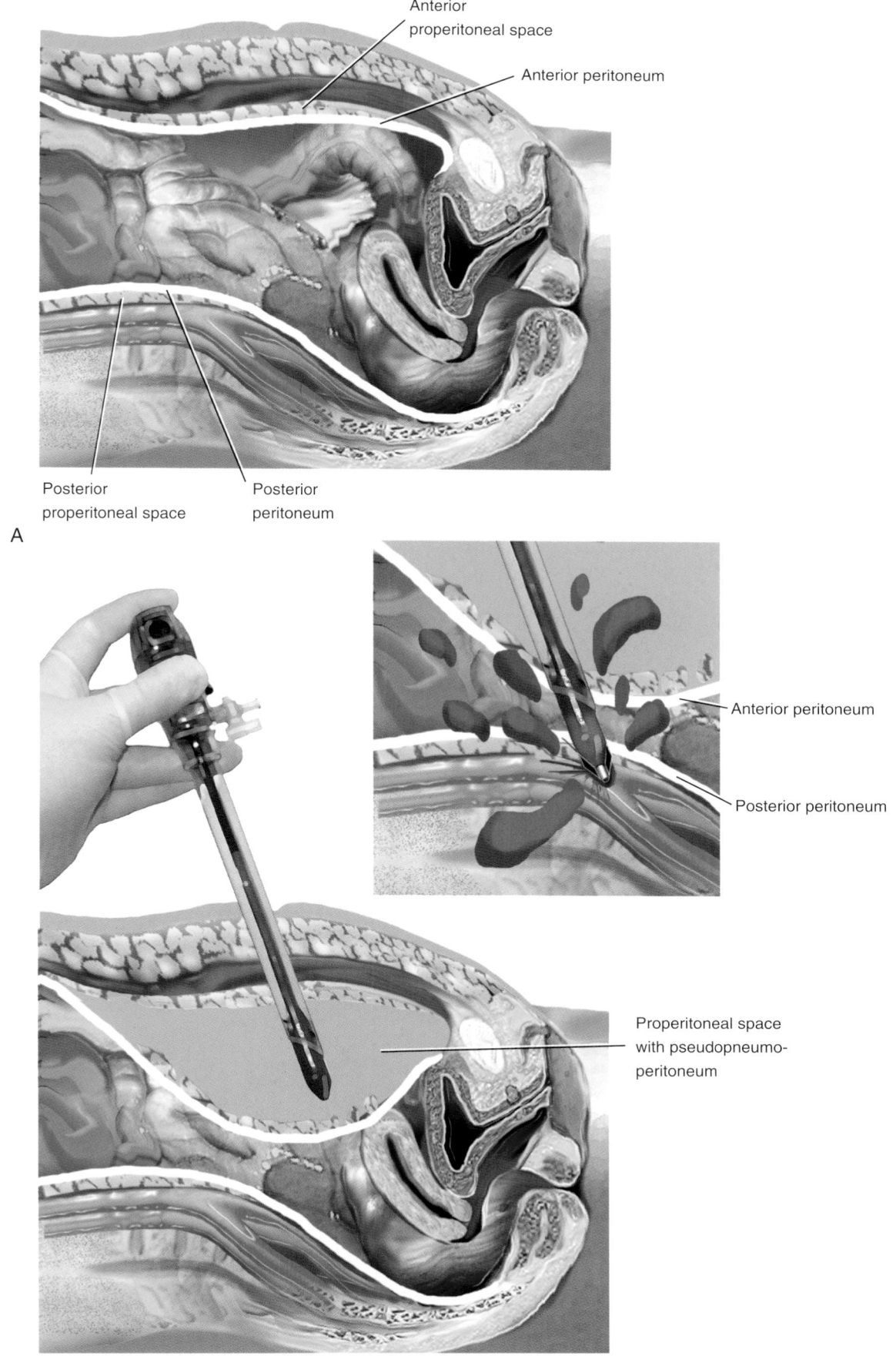

Anterior
properitoneal space

Anterior peritoneum

Posterior
properitoneal space

Posterior
peritoneum

A

Anterior peritoneum

Posterior peritoneum

Properitoneal space
with pseudopneumo-
peritoneum

B

**FIGURE 122–9 A.** A similar situation is shown here as in Fig. 122–8. **B.** In this case, a disposable trocar is depicted. Because the pseudopneumoperitoneal space is not capacious as compared with a true pneumoperitoneum, the shield fails to deploy, the trocar remains armed, and the sharp cutting blade penetrates into the posterior peritoneum, lacerating one of the large retroperitoneal vessels.

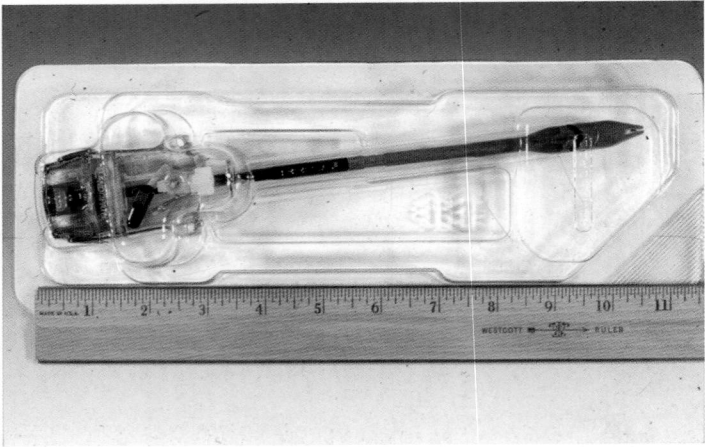

**FIGURE 122–10** The long disposable trocar measures 11 inches in length and is a risky device. It should not be used because it increases the chance of major vascular injury.

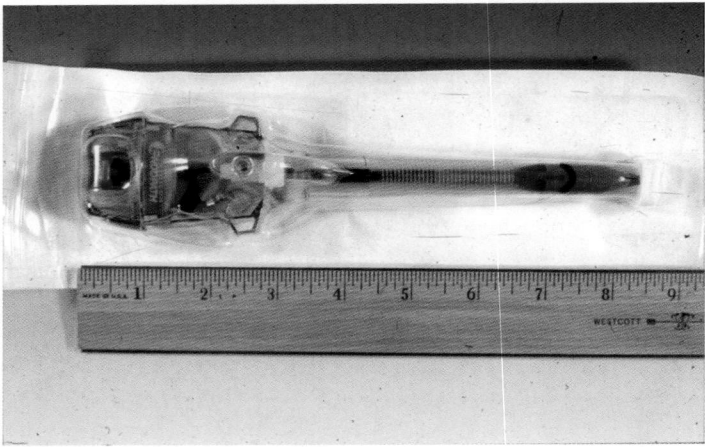

**FIGURE 122–11** The standard disposable trocar is 8 inches long and is capable of entering the abdominal cavity, even in obese women.

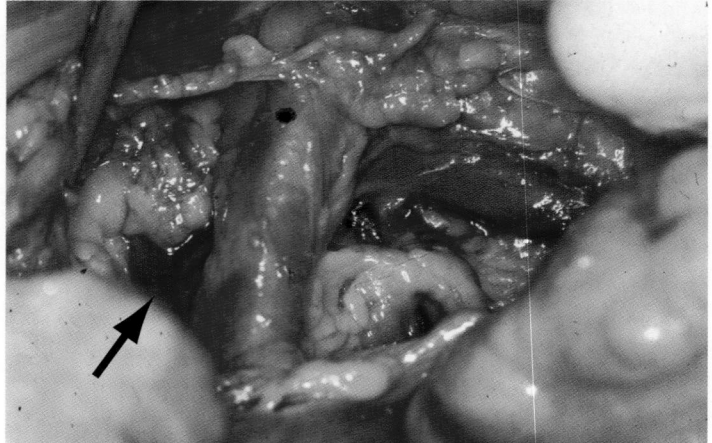

**FIGURE 122–12** Close-up view of the mid and right retroperitoneum. The dot marks the right common iliac artery. The left common iliac vein crosses the midline from left to right over the L5 vertebral body. The *arrow* points to the right common iliac vein, which forms the inferior vena cava after it unites with the left common iliac vein just lateral to the proximal portion of the right common iliac artery.

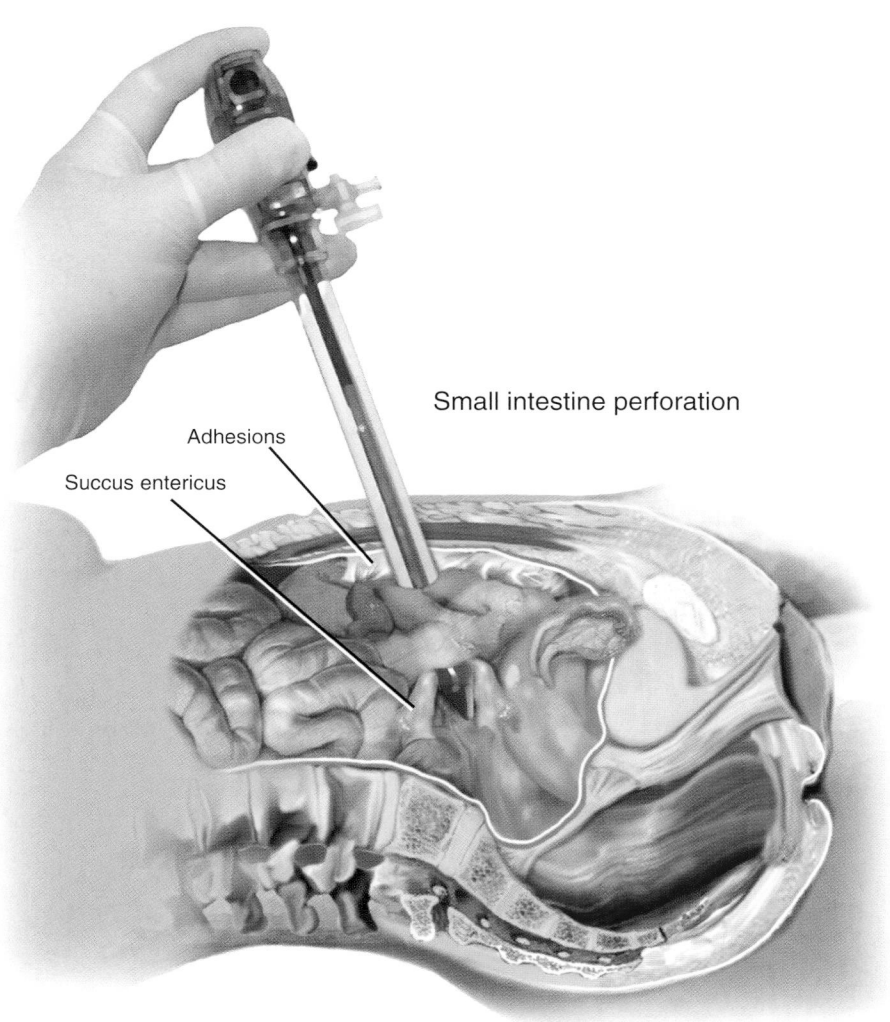

A

**FIGURE 122–13  A.** This figure illustrates the uncommon circumstance of adhesions fixing a segment of small intestine to the anterior abdominal wall. The trocar penetrates the loop of bowel. The injury will not be detected unless the surgeon carefully observes as the sheath and the laparoscope are simultaneously withdrawn at the end of the procedure.

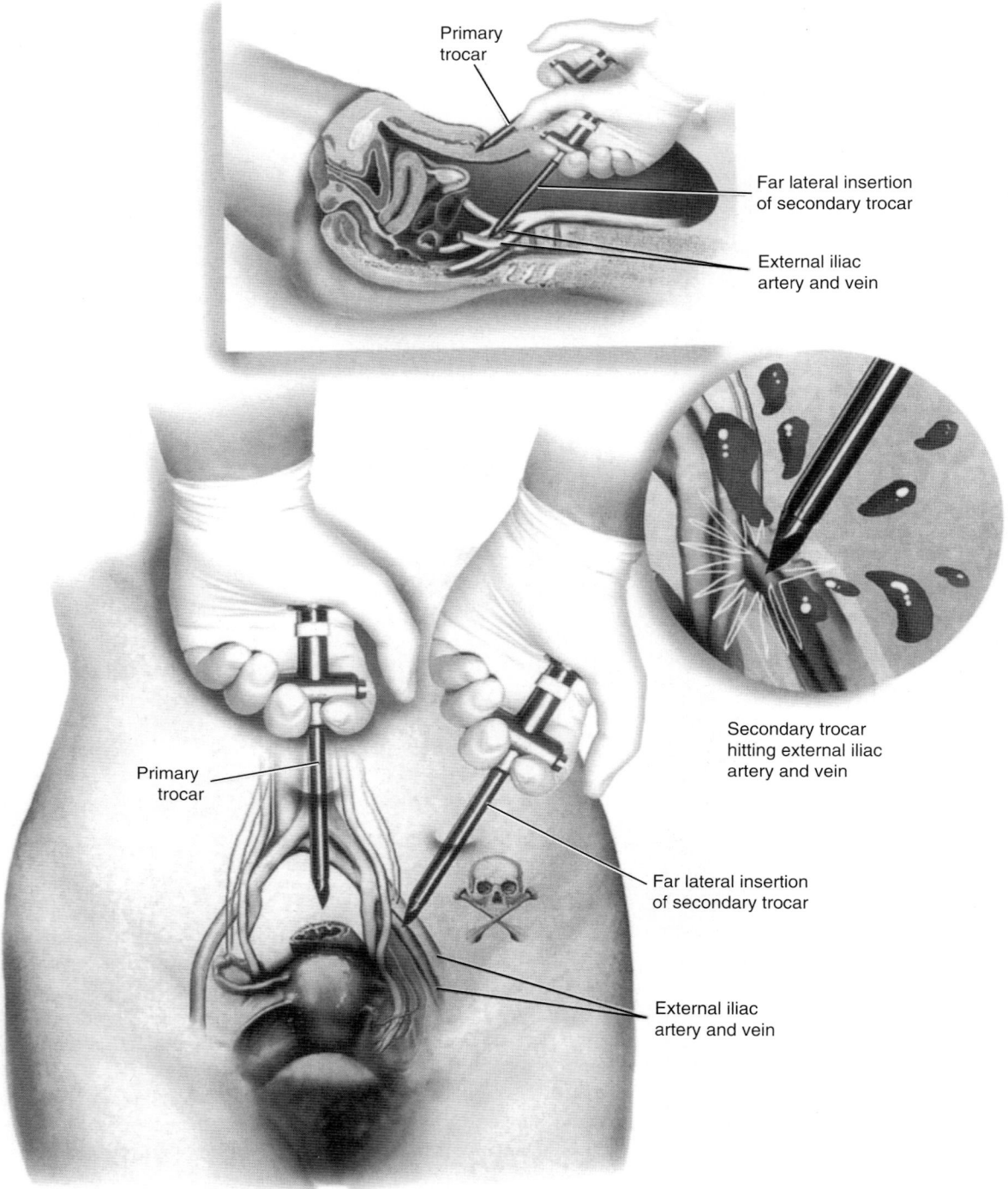

Primary
trocar

Far lateral insertion
of secondary trocar

External iliac
artery and vein

Secondary trocar
hitting external iliac
artery and vein

Primary
trocar

Far lateral insertion
of secondary trocar

External iliac
artery and vein

B

**FIGURE 122–13, cont'd  B.** Secondary trocars uncommonly cause major laparoscopic injuries because they are placed under direct vision. However, far lateral placement may cause injury to the external iliac vein or artery. (Baggish MS: J Gynecol Surg 19:63-73, 2003.)

## Operative Procedure

Injuries secondary to dissection are more likely to happen during laparoscopic operations than during laparotomy. Vision, particularly peripheral vision, is limited during laparoscopic procedures. Although the technique of bringing the laparoscope closer to the operative field magnifies the structures, the absence of a wide, panoramic, three-dimensional view limits depth perception and the ability to see surrounding structures. Finally, suturing and knot-tying are more difficult and more time consuming during laparoscopic procedures than during open techniques; thus energy devices (see Chapter 5) are more frequently employed during laparoscopy. High-power bipolar cutting and coagulating devices such as Plasma Kinetic Forceps (Gyrus ACMI, Southborough, Massachusetts) and LigaSure instruments (Covidien, Boulder, Colorado) are commonly used to obtain hemostasis; they do introduce the risk of thermal injury (Fig. 122–14A through D). Bipolar devices cause damage to structures by (1) spreading heat peripherally from the point of contact, and (2) directly grasping and cooking the wrong structure. Monopolar electrosurgical instruments are especially risky for high-frequency leaks, capacitive coupling, direct coupling, and insulation failure. Lasers and harmonic scalpel devices are also risky for creating thermal injuries beyond their intended target (Fig. 122–14E, Table 122–7). A seminal fact relates to minimally invasive operative procedures. The clinical pathway after laparoscopic surgery during the postoperative period is one of progressive clinical improvement. Each hour and each day should be marked by fewer symptoms and progressively improving signs. Deviation from the pathway should immediately signal the gynecologist to vigorously search for evidence of a complication related to his or her surgery (Fig. 122–15A, B). Early diagnosis of an injury will ameliorate the collateral damage. Failure to place a possible laparoscopic complication at the top of the differential diagnosis is an invitation to experience the most serious consequences (Tables 122–8, 122–9, and 122–10).

## Ureteral Injury

The third major complication associated with laparoscopic surgery is ureteral injury. The techniques used to avoid this type of injury are discussed in Chapter 37. Rarely are these complications caused by a trocar, although the ureter occasionally has been damaged as a collateral injury secondary to a major vessel or intestinal wound. Ureteral injuries generally will not result in mortality unless they are bilateral and neglected. However, an unrecognized ureteral obstruction or laceration may result in permanent kidney damage, leading to subsequent nephrectomy.

Ureteral injury is associated with the operative procedure and the sundry tools utilized for the purpose of hemostasis (Fig. 122–16A). Another major factor is related to lack of knowledge on the part of the surgeon relative to pelvic anatomy. Without this precise knowledge, surgeons are reluctant to explore the retroperitoneal space and isolate the ureter. As was noted in previous chapters, the ureter is vulnerable in three (Fig. 122–16B) principal locations: (1) where it crosses the common iliac vessels in concert with the ovarian blood supply, (2) where the uterine vessels cross over the ureter, and (3) where it enters the bladder, as well as within its intravesical course (Fig. 122–16C). Ancillary devices associated with ureteral injury include staplers, lasers, harmonic scalpels, and high-energy bipolar devices (LigaSure, plasma, kinetic forceps) (Fig. 122–16D). Less commonly, endo loops, sutures, and blunt dissection are associated with ureteral damage. The laparoscopic stapler is both wide and excessively long and accounts for an inordinately high number of ureteral injuries. This instrument typically obstructs and severs the ureter (Fig. 122–16E).

When a ureter or for that matter the bladder is lacerated or cut, urine spills into the abdominal cavity (Fig. 122–16F). The urine is partially absorbed via the peritoneum, leading to blood chemical derangements. The distention created by the accumulated fluid may be massive. A paracentesis should be performed to draw off the fluid, and a sample should always be sent to the laboratory for a creatine determination. An elevated creatine will cinch the diagnosis of urinoma.

Early recognition of ureteral obstruction or laceration is central to mitigate permanent kidney damage (Figs. 122–17 and 122–18). Symptoms of ureteral obstruction may range from severe abdominal and flank pain to minimal discomfort. Although any number of tests may be performed to enable a diagnosis to be made, the retrograde pyelogram is the most direct and important study (Fig. 122–19A through C). Once the diagnosis is secured, depending on the circumstances, treatment will take the form of passage of a stent or nephrostomy. Subsequent ureteroneocystotomy with or without psoas hitch will relieve the complication.

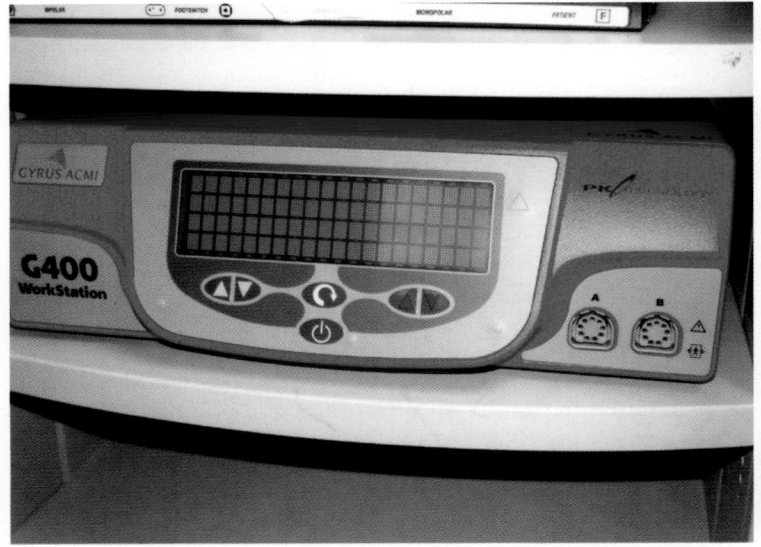

A

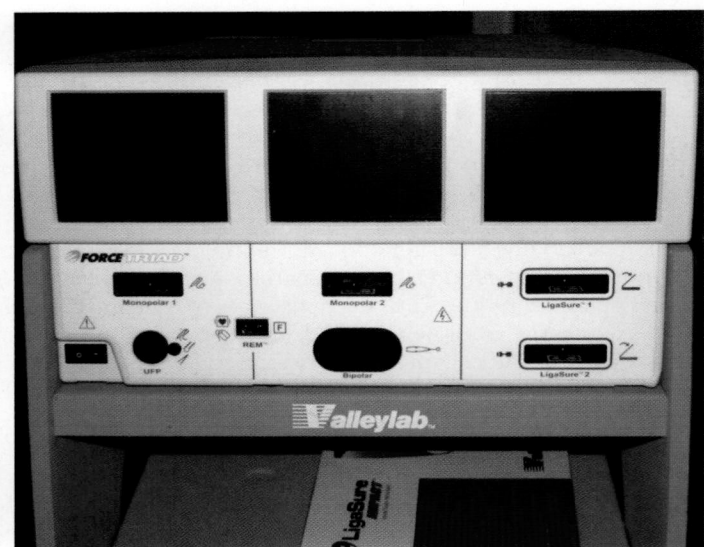

B

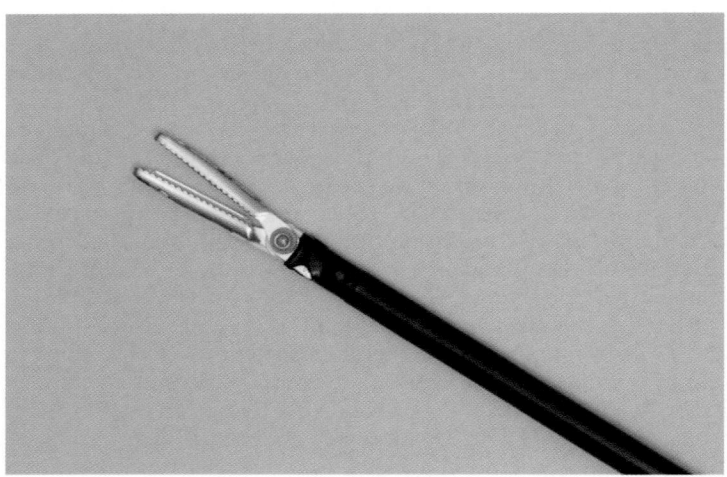

C

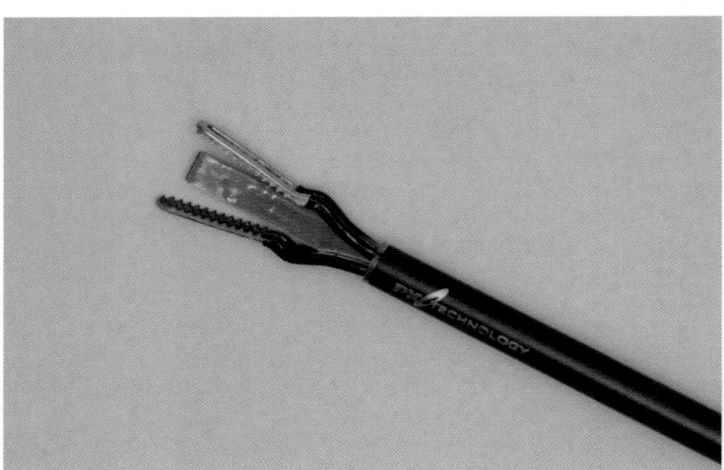

D

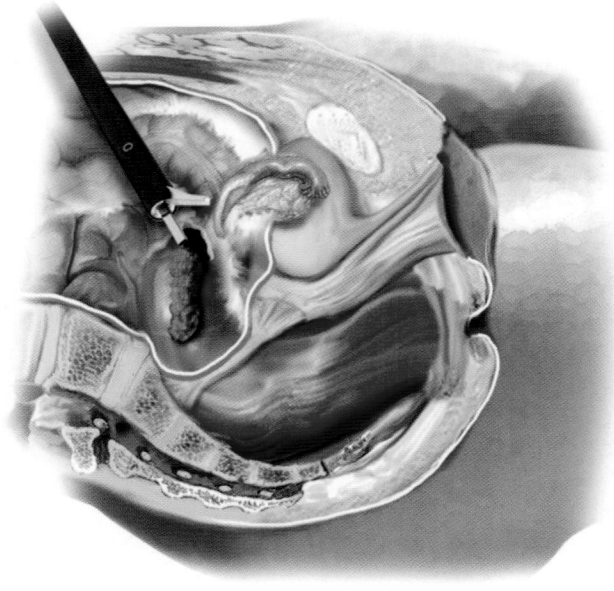

E

**FIGURE 122–14  A.** This high-power bipolar generator permits efficient bipolar coagulation and cutting. **B.** This contemporary multipurpose electrosurgical unit has monopolar, bipolar, and high output polar coagulation and cutting capability. **C.** This alligator-type Plasma Kinetic Forceps is utilized for hemostasis during robotic and major laparoscopic surgical procedures. **D.** This bipolar device (tripolar) coagulates tissue by extension of a sharp knife blade to instantly cut the thermally altered tissue. **E.** A harmonic cutting scissor-like device cuts into the sigmoid colon, creating a perforation and allowing fecal contents to spill into the peritoneal cavity.

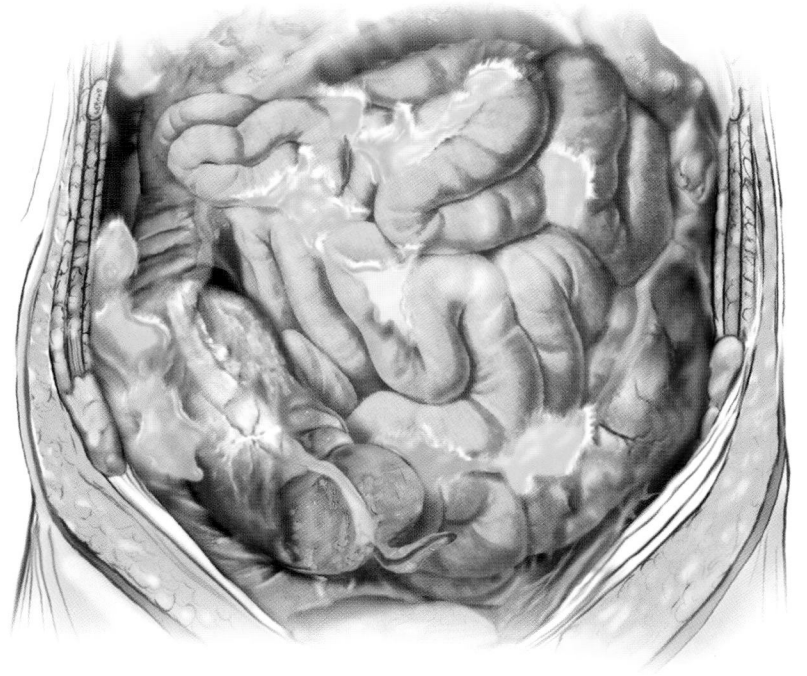

A

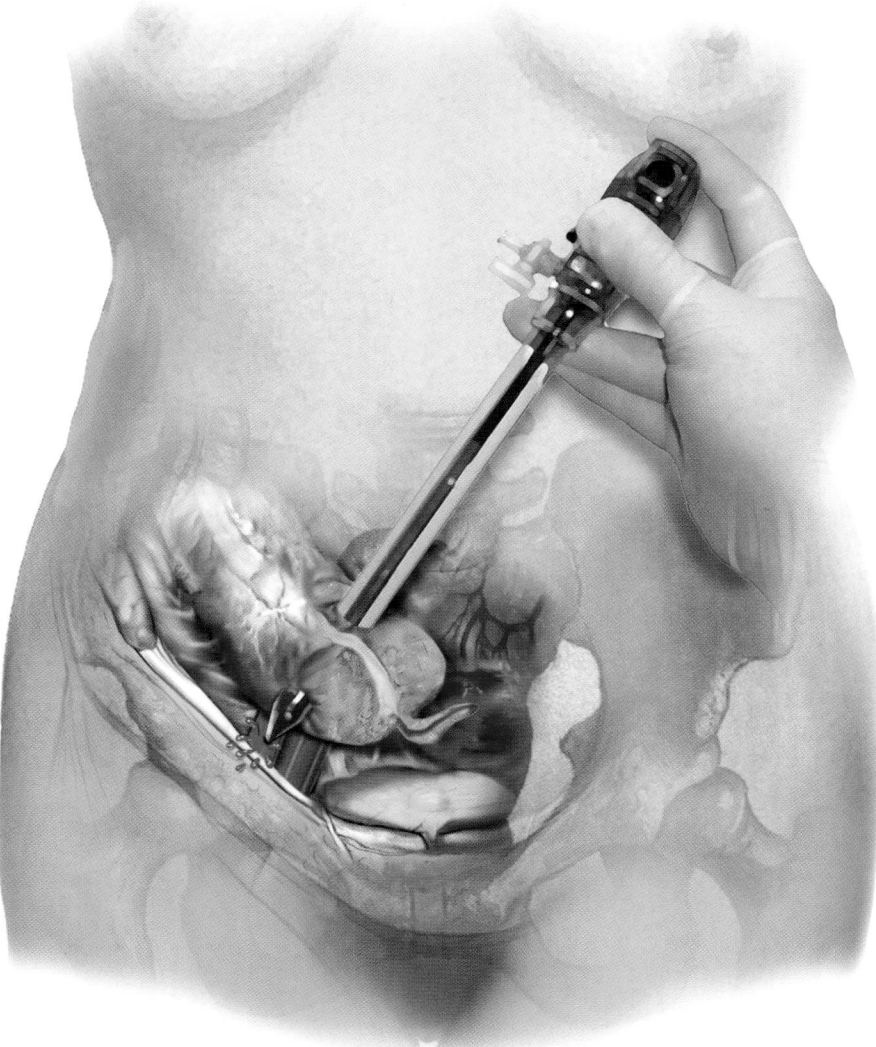

B

**FIGURE 122–15  A.** The results of intestinal perforation include peritonitis and multiple-interloop abscess formation. **B.** A collateral injury is illustrated here. The deviant trocar thrust not only perforates the cecum but additionally lacerates the right common iliac artery.

### TABLE 122–7 ■ Energy Devices Associated With Intestinal Injury

| Device | No. of Cases | Percentage |
|---|---|---|
| Monopolar | 9 | 43 |
| Bipolar | 6 | 29 |
| Laser | 1 | 5 |
| Harm scalpel | 5 | 23 |
| **Total** | **21** | |

Baggish MS: J Gynecol Surg 23:83-95, 2007. Ob-Gyn Management 16:70-87, 2004. With permission.

### TABLE 122–8 ■ Ten Ways to Lower the Risk of Intestinal Injury

- Avoid laparoscopy when severe adhesions are anticipated, such as when the patient has a history of multiple laparotomies, or when significant adhesions have been documented.

- Be aware that laparoscopy carries additional risks beyond those of the primary surgical procedure, owing to factors peculiar to endoscopic technique and instrumentation.

- Consider open laparoscopy or insert the primary trocar at an alternative location, such as the left upper quadrant, when the patient has a history of laparotomy.

- Avoid blunt dissection for anything other than mild (filmy) adhesions. Sharp dissection associated with hydrodissection is the safest method of adhesiolysis. Clear visualization of the operative site is the sine qua non for precise dissection.

- Avoid monopolar electrosurgical devices for laparoscopic surgery whenever possible. Also remember that bipolar and ultrasonic devices can cause thermal injury by heat conduction as well as by direct application. Laser energy will continue beyond the target unless provision is made to absorb the residual energy.

- At the conclusion of any laparoscopic procedure, especially after adhesiolysis or bowel dissection, inspect the intestines and include the details in the operative report.

- After any laparoscopic procedure, if the patient does not improve steadily, the first presumptive diagnosis to be excluded is injury secondary to the procedure or technique.

- The major symptom of intestinal perforation is abdominal pain, which does not ease without increasing quantities of analgesics.

- Investigate any bowel injury thoroughly to determine viability at the site of injury. Whenever possible, repair all injuries intraoperatively.

- After intestinal perforation, the risk of sepsis is high. Look for early signs such as tachycardia, subnormal body temperature, depressed white blood cell (WBC) count, and the appearance of immature white cell elements.

Baggish MS: J Gynecol Surg 23:83-95, 2007. Ob-Gyn Management 16:70-87, 2004. With permission.

### TABLE 122–9 ■ Recommended Management for Gynecologists

1. Call for vascular surgeon *STAT* and indicate this is an emergency.
2. Do not observe retroperitoneal hematoma.
3. Open abdomen via vertical incision.
4. Do not attempt to clamp the bleeding vessel, but do apply direct pressure with sponge stick.
5. Get emergency type and crossmatch for minimum of 6 units (whole blood is preferable).
6. Get baseline Hgb, Hct, platelets, fibrinogen, and fibrin split products.
7. Get accurate outputs and blood loss estimates, and have anesthesia personnel keep careful records of fluid(s) given.
8. Advise anesthesia staff to obtain additional help.
9. Use a circulator to manage *STATs*.

Baggish MS: J Gynecol Surg 19:63-73, 2003. With permission.

### TABLE 122–10 ■ Fatalities Always Involved Venous Injuries (7/31; 23%)

| | |
|---|---|
| Right common iliac vein | 3 |
| Vena cava and left common iliac vein | 1 |
| Left common iliac vein | 1 |
| Right hypogastric veins | 1 |
| Right external iliac vein and right hypogastric vein | 3 |

Baggish MS: J Gynecol Surg 19:63-73, 2003. With permission.
Note: Three fatalities were associated with long disposable trocars.

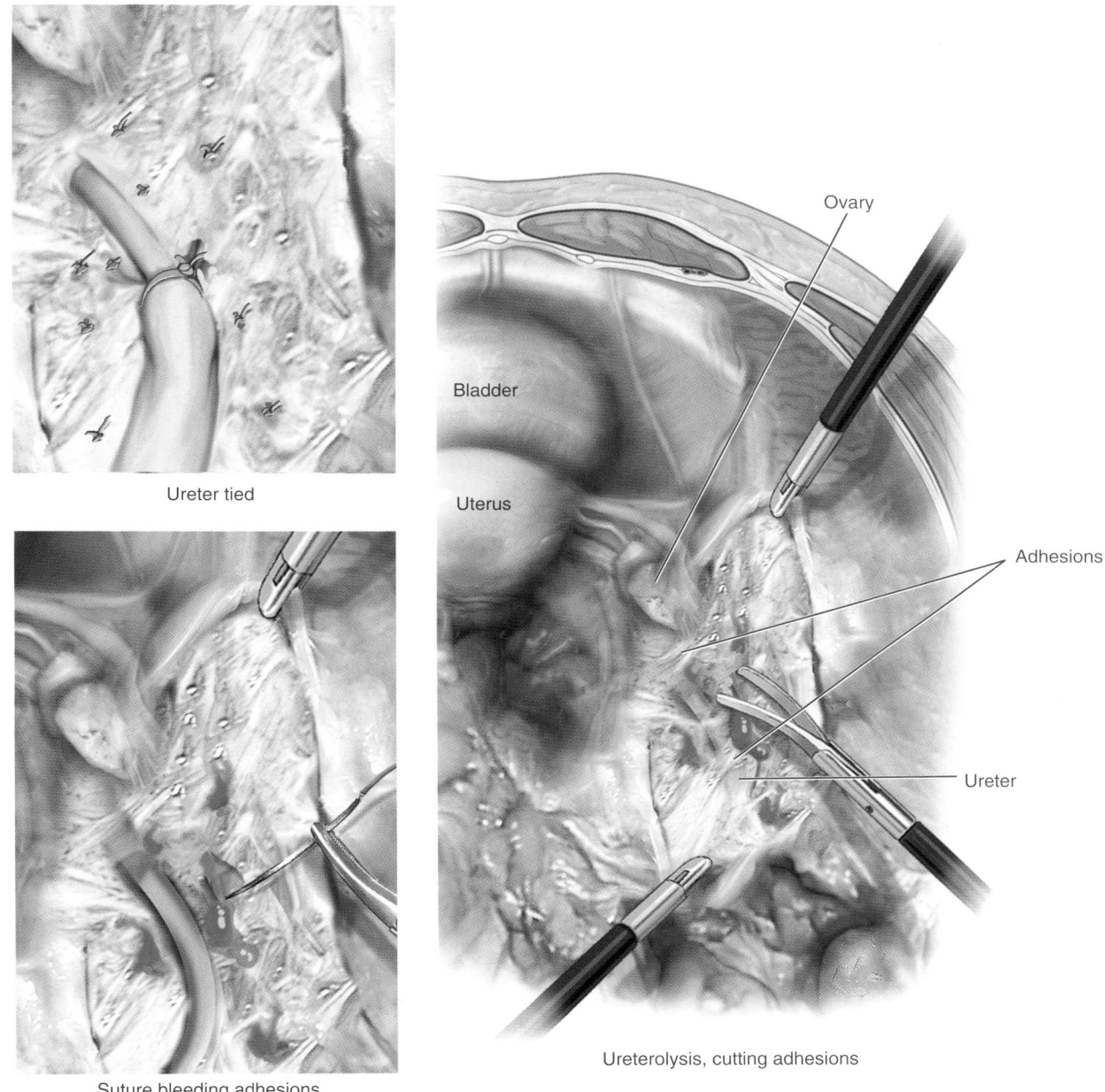

Ureter tied

Suture bleeding adhesions

Ovary

Bladder

Uterus

Adhesions

Ureter

Ureterolysis, cutting adhesions

A

**FIGURE 122–16  A.** The ureter is vulnerable to laceration or ligation during adhesiolysis. When adhesions are lysed, bleeding can ensue. Sutures placed to enable hemostasis can impinge upon or totally seal off the ureter if the latter is not secured.

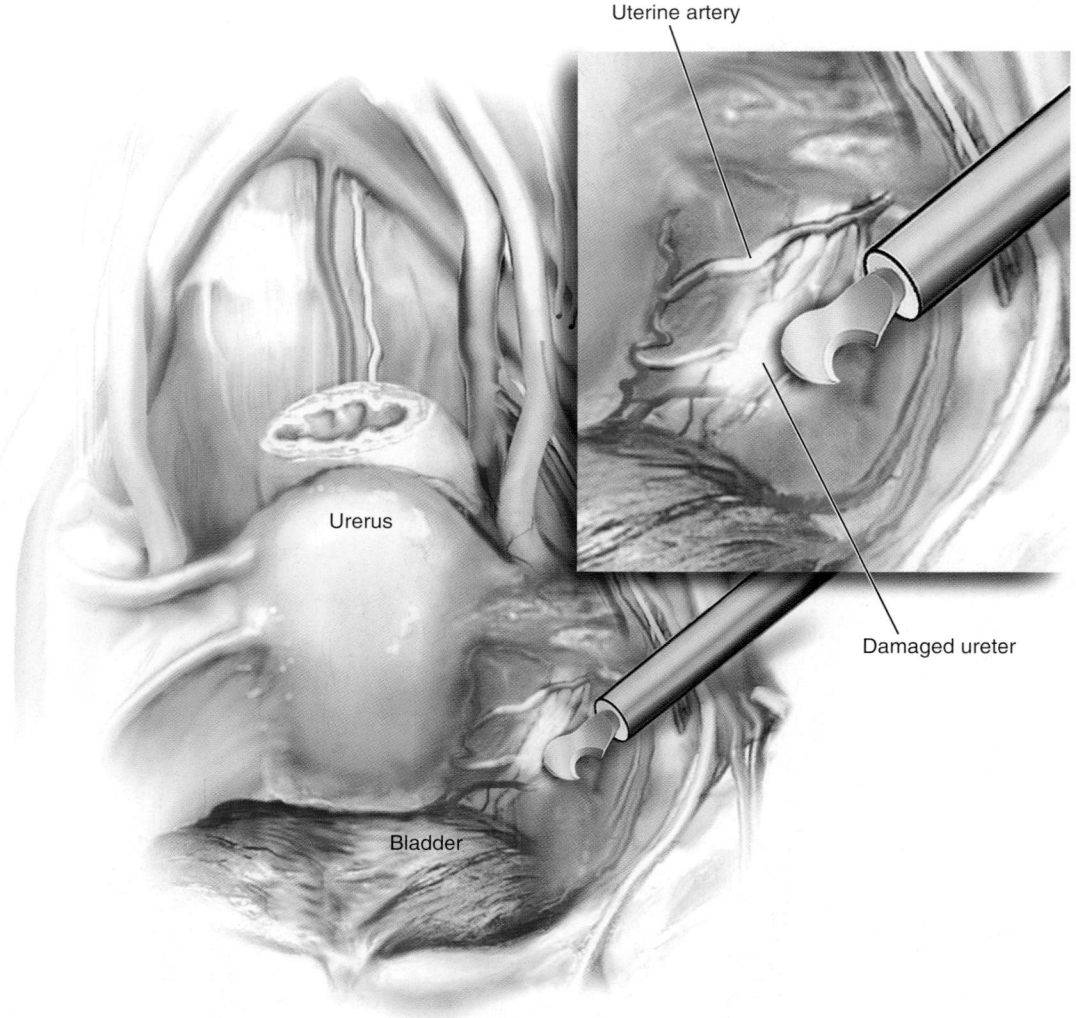

Uterine artery

Damaged ureter

Urerus

Bladder

Anterior view

B

**FIGURE 122–16, cont'd  B.** The harmonic scalpel creates hemostasis and cuts tissue. The hemostatic action generates heat through a variety of mechanisms, including friction. In the process of sealing and severing the uterine blood supply, the ureter may be thermally damaged as illustrated here.

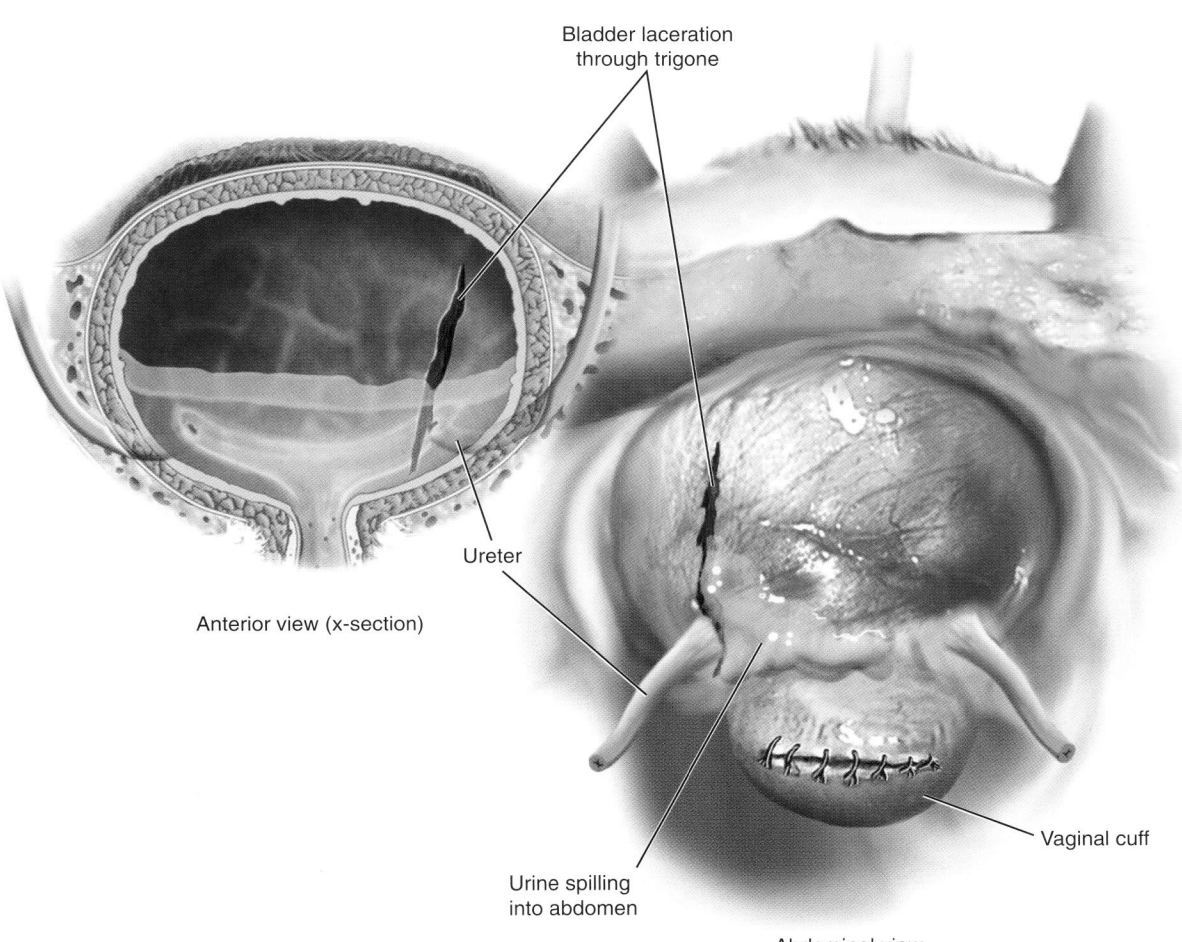

Bladder laceration
through trigone

Ureter

Anterior view (x-section)

Vaginal cuff

Urine spilling
into abdomen

Abdominal view

C

**FIGURE 122–16, cont'd  C.** A bladder laceration that extends through the trigone is a very serious injury that requires expert management. Damage to the intravesical ureter or to the ureter at the ureterovesical junction must be ruled out. This will involve cystoscopic examination and retrograde pyelography. During the repair, ureteral stenting is recommended even if the ureter has not sustained injury.

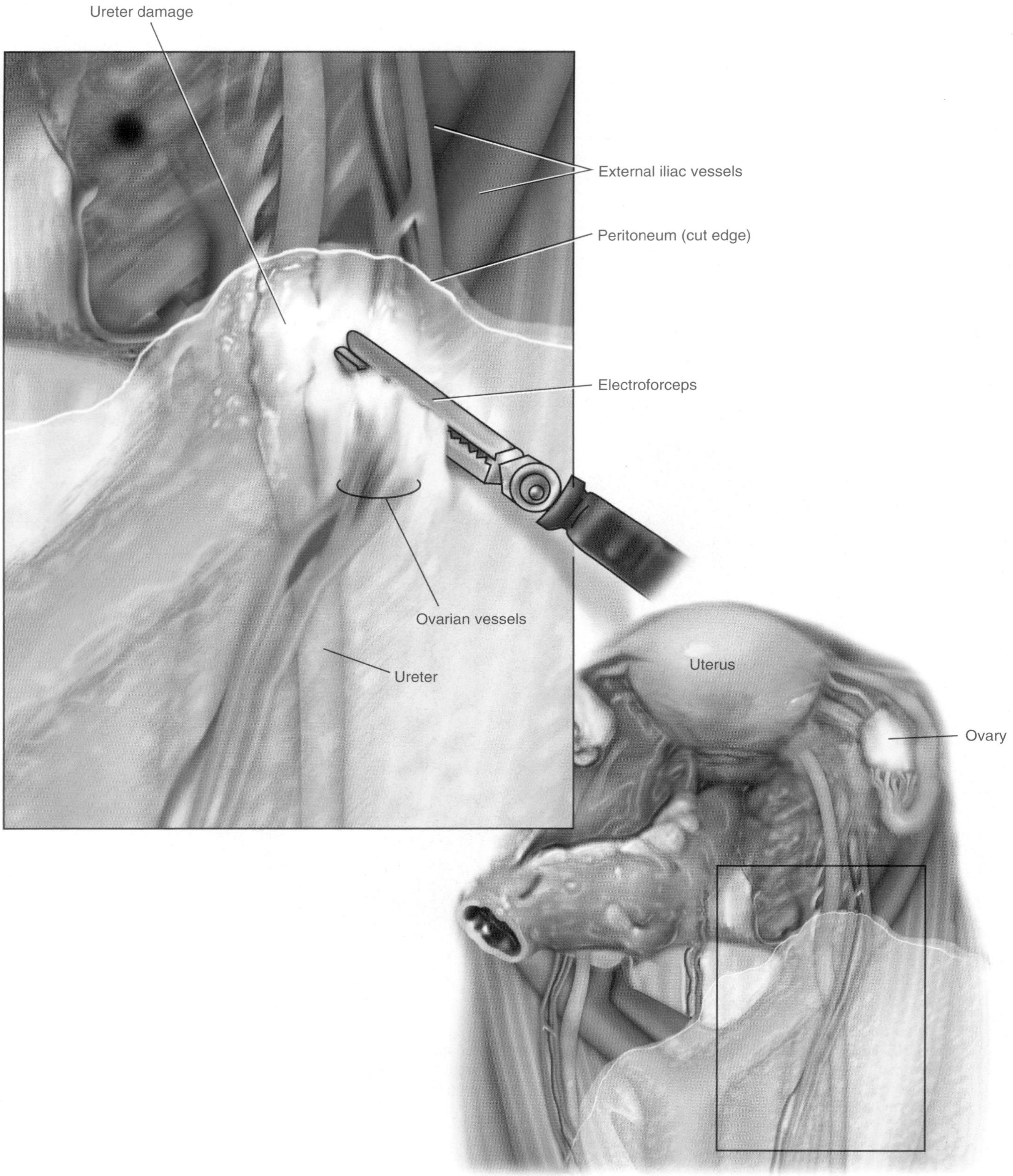

Ureter damage

External iliac vessels

Peritoneum (cut edge)

Electroforceps

Ovarian vessels

Ureter

Uterus

Ovary

D

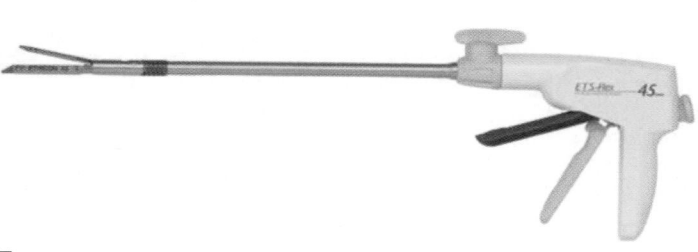

E

**FIGURE 122–16, cont'd  D.** High-energy bipolar coagulation can and will create ureteral injury via thermal conduction through neighboring tissues. In the case illustrated here, a bipolar forceps coagulates the ovarian vessels, but heat spreads to encompass the nearby ureter, creating significant damage to that structure. **E.** The laparoscopic stapling device can cause ureteral injury when the instrument is applied across a vascular pedical without first securing the ureter. The long, broad jaws and staple cartridge do not permit discrete applications.

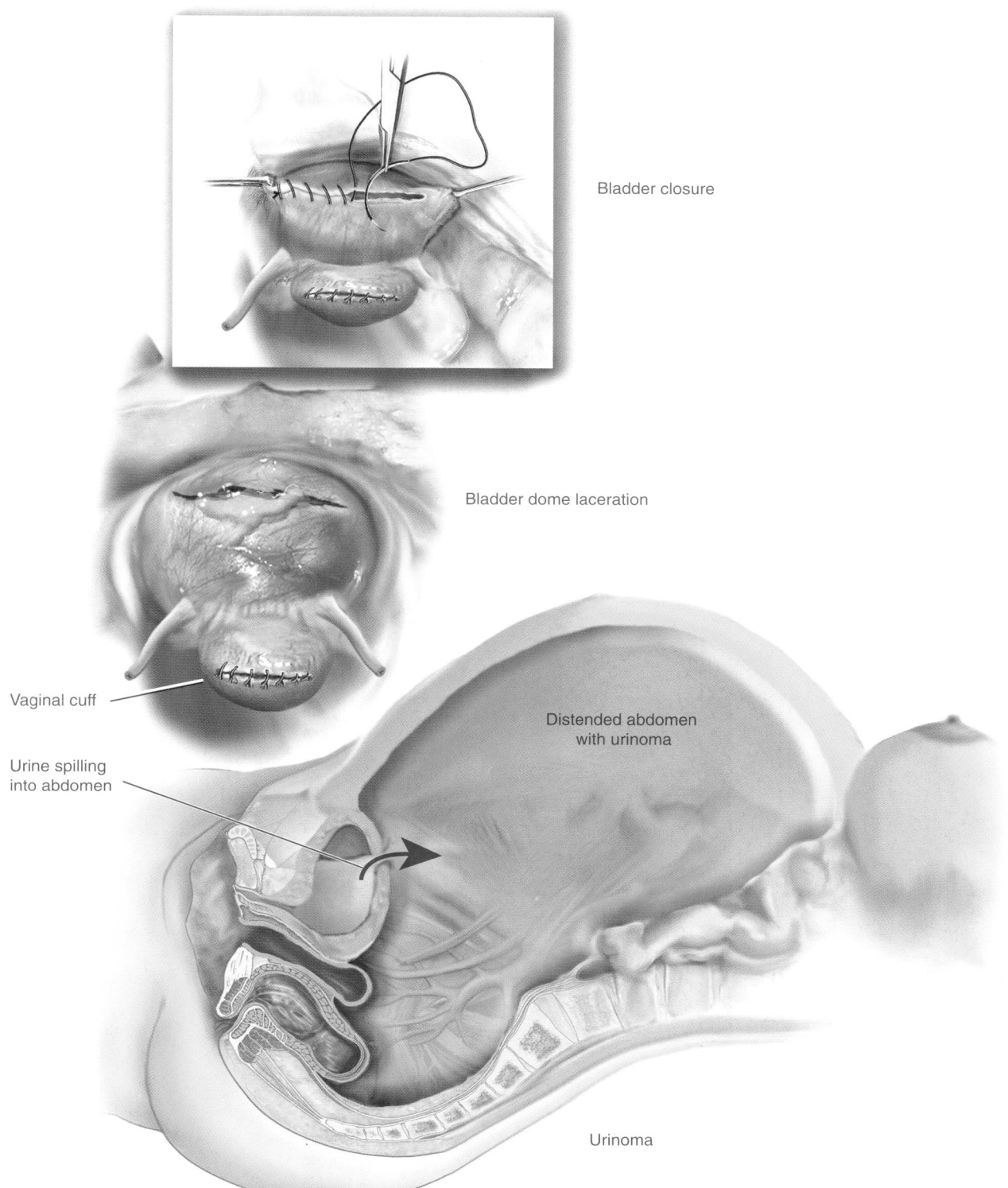

Bladder closure

Bladder dome laceration

Vaginal cuff

Urine spilling into abdomen

Distended abdomen with urinoma

Urinoma

F

**FIGURE 122–16, cont'd  F.** This drawing illustrates a laceration in the superior portion of the bladder's anterior wall (dome). The laceration was missed at the time of hysterectomy, and the patient developed a large urinoma. The laceration was subsequently repaired via a continuous through and through 2-0 chromic suture.

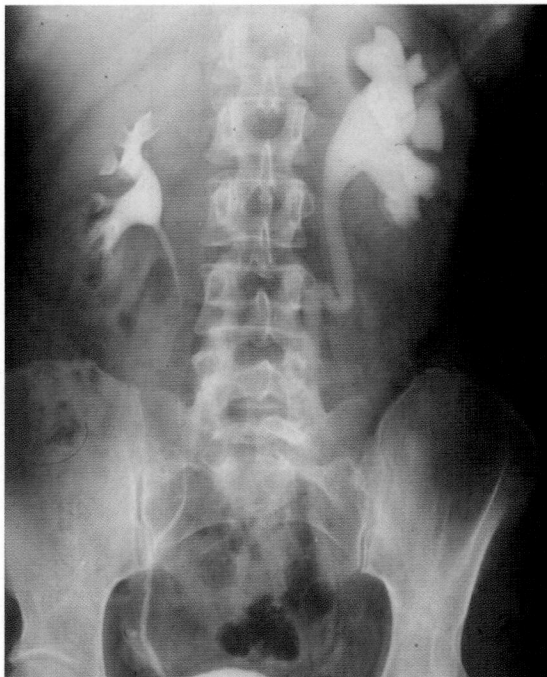

**FIGURE 122–17** Ureteral injury is demonstrated by an IVP note that the left ureter is dilated. The left kidney shows hydronephrosis.

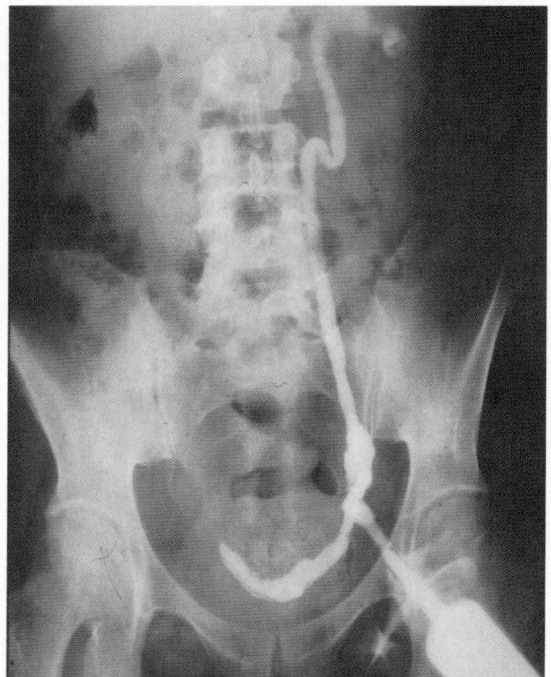

**FIGURE 122–18** A further complication is demonstrated in this picture. The patient chronically seeped urine through a drain site situated in the left lower quadrant. When radiographic dye was instilled through the drain site, a ureterocutaneous fistula was diagnosed.

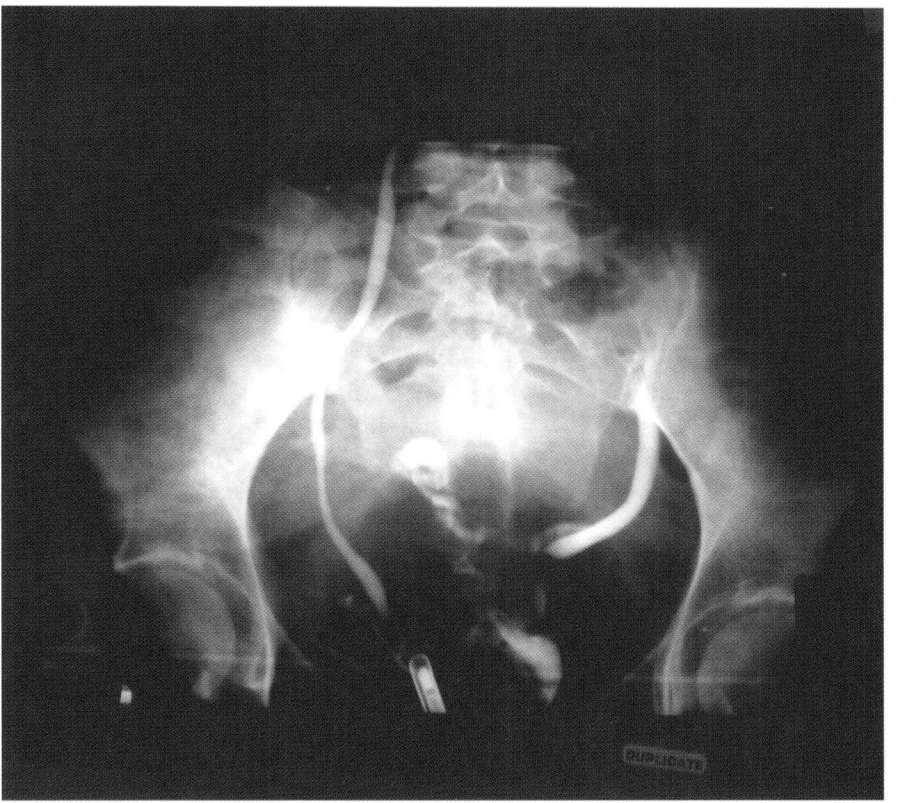

A

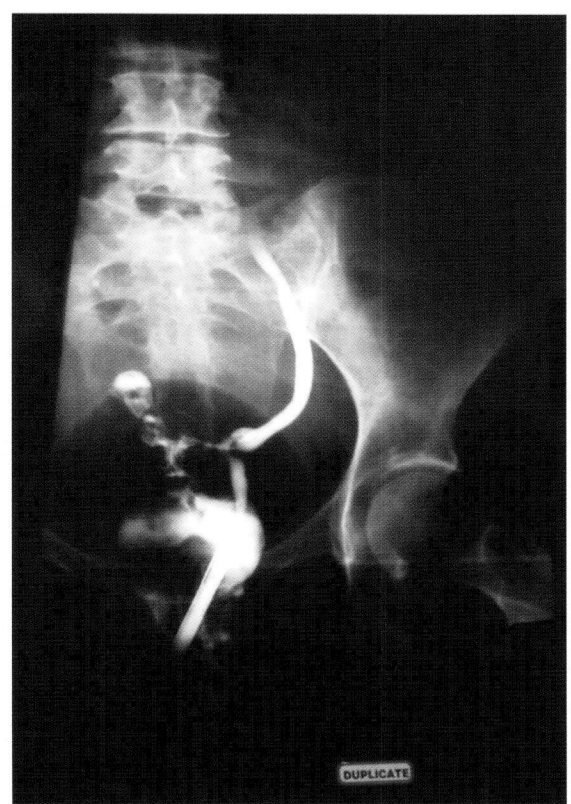

B

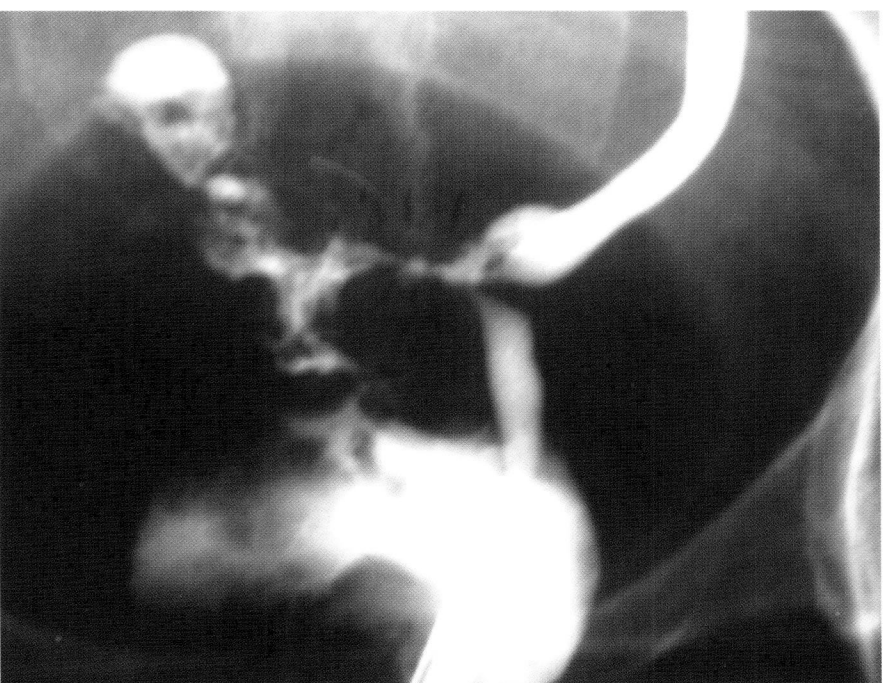

C

**FIGURE 122–19 A.** A retrograde urogram and intravenous pyelogram (IVP) were performed in this case. Note the normal right ureter. The left ureter shows disruption and extravasation of dye. The ureter was in fact severed. **B.** Retrograde urogram of the left ureter showing disruption and displacement of the ureter, as well as extravasation of dye. **C.** Close-up view of the left ureter shown in Fig. 122–19A and B.

# SECTION C

## Cystourethroscopy

UNIT 5 ■ SECTION C

1363

# CHAPTER 123

# Cystourethroscopy

*Alfred E. Bent* ■ *Geoffrey W. Cundiff*

## Instrumentation

The rigid urethroscope is a modification of the cystoscope, designed exclusively for evaluation of the urethra (Fig. 123–1). Because it is primarily a diagnostic instrument, it does not have a bridge. The telescope is shorter and has a 0° viewing angle, which provides a circumferential view of the urethral lumen as the mucosa in front of the urethroscope is distended by a distention medium. The 0° lens is essential for adequate ure-throscopy. The urethroscope sheath is designed to maximize distention of the urethral lumen. Sheaths are available in 15F and 24F calibers. If tolerated, the larger sheath is useful because it provides the best view of the urethral lumen by providing more rapid fluid flow for maximal distention. It also allows easier visibility of any abnormalities such as urethral diverticula.

The rigid cystoscope has three components: the telescope, the bridge, and the sheath (Fig. 123–2A through C). Each component serves a different function and is available with various options to facilitate its role under different circumstances. The telescope transmits light to the bladder cavity, as well as an image to the viewer. Telescopes designed for cystoscopy are available with several viewing angles, including 0° (straight), 30° (forward oblique), 70° (lateral), and 120° (retroview). The different angles facilitate the inspection of the entire bladder wall. Although the 0° lens is essential for adequate urethroscopy, it is insufficient for cystoscopy. The 30° lens provides the best view of the bladder base and posterior wall, and the 70° lens permits inspection of the anterior and lateral walls. The retroview of the 120° lens is not usually necessary for cystoscopy of the female bladder but can be useful for evaluating the urethral opening into the bladder. In diagnostic cystoscopy, the 30° telescope usually is sufficient, although a 70° telescope may be required in the presence of elevation of the urethrovesical junction, such as after colposuspension procedures. The angled telescopes have a field marker, which is a blackened notch on the outside of the visual field opposite the angle of the deflection that helps facilitate orientation. The cystoscope sheath provides a vehicle for introducing the telescope and distending media into the bladder cavity. Sheaths are available in various calibers, ranging from 17F to 28F for use in adults. When placed within the sheath, the telescope, which is a 15F instrument, only partially fills the lumen, leaving an irrigation working channel. The smallest sheath is better tolerated for diagnostic purposes, whereas usually at least a 19F sheath is required for placement of instruments into the irrigation working channel. The proximal end of the sheath has two working ports: one for introduc-tion of the distending media and another for removal. The distal end of the cystoscope sheath is fenestrated to permit use of instrumentation in the angled field of view. It is also beveled, opposite the fenestra, to increase the comfort of the introduc-tion of the cystoscope into the urethra. The bridge serves as a connector between the telescope and sheath and forms a water-tight seal. It also may have one or two ports for introduction of instruments into the irrigation working channel. The Albarran bridge is a variation with a deflector mechanism at the end of the inner sheath. When placed in the cystoscope sheath, the deflector mechanism is located at the distal end of the inner sheath within the fenestra of the outer sheath. In this location, elevation of the deflector mechanism assists the manipulation of instruments within the field of view.

Unlike the rigid cystoscope, the flexible cystoscope combines the optical systems and irrigation working channel in a single unit (Fig. 123–2D). The coated tip is 15F to 18F in diameter and 6 to 7 cm in length; the working unit makes up half the length. The flexibility of the fibers permits incorporation of a distal tip-deflecting mechanism, controlled by a lever at the eyepiece that will deflect the tip 290° in a single plane.

Any light source that provides adequate illumination via a fiberoptic cable is sufficient. A high-intensity xenon light source is often recommended for use in video monitoring or photog-raphy, but with recent innovations, the newest cameras require less light. Video recording and still-picture capabilities are very important for documentation, as well as teaching. Three types of distention media are available: nonconductive fluids, conduc-tive fluids, and gases. Cystourethroscopy is feasible with carbon dioxide, but most practitioners prefer the use of water or saline to distend the bladder and urethra. A liquid medium prevents the carbon dioxide from bubbling and washes away blood or debris that can limit visualization. Moreover, the bladder volumes achieved using a liquid medium more accurately approximate physiologic volumes.

Instrument care requires the removal of blood and debris from the equipment promptly to avoid accumulation in crev-ices and pitting of metal surfaces. The most common method of sterilization is immersion in a 2% activated glutaraldehyde solution (Cidex, or Surgifix, Inc, Arlington, Texas). Cystoure-throscopic equipment should be soaked for 20 minutes and then transferred to a base of sterile water until ready for use.

Operative instruments may be passed through operative channels in accordance with the size of the operative sheath. The most useful of these are a grasper, a biopsy forceps, and a cautery electrode (Fig. 123–3A through C).

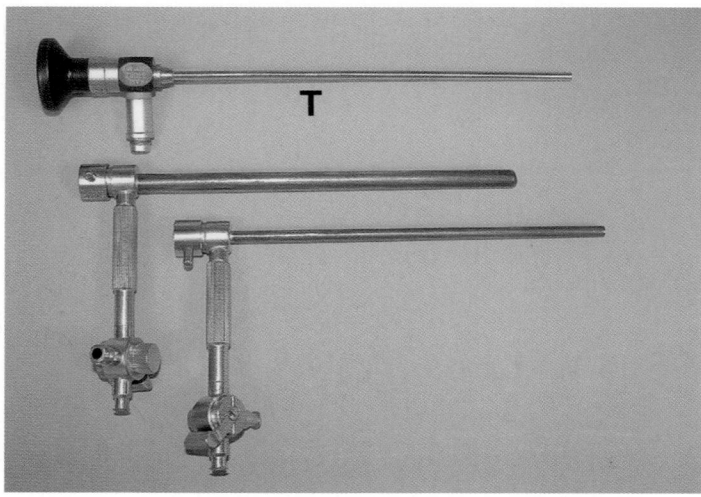

**FIGURE 123–1** Components of the urethroscope. The 0° telescope (T) is shown at the top. Below are two sheaths (15F and 24F).

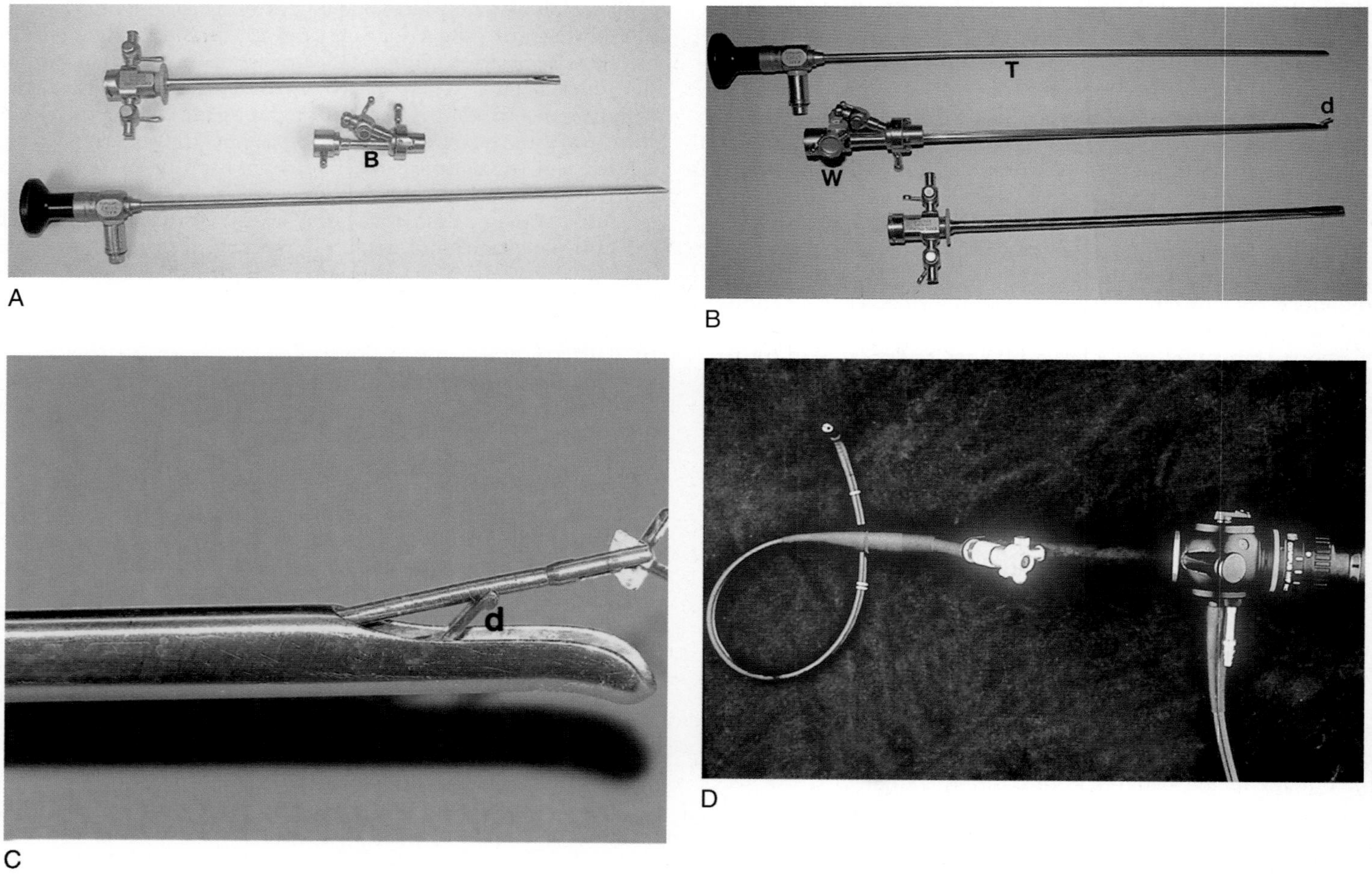

A

B

C

D

**FIGURE 123–2** Components of a rigid cystoscope. **A.** Above is the sheath (17F) with water intake valves on the right and left. In the center is a bridge with an operating channel that attaches to the above sheath. Lowermost is a telescope, which can range from 30° to 70°. In this case, the telescope has a 70° lens. **B.** This rigid cystoscopic system consists of a telescope (T), an operative sheath with a bridge and terminal deflector (d), and an operative sheath without the deflector. The deflector (d) is controlled by the wheel (W) device mounted onto the proximal portion of the sheath. **C.** Close-up of the deflector (d). Note how the deflector permits manipulation of the biopsy forceps. **D.** Unlike the rigid cystoscope, the flexible device combines optical, irrigation, and operating channels in a single unit.

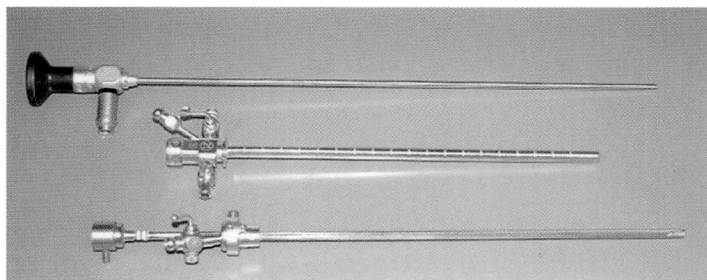

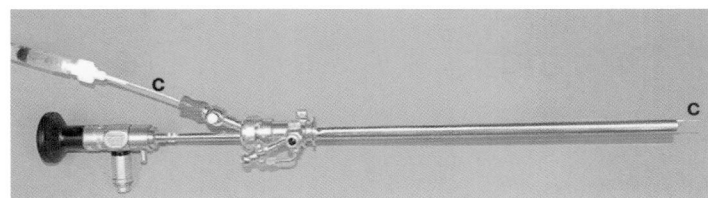

**FIGURE 123–3** Components of operative hysteroscopic sheaths. **A.** The telescope is usually 0° or 30°. In this case, the telescope has a 12° lens. **B.** Accessory instruments that are passed via the channel and into the bladder include (*from left to right*) alligator grasping forceps, biopsy forceps, and a coagulating electrode. **C.** An injection needle has been placed through the channel, and a collagen implant (Contigen) (c) will be injected. (**B** from Cundiff GW, Bent AE: *In* Endoscopic Diagnosis of the Female Lower Urinary Tract. WB Saunders, UK London, 1999, with permission.)

## Indications and Techniques

Indications for visualizing the anatomy of the female urethra and bladder include recurrent urinary tract infection, irritative bladder and urethral symptoms, hematuria, urogenital fistula, urethral or bladder diverticulum, complicated urinary stress incontinence, unresolved overactive bladder, suspected interstitial cystitis, calculus, suspected bladder or urethral cancer, obstructive voiding symptoms, suspected foreign body, assessment of ureteral function, and staging for cervical cancer. The procedure is performed in the office or ambulatory clinic. The patient is examined in the lithotomy position, and generally no analgesia is used. Topical anesthesia may be applied but usually is needed only on the cystoscopic sheath to allow it to slide along the tissues. The urethra is visualized using a 0° telescope with the infusion fluid (sterile water or saline) running briskly, by passing the instrument through the distal urethra and advancing it slowly to the bladder neck. The bladder is visualized by passing the 30° or 70° telescope with attached bridge and 17F sheath through the urethra in a smooth motion in a direction toward the umbilicus. The bladder is systematically examined at each hour of an imaginary clock, and then the trigone and ureters are visualized carefully (Fig. 123–4).

## Urethroscopy (Normal and Abnormal Findings)

The urethral mucosa is visualized as the instrument is passed through the urethra toward the bladder neck (Figs. 123–5 through 123–7). The effects of hold, cough, and strain maneuvers are observed at the bladder neck. The urethrovesical junction normally closes (Fig. 123–8). Voiding or urethral opening secondary to detrusor activity causes the urethra to open widely (Fig. 123–9). A similar picture is noted if the bladder neck is visualized in a patient with detrusor instability (Fig. 123–10). With the bladder relatively full and a finger compression beyond the end of the scope, the scope is slowly withdrawn as the infusing fluid distends the urethra. Periurethral glands (Fig. 123–11A through C) and exudate from the glands may be observed (Fig. 123–12). Other benign findings include inclusion cysts (Fig. 123–13A, B) and fronds and polyps (Fig. 123–14A through C).

Pathologic changes include urethral prolapse (Fig. 123–15A, B), caruncle (Fig. 123–16), inflammation (Fig. 123–17A through C), diverticulum (Fig. 123–18A through C), fistula (Fig. 123–19), and an ectopic ureter opening at the bladder neck (Fig. 123–20).

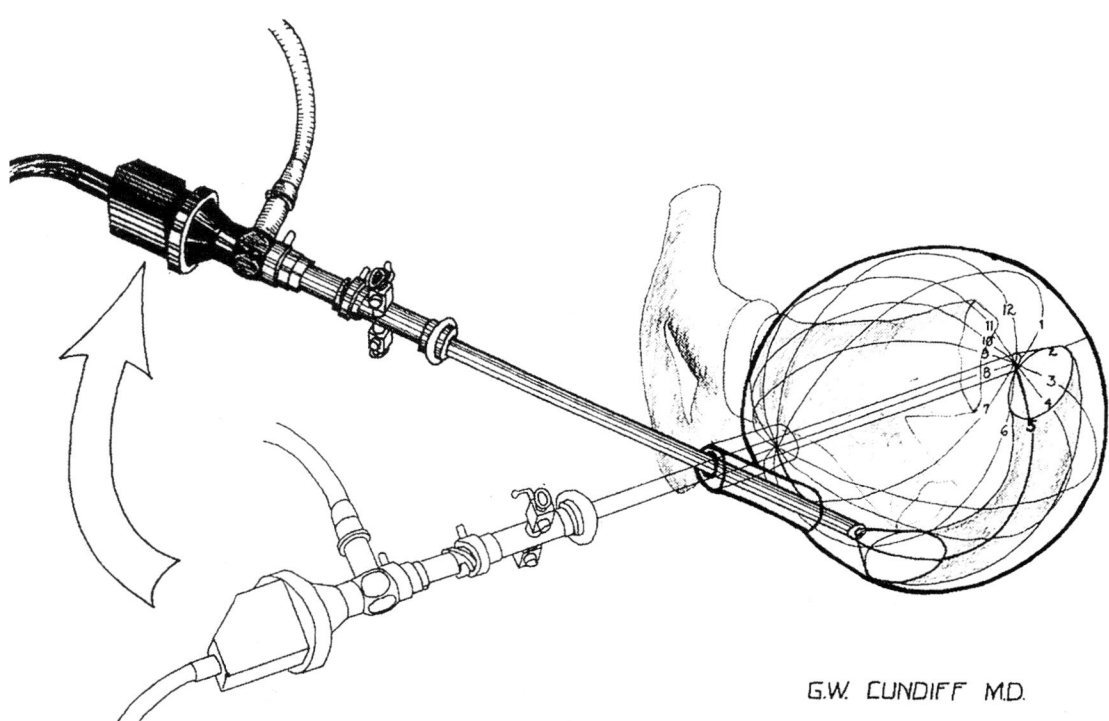

G.W. CUNDIFF M.D.

**FIGURE 123–4** Cystoscopic evaluation of the bladder. The bladder cavity is evaluated by making 12 sweeps along each hour of the clock from the bladder dome to the urethrovesical junction. The 5 o'clock examination is being performed, so the light cord is at 11 o'clock, or 180° opposite the direction the lens is looking. (From Cundiff GW, Bent AE: *In* Endoscopic Diagnosis of the Female Lower Urinary Tract. WB Saunders, UK London, 1999, with permission.)

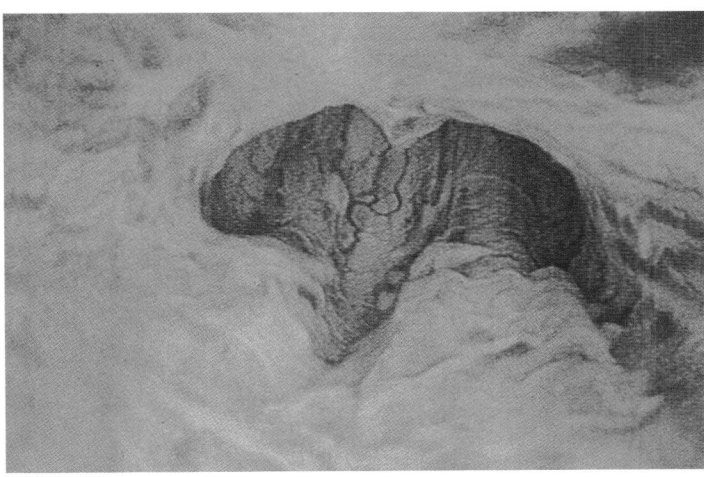

**FIGURE 123–5** Normal urethra. (From Cundiff GW, Bent AE: *In* Endoscopic Diagnosis of the Female Lower Urinary Tract. WB Saunders, UK London, 1999, with permission.)

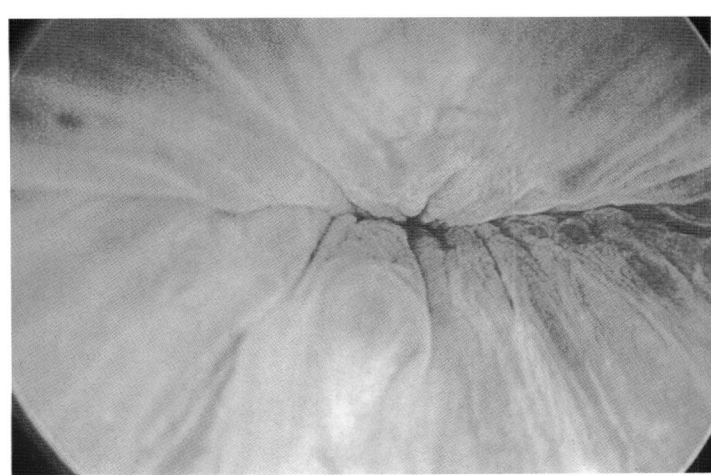

**FIGURE 123–6** Coaptation of urethra. (From Cundiff GW, Bent AE: *In* Endoscopic Diagnosis of the Female Lower Urinary Tract. WB Saunders, UK London, 1999, with permission.)

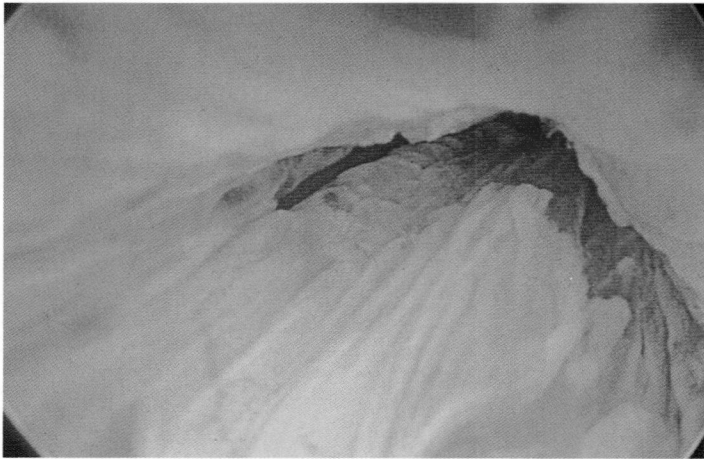

**FIGURE 123–7** Urethral metaplasia. (From Cundiff GW, Bent AE: Endoscopic Diagnosis of the Female Lower Urinary Tract. WB Saunders, UK London, 1999, with permission.)

A

B

C

D

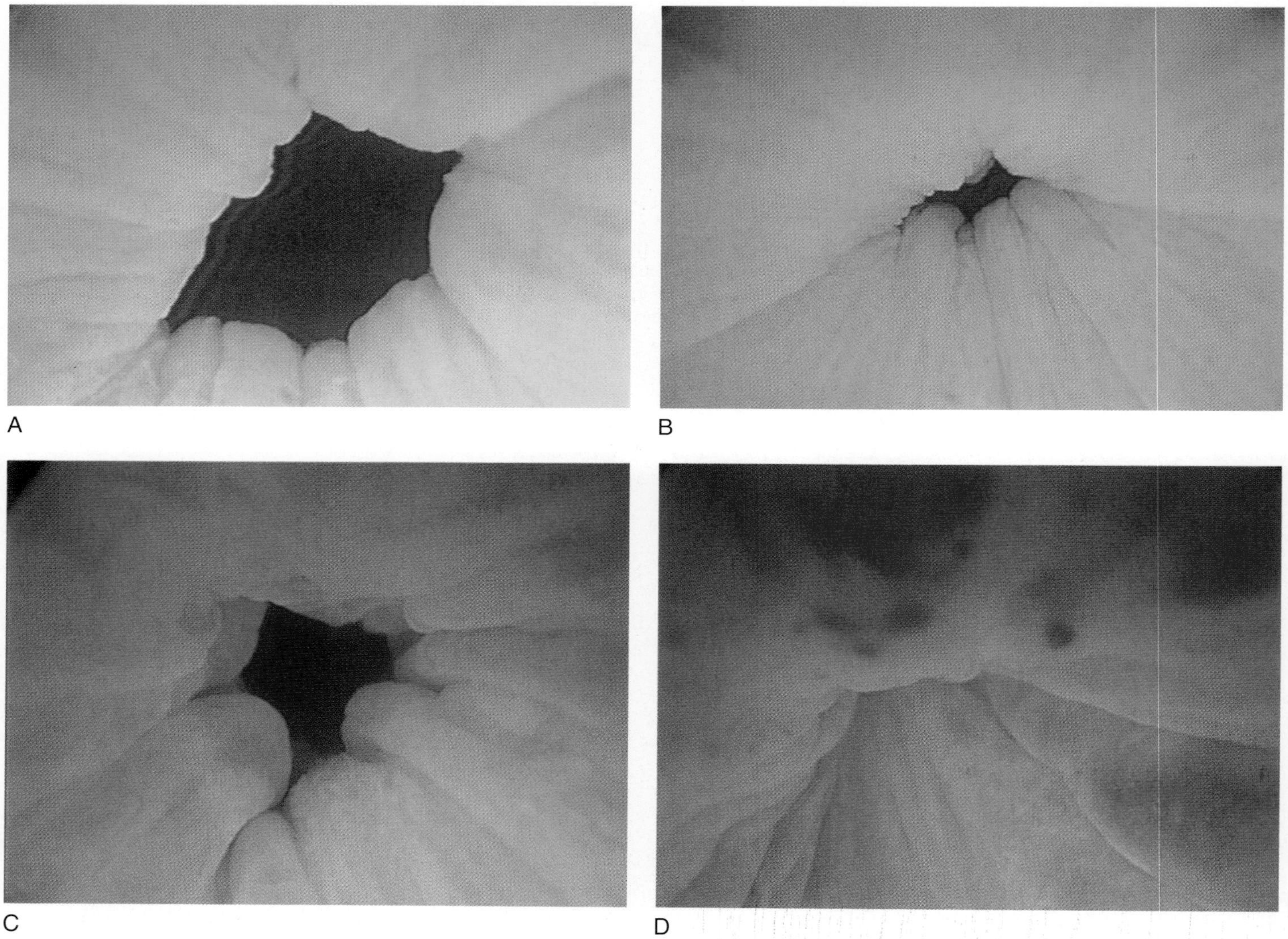

**FIGURE 123–8** Maneuvers at the bladder neck. **A.** Open urethrovesical junction. **B.** Closed urethrovesical junction. **C.** Open urethrovesical junction. **D.** Closed urethrovesical junction. (From Cundiff GW, Bent AE: *In* Endoscopic Diagnosis of the Female Lower Urinary Tract. WB Saunders, UK London, 1999, with permission.)

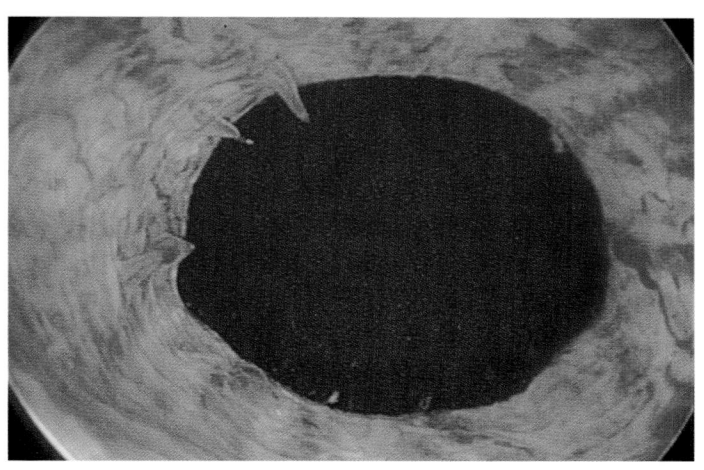

**FIGURE 123–9** Urethra during voiding. (From Cundiff GW, Bent AE: *In Endoscopic Diagnosis of the Female Lower Urinary Tract*. WB Saunders, UK London, 1999, with permission.)

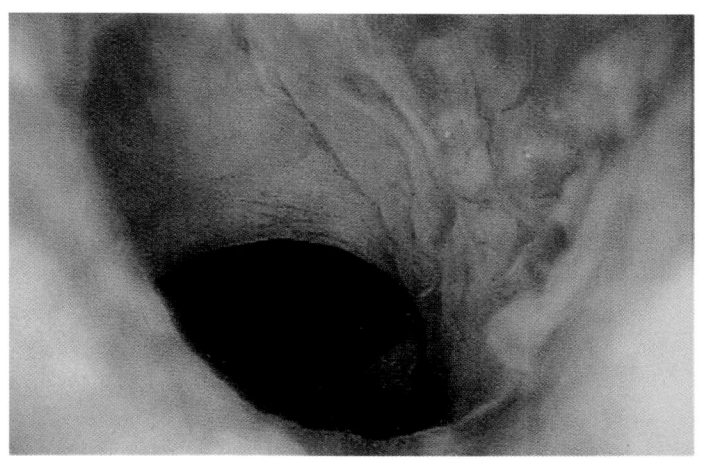

**FIGURE 123–10** Urethra in a patient with detrusor instability.

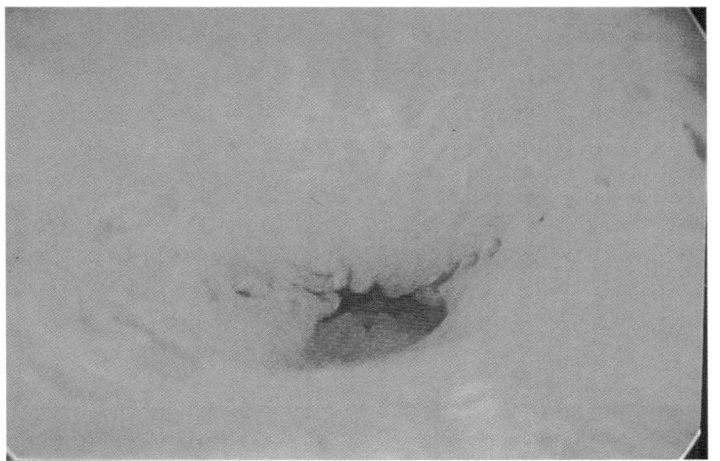

A

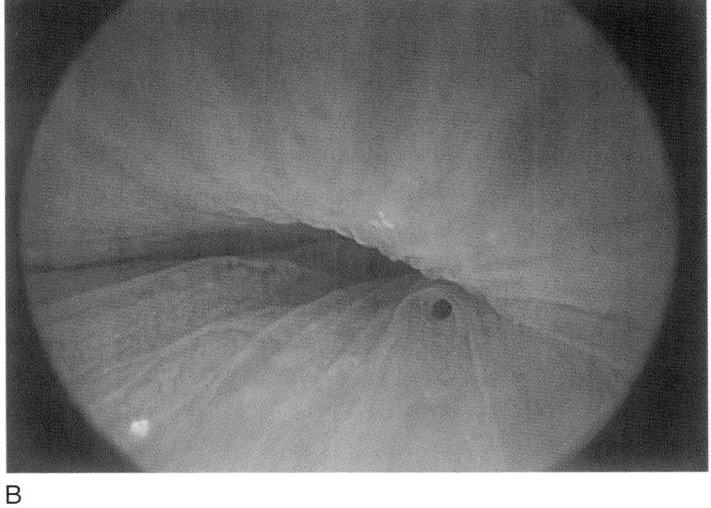

B

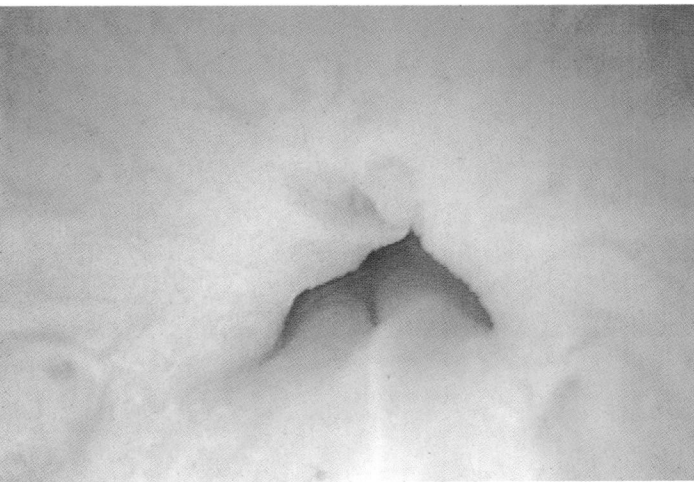

C

**FIGURE 123–11 A.** Periurethral gland openings, with several opening circumferentially. **B.** Large openings at 3 o'clock. **C.** Openings at 12, 4, and 8 o'clock.

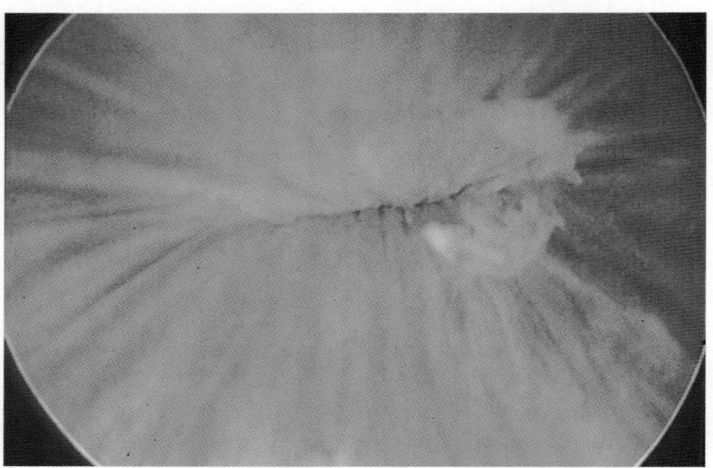

**FIGURE 123–12** Exudate from periurethral glands. (From Cundiff GW, Bent AE: *In* Endoscopic Diagnosis of the Female Lower Urinary Tract. WB Saunders, UK London, 1999, with permission.)

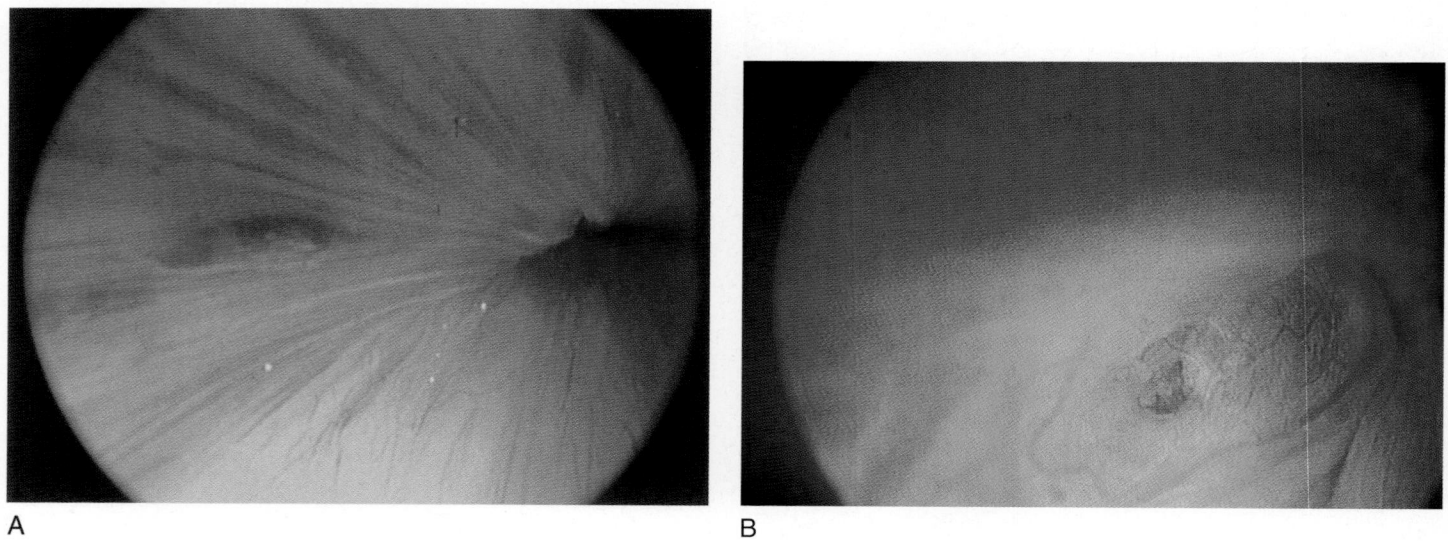

A    B

**FIGURE 123–13 A.** Urethral inclusion cysts. **B.** Urethral inclusion cyst at 7 o'clock.

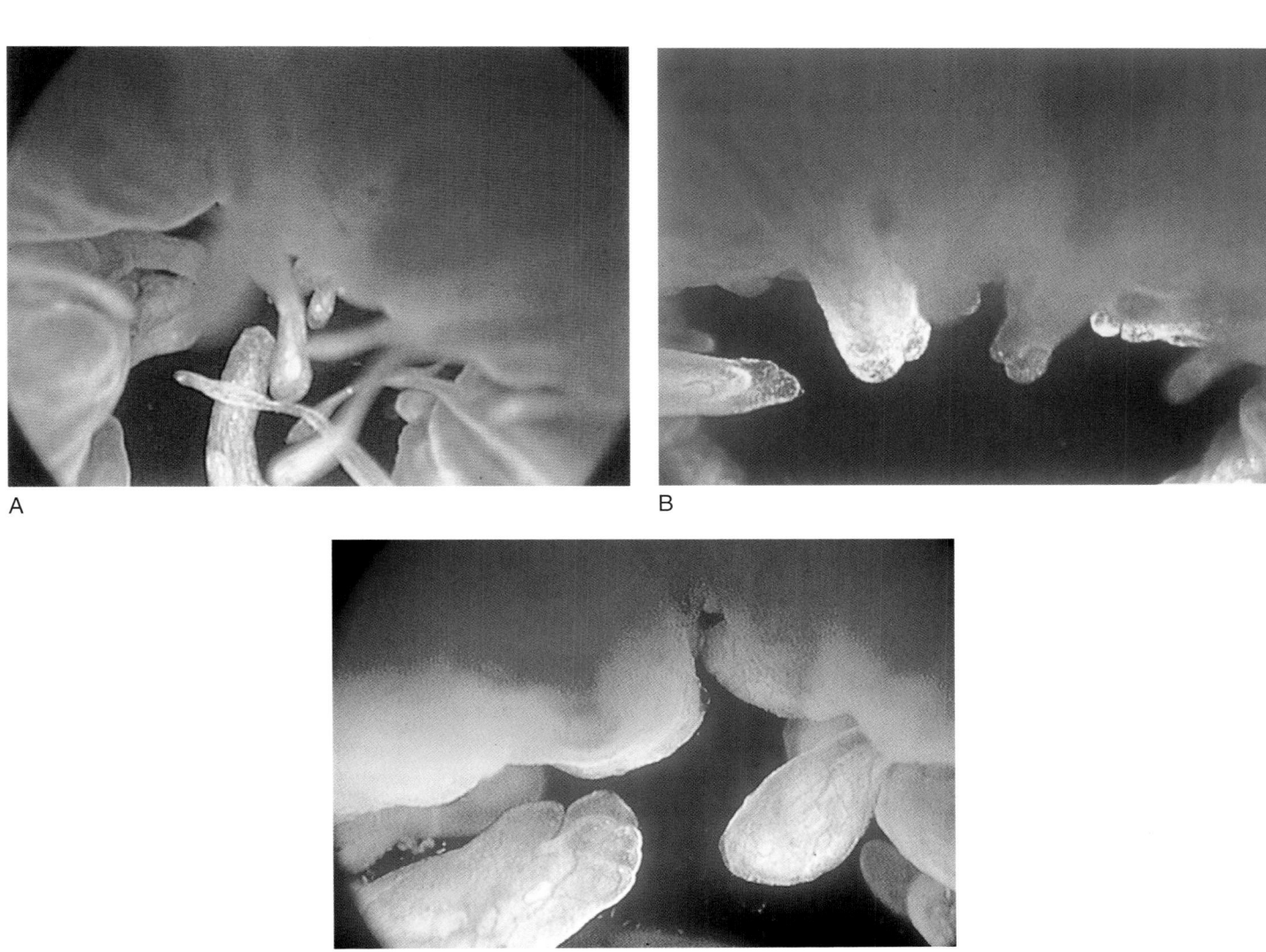

**FIGURE 123–14  A.** Fronds and polyps of urethra. **B.** Polyps at urethrovesical junction. **C.** Magnified view of urethral polyps.

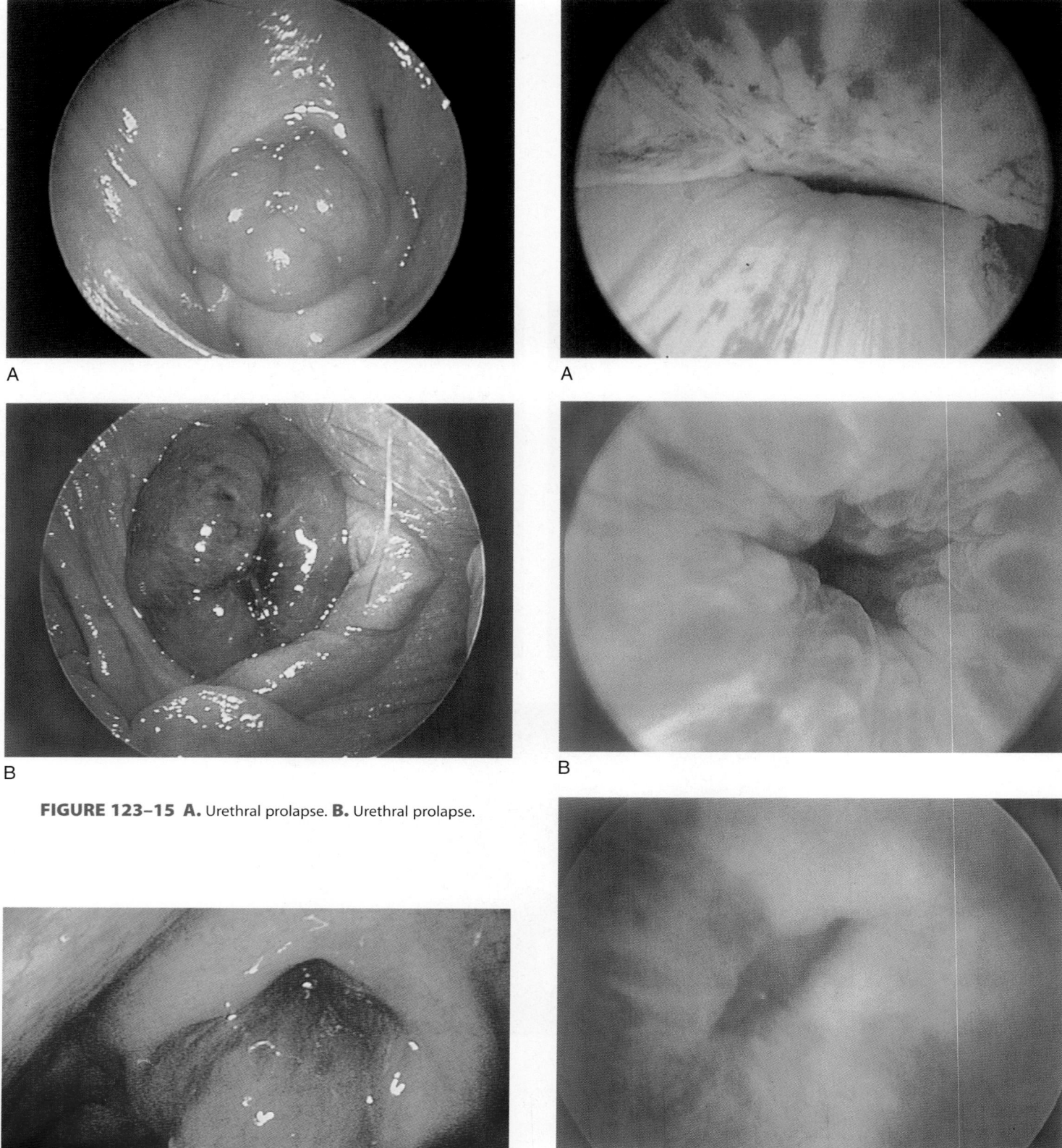

A

B

**FIGURE 123–15 A.** Urethral prolapse. **B.** Urethral prolapse.

A

B

C

**FIGURE 123–16** Urethral caruncle. (From Cundiff GW, Bent AE: *In Endoscopic Diagnosis of the Female Lower Urinary Tract.* WB Saunders, UK London, 1999, with permission.)

**FIGURE 123–17 A.** Urethral inflammation. **B.** Urethral inflammation. **C.** Severe urethral inflammation.

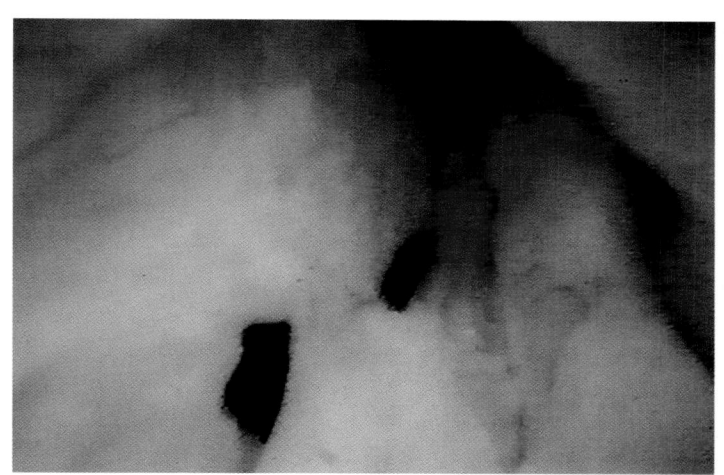

A

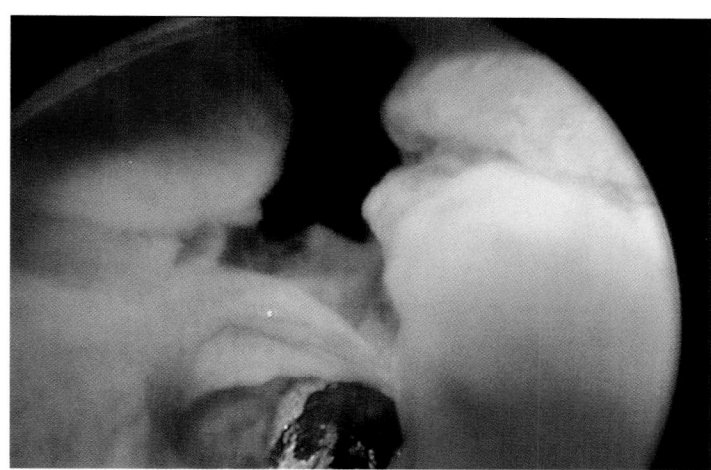

B

C

**FIGURE 123–18**  Urethral diverticulum. **A.** Chandelier diverticular openings. **B.** Urethral lumen at top with sound in diverticulum at 6 o'clock. (From Cundiff GW, Bent AE: *In* Endoscopic Diagnosis of the Female Lower Urinary Tract. WB Saunders, UK London, 1999, with permission.) **C.** Large midurethral diverticulum.

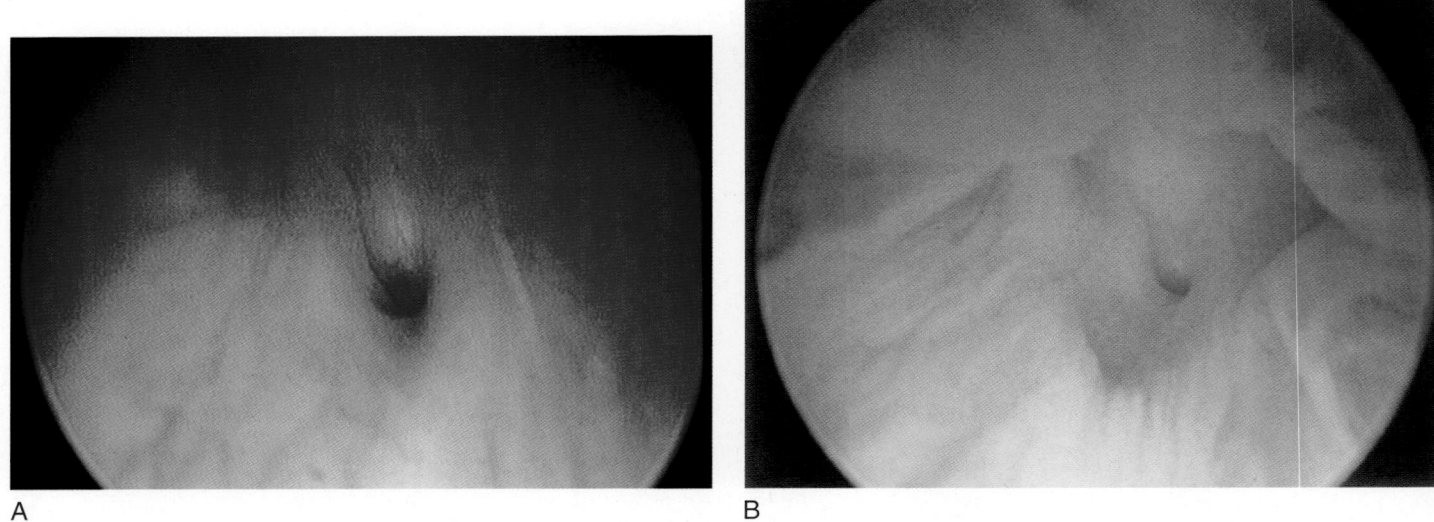

A                                    B

**FIGURE 123–19  A** and **B.** Urethrovaginal fistula.

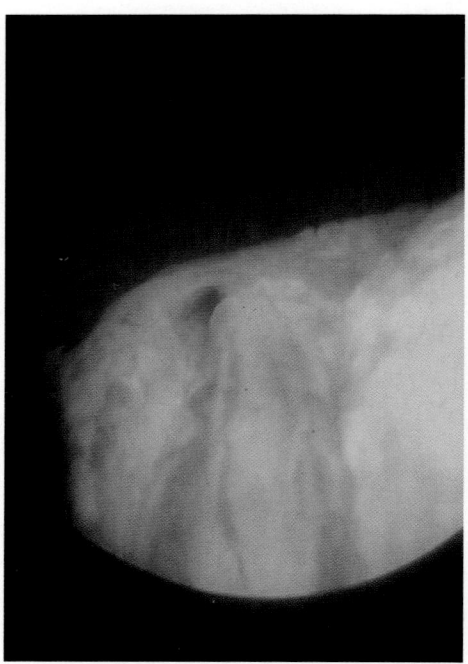

**FIGURE 123–20** Ectopic ureter. Ureteral orifice opening at the urethrovesical junction.

## Cystoscopy (Normal and Abnormal Findings)

The field of view is 180° opposite the light cord. A vaginally placed finger is occasionally needed to visualize the structures at the base of the bladder, especially in cases of marked prolapse with cystocele. The bladder should easily hold from 350 to 500 mL of fluid. The air bubble at 12 o'clock (Fig. 123–21) is observed first, then the clock faces from 1 to 5, then 11 back to 7. Finally, the trigone and ureteral opening are observed (Fig. 123–22A through D). The function of the ureters may be observed, especially if the patient has ingested some phenazopyridine (Pyridium) (Fig. 123–23). These other benign findings may be observed: uterus indenting the bladder (Fig. 123–24), paravaginal defect (Fig. 123–25), double ureters (Fig. 123–26), ureterocele (Fig. 123–27), cystitis cystica (Fig. 123–28A through C), bladder wall cysts (Fig. 123–29), bladder pigmentation (Fig. 123–30), prominent bladder venous channels (Fig. 123–31), bladder trabeculation (Fig. 123–32), and old scars (Fig. 123–33A through C). Pathologic changes that can be seen include trigonitis (Fig. 123–34), inflammation (Fig. 123–35A through E), cystitis glandularis (Fig. 123–36), interstitial cystitis (Fig. 123–37), foreign body (Fig. 123–38A through F), fistula (Fig. 123–39), and cancer (Fig. 123–40A through D).

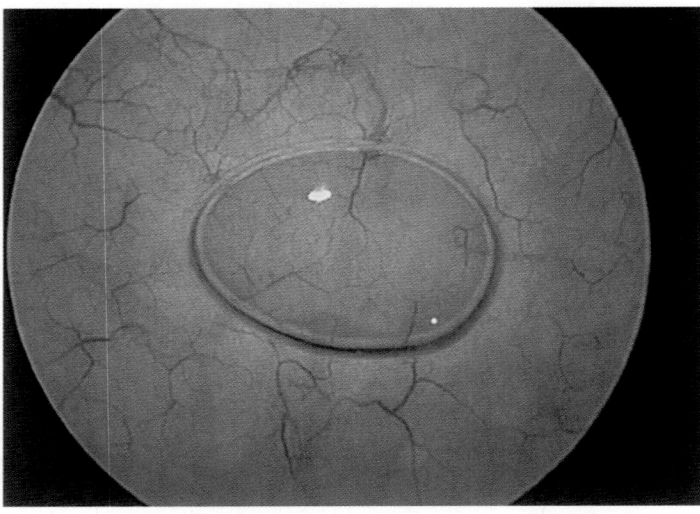

**FIGURE 123–21** Air bubble at the dome of bladder.

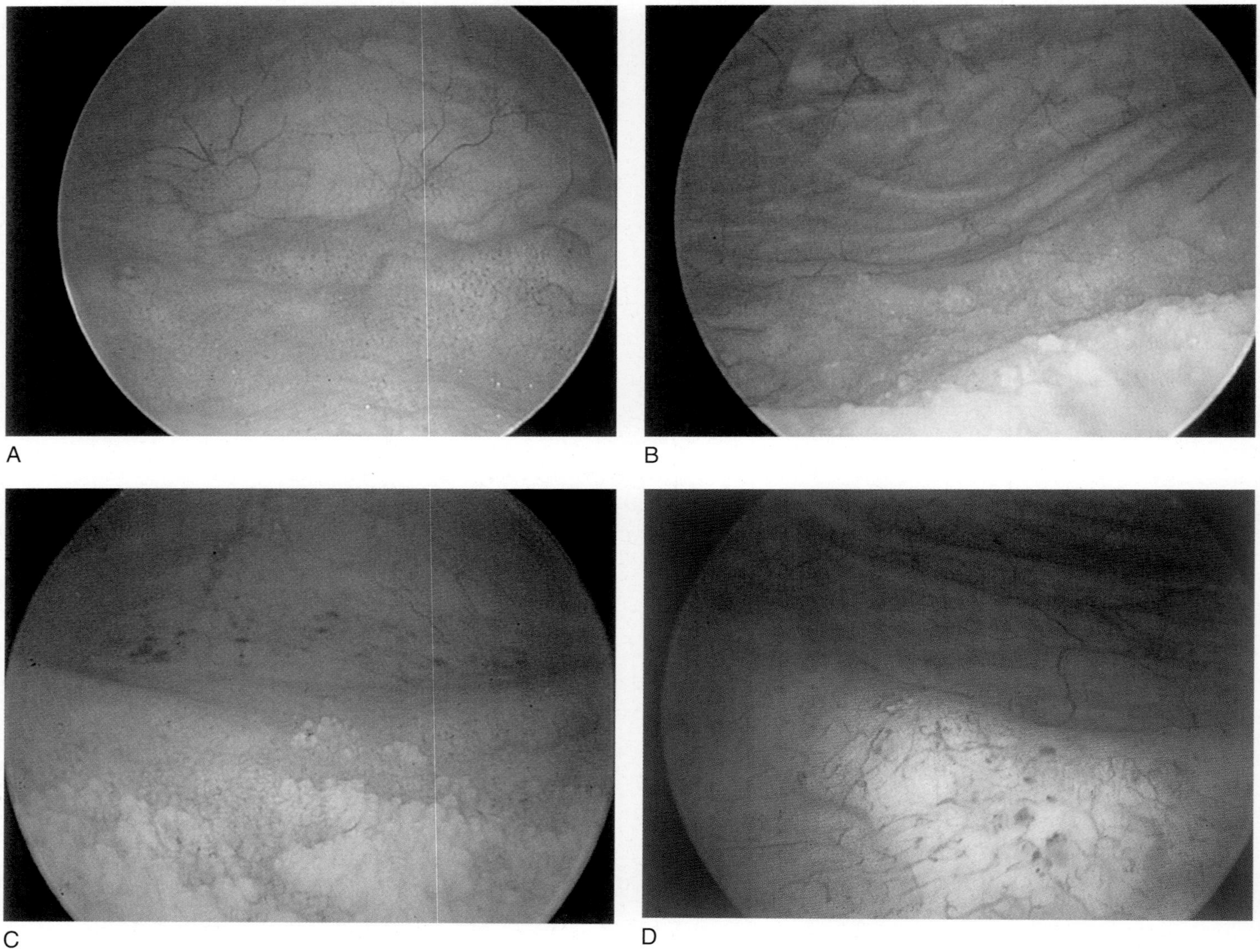

A

B

C

D

**FIGURE 123–22** Trigone and ureters. **A.** Normal trigone. **B.** Granular trigone with the ureters at the lateral margins. **C.** Granular trigone. **D.** Pigmentation in the trigonal area.

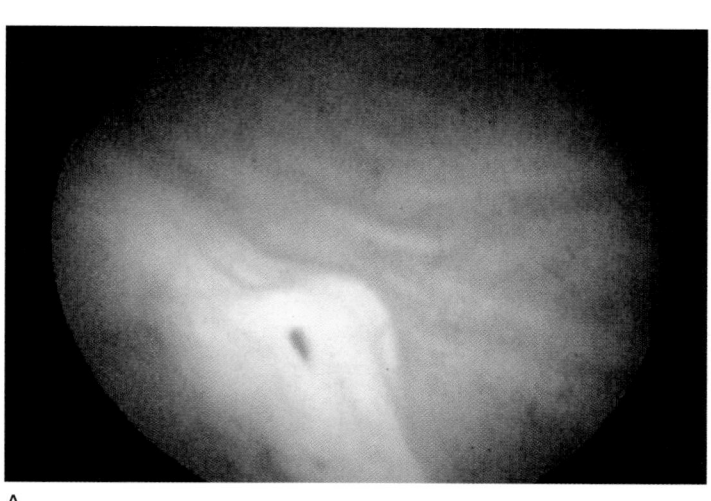

A

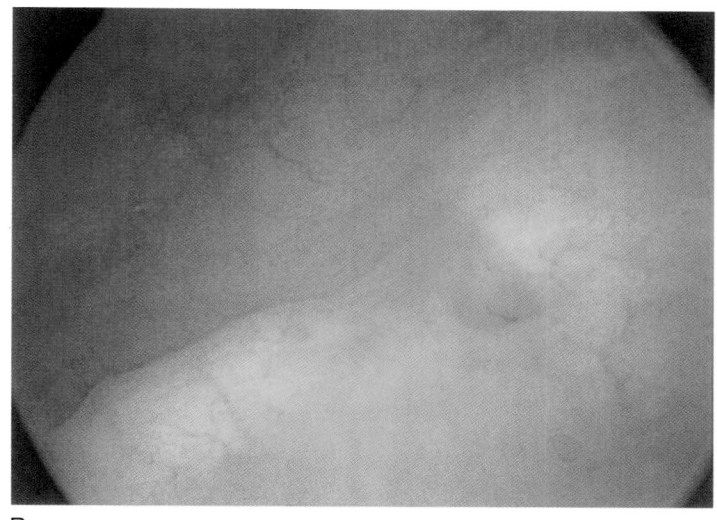

B

**FIGURE 123–23**  Ureteral function. **A.** Right ureter. **B.** Left ureter with Pyridium staining. (From Cundiff GW, Bent AE: *In* Endoscopic Diagnosis of the Female Lower Urinary Tract. WB Saunders, UK London, 1999, with permission.)

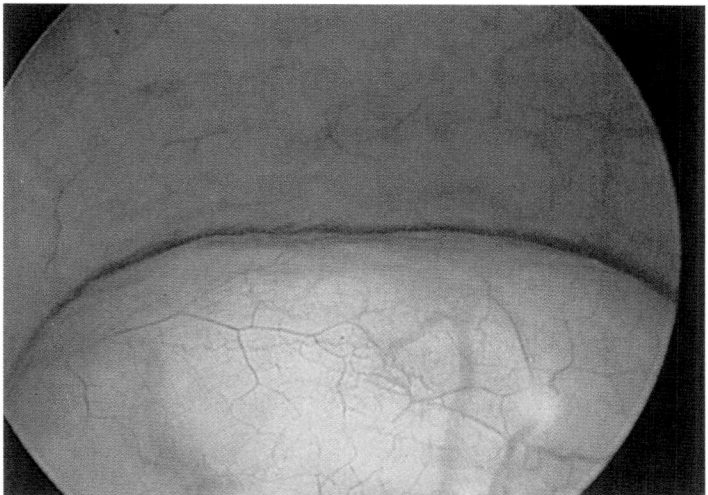

**FIGURE 123–24**  Uterus pressing into the inferior posterior wall of the bladder.

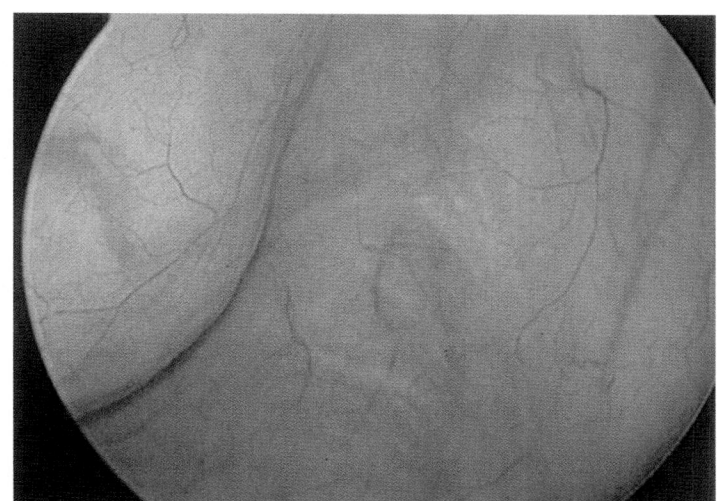

**FIGURE 123–25**  Right paravaginal defect.

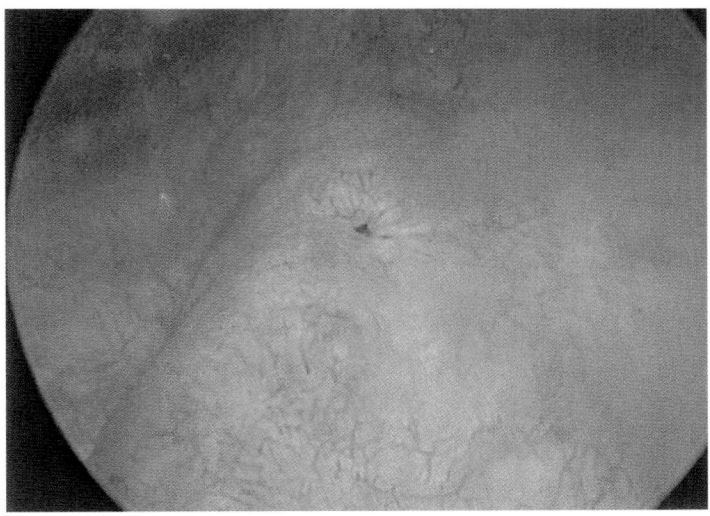

**FIGURE 123–26**  Double ureters.

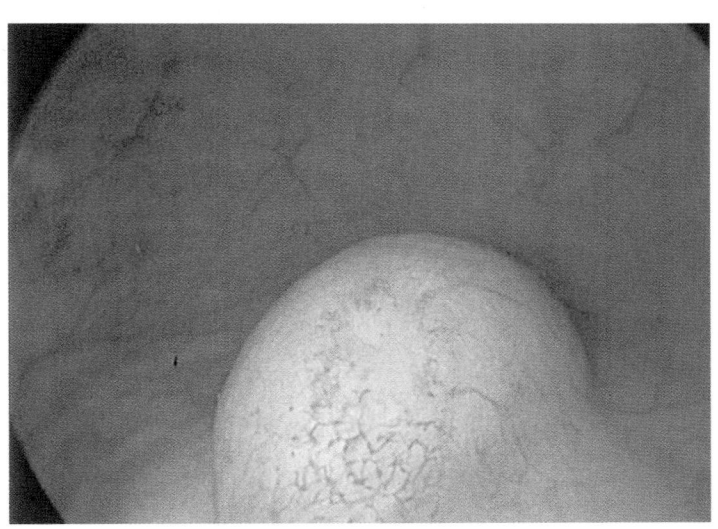

**FIGURE 123–27**  Ureterocele.

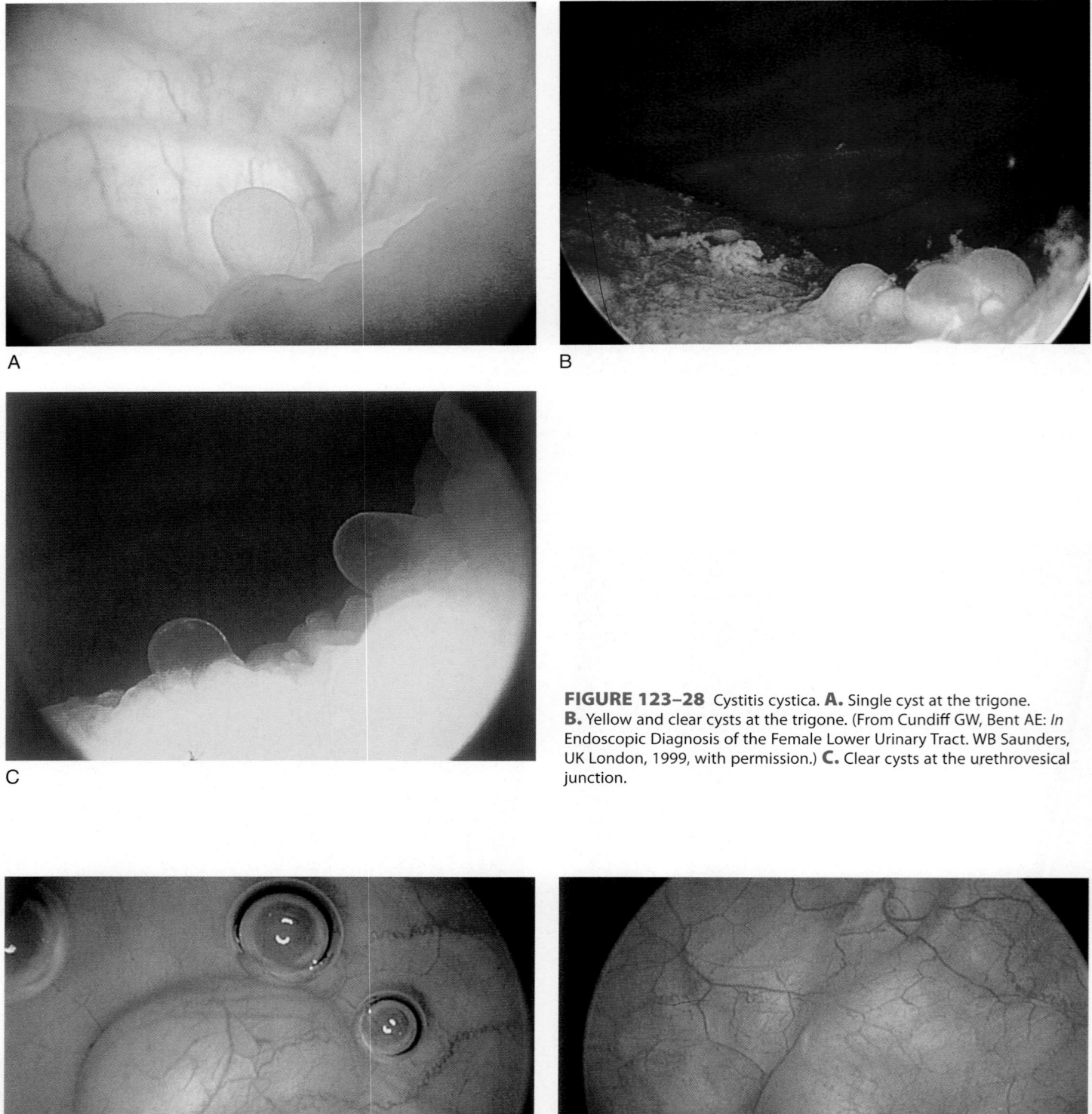

A

B

C

**FIGURE 123–28** Cystitis cystica. **A.** Single cyst at the trigone. **B.** Yellow and clear cysts at the trigone. (From Cundiff GW, Bent AE: *In Endoscopic Diagnosis of the Female Lower Urinary Tract.* WB Saunders, UK London, 1999, with permission.) **C.** Clear cysts at the urethrovesical junction.

A

B

**FIGURE 123–29  A** and **B.** Bladder wall cysts.

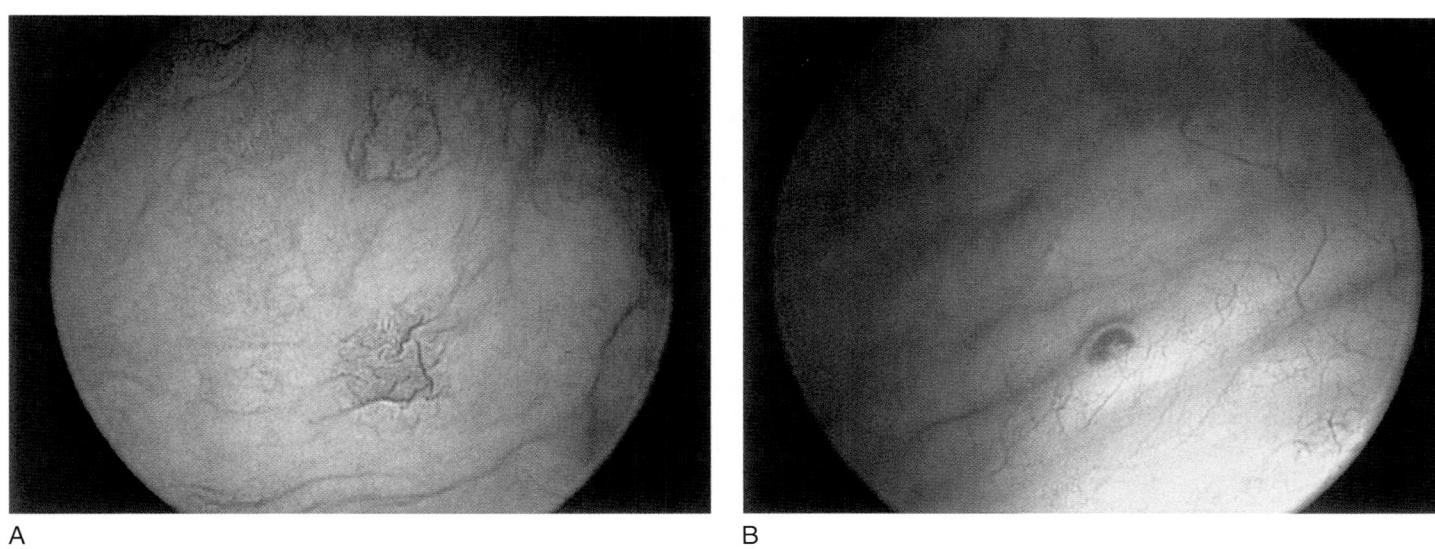

A        B

**FIGURE 123–30 A** and **B.** Bladder wall pigmentation.

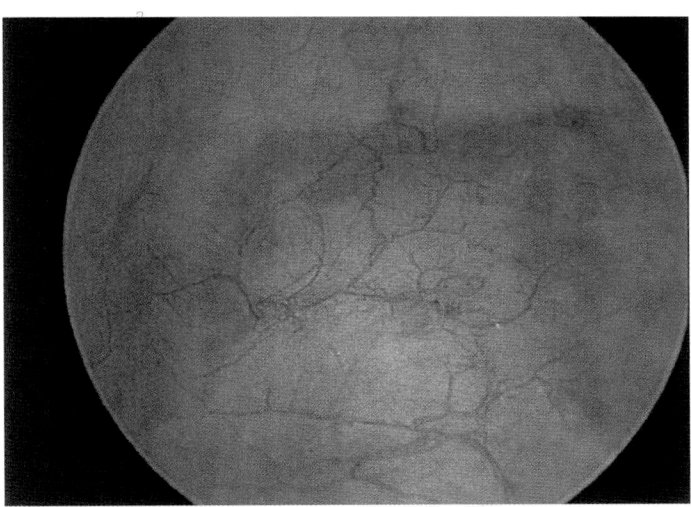

**FIGURE 123–31** Bladder wall venous channel.

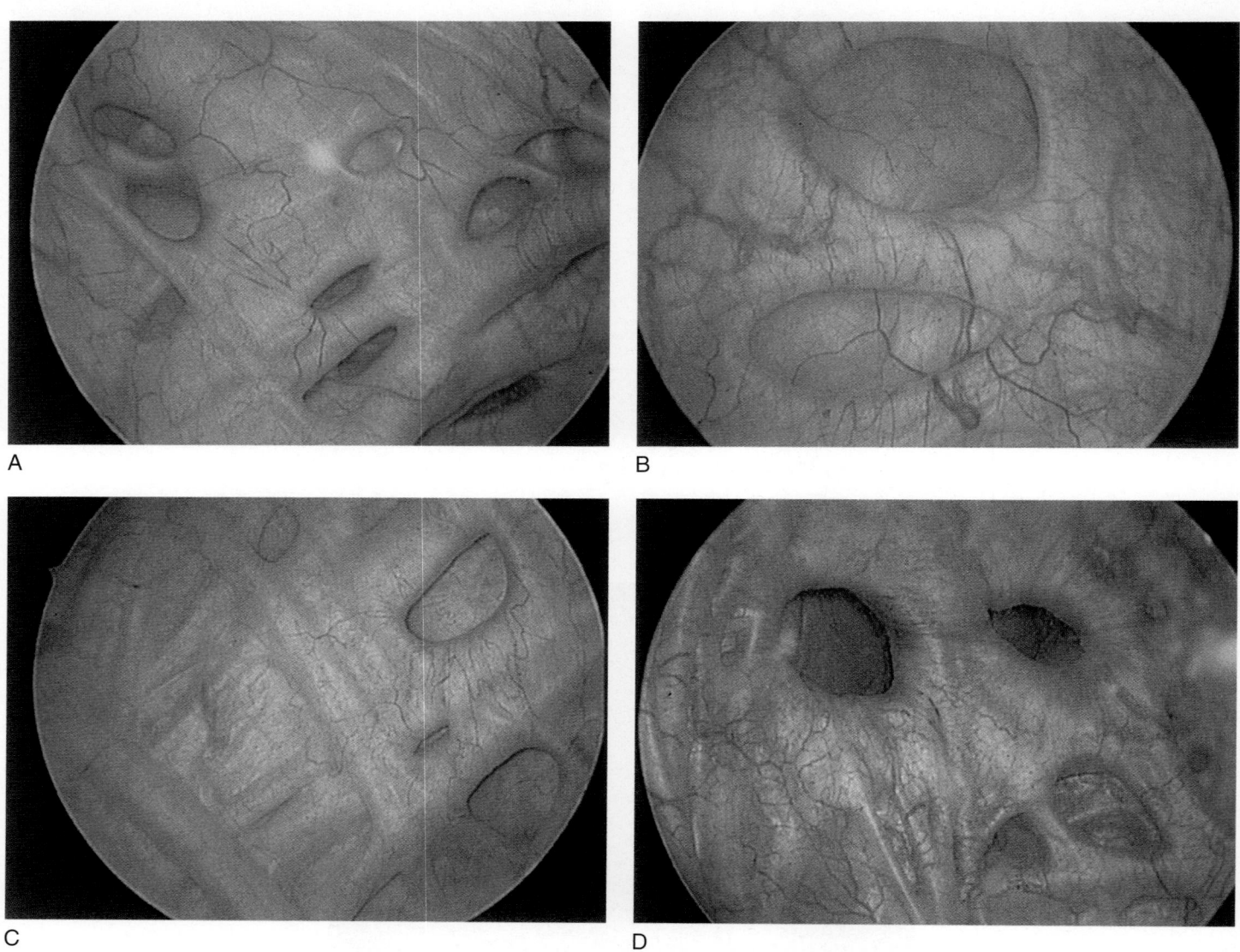

**FIGURE 123–32  A** through **D.** Trabeculation of bladder wall.

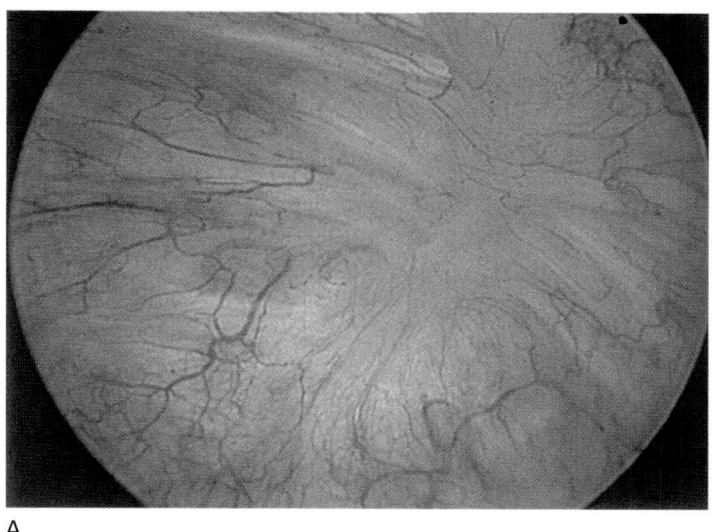

A

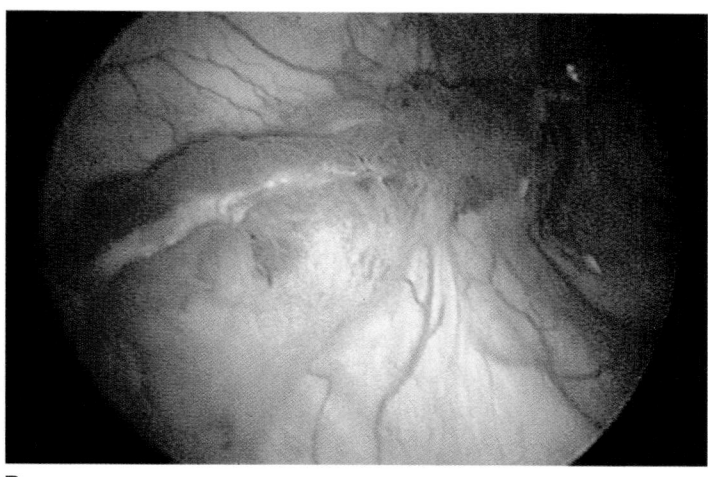

B

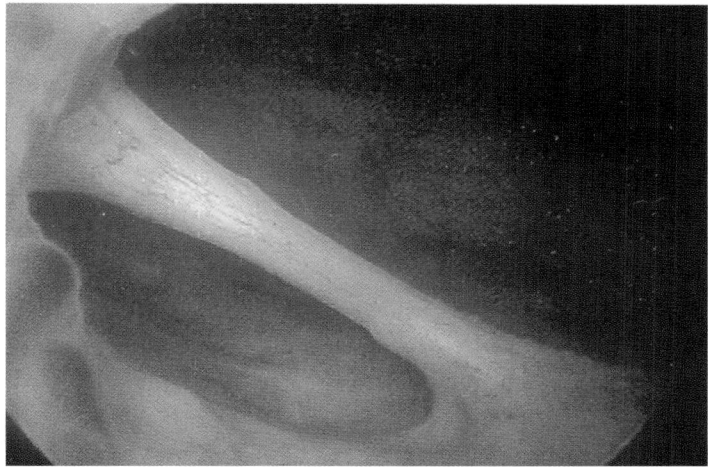

C

**FIGURE 123–33 A** and **B.** Bladder wall scars. **C.** Prominent synechia of the bladder.

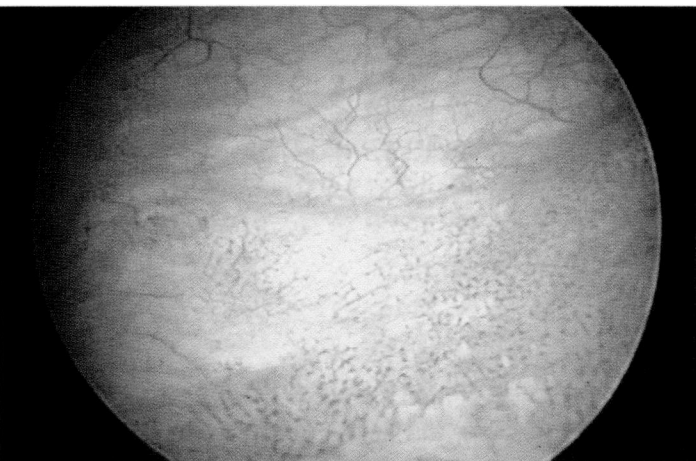

**FIGURE 123–34** Trigonitis. (From Cundiff GW, Bent AE: *In* Endoscopic Diagnosis of the Female Lower Urinary Tract. WB Saunders, UK London, 1999, with permission.)

UNIT 5 ■ SECTION C

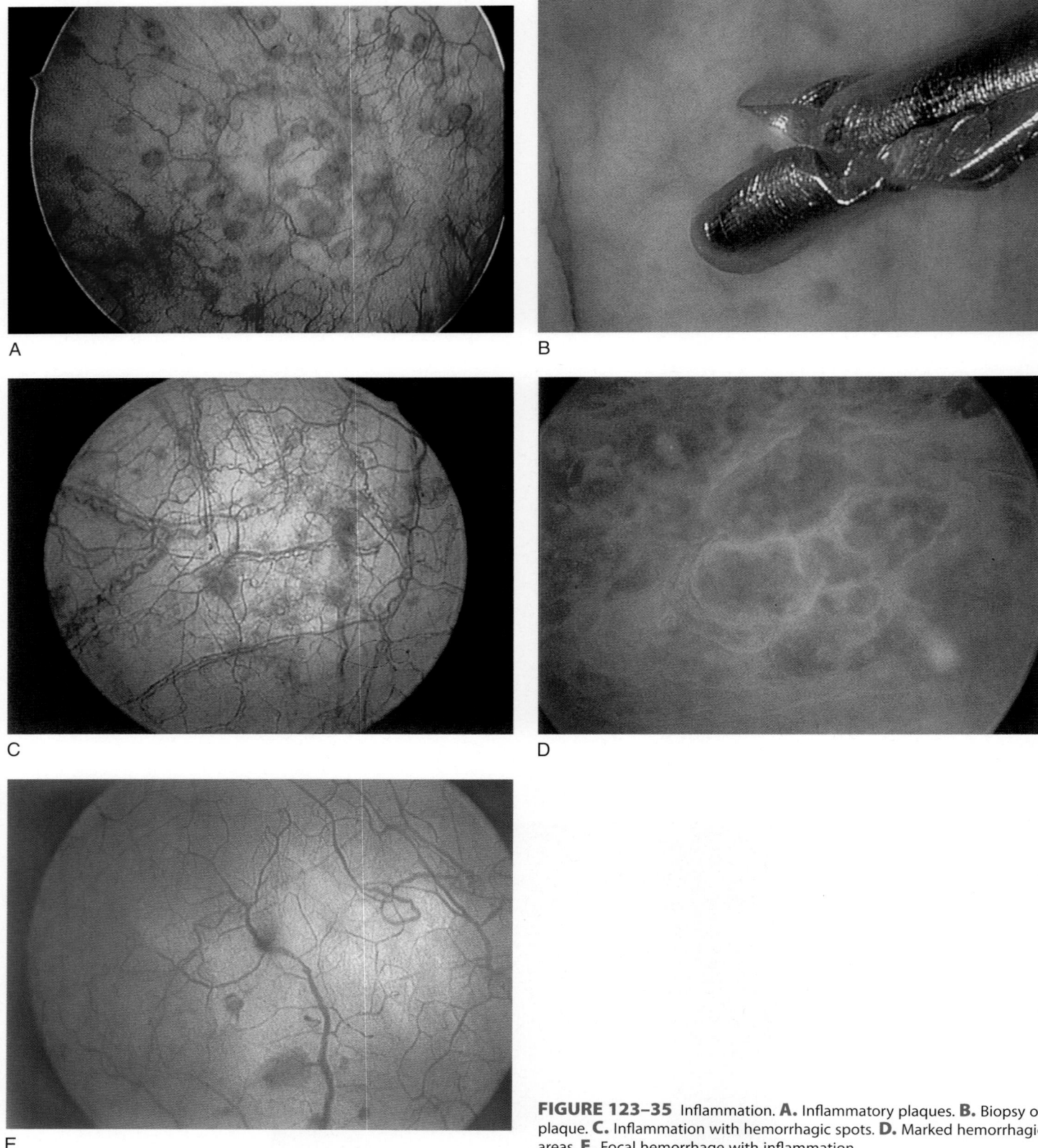

A

B

C

D

E

**FIGURE 123–35** Inflammation. **A.** Inflammatory plaques. **B.** Biopsy of plaque. **C.** Inflammation with hemorrhagic spots. **D.** Marked hemorrhagic areas. **E.** Focal hemorrhage with inflammation.

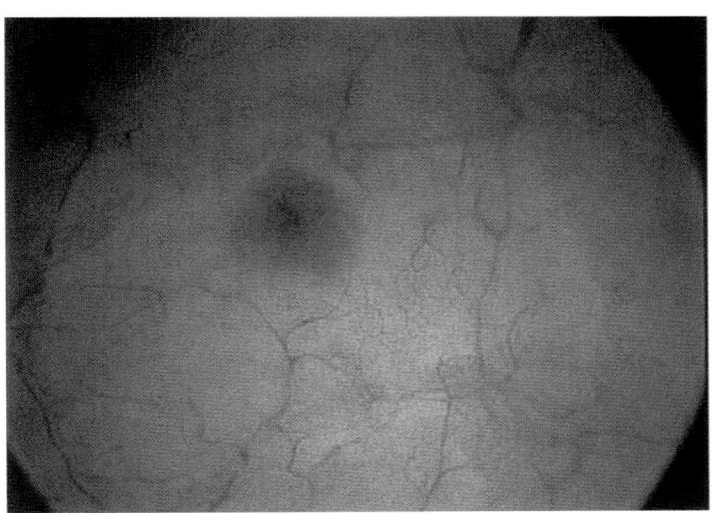

**FIGURE 123–36**  Cystitis glandularis.

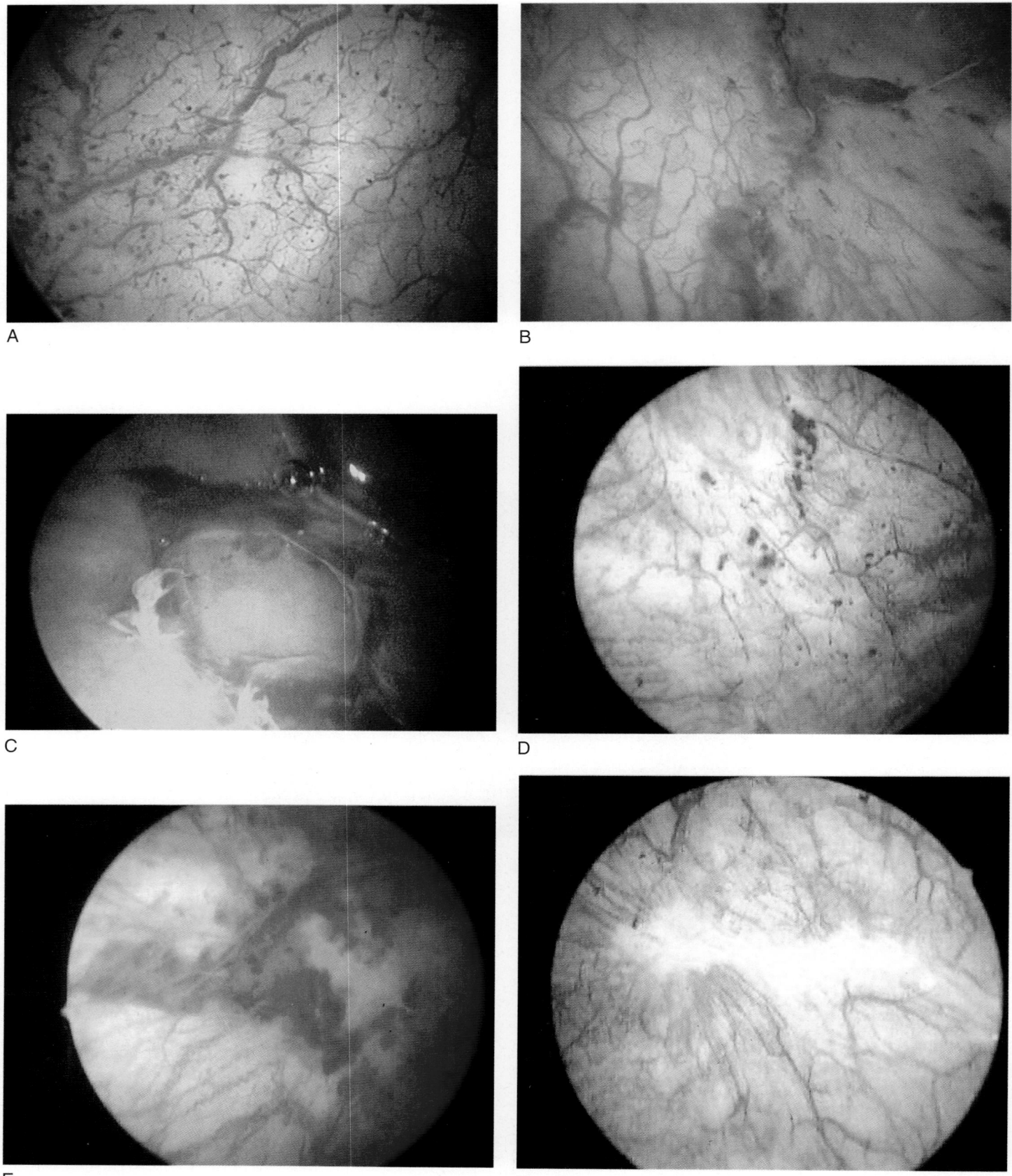

**FIGURE 123–37** Interstitial cystitis. **A.** Petechiae and glomerulations. **B.** Hemorrhagic areas after bladder distention. **C.** Mucosal rupture after distention. (From Cundiff GW, Bent AE: *In* Endoscopic Diagnosis of the Female Lower Urinary Tract. WB Saunders, UK London, 1999, with permission.) **D.** Note the petechiae and glomerulation in cyte mucosa of the bladder. **E.** Linear hemorrhage. **F.** Interstitial cystitis showing Hunner's ulcer (white scar in center of the figure).

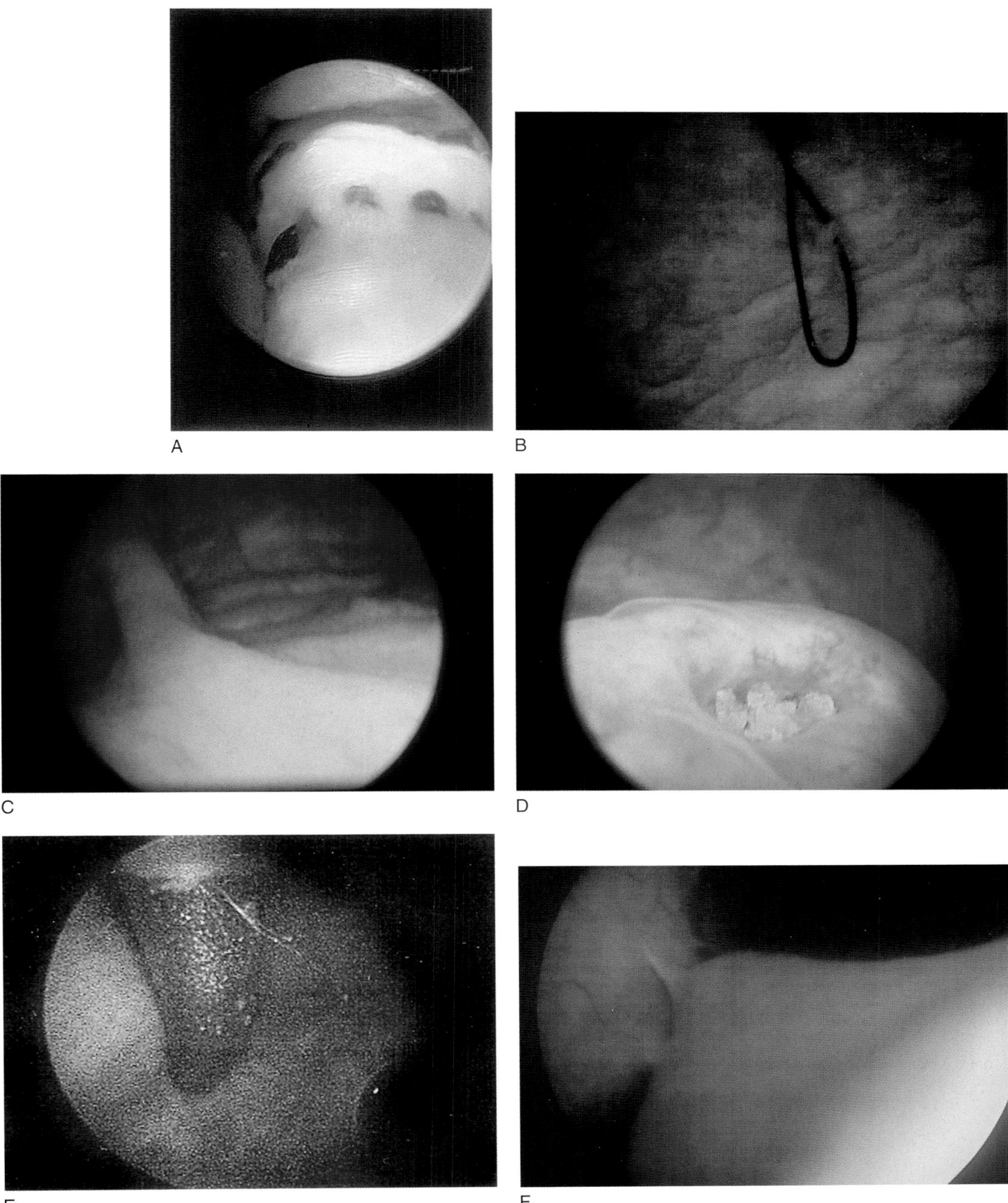

A

B

C

D

E

F

**FIGURE 123–38** Foreign bodies. **A.** ProteGen sling in urethra. **B.** Suture through the bladder wall. **C.** Fascia lata sling. **D.** Ureteral stones. **E.** TVT needle. (From Cundiff GW, Bent AE: *In* Endoscopic Diagnosis of the Female Lower Urinary Tract. WB Saunders, UK London, 1999, with permission.) **F.** Epithelialized suture.

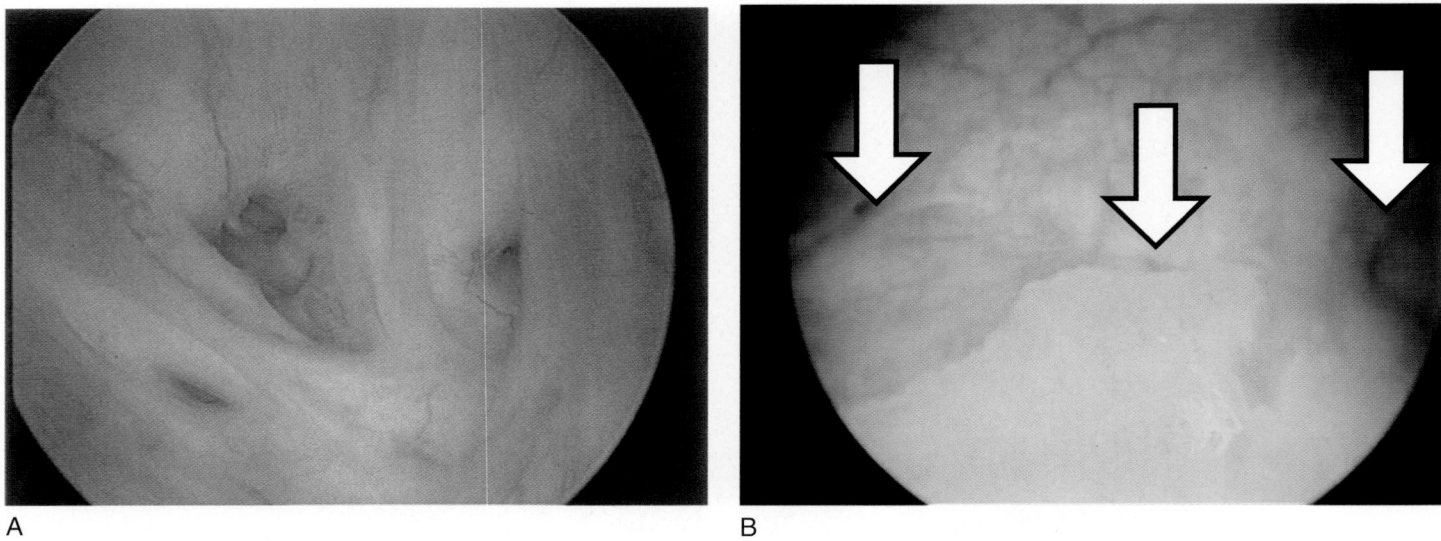

**FIGURE 123–39** Vesicovaginal fistula. **A.** Bladder side. **B.** Vesicovaginal fistula arising from the midportion of the trigone (*center arrow*); right and left arrows denote ureteral orifices.

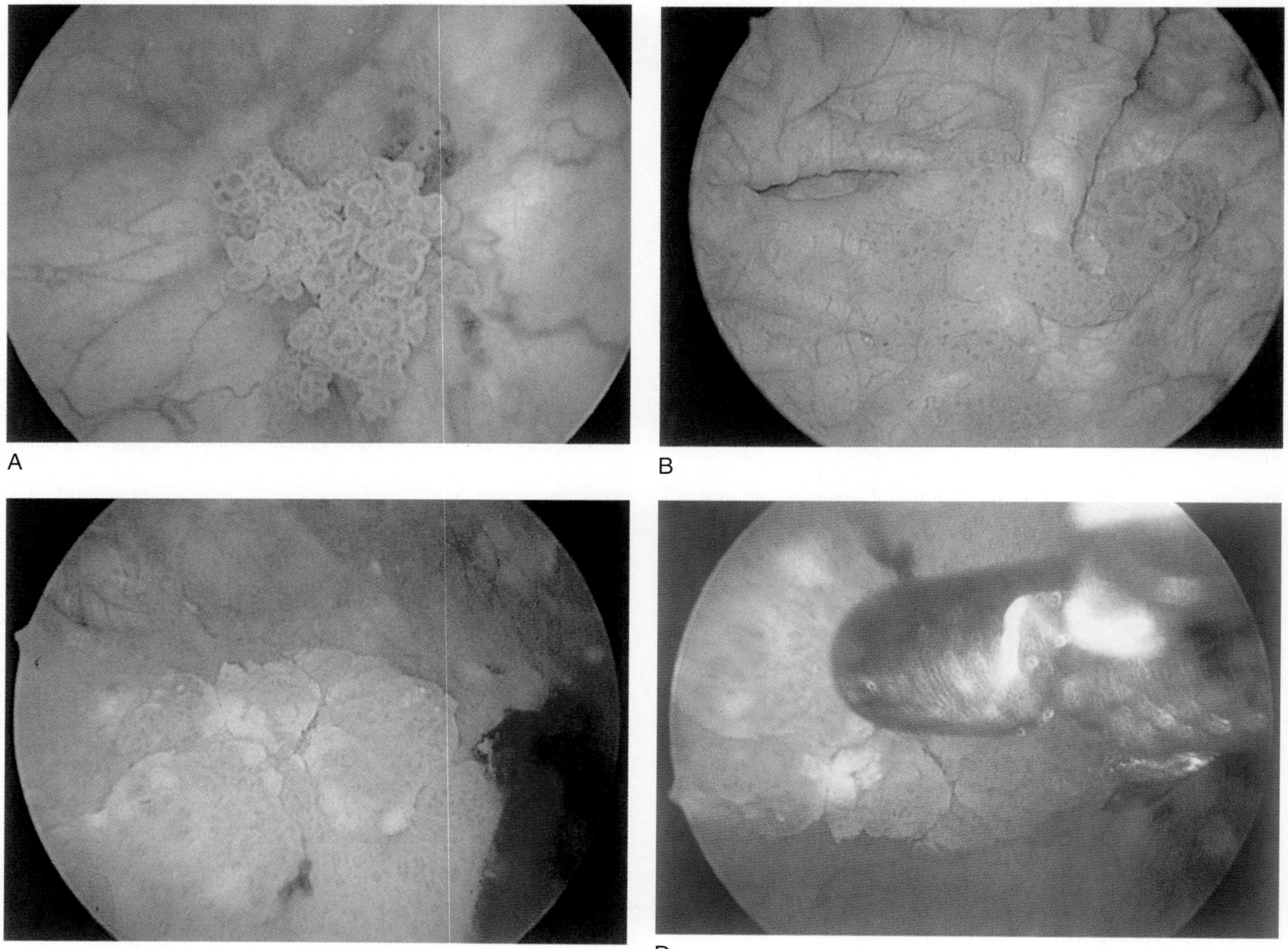

A

B

C

D

**FIGURE 123–40 A** through **C.** Bladder cancers. **D.** Directed biopsy of bladder cancer.

## Operative Cystoscopy

### Bladder Biopsy

Biopsy of the bladder is carried out in the office or outpatient setting. The bladder wall may be anesthetized by placing 50 mL of 4% lidocaine solution in the bladder for 5 minutes. The second aid is to place a bladder pillar block using 5 mL of 1% lidocaine injected 3 mm submucosally at the bladder pillars (Fig. 123–41). Bladder biopsy may require a 22F sheath to accommodate a biopsy instrument. The instrument is advanced until seen in the field of view. Gross movements are made by moving the scope, and finer ones are made by moving the biopsy instrument.

### Ureteral Catheterization

Ureteral patency is assessed in the operating room by injecting indigo carmine dye (2.5 to 5.0 mL) intravenously and then observing the dye-stained urine exiting from the ureters after 5 or more minutes (Fig. 123–42). Jets of urine are seen at the time of regular cystoscopy, indicating functioning ureters. At the time of surgery, it is imperative that the surgeon be certain that the ureters and bladder are intact. Failure to see dye on either side requires catheterization of that ureter and appropriate management to relieve the blockage. Ureteral catheterization is usually performed with the catheter threaded through the operating channel of the cystoscope, with an Albarran bridge in place. Once the ureteral orifice is visualized, the catheter (Fig. 123–43) is advanced into view, and then by rotation of the scope, the catheter is oriented in the axis of the ureteral lumen. The scope is advanced to gently start the catheter into the ureter, and then the catheter is manually advanced to the desired location (Fig. 123–44A, B).

### Injection of Bulk-Enhancing Agents

Collagen injection therapy is an outpatient or office procedure. Equipment includes a nonbeveled sheath (size 20F to 21F), with a 12° to 25° lens. The injection is most readily performed by the transurethral route. The collagen injection needle is placed in the assembled cystoscope with the needle lumen filled with 0.4 mL of 1% lidocaine. The needle is inserted approximately 2 cm from the bladder neck at 3 o'clock and is advanced 1 cm (Fig. 123–45). The injection is then performed, depositing the material 1 cm distal to the bladder neck. The needle is flushed with lidocaine and then is removed from the urethral wall. A second injection of 2.5 mL of collagen is performed at 9 o'clock. Usually 5 to 7.5 mL of collagen provides excellent coaptation of the urethrovesical junction (Fig. 123–46). A specially designed endoscopic system facilitates transurethral injection of bulk-enhancing agents. Periurethral collagen injection may also be performed. The periurethral area is anesthetized by injecting 1% lidocaine with indigo carmine along the lateral side of the urethra. The short 22-gauge collagen injection needle is then advanced through the periurethral tissues until it rests just distal to the bladder neck, and as the lidocaine/indigo carmine mixture is injected, the bulging and blue color are visible under the urethral mucosa (Fig. 123–47A through G). The rest of the injection is similar to the technique for transurethral injection in that the bladder neck is observed during the injection, and it closes gradually as the collagen material accumulates just distal to the bladder neck. Follow-up endoscopy usually shows evidence of old collagen.

UNIT 5 ■ SECTION C

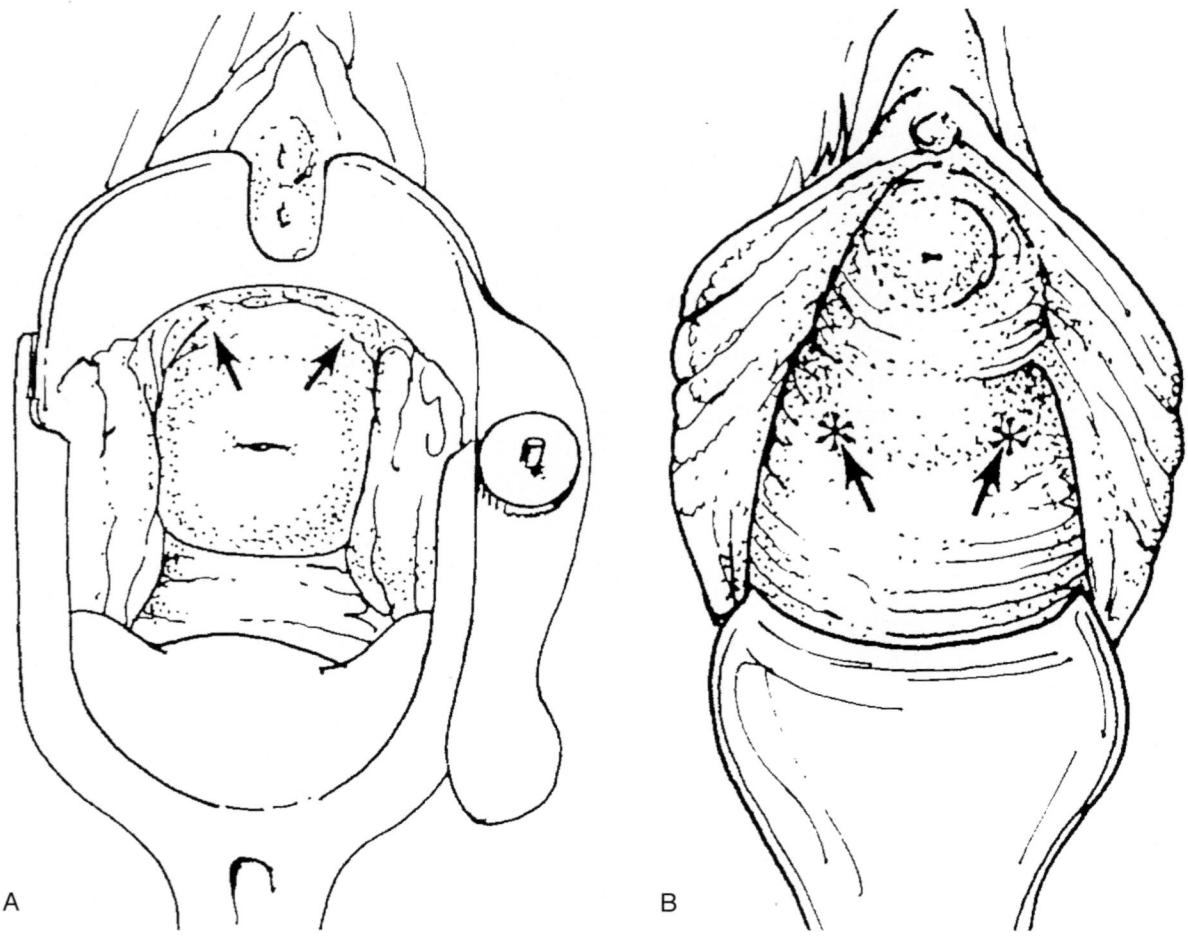

**FIGURE 123–41** Bladder pillar block. **A.** Injection at 2 and 10 o'clock with the cervix in situ. **B.** Injection at approximately 4 and 8 o'clock in the absence of the cervix. (From Ostergard DR: Bladder pillar block anesthesia for urethral dilatation in women. Am J Obstet Gynecol 1980;136:187–188, with permission.)

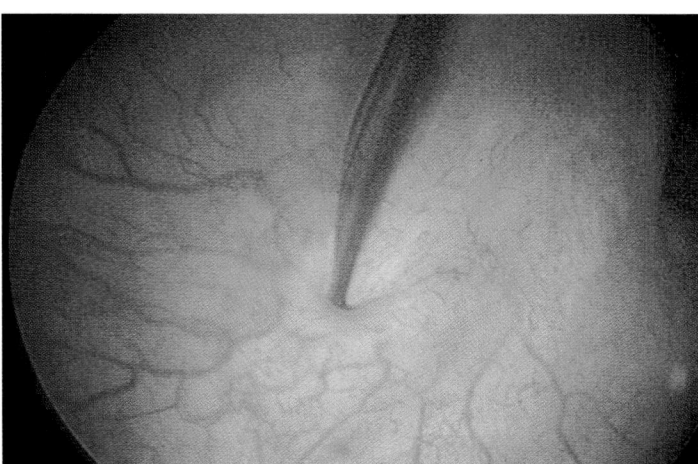

**FIGURE 123–42** Ureteral patency. Indigo carmine–stained urine spurting from the ureter. (From Cundiff GW, Bent AE: *In* Endoscopic Diagnosis of the Female Lower Urinary Tract. WB Saunders, UK London, 1999, with permission.)

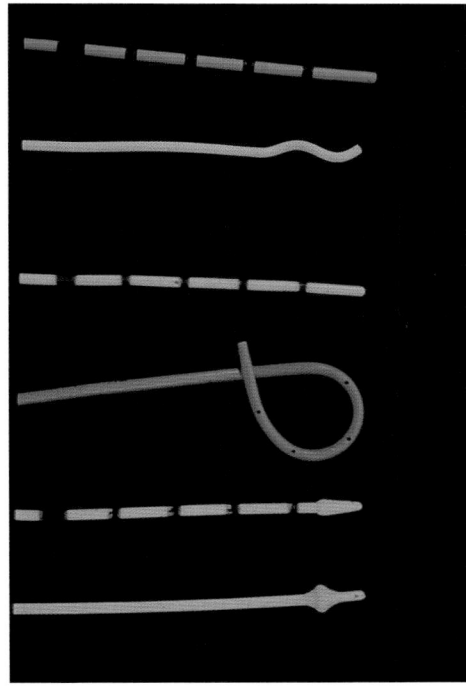

**FIGURE 123–43** Ureteral catheters. *From top to bottom:* general purpose, whistle tip, filiform, double J, acorn, and Rutner catheters. (From Cundiff GW, Bent AE: *In* Endoscopic Diagnosis of the Female Lower Urinary Tract. WB Saunders, UK London, 1999, with permission.)

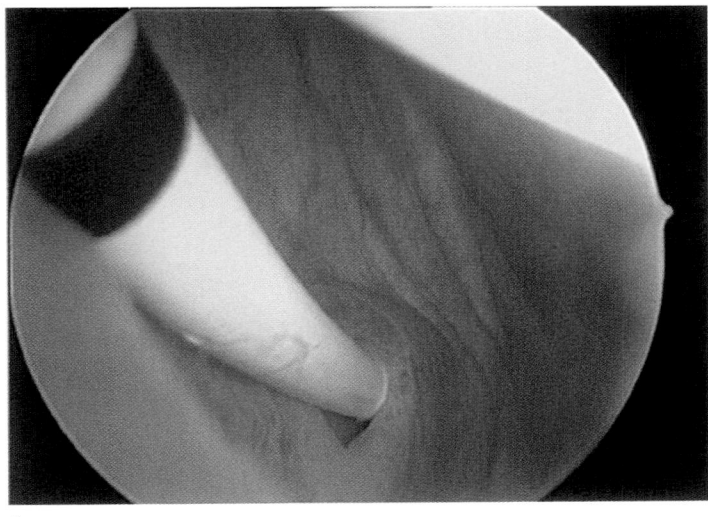

A

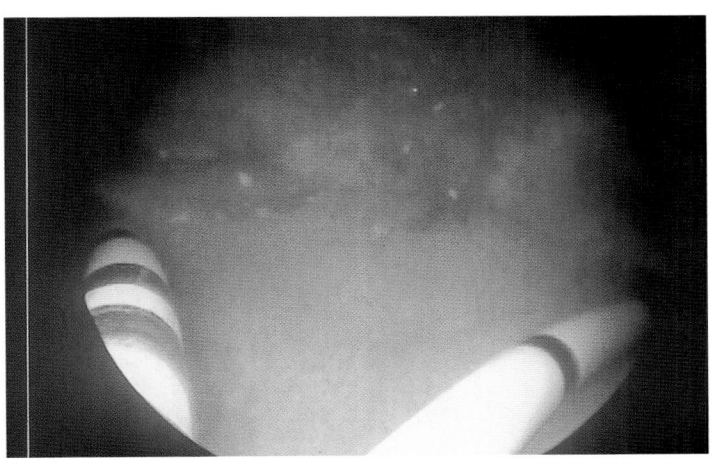

B

**FIGURE 123–44 A.** Ureteral catheter in situ. **B.** Bilateral ureteral catheters in situ.

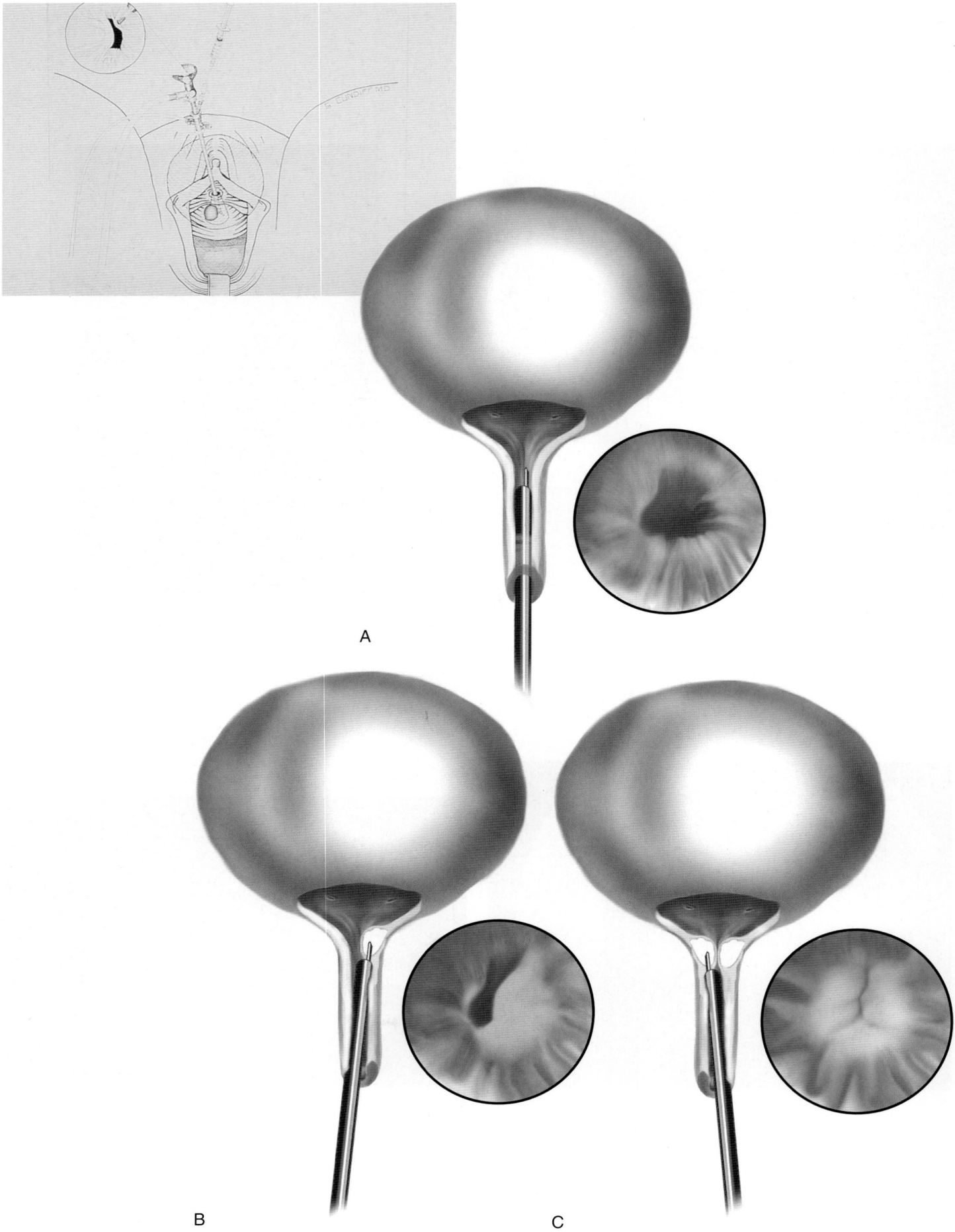

A

B

C

**FIGURE 123–45  A.** The needle is positioned at the urethrovesical junction. (From Cundiff GW, Bent AE: *In* Endoscopic Diagnosis of the Female Lower Urinary Tract. WB Saunders, UK London, 1999, with permission.) **B.** The needle penetrates the mucosa on the left, and the collagen is injected. **C.** The needle penetrates the mucosa on the right, and the collagen is injected. The **inset** shows the ballooned urethral wall coapting.

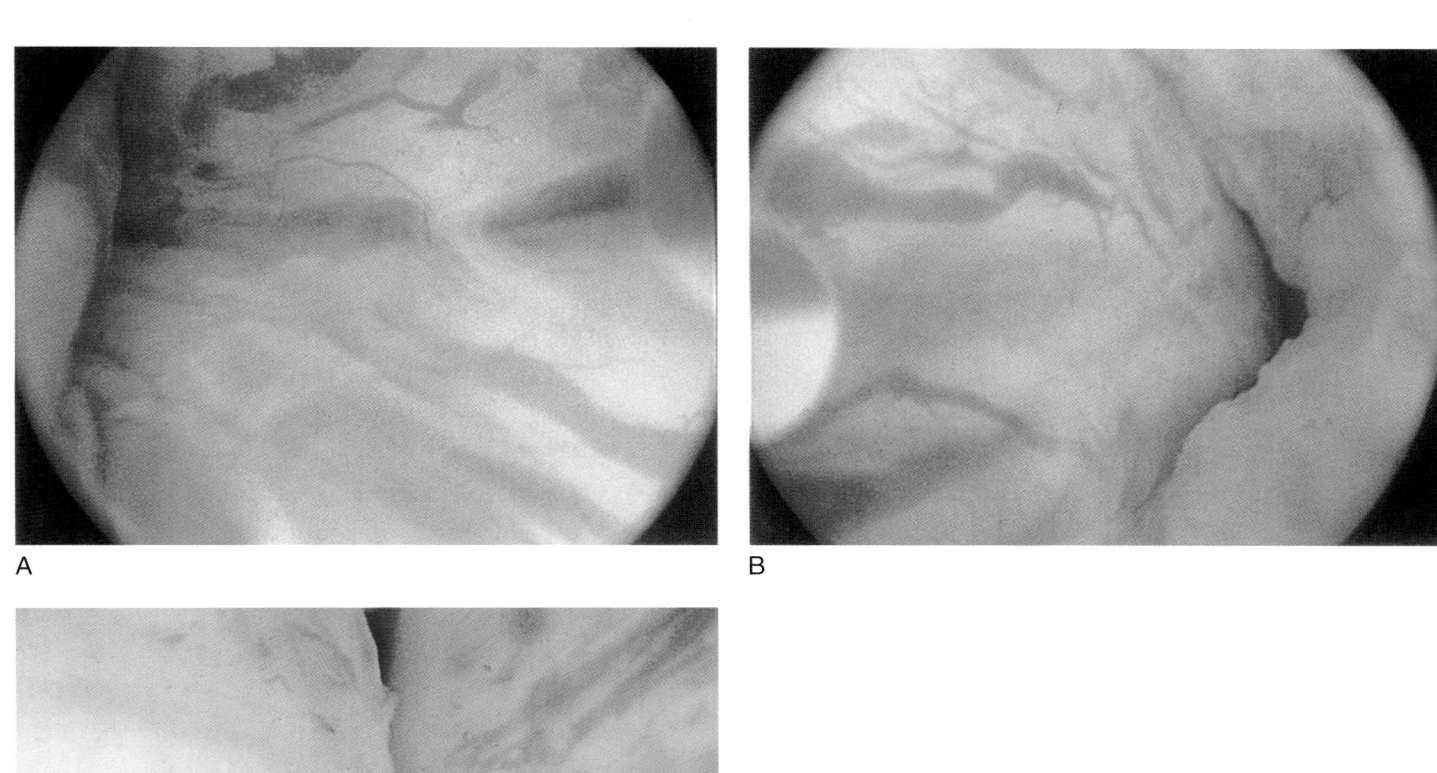

A

B

C

**FIGURE 123-46** Transurethral collagen injection. **A.** 3 o'clock position. **B.** 9 o'clock position. **C.** Occluded bladder neck. (From Cundiff GW, Bent AE: *In* Endoscopic Diagnosis of the Female Lower Urinary Tract. WB Saunders, UK London, 1999, with permission.)

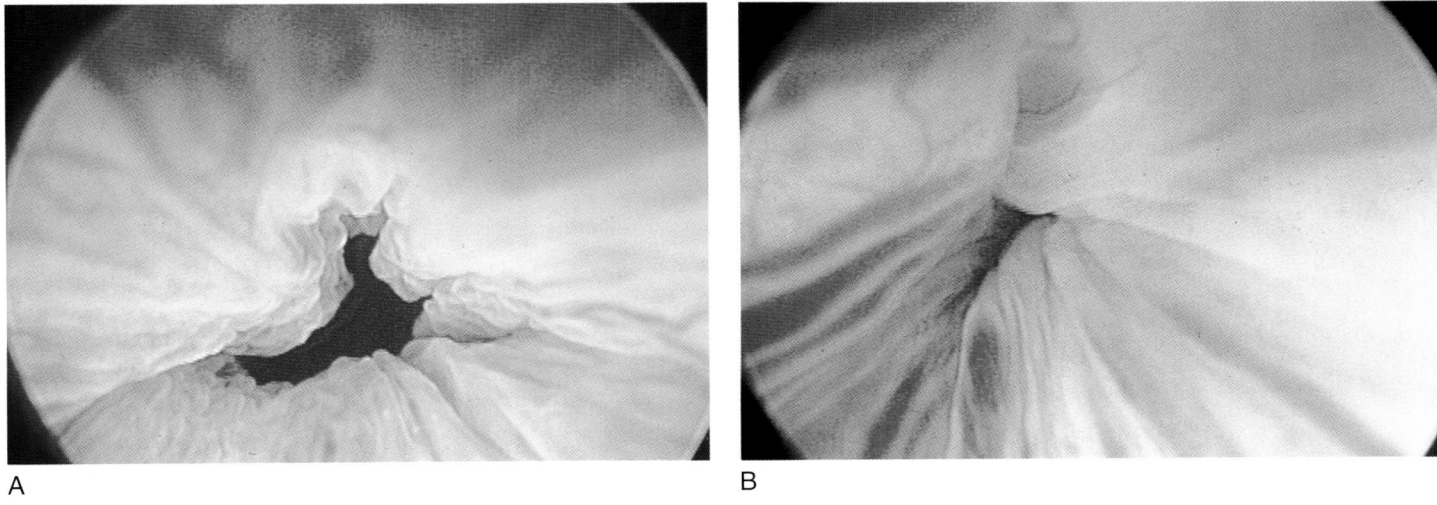

A

B

**FIGURE 123-47** Periurethral collagen injection. The scope is a 0° urethroscope that is positioned distal to the bladder neck. **A.** Open urethrovesical junction. **B.** Left side being injected.

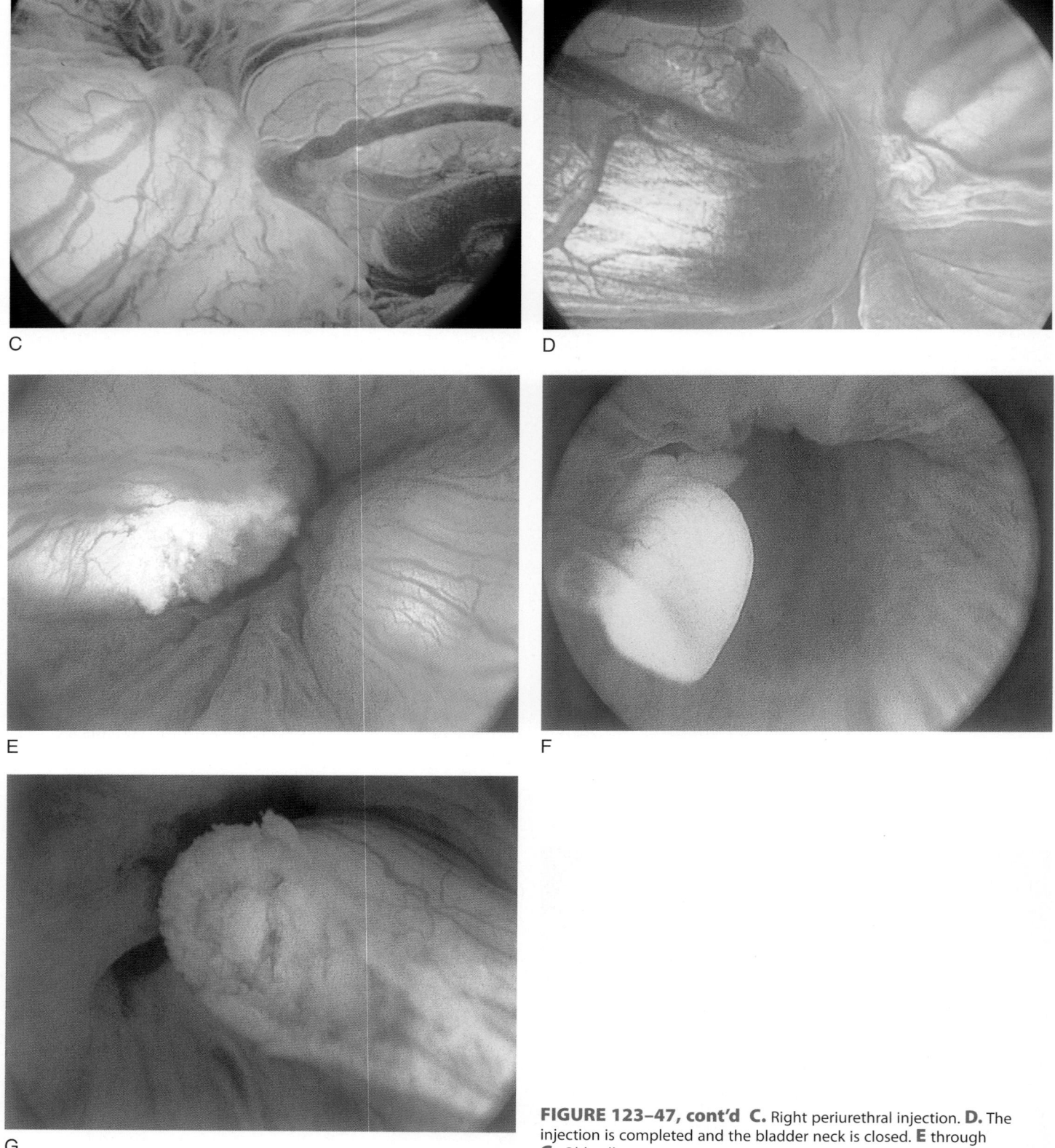

**FIGURE 123–47, cont'd** **C.** Right periurethral injection. **D.** The injection is completed and the bladder neck is closed. **E** through **G.** Old collagen.

## Suprapubic Telescopy

Suprapubic telescopy is an alternative to transurethral cystoscopy for evaluating the lower urinary tract during open abdominal pelvic surgery. Telescopy is an extraperitoneal technique that begins with closure of the anterior peritoneum to prevent contamination of the peritoneal cavity with spilled urine. Five cubic centimeters of intravenous indigo carmine is given to help identify the ureteral orifices. The bladder is filled in a retrograde fashion through a triple-lumen transurethral Foley catheter to at least 400 mL. A purse string suture is placed through the extraperitoneal dome of the bladder with a 3-0 absorbable suture. The suture should be placed through the muscularis layer of the bladder wall. A stab incision is made with a knife in the middle of the purse string; this is followed by immediate insertion of a 30° telescope through the stab wound. Drawing up of the purse string sutures prevents leakage without limiting movement of the telescope (Fig. 123–48). Because distention of the bladder is achieved through the transurethral catheter, the sheath and bridge are unnecessary, and the telescope is inserted alone. A 30° telescope provides the best view of the trigone and ureteral orifices while also permitting a thorough bladder survey. Orientation can be achieved by identifying the transurethral Foley catheter bulb and locating the trigone beneath the bulb (Fig. 123–49). If suprapubic catheterization is planned, the catheter can be placed through the same stab incision when telescopy is completed (Fig. 123–50).

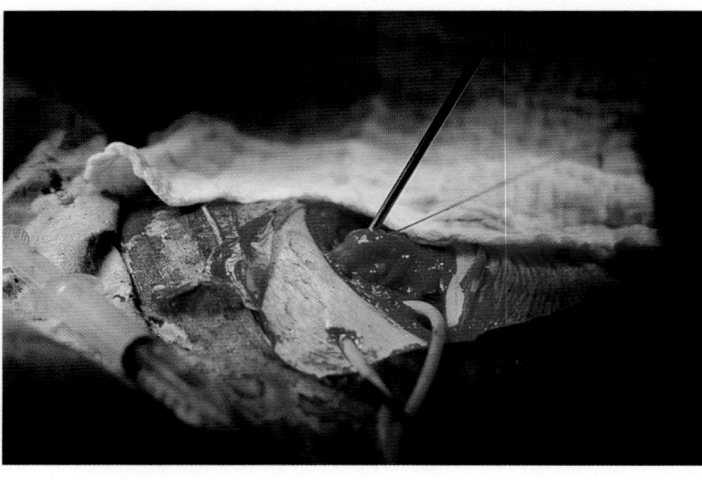

**FIGURE 123–48** Technique of suprapubic telescopy. Note that drawing up on the purse string prevents leakage during telescopy.

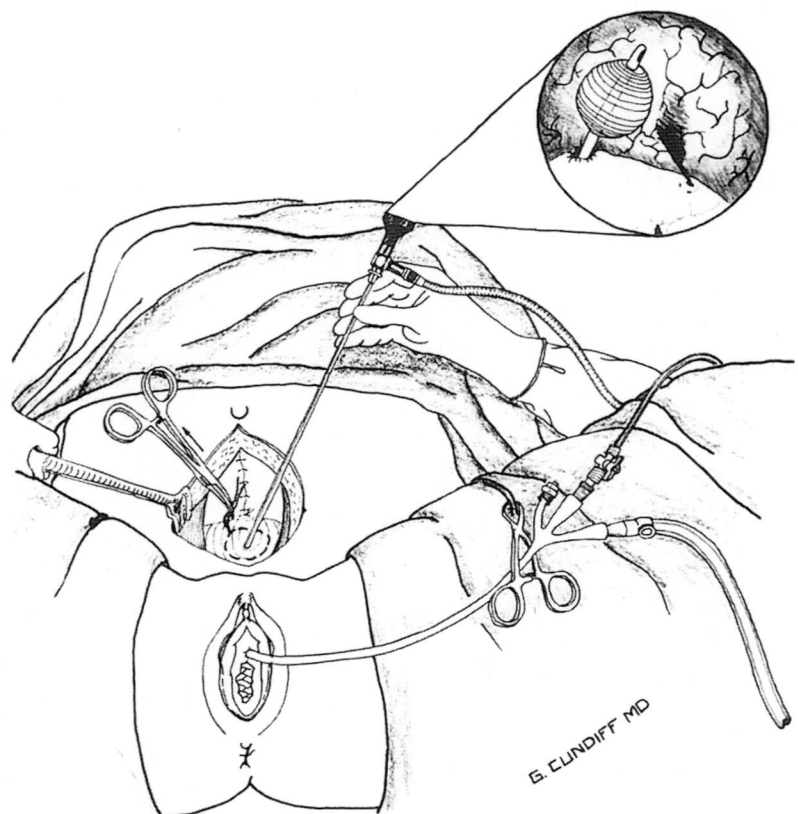

**FIGURE 123–49** Suprapubic telescopy. The bladder is filled retrogradely through a transurethral triple-lumen Foley catheter to a volume of 400 mL. A purse string absorbable suture is placed into the muscularis layer of the dome of the bladder, and a stab incision is made within the purse string for insertion of the telescope. The purse string is tightened sufficiently to prevent leakage without limiting movement of the telescope. Orientation can be achieved by identifying the transurethral Foley catheter bulb. The trigone is beneath the bulb with the urethral and ureteral orifices at its apices. (From Cundiff GW, Bent AE: *In Endoscopic Diagnosis of the Female Lower Urinary Tract.* WB Saunders, UK London, 1999, with permission.)

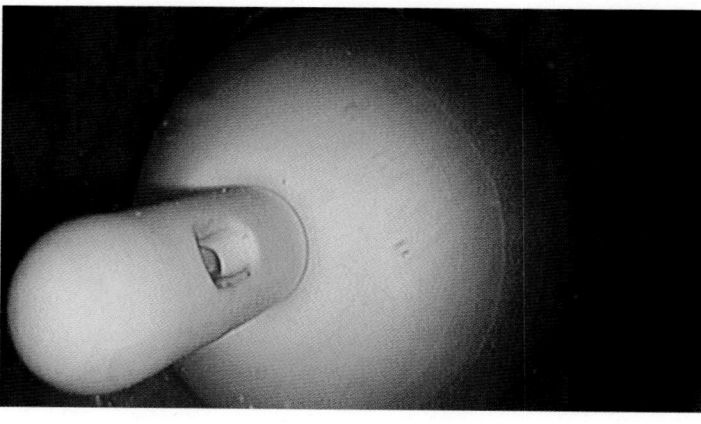

**FIGURE 123–50** The Foley catheter as viewed with a suprapubic cystoscope.

# INDEX

Page numbers followed by *f* indicate figures; *t*, tables.

INDEX